Netter's
Internal
Medicine

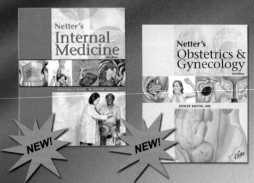
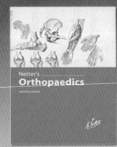
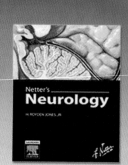
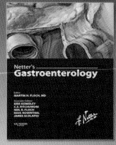
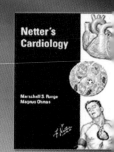
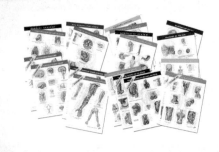
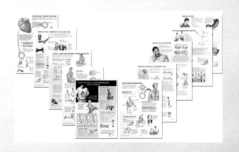
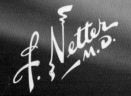

Netter's
Internal
Medicine

2nd Edition

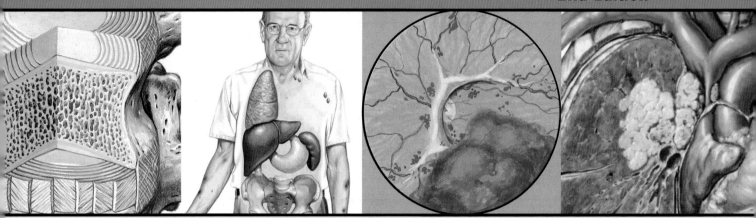

MARSCHALL S. RUNGE, MD, PhD

M. ANDREW GREGANTI, MD

Illustrations by Frank H. Netter, MD

CONTRIBUTING ILLUSTRATORS
Carlos A.G. Machado, MD
John A. Craig, MD
James A. Perkins, MS, MFA
Joe Chovan

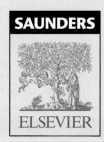

SAUNDERS

ELSEVIER

SAUNDERS
ELSEVIER

1600 John F. Kennedy Blvd.
Ste 1800
Philadelphia, PA 19103-2899

NETTER'S INTERNAL MEDICINE, 2nd Edition ISBN: 978-1-4160-4417-8

Previous edition copyrighted 2003

Library of Congress Cataloging-in-Publication Data (in PHL)

Netter's internal medicine / edited by Marschall S. Runge, M. Andrew Greganti; illustrations by Frank H. Netter; contributing illustrators, Carlos A.G. Machado . . . [et al.].—2nd ed.
    p.; cm.
   Includes bibliographical references and index.
   ISBN 978-1-4160-4417-8
  1. Internal medicine. I. Runge, Marschall Stevens, 1954- II. Greganti, M. Andrew. III. Netter, Frank H. (Frank Henry), 1906-1991. IV. Title: Internal medicine.
[DNLM: 1. Internal Medicine—Atlases. WB 17 N474 2009]
RC46.N486 2009
616—dc22
                                                           2007025788

Acquisitions Editor: Elyse O'Grady
Developmental Editor: Marybeth Thiel
Publishing Services Manager: Linda Van Pelt
Project Manager: Priscilla Crater
Design Direction: Lou Forgione
Editorial Assistant: Liam Jackson

Printed in China

Last digit is the print number: 9 8 7 6 5 4 3 2 1

Acknowledgments

This second edition of *Netter's Internal Medicine* benefited enormously from the hard work and talent of many dedicated individuals.

First, we thank the contributing authors of the University of North Carolina School of Medicine, Chapel Hill. Without their intellect, dedication, and drive for excellence, *Netter's Internal Medicine* could not have been published. We had a solid foundation on which to build the second edition, thanks to the hard work of the first edition contributing authors, many of whom we were fortunate to have continue on to this edition.

Special recognition goes to Dr. Carlos A.G. Machado, who coordinated and oversaw much of the artwork, adding to the major contributions of Drs. Frank Netter and John Craig. All are uniquely talented physician-artists who through their work brought to life important concepts in medicine in the new and updated figures included in this text. We also thank Joe Chovan and Jim Perkins for their contributions.

Anne Lenehan, Elyse O'Grady, and Marybeth Thiel at Elsevier were instrumental in helping us take a very good first edition and make it more comprehensive and more focused at the same time.

We are also indebted to Ms. Angela R. Rego, whose superb organizational skills were invaluable. Ms. Carolyn Kruse deserves special thanks for her tireless efforts in coordinating the first-pass editing process, an especially difficult task in a multi-authored textbook.

We would especially like to acknowledge our families: our wives—Susan Runge and Susan Greganti—whose constant support, encouragement, and understanding made completion of this text possible; our children—Thomas, Elizabeth, William, John, and Mason Runge; and Paul Greganti, Taylor Greganti, and Katie Hall—who inspire us and remind us that there is life beyond the word processor; and finally our parents—whose persistence, commitment, and work ethic got us started on this road many, many years ago.

About the Editors

Marschall S. Runge, MD, PhD, was born in Austin, Texas and graduated from Vanderbilt University with a BA in General Biology and a PhD in Molecular Biology. He graduated from the Johns Hopkins School of Medicine and trained in internal medicine at the Johns Hopkins Hospital. He was a cardiology fellow and junior faculty member at the Massachusetts General Hospital. Dr. Runge's next position was at Emory University, where he directed the Cardiology Fellowship Training Program. He then moved to the University of Texas Medical Branch in Galveston where he was Chief of Cardiology and Director of the Sealy Center for Molecular Cardiology. He came to the University of North Carolina in 2000 as Chairman of the Department of Medicine. Since 2006, Dr. Runge has also served as Vice Dean for Clinical Affairs at the UNC School of Medicine. Dr. Runge is board certified in internal medicine and cardiovascular diseases and has spoken and published widely on topics in clinical cardiology and vascular medicine. He maintains an active clinical practice in cardiovascular diseases and medicine in addition to his teaching and administrative activities in the Department of Medicine.

M. Andrew Greganti, MD, was born in Cleveland, Mississippi, graduated from Millsaps College with a BS in Chemistry and later received his medical degree from the University of Mississippi School of Medicine. He trained in Internal Medicine at the University of Rochester School of Medicine, Strong Memorial Hospital. After two years on the faculty of the University of Mississippi School of Medicine, he joined the faculty at UNC in the Division of General Medicine and Clinical Epidemiology in 1977, and has been Professor of Medicine since 1990. During his tenure at UNC, he has been Director of the Internal Medicine Residency Training Program and the Medicine-Pediatrics Residency Training Program, and has served as Division Chief of the Division of General Medicine and Clinical Epidemiology. He has also served as Associate Chairman and Interim Chairman of the Department of Medicine. He is currently Vice Chairman of the Department of Medicine and a member of the UNC Health Care System Board of Directors. He is board certified in internal medicine, and lectures as well as publishes on clinical topics in internal medicine and medical education. Known as the "doctor's doctor" at UNC, Dr. Greganti is one of the School of Medicine's busiest clinicians and a resource for many in the institution, regionally, and nationally.

Preface

The first edition of *Netter's Internal Medicine* was an effort to bring the ever-increasing amount of medical information to clinicians in a concise and highly visual format. The challenge that clinicians face in "keeping up" on the medical literature has continued to grow in the five years since publication of the first edition. This need to process the ever-expanding medical information base and apply new findings in the optimal care of patients is acute in all areas of medicine, but is perhaps most challenging in disciplines that require practitioners to understand a very broad spectrum of illnesses, as in internal medicine. The explosion of medical knowledge is also a very real educational issue for learners at all levels (students, residents, and practicing physicians), who must rapidly determine what is and is not important, organize the key information, and then apply these principles effectively in clinical settings.

For this second edition of *Netter's Internal Medicine*, our goal was to produce an improved text, one that keeps these issues in clear focus, and a text that fills in important clinical areas that were not well covered in the first edition, or in many internal medicine texts. To accomplish this expansion in the text, while maintaining a concise text that could be used as a ready reference, we again avoided exhaustive treatment of topics. We also have made every effort to present the essential information in a "reader-friendly" format that increases the reader's ability to learn the key facts without getting lost in details that can obfuscate the learning process.

After a careful review of reader comments about the first edition, we made some substantial changes to increase our likelihood of success in achieving our educational goals. Chapters were added to address reader concerns about the lack of coverage of a number of important topics commonly encountered in clinical practice, such as "Overview of Preventive Medicine," "Practicing in the Modern Environment: Improving Outcomes and Patient Safety," "Atrial Fibrillation," "Electrocardiography," "Gastrointestinal Bleeding," "Multiple Myeloma," and the "Autoinflammatory Syndromes," among others. The chapter format subheadings "Optimum Treatment" and

"Avoiding Treatment Errors" are new additions to address increasing concerns about therapeutic errors that can lead to patient harm. Algorithms have been color coded for quick reference. "Additional Resources" and "Evidence" based references are annotated to guide the reader to a more in-depth review if considered necessary. As in the first edition, the contributing authors have taken advantage of the genius of Frank Netter by carefully selecting the best of his artwork to illustrate the most important clinical concepts covered in each chapter. When Netter artwork was unavailable or difficult to apply to illustrate modern clinical concepts, as in the first edition, we utilized the great artistic talents of Carlos A.G. Machado, MD, to create new artwork or to skillfully edit and update some of Frank Netter's drawings. The combination of Dr. Machado's outstanding skills as a medical artist as well as his knowledge of the medical concepts being illustrated were invaluable assets. This new edition is also available in a premium online version, which includes image downloading capabilities and some printable patient handouts. The online offering makes the content even more accessible and portable and allows readers to use the magnificent art from this book in their personal presentations.

As in the first edition, we chose to use authors from the University of North Carolina School of Medicine at Chapel Hill. This allowed us to select authors who are clinical authorities. All have active clinical practices that require daily use of the information base covered in their chapters. In the selection process, we chose the very best clinicians, not necessarily the most published investigators in all fields. The result is a text that is truly clinically useful—and less of a compendium than is commonly the case in internal medicine texts. While all of these second edition authors are practicing clinicians, many are also well known for their national and international contributions. All are well aware of the approach to patient management utilized by their peers at other institutions and in other practice settings. We are convinced, based on our experience with the first edition, that keeping the text within our institution, in large part within the Department of Medicine, has allowed us to maintain our focus and to accomplish our goal of providing a useful text for practicing clinicians.

We believe that the changes we have made in the second edition have substantially improved *Netter's Internal Medicine* and will assure that it will remain a highly useful resource for all physicians, both generalists and subspecialists, who need to remain current in internal medicine—from the young to the old, from trainees to experienced practitioners. Whether we have succeeded will obviously remain in the hands of our readers. Based on our experience with the revision of the first edition, we welcome the comments, suggestions, and criticism of readers that will help us improve future editions of this work.

Marschall S. Runge, MD, PhD
Chairman, Department of Medicine
The University of North Carolina
School of Medicine, Chapel Hill

M. Andrew Greganti, MD
Vice Chairman, Department of Medicine
The University of North Carolina
School of Medicine, Chapel Hill

Algorithms have been color coded for quick reference.

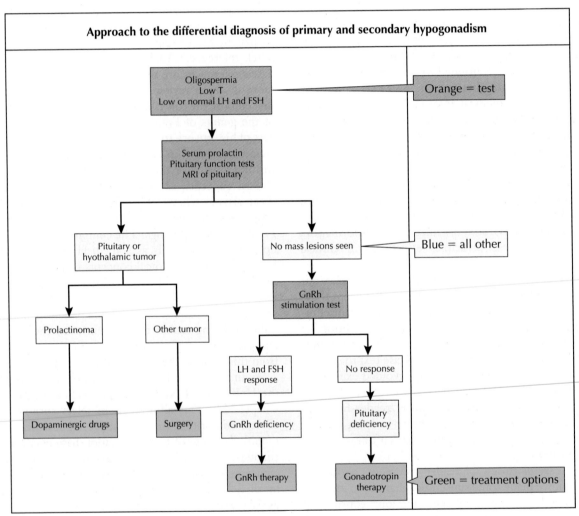

Approach to the differential diagnosis of primary and secondary hypogonadism

Oligospermia / Low T / Low or normal LH and FSH

Orange = test

Serum prolactin / Pituitary function tests / MRI of pituitary

Pituitary or hyothalamic tumor

No mass lesions seen — Blue = all other

GnRh stimulation test

Prolactinoma / Other tumor

LH and FSH response / No response

Dopaminergic drugs / Surgery / GnRh deficiency / Pituitary deficiency

GnRh therapy / Gonadotropin therapy — Green = treatment options

Frank H. Netter, MD

Frank H. Netter was born in 1906, in New York City. He studied art at the Art Student's League and the National Academy of Design before entering medical school at New York University, where he received his MD degree in 1931. During his student years, Dr. Netter's notebook sketches attracted the attention of the medical faculty and other physicians, allowing him to augment his income by illustrating articles and textbooks. He continued illustrating as a sideline after establishing a surgical practice in 1933, but he ultimately opted to give up his practice in favor of a full-time commitment to art. After service in the United States Army during World War II, Dr. Netter began his long collaboration with the CIBA Pharmaceutical Company (now Novartis Pharmaceuticals). This 45-year partnership resulted in the production of the extraordinary collection of medical art so familiar to physicians and other medical professionals worldwide.

Icon Learning Systems acquired the Netter Collection in July 2000 and continued to update Dr. Netter's original paintings and to add newly commissioned paintings by artists trained in the style of Dr. Netter. In 2005, Elsevier Inc. purchased the Netter Collection and all publications from Icon Learning Systems. There are now over 50 publications featuring the art of Dr. Netter available through Elsevier Inc.

Dr. Netter's works are among the finest examples of the use of illustration in the teaching of medical concepts. The 13-book *Netter Collection of Medical Illustrations*, which includes the greater part of the more than 20,000 paintings created by Dr. Netter, became and remains one of the most famous medical works ever published. *The Netter Atlas of Human Anatomy*, first published in 1989, presents the anatomical paintings from the Netter Collection. Now translated into 16 languages, it is the anatomy atlas of choice among medical and health professions students the world over.

The Netter illustrations are appreciated not only for their aesthetic qualities, but, more important, for their intellectual content. As Dr. Netter wrote in 1949, ". . . clarification of a subject is the aim and goal of illustration. No matter how beautifully painted, how delicately and subtly rendered a subject may be, it is of little value as a *medical illustration* if it does not serve to make clear some medical point." Dr. Netter's planning, conception, point of view, and approach are what inform his paintings and what makes them so intellectually valuable.

Frank H. Netter, MD, physician and artist, died in 1991.

Contributors

All the contributors are associated with the University of North Carolina School of Medicine at Chapel Hill.

Marschall S. Runge, MD, PhD
Charles Addison and Elizabeth Anne Sanders Distinguished Professor
Professor and Chairman, Department of Medicine
Division of Cardiology

M. Andrew Greganti, MD
John Randolph and Helen Barnes Chambliss Distinguished Professor of Medicine
Professor and Vice Chairman, Department of Medicine
Division of Geriatric Medicine
Program on Aging

Adaora A. Adimora, MD, MPH
Associate Professor of Medicine
Adjunct Associate Professor of Epidemiology
Division of Infectious Diseases

Maha Alattar, MD
Assistant Professor of Neurology
Division of Sleep and Epilepsy
Section of Adult Neurology

Robert M. Aris, MD
Associate Professor of Medicine
Director, Pulmonary Hypertension Program
Division of Pulmonary and Critical Care Medicine

Victoria Lin Bae-Jump, MD, PhD
Fellow and Instructor, Division of Gynecologic
    Oncology

Maria Q. Baggstrom, MD
Assistant Professor of Medicine
Division of Oncology
Washington University School of Medicine
St. Louis, Missouri

A. Sidney Barritt, MD
Instructor of Medicine
Division of Gastroenterology and Hepatology

Marc K. Bassim, MD
Chief Resident and Clinical Instructor, Department of
    Otolaryngology/Head and Neck Surgery

Toby Bates, DO
Instructor of Medicine
Division of Rheumatology, Allergy and Immunology
Thurston Arthritis Research Center

Anne W. Beaven, MD
Post-doctoral Fellow
Division of Hematology and Oncology

Robert G. Berger, MD
Professor of Medicine
Director, Medical Informatics
Associate Chief of Staff, University of North Carolina
    Hospitals
Division of Rheumatology, Allergy and Immunology
Thurston Arthritis Research Center

Lee R. Berkowitz, MD
Professor of Medicine
Associate Chair for Education
Division of Hematology and Oncology
Lineberger Comprehensive Cancer Center

Stephen A. Bernard, MD
Professor of Medicine
Co-Director, Palliative Care Program
Division of Hematology and Oncology

William S. Blau, MD, PhD
Professor of Anesthesiology
Chief, Division of Pain Medicine
Director, Acute Pain Service

John F. Boggess, MD
Associate Professor of Obstetrics and Gynecology
Division of Gynecologic Oncology

Mary C. Bowman, MD, PhD
Instructor of Medicine
Division of Infectious Diseases

Mark E. Brecher, MD
Professor of Pathology and Laboratory Medicine
Vice Chair, Department of Pathology and Laboratory
    Medicine
Chair, McLendon Clinical Laboratories
Director, Transfusion Medicine Service and Transplant
    Laboratories

Philip A. Bromberg, MD
Distinguished Professor of Medicine
Scientific Director, Center for Environmental Medicine,
    Asthma and Lung Biology
Division of Pulmonary and Critical Care Medicine

Sue A. Brown, MD
Assistant Professor of Medicine
Division of Endocrinology
University of Virginia
Charlottesville, Virginia

Vickie Brown, RN, MPH
Associate Director, Hospital Epidemiology
Department of Hospital Epidemiology
University of North Carolina Health Care System

Paul C. Bryson, MD
Resident, Department of Otolaryngology/Head and
    Neck Surgery

Robert A. Buckmire, MD
Associate Professor of Otolaryngology/Head and Neck
    Surgery
Chief, Division of Voice and Swallowing
    Disorders
Director, University of North Carolina Voice
    Center

Elizabeth Bullitt, MD
Professor of Surgery
Division of Neurosurgery

Craig Burkhart, MD
Resident, Department of Dermatology

M. Janette Busby-Whitehead, MD
Professor of Medicine
Chief, Division of Geriatric Medicine
Director, Program on Aging

John B. Buse, MD, PhD
Professor of Medicine
Chief, Division of Endocrinology and Metabolism

Debra L. Bynum, MD
Assistant Professor of Medicine
Division of Geriatric Medicine
Program on Aging

Lisa A. Carey, MD
Associate Professor of Medicine
Medical Director, University of North Carolina Breast
    Center
Division of Hematology and Oncology
Lineberger Comprehensive Cancer Center

Timothy S. Carey, MD, MPH
Professor of Medicine
Director, Cecil G. Sheps Center for Health Services
    Research
Division of General Internal Medicine and Clinical
    Epidemiology

Culley C. Carson III, MD
Rhodes Distinguished Professor of Surgery
Chief, Division of Urologic Surgery

Patricia P. Chang, MD, MHS
Assistant Professor of Medicine
Director, Heart Failure and Transplant Service
Division of Cardiology

Sanjay Chaudhary, MD
Instructor of Medicine
Division of Rheumatology, Allergy and Immunology
Thurston Arthritis Research Center

David R. Clemmons, MD
Professor of Medicine
Division of Endocrinology and Metabolism

James M. Coghill, MD
Post-doctoral Fellow
Division of Hematology and Oncology

Romulo E. Colindres, MD, MSPH
Professor of Medicine
Division of Nephrology and Hypertension
University of North Carolina Kidney Center

AnnaMarie Connolly, MD
Associate Professor of Obstetrics and Gynecology
Division of Urogynecology and Reconstructive Pelvic
    Surgery

Benjamin J. Copeland, MD, PhD
Practicing Otolaryngologist
Otolaryngology Associates
Carmel, Indiana

Todd Correll, PharmD
Clinical Pharmacy Specialist (ID-HIV)
University of North Carolina School of Pharmacy
University of North Carolina Hospitals

Cynthia J. Denu-Ciocca, MD
Assistant Professor of Medicine
Division of Nephrology and Hypertension
University of North Carolina Kidney Center

Thomas S. Devetski, OD
Practicing Optometrist
Alamance Eye Center
Burlington and Chapel Hill, North Carolina

Darren A. DeWalt, MD, MPH
Assistant Professor of Medicine
Division of General Internal Medicine and Clinical
    Epidemiology
Cecil G. Sheps Center for Health Services Research

Luis A. Diaz, MD
Professor of Dermatology
Chairman, Department of Dermatology

James F. Donohue, MD
Professor of Medicine
Chief, Division of Pulmonary and Critical Care
    Medicine

Mary Anne Dooley, MD, MPH
Associate Professor of Medicine
Division of Rheumatology, Allergy and Immunology
Thurston Arthritis Research Center

Jean M. Dostou, MD
Assistant Professor of Medicine
Division of Endocrinology and Metabolism

Douglas A. Drossman, MD
Professor of Medicine and Psychiatry
Co-Director, University of North Carolina Center for
    Functional GI and Motility Disorders
Division of Gastroenterology and Hepatology

Carla Sueta Dupree, MD, PhD
Associate Professor of Medicine
Medical Director, University of North Carolina
    Hospitals Heart Center at Meadowmont
Associate Director, Heart Failure Program
Division of Cardiology

Rose J. Eapen, MD
Resident, Department of Otolaryngology/Head and
    Neck Surgery

Charles S. Ebert, Jr., MD, MPH
Resident, Department of Otolaryngology/Head and
    Neck Surgery

Nurum F. Erdem, MD, MPH
Assistant Professor of Medicine
Division of Geriatric Medicine
Program on Aging

Joseph J. Eron, MD
Professor of Medicine
Director, Adult Clinical Trials Unit
Division of Infectious Diseases

Ronald J. Falk, MD
Doc J. Thurston Professor of Medicine
Chief, Division of Nephrology and Hypertension
Director, University of North Carolina Kidney Center

Mary Katherine Farmer-Boatwright, MD
Instructor of Medicine
Division of Rheumatology, Allergy and Immunology
Thurston Arthritis Research Center

Elizabeth A. Fasy, MD
Assistant Professor of Medicine
Division of Endocrinology, Metabolism and Lipids
Emory University
Atlanta, Georgia

Alan G. Finkel, MD
Professor of Neurology
Director, University of North Carolina Headache Clinic
Section of Adult Neurology

William F. Finn, MD
Professor of Medicine
Division of Nephrology and Hypertension
University of North Carolina Kidney Center

David P. Fitzgerald, MD
Instructor of Medicine
Division of Infectious Diseases

Carol A. Ford, MD
Associate Professor of Pediatrics and Medicine
Director, NC Multisite Adolescent Research Consortium
    for Health (NC MARCH)
Division of General Pediatrics and Adolescent
    Medicine

Catherine A. Forneris, PhD
Associate Professor of Psychiatry
Division of Adult Psychiatry

Amy M. Fowler, MD
Assistant Professor of Ophthalmology

W. Craig Fowler, MD
Associate Professor of Ophthalmology

Wesley Caswell Fowler, MD
Practicing Neurosurgeon
Mountain Neurosurgical and Spine Center
Asheville, North Carolina

Michael W. Fried, MD
Professor of Medicine
Director of Hepatology
Division of Gastroenterology and Hepatology

Don A. Gabriel, MD, PhD
Professor of Medicine
Division of Hematology and Oncology
Lineberger Comprehensive Cancer Center

Shannon Galvin, MD
Assistant Professor of Medicine
Division of Infectious Diseases

Lisa M. Gangarosa, MD
Associate Professor of Medicine
Division of Gastroenterology and Hepatology

James C. Garbutt, MD
Professor of Psychiatry
Medical Director, Alcohol and Substance
  Abuse Program, University of North Carolina
  Hospitals
Research Scientist, Bowles Center for Alcohol Study
Division of Adult Psychiatry

Cynthia Gay, MD, MPH
Assistant Professor of Medicine
Division of Infectious Diseases

Susan A. Gaylord, PhD
Assistant Professor of Physical Medicine and
  Rehabilitation
Director, University of North Carolina Program on
  Integrative Medicine

Leonard S. Gettes, MD
Distinguished Professor of Medicine
Division of Cardiology

Andrew J. Ghio, MD
Associate Professor of Medicine
University of North Carolina Division of Pulmonary and
  Critical Care Medicine
Research Medical Officer
National Health and Environmental Effects Research
  Laboratory
Clinical Research Branch, Human Studies Division
United States Environmental Protection Agency
Chapel Hill, North Carolina

John H. Gilmore, MD
Professor of Psychiatry
Vice Chair, Research and Scientific Affairs
Director, University of North Carolina Schizophrenia
  Research Center

Paul A. Godley, MD, PhD, MPP
Associate Professor of Medicine
Adjunct Associate Professor of Epidemiology and
  Biostatistics
Division of Hematology and Oncology
Lineberger Comprehensive Cancer Center

Lee R. Goldberg, MD
Practicing Cardiologist
Tucson Heart Hospital
Tucson Medical Center
Tucson, Arizona

Richard M. Goldberg, MD
Professor of Medicine
Chief, Division of Hematology and Oncology
Lineberger Comprehensive Cancer Center

Matthew N. Goldenberg, MD
Chief Resident and Clinical Instructor, Department of
  Psychiatry

Brian P. Goldstein, MD, MBA
Associate Professor of Medicine
Division of General Internal Medicine and Epidemiology
Executive Associate Dean for Clinical Affairs, University
  of North Carolina School of Medicine
Chief of Staff, University of North Carolina Hospitals

Robert S. Greenwood, MD
Professor of Neurology and Pediatrics
Chief, Section of Child Neurology

Ian S. Grimm, MD
Associate Professor of Medicine
Director, Gastrointestinal Endoscopy
Division of Gastroenterology and Hepatology

Steven H. Grossman, MD
Associate Professor of Medicine
Division of Nephrology and Hypertension
University of North Carolina Kidney Center

Robert E. Gwyther, MD, MBA
Professor of Family Medicine
Director, Medical Student Programs

John J. Haggerty, Jr., MD
Professor of Psychiatry
Director, Division of Social and Community Psychiatry

Russell P. Harris, MD, MPH
Professor of Medicine
Director, Program on Prevention
Director, MD-MPH Program
Division of General Internal Medicine and Clinical
    Epidemiology

William D. Heizer, MD
Professor of Medicine
Division of Gastroenterology and Hepatology

Ashley G. Henderson, MD
Instructor of Medicine
Division of Pulmonary and Critical Care Medicine

David C. Henke, MD, MPH
Associate Professor of Medicine
Division of Pulmonary and Critical Care Medicine

Michael A. Hill, MD
Professor of Psychiatry
Director, Adult Inpatient Program
Medical Director, Geropsychiatry Inpatient Unit
Division of Adult Psychiatry

Alan L. Hinderliter, MD
Associate Professor of Medicine
Division of Cardiology

Albert R. Hinn, MD
Associate Professor of Neurology
Section of Adult Neurology

Gerald A. Hladik, MD
Associate Professor of Medicine
Division of Nephrology and Hypertension
University of North Carolina Kidney Center

Hal M. Hoffman, MD
Associate Professor of Pediatrics and Medicine
Division of Allergy, Immunology, and Rheumatology
University of California, San Diego, Medical School
La Jolla, California

Mina C. Hosseinipour, MD, MPH
Assistant Professor of Medicine
Division of Infectious Diseases
University of North Carolina Project-Lilongwe,
    Malawi

James F. Howard, Jr., MD
Distinguished Professor of Neuromuscular Disease
Professor of Neurology and Medicine
Chief, Division of Neuromuscular Disorders
Section of Adult Neurology

David Y. Huang, MD, PhD
Assistant Professor of Neurology
Director, Inpatient and Emergency Neurology
Associate Director, University of North Carolina
    Hospitals Stroke Center
Section of Adult Neurology

Xuemei Huang, MD, PhD
Assistant Professor of Neurology
Acting Chief, Division of Movement Disorders
Medical Director, National Parkinson's Foundation
    Center of Excellence
Section of Adult Neurology

Burton R. Hutto, MD
Professor of Psychiatry
Division of Adult Psychiatry

Kim L. Isaacs, MD, PhD
Professor of Medicine
Associate Director, University of North Carolina
    Inflammatory Bowel Disease Center
Division of Gastroenterology and Hepatology

Bruce F. Israel, MD
Practicing Physician—Infectious Diseases
Asheville Infectious Disease Consultants
Asheville, North Carolina

Thomas S. Ivester, MD
Assistant Professor of Obstetrics and Gynecology
Division of Maternal-Fetal Medicine

Heidi T. Jacobe, MD
Assistant Professor of Dermatology
University of Texas Southwestern Medical Center
Dallas, Texas

Peter Lars Jacobson, MD
Professor of Neurology
Director, University of North Carolina Neurology
    Palliative Care Program
Section of Adult Neurology

Lukas Jantac, MD
Instructor of Medicine
Division of Cardiology

Jaspaul S. Jawanda, MD
Assistant Professor of Medicine
University of North Carolina Division of Infectious
    Diseases
First Health Infectious Diseases
Moore Regional Hospital
Pinehurst, North Carolina

Sandra M. Johnson, MD
Associate Professor of Ophthalmology
Director of Glaucoma
Medical College of Georgia
Augusta, Georgia

Beth L. Jonas, MD
Assistant Professor of Medicine
Division of Rheumatology, Allergy and Immunology
Thurston Arthritis Research Center

Joanne M. Jordan, MD, MPH
Associate Professor of Medicine and Orthopedics
Division of Rheumatology, Allergy and Immunology
Thurston Arthritis Research Center

Jonathan J. Juliano, MD, MSPH
Instructor of Medicine
Division of Infectious Diseases

Kevin A. Kahn, MD
Associate Professor of Neurology
Residency Program Director
Section of Adult Neurology
University of North Carolina Headache Clinic

Andrew H. Kaplan, MD[†]
Associate Professor of Medicine
Division of Infectious Diseases

Nigel S. Key, MB, ChB
Harold R. Roberts Distinguished Professor
Director, Harold R. Roberts Comprehensive Hemophilia
    Diagnostic and Treatment Center
Chief, Hematology Section
Division of Hematology and Oncology

William Y. Kim, MD
Instructor of Medicine
Division of Hematology and Oncology
Lineberger Comprehensive Cancer Center

John S. Kizer, MD
Professor of Medicine
Division of Geriatric Medicine
Program on Aging

Caroline M. Klein, MD, PhD
Assistant Professor of Neurology
Section of Adult Neurology

Philip J. Klemmer, MD
Professor of Medicine
Division of Nephrology and Hypertension
University of North Carolina Kidney Center

Karen Kölln, MD
Resident, Department of Otolaryngology/Head and
    Neck Surgery

Mark J. Koruda, MD
Professor of Surgery
Chief, Division of Gastrointestinal Surgery

James E. Kurz, MD
Associate Professor of Medicine and Pediatrics
Division of General Internal Medicine and Clinical
    Epidemiology

Jeffrey LaCour, MD
Resident, Department of Otolaryngology/Head and
    Neck Surgery

Alim M. Ladha, MD
Surgical Resident, Division of Neurosurgery

W. Derek Leight, MD
Resident, Department of Otolaryngology/Head and
    Neck Surgery

Peter A. Leone, MD
Associate Professor of Medicine
Medical Director, North Carolina HIV/STD Prevention
    and Care Branch, North Carolina DHHS
Division of Infectious Diseases

B. Anthony Lindsey, MD
Professor of Psychiatry
Vice Chair for Clinical Affairs
Division of Adult Psychiatry

Ryan D. Madanick, MD
Assistant Professor of Medicine
Division of Gastroenterology and Hepatology

Lawrence K. Mandelkehr, MBA
Director, Performance Improvement
University of North Carolina Hospitals

[†] Deceased.

J. Douglas Mann, MD
Professor of Neurology
Section of Adult Neurology

Silva Markovic-Plese, MD
Associate Professor of Neurology
Section of Adult Neurology

Allen F. Marshall, MD
Resident, Department of Otolaryngology/Head and
   Neck Surgery

William D. Mattern, MD
Emeritus Professor of Medicine
Division of Nephrology and Hypertension

Celeste M. Mayer, PhD, RN
Patient Safety Officer
University of North Carolina Hospitals

Travis A. Meredith, MD
Sterling A. Barrett Distinguished Professor of
   Ophthalmology
Professor and Chairman, Department of
   Ophthalmology

William C. Miller, MD, PhD, MPH
Associate Professor of Medicine and Epidemiology
Division of Infectious Diseases

Beverly S. Mitchell, MD
George E. Becker Professor of Medicine
Deputy Director, Stanford Comprehensive Cancer
   Center
Division of Oncology
Stanford University School of Medicine
Stanford, California

Stephan Moll, MD
Associate Professor of Medicine
Director, Thrombophilia Program
Division of Hematology and Oncology

Douglas R. Morgan, MD, MPH
Assistant Professor of Medicine
Division of Gastroenterology and Hepatology

Dean S. Morrell, MD
Associate Professor of Dermatology
Director, Residency Training Program

M. Cristina Muñoz, MD
Assistant Professor of Obstetrics and Gynecology
Division of Women's Primary Health Care

Patrick H. Nachman, MD
Associate Professor of Medicine
Division of Nephrology and Hypertension
University of North Carolina Kidney Center

Kelly C. Nelson, MD
Resident, Department of Dermatology

Carla M. Nester, MD, MSA
Instructor of Medicine
Division of Nephrology and Hypertension
University of North Carolina Kidney Center

Linda M. Nicholas, MD, MS
Professor of Psychiatry
Co-Director, Outpatient Services
Medical Director, Adult Diagnostic and Treatment
   Clinic

E. Magnus Ohman, MB
Professor of Medicine
Director, Program for Advanced Coronary Disease
Division of Cardiovascular Medicine
Duke University Medical Center
Durham, North Carolina

Bert H. O'Neil, MD
Assistant Professor of Medicine
Division of Hematology and Oncology
Lineberger Comprehensive Cancer Center

David A. Ontjes, MD
Professor of Medicine
Division of Endocrinology and Metabolism

Robert Z. Orlowski, MD, PhD
Associate Professor of Medicine
Division of Hematology and Oncology
Department of Pharmacology
Lineberger Comprehensive Cancer Center

Daniel J. Parsons, MD, MPH
Assistant Professor of Dermatology

Dhavalkumar D. Patel, MD, PhD
Head, Autoimmunity & Transplantation Research Basel
Novartis Institute for BioMedical Research
Basel, Switzerland

Cam Patterson, MD
Ernest and Hazel Craige Distinguished Professor of
   Cardiovascular Medicine
Professor of Medicine, Pharmacology, and Cell and
   Developmental Biology
Chief, Division of Cardiology
Director, Carolina Cardiovascular Biology Center
Associate Chair for Research, Department of Medicine

Kristine B. Patterson, MD
Assistant Professor of Medicine
Division of Infectious Diseases

Amanda Peppercorn, MD
Assistant Professor of Medicine
Division of Infectious Diseases

Harold C. Pillsbury III, MD
Thomas J. Dark Distinguished Professor of
    Otolaryngology/Head and Neck Surgery
Professor and Chairman, Department of
    Otolaryngology/Head and Neck Surgery

W. Kimryn Rathmell, MD, PhD
Assistant Professor of Medicine
Division of Hematology and Oncology
Lineberger Comprehensive Cancer Center

Daniel S. Reuland, MD
Assistant Professor of Medicine
NRSA Primary Care Research Fellow
Division of General Internal Medicine and Clinical
    Epidemiology

Yehuda Ringel, MD
Assistant Professor of Medicine
Division of Gastroenterology and Hepatology

M. Patricia Rivera, MD
Associate Professor of Medicine
Co-Director, Multidisciplinary Thoracic Oncology
    Program
Co-Director, Pulmonary/Critical Care Fellowship
    Program
Division of Pulmonary and Critical Care Medicine

Craig N. Rosebrock, MD
Instructor of Medicine
Division of Pulmonary and Critical Care Medicine

Pinchas Rosenberg, MD
Fellow and Instructor, Department of Ophthalmology

Robert A.S. Roubey, MD
Associate Professor of Medicine
Division of Rheumatology, Allergy and Immunology
Thurston Arthritis Research Center

David S. Rubenstein, MD, PhD
Associate Professor of Dermatology

Susan Riggs Runge, MD
Assistant Professor of Dermatology

Mark Russo, MD, MPH
Medical Director, Liver Transplantation
Carolinas Medical Center
Charlotte, North Carolina

William A. Rutala, PhD, MPH
Professor of Medicine
Division of Infectious Diseases
Director, Hospital Epidemiology, Occupational Health
    and Safety Program
University of North Carolina Health Care System

William E. Sanders, Jr., MD, MBA
Associate Professor of Medicine
Director, Clinical Cardiac Electrophysiology and Pacing
Division of Cardiology

Hanna K. Sanoff, MD
Assistant Professor of Medicine
Division of Hematology and Oncology

Scott L. Sanoff, MD
Instructor of Medicine
Division of Nephrology and Hypertension
University of North Carolina Kidney Center

Yolanda V. Scarlett, MD
Assistant Professor of Medicine
Division of Gastroenterology and Hepatology

Emily J. Schwarz, MD, PhD
Resident, Department of Dermatology

Brent A. Senior, MD
Associate Professor of Otolaryngology/Head and Neck
    Surgery
Chief, Division of Rhinology, Allergy and Sinus Surgery

Jonathan S. Serody, MD
Elizabeth Thomas Associate Professor of Medicine,
    Microbiology and Immunology
Division of Hematology and Oncology
Program in Stem Cell Transplantation

Nicholas J. Shaheen, MD, MPH
Associate Professor of Medicine and Epidemiology
Director, Center for Esophageal Diseases and
    Swallowing
Division of Gastroenterology and Hepatology

Thomas C. Shea, MD
Professor of Medicine
Director, Bone Marrow and Stem Cell Transplant
    Program
Division of Hematology and Oncology
Lineberger Comprehensive Cancer Center

Richard G. Sheahan, MD
Consultant Cardiologist/Electrophysiologist
Beaumont Hospital & Royal College of Surgeons in
    Ireland
Dublin, Ireland

William W. Shockley, MD
W. Paul Biggers Distinguished Professor of
    Otolaryngology/Head and Neck Surgery
Chief, Division of Facial Plastic and Reconstructive
    Surgery
Vice Chair, Department of Otolaryngology/Head and
    Neck Surgery

Roshan Shrestha, MD
Medical Director of Liver Transplantation
Piedmont Liver Transplant Program
Atlanta, Georgia

Emily E. Sickbert-Bennett, MS
Public Health Epidemiologist
Department of Hospital Epidemiology
University of North Carolina Health Care System

Micah J. Sickel, MD, PhD
Fellow and Instructor, Program in Child and Adolescent
    Psychiatry

Linmarie Sikich, MD
Associate Professor of Psychiatry
Director, Adolescent, School-Age Psychiatric
    Intervention Research Evaluation Program
Division of Child Psychiatry

Ross J. Simpson, Jr., MD, PhD
Professor of Medicine
Director, Lipid and Prevention Clinics
Division of Cardiology

Sidney C. Smith, Jr., MD
Professor of Medicine
Director, Center for Cardiovascular Science and
    Medicine
Division of Cardiology

Mark A. Socinski, MD
Associate Professor of Medicine
Director, Multidisciplinary Thoracic Oncology
    Program
Division of Hematology and Oncology
Lineberger Comprehensive Cancer Center

P. Frederick Sparling, MD
J. Herbert Bate Professor of Medicine and Microbiology
    and Immunology, Emeritus
University of North Carolina Division of Infectious
    Diseases
University of North Carolina Center for Infectious
    Diseases
Professor of Medicine, Duke University School of
    Medicine
Duke Human Vaccine Institute

Thomas E. Stinchcombe, MD
Assistant Professor of Medicine
Division of Hematology and Oncology
Lineberger Comprehensive Cancer Center

George A. Stouffer, MD
Professor of Medicine
Director, C.V. Richardson Cardiac Catheterization
    Laboratory
Director, Interventional Cardiology
Division of Cardiology

Teresa K. Tarrant, MD
Assistant Professor of Medicine
Division of Rheumatology, Allergy and Immunology
Thurston Arthritis Research Center

Mark Taylor, MD
Practicing Oncologist
Summit Cancer Center
Savannah, Georgia

Michael J. Thomas, MD, PhD
Practicing Endocrinologist
Carolina Endocrine, P.A.
Raleigh, North Carolina

Nancy E. Thomas, MD, PhD
Associate Professor of Dermatology

John M. Thorpe, Jr., MD
McAllister Distinguished Professor of Obstetrics and
    Gynecology
Division of Maternal-Fetal Medicine
Division of Women's Primary Care
Director, North Carolina Program on Women's Health
    Research

Stephen L. Tilley, MD
Assistant Professor of Medicine
Division of Pulmonary and Critical Care Medicine

Jenny P. Ting, PhD
Professor, Department of Microbiology and Immunology
Lineberger Comprehensive Cancer Center

Robert S. Tomsick, MD
Associate Professor of Dermatology

Charles M. van der Horst, MD
Professor of Medicine
Associate Director, Division of Infectious Diseases

Bradley V. Vaughn, MD
Professor of Neurology and Biomedical Engineering
Chief, Division of Sleep and Epilepsy
Section of Adult Neurology

Pamela G. Vick, MD
Adjunct Assistant Professor of Anesthesiology
Division of Pain Medicine

Robert J. Vissers, MD
Adjunct Associate Professor
Oregon Health Sciences University
Medical Director, Department of Emergency Medicine
Emanuel Hospital
Portland, Oregon

Peter M. Voorhees, MD
Assistant Professor of Medicine
Division of Hematology and Oncology
Lineberger Comprehensive Cancer Center

Tracy Y. Wang, MD, MS
Instructor of Medicine
Division of Cardiovascular Medicine
Duke University Medical Center
Durham, North Carolina

Lea C. Watson, MD, MPH
Assistant Professor of Psychiatry
Division of Adult Psychiatry

David J. Weber, MD, MPH
Professor of Medicine, Pediatrics, and Epidemiology
Division of Infectious Diseases
Medical Director, Hospital Epidemiology and
    Occupational Health
University of North Carolina Health Care System

Robert S. Wehbie, MD, PhD
Associate Professor of Medicine
University of North Carolina Division of Hematology
    and Oncology
Cancer Centers of North Carolina
Raleigh, North Carolina

Mark C. Weissler, MD
Joseph P. Riddle Distinguished Professor of
    Otolaryngology/Head and Neck Surgery
Chief, Division of Head and Neck Oncology

Ellen C. Wells, MD
Associate Professor of Obstetrics and Gynecology
Chief, Division of Urogynecology and Reconstructive
    Pelvic Surgery

Young E. Whang, MD, PhD
Associate Professor of Medicine and Pathology and
    Laboratory Medicine
Division of Hematology and Oncology
Lineberger Comprehensive Cancer Center

Park W. Willis IV, MD
Sarah Graham Distinguished Professor of Medicine and
    Pediatrics
Director, Cardiac Ultrasound Laboratories
Division of Cardiology

John B. Winfield, MD
Herman and Louise Smith Distinguished Professor of
    Medicine in Arthritis, Emeritus
Senior Member, University of North Carolina
    Neurosensory Disorders Center

Gary S. Winzelberg, MD, MPH
Assistant Professor of Medicine
Division of Geriatric Medicine
Program on Aging

David A. Wohl, MD
Associate Professor of Medicine
Division of Infectious Diseases
AIDS Clinical Trials Unit

Leslie P. Wong, MD
Practicing Nephrologist
Minor & James Medical
Seattle, Washington

Diem N. Wu, MD
Assistant Professor of Dermatology

Steven Zacks, MD, MPH
Assistant Professor of Medicine
Division of Gastroenterology and Hepatology

Contents

SECTION V

Disorders of Endocrinology and Metabolism

SECTION VI

Disorders of the Gastrointestinal Tract

SECTION XI

Sexually Transmitted Diseases

SECTION XII

Disorders of the Reproductive System

SECTION XIII

Neurologic Disorders

SECTION XIV

Disorders of the Kidney and Urinary Tract

SECTION XV

Disorders of the Immune System, Connective Tissue, and Joints

SECTION XVI

Ocular Diseases

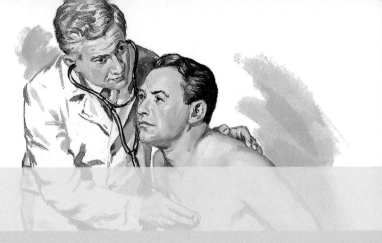
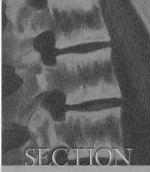

Common Clinical Challenges

Brian P. Goldstein ▪ Lawrence K. Mandelkehr ▪ Celeste M. Mayer

1

Practicing in the Modern Environment: Improving Outcomes and Patient Safety

Introduction

In this first decade of the 21st century, medicine in the United States remains a learned profession. Patients, and the public at large, continue to hold doctors in relatively high regard. Physicians preside over an ever-expanding array of diagnostic and therapeutic tools that are more targeted and therefore more successful, and many tests and procedures are less invasive than those available in the past. In general, the care available to individuals has never been more potentially powerful or more efficacious.

At the same time, Americans have lately become much more conscious of practitioners' imperfections, and they are especially aware of the shortcomings of the system that they must navigate to obtain care. The public now knows that the health care system often falls short of its potential; that medical care sometimes causes avoidable harms; and that the system includes wide variations in practice and cost without apparent differences in benefit to patients. Caregivers, and the organizations in which they practice, are increasingly tasked to demonstrate that their respective practices meet available standards and avoid potential harms.

As doctors well know, we remain limited in our ability to collect valid and reliable data and to appropriately compare different types of practice behaviors and different types of patients. Just as important, reimbursement models are fundamentally misaligned from the goals of optimizing performance and patient safety. Public and private pressures to change practice are, for now, modest, and physicians will face these demands while continuing to cope with others that at times will seem more pressing—such as billing regulations, staff shortages, and declining income. Despite these additional pressures, scrutiny of physician practice by the government, by payors and their customers (employers), and by the public is here to stay.

Before the mid-1990s, payors, policy makers, and the profession gave scant attention to the shortcomings of the health care system. To be sure, the U.S. tort system has long permitted compensation for individual victims of negligence. For a plaintiff to be compensated, a defendant must be judged as failing to meet a standard of care and therefore blamed for "more likely than not" causing harm. Medicine weathers periodic crises of rising insurance premiums, and a few states have enacted reforms, but the U.S. malpractice system remains fundamentally unchanged in structure, and it has contributed little if anything to the real evolution of the scrutiny of clinical practice.

The attention to the quality and safety of medical care is the result of several other trends. From roughly the 1960s to the 1980s, what we now call health services researchers gradually standardized the methods for evaluating the structure of health care delivery models, the processes of care delivery, and clinical outcomes. Advances in information technology have gradually brought the computing power to apply these methods for evaluating care, processes, and outcomes. Federal support for the evaluation of medical practice was boosted by the creation in 1990 of the Agency for Health Care Policy and Research (now the Agency for Health Research and Quality). Meanwhile, a multitude of groups—from employers who fund health insurance, to federal and state governments who also pay for an increasing share of health care, to managed care insurers and coalitions of consumer groups—all have steadily turned more of their attention to the quality of health care services and to the value of the services received in proportion to their cost.

Most recently, the medical profession has aggressively (if somewhat belatedly) lent its voice to the need for systemic change in the way doctors, hospitals, and others provide medical care. The Institute for Healthcare Improvement (IHI) is a private not-for-profit organization founded in 1991 by a pediatrician, Donald Berwick, MD, and has always included physicians in its leadership. IHI began as a lonely voice within the health care professions advocating for fundamental changes in care delivery. Over the ensuing years, IHI has been joined by a growing chorus of voices from "official" medicine, including many specialty societies, the American Medical Association, and the Institute of Medicine (IOM). Indeed, the IOM's serial reports on the flaws and the potential for improvements to the health care system represent a watershed in both raising national consciousness about these matters and stimulating real movement toward change, both within the profession and in public policy.

In this decade, widespread measurement of care has become a reality. The Joint Commission (TJC) has adopted a broadening set of performance measures that hospitals are required to collect and report. The data are posted to a public website. The Centers for Medicare and Medicaid Services (CMS) has now joined TJC in this effort; as of 2005, hospitals that wish to receive their full annual inflation update from CMS must report their performance measures. CMS has proposed the long-anticipated conversion of its program from "pay for accurate reporting" to "pay for performance," with some fraction of a hospital's payments adjusted according to its success in improving care as determined by these measures. The Leapfrog Group, a consortium of large employers founded in 1998 to press for changes in health care delivery, has its own scorecard to track hospitals' performance. Participation in the Leapfrog survey is voluntary, but payors and the public increasingly look to this data set for information about hospital performance. The Leapfrog and the TJC/CMS instruments measure processes (e.g., whether a hospital ensured that an aspirin was prescribed after an acute myocardial infarction) as opposed to clinical outcomes (e.g., the proportion of patients with a prior acute myocardial infarction who have a second heart attack). Process measures tend to be easier to track because they typically represent a behavior that is occurring at a snapshot in time, whereas outcomes may take much longer to assess. It is also easier to achieve expert consensus on the validity of a process

measure. Process measures also avoid the complications of socioeconomic mix of the population and severity adjustment. Hospital-based measures of outcomes tend to be reported to discipline-specific or specialty-specific national databases, or as research findings. Examples include the Vermont-Oxford database for neonatal care, the Society for Thoracic Surgeons database, and data sets collected by hospital-sponsored groups such as the University Health-System Consortium.

Physician-specific measurement has been slower to take shape in the United States but is now emerging as another important component of the field. CMS initiated in 2006 a voluntary reporting system for a finite set of process measures in the doctor's office. In December 2006, President Bush signed the Tax Relief and Health Care Act of 2006, mandating establishment of a physician quality reporting system and authorizing a payment incentive (at least initially). At this time, physician participation in the CMS quality reporting initiative is still voluntary, but beginning in the second half of 2007, physicians who share data about their care of certain conditions will receive a 1.5% financial incentive from Medicare. Private insurers have also initiated a few programs to encourage individual physicians to report data about their practice. An example is the Bridges to Excellence program, which offers bonus payments to doctors who meet standards for the care of several chronic diseases. Efforts to more closely align provider payments with quality and safety measures remain the exception but will continue to expand.

Other important contributors to the movement toward transparency and accountability in the health care system have focused less on tying performance to accreditation or payment, and more on emphasizing peer-stimulated and evidence-supported incremental change. A prominent example is the 2005 IHI 100,000 Lives Campaign. Participating hospitals (3,000 ultimately enrolled) and their medical staff volunteered to commit resources to implement a series of practices that the medical literature has unequivocally shown will reduce in-hospital deaths. The IHI evidence suggests that most hospitals were successful in improving clinical outcomes and safety in one or more of the six suggested interventions. Most participants continue to work on these interventions. In December 2006, the IHI launched a new drive to reduce avoidable morbidity in hospitalized patients. Another organization, the National Quality Forum (NQF), has focused on creating, codifying, and disseminating standards of clinical practice that represent the best clinical evidence (and expert consensus). The NQF serves a valuable function by accelerating the endorsement of consensus-based national standards for measurement and public reporting of data about specific clinical diagnostic and therapeutic interventions. Other groups, such as Leapfrog, TJC, CMS, and specialty societies, can adopt these standards rather than having to create their own and can thereby focus on helping providers to improve care.

Although the ultimate impact of the initiatives outlined on the quality of care rendered to individual patients remains to be established, few can dispute that the central goal of improving our health care delivery system is worth any effort required. The hesitancy of some providers to embrace and participate in quality-enhancing initiatives often reflects the time constraints of a busy clinical practice rather than a lack of interest. To deal with the realities of the modern time- and resource-constrained clinical practice environment, policymakers must acknowledge the need for clinicians to have more infrastructure support to comply with new guidelines. In many cases, that will require an increase in hospital and professional fees to cover the additional overhead costs.

Additional Resources

Donabedian A: Evaluating the quality of medical care. Milbank Mem Fund Q 44:166-206, 1966.
This article provides a good general review.

Donabedian A: Explorations in Quality Assessment and Monitoring, vols I-III. Ann Arbor, MI, Health Administration Press, 1980, 1985.
This text is considered the "bible" of the preferred methodologic approach for health services research.

Institute for Healthcare Improvement. Available at: http://www.ihi.org. Accessed February 4, 2007.
The IHI's website is an excellent source of information about U.S. and international care improvement activities. Some areas of the site are for members only, and some publications are available for sale, but a great deal of the information is free and available.

Kohn LT, Corrigan JM, Donaldson MS (eds), for the Committee on Quality of Health Care in America, Institute of Medicine: To Err is Human: Building a Safer Health System. Washington, DC, National Academy Press, 2000.
This first report of the Committee on the Quality of Health Care in America is the source of the oft-quoted figure of "98,000 deaths from medical errors each year." This figure is based on scant data, but the assertion drew attention to the remainder of this document, which focuses on all parties' obligation to prevent and mitigate harm in the course of trying to do good for patients.

National Quality Forum. Available at: http://www.qualityforum.org. Accessed February 4, 2007.
The NQF has evolved as the best developer of consensus standards for medical care. Expect its publications to continue to serve as the basis for P4P programs and Joint Commission goals.

U.S. Department of Health and Human Services, Centers for Medicare and Medicaid Services: Physician Voluntary Reporting Program. Available at: http://www.cms.hhs.gov/PQRI. Accessed February 4, 2007.
This website reviews the requirements, expectations, and general organization of this program.

EVIDENCE

1. Committee on Quality of Health Care in America, Institute of Medicine: Crossing the Quality Chasm: A New Health System for the 21st Century. Washington, DC, National Academy Press, 2001.
An excellent summary of the state of the health care system at the start of this century, and still the definitive consensus summary of the fundamental changes that physicians and health care organizations can make to improve care. The document's Six Aims for Improvement are the most widely cited definition of quality: health care should be safe, effective, patient centered, timely, efficient, and equitable.

2. U.S. Department of Health and Human Services: Hospital Compare—A quality tool for adults, including people with Medicare. Available at: http://www.hospitalcompare.hhs.gov/. Accessed February 4, 2007.
This consumer-friendly website provides data submitted by more than 90% of U.S. hospitals, allowing the viewer to make comparisons among these hospitals.

Russell P. Harris

2

Overview of Preventive Medicine

Introduction

High-quality health care requires not only treatment of medical conditions but also attention to effective preventive care. Prevention is defined as the reduction of risk for future adverse health events. A number of disparate services are regarded as prevention, including immunizations, screening, individual and group interventions for lifestyle change, and prophylaxis. As many as 50% of deaths in the United States are potentially preventable with current knowledge.

Like other medical care, preventive services can cause harm as well as benefit. Unlike treating serious medical problems, the risk that is addressed by prevention is small when seen in individual terms. For example, the probability of an asymptomatic 50-year-old woman having breast cancer detectable by her next mammogram is 4 to 5 in 1000, and the probability that her life will be extended by this mammogram is less than 1 in 1000. But, because so many people are involved, the absolute number of lives affected by preventive care can be large. For example, the lives of some 10,000 women each year in the United States either are or could be extended by breast cancer screening. Thus, it is most useful to think of the benefits and harms of prevention in terms of a practice's total patient population. High levels of participation are needed to maximize the number of patients who benefit.

For many health conditions, there is no effective prevention strategy yet available. This is sometimes frustrating and can lead proponents to recommend various untested or less than adequately tested preventive services. Because these services may ultimately be shown to lead to net harm rather than net benefit, and because performing ineffective services may take time and effort away from more effective services, it is important for clinicians to utilize two criteria to prioritize preventive services that (1) address an important health condition for the specific patient, and (2) have been shown to lead to more benefit than harm.

Although clinicians may be overwhelmed by the number of *proposed* preventive care services, only a limited number of these services actually meet these criteria. Analyzing the tradeoffs between benefits and harms for each service is complex, however. We suggest that clinicians closely follow the recommendations of the U.S. Preventive Services Task Force (USPSTF), a nonfederal panel of prevention experts, to help understand which preventive services to prioritize. For immunizations, the best recommendations are those by the Advisory Committee on Immunization Practices (ACIP), convened by the Centers for Disease Control and Prevention (CDC).

The next section briefly discusses the "prevention strategies" available to clinicians. The following sections discuss common conditions and proposed preventive services, examining which meet our criteria and should be prioritized by clinicians. Table 2-1 gives an overview of suggested priority preventive services for adults. Table 2-2 gives some selected services that should not be prioritized, and Table 2-3 provides some that should not be provided at all unless there are special circumstances.

Table 2-1 Priority Preventive Services for Adults

Priority Health Problem	Priority Population	Effective Service/Comments
Immunization-preventable disease	All ages	Various immunizations; see: http://www.cdc.gov/nip/recs/adult-schedule.htm
Tobacco-related problems (e.g., CVD, lung cancer, emphysema)	All ages	Screening and appropriate counseling of current smokers, plus preventive counseling of adolescents
Cardiovascular disease	Smoking and blood pressure screening at all ages; focus lipid screening on men ages 45 years and older; women ages 55 years and older; focus screening for diabetes on people with hypertension or dyslipidemia	Screening for and appropriately treating CVD risk factors: dyslipidemia, smoking, blood pressure, diabetes Note that aggressiveness of treatment depends on the level of global CVD risk No need to screen people for diabetes who do not have hypertension or dyslipidemia
Cardiovascular disease	Focus on men ages 45-75 years and women ages 55-75 years	Low-dose aspirin for people with more than 10% 10-year risk
Rupture of abdominal aortic aneurysm	Current or previously smoking men ages 65-75 years	Abdominal ultrasound, screen once only unless abnormal No need to screen nonsmokers and women
Colorectal cancer	Men and women, ages 50-75 years if healthy	Screening with one of four approaches: home fecal occult blood (FOBT) cards done annually; sigmoidoscopy every 5 years; both FOBT and sigmoidoscopy; colonoscopy every 10 years
Breast cancer	Women ages 50-75 years; women ages 40-50 years who have considered pros and cons of screening	Mammography and clinical breast examination by a health care provider every 1-2 years (note: women over age 50 years with a negative and no abnormal mammogram within the previous 2 years can be screened every 2 years)
Cervical cancer	Sexually active women under age 65 years with an intact cervix	Papanicolaou smear every 3 years unless recent positive test No need to screen women without a cervix, women not sexually active, women older than 65 years if previous negative screening
Depression	All adults	Two-question screening test: (1) "Over the past 2 weeks, have you felt down, depressed, or hopeless?" (2) "Over the past 2 weeks, have you felt little interest or pleasure in doing things?" Diagnostic interview and appropriate treatment/follow-up needed for positive screening test
Falls and fractures	Men and women ages 65 years and older	Screen for adequate vitamin D intake and counsel if too low Screen for previous falls and assess fall risk factors if positive Minimize psychoactive drugs Screen people ages 65 years and older for osteoporosis and appropriately treat people in osteoporotic range No need to screen people younger than 65 years unless they have important risk factors
Automobile crashes	All adults	Screen for alcohol misuse and counsel if detected Counsel to wear lap and shoulder restraints
Obesity	All adults	Screen for obesity by calculating BMI and for level of physical activity Discuss diagnosis of obesity and low physical activity with patient and consider approaches for change, including referral to intensive community programs
Sexually transmitted infections (e.g., chlamydia and gonorrhea)	Sexually active women ages 15-26 years and older women with risk factors	Screen and appropriately treat: (1) chlamydia in all groups meeting criteria; (2) gonorrhea, focusing on women living in high-prevalence areas
HIV	All ages	Screen and appropriately treat: patients who ask about screening; patients with any risk factors; patients who live in areas with average or high levels of HIV infection The only people excluded are people without risk factors living in low-risk areas
Visual problems	Adults ages 65 years and older	Screen by asking about visual function and by Snellen chart; refer to ophthalmologist if positive
Hearing problems	Adults ages 65 years and older	Screen by whispered-voice test or HHIE questionnaire; refer for audiology if positive

BMI, body mass index; CVD, cardiovascular disease; HHIE, Hearing Handicap Inventory for the Elderly; HIV, human immunodeficiency virus.

Table 2-2 Preventive Services That Should Not Be Prioritized*

Preventive Service	Population	Comments
Routine prostate-specific antigen and digital rectal exam to screen for prostate cancer	Adult men	May discuss with men ages 50-70 years and provide to those who understand pros and cons and still want to be tested
Routine total-body skin exam for melanoma	Adults	Should refer for suspicious lesions detected in usual exam for other reasons
Routine examination of the oral cavity for oral cancer	Adults	Should refer for suspicious lesions detected in usual exam for other reasons
Routine screening for family/domestic violence	Adults	Should maintain a high index of suspicion in women with depression or vague symptoms
Routine screening for dementia/cognitive impairment	Adults	Should maintain a high index of suspicion in people with cognitive change or poor judgment
Routine screening for glaucoma	Adults	Should maintain a high index of suspicion in older, African American men with eye complaints
Routine screening for thyroid dysfunction	Adults	Should maintain a high index of suspicion in older women with nonspecific complaints

* Note that all these suggestions refer to usual-risk people with no known symptoms. They do not refer to people at high risk or with special-risk situations. People with symptoms should be examined and tested appropriately—this is not screening.

Table 2-3 Preventive Services That Should Generally Not Be Provided*

Preventive Service	Population
Urine analysis for blood to screen for bladder cancer	Adults
Supplements for beta carotene, vitamins E, A, and C	Adults with normal diet
Postmenopausal hormone therapy	Postmenopausal women
Screening ECG, exercise ECG, coronary calcium, ankle-brachial index for existing coronary heart disease or risk for future coronary heart disease	Adults
CA-125 and ultrasound to screen for ovarian cancer	Adult women
Ultrasound or CT to screen for pancreatic cancer	Adults
Testicular examination to screen for testicular cancer	Adult men
Routinely teaching breast self-examination to screen for breast cancer	Adult women
Routine urinalysis to screen for asymptomatic bacteriuria	Adults
Routine screening for hepatitis C	Adults
Routine chest x-ray or spiral CT to screen for lung cancer	Adults
Duplex carotid ultrasound for carotid artery stenosis	Adults
Whole-body CT scan	Adults

* Note that all these suggestions refer to usual-risk people with no known symptoms. They do not refer to people at high risk or with special-risk situations. People with symptoms should be examined and tested appropriately—this is not screening.
CT, computed tomography; ECG, electrocardiography.

Prevention Strategies

Immunizations

Six immunizations are currently recommended by the ACIP for routine use in adults:

- Tetanus, diphtheria booster every 10 years (for people ages 19 to 64 years, at least one booster should be tetanus, diphtheria, and acellular pertussis)
- Influenza (inactivated intramuscular) vaccine once each year for people ages 50 years and older (and special groups under age 50 years; live vaccine [FluMist] can be offered to healthy, nonpregnant patients ages 5 to 49 years)
- Pneumococcal vaccine once after age 65 years (and special groups under age 65 years)
- Measles, mumps, and rubella if born in 1957 or afterward and not previously immunized
- Varicella for people born in 1966 or afterward who have never had varicella infection or previous immunization
- Human papillomavirus vaccine for females ages 9 to 26 years

Another vaccine approved by the Food and Drug Administration is a high-potency varicella vaccine for adults age 60 years and older to prevent herpes zoster. Other vaccines (e.g., hepatitis A and B and meningococcal vaccine) are recommended for special groups. The complete ACIP adult immunization recommendation table can be accessed from the CDC website.

Screening

Screening is a widespread strategy that is often misunderstood. We are screening all the time. The "annual physical" is actually a series of screening questions, examinations, and tests—searching for disease (or risk factors) in people with no recognized symptom or sign of the condition. The basic idea of screening is that earlier treatment may lead to better health than later treatment (after symptoms or signs appear). The problem is that, as intuitive as this idea seems, it is only sometimes correct. Sometimes, in fact, screening can lead to more harm than benefit.

There are at least three ways that screening can lead to harm: through adverse effects of (1) the screening test itself; (2) false-positive screening tests; and (3) detection of conditions that require surveillance or treatment but would never have progressed to cause clinical problems (sometimes called *pseudodisease*).

Adverse Effects of Screening Tests

Most screening tests have few adverse effects. Some tests, however, can cause complications. A study published in 2006, for example, found a serious complication rate of 5 per 1000 people receiving a colonoscopy. Any complication of screening tests must be counted against the number of people whose lives are extended by screening.

Adverse Effects of False-Positive Tests

Because screening is conducted in people who have a small (though not zero) risk for a condition, most screening tests result in more false-positive results than true-positive results. For example, less than 10% of "positive" mammograms lead to a diagnosis of breast cancer; more than 90% are falsely positive. People with false-positive screening tests often experience considerable anxiety until they have a negative confirmatory test. If the confirmatory test is itself not completely sensitive (e.g., prostate biopsy for an elevated prostate-specific antigen screening test), this anxiety can be prolonged. In addition, if the confirmatory test carries some discomfort or risk (e.g., laparoscopy for a positive ovarian cancer screening test or lung biopsy for a positive spiral computed tomography screening test), then the person with a false-positive screening test has a higher probability of being harmed. These possible harms must be counted against the number of people whose lives are extended by screening.

Adverse Effects of Detection of Pseudodisease

Studies of large groups of people tell us that some conditions detected by screening would never cause clinical problems for the patient. Some of these conditions include in situ cancers (e.g., ductal carcinoma in situ of the breast), "pre" conditions (e.g., "prediabetes" or "prehypertension"), benign conditions that only sometimes progress (e.g., colonic polyps or cervical intraepithelial neoplasia type I or II), or slowly progressive conditions (e.g., many prostate cancers). Detection of such conditions often leads to increased anxiety for the patient. Even more concerning, because we are often unable to determine which people

with these conditions will suffer clinical problems and which will not, we usually subject most or all to treatment. For those who would never have had clinical problems, this amounts to overtreatment and may cause undue suffering from adverse treatment effects (e.g., radical prostatectomy for prostate cancer, leading to impotence or incontinence).

Lifestyle Change

Such lifestyle issues as tobacco use, obesity, lack of physical activity, alcohol abuse, not using car restraints or bicycle helmets, and unsafe storage of firearms contribute to many deaths in the United States. Changing such unhealthy lifestyles would have potentially large benefit for the health of the public. Studies are clear that, properly done, counseling by clinicians can help patients stop smoking cigarettes and reduce problematic alcohol intake. Changing such behaviors as physical inactivity and unhealthy weight gain, however, is more difficult to accomplish in the context of a clinical office visit. Growing evidence suggests that broader programs that target groups with behavioral and social interventions as well as information can have positive effects on unhealthy lifestyles. Such programs may be developed and offered within the community or by health plans. Clinicians should consider referring appropriate patients to these programs. Appropriate patients would include those who have an interest in changing lifestyle. Clinicians can use motivational interviewing techniques to encourage patients to make these changes.

Prophylaxis

Prophylaxis is intervening with a treatment such as medication to prevent an adverse health event. Examples include "treatment" of hypertension and hyperlipidemia to prevent cardiovascular events. Many considerations are relevant in trying to maximize benefit and minimize harm from prophylactic interventions. Some of these include the following:

- At what level of risk to begin treatment
- How intensively to treat
- What should be the target of treatment
- What are the adverse effects of the treatment

In general, people at higher risk have more to benefit and can be treated more aggressively. Often, however, our approaches to defining an individual at sufficiently increased risk to warrant treatment are inadequate. Also, the safety of prophylactic interventions is an important limitation to widespread use of prophylaxis. If even a small percentage of the large number of treated people suffer an adverse effect of the treatment, this may outweigh any benefit. This is the case, for example, for tamoxifen prophylaxis to prevent breast cancer for most women.

Common Conditions and Proposed Preventive Services

Note that the recommendations below are for usual-risk patients, not for patients with special conditions at very high risk.

Cardiovascular Disease

A small number of preventive activities, widely performed, could effectively reduce the large burden of cardiovascular disease. These include appropriate treatment of risk factors, counseling for smoking cessation, and aspirin prophylaxis. The approach begins with an assessment of a patient's "global cardiovascular risk." People at high global risk should be offered aggressive risk factor control (see USPSTF recommendations on hypertension, lipids, aspirin, and smoking cessation). People at even moderate risk should still consider aspirin, smoking cessation, and moderate control of other risk factors. The most important risk factors to consider are those in the Framingham model: blood pressure, cholesterol, smoking, diabetes, age, and gender.

In addition to prevention of coronary artery disease and stroke, a single screening for large (>5.5 cm) abdominal aortic aneurysm (AAA) among men ages 65 to 75 years who have ever smoked could reduce the number of deaths from AAA rupture.

Cancer

The cancers that cause the largest number of deaths in the United States are lung, colorectal, breast, and prostate. Screening is clearly effective in reducing mortality for colorectal and breast cancers. The most effective way to reduce mortality for lung cancer is smoking cessation. We do not yet have a clearly effective way to reduce mortality from prostate cancer. Trials of screening are underway but will not be completed for another several years.

There are four effective ways to screen for colorectal cancer: home fecal occult blood test (FOBT) cards done annually; flexible sigmoidoscopy every 5 years; both FOBT and sigmoidoscopy; and colonoscopy every 10 years. The ideal approach is the one that the patient is most comfortable with.

Optimal breast cancer screening includes both screening mammography and clinical breast examination. Women over age 50 years who have had no abnormal screening test in the past several years may be screened every other year. Women in their 40s may be given the option of screening, although the benefit from screening is small at that age.

In addition to these cancers, screening for cervical cancer is clearly effective. A woman who has had her cervix removed for nonmalignant reasons need not be screened. Women with repeated negative screening tests can be screened every 3 years rather than annually. Women with recent negative screening tests need not be screened after age 65 years.

Depression

Brief screening for depression, coupled with evaluation and possible treatment of people who are found to be depressed, is effective in improving the quality of life. Asking two questions ("Over the past 2 weeks, have you felt down, depressed, or hopeless?" and "Over the past 2 weeks, have you felt little interest or pleasure in doing things?") is sufficient to detect many cases of subclinical depression.

Injury Prevention

Clinicians should consider three major areas in preventing injuries: prevention of falls and bone fractures; prevention of motor vehicle crashes; and prevention of domestic violence.

Multifactorial risk assessment and control programs and exercise interventions effectively reduce falls in older people. These programs assess such issues as postural hypotension, gait unsteadiness, psychotropic medication use, strength, nutrition, and auditory and visual problems. Routinely asking about previous falls and targeting more intensive examinations for those who have a recent fall is also a reasonable strategy.

Screening women older than 65 years for osteoporosis is another important strategy. Bisphosphonate therapy of women with osteoporosis reduces fractures. Because of the low fracture risk, screening younger women—unless they have special risk factors—is not indicated.

Use of car lap and shoulder restraint systems reduces motor vehicle crashes. These are most widely used when they are automatic and require no individual decision. Clinician counseling can reduce inappropriate alcohol use; clinicians should screen for this problem.

The evidence is insufficient to determine whether screening for family and domestic violence is useful; we don't recommend it at this time. However, being alert to the sometimes subtle signs and symptoms of family violence can help find women who are being abused physically or emotionally. Women who are found to be suffering domestic violence should be given information about local resources for assistance.

Lifestyle-Related Problems

Obesity and physical inactivity are major and growing problems in our society. Intentional weight reduction and increased physical activity are associated with reductions in diabetes risk, hypertension, and mortality. Although brief counseling infrequently affects these lifestyles, more intensive programs that include behavioral and social components can be effective. We recommend that clinicians familiarize themselves with community and health plan programs for obese and physically inactive patients and refer appropriate patients to these programs.

Sexually Transmitted Infections

Women at increased risk for chlamydia and gonorrhea infection should be screened. For chlamydia, this includes women ages 15 to 25 years and older women with behavioral risk factors such as multiple sexual partners. For gonorrhea, this includes younger, sexually active women living in high-risk areas.

The recommendation for screening for human immunodeficiency virus (HIV) infection includes more people now than in the past. This is because of both the availability of tests with very few false-positive results and the availability of effective treatment. Screening now should be considered for men and women who have other sexually transmitted infections, have behavioral risk factors (e.g., men who have sex with men, multiple sexual partners), or live in high or moderate prevalence areas.

Substance Abuse–Related Problems

Alcohol misuse is common and an important cause of morbidity and mortality in our society. Screening and brief counseling and follow-up for alcohol misuse in office settings have been shown to reduce alcohol consumption.

Tobacco use causes more than 400,000 deaths each year in the United States. Screening and brief counseling for smoking cessation increases long-term quit rates. Use of such adjunctive treatments as nicotine replacement and bupropion treatment can reduce quit rates further.

Vision and Hearing Problems

People over age 65 years frequently develop problems with vision and hearing. These problems may develop so slowly that patients are not aware that they are present. Thus, simple screening with questions about function (including the Hearing Handicap Inventory for the Elderly questionnaire for hearing), brief testing of visual acuity, and the whispered-voice test for hearing can detect people who would benefit from referral for further evaluation.

What Not to Do

If clinicians focus primarily on getting the previously described services done, they will be making an important contribution to the health of their patients. Other services may be highly recommended by others but frequently either cause important injuries or are backed by insufficient evidence of benefit. Table 2-3 gives a selected list of commonly discussed services that we recommend *not* be generally provided unless there are special circumstances.

The Health Maintenance Examination ("Annual Physical")

Much of the periodic health maintenance examination is screening. This examination is an insufficient approach to delivering preventive care for at least two reasons: (1) many people do not get a periodic exam, and (2) some services, such as controlling blood pressure, elevated lipids, and counseling for smoking cessation, cannot be effectively delivered in a single visit. In addition, the usual activities on this visit—a comprehensive review of systems and a complete physical examination—are poor screening tests for many patients.

On the other hand, a focused examination that takes into account the problems for which a patient is at highest risk, and the most effective preventive services for reducing that risk, can be an efficient way of delivering some preventive services to some people. This type of visit can also have other benefits, including developing the patient-clinician relationship and helping the patient understand better how to use the health care system.

Conclusion

Although preventive care is not the panacea that some have suggested, it can make a substantial contribution to the health of patients. It is best to know one's patients well: what are the health conditions for which they are at greatest risk? Then it is important to understand the science of prevention: what services can most effectively reduce that risk?

In the past, some have used a haphazard approach of delivering prevention to each patient, emphasizing whatever is "hot" and interesting (and there is time for). We prefer instead a thoughtful, proactive approach of determining ahead of time what you will recommend for each patient, and then finding systematic approaches within the practice to make sure all patients receive good information and encouragement to adhere to the preventive services that are appropriate for them. This approach is likely to help keep your patients healthy as long as possible.

Additional Resources

Centers for Disease Control and Prevention. Advisory Committee on Immunization Practices. Available at: http://www.cdc.gov/nip/acip/. Accessed December 20, 2006.

This is the website for the nationally endorsed set of recommendations for immunizations. The recommendations are updated regularly. The complete table of ACIP recommendations for adult immunizations can be accessed at http://www.cdc.gov/nip/recs/adult-schedule.htm.

The Community Guide. Recommendations of the Community Task Force on Preventive Health Practices. Sponsored by CDC's National Center for Health Marketing and the Community Guide Partners. Available at: http://www.thecommunityguide.org. Accessed January 9, 2007.

This website provides the recommendations of the Community Task Force, an evidence-based group convened by the CDC to examine community-level interventions for prevention.

Med-Decisions.com. Available at: http://www.med-decisions.com. Accessed December 20, 2006.

This website provides a simple and clinically useful approach to determining global risk for coronary heart disease.

EVIDENCE

United States Preventive Services Task Force. Available at: http://www.preventiveservices.ahrq.gov. Accessed January 28, 2007.

This is the website for the most evidence-based recommendations on preventive care. Recommendations are updated regularly, and the website contains key references for the recommendations in this chapter.

National Cancer Institute. Statements of the "Physician Data Query" (PDQ) Screening and Prevention Board of the NCI. Available at: http://www.cancer.gov/cancertopics/pdq/prevention or http://www.cancer.gov/cancertopics/pdq/screening. Accessed January 9, 2007.

This website gives regularly updated, evidence-based statements about issues in cancer screening and prevention.

John S. Kizer

3

Diagnostic Testing: The Example of Thromboembolism (PE/DVT)

Introduction

Testing is a strategy to improve diagnostic certainty. It is necessary because of the statistical improbability of any disease presenting according to classic descriptions. The diagnostic certainty needed by a clinician depends on the seriousness of the illness in question and the hazards of therapy—the notion of an action threshold. For example, a benign illness with a benign therapy (acetaminophen for viral pharyngitis) requires little certainty to take action, whereas a more serious disease, thromboembolism (pulmonary embolism and deep venous thrombosis [PE/DVT]), with a more hazardous therapy requires greater diagnostic certainty.

Typically, clinicians ask whether a test was positive or negative so that they can "rule out" or "rule in" a disease. Tests, however, are not dichotomous variables; they convey increasing levels of information the further they deviate from "normal." For example, a patient with 4-mm ST-segment depression and crushing chest pain during an electrocardiographic (ECG) exercise test is much more likely to have coronary artery disease than a patient with 2-mm ST-segment depression and no pain, even though both tests are "positive." Conversely, vitamin B_{12} deficiency is just as likely to be present at levels of 192 ng/mL and 194 ng/mL, even though the former is "abnormal" and the latter is "normal" by laboratory nomograms. By extrapolation, one can never state that a patient does or does not have a disease, only the probability that the patient has a disease. The physician then must decide whether a threshold for action has been crossed.

PE/DVT is particularly vexing because of the attendant morbidity, the difficulty in diagnosis, and the confusing array of diagnostic tests. Many diagnostic algorithms have been proposed, but they are cumbersome and still require the dichotomous notion of cutoffs: if "negative," go to A;

if "positive," go to B. Diagnostic methods that permit one to acquire realistic estimates of disease and to decide whether an action threshold has been crossed would be more useful. Such methods would circumvent cumbersome algorithms and enable clinicians to think of a continuum of risk. It is likely that concrete assessments of risk are understood more universally by clinicians than vaguer terms, such as *low probability* and *high risk*. For example, the perioperative risk for myocardial infarction in a high-risk population is 4% to 5%.

Glossary of Terms

Sensitivity: Rate of detection of those with disease, also true-positive rate
Specificity: Rate of detection of those without disease, also true-negative rate
False-positive rate: (1 − specificity)
False-negative rate: (1 − sensitivity)
Probability (or chance): Occurrence of given event expressed as fraction of all possible events. For

example, when tossing a coin twice, the probability of getting heads is 2/(2+2) = 2/4 = 50%

Odds: Number of occurrences of one event expressed as a ratio to the number of occurrences of a second event. For example, for two heads and two tails, the odds are 2/2 or 1/1 for heads. Thus, an odds ratio of 1/1 = probability of 1/2 (50%). (Note that odds may not be multiplied together.)

Positive likelihood ratio (+LLR): True-positive rate divided by false-positive rate

Negative likelihood ratio (−LLR): False-negative rate divided by true-negative rate

Pretest probability of disease: The probability that a patient has a given disease before testing. The pretest probability of disease for a specific patient is also equal to the prevalence of the disease in a population of similar patients.

Pretest odds: As for pretest probability, but calculated as an odds

Post-test probability: With positive test, also positive predictive value. Given a positive test, the probability that a patient has the disease for which he was tested

Post-test probability: With negative test, also negative predictive value

Post-test odds with positive test: As for post-test probability, but expressed as an odds. Post-test odds = pretest odds × LLR1 × LLR2 × LLR . . . n = post-test odds

Post-test odds with negative test: Similar to above

The Case for Likelihood Ratios

Traditionally, tests with high sensitivities have been advocated to "rule out" disease and tests with high specificities are considered to "rule in" disease. Consider, however, the following two tests. If negative, which test best excludes disease in a patient with a 50% chance (pretest odds, 1/1) of having the disease?

	Sensitivity	Specificity	+LLR	−LLR
Test A	90%	10%	1.0	1.0
Test B	80%	30%	1.1	0.7

Test A pretest odds (1/1) × −LLR (1.0) = post-test odds (1/1) = post-test probability of 50% (no change).
Test B pretest odds (1/1) × −LLR (0.7) = post-test odds (0.7/1) = post-test probability of 0.7/1.7 = 41%. Therefore, test B is a better test. Thus, an LLR can fully express the value of a test in a single number. As a guide, +LLRs near 10 and −LLRs near 1/10 are quite good and will affect decisions substantially.

Remember, according to Bayes' theorem, testing at very high pretest probabilities of disease or at very low pretest probabilities may not greatly affect a clinical decision. For example, what is the probability of breast cancer in a 40-year-old woman whose screening mammogram is read as suspicious? Pretest probability of breast cancer (prevalence) in 40-year-old = 1/4000 = pretest odds of 1/3999. +LLR for screening mammogram in 40-year-old = 80. Post-test odds = 1/3999 × 80 = 80/3999. Probability is 80/4079, or 1.9%. Thus, 98% of women such as this do not have breast cancer even if they have a suspicious mammogram.

As a corollary, expressing test performance as an "accuracy" (a positive or negative predictive value) is of little use because these terms are composites of pretest probability (highly dependent on the clinical scenario) and LLR (the only invariant measure of test performance).

Estimates of Pretest Probability of Thromboembolism (DVT/PE)

Calculating the post-test probability of disease depends, therefore, on knowledge of the LLR for a test and a reasonably accurate assessment of pretest probability (prevalence).

Pulmonary Embolism

The two best known scoring tools for pretest assessment of risk for PE are the Geneva score (outpatients) and the Wells score (inpatients and outpatients). Concordance between the two is excellent, but the latter is simpler, more widely used, and possibly more accurate:

Previous PE/DVT	1.5 points
Heart rate >100 beats/minute	1.5
Recent surgery or immobilization	1.5
Clinical signs of DVT	3.0
Other diagnoses less likely	3.0
Malignancy	1.0
Hemoptysis	1.0

Values ≤1 (<5% probability); 2 to 6 (20% to 30%); ≥7 (50% to70%). Others have suggested dichotomizing the results into low (0 to 4) and high (≥5) probabilities, but this modification lessens its discriminant power.

Deep Venous Thrombosis

Similarly, the simplified Wells prediction score for DVT has proved useful as a clinical tool for evaluation of outpatients, although its validity in primary care may require further study.

Cancer in past 6 months, treated or not	1 point
Paralysis, casting, or splinting of lower leg	1
Bedridden 3 days, major surgery past 3 months	1
Tenderness along the deep venous system	1
Entire leg swelling	1
Pitting edema confined to the affected leg	1
Calf swelling >3 cm larger than contralateral leg	1

Table 3-1 Testing for Pulmonary Embolism

Test	+LLR	−LLR
Arterial blood gas, A-a gradient, etc.	~1	~1
V/Q scan High probability	17	
Intermediate	1.1	
Low	0.7	
Normal or near normal	0.1	
Multidetector chest CT	7.8	0.24
Chest magnetic resonance imaging	Unknown	
Pulmonary angiography	50	0.02
D-Dimer Low sensitivity	1.7-5.0	0.15-0.35
High sensitivity	1.5-2.4	0.06-0.10

A-a, alveolar-arterial; CT, computed tomography; V/Q, ventilation-perfusion.

Table 3-2 Testing for Deep Venous Thrombosis

Test (Symptomatic Patients)	+LLR	−LLR
Duplex and color-flow ultrasonography	24	0.04
Impedance plethysmography	10	0.06
D-Dimer (as above)		

Superficial collateral veins (not varicosities)	1
Previous documented DVT	1
Other diagnosis equally as likely as DVT	−2

Values ≤0 (2% to 5% probability); 1 to 2 (30%); ≥3 (50% to 60%).

Laboratory Testing for DVT/PE

See Tables 3-1 and 3-2.

The LLRs for chest computed tomography (CT) presented in the table are less optimistic than those proposed by the Prospective Investigation of Pulmonary Embolism Diagnosis (PIOPED) II investigators because the investigators omitted any indeterminate scan from their calculations, a method that falsely inflates the sensitivities and specificities of a test. Thus, despite its wide use, the performance characteristics of chest CT are inferior to those of the ventilation-perfusion (V/Q) scan. In the presence of chronic lung disease, however, the LLRs for V/Q scans are degraded, perhaps by half, because of the presence of more indeterminate scans, rendering CT scans and V/Q scans of equal value in this setting.

Confidence in the D-dimer test is justified by the growing precision of estimates of its sensitivity and specificity, but it should be emphasized that this test is not applicable in sick inpatients, in whom the LLRs are less favorable because of low-grade clotting in venous access sites. Use of the D-dimer to estimate the risk for recurrence has been proposed but not extensively verified.

Strategies for Testing

Strategies for the diagnosis of PE rely heavily on an understanding of the disease. First, immediate evidence of a proximal venous thrombosis is often lacking in those presenting with PE, presumably because the clot is now in the lung. Second, in the stable patient with a recent PE, the goal of therapy is not to treat the current PE but to prevent a recurrence. Third, if the deep venous system (defined as the veins from the popliteal fossa proximally) remains empty of clot, the risk for recurrent PE is very low. These findings, coupled with the realization that calf vein thrombi rarely embolize unless they propagate proximally, have focused diagnostic strategies on proximal DVT in patients who cannot easily be shown to have a PE. Fourth, because these strategies for diagnosis have been validated only in the outpatient setting, caution should be exercised in applying them to sick inpatients. Finally, there is no firm evidence that each of these tests and prediction rules is statistically independent.

In the patient whose presentation suggests PE, the initial strategy is to perform a V/Q or CT scan because the pretest probability of finding clot in the chest is higher than finding it in the leg. For similar reasons, when DVT is suspected, investigation begins with studies of the leg (Boxes 3-1 and 3-2).

For both PE and DVT, the calculated action threshold is about 5% (the probability of disease at which the net benefits of therapy begin to exceed the net harm of no therapy). Therefore, because the goals of therapy are identical, the purpose of testing is to reduce the probability of venous thromboembolism to below 5%. If this threshold cannot be reached by any combination of tests, then one is forced to treat.

Further Testing

For the diagnosis of PE, when the V/Q scan (or CT scan) fails to lower the post-test probability of thromboembolism to below the action threshold of 5% to 10%, further

---

Box 3-1 Pulmonary Embolism

High-risk patient (75% probability) and the initial test is:

- Positive V/Q scan: pretest odds (3/1) × +LLR (17) = post-test odds (51/1) or post-test probability of 98%. Action: treat
- Positive CT scan: (3/1) × (7.8) = post-test odds (23/1) = post-test probability of 96%. Action: treat
- Normal V/Q scan: (3/1) × (0.1) = post-test odds (0.3/1) or post-test probability of 23%, well above action threshold. Action: test further for DVT (see below)
- Negative CT scan: post-test probability of 38%. Action: test further

Moderate-risk patient (33% probability) and the initial test is:

- Positive V/Q scan: pretest odds (1/2) × +LLR (17) = post-test odds (17/2) or post-test probability of 89%. Action: treat
- Normal scan: (1/2) × (0.1) = post-test odds (0.1/2) = post-test probability of 5%. Action: no treatment

- Negative CT: Post-test probability of 9%. Action: test further
- Negative D-dimer: post-test probability (using conservative LLR) of 5%

Low-risk patient (5%) and the initial test is:

- Positive V/Q scan: pretest odds (5/95) × +LLR (17) = post-test odds (85/95) or post-test probability of 47% Action: test further for DVT because negative study can reduce probability below action threshold. (see DVT, below)
- Negative V/Q scan: (5/95) × (0.1) = post-test odds (0.5/95) or probability of 0.5%. Action: no treatment
- Negative CT scan: (5/95) × (.24) = post-test odds (1.2/95) or probability of 1%. Action: no treatment
- Negative D-dimer: (5/95) × (0.1) = post-test odds (0.5/95) or probability of 0.5%. Action: no treatment

Low- or intermediate-probability V/Q scans have no impact on decision because the LLRs are near unity.

CT, computed tomography; DVT, deep venous thrombosis; LLR, likelihood ratio; V/Q, ventilation-perfusion.

Box 3-2 Deep Venous Thrombosis

High-risk patient (85%) and the initial test is:

- Positive US: pretest odds (85/15) × (24) = post-test odds (2040/15) or post-test probability of 99%. Action: treat
- Negative US: (85/15) × (0.04) = post-test odds (3.4/15) or post-test probability of 18%. Action: no further testing required

Moderate-risk patient (33%) and the initial test is:

- Positive US: pretest odds (1/2) × (24) = post-test odds (24/2) or probability of 92%. Action: treat
- Negative US: (1/2) × (0.04) = post-test odds (0.04/2) or post-test probability of 2.0%. Action: no treatment
- Negative D-dimer: (1/2) × (0.1) = post-test odds = 0.1/2 or post-test probability of 5%. Action: no treatment

Low-risk patient and the initial test is:

- Positive US: pretest odds (5/95) × (24) = post-test odds (120/95) or probability of 56%. Action: treat. (Only venography can lower probability below action threshold.)
- Negative US: (5/95) × (0.04) = post-test odds (0.2/95) or probability of 0.2%
- Negative D-dimer: (5/95) × (0.1) = post-test probability of 0.5%. If the initial test is the D-dimer, and it is positive (post-test probability of disease about 10%), then further testing with US is needed

US, ultrasound.

Box 3-3 Further Testing for Equivocal Results

High-risk patient (75%) for PE, with negative V/Q scan (see Box 3-1) post-test probability of 23%:

- If US now positive: odds (0.3/1) × (24) = post-test odds (7.2/1) or probability of 88%. Action: now treat
- If US now negative: odds (0.3/1) × (0.04) = post-test odds (0.012/1) or probability of 1.2%. Action: no treatment

For the diagnosis of DVT, further testing with the D-dimer assay can alter the estimate of disease.

High-risk patient (85%) for DVT, with negative US (see Box 3-2) post-test probability of 18%

- If D-dimer now negative: odds (3.4/15) × (0.1) = post-test odds (0.34/15) or probability of 2.2%. Action: no treatment

DVT, deep venous thrombosis; PE, pulmonary embolism; US, ultrasound; V/Q, ventilation-perfusion.

EVIDENCE

1. Hull RD, Raskob GE, Ginsberg JS, et al: A noninvasive strategy for the treatment of patients with suspected pulmonary embolism. Arch Intern Med 154:289-297, 1994.

   An empirical trial of noninvasive strategy for assessment and treatment of suspected PE is presented.

2. Kearon C, Ginsberg JS, Douketis J, et al: A randomized trial of diagnostic strategies after normal proximal vein ultrasonography for suspected deep venous thrombosis: D-Dimer testing compared with repeated ultrasonography. Ann Intern Med 142(7):490-496, 2005.

   The authors describe a pragmatic trial to examine combined strategies for the diagnosis of DVT.

3. PIOPED Investigators: Value of the ventilation-perfusion scan in acute pulmonary embolism: Results of the PIOPED. JAMA 263:2753-2759, 1990.

   This paper describes the original large trial of diagnostic accuracy of V/Q scanning for diagnosis of pulmonary embolism.

testing with ultrasound can better estimate the probability of thromboembolism (Box 3-3).

Additional Resources

Black ER, Bordley DR, Tape TG, Panzer RJ: Diagnostic strategies for common medical problems, 2nd ed. Philadelphia, American College of Physicians, 1999.

   The authors discuss methods for the use of LLRs and pretest probability estimates for many medical problems.

4. PIOPED II Investigators: Multidetector computed tomography for acute pulmonary embolism. N Engl J Med 354:2317-2327, 2006.

This report is the only large, well-designed clinical trial to examine the diagnostic accuracy of CT for PE.

5. Wells PS, Owen C, Doucette S, et al: Does this patient have deep venous thrombosis? JAMA 295:199-207, 2006.

The authors provide a systematic review of studies of D-dimer and clinical rules to predict DVT.

M. Andrew Greganti ▪ Marschall S. Runge

4

Obesity

Introduction

Obesity is a complex multifactorial disorder that results in the accumulation of excess adipose tissue, increases the risk for morbidity and mortality, and lessens life expectancy markedly (Figs. 4-1 and 4-2). Definitions of the terms *overweight*, *obesity*, and *severe* or *morbid obesity* vary among authoritative sources and depend on gender and ethnic background. Generally, overweight and obesity are defined based on body mass index (BMI), the weight in kilograms divided by the height in meters squared. Overweight in whites is defined as a BMI of 25 to 29.9 kg/m² and obesity as a BMI greater than 30 kg/m². Severe or morbid obesity refers to those patients with a BMI of greater than 40 kg/m². Some studies have demonstrated that the waist-to-hip ratio, which defines the degree of visceral obesity, correlates better with cardiovascular and other morbidity; however, the BMI-based definition is the common standard used in most clinical guidelines (see Fig. 4-1).

The developed world currently faces an epidemic of obesity. Based on National Health and Nutrition Examination Survey (NHANES) data comparing 1999 to 2000, 2001 to 2002, and 2003 to 2004 data for the United States, the prevalence of obesity among men increased significantly from 1999 to 2000 (27.4%) to 2003 to 2004 (31.1%). Data from 2003 to 2004 documented that 32.1% of adults in the United States were obese. The prevalence of morbid obesity among American men in 2003-2004 was 2.8% and among American women, 6.9%. Perhaps even more worrisome is the increasing prevalence of overweight children and adolescents: 17.1% in 2003 to 2004. The percentages are even higher in Hispanic Americans and African Americans. The current epidemic in obesity and obesity-related illnesses likely represents the fastest-growing health risk for men, women, and children in the United States. Although obesity is most prevalent in the United States, its rapidly increasing incidence is becoming a worldwide problem, with similar trends in most European countries.

Etiology and Pathogenesis

Obesity results from the complicated interaction of environmental and genetic factors and an imbalance between caloric intake and expenditure. Both increased caloric intake and decreased exercise are hallmarks of obesity (Fig. 4-3). The factors that affect adult obesity probably begin in utero with maternal caloric intake influencing later body size and composition. Maternal smoking and diabetes mellitus increase the risk for obesity in later life. Breastfeeding decreases the risk for childhood obesity and obesity later in life. Having an obese parent more than doubles the risk for obesity as an adult.

Although genetic factors are undoubtedly important, most experts believe that the marked increase in obesity in the United States during the past 40 years is caused by a convergence of two primary factors:

1. Only 20% of the population exercises enough to be considered physically fit. The percentage of adult Americans who engage in physical activity decreases with age, and the associated decrease in energy expenditure predicts weight gain. Multiple influences have resulted in a generation of Americans who do not regularly exercise. These include the movement from a rural and agricultural to a metropolitan society, the reduced emphasis on exercise in the formative years (particularly primary and secondary school), and the ever-increasing "pace of life" cited by many Americans. Another important relationship is that the daily length of time spent watching television predicts obesity and the risk for diabetes mellitus: every 2-hour increment is associated with a 14% increased risk for diabetes mellitus and a 23% increased risk for obesity.

Figure 4-1 Obesity I.

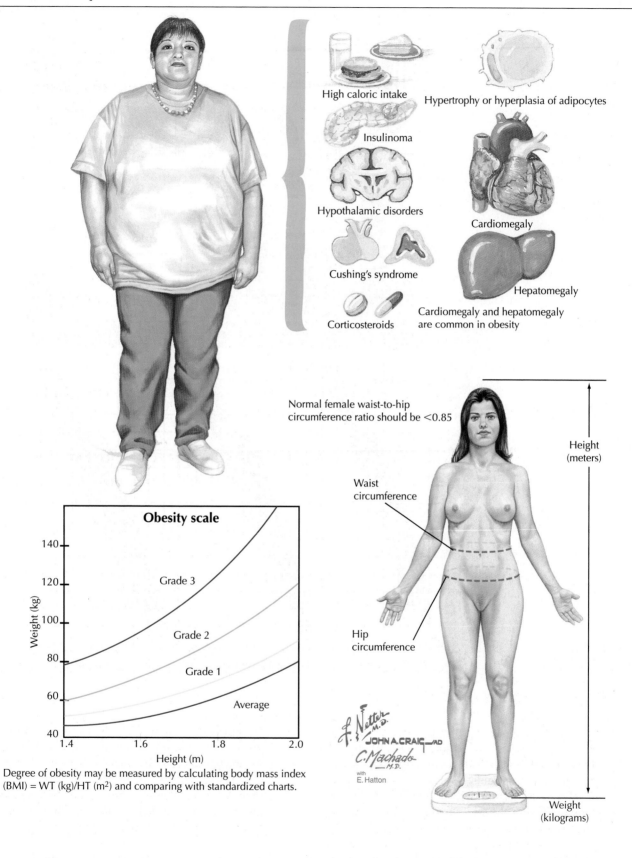

High caloric intake

Insulinoma

Hypothalamic disorders

Cushing's syndrome

Corticosteroids

Hypertrophy or hyperplasia of adipocytes

Cardiomegaly

Hepatomegaly

Cardiomegaly and hepatomegaly
are common in obesity

Normal female waist-to-hip
circumference ratio should be <0.85

Waist
circumference

Hip
circumference

Height
(meters)

Weight
(kilograms)

Obesity scale

Grade 3

Grade 2

Grade 1

Average

Weight (kg)

Height (m)

Degree of obesity may be measured by calculating body mass index
(BMI) = WT (kg)/HT (m²) and comparing with standardized charts.

Figure 4-2 Obesity II.

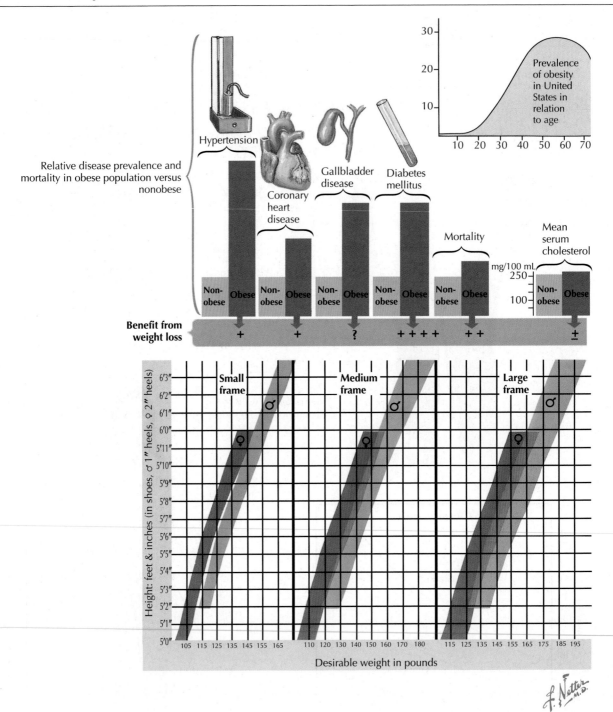

2. Dietary changes are equally important. The overwhelming influence of readily available high-fat foods through fast-food restaurants and vending machines (even in public schools), plus the emphasis on increased consumption of simple carbohydrates as exemplified by the traditional Food Pyramid of the American Dietetic Association, has contributed to the imbalance between caloric intake and expenditure. Population studies have clearly documented the direct relationship between the percentage of dietary fat and body weight. The ability to restrain caloric intake, a trait more commonly observed in higher socioeconomic classes, plays a role in obesity and explains, in part, the increased prevalence of obesity in lower socioeconomic classes. The habits of eating more than 50% of daily calories at night and of nocturnal binge-eating also contribute to obesity.

The increasing emphasis on the role of genetic predisposition reflects the impact of recent studies of the molec-

Figure 4-3 Obesity and Calories.

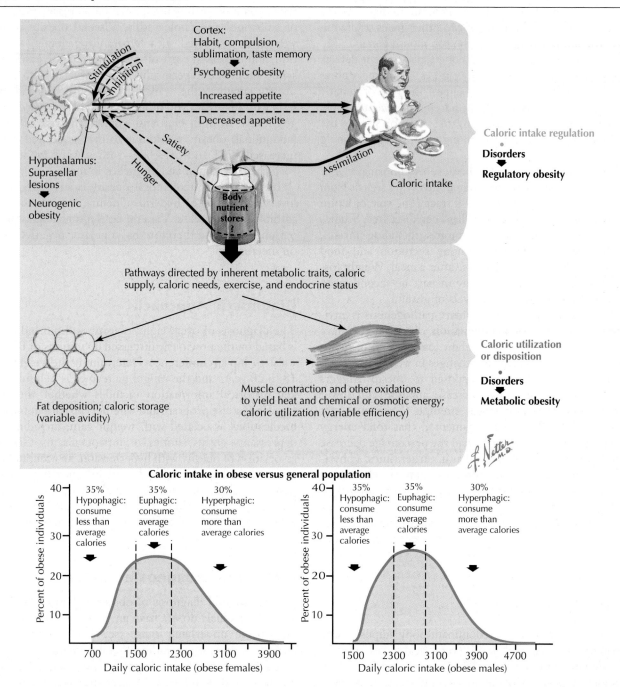

Caloric intake in obese versus general population

ular genetics of obesity in animals. Five single-gene defects have been identified in rodents. One of the most completely studied is the *ob* or *Lep* gene, which codes for the protein leptin produced in fat cells, gut, and placenta. Increases in adipose tissue result in leptin secretion, which signals the brain to decrease appetite, reduce energy intake, and increase energy expenditure. Leptin may act by decreasing neuropeptide Y secretion in the arcuate nucleus. Neuropeptide Y is a potent stimulator of food intake. Leptin deficiency has been reported in two consanguineous families. Treatment of affected individuals in these

families with physiologic doses of leptin resulted in decreased food intake and weight loss. Leptin receptor deficiency has also been reported in humans, a condition that is manifest by resistance to leptin. Based on these observations, leptin administration in limited clinical trials has not produced significant weight loss in the general population.

The agouti gene defect causes obesity in mice based on its signaling protein competing with the binding of melanocyte-stimulating hormone (MSH) to the melanocortin-4 receptor in the hypothalamus. This receptor decreases food intake, and its absence produces hyperphagia. The role of the agouti signaling protein in human obesity remains unclear, as does that of two other genes studied in mice: the fat mouse gene and the tub mouse gene.

In the general population, although specific gene defects have yet to be identified, family studies, including studies of twins and adoptees, clearly suggest the role of genetic factors in human obesity. The β_3-adrenergic receptor gene, the peroxisome proliferator-activated receptor-$\gamma 2$, and the melanocortin-4 receptor are among candidate genes being studied.

Obesity may also develop because of abnormalities of an intricate feedback control system involving signals from fat stores and the gastrointestinal tract. The role of leptin in signaling from adipose tissue has been discussed. Studies have implicated several gut hormones, including ghrelin, which stimulates growth hormone secretion and food intake. Levels of ghrelin decrease after a meal. Weight loss after gastric bypass surgery may in part be secondary to below-normal postoperative levels of ghrelin.

Whether the underlying primary pathogenesis is environmental, genetic, or a combination, obese patients have great difficulty maintaining weight loss because of metabolic changes that accompany changes in weight. In effect, weight loss in a person predisposed to obesity triggers feedback mechanisms that increase appetite and lower energy expenditure as the body attempts to return weight to baseline. Studies have documented that total energy expenditure drops 15% more than the percentage decrease in body weight. One theory is that in earlier times, a physiologic system may have protected humans when food accessibility was limited, leading to a survival advantage. Today, with high-fat food readily available, this physiology is clearly maladaptive, and it may explain the many frustrations faced by obese patients who fail repeatedly in their attempts to sustain weight loss.

Clinical Presentation

Obesity presents in two predominant body adipose tissue distributions, each with a different health risk profile. Abdominal, central, or visceral obesity is marked by an increased deposition of fat in visceral areas. It is more common in men, manifests as an increased waist-to-hip circumference ratio, and is often referred to as having an "apple shape." Women most often have a "pear-shaped" fat distribution, with a preponderance of adipose tissue in the gluteofemoral areas and an associated decrease in waist-to-hip circumference (see Fig. 4-1). The well-known metabolic consequences and risks of increased visceral fat (abdominal obesity) include hyperinsulinemia, insulin resistance, glucose intolerance, adult-onset diabetes mellitus, and lipid abnormalities—an increase in very-low-density lipoproteins (VLDLs) and low-density lipoproteins (LDLs) and a decrease in high-density lipoproteins

(HDLs). The relationship of abdominal obesity to hypertension is well documented, as is the increased prevalence of gallstones and cholecystitis. Visceral obesity in some women is associated with hyperandrogenemia, anovulation, and increased cortisol secretion (the polycystic ovary syndrome). The hyperinsulinemia associated with visceral obesity enhances the availability of androgens and manifests with hirsutism and other features of increased androgen levels. In both men and women, the risk of visceral (abdominal) obesity is additive to that associated with an increased BMI and correlates with a waist greater than 35 inches in women and 40 inches in men.

In contrast, gluteofemoral obesity is associated with a lower prevalence of hyperinsulinemia, hypertension, and cardiovascular disease. Visceral fat is mobilized faster than peripheral fat and therefore has a greater negative impact on metabolism.

Diagnostic Approach

The diagnosis of overweight, obesity, and morbid obesity is based on the previously discussed definitions of BMI and waist-to-hip circumference. Determining the weight at age 18 to 20 years and the weight gain since is helpful. Other key historical information includes whether there is a regular exercise program and whether the patient takes any medications associated with weight gain, including antidepressants, antipsychotics, or anticonvulsants. Given the association of obesity with hypertension, an accurate blood pressure reading is critical. Evaluation should include the following laboratory tests: fasting blood glucose, hemoglobin A1C, thyroid-stimulating hormone, total cholesterol, HDL cholesterol, LDL cholesterol, and triglycerides.

Differential Diagnosis

The differential diagnosis of obesity is limited, and most obese individuals do *not* have an endocrinologic or other identifiable underlying cause (see Fig. 4-1). However, endocrine diseases, including hypothyroidism and hypercortisolism, warrant consideration. These causes are usually readily excluded on physical examination and routine laboratory testing. The gluteofemoral distribution of adipose tissue in hypercortisolism and the associated buffalo hump, abdominal striae, and proximal muscle weakness provide helpful clues to cortisol excess. Obesity is often associated with a positive history in multiple family members. Moreover, obese persons often trace their problem to early childhood or puberty. Damage to the ventromedial hypothalamus secondary to trauma, inflammation, surgery in the posterior fossa, or increased intracranial pressure may result in the rare syndrome of hyperphagic obesity. The polycystic ovary syndrome is associated with obesity in more than half of women with this diagnosis.

Figure 4-4 Treatment of Obesity.
DM, diabetes mellitus; HTN, hypertension; Hyperlipid, hyperlipidemia; Rx, therapy.

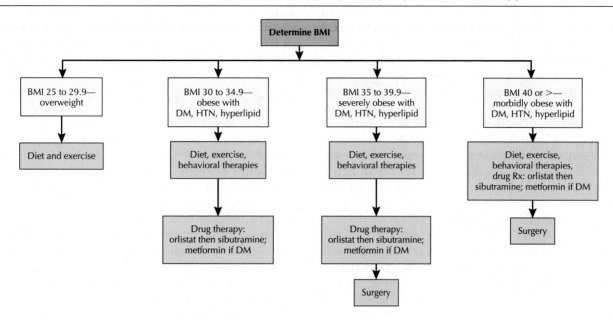

Management and Therapy

The treatment of obesity is one of the most frustrating problems for patients and health care providers alike, reflecting the less than 10% rate of a sustained response to therapy and the unrealistic expectation of some patients who feel that they should lose 20% to 30% of their total body weight. A goal of a 5% to 15% reduction is probably more rational and likely to be achieved and sustained. This amount of weight loss will decrease the health risk profile of most patients, including the risk for diabetes mellitus, hyperlipidemia, and hypertension. Figure 4-4 provides an overview of therapeutic options.

Diet and Exercise Therapy

Caloric restriction is an absolute requirement of any successful weight-reduction program and may be achieved by following general guidelines for healthful eating or by adopting a more restrictive food or liquid diet. Successful weight reduction requires that the total calories consumed remain below the total calories expended. Because of their increased lean body mass, men expend more calories and lose more weight than women of similar BMI. Older obese patients expend less energy and lose weight more slowly.

The optimal balance among carbohydrate, fat, and protein content remains controversial. Most guidelines recommend that the daily dietary fat content remain at 30% or below of the total caloric intake. Recent research has emphasized that low-fat foods often contain elevated levels of unhealthy carbohydrates that produce hyperinsulinemia, increasing the risk for cardiovascular compli-

cations. Furthermore, the subtle swings in plasma glucose concentrations (in nondiabetic patients) that result from diets high in junk food and simple carbohydrates accentuate difficulties in appetite control in obese individuals. Diets high in healthy carbohydrates, including fruit, vegetables, and grains, do not produce appetite control problems. These observations have led to an emphasis on low-calorie, high-fiber (healthy carbohydrate), low-fat, and high-protein diets that do not stimulate high levels of insulin secretion. Low-carbohydrate, high-fat diets initially raised concerns about the potential to produce a high-risk serum lipid profile; however, several randomized trials have demonstrated that such diets are safe and are more effective than low-fat diets in achieving short-term weight loss. If a higher-fat content diet is chosen, it is important to make sure that monounsaturated and polyunsaturated fats are selected. Long-term adherence to low-carbohydrate diets is difficult for many patients. In the final analysis, the critical issue is not the diet but whether the patient adheres to any prescribed diet, no matter what the specific food class balance is.

Obese patients with a BMI of more than 30 may require a more aggressive approach to dietary caloric restriction—800 calories or less per day. There is no evidence that diets of less than 800 calories per day are any more effective in the long-term; however, they do achieve more rapid weight loss initially. When very-low-calorie diets are discontinued, rapid weight gain often occurs—an obvious disadvantage. The key to this degree of restriction is to ensure a high biologic value protein intake of at least 1.5 grams per kilogram of ideal body weight and adequate amounts of vitamins, minerals, electrolytes, and essential fatty acids.

These diets are contraindicated during pregnancy and lactation, in patients with bulimia, and in patients with anorexia nervosa. They are also relatively contraindicated in patients with chronic medical diseases, including type I diabetes mellitus, chronic liver disease, chronic renal disease, and coronary heart disease manifested by arrhythmias or unstable angina, and in patients on chronic corticosteroid therapy. Complications include constitutional complaints of fatigue, weakness, and constipation or diarrhea. Gallstones and gout may also occur in the setting of rapid weight reduction, secondary to rapid cholesterol mobilization from fat stores and protein breakdown, respectively. One advantage of the more restrictive diets is that rapid weight loss produces more immediate positive feedback.

Many patients prefer to enroll in commercial and self-help programs such as Weight Watchers, OPTIFAST, and Take Off Pounds Sensibly. With the exception of a single randomized, controlled trial of Weight Watchers that reported a loss of 3.2% of initial weight at 2 years, the evidence to support the use of these programs is suboptimal.

Caloric restriction is more likely to be successful when combined with behavioral therapy and exercise. Group-focused weight reduction programs have the advantage of peer support, especially if the group remains intact over time and is led by a professional who has experience dealing with the nuances of eating behaviors. Participation in a group program provides reinforcement when behavioral change is successful and support when it is unsuccessful. The group leaders must teach self-monitoring, including maintaining a diary of what is eaten under what circumstances and under which outside stressors. This allows more effective stimulus control, for example, avoiding eating while watching television or other activities if doing both activities together predictably results in higher caloric intake. For many obese people, stress is a major stimulus for overeating, a problem that necessitates the teaching of more productive approaches to stress control, such as exercise and meditation.

Exercise is key, but its impact is limited by the previously described tendency for the body to do everything possible to maintain weight in the setting of weight reduction. The energy expended for a given level of physical activity is less after weight loss occurs. Patients frequently become discouraged when they find that any weight decrease requires a disproportionately large amount of exercise. Aerobic exercise has remained a key component of successful programs and is often supplemented by anaerobic strength training to build lean body mass. At least 30 minutes of exercise 3 days a week is recommended, with a maximum of 1 hour daily 6 days a week. Incorporating more exercise into daily activities, such as taking stairs rather than elevators, is also helpful.

Although exercise alone rarely results in sustained weight loss, the importance of exercise should not be underemphasized. Exercise may be an important surrogate for an individual's motivation to lose weight. In a recent study of 32,000 dieters by *Consumer Reports*, individuals who lost at least 10% of their starting weight and kept it off for 1 to 5 years credited exercise, not food deprivation, as the key to their sustained weight loss.

Pharmacologic Therapy

The use of drugs to treat obesity remains a hope for the future for many obese patients and is usually the next step when dietary therapy fails. Until recently, the drug therapies studied did little more than illustrate the limitations of pharmacologic approaches. In general, the literature had documented a discouraging series of initial successes followed by failure, either because of poorly sustained effectiveness or intolerable side effects. Fortunately, some recently published data offer room for guarded optimism.

Amphetamines were among the first drugs tried to suppress appetite. Although associated with short-term weight reduction, amphetamines were found to have an intolerable side-effect profile and a very high addictive potential. Subsequently, trials of amphetamine-like appetite suppressants (phentermine and others) failed to show sustained benefits.

The short-lived enthusiasm for the combination of phentermine and fenfluramine (the "Phen-fen" diet) was based on reports of a 16.5% reduction in body weight compared with 4.3% in the placebo group over 34 weeks of therapy. Weight reduction leveled off after 6 months, and continuous therapy was necessary to prevent regaining what had been lost. No worrisome side effects were noted initially; in fact, proponents emphasized that the known side effects of one agent seemed to cancel those of the other. Initial questions about this therapy were raised by a 1997 report from the Mayo Clinic that described 24 cases of an unusual valvular disorder resembling the valvular disease associated with carcinoid syndrome. Despite early conflicting reports in the literature, valvular thickening, left-sided valvular regurgitation, and pulmonary hypertension are now believed to be related to this therapy. These observations led to the U.S. Food and Drug Administration (FDA) recall of both fenfluramine and dexfenfluramine, another agent like fenfluramine that increases serotonin release and decreases reuptake. Dexfenfluramine had become one of the most commonly used agents outside of the United States and had enjoyed an anecdotal record of success in weight loss.

Sympathomimetic agents that have been studied include phentermine, benzphetamine, phendimetrazine, diethylpropion, sibutramine, and phenylpropanolamine. Except for sibutramine, they have short plasma half-lives. Phenylpropanolamine and diethylpropion have been shown to be effective in short-term studies; however, a positive long-term benefit on health outcomes has not been demon-

strated. Moreover, the association of phenylpropanolamine with a small but significant risk for hemorrhagic stroke in women has resulted in its removal from the market. Diethylpropion is a Schedule IV drug that is now approved only for short-term use—up to 12 weeks.

Sibutramine, a centrally acting neurotransmitter reuptake inhibitor that effectively inhibits norepinephrine, serotonin, and to a lesser extent, dopamine reuptake, has shown encouraging results for the treatment of obesity. In a multicenter trial with doses ranging from 5 to 30 mg/day, there was a clear dose response, with subjects in the 30-mg group losing 9.5% of body weight while the placebo group lost 1%. Subjects in a maintenance trial after diet-induced weight loss had a further loss of 5.2 kg over 1 year. The placebo group gained weight. Another trial documented similar evidence for maintenance of weight loss in subjects treated with 10 mg of sibutramine daily for 15 months after diet-induced weight loss. Additional benefits include reductions in total and LDL cholesterol, triglycerides, and uric acid. There is also an associated increase in HDL cholesterol. Patients with diabetes mellitus have significant decreases in glucose and hemoglobin A1C. Negative effects include nausea, constipation, dry mouth, insomnia, and an increase in pulse rate in some patients. A hypertensive response does occur in some patients but is relatively mild and rarely requires withdrawal of therapy. Use of sibutramine should be avoided in patients with coronary disease, congestive heart failure, cardiac arrhythmia, and stroke.

Antidepressants like sertraline and fluoxetine in the selective serotonin reuptake inhibitor group have shown short-term benefit in some patients. Fluoxetine at a dose of 60 mg in a placebo comparison study produced a weight loss of 4.8 kg at 6 months; however, 50% of this was regained in the second 6 months.

Orlistat is an inhibitor of pancreatic lipase that results in the malabsorption of 30% of all fat consumed when used at the higher end of its dose range. The associated negative gastrointestinal effects of fat malabsorption provide an added incentive to limit fat intake. In a 4-year, double-blind, randomized, placebo-controlled trial of more than 3000 patients, the orlistat-treated group lost 11% of baseline weight, whereas the placebo group lost 6% at the end of 1 year. In another study, in addition to weight loss, positive benefits included reduced LDL cholesterol, increased HDL cholesterol, decreased fasting insulin levels, improved glycemic control, and reduced blood pressure. Remarkably, the negative gastrointestinal effects did not result in a high dropout rate. The risk for malabsorption of fat-soluble vitamins requires supplementation with a multivitamin taken separately from orlistat.

Recently, an FDA panel has recommended that orlistat be made available in a reduced dosage (60 mg versus 120 mg for the prescription strength) for over-the-counter (OTC) purchase. The panel stated that the most positive effect of orlistat on weight loss will be obtained at reduced dose, although the best studies have shown a dose-response relationship.

The modern pharmacotherapy of diabetes mellitus has led to some success in weight reduction and in the control of associated risk factors. Metformin, a commonly used hypoglycemic agent, reduces hepatic gluconeogenesis, inhibits intestinal glucose transport, and enhances glucose uptake in muscle and adipose tissue. In contrast to exogenous insulin and insulin-stimulating oral agents, it causes weight loss, in part because it diminishes appetite. Glucose control in insulin-dependent and insulin-independent diabetic patients improves, as do lipid profiles. Lactic acidosis, a known risk, is uncommon when patients with renal and hepatic dysfunction are excluded. The thiazolidinediones, including pioglitazone, have similar positive effects secondary to increasing insulin sensitivity in peripheral tissues. Patients are often able to reduce their insulin dose and have an associated reduction in body weight. However, long-term negative effects, including edema and hypertriglyceridemia, may complicate therapy with these agents.

A new experimental drug, rimonabant, blocks the endocannabinoid system at the cannabinoid-1 receptor, which regulates appetite and body weight. Animals with a deletion of this receptor have a lean habitus and are resistant to diet-induced obesity and dyslipidemia. The initial placebo-controlled trial data documented that rimonabant at high dose (20 mg) produced 5% to 10% weight reduction substantially more often than placebo. These positive results, albeit early in the investigative process, warrant close scrutiny of this drug class in the future. Rimonabant has also shown promise in smoking cessation.

Optimum Treatment

The lack of an obvious first choice in the therapy of obesity excludes any dogmatic recommendation; nevertheless, many experts would agree that diet and exercise deserve an initial trial in patients with a BMI of 25 to 34.9 kg/m². If this approach fails, orlistat is the next line of therapy in patients with hypertension, cardiovascular disease, or dyslipidemia. Metformin therapy should be used initially in obese patients with diabetes mellitus. In obese patients who are otherwise healthy, sibutramine therapy is a rational first choice if dietary measures and exercise fail.

Surgical Therapy

Surgery should be considered in patients with a BMI of more than 40 kg/m² and in those with a BMI of more than 35 kg/m² who have failed other attempts at weight reduction and who have health complications such as sleep apnea, cardiac failure, uncontrolled diabetes mellitus, or severe venous stasis. The goal of surgery is to improve metabolic and organ function and to decrease the morbidity and mortality associated with severe obesity. Noncompliant patients must be excluded, given the need for careful

adherence to a compulsory regimen to supplement vitamins and other critical nutrients.

Two different surgical approaches have been developed: those that limit the reservoir size of the stomach (restrictive) and those that decrease the effectiveness of nutrient absorption (malabsorptive). Small intestinal bypass procedures that induce malabsorption have been largely abandoned because of an unacceptable risk for life-threatening metabolic complications and have been largely replaced by vertical banded gastroplasty, laparoscopic adjustable gastric banding, and gastric bypass procedures. Figure 4-5 presents an overview of the surgical approaches to be considered.

Gastric stapling (vertical banded gastroplasty) reduces gastric reservoir size and restricts the gastric outlet. Patients have an excess weight loss of 66% at 2 years and 55% at 9 years. The procedure fails in patients who gorge on liquid carbohydrates that can pass through the restricted gastric outlet, reversing weight loss in the process. Surgical revision has been required in a substantial number of patients (20% to 56%) for outlet band erosion, staple line disruption, stomal stenosis, gastroesophageal reflux, recurrent emesis, and gastric pouch enlargement.

Laparoscopic adjustable gastric banding involves the placement of an adjustable prosthetic band around the entrance to the stomach. This results in a restricted gastric inlet that can be further restricted by injection of saline into an accessible subcutaneous port. In general, the procedure is less prone to the complications of vertical banded gastroplasty. Study results vary, but some data document an excess weight loss of 15% to 20% at 3 months, 40% to 53% at 1 year, and 45% to 58% at 2 years. Frequent band adjustments are necessary to control the rapidity and degree of weight loss. Studies have documented improvements in diabetes mellitus, hypertension, and sleep apnea.

Gastric bypass is both a restrictive and a malabsorptive procedure involving the creation of a gastric pouch that empties into a gastrojejunostomy, the jejunal segment of which is connected to the excluded gastric segment, duodenum, and biliary-pancreatic secretions by a Roux loop. The altered bowel anatomy excludes some small bowel absorptive area. Malabsorption and the dumping syndrome result in weight reduction but with the concomitant risk for vitamin and mineral malnutrition unless a careful supplemental regimen is followed. Excess weight loss at 1 year averages 62% to 68%, and 50% to 75% at 2 years.

Mortality in the hands of an experienced bariatric surgeon is about 1%. Morbidity includes wound dehiscence or infection, anastomotic leaks, stomal stenosis, marginal ulcers, pneumonia, thrombophlebitis, and pulmonary emboli. At least some of the higher-than-expected risk relates to the risk associated with anesthesia and surgery in the morbidly obese. Refractory vomiting may occur with or without stomal stenosis. Esophageal dilation, esophageal reflux or ulceration, and pouch ulceration may

complicate gastroplasty. Folate, iron, vitamin B$_{12}$, and other micronutrient deficiencies are unique to gastric bypass and require careful follow-up and patient compliance. Even in the face of substantial morbidity risk, bariatric surgery offers hope for a selected group of patients, and studies continue to show advantages over diet and drug therapies.

Avoiding Treatment Errors

One of the most critical aspects in selecting a therapeutic approach that is both safe and effective is to predict the patient's level of compliance. The lack of highly effective therapies increases the likelihood that risk will exceed benefit, especially in patients who are not compliant. This is certainly true in the case of bariatric surgery, in which noncompliance after gastric bypass procedures can result in major morbidity, and even mortality. Substantial morbidity can also result in noncompliant patients who misuse pharmacologic agents that have significantly negative effects on blood pressure and cardiac function. Patients must adhere to a carefully outlined therapeutic regimen and must be committed to close medical follow-up.

Future Directions

Pharmacologic therapies will offer great promise in the coming years. Agents similar to rimonabant that block specific receptors important in the control of appetite and satiety are likely to provide a progressively more specific designer drug approach.

Although further studies are being done on existing therapeutic approaches, it must be recognized that some of these therapies may become available to the general public as OTC drugs. OTC access may, indeed, prove the safety and efficacy of these therapies, or the approaches may turn out not to be effective. Physicians and health care providers may be faced with previously unknown metabolic and electrolyte (or other) problems associated with the use of OTC drugs that principally reduce the urge to eat or reduce the absorption of food. Health care providers will need to be attentive to the use of OTC medication in obese and formerly obese patients by screening for the known side effects of these drugs.

On a brighter side, although slow in coming, there is hope that advances in genetic understanding may lead to improved pharmacologic therapy for weight loss. Leptin and its congeners are currently under study and, although limited by the need for subcutaneous or intravenous administration, may prove useful in preventing weight regain in patients who have lost weight using another therapy. The vast information now available as a result of the completion of the human genome project will likely stimulate new pharmacotherapies. The likelihood that purely genetic-based approaches will offer any significant success for obese patients is low at this time, because of

Figure 4-5 Surgical Options.

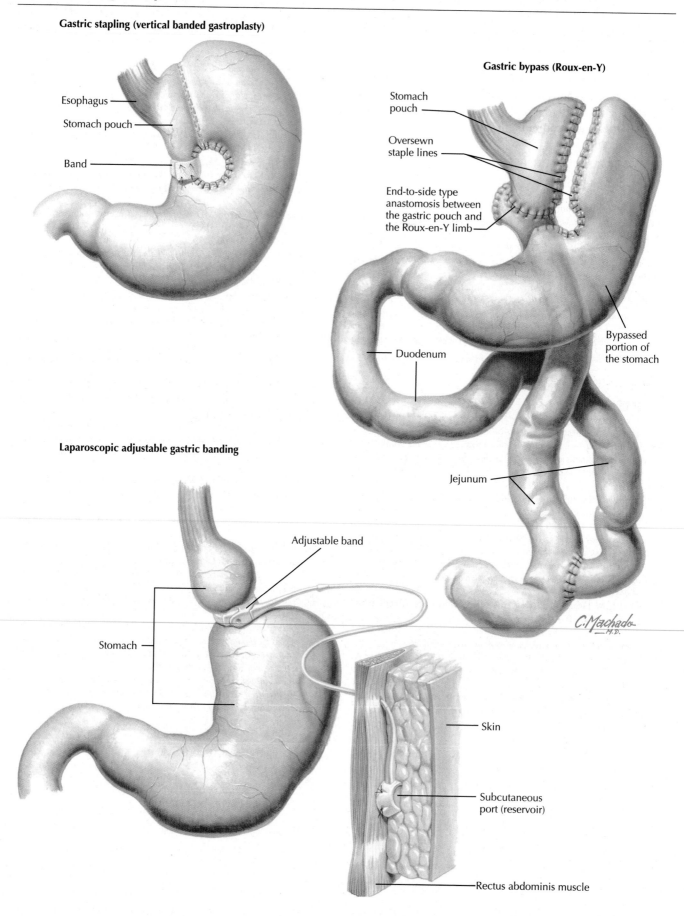

Gastric stapling (vertical banded gastroplasty)

Esophagus

Stomach pouch

Band

Gastric bypass (Roux-en-Y)

Stomach pouch

Oversewn staple lines

End-to-side type anastomosis between the gastric pouch and the Roux-en-Y limb

Duodenum

Bypassed portion of the stomach

Jejunum

Laparoscopic adjustable gastric banding

Adjustable band

Stomach

Skin

Subcutaneous port (reservoir)

Rectus abdominis muscle

C. Machado
—M.D.

the complicated relationship of this polygenic disease and the many environmental factors that can affect weight gain or loss. Recently, the National Human Genome Project, in collaboration with the National Institute for Environmental Health Sciences, has undertaken the Genes and Environment Initiative (GEI). The GEI offers promise to better understand the specific mediators of obesity (at all levels from the cell to the organism) and the interplay between these environmentally driven factors and the human genome.

Additional Resources

Centers for Disease Control and Prevention: Overweight and obesity. Available at: http://www.cdc.gov/nccdphp/dnpa/obesity/. Accessed August 22, 2006.

This well-organized CDC website provides a broad overview of the problem of obesity structured in a manner that is easily understandable for the lay public.

Willett WC, Dietz WH, Colditz GA: Guidelines for healthy weight. N Engl J Med 341:427-434, 1999.

This article provides useful information on healthy weight guidelines and emphasizes the importance of preventing weight gain and overweight in healthy-weight persons and on preventing further weight gain in those who are already overweight.

EVIDENCE

1. Aronne LJ: Obesity. Med Clin North Am 82:161-181, 1998.

   This useful review points out that obesity is a chronic disease that requires long-term treatment, which is successful only if the patient is willing to make major changes in eating habits, exercise, and overall lifestyle.

2. Berkowitz RI, Fujioka K, Daniels SR, et al: Effects of sibutramine treatment in obese adolescents: A randomized trial. Ann Intern Med 145:81-90, 2006.

   This article describes a comparison study of sibutramine versus placebo in obese adolescents enrolled in a behavior therapy program. The authors document that sibutramine, when added to behavior therapy, reduces body mass index and weight more than placebo and improves the profile of metabolic risk factors in obese adolescents.

3. Bray GA: Health hazards of obesity. Endocrinol Metab Clin North Am 25:907-919, 1996.

   The author provides a thorough review of the multiple medical complications of obesity that increase morbidity and mortality.

4. Buchwald H, Avidor Y, Braunwald E, et al: Bariatric surgery: A systematic review and meta-analysis. JAMA 292:1724-1737, 2004.

   This meta-analysis documents the high level of effectiveness of bariatric surgery in achieving weight loss in morbidly obese patients and in improving the associated morbidities of diabetes mellitus, hyperlipidemia, hypertension, and obstructive sleep apnea.

5. Flegal KM, Graubard BI, Williamson DF, Gail MH: Excess deaths associated with underweight, overweight, and obesity. JAMA 293:1861-1867, 2005.

   Using National Health and Nutrition Examination Survey (NHANES) data, the authors document that underweight and obesity are associated with increased mortality when compared with the normal weight category, but that the impact of obesity on mortality may have decreased over time.

6. Fontaine KR, Redden DT, Wang C, et al: Years of life lost due to obesity. JAMA 289:187-193, 2003.

   Using National Health and Nutrition Examination Survey (NHANES) data, the authors document the years of life lost secondary to obesity, noting the greatest impact on life expectancy in the younger age groups.

7. Ogden CL, Carroll MD, Curtin LR, et al: Prevalence of overweight and obesity in the United States 1999-2004. JAMA 295:1549-1555, 2006.

   This article provides useful prevalence data for overweight and obesity. Using the National Health and Nutrition Examination Survey (NHANES) data from 1999 to 2004, the authors document the increasing prevalence of overweight in children and adolescents, and of obesity in adult men, over the 6-year interval.

8. Rosenbaum M, Leibel RL, Hirsch J: Obesity. N Engl J Med 337:396-407, 1997.

   This article reviews the pathophysiology of obesity, genetic factors, and therapeutic approaches, including diet and exercise, drug therapy, and surgical therapy.

9. Tsai AG, Wadden TA: Systematic review: An evaluation of major commercial weight loss programs in the United States. Ann Intern Med 142:56-66, 2005.

   This review provides data on the efficacy of the major commercial and organized self-help weight-loss programs in the United States, noting that the evidence to support the use of these is suboptimal and that controlled studies are needed.

10. West DB: Genetics of obesity on humans and animal models. Endocrinol Metab Clin North Am 25:801-813, 1996.

    The author emphasizes the importance of defining the genetic mechanisms of obesity to allow more specific preventive and therapeutic approaches.

11. Williamson DA, Perrin LA: Behavioral therapy for obesity. Endocrinol Metab Clin North Am 25:943-954, 1996.

    These authors emphasize the importance of behavioral therapy in maintaining weight loss.

12. Yanovski SZ, Yanovski JA: Obesity. N Engl J Med 346:591-602, 2002.

    This article provides a very helpful perspective on the drug therapy of obesity, including a historical overview.

13. Zachwieja JJ: Exercise as treatment for obesity. Endocrinol Metab Clin North Am 25:965-988, 1996.

    The author emphasizes the importance of an exercise program that promotes the expenditure of 300 kcal per day in maintaining weight loss induced by dietary caloric restriction.

Pamela G. Vick ▪ William S. Blau

5

Evaluation and Treatment of Chronic Pain

Introduction

Millions of people are affected by both acute and chronic pain conditions costing in excess of $100 billion for treatment and lost work productivity. *Pain*, as defined by the International Association for the Study of Pain, is an unpleasant sensory or emotional experience associated with actual or potential tissue damage, or described in terms as such damage. Pain is subjective, and not all pain is equal. There is no useful clinical test that can quantify pain. A patient's pain experience is a result of interrelated physical and psychological factors, including physiologic response to actual or potential tissue damage, previous pain experience, beliefs about pain, coping style, emotions, and family and social influences. Chronic pain is a persistent pain that is refractory to treatments based on specific remedies, or to the routine methods of pain control such as non-narcotic analgesics. In the chronic setting, pain becomes a disease rather than merely a symptom. The best strategy for the management of the patient with chronic pain employs a multidisciplinary approach with pharmacologic, interventional, physical, and psychological therapies. Each patient is an individual whose response to therapy may be unpredictable, and sequential trials of alternative therapies are often required to arrive at an optimal treatment plan. Some types of intractable pain are resistant to virtually every available therapy.

Etiology and Pathogenesis

Pain transduction involves free nerve endings in the integument, viscera, and periosteum. Nociceptor responses are triggered directly by exogenous tissue trauma, but are also influenced by many endogenous factors whose precise mechanisms are unknown. Three classes of endogenous mediators are involved: (1) those that activate nociceptive afferents and produce pain by local application (e.g., bradykinin, acetylcholine, potassium); (2) those that facilitate pain by sensitizing nociceptors but are ineffective in evoking pain themselves (e.g., prostaglandins); and (3) those that produce local extravasation (e.g., substance P). These mediators contribute to primary hyperalgesia, in which pain thresholds in traumatized tissue are lowered.

Nociceptive transmission involves primarily unmyelinated C and thinly myelinated A delta nerve fibers. The cell bodies are located in the dorsal root ganglia, with first-order synapse within the marginal layers of the spinal cord dorsal horn. Substance P, glutamate, calcitonin gene–related peptide, cholecystokinin, and vasoactive intestinal polypeptide have all been implicated in synaptic pain transmission. Spinothalamic, spinoreticular, and spinomesencephalic pathways are the primary routes of transmission to the brain, where pain is ultimately perceived. The hypothalamus, medial thalamus, and limbic systems are involved in the motivational and affective features of pain (Fig. 5-1).

The periaqueductal gray and descending inhibitory pathways selectively inhibit pain transmission at the level of the spinal cord. Norepinephrine, serotonin, enkephalin, and endorphins are the predominant inhibitory neurotransmitters.

Chronic pain may involve ongoing peripheral nociception, as in osteoarthritis or pain associated with intervertebral disk degeneration. In many other cases, persistent neuropathic pain may result from pathologic alteration in the pain signaling processes themselves, for example, in diabetic or postherpetic neuralgia. In either case, pain may become self-perpetuating to some extent as a consequence of *N*-methyl-D-aspartate-mediated plasticity in the central nervous system, leading to central sensitization.

Figure 5-1 Pain Transmission.

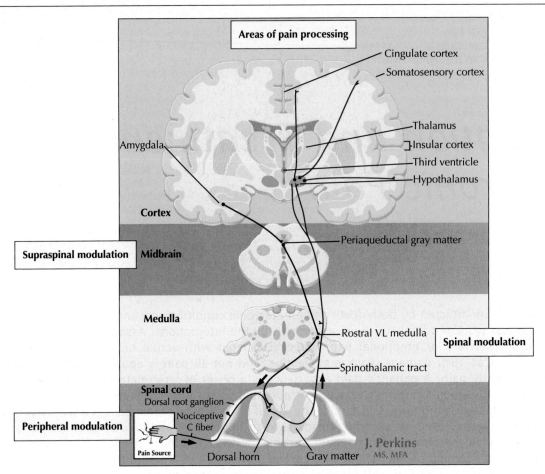

Pain Classification

Pain severity may be classified using various scales, such as verbal (mild, moderate, severe), numeric (0 to 10, where 0 = no pain and 10 = worst imaginable), visual analogue, faces (most appropriate for pediatric assessment), or more elaborate questionnaires (e.g., McGill Pain Questionnaire). Ultimately, all clinically useful scales are subjective and rely upon the report of the patient.

Current schemes for classification of pain according to the underlying pathophysiology remain relatively unsophisticated. Nociceptive pain arises from ongoing stimulation of peripheral nociceptors, as in the case of chronic or recurrent trauma or degenerative disease; the source may be somatic or visceral. Neuropathic pain is associated with some of the most severe pain disorders (Box 5-1). Typical descriptors include burning, tingling, shooting, numbing, and constricting. Cutaneous sensory abnormalities may range from anesthesia to hyperalgesia or allodynia (painful response to a nonpainful stimulus). Some varieties of neuropathic pain depend on tonic activity of the sympathetic nervous system (sympathetically maintained pain), so that pain and other symptoms may be abolished by sympathetic blockade with local anesthetics. Complex regional pain syndrome (reflex sympathetic dystrophy and causalgia) is characterized by persistent spontaneous pain after an injury, accompanied by sudomotor abnormalities, edema, and alterations in skin color and texture; it is often sympathetically maintained.

Anesthesia dolorosa is the clinical finding that defines a deafferentation pain syndrome—spontaneous pain in an area otherwise devoid of sensation. Phantom limb pain may be understood as an extreme example of deafferentation. The presence of pain in the absence of intact nerve conduction pathways implicates a problem with sensory integration at the level of the central nervous system. Other central pain disorders may follow direct tissue injury to the central nervous system (e.g., post–spinal cord injury pain, post-thalamic stroke syndrome) or may be functional (psychogenic).

Cancer-related pain is sometimes considered a separate category, although this is somewhat artificial because it is defined by the context rather than the pathophysiology. In fact, cancer pain can be caused by any one or more of the previously described categories of pain.

Clinical Presentation

Patients may present with one or more types of pain, and the precise pain diagnosis may remain obscure. Some clinical features distinguish common neuropathic pain syndromes (Table 5-1).

Box 5-1	Etiology of Painful Neuropathies: Major Categories

Toxic or Metabolic
Endocrine (e.g., diabetic)
Chemotherapy (e.g., isoniazid)
Chemical exposure associated
Nutritional (e.g., beriberi)

Post-traumatic
Complex regional pain syndrome types I and II

Compressive
Nerve entrapment syndromes (e.g., carpal tunnel syndrome)

Autoimmune
Vasculitic
Demyelinating
Paraneoplastic
Parainfectious

Infectious
Viral (e.g., HIV, herpes zoster)
Spirochetal (e.g., Lyme disease)
Guillain-Barré disease

Hereditary
Fabry's disease
Amyloid

Diagnostic Approach

Different algorithms can be used to develop the best treatment options for chronic pain patients. A 10-step process can be used for long-term opioid therapy in chronic pain (Box 5-2).

Management and Therapies

Chronic pain syndromes often involve significant emotional and behavioral issues, often lead to significant functional impairments, and are accompanied by significant sleep disturbance. These aspects of the patient's disease must not be neglected, and it is often necessary to enlist the assistance of specialists in psychology, psychiatry, physiatry, physical or occupational therapy, and others.

Medical treatment of the pain often begins with pharmacologic therapy. There are only two classes of general-purpose primary analgesics in use: nonsteroidal anti-inflammatory drugs (NSAIDs) and opioids. The utility of these classes of drugs is limited by toxicity, side effects, inefficacy for many varieties of chronic pain or pain with activity, tolerance, physical dependence, and risk for addiction or withdrawal.

Adjuvants such as antidepressants or anticonvulsants enhance the effectiveness of a primary analgesic, limit the side effects, treat concurrent symptoms that can increase pain, and provide analgesia for certain types of pain. They may be used alone or in combination with primary analgesics. Some adjuvants also have sedating or anxiolytic side effects that can be useful in treating insomnia or anxiety. Adjuvants should be started in low doses and titrated slowly to minimize side effects and maximize benefit. It is important to provide medication trials of adequate duration. Sometimes maximal analgesic effects are not seen for 4 to 6 weeks after therapeutic levels are reached. Educate the patient about the potential delay in action of these drugs. Patients should also be informed that serial drug trials may be required before an adequate combination is found.

Table 5-1 Clinical Features of Common Neuropathic Pain Syndromes	
Diagnosis	**Typical Clinical Features**
Painful diabetic neuropathy	Symmetrical sensory loss and burning pain in lower legs
Lumbosacral radiculopathy	Lancinating pain radiating into the anterior thigh (L2, L3) or lower leg (L4-S1) with motor weakness or sensory loss
Postherpetic neuralgia	Unilateral pain, sensory loss, or allodynia in the dermatome where herpes zoster had previously erupted
HIV-related neuropathy	Symmetrical painful paresthesias, most prominent in the toes and soles of the feet
Complex regional pain syndromes	Regional (e.g., limb) pain with edema, cutaneous blood flow, and sweating abnormalities
Postsurgical neuropathic pain	Peri-incisional sensory loss, pain, and allodynia for more than 3 months after surgery, phantom limb pain after amputation or mastectomy

From Gilron I, Watson CP, Cahill CM, Moulin DE: Neuropathic pain: A practical guide for the clinician. CMAJ 175(3):265-275, 2006.

Box 5-2   Ten-Step Process for Long-Term Opioid Therapy in Chronic Pain

Step I: Perform comprehensive initial evaluation

Step II: Establish diagnosis
X-rays, magnetic resonance imaging, computed tomography scan

Step III: Establish medical necessity
Physical diagnosis
Therapeutic interventional pain management
Physical modalities
Behavior therapy

Step IV: Assess risk-to-benefit ratio
Treatment is beneficial

Step V: Establish treatment goals

Step VI: Obtain informed medical consent and agreement

Step VII: Institute initial dose adjustment (up to 8-12 weeks)
Start low dose
Utilize opioids, nonsteroidal anti-inflammatory drugs, and adjuvants
Discontinue because of side effects
    Lack of analgesia
    Side effects
    Lack of functional improvement

Step VIII: Assess stable phase
Assess for the four A's
    Analgesia
    Activity
    Aberrant behavior
    Adverse effect

Step IX: Monitor adherence
Prescription monitoring program
Random drug screen
Pill counts

Step X: Assess outcomes
Successful: continue
    Stable doses
    Analgesia, activity
    No abuse, side effects
Failed: discontinue if
    No analgesia
    Noncompliance
    Abuse
    Side effects
    Complications

Adapted from Trescot AM, Boswell MV, Atluri SL, et al: Opioid guidelines in the management of chronic non-cancer pain. Pain Physician 9:1-39, 2006.

Nonsteroidal Anti-inflammatory Drugs (Acetaminophen)

NSAIDs are most effective for mild to moderate inflammatory pain, postsurgical pain, and pain associated with trauma, arthritis, and cancer (Table 5-2). The analgesic effect is potentiated when used in conjunction with opiates or other adjuvants. NSAIDs differ from opiate analgesics in the following ways: (1) there is a ceiling effect to analgesia; (2) they do not produce tolerance, physical dependence, or psychological dependence; (3) they have the potential for significant end-organ toxicity; and (4) the primary mechanism of action is inhibition of cyclooxygenase (COX), preventing the formation of prostaglandins that sensitize peripheral nerves and central sensory neurons to painful stimuli. COX-2-specific inhibitors have been developed that decrease the risk for gastrointestinal bleeding and do not inhibit platelet aggregation. However, evidence suggests an increased risk for myocardial infarction and stroke with the COX-2 inhibitors. Thus, the NSAIDs as a class are being reevaluated for safety. In the United States, there is a black box warning on all NSAIDs, and their use is contraindicated in patients undergoing coronary artery bypass grafting.

Opiates

Opiate therapy is indicated when chronic cancer or nonmalignant pain does not respond to nonopiate therapy alone (Table 5-3). Opiates have a central and peripheral site of action, particularly in the presence of inflammation. Many opiates available are in combination with nonopioids; this latter component is the limiting factor. For example, the upper dose limits for acetaminophen preparations is 4000 mg/day in adults and 90 mg/kg/day in children weighing less than 45 kg. For daily pain, long-acting drug formulations are preferred.

The undertreatment of pain is often caused by the misconception that opiate therapy will lead to unmanageable tolerance and physical and psychological dependence. Tolerance can occur, but it is not the most likely cause of increased narcotic requirement. Disease progression or new pain syndrome should be excluded. Physical dependence and withdrawal symptoms can be prevented by careful monitoring and slow withdrawal and tapering of narcotics. Psychological dependence is rare if narcotics are prescribed correctly. Pseudoaddiction is a pattern of drug-seeking behavior in an attempt to gain pain relief and may be perceived as addiction. It is often the result of uncontrolled pain due to inadequate treatment. This behavior stops once pain relief is adequately relieved. The long-term use of opioid analgesics is often appropriate for the control of otherwise intractable pain, but it requires close monitoring and an ongoing patient-physician relationship.

Antidepressants

Tricyclic antidepressants have been used as first-line therapy for a variety of neuropathic pain disorders and may be helpful in managing sleep disturbance associated with chronic pain. Atypical antidepressants, serotonin reuptake inhibitors, and monoamine oxidase inhibitors may also have a role, although the results of clinical trials of their efficacy as analgesics have been equivocal (Table 5-4).

Table 5-2 Commonly Used Nonsteroidal Anti-inflammatory Drugs and Doses

Drug	Average Dose (mg)	Dosing Interval (hr)	Maximum Daily (mg)	Comments
Ibuprofen	200-400	4-6	3200	
Naproxen	500 initial, 250 subsequent	8-12	1250	
Indomethacin	25	8-12	100	
Choline magnesium trisalicylate	1000-1500	8-12	1500	Does not increase bleeding time
Nabumetone	1000-1500	12-24	2000	Absorption increased with food
Diclofenac sodium	50-100	6-8	200	
Celecoxib	200	12	400	Cyclooxygenase-2 selective
Acetaminophen	500-1000	4-6	4000	Hepatotoxicity can occur if maximum dose exceeded

Table 5-3 Commonly Used Long-Acting Opiates and Doses

Drug	Equianalgesic Dose (Oral)	Start PO	Comments
Morphine (MS Contin, Oramorph, Kadian)	30 mg	15-30 mg/d	For all opioids, use caution in patients with impaired ventilation, asthma, increased intracranial pressure, or liver failure.
Oxycodone (OxyContin)	20 mg	20-40 mg/d	
Methadone	Use extreme caution when converting because of variability of patient response.	10-20 mg/d	Long plasma half-life (>12 hr); accumulates over several days; do not escalate dose rapidly.
Fentanyl (Duragesic transdermal patch)	Transdermal fentanyl patch 25 µg/hr roughly equals 45 mg/day of sustained release morphine.	25-µg/hr patch	12-hr delay in onset and offset of patch

Table 5-4 Commonly Used Antidepressants and Doses

Drug	Dose	Side Effects
Tricyclic		Anticholinergic and α-adrenergic blocking effects, cardiotoxicity, orthostatic hypotension, narrow angle glaucoma, lower seizure threshold
Amitriptyline	10-100 mg	
Nortriptyline	25-60 mg	
Desipramine	25-100 mg	
Doxepin	25-100 mg	
Atypical		Priapism
Trazodone	25-300 mg	Little anticholinergic effect
SSRIs		Insomnia, restlessness, gastrointestinal distress, tremor, primary ejaculatory delay, nausea
Fluoxetine	20-60 mg	
Paroxetine	10-40 mg	
Sertraline	50-200 mg	
SNRIs		
Duloxetine	60 mg/d (max, 120 mg/d)	Sedation, ataxia, nausea, dry mouth, hyperhidrosis
Venlafaxine	150-225 mg/d (max, 375 mg/d)	Hypertension, ataxia, sedation, insomnia, nausea, anxiety, anorexia

SNRI, serotonin-norepinephrine reuptake inhibitor; SSRI, selective serotonin reuptake inhibitor.

Table 5-5 Commonly Used Anticonvulsants and Doses

Drug	Daily Dose	Side Effects
Gabapentin	Start 300 mg every hour as needed; titrate to 900-1200 mg three times a day	Sedation, ataxia, edema, tremor, psychomotor slowing, difficulty concentrating
Pregabalin	Start 50 mg/d in divided doses every 8 hr; titrate to 300-600 mg/d (max, 600 mg/d)	Sedation, ataxia, edema, weight gain, diplopia, dry mouth
Topiramate	Start 50 mg every hour as needed; titrate to max dose 200 mg twice a day	Sedation, fatigue, psychomotor slowing, difficulty concentrating, paresthesias, kidney stones
Lamotrigine	Start 25 mg every hour as needed; titrate to 300-500 mg twice a day	Rash, drug interaction with other anticonvulsants
Carbamazepine	Start 200 mg every hour as needed; titrate to 400-2400 mg/day	Sedation, ataxia, hepatitis, aplastic anemia, slow intracardiac conduction
Valproate	5-10 mg/kg/d; titrate to 15-60 mg/kg/d	Sedation, transient elevation AST/ALT, thrombocytopenia, platelet dysfunction at higher doses

ALT, alanine transaminase; AST, aspartate aminotransferase.

Duloxetine has been approved for diabetic peripheral neuropathy.

Anticonvulsants

Anticonvulsants may relieve lancinating pain arising from peripheral nerve syndromes such as trigeminal neuralgia, postherpetic neuralgia, diabetic neuropathy, cancer pain, and post-traumatic neuralgia. These drugs are also effective as mood-stabilizing drugs and in migraine prophylaxis (Table 5-5).

Other Adjuvants

Antispasmodics are beneficial for pain of musculature origin. Their use for long-term therapy is limited by somnolence and the potential for abuse and dependency. Baclofen is most useful in treatment of spasticity of spinal cord origin. Patients with spinal cord injury and multiple sclerosis typically respond best. Tizanidine is a centrally acting α_2-adrenergic agonist. It is effective in the treatment of both spasticity and painful muscle spasm.

Tramadol binds with modest activity to μ opiate receptors and has weaker affinity for σ and κ receptors. It also inhibits the reuptake of norepinephrine and serotonin. Side effects include dizziness, nausea, constipation, dry mouth, and headache. It should be used with caution in patients with increased intracranial pressure and renal disease.

Mexiletine, an oral local anesthetic, has been used safely in neuropathic pain disorders such as myotonia, chronic painful diabetic neuropathy, and spasticity. Contraindications to use include preexisting second- or third-degree heart block, chronic hypotension, congestive heart failure, and hepatic injury.

Capsaicin is the most commonly used topical medication for neuropathic pain, particularly diabetic neuropathy, postherpetic neuralgia, and postmastectomy pain. Many patients report good pain relief, but many are unable to tolerate the burning at the application site.

Physical Interventions

Exercise, massage, applications of heat and cold, transcutaneous electrical stimulation, and acupuncture are physical interventions that are used in addition to medication therapy. These are particularly helpful in myofascial or localized pain disorders.

Various types of injections and nerve blocks can be employed as important diagnostic and therapeutic tools. Trigger-point injections are effective in myofascial pain disorders to help facilitate exercise and restoration of normal muscle function. Epidural steroid injection and selective nerve root blocks are effective for radicular neuropathic pain problems and spinal stenosis. Facet joint injections and medial branch nerve blocks are useful in mechanical back and neck pain.

Sympathetic nerve blocks (stellate ganglion, celiac plexus, lumbar sympathetic) can be diagnostic and therapeutic for sympathetically maintained pain and can facilitate rehabilitation-oriented therapy. A patient who experiences profound but temporary benefit from nerve blocks may be considered for chemical or surgical neurolysis. Such procedures are generally not permanent and are not without risk; they are best considered only as a last resort, especially for patients with limited life expectancy.

More aggressive interventional pain therapies include radiofrequency denervation, spinal cord stimulation, or intrathecal pumps.

Avoiding Treatment Errors

An individualized program is important in chronic pain management. The best available treatment options are based on an understanding of the pain mechanism, medical history, and available medications. The side effects of some drugs, particularly sedative medications, can be advantageous. Chronic pain management also requires ongoing patient evaluation, patient education, and diagnostic evaluation of any treatable underlying conditions. Analgesia, tolerability, and other benefits such as improved sleep or quality of life should be monitored. Patient education should include a discussion about the natural history of the condition and realistic treatment expectations. Functional goals such as improvement in sleep, activity, and quality of life should be emphasized. Reassessment and titration of medications should be tailored to improve functionality and quality of life. If one treatment regimen is not beneficial, the pain problem should be reevaluated, use other adjuvants or a different opiate should be considered, or the patient should be evaluated for possible interventional or injection therapies.

Future Directions

Until such time as we have the means to effectively eliminate chronic pain, newer cost-effective models of multidisciplinary assessment and care of patients are needed. Our understanding of neuropathic pain mechanisms and pathophysiology is still in its infancy but is advancing rapidly; more novel analgesic drugs are under investigation than ever before in history. Custom-designed analgesics seek to affect pain processes on a cellular level: to block nociception, counteract the processes of neuropathic pain, and prevent central sensitization. New interventional techniques will continue to be developed and explored as means to treat the sources of intractable pain. Chronic pain prevention is an area ripe for research and clinical development.

Additional Resources

American Pain Society: Principles of analgesic use in the treatment of acute pain and cancer pain. Available at: http://www.ampainsoc.org/pub/principles.htm. Accessed November 17, 2006.

This is an excellent resource for concise information about drug selection, dosing, the treatment of breakthrough pain, and minimization of side effects.

EVIDENCE

1. Gilron I, Watson CP, Cahill CM, Moulin DE: Neuropathic pain: A practical guide for the clinician. CMAJ 175(3):265-275, 2006.

   This article gives an excellent description of the pathophysiology, clinical features, and pharmacology indicated for the treatment of neuropathic pain. A primary care algorithm is also provided to assist with neuropathic pain management.

2. Trescot AM, Boswell MV, Atluri SL, et al: Opioid guidelines in the management of chronic non-cancer pain. Pain Physician 9:1-39, 2006.

   These guidelines were established after systematic review and analysis of the available literature on opioid use in the management of chronic non-cancer pain. These evidence-based guidelines should help provide consistency in opioid philosophy and treatment among diverse chronic pain groups.

M. Andrew Greganti

Chronic Fatigue Syndrome

Introduction

The chronic fatigue syndrome (CFS) was first operationally defined in 1988 to describe patients who present, usually after a viral illness, with incapacitating fatigue of such severity that continuation of regular activities is impossible. Associated symptoms include generalized muscle pain and weakness, poor concentration, irritability, and postexertional fatigue lasting longer than 24 hours. The onset is most often abrupt, occurring over a few hours to a few days, and disruptive of an otherwise productive life, often of a previously highly motivated and energetic individual. Medical experts have not provided an acceptable explanation based on an underlying organic or nonorganic disease process such as anxiety or depression. The lack of a definitive explanation has led to the frustration of patients and physicians alike, and CFS has become one of several so-called medically unexplained diseases.

Historical Overview and General Perspective

Medical authors have described patients with chronic fatigue at least since the late 1800s when the term *neurasthenia* defined a similar condition of uncertain cause characterized by severe physical and mental fatigue, protracted postexertional fatigue, nervous dyspepsia, and mood abnormalities. The syndrome seemed to present more commonly in women and hard-working professionals. It was often ascribed to the impact of life stresses on the nervous system. Over time, the term neurasthenia has given way to a variety of others, each defining a similar clinical syndrome often developing in localized cluster outbreaks or epidemics: *Iceland disease, Royal-Free disease, epidemic neuromyasthenia, myalgic encephalomyelitis, postviral fatigue syndrome, chronic brucellosis, chronic Epstein-Barr virus infection,* and *Lake Tahoe disease,* among others. The presentation of clusters of cases led to an infectious disease hypothesis and the designation of the syndrome as postinfectious or postviral. Much of the research on CFS over the past 50 to 60 years has focused on a possible viral etiology.

CFS has become one of several highly prevalent conditions that defy a clear-cut etiologic and pathogenetic explanation and challenge the dualistic model of medical illness. This model assumes that the mind and body are separate and categorizes every illness as mental or physical. The often-heated debate of recent years stems from moralistic prejudices that associate those illnesses characterized as "mental" with personal weakness and inferiority. In contrast, "physical" illnesses do not imply personal fault.

The dualistic model of illness has produced two approaches, each representing an attempt to explain the somatic and psychological symptoms that characterize CFS. The medical approach defines such syndromes as chronic fatigue, irritable bowel, and fibromyalgia as organic diseases with functional, rather than structural, abnormalities. The psychiatric approach regards these diseases as psychological disorders with somatic manifestations. Under this model, the somatic symptoms of CFS represent underlying depression and anxiety being manifest in an atypical somatoform manner. The focus on psychological factors was supported by a 1970 reanalysis of previously reported outbreaks of benign myalgic encephalomyelitis that concluded that the epidemics were secondary to a mass hysterical reaction. The debate continues as patients and their physicians search for answers.

Epidemiology

Not surprisingly, the lack of consensus on the definition of CFS and the lack of a diagnostic test have produced great variability in prevalence estimates, ranging from 2.3 to 600 cases per 100,000 population. Using the Centers for Disease Control and Prevention (CDC) criteria published in 1988, the crude prevalence in four surveillance sites in persons older than 18 years was 2.3 to 7.4 cases per 100,000. These estimates are conservative because of the exclusion of patients with preexisting affective, anxiety, and somatization disorders. A more recent study of the prevalence and incidence of CFS in Wichita, Kansas documented a point prevalence of 235 cases per 100,000 persons and a 1-year incidence of 180 per 100,000 persons. As previously noted, clusters are well documented; however, CFS usually occurs sporadically in adults—the mean age of presentation in five series using the CDC definition was 37.8 years. In the same five series, women comprised 76% of the patients. Based on limited demographic information, most of those affected are white, middle class, and well educated—hence the label, yuppie flu. As in the case of irritable bowel syndrome and other similar entities, more aggressive case finding could lead to a higher estimate of prevalence.

Etiology and Pathogenesis

A specific etiology has evaded investigators. Since CFS usually develops acutely after a respiratory or gastrointestinal infection, researchers have focused many of their efforts on the search for an infectious pathogen. Other pathogenic mechanisms have also been considered.

Viruses

Studies have implicated a number of viruses, including enteroviruses, particularly Coxsackie B. Other viruses considered include human herpes virus 6, herpes simplex types 1 and 2, human T-cell lymphotropic virus-2, retroviruses, and the Epstein-Barr virus (EBV). The proposed theory is that initial infection with a viral pathogen can induce long-term immune dysfunction in susceptible hosts. Chronic EBV infection has received the most attention. Several epidemics of CFS have seemed to follow the pattern of an extended illness after acute infectious mononucleosis. This association has depended on the serologic markers of EBV infection. Recent studies have documented that there is no greater incidence of EBV seropositivity in CFS patients than in the general population. It now seems unlikely that EBV or another virus will be the highly sought-after underlying pathogen.

Chronic Lyme Disease and Other Infections

Initial excitement about the Lyme disease spirochete as a causative agent has also waned. As in the case of viral agents, investigators have had great difficulty confirming a definite pathogenic association. The same holds for studies of other pathogens, including *Brucella abortus, Campylobacter jejuni, Mycoplasma pneumoniae,* and *Toxoplasma gondii,* among others.

Immune System Dysfunction

The literature has documented a number of immune system abnormalities, including peripheral blood lymphopenia, decreased lymphocyte proliferation in response to mitogens, abnormal numbers of helper and suppressor T cells, impaired killer cell activity, impairment of delayed skin test sensitivity, immunoglobulin G subclass deficiencies, and excessive production of interferon-α by mononuclear cells. Studies have not yielded consistent and reproducible results, and more data are needed to define more specific associations.

Psychological Causes

The proportion of CFS patients who have a previous history of psychiatric disorders or symptoms compatible with depression, anxiety, and somatoform disorders varies between 42% and 82% in some studies. The association with nonpsychotic depression is especially notable and has led to debate about what is primary and what is secondary; that is, is depression a reaction to the syndrome, or is it the primary cause? Another basic question is whether psychiatric disorders can produce the observed dysregulation and impairment of immunity.

Clinical Presentation

The most recent case definition, based on an international consensus of investigators, represents an attempt to provide a useful working definition pending the development of a better understanding of the etiology and pathogenesis of CFS. Box 6-1 lists the diagnostic criteria.

The overlap of the symptoms listed and those of depression and anxiety is obvious (Fig. 6-1). Clinical diagnosis is complicated further by the fact that a large proportion of CFS patients have a previous history of major depression. In those patients who meet the criteria of both CFS and major depression, the onset of the two disorders commonly coincides. Despite this strong association, as many as half of the patients diagnosed with CFS cannot be categorized operationally under the diagnosis of a major depressive disorder. The consideration of anxiety as an underlying disorder in addition to depression still does not fully explain the full complement of symptoms experienced by many patients with CFS.

Most patients do not have definitively abnormal physical findings, at least ones that are specific. Some experience low-grade fever (37.6° C to 38.6° C). Others have a nonexudative pharyngitis with palpable or tender cervical lymph nodes. Axillary adenopathy has also been observed.

Box 6-1 Case Definition of Chronic Fatigue Syndrome

Inclusion Criteria

Clinically evaluated, medically unexplained fatigue of at least 6 months' duration that is:
 Of new onset (not lifelong)
 Not a result of ongoing exertion
 Not substantially alleviated by rest
 Causing a substantial reduction in previous level of activity
The occurrence of four or more of the following symptoms:
 Subjective memory impairment
 Sore throat
 Tender lymph nodes
 Muscle pain
 Joint pain
 Headache
 Unrefreshing sleep
 Postexertional malaise lasting more than 24 hours

Exclusion Criteria

Active, unresolved, or suspected disease
Psychotic, melancholic, or bipolar depression (but not uncomplicated major depression)
Psychotic disorders
Dementia
Anorexia and bulimia nervosa
Alcohol or other substance misuse
Severe obesity

From Fakuda K, Straus SE, Hickie I, et al: The chronic fatigue syndrome: A comprehensive approach to its definition and study. Ann Intern Med 121:953, 1994.

Differential Diagnosis

Diseases that can present as fatigue include anemia, hypothyroidism, Addison's disease, chronic liver disease, hypercalcemia, low cardiac output states, neuromuscular diseases, sleep disorders, and depression.

Diagnostic Approach

The diagnosis depends on a careful review of the patient's history. In general, laboratory testing is not helpful given the lack of a sensitive and specific test and the associated poor likelihood ratios. The utility of laboratory testing lies in the need to exclude other diagnoses that can present as fatigue. Depression is an especially difficult diagnosis to exclude. Recommended testing includes the following: complete blood count, erythrocyte sedimentation rate, electrolyte profile, calcium, phosphorus, serum creatinine, urinalysis, glucose, liver function tests, thyroid-stimulating hormone, and creatine kinase. Testing for antinuclear antibodies and rheumatoid factor is rational in patients with especially severe arthralgias and myalgias. Excluding adrenal insufficiency with morning and evening cortisol levels should be considered. Evaluation for an underlying sleep disorder is also rational, especially if there is evidence of daytime somnolence. Testing for antibodies to EBV and enteroviruses is not recommended. Similarly, immune function testing is of no diagnostic value given the variability of the results. The basic approach is to exclude other causes of fatigue first. This avoids labeling a patient with CFS prematurely.

Management and Therapy

In general, the goals of therapy are to provide emotional support, to relieve the patient's symptoms and overall distress, and to protect the patient from the harm of an increasing array of poorly evaluated and documented therapies. Given the lack of a definitive etiology, the focus must be on symptomatic therapy. Accepting the patient's symptoms and disability as "real" is an essential first step. CFS patients, after interacting with the medical system on several occasions, understand that medical science places them in an "unexplained" category, one that often questions whether they are really sick. Discussion of possible underlying anxiety or depression regularly evokes overt hostility because such diagnoses equate with personal weakness and inferiority and, in effect, with the lack of "real" illness. It is helpful to emphasize that, in the face of insufficient knowledge about etiology, the patient and the physician must deal with a variety of possible underlying etiologies, but both must focus on treating the symptoms no matter what the cause. This requires them to abandon the dualistic model and to accept the inseparability of the mind and body in every disease process. Patients are much more willing to accept depression and anxiety as components of their disease process after being reassured that "it is not all in your head." They are also more willing to acknowledge that there is no quick fix given the complex interrelationships involved.

Optimum Treatment

As is often the case for diseases without definitive etiologies, therapy must be individualized. It is essential to provide the patient and the family with educational materials about the nature of the syndrome, while avoiding unproductive arguments about what is and is not a likely etiology in the patient's case. Identifiable depression and anxiety must be treated with antidepressant drugs. Serotonin reuptake inhibitors with anxiolytic characteristics are often helpful. These agents may also help with insomnia that can only worsen fatigue. The physician should gently encourage the patient to return to normal functioning and to remain physically active. Exercise programs should be graded in intensity and allow for patient input about what is and is not tolerated. Forcing poorly tolerated exercise can decrease rapport and patient self-confidence in the ability to recover function. Some studies have documented that cognitive behavioral therapy over extended intervals and with skilled therapists can help the patient develop coping skills in the face of a chronic illness. Supportive

Figure 6-1 Chronic Fatigue Syndrome: Signs and Symptoms.

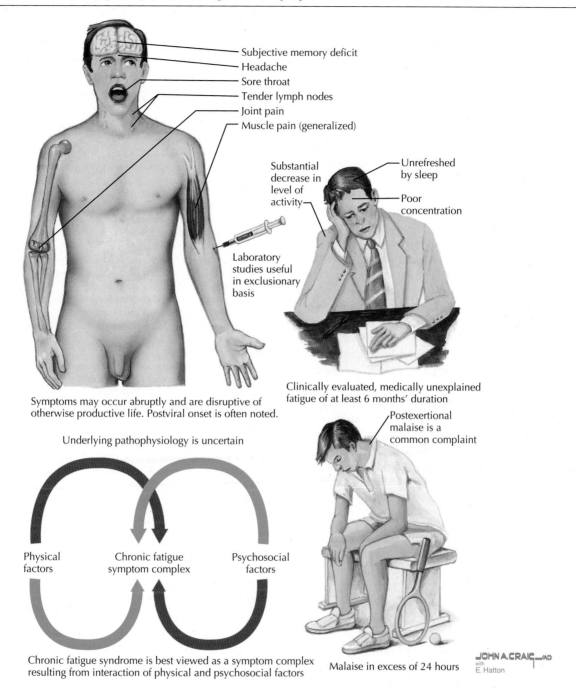

Subjective memory deficit
Headache
Sore throat
Tender lymph nodes
Joint pain
Muscle pain (generalized)

Substantial decrease in level of activity

Laboratory studies useful in exclusionary basis

Unrefreshed by sleep

Poor concentration

Symptoms may occur abruptly and are disruptive of otherwise productive life. Postviral onset is often noted.

Clinically evaluated, medically unexplained fatigue of at least 6 months' duration

Underlying pathophysiology is uncertain

Physical factors　　Chronic fatigue symptom complex　　Psychosocial factors

Postexertional malaise is a common complaint

Chronic fatigue syndrome is best viewed as a symptom complex resulting from interaction of physical and psychosocial factors

Malaise in excess of 24 hours

JOHN A. CRAIG—AD
with
E. Hatton

psychotherapy can help restore patient confidence and self-esteem.

Avoiding Treatment Errors

There is no convincing evidence that the use of intravenous or oral antibiotics, antivirals, or intramuscular or intravenous γ-globulin therapy is effective. The abiding concern is that such therapies can lead to iatrogenic complications, including renal dysfunction, intravenous-line infections, and allergic reactions.

Often, therapy is impaired by differences between the patient's and the physician's views on underlying disease mechanisms and therapy. Patients and their family members may have strong opinions based on the lay literature, Internet information, and information from self-help groups. Differences arise when the provider has to complete an official report about disability and is torn between helping the patient and avoiding a self-fulfilling prophecy that CFS is a hopeless disease process. The physician should not immediately reject the patient's ideas in any of these areas. Special time must often be set aside to allow extended discussion with the patient and the patient's family. The need for such "special time" is one of many aspects that make the management of CFS patients challenging and leads to avoidance of this patient group by health care providers.

Prognosis

The current literature does not provide reliable information about prognosis; however, there is clearly substantial variation among patients. The disease seems to be highly variable with day-to-day fluctuations and periods of incapacitating relapses occurring after periods of improvement. The duration of the disease is also variable, ranging from 1 to 5 years or more. Twenty-six to 57% of patients improve or recover after varying periods of follow-up. The risk for morbidity is high, especially in patients who have the disease indefinitely. In contrast, mortality is rare. Iatrogenic illness is a major risk brought on by frustrated attempts of both patients and their physicians to try any therapy, no matter how poorly documented. Patients fare worse when they insist that only an organic explanation is viable and fail to accept the biopsychosocial model of disease that espouses an intricate mind-body connection. This situation is greatly exacerbated by a health care system that insists on separating medical and psychiatric services, in effect catalyzing the dualistic approach. The exclusion of psychotherapeutic options by patients greatly limits what can be done to palliate their disease process. Unfortunately, the hesitancy of busy physicians, even those with the necessary training and experience, to take on so-called problem patients also perpetuates the dualistic model.

Future Directions

The need to move from the highly descriptive term, chronic fatigue syndrome, which defines a very heterogeneous group of patients, to one or several that define a more homogeneous group or groups, remains a central issue. Like other syndromes that are medically unexplained, CFS reminds us that our current classification model of disease perpetuates the dualistic mind-body separation and leads to the suboptimal care of this large group of patients. The publicity surrounding CFS has made the need to move toward the biopsychosocial model more apparent to patients, their physicians, and hopefully, those who fund research. There is no other alternative until a more specific etiology of CFS is defined. The need for more research that addresses underlying disease mechanisms and more useful ways to classify diseases that cross the mind-body divide is clear.

Additional Resources

Buchwald D: Fibromyalgia and chronic fatigue syndrome: Similarities and differences. Rheum Dis Clin North Am 22:219-243, 1996.

The author points out the demographic and clinical similarities between CFS and fibromyalgia and emphasizes that further clarification of the similarities and differences between these two entities may be useful in studies of prognosis and in defining subsets of patients who may benefit from specific therapies.

Centers for Disease Control and Prevention: Chronic fatigue syndrome. Available at: http://www.cdc.gov/cfs/. Accessed July 9, 2006.

This useful website maintains up-to-date information on diagnosis, therapy, and new research findings, organizing the information for both patients and health care professionals.

Klonoff DC: Chronic fatigue syndrome. Clin Infect Dis 15:812-823, 1992.

This is a helpful review of the history, definition, epidemiology, etiology, clinical presentation, and treatment of CFS.

Reeves WC, Wagner D, Nisenbaum R, et al: Chronic fatigue syndrome: A clinically empirical approach to its definition and study. BMC Med 3:19, 2005.

This article documents that CFS can be defined using readily available instruments that evaluate the major components specified in its 1994 case definition. Using this approach, CFS patients are clinically distinct from patients with unexplained fatigue. The authors urge that future research studies define CFS in this manner.

Resource for myalgic encephalomyelitis, chronic fatigue syndrome, and fibromyalgia. Available at: http://www.supportme.co.uk/. Accessed July 9, 2006.

This patient-oriented website provides information for the lay user, including a library of references that can be accessed.

Schluederberg A, Straus SE, Peterson P, et al: NIH conference. Chronic fatigue syndrome research: Definition and medical outcome assessment. Ann Intern Med 117:325-331, 1992.

This paper presents the results of a workshop at the NIH to address critical issues in research concerning CFS. Case definitions, confounding diagnoses, and medical outcome assessment are considered.

Sharpe M: Chronic fatigue syndrome. Psychiatr Clin North Am 19:549-573, 1996.

The author points out that the attempt to define CFS as either a strictly medical or psychiatric condition is not clinically useful. Helpful recommendations on patient management are provided.

Straus SE: The chronic mononucleosis syndrome. J Infect Dis 157:405-412, 1988.

This useful review of the early perspective on CFS set the standard for later studies.

EVIDENCE

1. Fukuda K, Straus SE, Hickie I, et al: The chronic fatigue syndrome: A comprehensive approach to its definition and study. International Chronic Fatigue Syndrome Study Group. Ann Intern Med 121:953-959, 1994.

   The authors propose a conceptual framework and a set of guidelines in an attempt to provide a comprehensive, systematic, and integrated approach to the evaluation, classification, and study of patients with unexplained fatigue.

2. Holmes GP, Kaplan JE, Gantz NM, et al: Chronic fatigue syndrome: A working case definition. Ann Intern Med 108:387-389, 1988.

   The authors propose a new name, chronic fatigue syndrome, for what was previously described as the chronic Epstein-Barr virus syndrome. The article presents a working definition of CFS to improve the comparability and reproducibility of clinical research and to provide a basis for the clinical evaluation of patients.

3. Reyes M, Nisenbaum R, Hoaglin DC, et al: Prevalence and incidence of chronic fatigue syndrome in Wichita, Kansas. Arch Intern Med 163:1530-1536, 2003.

   This paper presents the results of a study of the prevalence and incidence of CFS in the general population of Wichita, Kansas in an attempt to provide more accurate population-based epidemiologic data.

Robert J. Vissers

7

Poisoning and Drug Overdose

Introduction

Intentional overdose in suicidal adults is the most common cause of poisoning that leads to hospitalization or death. Ingestion of substances in the home by children younger than 6 years accounts for most reported poisonings; however, the morbidity is much lower. The incidence has more than doubled in the past decade, particularly in the teenage and elderly populations. Other poisoning scenarios include parenteral drug abuse, chemical exposure, medication interactions, and envenomations. Diagnosis can require the recognition of toxic syndromes and appropriate utilization of laboratory studies. Specific treatments using decontamination methods and antidotes may be required for some poisonings, although most are treated with supportive measures.

Etiology and Pathogenesis

Pharmaceuticals, particularly analgesics and over-the-counter preparations, are involved most frequently, followed by cleaning products, cosmetics, and plants. Ingestion is the most common route of exposure, but poisonings can occur through dermal, inhalational, mucosal, and parenteral exposures or through envenomation.

The mechanism of toxicity varies with the substance. Effects may be limited to the site of exposure and represent nonspecific chemical reactions. Systemic effects are the result of interactions between the toxin and specific target sites, such as receptors or organs. Most deaths occur before arrival at the hospital, often as a result of central nervous system and respiratory depression. Other life-threatening mechanisms include dysrhythmias, hypotension, and organ necrosis.

Clinical Presentation

Presentations are extremely variable, not only between different substances but also for a specific toxin. Signs and symptoms depend on the time from ingestion, the amount taken, and the interaction of coingestants. This variability in clinical presentation demands a thorough history and physical examination, and the consideration of a possible toxic ingestion in the differential diagnosis of all patients with an unexplained sudden change in their physiologic status. Poisoned patients can deteriorate quickly, and as a result, frequent reassessments and close monitoring are essential.

Identification of potential toxins and the time of ingestion are critical for diagnosis and management (Fig. 7-1). Most patients will admit to the substances ingested; however, the accuracy of the amount taken is notoriously unreliable. In addition, patients may be unable to give a history because of altered consciousness. Always assume a worst-case scenario regarding the amount taken (assume the bottle was full) and the probable presence of other coingestants. Collateral history from family members, friends, and prehospital personnel is often helpful. Intentional overdoses are associated with a much higher potential mortality than accidental overdose.

A complete physical examination of all systems, followed by frequently repeated vital signs and examinations, serves several purposes: (1) the identification of toxic syndromes (or *toxidromes*) and complications associated with the toxin; (2) the detection of underlying disease states or coexisting trauma; and (3) careful monitoring of the response to therapy (Table 7-1; Fig. 7-2).

Both sympathomimetic and anticholinergic drugs can cause central nervous system excitation, mydriasis, and an

Figure 7-1 Some Common Poisonous Plants.

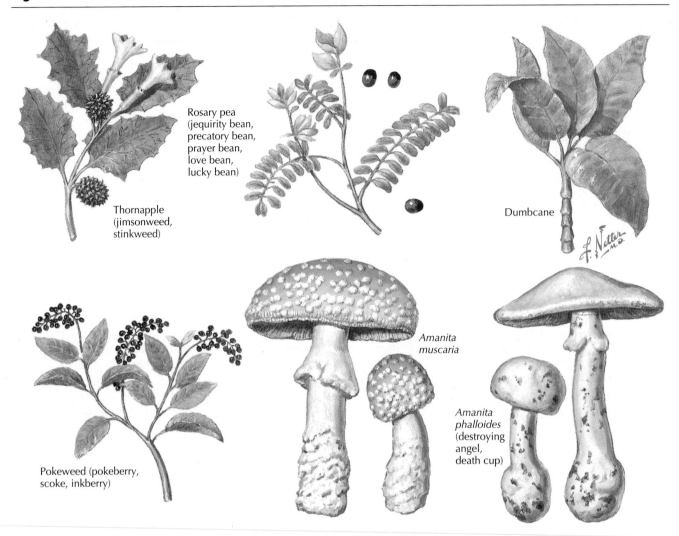

Thornapple
(jimsonweed,
stinkweed)

Rosary pea
(jequirity bean,
precatory bean,
prayer bean,
love bean,
lucky bean)

Dumbcane

Amanita muscaria

Amanita phalloides (destroying angel, death cup)

Pokeweed (pokeberry, scoke, inkberry)

Table 7-1 Toxic Syndromes		
Syndrome	**Clinical Manifestations**	**Associated Toxins**
Sympathomimetic	CNS excitation, seizures, tachycardia, hypertension, mydriasis, diaphoresis	Cocaine, caffeine, theophylline, amphetamines
Anticholinergic	Delirium, hallucinations, dry mucosa, mydriasis, decreased bowel sounds, dry skin, tachycardia, seizures	Atropine, tricyclic antidepressants, antihistamines, phenothiazines
Cholinergic	CNS excitation or depression, bradycardia or tachycardia, miosis or mydriasis, diarrhea, salivation, diaphoresis, lacrimation, paralysis	Organophosphates, pilocarpine, acetylcholine
Opiate	CNS depression, miosis, hypoventilation, hypotension, response to naloxone	Heroin, codeine, propoxyphene, pentazocine, oxycodone
Serotonin	Altered mental status, increased muscle tone, hyperreflexia, hyperthermia, tremors	MAOI + SSRI, MAOI + meperidine, SSRI + tricyclic, SSRI overdose

CNS, central nervous system; MAOI, monoamine oxidase inhibitor; SSRI, selective serotonin reuptake inhibitor.

Figure 7-2 The Pupils in Poisoning.

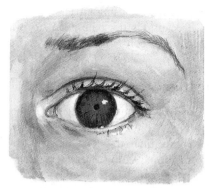

Miosis (pinhole pupils)
Seen in poisoning by morphine and
morphine derivatives, some types of
mushrooms, cholinesterase inhibitors,
parasympathomimetics, nicotine, chloral
hydrate, sympatholytics, and some other
compounds

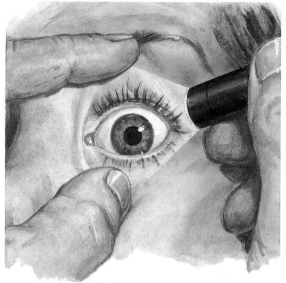

Mydriasis (pupils dilated and not reactive)
Seen in poisoning by barbiturates, carbon monoxide, methyl
and other alcohols, oxalic acid, cocaine, belladonna
derivatives, camphor, cyanide, sympathomimetics,
parasympatholytics, and a number of other compounds

elevation of blood pressure, pulse rate, respiratory rate, and temperature. Anticholinergic agents may be distinguished by the findings of dry skin and mucous membranes, diminished bowel sounds, urinary retention, skin flushing, and decreased visual acuity. Poisoning with a cholinergic agent produces a mixture of muscarinic and nicotinic effects. The muscarinic effects produce a hypersecretory state of salivation, lacrimation, urination, defecation, gastrointestinal hyperactivity, and emesis—thus the acronym, *sludge*. Nicotinic effects include mydriasis, hypertension, tachycardia, muscle fasciculations, and weakness. Patients may present atypically when multiple toxins are involved.

Differential Diagnosis

The differential is extensive and varies with the presentation. Poisonings need to be considered in patients with unexplained, acute alterations of mental status, seizures, or dysrhythmias.

Diagnostic Approach

Laboratory

Drug screens have limited utility in acute management. It is preferable to request specific drug assays in probable ingestions and when identification affects patient management. Specific quantitative toxicologic tests that may assist in management include acetaminophen, carboxyhemoglo-

bin, digoxin, ethanol, ethylene glycol, methanol, iron, lithium, methemoglobin, salicylates, and theophylline.

Routine screening for acetaminophen is indicated in all intentional overdoses because of the frequency of acetaminophen overdose, its asymptomatic presentation, and the associated preventable hepatic toxicity. A similar consideration may be given to screening for acetylsalicylic acid and ethanol; however, the evidence is not as compelling. An increased anion gap or an elevated osmolal gap suggests the presence of specific toxins (Box 7-1).

Liver function tests can be useful in acetaminophen toxicity. Calcium oxalate crystals in the urine are associated with ethylene glycol ingestion.

Electrocardiography and Radiography

An electrocardiogram is rarely diagnostic but can identify complications, particularly for toxins associated with sodium channel blockade. Widening of the QRS in tricyclic antidepressant overdoses is associated with seizures and dysrhythmias. Abdominal radiographs can occasionally demonstrate, but not rule out, some radiopaque ingestions (iron, phenothiazines, cocaine condoms, enteric coated tablets, heavy metals).

Management and Therapy

Most ingestions are successfully treated through supportive care as opposed to specific antidotal therapy. Support

> **Box 7-1** Toxins Associated with Laboratory Abnormalities
>
> **Increased Anion Gap Acidosis**
> Ethanol
> Methanol
> Ethylene glycol
> Paraldehyde
> Iron
> Isoniazid
> Salicylates
>
> **Increased Osmolal Gap***
> Ethanol
> Methanol
> Ethylene glycol
> Mannitol
> Isopropyl alcohol

*Osmolal gap = measured osmolality − [2X Na (Meq/L) + glucose (mg/dL)/18 + BUN (mg/dL)/2.8 + ethanol (mg/dL)/4.3].

of the airway, breathing, and circulation should take first priority. Ventilatory failure may occur secondary to respiratory depression, pulmonary edema, bronchoconstriction, or paralysis. Endotracheal intubation is often necessary to maintain the airway and to facilitate oxygenation and ventilation. Hypotension usually reflects venous pooling as opposed to myocardial depression; therefore, initial therapy consists of intravenous fluid boluses and Trendelenburg positioning. Norepinephrine is a good choice for inotropic support because α blockade is a common cause of hypotension in poisonings.

Altered Mental Status and Coma

Altered mental status is a frequent complication of poisoning. Attributing the symptoms to alcohol alone is a potential pitfall because many ingestions involve multiple toxins. Computed tomography scanning is indicated in patients with focal neurologic deficits or a history of head trauma. All patients who present with coma or altered sensorium should have an immediate bedside glucose check. Intravenous dextrose 50% is the most effective acute therapy for hypoglycemia. All malnourished and ethanol-abusing patients should receive thiamine, 100 mg intravenously. Intravenous naloxone, 2 mg, is recommended in all patients with coma of unknown etiology. Titrated doses of 0.4 mg should be considered in patients who are at high risk for withdrawal. If an opioid overdose is strongly suspected (see toxidromes discussed earlier), up to 10 mg may be required to reverse some opioids (propoxyphene, pentazocine, codeine). Flumazenil is a competitive antagonist of benzodiazepines. Intractable seizures and ventricular dysrhythmias may complicate its administration in patients with a history of ethanol or benzodiazepine abuse, or a history of seizures. Its indiscriminate use in comatose patients is not recommended.

Surface Decontamination

Surface decontamination requires removal of clothing and flushing the patient's skin with copious amounts of water. There is no indication for using an acid or base neutralizing solution. Precautions must be taken to protect caregivers from secondary contamination.

Gastrointestinal Decontamination

Gastrointestinal decontamination refers to interventions that empty the gastrointestinal tract, remove the toxin from the gastrointestinal tract, or bind to the toxin to prevent its absorption. Syrup of ipecac is an emetic agent that no longer has an indication in the hospital setting, and it has been removed from the market because of abuse by bulimics. Orogastric or nasogastric lavage is now rarely used because of its questionable efficacy in most ingestions and the potential for complications (Fig. 7-3). It may be beneficial in some patients who present within 1 hour of ingestion of a life-threatening toxin. Lavage is contraindicated in alkali ingestions and in nonintubated patients who are unable to protect their airway. It is performed through a large-bore, (36- to 40-French) tube. Patients should be placed in a left lateral decubitus, Trendelenburg position. Aspiration of the stomach is performed after confirmation of tube placement, and gastric lavage is repeated in 300-mL aliquots until return is clear. Whole-bowel irrigation uses large amounts of surgical bowel cleansing solution, administered through a nasogastric tube, to speed gastrointestinal transit time and reduce absorption of the toxin. It is indicated for toxins poorly bound to charcoal (iron, lithium), sealed containers (body-packers), and sustained-release products. Contraindications include bowel ileus, obstruction, or perforation. Activated charcoal has a remarkable ability to bind toxins because of its large surface area. In the past, it was recommended in most poisonings; however, its use is now being restricted to cases most likely to be beneficial (see later). Activated charcoal can obscure endoscopy in caustic ingestions and does not bind well to lithium, iron, alcohols, and strong acids and bases. The recommended dose of 1 g/kg given orally or nasogastrically may be combined with the cathartic sorbitol to reduce constipation and make the ingestion more palatable. Multiple dosing and the addition of cathartics are probably not useful.

Enhanced Elimination

Forced diuresis is no longer recommended because of unproven efficacy and the potential for volume overload. Alkalinization of the urine (urine pH 7 to 8) may enhance the elimination of some toxins (salicylates, phenobarbital). Urinary acidification is not recommended for any poisoning because of the potential to exacerbate renal failure in the presence of rhabdomyolysis. Dialysis is useful only for

Figure 7-3 Gastric Lavage: Specialized Equipment.

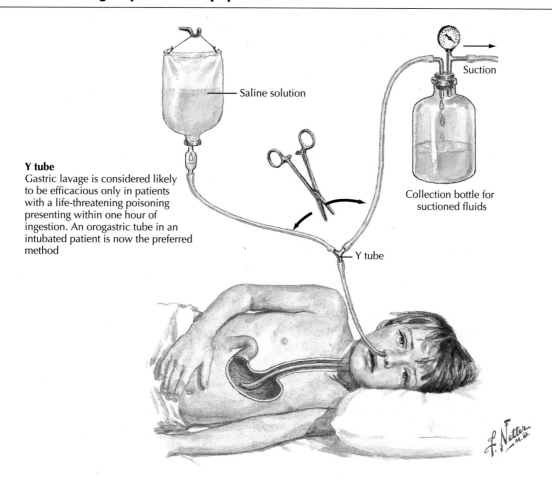

Saline solution

Suction

Collection bottle for suctioned fluids

Y tube
Gastric lavage is considered likely to be efficacious only in patients with a life-threatening poisoning presenting within one hour of ingestion. An orogastric tube in an intubated patient is now the preferred method

Y tube

a limited number of toxins, ideally those that are water soluble and have a low volume of distribution and low protein binding (amphetamines, chloral hydrate, ethylene glycol, lithium, methanol, phenobarbital, salicylates, theophylline). The decision to dialyze is based on serum levels, deterioration despite supportive care, the presence of renal failure, and comorbidities.

Antidotes

Specific antidotal therapy is available for very few poisonings; however, there are a few toxins for which antidotal therapy can be life saving (Table 7-2). The therapeutic half-life of the antidote may be shorter than the toxin, requiring repeat dosing or infusions (e.g., naloxone for a methadone overdose).

Management Resources

Regional poison center consultation is usually available 24 hours a day. Experienced nurses are commonly first-line consultants; however, a toxicologist is often on call and available for assistance with complex cases. POISINDEX

Table 7-2	Toxins with a Specific Antidotal Therapy
Toxin	**Antidote**
Acetaminophen	*N*-acetylcysteine
β-Blockers	IV glucagons
Calcium channel blockers	IV calcium, glucagons
Cholinesterase inhibitors	Atropine, pralidoxime
Cyanide	Cyanide kit
Cyclic antidepressants	Sodium bicarbonate
Carbon monoxide	Oxygen
Digitalis	Digibind
Ethylene glycol	Ethanol, 4-methylpyrazole
Fluoride	IV calcium, magnesium
Hypoglycemics	IV glucose
Isoniazid	IV pyridoxine
Iron	Deferoxamine
Methanol	Ethanol, 4-methylpyrazole
Methemoglobin producers	IV methylene blue
Narcotics	Naloxone, Naltrexone
Salicylates	Sodium bicarbonate

is a computer database available in most emergency departments and online. Nomograms are available for toxins such as acetaminophen; however, specific criteria, such as accurate timing, a single ingestion, and the absence of a slow-release formulation must be met for them to be clinically useful. Early administration of *N*-acetylcysteine may be life saving in acetaminophen overdose.

Optimum Treatment

The toxicology literature remains primarily case based. However, some recent clinical studies have changed the treatment of poisoned patients, particularly with regard to the questionable efficacy of gastric decontamination. Gastric lavage is now rarely, if ever, indicated. Activated charcoal can no longer be recommended as routine in poisoned patients. Its use should be restricted to those cases with potential for clinical benefit, such as patients presenting early after ingestion or for drugs with delayed emptying (anticholinergic, opioids, or sustained-release drugs). Whole-bowel irrigation may be useful in severe lithium or metal poisonings and to assist with evacuation of drug packets from body-packers.

In some circumstances, specific therapy such as antidotes and dialysis may be life saving. However, most poisonings are managed with supportive care, attention to airway maintenance, and cardiovascular support.

Avoiding Treatment Errors

A toxicology screen rarely guides patient management and disposition. Many commonly ingested substances are not screened for, and most screening tests are fraught with significant false-positive and false-negative result rates. Routine drug screening cannot be recommended in all cases of poisoning. Rather, discrete drug levels should be requested based on clinical suspicion. Acetaminophen is one of the rare drugs that should be routinely screened for in most intentional adult ingestions because of its frequency, delayed clinical manifestations, and potential to change clinical outcome. A 6-hour observation period for minimally symptomatic patients is usually adequate; however, extended-release preparations may require longer monitoring and admission.

Future Directions

Fab fragment antidotes are drug-specific antibody fragments that bind drug or protein antigen to prevent toxicity. The antibody-toxin is then excreted in the urine. Fab fragment therapy exists for digoxin and crotalid envenomations and is being developed for a number of other toxins. An alcohol dehydrogenase inhibitor, 4-methylpyrazole (4-MP), is available as an antidote to methanol and ethylene glycol poisoning. It does not cause the sedation that is associated with traditional ethanol therapy. Hallucinogenic designer drugs, such as Ecstasy and γ-hydroxybutyrate, present new challenges in identification and management. Traditional herbal therapies can also be associated with significant toxicities, and databases are available to assist in their identification and management. There is a need for heightened disaster preparedness for mass toxin exposures associated with chemical warfare and terrorism.

Additional Resources

POISINDEX. Available at: http://www.micromedex.com/products/poisindex/. Accessed June 4, 2007.
   This comprehensive, online poisoning reference can be accessed through most medical libraries or through the Internet.
Goldfrank L, Flomenbaum N, Lewin N, et al (eds): Goldfrank's Toxicologic Emergencies, 7th ed. New York, McGraw-Hill, 2002.
   This comprehensive and detailed text on diagnosis and management of acute poisonings is now in its seventh edition.

EVIDENCE

1. American Academy of Clinical Toxicology, European Association of Poisons Centres and Clinical Toxicologists: Position statements: Ipecac syrup, gastric lavage, single-dose activated charcoal, cathartics, whole bowel irrigation. Clin Toxicol 35:699, 1997.
   This comprehensive review of the literature both for and against gastrointestinal decontamination represents an important position that supports the increasingly limited role of these modalities.
2. Eldridge DL: Utilizing diagnostic investigations in the poisoned patient. Med Clin North Am 89:1079-1105, 2005.
   This recent review of diagnostic tools in the undifferentiated poisoned patient provides a well-referenced overview.
3. Hartington K, Hartley J, Clancy M: Measuring plasma paracetamol concentrations in all patients with drug overdoses: Development of a clinical decision rule and clinicians willingness to use it. Emerg Med J 19:408-411, 2002.
   This is one example of many studies that were used as a rationale for the suggested screening labs in the undifferentiated, poisoned patient.
4. Kulig K: General approach to the poisoned patient. In Marx JA, Hockberger RS, Walls RM, et al (eds): Rosen's Emergency Medicine, Concepts and Clinical Practice, 6th ed. St. Louis, Mosby, 2006, pp 2325-2331.
   This recent book chapter from an authoritative emergency medicine textbook nicely summarizes the approach to the poisoned patient. It is authored by a recognized leader in toxicology and incorporates recent toxicology literature and practice.
5. Merigian KS, Woodard M, Hedges JR, et al: Prospective evaluation of gastric emptying in the self-poisoned patient. Am J Emerg Med 8:479-483, 1990.
   This classic study demonstrates the limited utility of gastric emptying in the poisoned patient.
6. Perrone J, De Roos F, Jayaraman S, Hollander JE: Drug screening versus history in detection of substance use in ED psychiatric patients. Am J Emerg Med 19:49-51, 2001.
   This is one example of many studies that were used as a rationale for the suggested screening labs in the undifferentiated, poisoned patient.

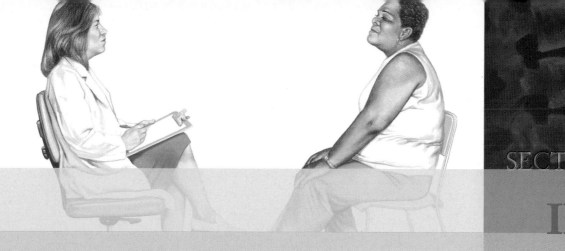

Disorders of the Upper Respiratory Tract and Oropharynx

Daniel S. Reuland

8

Pharyngitis

Introduction

Pharyngitis accounts for 1% to 2% of visits to outpatient clinics, physicians' offices, and emergency rooms. Between 10% and 20% of these cases are caused by infection with group A β-hemolytic streptococcus (GABHS). Identifying and treating this subset is the principal goal in routine clinical practice.

Etiology and Pathogenesis

Respiratory viruses such as adenovirus and rhinovirus cause most cases of pharyngitis. Pharyngitis is also seen as part of the acute infectious mononucleosis syndrome, primarily in adolescents and young adults. Other viral etiologies include primary HIV infection, herpes simplex virus, and Coxsackie A virus.

The most important common bacterial pathogen, GABHS or *Streptococcus pyogenes* (strep), is generally more common in urgent care and emergency department settings, especially during the winter. The organisms are spread by droplets from patients with pharyngitis or from asymptomatic nasopharyngeal carriers. They elaborate a variety of enzymes, including streptolysin, streptokinase, deoxyribonuclease, and hyaluronidase, that promote direct invasion of tissue. GABHS can also produce exotoxins, which are central in the pathogenesis of scarlet fever and the streptococcal toxic shock syndrome. Other streptococci from groups C and G can cause pharyngitis, although without the complications that can follow GABHS infection.

Clinical Presentation

Although no single clinical finding reliably distinguishes between viral sore throats and those caused by GABHS, combinations of clinical findings and laboratory test results can be used to make rational treatment decisions. The following four clinical features tend to be associated with pharyngitis caused by GABHS:

- History of fever
- Tonsillar exudates
- Anterior cervical adenopathy
- Absence of cough

A clinical algorithm for estimating the likelihood of GABHS infection in patients with sore throat that uses these four clinical findings has been developed and validated. (See "Diagnostic Approach").

Complications of Streptococcal Pharyngitis

Complications of streptococcal pharyngitis are classified as either *suppurative* or *nonsuppurative*.

Suppurative Complications

Suppurative complications such as *peritonsillar* or *retropharyngeal abscess* occur in just 1% to 2% of cases but require prompt recognition and treatment to avoid major morbidity and even mortality. Symptoms are severe and typically include fever and systemic toxicity. The pain is such that patients are often unable to take liquids, resulting in dehydration. In peritonsillar abscess, the voice becomes altered and muffled, and there is swelling of the anterior tonsillar pillar and medial displacement of the tonsil (Fig. 8-1). Streptococcal *bacteremia* with shock is a rare but serious complication of pharyngeal GABHS infection. Early treatment of GABHS-associated pharyngitis with antibiotics appears to reduce the incidence of these complications.

The term *Ludwig's angina* (see Chapter 16, Fig. 16-1) refers to other parapharyngeal space infections, including the submandibular, sublingual, and submaxillary spaces. These are sometimes polymicrobial and associated with foreign bodies or poor dental hygiene. Epiglottitis, caused by GABHS or *Haemophilus influenzae*, is rare in adults but can progress rapidly and lead to airway obstruction.

Figure 8-1 Infections of the Pharynx.

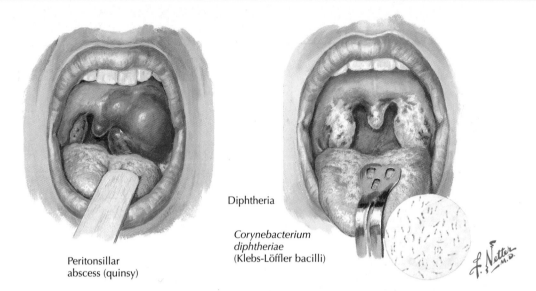

Peritonsillar
abscess (quinsy)

Diphtheria

*Corynebacterium
diphtheriae*
(Klebs-Löffler bacilli)

Suspicion for any of these conditions is an indication for urgent referral to an otolaryngologist.

Scarlet fever occurs primarily in children and is associated with certain toxin-elaborating strains of GABHS. It presents with a fine, erythematous, papular rash that starts on the trunk. Facial flushing with perioral pallor, petechiae, and palmar desquamation may be seen. It is generally self-limited.

Nonsuppurative Complications

Acute rheumatic fever is the most serious of the nonsuppurative complications of streptococcal pharyngitis. Antibiotics reduce the risk by more than two thirds. However, given the very low absolute risk for this complication in the developed world, antibiotic prescribing solely to prevent rheumatic fever is controversial. *Poststreptococcal glomerulonephritis*, the other main nonsuppurative complication, occurs with varying severity, although it is usually self-limited. It is not known whether antibiotic treatment of GABHS reduces the risk for this complication.

Differential Diagnosis

Pharyngitis may be caused by oropharyngeal candidiasis (*thrush*) in immunocompromised hosts and in those receiving broad-spectrum antibiotics or corticosteroids (both systemic and inhaled). Gonococci occasionally cause pharyngitis in patients engaging in orogenital sex. Although rarely diagnosed, other organisms associated with pharyngitis include *Mycoplasma pneumoniae*, *Chlamydia pneumoniae*, *Treponema pallidum* (primary or secondary syphilis), *Yersinia enterocolitica*, and fusobacteria. Certain spirochetes and anaerobes can cause a membranous pharyngitis associated with a foul odor known as Vincent's angina. Diphthe-

ria, caused by *Corynebacterium diphtheriae*, presents with a grayish membrane on the tonsils, pharynx, uvula, and nares and requires prompt recognition and therapy (see Fig. 8-1). Outbreaks can occur in unimmunized populations. Pharyngitis is also part of the acute retroviral syndrome, along with fever, arthralgias, and lymphadenopathy, associated with primary HIV infection.

Diagnostic Approach

Table 8-1 offers an evidence-based approach to diagnosis and treatment of patients presenting with pharyngitis. The prevalence (i.e., pretest probability) of GABHS in a typical office practice is about 10%. In emergency departments, the prevalence is about 20%. The Centor score is used for refining this pretest estimate of the probability of streptococcal disease and is obtained by assigning one point for the presence of each clinical finding: history of fever, tonsillar exudates, anterior cervical lymphadenopathy, and absence of cough.

Use of Laboratory Tests

Office-based antigen tests have sensitivities of about 85% and specificities of about 95%. They offer rapid results that improve the diagnostic accuracy over clinical assessment alone. Throat cultures, when performed by reference laboratories, have sensitivities of 90% and specificities approaching 99%. Some controversy surrounds whether or not negative antigen tests should be confirmed by culture. The Infectious Diseases Society of America recommends laboratory confirmation, whereas the American College of Physicians endorses several options, including empiric treatment of patients with Centor scores of 3 and 4. One reasonable compromise is to consider performing a confirmatory throat culture when the clinical suspicion

Table 8-1 Suggested Office-Based Approach to the Patient with Pharyngitis

Centor Score*	Post-test Probability of Streptococcal Infection (%)	Action
0	1	Supportive care
1	4	Supportive care
2	9	Antigen testing, antibiotics if positive
3	21	Empiric antibiotics *or* antigen testing, antibiotics if positive
4	43	Empiric antibiotics

* The Centor score is obtained by assigning 1 point for each of the following clinical findings: history of fever, tonsillar exudates, anterior cervical lymphadenopathy, absence of cough. Note that post-test probabilities will be higher (approximately double) in emergency department settings.

for strep is moderately high (i.e., a strep score of 3) and the initial antigen test is negative.

Management and Therapy

Although guidelines vary somewhat, empiric antibiotic therapy is generally recommended for patients with acute pharyngitis and a Centor score of 4 as well as for those with intermediate scores (2 or 3) and a positive rapid antigen test (see Table 8-1). Lower thresholds for antibiotic therapy should be considered for patients having a household contact with current documented strep infection as well as for those with a history of rheumatic fever.

Optimum Antibiotic Treatment

Penicillin is still the antibiotic treatment of choice for adults, although use of cephalosporins is associated with fewer treatment failures in children. Penicillin V at a dose of 500 mg taken 3 times daily for 10 days shortens the course of the illness. When adherence is a problem, benzathine penicillin given intramuscularly is highly effective, although the risk for anaphylaxis is higher. In penicillin-allergic patients, erythromycin, azithromycin, clarithromycin, clindamycin, or an oral cephalosporin is a reasonable alternatives.

Symptomatic Treatment

Regardless of etiology, patients with pharyngitis require symptom relief. Acetaminophen, aspirin, and nonsteroidal anti-inflammatory drugs are probably similarly effective in relieving symptoms. There is limited evidence on the effectiveness of other treatments such as corticosteroids. At least one small study has shown a reduction in duration of symptoms in children with moderate to severe pharyngitis treated with oral dexamethasone. However, no evidence supports routine use of these agents to treat pharyngitis in adults.

Avoiding Treatment Errors

Using the treatment algorithm in Table 8-1 should reduce both overtreatment of viral infections and undertreatment of GABHS infections. Maintaining an index of suspicion

for complications, including peritonsillar or retropharyngeal abscess, is important.

Future Directions

Given that the overall benefit of antibiotic treatment for GABHS-associated pharyngitis is low, studies distinguishing populations at higher or lower risk for complications would help refine estimates of benefit in certain settings. Specifically, studies of prognosis in developing countries as well as in more crowded or socioeconomically depressed areas in developed countries would help define risks for complications of streptococcal pharyngitis in these populations. Studies using rigorously defined, patient-centered outcome measures, including those that measure *severity* as well as the duration of symptoms, may help assess the true degree of benefit from antibiotic treatment in streptococcal pharyngitis.

Additional Resources

Del Mar CB, Glasziou PP, Spinks AB: Antibiotics for sore throat. Cochrane Database Syst Rev 4:CD000023, 2006.
  This recently updated systematic review focuses specifically on assessing the benefits of antibiotics for sore throat, including symptom reduction and suppurative and nonsuppurative complications. The authors conclude that antibiotics confer modest benefits for sore throat sufferers in the context of modern Western society.

Thomas M, Del Mar C, Glasziou P: How effective are treatments other than antibiotics for acute sore throat? Br J Gen Pract 50(459):817-820, 2000.
  The authors present a systematic review of nonantibiotic treatment trials for sore throat.

EVIDENCE

1. Cooper RJ, Hoffman JR, Bartlett JG, et al: Principles of appropriate antibiotic use for acute pharyngitis in adults: Background. Ann Intern Med 134(6):509-517, 2001.
  This position paper summarizes an extensive systematic review of evidence regarding diagnosis, treatment, and complications of acute pharyngitis in adults.
2. Snow V, Mottur-Pilson C, Cooper RJ, et al: Principles of appropriate antibiotic use for acute pharyngitis in adults. Ann Intern Med 134(6):506-508, 2001.
  This companion article presents a focused practice guideline on how clinicians can distinguish pharyngitis caused by GABHS from pharyngitis resulting from other causes.

Daniel S. Reuland ▪ Brent A. Senior

9

Rhinosinusitis

Introduction

Rhinosinusitis, characterized by inflammation of the maxillary and ethmoid sinuses, accounts for about 25 million office visits annually in the United States. It is the fifth most common reason physicians prescribe antibiotics. For practical purposes, *sinusitis* and *rhinosinusitis* are interchangeable terms, although many experts now prefer the latter because the nasal structures that are contiguous with the paranasal sinuses are also invariably inflamed along with the sinuses.

Etiology and Pathogenesis

The normal sterility of the sinuses is maintained by continuous mucociliary clearance. A variety of physiologic and anatomic abnormalities can lead to loss of patency of the sinus ostia and the ostiomeatal complex, the region of common sinus drainage in the anterior middle meatus. This mechanism is thought to be common to the pathogenesis of most cases of bacterial sinusitis (Fig. 9-1), both acute and chronic. Although viral upper respiratory infection (URI) is the most common antecedent, allergic and vasomotor rhinitis can also predispose to bacterial sinusitis. Anatomic factors that may play a role include deviated nasal septum and enlarged, pneumatized nasal turbinates (concha bullosae). Nasal polyps arising in the presence of chronic inflammation in the sinuses may also lead to more infection. Foreign bodies such as nasotracheal and nasogastric tubes are significant in the hospitalized patient.

Cigarette smoking and certain intranasal drugs can impair ciliary action, predisposing to sinusitis. Any of these conditions may increase edema at the sinus ostia or impair clearance from the sinuses. A relatively distinct pathogenetic mechanism is the occasional extension of a dental abscess into the maxillary sinuses that may spread into adjacent sinuses.

Cultures obtained by maxillary sinus puncture, as well as endoscopically directed cultures obtained from the middle meatus, show that the most common bacterial pathogens, if present, are *Streptococcus pneumoniae* and *Haemophilus influenzae*; however, other streptococci and *Moraxella catarrhalis* are sometimes isolated.

In patients with uncontrolled diabetes, neutropenia, or other immune-compromised states, pathogens such as *Aspergillus, Rhizopus (Mucor), Candida, Alternaria, Pseudomonas, Nocardia, Legionella*, atypical mycobacteria, and certain parasites are unusual but important etiologic considerations. Nosocomial sinusitis associated with nasotracheal or nasogastric tubes is frequently polymicrobial. In this setting, *Staphylococcus aureus*, enteric gram-negative bacteria, and anaerobes, particularly anaerobic streptococci and *Bacteroides*, may be present.

Culture studies of chronic rhinosinusitis reveal a different bacteriology. Anaerobes have been associated with some cases of chronic rhinosinusitis, although their pathologic role is unclear. Similarly unclear is the high rate of coagulase-negative staphylococcus as well as *S. aureus* frequently isolated in the presence of frank purulence. In the setting of previous surgery, cultures reveal a greater prominence of gram-negative bacteria, including *Pseudomonas aeruginosa*, in up to 30% of cases.

Recent studies have suggested several different associated mechanisms that may contribute to the development of chronic rhinosinusitis, distinguishing it from acute disease and suggesting novel treatment modalities. Theories suggested include staphylococcal superantigen, chronic osteitis, biofilms, and an abnormal response to the presence of fungus in the nose.

Clinical Presentation

Patients with a "common cold" (viral rhinosinusitis or URI) usually have some combination of the following symptoms: sneezing, rhinorrhea, congestion, facial pressure, postnasal drip, hyposmia or anosmia, sore throat, cough, ear fullness, fever, and myalgia. Color of the mucus discharge is not an accurate indicator of bacterial infection.

who have symptoms lasting longer than 7 days, maxillary pain or tenderness in the face or teeth, and purulent nasal secretions, as well as for those who fail to respond to decongestants or who have severe symptoms. These recommendations apply to most routine cases in immunocompetent patients. Early antibiotic therapy along with aggressive diagnostic evaluation and referral is indicated for any patient with signs of toxicity or evidence of complications. Referral to an otolaryngologist is also indicated when sinusitis is either recurrent or refractory to empiric treatment.

Optimum Therapy

Antibiotic Treatment for Acute Bacterial Rhinosinusitis

Three recent meta-analyses have concluded that newer, broad-spectrum antibiotics are no more effective than narrow-spectrum agents. When an antibiotic is prescribed, it should be the agent with the narrowest spectrum that is active against the most common bacterial pathogens, *S. pneumoniae* and *H. influenzae*. Newer consensus guidelines from the American Academy of Otolaryngology and the Centers for Disease Control and Prevention suggest that amoxicillin with or without clavulanate and the cephalosporins cefpodoxime and cefuroxime appear to be as effective as newer, more expensive agents when used as first-line therapies in patients who have not received an antibiotic in the preceding 4 to 6 weeks. Trimethoprim-sulfamethoxazole (TMP-SMX), doxycycline, and macrolides are alternatives for penicillin-allergic patients. In those who have received recent antibiotic therapy, newer quinolones may be appropriate. The optimal duration of therapy is unknown, but 7- to 14-day regimens are typically used. In one study, 3 days of TMP-SMX was as effective as 10 days of therapy. Given the rapid increase of antibiotic resistance among *S. pneumoniae* and *H. influenzae*, the clinician may also want to consider current recommendations for therapy against these organisms when making treatment decisions, particularly if the prevalence of resistant organisms or the risk for complications is high.

Nonantibiotic Therapy

Because complications are rare and rhinosinusitis usually resolves without antibiotic treatment, ambulatory patients with acute, uncomplicated rhinosinusitis can often be treated with analgesics, decongestants, and topical heat for discomfort. Topical decongestants are thought to decrease edema at the sinus ostia and ostiomeatal complex. The problem of short-term rebound is minimized when these medications are used for fewer than 4 days. Antihistamines are said to promote thickening of the secretions and therefore are discouraged, at least initially, although evidence for this is limited. Inhalation of warm, humid vapor may be helpful, as may nasal saline irrigation.

Avoiding Treatment Errors

Physicians tend to prescribe antibiotics in about 90% of cases of sinusitis, even though most cases resolve spontaneously. Clearly, overprescribing of antibiotics to treat what is most often a viral infection is the most common treatment error. This is not entirely avoidable given the difficulty in distinguishing between viral and bacterial etiologies. However, reminding patients of both the increasing problem of antibiotic resistance and the relatively modest benefits of antibiotics for acute rhinosinusitis may help reduce overprescribing in routine clinical practice.

Future Directions

Because no simple, accurate office-based test is currently available to diagnose sinusitis, studies aimed at improving our ability to use clinical findings to make appropriate decisions would be helpful. Particular attention needs to be paid to assessing clinical outcomes at different time points, as well as incorporating symptom severity and patient-assigned utilities to help apply this increasing body of evidence to clinical practice. More studies are needed to assess the prevalence of drug-resistant organisms and the implications for therapy.

Additional Resources

Hickner JM, Bartlett JG, Besser RE, et al: Principles of appropriate antibiotic use for acute rhinosinusitis in adults: Background. Ann Intern Med 134(6):498-505, 2001.
   This article presents a detailed review of the high-quality evidence pertaining to diagnosis and treatment of rhinosinusitis. It is extremely well referenced and includes evidence grades for all principles and recommendations.
Williams JW Jr, Aguilar C, Makela M, et al: Antibiotic therapy for acute sinusitis: A systematic literature review. The Cochrane Collection Web Site. Available at: http://www.cochrane.org. Accessed October 4, 2006.
   This thorough review of the evidence supports the use of antibiotics for acute maxillary sinusitis. This website also includes reviews addressing related topics such as functional endoscopic sinus surgery for chronic sinusitis and protocols for ongoing reviews such as intranasal steroids for acute sinusitis.
Zucher DR, Balk E, Engels E, et al: Diagnosis and treatment of acute bacterial rhinosinusitis. Agency for Health Care Policy and Research Publication No. 99-E016: Evidence Report/Technology Assessment Number 9. Available at: http://www.ahrq.gov/clinic/sinussum.htm. Accessed October 4, 2006.
   This is another comprehensive review of evidence, along with a decision- and cost-effectiveness analysis. There is also a detailed outline of future research questions at the end.

EVIDENCE

Van Buchem FL, Knottnerus JA, Schrijnemaekers VJ, Peeters MF: Primary-care-based randomised placebo-controlled trial of antibiotic treatment in acute maxillary sinusitis. Lancet 349(9053):683-687, 1997.
   This is one of several examples of well-designed, randomized clinical trials demonstrating the modest utility of empiric antibiotics and the absent utility of radiography in managing primary care patients with rhinosinusitis.

David C. Henke

Rhinitis: Allergic and Idiopathic

Introduction

Rhinitis presents clinically as nasal congestion. Other symptoms include discharge, itching, sneezing, and sinus pressure attributed to upper airway mucosal inflammatory hyperreactivity. The inflammatory process often progresses to involve the paranasal sinus cavities and the eustachian tubes, producing frontal headaches and a popping sensation in the ears. The associated postnasal mucus discharge can also cause cough and often aggravates lower airway symptoms such as wheezing in asthmatics. Most people experience rhinitis symptoms during their lives.

Several syndromes are associated with chronic rhinitis, including allergic, idiopathic, and secondary rhinitis. Allergic rhinitis is triggered by exposure to allergen, but symptoms can be perennial when exposure is chronic. Classically, there are also associated ocular symptoms, including excess tearing and itching. Idiopathic rhinitis, previously called vasomotor rhinitis or nonallergic noninfectious perennial rhinitis, shares many features with allergic rhinitis, including nasal mucosal hyperreactivity, but lacks the associated skin test sensitivity. Acute and self-limited infectious rhinitis, "the common cold," is not reviewed here.

Allergic rhinitis is the fifth most prevalent chronic condition in the United States, affecting more than 24 million people. The prevalence of allergic rhinitis has increased 25% in the past two decades. Related diagnoses such as nasal polyps, deviated nasal septum, and chronic disease of the tonsils and adenoids affect an additional 5.3 million Americans. The direct costs of allergic rhinitis in the United States are estimated to be $1.23 billion annually. These figures do not include over-the-counter pharmacotherapy costs, nor do they allow for the costs associated with the introduction of new generations of antihistamines, diagnostic testing, or immunotherapy. In patients with asthma and allergic rhinitis as opposed to asthma alone, the cost of care increases by 46%.

Etiology and Pathogenesis

Nonallergic and allergic rhinitis is associated with the release of histamine, prostaglandins, leukotrienes, and cytokines from mast cells, basophils, and eosinophils. In allergic disease, the release of mediators is associated with the cross-linking of immunoglobulin E (IgE) on the mast cell by allergen (Figs. 10-1 and 10-2). A similar cellular reaction occurs in nonallergic rhinitis by an undefined mechanism.

The clinical expression of allergic rhinitis has been linked to whether the immune response is driven by Th1 or Th2 lymphocytes as determined by the interactions between the T cells and antigen-presenting cells (see Fig. 10-2). If the antigen-presenting cell (e.g., the dendritic cell) triggers the expression of Th2 cells, a number of factors, including interleukin-4 (IL-4), IL-5, IL-9, and IL-13, histamine-releasing factor, and neuropeptides, are released. These factors interact with other mediators, including interferon-γ, IL-11, IL-12, and leukotrienes. The response leads to IgE production, the accumulation of eosinophils and basophils in the lung and upper airway, mast cell proliferation, airway hyper-responsiveness, mucus overproduction, and the exudation of bloodstream-derived proteins into the airways. A specific association of a new subclass of natural killer T (NKT) cells, CD1d-restricted NKT cells, with asthma may prove relevant to developing a better understanding of rhinitis, because the conditions are closely linked.

Figure 10-1 Extrinsic Asthma: Mechanism of Type 1 (Immediate) Hypersensitivity.
APC, antigen-presenting cell.

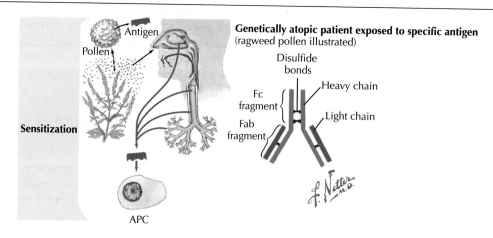

Figure 10-2 Allergic Inflammation.
APC, antigen-presenting cell; IFN-γ, interferon-γ; IgE, immunoglobulin E; IL, interleukin.

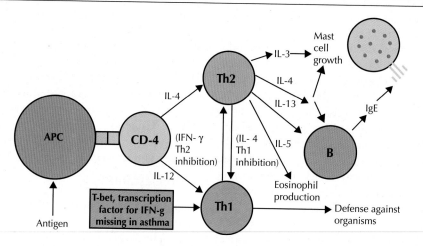

Both genetic and environmental factors appear to play a role in selecting for a Th2 inflammatory response. In nonatopic individuals, there is a switch to a Th1 response to allergen shortly after birth. There is an association between an allele of HLA-DR and a polymorphism for IgE and atopy. Atopic disease also appears to be associated with (1) the Western lifestyle, even when lived in a third-world environment; (2) excessive hygiene; (3) antibiotics in the first 2 years of life; and (4) vaccination (Fig. 10-3).

There is some evidence to support the notion that microorganisms can influence T-cell responses. For example, products of *Aspergillus fumigatus* evoke Th2-mediated IgE production. In contrast, interferon-γ from Th1 cells and IL-18 from macrophages potentially inhibit the production of IgE. Immunotherapy and bacterial cytosine guanosine (C-p-G) DNA repeats, especially when used as adjuvants, may switch the Th2 to the Th1 phenotype.

The increased prevalence in allergic rhinitis has also been linked to higher concentrations of pollen that in turn have been attributed to increased atmospheric CO_2. It has also been associated with the development of energy-efficient buildings that slow the exchange of outside air and promote the concentration of indoor allergens.

Clinical Presentation

The various forms of rhinitis are diagnosed by recognizing the patient's symptom patterns and associations and to a lesser extent by physical examination and laboratory testing. Symptoms include sneezing, watery eyes, pruritic eyes and ears, popping in the ears, sinus pain, and rhinorrhea. It is important to establish the duration, chronicity, and temporal patterns of the symptoms. Triggers such as exposures to flowering plants, mold-rich environments, and animal dander, exacerbations during the spring and

Figure 10-3 Factors Favoring the Th1 and Th2 Phenotypes.

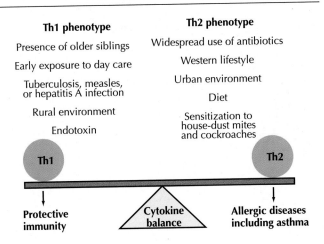

Th1 phenotype	Th2 phenotype
Presence of older siblings	Widespread use of antibiotics
Early exposure to day care	Western lifestyle
Tuberculosis, measles, or hepatitis A infection	Urban environment
Rural environment	Diet
Endotoxin	Sensitization to house-dust mites and cockroaches

fall, and a positive family history suggest allergic rhinitis. But there are many other considerations when evaluating nasal congestion. Symptoms secondary to illicit drug use include upper airway irritation.

The frequent use of nasal decongestants may provide the clue to the diagnosis of rhinitis medicamentosa. Possible reactions to β blockers and nonsteroidal anti-inflammatory drugs (NSAIDs) in asthmatic individuals should be investigated. An occupational and hobby history may reveal exposure to nasal irritants and potentially carcinogenic wood dusts. Food allergies rarely cause adult rhinitis, but do so more commonly in children. Allergic rhinitis can cause the upper airway resistance syndrome (UARS), which leads to hypersomnolence. These patients may not have frank obstructive sleep apnea.

A physical examination revealing an "allergic crease" from frequent nose rubbing, reddened and inflamed upper airway mucosa, periorbital edema, and a bluish periorbital discoloration secondary to venous stasis ("allergic shiners") supports the diagnosis of chronic rhinorrhea. Polyps, foreign bodies, septal deviations or perforation, tumors, conjunctivitis, serous otitis, vasculitic rash, urticaria, and wheezing suggest specific etiologies and require careful consideration. Sinus pain, purulent drainage, and fever indicate complicating infection. The diagnosis of idiopathic rhinitis is one of exclusion.

Laboratory testing and physical examination are needed to diagnose local and systemic disorders that can mimic allergic rhinitis. Rhinitis has been linked to cystic fibrosis, tumors, foreign bodies, atrophic rhinitis, hypothyroidism, HIV infection, conditions associated with hormonal fluctuations such as pregnancy, Wegener's granulomatosis, sarcoidosis, and allergic granulomatosis of Churg-Strauss syndrome.

The diagnosis of allergic rhinitis is established by demonstrating specific IgE either by in vivo scratch skin test or by in vitro radioallergosorbent test (RAST). Such testing

is important when designing avoidance strategies and immunotherapy. A blood count differential demonstrating hypereosinophilia, an elevated IgE, and pulmonary function testing revealing reversible airflow obstruction, bronchial hyperreactivity, and an elevated diffusing capacity for carbon monoxide (DLCO) can be useful to confirm the diagnosis of allergic rhinitis associated with asthma.

Management and Therapy

Optimum Treatment

Conservative interventions include topical or systemic decongestants, topical corticosteroids, anticholinergics, antihistamines, allergen and irritant avoidance strategies, immunotherapy, and mechanical devices such as continuous positive airway pressure (CPAP) when UARS is diagnosed. Surgery warrants consideration if these measures fail and there is anatomic pathology such as nasal polyps that account for the patient's persistent symptoms. Optimizing therapy for allergic rhinitis is patient specific. However, the first goal in all patients is to control symptoms employing one or more of these therapies. Controlling symptoms is especially important when allergic rhinitis is a trigger for a patient's asthma. When symptom control is achieved, a systematic tapering of therapies should begin to reduce or eliminate systemic therapies first with the long-term goal of minimizing unwanted medicine side effects. Generally, however, it is difficult to completely stop systemic antihistamines, especially when immunotherapy is not a part of the intervention.

Decongestants

Topical decongestants are therapeutic but cause rhinitis medicamentosa when overused. Rhinitis medicamentosa is treated by slowly tapering the medication and using topical nasal steroids. When employed as therapy, topical decongestants should be used sparingly and for no longer than 7 days. Systemic decongestants work well as nasal decongestants but are associated with tremor, oral dryness, palpitations, and insomnia. They also can aggravate cardiac disease, hypertension, diabetes, glaucoma, thyrotoxicosis, and bladder obstruction. Neither topical nor systemic decongestants significantly influence pruritus, sneezing, or rhinorrhea. The combination of decongestants and antihistamines is more effective than either agent alone (Boxes 10-1 and 10-2).

Corticosteroids

Corticosteroids reduce inflammation, promote vascular constriction, and diminish hyperactivity and vascular permeability. Topical application is the preferred route of administration because it avoids many of the unwanted systemic effects associated with oral and parenteral corticosteroids. The vasoconstrictive property of topical nasal steroids also provides a rapid therapeutic decongestant

Box 10-1 Antihistamines

Generic Name

First Generation

Chlorpheniramine
Diphenhydramine
Hydroxyzine
Triprolidine

Second Generation

Cetirizine
Fexofenadine
Loratadine
Desloratadine

Topical

Azelastine (nasal)
Levocabastine (ophthalmic)
Olopatadine (ophthalmic)

Adapted from Corey JP, Houser SM, NgBA: Nasal congestion: A review of its etiology, evaluation, and treatment. Ear Nose Throat J 79:690-693, 2000.

Box 10-2 Antihistamine-Decongestant Combinations*

- Acrivastine and pseudoephedrine
- Azatadine and pseudoephedrine
- Fexofenadine and pseudoephedrine
- Loratadine and pseudoephedrine
- Triprolidine and pseudoephedrine

*The U.S. Food and Drug Administration has taken steps to remove highly addictive phenylpropanolamine (PPA), historically used as an oral decongestant, from all drug products and has issued a public health advisory concerning PPA.

Adapted from Corey JP, Houser SM, NgBA: Nasal congestion: A review of its etiology, evaluation, and treatment. Ear Nose Throat J 79:690-693, 2000.

Box 10-3 Topical Intranasal Steroids

- Beclomethasone
- Budesonide
- Fluticasone
- Mometasone
- Triamcinolone

Adapted from Corey JP, Houser SM, NgBA: Nasal congestion: A review of its etiology, evaluation, and treatment. Ear Nose Throat J 79:690-693, 2000.

effect. However, mucosal drying can produce nasal irritation, bleeding, septal perforations, and candidiasis. Patients should titrate topical steroids to control symptoms and should avoid excessive mucosal drying; one alternative is to use products available in aqueous formulation. Topical steroids are superior to antihistamines in controlling nasal symptoms (Box 10-3).

Antihistamines

Oral H_1 blockers are employed in the therapy for allergic rhinitis (see Box 10-1). H_1 blockers are in fact one of the most successful and widely used therapies. Sedation is a major limiting factor. The latest generation of antihistamines (acrivastine, cetirizine, fexofenadine, loratadine, and desloratadine) is less sedating and does not cause delayed cardiac repolarization (QT prolongation on electrocardiogram), thus avoiding the potential complication of sudden cardiac death caused by torsades de pointes associated with astemizole and terfenadine. The newer antihistamines (azelastine, levocabastine, and olopatadine) are available in topical formulations. Azelastine inhibits histamine release, as well as other inflammatory mediator production,

although use is associated with drowsiness. Levocabastine and olopatadine are available as topical ocular agents with a rapid onset of action and no sedating effects (see Box 10-1).

Antileukotriene Agents

The arachidonic acid metabolites, leukotrienes, are important mediators thought to play a role in many inflammatory diseases. The leukotriene D4 receptor blocker, montelukast, has been shown to be effective in controlling allergic rhinitis. It is more widely prescribed than zileuton, a 5-lipoxygenase inhibitor that inhibits the formation of all leukotrienes, because it is dosed once a day, as opposed to more frequent dosing with zileuton, and because it lacks the liver toxicity associated with zileuton (see Chapter 20).

Mast Cell Stabilizers

Cromolyn and its more potent derivative, nedocromil, increase intracellular cyclic adenosine monophosphate, thereby raising the threshold for mast cell degranulation and release of histamine. They ameliorate allergic symptoms, although to a less extent than topical steroids. Cromolyn is available over the counter; nedocromil is available as an ophthalmic preparation but is not yet available in a topical nasal application. A drawback to the use of mast cell stabilizers is the need to use them multiple times each day.

Anticholinergics

Ipratropium bromide inhibits secretions from vagally innervated serous and seromucous glands by antagonizing acetylcholine at the cholinergic receptor. The drug is poorly absorbed, not associated with rebound rhinorrhea, and well tolerated. Ipratropium is effective in reducing rhinorrhea but has less effect on nasal congestion and sneezing.

Immunotherapy

Immunotherapy is reserved for patients with severe symptoms of allergic rhinitis who suffer much of the year or who cannot be managed with medications and avoidance strategies. The exact therapeutic mechanism is unknown. It is now thought that there is a switch in T-helper (Th) cell antigen processing away from pathways associated with IgE production. In general, this therapy is continued

for about 6 years and then stopped. After discontinuing, there is often a honeymoon period, of variable duration, during which no therapy of any type may be required. Patients with severe asthma are considered at greatest risk for significant adverse reactions to immunotherapy, including anaphylaxis and death.

Avoiding Treatment Errors

There are two issues regarding the treatment of allergic rhinitis. The first focuses on the absolute requirement that the diagnosis is correct because other treatable serious conditions, such as cystic fibrosis, sarcoidosis, and vasculitis, as mentioned earlier, are associated with chronic rhinitis. The second is the need to avoid aggravating other medical conditions patients may have with therapy, as mentioned associated with systemic decongestants.

Future Directions

Discriminating between allergic and idiopathic rhinitis is difficult. Fas, a cell surface molecule that induces apoptosis, has been linked to rhinitis. The serum soluble Fas (Sfas) level is normal in idiopathic rhinitis, a condition attributed to an imbalance in the autonomic nervous system. It is reduced in allergic rhinitis. Allergic rhinitis, to date, is the only disease associated with reduced levels.

The anti-IgE antibody, omalizumab, has clinical efficacy in allergic rhinitis and asthma, but its use for allergic rhinitis is unlikely until the cost of the drug, average $12,000 per annum, has been reduced. Agents that block interleukins are also of therapeutic interest. A soluble IL-4 receptor, for example, has demonstrated effectiveness in asthma and may prove useful in treating allergic rhinitis. Anti IL-5 lowered circulating eosinophils in asthmatics but had no clinical effect.

Future therapies may employ CpG bacterial DNA repeats as adjuvants with vaccines and in immunotherapy with the goal of altering allergen processing to avoid or cure an atopic condition. They are also likely to increasingly focus on the functions of the immunoregulatory CD1d-restricted NKT cell.

Additional Resource

American Academy of Allergy, Asthma and Immunology. Patient Fact Sheet on Allergic Rhinitis. Available at: http://www.aaaai.org/patients/resources/fact_sheets/allergic_rhinitis.pdf.
This fact sheet is suitable as a patient handout.

EVIDENCE

1. Akbari O, Faul JL, Hoyte EG, et al: CD4+ invariant T-cell-receptor+ natural killer T cells in bronchial asthma. N Engl J Med 354(11):1117-1129, 2006.
   This is the initial description of a new class of lymphocyte, which is resistant to modulation by steroids and linked to asthma.
2. Borish LC, Nelson HS, Lanz MJ, et al: Interleukin-4 receptor in moderate atopic asthma. A phase I/II randomized, placebo-controlled trial. Am J Respir Crit Care Med 160:1816-1823, 1999.
   This article presents a review of the role of interleukins and some other inflammatory mediators in asthma and a report of therapeutic effectiveness of the IL-4 receptor that binds and sequesters circulating IL-4.
3. Kato M, Hattori T, Ito H, et al: Serum-soluble Fas levels as a marker to distinguish allergic and nonallergic rhinitis. J Allergy Clin Immunol 103:1213-1214, 1999.
   This study is an example of an ongoing search to identify biologic markers for specific diseases with similar clinical presentations.
4. Kay AB: Allergy and allergic diseases. First of two parts. N Engl J Med 344:30-37, 2001.
   This is the first part of a two-part review of the state of the art, describing immunologic pathways involved in allergic disease.
5. Kay AB: Allergy and allergic diseases: Second of two parts. N Engl J Med 344:109-113, 2001.
   This is the second part of a two-part review of the state of the art, describing immunologic pathways involved in allergic disease.
6. Naclerio R, Solomon W: Rhinitis and inhalant allergens. JAMA 278:1842-1848, 1997.
   This is a good review of pathologic allergic rhinitis and its treatment.
7. Van Cauwenberge P, Watelet JB: Epidemiology of chronic rhinosinusitis. Thorax 55(Suppl 2):S20-S21, 2000.
   This lucid review of the proposed immunologic mechanisms directing the "uncommitted" biologic response toward immunity (the desired outcome) or allergic disease includes a review of the hygiene hypothesis, which suggests that the exposure to infectious agents in the first few weeks of life may be critical to encouraging the immune system to respond to the environment later in life by developing immunity rather than allergic disease.
8. Weiss KB, Sullivan SD: The health economics of asthma and rhinitis. I. Assessing the economic impact. J Allergy Clin Immunol 107:3-8, 2001.
   The authors define the human and economic impacts of rhinitis.
9. Yawn BP, Yunginger JW, Wollan PC, et al: Allergic rhinitis in Rochester, Minnesota residents with asthma: Frequency and impact on health care charges. J Allergy Clin Immunol 103:54-59, 1999.
   This is another perspective on the epidemiology and the limitations of present technology to understand the full extent of the impact of rhinitis.

Rose J. Eapen ▪ William W. Shockley

11

Common Oral Lesions

Introduction

The oral cavity, along with the nasal cavity, represents the initial point of contact for pathogens and irritants entering the respiratory and digestive systems. The borders for this region extend from the vermilion border of the lips to the junction of the hard and soft palate and the circumvallate papillae of the tongue. The oral cavity includes the lips, buccal and gingival mucosa, teeth, hard palate, floor of the mouth, retromolar trigone, and the anterior two thirds of the tongue. Complete examination of the oral cavity should include visualization of all mucosal surfaces and palpation of the buccal surfaces, tongue, palate, and floor of the mouth. A wide variety of disease processes can present in the mouth as similar lesions, creating a diagnostic challenge in the evaluation of the oral cavity.

Recurrent Aphthous Ulcers

Recurrent aphthous ulcers (RAUs) are the most common oral mucosal ulcers in North America, affecting 5% to 66% of the adult population (Fig. 11-1). RAUs are more common in higher socioeconomic classes and typically present in the second decade of life. Their etiology remains uncertain. Nutritional deficiencies, hormonal changes, bacterial and viral infections, food hypersensitivities, stress, and genetic predisposition have all been postulated as causative factors.

Depending on the presentation, RAUs are classified as *major, minor,* or *herpetiform.* All types are generally found on the nonkeratinized, mobile mucosa of the buccal region, lips, and floor of the mouth. RAUs are not associated with fever or other systemic reactions. Recurrence is most frequent in younger patients, and 30% of patients may have constant disease for months to years.

Major RAUs, the most severe form, affects 7% to 20% of patients. Lesions of this type are greater than 10 mm in diameter and may last from weeks to months. They may coalesce into large, irregular ulcers that produce scars when healed. These ulcers are found on soft, movable mucosa but may also be located posteriorly, on the soft palate, tonsils, and pharynx.

Minor RAUs are most common, accounting for 70% to 87% of all aphthous ulcers. They measure less than 10 mm in diameter and present as discrete, shallow, painful ulcers with central fibrous exudate surrounded by an erythema-

tous border. They are usually located on the buccal mucosa. The duration of the ulcer is 1 to 2 weeks and is followed by spontaneous healing without scarring.

Herpetiform RAUs make up 7% to 10% of all RAU lesions. These ulcers measure less than 5 mm and occur in groups of 10 to 100. They can also coalesce into larger ulcers and are found throughout the oral cavity. The ulcers are usually located on the dorsal tongue and palate and heal spontaneously over 1 to 4 weeks.

Differential diagnosis includes infectious (herpes viruses, HIV), rheumatic disease (Behçet's syndrome, Reiter's syndrome), cutaneous disease (erythema multiforme), gastrointestinal disease (gluten-sensitive enteropathy), and drugs (nonsteroidal anti-inflammatory drugs, β blockers, nicorandil, alendronate). Diagnosis is based primarily on a thorough history and physical exam. Patients with lesions that do not resolve after 3 weeks of therapy should be referred to a specialist for biopsy and further management.

Optimum Treatment

There are many available treatments, and their use should be guided by severity of disease, frequency of ulceration, and potential adverse effects of the medication used to treat the ulcers. New U.S. Food and Drug Administration–approved therapies include 0.1% triamcinolone dental paste, which works to decrease inflammation, and 5% amlexanox paste, which also mediates the inflamma-

Figure 11-1 Common Oral Lesions.

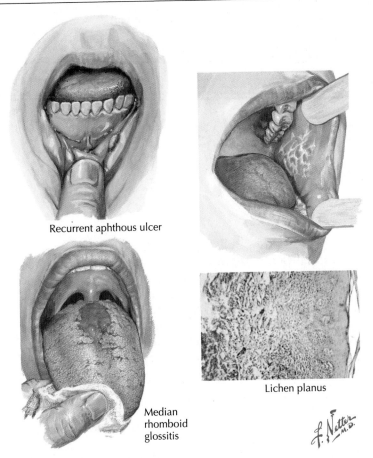

Recurrent aphthous ulcer

Median rhomboid glossitis

Lichen planus

tory cascade specifically acting against interleukin-3. These are applied to the ulcer two to four times daily until healing occurs. Topical corticosteroids are also used in treatment. When applied directly to the dried ulcer or area of prodromal pain and paresthesia, they reduce the duration of the lesion, but they do not affect the frequency of recurrence. Intralesional steroid injections and systemic corticosteroids are reserved for more persistent cases of major RAUs. Thalidomide has been shown to decrease lesion duration and disease-free time in refractory RAUs. However, this treatment has severe side effects—teratogenicity and peripheral neuropathy—which have limited its use.

Infectious Lesions

Viral Stomatitis

Herpes Simplex

Herpes simplex is the most common organism causing viral stomatitis. Initial exposure to herpes simplex virus (HSV) usually occurs during childhood. After resolution of the initial infection, the virus remains latent in the trigeminal ganglion. Primary infection is often asymptomatic. When symptoms occur, they typically include the sudden onset of 1- to 2-mm vesicles bordered by an inflammatory, erythematous base associated with fever. These lesions rupture to form ulcers. Primary oral HSV lesions tend to involve the buccal mucosa. Recurrent disease is usually confined to keratinized areas, like the lips or perioral areas. The ulcers undergo spontaneous healing in 10 to 14 days. Recurrent oral herpes is not associated with fever and may be incited by exposure to sunlight, trauma, and emotional stress. Most patients develop pain, burning, and tingling about 24 hours before the appearance of recurrent lesions. The differential diagnosis of these lesions is similar to that of aphthous ulcers. The diagnosis is generally clinical but may be confirmed by identifying multinucleated giant cells on a Tzanck smear. Viral culture from lesions is the gold standard for diagnosis.

OPTIMUM TREATMENT. Most immunocompetent individuals with recurrent herpes labialis do not require treatment other than the occasional use of local analgesics. Steroid treatment is contraindicated. Systemic acyclovir may shorten episodes and increase disease-free intervals but works when the virus is most active, which is usually

before the characteristic lesions appear. Other antiviral agents like valacyclovir are similarly effective.

Primary Varicella-Zoster

Primary varicella-zoster virus (VZV) infection occurs during childhood when the human herpesvirus 3 causes chickenpox. Infection with VZV can appear as grouped vesicles or erosions on the hard palate, buccal mucosa, tongue, and gingiva. The virus then remains dormant in sensory ganglia and is sometimes reactivated, causing shingles. Shingles presents as an eruption of multiple 1- to 2-mm painful vesicles that soon burst resulting in ulcerative lesions. These lesions present in a classic unilateral dermatomal pattern. In the head and neck, there are varied presentations of zoster ranging from facial nerve paralysis in Ramsay Hunt syndrome to uveitis, keratoconjunctivitis, and optic neuritis in zoster ophthalmicus. Eruptions generally indicate an immunosuppressed state, which may require further investigation.

OPTIMUM TREATMENT OF PRIMARY VZV. Varicella treatment is generally supportive in immunocompetent hosts, and acyclovir is the drug of choice for varicella infection in adults and immunosuppressed patients. Valacyclovir and famciclovir are also effective. Corticosteroids are contraindicated in initial VZV infection. Vaccination is recommended in all children between 12 months and 13 years of age. Vaccination is also recommended in adults with ongoing risk for exposure (e.g., day care employees), those who are household contacts of immunosuppressed hosts, and women of childbearing age. Vaccination is not recommended for immunocompromised hosts because the vaccine is made up of live attenuated VZV.

OPTIMUM TREATMENT OF RECURRENT VZV. Treatment of recurrent herpes zoster includes acyclovir, valacyclovir, or famciclovir, as well as corticosteroids. Antiviral therapy should be initiated within 72 hours of clinical presentation in patients older than 50 years to maximize the potential benefits of treatment.

Coxsackie A

Herpangina is associated with Coxsackie A virus types A1 to A6, A8, A10, and A22. It affects children aged 3 to 10 years and presents as small aphthous lesions on the soft palate and tonsillar pillars associated with fever and odynophagia. This disease is self-limited and requires only supportive therapy.

Hand, foot, and mouth disease (HFM) is associated with Coxsackie A virus type A16. HFM occurs most frequently in the spring and early summer in children younger than 5 years. It presents with small aphthous lesions seen on the buccal mucosa and tongue, as well as oval pale papules with a rim of erythema on the palms and soles. These lesions tend to spare the lips and gingiva, in contrast to HSV. This disease is self-limited and requires only supportive therapy.

Fungal Stomatitis

Oral Candidiasis

Candida species, the most common cause of oral fungal infections, are present in the oral cavity of 30% to 60% of healthy adults; therefore, their isolation does not necessarily indicate a pathologic process. However, the numbers of true candidal infections are rising, secondary to iatrogenic infection. Factors that predispose patients to candidal infection are age extremes, an immunocompromised state, malnourishment, concurrent infections, broad-spectrum antibiotic treatment, radiation-induced mucositis, and xerostomia. *Oral candidiasis* classically presents as pseudomembranous candidiasis, or thrush. These white, plaque-like lesions can be present on the buccal mucosa, palate, tongue, or oropharynx and scrape away easily, leaving a raw, hemorrhagic undersurface. *Hyperplastic candidiasis* presents as a white, plaque-like lesion that cannot easily be removed. *Chronic atrophic candidiasis* is the most common form of oral candidiasis and is found in up to 60% of denture-wearing patients. It presents as an erythematous, cobblestone patch on the mucosa under dentures. *Median rhomboid glossitis* (see Fig. 11-1) is confined to the dorsal tongue. It presents as an asymptomatic, erythematous, well-demarcated area of papillary atrophy found just anterior to the circumvallate papillae. *Angular cheilitis* presents as painful, bleeding, ulcerative patches at the oral commissures. Diagnosis of oral candidiasis is based on clinical presentation. The differential diagnosis includes a wide range of oral lesions from systemic infections to squamous cell carcinoma. In patients with recurrent or extensive disease, immunologic status should be evaluated with HIV testing. The diagnosis of oral candidiasis is confirmed by obtaining a potassium hydroxide (KOH) prep. Microscopic evaluation of scrapings from the white patches or erosive areas of the mucosa should reveal budding yeasts with or without pseudohyphae. Failure of these lesions to respond to adequate therapy after 1 to 2 weeks should result in referral to a specialist for possible biopsy.

OPTIMUM TREATMENT. Therapy consists of topical and systemic antifungals. Oral rinses with nystatin or clotrimazole solution 4 to 5 times per day are used for treatment of oral mucosal lesions. Denture-related lesions require treatment of the dentures with an antifungal soak or ointment as well as direct application of antifungal ointment or cream to the lesion. Angular cheilitis responds best to direct topical application of antifungal ointment to the lesion. Systemic fluconazole, ketoconazole, or itraconazole is used to treat severe or refractory lesions.

Noninfectious Oral Lesions

Lichen Planus

Oral lichen planus (OLP) (see Fig. 11-1) is a common disorder affecting about 2% of adults. Its etiology is unknown,

but it has been determined to result from a T-cell-mediated immune response directed against the basal epithelial cell. Histologic characteristics of OLP include epithelial basal cell destruction and infiltration of the adjacent tissue with lymphocytes. There are many forms of these lesions that are characterized by their appearance. The *reticular* form is the most common type of OLP and is present in most patients studied with this disease. It is seen most often as lace-like striae of Wickham on the buccal mucosa. *Erosive* OLP is the next most common form and presents as painful, ulcerative lesions affecting the gingiva, buccal mucosa, and lateral tongue. Poorly fitting dentures can be an inciting factor in OLP. Candidal superinfection can present in one third of OLP lesions, necessitating antifungal treatment. Evaluation of the patient's medications is also essential because some drugs can result in lichenoid eruptions. OLP may require biopsy for definitive diagnosis. It is important to monitor these lesions over time because there is a small risk for malignant transformation. In most reported cases, the erosive subtype most frequently underwent malignant transformation.

Symptomatic OLP is treated first with topical steroids. Refractory cases usually respond to systemic steroids. Treatment with immunomodulating medications such as cyclosporine and azathioprine may be required in severe cases.

Leukoplakia

Oral leukoplakia is a precancerous lesion that presents as white patches or plaques on the oral mucosa. These lesions are composed of hyperplastic squamous epithelium. Leukoplakia itself is a benign reactive process. However, some lesions will progress to carcinoma within 10 years. Different studies have shown varying progress to carcinoma. Lesions located in trauma-prone regions of the oral cavity, such as the cheek and dorsum of the tongue, are at less risk for malignant transformation. Any suspicious lesions should undergo biopsy to evaluate for dysplasia. If malignancy is identified, the patient should be referred to a specialist for further management, including possible resection or chemotherapy. Cyclooxygenase-2 (COX-2) inhibitors are being investigated as a treatment of leukoplakia.

Hairy Leukoplakia

Hairy leukoplakia is a benign mucosal lesion of the lateral tongue found in up to one third of HIV-positive patients. These painless lesions are caused by epithelial infection with the Epstein-Barr virus. They present as irregular, white areas of mucosal thickening on the lateral tongue. Diagnosis is based on clinical presentation, and occasionally a biopsy is needed for confirmation. No specific treatment is indicated; however, patients presenting with hairy leukoplakia should undergo testing for HIV.

Oral Papilloma and Verruca Vulgaris

Oral papilloma and verruca vulgaris lesions are easily recognized in the oral cavity. Both lesions are caused by infection with strains of human papillomavirus. Papillomas present as pedunculated, cauliflower-like masses of squamous epithelium similar to papillomas seen at other sites (Fig. 11-2). Verrucae vulgaris present as hyperkeratotic, hard, round lesions similar to those seen on the skin of the hands and feet. Differential diagnosis includes condyloma acuminatum and verrucous carcinoma. Excisional biopsy is the treatment of choice.

Torus Palatinus and Torus Mandibularis

Tori are benign exostoses of the hard palate and mandible that present as smooth, hard lesions of the midline hard palate or the lingual surface of the mandible. Patients are often unaware of their presence. Diagnosis is based on physical exam. No treatment is necessary, but tori occasionally must be removed to accommodate dentures (see Fig. 11-2).

Fordyce Granules

Fordyce granules are ectopic sebaceous glands that appear as clusters of yellowish spots on the buccal mucosa, typically found just inside the oral commissure. Diagnosis is based on physical exam, and no treatment is necessary.

Amalgam Tattoo

Silver alloys used during dental procedures may become implanted in the surrounding gingiva, appearing as blue-black macules. The most common site for amalgam tattoos is the mandibular arch. Differential diagnosis for this lesion includes nevi and melanoma. Diagnosis is based on physical exam. Confirmation can be obtained with the appearance of fine, radiopaque densities on dental films. Excisional biopsy should be performed for suspicious pigmented lesions.

Mucoceles

Mucoceles form when saliva extrudes from a minor salivary gland into surrounding tissue. Trauma is thought to cause most mucoceles. They may present anywhere in the oral cavity but are seen most commonly on the lower lip. They present as a blue, round lesion with overlying smooth mucosa. They may burst and recur or become infected and purulent. Excision is the treatment of choice for persistent mucoceles. Marsupialization typically results in recurrence (see Fig. 11-2).

Figure 11-2 Common Oral Lesions.

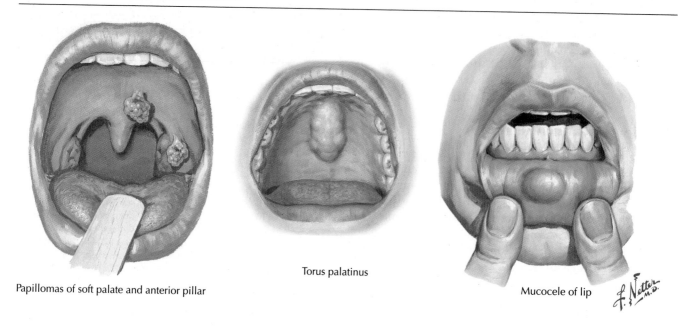

Papillomas of soft palate and anterior pillar

Torus palatinus

Mucocele of lip

Figure 11-3 Common Oral Lesions.

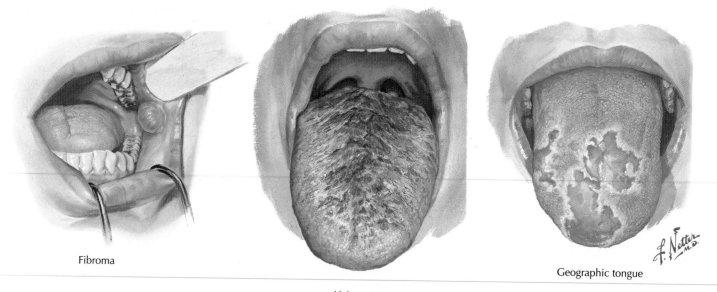

Fibroma

Hairy tongue

Geographic tongue

Fibromas

Fibromas are soft, tan or pink lesions found at sites of repetitive trauma, typically on the buccal mucosa or lateral tongue. Recurrent trauma results in chronic inflammation and fibrous hyperplasia. Excisional biopsy is diagnostic and therapeutic (see Fig. 11-3).

Hairy Tongue

Hairy tongue is a benign condition caused by accumulation of keratin and commensal bacteria on filiform papillae of the tongue. Hairy tongue has a characteristic appearance and is treated by reassuring the patient of the benign nature of the condition. Some improvement of appearance can be achieved by daily scraping of excess keratin and debris off the area (Fig. 11-3).

Geographic Tongue

Geographic tongue, or benign migratory glossitis, is a benign condition characterized by areas of smooth atrophy on the tongue, with loss of papillae. This leads to ulcer-like

lesions that appear as erythematous patches on the dorsal tongue with circumferential white polycyclic borders. The diagnosis is made using clinical presentation, and biopsy is not necessary. The painless lesions spontaneously regress, only to appear on other parts of the tongue. Etiology is unknown, and no treatment is necessary (see Fig. 11-3).

Avoiding Treatment Errors

A careful physical examination of the oral cavity will remain the key element in the evaluation and treatment of patients with oral lesions. These lesions need close monitoring to ensure that the initial diagnosis is correct. In some of these lesions, there is the potential for malignant transformation, mandating the need for routine follow-up after initial diagnosis. Biopsy is also a helpful tool for diagnosis and monitoring of premalignant lesions.

Future Directions

Research will continue in an attempt to define the specific etiology of aphthous ulcers, oral lichen planus, and other less well-understood lesions. The ultimate goal is to develop more specific therapies.

Additional Resources

Aragon S: Stomatitis. In Bailey B, Calhoun K, Derkey CS, et al (eds): Head and Neck Surgery—Otolaryngology. Philadelphia, Lippincott Williams & Wilkins, 2001.

  This text provides a review of the diagnosis and treatment of oral pathology.

Marx RE, Stern D: Oral and Maxillofacial Pathology: A Rationale for Diagnosis and Treatment. Chicago, Quintessence Publishing, 2002.

  This text is comprehensive in its review of oral lesions and provides detailed diagnosis and treatment for each lesion, as well as photographs.

EVIDENCE

1. Allen CM, Blozis GG: Oral mucosal lesions. In Cummings CW, Fredrickson JM, Harker LA (eds): Otolaryngology—Head and Neck Surgery, 3rd ed. St Louis, Mosby-Year Book, 1527-1545, 1998.

     This chapter provides an excellent in-depth review of the physical diagnosis and treatment of oral lesions.

2. Hairston BR, Bruce AJ, Rogers RS III: Viral diseases of the oral mucosa. Dermatol Clin 21:17-32, 2000.

     This paper represents an excellent review of the oral manifestations of viral diseases.

3. Ingafou M, Leao JC, Porter SR, Scully C: Oral lichen planus: A retrospective study of 690 patients. Oral Dis 12:463-468, 2006.

     The authors present a retrospective review of 690 consecutive patients found to have clinical and histopathologic features of OLP.

4. Letsinger JA, McCarthy MA, Jorizzo J: Complex aphthosis: A large case series with evaluation algorithm and therapeutic ladder from topicals to thalidomide. Am Acad Dermatol 52:500-508, 2005.

     The authors discuss the identification and treatment of 54 patients diagnosed with complex aphthosis from 1995 to 2001.

5. Lynch DP: Oral viral infections. Clin Dermatol 18:619-628, 2000.

     This article reviews oral viral infections with oral manifestations, images, and treatment.

6. Miles DA, Howard MM: Diagnosis and management of oral lichen planus. Dermatol Clin 14:281-290, 1996.

     The authors review oral lichen planus, providing detailed descriptions of subtypes.

7. Scully C: Aphthous ulceration. N Engl J Med 2:165-172, 2006.

     The author presents a clinical practice review of aphthous ulceration with an excellent differential diagnosis of oral lesions and a current review of treatment.

8. Sudbo S, Reith A: The evaluation of predictive oncology and molecular-based therapy for oral cancer prevention. Int J Cancer 115:339-345, 2005.

     The article provides a good review of novel treatment of early carcinogenesis with COX-2 and epidermal growth factor receptor inhibitors.

9. Woo SB, Sonis ST: Recurrent aphthous ulcers: a review of diagnosis and treatment. J Am Dent Assoc 127:1202-1213, 1996.

     This paper presents a review of recurrent aphthous ulcer diagnosis and treatment.

James E. Kurz

12

Acute Otitis Externa

Introduction

Acute otitis externa (AOE), commonly known as swimmer's ear, is defined as an acute inflammation of the external auditory canal. Nearly 95% of AOE is bacterial in origin but AOE can also be caused by fungal infections, allergic disorders, and dermatologic conditions.

Etiology and Pathogenesis

The pathogenesis of AOE is best understood with an appreciation of the anatomy of the external auditory canal (Fig. 12-1). The canal begins proximally at the tympanic membrane (TM) and extends distally to the external acoustic meatus. The proximal third of the canal is thinly lined with epithelium and dermis, which is immediately adjacent to the underlying periosteum; inflammation here is quite painful because of its proximity to the surrounding bone. The distal two thirds of the canal is surrounded by the cartilage supporting the external ear structures and is lined with thicker skin that contains cerumen glands, sebaceous glands, and hair follicles that collectively serve as the canal's defense system. Cerumen is hydrophobic and acidic, maintaining a dry environment that is hostile to skin flora and other bacterial pathogens. The epithelium lining the canal is continually sloughing and migrates distally to keep the ear cleansed of debris and excess cerumen. Anything that disrupts this cerumen-epithelial barrier, such as prolonged moisture, aggressive cerumen removal, indwelling hearing aids, and even eczema or psoriasis, can start the inflammatory process that allows organisms to invade. Exposure to water for long periods of time, as with swimmer's ear, for example, causes maceration of the epithelium and disrupts the protective cerumen barrier. This disruption alters the environment from a dry acidic one to a moist, nonacidic environment that allows bacteria to grow and infect. Once infection sets in, the canal becomes inflamed and fills with purulent fluid and debris that further obstruct the canal to create and maintain a warm, moist, alkaline environment for pathogens to grow. Unless fluid and debris can drain from the canal, and unless inflammation and edema can be reduced, the infection will spread to adjacent ear structures and cranial structures and can evolve into a life-threatening infectious process.

More than 90% of cases of AOE are caused by *Staphylococcus aureus* and *Pseudomonas aeruginosa*, either as individual pathogens or together in a polymicrobial process. These pathogens thrive in a moist, alkaline environment, which is why treatment is based on removal of debris and fluid from the canal, reduction of edema, and restoration of the canal's dry, acidic environment. Much less frequently, fungi can cause external otitis, as can eczema and other skin conditions.

Clinical Presentation

Patients with AOE present with the rapid onset of ear pain, sometimes with an antecedent history of itching or fullness. The key physical exam finding is tenderness with compression of the tragus or pain when pulling outward and upward on the auricle (pinna). In the earliest stages, otoscopy may show only erythema of the canal wall, but as the canal becomes more inflamed, the walls appear edematous and purulent with visible debris and discharge that is usually white, gray, or greenish in color. The TM should be visualized if possible by gentle removal of debris with a soft curette or by gentle irrigation if needed. The TM may appear clear but can also appear opaque, irregular, white, or gray; it should be intact and mobile on insufflation, indicating that no middle ear effusion is present and that it is not perforated.

If the patient is febrile, or if the soft tissue surrounding the auricle is red and swollen, then a periauricular cellulitis exists that will require systemic antibiotics. Periauricular cellulitis in a patient who is immunosuppressed, is febrile, or otherwise appears toxic might indicate malignant (nec-

Figure 12-1 Acute Otitis Externa.

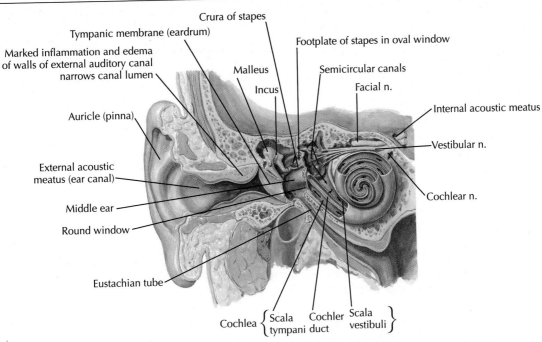

Crura of stapes

Tympanic membrane (eardrum)

Marked inflammation and edema of walls of external auditory canal narrows canal lumen

Footplate of stapes in oval window

Malleus

Semicircular canals

Incus

Facial n.

Auricle (pinna)

Internal acoustic meatus

External acoustic meatus (ear canal)

Vestibular n.

Middle ear

Cochlear n.

Round window

Eustachian tube

Cochlea { Scala tympani / Cochler duct / Scala vestibuli }

In otitis externa, inflammation, edema, and discharge are limited to external auditory canal and its walls

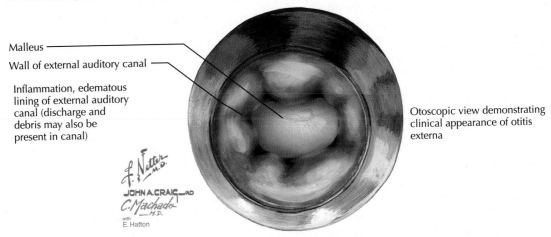

Malleus

Wall of external auditory canal

Inflammation, edematous lining of external auditory canal (discharge and debris may also be present in canal)

Otoscopic view demonstrating clinical appearance of otitis externa

rotizing) otitis externa and requires intravenous antibiotics and urgent evaluation by an otolaryngologist.

Differential Diagnosis

It is important to distinguish AOE from other causes of ear pain or drainage because the treatments are quite different and delay of diagnosis can lead to serious complications (Box 12-1). One of the more common causes of local ear pain is furunculosis, in which a tender red nodule, papule, or pustule is visible on the inner auricle or within the distal auditory canal. Pain from acute sinusitis and dental infections can be referred to the ear, as can the pain from the temporomandibular joint. Pain from cervical or cranial neuropathies is neuropathic in quality and may occur in short, stabbing volleys (trigeminal neuralgia) that

are distinct from the steady, gnawing pain of AOE. Acute otitis media with perforation causes ear drainage, but pain is a much less prominent feature once the TM ruptures and the ear starts to drain. A cholesteatoma can be associated with chronic drainage and appears on otoscopy as a cheesy mass adjacent to the wall of the canal, often near the TM. *Candida* and *Aspergillus* species cause otomycosis; this fungal infection of the external canal usually occurs after prior treatment for AOE but is also seen in diabetic and the elderly patients. Otomycosis usually presents with chronic itching and drainage rather than pain.

Noninfectious etiologies of external ear problems include dermatologic conditions such as eczema, psoriasis, and contact dermatitis. Dermatologic processes more commonly present with itching and flaking rather than pain. Carcinomas are rare causes of persistent ear drainage

Box 12-1	Differential Diagnosis of Ear Pain or Drainage

Infectious
Acute otitis media with perforation
Furunculosis
Otomycosis
Chronic otitis externa
Chronic suppurative otitis media
Sinusitis
Shingles
Necrotizing (malignant) otitis externa

Noninfectious
Atopic dermatitis
Psoriasis
Contact dermatitis
Carcinoma
Cholesteatoma

Other Painful Conditions
Temporomandibular joint dysfunction
Trigeminal or occipital neuralgia
Dental carries

but should be considered if drainage is not improving with appropriate AOE treatment.

Diagnostic Approach

The diagnosis of AOE is clinical. Because most cases of AOE are caused by *P. aeruginosa* and *S. aureus*, there is no reason to culture the fluid except in unusual circumstances such as treatment failures (in which case fungal infection is possible), immunocompromised hosts, chronically draining ears, and severe cases associated with cellulitis or high fever. Blood work or radiologic studies are rarely necessary in AOE. If the patient is febrile and appears ill, however, malignant otitis externa must be considered; in such cases, a sedimentation rate may be markedly elevated, and computed tomography or magnetic resonance imaging may be indicated to make the diagnosis.

Management and Therapy

The fundamentals of treatment of AOE are (1) adequate aural toilet to allow adequate delivery of drug to the site of infection; (2) topical agents effective against the primary pathogens; (3) adequate pain relief; (4) an awareness of factors that may modify management such as a perforated TM, a history of recurrent infections, the presence of tympanostomy tubes, and immunocompromised states such as diabetes; and (5) an awareness of alternative diagnoses and potential complications.

Optimum Treatment

For treatment to work, the drug must be delivered to the site of infection, and topical therapy works best. Debris and discharge may need to be removed from the canal (aural toilet) so that the drug can reach the proximal canal.

Aural toilet is accomplished with gentle use of a soft curette, cotton swab, or a microcurette under direct visualization through the otoscope. Gentle irrigation, preferably with half-strength hydrogen peroxide, can also help remove debris, but it is best to first confirm that the TM is not perforated so as not to flush infected material into the middle ear. If the canal remains obscured by debris or edema such that the TM cannot be visualized, and there is concern as to whether topical agents can reach the proximal canal, a wick or stent should be inserted to allow adequate delivery of drug to the proximal canal.

Topical therapy is strongly recommended over systemic therapy for AOE because it allows for much higher concentrations of drug at the site of infection. Systemic reviews of topical therapy have shown that acidifying agents (e.g., acetic acid and boric acid), antiseptic agents, and antibiotics all have similar efficacy in treating AOE. The addition of topical steroids hastens resolution of pain and discharge, and some studies have shown that topical steroids can also be used alone. The choice of therapy should take into account effectiveness, cost, ease of administration (compliance), and possible side effects.

The first choice of most clinicians is an inexpensive topical antibiotic combined with a steroid such as the combination of neomycin, polymyxin B, and hydrocortisone (available as combination therapy). Topical aminoglycosides such as gentamycin and tobramycin are also effective and inexpensive but do not come combined with a steroid preparation. Acidifying agents such as acetic acid inhibit growth of *P. aeruginosa* and *S. aureus* and have been found to be just as effective as antibiotics. The primary disadvantage of these agents is patient adherence because they must be instilled 4 times a day. Additionally, neomycin-containing products are more apt to cause contact dermatitis and allergic reactions, particularly in patients with underlying eczema. There is also the rare risk for ototoxicity if aminoglycosides reach the middle ear through a perforated TM. For these reasons, topical quinolones have gained favor as drugs of choice for AOE but are significantly more expensive. Ofloxacin otic solution only has to be used once a day but is more commonly linked to subsequent otomycosis. Ciprofloxacin, with or without a steroid combination (ciprofloxacin plus dexamethasone or ciprofloxacin with hydrocortisone) is dosed twice a day. Duration of therapy for antibacterial agents is 7 days. Longer durations of 10 to 14 days may be better for acidifying agents or steroids used alone.

Adequate pain management is strongly recommended in clinical practice guidelines and will not interfere with the clinician's ability to follow the response to therapy. Mild to moderate pain can be treated with acetaminophen or nonsteroidal anti-inflammatory agents, but one should not hesitate to prescribe stronger pain medication, including narcotic agents such as codeine, because the pain of AOE can be severe. Topical analgesics are not very effective and are of too short duration of action to be of much use.

Need for Systemic Antibiotics

Systemic antibiotics may be needed in circumstances such as an immunocompromised host (HIV, diabetes), involvement of infection beyond the external canal, or inability of antibiotic to reach the proximal canal through a wick or stent. In these cases, a quinolone antibiotic with activity against *Pseudomonas* species and *S. aureus*, such as ciprofloxacin, is preferred. β-Lactams that are effective against *Staphylococcus* species (e.g., amoxicillin-clavulanate, dicloxacillin, cephalexin) can be used and are much less expensive but are not effective against *Pseudomonas* species. Cultures are advised to guide therapy when there is a high level of clinical uncertainty. If the patient does not improve within 48 hours, treatment with a quinolone is indicated. Malignant otitis must be treated urgently with intravenous antibiotics and may require surgical débridement.

Treatment of Other Etiologies

Otomycosis (fungal infection of the external auditory canal) should be considered if the patient has drainage and itching after appropriate treatment for AOE, usually after trials of two different topical therapies, or if drainage recurs soon after successful treatment. Otomycosis is not usually painful. Cultures of the fluid can help make the diagnosis. Treatment is based on adequate aural toilet and use of topical antifungals such as clotrimazole solution twice a day (available over the counter, often as a preparation sold for tinea pedis or cruris). Patients with tympanostomy tubes and a draining ear likely have otitis media but are at risk for otitis externa and tube occlusion; treatment is a topical quinolone and steroid, usually ciprofloxacin combined with dexamethasone. Eczema and psoriasis are treated with topical steroid solutions or creams.

Avoiding Treatment Errors

The most common error in treating AOE is inadequate aural toilet so that the topical agent cannot reach the proximal auditory canal. If there is significant edema or debris that cannot be removed, the patient should be referred to an otolaryngologist, who can remove debris and place a wick or stent if necessary. A patient who appears toxic with a high fever may have malignant otitis and needs immediate hospitalization for intravenous antibiotic administration. One should not hesitate to consult an otolaryngologist in cases of severe AOE or when the patient is not responding as expected to initial therapy.

Prevention

Patients need to be educated that ear wax protects the ear canal and that cleaning the ears either with Q-tips or solutions is unnecessary and can lead to infections. In patients with recurrent cerumen impactions, 2 drops of mineral oil once a week will keep the cerumen soft so that it will naturally discharge from the ears. Swimmers who have a tendency to get recurrent infections can dry the area after swimming by tilting the ear down and using a towel roll to wick water from the external canal. Cotton swabs should not be inserted in the canal. After swimming, one can also use ear drops with acetic acid mixed with isopropyl alcohol (available over the counter or mixed at home using half white vinegar and half rubbing alcohol), which helps dry the canal and keep it acidic. Ear plugs are also effective in preventing recurrent infections.

Future Directions

The multiple treatments available for treating AOE all show similar efficacy in randomized trials, but this similarity may be a result of inadequately designed or powered studies; some studies have shown non–statistically significant trends in favor of certain antibiotics, especially quinolones combined with steroids. Larger, properly conducted randomized trials are still needed to determine the optimal therapy for AOE. Additionally, our aging population and the increasing prevalence of diabetes will make atypical presentations more common, particularly in the incidence of otomycosis and more severe presentations of bacterial otitis externa.

Additional Resources

American Academy of Pediatrics. Ear infections: Swimmer's ear. Available at: http://www.aap.org/healthtopics/earinfections.cfm. Accessed November 16, 2006.

This free online 2-minute audio describes how to prevent swimmer's ear after water exposure.

WebMD: Ear canal problems (swimmer's ear). A-Z Healthguide. Available at: http://www.webmd.com/hw/ear_disorders/hw87616.asp. Accessed December 15, 2006.

This Internet article gives tips to patients on identifying an infection and whether treatment may safely be tried at home, what treatment is appropriate, and when to seek medical care.

EVIDENCE

1. Goguen LA: External otitis. In Rose BD (ed): UpToDate. Available at: http://www.utdol.com/utd/content/topic.do?topicKey=pc_id/2947&type=A&selectedTitle=5~9. Accessed August 30, 2006.

   This website provides a basic review of the pathogenesis and treatment of AOE.

2. Rosenfeld RM, Brown L, Cannon CR, et al: Clinical practice guideline: Acute otitis externa. Otolaryngol Head Neck Surg 134(4 Suppl):S4-S23, 2006.

   The authors describe evidence-based clinical practice guidelines for the diagnosis and treatment of AOE.

3. Rosenfeld RM, Singer M, Wasserman JM, Stinnett SS: Systematic review of topical antimicrobial therapy for acute otitis externa. Otolaryngol Head Neck Surg 134(4 Suppl):S24-S48, 2006.

   The authors provide a systemic review of the literature on the treatment of AOE and include a meta-analysis of randomized controlled trials comparing different treatment regimens.

James E. Kurz

13

Acute Otitis Media

Introduction

Acute otitis media (AOM) is an acute inflammatory process of the middle ear. It is the single most common diagnosis of pediatric sick visits in the United States and the most common diagnosis for which antibiotics are prescribed to children. More than half of all children have AOM by their first birthday, and 80% have it at least once by age 3 years. Although most cases of AOM occur in childhood, more than 16% of cases occur after age 15 years.

Etiology and Pathogenesis

AOM is defined by the accumulation of fluid in the middle ear accompanied by signs of acute inflammation. The process by which this occurs requires an appreciation of the anatomy of the middle ear (Fig. 13-1). A properly functioning eustachian tube (pharyngotympanic tube) ventilates the middle ear, keeping the middle ear chamber in equilibrium with atmospheric pressure. If the tube becomes obstructed, most often because of swelling, secretions, and congestion from a viral upper respiratory infection (URI), the middle ear pressure becomes relatively negative and draws fluid into the chamber, creating an effusion. Bacteria then grow in this middle ear fluid and start an inflammatory, purulent process (Fig. 13-2). Dysfunction of the eustachian tube, and thus middle ear effusion and infection, is much more common in children because the tube is oriented more horizontally than that of adults, and gravity has less effect on its drainage. It is also narrower than that of adults, and the surrounding tissue is less supportive. On average, it takes about 4 days from the onset of viral symptoms for an inflammatory middle ear infection to develop.

Historically, the most common bacterial organisms isolated from middle ear fluid in AOM are *Streptococcus pneumoniae* (40%), nontypable *Haemophilus influenzae* (20%), and *Moraxella* species (10%). Group A streptococcus is much less common and usually occurs in older children. Since the introduction of the heptavalent pneumococcal conjugate vaccine (PCV7), however, studies of middle ear fluid show a decrease in the percentage of *S. pneumoniae*

isolates to 30%, whereas the incidence of *H. influenzae* has increased to 50%. Although the percentage of penicillin-resistant pneumococci isolated from infected effusions has diminished, the incidence of AOM has not changed.

Viruses, usually rhinoviruses, can also be isolated as the sole microorganisms in about 15% of cases of AOM and may play a role in treatment failures. Respiratory syncytial virus and adenovirus cause distinct clinical syndromes, which help distinguish these infections from bacterial AOM.

Clinical Presentation

AOM is almost always preceded by several days of viral URI symptoms followed by the acute onset of ear pain or fussiness. On examination, the tympanic membrane (TM) appears red or whitish and often is bulging. The normal light reflex and landmarks are absent, and the TM is immobile or minimally mobile on pneumatic otoscopy. An air-fluid level may be noted behind the eardrum. Purulent or bloody discharge in the canal usually indicates that the TM has perforated and may correlate with a history of sudden pain relief at the time of perforation. Otorrhea may also be noted in the patient with AOM with functioning tympanostomy tubes.

The American Academy of Pediatrics and American Academy of Family Physicians have published diagnostic criteria for AOM, shown in Box 13-1. AOM is definitively diagnosed if all three diagnostic criteria are fulfilled.

Figure 13-1 External Ear and Tympanic Cavity.

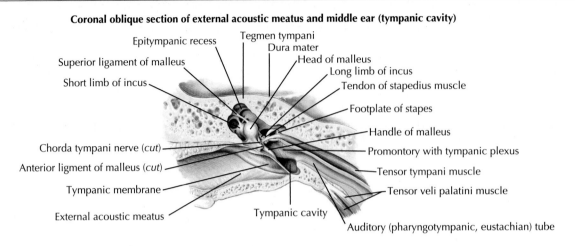

Coronal oblique section of external acoustic meatus and middle ear (tympanic cavity)

Epitympanic recess
Superior ligament of malleus
Short limb of incus
Tegmen tympani
Dura mater
Head of malleus
Long limb of incus
Tendon of stapedius muscle
Footplate of stapes
Handle of malleus
Chorda tympani nerve (*cut*)
Anterior ligment of malleus (*cut*)
Tympanic membrane
External acoustic meatus
Promontory with tympanic plexus
Tensor tympani muscle
Tensor veli palatini muscle
Tympanic cavity
Auditory (pharyngotympanic, eustachian) tube

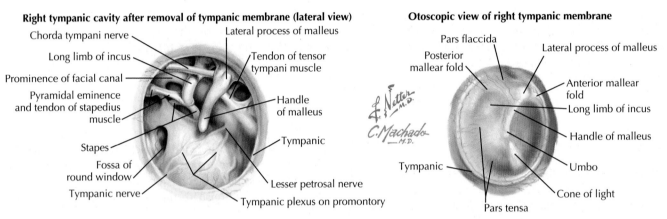

Right tympanic cavity after removal of tympanic membrane (lateral view)

Chorda tympani nerve
Long limb of incus
Prominence of facial canal
Pyramidal eminence and tendon of stapedius muscle
Stapes
Fossa of round window
Tympanic nerve
Lateral process of malleus
Tendon of tensor tympani muscle
Handle of malleus
Tympanic
Lesser petrosal nerve
Tympanic plexus on promontory

Otoscopic view of right tympanic membrane

Pars flaccida
Posterior mallear fold
Lateral process of malleus
Anterior mallear fold
Long limb of incus
Handle of malleus
Tympanic
Umbo
Cone of light
Pars tensa

F. Netter M.D.
C. Machado M.D.

Box 13-1 Diagnostic Criteria for Acute Otitis Media

1. Acute, often abrupt onset of signs of middle ear inflammation such as pain, or other signs of discomfort, fever, or hearing loss, *and*
2. The presence of a middle ear effusion based on visualization of the TM that is either bulging, has limited mobility on insufflation, is noted to contain an air-fluid level behind the TM, or reveals purulent fluid in the ear canal, *and*
3. Signs and symptoms of middle ear inflammation such as diffuse redness of the TM or significant otalgia bad enough to interfere with normal activities or sleep

Adapted from the American Academy of Pediatrics and American Academy of Family Physicians Subcommittee on Management Acute Otitis Media: Diagnosis and management of acute otitis media. Pediatrics 113(5):1451-1465, 2004.

Differential Diagnosis

Serous otitis, or otitis media with effusion, is a noninflammatory condition that is distinct from AOM. The TM will be immobile but will otherwise appear clear, as will the effusion. Serous otitis is common after AOM is successfully treated and can persist for several weeks after treatment. In the setting of a URI, the effusion will usually resolve once the viral symptoms resolve. Neither situation requires the use of antibiotics. The evaluation and management of chronic otitis media with effusion is beyond the scope of this chapter but can be found in the clinical practice guideline published by the American Academy of Pediatrics (see "Evidence").

A list of other differential diagnoses appears in Box 13-2. Some of the more common infectious causes of ear pain include acute otitis externa and acute sinusitis. Some of the most common noninfectious causes include eustachian tube dysfunction after flying (barotitis media), cerumen impaction, foreign bodies, temporomandibular joint syndrome, and referred pain from neuropathies such as occipital and trigeminal neuralgia. Bullous myringitis is an unusual cause of AOM resulting in *Mycoplasma pneumoniae* and appears as multiple bullae on the TM, often with hemorrhage; this is one of the few situations in which a macrolide antibiotic is the preferred treatment. One cause of acute hearing loss that deserves mention is "sudden sensorineural hearing loss"; recent evidence implicates varicella virus as the cause and requires rapid treatment with oral steroids and antivirals.

Figure 13-2 Acute Otitis Media.

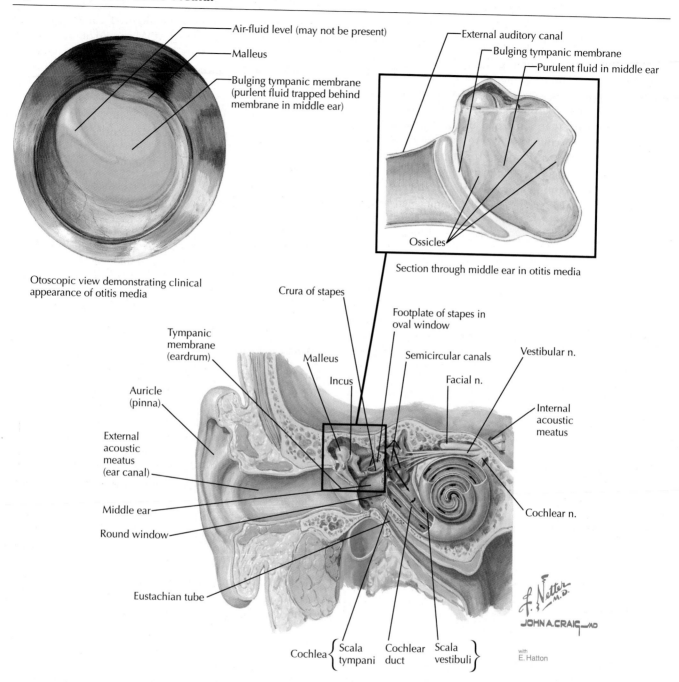

Air-fluid level (may not be present)

Malleus

Bulging tympanic membrane (purlent fluid trapped behind membrane in middle ear)

External auditory canal

Bulging tympanic membrane

Purulent fluid in middle ear

Ossicles

Section through middle ear in otitis media

Otoscopic view demonstrating clinical appearance of otitis media

Crura of stapes

Footplate of stapes in oval window

Tympanic membrane (eardrum)

Malleus

Incus

Semicircular canals

Facial n.

Vestibular n.

Auricle (pinna)

Internal acoustic meatus

External acoustic meatus (ear canal)

Middle ear

Round window

Cochlear n.

Eustachian tube

Cochlea { Scala tympani   Cochlear duct   Scala vestibuli }

with
E. Hatton

Complications of AOM can be quite serious and include mastoiditis, meningitis, sinus vein thrombosis, cholesteatoma, chronic serous otitis media, hearing loss and speech delay, and chronic suppurative otitis media with perforation.

Diagnostic Approach

AOM is a clinical diagnosis, and visualization of the TM is required to make the diagnosis. If the view is obstructed by cerumen or debris, a reasonable attempt should be made to remove the obstruction using a soft curette or gentle irrigation. Irrigation should be avoided if there is suspicion of a perforation (such as purulent or bloody fluid in the canal) because purulent debris could be flushed into the middle ear cavity. In practice, unfortunately, the TM cannot always be well visualized. In these cases tympanography or acoustic reflectometry can objectively assess the mobility of the TM and the presence or absence of an effusion. Cultures are rarely necessary except perhaps in the case of a chronically draining ear. Blood tests and radiologic tests are not necessary unless there is concern for mastoiditis or other extension of infection into surrounding structures.

Management and Therapy

The goal of treatment of AOM is to reduce pain and relieve symptoms, prevent complications, and minimize adverse effects of treatment. Prospective studies have shown that most children older than 2 years with AOM improve regardless of whether they receive antibiotics. As a result of this observation, there has been a trend toward observation rather than antibiotic treatment, particularly in many European countries, where most cases of AOM are not treated with antibiotics. Proponents of antibiotics recommend their use not so much to treat AOM but to prevent its complications, citing that the incidence of mastoiditis and secondary meningitis has diminished significantly in the postantibiotic era. Additionally, there is good evidence that antibiotics are superior to placebo in children younger than 2 years.

Optimum Treatment

Treatment options are age dependent. All children younger than 6 months with suspected AOM should be treated with antibiotics, with special consideration given to children younger than 2 months, who are more likely to have a systemic neonatal infection seeding the ear. Children from 6 months to 2 years of age with a clear diagnosis of AOM (one that fulfills all three criteria in Box 13-1) should be treated with antibiotics to prevent potential complications. In children 6 months to 2 years in which the diagnosis is uncertain and the child does not appear ill, one can observe closely for 48 hours and treat if they do not improve spontaneously. Children older than 2 years and adults who do not appear ill or have a high fever can be observed and provided pain relief, but follow-up must be available within 48 hours in case they worsen or do not improve. These recommendations are contained in the American Academy of Pediatrics and American Academy of Family Physicians clinical practice guidelines and are summarized in Table 13-1.

Choice of Antibiotic

Amoxicillin remains the drug of choice for AOM in all age groups beyond 2 months of age at a high dose of 80 to 90 mg/kg/day divided into two doses. This dose is higher than the traditional dose of 40 mg/kg/day and is active against most resistant strains of *S. pneumoniae*. In adults, amoxicillin is also recommended as the initial drug of choice, although high doses are not usually necessary because penicillin-resistant pneumococci are less prevalent in adults.

Amoxicillin should not be used as first-line therapy in cases in which amoxicillin resistance is likely. One such clinical scenario is AOM associated with purulent conjunctivitis, which is usually caused by nontypable *H. influenzae*. Additionally, if the patient was treated for AOM within the past 30 days with amoxicillin, or did not respond initially to amoxicillin, another antibiotic with broader coverage

---

Box 13-2   Differential Diagnosis of Acute Otitis Media

Acute Ear Pain
With Upper Respiratory Symptoms
Sinusitis (allergic or viral)
Pharyngitis
Allergic rhinitis
Parotitis
Mastoiditis
Otitis externa
Bullous myringitis
Without Upper Respiratory Symptoms
Foreign body or trauma
Temporomandibular joint dysfunction
Dental caries
Referred neuropathic pain (trigeminal or occipital neuralgia)
Herpes zoster (note that pain may appear before the rash)
Furunculosis
Barotitis media

Table 13-1   Criteria for Initial Antibacterial Treatment or Observation in Children with Acute Otitis Media

Age	Certain Diagnosis	Uncertain Diagnosis
<6 mo	Antibacterial therapy	Antibacterial therapy
6 mo to 2 y	Antibacterial therapy	Antibacterial therapy if severe; observation optional if not*
>2 y	Antibacterial therapy if severe; observation optional if not*	Observation optional*

* Observation for 48 to 72 hours is an appropriate option only when follow-up can be ensured, so that antibiotics can be started if symptoms persist or worsen. Nonsevere illness is defined as mild otalgia and temperature <39° C. A certain diagnosis depends on a history of acute onset, middle ear effusion, and signs of middle ear inflammation.

Modified from American Academy of Pediatrics and American Academy of Family Physicians Subcommittee on Management Acute Otitis Media: Diagnosis and management of acute otitis media. Pediatrics 113(5):1451-1465, 2004. Modified from the New York State Department of Health dnd the New York Region Otitis Project Committee.

should be used. The next best choices in children are amoxicillin-clavulanate, a second- or third-generation cephalosporin, or clindamycin (unless *H. influenzae* is suspected). In adults, in whom the theoretical effects of quinolones on bone and cartilage growth are not a concern, quinolones with good pneumococcal coverage such as levofloxacin or moxifloxacin (not ciprofloxacin) may also be used. Macrolides and sulfa drugs were commonly used in the past but are no longer advised for treatment of AOM because of rising bacterial resistance. One exception is the rare case of bullous myringitis caused by *Mycoplasma* species that should be treated with a macrolide. *H. influenzae* and *Moraxella* species will also respond to broad-spectrum macrolides such as azithromycin.

In children who appear toxic with a high fever (>39° C) or who have been vomiting or might otherwise not tolerate medication by mouth, intramuscular ceftriaxone, 50 mg/kg, is appropriate in a one-time dose and may be repeated in 24 to 48 hours if there is not significant improvement. In cases of persistent purulent otitis media that have not responded to two or three courses of oral antibiotics, ceftriaxone can be administered daily for 3 consecutive days. If this is ineffective, tympanostomy tubes may be indicated.

The duration of oral antibiotic therapy for AOM has traditionally been 10 days; however, recent studies have concluded that a 5-day course of treatment is as effective in older children (>2 years) and in adults without a history of recurrent AOM.

In all cases, pain control should be a priority, although the optimal regimen for such is not established. Analgesics such as acetaminophen or ibuprofen are preferred. Narcotics such as codeine may be indicated in severe cases. Topical agents such as benzocaine can provide brief relief and can be helpful in addition to oral pain relievers. Decongestants, antihistamines, and steroids have not shown much benefit in treatment of AOM and come at the cost of increased side effects.

Tube Otorrhea

Patients with a draining ear who have tympanostomy tubes in place likely have AOM with appropriate drainage through the tubes into the external canal. Topical therapy with ciprofloxacin drops with or without a steroid combination is indicated to prevent the external canal from getting infected and to maintain tube patency. Oral antibiotics are not necessary because the tubes are doing their job in allowing the middle ear chamber to drain; only if the tubes are blocked or the patient appears ill or has a high fever are systemic antibiotics indicated.

Avoiding Treatment Errors

The most common treatment error in AOM is overtreatment. Because AOM is a diagnosis based on examination of the patient, treating it over the phone or without examining the patient is inappropriate. A red TM that is mobile indicates there is no effusion and is not AOM. Likewise, a clear TM and clear effusion is not AOM and will generally not respond to antibiotics.

Many patients with AOM can be observed without antibiotics; however, a patient with AOM who appears ill, has a purulent bulging TM, or is younger than 2 years should be treated with antibiotics because this subset of patients is most at risk for complications of AOM. Mastoiditis should always be suspected in any patient with a high fever or who otherwise appears toxic. Mastoiditis is caused by extension of the purulent middle ear process into the mastoid air cells. It will present with redness, tenderness, and swelling behind the auricle severe enough that the auricle may protrude outward away from the skull. It requires prompt treatment with intravenous antibiotics and sometimes surgical débridement.

Prevention

Breast-feeding in the first 6 months of life has been shown to decrease the risk for AOM. Other studies have shown that the influenza vaccine can reduce the risk for AOM during cold and flu season in children older than 2 years. Day care exposure remains the single greatest risk factor for respiratory infections and AOM.

Future Directions

Better randomized clinical trials are needed to identify which antibiotics are most effective and which patients benefit most from antibiotic treatment versus observation. Particularly with the widespread use of the PCV7 vaccine, nontypeable *H. influenzae* is emerging as the predominant organism causing AOM. Thus, amoxicillin may soon be obsolete as the first choice of treatment, losing favor to drugs with better *H. influenzae* coverage such as amoxicillin-clavulanate or second- and third-generation cephalosporins. For prevention, the PCV7 vaccine has been somewhat unimpressive, but ongoing trials of a 9- and an 11-valent conjugate vaccine may show more benefit in preventing AOM and its complications. Additionally, affordable and easy-to-use tools to help clinicians objectively determine the presence of an effusion are needed to make better diagnoses and better determination on whom to treat.

Additional Resources

Block SL, Correa AG: Update in management of pediatric acute otitis media and acute bacterial sinusitis. Contemp Pediatr Suppl 23(12): 1-12, 2006. Available at: http://www.contemporarypediatrics.com/contpeds/data/articlestandard/contpeds/502006/393168/article.pdf. Accessed January 3, 2007.
This supplement provides good guidance for clinicians and discusses how amoxicillin may soon be phased out as first choice for treatment of AOM.

Centers for Disease Control and Prevention: Get smart: Know when antibiotics work. Available at: http://www.cdc.gov/drugresistance/community/know-and-do.htm. Accessed December 15, 2006.

The CDC presents a good discussion for parents and patients on why antibiotics are usually not indicated for upper respiratory infections.

New York State Department of Health: Observation option toolkit for acute otitis media. Available at: http://www.health.state.ny.us/nysdoh/antibiotic/toolkt.pdf. Accessed December 14, 2006.

This Internet article provides information sheets for health care providers and parents with guidelines for observing some children with AOM rather than treating with antibiotics.

EVIDENCE

1. American Academy of Pediatrics and American Academy of Family Physicians subcommittee on Management Acute Otitis Media. Clinical Practice Guideline: Diagnosis and management of acute otitis media. Pediatrics 113(5):1451-1465, 2004.

    These clinical practice guidelines address the proper diagnosis and management of AOM. They can also be accessed online at the American Academy of Pediatrics website, http://www.AAP.org.

2. American Academy of Family Physicians; American Academy of Otolaryngology-Head and Neck Surgery; American Academy of Pediatrics Subcommittee on Otitis Media with Effusion. Clinical Practice Guideline: Otitis media with effusion. Pediatrics 113(5):1412-1429, 2004.

    These evidenced-based guidelines address the management of chronic otitis media with effusion. This is an ever-changing topic that was beyond the scope of this chapter. Up-to-date guidelines can be found at the American Academy of Pediatrics website at http://www.AAP.org.

3. Klein JO, Pelton S: Epidemiology, pathogenesis, diagnosis, and complications of acute otitis media: Treatment of acute otitis media. In Rose BD (ed): UpToDate. Waltham, MA. Accessed August 31, 2006.

    The authors provide a general overview and recommendations for the diagnosis and treatment of AOM.

4. The Cochrane Collection Web Site. Acute otitis media. Available at: http://www.cochrane.org, search "acute otitis media." Accessed November 16, 2006.

    This is an excellent source of evidence for diagnosis and management of AOM. The site provides several summaries of evidence-based reviews ranging from use of decongestants to studies of observation versus antibiotics for AOM.

Mark C. Weissler ▪ Charles S. Ebert, Jr.

14

Hoarseness

Introduction

Hoarseness describes a rough or harsh voice caused by improper vibration of the epithelial covering of the vocal cord. Anything that causes stiffening or improper coaptation of the vocal cords will result in an abnormal voice. If the vocal cords do not coapt properly because of paralysis or bowing, there will often be a breathy and weak nature to the hoarseness, whereas inflammation in and around the vocal cords will result in a coarse sounding voice. Any hoarseness persisting for 2 weeks or more warrants direct examination of the vocal cords by an otolaryngologist (Fig. 14-1).

Etiology, Pathogenesis, and Clinical Presentation

Because hoarseness is the final common pathway for anything that impairs vocal cord vibration, a myriad of entities may cause it (Box 14-1 and Figs. 14-2 to 14-4). Gastroesophageal reflux disease (GERD), laryngopharyngeal reflux (LPR), postnasal drip, and chronic cough are common causes of voice changes. Carcinoma of the glottic larynx is of greatest concern in the adult patient. In otherwise healthy children, nodules of the vocal cords caused by excessive voice use ("screamers' nodules") are common. An abnormal cry in the neonate warrants examination for a congenital or acquired abnormality of the vocal cords.

The threshold for what a patient identifies as hoarseness varies with how the voice is used. Professional voice users such as singers, teachers, ministers, and actors may not tolerate even mild degrees of voice disturbance occurring only under certain circumstances.

Diagnostic Approach

Indirect laryngoscopy (see Fig. 14-1) is the mainstay of evaluation. A mirror may be used, but a better examination can be performed using a flexible or rigid fiberoptic telescope. In this manner, the structure and function of the vocal cords can be evaluated in patients of all ages. For subtle cases, and most particularly for the professional voice user with subtle voice problems, fiberoptic laryngoscopy with videostroboscopy is essential. By timing a strobe light to the frequency of the vocalization, this examination allows visualization of the mucosal wave and is the only method that allows the examiner to appreciate subtle abnormalities in the vibration of the surface epithelium of the vocal cord.

When clinical examination reveals abnormalities that warrant a biopsy, direct laryngoscopy under general anesthesia in the operating room is indicated. Blood tests (e.g., thyroid-stimulating hormone, free T_4) and imaging (e.g., chest x-ray, computed tomography [CT] of the neck) may be appropriate in certain clinical situations. If the airway is in any way impaired, emergent evaluation by an otolaryngologist is indicated.

Management and Therapy

Referral to an otolaryngologist for visualization of the vocal cords is indicated for any patient with hoarseness persisting longer than 2 weeks (Fig. 14-5). Treatment depends on the specific clinical situation, but common interventions consist of voice rest; cessation of tobacco use; treatment for gastroesophageal reflux, chronic rhinosinusitis, and cough; and referral to a speech pathologist for therapy and vocal coaching. Most inflammatory conditions and those caused by voice abuse are best treated nonsurgically if possible. Biopsy may be necessary to exclude malignancy. Before therapeutic surgical intervention for benign disease, it is essential to control the underlying conditions causing the inflammation.

Smoking cessation is often difficult to achieve. The mainstay of treatment is to get all members of the house-

Figure 14-1 Examination of the Larynx.

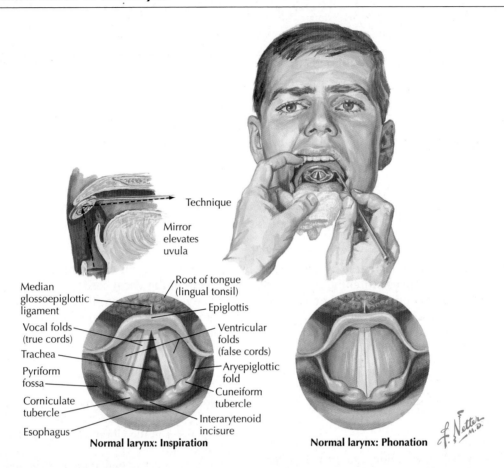

Technique

Mirror elevates uvula

Root of tongue (lingual tonsil)

Median glossoepiglottic ligament

Epiglottis

Vocal folds (true cords)

Ventricular folds (false cords)

Trachea

Pyriform fossa

Aryepiglottic fold

Cuneiform tubercle

Corniculate tubercle

Interarytenoid incisure

Esophagus

Normal larynx: Inspiration

Normal larynx: Phonation

Box 14-1   Causes of Hoarseness

Inflammation, Edema, or Swelling

Tobacco smoking
Gastroesophageal reflux
Alcohol use
Diet
Lifestyle
Chronic rhinosinusitis and postnasal drip
Allergy
Chronic cough
Asthma
Associated with angiotensin-converting enzyme inhibitors
Gastroesophageal reflux
Chronic rhinosinusitis
Voice abuse or overuse
Screamers' nodules in children
Amateur or professional singers without proper technique
   or coaching
Myxedema
Infections
Viral
Bacterial
Fungal
Postintubation

Stiffness

Scarring from previous surgery
Scarring from previous severe inflammation
Due to any of the above inflammatory conditions

Mass Lesion

Nodule
Cyst
Granuloma
Neoplasms
Squamous cell carcinoma
Granular cell tumor
Certain fungal infections

Bowing of the Vocal Cords

Presbylarynges
Atrophy due to chronic inhaled steroid use

Paralysis or Paresis

Postviral
Lesion along course of vagus nerve from brainstem to arch
   of aorta
Iatrogenic
   Thyroidectomy
   Anterior approach to cervical spine for laminectomy
Stroke
Arnold-Chiari malformation in neonates
Other congenital malformations

Figure 14-2 Inflammation of the Larynx.

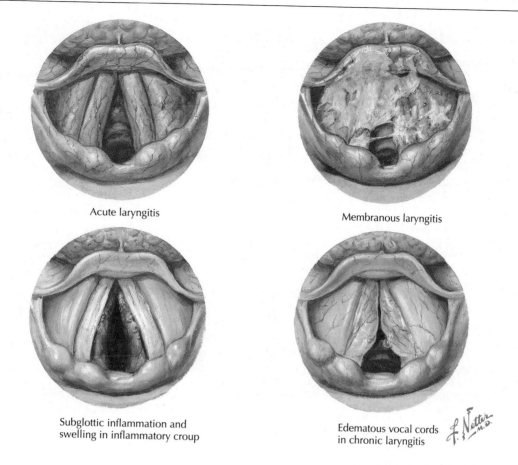

Acute laryngitis

Membranous laryngitis

Subglottic inflammation and
swelling in inflammatory croup

Edematous vocal cords
in chronic laryngitis

hold to stop smoking and to do so together on a defined timetable. Nicotine substitutes can be helpful, as can bupropion. Alternative medicine approaches such as acupuncture and hypnosis can benefit some patients.

Gastroesophageal Reflux Disease and Laryngopharyngeal Reflux

LPR is increasingly implicated in chronic inflammation of the upper aerodigestive tract. In up to 50% of cases, it is not associated with classic heartburn or GERD symptoms. Initial therapy consists of lifestyle changes, including avoidance of substances known to exacerbate reflux such as caffeine, alcohol, peppermint, and hot spicy foods or those that are associated with symptoms; avoidance of eating for 3 hours before bedtime; elevation of the head of the bed; regular exercise, and weight loss. If such measures are unsuccessful, addition of an over-the-counter H_2 receptor blocker or proton pump inhibitor is indicated. If this is still not successful, initiation of prescription-strength H_2 blockers or proton pump inhibitors is indicated. If the diagnosis remains in question, a 24-hour pH probe study with a concurrent diary performed while off antireflux medication can be helpful, although even this test is not

absolutely accurate if the patient is not symptomatic at the time. Esophageal manometry and a barium swallow are also often performed. If these tests are positive, and medical therapy has been unsuccessful, referral for consideration of surgical fundoplication, which can usually be performed laparoscopically, is indicated.

Chronic Rhinosinusitis and Postnasal Drip

Allergy and sensitivities to pollutants account for most of these cases. Treatment with avoidance, antihistamines, leukotriene inhibitors, topical intranasal corticosteroids or antihistamines, and inhaled cromolyn form the basis of medical management. Antihistamines with a minimum anticholinergic effect are preferable for this indication because the dryness associated with systemic antihistamines can aggravate vocal problems. In severe cases, formal intradermal allergy testing or radioallergosorbent testing and subsequent desensitization may be indicated. Hypertonic buffered saline nasal irrigations and gargle can also prove beneficial. Ipratropium is the treatment of choice for vasomotor rhinitis with postnasal drip. Patients not responding to medical management should undergo a CT

Figure 14-3 Lesions of the Vocal Cords.

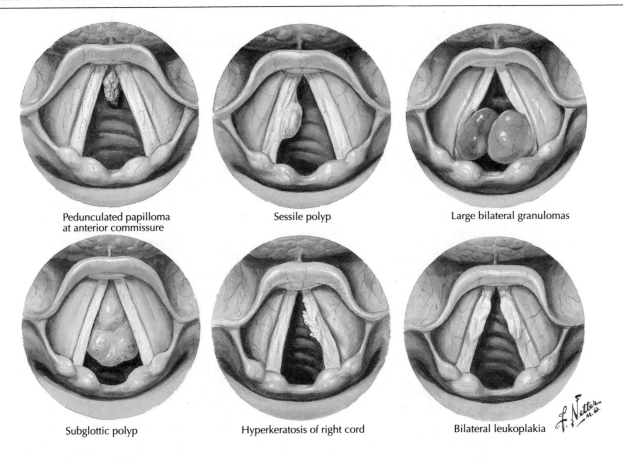

Pedunculated papilloma
at anterior commissure

Sessile polyp

Large bilateral granulomas

Subglottic polyp

Hyperkeratosis of right cord

Bilateral leukoplakia

Figure 14-4 Cancer of the Larynx.

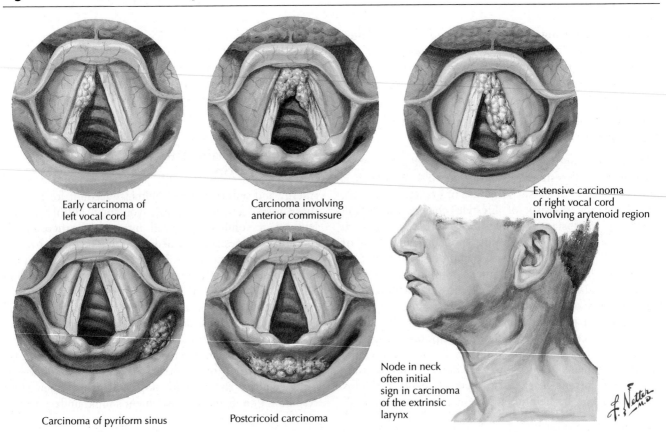

Early carcinoma of
left vocal cord

Carcinoma involving
anterior commissure

Extensive carcinoma
of right vocal cord
involving arytenoid region

Carcinoma of pyriform sinus

Postcricoid carcinoma

Node in neck
often initial
sign in carcinoma
of the extrinsic
larynx

Figure 14-5 Treatment Algorithm for Hoarseness.

CHF, congestive heart failure; COPD, chronic obstructive pulmonary disease; CT, computed tomography; ENT, ear, nose and throat specialist/otolaryngologist; GERD, gastroesophageal reflux disease; LPR, laryngopharyngeal reflux; PND, postnasal drip; PPI, proton pump inhibitor; URI, upper respiratory infection.

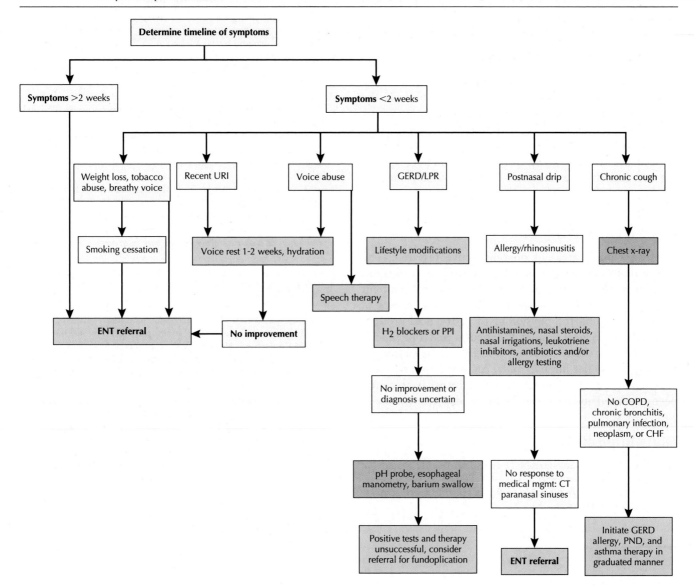

scan of the paranasal sinuses and referral to an otolaryngologist (rhinologist). In some cases, endoscopic surgery to correct obstructions to drainage of the paranasal sinuses can be helpful.

Chronic Cough

The most frequent causes, after excluding chronic bronchitis and chronic obstructive pulmonary disease, cardiac failure, pulmonary infection, and neoplasm, are gastroesophageal reflux, allergy, medications (especially angiotensin-converting enzyme inhibitors), chronic sinusitis with postnasal drip, and reactive airways disease. A chest x-ray should be performed on all patients with persistent

unexplained cough. If the chest film is normal, therapy for GERD, allergy, postnasal drip, and asthma may be instituted one at a time, in a graduated and exploratory manner. Alternatively, formal allergy testing, a methacholine challenge test for reactive airways disease, 24-hour pH probe testing with manometry and a barium swallow or upper endoscopy, and a CT scan of the paranasal sinuses can be undertaken also in a stepwise fashion, to determine a specific etiology.

Optimum Treatment

The treatment of most patients is usually well defined after the evaluation outlined and can be provided by the patient's primary care physician or otolaryngologist. However, optimal management for the professional voice user may require consultation with a speech therapist to improve vocal hygiene and avoid maladaptive behaviors such as hyperfunctional voice disorder or inappropriate vocal volume or fundamental frequency.

Avoiding Treatment Errors

The most noteworthy potential treatment error in someone with hoarseness is misdiagnosis of a carcinoma of the larynx. For this reason, any patient with symptoms lasting more than 2 weeks should have the larynx visualized by an otolaryngologist or head and neck surgeon. Any abnormality seen on fiberoptic laryngoscopy evaluation not responding to conservative medical therapy should undergo biopsy.

Future Directions

There are many areas of ongoing active research. The neuromuscular control and reflex control of vocal cord function is under study and may lead to new treatment strategies for cough and vocal problems. The causes of GERD, including the physiology of gastric acid production and esophageal sphincter function and the precise substances that cause irritation, especially in the larynx and pharynx, are under intense study. An association between reflux and upper aerodigestive tract malignancy has recently been proposed and deserves further study.

Additional Resources

Banfield G, Tandon P, Solomons N: Hoarse voice: An early symptom of many conditions. Practitioner 244:267-271, 2000.
  This article reviews the differential diagnosis of hoarseness from the primary care physician's perspective.

Berke GS, Kevorkian KF: The diagnosis and management of hoarseness. Compr Ther 22:251-255, 1996.
  This good general reference article reviews the diagnosis and management of hoarseness from the primary care physician's perspective.
Garrett GG, Ossoff RH: Hoarseness: Contemporary diagnosis and management. Compr Ther 21:705-710, 1995.
  This good general reference from the otolaryngology, head and neck surgery perspective reviews the evaluation of the patient with hoarseness and cautions that this may represent serious disease.
Maragos NE: Hoarseness. Prim Care 17:347-363, 1990.
  This general reference article reviews the abnormal production of voice often classified as hoarseness.
Miller RH, Nemecheck AJ: Hoarseness and vocal cord paralysis. In Bailey BJ (ed): Head and Neck Surgery; Otolaryngology, 2nd ed. Philadelphia, Lippincott-Raven, 1998, pp 741-751.
  This comprehensive reference from the otolaryngology, head and neck surgery perspective reviews the relevant anatomy and differential diagnoses for the evaluation and management of patients with hoarseness and vocal cord paralysis.
Rosen CA, Anderson D, Murry T: Evaluating hoarseness: Keeping your patient's voice healthy. Am Fam Physician 57:2775-2782, 1998.
  This good general reference from the primary care physician's perspective includes clinical photographs as well as discussion of the pertinent anatomy involved in the evaluation of the patient with hoarseness.

EVIDENCE

1. Meyer TK, Olsen E, Merati A: Contemporary diagnostic and management techniques for extraesophageal reflux disease. Curr Opin Otolaryngol Head Neck Surg 12(6):519-524, 2004.
   The authors provide a good review from an otolaryngology, head and neck surgery perspective of recent advances in the diagnosis and treatment of extraesophageal reflux.
2. Wilson JA: What is the evidence that gastroesophageal reflux is involved in the etiology of laryngeal cancer? Curr Opin Otolaryngol Head Neck Surg 13(2):97-100, 2005.
   The author provides a good review from an otolaryngology, head and neck surgery perspective of the current literature on the possible mechanisms and role of gastroesophageal reflux in the etiology of laryngeal cancer in patients without known risk factors of tobacco abuse and alcohol use.

Paul C. Bryson ▪ Robert A. Buckmire

15

Vocal Cord Dysfunction

Introduction

Vocal cord dysfunction (VCD) was first described in the medical literature by Patterson and colleagues in 1974 as "Munchausen's stridor" and has subsequently been referred to as factitious asthma, paradoxical vocal fold motion (PVFM), steroid-resistant asthma, laryngeal dyskinesia, functional laryngeal stridor, and functional airway obstruction in the otolaryngology, pulmonology, and emergency medicine literature. Clinically, VCD manifests as episodic, involuntary adduction of the true vocal folds during respiration (primarily inspiration). The varying degree of paradoxical glottal adductory motion causes a spectrum of respiratory complaints ranging from cough to frank respiratory embarrassment. As a clinical entity, VCD is relatively uncommon; however, the impact of this diagnosis can be substantial because patients often experience repeated emergency room visits, hospitalizations, multiple trials of ineffective medications, and potentially invasive measures such as endotracheal intubation or tracheostomy in an attempt to manage their clinical picture of airway obstruction.

The diagnosis of VCD is most often considered in the clinical settings of a patient with severe or chronic respiratory symptoms that prove refractory to common therapeutic interventions. Common presenting complaints include dyspnea or chronic cough without amelioration on standard asthmatic medications. The economic impact of these refractory symptoms is significant. These patients are routinely subjected to numerous tests (chest radiographs, computed tomography scans, bronchoscopy, and spirometry) and multiple pharmacologic therapies (antitussives, antihistamines, bronchodilators, and steroid medications) before receiving the diagnosis of VCD.

Etiology and Pathogenesis

The myriad, descriptive terminology for VCD underscores the lack of a single definitive cause for this disorder. In fact, the cause of VCD is often thought to be multifactorial. Many potential contributing etiologies have been advanced and include brainstem abnormalities, psychiatric or conversion disorders, laryngeal respiratory dystonia, physical exertion, exposure to environmental respiratory irritants, and chronic upper airway irritation or inflammatory processes (i.e., laryngopharyngeal reflux, allergy, and sinusitis). All these factors may lead to a final common pathway of an abnormal glottic closure reflex and subsequent vocal fold adduction (Fig. 15-1) during inspiration, causing symptoms of airway obstruction.

The link between VCD and psychiatric disorders has been well established. In a series of 10 patients with VCD, Altman and associates found that 70% had a diagnosis of anxiety, depression, or personality disorder. Patterson's original article supports this finding, as do several case reports in the literature. The theory that a subset of VCD may represent a form of laryngeal, respiratory dystonia is supported by series within the otolaryngology and neurology literature citing clinical responses to intralaryngeal botulinum toxin injected into the thyroarytenoid-vocalis muscles. Laryngeal hypersensitivity from gastroesophageal reflux, uncontrolled allergic rhinosinusitis, and even occupational exposure has also been observed in patients with VCD. Indeed, the presence of reflux as a contributing factor has been reported in as many as 70% of VCD patients in some series. It is hypothesized that the threshold for the laryngeal adductory reflex may be reduced in these patients.

Proposed classification schemes for VCD have focused on etiology (brainstem, upper and lower motor neurons, gastroesophageal reflux, malingering, psychogenic), further subclassifying by the degree of laryngeal overactivity (i.e., chronic cough and episodic laryngospasm).

Figure 15-1 Larynx in Abduction and Adduction.
This diagram illustrates the technique of indirect laryngoscopy and the appearance of the larynx in abduction (*lower left*) and in adduction (*lower right*).

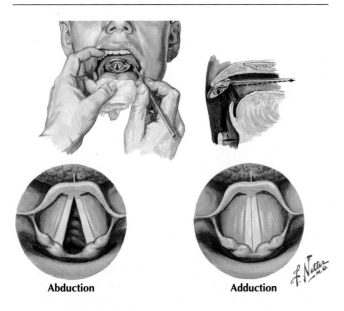

Abduction   Adduction

<table>
<tr><td>Box 15-1</td><td>Differential Diagnosis of Vocal Cord Dysfunction</td></tr>
</table>

Exercise-induced asthma
Airway foreign body
Allergic anaphylaxis
Anxiety attack
Vocal fold polypoid degeneration
Bilateral vocal fold immobility
Supraglottitis
Sensitivity to airborne irritants
Chronic cough
Supraglottic lesions
Extrathoracic airflow obstruction (i.e., subglottic stenosis)

Clinical Presentation

Patients who present with VCD are typically female and frequently have a past diagnosis of asthma and some type of psychiatric diagnosis (depression or anxiety). The most common complaints are of episodic hoarseness, throat tightness, chronic cough, aphonia, dysphonia, and dyspnea. Many patients may describe certain triggers such as stress, exercise, cold air, discrete odors, or respiratory irritants. Additionally, many patients may comment that they have begun treatment for asthma (without much benefit), suffer from acid reflux, or take allergy medications. It is reported that about 10% of patients with recalcitrant asthma have VCD.

Clinically, there is a recognized subset of VCD patients who are young, high-achieving, female athletes with isolated respiratory exacerbations precipitated by strenuous physical exercise. These patients are often misdiagnosed as having exercise-induced bronchospasm (EIB). Distinctive features differentiating EIB from VCD include cessation of the VCD-associated dyspnea with cessation of exercise and the failure of standard bronchodilators to abort the VCD symptoms. Some authors have advocated the use of exercise laryngoscopy to identify the diagnostic laryngeal behavior that is present only during strenuous exercise.

In symptomatic VCD patients without concomitant pulmonary disease, pulmonary function tests (PFTs) reveal spirometric measures within normal reference ranges and, potentially, flattening of the inspiratory flow loop. PFTs should also fail to show bronchial hyperresponsiveness to methacholine challenge. Oxygen saturation during dyspneic episodes is within normal ranges, in contrast to that in patients experiencing a significant asthma exacerbation.

Physical examination usually reveals an anxious, stridorous (upper airway inspiratory noise) patient with normal neurologic and pulmonary findings. The patient typically has more difficulty on inspiration than expiration. Flexible fiberoptic laryngoscopy demonstrates vocal fold adduction on inspiration with a classic appearance of a small posterior inspiratory glottic chink. Not uncommonly in the emergency department setting, a patient's respiratory status may clinically worsen and warrant invasive airway management such as endotracheal intubation or tracheostomy. In a 20-patient cohort across two published studies, 12 patients underwent an invasive airway intervention (5 of 20 received tracheotomies).

Differential Diagnosis

The differential diagnosis for vocal cord dysfunction is shown in Box 15-1.

Diagnostic Approach

Because PVFM is often misdiagnosed as asthma or chemical sensitivity, it is important to obtain a thorough history, including the success of previous medical therapy, PFT results, and the frequency of attacks. Routine laboratory studies, such as basic metabolic panel and complete blood count, are typically normal but should certainly be checked to rule out concomitant disease processes. Chest radiographs appear normal without hyperinflation. In anxious patients with tachypnea, the arterial blood gas findings may demonstrate respiratory alkalosis. Additionally, PFTs (typically done on an outpatient basis) do not show significant improvement with bronchodilators and in some cases show a diminished maximum inspiratory flow.

The most useful diagnostic tool is flexible fiberoptic laryngoscopy. This allows the examiner to clearly assess the mobility of the vocal folds throughout the respiratory cycle as well as to rule out obstructing lesions or anatomic laryngeal abnormalities. Supraglottic laryngeal neoplasms

Figure 15-2 Action of Intrinsic Muscles of Larynx.
This diagram illustrates the intrinsic muscles of the larynx. The abductor of the larynx is the posterior cricoarytenoid muscle.

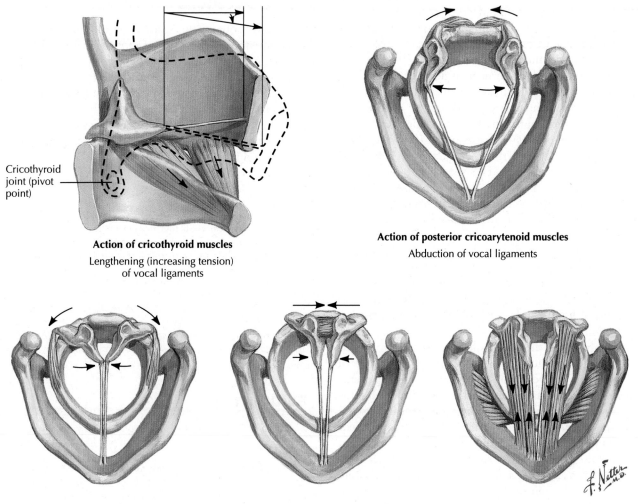

Cricothyroid joint (pivot point)

Action of cricothyroid muscles
Lengthening (increasing tension)
of vocal ligaments

Action of posterior cricoarytenoid muscles
Abduction of vocal ligaments

Action of lateral cricoarytenoid muscles
Adduction of vocal ligaments

Action of transverse and oblique arytenoid muscles
Adduction of vocal ligaments

Action of vocalis and thyroarytenoid muscles
Shortening (relaxation) of vocal ligaments

can easily mimic the symptoms of VCD. The resultant intermittent and variable glottic obstruction is caused by their close anatomic relationship above the glottis. Even benign glottic lesions have, on occasion, mimicked these symptoms. Large, edematous, overly mobile vocal folds such as those seen with polypoid degeneration (Reinke's edema) may cause similar symptomatology secondary to the Bernoulli effect, causing intermittent ball-valving of these lesions into the subglottic airway.

Laryngoscopy in patients with VCD confirms paradoxical adduction during inspiration, causing substantial functional airway obstruction, in association with the clinical complaints and laboratory findings mentioned earlier. Because of the episodic nature of this disorder, however, asymptomatic patients examined laryngoscopically may not exhibit pathologic laryngeal motion. In this baseline setting, some authors have reported the use of exacerbating stimuli or eliciting behaviors (based on patient history) during laryngoscopy in an attempt to increase the diagnostic sensitivity of the exam.

Management and Therapy

Optimum Treatment

Treatment of VCD can be divided into acute and long-term therapies. Initial management should focus on maintenance of a secure and safe airway. This includes supportive measures such as supplemental oxygen, continuous pulse oximetry, nebulized racemic epinephrine, heliox therapy, or continuous positive airway pressure. Invasive airway management with endotracheal intubation or awake tracheostomy is also well recognized in the literature, although with early diagnostic recognition, it can often be avoided.

Once the diagnosis of VCD is established, maneuvers such as sniffing, whistling, or breath-holding may help break the paradoxical vocal fold behavior. Additionally, relaxation techniques may help resolve the airway distress. In specific circumstances, a low dose of sedative-anxiolytic medications is useful in managing psychogenic contributing factors during acute exacerbations.

A personalized, multidisciplinary approach offers the best opportunity for long-term treatment. Medical management should include treatment of underlying psychiatric disorders (including psychological counseling), treatment of reflux, and management of allergic rhinitis. When these conditions are accounted for, the most acknowledged course of treatment involves behavioral speech therapy techniques. The speech pathologist can offer the patient respiratory re-education and relaxation techniques to remove the patient's focus from the inspiratory phase of breathing. Some therapists may also employ the use of laryngeal image biofeedback. First presented by Bastian and Nagorsky, this method employs the flexible fiberoptic laryngoscope and allows the patient to visualize the larynx in real time while performing various exercises with the speech pathologist. These investigators have shown this technique to be a useful instrument for patient re-education.

Although speech therapy has been shown to be beneficial for some patients, there appears to be a group of patients who have true respiratory dystonia. These patients are reasonable candidates for a trial of intralaryngeal botulinum toxin injection (into adductory laryngeal muscles; Fig. 15-2). Patients with psychiatric disorders that prevent them from participating in multidisciplinary treatment plans may also require long-term tracheotomy to mechanically bypass the laryngeal site of airway obstruction. There is yet another subgroup of PVFM patients who have central or brainstem etiologies for whom the previously described treatments are likely to be ineffective. These patients more frequently remain tracheotomy dependent.

Avoiding Treatment Errors

Vocal cord dysfunction remains a rare clinical entity. The clinician's primary focus should be the maintenance of a safe and secure airway. To avoid treatment errors in these patients, one must have a high index of suspicion when presented with patients who fit the historical and physical exam findings described.

Treatment errors include overly aggressive treatment and undertreatment. Overtreatment often results in endotracheal intubation or tracheotomy in an attempt to avoid what the clinician perceives as imminent loss of the patient's airway. Undertreatment arises from a failure to recognize this clinical entity and to appropriately address potential exacerbating factors such as laryngopharyngeal reflux, allergic rhinitis, and mental illness (including depression and anxiety). Otolaryngologic consultation for flexible fiberoptic laryngoscopy during an attack may lead to earlier diagnosis.

Future Directions

Future directions in the study of vocal cord dysfunction will require the development of a formal medical definition of this clinical entity, including inclusionary and exclusionary criteria. Further research into the neurologic underpinnings of the paradoxical vocal fold activity is necessary. Additionally, refinement of long-term therapy merits randomized, controlled trials examining treatment modalities such as pharmacotherapy, laryngeal biofeedback, and botulinum toxin injection.

Additional Resources

Blager FB: Paradoxical vocal fold movement: Diagnosis and management. Curr Opin Otolaryngol Head Neck Surg 8:180-183, 2000.
A review of the diagnosis and treatment of paradoxical vocal fold motion is presented.
Morrison M, Rammage L, Emami AJ: The irritable larynx syndrome. J Voice 13(3):447-455, 1999.
The authors discuss muscular tension dysphonia, episodic laryngospasm, globus, and chronic cough. They propose a unifying hypothesis that involves neural plasticity of brainstem laryngeal control networks through which each of the latter etiologies, plus central nervous system viral illness, can play a role.

EVIDENCE

1. Altman KW, Mirza N, Ruiz C, Sataloff RT: Paradoxical vocal fold motion: Presentation and treatment options. J Voice 14(1):99-103, 2000.
A case series of 10 patients treated and followed over six years is described. There is a good review of the literature and a description of the author's experience with biofeedback and botulinum injection.
2. Altman KW, Simpson CB, Amin MR, et al: Cough and paradoxical vocal fold motion. Otolaryngol Head Neck Surg 127(6):501-511, 2002.
The authors review the medical literature on the etiologies of chronic cough and its relationship to gastroesophageal reflux, vagal neuropathy, and paradoxical vocal fold motion.
3. Bastian RW, Nagorsky MJ: Laryngeal image biofeedback. Laryngoscope 97(11):1346-1349, 1987.
The technique of laryngeal image biofeedback is described, including its effectiveness in a series of 20 patients.
4. Ferris RL, Eisele DW, Tunkel DE: Functional laryngeal dyskinesia in children and adults. Laryngoscope 108(10):1520-1523, 1998.
A 20-year case series of patients with functional laryngeal dyskinesia is presented. The authors describe patient characteristics and treatment strategies.
5. Maschka D, Bauman NM, McCray PB, et al: A classification scheme for paradoxical vocal fold motion. Laryngoscope 107(11 Pt 1):1429-1435, 1997.
A classification scheme for paradoxical vocal fold motion is described.
6. Patterson R, Schatz M, Horton M: Munchausen's stridor: Nonorganic laryngeal obstruction Clin Allergy 4(3):307-310, 1974.
This is the original article describing the clinical entity of paradoxical vocal fold motion.

Mark C. Weissler ▪ Charles S. Ebert, Jr.

16

Neck Masses in Adults

Introduction

The causes of neck masses include congenital disorders, infection, and neoplastic lesions (Fig. 16-1 and Box 16-1), among others. With careful attention to patient history, physical examination, and properly selected laboratory and imaging tests, the physician can usually arrive at a correct diagnosis quickly and efficiently.

Etiology, Pathogenesis, and Clinical Presentation

Age

The patient's age may give a clue to the diagnosis. Neck masses in infants and children are usually branchial cleft abnormalities, thyroglossal duct cysts, hemangiomas, lymphangiomas, or benign lymphadenopathy. Adolescents and young adults with significant cervical lymphadenopathy, malaise, and pharyngitis often have infectious mononucleosis. Single large, inflamed anterolateral neck masses that develop after upper respiratory infections in this age group suggest branchial cleft cysts. Multiple rubbery, low neck masses, night sweats, fever, and malaise may indicate Hodgkin's disease. Metastatic cancer, primary salivary gland infections or neoplasms, and lymphomas are common causes of neck masses in older adults (see Box 16-1).

History

The history helps to limit the differential diagnosis. Infectious processes usually develop over hours to days and have associated pain, redness, warmth, and fever. Patients often have a preceding upper respiratory tract or dental infection. Infected congenital cysts may have enlarged on earlier occasions and resolved with antibiotic therapy. Submandibular gland infection often waxes and wanes, is exacerbated by eating, and causes a foul taste in the mouth as the gland decompresses. Hodgkin's disease is associated with night sweats, malaise, itching, and fever. Patients with cat-scratch disease give a history of cat contact.

Metastatic squamous cell carcinoma of the upper aerodigestive tract usually occurs in patients with a history of heavy smoking, many of whom also abuse alcohol. Odyno-phagia, dysphagia, dyspnea, otalgia, voice change, and weight loss are indicative of the primary malignancy. Patients with metastatic disease from distant sites may report symptoms of the primary tumor, such as cough, hemoptysis, abdominal pain, hematochezia, abnormal uterine bleeding, or difficulty urinating. Salivary gland neoplasms are usually painless and grow slowly, although high-grade malignancies may enlarge rapidly. Parotid gland malignancies sometimes cause facial nerve paralysis. Schwannomas, paragangliomas, dermoids, and other benign neoplasms typically grow slowly, cause few symptoms, and are noticed only coincidentally.

Physical Examination

The head and neck exam should include thorough visualization of the ears, nose, oral cavity, oropharynx, nasopharynx, hypopharynx, and larynx. In certain instances, general anesthesia may be required to perform an adequate exam in children. The fiberoptic laryngoscope is helpful in patients with brisk gag reflexes. Auscultation of the chest and over the neck mass may yield important data. Palpation for cervical, axillary, and inguinal lymphadenopathy and for liver or spleen enlargement may strengthen a suspicion of lymphoma. Breast, rectal, and pelvic exams are appropriate in many cases.

Mass consistency and location are critical in the neck examination. Metastatic squamous cell carcinoma feels firm and becomes fixed when advanced. Lymphoma or simple lymphadenopathy feels rubbery or soft, whereas branchial and other cysts are fluctuant. Infected lymph nodes or congenital cysts become tense. Infected masses become attached to the overlying skin as they begin to "point," are often warm and tender, and have erythema-

Figure 16-1 Neck Masses in Adults.

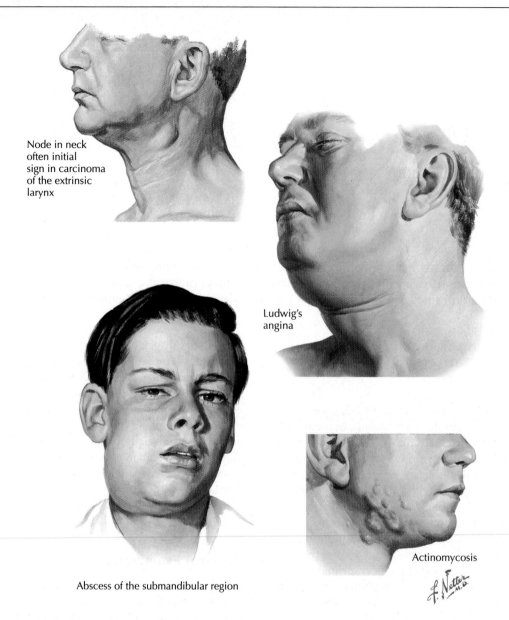

Node in neck often initial sign in carcinoma of the extrinsic larynx

Ludwig's angina

Abscess of the submandibular region

Actinomycosis

tous overlying skin. Capillary hemangiomas are generally flat and appear pink to red, whereas cavernous hemangiomas are raised, are purple to blue, and feel soft and cystic.

Thyroglossal duct cysts lie in or near the midline of the neck; most present below the level of the hyoid bone. Masses in the midline of the submental area can be dermoid cysts or teratomas; plunging ranulae may also present in this area. Masses in the submandibular region may develop secondary to sialadenitis, submandibular gland neoplasia, or enlarged submandibular lymph nodes from infection or metastatic tumor (most commonly squamous cell carcinoma of the oral cavity).

Posterior triangle lymph nodes suggest squamous cell carcinoma of the nasopharynx. The upper jugular lymph nodes are most commonly enlarged in cases of pharyngitis

and are often the first site of metastasis for oropharyngeal cancers. Enlarged supraclavicular lymph nodes suggest Hodgkin's disease or metastases from the thorax or abdomen. Masses in the lower anterior neck often indicate thyroid disease.

Differential Diagnosis

The differential diagnosis of a neck mass is extensive. One helpful way to categorize possible pathologic processes combines tissue of origin and disease type (see Box 16-1).

Congenital Lesions

Congenital neck masses may become apparent in infancy or later in life. Branchial cleft anomalies and thyroglossal duct cysts are most common. Branchial sinuses, or fistulas, present at birth as small draining puncta along the anterior border of the sternocleidomastoid muscle or in the preauricular area. Branchial cleft cysts present in young adults, typically during or after an acute upper respiratory infection. The cyst develops as a painful, warm, soft, or fluctuant area in the neck along the anterior border of the sternocleidomastoid muscle; deep neck abscess or cellulitis may complicate this problem. Surgical excision is usually required. Thyroglossal duct cysts occur in or near the midline of the neck, slightly below the level of the hyoid bone, and move superiorly with tongue protrusion. They represent thyroid gland remnants left during the gland's descent from its origin near the foramen cecum of the tongue to its normal paratracheal location. Dermoid cysts often develop in the submental area. These congenital cysts may present acutely when they become infected (usually during or after an upper respiratory infection) or chronically (as cystic neck masses) during young adult life.

Capillary and cavernous hemangiomas are benign tumors, generally obvious at or shortly after birth. Capillary hemangiomas (port wine stains) do not regress significantly with age. Recently, pigment-seeking laser therapy has yielded good results. Cavernous hemangiomas may regress significantly with age and therefore, call for a "watch and wait" approach. Overly aggressive early treatment may result in unnecessary damage to involved normal structures. Surgery is reserved for bleeding lesions or lesions obstructing the airway or digestive tract and hemangiomas that have not regressed significantly by the preschool years.

Cavernous lymphangiomas, or cystic hygromas, appear as soft, fleshy masses. Although benign, lymphangiomas in infants are often infiltrative and may cause obstructive symptoms requiring surgical excision. Total extirpation is not usually possible, so involved normal structures should not be sacrificed at surgery. Adults often manifest less infiltration, permitting more definitive surgical excision.

Neoplastic Lesions

Squamous cell carcinoma of the upper aerodigestive tract metastatic to cervical lymph nodes is the most common cause of a unilateral neck mass in middle-aged or older men with a history of tobacco use. Other common neoplasms include tumors of the parotid and submandibular salivary glands, Hodgkin's and non-Hodgkin's lymphomas, neurogenic tumors (schwannomas and neurofibromas), and paragangliomas (carotid body tumors and glomus tumors).

Squamous cell carcinomas metastatic to the neck often originate in the oral cavity, pharynx, or larynx but may come from the skin or more distant sites. Involved lymph nodes usually feel firm, and although initially mobile, they become fixed to surrounding structures as cancer breaks through their capsules. In advanced cases, there is multiple or bilateral node involvement. Usually, radical surgery with or without radiotherapy and chemotherapy is necessary (see Fig. 16-1).

Salivary gland tumors develop in older individuals. About 80% of parotid gland neoplasms, mostly pleomorphic adenomas, are benign. The most common malignant parotid gland tumor is the mucoepidermoid carcinoma. About 50% of submandibular gland neoplasms are benign. The most common benign submandibular gland neoplasm is the pleomorphic adenoma; the most common malignant tumor is adenoid cystic carcinoma. Surgical excision is usually necessary, with additional postoperative radiation for high-grade malignancies.

Involved cervical lymph nodes in Hodgkin's disease feel softer and more rubbery than those of squamous cell carcinoma. This lymphoma often causes enlargement of multiple nodes in the lower neck. Non-Hodgkin's lymphoma generally presents in older patients. Enlarged nodes are often matted and multiple, again having a rubbery rather than a hard infiltrative feel. It sometimes involves the tissue of the Waldeyer ring (palatine tonsils, lingual tonsils, and adenoids). Diagnosis is confirmed by biopsy. Treatment consists of radiation therapy, chemotherapy, or both.

Schwannomas usually grow on the vagus nerve or cervical sympathetic trunk. Neural function usually remains normal, as the lesion enlarges very slowly over many years. Surgical removal is frequently recommended. Neurofibromas in the neck, often multiple, can coexist with neurofibromas elsewhere and may involve any nerves. Surgeons generally reserve excision for solitary lesions or those causing obstructive symptoms or severe deformity. Most neurogenic tumors are benign; however, malignant degeneration has been described, usually marked by a rapid growth phase or loss of nerve function.

Paragangliomas are usually benign and occasionally multiple; these highly vascular neoplasms often produce bruits. Carotid body tumors typically splay the internal and external carotid arteries. Glomus jugulare and glomus vagale tumors, originating in specialized paraganglion tissue along the internal jugular vein and the vagus nerve, respectively, often erode the temporal bone and present high in the neck behind the angle of the mandible. Surgical removal is generally recommended.

Infectious Neck Masses

These may be indolent or fulminant. Simple lymphadenopathy often occurs with acute viral or bacterial pharyngitis, sinusitis, or tooth infections. Generally, these nodes feel soft and shrink over days to weeks after the acute infection resolves. Suppurative lymphadenopathy occurs when the center of a node necroses and an abscess develops. Most abscesses require antibiotic therapy and surgical drainage; untreated suppurative lymphadenopathy can lead to deep neck infections with potential for spread to the mediastinum that may be fatal.

Certain infection paths are common enough to have their own identity. Ludwig's angina begins with an infection in the oral cavity of dental origin. Sublingual inflammation and swelling retrodisplace and elevate the tongue, possibly leading to acute upper airway obstruction (see Fig. 16-1). Bezold's abscess develops when a mastoid infection breaks out inferiorly into the deep neck. Deep neck space infections require emergency hospitalization, intravenous antibiotics, and usually surgical drainage.

The parotid and submandibular glands may become infected. Acute parotid sialadenitis afflicts elderly individuals most commonly, especially when they get dehydrated; it may also reflect sialolithiasis. Cystic degeneration of the parotid gland has been described in patients with HIV infection. Acute submandibular sialadenitis often follows sialolithiasis. Patients often note intermittent submandibular swelling associated with eating. Parotitis is usually treated with hydration, intravenous antibiotics, local heat, massage, and sialogogues. Recurrent submandibular sialadenitis is usually treated with resection of the submandibular gland during a quiescent period (see Fig. 16-1).

Other infectious processes include atypical tuberculosis (scrofula), best treated by surgical excision of the involved lymph nodes; cat-scratch disease, which frequently requires surgical drainage; and actinomycosis, which often causes multiple chronically draining sinus tracts with sulfur granules of matted organisms (see Fig. 16-1). Many patients with HIV infection develop cervical lymphadenopathy; this complication does not generally require specific treatment unless rapid expansion suggests lymphomatous involvement.

Other Common Neck Masses

These include prominent normal structures, such as the (pulsatile) carotid bulb or the (hard) transverse process of the first cervical vertebra. Careful palpation should delineate these bilateral (although frequently asymmetric) structures. Carotid aneurysm, although uncommon, should be suspected if the patient has an expanding neck mass or a history of cervical trauma. Thyroid masses are quite common. Diffuse nodular thyroid enlargement present for many years suggests simple goiter. Solitary thyroid nodules, although usually benign, may represent thyroid cancer and, thus, demand evaluation. Epidermal and dermal inclusion cysts are very superficial and often result from recurrent cutaneous inflammation.

Diagnostic Approach

Laboratory Studies

A variety of studies may prove useful. A heterophil antibody test may reveal mononucleosis in the young patient with pharyngitis and cervical adenopathy out of proportion to that expected in cases of simple upper respiratory infection. Serologic tests for HIV infection may help in the evaluation of an at-risk patient with multiple enlarged cervical lymph nodes or parotid gland enlargement. Intradermal antigen testing for tuberculosis and a control substance, thyroid function tests, and a complete blood cell count with differential can each provide useful data in appropriate situations.

Imaging Studies

Chest x-rays may show lung carcinoma, metastases, findings consistent with lymphoma or tuberculosis, or tracheal deviation. Computed tomography (CT) scanning (or possibly magnetic resonance imaging) can delineate cervical anatomic relationships and reveal a pathologic process, such as a primary aerodigestive tract cancer. Although used less frequently since the advent of fine-needle cytologic examination, thyroid scanning still proves useful in some cases. Anteroposterior and lateral neck x-rays can show tracheal deviation or encroachment on the airway (before or instead of CT scans).

Further Diagnostic Workup

Patients should undergo complete clinical evaluation before any biopsy; the otolaryngologist with head-and-neck surgical training can best evaluate patients with neck masses of concern. Cytologic examination of neck masses by fine-needle aspiration is very helpful. More than 90% sensitive and specific, cytology often aids in counseling patients preoperatively or in directing further diagnostic maneuvers.

Patients with masses that represent metastases should undergo direct laryngoscopy, pharyngoscopy, esophagoscopy, and bronchoscopy under anesthesia before any excisional neck biopsy. If endoscopy reveals no obvious primary lesion, especially if previous cytologic evaluation documented squamous cell carcinoma in the neck, biopsies of the tongue base, the tonsils, and the nasopharynx should be obtained. If negative, the surgeon can perform an open neck biopsy and obtain frozen sections. If no primary tumor is found, but the open neck biopsy reveals unequivocal squamous cell carcinoma, a neck dissection is performed at the time of biopsy. There is a 20% incidence of second primary tumors in patients with upper aerodigestive tract malignancies.

If open neck biopsy does not reveal squamous cell carcinoma, the surgeon and pathologist should be ready to thoroughly evaluate the tissue specimens. Cultures for aerobes, anaerobes, acid-fast bacteria, and fungi should be obtained, and material should be processed for immunohistochemical or electron microscopic study if indicated by the frozen section findings.

Management and Therapy

Optimum Treatment

Optimal therapy demands that a patient presenting with a neck mass have a thorough examination of the upper aerodigestive tract. If no obvious benign reason for the mass is found, a fine-needle aspirate and other diagnostic workup as outlined, is indicated.

Avoiding Treatment Errors

Major errors in treatment include delay in diagnosis of a cancer of the upper aerodigestive tract and inappropriate open incisional biopsy without a thorough examination for a primary tumor. Doing so may result in spread of the tumor or contiguous tissue, which may be detrimental to the patient. Fine-needle aspiration is the preferred initial method of histologic examination.

Future Directions

New treatment modalities for head and neck cancer are needed. The mainstay of treatment for many years has been surgical excision and radiation. New organ preservation protocols using combinations of chemotherapy and radiation are becoming more popular. New treatments such as gene therapy, adenovirus vectors, antiangiogenesis factors, and immune modulators are on the horizon.

Additional Resources

Alvi A, Johnson JT: The neck mass: A challenging differential diagnosis. Postgrad Med 97:87-90, 93-94, 97, 1995.

This good general reference discusses the importance of accurate history taking with the use of diagnostic tests to evaluate patients with neck masses.

Schwetschenau E, Kelley DJ: The adult neck mass. American Academy of Family Physicians Website. Available at: http://www.aafp.org/afp/20020901/831.html. Accessed July 30, 2006.

This current overview of the evaluation of the adult neck mass from the primary care physician's perspective provides clinical photographs and nodal drainage patterns.

Armstrong WB, Giglio MF: Is this lump in the neck anything to worry about? Postgrad Med 104:63-64, 67-71, 75-76, 1998.

This good general reference provides an overview of the process of working up neck masses. Obtaining histories and performing thorough physical exams are important parts of this process as well as referral to an otolaryngologist when there is uncertainty of diagnosis.

Park YW: Evaluation of neck masses in children. Am Fam Physician 51:1904-1912, 1995.

This good general reference includes a thorough discussion of the evaluation and differential diagnosis of neck masses in children.

Schuller DE, Nicholson RE: Clinical evaluation and surgical treatment of malignant tumors of the neck. In Thawley SE, Panje WR, Batsakis JG, Lindberg RD (eds): Comprehensive Management of Head and Neck Tumors, 2nd ed. Philadelphia, WB Saunders, 1999, pp 1395-1415.

A more thorough discussion from an otolaryngology, head and neck surgery perspective, this chapter is a comprehensive overview of the evaluation and surgical management of head and neck malignancy.

Sobol SM, Bailey SB: Evaluation and surgical management of tumors of the neck: Benign tumors. In Thawley SE, Panje WR, Batsakis JG, Lindberg RD (eds): Comprehensive Management of Head and Neck Tumors, 2nd ed. Philadelphia, WB Saunders, 1999, pp 1416-1449.

A more thorough discussion from an otolaryngology, head and neck surgery perspective, this chapter is a comprehensive overview of the evaluation and surgical management of benign tumors of the head and neck.

EVIDENCE

1. Goldstein DP, Irish JC: Head and neck squamous cell carcinoma in the young patient. Curr Opin Otolaryngol Head Neck Surg 13(4):207-211, 2005.

   This is a brief and concise overview, from an otolaryngology, head and neck surgery perspective, of a new demographic of patients (those ≤45 years of age) who develop squamous cell carcinoma of the head and neck. This article contrasts this age group of patients with the traditional demographic and reviews the evidence of treatment patterns.

2. Back G, Sood S: The management of early laryngeal cancer: Options for patients and therapists. Curr Opin Otolaryngol Head Neck Surg 2:85-91, 2005.

   This article, from an otolaryngology, head neck surgery perspective, evaluates the current evidence for optimal treatment of early-stage laryngeal cancer. Multiple therapeutic modalities are available, and treatment choice should take into account post-treatment morbidity, patient quality of life, patient preference, and voice quality.

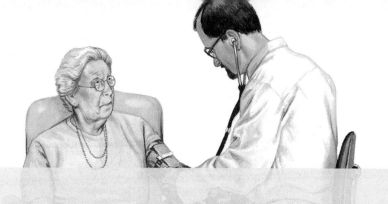
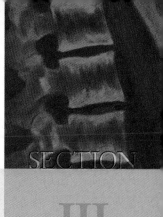

Disorders of the Respiratory System

Robert M. Aris

Cough

Introduction

Cough is the number one reason patients seek medical attention. Although an occasional cough is normal, excessive coughing or chronic coughing that produces blood or thick, discolored mucus is not. Cough is a symptom; its causes exist on a continuum from acute (<3 weeks) to subacute (3 to 8 weeks) to chronic (>8 weeks), and the duration is not linked to the potential seriousness of the underlying condition. Interestingly, smokers rarely report cough as a symptom and may consider it a normal phenomenon. Although they are excluded from most studies of chronic cough, making it difficult to cite an exact figure for how commonly it occurs, smoking and its related diseases are a major cause of acute and chronic cough.

Serious and potentially life-threatening causes include pneumonia, congestive heart failure (CHF), pulmonary embolism, and severe exacerbations of asthma or chronic obstructive pulmonary disease (COPD). Nonserious acute cough stems most commonly from viral upper respiratory infections (URIs) but may also be caused by mild exacerbations of chronic underlying lung diseases or environmental or occupational exposures. URIs are usually viral in nature and are considered benign and self-limiting. Pneumonic cough, usually with purulent sputum and associated fever or chills, chest pain, and dyspnea, is beyond the scope of this chapter (see Chapter 18).

Subacute cough, lasting 3 to 8 weeks, most commonly is postinfectious in nature following a common URI. Because this type of cough is self-limited, it is important not to initiate a complex workup if suspected. Other causes of subacute cough, including asthma, upper airway cough syndrome (previously known as postnasal drip), and gastroesophageal reflux disease (GERD), overlap with the causes of chronic cough and require similar diagnostic workups and treatments. Cough may, by itself, have clinical complications ranging from conjunctival bleeding, epistaxis, tussive or post-tussive syncope or vomiting, stress urinary incontinence, rib fractures, cervical disk herniation, abdominal hernias, esophageal rupture, cardiac arrhythmias and infarction, pulmonary barotrauma, and even cerebral air embolism. In addition, chronic cough takes a toll on quality of life, with significant effects on social relationship, sleep, concentration, mood, and daily activities affecting up to 80% of chronic cough patients. Therefore, chronic cough warrants a thorough evaluation.

Etiology and Pathogenesis

Asthma, upper airway cough syndrome, and GERD are the most common causes of subacute and chronic cough and account for about 75% of all cases. Each can present with cough as the only symptom. Between 75% and 90% of cases of chronic cough are a result of a single cause, 5% to 20% are a result of two causes (e.g., allergic rhinitis and asthma together), and less than 5% are a result of three or more causes simultaneously. Whooping cough (*Bacillus pertussis*) has made a strong resurgence, increasing 10-fold to a prevalence of about 1% in the United States (with a similar prevalence in Western Europe) in the past decade.

Whooping cough now needs to be considered in the differential diagnosis of both adolescents and adults with severe cough, whereas, in the past, it had largely been a disease in infants. In some modern series, it accounts for as much as 20% of the cases of prolonged (≥8 weeks) cough.

Statistics regarding the etiology of cough depend, in part, on the source of the information. Experience from general practice suggests that more than 90% of patients with chronic cough had either asthma or upper airway disease. In contrast, specialists in pulmonary medicine find that about 50% of their cough patients have COPD, bronchiectasis, pulmonary fibrosis, or lung cancer. Usually, smokers are excluded from chronic cough studies, a practice that leads to an underestimate of smoking-related diseases. Interestingly, women are referred to specialists more often than men, and this may be explained by differences in smoking habits or the social consequences of the symptom. Women also appear to have an intrinsically heightened cough response. More than 100 diseases are associated with chronic cough, but most are uncommon. Occupational diseases (especially in miners and tunnel and concrete manufacturing workers) are becoming increasingly linked to chronic cough. In addition, indoor and outdoor air pollutants (ozone, nitrogen dioxide, sulfur dioxide, and particulates) are becoming recognized as the cause of chronic cough. Although the prevalence of air pollution–induced or occupational cough is not known, the clinician should remain vigilant to the role of environmental factors in chronic cough. Finally, a higher percentage of patients being referred for cough in recent studies have unexplained cough (despite a full workup), a problem once referred to as "habit" or "psychogenic" cough.

Clinical Presentation

Chronic productive coughs with purulent sputum are usually seen in chronic bronchitis and bronchiectasis and, less commonly, from lung abscesses. Productive coughs with white to off-white sputum may be seen in asthma or postnasal drip. In the latter conditions, the secretions are usually from the upper respiratory tract. Dry chronic coughs usually result from asthma (many sufferers never report wheezing), interstitial lung disease (ILD), CHF, and the use of angiotensin-converting enzyme (ACE) inhibitors. Whooping cough should be considered when coughing paroxysms or an inspiratory "whoop" is present, especially in those exposed to a confirmed case. Childhood vaccination may not prevent whooping cough in adults but may lessen its severity.

Physical examination may detect some causes of chronic cough, including chronic airway obstruction if expiratory rhonchi or wheezes are present. CHF and ILD present with wet or dry inspiratory crackles, respectively. Inflamed nasal mucosa indicates the diagnosis of chronic rhinosinusitis. Lower extremity edema and an abnormal heart exam point to the diagnosis of CHF, whereas extremity clubbing may lead to the diagnoses of lung malignancy, ILD, or bronchiectasis.

Differential Diagnosis

An adequate history is vital in establishing a diagnosis. In smokers, the cough is considered a consequence of cigarette-related disease until proved otherwise. The most common causes of chronic cough in nonsmokers are asthma, upper airway cough syndrome, and GERD (Table 17-1). Chronic bronchitis is the most common diagnosis in smokers. Determining the precipitating factors for cough provides useful clues to the underlying cause. The

Table 17-1 Etiology of Chronic Cough with a Normal Chest Radiograph

Cause	Prevalence (%)
Upper airway cough syndrome (previously postnasal drip)	28-41
Asthma	24-33
GERD	10-21
Chronic bronchitis	5-10
Unexplained cough (previously "habit" or psychogenic)	10
Bronchiectasis	4
ACE inhibitors, tracheomalacia, eosinophilic bronchitis, etc.	5

ACE, angiotensin-converting enzyme; GERD, gastroesophageal reflux disease.

timing of cough may be important (e.g., it might occur postprandially in aspiration-induced cough or GERD, or nocturnally in asthma or CHF). Patients with chronic bronchitis or bronchiectasis often cough most vigorously after awakening because secretions have pooled in the lung during sleep. Often, response to specific antitussive therapy is critical to make the final diagnosis of cough (e.g., response to antihistamine or decongestants implicates either the common cold or upper airway cough syndrome, grades A and B*).

Diagnostic Approach

Diagnostic tests are unnecessary if the history or physical examination suggests benign or self-limited causes. Symptoms and signs suggestive of URI (i.e., cold) or upper airway cough syndrome (postnasal drip) warrant a therapeutic trial with an over-the-counter (first-generation) antihistamine-decongestant or a nonsteroidal anti-inflammatory drug before diagnostic testing (grade A). A cough caused by an ACE inhibitor, regardless of the temporal association between the two, is best managed with a trial off the drug or, if mild, observation while therapy continues (grade B). A chronic postinfectious cough is best managed with simple observation because it will probably spontaneously remit, but a short antitussive (inhaled anticholinergic agent or corticosteroid) therapy trial may be helpful (grade B). Otherwise, diagnostic tests should be directed by the history and physical examination. A chest radiograph is essential early in the investigation and has the potential to diagnose many serious parenchymal lung diseases (e.g., bronchogenic malignancy, CHF, ILD, lung abscess, or emphysema with a bronchitic component; Box 17-1 and Fig. 17-1). Symptoms suggestive of asthma or chronic bronchitis are more effectively evaluated with pulmonary function tests (PFTs) than chest

*The grading scale for diagnostics and treatments is evidence based: A, strong; B, moderate; C, weak; D, negative; I, inconclusive.

Figure 17-1 Causes of Chronic Cough with a Normal Chest X-Ray.

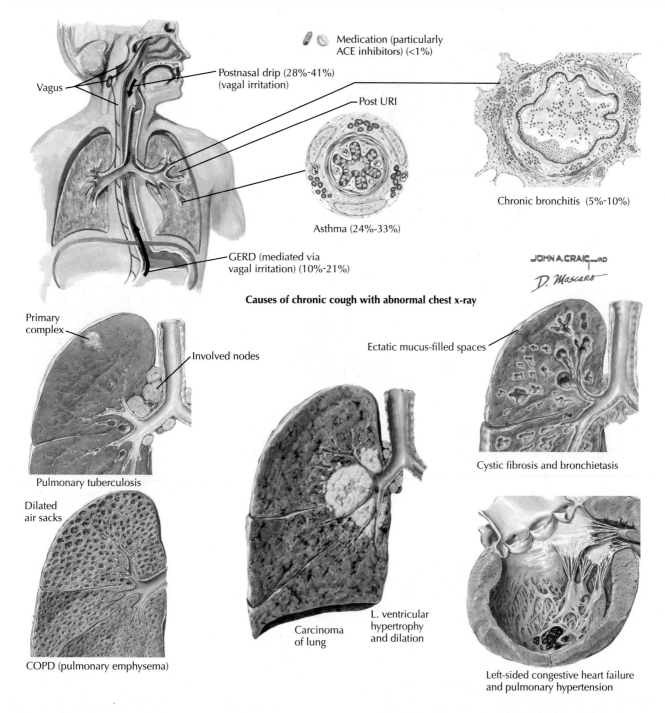

Medication (particularly ACE inhibitors) (<1%)

Vagus

Postnasal drip (28%-41%) (vagal irritation)

Post URI

Chronic bronchitis (5%-10%)

Asthma (24%-33%)

GERD (mediated via vagal irritation) (10%-21%)

JOHN A.CRAIG—AD

D. Mascaro

Causes of chronic cough with abnormal chest x-ray

Primary complex

Involved nodes

Ectatic mucus-filled spaces

Pulmonary tuberculosis

Cystic fibrosis and bronchietasis

Dilated air sacks

Carcinoma of lung

L. ventricular hypertrophy and dilation

COPD (pulmonary emphysema)

Left-sided congestive heart failure and pulmonary hypertension

radiography. Patients with chronic cough from advanced lung disease related to the airways or parenchyma should undergo both an anatomic (chest radiograph) and physiologic (i.e., PFTs) workup. Eosinophilic bronchitis should be considered in patients with normal PFTs and sputum or bronchial wash eosinophilia. Whooping cough can be diagnosed clinically or by culture of the organism from nasopharyngeal aspirates or by using polymerase chain reaction techniques, but the latter two are problematic (special culture media needed and good quality controls)

and have the highest yield early in the illness before patients are likely to seek medical attention.

A recommended diagnostic protocol is outlined below, but individualization based on the history and physical examination is important (Fig. 17-2). A chest radiograph is usually the most sensitive test. If a cause is identified from the chest radiograph, the workup proceeds on the basis of the abnormality (see Box 17-1). Sputum cultures are necessary if infection is suspected. Bronchoscopy or lung biopsy can confirm the presence of a malignant or an

Figure 17-2 Diagnostic Testing in Chronic Cough.

Chest x-ray

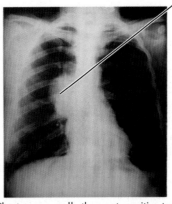

Hilar tumor demonstrated on chest x-ray

Sputum studies

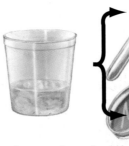

Sputum cultures should be obtained if infection is suspected

Chest x-ray usually the most sensitive test; if cause identified by chest x-ray, workup proceeds on basis of abnormality

JOHN A. CRAIG—AD

Endoscopic appearance of tumor in bronchial lumen

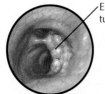

Bronchoscopy and lung biopsy

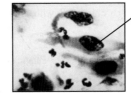

Malignant cells demonstrated on exam of scrapings

Endoscopic biopsy of bronchial lesion

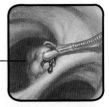

Bronchoscopy or lung biopsy can confirm presence of malignant or inflammatory entity

Pulmonary function testing (spirometry)

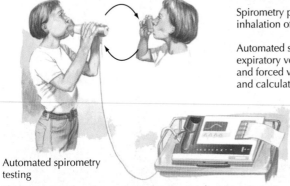

Spirometry performed before and after inhalation of short-acting bronchodilator

Automated spirometry measures forced expiratory volume in 1 second (FEV_1) and forced vital capacity (FVC) and calculates FEV_1/FVC ratio

Peak flow studies

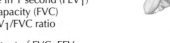

Printout of FVC, FEV_1, and FEV_1/FVC ratio

Test performed 3 times and results compared with best

If asthma remains a possibility after a normal exam and spirometry, home peak flow monitoring may demonstrate classic variability seen in asthma

Automated spirometry testing

If x-ray is normal or shows signs of quiescent disease, spirometry before and after bronchodilator use is updated if airway disease (asthma) suspected

---

Box 17-1   Common Diseases Causing Subacute and Chronic Cough Associated with an Abnormal Chest Radiograph

Bronchogenic carcinoma
Interstitial lung disease (e.g., pulmonary fibrosis, sarcoidosis)
Emphysema and chronic bronchitis
Congestive heart failure
Cystic fibrosis and bronchiectasis
Tuberculosis and nontuberculous mycobacterial infection
Alveolar hemorrhage syndromes
Pulmonary hypertension

---

inflammatory entity. When the chest radiograph is normal or shows signs of a quiescent disease, spirometry before and after bronchodilator therapy should be obtained if airway diseases (e.g., COPD and asthma) are suspected. Many patients with asthma show some evidence of airflow obstruction (forced expiratory volume in 1 second [FEV_1] <80% of predicted; FEV_1/forced vital capacity [FVC] ratio <80% of predicted; low forced expiratory flow 25% to 75%; or a large [>10% increase in FEV_1] bronchodilator response). Additional PFTs, including diffusing capacity and lung volume measurements, may be useful in a subset of patients with normal spirometry or to better define the extent of disease in those with abnormal spirometry. If the chest radiograph is normal in a smoker or an individual exposed to occupational or seasonal antigens or environmental irritants, the patient should be encouraged to avoid the irritating factor before additional diagnostic testing. Unfortunately, many patients cannot or will not avoid potential irritants, and PFTs may prove useful in defining the disease and its severity (if only to reinforce the need for irritant avoidance).

If the history, physical examination, chest radiograph, and spirometry do not suggest a cause for the chronic cough, pulmonary consultation may be indicated. If asthma remains a possibility with a normal examination and spirometry, home peak flow monitoring or methacholine challenge testing may be helpful to make the diagnosis. High-resolution chest computed tomography (CT) is the best diagnostic test if clinical suspicion for ILD exists based on the chest x-ray or restriction is present on PFTs (total lung capacity <80% predicted or FVC <80%). High-resolution CT is also useful to diagnose bronchiectasis because chest x-rays are insensitive. If GERD is suspected on the basis of symptoms, 24-hour esophageal pH monitoring may prove diagnostic, but many clinicians opt for a trial of therapy to reduce gastric acidity to determine whether the cough improves. Sinus x-rays are rarely helpful when symptoms are not present. If patients give a history of an upper airway source of cough (e.g., a tickle in the throat), laryngoscopy may exclude vocal cord nodules and lesions. Bronchoscopy or cardiac evaluation for left ventricular function is used as a last resort, but the diagnostic yield is low if other testing is negative.

Management and Therapy

The majority (>80%) of patients with subacute and chronic cough benefit from treatment. Because chronic cough has more than one cause in at least 20% of patients, add-on therapy should be considered if there is a poor response to the initial, cause-directed therapy. The management principles for intractable cough of unknown cause are not well defined. Some causes of cough are etiologically related to or trigger other causes of cough. For example, many patients with asthma have been found to have GERD, and in turn, chronic cough from any cause has been found to precipitate GERD. Thus, the potential for a self-perpetuating cycle exists.

Optimum Treatment

Specific Antitussive Therapy

Specific antitussive therapy has a high likelihood of success (>80%) because a specific cause for chronic cough is usually found (>80% based on previous studies). Common colds and upper airway cough syndrome treatments were men-

tioned previously. Allergic rhinitis can be treated with intranasal corticosteroids or combination antihistamine-decongestants (grade B). Asthma therapy guidelines focus on obtaining disease control with inhaled corticosteroids and leukotriene modifiers (e.g., montelukast) (grade A, see Chapter 20) and providing acute relief with bronchodilators. Infectious sinusitis should be treated with antibiotics.

Patients with chronic cough from GERD should use an antireflux regimen (weight loss; elevation of the head of the bed on blocks; avoidance of bedtime snacks, caffeine, and theophylline and antireflux medication) (grade B, see Chapter 50). A trial of medications is appropriate without additional diagnostic testing even if there are no reflux symptoms. H_2 receptor antagonists and proton pump inhibitors are effective in reducing cough in roughly half of the patients. Case reports of the prokinetic agent, metoclopramide, indicate that it is also effective. Other antireflux agents such as antacids and cytoprotective agents (e.g., sucralfate) have been disappointing in the management of cough. Patients with aspiration-induced cough (oral-pharyngeal dysphagia) should be diagnosed by a speech therapist with a swallowing evaluation and treated with either dietary modification or, when especially severe and intractable, gastric tube feedings (grade B).

Chronic bronchitis, chronic cough, and sputum expectoration occurring on most days for at least 3 months and for at least 2 consecutive years is successfully treated with smoking cessation alone in more than 90% (grade A). More than half the time, cough disappears within a month of cessation. For infectious exacerbations of chronic bronchitis or bronchiectasis, antibiotics and bronchodilators are the mainstay of therapy (grade A). There is no role for prophylactic antibiotics or expectorants in stable patients with chronic bronchitis (grade I). Chronic cough from COPD should be treated accordingly (see Chapter 22). The treatment of cough caused by potentially severe diseases, including ILD, CHF (see Chapter 34), and tuberculosis (see Chapter 103), should be directed at the underlying cause. Chest physiotherapy, hypertonic saline, and inhaled tobramycin may help cough in patients with chronic suppurative diseases (e.g., cystic fibrosis and bronchiectasis; grade B).

Eosinophilic bronchitis should be treated with inhaled corticosteroids (grade B). Patients with confirmed or probable whooping cough should receive a macrolide antibiotic for a week and should be isolated for 5 days from the start of treatment (grade A); early treatment within the first few weeks will diminish the coughing paroxysms and prevent spread of the disease; the patient is unlikely to respond to treatment beyond this period. In adults with chronic unexplained cough, common psychosocial problems such as anxiety, depression, domestic violence, and abuse or neglect are often associated with somatization disorders that should be evaluated by a psychotherapist (strongly recommended on the basis of expert opinion).

Nonspecific Antitussive Therapy

Ipratropium bromide is effective in suppressing the cough reflex through the efferent limb or decreasing airway secretions. A trial of inhaled or oral corticosteroids is often used in patients with intractable cough. This therapy may be particularly valuable in undiagnosed asthmatic patients and in patients with eosinophilic bronchitis. Non-narcotic medications, such as dextromethorphan and levopromazine, are useful for acute or chronic bronchitis but are not recommended for cough caused by the common cold or URI because of lack of proven efficacy (grade D). Narcotics (e.g., codeine, morphine) are not very effective antitussive agents and should be used judiciously. Guaifenesin and mucolytic drugs are of unclear benefit. It should be remembered that patients in the placebo arm of many cough studies improve, suggesting a strong "treatment" effect irrespective of drug used.

Avoiding Treatment Errors

Because chronic cough is, in and of itself, a nuisance symptom, the main potential treatment error is to misdiagnose the underlying disease. Thus, for a persistent cough, the diagnostic approach recommended previously is designed to detect important diseases.

Future Directions

Because cough is a common symptom of underlying respiratory and nonrespiratory disease, much of the future research in this area will address the underlying pathologic processes rather than the symptom itself. Studies measuring exhaled nitric oxide and inflammatory mediators in breath condensate or bronchoalveolar lavage samples may shed important light on the role of lung inflammation in the pathogenesis of chronic cough.

EVIDENCE

1. Birring SS, Berry M, Brightling CE, Pavord ID: Eosinophilic bronchitis: Clinical features, management and pathogenesis. Am J Respir Med 2(2):169-173, 2003.
   This article reviews the relatively new disorder, eosinophilic bronchitis.
2. Chang AB, Lasserson TJ, Kiljander TO, et al: Systematic review and meta-analysis of randomized controlled trials of gastro-oesophageal reflux interventions for chronic cough associated with gastro-oesophageal reflux. BMJ 332(7532):11-17, 2006.
   This is an up-to-date review of the value of proton pump inhibition in treating cough.
3. Crowcroft NS, Pebody RG: Recent developments in pertussis. Lancet 367(9526):1926-1936, 2006.
   This review article covers the resurgence of pertussis in the modern era.
4. Dicpinigaitis PV: Angiotensin-converting enzyme inhibitor-induced cough: ACCP evidence-based clinical practice guidelines. Chest 129(1 Suppl):169S-173S, 2006.
   This is a review article on ACE inhibition and cough.
5. Irwin RS, Baumann MH, Bolser DC, et al: Diagnosis and management of cough executive summary: ACCP evidence-based clinical practice guidelines. Chest 129(1 Suppl):1S-23S, 2006.
   The authors provide a summary of the most comprehensive, up-to-date, evidenced-based guidelines for the diagnosis and management of cough.
6. Pratter MR: Chronic upper airway cough syndrome secondary to rhinosinus diseases (previously referred to as postnasal drip syndrome): ACCP evidence-based clinical practice guidelines. Chest 129(1 Suppl):63S-71S, 2006.
   This article reviews UACS, or the more commonly used term, postnasal drip and cough.

David J. Weber ▪ Amanda Peppercorn ▪ William A. Rutala

18

Community-Acquired Pneumonia

Introduction

Community-acquired pneumonia (CAP) is an important source of morbidity and mortality in the United States. Each year, CAP results in about 10 million physician visits, 500,000 hospitalizations, and 45,000 deaths. About 258 cases of CAP per 100,000 population and 962 cases per 100,000 persons older than 65 years require hospitalization. The mortality rate of persons hospitalized is about 14% (range, 2% to 30%).

The following recommendations for the diagnosis and treatment of CAP are largely drawn from guidelines published by the Infectious Diseases Society of America (IDSA) and the American Thoracic Society (ATS), including an update published in 2007.

Etiology and Pathogenesis

Community-acquired pneumonia is an acute infection of the pulmonary parenchyma associated with symptoms of infection and accompanied by the presence of a new infiltrate on a chest radiograph or auscultatory findings consistent with pneumonia (such as altered breath sounds or localized rales). When CAP occurs in a patient who is hospitalized or who is a resident of an extended care facility, the infection is designated as "hospital" and "health care–associated pneumonia" and is treated according to different principles and guidelines. CAP in the normal host is caused by a variety of pathogens, with *Streptococcus pneumoniae* the most commonly identified (Table 18-1). The epidemiology, etiology, pathogenesis, and treatment of CAP differ from health care–associated pneumonia, pneumonia in the immunocompromised host, and pneumonia associated with travel outside the United States.

The lower respiratory tract is constantly exposed to microbes that are present in the upper airways through microaspiration. Usually, the lower airways remain sterile because of the pulmonary defense mechanisms, including the cough reflex and mucociliary clearance. The development of CAP indicates either a defect in defenses (e.g., damage to epithelial cells from smoking), exposure to an especially virulent microbe, or an overwhelming inoculum. Although microaspiration is the most common mechanism that allows pathogens to reach the lung, hematogenous spread from a distant infected site, direct spread from a contiguous focus, and macroaspiration are other important mechanisms.

Clinical Presentation

Pneumonia should be suspected in patients with newly acquired lower respiratory symptoms such as cough, sputum production, pleuritic chest pain, and shortness of breath. Fever and chills are common. Elderly and immunocompromised patients may not manifest the classic symptoms of CAP such as fever and cough; if such patients exhibit a significant medical deterioration (e.g., decreased responsiveness, poor appetite, low-grade fever), CAP should remain high on the differential list.

Cough is the hallmark of pneumonia. Initially, it may be nonproductive, only to become productive with disease progression. The sputum may be yellow to green as a result of the action of myeloperoxidase produced by neutrophils. Green sputum occurs most commonly as a result of bacterial infection, but it may result from invasive viral illness. Occasionally, pigment-producing *Pseudomonas* species may present with green-colored sputum. The neutropenic patient will not produce purulent sputum even with a life-threatening pneumonia because of the inhibi-

Table 18-1 Most Common Etiologies of Community-Acquired Pneumonia

Patient Type	Etiology
Outpatient	*Streptococcus pneumoniae*
	Mycoplasma pneumoniae
	Haemophilus influenzae
	Chlamydophila pneumoniae
	Respiratory viruses*
Inpatient	*S. pneumoniae*
	M. pneumoniae
	C. pneumoniae
	H. influenzae
	Legionella spp.
	Aspiration (mixed flora, especially anaerobes)
	Respiratory viruses*
Inpatient (ICU)	*S. pneumoniae*
	Staphylococcus aureus
	Legionella spp.
	Gram-negative bacilli
	H. influenzae

*Influenza A and B, adenovirus, respiratory syncytial virus (RSV), and parainfluenza.

Adapted from Mandell LA, Wunderink RG, Anzueto A, et al: Infectious Diseases Society of America/American Thoracic Society Consensus Guidelines on the management of community-acquired pneumonia in adults. Clin Infect Dis 44(Suppl 2):S27-S72, 2007.

tion of an inflammatory response to the pathogen. Signs of pneumonia include elevated temperature, elevated respiratory and heart rates, hypoxia, use of accessory muscles, and general ill appearance. Auscultatory signs are secondary to alveolar infiltration and include dullness to percussion, decreased breath sounds, rales, and egophony.

Pneumonia is traditionally divided into typical and atypical categories. Typical pneumonia is caused by extracellular bacterial pathogens such as *Streptococcus pneumoniae*, *Haemophilus influenzae*, *Klebsiella pneumoniae*, and *Staphylococcus aureus* (Figs. 18-1, 18-2, and 18-3). Its characteristics include sudden onset, prominent pulmonary symptoms and signs, purulent sputum, and clinical and radiographic evidence of lobar consolidation. Atypical pathogens consist of viruses and intracellular bacteria such as *Legionella* (Fig. 18-4) and *Mycoplasma* species and *Chlamydophila pneumoniae* (formerly *Chlamydia pneumoniae*). Pneumonia caused by atypical pathogens is often characterized by a stepwise fever curve, prolonged prodrome, frequent extrapulmonary symptoms and signs, nonpurulent sputum (i.e., dry cough), and diffuse infiltrates on chest radiography, often in an interstitial pattern. Extrapulmonary symptoms include headache and bullous myringitis (blood blebs on the tympanic membrane) with *Mycoplasma* species, headache and myalgias with viral influenza, and gastrointestinal symptoms (e.g., nausea, vomiting, diarrhea) with *Legionella* species. Often, the differentiation of typical from atypical

pneumonia is not clear because patients present with overlapping symptoms.

Differential Diagnosis

The differential diagnosis of lower respiratory tract illness is extensive and includes both upper and lower respiratory tract infections as well as noninfectious disorders. Important noninfectious etiologies that can mimic pneumonia include aspiration of blood or gastric contents, pulmonary emboli with or without pulmonary infarction, congestive heart failure, cryptogenic organizing pneumonia, primary pulmonary malignancy, metastatic cancer, acute respiratory distress syndrome, drug toxicity, pulmonary hemorrhage, sarcoidosis, and vasculitis (e.g., Wegener's granulomatosis). Many of these disorders are associated with fever, including aspiration of gastric contents, malignancy, pulmonary emboli with infarction, and vasculitis.

Diagnostic Approach

The diagnosis of CAP requires a combination of clinical and laboratory assessments (including microbiologic data). Differentiation of CAP from upper respiratory tract infection (URI) is important because most URIs and acute bronchitis are of viral origin and do not require antiinfective therapy. However, rapid testing for influenza A and B is indicated during epidemic periods because a positive result warrants treatment with a neuraminidase inhibitor (i.e., oseltamivir, zanamivir). Patients with bacterial pneumonia require appropriate antibiotic therapy. Obtaining a chest radiograph in persons with symptoms and signs suggestive of lower respiratory tract infection helps to substantiate the diagnosis of pneumonia. In addition, a chest radiograph is often useful for determining the etiologic diagnosis and the prognosis; it also raises suspicion for alternative diagnoses or associated conditions. For example, chest radiographs in patients with *Pneumocystis jiroveci* (formerly *Pneumocystis carinii*) pneumonia are normal at the time of presentation (false-negative results) in up to 30% of infected patients.

A few clinical pearls are helpful in evaluating a patient with pneumonia. First, viral infections are most common in the late fall through early spring and generally occur during community epidemics. Awareness of both local (e.g., influenza), national, and worldwide (e.g., severe acute respiratory syndrome) outbreaks is important. Second, clinicians must know the local epidemiology because several pathogens (e.g., *Histoplasma capsulatum*, *Coccidioides immitis*) occur only in selected areas of the United States. Third, *M. tuberculosis* and *B. pertussis* (whooping cough) deserve consideration in patients with prolonged (i.e., >2 to 3 weeks) cough. Fourth, *Pneumocystis* species should remain high on the differential diagnostic list of pneumonia in the immunocompromised host, especially persons with HIV infection, use of corticosteroids, or hematologic malignan-

Figure 18-1 Pneumococcal Pneumonia.

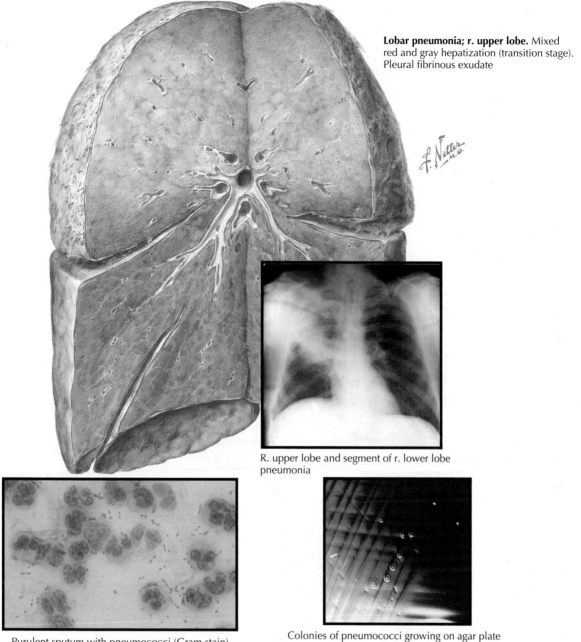

Lobar pneumonia; r. upper lobe. Mixed red and gray hepatization (transition stage). Pleural fibrinous exudate

R. upper lobe and segment of r. lower lobe pneumonia

Purulent sputum with pneumococci (Gram stain)

Colonies of pneumococci growing on agar plate

cies. Fifth, community-associated methicillin-resistant *S. aureus* (CA-MRSA) is increasingly recognized as a source of severe, often necrotizing, pneumonia, especially following a viral pneumonia such as influenza.

Management and Therapy

Optimal Therapy

The key decision concerning treatment is whether to treat in the outpatient setting or in the hospital. Most patients,

about 75%, can safely undergo therapy with oral antibiotics on an outpatient basis. Failure of recommended empiric therapy in appropriate outpatients is uncommon. The IDSA/ATS guideline recommends using a severity of illness score such as the CURB-65 criteria (confusion, elevated urea, elevated respiratory rate, low blood pressure, and age of at least 65) or prognostic models such as the Pneumonia Severity Index (PSI) as an aid in identifying patients who may be candidates for outpatient therapy. Hospitalization should be strongly considered for patients with two or more CURB-65 criteria: confusion, urea

Figure 18-2 Klebsiella (Friedländer's) Pneumonia.

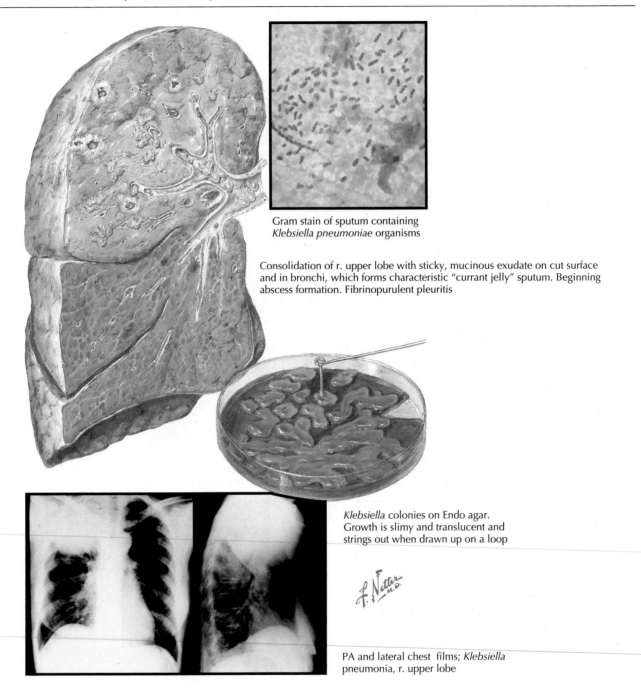

Gram stain of sputum containing
Klebsiella pneumoniae organisms

Consolidation of r. upper lobe with sticky, mucinous exudate on cut surface
and in bronchi, which forms characteristic "currant jelly" sputum. Beginning
abscess formation. Fibrinopurulent pleuritis

Klebsiella colonies on Endo agar.
Growth is slimy and translucent and
strings out when drawn up on a loop

PA and lateral chest films; *Klebsiella*
pneumonia, r. upper lobe

≥7 nmol/L, respiratory rate ≥30/min, systolic blood pressure ≤90 mm Hg, diastolic blood pressure ≤60 mm Hg, and age ≥65 years. The PSI is more complex, requires a two-step screening process, and places patients into five risk categories. Step 1 requires assessment of 11 risk factors including age, 5 coexisting medical conditions, and 5 abnormalities on physical exam. If any of these 11 risk factors are present, patients are screened using a point scoring system that includes 20 risk factors (age, gender, 5 coexisting diseases, 5 abnormal physical exam findings, and

7 laboratory or radiographic findings). Although much more complex, the PSI score has been more extensively studied and validated than the CURB-65 criteria. The current recommendations are as follows: patients falling into class I (mortality 0.1%) and II (mortality 0.6%) can be treated as outpatients; patients in risk class III (mortality 2.8%) are considered for treatment in an observation unit or with short-term hospitalization, and risk class IV (mortality 8.5%) or V (mortality 31.1%) patients are treated as inpatients. These prediction rules are meant to contribute

Figure 18-3 Staphylococcal Pneumonia.

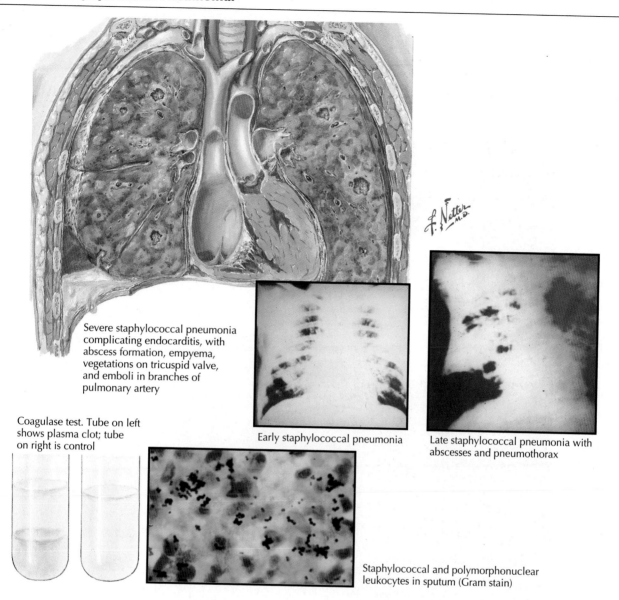

Severe staphylococcal pneumonia complicating endocarditis, with abscess formation, empyema, vegetations on tricuspid valve, and emboli in branches of pulmonary artery

Coagulase test. Tube on left shows plasma clot; tube on right is control

Early staphylococcal pneumonia

Late staphylococcal pneumonia with abscesses and pneumothorax

Staphylococcal and polymorphonuclear leukocytes in sputum (Gram stain)

to rather than supersede the physicians' judgment. Outpatient treatment requires that the patient be able to comply with therapy and to absorb oral antibiotics. Patients with cognitive impairment, history of substance abuse, nausea and vomiting, or underlying disorders that increase the risk for morbidity but are not included in the scoring systems often require hospitalization. The second-level decision is whether to admit the patient directly to an intensive care unit (ICU) or high-level monitoring unit rather than to a general medical ward. About 10% of hospitalized patients with CAP require ICU admission. Patients with a major criterion or with three or more minor criteria warrant direct ICU admission (Box 18-1).

Clinicians should make every effort to establish an etiologic diagnosis. Doing so permits optimal antibiotic selection specifically directed at the causative agent. Second, it

provides a rational basis for a change from parenteral to oral therapy and for a change in therapy necessitated by an adverse drug reaction. Third, a specific diagnosis permits antibiotic selection that limits the consequences of antibiotic use in terms of cost, inducible resistance, and adverse drug reactions. Finally, this allows identification of pathogens of potential epidemiologic significance, such as *Legionella* species, *B. pertussis*, and CA-MRSA. A detailed history may be helpful in suggesting a diagnosis (Table 18-2).

After a clinical diagnosis has been made, a microbiologic diagnosis using bacteriologic cultures of sputum and blood should be attempted in hospitalized patients. Ideally, initial studies should include a sputum sample from a deep-cough specimen for Gram stain (and culture) to aid in initial selection of antimicrobial therapy. Sputum is acceptable for culture if, under low-power microscopy, there are

Figure 18-4 Legionnaires' Disease.

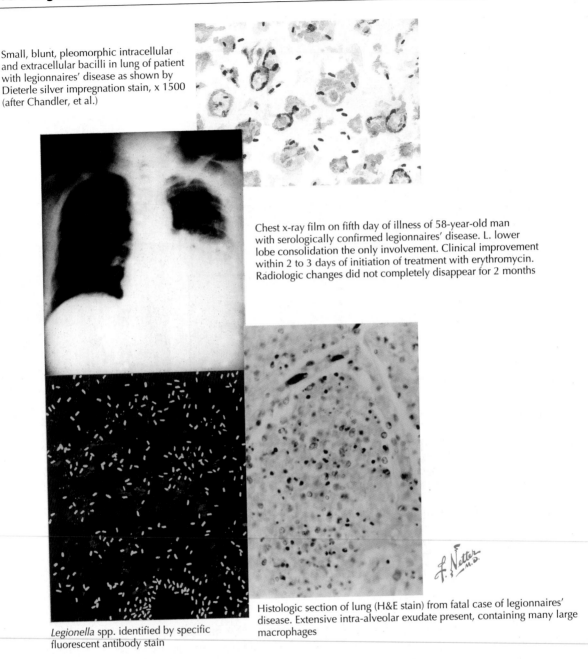

Small, blunt, pleomorphic intracellular and extracellular bacilli in lung of patient with legionnaires' disease as shown by Dieterle silver impregnation stain, x 1500 (after Chandler, et al.)

Chest x-ray film on fifth day of illness of 58-year-old man with serologically confirmed legionnaires' disease. L. lower lobe consolidation the only involvement. Clinical improvement within 2 to 3 days of initiation of treatment with erythromycin. Radiologic changes did not completely disappear for 2 months

Legionella spp. identified by specific fluorescent antibody stain

Histologic section of lung (H&E stain) from fatal case of legionnaires' disease. Extensive intra-alveolar exudate present, containing many large macrophages

more than 25 polymorphonuclear cells and less than 10 to 25 squamous epithelial cells. The Gram-stain appearance of *S. pneumoniae* (lancet-shaped gram-positive diplococci), *H. influenzae* (small gram-negative coccobacilli), and *S. aureus* (clusters of gram-positive cocci) are sufficiently distinctive to allow a tentative diagnosis. Blood culture results are positive in 5% to 14% of patients hospitalized with pneumonia. Additional diagnostic tests including rapid tests for respiratory syncytial virus and influenza, special smears (acid-fast smears) and culture for *M. tuberculosis*, urine antigen for *Legionella* species, and serologic tests for

Mycoplasma pneumoniae or *Legionella* or *Chlamydophila* species may be indicated, depending on the presence of epidemiologic clues, chest radiographic pattern, severity of illness, and host defense abnormalities. Many additional tests are available to diagnose less common pathogens.

Computed tomography (CT) or magnetic resonance imaging (MRI) is rarely required for the routine diagnosis of CAP. However, a CT scan, especially using high-resolution CT, is more sensitive than plain films for the evaluation of interstitial disease, bilateral disease, cavitation, empyema, and hilar adenopathy. Thus, a chest radio-

> **Box 18-1** Criteria for Severe Community-Acquired Pneumonia
>
> **Major Criteria**
> - Invasive mechanical ventilation
> - Septic shock with need for vasopressors
>
> **Minor Criteria[a]**
> - Respiratory rate[b] ≥30 breaths/min
> - PaO$_2$/FiO$_2$, ratio[b] ≤250
> - Multilobar infiltrates
> - Confusion, disorientation
> - Uremia (BUN level ≥20 mg/dL)
> - Leukopenia[c] (WBC ≤4000 cells/mm^3)
> - Thrombocytopenia (platelet count <100,000 cells/mm^3)
> - Hypothermia
> - Hypotension
>
> [a]Other criteria to consider include hypoglycemia (in nondiabetic patients), acute alcoholism and alcohol withdrawal, hyponatremia, unexplained metabolic acidosis or elevated lactate level, cirrhosis, and asplenia.
> [b]A need for noninvasive ventilation can substitute for respiratory rate ≥30 breaths/min or PaO$_2$/FiO$_2$, ratio[b] ≤250.
> [c]As a result of infection alone.
> *Adapted from Mandell LA, Wunderink RG, Anzueto A, et al: Infectious Diseases Society of America/American Thoracic Society Consensus Guidelines on the management of community-acquired pneumonia in adults. Clin Infect Dis 44(Suppl 2):S27-S72, 2007.*

graph is the preferred method for initial imaging, with CT scan or MRI reserved for further anatomic definition (e.g., detecting cavitation, adenopathy, or mass lesions). If radiographic studies demonstrate an effusion, consideration should be given to a diagnostic aspiration to exclude an empyema, which would require drainage.

Bronchoscopy is rarely indicated in immunocompetent patients with CAP. It should be considered in patients with a fulminant course without a clear etiology who require admission to the ICU or who have complex pneumonia unresponsive to antimicrobial therapy. Bronchoscopy is particularly useful for the detection of selected pathogens, such as *Pneumocystis*, *Mycobacterium*, and *Legionella* species and cytomegalovirus. Standard hematologic tests, chemistries, and oxygen saturation help assess the physiologic status of hospitalized patients and the need for intensive care.

Empiric antimicrobial therapy is guided by knowledge of likely pathogens (see Tables 18-1 and 18-2) and local resistance patterns. Therapy guidelines have undergone recent changes due to the increase in antimicrobial resistance of common pathogens (e.g., *S. pneumoniae*). Therapy may need to be altered or modified by host factors including age, pregnancy, liver or renal dysfunction, use of other medications that interact with planned antimicrobial therapy, and drug allergies. When possible, the least expensive effective therapy should be chosen. For oral therapy, important considerations include the frequency of dosing (better compliance is achieved with once- or twice-daily administration), taste, and the frequency of gastrointestinal irritation.

Antimicrobial therapy should be initiated promptly after the diagnosis is established with radiography, and ideally after Gram stain results are available to facilitate antimicrobial selection. For patients admitted to an inpatient unit through the emergency department, therapy should be initiated in the emergency department (preferably after blood culture specimens have been obtained). Antibiotic therapy should not be withheld from acutely ill patients because of delays in obtaining appropriate specimens or the results of Gram stains and cultures. The empiric therapy recommended by the IDSA and ATS is summarized in Box 18-2. If an etiologic agent is isolated, therapy should be altered based on the known susceptibilities of the pathogen or in vitro testing. Drug resistance is a growing problem with *S. pneumoniae* (especially resistance to β-lactam antibiotics, macrolides, and tetracyclines) and *S. aureus* (especially resistance to β-lactam antibiotics, macrolides, quinolones). The duration of therapy is based on the pathogen, response to therapy, comorbid illness, and complications. Patients should receive therapy for at least 5 days (longer therapy required for *S. aureus* and enteric gram-negative bacteria). In general, hospitalized patients can be switched from intravenous therapy to oral therapy when they are hemodynamically stable and improving clinically, are able to ingest medications, and have a normally functioning gastrointestinal tract. Criteria for clinical stability include temperature ≤37.8° C, heart rate ≤100 beats/min, respiratory rate ≤24 breaths/min, systolic blood pressure ≥90 mm Hg, arterial oxygen saturation ≥90% or PO$_2$ ≥60 mm Hg on room air, ability to maintain oral intake, and normal mental status.

Avoiding Treatment Errors

CAP is not difficult to diagnose in patients presenting with typical symptoms of fever, cough, sputum production, and shortness of breath. However, it is important to realize that pneumonia in elderly patients may present as confusion, lethargy, and poor feeding.

Both overtreatment and undertreatment for suspected pneumonia are common. Antibiotics should only be prescribed for patients with proven or highly suspected bacterial pneumonia. Although most patients can be treated as outpatients, many are inappropriately admitted to the hospital. However, the failure to admit appropriate patients should also be avoided. The CURB-65 criteria and PSI score are helpful guides in making admission decisions.

Empiric therapy is successful in most patients; nevertheless, a complete history and appropriate laboratory tests should be obtained for hospitalized patients to define the most appropriate therapy. A wider spectrum of pathogens, including multidrug-resistant pathogens, must be considered in immunocompromised patients or residents in an

Table 18-2 Epidemiology Clues Related to Specific Pathogens with Selected Community-Acquired Pneumonia

Epidemiologic Clue	Pathogen (Disease)
	Associated with Specific Pathogen
Poor dental hygiene; risk for aspiration (e.g., seizure disorder)	Anaerobes
Cough >2 weeks with whoop or post-tussive vomiting	*Bordetella pertussis*
Exposure to birds (especially psittacine birds)	*Chlamydia psittaci* (psittacosis)
Exposure to infected farm animals or cats, especially parturient animals	*Coxiella burnetii* (Q fever)
Exposure to rabbits or infected ticks	*Francisella tularensis* (tularemia)
Exposure to bats or soil enriched with bird dropping in an endemic area	*Histoplasma capsulatum* (histoplasmosis)
Hotel or cruise ship stay in previous 2 weeks	*Legionella* spp. (legionnaires' disease)
Exposure to cats and less commonly to dogs	*Pasteurella multocida* (pasteurellosis)
Exposure to infected fleas or host animals (e.g., ground squirrels) in an endemic area, or to persons with pneumonic plague	*Yersinia pestis* (plague)
	Associated with Multiple Pathogens
Alcoholism	*Streptococcus pneumoniae, Klebsiella pneumoniae,* anaerobes, *Acinetobacter* spp., *Mycobacterium tuberculosis*
Bioterrorism	*Bacillus anthracis* (anthrax), *Yersinia pestis* (plague), *Francisella tularensis* (tularemia)
Chronic obstructive pulmonary disease or smoking	*Haemophilus influenzae, Pseudomonas aeruginosa, Legionella* spp., *S. pneumoniae, Moraxella catarrhalis, Chlamydophila pneumoniae*
HIV infection (early)	*S. pneumoniae, H. influenzae, M. tuberculosis*
HIV infection (late)	Above plus *Pneumocystis, Cryptococcus, Histoplasma* spp., *Aspergillus,* nontuberculous mycobacteria (especially *M. kansasii*), *Pseudomonas aeruginosa, H. influenza*
Influenza active in community	Influenza, *S. pneumoniae, S. aureus, H. influenzae*
Lung abscess	Community-associated methicillin-resistant *S. aureus,* oral anaerobes, endemic fungal pneumonia, *M. tuberculosis,* nontuberculous mycobacteria
Residence in an extended care facility	*S. pneumoniae,* gram-negative bacilli, *H. influenzae, Staphylococcus aureus,* anaerobes, viral influenza, *Mycobacterium tuberculosis*
Structural abnormalities of the lung (e.g., cystic fibrosis, bronchiectasis)	*Pseudomonas aeruginosa, Burkholderia cepacia, S. aureus*
Travel to or residence in Southwestern U.S.	*Coccidioides* species, Hantavirus
Travel to or residence in Southeast and East Asia	*Burkholderia pseudomallei,* avian influenza, severe acute respiratory syndrome

extended care facility, and for this reason there is a separate IDSA/ATS guideline to address this patient population.

The optimum treatment of CAP requires at least 5 days of antibiotic therapy. Although some regimens are successful using 5 days of therapy (e.g., levofloxacin 750 mg each day for 5 days), most antibiotic agents are approved for 7 to 14 days. Patients should be discharged only when they demonstrate clinical improvement. Influenza and pneumococcal vaccines should be offered to appropriate patients per recommendations by the Advisory Committee on Immunization Practices (ACIP).

Prevention

The annual impact of viral influenza is highly variable. During years in which the infection is epidemic, its impact on CAP is sizeable as a result both of primary influenza pneumonia and secondary bacterial superinfection. Persons 50 years of age or older, those at high risk for complications of illness, and all health care workers should receive the influenza vaccine as recommended by ACIP. The currently available 23-valent pneumococcal capsular polysaccharide vaccine is about 50% effective in preventing hospitalization and about 80% effective in preventing death from pneumococcal disease in immunocompetent adults. All adults who are older than 65 years and all younger persons who are at high risk for pneumococcal infection, such as those with HIV infection, should receive the pneumococcal vaccine.

Future Directions

Recommendations for the therapy of CAP are likely to require frequent modifications based on the emerging

Box 18-2 Empiric Therapy for Patients with Community-Acquired Pneumonia

Outpatients

- Previously healthy and no use of antimicrobials within previous 3 months
  - A macrolide: erythromycin, azithromycin, clarithromycin (strong recommendation)
  - Doxycycline (weak recommendation)
- Presence of comorbidities such as chronic heart, lung, liver, or renal disease; diabetes mellitus; alcoholism; malignancy; asplenia; immunosuppressing conditions or use of immunosuppressive drugs; or use of antimicrobials within the previous 3 months (in which case an alternative from a different class should be selected)
  - A respiratory fluoroquinolone (levofloxacin [750 mg], moxifloxacin) (strong recommendation)
  - A β-lactam (high-dose amoxicillin [e.g., 1 g 3 times per day] or amoxicillin-clavulanate [2 g 2 times per day] is preferred; alternatives include ceftriaxone, cefpodoxime, and cefuroxime [500 mg 2 times per day]) plus a macrolide (strong recommendation)
- In regions with a high rate (>25%) of infections with high-level (MIC ≥16 μg/mL) macrolide-resistant Streptococcus pneumoniae, consider use of alternative agents for patients without comorbidities (moderate recommendation)

Inpatients, non-ICU Treatment

- A respiratory fluoroquinolone (strong recommendation)
- A β-lactam plus a macrolide (strong recommendation)

Inpatients, ICU Treatment

- A β-lactam (cefotaxime, ceftriaxone, or ampicillin-sulbactam) plus either azithromycin or a fluoroquinolone (preferred) (for penicillin-allergic patients, a respiratory fluoroquinolone and aztreonam are recommended)

Special Concerns

- If pseudomonas is a consideration (moderate recommendation)
  - An antipneumococcal, antipseudomonal β-lactam (piperacillin-tazobactam, cefepime, imipenem, or meropenem) plus either ciprofloxacin or levofloxacin (750 mg), or
  - The above β-lactam plus an aminoglycoside and azithromycin, or
  - The above β-lactam plus an aminoglycoside and an antipseudomonal fluoroquinolone (for penicillin-allergic patients, substitute aztreonam for above β-lactam)
  - Generally preferred are: an extended-spectrum cephalosporin or β-lactam/β-lactamase inhibitor plus either fluoroquinolone or macrolide
- If community-associated methicillin-resistant S. aureus (CA-MRSA)
  - Add vancomycin or linezolid (moderate recommendation)

Adapted from Mandell LA, Wunderink RG, Anzueto A, et al: Infectious Diseases Society of America/American Thoracic Society Consensus Guidelines on the management of community-acquired pneumonia in adults. Clin Infect Dis 44(Suppl 2):S27-S72, 2007.

---

antimicrobial resistance of respiratory pathogens and the introduction of new antimicrobial agents. Physicians providing primary care can help minimize the evolution of antimicrobial resistance by judicious use of antibiotics for bacterial respiratory tract infections and by withholding antibiotics when viral pathogens are highly suspected.

Additional Resources

Bartlett JG, Dowell SF, Mandell LA, et al: Practice guidelines for the management of community-acquired pneumonia in adults. Infectious Diseases Society of America. Clin Infect Dis 31:347-382, 2000.

This is an older guideline from the Infectious Disease Society of America.

Cunha BA: The atypical pneumonias: Clinical diagnosis and importance. Clin Microbiol Infect 12(Suppl 3):12-24, 2006.

This is an excellent review of atypical pathogens, including three zoonotic pathogens (C. psittaci [psittacosis], F. tularensis [tularemia], C. burnetii [Q fever]) and three nonzoonotic pathogens (C. pneumoniae, M. pneumoniae, Legionella species).

File TM Jr: Clinical implications and treatment of multiresistant Streptococcus pneumoniae pneumonia. Clin Microbiol Infect 12(Suppl 3):31-41, 2006.

The authors provide a useful review on the antibiotic resistance mechanisms that may be present in S. pneumoniae and treatment recommendations for multidrug-resistant strains.

Mandell LA, Barlett JG, Dowell SF, et al: Update of practice guidelines for the management of community-acquired pneumonia in immunocompetent adults. Clin Infect Dis 37:405-433, 2003.

This is an update of the guideline from the Infectious Disease Society of America.

Metlay JP, Fine MJ: Testing strategies in the initial management of patients with community-acquired pneumonia. Ann Intern Med 138:109-118, 2003.

The authors review the test characteristics of the history, physical examination, and laboratory findings, individually and in combination, in diagnosing community-acquired pneumonia.

EVIDENCE

1. Centers for Disease Control and Prevention: Recommended adult immunization schedule—United States, October 2006–September 2007. MMWR 55:Q1-Q4, 2006.

   These are the most recent (at time of writing this chapter) immunization recommendations for adults.

2. Fine MJ, Auble TE, Yearly DM, et al. A prediction rule to identify low-risk patients with community-acquired pneumonia. N Engl J Med 336:243-250, 1997.

   The authors describe and validate the Pneumonia Severity Index for predicting mortality in patients with community-acquired pneumonia.

3. Lim WS, van der Eerden MM, Laing R, et al: Defining community acquired pneumonia severity on presentation to hospital: An international derivation and validation study. Thorax 58:377-382, 2003.

   The authors describe and validate the CURB-65 criteria for predicting mortality in patients with community-acquired pneumonia.

4. Mandell LA, Wunderink RG, Anzueto A, et al: Infectious Diseases Society of America/American Thoracic Society Consensus Guidelines on the management of community-acquired pneumonia in adults. Clin Infect Dis 44(Suppl 2):S27-S72, 2007.

   This comprehensive guideline provides recommendations for the management of CAP including diagnostic tests, antibiotic therapy, and overall management.

M. Patricia Rivera

Pleural Effusion and Pneumothorax

Introduction

Typically, pleural effusions and pneumothoraces are secondary manifestations of other underlying disease states, such as empyema with pneumonia or spontaneous pneumothorax with emphysema. Less commonly, the pleura can be the primary site of disease, as with mesothelioma. Although many different diseases may cause a pleural effusion (Box 19-1), the most common causes in the United States are pneumonia, congestive heart failure (CHF), and cancer. The diagnostic approach in a patient with a pleural effusion largely depends on the probable etiologies of the effusion in that patient. Much is known about the clinical patterns of pleural diseases, but surprisingly little is understood about their pathogenesis.

Etiology and Pathogenesis

The pleural space, 10 to 20 mm in diameter, is filled with a thin layer of pleural fluid that acts as a lubricant. Both the visceral and parietal pleura are lined with a single layer of mesothelial cells overlying a layer of connective tissue and derive their blood supply from the systemic capillaries.

Pleural fluid can originate in the interstitial spaces of the lung, the pleural capillaries, the intrathoracic lymphatics, or the peritoneal cavity. In normal individuals, the origin of most pleural fluid is the capillaries in the parietal pleura, and the amount of fluid produced each day is about 0.1 to 0.2 mL/kg of body weight. The pleural space is in communication with the lymphatic vessels by means of stomas in the parietal pleura. The capacity for lymphatic clearance of fluid is 20-fold to 30-fold greater than the rate of fluid influx. Normal fluid has a pH of 7.6, protein of less than 1.5 g/dL, and a cell count of about 1500 cells/mL with a predominance of monocytes.

Fluid accumulates when the rate of formation exceeds the rate of absorption; the most common cause is increased interstitial fluid in the lungs. Mechanisms for pleural fluid accumulation include increased hydrostatic pressure, decreased oncotic or pleural pressure, increased vascular permeability, transdiaphragmatic movement of ascitic fluid, and disruption of the thoracic duct. Obstruction of the lymphatics draining the parietal pleura and an eleva-

tion of systemic vascular pressures are the most common causes of decreased fluid absorption.

Clinical and Radiologic Presentation

Patients may present asymptomatically or with pleuritic chest pain, nonproductive cough, and dyspnea. Examination of the chest reveals decreased tactile fremitus and diminished or absent breath sounds. When pleural effusions diminish in size spontaneously or because of treatment, a pleural rub may develop.

Obliteration of the posterior costophrenic angle by a meniscus-shaped homogeneous shadow is a common finding on the upright chest radiograph. As more fluid accumulates, the diaphragm silhouette on the affected side is lost, and the fluid extends upward around the anterior, lateral, and posterior thoracic walls. The lateral decubitus radiograph helps to quantify the size of the effusion. Fluid that exceeds 10 mm in diameter from the inside margin of the rib to the outside margin of the lung is amenable to thoracentesis.

At times, substantial amounts of pleural fluid can be present in a subpulmonic location without spilling into the costophrenic sulci. The radiographic characteristics of a subpulmonic effusion include elevation of the diaphragm, lateral displacement of the dome of the diaphragm,

diaphragmatic flattening, and if the effusion is on the left side, a gap greater than 2 cm between the left hemidiaphragm and the gastric bubble.

When the patient is in the supine position, pleural fluid gravitates to the posterior parts of the thoracic cavity. The supine radiograph reveals blunting of the costophrenic angle, loss of the hemidiaphragm silhouette, and increased homogeneous density superimposed over the lung.

When the entire hemithorax is opacified because of a pleural effusion, the mediastinum shifts to the contralateral side. Shifting of the mediastinum toward the ipsilateral side implies either complete obstruction of the ipsilateral mainstem bronchus or a trapped lung as in mesothelioma. If no shift is evident, the mediastinum is likely fixed as a result of fibrosis or malignant infiltration.

Diagnostic Approach, Management, and Therapy

A diagnostic thoracentesis is performed when a clinically significant effusion (thickness of pleural fluid on the lateral decubitus radiograph greater than 10 mm) is present or when loculated fluid is demonstrated on ultrasound. If a patient has typical clinical signs of CHF and bilateral pleural effusions, and is afebrile, a trial of diuresis can be undertaken. If the effusions persist for more than 3 days, thoracentesis is indicated.

Appearance of the Pleural Fluid

The gross appearance of the pleural fluid often provides useful information. Turbid fluid is usually associated with a chylothorax, elevated levels of cholesterol (pseudochylothorax), or empyema. Chocolate-brown fluid suggests amebiasis with a hepatobiliary fistula. Clear or bloody viscous fluid (increased hyaluronic acid level) is suggestive of malignant mesothelioma. Yellow-green fluid is described with rheumatoid pleural effusions, and black fluid with *Aspergillus* species infection. A bloody effusion with a red blood cell count of more than $100,000/mm^3$ suggests trauma, malignancy, or pulmonary embolism. When the pleural fluid hematocrit exceeds 50% of that of the peripheral blood, a hemothorax is present, and chest tube thoracostomy should be considered (Fig. 19-1). A feculent odor indicates an anaerobic infection; an ammonia scent is associated with urinothorax.

Pleural Fluid Analysis

Routine tests performed on all effusions include protein, lactate dehydrogenase (LDH), glucose, pH, and differential cell count. Additional studies include Gram stain and culture, potassium hydroxide preparation and fungal culture, acid-fast bacteria smear and culture, and cytology. In the appropriate clinical context, additional studies such as amylase, triglycerides, cholesterol, rheumatoid factor, and antinuclear antibody may be helpful.

Differential white blood cell count is one of the most informative tests on pleural fluid. Neutrophils predominate (>50% of the cells) in pleural fluid resulting from acute inflammatory processes such as bacterial infection, pancreatitis, and pulmonary embolism. Lymphocyte predominance indicates that the patient most likely has a malignancy or tuberculosis, although predominance of lymphocytes can also be seen in pleural effusions after coronary artery bypass surgery. The most common cause of pleural fluid eosinophilia (>10% eosinophils) is the presence of air or blood in the pleural space; other causes include asbestos, drugs (dantrolene, nitrofurantoin, bromocriptine), parasitic infections (paragonimiasis, amebiasis), and Churg-Strauss syndrome. Pleural fluid eosinophilia is uncommon in patients with cancer or tuberculosis, unless the patient has undergone repeated thoracenteses. Basophilia (>10%) is most common with leukemic pleural involvement. The presence of mesothelial cells (>5%) excludes tuberculosis.

Specific tests may provide additional insight. A markedly elevated fluid protein (>7 g/dL) implies a paraproteinemia or multiple myeloma. A low pleural fluid glucose

Figure 19-1 Hemothorax.

Sources
1. Lung
2. Intercostal vessels
3. Internal thoracic
   (internal mammary) artery
4. Thoracicoacromial
   artery   } via wound
5. Lateral thoracic   track
   artery
6. Mediastinal great vessels
7. Heart
8. Abdominal structures (liver,
   spleen) via diaphragm

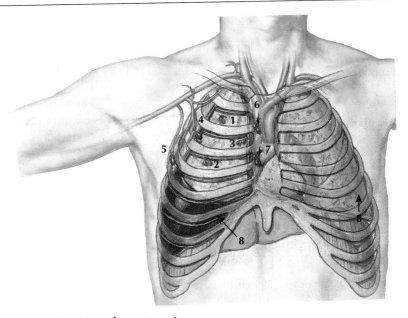

Degrees and management

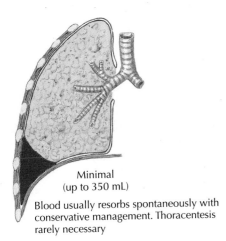

Minimal
(up to 350 mL)

Blood usually resorbs spontaneously with
conservative management. Thoracentesis
rarely necessary

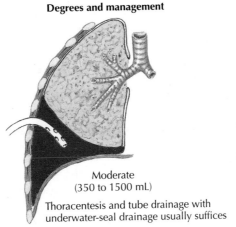

Moderate
(350 to 1500 mL)

Thoracentesis and tube drainage with
underwater-seal drainage usually suffices

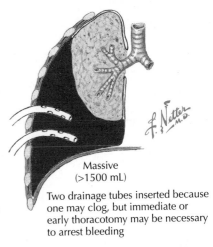

Massive
(>1500 mL)

Two drainage tubes inserted because
one may clog, but immediate or
early thoracotomy may be necessary
to arrest bleeding

level (<60 mg/dL) indicates rheumatoid disease, empyema, a complicated parapneumonic effusion, malignancy, esophageal rupture, and occasionally tuberculosis. Pleural fluid amylase above the upper limits for serum indicates one of four problems: pancreatic disease, esophageal rupture, malignancy, or ruptured ectopic pregnancy. A pH below 7.30 is seen in esophageal rupture, empyema, rheumatoid effusion, malignant effusion, lupus pleuritis, tuberculosis, and systemic acidosis. In the evaluation of collagen vascular disease, measurement of a rheumatoid factor and antinuclear antibodies often provides very useful information.

Transudate versus Exudate

A transudative effusion develops when systemic factors (hydrostatic or oncotic pressures) influencing the forma-

tion of fluid are altered. Vascular permeability is normal. Exudative effusions develop when the pleural surfaces or the capillaries in the location where the fluid accumulates are altered. Exudative pleural effusions meet at least one of the following criteria (Light's criteria): (1) fluid-to-serum protein ratio of more than 0.5; (2) fluid-to-serum LDH ratio of more than 0.6; and (3) pleural fluid LDH greater than two thirds the upper limit of normal for serum LDH. Transudative effusions meet none of the criteria.

A confounding factor encountered with the diagnostic separation of transudates and exudates is seen in diuretic-treated CHF, in which the fluid protein can be elevated in the range of 3 to 4 g/dL. In this instance, the pleural fluid–to–serum albumin gradient is useful; a gradient greater than 1.2 g/dL greatly increases the probability that the pleural fluid is a result of CHF.

Figure 19-2 Cryptococcosis (Torulosis).

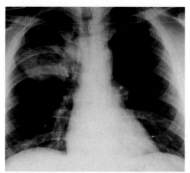

Pulmonary cryptococcosis presenting as a large mass-like lesion, easily mistaken for carcinoma

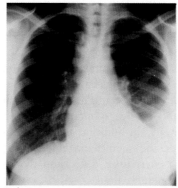

Pulmonary cryptococcosis. Mediastinal lymph nodes enlarged and pleural effusion on the left

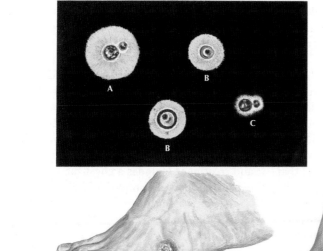

India ink preparation showing *C. neoformans*

A. Budding organism with thick capsule

B. Nonbudding organisms

C. Unencapsulated form (budding)

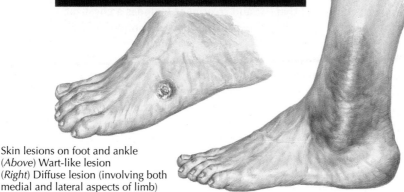

Skin lesions on foot and ankle
(*Above*) Wart-like lesion
(*Right*) Diffuse lesion (involving both medial and lateral aspects of limb)

Transudative Effusions

CHF is the most common cause of pleural effusions; most patients (88%) have bilateral effusions. Unilateral right- and left-sided effusions are reported in 8% and 4%, respectively. About 25% of patients with unilateral effusions attributable to CHF have concomitant pneumonia or pulmonary embolism. Patients with bilateral effusions and the accompanying physical findings of left ventricular dysfunction can safely be observed without thoracentesis. Failure of the effusion to respond to heart failure management or the presence of pleuritic chest pain or fever mandates evaluation of the pleural fluid. Other causes of transudative effusions are listed in Box 19-1.

Exudative Effusions

The differential diagnosis of exudative pleural effusions is extensive (see Box 19-1). The most common causes are infectious processes and malignancy (Fig. 19-2).

Parapneumonic effusions, associated with bacterial pneumonia or lung abscess, are the most common cause of exudative effusions in the United States. About 40% of cases of pneumonia have an associated pleural effusion. The bacteriology of empyema or complicated pleural effusions includes a predominance of gram-positive aerobes (*Streptococcus pneumoniae, Staphylococcus aureus*), gram-negative aerobes (*Klebsiella* species, *Pseudomonas* species, *Haemophilus influenzae*), and anaerobes (*Bacteroides* species,

Peptostreptococcus). *S. pneumoniae* is still responsible for most bacterial pneumonias, and an associated pleural effusion occurs in 40% to 53% of patients. Patients with anaerobic bacterial infections that involve the pleural space frequently present with a subacute illness. Many patients have a history of alcoholism, an episode of unconsciousness, or another factor that predisposes to aspiration. Typically, uncomplicated parapneumonic effusions have a pH greater than 7.30, glucose greater than 60 mg/dL, and LDH greater than 1000 IU/L and resolve spontaneously with appropriate antibiotic therapy. In addition to treatment with appropriate antibiotics, the main management decision is whether to insert a chest tube, a decision that is made after analysis of the pleural fluid obtained with a diagnostic thoracentesis. An empyema is pus in the pleural space and warrants immediate drainage with tube thoracostomy. A complicated parapneumonic effusion is defined by one or more of the following: pleural fluid pH greater than 7.0, glucose less than 40 mg/dL, LDH greater than 1000 IU/L, and Gram stain or culture positivity. These effusions are not likely to respond to antibiotic therapy alone, and drainage with tube thoracostomy (chest tube) is necessary. Inadequate drainage of an empyema or lack of clinical improvement requires aggressive management with computed tomography (CT) imaging and further intervention. The CT is useful to evaluate for the progressive development of a loculated effusion (pleural fluid that becomes encapsulated by adhesions anywhere between the parietal and the visceral pleura or in the interlobar fissures). Although individual studies of intrapleural installation of thrombolytics such as streptokinase have reported successful lysis of loculations and improved drainage through chest tube, a recent meta-analysis did not support routine use of fibrinolytics in all patients who required chest tube drainage for empyema or complicated parapneumonic effusions. Surgical options include decortication and open drainage.

Tuberculous pleural effusions are rare; typically, they present as an acute illness. Purified protein derivative skin test results are negative in about one third of patients. Fluid examination reveals a lymphocyte-predominant exudate. Mesothelial cells and eosinophils are uncommon. Typically, the fluid protein is greater than 5 g/dL, LDH is mildly elevated, and the glucose is less than 60 mg/dL. The acid-fast bacteria smears are rarely positive, and less than 40% of patients have positive pleural fluid cultures. Alternative tests to aid in the diagnosis of tuberculous pleurisy include adenosine deaminase (>40 U/L), interferon-γ (level of 140 pg/mL is comparable to an adenosine deaminase level of 40 U/L), or polymerase chain reaction for mycobacterial DNA. Pleural biopsy is reported to have a high diagnostic yield. Most tuberculous effusions resolve spontaneously; however, treatment with standard tuberculous therapy is indicated to prevent recurrent disease. Serial thoracentesis has not been shown to improve outcome.

Malignant pleural effusions are due most commonly to lung (30%) and breast (25%) cancer. Lymphoma is responsible for 20% of malignant effusions. Mechanisms for these effusions include direct pleural involvement by tumor, reduced pleural pressure associated with bronchial obstruction, pulmonary embolism, or sequelae of chemotherapy or radiation therapy. Malignant effusions are usually moderate in size and associated with dyspnea, show a lymphocyte predominance, and have red blood cell counts greater than 1,000,000/mm^3. Large tumor burden is associated with a low pH (<7.30) and glucose (<60 mg/dL) as well as shortened survival time. Pleural fluid cytology is diagnostic in about 65% of cases. The yield can increase when three separate fluid specimens are submitted. Closed pleural biopsy (CPB) is only diagnostic in about 50% of cases. Thoracoscopy provides a higher diagnostic yield of 93%. Therapeutic options include treating the underlying cancer, drainage with pigtail catheter or chest tube, and chemical pleurodesis.

Chylothorax is characterized by a milky-white effusion with an elevated triglyceride level caused by the accumulation of chyle in the pleural space from disruption of the thoracic duct. The most common cause of chylothorax is lymphoma (37% of cases). Other causes include metastatic cancer, surgical or nonsurgical trauma, lymphangiomyomatosis, and cirrhosis. Thoracentesis is used for diagnosis, and treatment includes a chest tube for drainage and lung expansion, bowel rest, parenteral nutrition, and treatment of the underlying disorder. If chylous drainage from the chest tube persists, repair of the thoracic duct needs to be considered.

Hemothorax is defined as a pleural fluid hematocrit exceeding 50% of the peripheral blood value. Trauma and iatrogenic vascular injury are the most common causes, but hemothorax is seen with a variety of disorders, including arteriovenous malformations, ascites, malignancy, coagulopathy, endometriosis, neurofibromatosis, pneumothorax, retroperitoneal hemorrhage, sequestration, and vascular anomalies. Treatment involves large-bore chest tube thoracostomy and thoracotomy if the bleeding persists.

Pneumothorax

Pneumothorax occurs when air escapes into the pleural space. Pneumothoraces can be divided into spontaneous (without antecedent trauma) and traumatic (result of direct or indirect trauma). Spontaneous pneumothoraces are further divided into primary (in otherwise healthy individuals) and secondary (a complication of underlying lung disease). Primary spontaneous pneumothoraces are caused by rupture of apical subpleural blebs. Most secondary spontaneous pneumothoraces are caused by chronic obstructive lung disease, although they have been associated with a variety of disorders (Box 19-2).

Dyspnea and pleuritic chest pain are the most common symptoms. If pneumothorax is suspected, an end-

Figure 19-3 Tension Pneumothorax.

Pathophysiology

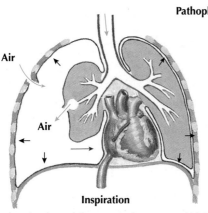

Air

Air

Inspiration

Air enters pleural cavity through lung wound or ruptured bleb (or occasionally via penetrating chest wound) with valve-like opening. Ipsilateral lung collapses, and mediastinum shifts to opposite side, compressing contralateral lung and impairing its ventilating capacity

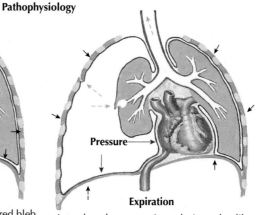

Pressure

Expiration

Intrapleural pressure rises, closing valve-like opening, preventing escape of pleural air. Pressure is thus progressively increased with each breath. Mediastinal and tracheal shifts are augmented, diaphragm is depressed, and venous return is impaired by increased pressure and vena caval distortion

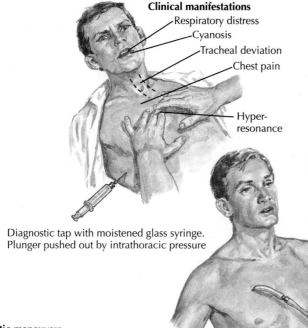

Clinical manifestations
- Respiratory distress
- Cyanosis
- Tracheal deviation
- Chest pain
- Hyper-resonance

Diagnostic tap with moistened glass syringe. Plunger pushed out by intrathoracic pressure

Left-sided tension pneumothorax. Lung collapsed, mediastinum and trachea deviated to opposite side, diaphragm depressed, intercostal spaces widened

To underwater seal

Therapeutic maneuvers
Large-bore needle inserted for emergency relief of intrathoracic pressure. Finger cot flutter valve, Heimlich valve, or underwater seal should be attached

Incision in 3rd interspace with introduction of thoracostomy tube attached to underwater-seal suction

---

expiratory chest radiograph is the most helpful diagnostic study. Simple observation will suffice as treatment in asymptomatic patients with small (<15% of hemithorax) primary spontaneous pneumothoraces. Supplemental oxygen accelerates the rate of air absorption. Needle aspiration is the initial treatment for symptomatic primary spontaneous pneumothorax. If it is unsuccessful, chest tube thoracostomy should be performed. Chest tube thoracostomy is the treatment of choice for secondary spontaneous pneumothoraces.

Tension pneumothorax, a one-way valve mechanism that results in a progressive rise in pleural pressure, occurs in 3% to 5% of patients with spontaneous pneumothorax and in 5% to 15% of those with barotrauma (patients on mechanical ventilation) (Fig. 19-3). The patient will look extremely distressed, and physical exam will reveal absence of breath sounds on the involved side associated with deviation of the trachea to the contralateral side. Displacement of the trachea and mediastinum along with impaired venous return results in cardiopulmonary distress. Placement of a

---

Box 19-2　Diseases Associated with Secondary
　　　　　　　Spontaneous Pneumothorax

Alveolar proteinosis
Asthma
Berylliosis
Chronic obstructive airways disease
Cystic fibrosis
Ehlers-Danlos syndrome
Histiocytosis X
Idiopathic pulmonary hemosiderosis
Lung cancer
Marfan syndrome
Metastatic sarcoma
Lymphangiomyomatosis
Paragonimiasis
Pneumocystis carinii pneumonia
Primary biliary cirrhosis
Sarcoidosis
Scleroderma
Silicosis
Tuberculosis
Rheumatoid lung disease

---

large-bore needle or an angiocatheter into the chest anteriorly in the 2nd rib space will decompress the tension. The mortality rate is approximately 30% when treatment is delayed.

Avoiding Treatment Errors

Appropriate initial selection of antibiotic therapy for patients with pneumonia and pleural effusion depends on whether the pneumonia is community or hospital acquired; antibiotic coverage is then guided by the results of pleural fluid cultures. If the patient is thought to have an anaerobic infection, penicillin and clindamycin are the drugs of choice. Prompt recognition of complicated parapneumonic effusions and empyema is of utmost importance because adequate drainage of the pleural space is at least as important in the cure as antimicrobial therapy. Chest tube insertion must occur as soon as it is determined that the patient has an empyema or complicated parapneumonic effusion; the longer the chest tube is delayed, the greater the chance of loculation and the more difficult the pleural drainage becomes. Malnourishment and immunocompromise, major complications in patients with chylothorax, are caused by removal of large amounts of protein, fats, and lymphocytes with repeated thoracentesis or prolonged chest tube drainage. Surgical correction of the thoracic duct needs to be considered if the chylous drainage persists. Tension pneumothorax is a medical emergency that must be treated immediately.

Future Directions

The workup of pleural effusions is often a lengthy process fraught with pitfalls, particularly when dealing with malignant pleural effusions. Several studies suggest that thoracoscopy increases the diagnostic yield in patients with benign and malignant pleural disease when thoracentesis and CPB results are nondiagnostic. Thoracoscopy is a minimally invasive and relatively safe procedure that will likely supplant CPB in the diagnostic workup of malignant pleural effusions.

Additional Resources

Sahn SA. Diagnostic evaluation of a pleural effusion in adults. Available at www.uptodateonline.com.
　　Reviews the basics of pleural fluid analysis and provides a practical approach to initial evaluation of pleural effusions.
Sahn SA. The undiagnosed pleural effusion. Available at www.uptodate online.com.
　　Reviews some of the nuances encountered in the diagnosis of pleural effusion when the initial basic evaluation does not yield a definitive diagnosis.
Light RW. Primary spontaneous pneumothorax in adults. Available at www.uptodateonline.com.
　　A helpful general review.

EVIDENCE

1. Diacon AH, Theron J, Schuurmans MM, et al: Intrapleural streptokinase for empyema and complicated parapneumonic effusions. Am J Respir Crit Care Med 170(1):49-53, 2004.
　　The authors provide a good review of the role of thrombolytic therapy in the management of empyema.
2. Light RW: Clinical practice. Pleural effusion. N Engl J Med 346(25):1971-1977, 2002.
　　This is an excellent review on the clinical approach to pleural effusions.
3. Light RW: Pleural Diseases, 4th ed. Philadelphia, Lippincott Williams & Wilkins, 2001.
　　This excellent textbook is recommended for pulmonologists in training and in clinical practice. It provides a great reference for issues related to pleural diseases.
4. Sahn SA: Management of complicated parapneumonic effusions. Am Rev Respir Dis 148(3):813-817, 1993.
　　This article presents a good review.
5. Sahn SA: State of the art. The pleura. Am Rev Respir Dis 138(1):184-234, 1988.
　　This very thorough review of pleural diseases is best for pulmonologists in training.
6. Tokuda Y, Matsushima D, Stein GH, Miyagi S: Intrapleural fibrinolytic agents for empyema and complicated parapneumonic effusions: A meta-analysis. Chest 129(3):783-790, 2006.
　　The author provides an excellent review of data on thrombolytic therapy for empyema.

David C. Henke

Asthma

Introduction

Asthma is a syndrome with a chronic but variable clinical course and presentation. Its main features are (1) reversible airflow obstruction, (2) nonspecific airways hyperreactivity, and (3) airways inflammation. The nonspecific nature of the hyperreactivity is perhaps a reflection of airway inflammation. Symptoms are triggered by nonallergic stimuli such as smoke and strong odors and quantified by sensitivity to inhalational challenge to nonallergic stimuli such as histamine. Airway hyperreactivity predisposes patients to symptoms in a variety of environments.

Both children and adults develop asthma. The remission rate in adults is 10% to 15% but is more than 50% in children. Despite advances in the understanding of asthma and better medications, asthma morbidity and mortality have increased. During the past 110 years, our understanding of asthma has changed greatly. It was long considered a disease of "twitchy" airways and a minor ailment that, according to Osler, allowed the patient to "pant into old age." Now, asthma is considered a disease of chronic fluctuating airways inflammation with a lethal potential of 5000 deaths annually in the United States. It is a major public health problem that results in 1.8 million emergency room visits per year, with about 10% of patients requiring hospitalization at a cost of $12 billion annually in the United States.

Etiology and Pathogenesis

Asthma manifests as inflammation in the lower airways. Over time, structural changes in the airway called *remodeling* result (i.e., muscle hypertrophy and thickening of the basement membrane) (Fig. 20-1). Acute asthma exacerbations cause airway muscle contraction, edema and sloughing of the airway mucosa, and the accumulation of mucus, cellular debris, and exudative secretions in the airway lumen. These changes degrade airway function, causing respiratory symptoms and even death by suffocation.

There are clinical and epidemiologic links between asthma and immunoglobulin E (IgE). Transcription factors, such as nuclear factor-KB and members of the signal transduction-activated transcription (STAT) factor family, act on genes encoding for inflammatory cytokines, such as interleukins (ILs), and appear to initiate and sustain airway (Fig. 20-2) inflammation. Corticosteroids are the most effective *controllers* of asthma. They inhibit these transcription factors and airway inflammation. Asthma refractory to corticosteroids has been linked to the tumor necrosis factor axis. However, the newly described subset of natural killer T (NKT) cells, CD1d-restricted NKT cells, with potent immunoregulatory functions and associated with asthma, are also resistant to modulation by corticosteroids.

A widely held mechanistic explanation is that inhaled antigen activates mast cells and T helper type 2 (Th2) lymphocytes, causing mediator release that promotes a persistent eosinophilic airway inflammation. There is no clear understanding of which biologic influences lead to chronic eosinophilic airway inflammation and hyperresponsiveness in asthma. Genetic factors (e.g., polymorphism for the IgE receptor, β receptor, matrix metalloproteinase, and CD14), environmental factors (e.g., excessive hygiene, vaccinations), and triggers (e.g., viral infection, exposures to tobacco smoke, pollutants, allergens) have all been implicated in the pathogenesis of asthma (see Fig. 10-3 in Chapter 10). Most asthmatic patients are atopic and have IgE-mediated disease, although there is evidence suggesting that intrinsic or nonatopic asthmatic patients may produce local, as opposed to circulating, IgE. Inflammation in atopic asthma can be demonstrated when the patient is challenged with inhaled allergen. The sensitive patient will show decline in pulmonary function demonstrated by obstruction of airflow with spirom-

Figure 20-1 Pathology of Asthma.

PAS, periodic acid–Schiff. *Courtesy of Nizar N. Jarjour, MD, University of Wisconsin, and with permission from Morgenroth K, Newhouse MT, Nolte D: Atlas of Pulmonary Pathology. PVG Pharmazeutische Verlagsgesellschaft, London, Butterworth Scientific, 1982, p 37.*

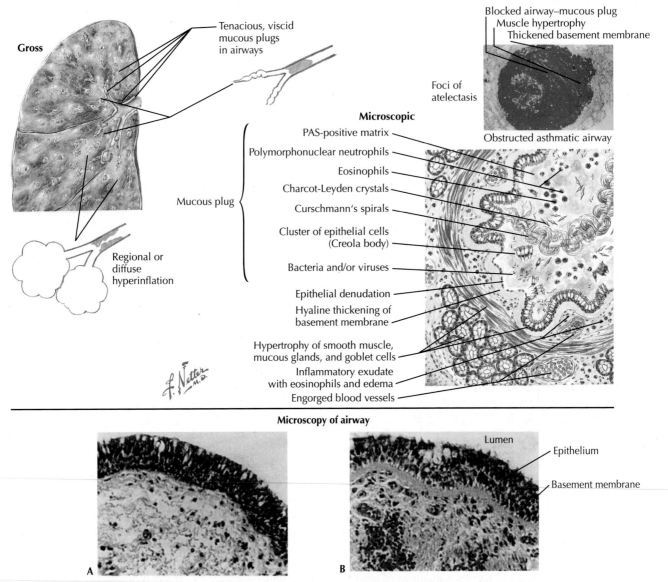

Gross

Tenacious, viscid mucous plugs in airways

Blocked airway–mucous plug
Muscle hypertrophy
Thickened basement membrane

Foci of atelectasis

Obstructed asthmatic airway

Microscopic

PAS-positive matrix
Polymorphonuclear neutrophils
Eosinophils
Charcot-Leyden crystals
Curschmann's spirals
Cluster of epithelial cells (Creola body)
Bacteria and/or viruses
Epithelial denudation
Hyaline thickening of basement membrane
Hypertrophy of smooth muscle, mucous glands, and goblet cells
Inflammatory exudate with eosinophils and edema
Engorged blood vessels

Mucous plug

Regional or diffuse hyperinflation

Microscopy of airway

Lumen
Epithelium
Basement membrane

A   B

(**A**) Normal airway after control of hyperreactivity following high doses of inhaled steroids.
(**B**) Asthmatic airway before therapy with high-dose inhaled steriods to control.

etry and decrease in the forced expiratory flow at 1 second (FEV_1) and in the peak expiratory flow rate (PEFR). There is an initial decline within about 20 minutes associated with histamine release from mast cells that is stimulated by allergen binding to IgE on the mast cell surface. This immediate reaction is blocked by antihistamines but not by steroids. Classically, a spontaneous recovery occurs, only to be followed by a second, later decline in flow rates. Steroid pretreatment inhibits this late phase reaction, which is manifest by the recruitment of inflammatory cells into and around the lower airway (Fig. 20-3).

The estimates of the rate of decline in pulmonary function vary from 22 to 35 mL/year in FEV_1 in those with no asthma to 38 to 160 mL/year in FEV_1 in those with asthma. Whether remodeling contributes to or causes the accelerated loss of pulmonary function is not known.

Clinical Presentation

The clinical presentation of asthma is nonspecific (Fig. 20-4). Prototypically, the chief complaint consists of the triad of wheezing, shortness of breath, and chest tightness.

Figure 20-2 Extrinsic Asthma: Mechanism of Type 1 (Immediate) Hypersensitivity.

APC, antigen-presenting cell; IFN-γ, interferon-γ; IL, interleukin. *Adapted with permission from Busse WW, Lemanske RF: Advances in Immunology: Asthma. N Engl J Med 344(5):353, 2001; and Schwartz RS: A new element in the mechanism of asthma. N Engl J Med 346(11):857, 2002. Copyright © 2001 and 2002, Massachusetts Medical Society. All rights reserved.*

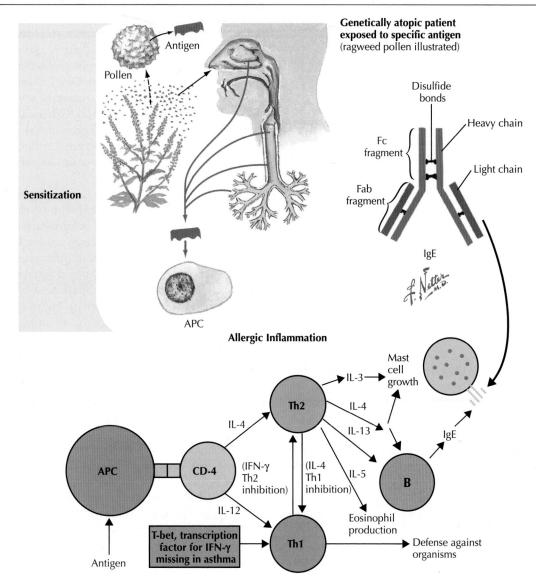

Symptoms vary in severity with time, sometimes changing in minutes or over many months, but commonly changing daily. Symptoms are typically worse at night. The hyperreactivity is associated with triggers such as respiratory infections and exposure to strong odors or cold air. Repeated allergen exposures lower the threshold for nonspecific hyperreactivity symptoms.

Occasionally, the sole presentation is dyspnea on exertion or cough. The cough with cough-variant asthma is usually unproductive. However, asthmatic patients can occasionally produce copious sputum laden with eosino-phils and eosinophilic debris, mucus casts of the small airways (Curschmann's spirals), airway epithelial cells (sometimes in clumps referred to as *Creola bodies*), and Charcot-Leyden crystals (protein from eosinophils) (Fig. 20-5). Thirty percent or more of patients with chronic cough have asthma.

Acute exacerbations generally present, by patient history, as a sudden onset of respiratory distress. Following the resolution of the acute event, a history, either from the patient or from others who have observed the patient, often reveals that signs of disease activity have been present

Figure 20-3 Antigen Challenge.
FEV₁, forced expiratory volume in 1 second.

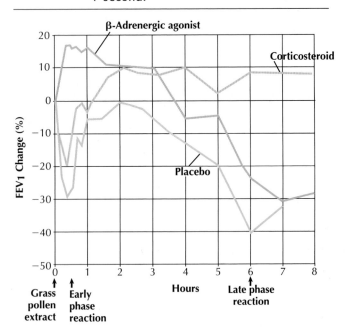

intermittent asthma, requiring bronchodilator therapy less than twice weekly, and *persistent asthma*, graded as mild, moderate, or severe (Table 20-1). Commonly, individual asthmatic patients move among these levels of disease severity as the activity of their disease varies.

Steroid-dependent asthma, steroid-resistant asthma, and *difficult* or *brittle asthma* are other terms employed to describe categories of severe asthma. Asthma is also classified into groups by presumed cause: *intrinsic asthma* with no apparent allergic sensitization, and *extrinsic asthma* demonstrating elevated IgE and skin test reactions to allergens and seasonal variability (see Fig. 20-2). Other categories separate asthma by the type of trigger of the exacerbation: exercise-associated asthma, nocturnal asthma, and drug-induced asthma (e.g., angiotensin-converting enzyme inhibitors and β blockers).

Sensitivity to nonsteroidal anti-inflammatory drugs (NSAIDs) in asthma is associated with severe disease and nasal polyps (Samter's triad). The proposed mechanism is not linked to anti-NSAID antibody production. Rather, it is proposed that there is enhanced inflammatory leukotriene production when arachidonic acid metabolism to prostaglandins is blocked by the inhibition of cyclooxygenase and shunted to the 5-lipoxygenase pathway (Fig. 20-7). Treatment requires avoidance of all drugs classified as NSAIDs (not just salicylates, or aspirin), salicylate-containing foods (e.g., apricots, dates, and almonds to name but a few), and artificial yellow-red food dyes. Acetaminophen is considered safe. Desensitizing protocols have also been developed and are reported to be clinically beneficial but need to be carried out under careful medical supervision.

Asthmatic bronchitis is associated with an acute respiratory infection causing prolonged cough and sputum production. Allergic bronchopulmonary mycosis reflects a hypersensitivity to airway colonization with a fungus such as *Aspergillus* species. Occupational asthma refers to new-onset asthma caused by workplace exposures and asthma aggravated by exposure to factors in the work environment.

for many hours or days before the acute decompensation. However, actual sudden-onset respiratory failure and death are reported with asthma. At autopsy, these individuals demonstrate less mucous plugging and more neutrophilic, and less eosinophilic, airway infiltration. Death in this setting is associated with suffocation secondary to bronchospasm rather than mucous occlusion of the airways. Objective monitoring of signs of respiratory disease activity such as peak expiratory flows, nocturnal awakenings caused by shortness of breath, chest tightness, and cough can be useful as a guide to early intervention (Fig. 20-6). Occasionally, lung infection or pneumothorax is associated with acute decompensation. These conditions require early detection and therapy in severely affected asthmatic patients to ensure survival. Life-threatening signs include marked accessory muscle use, depressed mental status, diaphoresis, cyanosis, fatigue, pulsus paradoxus greater than 15 mm Hg, peak expiratory flows less than 100 L/min, and CO_2 retention.

Morbidity and mortality from asthma are increased in elderly patients. Generally, there is less reversible airflow obstruction and eosinophilia. IgE concentrations are also less impressively elevated. The signs and symptoms are similar to those of younger patients, and response to therapy is good. Conditions that exacerbate asthma, such as congestive heart failure, hypothyroidism, and gastroesophageal reflux, are more common in this population. Chronic sinus disease should be evaluated in all asthmatic patients with refractory disease.

Asthma has many clinical forms. The syndrome has been classified based on severity by the National Asthma Education and Prevention Program (NAEPP) guidelines:

Differential Diagnosis

The causes of cough, wheezing, and dyspnea are legion, and the adage that "all that wheezes is not asthma" is true (Box 20-1).

Establishing the diagnosis of asthma in the setting of chronic obstructive pulmonary disease (COPD), which shares many signs and symptoms with asthma, can be challenging. Also, asthmatic smokers often can develop fixed airflow obstruction. However, even when no reversible airflow obstruction is demonstrated with spirometry, a clinical trial of corticosteroids and bronchodilators is appropriate. Another consideration is bacterial infections causing bronchial hyperreactivity in asthmatic patients, for example, pertussis, mycoplasma, and chlamydia pneumo-

Figure 20-4 Clinical Features.

Bottom left photo, *From Stradling P: Diagnostic bronchoscopy, 3rd ed. Philadelphia, Elsevier, 1976, p 42.* **Bottom right photo,** *From Smalhout B, Hill-Vaughan AB: The suffocating child; bronchoscopy: A guide to diagnosis and treatment. Munich, Boehringer Ingelheim, 1979.*

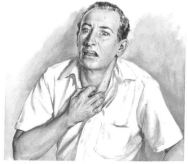

Features common to both extrinsic allergic and intrinsic asthma: Respiratory distress, dyspnea, wheezing, flushing, cyanosis, cough, flaring of alae, use of accessory respiratory muscles, apprehension, tachycardia, perspiration, hyperresonance, distant breath sounds and rhonchi, eosinophilia

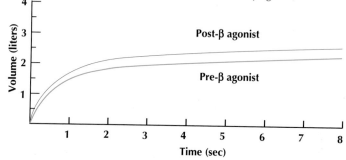

Spirogram demonstrating reversible airway obstruction by improvement of airflow after treatment with a bronchodilator (β agonist)

Post-β agonist

Pre-β agonist

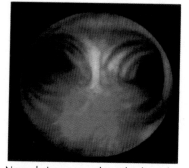

Normal airway seen through a broncho-scope looking at the main carina with the right main branches to the right

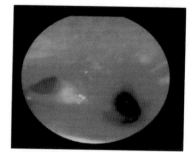

Asthmatic airway—same view as shown in the normal airway

nias. The functional disorder of vocal cord dysfunction is often initially confused with asthma and is diagnosed when inspection of the vocal cords reveals a characteristic paradoxical movement of the vocal cords with respiration (see Chapter 15). Underlying sinus disease, hypothyroidism, and gastroesophageal reflux aggravating asthma also warrant consideration.

Diagnostic Approach

Patients with undiagnosed asthma often present with complaints of episodic attacks of wheezing, cough, or shortness of breath. The suspected diagnosis is supported when examination documents wheezing and when the history of asymptomatic intervals and precipitating triggers is elicited. A chest x-ray is obtained to exclude other pulmonary pathology. Generally, the chest x-ray in asthma is normal. Radiographs may demonstrate hyperinflation during an acute attack, but this finding is more often associated with COPD. Atelectasis with mucous plugging is associated with asthma (see Fig. 20-1). Pneumothorax is more

common in asthmatic patients and can present as an asthma exacerbation.

Spirometry measurements before and after administering a bronchodilator are usually obtained to demonstrate reversible airflow obstruction and to determine the severity of the acute disease (see Fig. 20-4). Chronic cough associated with normal spirometry and an elevated D_{LCO} (carbon monoxide diffusion capacity) suggests the diagnosis of *cough asthma*. Skin scratch testing may be useful diagnostically and provides guidance when prescribing immunotherapy and designing avoidance strategies. Other observations supporting the diagnosis of asthma include variability in home monitoring of PEFRs, improving PEFRs on asthma therapy, hyperreactivity to challenge testing with histamine or methacholine, peripheral blood eosinophilia, elevated IgE, and the characteristic sputum previously described. Generally, the diagnosis is made correctly using only spirometry and chest radiography to support the physical examination and history. Failure to respond to asthma therapy should prompt a search for other causes.

Figure 20-5 Sputum in Bronchial Asthma.

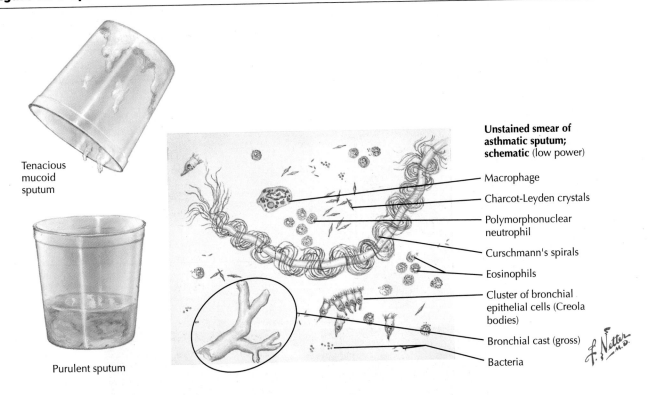

Tenacious
mucoid
sputum

Purulent sputum

**Unstained smear of
asthmatic sputum;
schematic** (low power)

Macrophage
Charcot-Leyden crystals
Polymorphonuclear
neutrophil
Curschmann's spirals
Eosinophils
Cluster of bronchial
epithelial cells (Creola
bodies)
Bronchial cast (gross)
Bacteria

Figure 20-6 Asthma Diary.

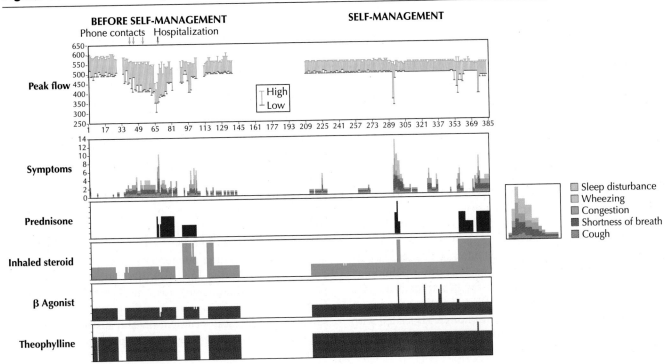

BEFORE SELF-MANAGEMENT   SELF-MANAGEMENT

Phone contacts Hospitalization

Peak flow

High
Low

Symptoms

Prednisone

Inhaled steroid

β Agonist

Theophylline

Sleep disturbance
Wheezing
Congestion
Shortness of breath
Cough

Table 20-1 Stepwise Approach for Managing Asthma in Adults and Children Older than Five Years of Age: Treatment

	Clinical Features before Treatment or Adequate Control		Medications Required to Maintain Long-Term Control
Classification	Symptoms/Day Symptoms/Night	PEF or FEV₁ PEF Variability	Daily Medications
STEP 1 Mild intermittent	<2 days/wk ≤2 nights/mo	>80% <20%	No daily medication needed. Severe exacerbations may occur, separated by long periods of normal lung function and no symptoms. A course of systemic corticosteroids is recommended.
STEP 2 Mild persistent	>2/wk but <1×/day >2 nights/mo	≥80% 20%-30%	*Preferred treatment:* Low-dose inhaled corticosteroids *Alternative treatment:* Cromolyn, leukotriene modifier, nedocromil, *or* Sustained-release theophylline to serum concentration of 5-15 µg/mL
STEP 3 Moderate persistent	Daily >1 night/week	>60%-<80% >30%	*Preferred treatment:* Low- to medium-dose inhaled corticosteroids and long-acting inhaled β₂ agonists *Alternative treatment:* Increase inhaled corticosteroids within medium-dose range, *or* Low- to medium-dose inhaled corticosteroids and either leukotriene modifier or theophylline *If needed* (particularly in patients with recurring severe exacerbations): *Preferred treatment:* Increase inhaled corticosteroids within medium-dose range and add long-acting inhaled β₂ agonists *Alternative treatment:* Increase inhaled corticosteroids within medium-dose range and add either leukotriene modifier or theophylline
STEP 4 Severe persistent	Continual Frequent	≤60% >30%	*Preferred treatment:* High-dose inhaled corticosteroids, *and* Long-acting inhaled β₂ agonists, *and, if needed,* Corticosteroid tablets or syrup long term (2 mg/kg/day, generally do not exceed 60 mg per day). (Make repeat attempts to reduce corticosteroids and maintain control with high-dose inhaled corticosteroids.)
QUICK RELIEF All patients	Short-acting bronchodilator: 2-4 puffs short-acting inhaled β₂ agonists as needed for symptoms. Intensity of treatment will depend on severity of exacerbation; up to 3 treatments at 20-min intervals or a single nebulizer treatment as needed. Course of systemic corticosteroids may be needed. Use of short-acting β₂-agonists >2×/wk in intermittent asthma (daily, or increasing use in persistent asthma) may indicate the need to initiate (increase) long-term control therapy.		

Adapted from The National Heart, Lung, and Blood Institute's National Asthma Education and Prevention Program, National Institutes of Health Expert Panel Report, December 2002.

Management and Therapy

Optimum Treatment

Asthma therapy focuses on the management of airway inflammation. The goal is to prevent exacerbations, minimize symptoms, and maintain near-normal lung function. Informed patient self-management with the goal of early intervention, allergen and inhaled irritant avoidance strategies, and repeated review of the proper techniques for employing inhaled medications are keys to controlling asthma. Anti-inflammatory agents (e.g., inhaled corticosteroids [ICS]) are the pharmacologic cornerstones for controlling asthma. ICS therapy should be initiated when asthma symptoms occur even once or twice during a week.

Figure 20-7 Leukotriene Modifiers.
AA, arachidonic acid; LT, leukotriene; NSAID, nonsteroidal anti-inflammatory drug; HETE, hydroxyeicosatetraenoic acid; PGs, prostaglandins; Tx, thromboxane.

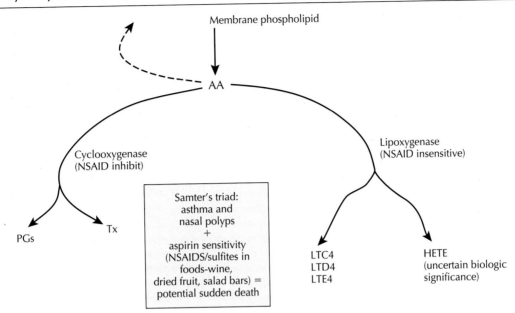

Bronchodilators such as β agonists, however, remain the cornerstone of acute management of exacerbations. Severe exacerbations may require monitoring in an intensive care unit and mechanical ventilation. Grading chronic asthma severity, however, is difficult. It is clear that physical examination, symptoms, and pulmonary function tests lack adequate predictive value. Even asthmatic patients with increasing PEFRs have died suddenly of their disease. Asthma deaths are equally distributed among asthmatic patients classified by NAEPP guidelines as mild, moderate, or severe. Classification of severity by monitoring β_2-agonist rescue use has identified *severe* asthmatic patients in the group defined as *mild* by NAEPP guidelines. A careful assessment of β_2-agonist use is easily accomplished with many patients and provides a practical management tool. Titrating anti-inflammatory therapy to eliminate sputum eosinophils or nonspecific bronchial hyperreactivity, as measured by inhaled histamine challenge testing, produces better asthma control compared with NAEPP guidelines.

Soon-to-be-released guidelines will therefore incorporate strategies to better address the potential for asthma exacerbations and define the present status of asthma disease activity. Integral to each individual patient plan will be accurately judging how responsive the patient will be to available therapies over the long run.

β_2 Agonists

β agonists reverse smooth muscle bronchospasm regardless of the stimulus, inhibit histamine and other mediator release from inflammatory cells, inhibit cholinergic neuro-transmission, inhibit airway vascular leakage, and increase mucociliary clearance. Although the anti-inflammatory effects of β agonists in asthma have been difficult to demonstrate clinically, no other class of drug is as effective at relieving the acute symptoms of asthma. Racemic albuterol (R-albuterol) is a commonly used short-acting bronchodilator drug. Levalbuterol, the active component in R-albuterol, is available and may prove superior to R-albuterol. Short-acting β agonists are used on an as-needed basis to relieve symptoms and not routinely in an effort to prevent them. The frequency of as-needed use, therefore, is a marker of disease control. A metered dose inhaler (MDI) with a spacer is as effective as wet nebulizer delivery of the drug when airflow is not extremely restricted. Parenteral β-agonist or wet-nebulizer delivery should be considered if there is little air movement and if the MDI technique is inadequate. Intravenous epinephrine poses a cardiovascular risk in adults.

Long-acting β agonists, such as salmeterol and formoterol, are used in conjunction with inhaled steroids as preventive agents. This combination is more effective than doubling the dose of steroid. In vitro work demonstrates enhanced transport of the steroid receptor into the nucleus in the presence of a β agonist. Whether this is an explanation for the clinical observation is not clear. Monotherapy with long- or short-acting β agonists does not control the clinical expression of persistent asthma, is associated with an increased risk for asthma death, and should not be used. There is a controversial U.S. Food and Drug Administration black-box warning that cautions patients and physicians against the use of any β-agonist therapy for asthma.

Steroids

Steroids are the most effective agents for preventing asthma symptoms through their role as inhibitors of inflammatory mediator production. They are the only class of medication demonstrated to decrease asthma mortality. Inhaled steroids are recommended to control chronic asthma when as-needed β-agonist rescue is required more than once or twice weekly. Potent inhaled steroids take days to weeks to produce significant clinical improvement. There is, however, reported effect in 2 hours with 4 puffs (1000 µg) of flunisolide every 10 minutes for 3 hours by MDI with spacer. This suggests a role for inhaled steroids in acute exacerbations.

Inhaled steroids dosing by NAEPP guidelines is established by PEFR measurements, the frequency of use of rescue short-acting albuterol, and symptoms (see Table 20-1). If, instead, inhaled corticosteroid dosing is based on normalization of hyperreactivity, defined by challenge testing with histamine, much higher doses of inhaled steroid are required. However, at these doses, asthma control is superior, and asthmatic lung remodeling improves (see Fig. 20-1).

A dose of 60 mg of prednisone orally to 125 mg of methylprednisolone intravenously is commonly used to initiate therapy in severely ill asthmatics. Generally, there is good bioavailability of steroids orally; however, intravenous administration is used to ensure delivery in the acute situation. The onset of action is uncertain, and variability is reported as 1 to 24 hours. Oral prednisone as outpatient therapy following a severe exacerbation is generally used at a dose of 40 mg orally each morning for 2 weeks. Morning dosing of systemic steroids is recommended to minimize adrenal suppression. Tapering schedules are the norm. However, this dose is generally tolerated without a taper for 3 weeks. Intramuscular dosing has not been studied as a long-term maintenance therapy but has rare indications—it may be useful for patients unable to comply with oral medications upon discharge from the emergency department.

Leukotriene Modifiers

Leukotrienes (LTs) are elevated in asthmatic patients and are linked to relevant inflammatory changes in the lung. (For a discussion of montelukast and zileuton, see Chapter 10.) This class of agents blocks aspirin-induced asthma. LT modifiers improve lung function in chronic asthma and decrease β-agonist rescue, inhaled corticosteroid use, and exacerbations requiring oral steroids. They are no longer recommended as first-line monotherapy in mild persistent asthma but may be useful additions to therapy when inhaled steroids alone fail or when inhaled steroids cannot be used. There is an unclear association between the use of LT modifiers to treat asthma and the risk for developing Churg-Strauss vasculitis. Although ICS are strongly preferred for any degree of persistent asthma, LT modifiers are an acceptable second-line choice when the use of ICS is not possible. Adding long-acting bronchodilators (β agonists) is recommended when inhaled steroids do not control symptoms; LT modifiers are an acceptable second choice when long-acting bronchodilators cannot be used. Triple therapy with inhaled steroids, long-acting β agonists, and LT modifiers is also prescribed for daily use to control asthma. Short-acting β agonists should be reserved for rescue therapy and monitored carefully as an index of asthma control. Neither short- nor long-acting bronchodilators should ever be used as monotherapy for persistent asthma.

Anti-immunoglobulin G Antibodies (Omalizumab)

Omalizumab is a humanized recombinant monoclonal anti-IgE antibody that binds only to circulating IgE, preventing IgE binding to mast cells and treating allergic asthma (Fig. 20-8). It does not bind to IgE bound to mast

Figure 20-8 Omalizumab Mechanism of Action in IgE-Mediated Asthma.
IgE, immunoglobulin E. *Adapted from Am J Health-Syst Pharm 61(14):1449-1459, 2004.*

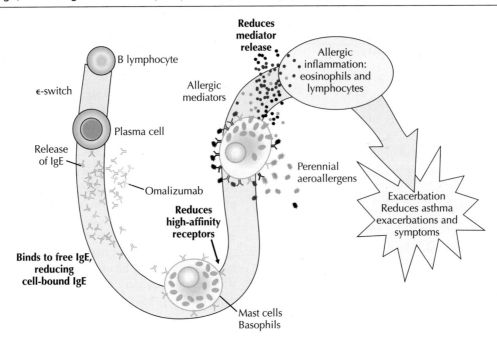

cells and is not associated with anaphylaxis. Omalizumab reduces early and late phase reactions to allergen challenge. In moderate to severe asthma, it reduced exacerbations and showed other clinical benefits. In more severe asthma, there was no reduction of exacerbations, but the drug again showed some clinical benefit. There are no guideline recommendations for its use at this time. Omalizumab is indicated in the treatment of poorly controlled asthma when other therapies have failed. The asthmatic patients selected for therapy should ideally have IgE levels of 30 to 700 IUs and be sensitive to at least one allergen by scratch skin testing or radioallergosorbent test (RAST).

Omalizumab is relatively expensive ($4000 to $20,000/year; average $12,000/year) compared with $1200/year for montelukast, $2160/year for combination fluticasone dipropionate and salmeterol, and $680/year for a theophylline preparation. Given the high costs involved, before starting omalizumab, health care providers should exclude specific causes of treatment failure, including compliance issues and poor understanding of inhaler technique.

Ipratropium Bromide

Ipratropium bromide is a bronchodilator, but is not as potent as β agonists in asthma; its most accepted role in asthma therapy is as a rescue in asthmatic patients receiving β blockers. It may prove useful in children and for severe adult exacerbations when routine agents fail.

Other Agents

Cromolyn and nedocromil are anti-inflammatory agents used primarily in children. Magnesium, 2 g intravenously over 15 minutes, is used in severely ill asthmatic patients to reverse bronchospasm. The phosphodiesterase inhibitor theophylline is a bronchodilator that also enhances respiratory muscle contraction and mucociliary clearance, decreases hypoventilation, and has anti-inflammatory properties. Its narrow therapeutic window and lack of dramatic efficacy limit its use. Mixtures of helium and oxygen, inhaled furosemide, inhaled anesthetics, tetracyclines—most recently telithromycin—and mucolytic agents have been reported to be beneficial.

Avoiding Treatment Errors

β Agonists should never be used as monotherapy for persistent asthma. Inhaled steroids are the cornerstone therapy for persistent asthma.

Before additional therapies are prescribed to improve management or asthma control, the issues of compliance and adequate inhaler technique must be resolved. Each patient interaction should include a review to ensure compliance and more importantly adequacy of inhaler technique. With good inhaler technique, 10% to 15% of the medication reaches the airway; with poor technique, no medication is inhaled.

It is important to remember that "all that wheezes" is not asthma and that the patient's environment may abound in disease triggers that, until addressed, will make control very difficult. Triggers are legion and include gastroesophageal reflux disease, sinus disease, cigarette smoke, medications, foods, food additives, industrial exposures, and season aeroallergens such as pollens and fungal blooms.

Future Directions

The focus for drug development in asthma is on interrupting its inflammatory cascade. Much effort is being made at the molecular level. Anti-IL-5, while able to reduce blood eosinophilia, had no effect on clinical disease. Soluble IL-4 receptor, on the other hand, shows clinical promise. Other efforts target other cytokines, transcription factors, arachidonic acid metabolites, platelet-activating factor, cell-adhesion molecules, phosphodiesterase-4, and T-cell markers. Also, a mutation on chromosome 10, involving the metalloproteinase matrix protein (MMP) ADAM-33, has been linked to bronchial hyperactivity and presumptively to airway smooth muscle hypertrophy. MMPs were formally thought to be involved only with remodeling of the extracellular matrix. Recent observations, however, suggest a role for MMPs in the clearing of cytokines and their receptors, and thus a role in immune modulation. Perhaps the most promising development in asthma research has been the link between asthma and the recently described subgroup of potent immunoregulatory CD1d-restricted NKT cells. These cells have become an interesting potential therapeutic target in asthma.

More importantly, efforts are emerging that may allow manipulation of the immune system to prevent the development of the asthmatic phenotype or to reverse the abnormal inflammatory response and prevent the chronic airway inflammation that we now call asthma. Interesting efforts include using bacterial DNA repeats, rather than aluminum sulfate, as adjuvants for vaccines to direct inflammatory responses away from pathways that produce pathologic chronic atopic inflammation.

Markers of asthmatic inflammation, for example, exhaled nitrous oxide (NO), may prove helpful in predicting exacerbations, grading disease severity, and judging therapeutic success.

Additional Resources

National Asthma Education and Prevention Program: Guidelines for the diagnosis and management of asthma. Available at: http://www.nhlbi.nih.gov/guidelines/asthma/execsumm.pdf.

This website includes a summary of the stepwise approach to managing infants, children, and adults with acute or chronic asthma, as well as usual dosages for long-term control medications. This summary is suitable for a patient handout.

National Asthma Education and Prevention Program (NAEPP) Expert Panel Report 3 (EPR 3): Guidelines for the diagnosis and management of asthma. Available at http://www.nhlbi.nih.gov/guidelines/asthma/asthgdln.htm.

This website provides the most recent guidelines on the diagnosis and management of asthma.

Swain AR, Dutton SP, Truswell A: Salicylates in foods. J Am Diet Assoc 85(8):950-960, 1985.

This site lists foods that contain salicylates.

EVIDENCE

1. Akbari O, Faul JL, Hoyte EG, et al: CD4+ invariant T-cell-receptor+ natural killer T cells in bronchial asthma. N Engl J Med 354(11):1117-1129, 2006.

    This is the first report of a newly described T cell, not regulated by steroids, that is linked to asthma.

2. Barnes PJ, Grunstein MM, Leff AR, Woolcock AJ (eds): Asthma, vol 1. Philadelphia, Lippincott-Raven, 1997.

    This offers a detailed review of asthma.

3. Berry MA, Hargadon B, Shelley M, et al: Evidence of a role of tumor necrosis factor alpha in refractory asthma. N Engl J Med 354(7):697-708, 2006.

    The authors describe a role for tumor necrosis factor-α in difficult-to-control asthma.

4. Busse WW, Lemnske RF Jr: Asthma. N Engl J Med 344:350-362, 2001.

    This article presents a lucid review of the immunohistopathology of asthma.

5. Horiuchi T, Castro M: The pathobiologic implications for treatment. Old and new strategies in the treatment of chronic asthma. Clin Chest Med 21:381-395, 2000.

    The authors provide a good review of asthma therapy with detailed mechanistic descriptions of the pharmacology of the most commonly employed asthma therapies.

6. Kay AB: Advances in immunology: Allergic diseases-first of two parts. N Engl J Med 344:30-37, 2001.

    The author presents a review of the most prominent theories of how allergy and allergic diseases arise.

7. Shapiro SD, Owen CA: ADAM-323 surfaces on an asthma gene. N Engl J Med 347:936-938, 2002.

    This is a description of a candidate gene for asthma. It focuses on matrix metalloproteinases and proposes a mechanistic model showing the part they are thought to play in health and asthma.

8. Strunk RC, Bloomberg GR: Omalizumab for asthma. N Engl J Med 354(25)2689-2695, 2006.

    This clinical problem-solving exercise focuses on defining the role of omalizumab in treating refractory asthma.

Ashley G. Henderson

Bronchitis: Acute and Chronic

Introduction

Bronchitis, the clinical term for inflammation of the bronchi, is divided into acute and chronic forms. It presents as cough, with or without sputum production, and has the potential for airway infection and no evidence of pneumonia on physical examination or chest x-ray.

Acute bronchitis (AB) and chronic bronchitis (CB) are distinct entities, although the original presentation of the patient can appear similar in both cases. The main distinguishing feature clinically is the duration of cough; however, AB must also be distinguished from acute exacerbations of CB because the underlying pathophysiology is different. Although both are diseases of the lower airways, CB is clinically defined as a productive cough for at least 3 months of the year for at least 2 years in a row. It is one component of the spectrum of chronic obstructive pulmonary disease that is discussed in more detail in Chapter 22. The remainder of this chapter focuses primarily on AB.

Epidemiology and Pathogenesis

AB affects about 5% of adults annually and is the ninth most common illness in outpatients in the United States. Cough is the most common symptom resulting in any outpatient visit, and AB is the number one cause of cough in this setting. Although concurrent airway infection is part of the definition, up to 90% of these infections are thought to be viral and do not warrant antibiotic treatment. In fact, AB is considered the number one cause of antibiotic abuse in this country. The usual viral causes include influenza A and B, parainfluenza, coronavirus, rhinovirus, respiratory syncytial virus, and human metapneumovirus. There are also some bacterial causes of AB, including *Mycoplasma pneumoniae*, *Chlamydophila pneumoniae*, *Bordetella pertussis*, and *Bordetella parapertussis*. In addition, patients with CB can develop acute exacerbations of their CB with *Streptococcus pneumoniae*, *Moraxella catarrhalis*, and *Haemophilus influenzae*, but these are not commonly proved to be a cause of uncomplicated AB. It is unclear whether these organisms are only colonizers or act as pathogens.

The cause of the cough is thought to be multifactorial, but histologically there is epithelial cell damage with release of proinflammatory mediators, which lead to transient bronchial hyperresponsiveness and airflow obstruction. Although some pathologic changes occur, the symptoms and the physical effects resolve completely in 3 to 6 weeks. Repeated attacks of AB can result in CB.

Clinical Presentation

Patients with AB present with a sudden onset of cough in the absence of fever, tachycardia, and tachypnea. By definition, patients should not have asthma, a common cold, or other upper respiratory tract infection. Uncomplicated AB is not an exacerbation of CB. Simple upper respiratory tract infections include rhinitis, laryngitis, pharyngitis, and sinusitis. They can be caused by both bacteria and viruses but are distinguished from AB by the lack of inflammation of the lower respiratory tract (trachea, bronchi, and bronchioles). The absence of lower tract inflammation explains why cough is rarely present in simple upper respiratory tract infections.

Some patients with AB may complain of soreness in the chest or mild shortness of breath, but the primary symptom is cough, with or without increased sputum production. AB warrants consideration in any patient who presents with a cough lasting more than 5 days. It is not unusual for a cough to last 10 to 20 days; however, the mean cough duration, taking all causes into account, is 18 days, with an occasional duration of 4 to 5 weeks. Only half of patients report purulent sputum. The physical exam is usually negative for a specific finding other than cough; hence, the presence of crackles or egophony on exam, especially when associated with fever, warrants further evaluation with chest x-ray to rule out pneumonia. If a patient presents with a fever and cough and a negative chest x-ray, influenza and pertussis are two potential causes of AB. Otherwise, other illnesses must be considered because 90% of AB cases are viral and only one virus—influenza—causes fever.

Influenza has the potential for high morbidity and mortality, and 93% of these patients present with a cough as well as weakness (94%), myalgia (94%), and fever (68%). During influenza season (primarily winter), the sudden onset of fever and cough suggests influenza.

Of the other viral infections that cause AB, coronavirus, rhinovirus, and adenovirus often present with an upper respiratory infection with the associated nasal congestion, rhinorrhea, and pharyngitis, as well as the cough.

Differential Diagnosis

Because the primary symptom of both acute and CB is cough, the differential diagnosis is large. The history and physical exam alone allow the exclusion of many of the diagnoses.

The differential of AB includes pneumonia or pneumonitis, asthma, upper airway cough syndrome (formerly postnasal drip syndrome), gastroesophageal reflux, CB with an acute exacerbation, and medication reaction. Many of these other diagnoses often last more than 3 weeks and are more likely to present with a chronic cough. Therefore, the primary differential diagnosis for the acute cough of AB is pneumonia and an acute exacerbation of CB. The associated mortality and required treatment for these diagnoses are different. As previously noted, fever is uncommon in AB unless it is associated with influenza or pertussis or unless it is complicated by pneumonia. Another cause of acute cough is severe acute respiratory syndrome (SARS) virus, which has a high morbidity and mortality rate and quickly develops into pneumonia.

Causes of subacute cough (3 to 6 weeks' duration) include upper airway cough syndrome, asthma, gastroesophageal reflux disease, pertussis, pneumonia, and an acute exacerbation of CB. Many of these diagnoses can be distinguished by history and physical examination alone. Upper airway cough syndrome often presents with upper airway congestion and the sensation of a "drip" in the posterior oropharynx and has often been present for longer than 6 weeks. Asthma is often intermittent or chronic, with acute "spells" of worsening shortness of breath or chest

pain, associated with wheezing and exacerbated by change in season, temperature, or climate. If the patient has a chronic cough and a smoking history but presents with an acute change in the baseline cough with increased sputum production or change in color, the underlying problem is probably an exacerbation of CB. Gastroesophageal reflux disease most often presents as a chronic cough, with a history of heartburn or a cough that exacerbates at nighttime or with meals. Pertussis is a cause of cough with fever, but it is often associated with a more prolonged cough, lasting as long as 10 to 12 weeks, and coughing paroxysms. Adults with pertussis often have a milder illness than children, do not always have the characteristic "whoop," and have post-tussive emesis in up to 40% of cases. As previously noted, pneumonia often presents with cough and fever and typical physical exam findings of tachycardia, lung crackles, or egophony. In contrast, only 30% of elderly patients aged 75 years or older with community-acquired pneumonia presented with a fever, and only 37% had tachycardia.

Excluding the specific laboratory diagnosis of influenza or pertussis, the specific cause of AB is often not determined (i.e., type of virus or bacterium), but it can occasionally be elucidated by a careful history. Exposure to ill contacts, duration of cough, associated symptoms, and vaccination history can be helpful. If AB associated with fever and pneumonia is excluded, then pertussis and influenza are the two main causes.

See Chapter 17 on cough for further discussion and differential diagnoses.

Diagnostic Approach

The routine use of laboratory tests to define the specific pathogen in AB is not cost effective; as a result, routine evaluation with sputum Gram stain and culture and routine serum tests is not recommended. The exceptions are influenza and pertussis, if clinically suspected. The rapid test for influenza is cost effective because it allows for the use of antiviral agents and improves the understanding of the epidemiology of outbreaks. Nevertheless, routine screening for influenza in AB is not recommended unless the patient presents with influenza-like symptoms during the influenza season. If pertussis is suspected, a routine complete blood count is helpful to look for the severe leukocytosis associated with this diagnosis. There are complicated serum and nasal culture recommendations based on the stage of the infection. Whether these tests are warranted can be debated because most cases of AB are not pertussis. Several diagnostic tests can determine other specific pathogens but are not cost effective in simple AB and are not recommended.

Obtaining a chest x-ray (if warranted by history and physical exam) to rule out pneumonia is usually helpful, especially given the significant morbidity and mortality rates associated with this diagnosis.

Management and Therapy

Optimum Treatment

Most cases of AB are viral or self-limited, and only symptomatic therapy is recommended.

Antimicrobial therapy is not indicated in most cases because multiple trials have demonstrated only minor reduction in the duration of cough (0.6 days) and no difference in the time of return to work, school, or usual activities at home on day 3 or 7. If a specific treatable pathogen is identified, antimicrobial therapy is more likely to be beneficial. The use of anti-influenza agents can reduce the duration of cough by 1 day if the agent is started within 48 hours of symptom onset, and treatment of pertussis is indicated to limit transmission. Although there are current recommendations to consider antimicrobial therapy for *M. pneumoniae* and *C. pneumoniae*, there are no data suggestive of improved outcomes with antimicrobial treatment.

Other therapies for AB include the use of antitussive agents, β_2 agonists, mucolytic agents, and corticosteroids. There are limited data and support for the use of β_2 agonists, mucolytics, and oral corticosteroids. A recent Cochrane Database review did not support the use of β_2 agonists based on five trials, including patients with airflow obstruction. There are also no significant clinical trials to support the use of antitussive agents, but they are routinely used for the acute symptomatic benefit of the patient.

The current guidelines released by the American College of Chest Physicians (ACCP) do not recommend the use of antibiotics. The ACCP recommends β_2 agonists only in the subgroups of patients with chronic airflow obstruction at baseline or wheezing at presentation. There is no role for mucolytic agents or anticholinergic agents. For the treatment of pertussis, both the ACCP and the Centers for Disease Control and Prevention recommend macrolides as first-line therapy and, for influenza, oseltamivir or zanamivir. Newer generations of influenza are resistant to amantadine and rimantadine.

Avoiding Treatment Errors

As previously stated, the major treatment error is the use of antimicrobial therapy for AB. Because of rising microbial resistance, physicians are encouraged to use only symptomatic therapy in patients with simple AB unless specific microbials are identified or suspected.

Future Directions

AB is highly prevalent in primary care practice. The careful history and physical examination remain the most helpful diagnostic tools. Other diagnostic modalities are likely to become available, including the use of the procalcitonin test to discriminate between patients with pneumonia and bronchitis. The chest physical exam remains the most useful tool to distinguish between these two types of pulmonary infection. The use of antibiotics is not recommended for most cases; however, more than 70% of patients who seek care receive antibiotics. This observation has led to a campaign to dissuade physicians from this practice. Limiting the overprescribing of antimicrobials should decrease the cost of health care and reduce the emergence of resistant pathogens.

EVIDENCE

1. American College of Chest Physicians: Diagnosis and management of cough: ACCP evidence-based clinical practice guidelines. Chest 129(1 Suppl):1S-23S, 2006.

    This paper is a summary of the most up-to-date review of diagnosis and management of cough as recommended by the American College of Chest Physicians.

2. Aris R: Cough. In Runge MS, Greganti MA (eds): Netter's Internal Medicine, 2nd ed. Philadelphia, Elsevier, 2009.

3. Braman SS: Chronic cough due to acute bronchitis: ACCP evidence-based clinical practice guidelines. Chest 129:95S-103S, 2006.

    The author summarizes the practice guidelines recommended and published by the American College of Chest Physicians in the diagnosis and management of acute bronchitis.

4. The Cochrane Collection. Available at: http://www.cochrane.org. Accessed April 18, 2007.

    This represents a large collection of meta-analyses available on multiple subjects and accessed on two topics: antibiotics for acute bronchitis and β_2 agonists for acute bronchitis. Both are collective meta-analyses and both were updated in 2006 with good summaries of multiple papers in the topic of interest.

5. Donohue J: Chronic obstructive pulmonary disease. In Runge MS, Greganti MA (eds): Netter's Internal Medicine, 2nd ed. Philadelphia, Elsevier, 2009.

6. Wenzel RP, Fowler AA 3rd: Acute bronchitis. N Engl J Med 355(20):2125-2130, 2006.

    This recent review was published with an overview and up-to-date data on acute bronchitis.

James F. Donohue

22

Chronic Obstructive Pulmonary Disease

Introduction

Chronic obstructive pulmonary disease (COPD) is a heterogeneous disorder that includes emphysema, chronic bronchitis, obliterative bronchiolitis, and asthmatic bronchitis. The definition of COPD includes the following: a disease state characterized by airflow limitation that is not fully reversible. The airflow limitation is usually progressive and is associated with an abnormal inflammatory response of the lungs to noxious particles or gases. COPD is a preventable and treatable disease with important systemic consequences.

Etiology and Pathogenesis

COPD affects more than 30 million people in the United States; only 10 million have been diagnosed, 6 million of whom are on therapy, whereas 20 million have impaired lung function. Cigarette smoking is the major risk factor for COPD. More than 20% of chronic smokers develop COPD, and more than 80% of cases in the United States can be attributed to smoking. Other important risk factors include occupational and environmental insults such as bronchitis related to the workplace and to air pollution.

COPD is characterized by chronic inflammation throughout the airways, parenchyma, and pulmonary vasculature. Macrophages, CD8 lymphocytes, and neutrophils are increased. Activated inflammatory cells release a variety of mediators, including leukotriene B4, interleukin-8, and tumor necrosis factor-α, all of which damage lung structures. Also important in the pathogenesis of COPD are an imbalance of proteinases and antiproteinases in the lung and oxidative stress. This inflammation is attributable to exposure to inhaled noxious particles and gases, including cigarette smoke and indoor air pollutants. These irritants directly inflame and damage the lungs. Oxidative stress results in further damage. For reasons poorly understood, inflammation and oxidative stress may persist long after smoking cessation occurs.

Pathologic changes are found in the central airways, pulmonary vasculature, peripheral airways, and lung parenchyma (Fig. 22-1). In the central airways, there are enlarged mucus-secreting glands and an increase in the number of goblet cells, plus a marked increase in inflammatory cells infiltrating the surface epithelium. Chronic inflammation also affects the peripheral airways, with repeated cycles of injury and repair of the airway walls leading to remodeling. Inflammatory nodules with exudate are the characteristic lesion in the small airways. Structural remodeling of the airway wall, with increased collagen content and scar tissue formation, results in narrowing and fixed obstruction. In the parenchyma, there is often centrilobular emphysema plus dilation and destruction of the respiratory bronchioles. In α_1-antitripysin deficiency, these changes are usually panlobular and involve the lower lobes. In cigarette smokers, centrilobular emphysema involves the upper lobes. The pulmonary arteries are thickened with increased smooth muscle mass, and infiltration of the vessel wall by inflammatory cells is noted.

Clinical Presentation

The clinical course of COPD is affected by multiple factors, including genetic susceptibility, low birth weight, maternal smoking, poor maternal nutrition, infections in the first years of life, asthma in childhood, exposure to inhaled irritants in the workplace, and environmental air pollution. Lung function in most nonsmoking adults decreases gradually throughout life, with a loss of 20 mL/year in forced expiratory volume in 1 second (FEV_1) in

Figure 22-1 Bronchitis.

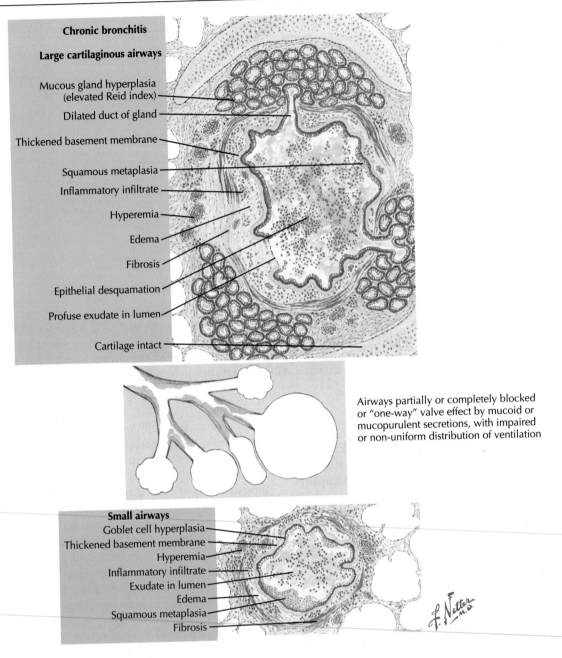

Chronic bronchitis

Large cartilaginous airways

Mucous gland hyperplasia (elevated Reid index)

Dilated duct of gland

Thickened basement membrane

Squamous metaplasia

Inflammatory infiltrate

Hyperemia

Edema

Fibrosis

Epithelial desquamation

Profuse exudate in lumen

Cartilage intact

Airways partially or completely blocked or "one-way" valve effect by mucoid or mucopurulent secretions, with impaired or non-uniform distribution of ventilation

Small airways

Goblet cell hyperplasia

Thickened basement membrane

Hyperemia

Inflammatory infiltrate

Exudate in lumen

Edema

Squamous metaplasia

Fibrosis

nonsmokers. Susceptible smokers may lose 60 mL/year in FEV_1, ex-smokers about 30 mL/year, and those who have α_1-antitrypsin deficiency may lose more than 100 mL/year. Young smokers at risk for future COPD often have frequent colds with lower respiratory symptoms that persist for weeks during their 20s and 30s (Fig. 22-2). Usually, middle-aged smokers begin to lose the ability to exercise, and laborers may lose the ability to work in their late 50s. There is a loss of quality of life and functional performance as the COPD patient approaches age 60 years. Many

patients can lose more than 10 years of life expectancy because of this disease. Smokers with COPD are also at increased risk for dying from lung cancer or coronary artery disease.

With far-advanced disease, structural changes result in chronic alveolar hypoxia, which in turn produces pulmonary hypertension and cor pulmonale (see Fig. 23-2). These patients, described as "blue bloaters," have cyanosis, edema, cardiomegaly, recurrent respiratory failure, hypoventilation, and carbon dioxide retention (Fig. 22-3).

Figure 22-2 Interrelationship of Chronic Bronchitis and Emphysema.

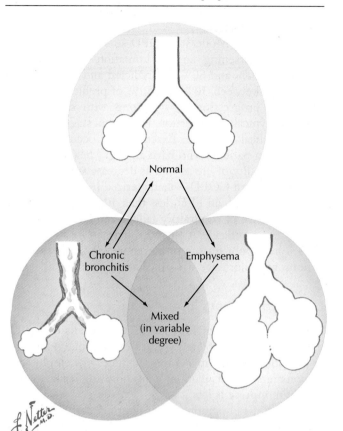

Normal

Chronic bronchitis

Emphysema

Mixed (in variable degree)

Figure 22-3 The Blue Bloater.

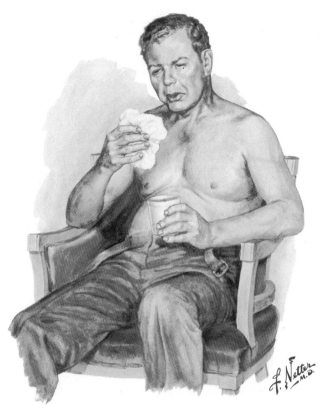

Patients at this stage require frequent hospitalization and have a poor prognosis. The more obese patients may have overlapping obstructive sleep apnea syndrome.

Patients in whom emphysema predominates are hyperinflated, resulting in severe dyspnea, and are called "pink puffers" (Fig. 22-4). They maintain relatively normal arterial oxygen and carbon dioxide tensions despite advanced lung disease but have clear evidence of systemic disease, including a cachectic appearance with marked weakness, fatigue, and poor muscle function. Pink puffers are usually thin and barrel-chested without cyanosis or edema, until the terminal stage of the disease. Most patients with COPD fall into a mixed bronchitis-emphysema clinical category (see Fig. 22-2).

Differential Diagnosis

There is a considerable overlap between COPD and asthma. Both conditions are characterized by obstruction, airway inflammation, and bronchial hyperresponsiveness, and there is an overlap in the response to inhaled β-adrenergic agonist bronchodilators. However, unlike obstruction in asthma, the obstruction in COPD is not completely reversible, and the inflammation is character-

ized predominantly by neutrophil, macrophage, and CD8 cellular infiltrates rather than eosinophils and CD4 lymphocytes. Hyperresponsiveness, although greater than that in the general population, is not nearly as marked as in asthma. Other obstructive lung diseases that may mimic COPD include bronchiectasis with dilation and inflammation of the airways complicated by recurrent respiratory infections. Cystic fibrosis, an inherited disease primarily affecting children and younger adults, is characterized by an abnormal sweat chloride test, susceptibility to repetitive infections with organisms like *Pseudomonas aeruginosa*, much thicker mucopurulent secretions, and a lack of a relationship to cigarette smoking. Obliterative bronchiolitis with obstruction of the small airways is another obstructive lung disease sometimes seen spontaneously, but it is also a complication of transplant rejection. This entity shares features with COPD, as does panbronchiolitis, a small airway obstructive disease primarily seen in Asia.

Diagnostic Approach

A diagnosis of COPD warrants consideration in any patient who has symptoms of cough, sputum production, or dyspnea or a history of exposure to risk factors. The diagnosis is usually confirmed by spirometry. The standards for staging by spirometry continue to evolve. The

Figure 22-4 The Pink Puffer.

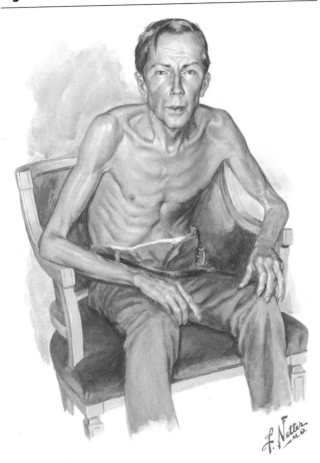

recent Global Initiative for Chronic Obstructive Lung Disease (GOLD) guidelines used the presence of a postbronchodilator FEV_1 of less than 80% of the predicted value in combination with an FEV_1/forced vital capacity (FVC) ratio of less than 70% to confirm the presence of airflow limitation that is not fully reversible. Clinical symptoms and signs, including progressive shortness of breath, hyperinflation, and increased forced expiratory time, are useful to support the diagnosis.

The diagnosis of COPD should be considered in a middle-aged patient with symptoms of cough, sputum production, or dyspnea or a history of exposure to risk factors. Women in their 50s are frequently misclassified as asthmatic. Spirometry confirms the diagnosis and is useful for assessing severity (Fig. 22-5). Bronchodilator testing of reversibility is indicated to rule out asthma. The management of COPD is largely symptom driven, and there is a correlation between the degree of airflow limitation and the presence of symptoms.

GOLD Guidelines

The recent GOLD guidelines classify patients with COPD in four stages:

Stage I: Mild COPD—with mild airflow limitation with an FEV_1/FVC ratio of less than 70% but with an FEV_1 greater than 80% of predicted. Some have cough and sputum production.

Stages II and III: Moderate COPD—*stage II* is characterized by worsening airflow limitation with an FEV_1 between 50% and 80% of predicted and *stage III* with an FEV_1 between 30% and 50% of predicted. Usually there is progression of symptoms with shortness of breath, typically on exertion. Patients in stages II and III seek medical attention. Exacerbations occur more frequently in patients who have an FEV_1 below 50% and impact quality of life as well as decrease survival.

Stage IV: Severe COPD—characterized by severe airflow limitations with an FEV_1 less than 30% of predicted or the presence of respiratory failure and clinical signs of right heart failure. Patients who have an FEV_1 less than 30% have poor quality of life, more frequent exacerbations, and shortened life expectancy.

Laboratory Tests

Spirometry reveals an FEV_1/FVC ratio of less than 70% that does not completely reverse to normal following bronchodilator therapy. Lung volumes in emphysema demonstrate hyperinflation, and diffusing capacity for carbon monoxide is low.

The chest radiograph appears normal early in COPD and is not useful in diagnosis. Lower-lobe lung markings are increased in chronic bronchitis, so-called dirty lungs. Findings in emphysema include hyperinflation with a low flattened diaphragm, enlarged anterior-posterior retrosternal space, hypovascularity, areas of hyperlucency, and bullae formation.

Arterial blood gases are usually measured in patients with COPD with more severe disease, usually when the FEV_1 is less than 40%. However, baseline values are commonly benchmarked for comparison during subsequent exacerbations. Mild hypoxemia is often seen during the early stages of COPD. In stages III and IV, because of ventilation-perfusion ratio abnormalities, severe arterial hypoxemia, respiratory acidosis, and hypoventilation are typical findings. The routine use of nocturnal oxygen has made secondary polycythemia a rare occurrence. Surprisingly, more than 20% of patients are chronically anemic.

Electrocardiogram findings are nonspecific in COPD. With severe disease, patients develop changes of right ventricular hypertrophy and atrial arrhythmias. Many have concurrent coronary artery disease.

All patients with COPD, particularly those with early onset or those with a family history of either lung or liver disease, should be screened for α_1-antitypsin deficiency, a clinical problem that occurs in 1% to 2% of patients with emphysema. Affected patients are those who have less than 15% of normal serum levels.

Figure 22-5 Pulmonary Function in Obstructive Disease.

$FEF_{25-75\%}$, forced expiratory flow, midexpiratory phase; FVL, forced vital capacity; FEV_1, forced expiratory volume in 1 second; MEFV, maximal expiratory flow volume; TLC, total lung capacity.

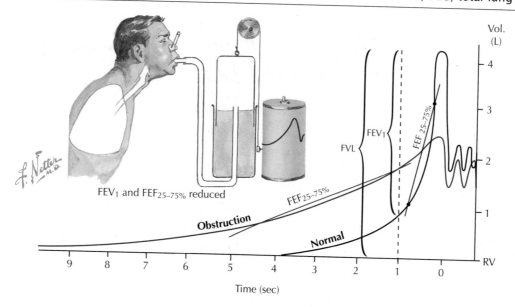

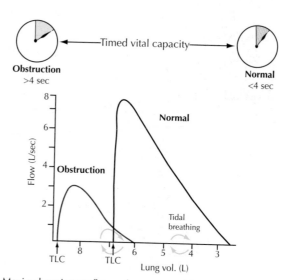

Maximal expiratory flow-volume curves. TLC increased in obstruction, but expiratory flow rate decreased. In severe obstruction, tidal breathing may coincide with MEFV curve

Management and Therapy

Optimum Treatment

Optimal management of COPD requires (1) educating patients and family; (2) retarding the progression of airflow limitation by early disease recognition and avoidance of risk factors; (3) minimizing airflow limitation by reducing the production and increasing the elimination of secre-tions; (4) performing bronchodilation; (5) correcting the secondary physiologic alterations including hypoxemia, hypercapnia, and pulmonary hypertension; and (6) opti-mizing functional lung capacity through exercise condi-tioning, muscle training, rest, nutrition, and psychosocial rehabilitation (Fig. 22-6). The overall approach to manag-ing stable COPD involves a stepwise increase in treatment, dependent on the severity of the disease. Smoking cessa-

Figure 22-6 Management of COPD.

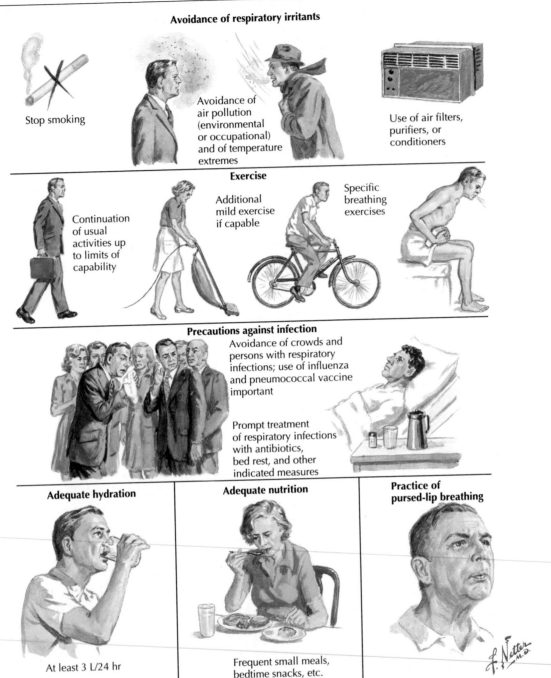

Avoidance of respiratory irritants

Stop smoking

Avoidance of air pollution (environmental or occupational) and of temperature extremes

Use of air filters, purifiers, or conditioners

Exercise

Continuation of usual activities up to limits of capability

Additional mild exercise if capable

Specific breathing exercises

Precautions against infection

Avoidance of crowds and persons with respiratory infections; use of influenza and pneumococcal vaccine important

Prompt treatment of respiratory infections with antibiotics, bed rest, and other indicated measures

Adequate hydration

At least 3 L/24 hr

Adequate nutrition

Frequent small meals, bedtime snacks, etc.

Practice of pursed-lip breathing

tion is of paramount importance. Counseling, nicotine replacement therapy, and newer agents like varenicline or bupropion should be offered.

Pharmacologic Therapy

Bronchodilator medications are central to the symptomatic management of COPD. They are administered on an as-needed basis or on a regular basis to prevent or reduce symptoms. The aerosol route using longer-acting bronchodilators is preferred. Frequently, bronchodilators such as long-acting β_2-agonists, anticholinergics, and theophylline are combined. For mild COPD, a short-acting as-needed bronchodilator like albuterol or ipratropium is often sufficient. For those with stages II, III, and IV disease, regular treatment with an inhaled long-acting β_2-agonist bronchodilator such as salmeterol and formoterol or an anticholinergic agent such as tiotropium bromide, either alone or combined, is usually recommended. A short-acting bronchodilator is often added for rescue. Short-acting β_2 agonists like albuterol can be used either regularly or on an as-needed basis, often in combination with ipratropium. These agents are frequently given by metered dose inhaler; however, elderly patients with COPD commonly have difficulty using these devices. Nebulized albuterol-ipratropium is often helpful in patients with more severe disease. With increasing doses of these agents, signs of cardiac toxicity require careful monitoring. Newer long-acting bronchodilators such as arformoterol and formoterol are now available in aerosol solution.

Anticholinergic medications include ipratropium bromide and tiotropium bromide, a new long-acting agent that is a 24-hour antimuscarinic antagonist. Anticholinergics are particularly useful in COPD, especially in patients who have smoked for many years and in those with a low FEV_1. These agents are poorly absorbed systemically, do not cross the blood-brain barrier, and do not adversely affect ciliary activity. The main side effects are dry mouth and cough. Because of their slow onset of action, they are not particularly useful in the rescue mode. However, these are excellent and safe medications in chronic maintenance programs for patients with COPD. Ipratropium can be administered either by metered dose inhaler or by a nebulized solution. It is also effective in acute respiratory failure. Usually long- and short-acting anticholinergics are not used concurrently. Tiotropium is often combined with a long-acting β agonist and at times with an inhaled corticosteroid (ICS).

Salmeterol and formoterol are 12-hour *long-acting bronchodilators* used as chronic maintenance therapy for patients with COPD. Both of these agents are highly effective and are safe in stable patients. The doses, in general, should not be increased. Formoterol has a more rapid onset of action. Salmeterol may be better tolerated. The risk of long-acting β_2 agonists (LABAs) in asthma does not seem to apply to COPD. These agents can easily be combined with theophylline, tiotropium, ipratropium bromide, or an ICS.

Theophylline was previously used in COPD as the first-line therapy but is now secondary therapy. This agent has some anti-inflammatory effects, improves the strength of diaphragmatic contractility, and improves mucociliary clearance and cardiac output. However, theophylline has substantial toxicity in patients with COPD. Elderly patients with preexisting abnormal cardiac function are at risk for cardiac arrhythmias, even if levels are in the high therapeutic range. Theophylline has important interactions with other drugs that are frequently used for COPD, such as macrolide antibiotics, ciprofloxacin, and cimetidine. Clearance may change with concomitant conditions like pneumonia, congestive heart failure, and liver disease. The recommended therapeutic level is 8 to 12 µg/dL. Most patients require a total dose of between 100 and 400 mg per/day.

Prolonged treatment with oral glucocorticosteroids is not recommended in COPD because of the associated severe side effects, including steroid myopathy, osteopenia, and cataracts. *Oral steroids* are very useful in acute exacerbations.

Prolonged treatment with *inhaled corticosteroids* does not modify the long-term decline in FEV_1 in patients with COPD. The GOLD guidelines recommend regular treatment with inhaled steroids in those with an FEV_1 less than 50% of predicted or in those with stage III or IV disease with frequent exacerbations requiring treatment with antibiotics and oral corticosteroids. In this setting, there is preservation of quality of life and a reduced number of exacerbations with ICS. A therapeutic trial of up to 3 months with inhaled corticosteroids may identify patients who would benefit. A recent 3-year study revealed an improvement in all-cause mortality when ICSs were added to LABAs in COPD.

Pulmonary Rehabilitation

Pulmonary rehabilitation is useful for all patients. This includes exercise training, nutrition counseling, and education in a program that usually improves exercise tolerance and overall health, especially in patients whose FEV_1 is below 1.5 L. The goals of pulmonary rehabilitation are to reduce symptoms, improve quality of life, decrease disability, and increase physical and emotional participation in everyday activities. The methods include anxiety management, relaxation, identifying and changing beliefs about exercise and health-related issues, and exercise management. Patients benefit with respect to both exercise tolerance and symptoms of dyspnea and fatigue. The minimum length of an effective rehabilitation program is 2 months, but the longer the program continues, the more effective the results are. There seems to be no effect on survival, and data on reduction in hospitalization rates are inconsistent.

Surgical Therapy

In carefully selected patients, *bullectomy* may reduce dyspnea and improve lung function. The procedure is based on a thoracic computed tomography scan showing a bulla with significant compression of adjoining lung, a large bulla occupying a substantial part of the thorax, or respiratory embarrassment due to an enlarging bulla. Often, a video-assisted thoracoscopy approach is selected.

The National Emphysema Therapeutic Trial of *lung volume reduction surgery* gave mixed results. For patients with very low lung function (FEV_1 <20%), low diffusing capacity (<20%), and diffuse disease, the mortality rate with surgery was greater than in the controlled population treated medically. However, in patients with predominant upper lobe emphysema and low baseline exercise tolerance, functional capacity and survival improved over 5 years of follow-up.

In carefully selected patients with advanced COPD, especially those with deficiency of α_1 antitrypsin, *lung transplantation* may improve quality of life and functional capacity. Selected patients are usually those with an FEV_1 of less than 35%, Pao_2 of 55 to 60 mm Hg, and $Paco_2$ of more than 50 mm Hg. Single-lung transplantations were previously offered, but double-lung transplantation is becoming more popular.

Treatment of Exacerbations

An acute exacerbation of COPD is defined as a subjective increase from baseline in some combination of dyspnea, sputum production, and sputum volume over a 2-day period. Exacerbations are often the defining clinical events in the life of a patient with COPD. There are multiple causes of an exacerbation, including infection, air pollution, exposure to allergens, and ozone. The most common symptoms are increased breathlessness accompanied by wheezing, chest tightness, increased cough and sputum, change in the color or tenacity of sputum, and fever. There may also be nonspecific systemic complaints, such as malaise, insomnia, fatigue, depression, and confusion. The outcome of an exacerbation is influenced by the disease's severity and the patient's previous exposure to antibiotics or recent use of oral corticosteroids. Simple lung function studies are helpful but are often very hard to perform. In the hospital setting, arterial blood gases are useful to guide oxygen therapy and prevent sedation in a patient with impending respiratory failure.

The differential diagnosis of an acute exacerbation includes congestive heart failure, pneumothorax, pleural effusion, pulmonary embolism, and arrhythmias, diagnoses that can be excluded using clinical assessment, chest radiography, electrocardiography, spiral computed tomography scan, and other diagnostic procedures. The presence of increased cough or purulent sputum is sufficient evidence to warrant antibiotic therapy. The most common pathogens are *Streptococcus pneumoniae*, *Haemophilus influenzae*, and *Moraxella catarrhalis*. More severely affected patients may have infections with gram-negative rods such as *Klebsiella* or *Pseudomonas*, which typically cause more severe lung involvement. Rarely, atypical bacteria such as mycoplasma, *Chlamydia pneumoniae*, or *Legionella* species, are the underlying pathogens. Many exacerbations are due to viruses, but the findings cannot be distinguished from bacterial infection. Similarly, air pollution due to ozone or particulates can cause exacerbations that are indistinguishable from those associated with bacteria.

Most exacerbations of COPD are treated at home. The dose or frequency of β agonists can be increased if no contraindication exists. An additional bronchodilator can be recommended. If the patient is using only metered dose inhalers, high-dose nebulized therapy deserves consideration.

Usually, patients with acute exacerbations of COPD benefit from *systemic corticosteroid therapy*, with alleviation of symptoms and improved lung function. For patients with moderate COPD, most controlled clinical trials have shown that short-term systemic corticosteroid therapy in combination with other effective therapies leads to small but clinically significant improvement and fewer treatment failures. The usual starting dose is about 30 to 40 mg of prednisone for 5 to 10 days with or without a taper. Increasing the dosage of inhaled corticosteroids is less effective.

Unless the patient is hospitalized or has pneumonia, sputum cultures are not usually necessary. The choice of *antibiotics* is based on the community patterns of bacterial resistance plus factors such as the patient's stage of disease and recent exposure to antibiotics and systemic corticosteroids. Antibiotics directed at the common pathogens are used. Second- and third-generation cephalosporins, newer macrolides, amoxicillin-clavulanate, or fluoroquinolones may be necessary for those who do not respond to simple oral antibiotics, or in cases of the known presence of β-lactamase-producing organism in the sputum.

Avoiding Treatment Errors

The first treatment error is to assume that exacerbations and chronic bronchitis are merely bacterial or viral infections and not an integral feature of the chronic underlying disease. A second error is to misdiagnose COPD as asthma and to use therapies appropriate for asthma but inappropriate for COPD, such as leukotriene receptor antagonists. Administering systemic corticosteroids on a chronic basis, even in the face of evidence that the side-effect profile of chronic oral steroids outweighs any benefits, is another ill-advised treatment decision. A fourth error is to avoid measuring pulmonary function and, as a result, fail to understand how severely impaired your patient is and the corresponding risk for elective surgery, as well as the corresponding prognosis.

Future Directions

Progress in COPD research is accelerating. Characterizations of human lung tissue by advanced molecular, biochemical, microbiologic, and histopathologic methods have revealed important observations on ongoing inflammation, oxidative stress, and apoptosis. Identification of novel biomarkers and clinical end points is essential for the development of new anti-inflammatory agents that might be highly effective. Knowledge of genetic determinants of COPD could lead to recognition of biochemical pathways that contribute to the disease and allow targeting of public health interventions to individuals at greatest risk. The causes and consequences of exacerbations need to be identified, and therapy directed at mucus gland metaplasia and excess mucus secretion is necessary. Finally, therapy that results in stimulation of alveolar regeneration is an exciting possibility for disease-modifying therapy of emphysema. Clinically, additional work is needed to identify better tools for disease monitoring, as well as more studies to validate or revise current clinical practice.

Additional Resources

American Thoracic Society/European Respiratory Society Statement: Standards for the Diagnosis and Management of Individuals with Alpha-1 Antitrypsin Deficiency. Am J Respir Crit Care Med 168(7):818-900, 2003.

The ATS/ERS guidelines closely follow the GOLD guidelines and emphasize matching treatment to level of obstruction as inhaled steroids are recommended for those with exacerbations.

Dahl M, Tybjaerg-Hansen A, Lange P, et al: Change in lung function and morbidity from chronic obstructive pulmonary disease in alpha-1 antitrypsin MZ heterozygotes: Longitudinal study of the general population. Ann Intern Med 136(4):270-279, 2002.

This study documents that most nonsmoking patients who are heterozygotes for α_1-antitrypsin deficiency do well.

EVIDENCE

1. Calverley PM, Anderson JA, Celli B, et al: Salmeterol and fluticasone propionate and survival in chronic obstructive pulmonary disease. N Engl J Med 356:775-789, 2007.

   This landmark study shows that the combination of fluticasone and salmeterol improves all-cause mortality, reduces exacerbations, improves quality of life, and changes the rate of decline in lung function.

2. Celli BR; Committee Members: Standards for the diagnosis and treatment of patients with COPD: A summary of the ATS/ERS Position Paper. Eur Respir J 23:932-946, 2004.

   This definitive summary outline of the levels of COPD and appropriate therapy at each stage provides useful information for both diagnosing and treating patients with COPD.

3. Global Initiative for Chronic Obstructive Lung Disease (GOLD). Available at: http://www.goldcopd.com/. Accessed April 14, 2007.

   This website includes the updated GOLD statement showing the levels of COPD.

4. Hogg JC, Chi F, Utokaparch S, et al: The nature of small-airway obstruction in chronic obstructive pulmonary disease. N Engl J Med 350:2645-2653, 2004.

   This paradigm-shifting paper notes the presence of active inflammation in the small airways of the lungs long after patients have stopped smoking cigarettes.

5. Mannino DM, Homa DM, Akinbami LJ, et al: Chronic obstructive pulmonary disease surveillance—United States, 1971-2000. MMWR Surveill Summ 51(6):1-6, 2002.

   This paper underscores the large number of patients with COPD who have not been physician diagnosed.

6. National Emphysema Treatment Trial Research Group: A randomized trial comparing lung volume reduction surgery with medical therapy for severe emphysema. N Engl J Med 348:2059-2073, 2003.

   Along with a subsequent 5-year follow-up study, this trial shows that patients with upper lobe emphysematous changes and low exercise tolerance who undergo surgery will have improvements in symptoms, quality of life, and survival.

Craig N. Rosebrock ▪ Stephen L. Tilley

Restrictive Lung Disease

Introduction

Diseases of the chest resulting from pathologies distal to the conducting airways produce restrictive lung disease (RLD). Collectively, this broad array of disorders manifests clinically as a reduction in the vital capacity (VC) of the lungs. Although less common than obstructive lung diseases such as asthma and chronic obstructive pulmonary disease, RLDs have the potential to progress to respiratory failure and death if not recognized and treated before fibrosis ensues. Therefore, it is essential that physicians are aware of this heterogeneous group of disorders because timely diagnosis and treatment can substantially influence morbidity and mortality.

Etiology and Pathophysiology

RLDs can be grouped into four distinct etiologic categories: chest wall disorders, pleural disease, neuromuscular disease, and diffuse parenchymal lung disease (DPLD). DPLD and interstitial lung disease (ILD) are used interchangeably in the literature; however, DPLD is a more appropriate term because many of these diseases involve the alveolar epithelium, alveolar space, and pulmonary vessels and are not truly limited to the interstitium of the lung. Refer to Chapter 19, which focuses on pleural disease, for a discussion of those disorders.

Although heterogeneous in their pathogenesis, all RLDs result in reductions in VC of the lungs. A restrictive pattern of spirometry is characteristic with reduced forced vital capacity (FVC), reduced forced expiratory volume in 1 second (FEV_1), and normal FEV_1/FVC ratios (>75%) (Fig. 23-1). Decreased compliance of the lungs in DPLDs and decreased compliance of the pleura and chest wall in pleural and chest wall diseases are mechanistically responsible for the reduction in VC observed in these disorders. Lung volume measurements show a reduction in total lung capacity (TLC), functional residual capacity (FRC), and residual volume (RV) (see Fig. 23-1). In contrast, compliance of the lungs, pleura, and chest wall is normal in neuromuscular diseases, and VC is reduced because of diaphragmatic weakness, which prevents full inflation of the lungs to a normal TLC. Because FRC is determined by the balance of forces between the chest wall and lungs, both of which are unaffected by neuromuscular disease,

FRC usually remains normal. The RV may be elevated in neuromuscular disease because of weakness of the expiratory muscles, resulting in the inability of the patient to forcefully exhale to a normal RV. These characteristic patterns of lung volumes are useful for the initial differentiation of RLDs. As weakness progresses or as compliance worsens with significant pleural fibrosis or chest wall deformity, hypercapnic respiratory failure can develop. Because the pulmonary parenchyma is normal in these patients, hypoxemia is uncommon unless a secondary process (e.g., atelectasis due to retention of secretions in patients with neuromuscular disease) is superimposed, or hypercapnia is severe.

In contrast to other RLDs, hypoxemia is a common feature of DPLDs. Hypoxemia results from ventilation-perfusion mismatching and diffusion impairment, and it is typically more severe with exertion as red blood cell transit through the pulmonary vascular bed is increased, reducing the available time for hemoglobin loading with oxygen. Hypercapnia is not seen in most DPLDs until end-stage disease is present.

Destruction of alveolar-capillary units by inflammation or fibrosis and hypoxemia act in concert to increase pulmonary vascular resistance. Right ventricular hypertrophy and dilation occur as a consequence of this increase in right ventricular afterload, and cor pulmonale ensues with associated peripheral edema (similar to changes occurring secondary to pulmonary emphysema; Fig. 23-2). Left ventricular diastolic dysfunction can occur from displacement of the septum into the left ventricular cavity as a

Figure 23-1 Restrictive Lung Disease Physiology.

Maximal expiratory flow volume curves in restrictive lung disease. TLC, residual volume, and vital capacity are all decreased in restriction. $FEF_{25-75\%}$ forced expiratory flow; FEV_1, forced expiratory volume in 1 second.

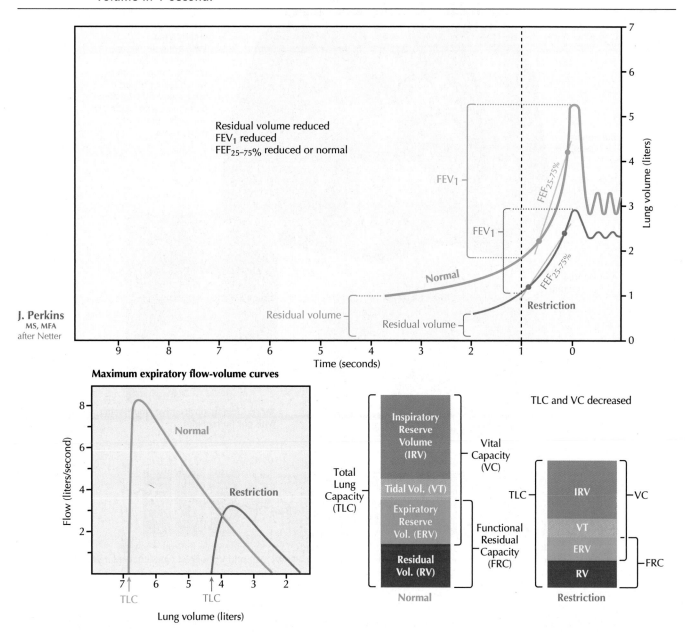

result of marked increases in right ventricular pressures, and pulmonary edema can result. The clinical implications of these pathophysiologic changes are discussed under "Management and Therapy."

Clinical Presentation

Patients with RLD most commonly complain of dyspnea on exertion. The degree of breathlessness usually depends on the etiology of restriction and the severity of lung dysfunction. Some patients notice only mild decreases in exercise tolerance. Patients with severe disease may present debilitated, unable to ascend a small flight of stairs without significant discomfort. As lung function worsens, patients may complain of dyspnea at rest. Patients with RLD, particularly DPLD, may also present with complaints of cough, which is usually nonproductive. Associated symptoms may include nonspecific chest discomfort depending on the etiology of disease. Because many diseases have similar presentations, a detailed history and thorough physical exam are critical to determining the etiology of restriction. Features of the history and physical exam that may aid in narrowing the differential diagnosis are covered under "Diagnostic Approach."

Figure 23-2 Cor Pulmonale.

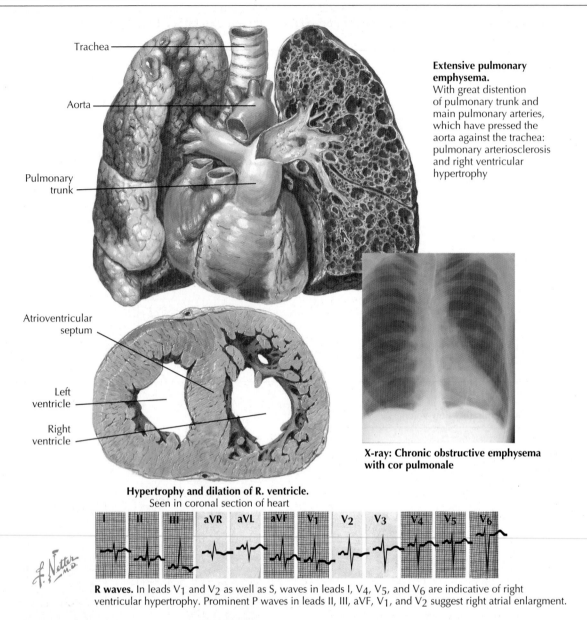

Trachea

Aorta

Pulmonary trunk

Extensive pulmonary emphysema. With great distention of pulmonary trunk and main pulmonary arteries, which have pressed the aorta against the trachea: pulmonary arteriosclerosis and right ventricular hypertrophy

Atrioventricular septum

Left ventricle

Right ventricle

X-ray: Chronic obstructive emphysema with cor pulmonale

Hypertrophy and dilation of R. ventricle.
Seen in coronal section of heart

R waves. In leads V_1 and V_2 as well as S, waves in leads I, V_4, V_5, and V_6 are indicative of right ventricular hypertrophy. Prominent P waves in leads II, III, aVF, V_1, and V_2 suggest right atrial enlargment.

When a neuromuscular disease is the cause of RLD (Box 23-1), patients can present with other neuromuscular complaints. Patients often complain of generalized weakness or fatigue. In some cases, they have objective findings of weakness on physical exam. If the diaphragm is affected, patients may experience worsening dyspnea while laying flat and may exhibit paradoxical breathing as evidenced by the abdominal wall moving inward instead of outward during inspiration. Physical exam may reveal musculoskeletal weakness; however, respiratory muscle weakness may occur in isolation.

Diseases of the chest wall (Box 23-2) usually are apparent on physical exam, and patients may present with more localized complaints. Included in this group are abdominal processes that interfere with the downward displacement of the diaphragm during inspiration. Tense ascites, an abdominal mass, and a massive pannus are common causes of restriction and may be evident at the bedside. Pectus excavatum is a common congenital disorder affecting the anterior chest wall. Patients with this deformity have a concave depression of the sternum. Younger patients rarely have symptoms. As they age, however, they may complain of mild dyspnea on exertion and pain at the site of deformity. Some patients with pectus excavatum develop mitral valve prolapse and complain of palpitations due to associated arrhythmias. Patients with deformities of the spine have specific findings on physical exam. An anteroposterior angulation is seen in patients with kyphosis. Patients with

---

Box 23-1 Neuromuscular Diseases Causing Restrictive Lung Disease

Upper or Lower Motor Neuron Lesions
- Amyotrophic lateral sclerosis
- Guillain-Barré syndrome

Diseases Affecting the Neuromuscular Junction
- Myasthenia gravis
- Botulism
- Lambert-Eaton syndrome

Muscle Diseases
- Duchenne's muscular dystrophy
- Becker's muscular dystrophy
- Mitochondrial myopathies
- Polymyositis and dermatomyositis
- Thyroid disease
- Drugs (steroids), toxins
- Glycogen storage disease

Box 23-2 Chest Wall and Pleural Diseases Responsible for Restrictive Lung Disease

- Congenital chest wall deformity (pectus excavatum)
- Ankylosing spondylitis
- Fibrothorax
- Abdominal process (ascites, abdominal mass, obesity)
- Chest tumor
- Kyphoscoliosis
- Flail chest
- Tension pneumothorax
- Hemothorax
- Pleural effusions and trapped lung

Box 23-3 Diffuse Parenchymal Lung Disease of Unknown Etiology

- Idiopathic interstitial pneumonias
  Usual interstitial pneumonia: idiopathic pulmonary fibrosis
  Nonspecific interstitial pneumonia
  Acute interstitial pneumonia
  Respiratory bronchiolitis-interstitial lung disease
  Desquamative interstitial pneumonia
  Lymphoid interstitial pneumonia
  Bronchiolitis obliterans organizing pneumonia: cryptogenic organizing pneumonia
- Sarcoidosis
- Lymphangioleiomyomatosis
- Pulmonary Langerhans cell histiocytosis: eosinophilic granuloma, histiocytosis X
- Wegener's granulomatosis
- Goodpasture's syndrome
- Chronic eosinophilic pneumonia
- Amyloidosis
- Churg-Strauss syndrome

---

scoliosis have lateral displacement or curvature of the spine. If severe rib distortion is present, a patient may report exercise intolerance, but patients are often asymptomatic at rest. With chest wall or spine deformities, children are usually asymptomatic because of the lack of rib rigidity. Adults may be asymptomatic as well until burdened with a superimposed insult such as bacterial pneumonia. RLD that is not manifest clinically when the patient is well can predispose to hypercapnic respiratory failure. Patients with morbid obesity often are asymptomatic at rest but may notice profound dyspnea with exertion due to the combination of deconditioning and pulmonary restriction.

The clinical presentation and physical findings associated with DPLD are important clues to the etiology of a patient's pulmonary disease. Most patients will present with shortness of breath with or without cough. Occasionally, early DPLD may be first brought to clinical attention by a chest x-ray (CXR) or chest computed tomography (CT) performed for other reasons. A sudden onset of respiratory failure, however, must be quickly diagnosed. Acute interstitial pneumonia, a form of idiopathic interstitial pneumonia (Box 23-3), presents with a prodrome of fever, malaise, and cough that precedes the development of hypoxemic respiratory failure by days to weeks. This entity must be recognized quickly because these patients may progress to respiratory failure and require mechanical ventilation. Chest pain is uncommon in most DPLDs, but when present, it is usually due to a systemic inflammatory disorder such as systemic lupus, mixed connective tissues disease, rheumatoid arthritis, or sarcoidosis. Patients with severe or progressive DPLD may develop pulmonary hypertension and present with complaints of dizziness, syncope, or lower extremity edema. Some DPLDs produce wheezing as the result of small airways involvement. Two examples are sarcoidosis and Churg-Strauss syndrome. Churg-Strauss syndrome is one of the pulmonary vasculitides that causes DPLD. This autoimmune disease has an asthma component, and affected patients may complain of wheezing.

Although the idiopathic interstitial pneumonias (see Box 23-3) are often limited to the lung, other DPLDs are part of a systemic illness in which additional organs are also affected. For example, DPLD may occur with many connective tissue diseases (Box 23-4), and other organ-specific complaints typical of the rheumatic process may be present and helpful in diagnosis. For example, patients with connective tissues diseases may complain of fatigue, weakness, joint pain, muscle pain, dry eyes, or dry mouth.

The physical exam findings in patients with DPLD are abnormal but nonspecific. The auscultatory examination of the chest usually reveals "Velcro" or dry inspiratory crackles. Interestingly, the lungs frequently sound clear in pulmonary sarcoidosis, despite the presence of significant parenchymal lung disease. Cyanosis and clubbing are

Box 23-4 Diffuse Parenchymal Lung Disease of Known Etiology

- Connective tissue disease associated
  Rheumatoid arthritis
  Mixed connective tissue disease
  Progressive systemic sclerosis
  Systemic lupus erythematosus
  Sjögren's syndrome
  Dermatomyositis and polymyositis
  Anklyosing spondylitis
- Inhaled organic antigens (hypersensitivity pneumonitis)
- Inhaled inorganic dusts (carbon, silicates, hard metals, coal dust)
- Drugs
  Amiodarone
  Methotrexate
  Nonsteroidal anti-inflammatory drugs
  Minocycline
  Sulfasalazine
  Ethambutol
  Isoniazid
  Bleomycin
  Cyclophosphamide
  Radiation
  Heroin
  Cocaine

usually late manifestations of disease and suggest advanced lung disease. Pulmonary hypertension also develops with advanced DPLD, and patients may present with a right-sided heart gallop or an abnormally accentuated P2. Elevated jugular venous pulse, hepatomegaly, and lower extremity edema may result from the development of right ventricular failure—cor pulmonale (see Fig. 23-2).

Extrapulmonary manifestations of disease can help to narrow the extensive differential of DPLD. Systemic hypertension may be seen in connective tissue diseases and vasculitides. Skin changes are common in connective tissues disorders like scleroderma. Sarcoidosis, neurofibromatosis, dermatomyositis, drug-induced DPLD, and systemic vasculitides may also have classic skin findings. When patients with DPLD report eye symptoms, sarcoidosis, ankylosing spondylitis, scleroderma, and the systemic vasculitides should be entertained. Objective findings of muscle weakness on physical exam may be a clue to an underlying connective tissue disease. The absence of extrapulmonary findings, however, should not exclude any particular etiology as the cause of DPLD because pulmonary disease can occasionally be the first manifestation of these systemic illnesses.

Diagnostic Approach

The evaluation of patients suspected of having RLD should include a detailed history with an extensive review of systems, physical exam, spirometry, and a posteroanterior (PA) and lateral CXR. An algorithm for approaching the patient with suspected RLD is presented in Figure 23-3. Vital signs should include a measurement of room air pulse oximetry. Pulse oximetry with exertion is a very useful test for detecting the presence of DPLD because exercise-induced hypoxemia is a common feature of these disorders. Although a comprehensive history and physical exam, imaging studies, and selected labs may suggest RLD, the diagnosis is based on pulmonary function testing. A diagnosis of restriction should be documented by spirometry and lung volumes before embarking on an extensive radiographic and pathologic workup. Patients with suspected lung disease should first have simple spirometry. If FEV_1, FVC, and the FEV1/FVC ratio are suggestive of restriction (see Fig. 23-1), then lung volumes and diffusion capacity (D_{LCO}) should be measured. Lung volumes are essential for the diagnosis and initial differentiation of RLDs because the volume compartments are differentially affected by the various classes of RLD.

In neuromuscular and chest wall disease, an extensive history, physical exam, and pulmonary function testing may be all that is necessary to generate a differential diagnosis (see Box 23-1). Patients with muscle weakness affecting the diaphragm typically have a decrease in TLC, a preserved FRC, and a mild increase in RV, as previously described. Muscle pressure measurements reveal a decrease in maximal inspiratory and expiratory pressures. Diffusion capacity is typically normal. A PA and lateral CXR may display an elevated hemidiaphragm in cases of diaphragm weakness or injury. Fluoroscopic visualization, however, is often necessary to document abnormal diaphragm movement. Nerve conduction studies and muscle biopsy may be necessary to diagnose neuromuscular disease. A diagnostic plan should be coordinated with an experienced neurologist.

Box 23-2 lists RLDs resulting from chest wall abnormalities. An isolated reduction in FRC is characteristic of obesity-induced RLD. With morbid obesity, TLC may also be reduced. In the absence of concomitant parenchymal lung disease, the D_{LCO} may be normal in patients with a restrictive ventilatory dysfunction from chest wall disease. Chest imaging will often reveal the underlying bony pathology responsible for chest wall disease. Serologic studies typically are not needed. If pleural plaques or chest wall tumors are present, tissue biopsy using CT guidance, video-assisted thoracoscopy, or open surgical procedures may be needed for definitive diagnosis. Depending on the etiology and severity of chest wall disease, patient care should be coordinated with a thoracic or orthopedic surgeon.

The list of causes of DPLD is extensive (see Boxes 23-3 and 23-4), and an approach to diagnosing these disorders is outlined below and in Figure 23-3. Individualization based on the clinical presentation and an extensive history is important. It is essential, as in any medical interview, that the clinician obtain a detailed history of disease onset and extensive review of systems. Information concerning

Figure 23-3 Diagnostic Algorithm.
COPD, chronic obstructive pulmonary disease; DDx, differential diagnosis; Dx, diagnosis; DLCO diffusion capacity; DPLD, diffuse parenchymal lung disease; ECG, electrocardiogram; HRCT, high-resolution computed tomography; PFTs, pulmonary function tests; VATS, video-assisted thoracoscopic surgery.

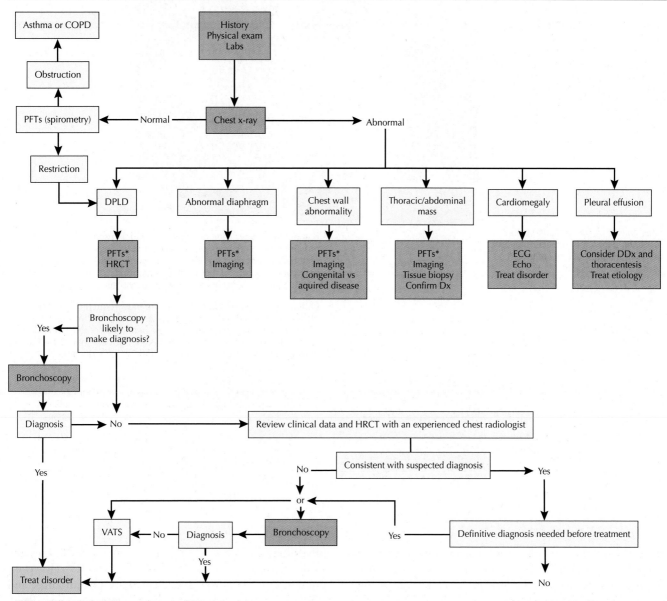

*PFTs = Full set including lung volumes and DLCO

smoking history is vital because some diseases, including respiratory bronchiolitis–interstitial lung disease (RB-ILD), desquamative interstitial pneumonia (DIP), and Langerhans cell histiocytosis, can improve with smoking cessation. The clinician must inquire about any current or previous occupational or recreational exposures (see Box 23-4) because avoidance of these factors can result in disease remission. Hypersensitivity pneumonitis (Fig. 23-4) is an important DPLD that may only be suspected by a detailed exposure history (e.g., pet bird). A complete list of current and previous medications is essential because a number of drugs have been associated with the develop-

ment of DPLD (see Box 23-4). A detailed family history may reveal clues to the diagnosis of diseases with well-established genetic components (e.g., sarcoidosis). Finally, a thorough physical exam may reveal clues to both the severity (e.g., signs of cor pulmonale) and etiology (e.g., skin findings such as lupus pernio, which may be suggestive of sarcoidosis) of DPLDs.

The CXR is an important diagnostic test when evaluating patients with suspected DPLD. The characteristic CXR in DPLD shows increased linear markings with or without small nodules—a reticular-nodular pattern. However, alveolar filling is seen in some of these disorders,

Figure 23-4 Hypersensitivity Pneumonitis.

Farmer's lung results from inhalation of dust from moldy hay containing thermophilic actinomycetes

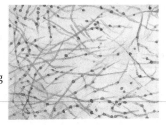

Slide culture of *Thermoactinomyces saccharii*, a thermophilic actinomycete that is principal souce of antigen in causation of bagassosis

Bailing dried sugar cane or "bagasse," widely used in manufacture of paper, wallboard, and building materials and as chicken litter. When moldy, dust may contain spores of thermophilic organisms, which act as antigens in causation of bagassosis.

Other related diseases in this group are mushroom picker's disease, pigeon breeder's disease, budgerigar (parakeet) fancier's disease, malt worker's lung, sequoiosis, maple bark disease, wheat thresher's lung, thatched roof disease, air conditioner disease (due to moldy dust or water from air conditioners), and fog fever of cattle.

Slide culture of *Micropolyspora faeni* (also known as *T. polyspora*), a thermophilic actinomycete that is a principal source of antigen producing farmer's lung, mushroom picker's disease, and fog fever of cattle

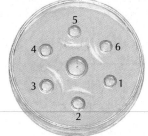

Precipitin reactions in bagassosis. Patient's serum in central well and extracts of bagasse from various sources in peripheral wells. Specimens 1 and 4, from fresh bagasse, show no precipitin bands.

emphasizing the basis for the change in nomenclature from ILD to DPLD. Chest imaging may show other findings associated with underlying disease such as hilar adenopathy or pleural abnormalities. Hilar adenopathy is a common feature of pulmonary sarcoidosis (Fig. 23-5). Normal CXRs have been reported in up to 10% of patients with DPLD; therefore, a normal CXR does not exclude the diagnosis. High-resolution computed tomography (HRCT) of the chest should be performed in all patients with suspected DPLD. HRCT is useful for (1) detecting subradiographic disease, (2) distinguishing active inflammation from fibrosis, and (3) suggesting a specific diagnosis. Some reports suggest that an accurate diagnosis can be made in a large percentage of cases when clinical data are combined with the radiographic pattern seen on HRCT.

The pathophysiologic features of DPLD are similar in that most of these diseases result in restrictive pulmonary physiology. Spirometry and lung volumes in DPLD usually show a pattern of decreased TLC, FRC, and RV. However, pulmonary sarcoidosis, hypersensitivity pneumonitis, and RB-ILD may present with a mixed restrictive-obstructive pattern, and pulmonary sarcoidosis can occasionally present as pure obstruction. A reduced D$_{LCO}$ is common in DPLD but is a nonspecific finding. Changes in D$_{LCO}$ and FVC, however, are strong predictors of prognosis early in disease. These values should be followed closely over the course of a patient's illness to monitor disease progression and response to therapy. The extent of lung involvement on HRCT correlates with a patient's functional capacity. Hypoxemia with an elevated alveolar-arterial oxygen gradient supports the diagnosis of DPLD. With early disease, an A-a gradient may become manifest only with exertion. Exercise pulse oximetry is a useful test for detecting DPLD and for monitoring disease progression and response to

Figure 23-5 Sarcoidosis.

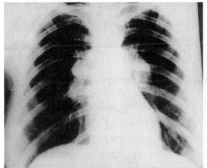

Radiologic stage I: Bilateral hilar lymph node enlargement

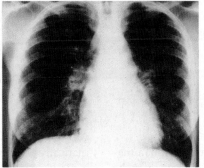

Stage II: Persistence of lymphadenopathy with reticular and nodular pulmonary infiltrations

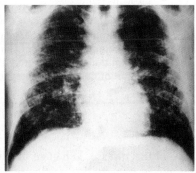

Stage III: Pulmonary infiltrations with no identifiable mediastinal lymphadenopathy

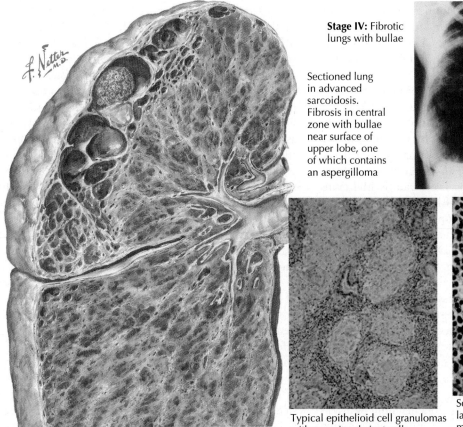

Stage IV: Fibrotic lungs with bullae

Sectioned lung in advanced sarcoidosis. Fibrosis in central zone with bullae near surface of upper lobe, one of which contains an aspergilloma

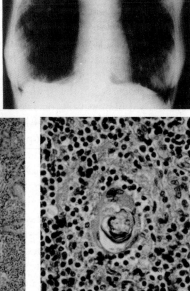

Typical epithelioid cell granulomas with occasional giant cells

Schaumann's body (concentrically laminated, calcified body) in a mediastinal lymph node giant cell

treatment. The physiologic workup will support the diagnosis DPLD but rarely is suggestive of a particular etiology.

Serologic studies are a useful part of the evaluation of patients with suspected DPLD. On initial evaluation, complete blood count with differential, reticulocytes, basic chemistries, urinalysis, and liver function tests (LFTs) should be ordered. Peripheral lymphopenia and elevated LFTs may be seen in sarcoidosis. An elevated serum angiotensin-converting enzyme (ACE) level may support the diagnosis of sarcoidosis; however, other granulomatous diseases can also produce an elevated ACE. Renal abnormalities may be present in pulmonary-renal syndromes such as Goodpasture's and Wegener's granulomatosis. Serum precipitins against antigens associated with hypersensitivity pneumonitis can be obtained if the history is

---

Box 23-5 Diseases that Mimic Diffuse Parenchymal Lung Disease

- Pulmonary infections
- Disseminated carcinoma (bronchoalveolar cell carcinoma, lymphangitic carcinomatosis)
- Cardiac disease (mitral stenosis, left ventricular failure)
- Chronic aspiration of gastric contents (severe gastric reflux)

---

suggestive of this disease. When an underlying inflammatory process is suspected, a sedimentation rate may be helpful. All patients with DPLD of undetermined etiology after initial evaluation should undergo testing for antinuclear antibodies (ANA), antineutrophilic cytoplasmic antibodies (ANCA), extractable nuclear antigen (ENA), creatinine kinase (CK), and aldolase because lung disease can occasionally be the first presenting features of connective tissue disease and vasculitides. When the serologic studies support a specific diagnosis, invasive studies may not be necessary for diagnosis.

Bronchoalveolar lavage (BAL) by fiberoptic bronchoscopy is a minimally invasive procedure that allows for sampling of the cells in the alveolar space. Evaluation of the lavage fluid for cell count, cultures for microorganisms, and cytology may be helpful in diagnosing some DPLDs. Elevated lymphocytes in the BAL suggests sarcoidosis, hypersensitivity pneumonitis, or bronchiolitis obliterans organizing pneumonia (BOOP). Elevated eosinophils in the BAL may be seen in eosinophilic pneumonia and Churg-Strauss syndrome. In addition, BAL may be useful in diagnosing diseases that mimic DPLD (Box 23-5).

When the clinical presentation, pattern of disease on HRCT, and serologic testing are nonspecific and inconclusive, lung biopsy may be necessary to determine the etiology of DPLD. Histopathologic evaluation of lung tissue is the most sensitive and specific way to determine the etiology of DPLD. An accurate diagnosis is necessary to initiate the proper treatment. The therapies for DPLD often have serious side effects, and treatment should not be initiated without a confident diagnosis. Fiberoptic bronchoscopy with BAL and transbronchial lung biopsy is the procedure of choice when sarcoidosis, eosinophilic pneumonia, or lymphangitic carcinomatosis is suspected. However, the small lung sample size obtained by this method is often inadequate for differentiating other DPLDs, particularly the idiopathic interstitial pneumonias (see Box 23-3). If transbronchial lung biopsy is nondiagnostic, or if an idiopathic interstitial pneumonia is suspected, surgical lung biopsy may be necessary. The histopathologic analysis, in combination with the clinical presentation and radiographic pattern on HRCT, ensures the highest level of diagnostic accuracy in patients with DPLD. Recently, it has been suggested that a diagnosis of idiopathic pulmonary fibrosis (IPF), the most common

DPLD of older adults, can be reasonably established without lung biopsy, if clinical presentation and HRCT are characteristic.

Management and Therapy

Optimum Treatment

Therapy for RLD is designed to halt or reverse the disease process responsible for producing restrictive physiology. Although simple physical measures can sometimes be dramatically effective for diseases affecting chest wall mechanics (e.g., weight loss for obesity), neuromuscular diseases are often progressive. Myasthenia gravis is an exception, and specific therapy for this disorder is discussed in Chapter 134.

Treatment of DPLD is tailored for each specific disease entity, highlighting the necessity of an accurate diagnosis of these disorders. For example, RB-ILD and DIP, two idiopathic interstitial pneumonias, may improve with smoking cessation. Immunosuppressive therapy is highly effective for pulmonary vasculitis and diseases in which acute or chronic inflammation is believed to drive disease pathogenesis (e.g., eosinophilic pneumonia, BOOP). However, diseases with active fibroblast proliferation such as IPF are poorly responsive to immunosuppressive therapy, and frequently side effects from these therapies in patients with IPF may outweigh the modest benefit that might be gained. For patients with IPF, and other DPLDs resulting in end-stage lung disease, lung transplantation should be considered. IPF is a uniformly fatal disease with a 2.5-year median survival; therefore, referral for lung transplantation evaluation should be considered early for these patients.

Nonspecific supportive care is an important component of treatment of RLDs including DPLD. Noninvasive positive pressure ventilation can be highly effective for neuromuscular disease and other nonparenchymal diseases affecting pulmonary mechanics. Oxygen therapy is essential to prevent hypoxemia and retard the development of cor pulmonale in these patients. Accordingly, assessment of oxygen requirements at rest, with exertion, and during sleep is warranted. Cor pulmonale should be treated initially with oxygen, which often prompts a spontaneous diuresis. If edema persists despite adequate oxygenation, diuretics can be added. Novel drugs initially developed for primary pulmonary arterial hypertension (PAH) may be available in the future for treating PAH and cor pulmonale secondary to DPLD.

Avoiding Treatment Errors

Sarcoidosis and IPF are the most common DPLDs affecting younger and older adults, respectively. Therefore, these disorders are sometimes treated by the primary care physician. One of the most common treatment errors related to sarcoidosis is the decision to initiate therapy in the first place. Most patients presenting with sarcoidosis, particularly Löfgren's syndrome (fever, bilateral hilar adenopathy, erythema nodosum), do not need treatment because the disease process has a high propensity for spontaneous remission. Another common treatment error in sarcoidosis is the use of high-dose prednisone. The granulomatous inflammation of sarcoidosis usually responds to an initial dose of 30 to 40 mg/day of prednisone, and can be suppressed with lower doses of 10 to 20 mg/day.

IPF responds poorly to corticosteroid therapy, and trials of high-dose prednisone are no longer indicated for patients with a definitive diagnosis. The need for oxygen therapy, particularly with exertion, should not be overlooked. Oxygen should be prescribed immediately if hypoxemia is present at rest, with exertion, or during sleep. Because novel antifibrotic agents with disease-modifying potential are on the horizon and currently available through clinical trials, consultation with a pulmonologist or IPF referral center should be considered given the lack of other truly effective therapies for this disease, other than lung transplantation. Because patients with IPF can deteriorate rapidly, early referral for lung transplantation evaluation is prudent.

Future Directions

Although the physiologic impairment produced by RLDs have been well recognized for many years, the pathogenesis of individual DPLDs remains poorly understood. Advances in our knowledge of IPF as a disorder of fibroblast proliferation rather than an inflammatory pneumoni-

tis has fueled interest in the development of antifibrotic drugs for this condition. A better understanding of the pathogenesis of specific DPLDs through modern genetic and molecular research with animal models and human tissue should identify new pathways and uncover novel therapeutic targets for this interesting group of diseases producing restrictive disease in the chest.

Additional Resources

UpToDate. Available at http://www.uptodate.com/. Accessed February 4, 2007.
   This website is an excellent source with frequently updated information.

EVIDENCE

1. King TE Jr: Clinical advances in the diagnosis and therapy of the interstitial lung diseases. Am J Respir Crit Care Med 172(3):268-279, 2005.
   This review article focuses on the idiopathic interstitial pneumonias and provides a clear presentation of diagnostic workup, disease prognosis, and new developments in clinical practice.
2. Martinez FJ: Idiopathic interstitial pneumonias: Usual interstitial pneumonia versus nonspecific interstitial pneumonia. Proc Am Thorac Soc 3(1):81-95, 2006.
   This review article concentrates on differentiating the various types of DPLD. Emphasis is placed on the importance of clinical history, pulmonary physiology, radiology, and bronchoscopy. It also provides a summary of recent studies on NSIP and UIP.
3. Shneerson JM, Simonds AK: Noninvasive ventilation for chest wall and neuromuscular disorders. Eur Respir J 20(2):480-487, 2002.
   This article provides a general overview of the use of noninvasive ventilation for treatment of acute or progressive respiratory failure due to neuromuscular and chest wall disorders.

Environmental Lung Disease

Introduction

Air pollution has presented a challenge to humans for millennia. This was initially of crustal and plant origin but later included particles generated from burning biomass in indoor spaces for heating and cooking. Larger anthropogenic contributions to ambient air pollution arrived with industrialization and accelerated with the development of automotive transport in the 20th century. Episodes of extremely high levels of ambient air pollution such as that in the Meuse Valley of Belgium in 1930 and Donora, Pennsylvania in 1948 were accompanied by acute elevations in morbidity and mortality in the exposed populations. Between 1948 and 1962, eight wintertime air pollution episodes occurred in London, England with the most clearly described being that in December of 1952. Excess deaths during this episode numbered 12,000 and were largely among infants and the elderly (with the majority of the latter suffering from chronic respiratory disease). Increasing concerns regarding the health consequences of air pollution in the United States culminated in the Clean Air Act of 1970 (and subsequent amendments). Despite reductions in air pollution, epidemiologic investigation during the 1980s and 1990s repeatedly demonstrated an association between the daily mean concentration of ambient particulate air pollution in cities both in the United States and worldwide with indices of acute morbidity and mortality. Likewise, associations between fluctuations in daily summertime ozone (O_3) levels and respiratory morbidity were demonstrated.

Etiology and Pathogenesis

Significant anthropogenic contributions to ambient air pollution result in large part from combustion of fossil fuels. This can include emissions from motor vehicle engines (mobile sources), power plants (stationary sources), and area sources (wood burning stoves, fireplaces, and grills). Tailpipe emissions are a major contributor of carbon monoxide (CO), nitrogen oxides (NO_x), hydrocarbons, diesel, and other airborne particles. Power plant emissions are largely responsible for atmospheric sulfur dioxide (SO_2), which is oxidized in the atmosphere to sulfuric acid and various particulate sulfates. Waste incinerators, smelters, steel mills, and other industrial activities may be responsible for emissions of a variety of acidic, organic, and metal compounds that cause local changes in air quality. Gaseous and particulate pollutants can undergo long-range transport in the atmosphere.

Particulate Matter

From the standpoint of adverse health effects, particulate matter (PM) is arguably the most important of the "Criteria Air Pollutants" defined in the Clean Air Act of 1970 (Table 24-1). PM is measured and reported in gravimetric units (micrograms) per cubic meter of ambient air and includes all PM that is respirable—that is, particles small enough to be inhaled into the lower respiratory tract by humans. The upper size limit for globular respirable particles is an aerodynamic diameter of 10 μm. Respirable PM is somewhat arbitrarily divided into size fractions, such as coarse (2.5 to 10 μm), fine (0.1 to 2.5 μm), and ultrafine (<0.1 μm); the last category includes so-called nanoparticles. Coarse particles are thought to arise mainly from the earth's crust and include compounds like aluminum silicates. They also contain biologic materials like endotoxin. Fine particles are thought to arise from

Table 24-1 U.S. Ambient Air Quality Standards (2006)*

PM$_{10}$	150 μg/m^3 (24 hr)	50 μg/m^3 (annual)
PM$_{2.5}$	65 μg/m^3 (24 hr)	15 μg/m^3 (annual)
Ozone	0.12 ppm (1 hr)	0.08 ppm (8 hours)
NO$_2$		0.053 ppm (annual)
SO$_2$	0.14 ppm (24 hr)	0.03 ppm (annual)
CO	35 ppm (1 hr)	9 ppm (8 hours)

*Lead is excluded from this list because it is not addressed in this chapter.

combustion processes in mobile and stationary sources. They include elemental carbon, organic carbon, metal compounds, and sulfates and nitrates. Some fine particles are primary emissions, but many represent particles generated from primary gaseous emissions by chemical or photochemical and physical processes occurring in the atmosphere. Fine particles do not sediment readily (unlike coarse particles) and therefore enjoy a long atmospheric lifetime. Ultrafine particles can be primary emissions from combustion processes and can also be generated de novo from volatile organic compounds undergoing oxidation in the atmosphere to poorly volatile oxy-organic species. Ultrafine particles agglomerate readily and contribute to the generation of more stable fine particles (sometimes referred to as the accumulation mode). Fine particles generally comprise a substantial fraction of the PM$_{10}$ mass. Ultrafine particles, on the other hand, contribute little to PM$_{10}$ mass. However, they account for most of the particle number, sometimes more than10^6/cm^3, and (in aggregate) have a very large surface area, a property that may confer a high degree of reactivity in biologic as well as physical systems. Decreasing the diameter of PM also reduces uptake by professional phagocytes and enhances penetration into other cells following their deposition on respiratory surfaces.

Time series analyses of short-term associations between fluctuations of daily gravimetric PM$_{10}$ levels in ambient air and daily nontraumatic mortality statistics, as well as indices of morbidity, have demonstrated significant associations in older adults. Death in older individuals appears to be a result of cardiovascular causes, including acute myocardial infarction, as well as respiratory causes. Morbidity is observed across the age spectrum and is primarily respiratory. There are several current hypotheses to account for PM-associated health effects and their causative agents. These hypotheses are not mutually exclusive.

1. Organic compounds and metals generate reactive oxygen species leading to oxidant stress in the lung and to systemic as well as local effects.
2. Biologic materials like endotoxin may act through high-affinity receptors (e.g., toll-like receptors) to prime the innate immune system and generate enhanced reactivity to other inhaled substances.

3. Ultrafine particles per se may provoke oxidant stress leading to proinflammatory and proliferative effects.
4. Particles (especially ultrafine) may cross the epithelium and gain access to the vascular system.

Some evidence for each of these mechanisms has been published; that for the direct passage of naked particles into the vascular system is least convincing.

With improved techniques for fractionation of the components of ambient air PM, observational studies have been able to assess temporal relations between these fractions and adverse health effects. Size fractionation has suggested that fine particles (PM$_{2.5}$) are the important agents, but some studies are not in accord with this exclusion of coarse PM.

Identification of the components of ambient air PM responsible for acute and subacute health effects, and of the mechanisms involved, is important to support the biologic plausibility of the reported associations and to pinpoint the source of the toxic components (and their precursors) for more effective monitoring and regulation. In addition, defining components and mechanisms could suggest approaches to identify susceptible individuals and to prevent effects in such persons. Unlike O$_3$, where indoor levels are substantially less than ambient concentrations and ambient air exposure avoidance strategies are effective, outdoor PM penetrates and persists indoors.

Ozone

O$_3$ is a second pollutant with a significant impact on human health. O$_3$ was first identified as a gaseous component of photochemical pollution (smog) in sunny Los Angeles, California during the 1940s. This gas is one of several photochemical oxidants formed in the troposphere as a secondary pollutant by the action of solar radiation on nitrogen dioxide (NO$_2$) in the presence of volatile organic compounds. Tropospheric O$_3$ pollution should be distinguished from that in the stratosphere, where O$_3$ prevents harmful ultraviolet radiation from reaching the surface of the earth. O$_3$ present at the Earth's surface, however, is detrimental to human health as well as to crops and materials.

O$_3$ pollution is worse from late spring to early fall, with levels typically rising in midmorning, several hours after the morning rush hour, peaking in the late afternoon, and declining in the evening. O$_3$ measurements are expressed as either ppb or μg/m^3 (1 ppm ≈ 2000 μg/m^3). Because the precursors of O$_3$ (i.e., NO$_2$ and organic compounds) share common origins with other pollutants, including PM and SO$_2$, the concentrations of these pollutants frequently correlate with each other.

O$_3$ causes ozonation and peroxidation of lipids in human lung epithelial lining fluid. Dietary antioxidant supplementation may provide some protection against O$_3$-induced acute reductions in lung function, but apparently not against the accompanying inflammatory response. Increased ventilation (exercise), exposure duration, and concentration enhance the health effects of O_3. These include substernal chest pain worsened by deep inspiration, decreased inspiratory capacity, increased bronchial reactivity to specific allergens as well as to methacholine or histamine, altered mucociliary clearance, and neutrophilic airways inflammation. These effects regress more or less rapidly after cessation of exposure. Whether repeated exposures to O_3 cause irreversible change is not clear. However, consecutive daily exposures to O_3 produce marked blunting of the initial spirometric effect and symptoms.

Nitrogen Oxides

During high temperature combustion, NO_x is generated. The significance of low concentrations of NO_x and the need for its regulation in ambient air derives from its role as an O_3 precursor rather than from direct effects on human health.

Sulfur Dioxide

Because of regulations included in the Clean Air Act of 1970, SO_2 concentrations in the United States have declined. This is a direct result of changing fuel quality (sulfur content) and use. High concentrations of SO_2 can still be observed in other parts of the world (e.g., China, where high sulfur coal is used for domestic cooking and heating).

Carbon Monoxide

CO is produced by an incomplete combustion of carbon. Individual exposure to CO occurs during motor vehicle travel, and concentrations of this gas can be high in road tunnels and indoor garages. National Ambient Air Quality Standards (NAAQS) are set to prevent levels of carboxyhemoglobin in the blood reaching 2.5% and above. An increase of 7 ppm CO in inspired air causes an equilibrium elevation of 1% blood carboxyhemoglobin above baseline (which is 0.5% to 1.0% in the healthy nonsmoker).

Clinical Presentation

We have chosen to discuss the individual criteria pollutants in this section. Nevertheless, interactive effects of different classes of pollutants and of other environmental agents (notably allergens) are receiving increasing attention.

Particulate Matter

The clinical presentation following exposure to elevated ambient air pollution PM levels includes an increased prevalence of respiratory symptoms (i.e., cough, phlegm, and wheeze) as well as hospitalizations for exacerbations of chronic obstructive pulmonary disease (COPD), bronchitis, and asthma. Elevation in ambient air PM levels can also be associated with increases in respiratory infections. Although not found in all studies, small, reversible decrements in pulmonary function as well as modest neutrophilia in the bronchoalveolar lavage have been described following controlled exposure of healthy volunteers to ambient air pollution particles. Such exposures also can elicit modest, acute changes in the peripheral blood, including elevations in white blood cell counts and increases in C-reactive protein, fibrinogen, and blood viscosity. The last two might possibly contribute to the epidemiologic association of ambient PM with thrombotic coronary artery events. Daily hospital admissions for cardiovascular diseases are also associated with PM levels, and the incidence of acute myocardial infarction has been reported to be increased within 2 hours of elevation in PM and to remain elevated for 24 hours.

Ozone

Exposure to low levels of O_3 can be accompanied by neutrophilic airways inflammation as early as within 1 hour (and can persist for 24 hours), even in the absence of either respiratory symptoms or lung function decrements. Prolonged controlled exposures of healthy, exercising volunteers to levels as low as 0.08 ppm caused pulmonary function changes (decreased inspiratory capacity and increased nonspecific airway reactivity) as well as evidence of airway inflammation. Spirometric reactivity to a given inhaled dose of O_3 appears to decrease with increasing age and possibly with antioxidant status and decreasing body mass index. However, most of the large range of interindividual response variability remains unexplained. Genetic polymorphisms may play a role. Ambient daily mean levels of O_3 above 0.02 ppm have been associated with increased daily hospitalizations for respiratory diseases, and levels above 0.05 ppm have been associated with increased respiratory symptoms, school and work absences, emergency department visits, physician visits, and medication use. Recent investigation suggests that mortality may increase with ambient O_3 exposure.

Although there is little evidence to support an induction of an atopic state or asthma by exposure to O_3, symptoms in patients with established asthma are clearly worsened. Panel studies in asthmatic children found an association of low ambient concentrations of O_3 with respiratory symptoms, increased bronchodilator use, and hospitalizations for asthma 1 day later.

Nitrogen Oxides and Sulfur Dioxide

Regarding the acute effects of exposure to NO_x and SO_2, healthy subjects can demonstrate reduced pulmonary

Figure 24-1 Air Quality Index for Pollution Based on Ozone and Particulate Matter Levels.
Adapted from U.S. Environmental Protection Agency at http://epa.gov/airnow.

Air-quality index	Air quality	Ozone (ppm)		Particulate matter (μ/g^3)		Health advisory
		8 hours	1 hour	PM 2.5	PM 10	
0 to 50	Good	0-0.064		0-15	0-50	None
51 to 100	Moderate	0.065-0.084		>15-40	>50-150	Unusually sensivite people should consider reducing prolonged or heavy exertion.
101 to 150	Unhealthy for sensitive groups	0.085-0.104	0.125-0.164	>40-65	>150-250	People with heart or lung disease, older adults, and children should reduce prolonged or heavy exertion.
151 to 200	Unhealthy	0.105-0.124	0.165-0.194	>65-150	>250-350	People with heart or lung disease, older adults, and children should avoid prolonged or heavy exertion. Everyone else should reduce prolonged or heavy exertion.
201 to 300	Very unhealthy	0.125-0.404	0.195-0.404	>150-250	>350-420	People with heart or lung disease, older adults, and children should avoid prolonged or heavy exertion. Everyone else should reduce prolonged or heavy exertion.

function and increased airway reactivity, but only at concentrations far greater than those ever observed in an outdoor environment. However, asthmatic people are more susceptible to bronchoconstrictive effects of NO_x and SO_2. The SO_2 effect has many similarities to exercise-induced bronchospasm and can provoke symptomatic bronchoconstriction during brief exposure to as little as 0.25 ppm.

Carbon Monoxide

Health effects of CO result from its high affinity for hemoglobin (which is 200 to 250 times that of O_2). Exposures to very high levels of CO can cause rapid uptake and acute poisoning, but such exposures are not encountered in outdoor settings. Carboxyhemoglobin levels between 2% and 4% cause a shortening of time to onset of exercise-induced angina, and somewhat higher levels cause increased ectopy in patients with coronary artery disease. A few studies have associated CO exposure with cardiac arrhythmia and with hospital admissions for heart disease and mortality, but ambient air CO levels may be surrogates for other pollutants rather than acting directly.

Diagnostic Approach

The air pollution–associated clinical events are essentially indistinguishable from the more common causes of these events. Therefore, the clinician must look for evidence of an association between the development of symptoms (or pathophysiologic changes) and exposure to elevated levels of ambient air pollution, especially in susceptible individuals. The mean daily levels of pollutants in a given region can be ascertained employing a U.S. Environmental Protection Agency website called AIRNOW.

Management and Therapy

Optimum Treatment

Therapies directed at adverse respiratory effects of air pollution include limiting outdoor activities (especially for O_3) and treatment of exacerbation of asthma and COPD. The latter can include bronchodilators, inhaled or systemic corticosteroids, and oxygen.

Empirical antibiotics, glucocorticosteroids, and bronchodilators are generally prescribed for patients with COPD exacerbations. The possible specific efficacy against air pollution–provoked health effects of chemopreventive and therapeutic efficacy of drugs like nonsteroidal anti-inflammatory agents (which blunt O_3-induced decrease in inspiratory capacity), leukotriene antagonists, and omalizumab, or enhancement of antioxidant metabolism, has not yet been sufficiently evaluated. In addition to individuals with asthma or COPD, patients with diabetes and cardiovascular disease are likely to benefit by following recommendations included in the Environmental Protection Agency AIRNOW air quality index (Fig. 24-1). Attempts at reduction to exposure to PM might include the following:

- Avoidance of residence in areas that frequently exceed the NAAQS
- Reduction of physical activities requiring exertion on days that pollution exceeds the NAAQS for PM or O_3

- Avoidance of exposure to environmental tobacco smoke
- Deferral of activities entailing exposure in environments affected by wildfires (e.g., Western United States)
- Avoidance of wood-burning stoves, fireplaces, and kerosene heaters
- Avoidance of specific household activities involving particle exposure (e.g., use of household cleansers and mulching)
- Consulting the AIRNOW internet site before travel to areas within the United States
- Avoidance of travel to international locations with high ambient air pollution levels

Future Directions

Control of air pollution by air quality monitoring, delineation of air quality standards, and imposition of controls on emissions from stationary and mobile sources has been the principal approach by which federal and state agencies have attempted to prevent adverse health effects. Individual avoidance of exposure to polluted ambient air is recommended. Future efforts will include identification of susceptible individuals (including determinants of genetic susceptibility). Chemoprophylaxis for such persons, including enhancement of antioxidant defenses, may follow.

Additional Resource

AIRNOW. Available at: http://epa.gov/airnow. Accessed November 26, 2006.

This Internet site predicts particle and ozone levels in the United States and is maintained by the U.S. Environmental Protection Agency.

EVIDENCE

1. Committee of the Environmental and Occupational Health Assembly of the American Thoracic Society: Health effects of outdoor air pollution. Am J Respir Crit Care Med 153(1):1-50 and 153(2):477-498, 1996.

This two part manuscript by the American Thoracic Society is the most comprehensive review on lung injury following environmental exposures.

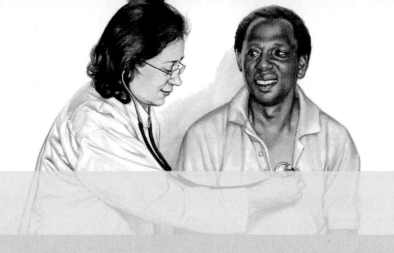
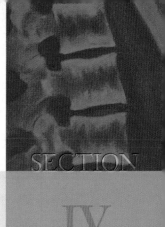

Disorders of the Cardiovascular System

Romulo E. Colindres ▪ Alan L. Hinderliter

Hypertension

Introduction

Hypertension is a major risk factor for cardiovascular disease (Fig. 25-1). Numerous large-scale prospective observational studies have demonstrated five major effects of hypertension, all of which contribute to the overall mortality and morbidity associated with hypertension. First, high blood pressure accelerates atherogenesis and increases the risk for cardiovascular events twofold to threefold. Second, the level of systolic and diastolic blood pressure is associated with cardiovascular events in a continuous, graded, and apparently independent fashion. In subjects 50 years and older, an elevated systolic blood pressure is a much more important cardiovascular risk factor than an elevated diastolic blood pressure (Fig. 25-2; see Fig. 25-1). Third, the risk for cardiovascular disease, beginning at 115/75 mm Hg, doubles with each increase of 20/10 mm Hg. Between a diastolic blood pressure of 110 mm Hg and 70 mm Hg, a persistently lower usual diastolic blood pressure of 5 mm Hg is associated with at least a 40% decrease in the incidence of stroke and a 21% decrease in the incidence of coronary heart disease. Fourth, hypertension often occurs in association with, and as a result of, other atherogenic risk factors, including dyslipidemia, glucose intolerance, hyperinsulinemia, and obesity. Fifth, the association of hypertension with other cardiovascular risk factors increases the risk for cardiovascular events in a multiplicative rather than additive fashion.

Pharmacologic treatment of hypertension reduces the incidence of stroke and coronary artery disease, and decreases mortality from cardiovascular causes in middle-aged and older adults (Fig. 25-3). The results of the randomized clinical trials of the treatment of hypertension indicate that the average percentage reductions in the incidence of stroke, myocardial infarction, and heart failure with drug treatment are 35% to 40%, 20% to 25%, and 50%, respectively. If anything, these trials likely underestimate the cardiovascular benefits of blood pressure control because numerous study patients assigned to active therapy stopped their treatment, whereas others assigned to placebo were prescribed medications. In addition, the average duration of treatment was only about 5 years, and most patients enrolled were at low risk for developing cardiovascular disease.

More recent clinical trials have focused on head-to-head comparisons of different antihypertensive drugs or combinations of drugs, to determine whether certain agents offer benefits beyond those attributable to lowering of blood pressure, particularly in older persons with cardiovascular risk factors. Meta-analyses of these trials have indicated that, with few exceptions, the most important factor in decreasing cardiovascular morbidity and mortality in hypertensive subjects is the magnitude of the blood pressure reduction rather than the drug or drugs used to achieve the reduction of the blood pressure. However, as indicated later, there are some compelling indications for the use of specific drug classes in appropriate patients. There is also evidence that β-adrenergic blockers may not be as effective as other medications in preventing cardiovascular complications in older people with hypertension.

Definition of Hypertension

Blood pressure is a continuous variable, and any level of blood pressure chosen to define hypertension will be arbitrary. Nevertheless, an operational definition of hypertension has long been advocated by clinicians as a guideline for treatment. Such a definition should theoretically be based on the estimated level of blood pressure above which the benefit of pharmacologic therapy in reducing cardiovascular risk exceeds the risk and inconvenience of therapy. The report of the Seventh Joint National Committee on the Prevention, Detection, Evaluation, and Treatment of

Figure 25-1 Hypertension as Risk Factor for Cardiovascular Disease.*

A, Adapted from Kannel WB: Blood pressure as a cardiovascular risk factor. JAMA 275:1571-1576, 1996.
B, Adapted from MacMahon S, Peto R, Cutler S, et al: Blood pressure, stroke, and coronary heart disease:
Part 1. Lancet 335:765-774, 1990.

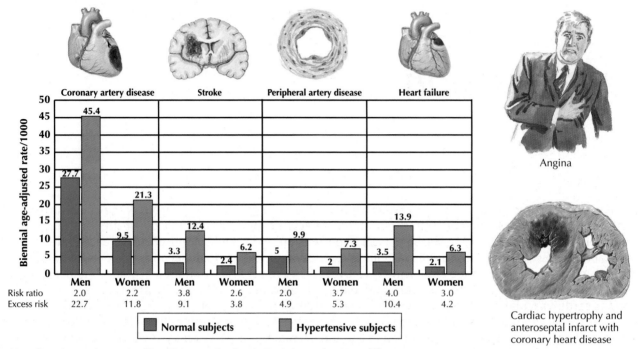

	Coronary artery disease		Stroke		Peripheral artery disease		Heart failure	
	Men	Women	Men	Women	Men	Women	Men	Women
Risk ratio	2.0	2.2	3.8	2.6	2.0	3.7	4.0	3.0
Excess risk	22.7	11.8	9.1	3.8	4.9	5.3	10.4	4.2

Values on chart: Coronary artery disease — Men: 27.7 / 45.4; Women: 9.5 / 21.3. Stroke — Men: 3.3 / 12.4; Women: 2.4 / 6.2. Peripheral artery disease — Men: 5 / 9.9; Women: 2 / 7.3. Heart failure — Men: 3.5 / 13.9; Women: 2.1 / 6.3.

Biennial age-adjusted rate/1000

■ Normal subjects   ■ Hypertensive subjects

Angina

Cardiac hypertrophy and anteroseptal infarct with coronary heart disease

*According to hypertensive status in subjects 35-64 years of age from the Framingham study at 36-year follow-up.

A

Level of blood pressure is associated with cardiovascular events in a continuous, graded, and apparently independent fashion**

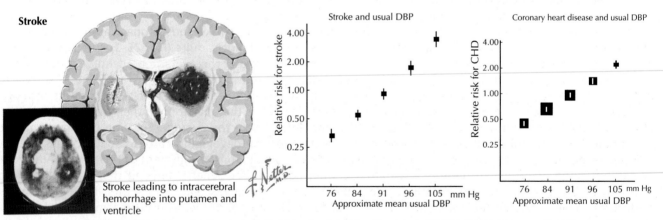

Stroke

Stroke leading to intracerebral hemorrhage into putamen and ventricle

Stroke and usual DBP

Relative risk for stroke

Approximate mean usual DBP
76   84   91   96   105   mm Hg

Coronary heart disease and usual DBP

Relative risk for CHD

Approximate mean usual DBP
76   84   91   96   105   mm Hg

**Relative risk for stroke and coronary heart disease as a function of usual diastolic pressure in 420,000 individuals 25 years or older with a mean follow-up period of 10 years.

B

High Blood Pressure (JNC VII) recommended the classification of blood pressure for adults shown in Table 25-1. As compared with the previous classification recommended by JNC VI, subjects with a blood pressure of 120/80 to 139/89 mm Hg are now designated as having prehypertension because they are at high risk for developing hypertension. Patients and clinicians need to be aware of this condition to ensure follow-up and institution of lifestyle modifications. Several observational studies have shown that subjects with prehypertension have increased cardio-

vascular morbidity, but it has yet to be demonstrated that antihypertensive drug therapy or even lifestyle modifications decrease morbidity in such subjects.

Similar, but subtly different, recommendations have been proposed by other organizations. The British Hypertension Society and the European Society of Hypertension classify as high-normal systolic blood pressures of 130 to 139 mm Hg and diastolic blood pressures of 80 to 89 mm Hg. However, both societies recommend lifestyle modifications for subjects having high-normal blood

Figure 25-2 Risk for Cardiovascular Events by Level of Systolic Blood Pressure: 30-Year Follow-up for Framingham Subjects, 65 to 95 Years Old.
Adapted from Wilson WF, Kannel WB. In Laragh JH, Brenner BT (eds): Hypertension, 2nd ed. New York, Raven Press, 1995, p 101.

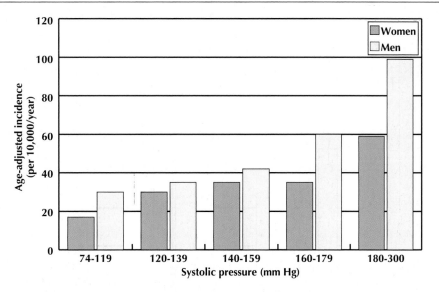

Figure 25-3 Effects of Antihypertensive Treatment on Stroke, Coronary Heart Disease, Total Cardiovascular Deaths, and All Other Deaths*.
CHD, Coronary heart disease; CVD, Cardiovascular disease. *Adapted from Cutler J, et al. Public issues in hypertension control: What has been learned from clinical trials? In Laragh JH, Brenner BT (eds): Hypertension, 2nd ed. New York, Raven Press, 1995.*

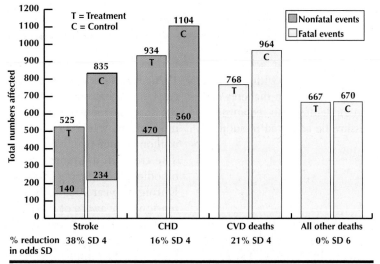

Table 25-1	Blood Pressure Classification		
Classification	**Systolic (mm Hg)**		**Diastolic (mm Hg)**
Normal	<120	*and*	<80
Prehypertension	120-139	*or*	80-89
Stage I hypertension	140-159	*or*	90-99
Stage II hypertension	≥160	*or*	≥100

Data from the National High Blood Pressure Education Program; National Heart, Lung and Blood Institute; National Institutes of Health and the Department of Health and Human Services.

Figure 25-4 Estimated Percentage of U.S. Adults with Hypertension by Sex, Race, and Ethnicity, 1999 to 2000.

Reprinted with permission from Fields LE, Burt VL, Cutler JA, et al: The burden of adult hypertension in the United States 1999 to 2000: A rising tide. Hypertension 44:398-404, 2004.

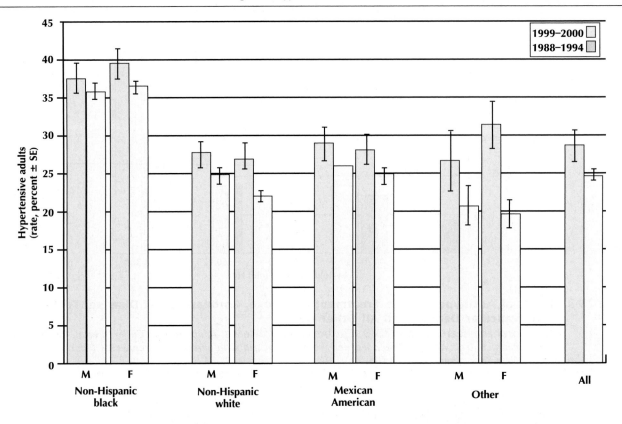

pressure. The U.S. guidelines suggest that achieving a blood pressure of less than 130/80 mm Hg with pharmacologic therapy is beneficial in patients with diabetes and kidney disease. The European guidelines also recommend that such levels of blood pressure be achieved in subjects with heart disease.

Epidemiology

Hypertension is a major health problem throughout the world. The prevalence of hypertension worldwide may be as high as 1 billion persons, and deaths attributed to hypertension now total about 7 million per year. The prevalence of hypertension is higher in developed countries, but it is increasing rapidly in developing countries as a consequence of longer life span, obesity, and changing dietary habits. In the United States, even those who are normotensive at 55 years have a 90% lifetime risk for hypertension. According to the World Health Organization, suboptimal blood pressure is the number one attributable cause of death throughout the world. Hypertension is the most common cause of preventable death in developed countries.

The U.S. National Health and Nutrition Examination Surveys (NHANES) have defined the characteristics of hypertension in subjects 18 to 76 years of age between 1976 and 2004. The overall prevalence of hypertension in the United States in 2004, based on measurement of blood pressure or reported use of prescribed antihypertensive medication, was 29.3%. About 30 million men and 35 million women had hypertension in that survey (Fig. 25-4). The trend in awareness, treatment, and control of high blood pressure during those years is shown in Table 25-2. During the year 2003 to 2004, 76% of patients with hypertension were aware of their condition, 65% were receiving treatment, and 37% had controlled hypertension, defined as a blood pressure of less than 140/90 mm Hg. There has been a gradual improvement of these parameters over the years in both genders, in all age groups, and in various ethnic groups, but only 57% of treated subjects had controlled hypertension. The percentage of patients with controlled hypertension is lower in some Western countries such as Canada and England, and is less than 10% in developing countries—a disappointing figure given the medications available to treat hypertension and efforts made to educate the public and physicians about the risks of high blood pressure. Hypertension is therefore a major worldwide public health problem and a highly prevalent major cardiovascular risk factor, the prevention and treatment of which should be prioritized.

Table 25-2 Trends in the Awareness, Treatment, and Control of High Blood Pressure in U.S. Adults

	National Health and Nutrition Examination Survey (%)				
	1976-1980	**1988-1991**	**1991-1994**	**1999-2000**	**2003-2004**
Awareness	51	73	68	70	76
Treatment	31	55	54	59	65
Control	10	29	27	34	37

Data are for adults 18 to 74 years of age with a systolic blood pressure equal to or greater than 140 mm Hg or a diastolic blood pressure equal to or greater than 90 mm Hg. Control is defined as a systolic blood pressure <140 mm Hg and a diastolic blood pressure <90 mm Hg.

Modified from The sixth report of the Joint National Committee on Prevention, Detection, Evaluation, and Treatment of High Blood Pressure. Arch Intern Med 157:2413-2446, 1997. Recent data are from Hypertension 49:69-75, 2007.

Figure 25-5 Factors Involved in the Control of Blood Pressure.
Reprinted with permission Kaplan NM, Kaplan's Clinical Hypertension. 8th ed. Philadelphia, Lippincott, Williams & Wilkins, 2002.

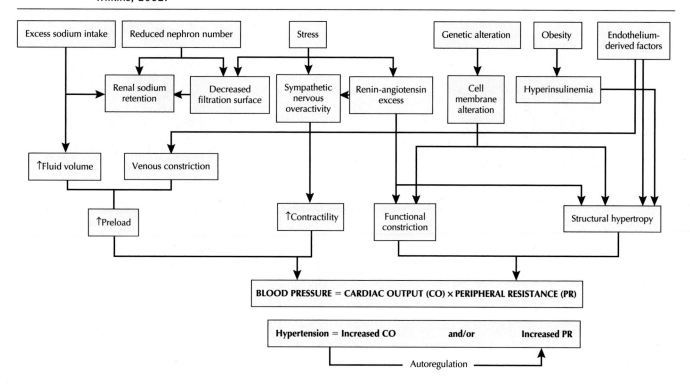

Etiology and Pathogenesis

Hypertension is a disorder of blood pressure regulation that most often results from an increase in total peripheral vascular resistance. Although increased cardiac output plays an etiologic role in the development of hypertension, most individuals with essential hypertension have normal cardiac output. This apparent paradox is explained by the phenomenon of autoregulation, whereby an increase in cardiac output causes a persistently elevated peripheral vascular resistance, with a resulting return of cardiac output to normal. Figure 25-5 shows the numerous mechanisms that can lead to hypertension.

Inappropriate activation of the renin-angiotensin system, decreased renal sodium excretion, and an increase in sympathetic nervous system activity, individually or in combination, are most likely involved in the pathogenesis of all types of hypertension. Hypertension has both genetic and environmental causes, including excess sodium intake, obesity, and stress. The inability of the kidneys to optimally excrete sodium, and thus regulate the plasma volume, leads to a persistent increase in blood pressure regardless of the specific underlying etiology.

Many elderly patients with elevated blood pressure have isolated systolic hypertension—a systolic pressure that exceeds 140 mm Hg with a normal diastolic pressure.

Figure 25-6 Wave Reflection and Isolated Systolic Hypertension.

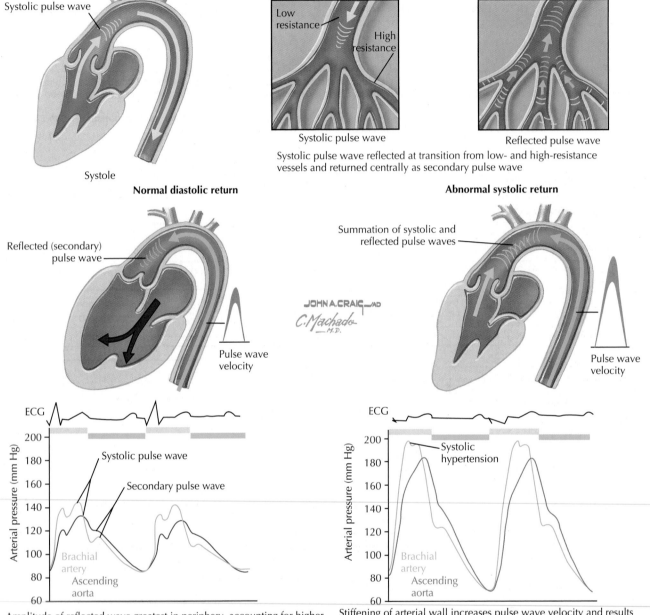

Pulse wave generation

Systolic pulse wave reflected at transition from low- and high-resistance vessels and returned centrally as secondary pulse wave

Amplitude of reflected wave greatest in periphery, accounting for higher systolic pressures in extremities than in aorta. Diastolic return of reflected wave to heart increases coronary perfusion and decreases afterload

Stiffening of arterial wall increases pulse wave velocity and results in systolic return of reflected wave with increase in systolic pressure (isolated systolic hypertension), decreased diastolic pressure, increased afterload, and left ventricular hypertrophy

Isolated systolic hypertension correlates with stiffening of large arteries, an increase in systolic pulse wave velocity causing an increase in systolic blood pressure, and increased myocardial work with decreased coronary perfusion (Fig. 25-6).

Clinical Presentation

Most patients with early hypertension have no symptoms attributable to high blood pressure. It is essential to detect and treat hypertension at this asymptomatic stage because by the time symptoms occur in individuals with long-term blood pressure elevation, hypertensive heart disease, atherosclerosis of the aorta and peripheral vessels, cerebrovascular disease, or renal insufficiency may be present.

The cardiac manifestations of hypertension result from both the hypertrophic effects of increased afterload and the acceleration of coronary atherosclerosis seen in hypertensive patients. Left ventricular hypertrophy is a powerful and independent risk factor for cardiovascular morbidity and mortality. Most hypertensive patients with left ventricular hypertrophy have concentric hypertrophy—an

Figure 25-7 Development of Congestive Heart Failure in Patients with Hypertension.
CHF, congestive heart failure; LV, left ventricular; LVH, left ventricular hypertrophy; MI, myocardial infarction. *Adapted from Vasan RS, Levy D: The role of hypertension in the pathogenesis of heart failure. A clinical mechanistic overview. Arch Intern Med 156:1789-1796, 1996.*

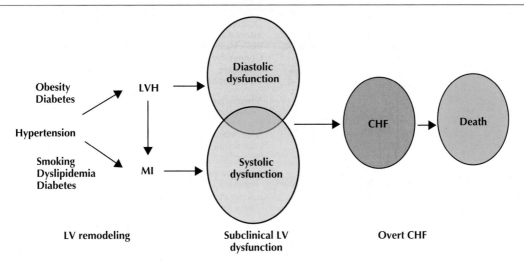

increase in wall thickness relative to chamber dimensions. In addition, myocardial fibrosis, stimulated in part by increased angiotensin II and aldosterone levels, causes decreased ventricular compliance and diastolic dysfunction and may result in congestive heart failure despite normal left ventricular systolic function. Sustained blood pressure elevations may ultimately lead to left ventricular decompensation and diminished cardiac output. Hypertension is an independent risk factor for coronary artery disease. The incidence of coronary events increases proportionally with increases in systolic or diastolic blood pressure. These two effects, left ventricular hypertrophy and accelerated atherosclerosis, combine to greatly enhance the risk for congestive heart failure and cardiovascular death in patients with hypertension (Fig. 25-7).

As many as half of patients with high blood pressure and heart failure have a normal left ventricular ejection fraction. Typically, these patients have long-standing hypertension and left ventricular hypertrophy, and their symptoms result from diastolic dysfunction. Compared with patients with heart failure and a decreased ejection fraction, patients with diastolic heart failure tend to be older and are more likely to be female and hypertensive. Although diastolic heart failure confers a lower risk for mortality, it is an important cause of morbidity and hospitalization.

Occasionally, asymptomatic hypertension may enter a phase called *malignant* or *accelerated* hypertension. This syndrome is characterized by greatly elevated systolic and diastolic blood pressures, severe neuroretinitis, proteinuria, microscopic hematuria, impairment of renal function, and a variety of symptoms caused by proliferative endarteritis and fibrinoid necrosis of small arteries and arterioles.

Differential Diagnosis

About 95% of patients with elevated arterial pressure have essential hypertension. In many such patients, obesity is a contributing factor. Obstructive sleep apnea is frequently associated with obesity and hypertension, but it has yet to be definitively proved that appropriate treatment of this condition consistently lowers blood pressure. The remaining 5% of patients with high blood pressure have secondary hypertension (Fig. 25-8). The prevalence of secondary hypertension is higher in the very old and in the very young. Although patients with secondary hypertension are few in number, it is important to identify such patients because their hypertension can often be cured or significantly improved by an interventional procedure, a specific drug therapy, or stopping a culprit drug.

Evidence of identifiable causes of hypertension should be sought in the initial history, physical examination, and laboratory studies. Further diagnostic evaluation for causes of secondary hypertension should be pursued when the presentation is atypical for essential hypertension, or when the initial evaluation suggests an identifiable cause (Box 25-1). Diagnostic methods used in evaluating specific causes of secondary hypertension are discussed in Chapters 26 and 27.

Diagnostic Approach

The initial evaluation of the hypertensive patient should include the following steps:

- Confirmation of the presence of hypertension
- Determination of the presence and extent of target organ disease

Figure 25-8 Causes of Hypertension.

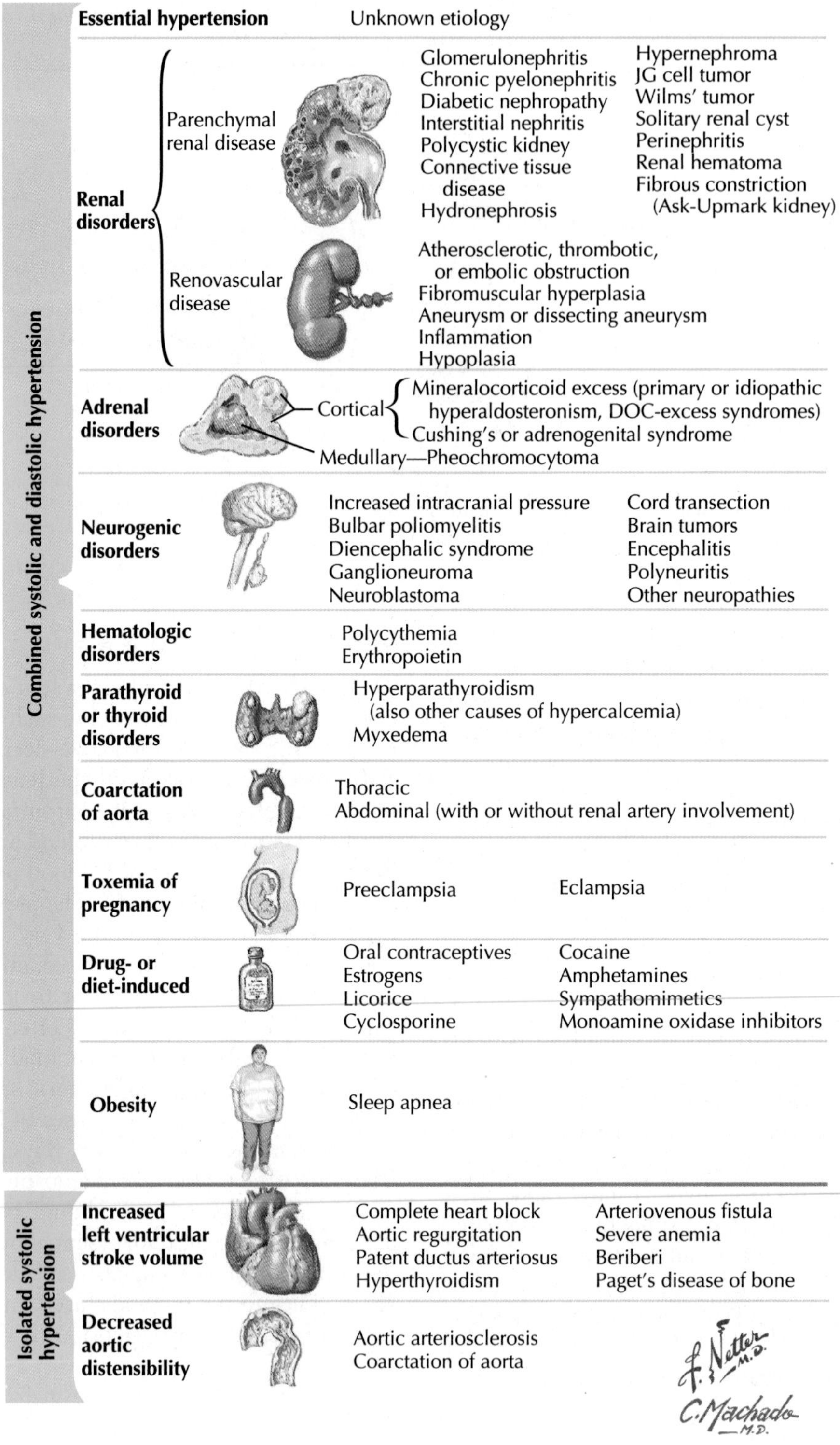

Combined systolic and diastolic hypertension

Essential hypertension — Unknown etiology

Renal disorders

Parenchymal renal disease:
Glomerulonephritis
Chronic pyelonephritis
Diabetic nephropathy
Interstitial nephritis
Polycystic kidney
Connective tissue disease
Hydronephrosis
Hypernephroma
JG cell tumor
Wilms' tumor
Solitary renal cyst
Perinephritis
Renal hematoma
Fibrous constriction (Ask-Upmark kidney)

Renovascular disease:
Atherosclerotic, thrombotic, or embolic obstruction
Fibromuscular hyperplasia
Aneurysm or dissecting aneurysm
Inflammation
Hypoplasia

Adrenal disorders

Cortical:
Mineralocorticoid excess (primary or idiopathic hyperaldosteronism, DOC-excess syndromes)
Cushing's or adrenogenital syndrome
Medullary—Pheochromocytoma

Neurogenic disorders

Increased intracranial pressure
Bulbar poliomyelitis
Diencephalic syndrome
Ganglioneuroma
Neuroblastoma
Cord transection
Brain tumors
Encephalitis
Polyneuritis
Other neuropathies

Hematologic disorders

Polycythemia
Erythropoietin

Parathyroid or thyroid disorders

Hyperparathyroidism (also other causes of hypercalcemia)
Myxedema

Coarctation of aorta

Thoracic
Abdominal (with or without renal artery involvement)

Toxemia of pregnancy

Preeclampsia   Eclampsia

Drug- or diet-induced

Oral contraceptives
Estrogens
Licorice
Cyclosporine
Cocaine
Amphetamines
Sympathomimetics
Monoamine oxidase inhibitors

Obesity

Sleep apnea

Isolated systolic hypertension

Increased left ventricular stroke volume

Complete heart block
Aortic regurgitation
Patent ductus arteriosus
Hyperthyroidism
Arteriovenous fistula
Severe anemia
Beriberi
Paget's disease of bone

Decreased aortic distensibility

Aortic arteriosclerosis
Coarctation of aorta

Box 25-1 Indications for Considering Testing for Identifiable Causes of Hypertension

- Age of onset of hypertension <20 years or >50 years
- Target organ damage at presentation
  Serum creatinine concentration >1.5 mg/dL
  Left ventricular hypertrophy by electrocardiography
- Presence of features indicative of secondary causes:
  Hypokalemia
  Abdominal bruit
  Labile pressures with tachycardia, sweating, and tremor
  Family history of renal disease
- Poor response to generally effective therapy

- Identification of cardiovascular risk factors and coexisting conditions that influence prognosis and therapy
- Exclusion or detection of identifiable causes of elevated blood pressure

These goals can usually be achieved with a comprehensive history, a thorough physical examination, and selected laboratory studies.

A comprehensive history is essential, and should include the following:

- The duration and severity of elevated blood pressure, and the results of prior medication trials
- The presence of diabetes, hypercholesterolemia, tobacco use, and other cardiovascular risk factors
- A history or symptoms of target organ disease, including coronary heart disease and heart failure, cerebrovascular disease, peripheral vascular disease, and renal disease
- Symptoms suggesting identifiable causes of hypertension
- The use of drugs or substances that may raise blood pressure
- Lifestyle factors, such as diet, leisure time physical activity, and weight gain, that may influence blood pressure control
- Psychosocial and environmental factors, such as family support, income, and educational level, including factors that could influence the efficacy of antihypertensive therapy
- Any family history of hypertension or cardiovascular disease

The physical examination should focus on determining the level of blood pressure and searching for evidence of target organ disease or identifiable causes of hypertension. Important facets of the examination include the following:

- Careful measurement of blood pressure
- Measurement of height and weight
- Funduscopic examination for hypertensive retinopathy
- Examination of the neck for carotid bruits, elevated jugular venous pressure, and thyromegaly

- Examination of the heart for abnormalities of the apical impulse or the presence of extra heart sounds or murmurs
- Examination of the abdomen for bruits, enlarged kidneys, and other masses
- Examination of the extremities for diminished arterial pulsations or peripheral edema

Laboratory studies are recommended to determine the presence of target organ damage and other cardiovascular risk factors and to exclude identifiable causes of hypertension. These include the following:

- Complete blood count
- Serum concentrations of potassium, creatinine, thyroid-stimulating hormone, fasting glucose, and high-density lipoprotein and total cholesterol
- Urinalysis for blood, protein, glucose, and microscopic examination
- An electrocardiogram

Detection and diagnosis of hypertension begins with the accurate measurement of blood pressure. Measurements should be acquired at each health care encounter, with follow-up determinations at intervals based on the initial blood pressure level. Accurate equipment and utilization of a standardized technique are critical. In many patients, home blood pressure monitoring may help in establishing baseline blood pressure levels or evaluating the response to therapy. Home blood pressures, when acquired with a reliable device in a systematic fashion and recorded accurately, correlate more closely with cardiovascular event rates than do office blood pressure measurements. Patients with white-coat hypertension, who may not require additional therapy, as well as those who remain at increased risk because of masked hypertension, can be identified with this technique. Twenty-four-hour ambulatory blood pressure monitoring may be useful in cases of unusual variability between visits, suspected white-coat hypertension, symptoms suggesting hypotensive episodes, or hypertension resistant to medication, or when there are large discrepancies between home and office measurements.

Management and Therapy

Optimum Treatment

The principal goal in treatment of hypertension is to reduce the risk for cardiovascular morbidity and mortality. The approach to therapy in an individual should be determined in part by the absolute risk for a cardiovascular event, based on the presence of major cardiovascular risk factors or target organ damage. Patients with diabetes mellitus, chronic kidney disease, or clinical cardiovascular disease are at particularly high risk for cardiovascular events. Pharmacologic therapy should be considered for these individuals when blood pressure is mildly elevated or in the prehypertensive range, with a treatment goal of

Table 25-3 Classification and Management of Blood Pressure for Adults

Classification	Systolic* (mm Hg)	Diastolic* (mm Hg)	Lifestyle Modification	Initial Drug Therapy Without Compelling Indication	Initial Drug Therapy With Compelling Indication
Normal	<120	and <80	Encourage		
Prehypertension	120-139	or 80-89	Yes	No antihypertensive drug indicated	Drug(s) for compelling indications‡
Stage 1 hypertension	140-159	or 90-99	Yes	Thiazide-type diuretics for most; may consider ACE-1, ARB, BB, CCB, or combination	Drug(s) for the compelling indications‡
Stage 2 hypertension	≥160	or ≥100	Yes	Two-drug combination for most† (usually thiazide-type diuretic and ACE-1, ARB, BB, or CCB)	Other antihypertensive drugs (diuretics, ACE-1, ARB, BB, CCB) as needed

*Treatment determined by highest blood pressure category.
†Initial combined therapy should be used cautiously in those at risk for orthostatic hypotension.
‡Treat patients with chronic kidney disease or diabetes to blood pressure goal of <130/80 mm Hg.
ACE-1, angiotensin-converting enzyme inhibitor; ARB, angiotensin receptor blocker; BB, β blocker, CCB, calcium channel blocker.
Data from the National High Blood Pressure Education Program; National Heart, Lung and Blood Institute; National Institutes of Health and the Department of Health and Human Services.

normalizing the pressure (i.e., <130/80 mm Hg). Lower-risk patients may benefit from a period of observation and lifestyle modification, using medical therapy if the average systolic pressure exceeds 140 mm Hg or diastolic pressure exceeds 90 mm Hg over months of monitoring. The management strategy recommended in the JNC VII report is outlined in Table 25-3.

Lifestyle modifications are an important component of the therapy for high blood pressure. All patients with hypertension, prehypertension, or a strong family history of hypertension should be encouraged to lose weight if overweight, participate in regular aerobic exercise, limit alcohol intake, and adopt a healthy diet. The Dietary Approaches to Stop Hypertension (DASH) eating plan, a diet rich in fruits, vegetables, and low-fat dairy products with reduced saturated fats, is as effective as single-drug therapy in many hypertensive individuals. Additional benefit can be realized by limiting dietary sodium intake. These lifestyle changes not only lower blood pressure but also enhance the effectiveness of antihypertensive drugs and favorably influence other cardiovascular risk factors. Smoking cessation further reduces cardiovascular risk and should be strongly encouraged.

Drug therapy is indicated if lifestyle modifications do not bring the blood pressure into the desired range. The optimal agent for initial therapy of uncomplicated patients with hypertension remains a subject of considerable controversy. Thiazide diuretics, β-adrenergic receptor blockers, angiotensin-converting enzyme (ACE) inhibitors, angiotensin-receptor blockers (ARBs), and calcium antagonists have all been viewed as appropriate first-line agents for the treatment of hypertension. Thiazide diuretics are inexpensive and generally well-tolerated, and

ALLHAT* and other comparative trials suggest that they are as effective as newer drugs in preventing stroke and myocardial infarction. Compared with ACE inhibitors, ARBs, and calcium antagonists, however, diuretics increase the risk for developing diabetes. The results of the ASCOT** study reinforce data from several previous trials suggesting that β-blockers are less effective than alternative therapies in preventing cardiovascular events, especially stroke, in elderly patients. Ultimately, however, most patients will require more than one antihypertensive drug, and achieving optimal blood pressure control is more important than the choice of the initial agent. In many patients, the appropriate antihypertensive drug is dictated by comorbid conditions. Table 25-4 lists agents that are preferred or relatively contraindicated in specific circumstances.

In general, medical therapy should be initiated at low doses in an effort to minimize side effects. Based on the patient's response, the dose of the initial agent can be titrated upward, or a small dose of a second agent can be added. Many experts favor using lower doses of two or even three antihypertensive drugs with a goal of minimizing dose-dependent side effects. Other experts favor up-titration of monotherapy, arguing that patient adherence to therapy will be better with less complicated regimens. It should be noted that with the advent of many once-daily antihypertensive medications, most patients can be treated with once-a-day therapies, even if this involves more than one antihypertensive agent.

*Antihypertensive and Lipid-Lowering Treatment of Prevent Heart Attack Trial.
**Anglo-Scandanavian Cardiac Outcomes Trial.

Table 25-4   Choice of Antihypertensive Agent Based on Coexistent Illnesses

Indications for Specific Drugs

Diabetes mellitus	ACE inhibitor or ARB
Congestive heart failure	ACE inhibitor or ARB, β-blocker, diuretic, aldosterone antagonist
Myocardial infarction	ACE inhibitor or ARB, β-blocker, aldosterone antagonist
Chronic coronary disease	ACE inhibitor, β-blocker
Renal insufficiency	ACE inhibitor or ARB

Contraindications to Specific Drugs

Pregnancy	ACE inhibitor, ARB
Renal insufficiency*	Potassium-sparing agent
Peripheral vascular disease	β-blocker
Gout*	Diuretic
Depression*	β-blocker, central α agonist
Reactive airway disease	β-blocker
Second- or third-degree heart block	β-blocker, nondihydropyridine calcium antagonist
Hepatic insufficiency	Labetalol, methyldopa

*Relative contraindications.
ACE, angiotensin-converting enzyme inhibitor; ARB, angiotensin receptor blocker.

Patients with stage 2 hypertension can be started on two drugs initially. Effective drug combinations utilize medications from different classes and result in additive blood pressure lowering effects, while minimizing dose-dependent adverse effects. Diuretics potentiate the effect of β-blockers, ACE inhibitors, and ARBs; other useful combinations include dihydropyridine calcium antagonists and β-blockers, or calcium antagonists and ACE inhibitors or ARBs. Long-acting formulations with 24-hour efficacy are preferred over shorter-acting agents because of greater patient adherence, as discussed previously, as well as because more consistent blood pressure control during the course of the day can be obtained with long-acting medications.

Lowering blood pressure is but one mechanism by which cardiovascular risk can be lowered in hypertensive patients. Irrespective of baseline cholesterol levels, statin therapy is effective in reducing the incidence of myocardial infarction and stroke in hypertensive patients, and most patients with high blood pressure benefit from treatment with a lipid-lowering agent. Low-dose aspirin also reduces the risk for cardiovascular events.

The goal of preventing cardiovascular morbidity and mortality is usually achieved with a gradual reduction of blood pressure, maintained over many years. Occasionally, a hypertensive crisis may occur, and blood pressure must be reduced urgently. A hypertensive crisis is defined as acute organ dysfunction of the cardiovascular or nervous system accompanied either by a marked absolute elevation of blood pressure or an abrupt increase in blood pressure in a previously normotensive individual. The initial therapy for hypertensive crisis may involve use of intravenous medications in an intensive care unit setting (Box 25-2).

Avoiding Treatment Errors

- Distinguish between severe, grade 2 hypertension and a hypertensive crisis. The latter mandates a decrease in

---

Box 25-2   Agents Used for Intravenous Drug Therapy of Hypertensive Emergencies

- Nitroprusside: preferred agent in most instances except acute coronary syndromes or pregnancy. Should be combined with β-blocker in some instances
- Nitroglycerine: use in acute coronary syndromes alone or combined with metoprolol or labetalol
- Labetalol: use as adjunctive therapy with nitroprusside or nitroglycerine. Use alone in less intensely monitored situations or treatment of postoperative hypertension
- Enalaprilat: use for scleroderma crisis or as adjunctive therapy in some high renin states
- Hydralazine: may use for treatment of preeclampsia, eclampsia
- Fenoldopam: same indication as for nitroprusside. Useful in postoperative or postprocedure hypertension in closely monitored situations
- Esmolol: use in case of need for immediate, very short-acting β-blocker effect. Use for supraventricular tachycardia

---

blood pressure and achievement of a certain blood pressure goal within minutes or hours. In grade 2 hypertension, blood pressure can be lowered within days and titration to the desired level may sometimes take weeks.

- Use thiazide diuretics as first-line therapy in certain salt-sensitive hypertensive patients such as African Americans and in patients requiring a combination of antihypertensive drugs, unless there is a clear contraindication to the use of such drugs.
- Institute lifestyle modifications as the first step in the treatment of hypertension, and continue these measures if drug therapy is ultimately required.
- Monitor patients for the metabolic effects of antihypertensive medications at initiation of therapy and periodically as needed.

- Look for an orthostatic fall in blood pressure in older patients and in those suspected of having autonomic dysfunction, such as subjects with long-standing diabetes mellitus. Titrate antihypertensive medication to avoid an excessive fall in blood pressure in the standing position.
- Treat isolated systolic hypertension with slow titration of antihypertensive medications, starting at a low dose of the drug: "Go low and slow."
- Avoid continuing to try to lower an elevated systolic blood pressure if the diastolic blood pressure is persistently lower than 65 mm Hg because of the risk for cardiac ischemia, particularly in patients with preexisting coronary artery disease.
- Avoid sudden withdrawal of certain antihypertensive medications such as β-blockers and clonidine to prevent acute coronary syndromes or rebound hypertension.
- Select antihypertensive drugs according to the individual clinical conditions of the patients and the associated comorbidities. Use specific antihypertensive medication for certain conditions unless contraindicated. For example, use ACE inhibitors and angiotensin II receptor blockers in patients with kidney disease, diabetes, or heart failure; use β-blockers for secondary prevention of myocardial infarction and in patients with heart failure due to left ventricular systolic dysfunction; use a combination of a thiazide diuretic and an inhibitor of the renin-angiotensin system for the secondary prevention of stroke.
- Avoid ACE inhibitors and angiotensin II receptor blockers in pregnant women.
- Avoid overtreatment of subjects with white-coat hypertension and undertreatment of patients with masked hypertension.

Future Directions

The past half-century has witnessed remarkable advances in the understanding of the pathophysiology, epidemiology, and natural history of hypertension, as well as dramatic advances in therapy. Nevertheless, many patients with hypertension are undiagnosed or inadequately treated, and high blood pressure remains an important contributor to coronary events, congestive heart failure, stroke, and end-stage kidney disease.

Future research and public health initiatives should be directed at achieving the following objectives:

- Ascertain the most effective antihypertensive agents in reducing cardiovascular end points in patients with uncomplicated hypertension.
- More accurately define treatment thresholds and optimal target blood pressures in patients with diabetes mellitus or with target organ damage.
- Determine the treatment threshold and optimal target blood pressure in elderly patients with isolated systolic hypertension.
- Develop more effective drugs for treating elderly patients with isolated systolic hypertension.
- Develop better strategies to improve patient compliance.
- Decrease the content of sodium and fat in American diets.
- Improve screening techniques and care delivery systems.
- Further define the roles of home and ambulatory blood pressure monitoring.

Additional Resources

British Hypertension Society. Available at: http://www.bhsoc.org. Accessed October 11, 2007.

Through this website, the British Hypertension Society provides a medical and scientific research forum to enable sharing of clinical information for the management of hypertension. Included in the website is information regarding cutting-edge research in the field, ongoing clinical trials, and important recent publications. The website also reviews recent guidelines, such as the partial update of the UK National Institute of Clinical Excellence and British Hypertension Society's Guidelines for Management of Hypertension in Adults published in June 2006. This document reviews the most recent clinical trials on the treatment hypertension in a brief but comprehensive manner.

Kaplan NM: Kaplan's Clinical Hypertension. 9th ed. Philadelphia, Lippincott Williams & Wilkins, 2006.

This thorough, detailed, yet succinct, eminently readable textbook on clinical hypertension was authored by Dr. Norman Kaplan. It reflects the vast clinical experience and wisdom of the author and offers up-to-date references on all topics.

Pickering TG, Hall JE, Appel LJ, et al: Recommendations for blood pressure measurement in humans and experimental animals. Part 1: Blood pressure measurement in humans. Hypertension 45:142-161, 2005.

This is a scientific statement by the American Heart Association with a major focus on the recommended techniques of blood pressure measurement in different clinical settings and circumstances. There is valuable and useful information in this statement for all who treat patients with hypertension and for those in charge of selecting and maintaining the equipment used to measure blood pressure in clinical facilities.

U.S. Department of Health and Human Services, National Heart, Lung, and Blood Institute. National High Blood Pressure Education Program. Available at: http://www.nhlbi.nih.gov/about/nhbpep/index.htm. Accessed October 11, 2007.

The National High Blood Pressure Education Program provides valuable educational information on hypertension for health care providers and the general public. All of the reports, guidelines, and publications sponsored by the Program are available, and educational materials such as slides, tables, and graphs can be downloaded. Some of the materials are available in Spanish.

EVIDENCE

1. ALLHAT Officers and Coordinators for the ALLHAT Collaborative Research Group: Major outcomes in high-risk hypertensive patients randomized to angiotensin-converting enzyme inhibitor or calcium channel blocker vs diuretic: The Antihypertensive and Lipid-Lowering Treatment to Prevent Heart Attack Trial (ALLHAT). JAMA 288:2981-2997, 2002.

This is the largest double-blind trial undertaken in hypertensive patients, and strongly influenced the recommendations of JNC VII. The trial compared treatment with amlodipine or lisinopril with a reference drug, chlorthalidone, and found no advantage of newer drugs over a thiazide-type diuretic in preventing fatal coronary heart disease or nonfatal myocardial infarction.

2. Appel LJ, Brands MW, Daniels SR, et al: Dietary approaches to prevent and treat hypertension: A scientific statement from the American Heart Association. Hypertension 47:296-308, 2006.

This scientific statement provides a concise review of dietary interventions to both prevent and treat hypertension. The DASH diet, reduced salt intake, weight loss, and moderation of alcohol consumption are promoted as dietary modifications that have an established role in blood pressure reduction.

3. Blood Pressure Lowering Treatment Trialists' Collaboration: Effects of different blood-pressure-lowering regimens on major cardiovascular events: Results of prospectively-designed overviews of randomized trials. Lancet 362:1527-1535, 2003.

This set of prospectively designed overviews with data from 29 randomized trials examines the comparative effects of different blood pressure–lowering regimens and the benefits of targeting lower blood pressure goals on the risk of major cardiovascular events and death. The overall conclusion is that treatment with any commonly used regimen reduces the risk for major cardiovascular events and that larger reductions in blood pressure produce larger reductions in risk.

4. Chobanian AV, Bakris GL, Black HR, et al: National High Blood Pressure Education Program Coordinating Committee: Seventh report of the Joint National Committee on Prevention, Detection, Evaluation, and Treatment of High Blood Pressure: JNC 7—Complete Version. Hypertension 42:1206-1252, 2003.

This report from the National High Blood Pressure Education Program provides a comprehensive guideline for hypertension prevention and management, and is a "must read" for all physicians who treat patients with high blood pressure. Differences from previous reports include an emphasis on systolic blood pressure as a cardiovascular disease risk factor, and introduction of the classification "prehypertension." Thiazide-type diuretics are recommended for most patients with uncomplicated hypertension, either alone or combined with drugs from other classes.

5. Chobanian AV, Bakris GL, Black HR, et al: The Seventh Report of the Joint National Committee on Prevention, Detection, Evaluation, and Treatment of High Blood Pressure: The JNC 7 Report. JAMA 289:2560-2572, 2003.

This condensed version of the JNC VII report highlights the major points of the National High Blood Pressure Education Program recommendations.

6. Dahlof B, Sever PS, Poulter NR, et al: The ASCOT Investigators. Prevention of cardiovascular events with an antihypertensive regimen of amlodipine adding perindopril as required versus atenolol adding bendroflumethiazide as required, in the Anglo-Scandinavian Cardiac Outcomes Trial-Blood Pressure Lowering Arm (ASCOT-BPLA): A multicentre randomised controlled trial. Lancet 366:895-906, 2005.

This large European study found an advantage of newer drugs (amlodipine ± perindopril, as required) over conventional blood pressure lowering therapy (atenolol ± bendroflumethiazide, as required) in reducing cardiovascular mortality. These results reinforced data from previous studies suggesting that β-blocker–based therapy is less effective than other first-line drugs in reducing cardiovascular events in older patients.

7. Fields LE, Burt VL, Cutler JA, et al: The burden of adult hypertension in the United States 1999 to 2000. A rising tide. Hypertension 44:498-404, 2004.

The purpose of this study was to estimate the absolute number of persons with hypertension in the year 2000 using data from the National Health and Nutrition Examination Survey of U.S. resident adults. The authors found that at least 65 million adults had hypertension in 1999 to 2000. A more recent survey has shown that the prevalence of hypertension in this population remains constant at about 29%. Because the adult population is now greater than in the year 2000, the burden of hypertension continues to rise in the United States.

8. Guidelines Committee: 2003 European Society of Hypertension—European Society of Cardiology guidelines for the management of arterial hypertension. J Hypertens 21:1011-1053, 2003.

Like the BHS report, this set of guidelines also recommends initiation of medical therapy based on a comprehensive assessment of other risk factors, target organ disease, diabetes, and associated clinical conditions.

9. Ong KL, Cheung BMY, Man YB, et al: Prevalence, awareness, treatment, and control of hypertension among United States adults 1999-2004. Hypertension 49:69-75, 2007.

This latest report from the National Health and Nutrition Examination Survey (NHANES) 1999-2004 examines changes in the prevalence, awareness, treatment, and control of hypertension in the United States. Although encouraging trends are noted, the overall prevalence of hypertension remains high (>29%), and the blood pressure control rate is only 37%.

10. Sever PS, Dahlof B, Poulter NR, et al: The ASCOT Investigators. Prevention of coronary and stroke events with atorvastatin in hypertensive patients who have average or lower-than-average cholesterol concentrations, in the Anglo-Scandinavian Cardiac Outcomes Trial-Lipid Lowering Arm (ASCOT-LLA): A multicentre randomised controlled trial. Lancet 361:1149-1158, 2003.

This study demonstrated the value of a statin in reducing the risk for coronary heart disease and stroke in patients with hypertension.

11. Williams B, Poulter NR, Brown MJ, et al: Guidelines for management of hypertension: Report of the Fourth Working Party of the British Hypertension Society, 2004—BHS IV: British Hypertension Society Guidelines. J Hum Hypertens 18:139-185, 2004.

This comprehensive guideline differs from the JNC VII report in several important respects: it recommends a more individualized threshold blood pressure for treatment with medications, based on the presence of target organ damage, cardiovascular complications, diabetes, and estimated 10-year risk of cardiovascular disease. The report recommends basing the choice of an initial blood pressure–lowering drug on the age and ethnicity of the patient. ACE inhibitors, angiotensin receptor blockers, or perhaps β blockers are recommended for young, nonblack patients without compelling indications, whereas calcium antagonists or thiazide-like diuretics are recommended as first-line therapy for older or black patients. The report recommends statin therapy for all people with high blood pressure complicated by cardiovascular disease or with a 10-year risk for cardiovascular disease of more than 20%, irrespective of blood lipid levels.

Romulo E. Colindres ▪ Steven H. Grossman

26

Hypertension Secondary to Renovascular Diseases

Introduction

Up to 20% of middle-aged men and women in the United States have high blood pressure. In 90% to 95% of these patients, the cause of the hypertension is unknown. This is termed *essential* or *primary hypertension*. The remaining 5% to 10% of the general population who have hypertension have an identifiable cause for the elevated blood pressure, with a defined pathophysiology and, in some instances, unique clinical or laboratory findings. This condition is called *secondary hypertension*. There is a strong incentive for diagnosing secondary forms of hypertension because, in many instances, the cause of the hypertension can be eliminated or treated with a specific drug, procedure, or surgical intervention. Furthermore, early diagnosis of these conditions is of paramount importance because most studies have shown that the longer secondary hypertension remains untreated, the less likely the hypertension can be cured. Secondary hypertension is more common in older people because of the higher incidence and prevalence of two frequent forms of secondary hypertension: renal parenchymal disease and atherosclerotic renal artery stenosis (RAS).

There are several primary diseases of the renal artery that cause RAS; the most common are atherosclerosis and fibromuscular dysplasia (FMD). Atherosclerotic RAS accounts for about 80% to 90% of cases, whereas FMD accounts for 10% to 20% of such cases. Atherosclerotic RAS is associated with atherosclerosis of the abdominal aorta and other arteries. The atheroma usually narrows the lumen of the proximal third of one or both renal arteries; the ostium is involved in about 75% of cases. FMD is characterized by fibrous changes in the wall of the distal two thirds of one or both renal arteries and their branches. This condition affects the media of the arteries in most subjects, although in some individuals, the disease involves only the intima or the adventitia of the vessel wall.

Etiology and Pathogenesis

Atherosclerotic RAS is caused by the same factors that cause generalized atherosclerosis obliterans: smoking, dyslipidemia, hypertension, glucose intolerance, genetic predisposition, and other factors. The etiology of the fibrous changes that occur in young patients with FMD is unknown. Possible causes include diseases of the vasa vasorum, genetic predisposition, and hormonal factors. There is evidence that smoking can worsen this condition. Hypertension secondary to atherosclerotic RAS or FMD is caused by a decrease in renal perfusion pressure and is termed *renovascular hypertension* (RVH). Renovascular hypertension occurs in the presence of one or more high-grade stenoses, defined as a 60% or greater reduction of the lumen of the main renal artery or its branches, and accounts for about 3% of cases of hypertension. High-grade RAS does not always cause hypertension, and even when hypertension and high-grade RAS coexist, the RAS may be incidental, and the subject may have essential or another type of secondary hypertension. RAS is more common than renovascular hypertension. Figure 26-1 depicts the events leading to hypertension in the presence of high-grade unilateral RAS. Bilateral atherosclerotic RAS, or atherosclerotic RAS in a solitary kidney, can cause a decrease in excretory function of the kidney with the development of chronic renal failure. This is called *ischemic nephropathy*.

Figure 26-1 Pathophysiology of Renovascular Hypertension in Unilateral Renal Artery Stenosis.

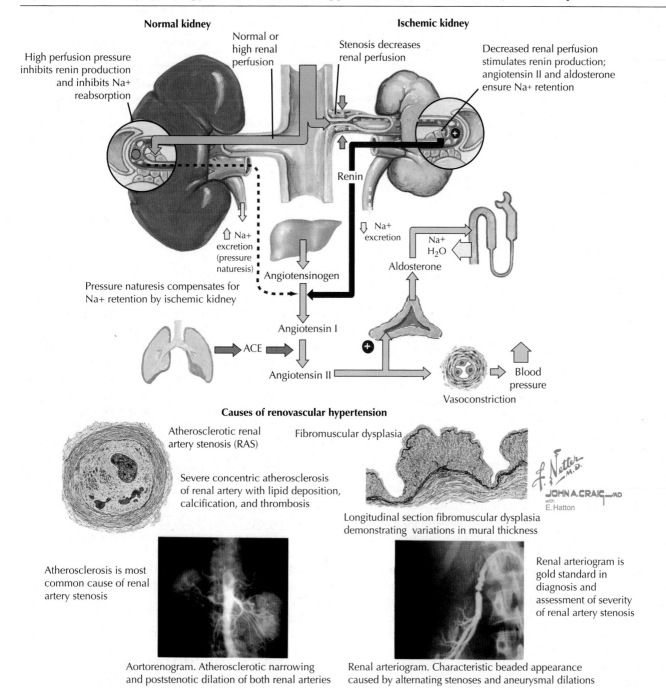

Normal kidney

Ischemic kidney

High perfusion pressure inhibits renin production and inhibits Na+ reabsorption

Normal or high renal perfusion

Stenosis decreases renal perfusion

Decreased renal perfusion stimulates renin production; angiotensin II and aldosterone ensure Na+ retention

Renin

↑ Na+ excretion (pressure natruresis)

⬇ Na+ excretion

Na+ H₂O

Aldosterone

Pressure natruresis compensates for Na+ retention by ischemic kidney

Angiotensinogen

Angiotensin I

ACE

Angiotensin II

Vasoconstriction

Blood pressure

Causes of renovascular hypertension

Atherosclerotic renal artery stenosis (RAS)

Fibromuscular dysplasia

Severe concentric atherosclerosis of renal artery with lipid deposition, calcification, and thrombosis

Longitudinal section fibromuscular dysplasia demonstrating variations in mural thickness

Atherosclerosis is most common cause of renal artery stenosis

Renal arteriogram is gold standard in diagnosis and assessment of severity of renal artery stenosis

Aortorenogram. Atherosclerotic narrowing and poststenotic dilation of both renal arteries

Renal arteriogram. Characteristic beaded appearance caused by alternating stenoses and aneurysmal dilations

Clinical Presentation

Atherosclerotic RAS may be silent or may cause renovascular hypertension, ischemic nephropathy, or both. Ischemic nephropathy can occasionally occur in the absence of hypertension. *Flash pulmonary edema*, acute pulmonary edema that develops abruptly, is a syndrome related to renovascular hypertension and ischemic nephropathy.

Atherosclerotic RAS occurs in older patients. About 90% of patients are or have been heavy smokers. Most have evidence of atherosclerosis in other vascular beds. There may be abrupt onset of hypertension, worsening of existing hypertension, or development of malignant hypertension after the age of 50 years. Physical examination may show advanced retinopathy, an abdominal or flank bruit, and pulse deficits or bruits over major arteries. Laboratory studies may show hypokalemia caused by elevated plasma renin activity (secondary aldosteronism) and elevation of serum creatinine concentration caused by ischemic nephropathy or other associated

Table 26-1   Screening Tests for Renal Artery Stenosis

Test	Type of Assessment	Features
Captopril renogram	Functional: ACE inhibitor–induced reduction of GFR	High sensitivity and specificity if kidneys of equal size, SCr <2 mg/dL. Prognostic value for improvement of HTN
MRA of the renal arteries	Anatomic: proximal renal arteries	No nephrotoxicity. Cannot use after stent placement
Doppler ultrasound of renal arteries	Anatomic, functional: proximal renal arteries	Highly variable results; technically difficult; operator dependent
Spiral CT angiography	Anatomic: proximal renal arteries	Large volume of contrast dye

ACE, angiotensin-converting enzyme; CT, computed tomography; GFR, glomerular filtration rate; HTN, hypertension; MRA, magnetic resonance angiography; SCr, serum creatinine concentration.

kidney diseases. There may be a large discrepancy in kidney size.

RAS caused by FMD presents as renovascular hypertension starting at a young age. The disease is more common in women younger than 50 years, and also occurs in children. An abdominal bruit may be present, but peripheral pulses are normal. Laboratory studies may show hypokalemia. A large discrepancy in kidney size is unusual. Fibromuscular dysplasia does not cause ischemic nephropathy or flash pulmonary edema.

Differential Diagnosis

The main differential diagnosis of renovascular hypertension caused by atherosclerotic RAS is essential hypertension and other types of secondary hypertension, particularly renal parenchymal disease. In older people with peripheral vascular disease or abdominal aortic disease, the prevalence of atherosclerotic RAS is as high as 38% to 55%. The prevalence of essential hypertension in this population is about 60%. Therefore, it is often difficult to establish whether atherosclerotic RAS in this setting is causing the hypertension or is an incidental occurrence, perhaps related to long-standing hypertension with consequent atherosclerosis. Correction of the stenosis in the latter situation would not lead to cure or improvement of hypertension. Renal failure caused by atherosclerotic RAS must be distinguished from renal failure resulting from renal parenchymal disease such as small vessel disease (nephrosclerosis or atheroembolic disease) or other diseases such as diabetic nephropathy. Characteristics of ischemic nephropathy include minimal proteinuria, scant urine sediment, and frequently a large discrepancy in kidney size with involvement of both renal arteries.

The differential diagnosis of renovascular hypertension caused by FMD includes other causes of hypertension in children or young women: essential hypertension, subtle renal disease, obesity-related hypertension, endocrine hypertension, and coarctation of the aorta.

Diagnostic Approach

The gold standard for the diagnosis of RAS is a renal arteriogram, which permits an assessment of the degree of stenosis and shows the characteristic atherosclerotic involvement of the proximal third of the renal artery in atherosclerotic RAS. The most common form of FMD, medial fibroplasia (75%), has characteristic areas of stenoses alternating with aneurysmal dilations ("string of pearls" image) in the distal renal artery, sometimes extending to the branches of the main renal artery. A renal arteriogram is an expensive and invasive test with associated discomforts and risks, and generally provides no information about the functional significance of the lesion. In view of these limitations, several screening tests for the detection of RAS or assessment of its functional significance have been developed (Table 26-1). The sensitivity and specificity of these tests vary from institution to institution according to the local expertise in performing the various studies. For example, Doppler ultrasound of the renal arteries is the preferred screening test in some institutions, yet others find this test to be cumbersome, unreliable, and operator dependent.

None of the anatomic screening tests is adequate to evaluate the distal renal artery; therefore, there is no adequate screening test for FMD, although a captopril renogram may suggest the presence of functionally significant RAS (Fig. 26-2).

Figure 26-3 shows the diagnostic scheme we use to evaluate subjects suspected of having RAS at our institution. The first step in the evaluation is to look for unsuspected renal parenchymal disease with renal sonography and urinalysis. We recommend measuring the resistive indexes over the kidney using Doppler studies at the same time as the kidney ultrasound is performed. This study is easier to perform and more reliable in our institution than Doppler ultrasound of the renal arteries. The resistive indexes appear to have some prognostic value in terms of the response to revascularization. Screening evaluation is

Figure 26-2 Captopril Renogram.

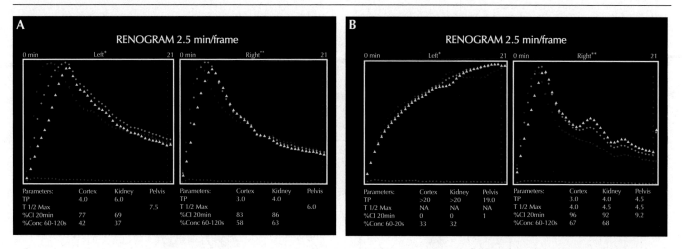

A

RENOGRAM 2.5 min/frame

0 min   Left*   21   0 min   Right**   21

Parameters:	Cortex	Kidney	Pelvis
TP	4.0	6.0	
T 1/2 Max			7.5
%Cl 20min	77	69	
%Conc 60-120s	42	37	

Parameters:	Cortex	Kidney	Pelvis
TP	3.0	4.0	
T 1/2 Max			6.0
%Cl 20min	83	86	
%Conc 60-120s	58	63	

B

RENOGRAM 2.5 min/frame

0 min   Left*   21   0 min   Right**   21

Parameters:	Cortex	Kidney	Pelvis
TP	>20	>20	19.0
T 1/2 Max	NA	NA	NA
%Cl 20min	0	0	1
%Conc 60-20s	33	32	

Parameters:	Cortex	Kidney	Pelvis
TP	3.0	4.0	4.5
T 1/2 Max	4.0	4.5	4.5
%Cl 20min	96	92	9.2
%Conc 60-120s	67	68	

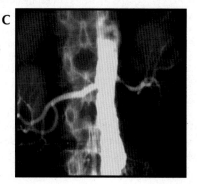

C

Uptake and excretion of Tc-99m mertiatide, given intravenously, by the left and right kidney before (**A**), and after (**B**), oral administration of 50 mg of captopril. Panel **B** shows slow uptake and no excretion of the radiopharmaceutical, suggesting functionally significant stenosis of the left renal artery. The aortogram (**C**) shows a high-grade atherosclerotic RAS of the left renal artery with poststenotic dilation in the same patient. The right renal artery is normal. Note the atherosclerotic changes of the abdominal aorta.

* Left kidney
** Right kidney

Figure 26-3 Evaluation for Renal Artery Stenosis in Subjects with Compatible Clinical Picture and Predicted Benefit of Revascularization.

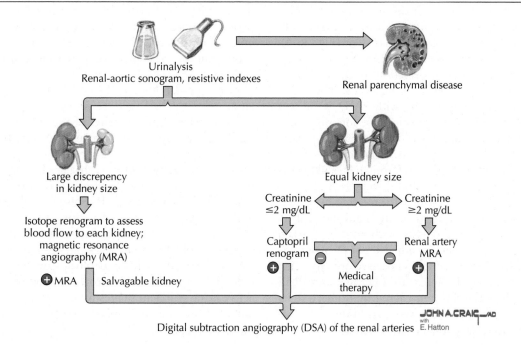

Urinalysis
Renal-aortic sonogram, resistive indexes

Renal parenchymal disease

Large discrepency in kidney size

Equal kidney size

Creatinine ≤2 mg/dL   Creatinine ≥2 mg/dL

Isotope renogram to assess blood flow to each kidney; magnetic resonance angiography (MRA)

Captopril renogram   Renal artery MRA

⊕ MRA   Salvagable kidney

Medical therapy

Digital subtraction angiography (DSA) of the renal arteries

JOHN A. CRAIG MD
with
E. Hatton

Figure 26-4 Balloon Angioplasty of Stenotic Renal Arteries.

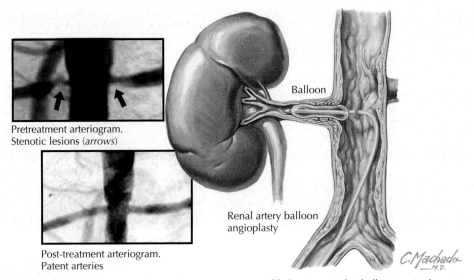

Pretreatment arteriogram.
Stenotic lesions (*arrows*)

Post-treatment arteriogram.
Patent arteries

Balloon

Renal artery balloon
angioplasty

Patients with hypertension and atherosclerotic renal artery stenosis most likely to respond to balloon angioplasty are those with onset of hypertension within the past 5 years, those without primary renal disease, and middle-aged men with atherosclerotic renal artery stenosis and malignant hypertension not caused by primary renal disease. A positive captopril renogram predicts cure or improvement of hypertension after revascularization

limited to patients who have a compatible clinical picture and who are likely to benefit from revascularization of the renal arteries. There is no functional test that predicts improvement of renal function after revascularization.

Management and Therapy

Optimum Treatment

The treatment of RAS can be divided into medical treatment and surgical or endovascular revascularization. Endovascular revascularization consists of balloon angioplasty with or without placement of a vascular stent (Fig. 26-4). Medical treatment for atherosclerotic RAS consists of antihypertensive therapy, smoking cessation, aspirin and other antiplatelet agents, and lipid-lowering drugs. The treatment of choice for young people with FMD is balloon angioplasty. If the balloon can reach the lesion, dilation is usually successful, and hypertension is cured or greatly improved in about 90% of patients. Randomized clinical trials of older patients with atherosclerotic RAS and hypertension have suggested that medical therapy is as effective as angioplasty and stent placement for treating hypertension. The patients with atherosclerotic RAS most likely to respond to balloon angioplasty with cure or marked improvement are those who have had onset of hypertension within the past 5 years and do not have primary renal disease, and middle-aged men with atherosclerotic RAS and malignant hypertension not caused by primary renal disease. We do not advocate revascularization for treatment of hypertension in patients with atherosclerotic RAS

unless the foregoing conditions are met or the patient does not respond to an optimal antihypertensive three- to four-drug regimen. A positive captopril scan is a good predictor of cure or improvement of hypertension after revascularization.

Revascularization for Treatment of Ischemic Nephropathy

Atherosclerotic RAS may be a cause of end-stage renal disease. Several studies have suggested that 11% to 22% of older people reaching end-stage renal disease have high-grade atherosclerotic RAS in at least one renal artery. No major clinical trials have compared medical treatment to balloon angioplasty of the renal artery for preserving or improving renal function. Only a minority of patients with atherosclerotic RAS and renal failure appear to derive long-term benefit from relief of the stenosis with angioplasty. Therefore, it is important to identify those subjects who are not likely to benefit from the procedure or who may be harmed by it. Factors that predict lack of improvement, or worsening of renal function with correction of high-grade atherosclerotic RAS are (1) low-grade stenosis with reduction in luminal diameter of less than 50% in at least one renal artery; (2) unilateral RAS unless the artery supplies a solitary kidney; (3) kidney length less than 8 cm; (4) presence of diabetic nephropathy or other known kidney diseases, or severe proteinuria accompanied by an active urine sediment suggestive of a primary renal disease; and (5) a high resistive index as determined with Doppler ultrasonography.

The National Heart, Lung, and Blood Institute of the National Institutes of Health is sponsoring an ongoing prospective, randomized, multicenter clinical trial called Cardiovascular Outcomes in Renal Atherosclerotic Lesions (CORAL). This study, involving 1080 subjects, will compare optimal medical therapy alone with angioplasty and stenting plus optimal medical therapy in patients with hemodynamically significant atherosclerotic renal artery stenosis and systolic hypertension.

Avoiding Treatment Errors

The main error to avoid in treating atherosclerotic RAS is performing angioplasty and stent placement in an artery with stenosis when there is limited functional or historical data to suggest that endovascular revascularization will be better than optimal medical therapy for the control of hypertension or improvement of kidney function. Under these conditions, the risk of the procedure may exceed the benefits. Before deciding to proceed with revascularization, one should review the history, response to medical therapy, laboratory findings, and anatomic information.

Future Directions

We believe that continued progress in the diagnosis and treatment of atherosclerotic RAS in the coming years will require the following:

- Continued technical improvement of balloon angioplasty and vascular stents
- Development of noninvasive imaging techniques for assessment of the distal renal artery and its branches
- Development of better functional tests to predict the effects of renal artery revascularization on blood pressure and renal function
- Development of markers to detect diseases of the small arteries and arterioles of the kidney
- Randomized clinical trials, such as the CORAL study, to compare the effect of revascularization of the renal arteries with intensive medical therapy on hypertension, cardiovascular disease, and the progression of chronic renal failure
- Development of new drugs to treat atherosclerosis and continued promotion of public health measures to decrease risk factors for atherosclerosis

Additional Resource

Cardiovascular Outcomes in Renal Atherosclerotic Lesions (CORAL). Available at: http://www.coralclinicaltrial.org. Accessed October 11, 2007.

This is the website of the CORAL study, the only ongoing, prospective, randomized study in the United States that is comparing angioplasty plus stent placement of atherosclerotic RAS and optimal medical therapy with optimal medical therapy alone. Information about the progress of the trial, enrollment, and participating centers can be obtained through this website.

EVIDENCE

1. Cooper CJ, Murphy TP, Matsumoto A, et al: Stent revascularization for the prevention of cardiovascular and renal events among patients with renal artery stenosis and systolic hypertension: Rationale and design of the CORAL trial. Am Heart J 152(1):59-66, 2006.

   The National Institutes of Health, after hearing from many experts on atherosclerotic renal artery stenosis, concluded that it is not known whether angioplasty and stent placement combined with optimal medical therapy is superior to optimal medical therapy alone for the prevention of cardiovascular morbidity and progressive kidney disease in patients with high-grade atherosclerotic RAS. Given this situation of "equipoise" regarding the best treatment for the condition, the NIH is sponsoring the study described in this publication.

2. Pedersen EB: New tools in diagnosing renal artery stenosis. Kidney Int 57(6):2657-2677, 2000.

   Many recent publications have dealt with the several tests available to screen for renal artery stenosis. This article by Pedersen is one of the most detailed and balanced reviews on this topic. Although some of the tests, such as magnetic resonance angiography, have been refined in the past few years, the recommendations and guidelines regarding diagnosis of RAS presented in this paper are still valid. The techniques, advantages, disadvantages, and predictive values of the several tests are described in detail.

3. Radermacher J, Chavan A, Bleck J, et al: Use of Doppler ultrasonography to predict the outcome of therapy for renal-artery stenosis. N Engl J Med 344(6):410-417, 2001.

   The authors relate their experience in treating RAS with renal artery angioplasty in a large cohort of patients with hypertension, kidney failure, or both. They found that a resistive index above 80 reliably identifies patients with RAS in whom angioplasty or surgery will not improve kidney function, blood pressure, or kidney survival.

4. Safian RD, Textor SC: Renal-artery stenosis. N Engl J Med 344(6):431-442, 2001.

   The authors provide a comprehensive review of the pathophysiology, clinical manifestations, diagnostic approaches and treatment of renovascular hypertension and ischemic nephropathy.

5. Textor SC: Ischemic nephropathy: Where are we now? J Am Soc Nephrol 15(8):1974-1982, 2004.

   An excellent review of ischemic nephropathy, defined as kidney failure directly caused by high-grade atherosclerotic renal artery stenosis of both renal arteries or of the artery to a solitary kidney, which describes the epidemiology, clinical manifestations, and presumed pathophysiology of the condition.

Romulo E. Colindres ▪ Steven H. Grossman

Hypertension Secondary to Diseases of the Adrenal Gland

Introduction

Diseases of the adrenal gland are clinically important causes of secondary hypertension. In this chapter, we review their clinical presentation, evaluation, and therapy. Renovascular hypertension, another cause of secondary hypertension, is reviewed in Chapter 26.

The adrenal cortex can cause hypertension through overproduction of aldosterone, deoxycorticosterone (DOC), and cortisol. The first two are mineralocorticoid hormones that cause increased salt and water retention by the kidney. Cortisol is a glucocorticoid. When hypersecretion is marked, it can stimulate mineralocorticoid receptors and can be associated with release of DOC and vasoconstrictors. Pheochromocytoma is a tumor of the adrenal medulla that produces excessive quantities of catecholamines.

Identifying causes of adrenal hypertension is important for the following reasons:

- Many of these disorders are curable or responsive to specific therapy.
- These conditions, particularly pheochromocytoma, are associated with the risk for severe hypertension and major cardiovascular complications, including sudden death; the consequences of aldosterone, aside from blood pressure elevation, on cardiovascular outcomes have become increasingly recognized.
- The prevalence of primary aldosteronism among individuals with hypertension is higher than the 1% or less previously estimated.
- New syndromes of mineralocorticoid hypertension have been described or defined in the past few years.
- Diagnostic tests for primary aldosteronism have been simplified.

PRIMARY ALDOSTERONISM AND MINERALOCORTICOID HYPERTENSION

Etiology and Pathogenesis

Table 27-1 shows the causes of mineralocorticoid hypertension and its associated syndromes, the most common of which is primary aldosteronism. The normal physiologic control of aldosterone secretion is by the renin-angiotensin system. Adrenocorticotropic hormone (ACTH) and serum potassium concentration are less important. Hyperaldosteronism is caused by autonomous secretion of the hormone, totally or largely independent of the control of the renin-angiotensin system.

Hypertension caused by aldosterone results from increased stimulation of mineralocorticoid receptors in the cortical collecting ducts of the kidney. This causes opening of sodium channels leading to increased tubular reabsorption of sodium, and secondary reabsorption of water. There is also increased secretion and urinary excretion of potassium and hydrogen ions. Salt and water retention causes an increase in plasma volume and an increase in cardiac output, resulting in increased blood pressure and suppressed renin production. Total exchangeable sodium

Table 27-1   Differential Diagnosis of Mineralocorticoid Hypertension

Cause	Pathophysiology
Primary aldosteronism*	Increased aldosterone secretion
DOC-secreting tumors[†]	Increased DOC secretion
Congenital adrenal hyperplasia[†]	Congenital deficiency of enzymes needed for cortisol synthesis. Increased ACTH secretion: increased DOC
Liddle's syndrome[†]	Congenital up-regulation of sodium channels in collecting ducts. Increased sodium reabsorption by kidney
11β-Hydroxysteroid dehydrogenase deficiency and inhibition[†]	Congenital deficiency (syndrome of AME) or inhibition (licorice) of the enzyme that converts cortisol to cortisone. Increased cortisol levels stimulate mineralocorticoid receptors
S81OL mutation in MR[†]	MR constitutively activated by steroids lacking 21 (OH) groups to progesterone
Ectopic ACTH syndrome[‡]	1. ↑ Secretion of DOC 2. ↑ Cortisol: cannot all be degraded to cortisone 3. ↑ Vasoconstrictors, vasodilators

*Causes of primary aldosteronism are discussed in the text.
[†] Aldosterone secretion inhibited, plasma renin activity suppressed.
[‡] Aldosterone secretion inhibited, plasma renin activity variable.
↑, increased; ↓, decreased; ACTH, corticotrophin; AME, apparent mineralocorticoid excess; ectopic ACTH syndrome, production of corticotrophin by a tumor outside the pituitary gland; DOC, deoxycorticosterone; MR, mineralocorticoid receptor.

is increased, but the process is limited by a subsequent decrease in sodium reabsorption from the proximal tubule and the terminal part of the nephron under the influence of atrial natriuretic peptide and other natriuretic factors, an effect known as *aldosterone escape*. The escape explains the lack of edema in primary aldosteronism and related syndromes. Other factors that may contribute to mineralocorticoid hypertension include central nervous system effects of aldosterone, increased sympathetic nerve activity, and release of vasoconstrictive agents such as antidiuretic hormone (Fig. 27-1).

About 30% of patients with primary aldosteronism have a surgically curable aldosterone-producing adenoma (APA), whereas two thirds have bilateral adrenal gland hyperplasia, a condition termed *idiopathic hyperaldosteronism*. Very rarely, the hyperplasia can be unilateral, a condition called *primary adrenal hyperplasia*. In glucocorticoid-remediable aldosteronism (GRA), ACTH controls secretion of aldosterone. This is an autosomal dominant disorder caused by a mutation in chromosome 8, so that aldosterone secretion is no longer under the control of angiotensin II but under the control of normal concentrations of ACTH. If ACTH secretion is inhibited with the glucocorticoid dexamethasone, aldosterone secretion decreases. Primary aldosteronism can also be caused by aldosterone-producing adrenal or ovarian carcinomas.

Clinical Presentation

The typical clinical features of primary aldosteronism are hypertension, hypokalemia, excessive urinary excretion of potassium, suppressed plasma renin activity (PRA), mild hypernatremia, and metabolic alkalosis. The symptoms of hypokalemia may include polyuria, polydipsia, muscle cramps, muscle weakness, and glucose intolerance. The hypokalemia is more severe in patients with APA than in those with idiopathic hyperaldosteronism. The hypertension may be severe and resistant to treatment.

The disease usually presents in middle age (generally, patients are 30 to 50 years old) and may be more common among women. The presence of the above symptoms in younger patients, or in those with a family history of hyperaldosteronism, suggests a congenital type of mineralocorticoid hypertension such as GRA or Liddle's syndrome. In most series, 10% to 20% of patients with primary aldosteronism may present with normokalemia. Patients with GRA frequently have a normal serum potassium concentration.

Differential Diagnosis

Primary aldosteronism should be suspected in the following circumstances:

- Hypertension with spontaneous (unprovoked) hypokalemia
- Hypertension with severe and refractory diuretic-induced hypokalemia (serum potassium concentration <3 mEq/L)
- Family history of hyperaldosteronism
- Unexplained hypertension, refractory to treatment
- Unexplained hypertension in children and young adults
- Incidentally discovered adrenal tumor

Patients with hypokalemia and hypertension should have measurement of PRA. A PRA greater than 3 ng/mL/hr

Figure 27-1 Primary Hyperaldosteronism and Mineralocorticoid Hypertension.

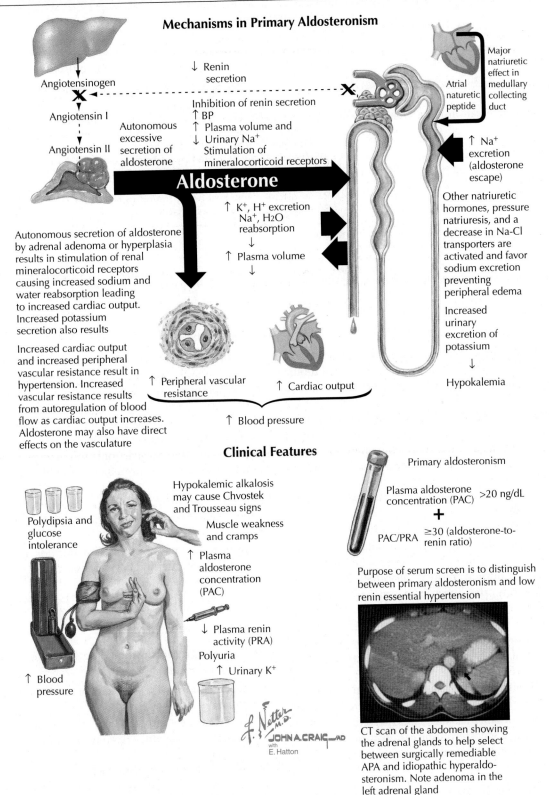

Mechanisms in Primary Aldosteronism

Angiotensinogen

Angiotensin I

Angiotensin II

↓ Renin secretion

Inhibition of renin secretion
↑ BP
↑ Plasma volume and
↓ Urinary Na^+
Stimulation of mineralocorticoid receptors

Autonomous excessive secretion of aldosterone

Aldosterone

↑ K^+, H^+ excretion
Na^+, H_2O reabsorption

↑ Plasma volume
↓

Major natriuretic effect in medullary collecting duct

Atrial natiuretic peptide

↑ Na^+ excretion (aldosterone escape)

Other natriuretic hormones, pressure natriuresis, and a decrease in Na-Cl transporters are activated and favor sodium excretion preventing peripheral edema

Increased urinary excretion of potassium
↓
Hypokalemia

Autonomous secretion of aldosterone by adrenal adenoma or hyperplasia results in stimulation of renal mineralocorticoid receptors causing increased sodium and water reabsorption leading to increased cardiac output. Increased potassium secretion also results

Increased cardiac output and increased peripheral vascular resistance result in hypertension. Increased vascular resistance results from autoregulation of blood flow as cardiac output increases. Aldosterone may also have direct effects on the vasculature

↑ Peripheral vascular resistance

↑ Cardiac output

↑ Blood pressure

Clinical Features

Polydipsia and glucose intolerance

Hypokalemic alkalosis may cause Chvostek and Trousseau signs

Muscle weakness and cramps

↑ Plasma aldosterone concentration (PAC)

↓ Plasma renin activity (PRA)

Polyuria

↑ Urinary K^+

↑ Blood pressure

Primary aldosteronism

Plasma aldosterone concentration (PAC) >20 ng/dL
+
PAC/PRA ≥30 (aldosterone-to-renin ratio)

Purpose of serum screen is to distinguish between primary aldosteronism and low renin essential hypertension

CT scan of the abdomen showing the adrenal glands to help select between surgically remediable APA and idiopathic hyperaldosteronism. Note adenoma in the left adrenal gland

F. Netter M.D.
JOHN A.CRAIG—AD
with
E. Hatton

suggests secondary hyperaldosteronism as seen with malignant hypertension, renal artery stenosis, primary renal disease, reninoma, and estrogen use. A value of less than 1 ng/mL/hr suggests low-renin essential hypertension or mineralocorticoid hypertension. Under these circumstances, screening and confirmatory tests for the presence of primary aldosteronism should be performed.

Diagnostic Approach

Figure 27-2 shows a diagnostic approach for subjects with hypertension and unprovoked or severe diuretic-induced hypokalemia. The same approach can be used in evaluating difficult-to-treat hypertension of unknown etiology with normal serum potassium concentration.

The first step of the evaluation is to distinguish primary aldosteronism from low-renin essential hypertension. The measurement of plasma aldosterone concentration (PAC) and PRA in peripheral venous blood has become the most useful screening test for primary aldosteronism. A PAC greater than 20 ng/dL combined with an aldosterone-to-renin ratio (ARR) greater than 30 has a sensitivity and specificity of more than 95% for primary aldosteronism in subjects with normal renal function. A very high ARR but normal PAC can be seen in some patients with low-renin essential hypertension or in rare forms of mineralocorticoid hypertension (see Table 27-1). Therefore, the test can only be considered indicative of primary aldosteronism if a high ARR coexists with a PAC greater than 20 ng/dL. False-positive results with high PAC are seen in patients with chronic renal failure and in patients taking large doses of spironolactone. Severe hypokalemia can cause a false-negative result by decreasing PAC. Diuretics and inhibitors of the renin-angiotensin system may theoretically produce false-negative results because of an increase in PRA, and β-blockers may produce false-negative results. Ideally, the test should be done off all antihypertensive medications, but this is neither practical nor generally safe for most patients. Several authors have reported that the test is robust even if patients are taking antihypertensive drugs, with the exception of aldosterone antagonists. Some centers recommend that PAC and PRA be measured in the early morning and in the seated position.

The diagnosis of primary aldosteronism can be confirmed by demonstrating that secretion of aldosterone is not suppressed after an infusion of a solution of isotonic sodium chloride or ingestion of a very-high-salt diet with or without administration of the mineralocorticoid fludrocortisone for several days. However, this confirmatory test is somewhat cumbersome and involves discomfort and risk for the patient. Many authors consider a positive screening test enough evidence of primary aldosteronism to proceed with a computed tomography (CT) scan or magnetic resonance imaging of the adrenal glands to distinguish between surgically curable APA and idiopathic hyperaldosteronism. In cases in which proof of nonsuppressibility is considered important, infusion of 2 liters of normal saline over 3 to 4 hours with measurement of PAC before and after is a reasonable approach. If the plasma aldosterone is not suppressed to less than 10 ng/dL, nonsuppressibility is confirmed.

Patients with APA have a high serum concentration of the aldosterone precursor 18-hydroxycorticosterone (18-[OH]-B). Thus, in addition to CT or MRI, we obtain a blood sample for measurement of 18-(OH)-B. The presence of a hypodense adrenal adenoma, larger than 1 cm in diameter, on CT or MRI and a serum concentration of 18-(OH)-B greater than 65 ng/dL is diagnostic of APA and is an indication for adrenalectomy. Ambiguous findings in the adrenal glands or low serum levels of 18-(OH)-B require measurement of ACTH-stimulated aldosterone concentration from each adrenal vein to look for increased unilateral production of aldosterone indicative of surgically curable primary aldosteronism. If GRA is suspected, genetic testing should be done. Some patients with long-standing hypertension who have ambiguous findings on the imaging studies can be treated with aldosterone antagonists without having adrenal vein sampling because even if an adenoma were present, adrenalectomy would not be expected to cure the hypertension, and the hypokalemia usually can be controlled pharmacologically.

Management and Therapy

The treatment of primary aldosteronism depends on the etiology of the condition as ascertained by diagnostic studies.

Optimum Surgical Treatment

Most patients with APA should undergo adrenalectomy, which can usually be performed by a laparoscopic approach. Patients should be treated with spironolactone, 100 to 200 mg/daily for 6 to 8 weeks before surgery, permitting correction of the hypokalemia and improvement of the hypertension. This therapy also decreases extracellular fluid volume and restores the responsiveness of the renin-angiotensin system. A decrease in blood pressure predicts a good response to surgery. About 65% to 70% of patients with an APA are cured of their hypertension; the remainder show improvement. The main postoperative complication is transient hypoaldosteronism with inability to conserve sodium, hypotension, and mild hyperkalemia. This can be prevented by prior treatment with spironolactone and can usually be treated with an increase in salt intake. Persistent hypertension suggests superimposed primary hypertension or nephrosclerosis caused by long-standing hypertension.

Optimum Medical Treatment

Medical treatment of bilateral adrenal hyperplasia is initiated with spironolactone, 50 to 200 mg/daily, with a

Figure 27-2 Diagnostic Approach to Patients with Suspected Primary Aldosteronism.

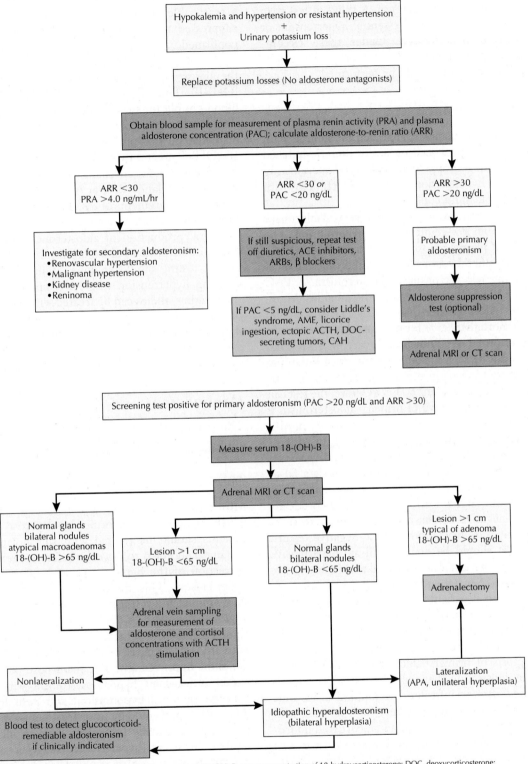

AME, syndrome of apparent mineralocorticoid excess; serum 18-(OH)-B, serum concentration of 18-hydroxycorticosterone; DOC, deoxycorticosterone; APA, aldosterone-producing adenoma; ARR, aldosterone-to-renin ratio; CAH, congenital adrenal hyperplasia; CT, computed tomography; ectopic ACTH, production of corticotropin by a tumor outside the pituitary gland; PAC, plasma aldosterone concentration; PRA, plasma renin activity. Definition; lateralization=aldosterone: cortisol concentration ration in an adrenal vein 4 times greater than that in the other adrenal vein, and/or an aldosterone: cortisol cocentration ratio from the vein of the unaffected adrenal that is less than the ratio in the vena cava. Urinary loss of potassium can be documented by measuring potassium excretion in a 24-hour collection of urine; excretion of more than 30 mEq per day in the presence of hypokalemia indicates potassium wasting. An alternative and simpler approach is to obtain a random sample of urine to calculate fractional excretion of potassium. A fractional excretion greater than 10% when hypokalemia is present indicates potassium wasting.

maximum dose of 400 mg. However, painful gynecomastia and erectile dysfunction in men and menstrual irregularities in women are common at high doses. Therefore, the goal should be to reduce the dose of spironolactone to 50 mg/daily, with the addition of amiloride, 5 to 15 mg/daily, or triamterene, 75 to 150 mg/daily, if needed. Eplerenone, a specific inhibitor of aldosterone receptors, has been approved in the United States for treatment of hypertension and heart failure but not specifically for treatment of primary aldosteronism. A dose of 50 mg once or twice daily may be used as an alternative to spironolactone in those experiencing antiandrogenic adverse effects with spironolactone.

Many patients will require additional antihypertensive therapy. Drugs of choice are thiazide diuretics, calcium channel blockers, and angiotensin-converting enzyme inhibitors. The diet should be low in sodium and rich in potassium. Patients with GRA or apparent mineralocorticoid excess can be treated with 1 to 2 mg/daily of dexamethasone to suppress ACTH secretion; however, there may be corticosteroid-related adverse effects, and hypertension may not be adequately controlled. Patients with Liddle's syndrome do not respond to spironolactone and should be treated with amiloride or triamterene and other antihypertensive drugs combined with salt restriction and potassium supplementation, as needed.

Avoiding Treatment Errors

Postoperative hyperkalemia can be avoided by preoperative treatment with spironolactone or eplerenone.

PHEOCHROMOCYTOMA

Etiology and Pathogenesis

Pheochromocytoma is a tumor arising from adrenomedullary chromaffin cells that produces excess secretion of catecholamines causing intermittent or sustained hypertension (Fig. 27-3). These tumors account for less than 0.5% of causes of hypertension. Although rare, pheochromocytomas are important because of their potential lethality.

Clinical Presentation

Hypertension is the most common presenting feature, occurring in greater than 90% of patients. The hypertension may be severe and is usually sustained, but it may be paroxysmal and associated with spells or may present as a hypertensive emergency. The paroxysms may cause the classic symptom triad of headache, sweating, and palpitation. Other common symptoms are pallor, nausea, tremor, weakness, anxiety, epigastric pain, chest pain, flushing, and dizziness. The paroxysms may be fleeting or last for hours and may occur spontaneously or be precipitated by activities such as lifting, straining, or stretching. The hyperten-

sion is sometimes resistant to pharmacologic treatment but usually responds to α-adrenergic blocking agents.

Pheochromocytomas may occur at any age. Ninety-eight percent of pheochromocytomas are in the abdomen or pelvis, and 90% are in the adrenal gland; 5% to 10% are multiple, less than 10% are malignant, and 10% are familial. Bilateral tumors are more likely to be familial. When extra-adrenal, the tumors are associated with chromaffin cells in paraganglia and are called paragangliomas (see Fig. 27-3). Pheochromocytomas may be inherited as part of the multiple endocrine neoplasia (MEN) syndromes. In MEN IIA, the pheochromocytoma is associated with medullary carcinoma of the thyroid gland and with parathyroid adenoma or hyperplasia. In MEN IIB, pheochromocytomas are also associated with neuromas of the lip and tongue, corneal nerve thickening, and marfanoid body features.

Pheochromocytomas may range in size from microscopic to kilograms in weight. The tumors are usually encapsulated. Only 10% of adrenal pheochromocytomas invade local structures or metastasize, whereas about 40% of extra-adrenal pheochromocytomas invade or metastasize.

Pheochromocytomas most often secrete norepinephrine and epinephrine, but rarely only one of these catecholamines. The finding of excess dopamine secretion suggests the presence of malignancy.

Differential Diagnosis

Pheochromocytoma should be considered in patients with primary hypertension and hyperadrenergic symptoms such as tachycardia, palpitations, sweating, anxiety, and panic attacks. Other syndromes with increased sympathetic nervous system activity and hypertensive crises include use of monoamine oxidase inhibitor antidepressants, clonidine or β-blocker withdrawal, use of drugs with sympathomimetic effects such as cocaine, increased intracranial pressure, thyrotoxicosis, and angina pectoris.

Diagnostic Approach

The key to diagnosis is a high index of suspicion. Most patients who have a pheochromocytoma with a typical clinical presentation will have a positive biochemical test result. However, one third of pheochromocytomas are found incidentally. The approach to screening tests depends on the level of clinical suspicion. If there is any suspicion and screening test results are equivocal, a different screening test should be considered. Measurement of free metanephrines (metanephrine and normetanephrine) in plasma has become the most convenient and accurate screening test, with a sensitivity of 99% and specificity of 89%. Measurement of 24-hour urinary metanephrines and free catecholamines has a diagnostic sensitivity of about 75% to 99% and specificity of about 70% to 93%. The

Figure 27-3 Pheochromocytoma.

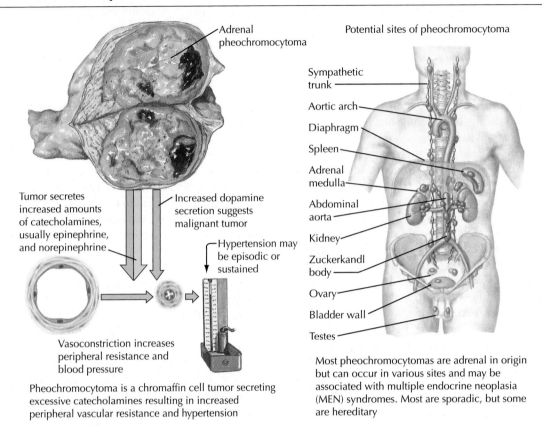

Adrenal pheochromocytoma

Potential sites of pheochromocytoma

Tumor secretes increased amounts of catecholamines, usually epinephrine, and norepinephrine

Increased dopamine secretion suggests malignant tumor

Hypertension may be episodic or sustained

Vasoconstriction increases peripheral resistance and blood pressure

Pheochromocytoma is a chromaffin cell tumor secreting excessive catecholamines resulting in increased peripheral vascular resistance and hypertension

Sympathetic trunk
Aortic arch
Diaphragm
Spleen
Adrenal medulla
Abdominal aorta
Kidney
Zuckerkandl body
Ovary
Bladder wall
Testes

Most pheochromocytomas are adrenal in origin but can occur in various sites and may be associated with multiple endocrine neoplasia (MEN) syndromes. Most are sporadic, but some are hereditary

Clinical features of pheochromocytoma

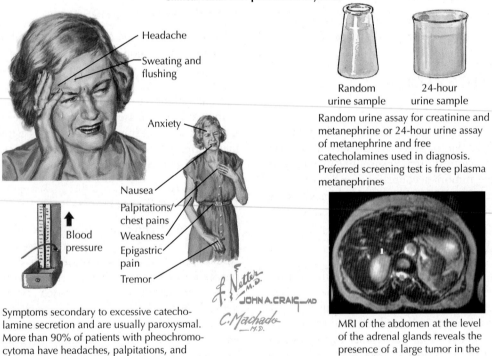

Headache
Sweating and flushing

Anxiety

Nausea
Palpitations/chest pains
Weakness
Epigastric pain
Tremor

Blood pressure

Random urine sample

24-hour urine sample

Random urine assay for creatinine and metanephrine or 24-hour urine assay of metanephrine and free catecholamines used in diagnosis. Preferred screening test is free plasma metanephrines

Symptoms secondary to excessive catecholamine secretion and are usually paroxysmal. More than 90% of patients with pheochromocytoma have headaches, palpitations, and sweating alone or in combination

MRI of the abdomen at the level of the adrenal glands reveals the presence of a large tumor in the right adrenal gland

Figure 27-4 Clinical Suspicion of Pheochromocytoma.
MIBG, iodine-131 metaiodobenzylguanidine.

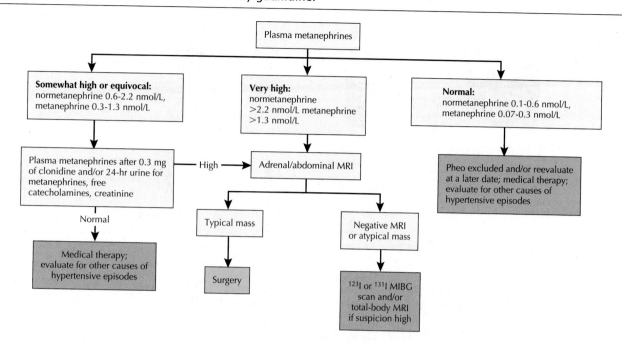

adequacy of the urine collection should be ascertained by measuring creatinine excretion. Plasma catecholamines are highly specific but inconvenient to perform and somewhat less sensitive than urinary measurements. The lower sensitivity may be related to episodic secretion in most patients. However, a value of more than 2000 pg/mL is rarely seen in the absence of a pheochromocytoma. Values between 1000 and 2000 pg/mL require further investigation. Figure 27-4 shows a diagnostic approach to the patient with suspected pheochromocytoma.

Once a pheochromocytoma is suspected clinically and biochemically, a radiographic approach to localization is initiated. CT or MRI depicts most pheochromocytomas; MRI is preferred because of higher specificity on T2-weighted images (see Fig. 27-3). Nuclear scanning with iodine-131 metaiodobenzylguanidine (MIBG) or total-body MRI may be used when CT or abdominopelvic MRI results are negative in the presence of suggestive biochemical results.

Management and Therapy

Optimum Treatment

Surgical removal is the definitive treatment for pheochromocytoma. During anesthesia and surgery, blood pressure may fluctuate widely. Blockade of α-adrenergic receptors blocks the effects of the high circulating catecholamine levels. Before elective surgery, oral phenoxybenzamine is prescribed and is switched to parenteral phentolamine the day of surgery and titrated to maintain blood pressure stability. Metyrosine has recently been approved for the short-term management of pheochromocytoma before surgery, for long-term management when surgery is contraindicated, and for treatment of chronic malignant pheochromocytoma. The drug blocks the conversion of tyrosine to dihydroxyphenylalanine, the rate-limiting step in the catecholamine biosynthetic pathway.

Once blood pressure control is attained, β-adrenergic blocking drugs are administered to control heart rate and prevent arrhythmias, but they should not be used as the only therapy because this would allow unopposed α-adrenergic stimulation. Patients with pheochromocytoma tend to be volume depleted because of pressure natriuresis. Therefore, volume repletion is important before and during surgery.

Avoiding Treatment Errors

Proper preoperative management reduces the risk for perioperative morbidity and mortality.

CUSHING'S SYNDROME

Clinical Presentation

Hypertension is present in 80% of patients with Cushing's syndrome (Fig. 27-5). The hypertension may be severe, and target organ damage is common. Most cases of Cushing's syndrome are caused by the administration of exogenous glucocorticoids, but hypertension is more common with the endogenous causes of hypercortisolism: primary hypersecretion of ACTH by the pituitary gland (Cushing's disease); adrenal adenoma, carcinoma, or hyperplasia; and ectopic secretion of ACTH by a nonen-

Figure 27-5 Cushing's Syndrome and Mineralocorticoid Hypertension.

*ANP, atrial naturetic peptide.

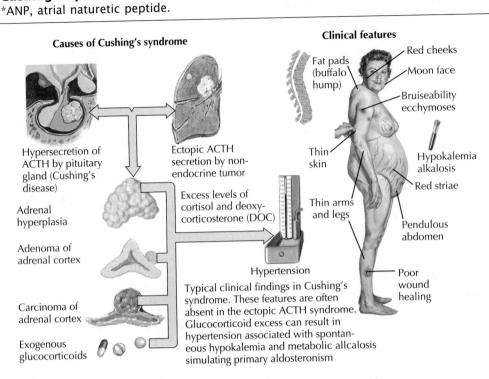

Causes of Cushing's syndrome

Hypersecretion of ACTH by pituitary gland (Cushing's disease)

Ectopic ACTH secretion by non-endocrine tumor

Adrenal hyperplasia

Adenoma of adrenal cortex

Carcinoma of adrenal cortex

Exogenous glucocorticoids

Excess levels of cortisol and deoxy-corticosterone (DOC)

Hypertension

Typical clinical findings in Cushing's syndrome. These features are often absent in the ectopic ACTH syndrome. Glucocorticoid excess can result in hypertension associated with spontaneous hypokalemia and metabolic allcalosis simulating primary aldosteronism

Clinical features

Fat pads (buffalo hump)

Red cheeks

Moon face

Bruiseability ecchymoses

Thin skin

Hypokalemia alkalosis

Red striae

Thin arms and legs

Pendulous abdomen

Poor wound healing

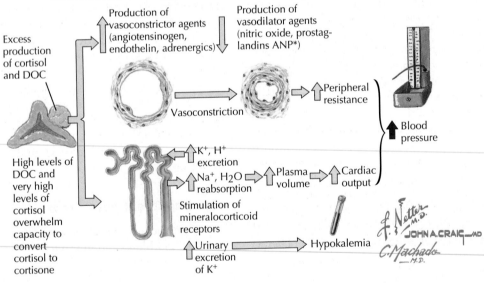

Possible mechanisms of hypertension associated with glucocorticoid excess

Excess production of cortisol and DOC

Production of vasoconstrictor agents (angiotensinogen, endothelin, adrenergics)

Production of vasodilator agents (nitric oxide, prostaglandins ANP*)

Vasoconstriction

Peripheral resistance

Blood pressure

High levels of DOC and very high levels of cortisol overwhelm capacity to convert cortisol to cortisone

K^+, H^+ excretion

Na^+, H_2O reabsorption

Plasma volume

Cardiac output

Stimulation of mineralocorticoid receptors

Urinary excretion of K^+

Hypokalemia

docrine tumor. ACTH secretion in this situation is greater than that with pituitary hypersecretion. Severe hypertension with hypokalemia and metabolic alkalosis is common with ectopic ACTH secretion.

The possible mechanisms of hypertension associated with glucocorticoid excess include stimulation of mineralocorticoid receptors with plasma volume expansion, increased cardiac output, and sodium shifts from the intra-cellular to the extracellular space. There is also an increase in peripheral vascular resistance caused by decreased production of vasodilator substances (nitric oxide, prostaglandins, atrial natriuretic peptide), and increased production of vasoconstrictor factors (angiotensinogen, adrenergic agents, endothelin). Increased levels of DOC and very high levels of cortisol are seen, particularly with ectopic ACTH secretion (see Fig. 27-5).

Differential Diagnosis

Patients presenting with hypertension, hypokalemia, and typical clinical features should be considered for evaluation. Patients with ectopic ACTH syndrome do not usually display the physical features associated with glucocorticoid excess. The main differentiation is from other causes of mineralocorticoid-associated hypertension. The approach to the diagnosis of Cushing's syndrome is presented in Chapter 44.

Management and Therapy

Optimum Treatment

Medical management of the hypertension associated with glucocorticoid excess is the same as that for low-renin essential hypertension, pending possible surgical approaches. Diuretics, including potassium-sparing diuretics, are first-line therapy. Additions or substitutions are based on the blood pressure response and individual patient characteristics. The management of Cushing's syndrome is discussed in Chapter 44.

FUTURE DIRECTIONS

The next few years will see rapid advances in the diagnosis, localization, management, and genetics of adrenal hypertension. The following are key areas of interest:

- Developing imaging studies to distinguish functional from nonfunctional masses of the adrenal cortex
- Determining the prevalence of normokalemic hyperaldosteronism
- Continuing the study of genetic types of primary hyperaldosteronism and pheochromocytoma
- Optimizing cost-effectiveness of diagnostic imaging for pheochromocytoma and determining the role of new techniques such as positron emission tomography in the diagnostic evaluation

Additional Resources

National Cancer Institute. Pheochromocytoma treatment. Available at: http:///www.cancer.gov. Accessed October 11, 2007.
This website provides a well-referenced summary of pheochromocytoma.

EVIDENCE

1. Bornstein SR, Stratakis CA, Chrousos GP: Adrenocortical tumors: Recent advances in basic concepts and clinical management. Ann Intern Med 130(9):759-771, 1999.
   This review of new aspects of adrenocortical tumor genesis and their clinical implications summarizes recent advances in the diagnosis and management of adrenocortical tumors.
2. Grumbach MM, Biller BM, Braunstein GD, et al: Management of the clinically inapparent adrenal mass ("incidentaloma"). Ann Intern Med 138(5):424-429, 2003.
   The National Institutes of Health Consensus Development Program convened to address the causes, prevalence, and natural history of clinically inapparent adrenal masses, or "incidentalomas"; the appropriate evaluation and treatment of such masses; and directions for future research. The panel recommended a 1-mg dexamethasone suppression test and measurement of plasma-free metanephrines for all patients with an adrenal incidentaloma.
3. Lenders JW, Eisenhofer G, Mannelli M, Pacak K: Phaeochromocytoma. Lancet 366(9486):665-675, 2005.
   In this comprehensive review of the genetics, biochemical testing, localization, and management of suspected pheochromocytomas, the authors indicate that measurement of free plasma metanephrines is the most sensitive test for the biochemical diagnosis of pheochromocytoma.
4. Mattsson C, Young WF Jr: Primary aldosteronism: Diagnostic and treatment strategies. Nat Clin Pract Nephrol 2(4):198-208, 2006.
   In this comprehensive review with critical appraisal of the predictive value of screening and confirmatory tests for primary aldosteronism, the authors favor confirmation of the diagnosis of primary aldosteronism by demonstrating that aldosterone production is not suppressed after isotonic saline infusion or a high-salt diet.
5. Young WF Jr: Clinical practice. The incidentally discovered adrenal mass. N Engl J Med 356(6):601-610, 2007.
   In these comprehensive recommendations for the approach to the incidentally discovered adrenal mass with emphasis on proof of function and suppressibility, the author indicates that subjects need not discontinue antihypertensive medications, except aldosterone antagonists, to screen for primary aldosteronism. The author favors measurement of urinary catecholamines and metanephrines to exclude pheochromocytoma.

Angina Pectoris

Introduction

Angina is the sensation caused by the myocardial ischemia that results when cardiac metabolic demand exceeds supply. It is generally defined as "pressure," "discomfort," or a "choking sensation" in the left chest that is precipitated by exertion, excitement, or cold weather, and relieved by rest or nitroglycerin. In some patients, the discomfort radiates into the left arm, into the jaw, or, more rarely, into the right arm (Fig. 28-1). When severe, it can be accompanied by dyspnea, diaphoresis, or nausea. Not all patients experience these classic symptoms, and in some individuals, myocardial ischemia may cause atypical symptoms, such as jaw pain, fatigue, arm discomfort, or upper abdominal pain. Myocardial ischemia can also be "silent" (not associated with symptoms), especially in diabetic patients.

Etiology and Pathogenesis

The most common cause of angina is obstruction of coronary arteries by atherosclerosis (Figs. 28-2 and 28-3). Atherosclerosis, the leading cause of death in the developed world, develops over a period of decades. Risk factors include hypertension, tobacco use, diabetes mellitus type 1, insulin-resistant states (such as diabetes mellitus type 2 and obesity), hypercholesterolemia, and family history of premature vascular disease.

Angina can also result from other less common conditions in which cardiac metabolic demand exceeds supply. These include coronary artery anomalies, coronary artery spasm (Prinzmetal's syndrome), aortic stenosis, anemia, hyperthyroidism, cocaine use, carbon monoxide poisoning, and hypertrophic cardiomyopathy.

Clinical Presentation

Coronary artery disease (CAD) generally manifests as chronic stable angina, unstable angina, acute myocardial infarction, unrecognized myocardial infarction, or sudden cardiac death. Patients with acute myocardial infarction can be further subdivided into those with ST elevation on electrocardiogram (ECG) and those without (commonly called non–ST elevation myocardial infarction).

Chronic Stable Angina

Fixed, stable, obstructive CAD causes a syndrome termed *chronic stable angina* that occurs when myocardial metabolic

demand exceeds a fixed threshold of supply. Angina is commonly precipitated by exertion, emotional excitement, mental stress, or exposure to cold, and resolves after the precipitating event has ceased. Angina generally occurs at the same level of exertion but may vary depending on time of day, recent meals, and ambient temperature.

The most commonly used classification for grading angina severity is the Canadian Cardiovascular Society scale. Patients in Class I experience angina with strenuous or protracted physical activity, whereas those in Class II occasionally have angina with normal daily activities such as climbing stairs or walking up a hill. Patients in Class III have marked limitation and commonly experience angina during activities of everyday living (e.g., walking across a room). Class IV symptoms occur at rest.

Unstable Angina or Non–ST Elevation Myocardial Infarction

Unstable angina, or non–ST elevation myocardial infarction, is generally due to formation of a nonocclusive thrombus at the site of rupture or erosion of the surface of an atherosclerotic plaque (see Fig. 28-3). This event exposes the blood to the highly thrombotic materials within the plaque, leading to thrombus formation. The thrombus can progress until it occludes the blood vessel or, alternatively, may embolize and occlude smaller, more distal vessels. Sudden onset of chest discomfort that is unrelated to a precipitating event is a hallmark of this

Figure 28-1 Angina Pectoris.

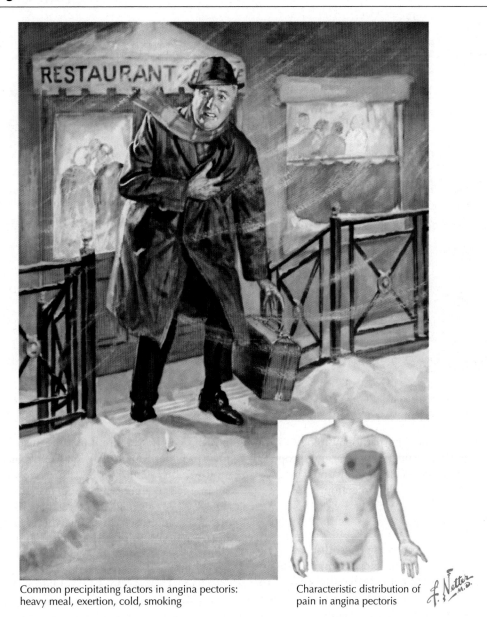

Common precipitating factors in angina pectoris: heavy meal, exertion, cold, smoking

Characteristic distribution of pain in angina pectoris

syndrome. Other patients initially have symptoms that occur with exertion, but over a period of days to weeks, the discomfort occurs with less and less exertion.

Acute Myocardial Infarction with ST Segment Elevation

Acute myocardial infarction with ST segment elevation is characterized by the abrupt onset of unremitting chest discomfort and is generally associated with dyspnea, diaphoresis, and a "sense of doom." It is typically caused by abrupt occlusion of a coronary artery by thrombus at the site of a ruptured atherosclerotic plaque. The ECG shows ST elevation in two or more leads corresponding to the territory of a coronary artery. Patients who are not treated

within 6 to 12 hours generally suffer significant myocardial damage.

Variant (Prinzmetal's) Angina

In Prinzmetal's angina, an uncommon disorder, coronary spasm develops, usually at the site of an atherosclerotic lesion. The hallmark is transient chest pain with ST elevation on ECG, often occurring at rest.

Syndrome X

Syndrome X includes patients with angina, evidence of exercise-induced ischemia, and normal epicardial coronary arteries. These patients are often female (about 70%), with

Figure 28-2 Types and Degrees of Coronary Atherosclerotic Narrowing or Occlusion.

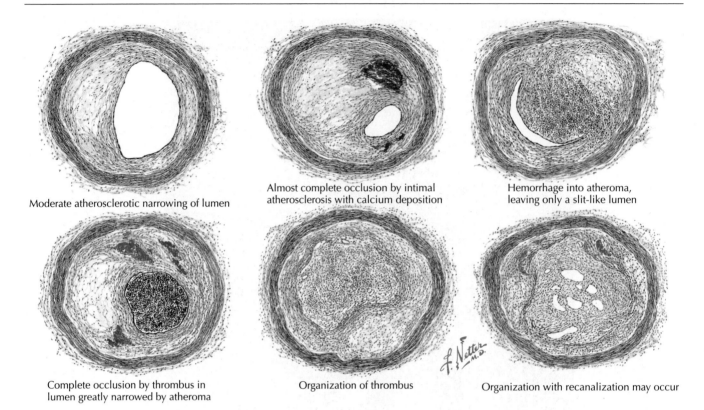

Moderate atherosclerotic narrowing of lumen

Almost complete occlusion by intimal atherosclerosis with calcium deposition

Hemorrhage into atheroma, leaving only a slit-like lumen

Complete occlusion by thrombus in lumen greatly narrowed by atheroma

Organization of thrombus

Organization with recanalization may occur

an average age of 50 years. The pathophysiology of this syndrome is incompletely understood; various proposed etiologies include microvascular dysfunction, incipient cardiomyopathy, and altered pain perception.

Differential Diagnosis

A number of disease states can cause chest discomfort. In some cases, the symptoms can closely mimic angina, although a careful history can help distinguish between the various conditions. Exertional symptoms are common in diastolic dysfunction, exertional hypertension, asthma, and pulmonary hypertension. Response to nitroglycerin can be observed in esophageal spasm and diastolic dysfunction. Other diagnoses mimicking angina or myocardial infarction include esophageal spasm, peptic ulcer, asthma, aortic dissection, mitral valve prolapse, pulmonary embolism, exertional hypertension, cholecystitis, musculoskeletal syndromes, anxiety (panic attack), pericarditis or pleuritis, congestive heart failure, diastolic dysfunction, and costochondritis. A diagnostic algorithm is outlined in Figure 28-4.

Diagnostic Approach

Chronic Stable Angina

In chronic stable angina, typical history and presence of risk factors are the most important information for diag-

nosis. The physical examination is usually not helpful but may provide evidence of left ventricular systolic or diastolic dysfunction (S_3 or S_4, respectively). During an attack of angina, patients tend to be still and may appear pale. The ECG is normal in more than half of patients with coronary atherosclerosis, but there may be evidence of prior myocardial infarction or ischemia (e.g., ST depression). The three most important determinants of prognosis in patients with chronic stable angina are age, number of diseased coronary arteries, and left ventricular function.

An exercise treadmill test can diagnose CAD by the development of ECG changes with exercise. In addition, symptoms during exercise, blood pressure response, and duration of exercise are all important in determining the post-test probability of CAD and whether the patient needs further evaluation. The treadmill test can be enhanced by assessing left ventricular wall motion (with echocardiography) or myocardial perfusion (with nuclear imaging). Pharmacologic stress testing can be used in patients who are unable to exercise.

The recent advent of 64-slice computed tomography (CT) scanners has enabled noninvasive coronary angiography. Patients are given an intravenous bolus of contrast dye, and then the coronary arteries are imaged. The usefulness of this test remains to be determined, but there are promising data, especially in excluding CAD in low-risk patients. CT angiography has several limitations, including significant radiation exposure, exposure to contrast

Figure 28-3 Atherogenesis: Unstable Plaque Formation.

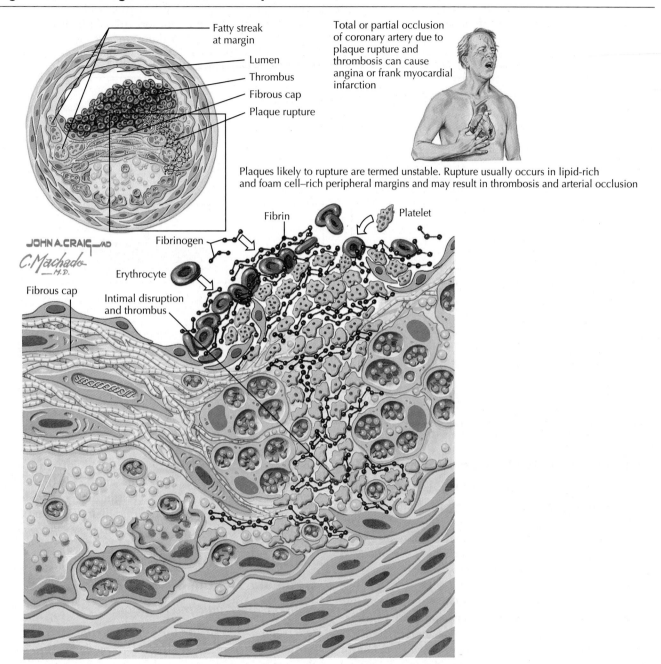

Fatty streak at margin

Lumen

Thrombus

Fibrous cap

Plaque rupture

Total or partial occlusion of coronary artery due to plaque rupture and thrombosis can cause angina or frank myocardial infarction

Plaques likely to rupture are termed unstable. Rupture usually occurs in lipid-rich and foam cell–rich peripheral margins and may result in thrombosis and arterial occlusion

Fibrin

Platelet

Fibrinogen

Erythrocyte

Fibrous cap

Intimal disruption and thrombus

JOHN A. CRAIG—MD
C. Machado —M.D.

dye, the need to be in sinus rhythm, and an ability to tolerate relative bradycardia.

Direct coronary angiography remains the gold standard for diagnosing CAD. This test, which involves direct injection of contrast dye into the coronary arteries, delineates the location and severity of obstructive coronary disease. As such, angiography is a necessary prerequisite for coronary revascularization through either percutaneous intervention or coronary artery bypass surgery. Left ventriculography, generally performed immediately before or after coronary angiography, provides important information regarding intracardiac pressures and left ventricular function.

Clinically assessing the functional importance of intermediate lesions (lesions that appear to obstruct 40% to 60% of the coronary lumen) may be difficult using coronary angiography alone. This limitation can be partially overcome by using intracoronary ultrasound or by measuring coronary flow velocity or intracoronary pressure changes during maximal hyperemia.

Figure 28-4 Assumptions for Diagnostic Algorithm.
This algorithm is highly simplified. Symptoms worrisome for myocardial ischemia will vary depending on the patient. The decision to perform angiography must be individualized and take into account the patient's wishes, renal status, age, etc. ECG, electrocardiogram. *Pretest probability of coronary artery disease can be estimated using information in Diamond GA, Forrester JS: Analysis of probability as an aid in the clinical diagnosis of coronary-artery disease. N Engl J Med 300(24):1350-1358, 1979.*

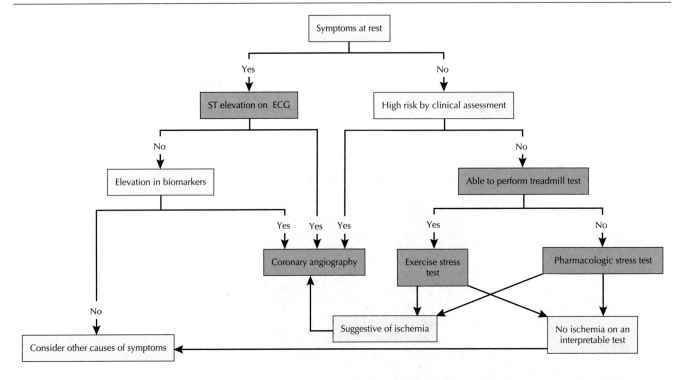

Acute Coronary Syndromes

Patients with unstable angina, non–ST elevation myocardial infarction, or ST elevation myocardial infarction are considered to have an acute coronary syndrome. The diagnosis is generally based on the constellation of typical symptoms (described earlier), ECG changes, and elevated levels of cardiac enzymes (in the case of myocardial infarction).

The ECG is essential in differentiating unstable angina or non–ST elevation myocardial infarction from ST elevation myocardial infarctions. In unstable angina, the ECG may be normal or may demonstrate T-wave inversion or ST depression. ST depression often indicates multivessel CAD and is associated with a worse prognosis in patients with unstable angina. In patients with ST elevation myocardial infarction, the ECG shows contiguous ST elevation involving the anterior (V1 to V4), lateral (V5, V6, I, AVL), or inferior (II, III, AVF) walls.

Myocardial Infarction

Highly sensitive blood tests for myocardial proteins have greatly enhanced our ability to diagnose myocardial infarction. Troponins and creatine kinase-MB (CK-MB) are intracellular cardiac proteins released into the bloodstream upon the death of myocytes. Plasma levels of these proteins

are useful both in detecting myocardial infarction and establishing prognosis. Troponins and CK-MB do not appear in plasma in significant levels until 8 or more hours after the onset of symptoms, limiting their diagnostic value in the very early stages of an acute coronary syndrome.

Management and Therapy

Optimum Treatment

Nonpharmacologic Interventions

Controlling risk factors for atherosclerosis is crucial. In particular, patients should be advised on the need to lower the intake of cholesterol and saturated fat in their diets, the importance of weight loss if obese, and the need to avoid tobacco. A regular exercise program should be prescribed for all patients in whom it is feasible. An exercise stress test can be used to determine safe levels of activity.

Transmyocardial revascularization, enhanced external counterpulsation, spinal cord stimulation, and sympathectomy are occasionally used in patients who have refractory angina despite optimal medical treatment.

Pharmacologic Interventions

Pharmacologic therapy for angina was traditionally directed at relieving symptoms. More recently, medications have been classified based on their effect on survival (Table

Table 28-1 Summary of Pharmacologic Treatment of Patients with Chronic Stable Angina

Medication	Dosage	Which Patients?	Effect on Cardiovascular Clinical Endpoints
Aspirin	80-325 mg every day	All patients with vascular disease	Decreases the risk for death, MI, and stroke
Statin drugs	Varies depending on particular drug	All patients with vascular disease	Decreases the risk for death in patients who have had a prior MI
Angiotensin-converting enzyme inhibitors	Varies depending on particular drug; initial dosage will depend on blood pressure	All patients with vascular disease (in particular, any patient with vascular disease and hypertension or diabetes)	In the HOPE trial, ramipril, 10 mg every day, reduced the rate of death, MI, and stroke in patients with vascular disease
β-Blockers	Begin at low dose (e.g., metoprolol, 12.5 mg twice a day) and titrate depending on heart rate and blood pressure	Patients with prior MI or with cardiomyopathy (caution is needed when initiating β-blockers in patients with congestive heart failure)	Decreases the risk for death in patients who have had a prior MI and improves outcomes in patients with dilated cardiomyopathy
Nitrates	Sublingual or buccal spray can be used as needed; longer-acting oral and transdermal formulations are available	Patients with anginal symptoms	None
Calcium channel blockers	Varies depending on particular drug; initial dosage will depend on blood pressure and heart rate	Patients with anginal symptoms	No beneficial effect on survival; nifedipine worsens survival in acute coronary syndromes; diltiazem worsens survival in left ventricular dysfunction
Warfarin	Varies depending on response; needs continual monitoring	Useful in selected patients with vascular disease	A meta-analysis demonstrates reduction in the risk for death, MI, or stroke if INR >2 and used with concurrent ASA; bleeding increased by 1.9-fold

ASA, aspirin; HOPE, Heart Outcomes and Prevention Evaluation; INR, international normalized ratio; MI, myocardial infarction.

28-1). Medications that improve survival and decrease cardiovascular events in patients with CAD include aspirin, hydroxymethyl glutaryl–coenzyme A (HMG-CoA) reductase inhibitors ("statins"), and angiotensin-converting enzyme inhibitors. In patients with prior myocardial infarction or left ventricular dysfunction, β-blockers also reduce mortality. Medications that treat symptoms without improving survival include nitrates and calcium channel blockers. The use of calcium channel blockers, with the exception of amlodipine and felodipine, should be avoided in patients with left ventricular dysfunction.

Low-density lipoprotein (LDL) cholesterol levels should be aggressively lowered, even in patients with ostensibly normal LDL levels, through the use of diet and statins. Recent guidelines suggest that LDL cholesterol should be less than 70 mg/dL in patients with CAD. Blood pressure should be closely monitored, with optimum levels below 140/90 mm Hg. In diabetic patients, optimum levels are even lower, with the goal of diastolic blood pressures at 80 mm Hg or less. Patients must be strongly encouraged to quit smoking and offered pharmacologic aids (e.g., nicotine patches, bupropion, varenicline) or support group help as needed. Antioxidant vitamins have not been shown to be beneficial.

Therapies that interrupt thrombus formation have an important role in acute coronary syndromes. In unstable angina or non–ST elevation myocardial infarction, aspirin and heparin reduce the rate of death and myocardial reinfarction. Glycoprotein IIb/IIIa inhibitors are useful in patients with high-risk features (e.g., elevated troponins or ST depression) who are undergoing percutaneous coronary intervention.

In ST elevation myocardial infarction, the goal of therapy is rapid restoration of blood flow using either thrombolytic therapy or a percutaneous coronary intervention such as balloon angioplasty. In hospitals with 24-hour availability of an experienced interventional cardiologist and staff, percutaneous intervention is the preferred treatment. In other hospitals, prompt administration of thrombolytic therapy, especially within 6 hours of the onset of symptoms, improves patient survival. Streptokinase and tissue plasminogen activator (tPA) have been extensively studied, but newer thrombolytic drugs derived from tPA, including reteplase and tenecteplase, have similar efficacy and are easier to administer (1 or 2 bolus injections).

Revascularization

Revascularization re-establishes unobstructed blood flow either through percutaneous intervention, in which the atherosclerotic blockage is relieved by angioplasty balloon inflation or stent placement, or by coronary artery bypass grafting, in which blood flow is diverted around atherosclerotic obstructions using an arterial (e.g., left internal mammary artery) or venous conduit. Revascularization prolongs survival in patients with significant left main CAD and multivessel CAD with impaired left ventricular function. The most common indication for revascularization, however, is relief of symptoms.

Avoiding Treatment Errors

One of the most common, major, preventable treatment errors is the misdiagnosis of acute myocardial infarction. It has been estimated that approximately 4% of patients with myocardial infarction presenting to emergency rooms are discharged home inappropriately. The mortality rate associated with a missed diagnosis of myocardial infarction is twice as high as that of patients who are admitted to the hospital. Misdiagnosis of myocardial infarction is a major medical malpractice issue and accounts for up to 20% of emergency department litigation expenses in the United States.

Another major problem to avoid is the undertreatment of ST elevation myocardial infarction. It has been estimated in various studies that 20% to 30% of patients with ST elevation myocardial infarction who would benefit from reperfusion therapy (either thrombolytic therapy or primary angioplasty) do not receive it. In these cases, the diagnosis is correct; however, appropriate therapy is withheld. Common misperceptions that lead to withholding of therapy include overestimation of the bleeding risk (especially intracerebral bleeding), comorbid conditions, and time to presentation.

Future Directions

Plasma levels of C-reactive protein, a marker of inflammation, are useful in determining the prognosis of patients with unstable angina or non–ST elevation myocardial infarction. Large population-based studies have also shown a correlation between C-reactive protein levels and CAD. Electron-beam CT and three-dimensional echocardiography may enhance the ability of noninvasive testing to detect CAD. In preliminary studies, inroads are being made into the identity of genetic polymorphisms that contribute to CAD. Further progress in this area may identify high-risk individuals who will benefit from specific, risk factor–modifying therapy initiated early in life.

Several new pharmaceuticals are being evaluated for use in patients with angina, including potassium channel blockers and agents that enhance nitric oxide production. Large-scale clinical studies are also testing the use of antibiotics and anti-inflammatory medications as means to slow the progression of atherosclerosis. Finally, the stimulation of myocardial angiogenesis through intracoronary injection of growth factors (e.g., vascular endothelial growth factor) or genes encoding angiogenic factors is an exciting area now entering clinical trials.

Additional Resources

American Heart Association Website. Available at: http://www.americanheart.org/presenter.jhtml?identifier=2158. Accessed October 15, 2006.

This site provides access to the most up-to-date versions of various guidelines (most developed in conjunction with the ACC).

European Society of Cardiology Website. Available at: http://www.escardio.org/knowledge/guidelines/Guidelines_list.htm?hit=quick. Accessed October 15, 2006.

This site provides access to the most up-to-date versions of various guidelines.

Gibbons RJ, Balady GJ, Bricker JT, et al: ACC/AHA 2002 guideline update for exercise testing: Summary article. A report of the American College of Cardiology/American Heart Association Task Force on Practice Guidelines (Committee to Update the 1997 Exercise Testing Guidelines). Circulation 106(14):1883-1892, 2002.

This report describes the appropriate use and interpretation of exercise stress testing as defined by an expert committee assembled by the ACC and AHA.

Thompson PD, Buchner D, Piña IL, et al: Exercise and physical activity in the prevention and treatment of atherosclerotic cardiovascular disease: A statement from the Council on Clinical Cardiology and the Council on Nutrition, Physical Activity, and Metabolism, American Heart Association. Circulation 107(24):3109-3116, 2003.

The importance of exercise and physical activity is outlined in this report.

EVIDENCE

1. Antman EM, Anbe DT, Armstrong PW, et al: ACC/AHA guidelines for the management of patients with ST-elevation myocardial infarction: A report of the American College of Cardiology/American Heart Association Task Force on Practice Guidelines (Committee to Revise the 1999 Guidelines for the Management of patients with acute myocardial infarction). J Am Coll Cardiol 44(3):E1-E211, 2004.

This article outlines the appropriate diagnosis and treatment of ST elevation myocardial infarction as defined by an expert committee assembled by the ACC and AHA.

2. Braunwald E, Antman EM, Beasley JW, et al: ACC/AHA guidelines for the management of patients with unstable angina and non–ST-segment elevation myocardial infarction: Executive summary and recommendations. A report of the American College

of Cardiology/American Heart Association Task Force on Practice Guidelines (Committee on the Management of Patients with Unstable Angina). Circulation 106(14):1893-1900, 2002.

This article outlines the appropriate diagnosis and treatment of non–ST elevation myocardial infarction as defined by an expert committee assembled by the ACC and AHA.

3. Eagle KA, Guyton RA, Davidoff R, et al: ACC/AHA 2004 guideline update for coronary artery bypass graft surgery: A report of the American College of Cardiology/American Heart Association Task Force on Practice Guidelines (Committee to Update the 1999 Guidelines for Coronary Artery Bypass Graft Surgery). Circulation 110:e340-e437, 2004.

This report describes the appropriate use of coronary artery bypass grafting as defined by an expert committee assembled by the ACC and AHA.

4. Fox K, Garcia MA, Ardissino D, et al: Guidelines on the management of stable angina: Executive summary. Task Force on the Management of Stable Angina Pectoris of the European Society of Cardiology. Eur Heart J 27(11):1341-1381, 2006.

This paper describes the appropriate treatment of chronic stable angina as defined by an expert committee assembled by the European Society of Cardiology.

5. Gibbons RJ, Abrams J, Chatterjee K, et al: ACC/AHA 2002 guideline update for the management of patients with chronic stable angina: Summary article. A report of the American College of Cardiology/American Heart Association Task Force on Practice Guidelines (Committee on the Management of Patients with Chronic Stable Angina). Circulation 107(1): 149-158, 2003.

This report outlines the appropriate treatment of chronic stable angina as defined by an expert committee assembled by the ACC and AHA.

6. Scanlon PJ, Faxon DP, Audet AM, et al: ACC/AHA guidelines for coronary angiography: Executive summary and recommendations. A report of the American College of Cardiology/American Heart Association Task Force on Practice Guidelines (Committee on coronary angiography) developed in collaboration with the Society for Cardiac Angiography and Interventions. Circulation 99(17): 2345-2357, 1999.

This paper describes the appropriate use of coronary angiography as defined by an expert committee assembled by the ACC and AHA.

Tracy Y. Wang ▪ E. Magnus Ohman

29

Myocardial Infarction

Introduction

Each year, about 32 million myocardial infarctions (MIs) occur worldwide, resulting in 12.5 million deaths. MI reflects myocyte necrosis and is clinically defined as a typical rise and fall in biochemical markers of myocardial necrosis (preferentially troponin) accompanied by ischemic symptoms and/or electrocardiogram (ECG) changes. The terms MI and acute coronary syndrome (ACS) are often mentioned in the same context. ACS encompasses the spectrum of myocardial ischemia, which includes myocardial infarction with ST-segment elevation (STEMI), myocardial infarction without ST elevation (NSTEMI), and unstable angina (UA). MI refers to the first two components of ACS wherein sufficient myocardial damage has occurred to release detectable quantities of troponin into the bloodstream.

Etiology and Pathogenesis

MI occurs as a result of an imbalance between myocardial oxygen supply and demand. Most MIs arise from the pathologic substrate of coronary artery atherosclerosis (Fig. 29-1). Localized vascular endothelial injury and inflammation, uptake and oxidation of low-density lipoprotein (LDL), and smooth muscle cell proliferation contribute to development of the atherosclerotic plaque that is sequestered from circulating blood by a collagenous fibrous cap. Disruption of the fibrous cap exposes this inflammatory mixture, leading to platelet activation, thrombin generation, and thrombus formation. Patients with STEMI typically have complete thrombus occlusion of the infarct artery on angiography, whereas NSTEMI/UA patients have partial stenoses of varying severity. Decreased epicardial coronary blood flow results in myocardial ischemia and necrosis that start in the more vulnerable endocardium and spread outward. This process is modulated by the extent of collateral flow and by determinants of myocardial oxygen demand. Subsequent anaerobic metabolism results in myocardial dysfunction with impairment of myocardial contractility and ventricular compliance, and electrical instability with conduction disturbances. Mechanical problems such as mitral regurgitation, free wall or ventricular septal rupture, and ventricular aneurysm can also occur as a result of myocardial structural disruption.

Other causes of MI include microembolization, dynamic obstruction (focal coronary artery spasm or abnormal constriction of intramural vessels), increased myocardial oxygen requirement (fever, tachycardia, thyrotoxicosis), and decreased myocardial oxygen delivery (hypotension, anemia, hypoxemia).

Clinical Presentation

The clinical presentation of MI can range from typical chest discomfort to nonspecific symptoms with varying degrees of severity. The most typical presentation is of chest pain that is described as an intense, substernal pressure, often radiating to either arm, the neck, the jaw, or the epigastrium. Accompanying symptoms include dyspnea, diaphoresis, nausea or vomiting, palpitations, weakness, and lightheadedness. Occasionally, these associated symptoms, rather than chest discomfort, may predominate. Atypical symptoms are common in elderly patients (particularly among women) and in diabetic patients. These individuals have a higher risk for adverse outcomes, so MI should be considered even in the presence of minor or atypical symptoms. More than 40% of patients have sudden cardiac death as their first symptom of MI.

Physical Examination

The physical examination should focus on identifying potentially correctable causes of myocardial ischemia, complications of ischemia, and signs pointing to an alternative diagnosis. Vital signs, including blood pressure measurements in both arms, are critical. Treatment of

Figure 29-1 Atherogenesis: Unstable Plaque Formation.

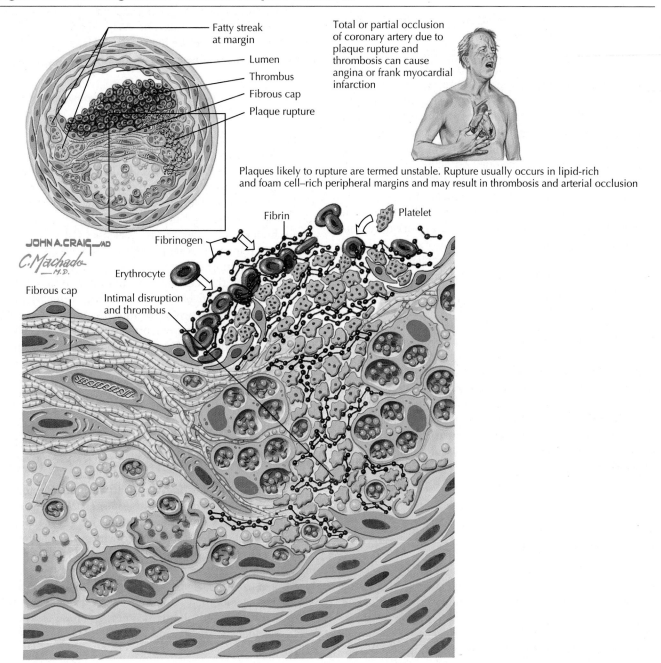

Fatty streak at margin

Lumen

Thrombus

Fibrous cap

Plaque rupture

Total or partial occlusion of coronary artery due to plaque rupture and thrombosis can cause angina or frank myocardial infarction

Plaques likely to rupture are termed unstable. Rupture usually occurs in lipid-rich and foam cell–rich peripheral margins and may result in thrombosis and arterial occlusion

Fibrin

Platelet

Fibrinogen

Erythrocyte

Fibrous cap

Intimal disruption and thrombus

uncontrolled hypertension, tachyarrhythmias, fever, or evident thyrotoxicosis reduces myocardial oxygen demand. Similarly, correction of bradycardia, hypotension, or hypoxemia improves oxygen supply. Bradycardia commonly occurs in inferior MIs as a result of atrioventricular node ischemia. Cardiopulmonary examination often reveals an S_4 gallop due to an ischemia-induced decrease in left ventricular compliance. Signs of congestive heart failure, including pulmonary rales, jugular venous distention, S_3 gallop, and hepatosplenomegaly, can be harbingers of cardiogenic shock, which is manifested by hypotension,

tachycardia, and cool extremities. A new systolic murmur may indicate mechanical complications such as mitral valvular incompetence or a ventricular septal defect.

The physical examination includes an assessment of cardiac risk. Findings of obesity, xanthelasma (indicative of hypercholesterolemia), nicotine stains on fingers (suggestive of smoking history), ophthalmologic evidence of hypertension, limb weakness, facial asymmetry or slurred speech (indicative of previous stroke), or differential pulses and bruits (suggestive of peripheral vascular disease) identify patients at higher risk for coronary artery disease.

Differential Diagnosis

Several conditions can mimic MI and may be life threatening if not diagnosed accurately.

Aortic dissection typically presents with a stabbing or ripping chest discomfort radiating to the back. Differential blood pressures between the right and left arm or a new diastolic murmur (aortic regurgitation) suggests aortic dissection, and the diagnostic suspicion is increased when a wide mediastinum is seen on chest radiography. Confirmation requires computed tomography (CT) or transesophageal echocardiographic imaging. An acute MI can occur concurrently with aortic dissection if the dissection involves a coronary ostium (more commonly that of the right coronary artery), resulting in its exclusion from the true aortic lumen. Excluding aortic dissection is important before administering thrombolytics or antithrombotic medications for acute MI. When the chief complaint is dyspnea associated with pleuritic chest discomfort, hemoptysis, and low oxygen saturation, pulmonary embolism should be suspected. This diagnosis is confirmed by ventilation-perfusion scanning or CT of the chest with contrast. Differential breath sounds suggest pneumothorax. Pericarditis pain is usually sharp, pleuritic, and positional and is better when sitting up or leaning forward. A friction rub or pulsus paradoxus suggests pericarditis.

Other conditions, including esophageal spasm, gastroesophageal reflux, peptic ulcer disease, acute cholecystitis, and costochondral pain, often present with similar symptoms and should be ruled out by a careful history and physical examination.

Diagnostic Approach

Electrocardiography

The ECG drives therapeutic decision making for the patient with MI and should be performed within 10 minutes of arrival. Evidence of a new left bundle branch block or new ST-segment elevation greater than 0.1 mV in two or more contiguous leads identifies patients who should be considered for acute reperfusion therapy (Fig. 29-2).

Patients without ST elevation do not benefit from acute reperfusion therapy, except for those with acute posterior MI with ST depression in leads V_1 to V_3, which is equivalent to ST elevation seen in posterior chest leads. Patients with NSTEMI or UA can have ST-segment depression and T-wave inversion. Acute symmetrical precordial T-wave inversion (≥0.2 mV) suggests acute ischemia from a critical stenosis of the left anterior descending coronary artery. A completely normal ECG in the setting of chest pain does not exclude the possibility of MI. The presence of bundle branch block, left ventricular hypertrophy, or ST-segment deviation on ECG predicts poor prognosis independently of clinical findings and cardiac biomarker elevation.

Findings such as a known left bundle branch block, a paced rhythm, left ventricular hypertrophy with strain, wide complex tachycardia, or Wolff-Parkinson-White syndrome can obscure the diagnosis of MI; comparison to a prior ECG if available can occasionally enhance diagnostic accuracy.

Biomarker Testing

Myocyte necrosis with subsequent loss of cell membrane integrity releases cardiac-specific biomarkers that are detectable in the peripheral circulation. Before the advent of troponin, creatine kinase-MB (CK-MB) was the principal biomarker available; however its use was hampered by low sensitivity and specificity. CK-MB becomes elevated 3 to 4 hours after onset of MI, peaks between 12 and 24 hours, and remains elevated for 36 to 48 hours. Troponin assays have demonstrated superior sensitivity and tissue specificity, such that current guidelines have declared troponins the preferred biomarker for diagnosing MI, and their use has been incorporated into the definition of MI. Troponin I and T measurements provide similar diagnostic and prognostic information. Troponin levels begin to rise 3 to 6 hours after symptom onset and remain elevated 7 to 14 days after infarction. Troponin elevation independently predicts higher mortality even among patients with normal CK-MB levels, and NSTEMI patients with troponin elevation may benefit from more aggressive therapies such as low–molecular-weight heparin, glycoprotein IIb/IIIa inhibitors, or an early invasive cardiac catheterization strategy.

Serial biomarker testing for up to 18 hours should be performed for all patients with suspected MI. However, for patients with STEMI, the decision for acute reperfusion therapy should not be delayed while awaiting results of biomarker testing. To permit earlier diagnosis before myocardial damage occurs, recent efforts have focused on markers of cardiac ischemia and plaque instability, including ischemia-modified albumin, malondialdehyde, and pregnancy-associated plasma protein A. These assays are not yet widely available and require large clinical trial validation.

Other Diagnostic Tools

Although the ECG and cardiac biomarkers are the most important tests for suspected MI, diagnostic imaging such as two-dimensional echocardiography, nuclear scintigraphy, or cardiac magnetic resonance imaging can provide complementary diagnostic and prognostic information. Bedside echocardiography is useful in detecting infarction in electrocardiographically silent areas such as the circumflex artery distribution; new wall motion abnormalities are diagnostic of ischemia. Echocardiography can provide further information regarding left ventricular function, size and location of infarction, valvular pathology, and

Figure 29-2 Localization of Myocardial Infarcts.

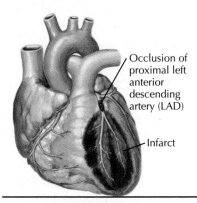

Anterior Infarct

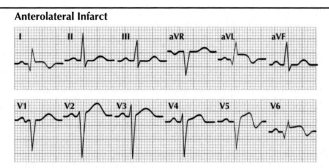

Occlusion of proximal left anterior descending artery (LAD)

Infarct

Significant Q waves and T-wave inversions in leads I, V_2, V_3, and V_4

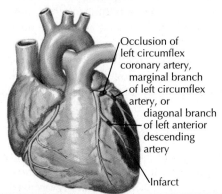

Anterolateral Infarct

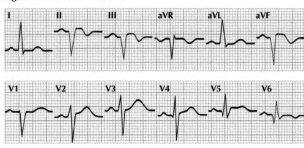

Occlusion of left circumflex coronary artery, marginal branch of left circumflex artery, or diagonal branch of left anterior descending artery

Infarct

Significant Q waves and T-wave inversions in leads I, aVL, V_5, and V_6

Diaphragmatic or Inferior Infarct

Occlusion of right coronary artery

Infarct

Significant Q waves and T-wave inversions in leads II, III, and aVF. With lateral damage, changes also may be seen in leads V_5 and V_6

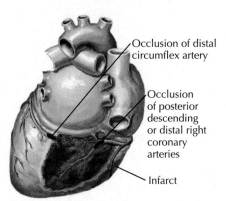

True Posterior Infarct

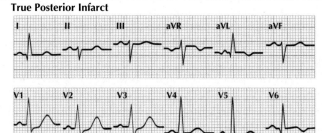

Occlusion of distal circumflex artery

Occlusion of posterior descending or distal right coronary arteries

Infarct

Since no ECG lead reflects posterior electrical forces, changes are reciprocal of those in anterior leads. Lead V_1 shows unusally large R wave (reciprocal of posterior Q wave) and upright T wave (reciprocal of posterior T-wave inversion)

mechanical complications such as mitral regurgitation or ventricular septal rupture. Radionuclide imaging, particularly during ongoing chest discomfort, can be useful but is limited by lack of 24-hour personnel or isotope availability. Recent enthusiasm about cardiac magnetic resonance imaging reflects its dual advantages of providing superior structural information as well as detecting ischemic, viable, or scarred vascular territories.

Management and Therapy

Optimum Treatment

Every patient presenting with symptoms and signs suggestive of MI should be triaged per a standardized protocol to expedite evaluation and therapy. All patients should receive an intravenous line, oxygen administered through nasal prongs, and continuous cardiac telemetry monitoring for arrhythmias. After targeted history and physical examination are performed, 160 to 325 mg of aspirin should be given. Aspirin is associated with a 24% reduction in early mortality. Patients with ongoing chest discomfort should receive 0.4 mg of sublingual nitroglycerin at 5-minute intervals unless they are hypotensive, are bradycardic, or have evidence of right ventricular infarction. Nitrates reduce preload and afterload and promote coronary vasodilation. β-Blockers reduce myocardial oxygen demand and, in the absence of hypotension, bradycardia, congestive heart failure, or a history of bronchospasm, should be given orally and titrated upward in dosing as clinical condition allows. Further treatment is stratified by the presence or absence of ST elevation on ECG.

ST Elevation Myocardial Infarction

All patients with ST elevation or new left bundle branch block should be considered for immediate reperfusion therapy. Restoration of coronary flow can be achieved pharmacologically with thrombolytic medications or mechanically with percutaneous coronary intervention (PCI).

Commonly used thrombolytic agents include intravenous streptokinase and recombinant tissue plasminogen activators such as tPA (alteplase), rPA (reteplase), and TNK (tenecteplase). Streptokinase is less costly and more commonly used worldwide. Recombinant agents are more efficacious and, in the cases of rPA and TNK, are more easily administered. All have been associated with significant reductions in 30-day and long-term mortality. Contraindications to thrombolysis include recent bleeding, stroke, intracranial hemorrhage, major surgery, or chronic warfarin anticoagulation. Adjunctive therapies include heparin and clopidogrel. Low–molecular-weight heparin has been shown to be superior to unfractionated heparin when combined with TNK. Clopidogrel use has been shown to significantly reduce mortality as well as recurrent infarction and stroke.

Primary PCI of the infarct-related artery is superior to thrombolysis in terms of both efficacy (reduced mortality) and safety (reduced bleeding complications). However, its use is limited by timely availability of qualified catheterization facilities and staff. Adjunctive glycoprotein IIb/IIIa inhibition has been found to enhance the outcome of primary PCI with lower rates of death, reinfarction, and need for urgent repeat revascularization. Clopidogrel use after stent implantation is routine. Recent evidence shows that delayed opening of an occluded infarct-related artery (>3 days from symptom onset) is not beneficial, emphasizing the need for timely reperfusion therapy.

Time to artery patency is a key determinant of both short- and long-term prognosis; hence, rapid triage and decision making are critical. A door-to-needle time of 30 minutes and a door-to-balloon time of 90 minutes are the longest acceptable time delays, and in the absence of contraindications, the selection of reperfusion strategy should be based on which method allows the most rapid means of restoring coronary flow. Primary PCI is the preferred reperfusion strategy in patients with cardiogenic shock.

Non–ST Elevation Myocardial Infarction

Although there is less urgency in managing patients with NSTEMI compared with those with ST elevation, early cardiac catheterization with appropriate revascularization (either PCI or surgical bypass grafting) has been shown to reduce mortality and morbidity, particularly in higher risk patients with recurrent ischemia, elevated troponin, heart failure symptoms, and new ST-segment changes on ECG. In general, antiplatelet and antithrombotic medications remain the cornerstone of NSTEMI therapy. Combination antiplatelet therapy with aspirin and clopidogrel is superior to aspirin alone. Low–molecular-weight heparin reduces mortality and major adverse cardiac events compared with unfractionated heparin in troponin-positive patients. Furthermore, in high-risk patients, use of glycoprotein IIb/IIIa inhibitors further reduces mortality and adverse outcomes, particularly among patients undergoing PCI. Patients with troponin-positive NSTEMI derive additional benefit from glycoprotein IIb/IIIa inhibition even after receiving aspirin, heparin, and clopidogrel. Although individual glycoprotein IIb/IIIa inhibitors are mostly interchangeable, in patients not proceeding to early revascularization, use of abciximab provides no significant benefit and is discouraged. In patients treated with an early invasive cardiac catheterization strategy, recent evidence shows that bivalirudin, used as an alternative to heparin plus glycoprotein IIb/IIIa inhibition, provides similar antiischemic benefits with a reduced rate of bleeding complications. Fondaparinux has also demonstrated comparable reductions in death, MI, and refractory ischemia, accompanied by a significantly lower bleeding rate when compared with low–molecular-weight heparin in patients with non–ST elevation ACS. However, concerns regarding an

Figure 29-3 Nondrug Therapy.

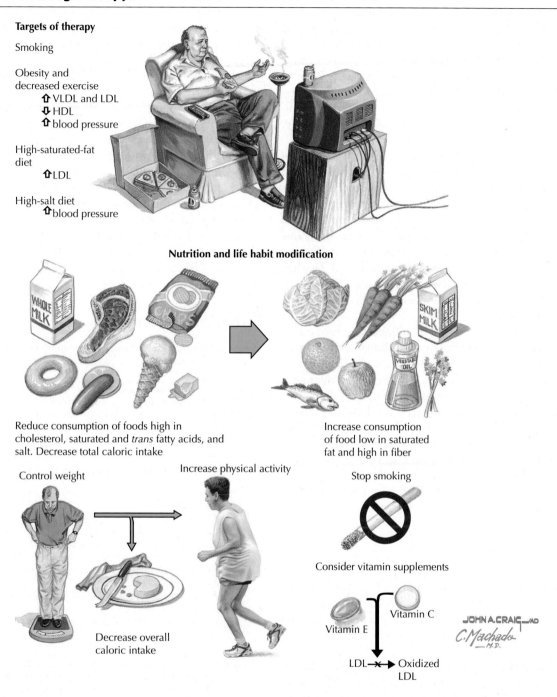

Targets of therapy

Smoking

Obesity and
decreased exercise
⬆ VLDL and LDL
⬇ HDL
⬆ blood pressure

High-saturated-fat
diet
⬆ LDL

High-salt diet
⬆ blood pressure

Nutrition and life habit modification

Reduce consumption of foods high in
cholesterol, saturated and *trans* fatty acids, and
salt. Decrease total caloric intake

Increase consumption
of food low in saturated
fat and high in fiber

Control weight

Increase physical activity

Stop smoking

Decrease overall
caloric intake

Consider vitamin supplements

Vitamin C

Vitamin E

LDL —✕→ Oxidized
LDL

JOHN A.CRAIG—MD
C.Machado
—M.D.

increased risk for catheter-related thrombosis have limited its use to patients who are managed with a conservative invasive strategy.

Coronary Revascularization

Recent advances, including use of drug-eluting stents and adjunctive antiplatelet therapies (clopidogrel, glycoprotein IIb/IIIa inhibitors), have increased the utilization and success rates of percutaneous coronary revascularization. Although indications for catheter-based therapies are continuing to expand, currently, coronary artery bypass graft-

ing provides more long-term survival benefit for high-risk patients with significant left main or multivessel coronary artery disease, particularly for those with abnormal left ventricular function or diabetes.

Secondary Prevention

Aggressive blood pressure and glycemic control, smoking cessation, dietary modification, and cardiac rehabilitation are key components of secondary prevention (Fig. 29-3). Aspirin therapy provides a 25% reduction in recurrent ischemic events. β-Blockers provide benefit in patients across all age groups treated with or without reperfusion. Angiotensin-converting enzyme (ACE) inhibitors improve survival in post-MI patients with or without left ventricular dysfunction. In the absence of hypotension, β-blockers and ACE inhibitors should be started during the hospitalization and are routine components of post-MI care. Patients with MI complicated by left ventricular dysfunction and heart failure who are already optimized on the aforementioned therapies receive further morbidity and mortality reduction with aldosterone blockade.

A fasting lipid profile should be obtained in the first 24 hours after admission. Recent studies have shown that intensive early post-MI lipid lowering with statins provides greater protection against death and other major cardiac events. This evidence has led to a revision of the National Cholesterol Education Program—Adult Treatment Panel III guidelines, which now recommend initiation of statin therapy in all post-MI patients irrespective of baseline LDL level. Statin therapy should be initiated before hospital discharge (to enhance compliance) and target an LDL goal of less than 70 mg/dL.

Postinfarction patients are at higher risk for sudden cardiac death due to ventricular arrhythmias. Antiarrhythmic drugs such as amiodarone have limited efficacy in preventing sudden death after MI. Recent randomized clinical trials have suggested that prophylactic implantation of implantable cardioverter defibrillators (ICDs) improves survival in patients with left ventricular dysfunction irrespective of the presence or absence of spontaneous or "provokable" ventricular arrhythmias. ICD implantation should be considered for patients with an ejection fraction of 30% or less who have been on optimal medical therapy for at least 6 weeks after the MI.

Avoiding Treatment Errors

A chest pain protocol should be in place to triage symptomatic patients, such that the appropriate diagnostic and therapeutic measures can be delivered in an expeditious manner. Keeping in mind that not all patients present with typical chest pain, a 12-lead ECG, in particular, is critical for rapid risk stratification. The phrase "time is muscle" is frequently used to describe the urgency of revascularization once coronary artery occlusion is suspected. Therapies for MI involve the use of antithrombotic medications, which carry the risk for bleeding. This bleeding risk can be minimized by proper dosing of medications (e.g., heparin, glycoprotein IIb/IIIa inhibitors), with careful attention to weight and creatinine clearance.

Future Directions

Current treatment paradigms for MI are founded on anticoagulating medications and invasive therapies that increase the risk for bleeding. Early trials of novel pharmacologic therapies such as fondaparinux and bivalirudin show reduction in both mortality and bleeding risk compared with standard therapies. Their long-term benefit and risk remain to be studied. New anti-ischemic agents, such as fatty acid oxidation inhibitors (ranolazine) and adenosine diphosphate receptor antagonists (prasugrel), are being studied for both acute and chronic treatment of coronary disease. Novel single-strand nucleic acid aptamers, providing the advantages of both high specificity to the target molecule (e.g., factor IXa) and availability of an antidote that allows controlled, rapidly reversible anticoagulation, are also being studied in patients with coronary disease. Studies evaluating newer-generation drug-eluting stents and coronary debulking devices are also ongoing in the hope of minimizing the need for open-chest surgical procedures. In this era of genomics, proteomics, and metabolomics, the ultimate goal is to deliver therapies for MI tailored to individual genetic and phenotypic profiles that will allow optimal outcomes without significant complications.

Additional Resources

Swap CJ, Nagurney JT: Value and limitations of chest pain history in the evaluation of patients with suspected acute coronary syndromes. JAMA 294(20):2623-2629, 2005.

The authors characterize aspects of the chest pain history that help to identify acute coronary syndrome.

Zimetbaum PJ, Josephson ME: Use of the electrocardiogram in acute myocardial infarction. N Engl J Med 348(10):933-940, 2003.

This report examines electrocardiographic features that help guide management and determine prognosis in patients with myocardial infarction.

EVIDENCE

1. Alpert JS, Thygesen K, Antman E, Bassand JP: Myocardial infarction redefined: A consensus document of the Joint European Society of Cardiology/American College of Cardiology Committee for the Redefinition of Myocardial Infarction. J Am Coll Cardiol 36(3):959-969, 2000.

   This consensus statement defines myocardial infarction in various clinical settings.

2. Antman EM, Anbe DT, Armstrong PW, et al: ACC/AHA guidelines for the management of patients with ST-elevation myocardial infarction: A report of the American College of Cardiology/American Heart Association Task Force on Practice Guidelines (Committee to Revise the 1999 Guidelines for the Management of patients with acute myocardial infarction). J Am Coll Cardiol 44(3):E1-E211, 2004.

   This guideline statement provides an overview of STEMI management.

3. Anderson JL, Adams CD, Antman EM, et al. ACC/AHA 2007 Guidelines for the Management of Patients With Unstable Angina/Non ST-Elevation Myocardial Infarction: Executive Summary. A report of the American College of Cardiology/American Heart Association Task Force on Practice Guidelines (Writing Committee to Revise the 2002 Guidelines for the Management of Patients With Unstable Angina/Non ST-Elevation Myocardial Infarction). J Am Coll Cardiol 50:1707-1732, 2007.

   This guideline update summarizes the evidence for current recommended therapies for NSTEMI/UA.

Leonard S. Gettes

30

Electrocardiography

Introduction

In 1902, the Dutch physiologist Willem Eintoven recorded the first electrocardiogram (ECG) from humans. Since then, the number of recording leads has increased from 3 to 12, and the recording instruments have evolved into sophisticated automated digital recorders capable of recording, measuring, and interpreting the electrocardiographic waveform. However, the basic principals underlying the ECG are unchanged. It records, from the body surface, the uncanceled voltage gradients created as myocardial cells sequentially depolarize and repolarize.

The ECG is the most commonly used technique to detect and diagnose heart disease and to monitor therapies that influence the electrical activity of the heart. It is noninvasive, virtually risk free, and relatively inexpensive. Since its introduction, a large database has been assembled correlating the ECG waveform recorded from the body surface to the underlying electrical activity of individual cardiac cells on the one hand, and to the clinical presentation of the patient on the other, thereby providing insight into the electrical behavior of the heart and its modification by physiologic, pharmacologic, and pathologic events.

Leads

Twelve leads are routinely used to record the body surface ECG. Three bipolar limb leads, leads 1, 2 and 3; three augmented limb leads, leads aVR, aVL, and aVF; and six unipolar chest leads, leads V_1 through V_6 (Fig. 30-1). In the bipolar limb leads, the negative pole for each of the leads is different, whereas in the unipolar chest leads, the negative pole is constant and created by the three limb leads. The positive chest lead is, in effect, an exploring lead that can be placed anywhere provided that the ECG reader knows its position. For instance, in children, the routine ECG often includes placing leads on the right side of the chest wall in positions referred to as V_3R and V_4R. Similar right-sided chest leads are often used in adults to diagnose right ventricular infarction, and one or more leads positioned on the back are sometimes used to diagnose posterior wall infarction.

The chest leads are relatively close to the heart and are influenced by the electrical activity directly under the recording electrode. This is in contrast to the limb leads in which the electrodes are placed outside of the body torso. Changes in the position of an individual chest lead or the relationship between the chest leads and the heart may cause significant changes in the ECG pattern. For instance, if the patient is in a sitting rather than a supine position, the relationship of the various chest leads to the heart and the ECG waveform will be affected. Similarly, if the lead is placed an interspace too high or too low, the ECG waveform recorded by that lead will change. For this reason, in assessing a patient with serial ECGs, it is very important that lead placement be consistent and reproducible. In contrast to the situation with chest leads, limb leads may be placed anywhere on the various limbs with little significant alteration of the ECG waveform.

Electrocardiographic Waveform

The ECG waveform consists of a P wave, a PR interval, the QRS complex, an ST segment, and T and U waves. The relationship of these waveform components to the underlying action potentials of the various cardiac tissues is shown in Figure 30-2. The P wave reflects depolarization of the atria, the QRS complex reflects depolarization of the ventricles, and the ST segment and T wave reflect repolarization of the ventricles. The U wave, which occurs after the T wave, is thought to be an electrical event coupled to contraction.

Depolarization of the sinus node occurs before the onset of the P wave, but the voltage gradients created are

Figure 30-1 Electrocardiographic Leads and Reference Lines.

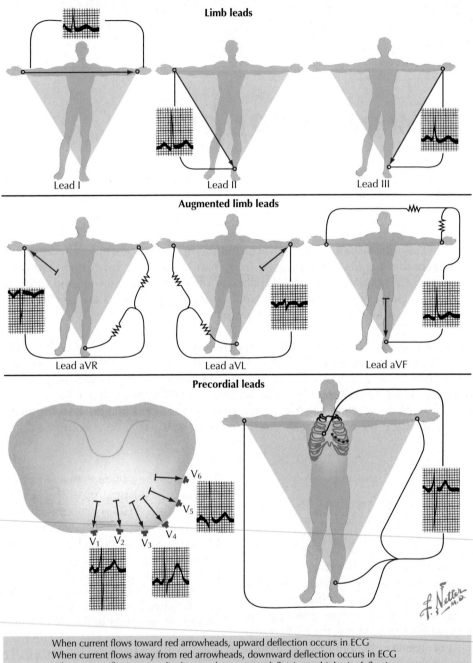

When current flows toward red arrowheads, upward deflection occurs in ECG
When current flows away from red arrowheads, downward deflection occurs in ECG
When current flows perpendicular to red arrows, no deflection or biphasic deflection occurs

too small to be recorded on the body surface by clinically used electrocardiographic machines. Therefore, the event is electrocardiographically silent. Similarly, the electrical activity of the atrioventricular (AV) junction and the His-Purkinje system, which occur during the PR interval, is electrocardiographically silent. Figure 30-3 is an example of the normal ECG.

P Wave

The P wave is caused by the voltage gradients created as the atrial cells sequentially depolarize. The shape and duration of the P wave are determined by the sequence of atrial depolarization and the time required to depolarize the cells of both atria. The sinus node is located at the

Figure 30-2 Relation of Action Potential from the Various Cardiac Regions to the Body Surface ECG.

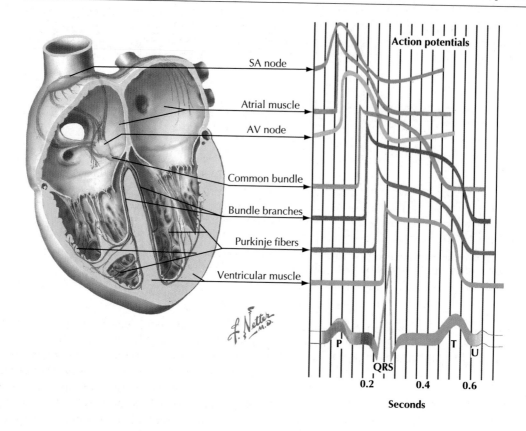

Figure 30-3 Normal ECG.

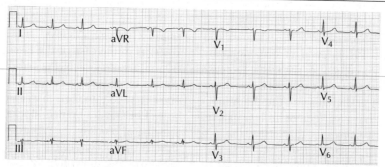

Example of a normal ECG recorded from a 24-year-old woman. Note that the P wave is upright in leads I and II and inverted in aVR. The QRS complex gradually changes from negative to V_1 to positive V_6. Note that the polarity of the T wave is similar to that of the QRS complex.

junction of the superior vena cava and the right atrium, and the direction of atrial depolarization is from right to left, from superior to inferior, and from anterior to posterior. This results in a P wave that is characteristically upright or positive in leads 1, 2, V_5, and V_6 and inverted or negative in lead aVR. In lead V_1, the P wave may be upright, biphasic, or inverted (see Fig. 30-3). The amplitude and duration of the normal sinus P wave may be affected by atrial hypertrophy and dilation and by slowing of interatrial and intra-atrial conduction by atrial fibrosis.

Impulses arising from an ectopic atrial focus are associated with P waves whose shape depends on the location of the focus. If the abnormal focus is in close proximity to the sinus node, the sequence of atrial activation will be normal or nearly normal, and the P wave will resemble the normal sinus P wave described earlier. The further the abnormal ectopic focus is from the sinus node, the more abnormal will be the sequence of atrial activation and the P-wave configuration. For instance, impulses originating in the inferior portion of the atrium or within the AV node will

Figure 30-4 Ectopic Atrial Rhythm.

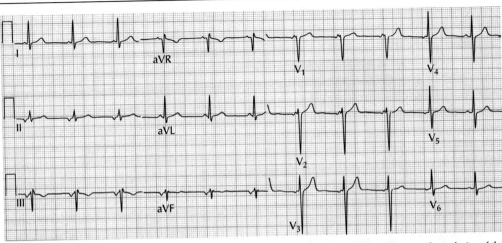

Electrocardiogram showing an ectopic atrial rhythm. It was recorded from a 59-year-old man. The polarity of the P wave is abnormal. It is inverted in leads II, III, and aVF and upright in lead aVR.

depolarize the atria in a retrograde, superiorly oriented direction and will be associated with the P waves that are inverted in leads 2, 3, and aVF and upright in aVR (Fig. 30-4).

PR Interval

The PR interval includes the P wave and the PR segment, that is, the segment from the end of the P wave to the onset of the QRS complex. Although appearing flat or isoelectric on the body surface ECG, the PR segment consists of atrial repolarization and depolarization of the AV node and His-Purkinje system. The PR interval is prolonged by factors that slow AV nodal conduction, such as a decrease in sympathic tone or an increase in vagal tone, by drugs that have these effects such as digitalis and the β-adrenergic blocking agents, and by a variety of inflammatory, infiltrative, and degenerative diseases that affect the AV junction. The PR interval is shortened when impulses reach the ventricles through an AV nodal bypass tract to cause ventricular preexcitation (as in the Wolff-Parkinson-White syndrome).

QRS Complex

The QRS complex reflects ventricular depolarization. The interventricular septum is the first portion of the ventricle to be depolarized. Thereafter, the ventricles depolarize simultaneously, with the impulse spreading from endocardium to epicardium and from apex to base. Because the left ventricle is 3 times the size of the right, its depolarization overshadows and largely obscures right ventricular depolarization. The QRS complex reflects this left ventricular dominance, and for this reason, the QRS complex is usually upright or positive in leads 1, V_5, and V_6, the left-sided and more posterior leads, and negative or inverted in aVR and V_1, the right-sided and more anterior leads. It is only in situations such as right bundle branch block and significant right ventricular hypertrophy that the electrical activity associated with right ventricular depolarization is identified on the ECG.

The QRS complex is altered in both shape and duration by abnormalities in the sequence of ventricular activation. These include the bundle branch blocks (Fig. 30-5), the fascicular blocks, ventricular preexcitation (Fig. 30-6), and nonspecific intraventricular conduction disturbances. The increase in QRS duration may range from a few milliseconds, as in the case of the fascicular blocks, to more than 80 milliseconds, as in the bundle branch blocks. The fascicular blocks reflect conduction slowing in one fascicle of the left bundle and are characterized by a shift in electrical axis. The bundle branch blocks are caused by conduction slowing or block in the right or left bundle branch, usually caused by fibrosis, calcification, or congenital abnormalities involving the conducting system. They are associated with more pronounced abnormalities in the sequence of ventricular activation and thus with more significant changes in the QRS configuration than are associated with the fascicular blocks. Nonspecific conduction abnormalities may occur without a change in QRS configuration and reflect slow conduction throughout the ventricles without a change in the sequence of activation. Such slowing may be caused by cardioactive drugs, an increase in extracellular potassium concentration, and diffuse intraventricular slowing of conduction due to fibrosis or scarring as frequently occurs in patients with severe cardiomyopathies.

The electrocardiographic criteria for the diagnosis of intraventricular conduction disturbances have been published. Important features include the following:

Figure 30-5 Bundle Branch Block.

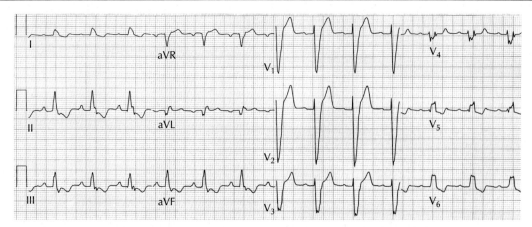

Electrocardiogram showing left bundle branch block. It was recorded from a 73-year-old man. Note that the QRS complex is diffusely widened and is notched in leads V₃, V₄, V₅, and V₆. Note also that the T wave is directed opposite to the QRS complex. This is an example of a secondary T-wave change.

Figure 30-6 Ventricular Preexcitation.

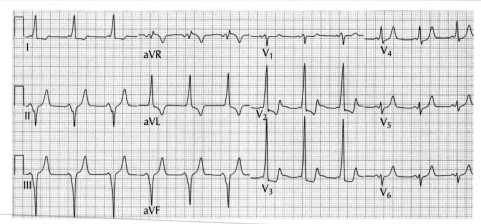

ECG showing ventricular preexcitation. It is recorded from a 28-year-old woman. Note the short PR interval (0.9 sec) and the widened QRS complex (0.134 sec). The initial portion of the QRS complex appears slurred. This is referred to as a *delta wave*. This combination of short PR interval and widened QRS complex with a delta wave is characteristic of ventricular preexcitation. Note also that the T wave is abnormal, another example of a secondary T-wave change.

1. The fascicular blocks not only alter the electrical axis in the frontal plane but also influence the initial portion of the QRS complex. As a result, they may obscure the diagnosis of a prior myocardial infarction while causing other changes that simulate an infarction.

2. Right bundle branch block does not affect the initial portion of the QRS complex because activation of the interventricular septum and the left ventricle are unaffected. Thus the electrocardiographic changes of a prior myocardial infarction or left ventricular hypertrophy can still be appreciated in an individual with a right bundle branch block.

3. Left bundle branch block and ventricular preexcitation do affect the initial portion of the QRS complex. Thus, the ECG changes associated with a prior myocardial infarction and hypertrophy are often obscured and cannot be diagnosed.

4. Abnormalities in the sequence of depolarization are always associated with abnormalities in the sequence of repolarization. This results in changes in the ST segment and T wave that are referred to as *secondary changes*. This is particularly prominent in the setting of left bundle branch block and ventricular preexcitation (see Figs. 30-5 and 30-6).

Figure 30-7 ECG Changes of LV Hypertrophy.

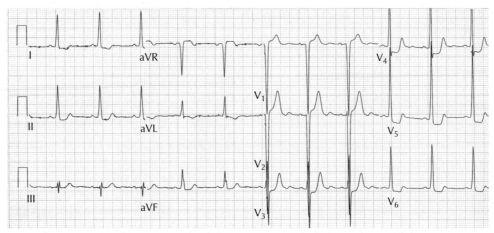

Example of the ECG changes of LV hypertrophy. It is recorded from an 83-year-old woman with aortic stenosis and insufficiency. Note the increase in QRS amplitude, the slight increase in QRS duration to 100 ms, and the ST-segment and T-wave changes.

5. Changes in intraventricular conduction may be rate dependent and present only when the rate is above a critical level or after an early atrial premature beat. In this situation, it is referred to as *rate-dependent aberrant ventricular conduction.*

The amplitude of the QRS complex is subject to a variety of factors: the thickness of the left ventricular and right ventricular walls, the presence of pleural or pericardial fluid, or an increased tissue mass. QRS amplitude is also affected by age, sex, and race. For instance, younger individuals have greater QRS voltages than older individuals, and men have greater QRS voltages than women. In left ventricular hypertrophy, the R wave in the left-sided leads (V$_5$ and V$_6$) and the S wave in the right-sided chest leads (V$_1$ and V$_2$) are increased. QRS duration may increase, reflecting the increased thickness of the left ventricle. There may also be changes in repolarization that cause changes in the ST segment and T wave (Fig. 30-7). Right ventricular hypertrophy is more difficult to diagnose electrocardiographically. Initially it causes cancellation of left ventricular forces, resulting in a decrease in S-wave amplitude in the right-sided leads V$_1$ and V$_2$ and a decrease in R-wave amplitude in the left-sided lead V$_5$ and V$_6$. With more advanced right ventricular hypertrophy, an increased R wave occurs in the right-sided leads and a deeper S wave is seen in the left-sided leads. Pericardial and pleural effusions decrease QRS voltage in all leads, as may infiltrative diseases such as amyloidosis.

ST Segment and T Wave

The ST segment and T wave reflect ventricular repolarization. During the ST segment, the ventricular action potentials are at their plateau voltage, and only minimal voltage gradients are generated. Therefore, the ST segment is at

the same level on the ECG as the TP and PR segments, during which time there are also no voltage gradients created because the action potentials are all at their resting levels. The T wave occurs as a result of the sequential repolarization of the ventricular cells. If the sequence of repolarization were the same as the sequence of depolarization, the T wave would be opposite in direction to the QRS complex. However, the sequence of repolarization is reversed relative to the sequence of depolarization, and as a result, the normal T wave is generally upright or positive in leads with an upright or positive QRS complex (leads 1, V$_5$, and V$_6$) and inverted or negative in leads with an inverted QRS complex (aVR and V$_1$) (see Fig. 30-3).

Abnormalities in repolarization are manifest by elevation or depression of the ST segment and changes in polarity of the T wave. As mentioned, such changes may occur as the result of an intraventricular conduction disturbance, in which case they are referred to as secondary. They may also occur as a result of electrolyte abnormalities or cardioactive drugs or as the manifestation of diseases such as hypertrophy, ischemia, or myocarditis, in which case they are considered to be primary.

Changes in T-wave polarity occurring in the absence of QRS and ST-segment changes are the most difficult ECG abnormalities to interpret because they are nonspecific and may be caused by a variety of nonpathologic as well as pathologic causes. The following guidelines have served as an approach to interpreting T-wave abnormalities:

1. In general, T-wave amplitudes should be equal to or greater than 10% of the QRS amplitude.
2. Inverted T waves in lead 1 are always abnormal and usually indicative of underlying cardiac pathology.
3. Minor T-wave changes such as T-wave flattening or slightly inverted T waves, particularly when they occur in the absence of known cardiac abnormalities or in

Figure 30-8 Changes Associated with Hypokalemia.

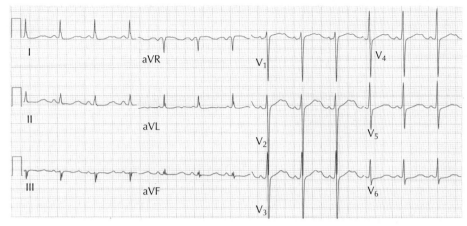

Example of the changes associated with hypokalemia. It is recorded from a 44-year-old man who was receiving long-term thiazide therapy. The QT interval is prolonged due to the presence of a U wave, which interrupts the descending limb of the T wave and is of equal amplitude to the T wave. In this patient, the serum potassium concentration was 2.7 mM.

populations at low risk for cardiac disease, are more likely to be nonspecific and nonpathologic than more marked T-wave changes or T-wave changes occurring in the presence of cardiac disease.

4. Flat or inverted T waves often occur in association with rapid ventricular rates and in the absence of other ECG changes. These changes are nonspecific and not indicative of underlying cardiac disease.

Elevation or depression of the ST segment indicates the creation of voltage gradients during the plateau phase of the ventricular action potentials and, unlike the T-wave changes referred to above, are most often a manifestation of cardiac disease. The most common causes of ST-segment elevation include acute transmural ischemia and pericarditis. High serum potassium and acute myocarditis may also occasionally cause ST-segment elevation and simulate ischemia, although this is quite rare. A normal variant referred to as *early repolarization* is not an uncommon cause of ST elevation, particularly in young males. These changes characteristically occur in the V leads, involve elevation of the junction of the ST segment with the end of the QRS complex, and may simulate acute ischemia or pericarditis.

Left ventricular hypertrophy, cardioactive drugs, low serum potassium, and acute nontransmural or subendocardial ischemia are the most common causes of ST-segment depression.

U Wave

When present, the U wave follows the T wave or may arise within the terminal portion of the T wave and be difficult to distinguish from a notched T wave. The precise etiology of the U wave is not clear, although most believe it is an electrical manifestation of mechanical events. An increase in the magnitude of the U wave or a change in its polarity may occur in several clinical entities. An increase in U-wave amplitude is frequently associated with hypokalemia (Fig. 30-8) and with some direct-acting cardiac drugs. Notching of the T wave resembling an increase in the U-wave amplitude and lengthening of the QT-U interval also often occurs in patients with congenital long QT syndromes (Fig. 30-9).

QT Abnormalities

The interval from the onset of the Q wave to the end of the T wave is referred to as the QT interval and includes the QRS complex, the ST segment, and the T wave. Changes in the duration of any of these components will alter the QT interval. The QT interval is rate dependent, becoming shorter at the more rapid rate and longer at slower heart rates. This reflects the rate-dependent changes in action potential duration. To accommodate this rate dependency, several correction factors have been applied to the measured QT interval and used to generate the term referred to as QTc on automated recording systems. In addition to changes in heart rate, the QT interval is influenced by the following:

1. Temperature
2. Drugs
3. Electrolyte abnormalities
4. Genetic factors
5. Neurogenic factors
6. Ischemia

There is an extensive and ever-increasing list of drugs that lengthen the QT interval by prolonging the ST segment or the T wave. For this reason, it is often

Figure 30-9 Congenital Long QT Syndrome.

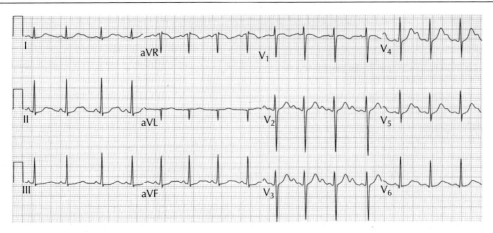

Recorded from a 16-year-old girl with syncopal episodes that were documented to be due to rapid ventricular tachycardia. It is an example of long QT syndrome. The T wave is notched and prolonged in much the same way as was shown in the patient with hypokalemia. However, in this patient, the serum potassium concentration was normal.

necessary to monitor the ECG when drugs recognized as having potential for lengthening the QT interval are initiated. The lengthening of the QT interval following administration of these drugs is clinically important because it may be a harbinger of a specific type of ventricular tachycardia, torsades de pointes, which may progress to ventricular fibrillation and cause sudden cardiac death.

Low serum potassium and low serum calcium are both associated with prolongation of the QT interval. However, their electrocardiographic patterns are different and distinctive. Low potassium causes ST-segment depression T-wave changes, a prominent U wave, and prolongation of the QT-U interval (see Fig. 30-8), whereas low calcium lengthens the ST segment without causing significant T-wave changes (Fig. 30-10). An increase in serum potassium and serum calcium shortens the QT interval by shortening the ST segment. In addition, high potassium shortens the duration of the T wave and makes it more symmetrical, giving it the appearance of a tented or peaked T wave (Fig. 30-11).

Abnormalities in one or more of the several genes that regulate the repolarizing currents are responsible for causing the congenital long QT syndromes and are a significant cause of sudden cardiac death in younger individuals due to ventricular arrhythmias. The ECG patterns associated with congenital long QT intervals are often difficult to distinguish from electrolyte abnormalities (see Fig. 30-9).

Marked QT prolongation and a deeply inverted T wave occur frequently within the first several days following an acute myocardial infarction, particularly when the infarction is due to occlusion of the left anterior descending coronary artery. This QT prolongation usually resolves, although the T-wave inversion may persist for long periods of time. Similar T-wave and QT-interval changes may

occur in the chest leads following an acute ischemic event but in the absence of an infarction (Fig. 30-12). This particular ECG pattern usually indicates a severely but not totally obstructed proximal portion of the left anterior descending coronary artery.

Some neurologic events, particularly intracranial hemorrhage and an increase in intracranial pressure, may cause T-wave inversion and dramatic lengthening of the QT intervals, very similar to that shown in Figure 30-12. When it occurs in this clinical setting, it is referred to as the *cerebrovascular accident pattern* and is thought to represent an imbalance of sympathetic stimulation. It is self-limited, and the ECG generally returns to normal within a few days.

Acute Ischemia and Infarction

Acute myocardial ischemia and infarction cause characteristic changes in the ST segment, QRS complex, and T wave, which permit early diagnosis and prompt treatment—either thrombolytic therapy or percutaneous coronary revascularization—that can reverse ischemia and prevent the loss of myocardial cells and subsequent scarring with its attendant effects on morbidity and mortality. For this reason, the ECG is the single most important test currently available for the early detection of acute ischemia and infarction.

The sequence of ECG changes associated with acute ischemia and infarction is as follows:

1. Peaking of the T wave
2. ST-segment elevation or depression
3. Development of abnormal Q waves
4. T-wave inversion

These changes can be understood by recognizing that acute ischemia or infarction is caused by occlusion of a

Figure 30-10 ST-Segment and QT-Interval Changes Associated with Hypocalcemia.

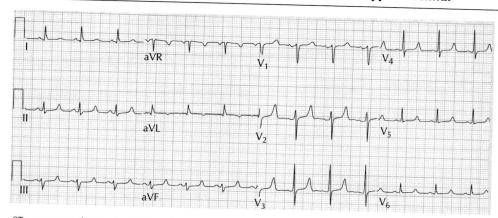

ST-segment and QT-interval changes associated with hypocalcemia. It is recorded from a 53-year-old man with chronic renal disease. The ST segment is prolonged, but the T wave is normal. The QT interval reflects ST-segment lengthening and is prolonged.

Figure 30-11 Changes Associated with Hyperkalemia.

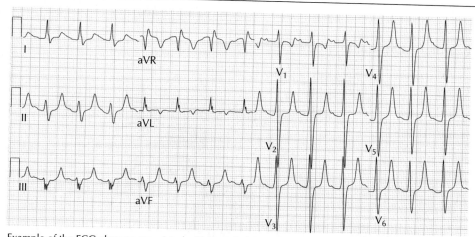

Example of the ECG changes associated with hyperkalemia. It is recorded from a 29-year-old woman with chronic renal disease. The P wave is broad and difficult to identify in some leads. The QRS is diffusely widened (0.188 sec), and the T wave is peaked and symmetrical. These changes are characteristic of severe hyperkalemia, and in this patient, the serum potassium concentration was 8.2 mM.

coronary artery and is localized to the myocardial region supplied by that artery. This produces a gradient of changes between the ischemic and nonischemic regions that are separated by a rather well-defined border zone (Fig. 30-13).

Peaking of the T waves in leads overlying the ischemic region is the earliest ECG manifestation of acute transmural ischemia and is transient. It is only rarely observed because the ECG is usually not recorded early enough to permit its detection unless the patient is in a hospital setting when ischemia first begins. ST elevation and depression are the most frequently observed early changes and occur within minutes of the onset of the acute event. The ST changes are caused by voltage gradients across the ischemic border that result in an electrical current,

referred to as an *injury current*, flowing across the ischemic borders. Whether these injury currents cause ST elevation or depression depends on whether the ischemic zone is transmural, extending from endocardium to epicardium, or is nontransmural and localized to the subendocardial region, and on the relationship of the recording electrodes to the ischemic border. In general, electrodes directly overlying a region of transmural ischemia will record ST elevation, whereas all other electrodes will record ST depression or no change in the ST segment.

Subendocardial ischemia, such as that associated with subtotal coronary occlusion, and that which is often brought on by exercise in patients with flow-limiting coronary artery obstruction, does not extend to the epicardium.

Figure 30-12 T-Wave Changes Induced by a Recent Ischemic Event.

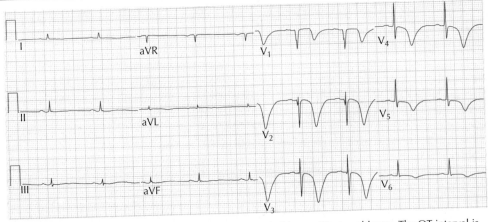

T-wave changes induced by a recent ischemic event, recorded from a 70-year-old man. The QT interval is prolonged, and the T waves are markedly inverted in the precordial leads (V_1 through V_6). These changes gradually evolved over several days, and coronary angiography recorded the day this tracing was taken revealed a subtotal occlusion of the left anterior descending coronary artery.

Figure 30-13 Myocardial Ischemia, Injury, and Infarction.

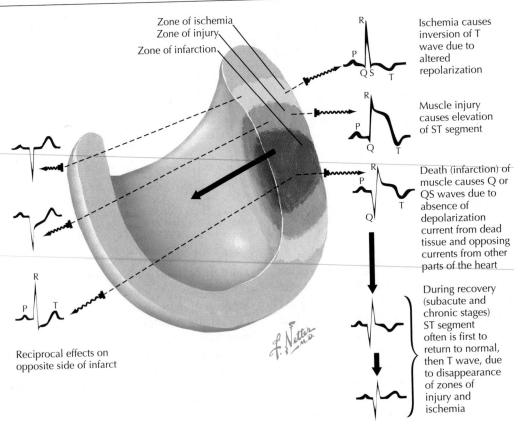

Zone of ischemia
Zone of injury
Zone of infarction

Ischemia causes inversion of T wave due to altered repolarization

Muscle injury causes elevation of ST segment

Death (infarction) of muscle causes Q or QS waves due to absence of depolarization current from dead tissue and opposing currents from other parts of the heart

During recovery (subacute and chronic stages) ST segment often is first to return to normal, then T wave, due to disappearance of zones of injury and ischemia

Reciprocal effects on opposite side of infarct

Figure 30-14 Abnormal Cardiac Rhythms.

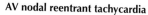

AV nodal reentrant tachycardia

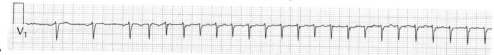

A

Lead V_1 recorded from a patient with abnormal cardiac rhythms. This tracing shows the onset of AV nodal reentrant tachycardia in a 47-year-old man. There are three sinus beats followed by an atrial premature beat, which initiates a run of AV nodal reentrant tachycardia, with a rate of 170 beats/min.

Atrial fibrillation

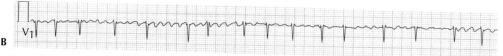

B

Example of atrial fibrillation in a 50-year-old woman. Note the undulating baseline and the irregularly irregular QRS complexes, with a rate of 105 beats/min.

Ventricular tachycardia

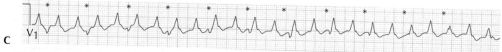

C

Ventricular tachycardia with a rate of 150 beats/min from a 56-year-old man. The QRS complex is widened, and there is AV disassociation. The P waves, with an atrial rate of 73 beats/min, are marked with an asterisk.

Complete AV block

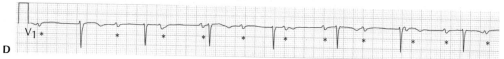

D

Complete AV block from a 78-year-old woman. The atrial rate is 70 beats/min, and the ventricular rate is 46 beats/min. There is no relation between the P waves (marked with an asterisk) and the QRS complexes.

Thus, none of the body surface leads directly overlie the ischemic region, and ST depression, rather than ST elevation, is recorded.

The development of abnormal Q waves indicates slowed or absent conduction through the ischemic region and implies the presence of severely depressed or infarcted tissue, whereas the T-wave changes that occur after the ischemic event reflect changes in repolarization and may persist for periods ranging from days to years.

These various ECG changes permit the localization of the ischemic or infracted region and, by inference, the identification of the occluded vessel.

Arrhythmias

The ECG is indispensable for the diagnosis of brady-arrhythmias and tachyarrhythmias. For instance, a heart rate greater than 100 beats/min may have multiple causes, including sinus tachycardia, atrial and AV junctional tachycardia (Fig. 30-14A), atrial flutter, atrial fibrillation (Fig. 30-14 B), and ventricular tachycardia (Fig. 30-14C). The rate and configuration of the P wave, its relation to the QRS complexes, and the shape and duration of the

QRS complex establish the correct diagnosis. Abnormally slow heat rates may also be caused by several entities, including sinus bradycardia or sinoatrial or AV block (Fig. 30-14D). Again, the diagnosis can be established by noting the rate, regularity, and configuration of the P wave and QRS complexes, the relation of the P wave to the QRS complexes, and the PR interval.

Irregular rhythms may be due to atrial and ventricular premature beats (Fig. 30-15A, B), atrial fibrillation (see Fig. 30-14B), and incomplete (second-degree) sinoatrial or AV block (Fig. 30-15C).

Future Directions

The ECG provides a window into the electrophysiologic properties of the heart and their modification by physiologic, pharmacologic, and pathologic factors. When correctly interpreted, it is of inestimable help in the diagnosis and treatment of a wide variety of cardiac diseases. It is of particular importance in the diagnosis of myocardial ischemia and arrhythmias. The use of the ECG recorded during daily activities and during stress further adds to its capabilities. The value of the ECG is greatly enhanced

Figure 30-15 Irregular Cardiac Rhythms.

Atrial premature beats

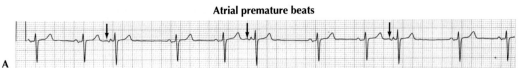

A

Atrial premature beats (shown with an *arrow*) recorded from a 77-year-old man. In this example, there is an atrial premature beat after every two sinus beats. This is referred to as *atrial trigeminy*. Note that the shape of the premature P wave is different from that of the sinus P waves, reflecting its ectopic location.

Ventricular premature beats

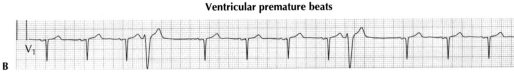

B

Ventricular premature beats recorded from a 30-year-old man with no known heart disease.

Type I second-degree AV block

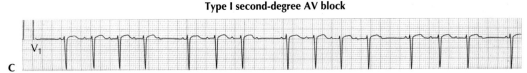

C

Type I second-degree AV block with Wenckebach periodicity recorded from a 74-year-old man. There is progressive prolongation of the PR interval, followed by a blocked or nonconducted P wave. This leads to irregular groups of QRS complexes. In this example, there is 5:4 and 4:3 AV block. The atrial rate is 110 beats/min, and the ventricular rate is 90 beats/min.

when pertinent patient information, such as symptoms, drug usage, and important laboratory findings, is provided to the reader. It is reasonable to anticipate that in the future, additional leads such as V_3R, V_4R, and V_{7-9} may be recorded; that new analytic measurements, particularly those dealing with the QRS complex and the T wave, will be developed; and that the library of diagnostic and prognostic statements will be expanded. However, it is important to stress that the automated interpretations provided by computerized ECG systems now and in the future may be incomplete or inaccurate, particularly when the tracing is abnormal, and require over-reading by qualified personnel.

Additional Resources

Kligfield P, Gettes LS, Bailey JJ, et al: Recommendations for the standardization and interpretation of the electrocardiogram. Part I: The electrocardiogram and its technology: A scientific statement from the American Heart Association Electrocardiography and Arrhythmias Committee, Council on Clinical Cardiology; the American College of Cardiology Foundation; and the Heart Rhythm Society Endorsed by the International Society for Computerized Electrocardiology. Circulation 115:1306-1324, 2007.

This is the first part of a series of reports designed to update ECG standards and interpretation. This paper focuses on the computerized, automated technology currently employed. It emphasizes areas that have clinical relevance.

Mason JW, Hancock EW, Gettes LS: Recommendations for the standardization and interpretation of the electrocardiogram. Part II: Electrocardiography diagnostic statement list: A scientific statement from the American Heart Association Electrocardiography and Arrhythmias Committee, Council on Clinical Cardiology; the American College of Cardiology Foundation; and the Heart Rhythm Society: Endorsed by the International Society for Computerized Electrocardiology. Circulation 115;1325-1332, 2007.

This is the second part of the ECG standards series. It provides a set of diagnostic statements that are more concise and streamlined than existing diagnostic statements. If accepted, these statements should eliminate differences in the various systems currently in use.

EVIDENCE

1. Chou TC: In Surawicz B, Knilans TK (eds): Chou's Electrocardiography in Clinical Practice: Adult and Pediatric, 5th ed. Philadelphia, WB Saunders, 2001.
   This is a complete text with excellent figures and extensive, up-to-date references.
2. Gettes LS: ECG Tutor [CD-ROM]. Armonk, NY, Future Publishing, 2000.
   This animated graphic CD-ROM illustrates the electrophysiologic basis for the ECG and the interpretive approach.
3. Surawicz B: Electrophysiologic Basis of ECG and Cardiac Arrhythmias. Philadelphia, Williams & Wilkins, 1995.
   The author provides an in-depth correlation of basic electrophysiologic phenomena to the waveform of the normal and abnormal body surface ECG.

George A. Stouffer ▪ Leslie P. Wong ▪ Marschall S. Runge

31

Peripheral Arterial Disease

Introduction

Peripheral arterial disease (PAD) refers to stenosis or occlusion in the arteries of the lower extremities. Most patients with PAD are asymptomatic. Symptomatic patients can present with mild symptoms, occurring only with extreme exertion to symptoms with moderate exertion, or with severe symptoms occurring at rest with ongoing limb ischemia. In the Framingham Study, and other population studies, PAD is generally a disease of aging. Intermittent claudication, occurring as a result of PAD, increases in prevalence in late middle age. The incidence of PAD is negligible in young adulthood but is present, depending on the definition used, in 10% to 30% of adults older than 50 years. PAD is a marker for the presence of coronary and cerebrovascular disease, and in many patients with PAD, the development and progression of atherosclerosis is a diffuse systemic process (Fig. 31-1). An estimated 60% of patients with PAD have coronary artery disease, cerebrovascular disease, or both. Stroke and myocardial infarction occur in patients with PAD at a rate about 3 times greater than in those without PAD, even among individuals with no vascular symptoms.

Recognizing the link between PAD of the extremities and atherosclerosis elsewhere has led to the integration of therapies that target not only claudication but also cardiovascular death and morbidity.

Etiology and Pathogenesis

Atherogenesis begins with injury to the vascular endothelium and formation of an atherosclerotic plaque. This process is potentiated by a local leukocyte-mediated inflammation and oxidized lipoprotein species, particularly low-density lipoproteins. Although many advances have been made in recent years, the precise molecular mechanisms by which smoking, hypercholesterolemia, diabetes, and hypertension accelerate atherosclerosis remain the focus of ongoing investigation.

The presence of endothelial dysfunction and fatty streaks (the predecessor of atherosclerotic plaques) is ubiquitous in Western countries, as documented by autopsy studies on young adults dying of other causes. According to current theories, plaques probably expand in increments owing to subclinical episodes of plaque rupture, although plaques likely also undergo gradual enlargement with accretion of cells and noncellular material in the lipid-rich core. Most commonly, the plaque core is surrounded by a complex fibrotic cap composed of calcium, connective tissue, and smooth muscle cells. Stable symptoms, such as those of claudication, result from an inability to increase blood flow at times of increased demand. Plaque rupture exposes the highly thrombogenic core to circulating blood elements, resulting in platelet activation and aggregation, along with activation of fibrinogen.

As noted, plaque rupture often only worsens an existing lesion without causing arterial occlusion or clinical symptoms. However, more significant episodes of plaque rupture result in worsening limb ischemia with effort, or ischemia at rest. These symptoms result from either thrombotic occlusion of a peripheral artery or embolization of a thrombus with occlusion of small distal arteries. Depending on the location of a thrombotic occlusion, urgent revascularization can be indicated.

The same factors that predispose to coronary atherosclerosis increase the likelihood of PAD. These include male gender, smoking, diabetes, hypertension, and hypercholesterolemia. Of these, the strongest association is between cigarette smoking and PAD.

Figure 31-1 Carotid Artery Stenosis.

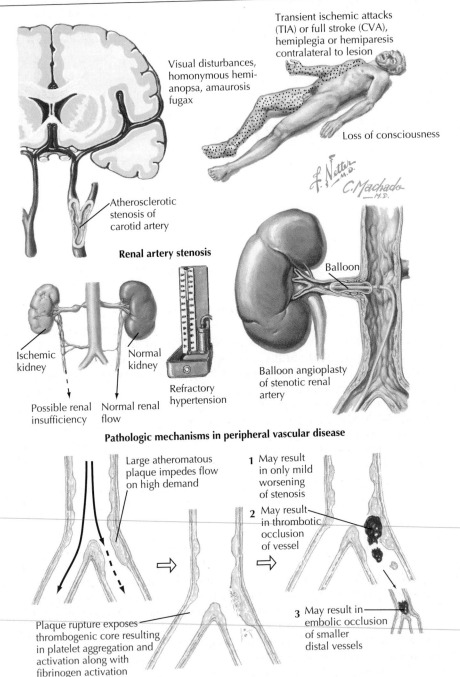

Transient ischemic attacks (TIA) or full stroke (CVA), hemiplegia or hemiparesis contralateral to lesion

Visual disturbances, homonymous hemianopsa, amaurosis fugax

Loss of consciousness

Atherosclerotic stenosis of carotid artery

Renal artery stenosis

Ischemic kidney

Normal kidney

Balloon

Possible renal insufficiency

Normal renal flow

Refractory hypertension

Balloon angioplasty of stenotic renal artery

Pathologic mechanisms in peripheral vascular disease

Large atheromatous plaque impedes flow on high demand

1 May result in only mild worsening of stenosis

2 May result in thrombotic occlusion of vessel

Plaque rupture exposes thrombogenic core resulting in platelet aggregation and activation along with fibrinogen activation

3 May result in embolic occlusion of smaller distal vessels

Clinical Presentation

PAD produces symptoms of claudication. Derived from the Latin word *claudatico*, "to limp," claudication describes pain in the lower extremities produced by inadequate blood flow during exercise. Claudication occurs when there is a reduction in arterial lumen that prevents a sufficient increase in blood flow when tissue oxygen demands increase with exercise. In these cases, exercise-induced local vasodilation is frequently also impaired. This combi-

nation results in local ischemia and production of lactic acid and other metabolites that are responsible for the pain associated with claudication.

Claudication is manifested by cramping pain in the lower extremities or buttocks that is reliably produced by a threshold level of exercise. This pain is relieved by a few minutes of rest. Elevation of the limb can worsen claudication, whereas holding the limb in a dependent position may help. Symptoms may be unilateral or bilateral, depending on the extent and location of atherosclerotic disease.

Calf claudication most commonly occurs because of femoral artery stenoses, whereas foot involvement suggests popliteal or proximal tibioperoneal arterial disease. Thigh and buttock pain are indicative of aortoiliac involvement. As PAD worsens in severity, claudication may occur at night and at rest.

In community cohort studies, ambulatory patients with PAD most commonly reported exertional leg pain atypical for claudication, no symptoms, or intermittent claudication, in that order. Classic claudication occurs in less than one third of patients with PAD. Some patients may experience only mild leg discomfort with exercise and not communicate this to their physician, misinterpreting these symptoms as a normal consequence of aging. Because even asymptomatic patients with PAD still incur a higher relative risk for adverse cardiovascular events, it is important to maintain a high index of suspicion for atypical symptoms of claudication.

Critical limb ischemia is a rare, but potentially fatal, complication of PAD. It is manifested by pain, typically described as a burning pain in the foot that occurs at rest. The pain worsens when the foot is elevated and is relieved when the feet are in a dependent position. In addition to pain, limb ischemia is manifested by nonhealing wounds or tissue necrosis. The development of critical limb ischemia usually requires multiple sites of severe obstruction in the arteries of the lower extremity.

The most useful findings on physical examination in patients with PAD are the presence of arterial bruits and decreased pulses in the lower extremity. In patients with symptoms at rest, additional findings may include cool skin, pallor, dependent rubor, atrophic skin and nails, delayed capillary refill, and ischemic ulcers. Ischemic ulcers tend to be painful and usually occur at the lateral malleolus, tips of the toes, metatarsal heads, or bunion area. In contrast, venous stasis ulcers are usually painless and occur on the medial malleolus. Ulcers, poor wound healing, and frank gangrene can develop with chronic critical ischemia (Fig. 31-2). The absence of any bruits (iliac, femoral, or popliteal) or pulse abnormalities reduces the likelihood of significant PAD.

Loss of femoral and all distal pulses bilaterally, referred to as Leriche's syndrome, is caused by occlusion at the aortoiliac bifurcation.

Differential Diagnosis

Distinguishing true claudication from its mimic, pseudoclaudication (a symptom of spinal stenosis), by clinical symptoms is very important because the diagnostic approach and treatment for the two entities are completely different. In distinction from the symptoms of claudication, pseudoclaudication is characteristically less reproducible based on a specific effort level. Rather than being relieved by cessation of exercise, pseudoclaudication typically is only relieved with sitting or other lumbar flexion

Box 31-1 Differential Diagnosis of Claudication
■ Osteoarthritis
■ Deep venous thrombosis
■ Ruptured Baker's cyst
■ Atheroembolism
■ Chronic venous insufficiency
■ Diabetic neuropathy
■ Reflex sympathetic dystrophy
■ Chronic compartment syndrome
■ Popliteal artery entrapment
■ Restless leg syndrome
■ Remote trauma
■ Radiation injury
■ Ergotamine abuse
■ Vasospasm
■ Vasculitis (e.g., thromboangiitis obliterans, Takayasu's disease)
■ Lymphangitis
■ Phlebitic syndrome after deep venous thrombosis

maneuvers that increase spinal canal volume (spinal stenosis is discussed in more detail in Section XV, "Disorders of the Immune System, Connective Tissue, and Joints"). One useful way to differentiate claudication from pseudoclaudication is to ask the patient what happens when he or she stands still after walking—the discomfort of pseudoclaudication will remain constant (improving only with a change of position such as sitting), whereas the discomfort of claudication will improve.

Alternative diagnoses should be actively sought in patients younger than 50 years and without predisposing risk factors. The extensive differential diagnosis is shown in Box 31-1.

Diagnostic Approach

A careful history and physical exam are essential for the correct diagnosis of PAD and should include a thorough elicitation of symptoms (Fig. 31-3). When PAD is suspected, an ankle-brachial index (ABI) should be measured. This is done by recording the systolic blood pressure by Doppler ultrasound in the brachial artery and comparing it with the pressure in the dorsalis pedis and posterior tibial arteries (Fig. 31-4). The ratio of the highest measurement of the lower extremity divided by arm pressure for each side of the body is calculated. An ABI ≤0.90 has a sensitivity of 95% and a specificity near 100% for identifying PAD. An ABI ≤0.70 is indicative of moderate PAD, with an ABI ≤0.40 consistent with severe PAD. Extremities that are ischemic at rest are generally associated with an ABI ≤0.20.

Sensitivity may be increased by measuring the ABI following exercise treadmill testing. Elderly patients and those with diabetes or renal insufficiency may have significant vessel calcification resulting in an artifactually elevated

Figure 31-2 Lower Extremity Arterial Occlusive Disease.

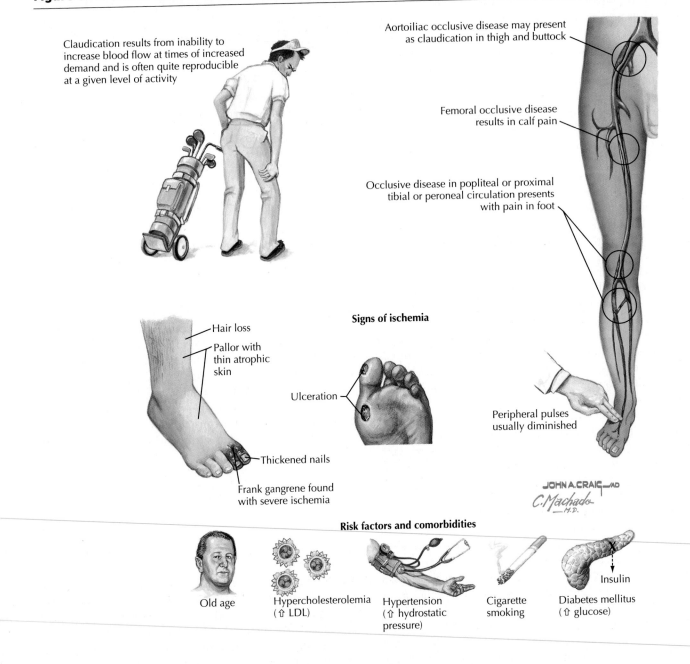

Claudication results from inability to increase blood flow at times of increased demand and is often quite reproducible at a given level of activity

Aortoiliac occlusive disease may present as claudication in thigh and buttock

Femoral occlusive disease results in calf pain

Occlusive disease in popliteal or proximal tibial or peroneal circulation presents with pain in foot

Signs of ischemia

Hair loss

Pallor with thin atrophic skin

Ulceration

Peripheral pulses usually diminished

Thickened nails

Frank gangrene found with severe ischemia

JOHN A. CRAIG—MD
C. Machado—M.D.

Risk factors and comorbidities

Old age

Hypercholesterolemia (⇧ LDL)

Hypertension (⇧ hydrostatic pressure)

Cigarette smoking

Insulin

Diabetes mellitus (⇧ glucose)

ABI >1.3. These patients are better evaluated with toe-brachial pressure index measurements. Arterial Doppler ultrasound studies and plethysmography are noninvasive modalities that are often useful in diagnosing PAD.

Contrast angiography remains the gold standard for complete assessment and definition of the arterial vasculature (see Fig. 31-4). Angiography is necessary if revascularization is being considered, but not essential for clinical diagnosis. The severity of symptoms or objective evidence of effort-related or rest ischemia and the goal of pursuing revascularization should be considered before proceeding with percutaneous or surgical revascularization. Because of the risks, however small, of arterial injury and contrast-induced nephrotoxicity, angiography should only be considered if revascularization is a viable option.

Computed tomographic angiography (CTA) and magnetic resonance angiography (MRA) have been touted as alternatives to angiography. A recent meta-analysis showed high accuracy in assessing lower extremity arterial disease, particularly with three-dimensional gadolinium-enhanced images. Although neither CTA nor MRA has supplanted traditional arteriography in the preoperative mapping of vessels, these promising tools merit further study (see Fig. 31-4).

Figure 31-3 Evaluation of Suspected Peripheral Arterial Disease.

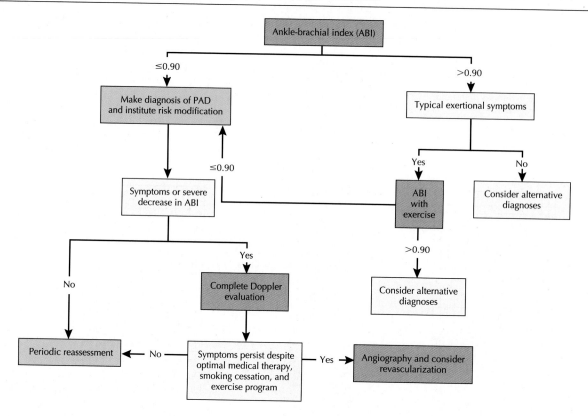

Management and Therapy

Exercise programs, smoking reduction, medical therapy, and reduction of cardiovascular risk factors are the cornerstones of treatment of PAD. Revascularization is indicated for rest ischemia or in cases of effort-induced ischemia that are refractory to maximal medical therapy.

Medical Management

Smoking is strongly related to the progression of atherosclerosis and is associated with a higher risk for amputation. Tobacco use is also linked to increased cardiovascular death and events. Smoking cessation programs and, if necessary, treatment with nicotine replacement or other medical approaches should be strongly considered.

Diabetes is a major cardiovascular risk factor and important in patients with PAD because diabetes is associated with a uniformly worse prognosis. Although large prospective trials have not shown a direct effect on PAD with intensive glycemic control in diabetes, given the benefit in reducing microvascular complications, a goal HbA1C (hemoglobin A1C) of less than 7% is warranted. Tight glycemic control may delay the development of peripheral neuropathy, which can complicate the treatment of PAD.

Hypertension is closely linked to development of atherosclerosis. Although lowering of blood pressure has not been clearly shown to reduce claudication, the mortality benefit in cardiovascular disease is clear. The recommendations of the sixth Joint National Committee on Hypertension outline a goal blood pressure of less than 130/85 mm Hg for most patients with PAD. Angiotensin-converting enzyme inhibitors should be considered first-line agents, along with diuretics and β-blockers. In recent years, the proposed detrimental effect of β-blockers on claudication has been shown to rarely present a problem.

Hypercholesterolemia is a key component of atherogenesis. Lipid-lowering therapy with hydroxymethyl glutaryl–coenzyme A (HMG-CoA) reductase inhibitors (statins) has been shown to improve claudication, induce stabilization of atherosclerotic lesions, and provide effective secondary prevention of cardiovascular events. Recent studies indicate that statin therapy not only reduces cardiac events but also reduces the risk for stroke and death from stroke. Early reports suggest that statins will improve outcomes in patients with PAD.

Antiplatelet agents are recommended in PAD. Treatment with aspirin (81 to 325 mg daily) reduces death and disability from stroke and myocardial infarction. The combination of aspirin and dipyridamole is not clearly better than aspirin alone. Ticlopidine is effective for reducing claudication severity and adverse cardiovascular events, but its use has declined because of its association with thrombotic thrombocytopenic purpura. Clopidogrel is slightly superior to aspirin in reducing ischemic complications related to vascular disease, but the absolute risk reduction

Figure 31-4 Peripheral Vascular Disease.

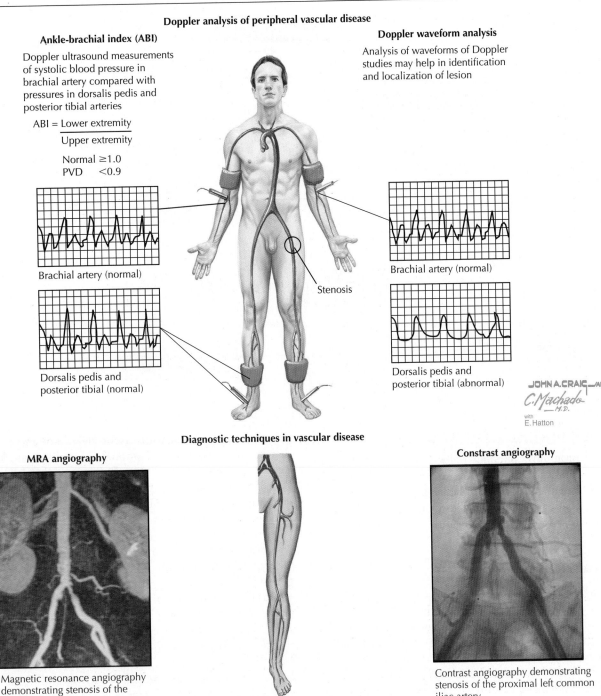

Doppler analysis of peripheral vascular disease

Ankle-brachial index (ABI)

Doppler ultrasound measurements of systolic blood pressure in brachial artery compared with pressures in dorsalis pedis and posterior tibial arteries

$$ABI = \frac{\text{Lower extremity}}{\text{Upper extremity}}$$

Normal ≥1.0
PVD   <0.9

Brachial artery (normal)

Dorsalis pedis and posterior tibial (normal)

Doppler waveform analysis

Analysis of waveforms of Doppler studies may help in identification and localization of lesion

Stenosis

Brachial artery (normal)

Dorsalis pedis and posterior tibial (abnormal)

JOHN A. CRAIG—MD
C. Machado—M.D.
with
E. Hatton

Diagnostic techniques in vascular disease

MRA angiography

Magnetic resonance angiography demonstrating stenosis of the proximal left common iliac artery

Constrast angiography

Contrast angiography demonstrating stenosis of the proximal left common iliac artery

is small, and the cost-effectiveness of clopidogrel versus aspirin is uncertain. In patients who cannot tolerate aspirin, clopidogrel is an effective alternative.

In intermittent claudication, exercise significantly improves maximal walking time, time until the appearance of claudication, and overall walking ability. The benefits of exercise appear to occur exclusive of a significant improvement in blood flow. With training, skeletal muscle oxidative capacity increases, and exercise-related inflammation decreases. Exercise also improves overall cardiorespiratory efficiency, reduces insulin resistance, and has a beneficial effect on lipids. This leads to increased functional capacity as measured by improved walking distance and quality of life. The optimal exercise program for patients with PAD involves walking to near-maximal pain several times per week. An exercise program should be

continued for at least 3 months before efficacy is assessed.

Anticlaudicatory agents can also be used to improve symptoms. Two drugs are approved for claudication: pentoxifylline and cilostazol. Trials of pentoxifylline have shown mixed results, and presently pentoxifylline is not routinely recommended. Cilostazol, an inhibitor of phosphodiesterase type 3, has demonstrated benefits in symptom relief, exercise capacity, and quality of life compared with placebo and pentoxifylline. The clinical benefits are modest relative to its cost, and cilostazol should probably be reserved for patients with disabling symptoms who are not candidates for revascularization. Cilostazol is contraindicated in congestive heart failure. Gingko biloba may have some small benefit. Vasodilators, chelation, vitamin E, testosterone, and estrogen have not shown any effect and are not currently indicated.

Revascularization

Revascularization should be considered for patients who have symptoms refractory to comprehensive medical management or in individuals who cannot tolerate medical therapy because of medication side effects. Two approaches are used: percutaneous intervention and surgical bypass. The choice depends on the length of the obstruction and location of the diseased arterial segment. Regardless of the technique chosen, early referral to an experienced interventional radiologist, interventional cardiologist, or a vascular surgeon is prudent.

Percutaneous Angioplasty

Percutaneous angioplasty (with or without endovascular stent placement) of the stenoses in diseased vessels has become more common in recent years as an alternative to traditional surgical bypass. Endovascular intervention is the treatment of choice for focal stenoses less than 3 cm long. Stenoses 3 to 5 cm long are also often amenable to percutaneous approaches (Fig. 31-5).

Percutaneous revascularization for PAD remains controversial in several areas. First, the comparison of percutaneous and surgical revascularization is understudied. Second, the use of stents has revolutionized coronary revascularization and will likely also improve percutaneous revascularization for PAD, although few studies have directly compared balloon angioplasty and stenting. Third, as for percutaneous revascularization in the coronary vasculature, technical improvements have greatly improved outcomes and safety. Finally, patient preference plays a large role. The lack of clear consensus on optimum therapy and individual variation in symptoms means various patients may opt for different therapies despite angiographically similar disease.

These factors, along with more rapid recovery than from surgery, have led to a dramatic increase in the use of percutaneous approaches. Until prospective, randomized studies are conducted, there will undoubtedly be considerable variation in practice for treating individuals with limiting symptoms from PAD.

Surgical Therapy

Surgical bypass of the atherosclerotic vessel should be considered for carefully selected patients. Because operative mortality rates range from 1% to 3%, the benefits of surgery must be carefully weighed against the risk involved. Ideally, candidates should be younger than 70 years, nondiabetic, and have little distal arterial involvement. Bypass is the intervention of choice for multifocal stenoses and segments more than 5 cm in length. Aortofemoral bypass for iliac disease results in more than 90% patency at 5 years. Infrainguinal procedures such as femoral-popliteal bypass share high long-term patency rates. Localized stenosis may be corrected by endarterectomy. Patients with PAD necessitating surgery often have coexisting coronary artery disease and must be screened appropriately before surgery.

Optimum Treatment

In patients with stable symptoms of PAD, optimal treatment includes:

- Smoking cessation
- Exercise program
- Blood pressure control
- Diabetes management
- Cholesterol management with HMG-CoA reductase inhibitors
- Antiplatelet therapy
- Revascularization if lifestyle-limiting symptoms persist despite optimal medical therapy

Avoiding Treatment Errors

There are several potential treatment errors to be avoided. Claudication is occasionally confused with pseudoclaudication. As noted previously, pseudoclaudication is characterized by pain and discomfort in the buttocks, legs, and feet and is positional (whereas claudication occurs with exertion). Another potential treatment error is failing to prescribe cholesterol-lowering therapy in patients with PAD. Most patients with PAD will die of myocardial infarction, and thus cholesterol-lowering therapy has the potential to improve survival as well as improve symptoms.

Future Directions

Many new medications are under investigation. Levocarnitine, prostaglandins, naftidrofuryl, defibrotide, and angiogenic factors may someday be added to the armamentarium for treatment of claudication. Advances in the

Figure 31-5 Percutaneous Peripheral Angioplasty, Surgical Bypass Procedures.

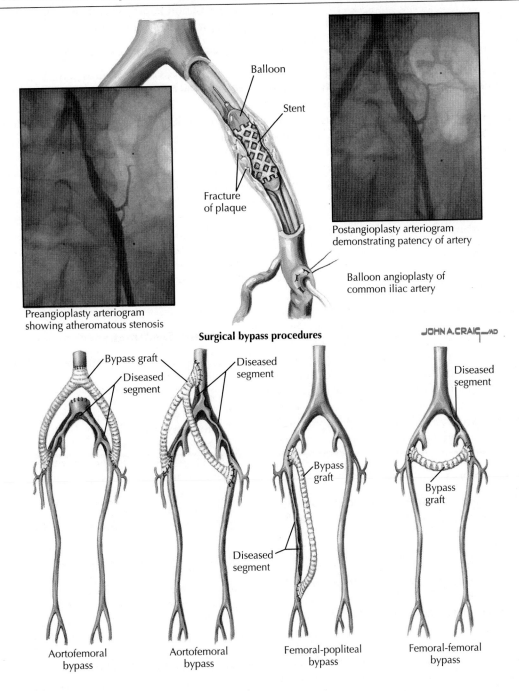

Balloon

Stent

Fracture
of plaque

Preangioplasty arteriogram
showing atheromatous stenosis

Postangioplasty arteriogram
demonstrating patency of artery

Balloon angioplasty of
common iliac artery

Surgical bypass procedures

JOHN A.CRAIG—AD

Bypass graft
Diseased
segment

Diseased
segment

Bypass
graft

Diseased
segment

Diseased
segment

Bypass
graft

Aortofemoral
bypass

Aortofemoral
bypass

Femoral-popliteal
bypass

Femoral-femoral
bypass

prevention and treatment of cardiovascular events will improve the prognosis of the patient with PAD. A growing body of experience with endovascular stenting may help clarify its role in therapy. Drug-eluting stents, laser recanalization, endoluminal radiation, and photoangioplasty are promising experimental modalities that may improve endovascular outcomes if proven in clinical trials. Because of these advances, individuals with symptomatic PAD will likely fare better in the coming years.

Additional Resources

Cochrane Collection Web Site. Available at: http://www.cochrane.org. Accessed November 27, 2006.
This website presents evidence-based medicine relevant to PAD.
eMedicine Website. Available at: http://www.emedicine.com. Accessed November 27, 2006.
This website provides an up-to-date review of PAD.
Hiatt WR: Medical treatment of peripheral arterial disease and claudication. N Engl J Med 344(21):1608-1621, 2001.

The author provides a general overview of medical therapy in patients with PAD.

Hirsch AT, Haskal ZJ, Hertzer NR, et al: ACC/AHA 2005 Practice Guidelines for the management of patients with peripheral arterial disease (lower extremity, renal, mesenteric, and abdominal aortic): A collaborative report from the American Association for Vascular Surgery/Society for Vascular Surgery, Society for Cardiovascular Angiography and Interventions, Society for Vascular Medicine and Biology, Society of Interventional Radiology, and the ACC/AHA Task Force on Practice Guidelines (Writing Committee to Develop Guidelines for the Management of Patients with Peripheral Arterial Disease). Endorsed by the American Association of Cardiovascular and Pulmonary Rehabilitation; National Heart, Lung, and Blood Institute; Society for Vascular Nursing; TransAtlantic Inter-Society Consensus; and Vascular Disease Foundation. Circulation 113(11):e463-e654, 2006.

This paper presents guidelines relevant to the diagnosis and treatment of patients with PAD.

Koelemay MJ, Lijmer JG, Stoker J, et al: Magnetic resonance angiography for the evaluation of lower extremity arterial disease: A meta-analysis. JAMA 285(10):1338-1345, 2001.

This meta-analysis examined the usefulness of magnetic resonance angiography in diagnosing PAD.

EVIDENCE

1. Golomb BA, Dang TT, Criqui MH: Peripheral arterial disease: Morbidity and mortality implications. Circulation 114(7):688-699, 2006.

This meta-analysis demonstrates the high prevalence of coronary artery disease and cerebrovascular disease in patients with PAD and emphasizes the important implications this has for survival and treatment.

2. Hankey GJ, Norman PE, Eikelboom JW: Medical treatment of peripheral arterial disease. JAMA 295(5):547-553, 2006.

The authors present a general overview of medical therapy in patients with PAD.

3. Hirsch AT, Criqui MH, Treat-Jacobsen D, et al: Peripheral arterial disease detection, awareness, and treatment in primary care. JAMA 286:1317-1324, 2001.

This study examined the prevalence of PAD in an ambulatory cohort of patients being seen in primary care clinics. PAD was detected in 29% of 6979 patients aged 50 years or older.

4. Khan NA, Rahim SA, Anand SS, et al: Does the clinical examination predict lower extremity peripheral arterial disease? JAMA 295(5):536-546, 2006.

The authors report on a study of the usefulness of the physical examination in identifying PAD.

5. Ouriel K: Peripheral arterial disease. Lancet 358(9289):1257-1264, 2001.

The author provides a general overview of PAD.

Lee R. Goldberg ▪ Park W. Willis IV

Congenital and Valvular Heart Disease

Introduction

Most patients with congenital or valvular heart disease come to medical attention when a routine examination detects cardiac abnormalities. Clinical presentation with symptoms of heart failure, an important arrhythmia, or infective endocarditis is less common. Although congenital heart disease is usually discovered in childhood, the diagnosis of atrial septal defect and minimally symptomatic, noncyanotic defects can, at times, be made for the first time in adulthood.

With the declining incidence of rheumatic fever in recent years, the most common etiologies for acquired valvular disease are now inherited conditions or age-related degenerative change. Most adult physicians will care for patients with valvular heart disease either before or after surgical repair, and this chapter focuses on these patients. Although patients with congenital heart disease should be referred to a specialist in this area, the increasing number of patients reaching adulthood with surgically corrected defects means that most adult physicians will also be exposed to this group of patients as well.

To accurately define structural disease and quantify hemodynamic abnormalities, the diagnostic approach must include transthoracic echocardiography, appropriately focused according to clinical findings, in addition to standard chest radiography and electrocardiography. Transesophageal echocardiography and cardiac catheterization may be necessary in difficult cases. This evaluation is important not only for consideration in treatment but also for important life choices. Participation in competitive athletics should be restricted in many conditions, and some patients require special consideration in the workplace. Family planning and management of pregnancy require a multidisciplinary approach.

One of the most common considerations in patients with valvular or congenital heart disease is prevention of infective endocarditis. Guidelines for the prevention of infective endocarditis have recently been revised. These guidelines emphasize maintenance of optimal oral health and hygiene in all patients with congenital and valvular heart disease. Antibiotic prophylaxis is recommended only for individuals at highest risk for adverse outcome from infective endocarditis. This includes those with previous infective endocarditis, those with prosthetic heart valves, and cardiac transplant recipients who develop valvulopathy. Individuals with unrepaired cyanotic congenital heart disease, including palliative shunts and conduits, should be treated. Antibiotic prophylaxis is also indicated for completely repaired congenital heart disease with prosthetic material or device, whether by surgery or catheter intervention, during the first 6 months after the procedure; those with residual defects at the site, or adjacent to the site, of a prosthetic patch or device should be treated indefinitely.

Antibiotic prophylaxis is recommended for all dental procedures that involve manipulation of gingival tissue or the periapical region of the teeth, or perforation of the oral mucosa. Patients undergoing procedures on the respiratory tract or infected skin, skin structures, or musculoskeletal tissue should also be treated. Antibiotic prophylaxis is not recommended, solely to prevent infective endocarditis, for genitourinary or gastrointestinal tract procedures. Those with rheumatic disease require prophylaxis for recurrent streptococcal infection.

AORTIC STENOSIS

Etiology and Pathogenesis

Congenital aortic stenosis most commonly involves a defect in the aortic valve. Congenitally bicuspid aortic valves, present in 1% to 2% of the general population, undergo accelerated degenerative change. In older individuals, age-related calcification and rheumatic disease cause acquired stenosis of normal, trileaflet valves.

Patients' nonvalvular congenital lesions can present with symptoms and examination findings indistinguishable from valvular aortic stenosis. Etiologies include the presence of either a discrete subaortic membrane or supravalvular aortic stenosis. Hypertrophic cardiomyopathy, which is covered elsewhere (see Chapter 33), can also present with symptoms and exam findings similar to those in patients with valvular aortic stenosis.

Aortic stenosis of any cause results in fixed outflow obstruction and left ventricular pressure overload. Compensatory left ventricular hypertrophy increases myocardial oxygen demand, and ischemia can develop, even in the absence of coronary artery disease. Although contractile performance is preserved, hypertrophy causes abnormal myocardial relaxation, decreased chamber compliance, and diastolic left ventricular dysfunction. For this reason, atrial contraction can be critical to diastolic filling and maintenance of cardiac output (Fig. 32-1).

Clinical Presentation

Aortic stenosis causes a midsystolic murmur, loudest in the second right intercostal space and transmitted to the neck. Signs of moderate or severe aortic stenosis include a diminished and slow-rising arterial pulse, a systolic thrill in the second right intercostal space or suprasternal notch, and a sustained apical impulse. An aortic ejection sound is present in most patients with congenital valvular disease. The second heart sound is usually normal, but reversed splitting can occur with severe obstruction.

Important symptoms of moderate or severe aortic stenosis are angina pectoris, syncope, and left heart failure. The prognosis is worst when patients with aortic stenosis present with left heart failure. The onset of atrial fibrillation can cause abrupt hemodynamic deterioration and precipitate symptoms in a previously asymptomatic individual.

Differential Diagnosis

Midsystolic murmurs can be innocent, particularly in childhood and adolescence or in high flow states (pregnancy, anemia, hyperthyroidism). Pathologic causes include any type of obstruction to ventricular outflow and dilation of the aortic root or main pulmonary artery.

Hypertrophic cardiomyopathy causes dynamic left ventricular outflow obstruction. In these patients, the carotid pulse is brisk and biferiens in contour, and the midsystolic murmur is characteristically loudest at the left sternal edge. Distinguishing between normal and abnormal midsystolic murmurs requires careful attention to the physical examination and, often, confirmation by echocardiography.

Diagnostic Approach

Although careful physical examination and electrocardiography can detect left ventricular hypertrophy in moderate or severe obstruction, precise quantification of aortic stenosis requires echocardiography for anatomic assessment and evaluation of left ventricular wall thickness, chamber size, and contractile performance. Simultaneous Doppler studies should be performed to measure left ventricular outflow velocity, mean transvalvular pressure gradient, and valve area. Invasive assessment in the cardiac catheterization laboratory may be recommended in symptomatic patients when noninvasive tests are inconclusive or there is discrepancy between clinical and echocardiographic findings.

Management and Therapy

Optimum Treatment

In asymptomatic patients, mild aortic stenosis is an indication for annual evaluation, patient education, and in the absence of a change in clinical status or physical examination, repeat echocardiography every 3 to 5 years. Patients with moderate aortic stenosis require annual clinical examination and should undergo noninvasive studies every 1 to 2 years. Those with severe aortic stenosis should be evaluated semiannually to determine whether the patient should undergo valve replacement. Echocardiography should be performed more frequently when signs or symptoms change.

Although patients with aortic stenosis frequently have clinical risk factor profiles and valvular tissue abnormalities in common with atherosclerosis, medical treatment has not been shown to prevent, or delay progression of, aortic stenosis. Nevertheless, risk modification is important to prevent concurrent coronary artery disease. Physical activity need not be limited in asymptomatic patients with mild aortic stenosis. Those with moderate to severe aortic stenosis should avoid competitive sports that involve high dynamic and static muscular demands.

Valve replacement is indicated for patients with symptomatic severe aortic stenosis. Older patients, or any patient with a significant risk for coronary atherosclerosis, should be evaluated by coronary angiography before undergoing surgery for aortic valve replacement. Left

Figure 32-1 Valvular Stenosis and Insufficiency I.

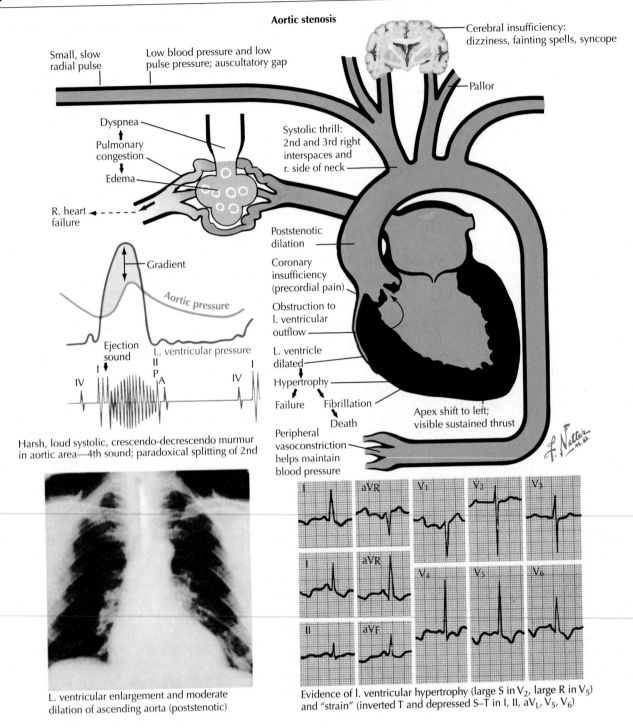

Aortic stenosis

Small, slow radial pulse

Low blood pressure and low pulse pressure; auscultatory gap

Cerebral insufficiency: dizziness, fainting spells, syncope

Pallor

Dyspnea

Pulmonary congestion

Edema

Systolic thrill: 2nd and 3rd right interspaces and r. side of neck

R. heart failure

Poststenotic dilation

Gradient

Aortic pressure

Coronary insufficiency (precordial pain)

Obstruction to l. ventricular outflow

Ejection sound

L. ventricular pressure

L. ventricle dilated

Hypertrophy

Failure   Fibrillation

Death

Apex shift to left; visible sustained thrust

Harsh, loud systolic, crescendo-decrescendo murmur in aortic area—4th sound; paradoxical splitting of 2nd

Peripheral vasoconstriction helps maintain blood pressure

L. ventricular enlargement and moderate dilation of ascending aorta (poststenotic)

Evidence of l. ventricular hypertrophy (large S in V₂, large R in V₅) and "strain" (inverted T and depressed S–T in I, II, aV_L, V₅, V₆)

ventricular contractile dysfunction is not a contraindication to surgery in patients with aortic stenosis, and operative results are satisfactory in symptomatic octogenarians. In selected cases, the Ross procedure is an alternative to valve replacement. Aortic balloon valvuloplasty is indicated in many children, but this technique is of limited utility in adults with calcified valves.

Avoiding Treatment Errors

Exercise testing is contraindicated in symptomatic patients with aortic stenosis. Associated systemic arterial hypertension must be treated cautiously because diuretic and vasodilating drugs can unfavorably alter well-compensated hemodynamics. Aortic valve replacement is not indicated for prevention of sudden death in asymptomatic patients with aortic stenosis.

AORTIC REGURGITATION (INSUFFICIENCY)

Etiology and Pathogenesis

Congenitally malformed leaflets, rheumatic disease, age-related degenerative change, and infective endocarditis cause valvular aortic regurgitation. In long-standing hypertension and aging, aortic regurgitation may occur secondary to aortic root dilation. Connective tissue abnormalities, including Marfan syndrome, are associated with cystic medial necrosis of the aorta. Complications in patients with Marfan syndrome include progressive aortic root dilation, aortic dissection, and aortic regurgitation.

Chronic aortic regurgitation causes compensatory left ventricular dilation and enhanced chamber compliance, resulting in accommodation of increasing end-diastolic volumes without a rise in filling pressure. In the long term, progressive left ventricular dilation ultimately results in left heart failure. Acute aortic regurgitation, most commonly caused by infective endocarditis, aortic dissection, or trauma, does not allow time for left ventricular chamber dilation, and large regurgitant volumes result in rapidly increasing diastolic filling pressure, pulmonary edema, and shock (Fig. 32-2). In patients who are surgical candidates, it is important to consider aortic valve replacement before the development of irreversible left ventricular dilation. Guidelines for making this determination are discussed later.

Clinical Presentation

Most patients have a high-pitched, early diastolic decrescendo murmur at the left sternal edge. If the murmur is loudest at the right sternal border, aortic root disease is usually present.

Moderate or severe aortic regurgitation causes systolic hypertension, a widened pulse pressure, biferiens carotid pulse, and displaced apical impulse. There is usually a midsystolic murmur caused by increased left ventricular stroke volume and turbulent flow through the outflow tract. A mid-diastolic (Austin Flint) murmur, mimicking mitral stenosis, is often audible at the mitral area. Symptoms of moderate or severe aortic regurgitation usually reflect left heart failure. Angina pectoris is less commonly a presenting symptom. Clinically silent aortic regurgitation can be detected by Doppler echocardiography.

In acute aortic regurgitation, left ventricular failure develops rapidly, and the physical signs of chronic disease are usually absent. In this circumstance, abnormal findings are limited to a soft first heart sound and short early diastolic murmur.

Differential Diagnosis

In patients with pulmonary hypertension and pulmonic regurgitation, an early diastolic decrescendo (Graham Steell's) murmur that can be difficult to distinguish from aortic regurgitation may be present. Pulmonic regurgitation after complete repair for tetralogy of Fallot causes a relatively low-pitched early diastolic decrescendo murmur.

Diagnostic Approach

Echocardiography is indicated at the time of diagnosis to identify cause, assess valve morphology and aortic root size, provide semiquantitative assessment of severity, and evaluate left ventricular dimension, wall thickness, and contractile performance. Serial measurement of left ventricular chamber size and contractile performance by echocardiography or radionuclide ventriculography is important in the long-term management of patients with chronic (mild to moderate) aortic regurgitation.

Management and Therapy

Optimum Treatment

In asymptomatic patients, mild aortic regurgitation calls for annual evaluation and, in the absence of a change in clinical status or physical examination, repeat echocardiography every 2 or 3 years. An interval change in left ventricular dimensions, or contractile performance, is an indication for 3- to 6-month follow-up to differentiate progressive disease from measurement variability. Patients with moderate or severe aortic regurgitation require annual examination and a noninvasive assessment of left ventricular function. For patients with symptoms of left heart failure in addition to moderate or severe aortic regurgitation, aortic valve replacement is indicated. In acute severe aortic regurgitation, urgent surgical intervention is required.

Left ventricular contractile dysfunction can compromise long-term prognosis and operative results. Numerous studies have demonstrated that even in the absence of symptoms, aortic valve replacement is indicated for patients with severe aortic regurgitation and echocardiographically derived left ventricular end-systolic dimension of 55 mm or greater, or left ventricular ejection fraction of 50% or less.

Patients with chronic aortic regurgitation secondary to disease of the aortic root, especially those with Marfan syndrome, require annual echocardiographic evaluation. The timing of surgical intervention in these individuals is usually based on the degree and rate of root dilation (>45 mm) rather than the magnitude of regurgitant flow or left ventricular contractile performance.

Long-term vasodilator therapy is indicated for patients with severe aortic regurgitation who have symptoms of left

Figure 32-2 Valvular Stenosis and Insufficiency II.

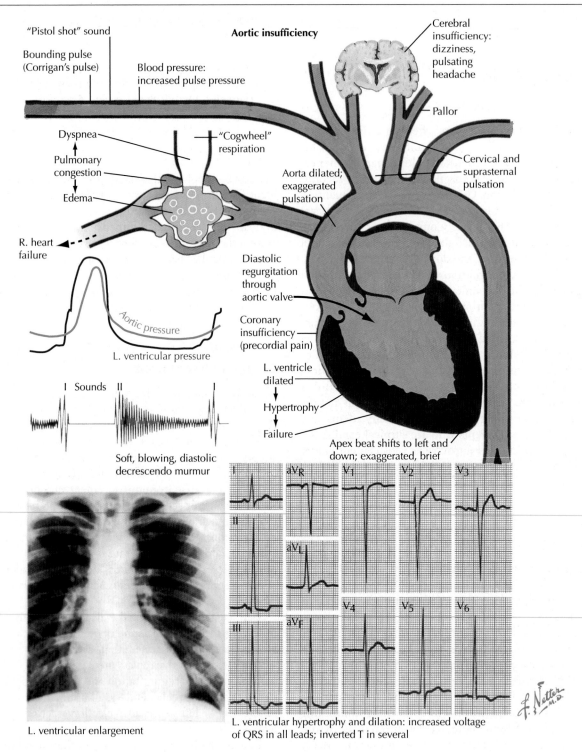

Aortic insufficiency

"Pistol shot" sound

Bounding pulse (Corrigan's pulse)

Blood pressure: increased pulse pressure

Cerebral insufficiency: dizziness, pulsating headache

Pallor

Dyspnea

Pulmonary congestion

"Cogwheel" respiration

Edema

R. heart failure

Aorta dilated; exaggerated pulsation

Cervical and suprasternal pulsation

Aortic pressure

L. ventricular pressure

Diastolic regurgitation through aortic valve

Coronary insufficiency (precordial pain)

L. ventricle dilated

Hypertrophy

Failure

I Sounds II

Soft, blowing, diastolic decrescendo murmur

Apex beat shifts to left and down; exaggerated, brief

L. ventricular enlargement

L. ventricular hypertrophy and dilation: increased voltage of QRS in all leads; inverted T in several

ventricular dysfunction when surgery is not recommended because of additional cardiac risk factors or noncardiac factors. Vasodilator therapy should also be considered in asymptomatic patients with severe aortic regurgitation, left ventricular dilation, and normal ejection fraction. β-Blocker therapy is indicated to slow progression of aortic root dilation in patients with Marfan syndrome.

Avoiding Treatment Errors

Vasodilator therapy, in lieu of observation and appropriate referral for surgery, is not indicated for long-term therapy in asymptomatic patients with mild to moderate aortic regurgitation and normal left ventricular ejection fraction, or in those who meet indications and are candidates for aortic valve replacement as outlined previously.

MITRAL STENOSIS

Etiology and Pathogenesis

Mitral stenosis is most commonly a manifestation of rheumatic heart disease characterized by commissural fusion and degenerative changes in the mitral apparatus. The obstruction in left ventricular inflow results in a compensatory increase in left atrial pressure, which can maintain left ventricular filling. However, over time, this increase in left atrial pressure results in left atrial chamber dilation, pulmonary venous congestion, and secondary pulmonary arterial hypertension. Irreversible pulmonary vascular disease can be a long-term complication of mitral stenosis (Fig. 32-3), although usually, with correction of mitral stenosis, increased pulmonary vascular pressures at least partially resolve.

Clinical Presentation

Abnormal physical findings precede the development of clinical symptoms. The earliest signs are an increase in the amplitude of the first heart sound, an opening snap, and a mid-diastolic murmur at the mitral area. About half of patients with mitral stenosis give a history of acute rheumatic fever. Symptoms of left heart failure commonly develop during pregnancy, with other hemodynamic stresses, with the development of atrial fibrillation, or simply with progression of mitral stenosis over time. The risk for systemic thromboembolism is high in patients with mitral stenosis and either chronic, or paroxysmal, atrial fibrillation.

Differential Diagnosis

Congenital malformations of the mitral valve and papillary muscles, cor triatriatum, and left atrial myxoma all can cause obstruction to left ventricular inflow, mimicking valvular mitral stenosis, even to the point of presenting with a mid-diastolic murmur at the mitral area. Mitral stenosis itself can mimic isolated severe pulmonary hypertension when decreased cardiac output causes the mid-diastolic murmur to be soft or absent in the setting of other physical examination, electrocardiographic, and radiographic evidence of pulmonary hypertension.

Diagnostic Approach

The initial echocardiographic evaluation should include an estimate of mitral valve area and pulmonary arterial systolic pressure. In patients with severe mitral stenosis, a detailed assessment of the mitral apparatus is necessary in considering whether percutaneous balloon mitral valvulo-plasty or surgical mitral valve replacement should be performed. Critical factors include the degree and extent of degenerative change, the degree of leaflet mobility, the magnitude of associated mitral regurgitation, and the presence or absence of a left atrial thrombus. Cardiac catheterization is indicated when noninvasive tests are inconclusive, discrepant, or discordant with clinical findings.

Management and Therapy

Optimum Treatment

Echocardiography is indicated for changing symptoms or signs. Patients with mild left heart failure have a favorable prognosis and can be successfully managed with dietary sodium restriction and diuretic therapy. β-Blocking drugs can improve diastolic filling of the left ventricle by slowing heart rate at rest and during exercise. Anticoagulation and antiarrhythmic drug therapy is required for patients with atrial fibrillation. Some studies suggest that surgery should be considered with the early onset of symptoms. Carefully selected patients with significantly limiting symptoms are candidates for percutaneous balloon valvuloplasty; for those with severe valvular calcification or significant mitral regurgitation, open commissurotomy or mitral valve replacement is required.

Avoiding Treatment Errors

It is of utmost importance that physicians recognize the high risk for left atrial thrombus formation and thromboembolic complications in patients with mitral stenosis and atrial fibrillation and carefully screen patients for even paroxysmal atrial fibrillation. Percutaneous mitral balloon valvotomy and mitral valve repair, or replacement, are not indicated for patients with mild mitral stenosis. Moderate to severe mitral regurgitation and left atrial thrombus are contraindications to percutaneous mitral balloon valvotomy.

MITRAL REGURGITATION (INSUFFICIENCY)

Etiology and Pathogenesis

Congenital mitral regurgitation is rare as an isolated abnormality. Acquired causes are much more common and include papillary muscle dysfunction secondary to ischemic heart disease, myxomatous disease and prolapse of the mitral valve, rheumatic heart disease, spontaneous rupture of chordae tendineae, and infective endocarditis.

Chronic mitral regurgitation causes left atrial dilation. Because large regurgitant volumes can be accommodated at normal pressure, patients with mild to moderate mitral regurgitation are most often asymptomatic. With moderate or severe mitral regurgitation, progressive left ventricular dilation can occur, leading to increasing limitation of

Figure 32-3 Valvular Stenosis and Insufficiency III.

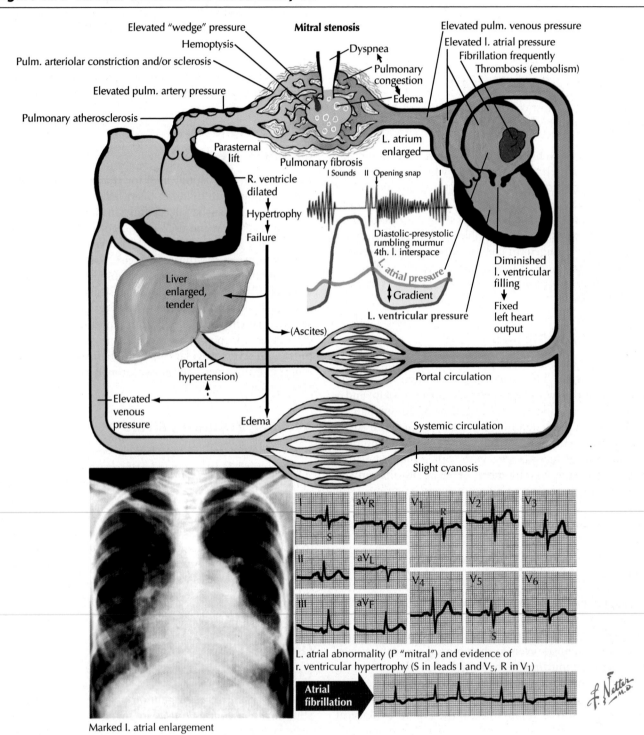

Mitral stenosis

Elevated "wedge" pressure

Hemoptysis

Pulm. arteriolar constriction and/or sclerosis

Elevated pulm. artery pressure

Pulmonary atherosclerosis

Dyspnea

Pulmonary congestion

Edema

Elevated pulm. venous pressure

Elevated l. atrial pressure

Fibrillation frequently

Thrombosis (embolism)

Parasternal lift

Pulmonary fibrosis

L. atrium enlarged

R. ventricle dilated

Hypertrophy

Failure

I Sounds II Opening snap I

Diastolic-presystolic rumbling murmur 4th. l. interspace

L. atrial pressure

Gradient

L. ventricular pressure

Liver enlarged, tender

Diminished l. ventricular filling

Fixed left heart output

(Ascites)

(Portal hypertension)

Portal circulation

Elevated venous pressure

Edema

Systemic circulation

Slight cyanosis

L. atrial abnormality (P "mitral") and evidence of r. ventricular hypertrophy (S in leads I and V5, R in V1)

Atrial fibrillation

Marked l. atrial enlargement

exercise tolerance. As noted later, it is very important that patients be carefully followed to avoid irreversible decrement in left ventricular function with significant, chronic mitral regurgitation. Acute mitral regurgitation does not allow time for left atrial dilation, and pulmonary venous pressure rises precipitously, causing irreversible pulmonary edema and shock (Fig. 32-4).

Clinical Presentation

The cardiac examination in patients with chronic mitral regurgitation characteristically shows a holosystolic murmur, loudest at the mitral area, and commonly transmitted to the axilla or left sternal edge. Clinically silent mitral regurgitation can be detected by Doppler echocar-

Figure 32-4 Valvular Stenosis and Insufficiency IV.

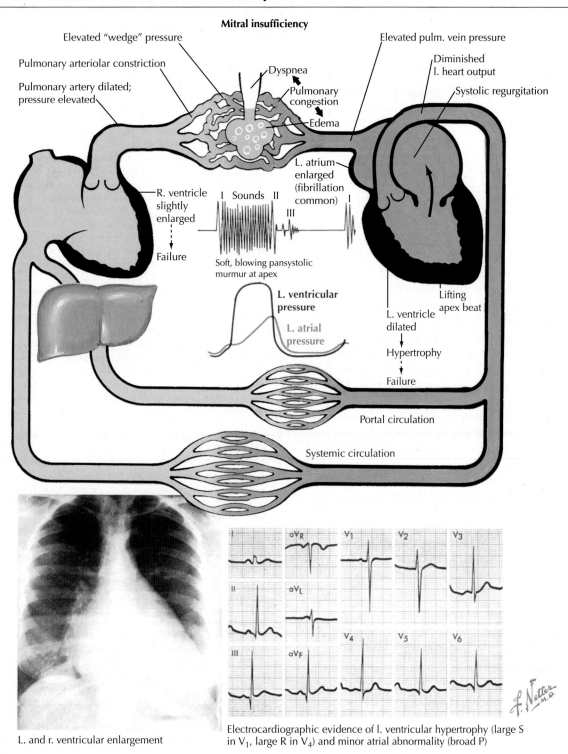

Mitral insufficiency

Elevated "wedge" pressure

Pulmonary arteriolar constriction

Pulmonary artery dilated; pressure elevated

Dyspnea

Pulmonary congestion

Edema

Elevated pulm. vein pressure

Diminished l. heart output

Systolic regurgitation

R. ventricle slightly enlarged

Failure

I Sounds II

III

I

Soft, blowing pansystolic murmur at apex

L. atrium enlarged (fibrillation common)

L. ventricular pressure

L. atrial pressure

L. ventricle dilated

Hypertrophy

Failure

Lifting apex beat

Portal circulation

Systemic circulation

L. and r. ventricular enlargement

oV_R   V_1   V_2   V_3

oV_L

oV_F   V_4   V_5   V_6

Electrocardiographic evidence of l. ventricular hypertrophy (large S in V_1, large R in V_4) and minor atrial abnormality (broad P)

diography. Moderate or severe chronic mitral regurgitation can cause lateral displacement of the apical impulse, wide splitting of S_2, and a third heart sound, S_3. Symptoms are related to left heart failure and atrial, or ventricular, arrhythmia. In acute mitral regurgitation, the systolic murmur is often abbreviated and can be soft or entirely absent.

Differential Diagnosis

The holosystolic murmur of tricuspid regurgitation can be misinterpreted as mitral regurgitation. One means to distinguish the two is that murmur of tricuspid regurgitation characteristically increases in amplitude on inspiration. A ventricular septal defect causes a holosystolic murmur, loudest at the left sternal border.

Diagnostic Approach

Chronic mitral regurgitation requires a thorough baseline assessment of left ventricular contractile performance by echocardiography, or radionuclide ventriculography for planning initial medical therapy and long-term follow-up.

Management and Therapy

Optimum Treatment

In asymptomatic patients, mild mitral regurgitation calls for annual examination, but repeat echocardiography is not necessary unless there is a change in functional status or physical examination. Those with moderate or severe mitral regurgitation require annual examination and echocardiography or radionuclide ventriculography to assess left ventricular performance. Patients with chronic severe mitral regurgitation can develop subclinical left ventricular contractile dysfunction, which compromises operative results and long-term prognosis. For this reason, even in the absence of symptoms, operative intervention is indicated for those with echocardiographically derived left ventricular end-systolic dimension of 40 mm or greater, or left ventricular ejection fraction of 30% to 60%.

Operative intervention is also indicated for symptomatic patients with acute or chronic severe mitral regurgitation. If the mitral apparatus is suitable, valve repair is the procedure of choice. Mitral valve replacement, with preservation of the chordal apparatus, is the next best option.

Treatment of comorbid conditions, especially systemic hypertension and coronary artery disease, can help to avoid unnecessarily accelerated progression of mitral regurgitation.

Avoiding Treatment Errors

Mitral valve surgery is not indicated for patients with mild or moderate mitral regurgitation. It is reasonable to consider mitral valve repair in asymptomatic patients with chronic severe mitral regurgitation and normal left ventricular function when the likelihood of successful surgery is greater than 90%. However, operation is not indicated when there is doubt regarding the feasibility of valve repair.

FUTURE DIRECTIONS

Because of improved operative outcomes in children and aging of the population, the number of patients with congenital and valvular heart disease will continue to grow. Improved medical management and evolving catheter-based interventions will delay, or replace, the need for cardiac surgery in some conditions. Evolving, less invasive operative techniques and increased utilization of autologous tissue, homografts, and more durable bioprosthetic valves will enhance surgical outcomes.

Additional Resources

Brickner ME, Hillis LD, Lange RA: Congenital heart disease in adults. First of two parts. N Engl J Med 342(4):256-263, 2000.
    The authors provide a comprehensive and well-written review of acyanotic congenital heart disease in adults.
Brickner ME, Hillis LD, Lange RA: Congenital heart disease in adults. Second of two parts. N Engl J Med 342(5):334-342, 2000.
    This second part of a thorough review of congenital heart disease in adults covers the evaluation and management of cyanotic lesions.
Dajani A, Taubert K, Ferrieri P, et al: Treatment of acute streptococcal pharyngitis and prevention of rheumatic fever: A statement for health professionals. Committee on Rheumatic Fever, Endocarditis, and Kawasaki Disease of the Council on Cardiovascular Disease in the Young, American Heart Association. Pediatrics 96(4 Pt 1):758-764, 1995.
    This comprehensive report details current approaches to primary prevention of acute rheumatic fever and also covers issues related to secondary prophylaxis for individuals after an initial attack.
Gutgesell HP, Gessner IH, Vetter VL, et al: Recreational and occupational recommendations for young patients with heart disease. A Statement for Physicians by the Committee on Congenital Cardiac Defects of the Council on Cardiovascular Disease in the Young, American Heart Association. Circulation 74(5):1195A-1198A, 1986.
    This statement provides specific recommendations useful in counseling young patients with heart disease.

EVIDENCE

1. Bonow RO, Carabello BA, Chatterjee K, et al: ACC/AHA 2006 guidelines for the management of patients with valvular heart disease: A report of the American College of Cardiology/American Heart Association Task Force on Practice Guidelines (Writing Committee to Revise the 1998 guidelines for the management of patients with valvular heart disease) developed in collaboration with the Society of Cardiovascular Anesthesiologists endorsed by the Society for Cardiovascular Angiography and Interventions and the Society of Thoracic Surgeons. J Am Coll Cardiol 48(3):e1-e148, 2006.
    This comprehensive and well-referenced document includes detailed discussions of level of evidence for each recommendation.
2. Bonow RO, Cheitlin M, Crawford M, Douglas PS: Task Force 3: Valvular heart disease. J Am Coll Cardiol 45(8):1334-1340, 2005.
    This is a useful consensus statement on recommendations for athletic competition in patients with congenital and valvular heart disease.
3. Wilson W, Taubert KA, Gewitz M, et al: Prevention of infective endocarditis. Guidelines from the American Heart Association. A guideline from the American Heart Association Rheumatic Fever, Endocarditis, and Kawasaki Disease Committee, Council on Cardiovascular Disease in the Young, and the Council on Clinical Cardiology, Council on Cardiovascular Surgery and Anesthesia, and the Quality of Care and Outcomes Research Interdisciplinary Working Group. Circulation. Available at: http://circ.ahajournals.org/cgi/reprint/CIRCULATIONAHA.106.183095. Accessed May 25, 2007.
    This statement updates guidelines from the American Heart Association for the prevention of infective endocarditis. The document presents an in-depth discussion of the rationale and available evidence supporting major changes in recommended practice.

Patricia P. Chang ▪ Carla Sueta Dupree

33

Cardiomyopathies

Introduction

Heart failure (HF) results from any of a large number of pathophysiologic processes that directly, or indirectly, result in myocardial dysfunction. Although some causes of HF reflect systemic metabolic (or other) abnormalities, most individuals with HF are also diagnosed with cardiomyopathy. The word cardiomyopathy stems from Greek roots: *kardia* (heart), *mys* (muscle), *pathos* (suffering). Cardiomyopathy broadly describes diseases of the myocardium associated with either systolic or diastolic ventricular dysfunction. Traditionally, cardiomyopathies have been categorized into one of three distinct types: dilated cardiomyopathy (DCM), hypertrophic cardiomyopathy (HCM), and restrictive cardiomyopathy (RCM). As defined by the World Health Organization in 1995, a fourth type of cardiomyopathy is more related to arrhythmias than to HF symptoms, namely, arrhythmogenic right ventricular dysplasia (ARVD) or arrhythmogenic right ventricular cardiomyopathy (ARVC).

A characteristic of all cardiomyopathies is altered cardiomyocyte structure or function of sufficient magnitude to cause clinical symptoms. The most common clinical presentation is heart failure symptoms and signs regardless of the type of cardiomyopathy, except for ARVC, in which the primary clinical manifestation is ventricular arrhythmias. This chapter describes the different types of cardiomyopathy and general treatment options.

Etiology, Pathogenesis, and Clinical Presentation

Dilated Cardiomyopathy

DCM is characterized by dilation and impaired contraction of the ventricle, primarily the left ventricle. This is the most common type of cardiomyopathy. Because of ventricular systolic dysfunction, gradual compensatory responses of the cardiomyocytes lead to cardiac remodeling (Fig. 33-1). Initially, cardiomyocytes respond to hemodynamic stress by becoming hypertrophied. With progressive left ventricular dysfunction and the neurohormonal changes that accompany low cardiac output (see Chapter 34), the poorly functioning ventricle gradually dilates. The increased ventricular size provides short-term relief, a compensatory effect termed the *Starling effect*. However, with progressive dilation, left ventricular function continues to worsen, resulting in DCM.

There are many etiologies for DCM (Box 33-1). The most common is ischemic heart disease ("ischemic cardiomyopathy"): coronary artery disease contributes about two thirds of all cases of heart failure. After a myocardial infarction, the infarct scar may expand to develop into a large area of nonfunctioning myocardium over hours to days;

global remodeling over days to months results in a dilated and globally poorly contractile ventricle (Fig. 33-2).

Other causes of DCM include valvular heart disease (*valvular cardiomyopathy*); infection; cardiotoxins (e.g., alcohol, chemotherapy such as anthracyclines and Herceptin); end-stage hypertension; abnormal metabolic state, such as endocrine abnormalities (e.g., hypothyroidism or thyrotoxicosis, diabetes, acromegaly, adrenal cortical insufficiency, pheochromocytoma), nutritional deficiencies, and infiltrative disease (e.g., copper deposition in Wilson's disease, iron deposition in hemochromatosis); other infiltrative diseases (e.g., amyloidosis, sarcoidosis, leukemia); autoimmune diseases, such as connective tissue diseases (e.g., scleroderma, systemic lupus erythematosus) and giant cell myocarditis; peripartum state (*peripartum cardiomyopathy*); and familial and genetic diseases (e.g., muscular dystrophies, MELAS (mitochondrial encephalopathy, lactic acidosis, stroke-like) syndrome, and other recently discovered associated chromosomal abnormalities). When no specific cause is found, the DCM is described as *idiopathic cardiomyopathy*. In recent years, it has become increasingly evident that a significant portion (perhaps as high as 30%) of idiopathic DCMs result from a genetic predisposition. A few familial conditions have already been described, such as

Figure 33-1 Cardiac Remodeling Secondary to Volume Overload.

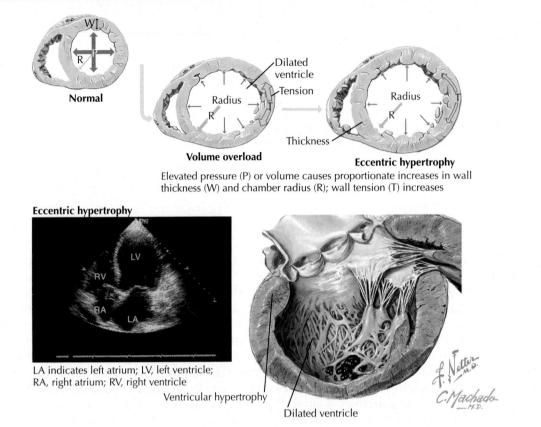

Elevated pressure (P) or volume causes proportionate increases in wall thickness (W) and chamber radius (R); wall tension (T) increases

LA indicates left atrium; LV, left ventricle; RA, right atrium; RV, right ventricle

Figure 33-2 Dilated Cardiomyopathy after Myocardial Infarction.

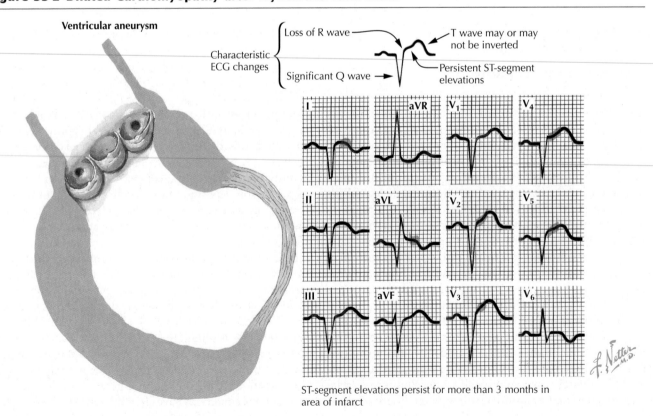

ST-segment elevations persist for more than 3 months in area of infarct

---

Box 33-1 Differential Diagnosis of
        Cardiomyopathies

Dilated Cardiomyopathy

Ischemic heart disease (coronary artery disease)
Hypertension*
Valvular heart disease
Infectious (e.g., viral, Chagas' disease, Lyme disease)
Cardiotoxins (e.g., alcohol, anthracycline,* excess
    catecholamines, heavy metals—lead, arsenic, cobalt)
Metabolic/endocrine (e.g., hypothyroidism,
    hyperthyroidism, diabetes mellitus, adrenal
    insufficiency, pheochromocytoma)
Connective tissue disease (e.g., systemic lupus
    erythematosus, scleroderma,* dermatomyositis,
    polyarteritis nodosa, rheumatoid arthritis)*
Infiltrative (e.g., Wilson's disease, hemochromatosis,*
    amyloidosis,* sarcoidosis*)
Metabolic/nutritional (e.g., magnesium deficiency,
    kwashiorkor, anemia, beriberi, selenium deficiency)
Peripartum cardiomyopathy
Giant cell myocarditis
Muscular dystrophies (e.g., Duchenne's, Becker-type,
    myotonic dystrophies)
Familial (e.g., X-linked)
Idiopathic

Hypertrophic Cardiomyopathy

Hypertension*
Asymmetric septal hypertrophy with obstruction
Genetic mutations of myocyte sarcomere proteins
Glycogen storage diseases

Restrictive Cardiomyopathy

Amyloidosis*
Sarcoidosis*
Hemochromatosis*
Endomyocardial fibrosis
Irradiation (e.g., radiation fibrosis)
Scleroderma*
Anthracycline toxicity*
Carcinoid heart disease
Genetic storage or infiltrative diseases (e.g., glycogen
    storage disease, Fabry's disease, Refsum's syndrome,
    Niemann-Pick's disease, Gaucher's disease, Hurler's
    syndrome, Hand-Müller-Christian's disease)
Familial (e.g., Noonan's syndrome, not otherwise
    specified)
Idiopathic

Arrhythmogenic Right Ventricular Cardiomyopathy

Arrhythmogenic right ventricular dysplasia

Unclassified Cardiomyopathies

Fibroelastosis
Left ventricular noncompaction
Mitochondrial diseases

---

*Diseases that can belong to more than one type of cardiomyopathy.

the muscular dystrophies (e.g., Duchenne's, Becker's), X-linked DCM (e.g., other dystrophin gene mutations), and autosomal dominant forms of familial DCM (e.g., lamin A/C gene mutation). It is likely that numerous other genetic predispositions to DCM will be elucidated in the future.

When the cardiomyopathy is thought to have been caused by an infectious agent—because of a viral-like prodrome—most often, no specific pathogen is identified. In this circumstance, the generic term *viral myocarditis* is commonly used. In cases deemed viral myocarditis or viral cardiomyopathy, a diffuse inflammatory response is often observed, with lymphocytes infiltrating the myocardium (Fig. 33-3). Specific pathogens associated with development of DCM include viruses such as Coxsackie B virus, enterovirus, adenovirus, parvovirus, HIV, and cytomegalovirus, and parasites such as trypanosomiasis in Chagas' disease (the most common cause of infectious cardiomyopathy in South America) and Lyme disease. Although no specific bacteria or fungi have been known to cause cardiomyopathy, acute ventricular systolic dysfunction has been seen in the setting of sepsis.

Hypertrophic Cardiomyopathy

HCM is characterized by left or right ventricular hypertrophy. The underlying pathophysiology is hypertrophied cardiomyocytes impairing normal relaxation or compliance of the ventricle, resulting in diastolic dysfunction. Phenotypically, the left (less commonly right) ventricular walls are markedly thickened, but the ventricular chamber size is normal or even small (Fig. 33-4). The electrocardiogram typically shows left ventricular hypertrophy. Ventricular systolic function is preserved and often hyperdynamic. Although HCM usually presents in this manner, over time, a hypertrophied ventricle may progress to the DCM phenotype in end-stage disease because of continued remodeling in the setting of chronic uncontrolled pressure or volume overload.

Unlike DCM, the potential etiologies of ventricular hypertrophy severe enough to produce HCM are few (see Box 33-1). The most common cause for HCM in older populations is severe hypertension (*hypertensive cardiomyopathy*). The ventricular hypertrophy is usually concentric and rarely causes an obstruction of blood flow through left ventricular outflow tract. There are clearly genetic (and possibly environmental) factors that predispose individuals to developing this level of left ventricular hypertrophy in the setting of hypertension because only a small percentage of patients with severe hypertension develop hypertensive HCM.

The second major cause of HCM is any of a rapidly growing number of mutations in genes important in the myocardial sarcomere. With an estimated prevalence of about 0.2% in the adult population, HCM is not rare and is the most common genetic cardiovascular disease. It is usually this cardiomyopathy that has caused unexpected sudden cardiac death in young athletes. Most young patients are asymptomatic and are diagnosed only after a screening electrocardiogram demonstrates abnormal left ventricular hypertrophy.

Figure 33-3 Diphtheritic and Viral Myocarditis.

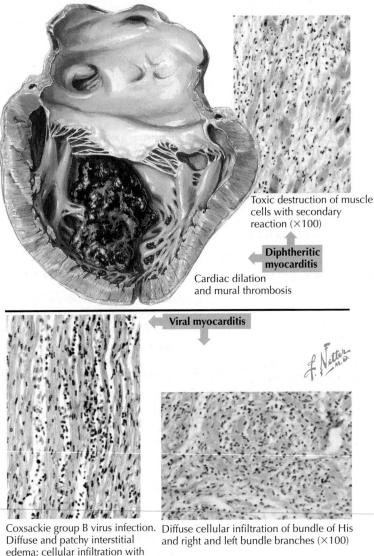

Toxic destruction of muscle cells with secondary reaction (×100)

Diphtheritic myocarditis

Cardiac dilation and mural thrombosis

Viral myocarditis

Coxsackie group B virus infection. Diffuse and patchy interstitial edema; cellular infiltration with only moderate muscle fiber destruction (×100)

Diffuse cellular infiltration of bundle of His and right and left bundle branches (×100)

Sarcomere-protein gene mutations account for most cases of genetically based HCM. More than 400 individual mutations have been identified in 11 sarcomere genes, including cardiac β- and α-myosin heavy chains; cardiac troponins T, I, and C; cardiac myosin-binding protein C; α-tropomyosin; actin; the essential and regulatory myosin light chains; and titin. Glycogen storage diseases have also been associated with HCM.

The specific degree and location of hypertrophy varies considerably among the different gene mutations and even within family members who all have a single specific mutation. This observed variation likely relates to other genetic variations and environmental factors yet to be elucidated that affect the precise phenotype that results from mutations associated with hypertropic cardiomyopathy.

Ventricular hypertrophy may be concentric or eccentric, such as asymmetric septal hypertrophy (ASH) or apical hypertrophy. When the septal hypertrophy causes systolic anterior motion of the anterior mitral leaflet with subsequent obstruction of the left ventricular outflow tract, a hemodynamically significant left ventricular outflow tract gradient (≥50 mm Hg) may be present at rest or provoked (Fig. 33-5). This left ventricular outflow tract obstruction is often a major contributor to symptoms of dyspnea, arrhythmias, and syncope. In this setting, the HCM may be called obstructive HCM, hypertrophic obstructive cardiomyopathy (HOCM), or, as initially described, idiopathic hypertrophic subaortic stenosis (IHSS) or ASH. Common complications are arrhythmias; atrial arrhythmias, most commonly atrial fibrillation, are often poorly tolerated, and ventricular tachycardia is often the cause of sudden death in young patients. However, HCM is predominantly a nonobstructive disease (75% of patients). Occasionally, young patients with HCM also have Wolff-

Figure 33-4 Heart Disease in Hypertension.

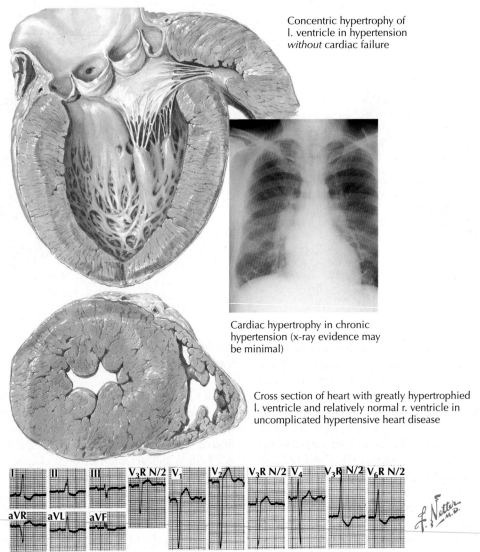

Concentric hypertrophy of l. ventricle in hypertension *without* cardiac failure

Cardiac hypertrophy in chronic hypertension (x-ray evidence may be minimal)

Cross section of heart with greatly hypertrophied l. ventricle and relatively normal r. ventricle in uncomplicated hypertensive heart disease

Electrocardiographic evidence of l. ventricular hypertrophy may or may not be present (tall R waves in V_4, V_5, and V_6; deep S waves in V_3R, V_1, V_2, III, and aVR; depressed ST and inverted T in V_5, V_6, I, II, aVL, and aVF)

Parkinson-White syndrome. Routine exercise testing is often used for risk stratification.

Restrictive Cardiomyopathy

Similar to HCM, the underlying pathophysiology of RCM is diastolic dysfunction with impaired relaxation (reduced compliance) of the ventricle. Unlike HCM, this diastolic dysfunction is not caused by ventricular hypertrophy. Instead, the intrinsic disease process affecting the myocardium results in a stiff ventricle with a restrictive diastolic filling pattern. Ventricular systolic function is usually preserved or only mildly reduced, ventricular chamber size is normal, and the wall thickness is usually either normal or mildly increased. The phenotypic hallmark of the heart is

often marked biatrial enlargement, in which the atria are disproportionately much larger than the ventricle. Histologic examination varies depending on the primary cause of the RCM. Interstitial fibrosis and myocardial disarray are common findings in all cases. Conduction system disease (e.g., atrioventricular block) may precede the clinical heart failure symptoms from ventricular diastolic dysfunction.

The most common causes of RCM include infiltrative diseases (e.g., amyloidosis and sarcoidosis; Fig. 33-6); non-infiltrative diseases—idiopathic fibrosis of unknown cause or "primary RCM"; and endomyocardial diseases (e.g., endomyocardial fibrosis, radiation fibrosis, anthracycline toxicity) (see Box 33-1). Idiopathic RCM is often associated with a familial or genetic predilection that may have been manifested prior to the diagnosis of RCM (as in

Figure 33-5 Anomalies of the Left Ventricular Outflow Tract.

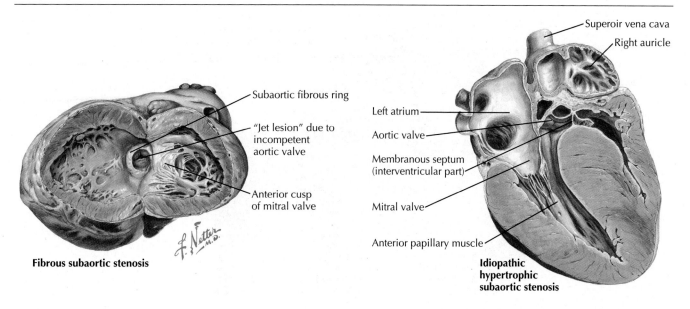

Subaortic fibrous ring

"Jet lesion" due to incompetent aortic valve

Anterior cusp of mitral valve

Fibrous subaortic stenosis

Superoir vena cava

Right auricle

Left atrium

Aortic valve

Membranous septum (interventricular part)

Mitral valve

Anterior papillary muscle

Idiopathic hypertrophic subaortic stenosis

Noonan's syndrome and various muscular dystrophies). In other circumstances, the only manifestation of the familial nature of the disease is RCM in affected family members.

Sarcoidosis and the multiple types of amyloidosis are both systemic diseases. In all cases, although the most common initial presentation is RCM, in later stages of the disease, DCM can develop. Primary amyloidosis (AL, or light-chain–associated amyloidosis) is caused by deposition of amyloid protein that is composed of immunoglobulin light chains produced by a monoclonal population of plasma cells. Secondary amyloidosis (AA, or amyloid-associated amyloidosis) is caused by production of a non-immunoglobulin amyloid protein. Familial amyloidosis is an inherited autosomal dominant trait resulting from a variant prealbumin protein, transthyretin. This is the only type of amyloidosis for which cardiac transplantation has been shown to offer promise. Results have been mixed (some patients have recurrent amyloid heart disease after transplantation). As the genetics of the familial amyloidosis syndromes become better understood, it is likely that the role of cardiac transplantation can be refined.

For RCM, unless the underlying cause is reversible (which is uncommon), this cardiomyopathy often portends the worst prognosis. As this disease progresses to end-stage, ventricular systolic function usually does not worsen significantly, and the clinical heart failure is often considered the most difficult to treat with more limited treatment options than DCM and HCM. It should also be noted that, at times, ascertaining whether an individual has RCM or a constrictive pericardial process can be difficult, requiring multiple, complementary hemodynamic and imaging modalities.

Arrhythmogenic Right Ventricular Cardiomyopathy

ARVD is a genetic disease characterized by morphologic and functional abnormalities of the right ventricle, resulting in ventricular tachycardia. The right ventricle is usually dilated with wall motion abnormalities, but the left ventricle often appears and functions normally. The hallmark feature is progressive fibrofatty replacement of right ventricular myocardium, initially in discrete regions and ultimately globally. Rarely, the left ventricle is involved. Advances in cardiac magnetic resonance imaging have made it possible to detect these morphologic changes at an early stage. On histologic examination, inflammatory lymphocytic infiltrates may also be present.

Unlike the other cardiomyopathies that often present with heart failure symptoms, the clinical manifestation of ARVD is commonly ventricular arrhythmias and occasionally sudden cardiac death, particularly in the young. The risk for sudden death in patients with ARVD is 1% per year. There is a male predominance and a strong genetic component. ARVD is now known as a disease of desmosomal dysfunction, resulting in a disruption of myocyte binding. In evaluating patients with suspected ARVD, the other major condition that needs to be excluded is the more common condition of idiopathic ventricular tachycardia arising from the outflow tract (e.g., right ventricular outflow tract tachycardia), where there is no structural heart abnormality. Treatment is targeted to control the ventricular arrhythmias with either medications or catheter ablation and defibrillator implantation. The only curative therapy is cardiac transplantation, which should be considered on an individual basis.

Figure 33-6 Idiopathic and Infiltrative Causes of Restrictive Cardiomyopathy.

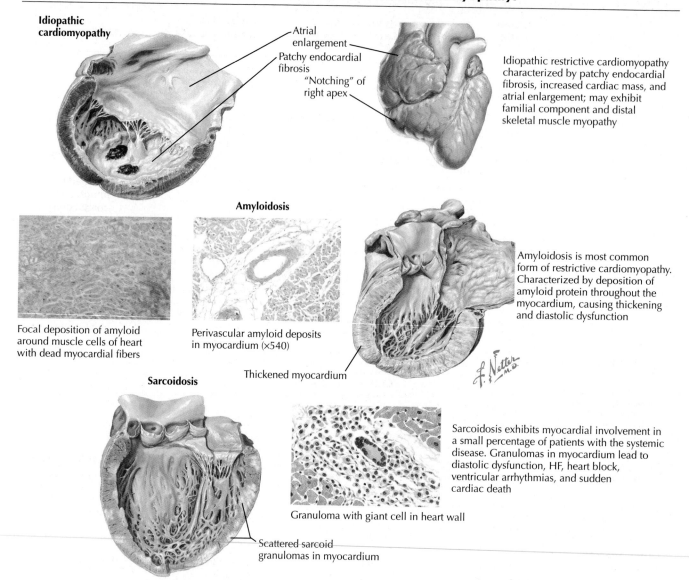

Idiopathic cardiomyopathy

Atrial enlargement

Patchy endocardial fibrosis

"Notching" of right apex

Idiopathic restrictive cardiomyopathy characterized by patchy endocardial fibrosis, increased cardiac mass, and atrial enlargement; may exhibit familial component and distal skeletal muscle myopathy

Amyloidosis

Focal deposition of amyloid around muscle cells of heart with dead myocardial fibers

Perivascular amyloid deposits in myocardium (×540)

Thickened myocardium

Amyloidosis is most common form of restrictive cardiomyopathy. Characterized by deposition of amyloid protein throughout the myocardium, causing thickening and diastolic dysfunction

Sarcoidosis

Granuloma with giant cell in heart wall

Sarcoidosis exhibits myocardial involvement in a small percentage of patients with the systemic disease. Granulomas in myocardium lead to diastolic dysfunction, HF, heart block, ventricular arrhythmias, and sudden cardiac death

Scattered sarcoid granulomas in myocardium

Unclassified Cardiomyopathies

There are scattered cases of cardiomyopathies that do not fit into any of the previously defined classifications. These include fibroelastosis, noncompaction of the left ventricle, and mitochondrial diseases.

Diagnostic Approach

Specific treatment should be directed toward the underlying cause of the cardiomyopathy if identified, especially if that cause can be reversed. Thus, the diagnostic evaluation begins with determination of the characteristics of an individual's cardiomyopathy. Is it global, regional, dilated, or restrictive (or both), and is coronary artery disease present?

(Table 33-1). For example, a thorough family history should be obtained, and obstructive coronary artery disease should be excluded because ischemic heart disease is the most common cause for heart failure. Some specific tests may be useful only for some etiologies of cardiomyopathy; for example, cardiac magnetic resonance imaging may only be useful for myocardial viability (ischemic cardiomyopathy), diffuse patchy defects (sarcoidosis), or fatty infiltration (ARVD). Endomyocardial biopsy is now rarely performed to determine the cause of the cardiomyopathy, but it may be helpful in diagnosing certain conditions that dictate specific therapies, such as giant cell myocarditis or acute fulminant myocarditis, in which immunosuppression could be considered in severe cases, acknowledging the generally unfavorable results from clinical trials.

Table 33-1 Diagnostic Approach for Unexplained Cardiomyopathy*

	Dilated Cardiomyopathy	Hypertrophic Cardiomyopathy	Restrictive Cardiomyopathy	ARVC
History				
Past medical history	Etiology	Etiology (HTN)	Etiology	Etiology
Family history	Familial	Familial	Familial	Familial
Cardiac Assessment				
Physical examination	$+S_3$, $\pm S_4$, $\pm$murmur, L- and R-sided HF	$\pm S_4$, $\pm$murmur, L-sided HF	$+S_3$, $\pm S_4$, murmur, R > L-sided HF, Kussmaul's sign	(Nonspecific)
Electrocardiography	Abnormal ST and T wave, old MI	Abnormal ST and T waves, LVH	Low voltage, abnormal ST and T, $\pm$atrial fibrillation	Repolarization and depolarization abnormalities, conduction abnormalities, $\pm$RBBB, PVCs
Echocardiography	Dilated LV; systolic dysfunction $\pm$ diastolic dysfunction; valve disease	Small LV size, LVH; diastolic dysfunction; initially normal LVEF, later systolic dysfunction; LVOT gradient	Normal LV size, $\pm$LVH, marked biatrial enlargement; diastolic dysfunction (restrictive filling), normal LVEF; mitral and tricuspid regurgitation	Dilated RV with systolic dysfunction; occasionally dilated LV with systolic dysfunction
Stress test	CAD	CAD if +HTN Risk stratification		Risk stratification
Coronary angiography or (rare) cardiac computed tomographic angiography	CAD	CAD if +HTN LVOT gradient		
Right heart catheterization	↓ Cardiac output, ↑ filling pressures	↑ Filling pressures, normal vs. ↓ cardiac output	↓ Cardiac output, restrictive filling (square root sign), ↑ filling pressures	↓ Cardiac output (right-sided)
Cardiac magnetic resonance imaging	Myocardial viability, fibrosis	—	Sarcoidosis	Fibrofatty replacement
Other Testing				
Blood tests	TSH Glucose, HbA1c ANA ± ENA HIV SPEP, UPEP Free copper, ceruloplasmin	Genetics	SPEP, UPEP ACE level ANA, Scl-70	Genetics
Serologies	Coxsackie B antibody titers Enterovirus PCR *Trypanosoma cruzi* antibody (IgM, IgG)			

* Rationale and/or common findings are listed by type of cardiomyopathy.

ACE, angiotensin-converting enzyme; ANA, antinuclear antibody; ARVC, arrhythmogenic right ventricular cardiomyopathy; CAD, coronary artery disease; ENA, extractable nuclear antigens; HbA1c, hemoglobin A1c; Ig, immunoglobulin; HTN, hypertension; L-sided HF, left-sided heart failure signs/symptoms; LV, left ventricle; LVEF, left ventricular ejection fraction; LVH, left ventricular hypertrophy; LVOT, left ventricular outflow tract; MI, myocardial infarction; PCR, polymerase chain reaction; PVCs, premature ventricular contractions; RBBB, right bundle branch block; R-sided HF, right-sided heart failure signs/symptoms; RV, right ventricle; Scl-70, Scl-70 antibody; SPEP, serum protein electrophoresis; TSH, thyroid-stimulating hormone; UPEP, urine protein electrophoresis.

Management and Therapy

Dilated Cardiomyopathy

The treatment goals for patients with cardiomyopathy generally reflect therapy for the resulting heart failure symptoms and for reducing the risk for disease progression and sudden cardiac death. Thus, treatment is directed toward management of heart failure symptoms and signs and to reversing the cardiac remodeling where possible. As detailed in Chapter 34 and in the Practice Guidelines from the American College of Cardiology/American Heart Association and the Heart Failure Society of America, standard treatment includes behavioral and lifestyle modifications, such as low-salt diet, fluid restriction, and minimizing coronary risk factors; medications, both oral and intravenous; electrophysiologic devices, such as implantable defibrillators and cardiac resynchronization therapy; and surgical therapies where indicated, such as revascularization, valve surgery, mechanical cardiac support, and cardiac transplantation. The best approach involves optimizing medications to at least target doses as tolerated and appropriate use of the various electrophysiologic device or surgical therapies available. Certain cardiomyopathies require more aggressive use of some therapies (e.g., defibrillators for ischemic cardiomyopathy, some hypertrophic cardiomyopathies, ARVD), and conversely, other therapies are not appropriate in a given type of cardiomyopathy (e.g., inotropes in ARVD, biventricular pacemakers in nondilated cardiomyopathies).

Hypertrophic Cardiomyopathy

Treatment of HCM is directed at regression or at least the prevention of progression of the ventricular hypertrophy and blood pressure control (because elevated blood pressure can promote further hypertrophy) for those with hypertension. Usual medications include β-blockers and calcium channel blockers (verapamil). Disopyramide has been useful in decreasing outflow gradient and improving exercise tolerance and is used occasionally for this indication. Pacemakers were more commonly used in the past in an effort to reverse remodeling, but this approach is now not considered to be efficacious. Arrhythmias are poorly tolerated and potentially even fatal. Defibrillator implantation should be considered in HCM patients at high risk for sudden death. Risk factors for sudden death include prior cardiac arrest, sustained ventricular tachycardia, frequent nonsustained ventricular tachycardia on serial Holter electrocardiographic monitoring, positive family history of premature HCM-related death, history of syncope, abnormal (hypotensive) blood pressure response to exercise, and severely increased left ventricular wall thickness (≥30 mm). Symptomatic patients with obstructive HCM should be considered for surgical myectomy of the septum or alcohol septal ablation.

Avoiding Treatment Errors

Avoiding treatment errors in this group of patients necessitates careful monitoring. For example, patients need to be assessed regularly for hyperkalemia, given the efficacy in heart failure of multiple agents that can elevate serum potassium levels (angiotensin-converting enzyme inhibitors, angiotensin receptor blockers, and aldosterone blockers). Patients should be assessed regularly for symptoms and signs of hypotension, given the potential for all the above medications and β-blockers to lower blood pressure. Finally, consideration should always be given to timely referral for specific therapies for refractory or stage D heart failure (e.g., ventricular assist device [VAD] or cardiac transplantation before disease is truly end-stage).

Cardiac Transplantation

Considered the only definitive cure for heart failure, more than 73,000 heart transplantation surgeries have been performed in more than 200 hospitals worldwide. In the United States, more than 2000 transplantations are performed per year in about 134 centers. This surgery requires a median sternotomy, cardiopulmonary bypass, recipient cardiectomy, and donor implantation. The most common anastomosis of the donor heart to the recipient cardiac tissues has been either a biatrial technique, in which the donor left and right atria are sutured to the respective remnant atria of the recipient (Fig. 33-7), or a bicaval technique, in which the anastomoses are between donor's and recipient's vena cava and left atria.

Although the first transplantations were performed more than 30 years ago (December, 1967 in South Africa by Dr. Christiaan Barnard, and January, 1968 at Stanford University by Dr. Norman Shumway), rejection and infection in immunosuppressed patients remained major problems and limited the number of operations. In 1983, with the availability of the first calcineurin inhibitor (cyclosporin A), the ability to manage rejection and immunosuppression improved dramatically, and the number of cardiac transplantations again increased. The numbers of transplantations have now reached a plateau (and have even slightly declined) since the mid-1990s (about 4000 per year) because of the limited availability of donor hearts. This limited availability has resulted in the need for stringent selection of patients for consideration of cardiac transplantation.

Current indications for cardiac transplantation are end-stage heart failure or cardiomyopathy, with New York Heart Association class III or IV symptoms, and failure of maximal medical therapy not due to patient noncompliance or inadequate treatment. Contraindications include advanced age; active infection; significant other organ dysfunction (unless cured by combined organ transplantation, e.g., heart-kidney); recent malignancy; excessive obesity; major chronic disabling disease; active mental illness; active or recent substance abuse; noncompliance; lack of social

Figure 33-7 Technique of Orthotopic Biatrial Cardiac Transplantation.

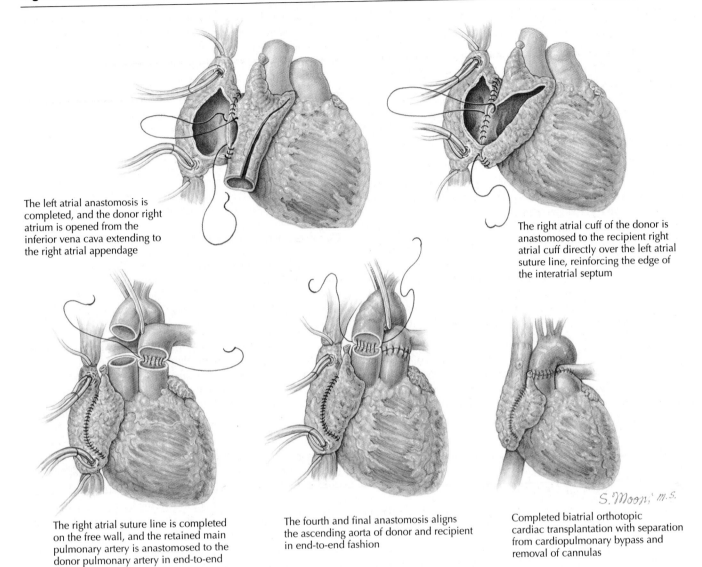

The left atrial anastomosis is completed, and the donor right atrium is opened from the inferior vena cava extending to the right atrial appendage

The right atrial cuff of the donor is anastomosed to the recipient right atrial cuff directly over the left atrial suture line, reinforcing the edge of the interatrial septum

The right atrial suture line is completed on the free wall, and the retained main pulmonary artery is anastomosed to the donor pulmonary artery in end-to-end fashion

The fourth and final anastomosis aligns the ascending aorta of donor and recipient in end-to-end fashion

Completed biatrial orthotopic cardiac transplantation with separation from cardiopulmonary bypass and removal of cannulas

S. Moon, M.S.

support; and lack of medical insurance. Invasive hemodynamics, including reversibility of secondary pulmonary hypertension, and peak exercise oxygen consumption are objectively measured to assess patient's eligibility and timing for transplantation. Median survival is about 10 years. Common complications and comorbidities include cardiac rejection, infection (opportunistic and nonopportunistic), hypertension, hyperlipidemia, renal dysfunction, diabetes, and coronary allograft vasculopathy. Care of the transplant recipient involves aggressive preventive care based on chronic immunosuppression, prophylactic antimicrobials as needed, timely health maintenance, and management of comorbidities.

Mechanical Cardiac Support

Because cardiac transplantation is not available or appropriate for everyone with end-stage cardiomyopathy, a number of other treatment modalities have been developed and are available to the end-stage patient. Intravenous inotropes have been used for both palliative care and as a bridge therapy for transplantation. Except for acute exacerbations treated in an intensive care setting, the use of intravenous inotropes is controversial because of their potential to exacerbate cardiac arrhythmias and the limited data supporting outpatient efficacy. Mechanical cardiac support for the failing heart has been available for decades for use as a bridge to transplantation or as a bridge to recovery. The first types of mechanical cardiac support were extracorporeal membrane oxygenators (ECMO) and percutaneous intra-aortic balloon pumps; both are short-term therapies. Surgically placed ventricular assistive devices (VADs) have evolved into sophisticated machines to unload and support the ventricle, many of which are now portable and can be used for at least a few years. Like ECMO and balloon pumps, VADs have served primarily

as a bridge to transplantation or as a bridge to recovery. Since 2002, left ventricular assistive devices are now available for destination therapy for the patient who is not eligible or not interested in heart transplantation. Thus, mechanical support has become an alternative to hospice. As mechanical devices continue to improve, it is possible that some patients who previously would have undergone cardiac transplantation will be considered, instead, for VAD placement. Limited studies have even indicated that left ventricular function can improve after sustained support with a VAD.

Future Directions

As medical technology continues to evolve, we anticipate future tools for both diagnostics and therapeutics for all types of cardiomyopathy. Genetic advances will allow easier diagnosis of otherwise unexplained cardiomyopathy presumed to be familial. Although purely investigational at the current time, treatment with novel drugs, stem cells, and total artificial hearts may provide even more hope to the patient with end-stage disease. Finally, as noted earlier, there will likely continue to be improvement in implantable devices for this group of patients.

Additional Resources

Heart Failure Society of America. Available at: http://www.hfsa.org. Accessed December 22, 2006.
  This website contains many helpful resources about heart failure for health professionals, patients, and their families.
International Society of Heart and Lung Transplantation. Available at: http://www.ishlt.org. Accessed December 22, 2006.
  This website contains many helpful resources about heart, heart-lung, and lung transplantation for health professionals, patients, and their families.
United Network of Organ Sharing. Available at: http://www.unos.org. Accessed December 22, 2006.
  This website contains many helpful resources about organ transplantation in the United States for health professionals, patients and their families.

EVIDENCE

1. Gronda E, Bourge RC, Costanzo MR, et al: Heart rhythm considerations in heart transplant candidates and considerations for ventricular assist devices: International Society for Heart and Lung Transplantation guidelines for the care of cardiac transplant candidates—2006. J Heart Lung Transplant 25(9):1043-1056, 2006.
  These guidelines provide current recommendations for optimizing nonpharmacologic treatment of patients being considered for heart transplantation based on available data and consensus opinion for electrophysiologic devices and mechanical ventricular assist device support (class I, IIa, IIb, III; levels A, B, C).
2. Heart Failure Society of America: Executive summary: HFSA 2006 Comprehensive Heart Failure Practice Guideline. J Card Fail 12(1):10-38, 2006.
  These guidelines provide current recommendations for treatment of chronic heart failure based on available data and consensus opinion (class I, IIa, IIb, III; levels A, B, C).
3. Ho CY, Seidman CE: A contemporary approach to hypertrophic cardiomyopathy. Circulation 113(24):e858-e862, 2006.
  This review provides an overview of hypertrophic cardiomyopathy from a genetics perspective.
4. Hunt SA, Abraham WT, Chin MH, et al: ACC/AHA 2005 Guideline Update for the Diagnosis and Management of Chronic Heart Failure in the Adult: A report of the American College of Cardiology/American Heart Association Task Force on Practice Guidelines (Writing Committee to Update the 2001 Guidelines for the Evaluation and Management of Heart Failure). Developed in collaboration with the American College of Chest Physicians and the International Society for Heart and Lung Transplantation, endorsed by the Heart Rhythm Society. Circulation 112(12):e154-e235, 2005.
  These guidelines provide current recommendations for treatment of chronic heart failure based on available data and consensus opinion (class I, IIa, IIb, III; levels A, B, C).
5. Jessup M, Banner N, Brozena S, et al: Optimal pharmacologic and non-pharmacologic management of cardiac transplant candidates: Approaches to be considered prior to transplant evaluation. International Society for Heart and Lung Transplantation guidelines for the care of cardiac transplant candidates—2006. J Heart Lung Transplant 25(9):1003-1023, 2006.
  These guidelines provide current recommendations for optimizing treatment of patients being considered for heart transplantation based on available data and consensus opinion (class I, IIa, IIb, III; levels A, B, C).
6. Kushwaha SS, Fallon JT, Fuster V: Restrictive cardiomyopathy. N Engl J Med 336(4):267-276, 1997.
  This review provides an overview as well as the diagnostic and therapeutic approach to patients with restrictive cardiomyopathy based on available data and consensus opinion.
7. Maron BJ: Hypertrophic cardiomyopathy: A systematic review. JAMA 287(10):1308-1320, 2002.
  This review provides an overview as well as the diagnostic and therapeutic approach to patients with hypertrophic cardiomyopathy based on available data and consensus opinion.
8. Mehra MR, Kobashigawa J, Starling R, et al: Listing criteria for heart transplantation: International Society for Heart and Lung Transplantation guidelines for the care of cardiac transplant candidates—2006. J Heart Lung Transplant 25(9):1024-1042, 2006.
  These guidelines provide current recommendations for evaluating patients for heart transplantation based on available data and consensus opinion (class I, IIa, IIb, III; levels A, B, C).
9. Miller LW, Lietz K: Candidate selection for long-term left ventricular assist device therapy for refractory heart failure. J Heart Lung Transplant 25(7):756-764, 2006.
  This review outlines current strategies for evaluating patients being considered for ventricular assist device support based on available data and consensus opinion.
10. Richardson P, McKenna W, Bristow M, et al: Report of the 1995 World Health Organization/International Society and Federation of Cardiology Task Force on the Definition and Classification of Cardiomyopathies. Circulation 93(5):841-842, 1996.
  This paper outlines the classification of cardiomyopathies based on expert consensus opinion.

Carla Sueta Dupree

Heart Failure

Introduction

Heart failure (HF), the accepted term for a constellation of syndromes previously referred to as congestive heart failure, is caused by cardiac dysfunction. Most commonly, HF results from myocardial muscle dysfunction with accompanying dilation or hypertrophy of the left ventricle (LV) and neurohormonal activation. HF can be divided into two primary types. Systolic HF is the inability of the ventricle to empty normally, with reduced ejection fraction (EF ≤40%), usually accompanied by ventricular dilation. HF with preserved systolic function (HF-PSF), sometimes referred to as *diastolic HF*, is the inability of the ventricle to relax or fill normally. In HF-PSF, ventricular size and systolic function (as measured by EF) are often normal, but left ventricular end-diastolic pressure is elevated.

HF affects 5 million Americans, with an incidence of 550,000 cases per year, increasing significantly with age. HF is the most common cause of hospitalization for patients 65 years of age and older, and the annual health care cost of patients with HF exceeds $29 billion. With appropriate therapy, patients with HF can be stabilized and have significant improvement in their symptoms. However, despite therapeutic advances, the mortality rate of patients with HF is about 50% at 5 years. It is likely that more broad use of evidence-based approaches for the treatment of patients with HF will lead to reduction in mortality. More aggressive efforts for risk factor modification, especially for coronary heart disease risk factors, are of importance given that HF following myocardial infarction is common. Recent studies have demonstrated that treating hypertension, vascular disease, or high-risk diabetics significantly reduces the development of HF.

Risk factors for developing HF include a history of hypertension, atherosclerosis, hyperlipidemia, diabetes, valvular disease, obesity, physical inactivity, excessive alcohol intake, exposure to cardiotoxins, family history of cardiomyopathy, sleep-disordered breathing, and smoking.

Etiology and Pathogenesis

Coronary artery disease (CAD) accounts for 50% of the incidence of HF worldwide. Patients with previous myocardial infarction can exhibit both decreased systolic performance and diastolic impairment due to interstitial fibrosis and scar formation. Hypertension is a common cause of HF, especially in African Americans and older women (Fig. 34-1). A common cause of initially unexplained HF (following exclusion of CAD) is idiopathic cardiomyopathy. Familial cardiomyopathies may account for up to one third of cardiomyopathies thought to be idiopathic. Other etiologies of dilated cardiomyopathy include thyroid disease, chemotherapy (doxorubicin or Herceptin), myocarditis, infection due to HIV, diabetes, alcohol, cocaine, connective tissue disease, peripartum cardiomyopathy, and arrhythmias. Hypertrophic and restrictive cardiomyopathies can cause HF, but this is less common. Refer to Chapter 33 for further information on these cardiomyopathies.

Systolic Heart Failure

Systolic dysfunction (EF ≤40%) results in a reduction in cardiac output that is perceived as "hypovolemia" by the kidneys and triggers activation of the renin-angiotensin system (RAS). With RAS activation, salt and water retention occurs. Initially, this results in increased preload, transiently improving cardiac output. Over longer periods of time, chronic activation of the RAS results in volume overload and symptoms of HF.

Declining blood pressure due to decreased cardiac output also triggers activation of the sympathetic nervous

Figure 34-1 Heart Failure with Preserved Ejection Fraction Due to Hypertension.

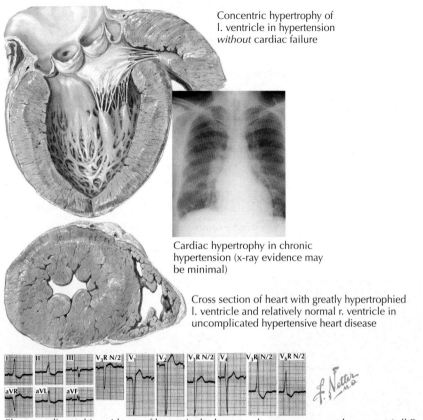

Concentric hypertrophy of
l. ventricle in hypertension
without cardiac failure

Cardiac hypertrophy in chronic
hypertension (x-ray evidence may
be minimal)

Cross section of heart with greatly hypertrophied
l. ventricle and relatively normal r. ventricle in
uncomplicated hypertensive heart disease

Electrocardiographic evidence of l. ventricular hypertrophy may or may not be present (tall R waves in V_4, V_5, and V_6; deep S waves in V_3R, V_1, V_2, III, and aVR; depressed ST and inverted T in V_5, V_6, I, II, aVL, and aVF)

system. This, along with RAS activation and increased circulating levels of endothelin and vasopressin, results in systemic vasoconstriction. The short-term benefit of vaso-constriction—increased perfusion of critical organs—is followed by worsening HF due to chronically increased LV afterload that ultimately causes worsening HF. Sympathetic nervous system activation can also precipitate ventricular arrhythmias, a common cause of death in patients with HF.

HF generally follows an injury to the myocardium (due to ischemia, a toxic effect, or an increased volume or pressure load on the LV). LV remodeling, a maladaptive response, follows, with resulting changes in cardiac size, shape, and function (Fig. 34-2). Myocyte length may increase, with a resulting increase in chamber volume, which preserves stroke volume. Myocyte hypertrophy also occurs, along with a loss of myocytes due to apoptosis or necrosis, and fibroblast proliferation and fibrosis. As the heart remodels, it becomes less elliptical and more spherical, hence more dilated. The mitral valve annulus may become dilated, resulting in mitral regurgitation and further increased wall stress.

The success of angiotensin–converting enzyme inhibitor (ACE-I), angiotensin II receptor blockers (ARB), β-

blockers, and aldosterone antagonists in reducing mortality in patients with HF almost certainly relates to their ability to interrupt the cycle of LV remodeling and dilation by blocking the neurohormonal activation that occurs early in HF. All have been shown to attenuate and even reverse remodeling.

Heart Failure with Preserved Ejection Fraction

HF-PSF accounts for 40% to 50% or more of HF cases and, until recently, resulted in considerable confusion and debate about treatment. It is now clear that the morbidity and mortality of patients with HF-PSF is similar to that of patients with HF due to systolic dysfunction. HF-PSF affects older patients, especially women. Ischemic heart disease and hypertension are the most common causes of isolated HF-PSF. In the typical patient with HF-PSF, the ventricular size is normal. However, ventricular dilation occurs in mitral and aortic regurgitation as well as in high-output HF caused by anemia or thiamine deficiency.

Restrictive and hypertrophic cardiomyopathies can result in similar clinical presentations (see Chapter 33), as can constrictive pericarditis. Indeed, distinguishing these

Figure 34-2 Cardiac Remodeling Secondary to Volume Overload.

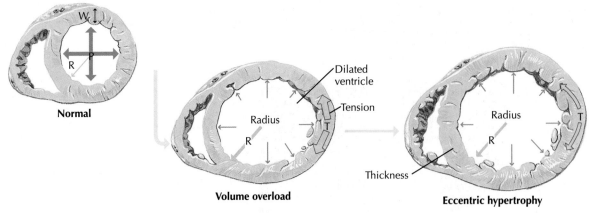

Elevated pressure (P) or volume causes proportionate increases in wall thickness (W) and chamber radius (R); wall tension (T) increases

LA indicates left atrium; LV, left ventricle; RA, right atrium; RV, right ventricle

Ventricular hypertrophy

Dilated ventricle

entities can be difficult, requiring extensive noninvasive and invasive hemodynamic assessment. The distinction is of importance, however. For instance, in patients with diastolic dysfunction related to the constraining effect of a thickened and rigid pericardium, surgical removal of the pericardium can produce profound relief of symptoms and findings of HF.

The pathophysiology of HF-PSF has not been entirely elucidated, nor is it precisely the same in all patients. The LV in typical patients with HF-PSF is characterized by hypertrophy, increased extracellular matrix, and abnormal calcium handling. Activation of the RAS and sympathetic nervous system is common in patients with HF-PSF.

Clinical Presentation

The presentation of patients with HF includes signs and symptoms of pulmonary congestion, systemic fluid reten-tion, exercise intolerance, or inadequate organ perfusion. Symptoms include dyspnea on exertion, exercise intoler-ance, orthopnea, paroxysmal nocturnal dyspnea, cough, chest pain, weakness, fatigue, nausea, abdominal pain, noc-turia, oliguria, confusion, insomnia, depression, and weight loss. Physical examination findings that should be system-atically assessed include engorged neck veins, rales, pleural effusion, displaced point of maximal intensity, right ven-tricular heave, S_3, S_4, murmurs, hepatomegaly, low-volume pulses, and peripheral edema.

The clinical presentation may be indistinguishable between patients with HF and HF-PSF (Fig. 34-3). The cardiac silhouette is usually enlarged in both circum-stances, with cardiomegaly due to ventricular dilation in HF with systolic dysfunction due to hypertrophy in patients with HF-PSF. Assessment of LV function is essential in designing the appropriate approach to therapy.

Figure 34-3 Left Heart Failure and Pulmonary Congestion.

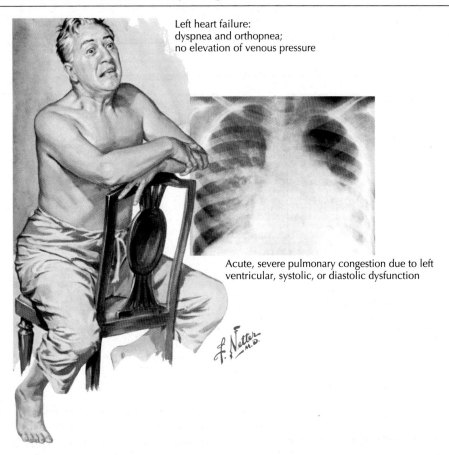

Left heart failure: dyspnea and orthopnea; no elevation of venous pressure

Acute, severe pulmonary congestion due to left ventricular, systolic, or diastolic dysfunction

Differential Diagnosis

The difficulty in arriving at a new diagnosis of HF lies in its vague symptoms and exam mimickers (Box 34-1). Symptoms of dyspnea and exercise intolerance can be attributed to many diagnoses: lung disease (including chronic obstructive lung disease, reactive airways diseases, thromboembolic pulmonary disease, pulmonary hypertension, and others), thyroid disease, arrhythmias, anemia, obesity, deconditioning, and cognitive disorders. Signs of volume overload are not specific to HF. Sodium-avid states of nephrosis and cirrhosis, as well as pericardial disease, can present with similar findings of jugular venous distention, hepatomegaly, and edema.

Box 34-1   Differential Diagnosis
■ Myocardial ischemia
■ Pulmonary disease
■ Sleep-disordered breathing
■ Obesity
■ Deconditioning
■ Thromboembolic disease
■ Anemia
■ Hepatic failure
■ Renal failure
■ Hypoalbuminemia
■ Venous stasis
■ Depression
■ Anxiety and hyperventilation syndromes

Diagnostic Approach

The diagnosis is made by taking a careful history, performing a directed exam, and assessing systolic and diastolic ventricular function. Laboratory evaluation and pulmonary function testing will eliminate most noncardiac diagnoses (Box 34-2). Measurement of serum brain natriuretic peptide (BNP >500 pg/mL) or N-terminal prohormone brain natriuretic peptide (pro-BNP >450 pg/mL in individuals <50 years old or ≥900 pg/mL in individuals >50

years old) can be very helpful in the acute setting. These markers correlate with elevated filling pressures and are particularly helpful in the evaluation of patients with dyspnea. Although an elevated level of BNP or pro-BNP does not rule out pulmonary causes of dyspnea, normal levels argue against HF as the predominant cause of dyspnea. Even though levels are generally higher in cases of systolic HF, these tests cannot distinguish between systolic HF and HF-PSF.

Figure 34-4 Echo-Doppler Criteria for Assessment of Diastolic Function.
A, Late peak mitral inflow velocity; DT, deceleration time of the E wave; E, early peak mitral inflow velocity; e′, velocity of annulus early diastolic motion. © *Copyright American Medical Association. From Bursi F, Weston SA, Redfield MM, et al: Systolic and diastolic heart failure in the community. JAMA 296(18):2209-2216, 2006.*

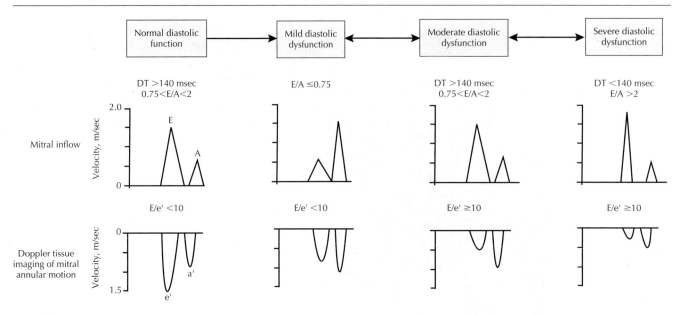

Box 34-2   Laboratory Evaluation

- Brain natriuretic peptide or N-terminal prohormone brain natriuretic peptide
- Serum electrolytes
- Blood urea nitrogen
- Creatinine
- Glucose
- Calcium
- Magnesium
- Lipid profile
- Complete blood count
- Serum albumin
- Liver functions tests
- Urinalysis
- Thyroid function
- Electrocardiogram
- Chest x-ray
- Additional directed tests (serum protein electrophoresis, urine protein electrophoresis)

Determining the Type and Degree of Left Ventricle Dysfunction

Echocardiography is the most common method for initial assessment of LV function. EF, valve function, hypertrophy, and diastolic function can all be rapidly assessed. Most patients with HF-PSF have impaired LV relaxation with or without reduced LV compliance and preserved EF. The most reproducible and validated method of diagnosing diastolic dysfunction combines echocardiographic two-dimensional M-mode Doppler measurements of mitral valve inflow with the sensitive, relatively load-independent measure of LV relaxation (e′ velocity) obtained by tissue Doppler imaging of the mitral annulus. This approach has resulted in four classifications of diastolic function: normal, mild dysfunction (impaired relaxation, normal filling pressure), moderate dysfunction (impaired relaxation or pseudonormal with moderately elevated filling pressure), and severe dysfunction (restrictive or advanced with reduced compliance) (Fig. 34-4).

Radionuclide ventriculography is often used to determine EF in obese patients and in those with significant chronic obstructive pulmonary disease. Magnetic resonance imaging is a newer imaging modality that provides EF, allows assessment of myocardial viability, and can identify infiltrative disease.

Defining the Etiology of Heart Failure

The degree of reversibility and, hence, the progression and management of HF differ depending on the underlying cause. Many underlying causes of HF are largely reversible. Treatment of uncontrolled hypertension, thyroid disease, and active ischemia may result in significant improvement in LV function. Conversely, patients with prior myocardial infarction and systolic dysfunction; patients who are older, are male, and have a marked reduction in LV function; and patients who have hyponatremia, anemia, renal dysfunction, or New York Heart Association (NYHA) class III or IV disease have a worse prognosis.

Ischemic heart disease should be excluded in every patient. Focal wall motion abnormalities do not always represent CAD, and conversely, global LV dysfunction does not rule out an ischemic cause. Testing options include cardiac catheterization, exercise or pharmacologic echocardiographic or nuclear stress testing. Patients with left bundle branch block should not be evaluated with stress echocardiography because the conduction delay can result in a false-positive test result. Newer imaging techniques include computed tomographic angiography, which can identify CAD, and cardiac magnetic resonance imaging, which can also provide assessment of viability.

Determining NYHA classification is important for assessing prognosis, medical management, indication for device placement, and for longitudinal follow-up and evaluation of response to therapy (Box 34-3).

Management and Therapy

As a first step, it is important to correct precipitating factors, such as dietary noncompliance, ischemia, uncontrolled hypertension, atrial fibrillation, hypoxemia, thyroid disease, anemia, and the presence and causes of medication nonadherence, including financial disability. An overall approach to management is shown in Figure 34-5.

Revascularization should be considered in ischemic patients. Observational studies suggest that patients with reversible ischemia, even with marked systolic dysfunction, improve with revascularization. The ongoing National Institutes of Health–sponsored Surgical Treatment for Intracerebral Hemorrhage (STICH) trial will provide evidence for the efficacy of revascularization with or without surgical ventricular restoration in patients with CAD and an EF of 35% or less.

Optimum Treatment for Systolic Heart Failure

For systolic HF, blockade of the RAS with ACE-I or ARB therapy is recommended in all patients. Improved survival, decreased frequency of hospitalization, and improved quality of life have been demonstrated in patients with NYHA class I to IV HF and in post–myocardial infarction patients treated with target doses of ACE-Is or ARBs (Table 34-1). Contraindications to ACE-I or ARB therapy

include moderate to severe aortic stenosis, bilateral renal artery stenosis, and hyperkalemia (K >5.5 mEq/dL).

ACE-I therapy can cause intractable cough or, rarely, angioedema. An ARB can generally be substituted for ACE-I therapy, although angioedema has been reported rarely with an ARB. Both agents have an equivalent effect on renal function. In patients with significant renal dysfunction and hyperkalemia (K >5.5 mEq/dL), the combination of isosorbide dinitrate (160 mg daily in four divided doses) and hydralazine (300 mg daily in four divided doses) is an alternative, although not as effective as ACE-I therapy. All patients with CAD should be treated with aspirin (81 to 325 mg/day) unless there is a contraindication.

β-blockers should be added to ACE-I therapy in all patients who do not have evidence of fluid overload. Improved survival and EF, reduction in sudden death, and hospitalizations have been demonstrated in patients with NYHA class II to IV symptoms, and in all post–myocardial infarction patients at target doses (see Table 34-1). Contraindications include severe reactive airway disease in patients receiving inhaled daily β-agonists, severe bradycardia, or advanced heart block. β-blockers should be started at a low dose and titrated up every 2 weeks. Most patients require diuretic therapy during β-blocker initiation and up-titration to prevent fluid overload. β-blockers should not be initiated or titrated in patients exhibiting volume overload; these patients should be treated for fluid overload first. Side effects (transient fatigue, weight gain, and diarrhea) are more common with the first few doses. If patients have difficulty tolerating the drug, dose titration can be slowed by increasing the time between titrations or by increasing the dose by a smaller amount. Although target doses should be the goal, lower doses (i.e. carvedilol 6.25 mg twice daily) also confers a mortality and morbidity benefit. Studies indicate that at least 80% of patients tolerate β-blocker therapy. ACE-I and β-blocker up-titration can be alternated, rather than titrating ACE-I to the target dose before adding a β-blocker.

Aldosterone antagonists can be added to therapy in patients with NYHA class III (previously class IV) or IV chronic HF, and in post–myocardial infarction patients with an EF less than 40%. Therapy should only be initiated in patients whose potassium is less than 5 mEq/mL, serum creatinine 2.5 mg/DL or less and creatinine clearance >30 ml/min. The serum potassium level often increases with treatment, especially in diabetic and older patients, and regular monitoring is necessary. Potassium and creatinine should be reassessed at least 1 week and 1 month after initiation or change in dose.

The combination of isosorbide dinitrate and hydralazine added to standard therapy of ACE-I or ARB and β-blocker therapy has been shown to provide additional mortality and morbidity benefit in African American patients. The target doses from the largest clinical trial were isosorbide dinitrate, 40 mg three times daily, and hydralazine, 75 mg three times daily.

Figure 34-5 Algorithm for Management.
ACE-I, angiotensin-converting enzyme-I; ARB, angiotensin II receptor blockers; BP, blood pressure; CAD, coronary artery disease; CRT, chronic resynchronization therapy (also called a biventricular pacemaker); EF, ejection fraction; HF, heart failure; ICD, implantable defibrillator; LV, left ventricle; MI, myocardial infarction; NYHA, New York Heart Association; QRSI, QRS integral.

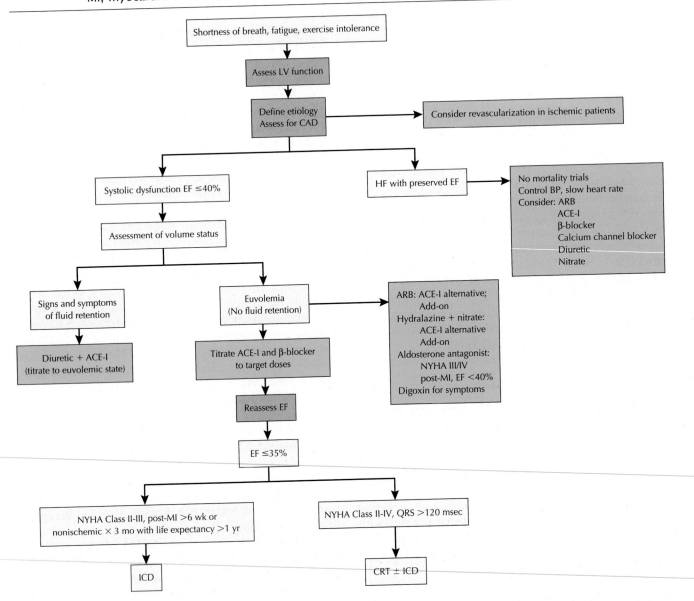

Diuretics such as hydrochlorothiazide, furosemide, and bumetanide are prescribed in most patients to alleviate fluid overload. Because they activate the RAS, the minimal effective dose should be used. In patients with severe HF, combination therapy (a loop diuretic and hydrochlorothiazide or metolazone) can be used, but potassium and magnesium levels must be carefully monitored.

Digoxin reduces hospitalization and improves symptoms. However, there is no survival benefit. Higher serum concentration (≥1.2 ng/dL) is associated with poor outcome. Therefore, low-dose digoxin, generally 125 μg daily, is recommended, with a goal concentration of less than 1 ng/dL. Digoxin doses should be reduced by half and monitored closely if amiodarone or warfarin is initiated.

Nitrates reduce preload and are prescribed as antianginal agents. At higher doses, systemic and pulmonary vasodilation occurs. Nitrate tolerance can be prevented acutely by increasing the dose and chronically by allowing a nitrate-free interval of at least 8 hours. The addition of hydralazine also mitigates nitrate tolerance.

Amlodipine and felodipine are used to treat hypertension and angina unresponsive to ACE-Is and β-blockers. Nifedipine, verapamil, and diltiazem should not be used in

Table 34-1 Drug Therapy for Systolic Heart Failure

	Starting Dose	Target Dose
Angiotensin Converting Enzyme Inhibitors		
Generic		
Enalapril	2.5-5 mg twice a day	10 mg twice a day
Lisinopril	2.5-5 mg once a day	20-40 mg once a day
Captopril*	6.25-12.5 mg three times a day	50 mg three times a day
Nongeneric		
Ramipril	2.5 mg every day to twice a day	5 mg twice a day/10 mg once daily
Trandolapril	1 mg once a day	4 mg once a day
Quinapril	5-10 mg twice a day	20 mg twice a day
Fosinopril	5-10 mg once a day	40 mg once a day
Perindopril	2 mg once a day	8-16 mg once a day
Angiotensin Receptor Blockers		
Nongeneric		
Valsartan	20-40 mg twice a day	160 mg twice a day
Candesartan	4-8 mg once a day	32 mg once a day
Losartan†	25 mg once a day	50-100 mg once a day
β-Blockers		
Nongeneric		
Carvedilol-CR	10 mg once a day	80 mg once a day
Generic		
Bisoprolol	1.25 mg once a day	10 mg once a day
Metoprolol tartrate immediate release†	12.5-25 mg twice a day	100 mg twice a day
Metoprolol succinate extended release	12.5-25 mg once a day	200 mg once a day
Carvedilol	3.125 mg twice a day	25 mg twice a day; if >85 kg, 50 mg twice a day
Aldosterone Antagonists		
Generic		
Spironolactone	12.5-25 mg once a day	25-50 mg once a day
Nongeneric		
Eplerenone	12.5-25 mg once a day	25-50 mg once a day

* Absorption is decreased by food.
† Not approved by the U.S. Food and Drug Administration for treatment of heart failure.

patients with systolic HF because of their negative effect on contractility.

Intravenous diuretic therapy should be considered in acute decompensated HF with volume overload. Continuous furosemide infusion can result in a steady diuresis, particularly in patients who are resistant to initial intravenous diuretics. Metolazone, spironolactone, or intravenous chlorthalidone (500 mg twice daily) can be added in refractory cases.

In the absence of symptomatic hypotension, one should consider nitroglycerin, nitroprusside, or nesiritide in patients who are refractory to diuretics. Nitrate therapy is particularly effective in acute myocardial infarction with pulmonary edema. Compared with nitroglycerin, nitroprusside is a more powerful afterload-reducing agent for the same degree of preload reduction. Nesiritide is a vasodilator and natriuretic agent that can be useful in hospitalized patients, particularly those who have been shown to be unresponsive to intravenous diuretics. Because a meta-analysis reported an increase in 30-day mortality in patients who received nesiritide, it is not a first-line agent.

Renal function should be monitored closely because worsening renal function has been reported.

Intravenous inotropes, such as dobutamine or milrinone, may be considered to relieve symptoms in patients with advanced systolic HF and diminished peripheral perfusion, referred to as *low-output syndrome*. Dobutamine is an inotrope with limited vasodilator activity. Milrinone, a phosphodiesterase inhibitor, is both an inotrope and vasodilator and, for this reason, may worsen hypotension in patients with severe HF. Nonetheless, both agents can be helpful but must be initiated carefully. Heart rate, assessment of angina, and heart rhythm must be monitored. If systolic pressure is less than 90 mm Hg or mean arterial pressure is less than 65 mm Hg, nitroglycerin, nitroprusside, milrinone, and nesiritide should be used with caution. Bolus dosing is usually not given. Although routine invasive hemodynamic monitoring is not recommended, placement of a Swan Ganz catheter is considered in patients whose filling pressures is unclear, who are refractory to standard therapy, who have symptomatic hypotension (i.e., systolic pressure <80 mm Hg) or worsening renal function,

or who need documentation of improved hemodynamics when an inotrope is considered for chronic therapy. Intermittent chronic administration of dobutamine or milrinone has not resulted in improved outcomes in patients with HF.

Device Therapy for Systolic Heart Failure

Implantable cardiac defibrillators (ICDs) are indicated in all patients who have survived a cardiac arrest. ICD placement also reduces mortality in NYHA class II and III patients with an EF of 35% or less, whether the HF is ischemic or nonischemic. Biventricular pacemakers improve survival and quality of life and reduce hospitalization in class III and IV patients with reduced EF and a prolonged QRS duration. These devices should be considered only in optimally treated patients, that is, those receiving ACE-I and β-blocker therapy. It is important to reassess LV function after reaching the target or maximum dose before device implantation because EF may have improved.

LV assist devices are most often used as a bridge to cardiac transplantation but are also approved as destination therapy for end-stage patients who are not transplantation candidates.

Treatment of Heart Failure with Preserved Ejection Fraction

There are no completed randomized trials indicating a medical regimen that improves survival in patients with HF-PSF, but several studies have demonstrated an improvement in symptoms and morbidity. Candesartan, an ARB, reduced subsequent HF hospitalizations in patients admitted for a cardiac reason whose EF was more than 40%. Nebivolol, a β1-selective β-blocker, significantly reduced the combined outcome of mortality or cardiovascular hospitalization in patients 70 years and older admitted with HF regardless of EF.

Blood pressure control is essential. ARB, β-blockers, ACE-I, calcium channel blockers, and aldosterone antagonists cause regression of LV hypertrophy. Agents that reduce preload, such as diuretics and nitrates, are commonly prescribed. Nitrates are also used to treat ischemia. Calcium channel blockers, particularly verapamil, improve ventricular relaxation. Agents that decrease heart rate (increasing diastolic filling time), including verapamil, diltiazem, and β-blockers, are usually beneficial. Smaller studies have demonstrated a benefit of daily, moderate exercise.

Maintaining atrial contraction is important. Atrial contraction contributes up to 50% of ventricular filling in patients with decreased compliance, explaining why the loss of atrial contraction in atrial fibrillation results in acute decompensation. Cardioversion treatment with antiarrhythmic agents or radiofrequency ablation are options that should be considered on an individualized basis.

Avoiding Treatment Errors

Prescribing an ACE-I plus ARB plus an aldosterone antagonist is not recommended because of the increased danger of hyperkalemia. Regular monitoring of potassium and renal function is strongly recommended in patients receiving any of these drugs.

Routine administration of nonsteroidal agents is not recommended in patients with HF because of the increased risk for fluid retention and worsening renal function. Nifedipine, verapamil, and diltiazem should not be used in patients with systolic HF because of their negative effect on contractility. Digoxin has not been shown to have a benefit in patients with HF-PSF unless they are in atrial fibrillation.

Drug Cost

HF patients take an average of 9 to 10 medications daily. The huge financial cost of medications often leads to medication nonadherence. Even if patients have insurance or receive Medicare Part D benefits, nongeneric medications can cost as much as $40 per prescription. It is important to determine how patients pay for their medications and to estimate their monthly drug bill. Prescribing generics when available will reduce cost (see Table 34-1). Mail-order companies may also offer reduced pricing.

Nonpharmacologic Strategies

Daily exercise, salt restriction of less than 2.5 to 3 g daily, fluid restriction, and daily weights should all be in the patient's care plan. Obese HF patients benefit from weight loss, and all benefit from discontinuation of alcohol and from smoking cessation. Every patient should receive an annual flu shot. Educate the patient and family about the symptoms and signs of the disease, prognosis, medications, and when to contact a health professional.

HF specialists can be helpful in the care of complex HF patients. Those who may benefit include patients who remain severely limited on an optimized medical regimen, do not tolerate medication up-titration, are transplantation candidates (refractory HF, EF <20%, without significant comorbid disease, compliant, psychologically stable with good social support), or are candidates for clinical trials or an LV assist device.

Treatment of Comorbid Disease

Aggressive management of hypertension, hyperlipidemia, diabetes mellitus, obstructive sleep apnea, and depression is part of routine care.

Future Directions

Passive mechanical devices are under development to prevent the progressive LV dilation and shape changes that

occur during the evolution of HF. The effects of intra-coronary injection of autologous bone marrow cells on LV function in patients with acute myocardial infarction have yielded contradictory results. Gene therapy approaches hold promise for the future with ongoing improvements in vector technology, cardiac gene delivery, and understanding of molecular pathogenesis. Disease prevention by aggressive modification of risk factors and early detection continue to have an enormous impact on cardiovascular disease leading to HF.

Additional Resources

American Heart Association. Available at: http://www.americanheart.org.

This website contains many helpful resources about heart failure for health professionals, patients, and their families.

Heart Failure Society of America. Available at: http://www.HFSA.org. Accessed December 22, 2006.

This website contains much helpful information about heart failure for health professionals, patients, and their families.

EVIDENCE

1. American Heart Association. Available at: www.americanheart.org. Accessed December 22, 2006.

This website provides the latest epidemiology data on the prevalence, incidence, mortality, hospitalization, and cost related to heart failure.

2. Bursi F, Weston SA, Redfield MM, et al: Systolic and diastolic heart failure in the community. JAMA 296(18):2209-2216, 2006.

This is a prospective study that describes the demographic and echocardiographic characteristics and prognosis of 556 heart failure patients living in Olmsted County, Minnesota. Heart failure with preserved ejection fraction was associated with a high mortality rate, comparable to that of patients with reduced ejection fraction. Echocardiographic classification of diastolic dysfunction is also reviewed.

3. Heart Failure Society of America: HFSA 2006 Comprehensive Heart Failure Practice Guideline. J Card Fail 12(1):e1-e12, 2006.

These guidelines provide current recommendations for treatment of heart failure based on evidence-based data and consensus opinion.

4. Hunt SA, Abraham WT, Chin MH, et al: ACC/AHA 2005 Guideline Update for the Diagnosis and Management of Chronic Heart Failure in the Adult: A report of the American College of Cardiology/American Heart Association Task Force on Practice Guidelines (Writing Committee to Update the 2001 Guidelines for the Evaluation and Management of Heart Failure). Developed in collaboration with the American College of Chest Physicians and the International Society for Heart and Lung Transplantation, endorsed by the Heart Rhythm Society. Circulation 112(12):e154-e235, 2005.

These guidelines provide current recommendations for treatment of heart failure based on evidence-based data and consensus opinion.

5. Owan TE, Hodge DO, Herges RM, et al: Trends in prevalence and outcome of heart failure with preserved EF. N Engl J Med 355(3):251-359, 2006.

This article reviewed the secular trends in the prevalence and mortality of 4596 heart failure patients followed at the Mayo Clinic over a 15-year period (1987-2001). The prevalence of heart failure with preserved ejection fraction increased over this period, while the mortality rate remained unchanged. In contrast, survival of patients with systolic heart failure improved over this time period but remained lower compared with that of patients with preserved ejection fraction.

Ross J. Simpson, Jr. ▪ Sidney C. Smith, Jr.

Hypercholesterolemia: Evaluation and Treatment

Introduction

Cholesterol is found in cell membranes and is a precursor of steroids and bile acids. It is a particularly important lipid because it is a major component of atherosclerotic plaques and because elevated blood cholesterol concentration is a major, and reversible, cause of coronary heart disease (CHD).

Cholesterol is primarily synthesized in the liver and is excreted as bile salts (Fig. 35-1). Individuals on the average Western diet absorb 20% to 40% of their cholesterol intake, on average about 300 to 700 mg daily. In average individuals, up to 1000 mg is recirculated each day by secretion and reabsorption as bile salts. Blood levels of cholesterol are determined by dietary intake of cholesterol, inheritance, physical activity, and intake of dietary fats, particularly saturated fats.

Cholesterol is transported in the blood as macromolecules of lipoproteins, with the nonpolar lipid core surrounded by a polar monolayer of phospholipids, the polar portion of cholesterol, and apolipoproteins. Specific lipoproteins differ in lipid core content, the proportion of lipids in the core, and the proteins on the surface. Lipoproteins are commonly classified by density as chylomicrons, chylomicron remnants, very-low-density lipoprotein (VLDL), low-density lipoprotein (LDL), intermediate-density lipoprotein (IDL), or high-density lipoprotein (HDL) cholesterol.

Triglycerides are esters of glycerol and long-chain, saturated, and desaturated fatty acids. They are found in all plasma lipoproteins but are the major constituent of chylomicrons, chylomicron remnants, VLDL, and IDL. Most triglycerides are contained in VLDL, which makes up 10% to 15% of the total cholesterol. The precise relationship of plasma triglycerides and atherosclerotic disease is uncertain because of the strong association of elevated triglycerides with low HDL as well as with other atherogenic factors (e.g., diabetes, smoking, and hypertension). If triglyceride-rich particles are present in sufficiently high concentration (>400 mg/dL), the plasma is turbid or opalescent. Severe elevations of triglycerides (1000 mg/dL) are associated with pancreatitis and eruptive xanthoma.

HDL cholesterol (HDL-C) is a family of lipoproteins that usually constitutes 20% to 30% of the total cholesterol. HDL-C shows a strong, inverse association with CHD risk and may facilitate reverse cholesterol transport from tissue. HDL-C is decreased by diets high in polyunsaturated fats, obesity, smoking, diabetes, and drugs (diuretics, anabolic steroids, and progestins). Physical activity and alcohol increase HDL-C. However, HDL-C concentration fluctuates considerably as a result of physiologic and analytic variation. Thus, a single measurement of the HDL-C may not be sufficient to determine a patient's usual HDL-C.

LDL cholesterol (LDL-C) makes up one half to two thirds of the total cholesterol and is thus the major determinant of the total serum cholesterol. As commonly measured, LDL is not a unique molecule but a population of particles similar in chemical and physical properties. For example, IDL cholesterol and lipoprotein (a) cholesterol, both of which appear to be atherogenic, generally constitute 2% to 4% of the total cholesterol and are encompassed in the LDL-C value.

LDL-C shows a strong and consistent epidemiologic, experimental, and clinical link to the rate of CHD (Fig. 35-2). Lowering of LDL-C cholesterol by diet, exercise, or pharmacologic therapy slows atherosclerotic vascular disease progression and lowers the risk for coronary events. This strong link of LDL-C cholesterol with CHD makes management of elevated LDL-C a critical focus for medical

Figure 35-1 Hypercholesterolemia: Cholesterol Synthesis and Metabolism.
APO, apolipoprotein.

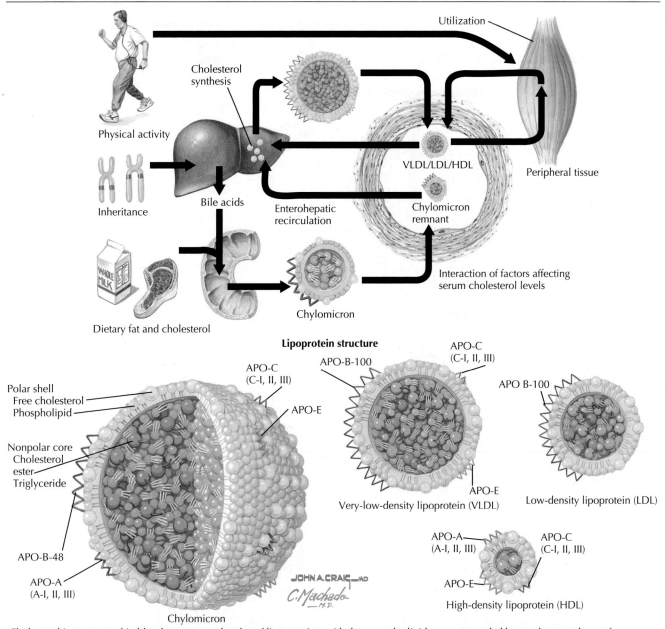

Cholesterol is transported in blood as macromolecules of lipoproteins, with the nonpolar lipid core surrounded by a polar monolayer of phospholipids and the polar portion of cholesterol and apolipoproteins (APO). Specific lipoproteins differ in lipid core content, proportion of lipids in core and proteins on the surface. Lipoproteins are classified by density as chylomicrons, very-low-density lipoprotein (VLDL), low-density lipoproteins (LDL), and high-density lipoproteins (HDL).

treatment. Although independent interventions to lower triglycerides and raise HDL-C should also be considered, therapies that lower LDL-C (e.g., statins and niacin) often positively affect triglycerides and HDL-C. However, to date, new pharmacotherapies aimed solely at raising HDL-C have been associated with increased adverse events.

Etiology and Pathogenesis

CHD may result from high LDL-C levels in patients without other risk factors for coronary artery disease, par-

ticularly children and young adults who have inherited a lack of sufficient cell membrane receptors to remove LDL-C from circulation. These forms of familial hypercholesterolemia, present in 1 in 500 individuals who are heterozygous and 1 in 1,000,000 who are homozygous, are characterized by a twofold to fourfold increase in LDL-C levels in heterozygotes and much greater increases in homozygotes. Familial combined hypercholesterolemia occurs in about 1 in 100 people and is characterized by overproduction of apolipoprotein B. In all these individuals, the coronary risk conferred by an elevated LDL-C is

Figure 35-2 Hypercholesterolemia as Risk Factor in Coronary Artery Disease.

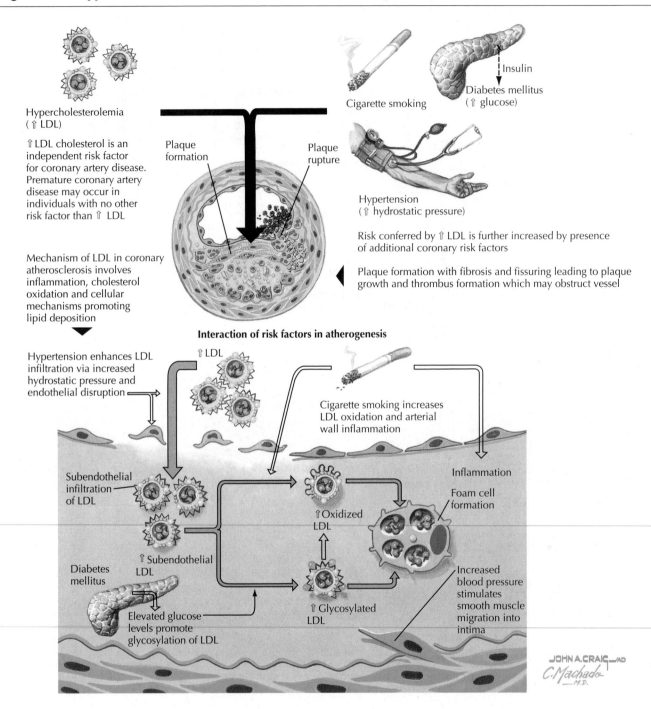

Hypercholesterolemia
(⇑ LDL)

⇑ LDL cholesterol is an independent risk factor for coronary artery disease. Premature coronary artery disease may occur in individuals with no other risk factor than ⇑ LDL

Mechanism of LDL in coronary atherosclerosis involves inflammation, cholesterol oxidation and cellular mechanisms promoting lipid deposition

Plaque formation

Plaque rupture

Cigarette smoking

Insulin

Diabetes mellitus (⇑ glucose)

Hypertension (⇑ hydrostatic pressure)

Risk conferred by ⇑ LDL is further increased by presence of additional coronary risk factors

Plaque formation with fibrosis and fissuring leading to plaque growth and thrombus formation which may obstruct vessel

Interaction of risk factors in atherogenesis

Hypertension enhances LDL infiltration via increased hydrostatic pressure and endothelial disruption

⇑ LDL

Cigarette smoking increases LDL oxidation and arterial wall inflammation

Inflammation

Subendothelial infiltration of LDL

Foam cell formation

⇑ Oxidized LDL

Diabetes mellitus

⇑ Subendothelial LDL

Elevated glucose levels promote glycosylation of LDL

⇑ Glycosylated LDL

Increased blood pressure stimulates smooth muscle migration into intima

JOHN A. CRAIG—AD
C. Machado—M.D.

further increased by the presence of additional coronary risk factors, as described later.

The mechanisms by which LDL-C accelerates coronary atherosclerosis are complex. Coronary atherosclerosis appears to be part of an inflammatory response to endothelial injury in which monocytes infiltrate the arterial intima and promote cholesterol oxidation and conversion of monocytes into tissue macrophages and eventually to lipid-laden foam cells (see Fig. 35-2). These cells initially deposit in fatty streaks below the endothelial layer. With further accumulation, an eccentric lipid-rich plaque develops. Smooth muscle cells form a fibrous cap over the lipid core that repeatedly fissures, leading to thrombus formation and plaque growth. Eventually, a major fissure occurs, and a thrombus partially or completely obstructs the coronary artery, leading to unstable angina, myocardial infarction, or sudden cardiac death. The forces that precipitate plaque rupture, and the means to detect the propensity of such an event in the immediate future, are being actively investigated.

Clinical Presentation

Individuals with lipid abnormalities may present in one of several ways, but ultimately hypercholesterolemia is a diagnosis made by laboratory analysis. Because cholesterol-lowering drugs are efficient in reducing coronary risk, any individual who presents with chronic or acute coronary syndromes, "high-risk" family history, or has diabetes mellitus or multiple cardiac risk factors is deemed to be at increased risk and should be screened. Historically, screening was underutilized, but with increased public emphasis, this has improved substantially.

In some settings, patients not known to be at increased risk but with hypercholesterolemia can be identified. Patients with familial hypercholesterolemia may present with physical findings that reflect long-standing hypercholesterolemia. These findings include subcutaneous cholesterol deposits, most frequently tendinous xanthomas or xanthelasmas. Arcus senilis, once thought to be indicative of hypercholesterolemia, is far less specific, particularly in elderly people. Patients may also be identified when turbid serum is found on routine blood work.

Differential Diagnosis

Secondary causes of elevated cholesterol are common. These include poorly controlled diabetes, hypothyroidism, and the nephrotic syndrome. Estrogen replacement therapy may elevate triglycerides, and HDL may be dramatically lowered by progestins and anabolic steroids.

Diagnostic Approach

The primary blood test required for diagnosis and treatment of elevated cholesterol measures the fasting total cholesterol, triglycerides, and HDL-C. These values are then used to calculate the LDL-C [total cholesterol – (HDL-C + triglycerides/5)]. This method is useful only if the triglycerides are lower than 400 mg/dL. Direct measures of LDL-C and estimation of LDL and other lipid fraction particle size and particle number are also available but are not commonly necessary or used. Blood samples should be measured after a 12-hour fast because chylomicrons interfere with the estimation of LDL-C.

Established CHD and atherosclerotic vascular disease in other vascular beds dramatically increase the risk associated with elevated LDL-C. In addition, diabetes mellitus is a coronary risk equivalent, and patients with known diabetes should be evaluated and treated as if they have diagnosed CHD because of the increased risk associated with diabetes. These clinical situations require aggressive management of LDL-C. For patients who are not in this highest-risk group, the goal of lipid management is to delay the complications of coronary artery disease, and less aggressive therapy is warranted. For these reasons, a search for the major, established risk factors for CHD should be performed. Any change in exercise capacity, chest pain, or angina should be assessed by appropriate historical information or diagnostic tests (e.g., treadmill, nuclear imaging, and cardiac angiography).

The accepted major risk factors for CHD include age older than 45 years in men and older than 55 years in women, a history of premature CHD in first-degree relatives (sudden death or coronary disease onset before age 55 years for men or 65 years for women), current smoking, presence and severity of hypertension, physical inactivity, and dietary patterns. Life habit risk factors including obesity (body mass index >30), physical inactivity, and an atherogenic diet should also be assessed. Screening for elevated glucose may be particularly appropriate if the metabolic syndrome (central obesity, hypertension, glucose intolerance with low HDL-C, elevated triglycerides, and modestly elevated LDL-C) is suspected. Assessment of proteinuria, serum creatinine, and liver function studies may also help guide therapy. Additional risk factors for CHD, including lipoprotein (a), homocysteine, and pro-thrombotic and proinflammatory factors (C-reactive protein), are not routinely measured but may be helpful in situations in which a family history or established CHD occurs in the absence of a markedly elevated LDL-C. These latter risk factors are emerging as potentially important causes of coronary disease.

Lowering the LDL-C should be the primary goal of therapy. For patients with CHD, other vascular disease, diabetes, or a 10-year Framingham risk for CHD events of more than 20%, the target LDL-C should be less than 100 mg/dL. In higher-risk patients, an optimal target LDL-C of 70 mg/dL is supported by more aggressive clinical trials and advisory groups. Ideal values of HDL-C are more than 40 mg/dL in men and more than 50 mg/dL in women, and triglycerides should be less than 150 mg/dL. For patients with increased triglycerides (>200 mg/dL), non–HDL-C may be used to guide therapy, with a target level of 30 mg/dL greater than the recommended LDL-C target.

Management and Therapy

Optimum Treatment

Appropriate diet and exercise are the cornerstones of cholesterol management (Fig. 35-3). All patients who have elevated cholesterol should receive dietary counseling and dietary reinforcement to help them achieve their cholesterol goals. Although there remains some controversy about the optimal diet to reduce the risk for CHD, the strongest data available today support either of two approaches. The modified step II American Heart Association (AHA) diet of less than 7% of calories from saturated fat and less than 200 mg/day of dietary cholesterol focuses on reduction in cholesterol intake and low total fat intake. Plant sterols and stanols of 2 g/day can be encouraged; these plant analogues of cholesterol displace cholesterol from bile salts and lower cholesterol, as do soluble fibers.

Figure 35-3 Hypercholesterolemia: General Management Measures.
PPAR, peroxisome proliferator-activated receptor.

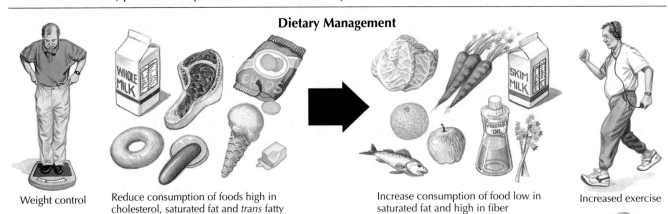

Dietary Management

Weight control

Reduce consumption of foods high in cholesterol, saturated fat and *trans* fatty acids, and salt. Decrease total caloric intake

Increase consumption of food low in saturated fat and high in fiber

Increased exercise

Fish oil supplements

Appropriate diet and exercise are cornerstones of cholesterol management. Dietary counseling and reinforcement and a planned program of physical activity are recommended

Actions of Lipid-Lowering Medications

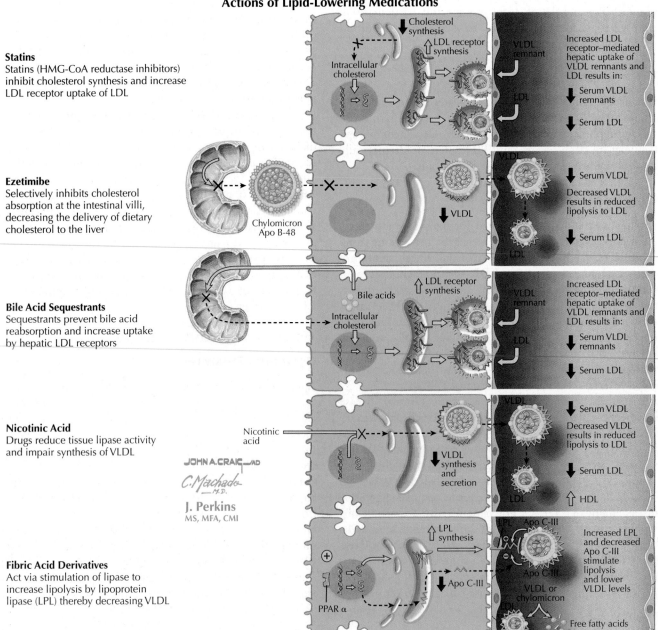

Statins
Statins (HMG-CoA reductase inhibitors) inhibit cholesterol synthesis and increase LDL receptor uptake of LDL

Ezetimibe
Selectively inhibits cholesterol absorption at the intestinal villi, decreasing the delivery of dietary cholesterol to the liver

Bile Acid Sequestrants
Sequestrants prevent bile acid reabsorption and increase uptake by hepatic LDL receptors

Nicotinic Acid
Drugs reduce tissue lipase activity and impair synthesis of VLDL

Fibric Acid Derivatives
Act via stimulation of lipase to increase lipolysis by lipoprotein lipase (LPL) thereby decreasing VLDL

An alternative approach to the AHA diet is the Mediterranean Diet, which encourages increased intake of fish and a variety of other foods that are low in saturated fats, but not as low as the American Heart Association diets in total fat. Low carbohydrate and low glycemic index diets have also gained popularity, and somewhat surprisingly, in initial studies no negative impact on plasma lipid profiles has been reported. A planned program of daily physical activity should be started and reinforced.

Fish oil (eicosapentaenoic acid and docosahexaenoic acid) is a promising dietary intervention that appears to reduce hepatic triglyceride synthesis. Dietary supplements of fish oil containing 2 to 5 g of omega-3 fatty acid may decrease triglycerides by up to 30% and VLDL by 40%, with resulting modest changes in LDL cholesterol and increases in HDL cholesterol. Gastrointestinal complaints (bloating, diarrhea), increased bleeding time, and effects of hypervitaminosis A and D (dermatitis or hypercalciumemia) may occur with high doses of fish oil. The routine use of high-dose vitamins or antioxidant supplements is not recommended.

Initiation of drug therapy is based on the absolute risk of a patient developing a CHD and the LDL-C value following diet therapy (see Fig. 35-3). If the 10-year Framingham risk is more than 20% or the patient has a CHD risk equivalent, drug therapy should be initiated if the LDL-C exceeds 100 mg/dL. If the patient has a 10-year risk of less than 20% and has two or more risk factors, drugs should be considered if the LDL-C exceeds 130 mg/dL. If the patient has only one other risk factor and the 10-year risk is less than 10%, drugs are often initiated if the LDL-C is 160 mg/dL or higher.

Drug therapy with hydroxymethyl glutaryl coenzyme A (HMG-CoA) reductase inhibitors (statins) is highly effective at lowering LDL-C. Statins inhibit cholesterol synthesis and increase LDL receptor uptake of LDL. In addition, statins lower triglycerides by up to 30% and can be expected to raise HDL-C by up to 15%. These drugs include lovastatin (10 to 80 mg/day), pravastatin (20 to 80 mg/day), simvastatin (10 to 80 mg/day), fluvastatin (20 to 80 mg/day), atorvastatin (10 to 80 mg/day), and rosuvastatin (10 to 40 mg/day). There is a predictable dose-response relationship with these drugs such that doubling the dose of the statin results in an approximate 6% additional LDL cholesterol reduction from the initial baseline level. These drugs are, in general, well tolerated. There is a small risk for myopathy with higher doses or when statins are combined with fibrates or with drugs that interfere with metabolism of the statin. A modest but dose-dependent increase in the probability of elevated liver enzymes also occurs. The therapeutic benefit of statins in lowering LDL cholesterol can be potentiated by bile acid sequestrants, plant stanols, and intestinal cholesterol-absorber blockers like ezetimibe.

Second-line medications include bile acid sequestrants: cholestyramine (4 to 16 g/day), colestipol (2 to 16 g/day), and colesevelam (4 to 6 tablets of 625 mg each/day). These drugs prevent bile acid reabsorption and increase uptake by liver LDL receptors. They can reduce LDL-C by up to 30% in a dose-dependent manner and can increase HDL-C by 5% but may also increase triglycerides. They should not be used in patients with dysbetalipoproteinemia or elevated triglycerides. They are not systemically absorbed, and side effects are generally limited to their potential to interfere with decreased absorption of other drugs, constipation, dyspepsia, and bloating.

Nicotinic acid reduces tissue lipase activity and impairs VLDL synthesis. It lowers LDL-C by up to 25%, decreases triglycerides by up to 50%, and raises HDL-C by up to 35%. Side effects include flushing, elevated blood glucose, hyperuricemia, abdominal pain, and hepatotoxicity. Nicotinic acid should not be used in patients with severe gout, peptic ulcer disease, or liver disease and should be used only with close monitoring in patients with diabetes or insulin resistance. Nicotinic acid is available in three forms: immediate release (target dose of 1.5 to 2 g/day), extended release (500 mg to 2 g/day), and sustained release (not recommended). Although nicotinic acid is highly effective and has a demonstrated safety record, compliance is not good unless supportive counseling is provided.

The fibric acid derivatives gemfibrozil (600 mg twice daily) and fenofibrate (48 to 145 mg/day) decrease VLDL and triglyceride levels by increasing lipolysis by lipoprotein lipase, thereby increasing catabolism of triglyceride-rich particles. They can be expected to lower LDL-C by up to 20%, to raise HDL-C by up to 20%, and to lower triglycerides by up to 50%. Side effects include dyspepsia, gallstones, and a propensity toward myopathy when combined with statins. These drugs are contraindicated in renal or hepatic disease. Ezetimibe (10 mg/day) is a selective inhibitor of cholesterol absorption at the intestinal villi and can reduce LDL-C by 20%; it can also be combined with statins to further reduce LDL-C.

Specific Dyslipidemia

When LDL-C is extremely high (>190 mg/dL), a genetic disorder should be suspected and family screening undertaken. Monogenetic familial hypercholesterolemia, familial defective apolipoprotein B100 synthesis, or polygenic hypercholesterolemia is likely. Therapy almost always requires a statin in high doses or a statin combined with another drug. Occasionally patients require plasma apheresis, particularly in the rare homozygous forms of hypercholesterolemia.

Treatment of other lipid factors may also be required. Elevated triglycerides may be caused by obesity, physical inactivity, cigarette smoking, excess alcohol intake, failure to fast before the lipid test, a high-carbohydrate (>60% of energy intake) diet, type II diabetes, chronic renal failure, and nephrotic syndrome. Certain drugs (corticosteroids, estrogens, retinoids, high-dose β-blockers) and genetic dyslipidemia may also be implicated. When the triglycerides exceed 500 mg/dL, triglyceride-lowering therapy should be undertaken to avoid pancreatitis or eruptive xanthomas. Dietary counseling is essential and should focus on very-low-fat diets (less than 15% of calories) and restrictions of sugars and simple carbohydrates. Fibrates, nicotinic acid, and fish oil dietary supplements, along with tight diabetic control, can all be helpful in treatment of hypertriglyceridemia.

Avoiding Treatment Errors

Combination therapy and high-dose statins may often be required in patients with severely elevated LDL-C to achieve guideline recommended levels. The combination of a statin with a fibric acid should be considered only in the most refractory circumstances because some such combinations carry an increased risk for serious side effects. In most patients, additional dietary considerations, or exercise or counseling to improve compliance, will further improve their lipid management.

Optimal and safe pharmacotherapy of lipid disorders requires careful and ongoing monitoring of the medical literature. Specific dosing recommendations often change and depend on a given patient's set of medical problems. Moreover, there is a high potential for drug interactions, and starting and maintenance doses may differ substantially.

Future Directions

New drugs and new therapies are rapidly being developed for managing dyslipidemia and diagnosing atherosclerosis earlier in its course. Diagnostic tests to more accurately predict the risk for developing coronary events include measurement of the C-reactive protein and multiple other serum and genetic biomarkers, measurement of lipid particle size and density, and use of electron-beam tomography to access calcium levels in the coronary arteries and high-resolution computed tomographic angiography. Other noninvasive tests to assess the extent of atherosclerosis and establish risk for future events include carotid Doppler ultrasound to determine intima-to-media thickness ratio, and the ankle-brachial index, a measurement of the extent of peripheral vascular disease that provides important cardiovascular prognostic information. Invasive techniques include intracoronary ultrasound to assess the plaque burden and lipid density and the possible propensity of coronary artery to plaque rupture.

Drugs that raise HDL-C remain under development despite initially disappointing results. One example of a new approach now available for treating patients is ezetimibe, a selective inhibitor of cholesterol absorption at the intestinal villi that can be readily combined with statins. Other promising therapies are in clinical trials, and it is likely that, in the future, lipid disorders will be managed more effectively with fewer side effects, thereby more effectively reducing cardiovascular risk.

Additional Resources

Baigent C, Keech A, Kearney PM, et al: Efficacy and safety of cholesterol-lowering treatment: Prospective meta-analysis of data from 90,056 participants in 14 randomised trials of statins. Lancet 366(9493):1267-1278, 2005.

The authors present an excellent systematic summary of effectiveness of lipid lowering therapy, including strong empirical support of ATP III recommendations.

Folsom AR, Chambless LE, Ballantyne M, et al: An assessment of incremental coronary risk prediction using C-reactive protein and other novel risk markers: The atherosclerosis risk in communities study. Arch Intern Med 166(13):1368-1373, 2006.

This article provides scientific balance on use of novel risk factors in guiding decisions on treatment.

Kris-Etherton P, Eckel RH, Howard BV, et al: AHA science advisory. Lyon diet heart study: Benefits of a Mediterranean-style, National Cholesterol Education Program/American Heart Association step I dietary pattern on cardiovascular disease. Circulation 103(13):1823-1825, 2001.

This landmark study shows the importance and practicality of diet therapy in preventing recurrent heart attacks.

Lammert F, Wang DQ: New insights into the genetic regulation of intestinal cholesterol absorption. Gastroenterology 129(2):718-734, 2005.

This paper highlights the importance and variation of cholesterol absorption in determining serum blood levels of cholesterol.

National Heart, Lung, and Blood Institute: National Cholesterol Education Program. Third Report of the Expert Panel on Detection, Evaluation, and Treatment of High Blood Cholesterol in Adults (Adult Treatment Panel III). Available at: http://www.nhlbi.nih.gov/guidelines/cholesterol/index.htm. Accessed May 31, 2007.

This website contains additional resources, including the full report of the panel, downloadable risk calculators, slide shows, and specific dietary and other information for patients.

Pearson TA, Laurora I, Chu H, Kafonek S: The Lipid Treatment Assessment Project (L-TAP): A multicenter survey to evaluate the percentages of dyslipidemic patients receiving lipid-lowering therapy and achieving low-density lipoprotein cholesterol goals. Arch Intern Med 160(4):459-467, 2000.

Lipid-lowering therapy is underused, and only a relatively small percentage of patients have achieved their guideline recommended levels of LDL-C.

EVIDENCE

1. Expert Panel on Detection, Evaluation, and Treatment of High Blood Cholesterol in Adults: Executive Summary of the Third Report of the National Cholesterol Education Program (NCEP) Expert Panel on Detection, Evaluation, and Treatment of High Blood Cholesterol in Adults (Adult Treatment Panel III). JAMA 285(19):2486-2497, 2001.

   The Expert Panel provides an excellent summary of the full report of the ATP III.

2. Gotto AM Jr: Contemporary Diagnosis and Management of Lipid Disorders, 2nd ed. Newtown, PA, Handbooks in Health Care, 2001.

   This is a well-written monograph by a true expert in lipid metabolism and treatment. It includes an easy-to-follow summary of complex lipid metabolism.

3. Grundy SM, Cleeman JI, Merz CN, et al: Implications of recent clinical trials for the National Cholesterol Education Program Adult Treatment Panel III guidelines. Circulation 110(2):227-239, 2004.

   This article updates the ATP III guidelines based on key clinical trials not available at the time of the panels meeting. These studies endorse the importance of focusing on LDL-C as the primary target and suggest the need for more aggressive LDL-C targets.

Richard G. Sheahan

Cardiac Arrhythmias

Introduction

Cardiac arrhythmias are abnormal and usually symptomatic changes in heart rhythm. Cardiac rhythm disturbances may involve abnormally fast (tachycardias) or slow (bradycardias) heart rates and may be either regular or irregular. Patients use various terms to describe symptoms associated with cardiac arrhythmia (which may also be asymptomatic), the most common of which is the term *palpitations* or a synonymous description. In general, the diagnosis and treatment of tachyarrhythmias is more complex than that of bradyarrhythmias.

Etiology and Pathogenesis

Tachycardias can be divided into two broad categories, supraventricular or ventricular tachycardia (VT), each of which can be due to any of several underlying etiologies.

Supraventricular tachycardia (SVT) is an often benign tachycardia that initiates above the bundle of His. Most SVTs involve two discrete pathways or limbs with different conduction and refractory properties. The pathways are composed of conducting cells, and in many cases, a portion of the pathways is due to the presence of conducting cells in an atypical anatomic location. Atrioventricular nodal reentrant tachycardia (AVNRT) has so-called fast and slow pathways, both of which are located in or very near the atrioventricular (AV) node. Atrioventricular reentrant tachycardia (AVRT) requires an accessory pathway that is present in another location from the AV node. Atrial tachycardia usually arises from a focal collection of rapidly depolarizing cells located in the right (or sometimes left) atrium. Atrial flutter occurs as a reentrant circuit usually in the right atrium.

Atrial fibrillation is the most common arrhythmia and can present with rapid, normal, or slow ventricular conduction. Atrial fibrillation occurs in a broad spectrum of patients with many underlying etiologies. The incidence of atrial fibrillation increases with age, and with the increased age of the population, age-related atrial fibrillation is common. Once a patient develops atrial fibrillation, it is very likely to recur.

Any SVT can become dangerous in settings in which myocardial function is impaired at high heart rates, including coronary artery disease, congenital heart disease, congestive heart failure (CHF), and hypertrophic cardiomyopathy. Atrial fibrillation also carries the risk for left atrial thrombus formation and thromboembolism—most commonly resulting in transient ischemic attack or cerebrovascular accident. For this reason, in addition to considering dangers relating to atrial fibrillation with a rapid ventricular response, care providers must also consider anticoagulation to prevent thromboembolic events.

VT usually originates from scar tissue in patients with a previous myocardial infarction or from abnormal ventricular tissue found in various forms of cardiomyopathy, including dilated, hypertrophic, or infiltrative pathologies. Rarely, exercise-induced VT (the so-called verapamil- or adenosine-sensitive VT) can occur in patients with normal hearts. Ventricular fibrillation (VF) usually occurs in the setting of ongoing ischemia. VF is uniformly fatal unless treated immediately. VT, although often lethal, may present in other ways if it is episodic and nonsustained, or is stable at heart rates below 150 beats per minute.

The long QT syndrome and Brugada's syndrome are examples of arrhythmias resulting from inherited channelopathies. Brugada's syndrome is characterized by ST elevation beginning at the terminal R wave with a slowly descending ST segment and continuing with a flat or negative T wave appearing spontaneously in leads V_1 to V_3. Both conditions are associated with sudden cardiac death.

Bradycardias result from either permanent or transient heart block at the level of the AV node or bundle of His, sinus arrest, or neurocardiogenic factors (as in vagally mediated bradycardias). The severity of a given bradycardia depends on how slow the heart rate is. This varies considerably with the type of bradycardia and the individual. Any heart rate less than 60 beats per minute in adults is bradycardia by definition. However, bradycardia can be normal in athletes and well-trained individuals. Many modest bradycardias require no therapy. Marked bradycardia can be life threatening and require hospitalization.

Clinical Presentation

In addition to palpitations, patients may present with other symptoms, including dyspnea, dizziness, lightheadedness, chest pain, syncope, weakness, fatigue, sudden cardiac death (SCD), or the consequences of injuries that result from the arrhythmia. Symptom severity depends on a complex interaction between the hemodynamic consequences of the arrhythmia and the underlying cardiac function. Syncope, per se, does not distinguish a benign from a malignant arrhythmia. The occurrence of palpitations, syncope, or presyncopal symptoms during exertion requires urgent evaluation.

SCD merits additional description because this is a term that has been used variably in recent years. SCD is most commonly defined as an abrupt loss of consciousness within 1 hour of the onset of acute symptoms resulting in natural death. If SCD is witnessed, it may be possible to resuscitate the individual. The most effective therapy is electrical cardioversion, in combination with other resuscitative efforts. Individuals who have been resuscitated and survived an episode of SCD are at highest risk for death from arrhythmia and should be immediately hospitalized and aggressively treated.

Diagnostic Approach

Patient Evaluation

In evaluating a cardiac arrhythmia, details of the presenting history, including the associated circumstances, family history of arrhythmia or SCD, medications (including recent dose changes or additions), recent illnesses or surgeries, and physical examination are crucial (Box 36-1). A baseline electrocardiogram (ECG) may help in identifying the abnormal arrhythmia and may exclude AV conduction abnormalities, preexcitation of Wolff-Parkinson-White (WPW) syndrome (delta wave, short PR interval, and a wider QRS complex), long QT syndrome, Brugada syndrome, and abnormalities in ventricular conduction. The laboratory tests chosen will vary from patient to patient and should be tailored accordingly. In almost every setting, one should screen for electrolyte abnormalities. In a patient with bizarre behavior, blood alcohol and urine toxicology screening should be performed. Elderly patients, in particular, should also be screened for toxic levels of prescribed medications.

> **Box 36-1   Evaluation of a Patient with a Cardiac Arrhythmia**
>
> - History and physical examination: family history of sudden death, medications
> - Electrocardiogram: baseline and during event
> - Laboratory may include complete blood cell count, electrolytes, blood glucose, serial cardiac enzymes, thyroid-stimulating hormone, digoxin, blood and urine drug screen, and alcohol levels
> - Echocardiogram to document cardiac function and rule out valvular abnormality and cardiomyopathy
> - Ambulatory Holter monitoring
> - Patient-activated monitoring device: may include event, loop, or insertable loop recorder
> - Procainamide provocative test
> - Electrophysiology study
>
> *Adapted from Sheahan RG: Syncope and arrhythmias: Role of the electrophysiological study. Am J Med Sci 322:37-43, 2001.*

Symptom Rhythm Correlation

A 12-lead ECG during the arrhythmia provides the gold standard of a symptom rhythm correlation. This is an elusive goal because symptoms are most commonly paroxysmal and occur infrequently. Holter monitoring over a 24- or 48-hour period can be used to document rhythms that occur almost daily. A loop recorder over a 1- to 2-month interval may record rhythms that occur once every 4 weeks. The use of these devices for longer periods is unlikely to yield a diagnosis due to decreasing patient motivation and contact dermatitis caused by the gel contained in the recording electrodes. In circumstances in which the diagnosis of a suspected arrhythmia is particularly elusive, an insertable loop recorder can be used to correlate symptoms with the cardiac rhythm. This is a recording device that is implanted under the skin in the anterior chest well and can be activated by the patient or automatically. The automated features record heart rates of less than 40 beats per minute or greater than 145 beats per minute, or ventricular asystole of greater than 3 seconds. The insertable loop recorder is an option for patients with infrequent but significant symptoms, after structural heart disease and other obvious causes have been excluded.

Ventricular arrhythmias require further evaluation of myocardial function and evaluation for significant coronary artery disease. An echocardiogram, nuclear ventriculogram, or magnetic resonance imaging can be used to detect segmental wall motion abnormalities, hypertrophic cardiomyopathy, dilated cardiomyopathy, arrhythmogenic right ventricular cardiomyopathy (ARVC), valvular abnormalities, and atrial dimensions (in atrial fibrillation). Coronary angiography is usually recommended to rule out significant coronary artery disease and myocardial ischemia as a cause for ventricular arrhythmias.

In patients presenting with syncope and left ventricular dysfunction (ejection fraction [EF] <35%), an implantable cardioverter defibrillator (ICD) is usually recommended because these patients are at a higher risk for sudden cardiac death. Revascularization, if required, should also be performed.

Management and Therapy

Optimum Treatment

Acute Management of Arrhythmias

Rhythm recognition in conjunction with the hemodynamic consequences of the arrhythmia determines the immediate therapeutic approach to managing acute sustained arrhythmias (Table 36-1). If a patient has SVT with a blood pressure less than 80 mm Hg and is presyncopal, then an immediate synchronized direct current (DC) cardioversion is required. While preparing for cardioversion, one can consider an intravenous bolus of adenosine (6 to 12 mg) to terminate the arrhythmia. Similarly, if a patient has VT and is hemodynamically unstable, immediate synchronized DC cardioversion is recommended. In conscious patients requiring electrical cardioversion, regardless of the underlying arrhythmia, anesthesia (conscious sedation) should be initiated before electrical cardioversion except in life-threatening circumstances. In patients with either SVT or VT who are hemodynamically stable and minimally symptomatic, pharmacologic therapy can be initiated (see later). Electrical cardioversion is contraindicated in a symptomatic patient with sinus tachycardia and hypotension.

In patients who present with hemodynamically *stable* SVT, the initial drug of choice is adenosine, infused as a rapid intravenous push in a large proximally located vein, followed by a fluid bolus. Intravenous diltiazem or metoprolol may also be used. One should avoid using an intravenous calcium channel blocker in a patient who is currently taking a scheduled dose of an oral β-blocker, and vice versa. In patients with known WPW syndrome and SVT, adenosine is the drug of choice, and diltiazem and metoprolol should be used only for special indications.

In patients who present with hemodynamically *unstable* VT requiring urgent synchronized DC cardioversion, it is important to immediately follow restoration of normal sinus rhythm with institution of intravenous antiarrhythmic therapy. Amiodarone, β-blocker, and magnesium are most commonly used.

In patients presenting with a hemodynamically *stable* VT, one should consider treatment with intravenous β-blockers, amiodarone, magnesium, or a combination of these. If 1 hour elapses without termination to sinus rhythm, a synchronized DC shock should be performed.

VF requires an emergent asynchronous DC shock followed by infusion of intravenous amiodarone, β-blocker, and magnesium.

The acute management of *atrial flutter* and *atrial fibrillation* with rapid ventricular response depends on the clinical presentation, as with SVT and VT. Hemodynamically stable patients can be treated medically. Intravenous diltiazem or esmolol are the drugs of choice because they provide graded, dose-related control of the ventricular response. When not effective, it is often because an inadequate dose has been used. Slowing the ventricular response to less than 90 beats per minute increases the diastolic filling time and improves cardiac output. Patients with atrial flutter or atrial fibrillation with rapid ventricular response who are hemodynamically unstable should undergo immediate synchronous DC cardioversion.

In significant *bradycardia* due to sinus arrest or complete heart block, a temporary transvenous pacemaker should be placed in the right ventricle until the condition resolves or a permanent pacemaker is placed (Fig. 36-1). Patients who present with second-degree AV block Mobitz types I and II should be monitored closely. Temporary pacing is ordinarily only necessary if these rhythms result in hemodynamic instability or progress (Fig. 36-2).

Sinus tachycardia most often reflects an underlying condition. A careful history and physical examination should provide clues as to the etiology. These include, but are not limited to, dehydration, anemia, fever, pain, anxiety, medications including bronchodilators, vomiting, diarrhea, and illicit drug use. Pharmacologic or other therapy for sinus tachycardia (or multifocal atrial tachycardia, which usually occurs in the setting of respiratory distress) should focus on treating the underlying disease rather than the resulting tachycardia.

Long-term Management

Initial therapies for *recurrent SVT* may include β-blockers or calcium channel blockers (see Table 36-1). Initiation of these agents will depend on the frequency of the episodes and the presence of comorbid conditions. An electrophysiology study and radiofrequency ablation (RFA) should be considered for recurrent episodes, intolerance to medications, or women in childbearing years who wish to become pregnant. RFA successfully eliminates the SVT in 90% to 95% of patients with a 5% recurrence rate.

For those with *AVNRT*, the ablation target is the "slow pathway," which is occasionally located in close proximity to the AV node. Ablation in this location is associated with a 1% to 2% risk for heart block, which may require pacemaker placement. Other complications related to this procedure are uncommon (occurring in about 1% of patients).

SVT in the presence of a *WPW* pattern is associated with a risk for sudden death (see Fig. 36-3), particularly in patients in whom atrial fibrillation develops with rapid antegrade conduction over the accessory pathway. Patients with WPW in whom atrial fibrillation develops can progress rapidly to VF. In these patients, who typically have a wide, rapid, irregular tachycardia, treatment options

Table 36-1 Acute and Long-term Management of Arrhythmias

Arrhythmia	Acute Care	Long-term Management
Sinus tachycardia (>100 beats/min)	Treat underlying cause	If inappropriate, β-blocker or calcium channel blocker. Consider POTS and midodrine or fludrocortisone, rehabilitation, rehabilitative aerobic training (e.g., swimming, walking)
Sinus bradycardia (<60 beats/min)	If asymptomatic, no intervention. If symptomatic and severe (rates <40 beats/min) with nonreversible cause, consider temporary pacing	If asymptomatic, no intervention. If symptomatic and severe (rates <40 beats/min) with nonreversible cause, consider permanent pacing
Premature atrial complexes	If asymptomatic, no intervention. Check potassium, magnesium	If asymptomatic, no intervention. Check potassium, magnesium. If symptomatic, consider β-blocker
Premature ventricular complexes	If asymptomatic, no intervention. Check potassium, magnesium	Echo to assess LV and RV function, and LV wall thickness. Normal echo: no intervention. β-Blocker for symptoms. Abnormal echo: evaluate etiology and add β-blocker. Consider PO magnesium PRN
Sinus node dysfunction	No intervention, unless unstable	Permanent pacemaker. Allows the use of β-blocker in patients with tachybrady syndrome
Prolonged PR interval	No intervention	No intervention unless symptomatic
Second degree AV block		
Mobitz type I (Wenckebach)	No intervention, unless unstable	Symptomatic patient, consider permanent pacemaker
Mobitz type II AV block	No intervention, unless unstable	Permanent pacemaker
Complete heart block	Possible temporary pacemaker	Permanent pacemaker
Supraventricular tachycardia (SVT)	Control SVT with adenosine	Consider EPS and RFA for recurrent episodes
Wolff-Parkinson-White syndrome and concealed accessory pathway	Control SVT with adenosine	WPW with SVT needs EPS and RFA, because of risk for sudden death
AV nodal reentrant tachycardia	Control SVT with adenosine, IV β-blocker, diltiazem	Consider EPS and RFA for recurrent episodes
Atrial tachycardia	Control SVT with adenosine, IV β-blocker, diltiazem	Consider EPS and RFA for recurrent episodes
Atrial fibrillation anticoagulation	Heparin in all. Determine time of symptom onset. Duration <48 hours may cardiovert (DC or IV antiarrhythmic agents); >48 hours, either TEE, and if negative for thrombus, cardiovert; or warfarin with INR 2.0-3.0 for 3 weeks and then cardioversion	Warfarin with INR 2.0 to 3.0 in all at-risk patients. Consider pharmacologic treatment or elective DC cardioversion. Soluble aspirin, 81-325 mg, for all other patients at low risk for stroke
Paroxysmal	Rate control	Recurrent episodes need antiarrhythmic agent. Pulmonary vein isolation ablation for drug failures
Persistent	Rate control	Cardioversion, addition of antiarrhythmic agent for recurrences. Pulmonary vein isolation ablation for drug failures
Permanent	Rate control	Rate control. If unsuccessful, consider pulmonary vein isolation or AV node ablation and permanent pacemaker
Atrial flutter	Rate control	RFA for recurrent episodes
Ventricular tachycardia	DC cardioversion if unstable or refractory to antiarrhythmic drugs	Echo to assess LV function. Ischemic evaluation +/− revascularization. EF <35% for ICD placement. Normal echo, consider RVOT or LV VT and ablation
Ventricular fibrillation	Emergent DC cardioversion	Rule out acute myocardial infarction. ICD placement in absence of acute myocardial infarction
Nonsustained ventricular tachycardia (3-30 beats)	Rate control	Rule out RV and LV dysfunction; EF <35%, needs ICD. If normal β-blockers, possible ablation.
Left ventricular dysfunction	Primary prevention of sudden cardiac death	Previous myocardial infarction or dilated cardiomyopathy, LV EF <35%, require ICD placement
Hypertrophic cardiomyopathy	Treat as for arrhythmia	ICD for at-risk individuals
Long QT syndrome	Resuscitate as for arrhythmia	β-blocker or permanent pacemaker at 85 beats/min/ICD
Brugada syndrome	Resuscitate as for arrhythmia	Symptomatic ICD placement. Asymptomatic and abnormal ECG, some favor EPS +/−ICD, but others favor observation

AV, atrioventricular; DC, direct current; EF, ejection fraction; EPS, electrophysiology study; ICD, implantable cardioverter-defibrillator; INR, international normalized ratio; LV, left ventricular; POTS, postural orthostatic tachycardia syndrome; RFA, radiofrequency ablation; RV, right ventricular; RVOT, right ventricular outflow tract; TEE, transesophageal echocardiography; VT, ventricular tachycardia; WPW, Wolff-Parkinson-White syndrome.

Figure 36-1 Atrioventricular Conduction Variations I.

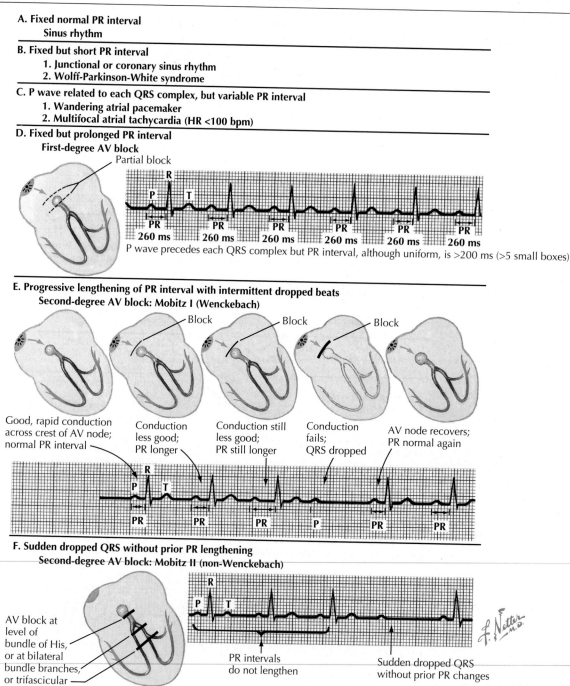

A. Fixed normal PR interval
Sinus rhythm

B. Fixed but short PR interval
1. Junctional or coronary sinus rhythm
2. Wolff-Parkinson-White syndrome

C. P wave related to each QRS complex, but variable PR interval
1. Wandering atrial pacemaker
2. Multifocal atrial tachycardia (HR <100 bpm)

D. Fixed but prolonged PR interval
First-degree AV block

Partial block

R

P T

PR PR PR PR PR PR
260 ms 260 ms 260 ms 260 ms 260 ms 260 ms

P wave precedes each QRS complex but PR interval, although uniform, is >200 ms (>5 small boxes)

E. Progressive lengthening of PR interval with intermittent dropped beats
Second-degree AV block: Mobitz I (Wenckebach)

Block Block Block

Good, rapid conduction across crest of AV node; normal PR interval

Conduction less good; PR longer

Conduction still less good; PR still longer

Conduction fails; QRS dropped

AV node recovers; PR normal again

R

P T

PR PR PR P PR PR

F. Sudden dropped QRS without prior PR lengthening
Second-degree AV block: Mobitz II (non-Wenckebach)

R

P T

AV block at level of bundle of His, or at bilateral bundle branches, or trifascicular

PR intervals do not lengthen

Sudden dropped QRS without prior PR changes

F. Netter

include intravenous procainamide or synchronized DC cardioversion. Blocking the AV node with agents such as verapamil and digoxin may accelerate the ventricular rate, and these drugs are contraindicated in WPW with atrial fibrillation and a rapid ventricular response.

Patients who present with WPW syndrome and SVT should undergo an RFA to reduce the risk for sudden death. In WPW syndrome, an accessory pathway allows antegrade (antidromic) and retrograde (orthodromic) conduction. Most SVTs associated with WPW syndrome are orthodromic. Antidromic tachycardia presents with wide complexes that resemble VT and should be treated as such unless there is a clear history of WPW syndrome.

Patients who have WPW may also have a concealed accessory pathway detectable only during an electrophysiology study. In these individuals, the tachycardia usually conducts retrograde over the accessory pathway and antegrade through the AV node.

The evaluation of patients who present with WPW on resting ECG without SVT is best done by a physician with

Figure 36-2 Atrioventricular Conduction Variations II.

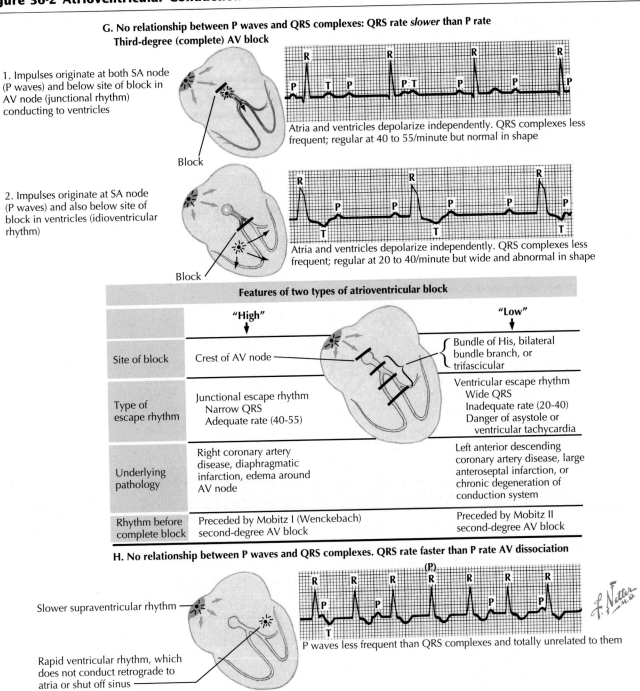

G. No relationship between P waves and QRS complexes: QRS rate *slower* than P rate
Third-degree (complete) AV block

1. Impulses originate at both SA node (P waves) and below site of block in AV node (junctional rhythm) conducting to ventricles

Block

Atria and ventricles depolarize independently. QRS complexes less frequent; regular at 40 to 55/minute but normal in shape

2. Impulses originate at SA node (P waves) and also below site of block in ventricles (idioventricular rhythm)

Block

Atria and ventricles depolarize independently. QRS complexes less frequent; regular at 20 to 40/minute but wide and abnormal in shape

Features of two types of atrioventricular block

	"High"	"Low"
Site of block	Crest of AV node	Bundle of His, bilateral bundle branch, or trifascicular
Type of escape rhythm	Junctional escape rhythm Narrow QRS Adequate rate (40-55)	Ventricular escape rhythm Wide QRS Inadequate rate (20-40) Danger of asystole or ventricular tachycardia
Underlying pathology	Right coronary artery disease, diaphragmatic infarction, edema around AV node	Left anterior descending coronary artery disease, large anteroseptal infarction, or chronic degeneration of conduction system
Rhythm before complete block	Preceded by Mobitz I (Wenckebach) second-degree AV block	Preceded by Mobitz II second-degree AV block

H. No relationship between P waves and QRS complexes. QRS rate faster than P rate AV dissociation

Slower supraventricular rhythm

Rapid ventricular rhythm, which does not conduct retrograde to atria or shut off sinus

P waves less frequent than QRS complexes and totally unrelated to them

expertise in this area. Many of these patients are at low risk and do not require further therapy. However others, particularly with a high-risk family history and significant symptoms without prior documentation of SVT or atrial fibrillation, are best treated with RFA.

Atrial tachycardia occurs in about 10% of SVTs. Ablation has, historically, been more difficult in these individuals. However, the latest mapping technology allows for accurate and easier localization of the focus and facilitates ablation.

In *atrial flutter*, the atrial rate is usually 300 beats per minute, with conduction occurring over the AV node at a 2 : 1, 3 : 1, 4 : 1, or 5 : 1 ratio. After the ventricular response is controlled, it is important to restore sinus rhythm chemically or electrically. Antiarrhythmic agents may be used to treat recurrent episodes. Current techniques allow successful and curative ablation for patients with recurrent episodes of atrial flutter.

Atrial fibrillation is a lifelong condition involving recurrent episodes. Atrial fibrillation presents in several ways:

Figure 36-3 Ventricular Rhythms I.

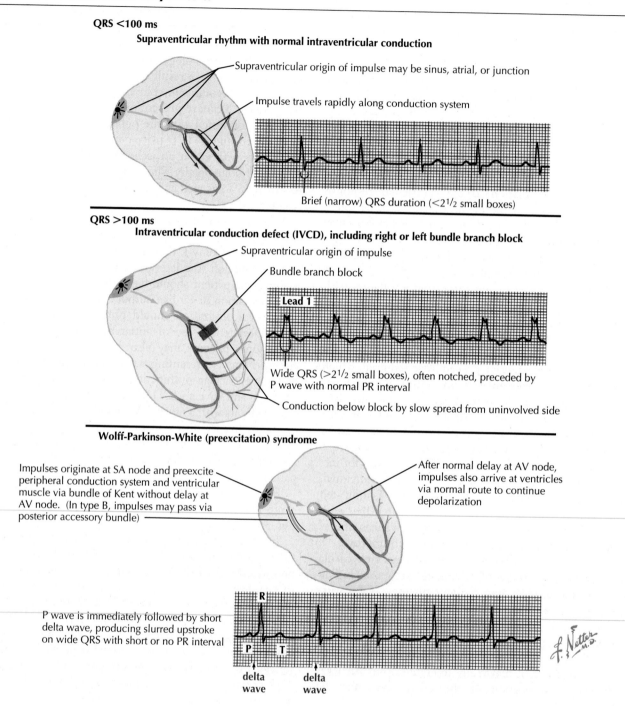

QRS <100 ms

Supraventricular rhythm with normal intraventricular conduction

Supraventricular origin of impulse may be sinus, atrial, or junction

Impulse travels rapidly along conduction system

Brief (narrow) QRS duration (<2½ small boxes)

QRS >100 ms

Intraventricular conduction defect (IVCD), including right or left bundle branch block

Supraventricular origin of impulse

Bundle branch block

Lead 1

Wide QRS (>2½ small boxes), often notched, preceded by P wave with normal PR interval

Conduction below block by slow spread from uninvolved side

Wolff-Parkinson-White (preexcitation) syndrome

Impulses originate at SA node and preexcite peripheral conduction system and ventricular muscle via bundle of Kent without delay at AV node. (In type B, impulses may pass via posterior accessory bundle)

After normal delay at AV node, impulses also arrive at ventricles via normal route to continue depolarization

P wave is immediately followed by short delta wave, producing slurred upstroke on wide QRS with short or no PR interval

R P T

delta wave   delta wave

paroxysmal (terminates spontaneously), persistent (needs cardioversion to terminate), or permanent (cannot be maintained in sinus rhythm, i.e., chronic). Patients with nonvalvular heart disease who have any one of several risk factors (older than 75 years, hypertension, diabetes, congestive heart failure, previous embolic episode) have a higher risk (>5% per year) for stroke and require chronic anticoagulation with an International Normalized Ratio (INR) between 2 and 3.

Antiarrhythmic agents are indicated to prevent recurrences of either paroxysmal or persistent atrial fibrillation. Therapeutic choices include amiodarone, sotalol, propafenone, flecainide, and dofetilide. The latter four drugs have proarrhythmic effects and require close monitoring. Digoxin, β-blockers (other than sotalol), and diltiazem do not convert atrial fibrillation to sinus rhythm, but conversion to normal sinus rhythm may occur with rate control. Pulmonary vein isolation is the ablation procedure of

choice for patients who have been unresponsive or intolerant of two or more antiarrhythmic agents. Premature atrial complexes originating from the atrial tissue in the pulmonary veins act as triggers for the initiation of atrial fibrillation, and occasionally as facilitators for the maintenance of atrial fibrillation. This procedure is associated with a greater than 70% freedom of atrial fibrillation at 1 year.

Permanent atrial fibrillation requires rate control using combinations of β-blockers, calcium channel blockers, and digoxin. Patients in whom intermittent bradycardia develops (tachy-brady syndrome) or who have a persistent tachycardia may require a permanent pacemaker with or without AV node ablation. If the ventricular response cannot be controlled or the medications cannot be tolerated, AV node ablation will prevent rapid ventricular response, and a permanent pacemaker will prevent bradycardia. After ablation and pacemaker placement, quality-of-life scores are greatly improved.

Patients who are active and have atrial fibrillation with a rapid ventricular response, and who get an inadequate therapeutic response to rate-control agents, should be considered for isolation and radiofrequency ablation of the pulmonary veins. For these patients with permanent atrial fibrillation, a more extensive procedure is required, which includes a left atrial roof ablation line, mitral annulus ablation line, coronary sinus isolation, tricuspid annulus ablation line, and isolation of the superior and inferior vena cava. Sinus rhythm can be restored in more than half of patients. Because atrial fibrillation can be due to numerous pathophysiologic factors and because multiple sites for initiation of atrial fibrillation often exist in a single individual, radiofrequency ablation has been challenging, as indicated by the success rates cited here. It is anticipated that with continued investigation and technologic advances, therapeutic outcomes in this area will continue to improve.

Inappropriate sinus tachycardia refers to sinus tachycardia occurring in the absence of provoking factors, including hyperthyroidism, fever, and systemic diseases. It is a frustrating and debilitating condition; patients complain of sudden rapid increases in heart rate with minimal or no physical activity. Initially, β-blocker or calcium channel blocker alone or in combination may be used. If symptoms persist despite use of maximally tolerated doses, an RFA of the superior portion of the sinus node may be considered.

In some individuals with inappropriate sinus tachycardia, head-up tilt testing will reveal a rapid increase in heart rate upon changing from a supine position to a 70-degree upright position. This condition is called *postural orthostatic tachycardia syndrome* (POTS). Ablation of the sinus node in the setting of POTS may worsen the condition. Preliminary studies suggest that an immunologic mechanism may be responsible for POTS.

The use of ICDs has significantly reduced arrhythmic death from *VT*. The largest potential target group includes patients with VT due to prior myocardial infarction. In the recent past, guidelines limited ICD implantation in this group of patients and were stringent, requiring demonstration of nonsustained VT in the setting of left ventricular dysfunction due to a previous myocardial infarction and a positive electrophysiology study for inducible VT before ICD placement. As a result of recent studies, ICD placement is now recommended in a much larger group of at-risk patients. Primary prevention of sudden cardiac death has been confirmed with the publication of a number of randomized studies. ICD placement is now recommended in patients with either an ischemic cardiomyopathy or a dilated cardiomyopathy who have a left ventricular EF of less than 35%, as well as in those presenting with VT or resuscitated VF.

VT most commonly presents in patients with left ventricular dysfunction (Fig. 36-4), although there are less common types of VT that present with normal left ventricular function (see later). If an abnormal EF is documented, the patient should have a cardiac catheterization with calculation of cardiac output and coronary angiography. Revascularization should precede placement of an ICD. Despite the use of antiarrhythmic agents and an ICD, some patients may also require RFA of the VT circuit. Patients presenting with syncope in the presence of left ventricular dysfunction should be considered to have VT and have an ICD placed.

In patients with a normal echocardiogram, the VT may originate from a focus located in the right ventricular outflow tract or the left ventricle, and may be verapamil or adenosine sensitive. RFA is a curative option for these patients.

Patients with *VF* that occurs outside the setting of an acute myocardial infarction should receive an ICD (see Fig. 36-4).

In those patients who have an ICD indication and a QRS duration of more than 120 milliseconds and CHF, a biventricular ICD should be placed. This has been shown to significantly improve the quality of life and exercise duration and decreases rehospitalization and mortality.

Symptomatic patients with *complete heart block, second-degree Mobitz type II AV block*, and *sinus pauses* should receive a permanent pacemaker. Asymptomatic patients with prolonged PR intervals, sinus bradycardia, or second-degree Mobitz type I AV block (Wenckebach) should not receive a pacemaker (see Fig. 36-2). Also, a *bifascicular block* (bundle branch block in the context of left anterior fascicular block or left posterior fascicular block) in asymptomatic individuals should be observed, rather than referred for pacemaker implantation. However, patients with bifascicular block, who present with syncope in the absence of any identifying cause, should undergo pacemaker placement.

Premature ventricular complexes without left ventricular dysfunction should be managed conservatively, as should *premature atrial complexes*. Because caffeine, sleep deprivation, and alcohol can all increase the frequency of premature ventricular and atrial complexes, patients should be

Figure 36-4 Ventricular Rhythms II.

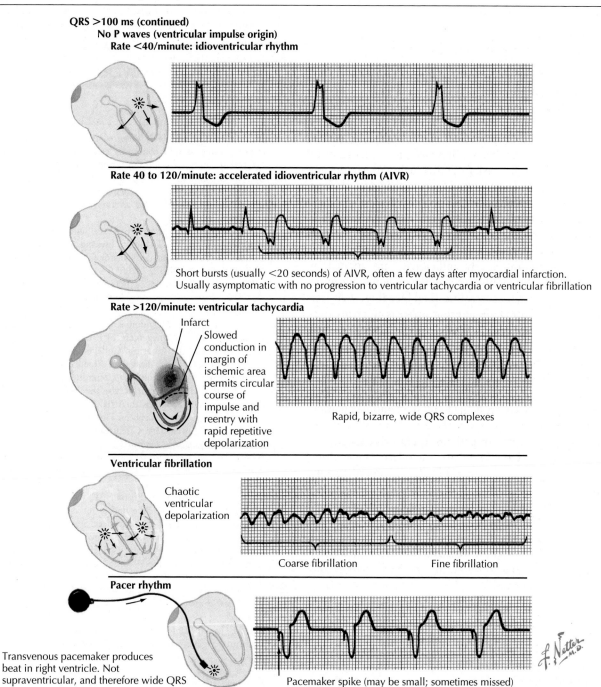

QRS >100 ms (continued)
No P waves (ventricular impulse origin)
Rate <40/minute: idioventricular rhythm

Rate 40 to 120/minute: accelerated idioventricular rhythm (AIVR)

Short bursts (usually <20 seconds) of AIVR, often a few days after myocardial infarction.
Usually asymptomatic with no progression to ventricular tachycardia or ventricular fibrillation

Rate >120/minute: ventricular tachycardia

Infarct
Slowed conduction in margin of ischemic area permits circular course of impulse and reentry with rapid repetitive depolarization

Rapid, bizarre, wide QRS complexes

Ventricular fibrillation

Chaotic ventricular depolarization

Coarse fibrillation   Fine fibrillation

Pacer rhythm

Transvenous pacemaker produces beat in right ventricle. Not supraventricular, and therefore wide QRS

Pacemaker spike (may be small; sometimes missed)

encouraged to cease or limit these. Regular exercise can reduce the frequency of premature ventricular and atrial complexes.

Congenital long QT syndrome is an inherited condition that presents with syncope or sudden death. Exercise-induced symptoms are a particular cause for concern. Frequently, a family history of similar episodes will be found. Management includes β-blockers, dual-chamber pacemaker with a lower rate at 85 beats per minute, or an ICD.

Patients with *Brugada syndrome* are at risk for sudden cardiac death. Symptomatic individuals should receive an ICD; asymptomatic individuals with an abnormal ECG pattern may undergo an electrophysiology study, and, if results are positive, may have an ICD placed.

More recently, the *short QT syndrome* and *catecholamine-induced polymorphic VT* have been recognized. These conditions are associated with sudden cardiac death and may need an ICD with or without an antiarrhythmic agent.

In all these instances, referral to a cardiac electrophysiologist is recommended for management.

Avoiding Treatment Errors

Many opportunities for error exist in the treatment of patients with symptomatic arrhythmias. In some circumstances, a failure to pursue adequate evaluation represents a preventable error. For instance, occasional patients with SVT are only diagnosed after years of being treated ineffectively for panic attacks. Similarly, it is important to recognize the increased risk for individuals with significant LV dysfunction and syncope. These individuals are best treated with ICD placement.

In elderly patients with atrial fibrillation, physicians may overestimate the relative risk of warfarin therapy versus its protective effect against thromboembolic events. In reality, although elderly individuals are indeed at increased risk for both falls (and if anticoagulated, bleeding due to their injury) and gastrointestinal bleeding, their risk for having a devastating life-altering stroke is much greater. Unless there is a history of falls or of gastrointestinal bleeding, most elderly patients with atrial fibrillation will benefit from anticoagulation with warfarin.

An INR below 2 is associated with an increased risk for stroke and is not associated with a decreased risk for hemorrhage. Once a decision is made to start anticoagulation for atrial fibrillation, an INR in the 2 to 3 range should be the goal for all patients. In patients at high risk for stroke, soluble aspirin and clopidogrel are not an acceptable alternative to therapeutic warfarin. Finally, in regard to rate control in atrial fibrillation, it is important to objectively assess the efficacy of the medical regimen being used.

Before the final decision-making analysis, whether for ICD placement, radiofrequency ablation, pharmacologic therapy, or warfarin therapy for atrial fibrillation in elderly patients, it is essential to define the patient's wishes and the family's preferences.

Future Directions

Further improvements in ablation technology for atrial fibrillation will greatly simplify the procedure and increase its safety and efficacy. ICD technology continues to evolve and improve the quality of life of patients who previously were at high risk for arrhythmic death. Cardiac resynchronization therapy with atrio-biventricular pacing in patients with CHF and prolonged intraventricular conduction (wide QRS complexes) is now a very effective therapy in this group of severely impaired and debilitated patients. Current device studies are examining the role of biventricular device placement in the prevention of CHF progression in patients receiving an ICD who have wide QRS complexes (the REsynchronization reVErses Remodeling in Sytolic left vEntricular dysfunction (REVERSE) study).

EVIDENCE

1. Antzelevitch C, Brugada P, Borggrefe M, et al: Brugada syndrome: Report of the second consensus conference. Endorsed by the Heart Rhythm Society and the European Heart Rhythm Association. Circulation 111:659-670, 2005.
   This article outlines the diagnostic and treatment strategies for patients with Brugada syndrome and screening strategy for their family members.
2. Bardy GH, Lee KL, Mark DB, et al: Sudden Cardiac Death in Heart Failure Trial (SCD-HeFT) Investigators. Amiodarone or an implantable cardioverter-defibrillator for congestive heart failure. N Engl J Med 352:225-237, 2005.
   This paper evaluates the role of ICD therapy in the primary prevention of SCD in patients with congestive heart failure, EF <35%, and NYHA class II and III.
3. Fuster V, Ryden LE, Cannom DS, et al: ACC/AHA/ESC 2006 Guidelines for the Management of Patients with Atrial Fibrillation: A report of the American College of Cardiology/American Heart Association Task Force on Practice Guidelines and the European Society of Cardiology Committee for Practice Guidelines (Writing Committee to Revise the 2001 Guidelines for the Management of Patients with Atrial Fibrillation). Developed in collaboration with the European Heart Rhythm Association and the Heart Rhythm Society. Circulation 114:e257-e354, 2006.
   These latest guidelines confirm the importance of anticoagulation as key in the management of stroke prevention. The article has an extensive reference base and provides a great overview of atrial fibrillation management.
4. Gregoratos G, Abrams J, Epstein AE, et al: Guidelines. ACC/AHA/NASPE 2002 guideline update for implantation of cardiac pacemakers and antiarrhythmia devices. Summary article: A report of the American College of Cardiology/American Heart Association Task Force on Practice Guidelines (ACC/AHA/NASPE Committee to Update the 1998 Pacemaker Guidelines). Circulation 106:2145-2161, 2002.
   This collaborative report provides details of when placement of a device is indicated. It also provides guidance on conditions when a device is not indicated.
5. Hsu LF, Jais P, Sanders P, et al: Catheter ablation for atrial fibrillation in congestive heart failure. N Engl J Med 351:2373-2383, 2004.
   This paper confirms the importance of restoring sinus rhythm in improving the functional status of patients with CHF and atrial fibrillation.
6. Weber BE, Kapoor WN: Evaluation and outcomes of patients with palpitations. Am J Med 103:86, 1997.
   This article reviews the diagnosis, etiology and 1-year prognosis of a consecutive series of patients admitted with palpitations.

Richard G. Sheahan ▪ Marschall S. Runge

Atrial Fibrillation

Introduction

Atrial fibrillation, the most common arrhythmia in adults and elderly people, occurs in response to a myriad of conditions. The irregular pulse found with mitral valve disease, described as *delirium cordis*, was once the most common manifestation of atrial fibrillation. With the decreasing prevalence of rheumatic fever, other causes of atrial fibrillation now far surpass mitral valve disease. Moreover, it is understood that patients with atrial fibrillation have substantially increased morbidity and mortality.

The prevalence of atrial fibrillation is increasing worldwide, particularly as populations age. Atrial fibrillation is uncommon in infants and children and becomes increasingly common with age. Of adults younger than 55 years, less than 0.1% have atrial fibrillation, whereas 4% of individuals older than 60 years and about 10% of those older than 80 years have atrial fibrillation. It is estimated that more than 2 million U.S. adults have atrial fibrillation; by the midpoint of the 21st century, that number may exceed 5.5 million, with more than 50% being older than 80 years. Patients with atrial fibrillation have a 1.5- to 2.0-fold increased mortality risk, compared with age- and disease-matched controls, and a markedly increased risk for embolic events and congestive heart failure (CHF), according to data from the Framingham Study.

Etiology and Pathogenesis

Many factors predispose the heart to atrial fibrillation (Box 37-1; Fig. 37-1), including structural abnormalities (such as valvular heart disease), systolic or diastolic dysfunction, CHF, hypertension, diabetes, and myocardial infarction. Other conditions associated with an increased prevalence of atrial fibrillation include acute or chronic alcohol ingestion, hyperthyroidism or hypothyroidism, and alterations in vagal or sympathetic tone. Of patients with atrial fibrillation, less than 10% are classified as having *lone atrial fibrillation*, that is, no clinical, electrocardiographic, or echocardiographic evidence of structural heart disease and none of the predisposing factors cited earlier.

No single electrical mechanism causes atrial fibrillation. Early investigators proposed multiple reentrant waves (or wavelets) to indicate that these small multiple waves initiate in the atrium, spreading and coalescing to form small circuits of reentrant electrical activity. The short and variable wavelengths of these activities preclude organized atrial electrical activity and result in atrial fibrillation. It has been found that rapid, repetitive impulse generation by atrial myocytes located near the orifice of the pulmonary veins stimulates atrial fibrillation. Moreover, atrial fibrillation begets atrial fibrillation. Anatomic remodeling, disruption of electrical circuits, and cellular damage and fibrosis result from chronic atrial fibrillation, all decreasing the likelihood of a return to normal sinus rhythm.

More recently, triggers, which initiate, and rotors, which maintain atrial fibrillation, have been identified. Ganglionic plexuses, a complex and extensive neuronal network, have been demonstrated in atrial tissue. Electrical activity from these plexuses can result in abnormal (fractionated) electrograms that are important in continued atrial fibrillation. Ablation of these electrograms is often associated with successful termination of atrial fibrillation.

Clinical Presentation

The clinical presentation of patients with atrial fibrillation varies. Some patients are asymptomatic. The diagnosis of atrial fibrillation may be made on a regular annual examination or as an incidental finding during the evaluation of a patient being seen for a different (sometimes related) illness. Others patients with atrial fibrillation note sensations that reflect the irregularity of the rhythm, often indistinguishable from frequent ventricular or atrial pre-

---

Box 37-1   Underlying Etiologies of Atrial Fibrillation

Cardiac

Mitral valvular heart disease
Systolic or diastolic dysfunction
Congestive heart failure
Hypertension
Diabetes
Myocardial infarction
Hypertrophic cardiomyopathy
Pericarditis
Wolff-Parkinson-White syndrome
Sick sinus syndrome
Congenital heart disease
Postcoronary artery bypass surgery

Noncardiac

Acute or chronic alcohol ingestion (holiday heart syndrome)
Hyperthyroidism or hypothyroidism
Alterations in vagal or sympathetic tone
Pulmonary embolism
Sepsis
Chronic obstructive pulmonary disease
Lone atrial fibrillation

---

mature contractions. These symptoms may range from noticeable but not bothersome to nerve-wracking. Occasionally, a patient presents for evaluation of bradycardia diagnosed by the patient or someone who recorded a slow radial pulse rate (that underestimates the true heart rate). Still others present with symptoms reflecting decreased cardiac output, which occurs when atrial fibrillation replaces normal sinus rhythm; these symptoms range from fatigue to shortness of breath at rest or with activity, to chest pain. Severe symptoms and physical examination findings of CHF occasionally are found in patients with new-onset atrial fibrillation. Finally, the first manifestation of atrial fibrillation may be the devastating effects of a cerebrovascular accident/transient ischemic attack (CVA/TIA).

Diagnostic Approach

The history, physical examination, electrocardiogram, and a variety of laboratory and cardiovascular tests are commonly employed in the initial evaluation of atrial fibrillation. Upon presentation, most patients can be classified into one of four categories, as recommended by a joint task force of the American College of Cardiology, the American Heart Association, and the European Society of Cardiology: paroxysmal, persistent, permanent, or lone atrial fibrillation. Treatment differs among the four groups.

1. *Paroxysmal atrial fibrillation* is described as episodes of atrial fibrillation that last less than a week (and often less than 24 hours), self-terminate, and are usually recurrent.

2. *Persistent atrial fibrillation* lasts more than a week, does not self-terminate, and may recur after cardioversion.

3. *Permanent atrial fibrillation* is diagnosed if atrial fibrillation has lasted more than a year, has been refractory to cardioversion, or both.

4. *Lone atrial fibrillation* can be paroxysmal, persistent, or permanent atrial fibrillation in the absence of structural heart disease.

In addition to classifying the atrial fibrillation, the history and physical examination should focus on clues to the underlying cause. Symptoms and examination findings relevant to the conditions that predispose to atrial fibrillation (as listed previously) should be sought. It is important to seek evidence for complications of atrial fibrillation, including presyncopal symptoms (especially with initiation or termination of atrial fibrillation), decreased cardiac output, and thromboembolism (including transient ischemic attacks, evidence of peripheral embolization, or both). An ophthalmoscopic examination may reveal retinal artery embolism in some patients with atrial fibrillation. Patients at highest risk for atrial fibrillation with rapid ventricular response, including those with accessory pathways (Wolff-Parkinson-White syndrome) or dilated cardiomyopathy, can present with frank syncope or even sudden cardiac death.

The electrocardiogram can confirm atrial fibrillation, heart rate, and the presence of underlying structural heart disease, such as chamber enlargement or (hypertrophy), prior myocardial infarction, and conduction abnormalities. The transthoracic echocardiogram is an essential part of a complete evaluation, particularly in patients being considered for cardioversion. Underlying structural contributors to atrial fibrillation and left atrial size, a predictor of short- and long-term success in cardioversion, should be examined by echocardiography. Transesophageal echocardiography is indicated in some settings to document, before cardioversion, the presence or absence of thrombi in the left atrium or the left atrial appendage. Laboratory testing should be performed to evaluate thyroid status and screen for electrolyte abnormalities. Additional testing may include functional assessment for coronary heart disease (exercise or pharmacologic stress testing with or without imaging) and even coronary angiography. Electrophysiology studies are not indicated as part of the initial evaluation but are indicated when radiofrequency ablation of potential atrial fibrillation sites is being considered. An electrophysiology study may also be considered for younger patients with a history of supraventricular tachycardia and a regular rhythm, which has now become more irregular. In this setting, the supraventricular tachycardia may be the trigger for the initiation of atrial fibrillation. Although uncommon, this is an example of tachycardia-induced tachycardia. In this circumstance, radiofrequency ablation of the supraventricular tachycardia can prevent subsequent episodes of atrial fibrillation.

Figure 37-1 Atrial Fibrillation.

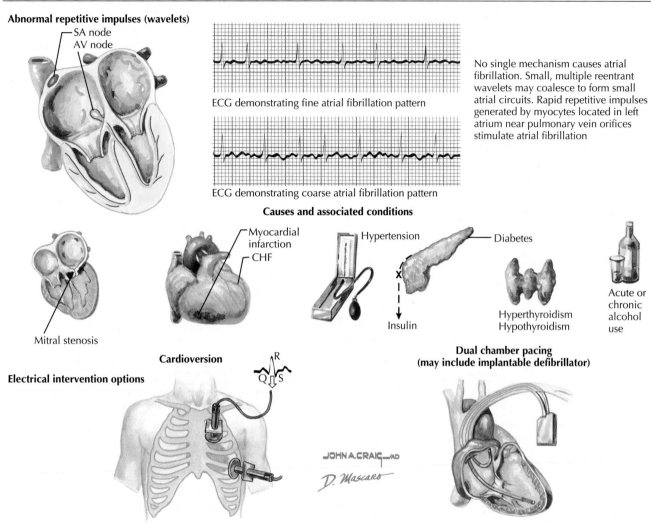

Abnormal repetitive impulses (wavelets)

SA node
AV node

ECG demonstrating fine atrial fibrillation pattern

ECG demonstrating coarse atrial fibrillation pattern

No single mechanism causes atrial fibrillation. Small, multiple reentrant wavelets may coalesce to form small atrial circuits. Rapid repetitive impulses generated by myocytes located in left atrium near pulmonary vein orifices stimulate atrial fibrillation

Causes and associated conditions

Mitral stenosis

Myocardial infarction
CHF

Hypertension

Insulin

Diabetes

Hyperthyroidism
Hypothyroidism

Acute or chronic alcohol use

Electrical intervention options

Cardioversion

JOHN A. CRAIG—MD
D. Mascaro

Dual chamber pacing (may include implantable defibrillator)

Emergent cardioversion is considered in two circumstances: (1) when onset of atrial fibrillation results in hemodynamic instability in a previously stable patient (manifest as hypotension, angina/myocardial ischemia, or rapid onset of CHF) or (2) when patient with borderline hemodynamic status suddenly develops atrial fibrillation. Elective cardioversion is indicated unless severe circumstances

Permanent dual chamber pacing should be considered in those with bradycardia and paroxysmal atrial fibrillation (to help maintain sinus rhythm) or in patients with persistent atrial fibrillation in whom use of AV-node-suppressing drugs (to prevent rapid ventricular response) results in significant bradycardia at rest

Management and Therapy

Treatment of atrial fibrillation largely depends on symptoms and the cause of the atrial fibrillation (Figs. 37-2 to 37-4). Are the symptoms related to atrial fibrillation tolerable or intolerable to the patient? Has atrial fibrillation resulted in an unfavorable hemodynamic picture that may have long-term consequences? Have embolic events occurred, and what is the long-term risk for thromboembolism? Consideration of important issues related to each of these areas can help guide treatment options.

Optimum Treatment

Acute Management of Atrial Fibrillation

Initial management of atrial fibrillation is dependent on ventricular response, blood pressure, evidence of ischemia,

shortness of breath, and cardiogenic shock. Figure 37-2 provides a schematic to management. Once the patient has been stabilized, subsequent evaluation and management depend on age, heart rate, symptoms, etiologic considerations, hypertension, myocardial ischemia, diabetes mellitus, thyroid disease, cerebrovascular accidents, and pulmonary considerations (see Box 37-1 and Figs. 37-2 to 37-4).

Nonacute Management of Atrial Fibrillation

Four major issues must be considered in determining the treatment of atrial fibrillation: conversion from atrial fibrillation to normal sinus rhythm, maintenance of normal sinus rhythm, rate control in patients with chronic atrial

Figure 37-2 Long-term Management of Paroxysmal Atrial Fibrillation.
ARB, angiotensin receptor blocker; CHF, congestive heart failure; ECG, electrocardiogram; EF, ejection fraction; LA, left atrial; LV, left ventricular.

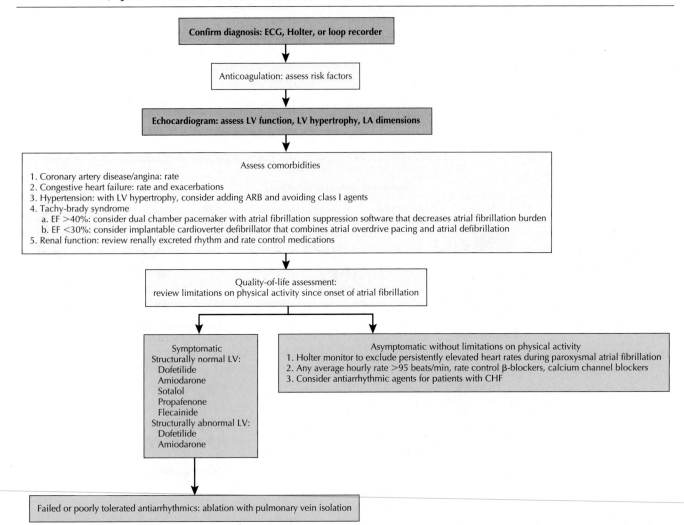

fibrillation, and prevention of thromboembolic complications (Fig. 37-5). These four issues are discussed with special emphasis on controversial factors.

Cardioversion

Cardioversion for atrial fibrillation should be considered in two settings. In patients who present acutely with hemodynamically unstable atrial fibrillation, immediate cardioversion may be indicated. Remember the sinus tachycardia concept: atrial fibrillation with a rapid response may be triggered by an underlying cause. Initially, this cause should be sought and, if necessary, addressed. Other causes of hypotension and tachycardia should be excluded, including hypovolemia, septic shock, acute hemorrhage, profound anemia, and acute myocardial infarction leading to cardiogenic shock. Usually, patients who are hypotensive from atrial fibrillation with a rapid ventricular rate also have underlying cardiovascular disease. After reversible

factors have been addressed, these patients should undergo electrical cardioversion immediately. Rate control with intravenous short-acting β-blockers (esmolol) or calcium channel blockers (diltiazem) can be considered, but in the setting of marked hypotension, these should be cautiously initiated. However, because there is no atrial contraction in atrial fibrillation, the left ventricle (LV) fills passively. Therefore, in patients with a rapid ventricular response, slowing of the ventricular rate allows a more prolonged diastolic filling time and thus may improve cardiac output. In hemodynamically stable patients with myocardial ischemia, either intravenous β-blockers (including esmolol or metoprolol) or calcium channel blockers (diltiazem or verapamil) can be used safely before cardioversion. Neither β-blockers nor calcium channel blockers are effective agents for cardioversion, although spontaneous cardioversion may occur when the heart rate is slowed pharmacologically. There is a growing indication for certain type III

Figure 37-3 Long-term Management of Persistent Atrial Fibrillation.

ARB, angiotensin receptor blocker; CHF, congestive heart failure; DC, direct current; ECG, electrocardiogram; EF, ejection fraction; INR, International Normalized Ratio; LA, left atrial; LV, left ventricular.

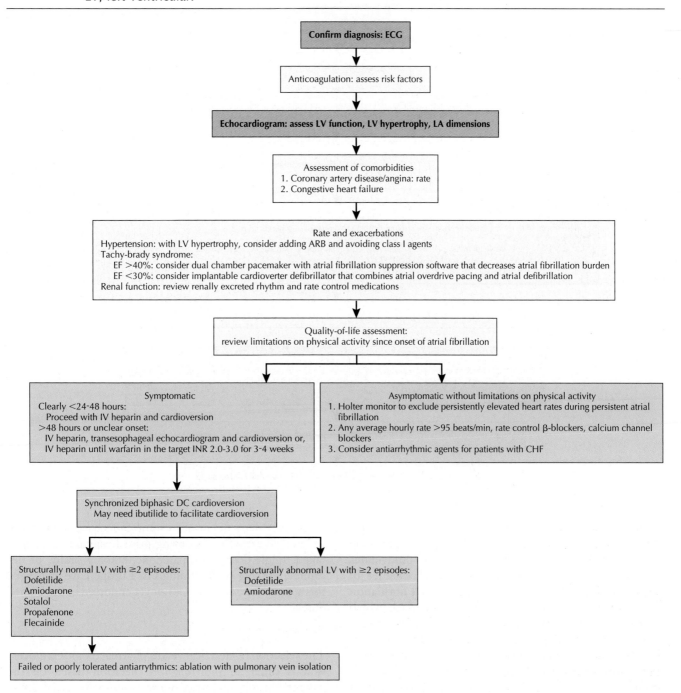

antiarrhythmic drugs in the urgent treatment of atrial fibrillation. Intravenous ibutilide and amiodarone are safe in this setting, when used with proper monitoring. In some circumstances, class IA agents (intravenous procainamide principally) are recommended in the acute setting, but the advent of ibutilide and amiodarone have largely displaced their use.

The second setting in which cardioversion is considered for atrial fibrillation is in symptomatic (or sometimes even asymptomatic) but stable patients. In this setting, before cardioversion, it is essential to consider the need for anti-coagulation (see "Anticoagulation in Atrial Fibrillation"). In general, in uncomplicated cases when the duration of atrial fibrillation is clearly less than 24 hours, anticoagula-

Figure 37-4 Long-term Management of Permanent Atrial Fibrillation.

ARB, angiotensin receptor blocker; ECG, electrocardiogram; LV, left ventricular; LA, left atrial; EF, ejection fraction.

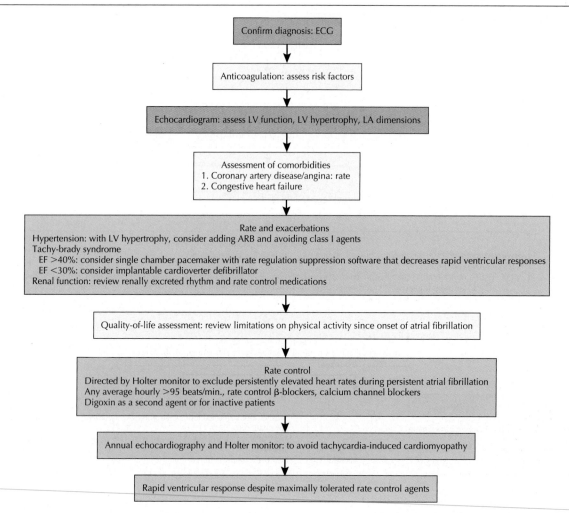

tion is not required before cardioversion. When the duration of atrial fibrillation is more than 48 hours, it is generally recommended that the patient be started on intravenous heparin. Differences of opinion exist about whether to anticoagulate patients who have been in atrial fibrillation for 24 to 48 hours. The more conservative approach (which we adhere to) is to anticoagulate, the same as for patients in whom the duration of atrial fibrillation has been more than 48 hours. An alternative approach uses transesophageal echocardiography to screen for thrombi in the atria or the atrial appendages and proceed with cardioversion if no thrombi are present. In this case, anticoagulation with warfarin for 3 to 4 weeks (International Normalized Ratio [INR], 2.0 to 3.0) is initiated at the time of cardioversion and for at least 1 month afterward. These issues are discussed in the following subsections.

A trend in Europe, but less so in the U.S. is the so-called "pill in the box" strategy in patients at low risk for proarrhythmia is a safe and effective way of pharmacologic cardioversion. Patients who either are on telemetry in the emergency department or in some cases have been shown to have no arrhythmias during prior hospitalizations may take a single dose of propafenone, 600 mg orally, or flecainide, 300 mg orally. Studies in Europe have suggested this approach is safe, but it is not yet endorsed in the United States.

Rhythm Control

The selection of electrical versus pharmacologic cardioversion is often an individualized decision based on the patient's history and predisposing factors for atrial fibrillation. For instance, patients with paroxysmal or persistent atrial fibrillation are likely to require antifibrillatory medication to maintain sinus rhythm. Obviously, these patients need to be maintained on anticoagulants before chemical cardioversion. The pharmacologic choices for cardioversion are principally amiodarone, sotalol, and dofetilide. All have advantages and disadvantages. For patients with paroxysmal atrial fibrillation, amiodarone can safely be initiated in the outpatient setting and is probably the most

Figure 37-5 Complications of Atrial Fibrillation.

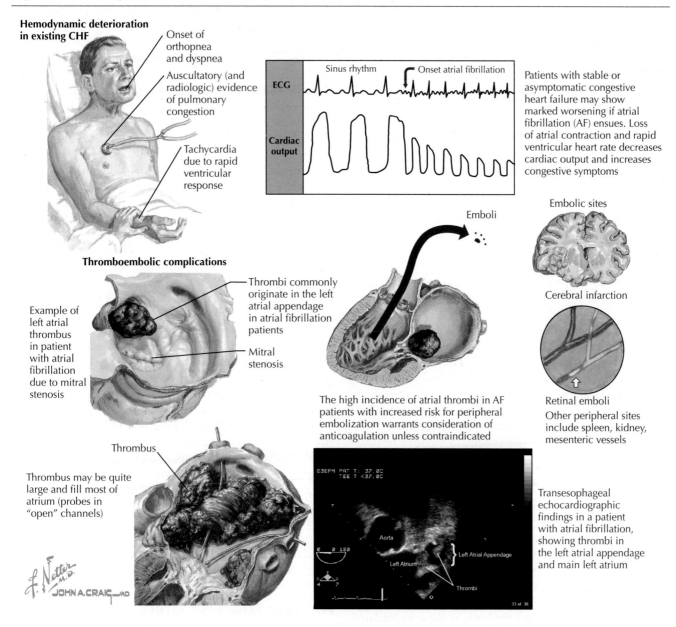

Hemodynamic deterioration in existing CHF

Onset of orthopnea and dyspnea

Auscultatory (and radiologic) evidence of pulmonary congestion

Tachycardia due to rapid ventricular response

Sinus rhythm — Onset atrial fibrillation

ECG

Cardiac output

Patients with stable or asymptomatic congestive heart failure may show marked worsening if atrial fibrillation (AF) ensues. Loss of atrial contraction and rapid ventricular heart rate decreases cardiac output and increases congestive symptoms

Emboli

Embolic sites

Thromboembolic complications

Thrombi commonly originate in the left atrial appendage in atrial fibrillation patients

Example of left atrial thrombus in patient with atrial fibrillation due to mitral stenosis

Mitral stenosis

Cerebral infarction

The high incidence of atrial thrombi in AF patients with increased risk for peripheral embolization warrants consideration of anticoagulation unless contraindicated

Retinal emboli
Other peripheral sites include spleen, kidney, mesenteric vessels

Thrombus

Thrombus may be quite large and fill most of atrium (probes in "open" channels)

Transesophageal echocardiographic findings in a patient with atrial fibrillation, showing thrombi in the left atrial appendage and main left atrium

83BPM PAT T: 37.0C
TEE T <37.0C

Aorta

Left Atrial Appendage

Left Atrium

Thrombi

0 180

33 of 36

JOHN A. CRAIG—MD

---

effective antifibrillatory agent. Even at the low doses used for atrial fibrillation prophylaxis (about 200 mg/day), the side-effect profile of amiodarone requires annual or semi-annual screening for thyroid and hepatic dysfunction and for the rare occurrence of diminishing pulmonary function from early pulmonary fibrosis. Sotalol is also effective and can be particularly beneficial in patients who require β blockade for other reasons, but sotalol should be initiated in an inpatient setting because of unpredictable QT prolongation in some individuals. Dofetilide is a promising agent, but its use also requires 3 days of telemetry monitoring for QT prolongation and torsades de pointes. The initial dofetilide dosage is based on renal function. Subsequent doses are determined by QT response to the previous dose until a steady state is reached.

The decision to use medications in an effort to maintain normal sinus rhythm is common. Indeed, less than one third of patients who are successfully cardioverted maintain normal sinus rhythm for more than a year without antifibrillatory therapy. Many predictors of the potential need for antifibrillatory therapy are known. Sometimes the use of β-blockers can blunt adrenergic drive sufficiently to prevent recurrence of atrial fibrillation, although this is the exception. Many cardiologists favor an initial trial of electrical cardioversion alone in low-risk patients with atrial fibrillation, reasoning that the third of patients who do not require antifibrillatory therapy will be spared the expense and the associated risks. In patients who have an increased risk for recurrent atrial fibrillation, or who have had a second electrical cardioversion, use of the medications discussed previously (and in Figs. 37-2 and 37-3) is generally indicated for maintenance of normal sinus rhythm. However, this practice has come into question and is discussed later in the section, "Rate versus Rhythm Control."

The issue of measuring quality of life (QOL) in patients with atrial fibrillation is fraught with methodologic difficulties. Using an intention to treat analysis does not adequately control for the rhythm at time the QOL questionnaire is completed. Likewise, using the rhythm at the time of the QOL questionnaire completion makes comparisons between different treatment strategies extremely difficult to interpret. Several studies have now shown that patients in sinus rhythm have improved QOL scores compared with patients in atrial fibrillation at the time of QOL questionnaire completion.

Rate Control

Many patients with chronic atrial fibrillation are not successfully treated with cardioversion or antiarrhythmic agents, are unwilling to undergo cardioversion, are unable to tolerate antiarrhythmic agents, or have factors that predict that treatment will fail and are minimally symptomatic except at rapid heart rates. For them (see Fig. 37-4), pharmacologic rate control should be considered. β-Blockers, calcium channel blockers, or both can often control rapid heart rates with or without digoxin. Digoxin is particularly useful in controlling atrioventricular (AV) conduction in patients who are minimally active or bedridden from comorbidities. However, because there is considerable overlap between atrial fibrillation and conduction abnormalities, including sinus node dysfunction (sick sinus syndrome), an appropriate balance between tachycardia and bradycardia may be difficult to obtain. These patients may require a permanent pacemaker to prevent bradycardic episodes while being treated with β-blockers, calcium channel blockers, or antifibrillatory medications for tachycardia. Although the initial promise of permanent dual-chamber pacing (or even atrial pacing alone) to prevent atrial fibrillation has not been fulfilled, in patients with episodic atrial fibrillation, dual-chamber pacing with an atrial fibrillation suppression algorithm should be considered when a pacemaker is indicated. Use of ventricular pacing is likely to convert episodic atrial fibrillation into chronic atrial fibrillation. Another special case, discussed later (see "Atrioventricular Node Ablation and Permanent Pacing"), is the patient whose rapid ventricular response is resistant to pharmacologic control or for whom the pharmacologic approach results in intolerable side effects.

Anticoagulation in Atrial Fibrillation

Anticoagulation considerations include anticoagulation during restoration of normal sinus rhythm, chronic anticoagulation, and cessation and restoration of anticoagulation for patients with atrial fibrillation who are undergoing surgical procedures. Consensus panels from the American College of Cardiology, the American Heart Association, the European Society of Cardiology, and the American College of Chest Physicians have concurred on the use of anticoagulation therapy in the pericardioversion period. In patients with atrial fibrillation of unknown duration, valvular heart disease, evidence of LV dysfunction, or prior thromboembolism, or for whom cardioversion is entirely elective, therapeutic anticoagulation with warfarin (with an INR of 2.0 to 3.0) for 3 to 4 weeks before cardioversion is strongly recommended. Anticoagulation should be continued at the same level for at least 4 weeks after cardioversion. An alternative approach in low-risk patients (lacking any of the criteria listed here) is to assess for atrial or atrial appendage thrombi by transesophageal echocardiography. Lacking thrombi, or a low-flow state (also referred to as "smoke" or spontaneous echocardiographic contrast), the patient can be safely cardioverted without antecedent anticoagulation with warfarin, although many use heparin or low–molecular-weight heparin before cardioversion. These patients do require anticoagulation for 4 to 6 weeks after cardioversion.

Long-term anticoagulation with warfarin is advocated in patients in several settings. Irrespective of the type of atrial fibrillation (paroxysmal, persistent, or permanent), patients at high risk for stroke should be anticoagulated for life. Because many patients have recurrent atrial fibrillation, some episodes of which may not be recognized by the patient, anticoagulation is indicated. Other symptomatic patients may also experience asymptomatic episodes of atrial fibrillation that predispose to embolic events, even when they are in sinus rhythm. Finally, in patients with chronic atrial fibrillation, five large prospectively randomized studies demonstrated that warfarin reduced the risk for stroke by 45% to 82%. The use of aspirin remains controversial for patients at low risk for stroke (lone atrial fibrillation) or for patients with increased risk for bleeding in whom warfarin may be contraindicated.

Avoiding Treatment Errors

The three most common types of errors in treatment of patients with atrial fibrillation are (1) failure to recognize an underlying, potentially reversible cause of atrial fibrillation; (2) failure to consider potential drug interactions that could lead to bradycardia in patients with atrial fibrillation treated with AV node blocking drugs; and (3) failure to rigorously monitor and adjust anticoagulant therapy, leading to either excess bleeding or thrombus formation. Although these complications cannot be completely avoided, with careful and conscientious physician oversight, the risk for one of these complications can be minimized. All patients with atrial fibrillation should have a comprehensive evaluation before initiation of therapy. Upon initiation of therapy with AV node blocking drugs, all concurrent therapies should be reviewed, and patients should be followed closely. Finally, difficulty with anticoagulant therapies can largely be avoided by using standardized protocols and, for difficult to control patients, referral to an anticoagulation clinic.

Special Issues

Because atrial fibrillation represents a diverse group of etiologies and risks, several special issues merit further discussion.

Lone Atrial Fibrillation

By definition, *lone atrial fibrillation* occurs in individuals younger than 60 years who lack evidence of other cardiovascular diseases, including structural heart disease, hypertension, or diabetes. This definition has been refined with the use of echocardiography to confirm the lack of structural heart disease, even including mild mitral valve regurgitation, left atrial enlargement, and LV hypertrophy. The general experience in patients with lone atrial fibrillation is that their risk for stroke is low, anticoagulation is unnecessary for stroke prophylaxis, and further treatment for atrial fibrillation is probably also not necessary. As lone atrial fibrillation has become more clearly defined, this trend holds. Questions that remain include: How often should individuals carrying the diagnosis of lone atrial fibrillation have echocardiography to be certain that structural abnormalities are still absent? Should patients with lone atrial fibrillation be given aspirin? There are no studies that answer these questions. In general, patients with lone atrial fibrillation should be seen at least annually to document that stroke risk factors, including hypertension and diabetes, are still absent, and echocardiography and Holter monitoring should be performed annually to ascertain that there is no evidence of tachycardia-induced cardiomyopathy. The results of studies are mixed on the role of aspirin in patients with lone atrial fibrillation, and there is no consensus for its use. However, given the epidemiologic data supporting the use of low-dose aspirin (81-325 mg per day, as tolerated) in lessening long term risk for stroke and myocardial infarction in patients from age 40 on, low-dose aspirin is often recommended in patients with lone atrial fibrillation.

Nonpharmacologic Approaches to Preventing Atrial Fibrillation

Surgical and percutaneous approaches exist for the treatment of atrial fibrillation (Fig. 37-6; and see Figs. 37-2 to 37-4). In the past, two landmark surgical approaches led the way for the current understanding of the critical role of the pulmonary veins in the initiation and maintenance of atrial fibrillation. The best-studied surgical approaches are the corridor and maze procedures. In the *corridor procedure*, a corridor of atrial tissue is surgically isolated between the sinus and the AV nodes from the rest of the atria, providing chronotropic rate control and demonstrating an increased ability to maintain normal sinus rhythm. In the *maze procedure*, small incisions are made to effectively interrupt reentrant atrial arrhythmias and prevent sustained atrial fibrillation, while providing one pathway from the sinus node to the AV node and simultaneously activating the right and left atria. The concept behind both of these procedures is maintenance of normal sinus rhythm and atrial systole. Although both procedures are effective, they both require open chest surgery, usually require continued anticoagulation, are complicated by the frequent need for permanent pacing, and, hence, are indicated only for a small portion of patients with atrial fibrillation, principally those with a planned cardiac surgical procedure for other reasons (coronary or valvular heart disease). Currently, a modified procedure is employed that isolates the pulmonary veins and adds an ablation line from the veins to the mitral valve annulus.

Radiofrequency catheter ablation of atrial fibrillation isolates foci of early depolarizing atrial cells in the cuffs of the pulmonary veins and has a success rate of 70% to 80% of individuals who are free of atrial fibrillation and off all antiarrhythmic agents. Recurrent atrial fibrillation, risk for thromboembolic episodes, cardiac tamponade, infrequent pulmonary vein stenosis, and rarely an atrioesophageal fistula make the procedure technically challenging. The use of advanced mapping techniques has undoubtedly improved the efficacy of radiofrequency catheter ablation, which is recommended in cases in which pharmacotherapy has failed or is not tolerated and other approaches are unsuitable. Imaging of the left atrium using computed tomographic angiography or magnetic resonance angiography can now be merged with data obtained by electrophysiologic mapping to provide a three-dimensional view that improves the accuracy of ablation. Newer catheter technologies and a better understanding and identification of electrogram targets will allow for an easier and more reliable ablation procedure. In the future, stereotactic technology will likely make atrial fibrillation ablation procedures faster and more effective.

Frequently because of coexistent sinus node dysfunction, tachy-brady syndrome, or excessive bradycardia caused by medications, a permanent pacemaker is indicated. For patients with paroxysmal or persistent atrial fibrillation (see Figs. 37-2 and 37-3), a pacemaker that combines atrial suppression software should be considered. These pacemakers prevent atrial sensing by pacing at rates faster than the underlying atrial rhythm. In clinical trials, these pacemakers reduced atrial fibrillation burden by up to 25%. Dual-chamber pacemakers are superior to ventricular pacemakers in preventing the development of atrial fibrillation.

Rate versus Rhythm Control

On the basis of hemodynamic studies, it has been assumed that patients with normal sinus rhythm fare better than do

Figure 37-6 Surgical Management of Atrial Fibrillation.

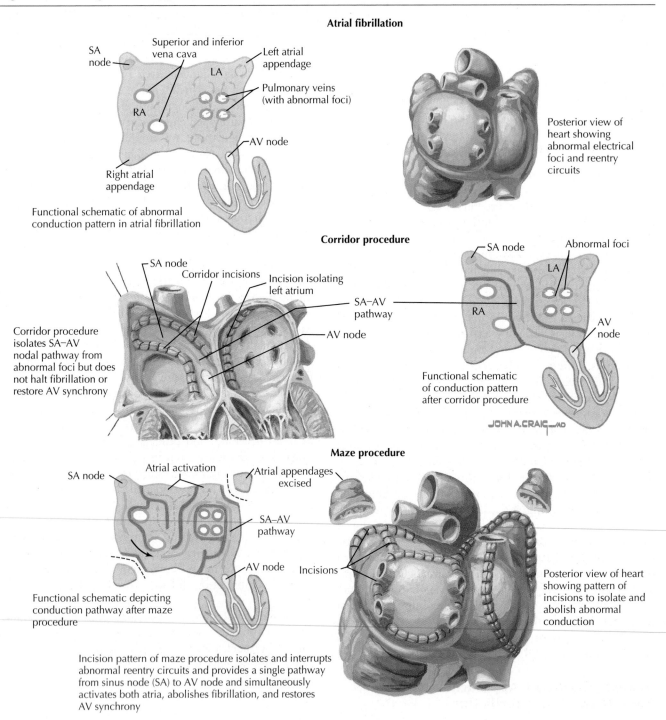

Atrial fibrillation

SA node
Superior and inferior vena cava
Left atrial appendage
LA
Pulmonary veins (with abnormal foci)
RA
AV node
Right atrial appendage

Functional schematic of abnormal conduction pattern in atrial fibrillation

Posterior view of heart showing abnormal electrical foci and reentry circuits

Corridor procedure

SA node
Corridor incisions
Incision isolating left atrium
SA–AV pathway
AV node

Corridor procedure isolates SA–AV nodal pathway from abnormal foci but does not halt fibrillation or restore AV synchrony

SA node
Abnormal foci
LA
RA
AV node

Functional schematic of conduction pattern after corridor procedure

JOHN A. CRAIG—MD

Maze procedure

SA node
Atrial activation
Atrial appendages excised
SA–AV pathway
AV node
Incisions

Functional schematic depicting conduction pathway after maze procedure

Incision pattern of maze procedure isolates and interrupts abnormal reentry circuits and provides a single pathway from sinus node (SA) to AV node and simultaneously activates both atria, abolishes fibrillation, and restores AV synchrony

Posterior view of heart showing pattern of incisions to isolate and abolish abnormal conduction

those with atrial fibrillation but well-controlled ventricular rates. Two studies call into question this conventional wisdom. In both, rhythm control did not provide a survival advantage over rate control in terms of symptoms, risks for stroke, or other morbidities. The groups were highly selected and minimally symptomatic, and there was considerable crossover, such that a statistically significant portion of the rate control group was actually in normal sinus rhythm at the conclusion of the study, creating a significant negative impact on the power of the study. In addition, patients at higher risk for hemodynamic compromise were largely excluded from these studies. Although we await a final answer to the debate on rate versus rhythm control, these studies clearly demonstrate that rhythm control is a more viable option than it was previously considered to be.

Atrioventricular Node Ablation and Permanent Pacing

Consistent with the idea that rhythm control is a useful approach, several studies demonstrated remarkable symptom reduction in patients with atrial fibrillation and refractory rapid ventricular response by making these patients pacemaker dependent. In essence, the patient undergoes radiofrequency catheter ablation of the AV node and implantation of a permanent pacemaker. Depending on the likelihood of restoring normal sinus rhythm, a dual-chamber pacemaker may be used, or in cases where that likelihood is low, a single-chamber ventricular pacemaker is implanted. Studies support the rationale that the rapid ventricular response resulting from atrial fibrillation can be effectively eliminated for selected patients. There may also be a reversal of tachycardia-induced cardiomyopathy, with improvement in LV ejection fraction. Uniformly for patients with permanent atrial fibrillation, QOL scores and exercise tolerance improve and rehospitalization and resource utilization decrease following AV node ablation and permanent pacemaker placement.

Currently, the procedure of "ablate and pace" is reserved for patients with permanent atrial fibrillation, who are not candidates or do not wish to have pulmonary vein isolation performed. Many will already have a single-lead ventricular (VVI) pacemaker. In patients undergoing a de novo procedure, a few small studies have shown that biventricular pacing is superior to right ventricular pacing only.

Congestive Heart Failure

Atrial fibrillation occurs in 15% to 30% of patients with CHF. In these patients, atrial fibrillation can lead to hemodynamic deterioration and rehospitalization, with worsening of symptoms in patients with existing heart failure. The rapid heart rate and loss of atrial contraction can precipitate an exacerbation of CHF in patients with asymptomatic stable LV dysfunction. These changes can be reversed with rate control or reversion to sinus rhythm. It appears that patients with more severe CHF (New York Heart Association class III and IV) and atrial fibrillation have higher all-cause mortality and pump failure deaths. In patients with milder forms of CHF (New York Heart Association class I and II), however, atrial fibrillation was not associated with an increase in mortality or rehospitalization. Class I antiarrhythmic agents are independently associated with an increased mortality in patients with CHF and atrial fibrillation and should be avoided. Amiodarone and dofetilide are safe for patients with CHF. Optimal pharmacologic therapy may play a favorable role in influencing the outcomes for these patients. Even in patients at highest risk with atrial fibrillation and severe CHF, it has not been shown that maintenance of sinus rhythm with antiarrhythmic agents improves survival. Since the emergence of isolation of the pulmonary veins even for patients with permanent atrial fibrillation of several years' duration, this

procedure has been shown to improve QOL, LV ejection fraction, and symptoms.

Implantable Atrial Defibrillation

Between 20% and 30% of patients have coexisting atrial fibrillation at the time of placement of an implantable cardioverter-defibrillator (ICD). Seventeen months after placement of an ICD, up to 45% of patients have atrial fibrillation. The latest ICDs also incorporate atrial conversion therapy, which includes atrial overdrive antitachycardia pacing, atrial high-frequency burst pacing, and atrial defibrillation. These devices are safe and efficacious. Therefore, an ICD with atrial therapies should be considered for patients with atrial fibrillation or the potential to develop atrial fibrillation.

Coronary Artery Bypass Surgery

Atrial fibrillation is frequently seen in patients after coronary artery bypass graft (CABG) surgery. Up to 40% of patients are estimated to develop atrial fibrillation, usually beginning after postoperative day 1 and lengthening the hospital stay. Older patients and those who have β-blockers withdrawn before surgery are more likely to develop atrial fibrillation. Use of β-blockers or amiodarone preoperatively decreases the frequency of postoperative atrial fibrillation. Interestingly, atrial fibrillation is a transient phenomenon; most patients are in sinus rhythm when discharged. Only a minority, less than 5%, are in atrial fibrillation 30 days after surgery.

Ablation has been performed during CABG in patients undergoing mitral valve surgery. The four pulmonary veins are isolated with either radiofrequency ablation or cryoablation. In some circumstances, the ablation line is extended to the mitral valve annulus, with reportedly fewer episodes of recurrence of atrial fibrillation. Early studies showing sinus rhythm maintenance have been encouraging, even in patients with permanent atrial fibrillation before surgery.

Postmortem studies have identified the left atrial appendage as the most likely source for the development of thrombus in patients with atrial fibrillation. This has been confirmed in a large series of patients who underwent transesophageal echocardiogram before cardioversion. Percutaneous approaches have been developed that aim to isolate the left atrial appendage from the left atrium in an attempt to prevent the development of thrombus in patients who cannot take warfarin. During CABG or valve surgery, many surgeons either remove the appendage or oversuture the orifice of the appendage, thereby preventing flow and stasis in the appendage.

Hypertension

Two recent antihypertensive studies, Losartan Intervention for End Point Reduction in Hypertension (LIFE) and

Valsartan Antihypertensive Long-term Use Evaluation (VALUE), have shown prospective observational data suggesting a significant decrease in the prevalence of atrial fibrillation in patients treated with the angiotensin receptor blockers (ARBs) losartan and valsartan. These agents were compared with atenolol in the LIFE study and amlodipine in the VALUE study. In both studies, there was either a similar or slightly better control of blood pressure with atenolol and amlodipine. However, despite adequate blood pressure control, significantly fewer patients taking ARBs developed atrial fibrillation. Several possible explanations may account for these observations. The antifibrotic and anti-inflammatory effects associated with ARBs, as well as a more favorable effect on LV remodeling, may facilitate a reverse remodeling of the left atrium, thereby decreasing the propensity to develop atrial fibrillation. This hypothesis is being tested prospectively in the Atrial Fibrillation Clopidogrel Trial with Irbesartran for Prevention of Vascular Events (ACTIVE) irbesartan trial.

Future Directions

Advances in the treatment of atrial fibrillation hold promise. Newer antifibrillatory agents are in development, as are anticoagulants that will be easier to administer and safer than warfarin. Although the oral thrombin inhibitor ximelagatran was shown to be comparable to warfarin in anticoagulant efficacy, there was an unexplained and unexpected elevation in liver function tests. Newer oral thrombin inhibitors are currently being studied. Exciting nonpharmacologic therapies are undergoing testing and early clinical use, including implantable atrial defibrillators and pacemakers (with the rationale that early conversion of atrial fibrillation to normal sinus rhythm facilitates maintenance of normal sinus rhythm), newer mapping, and more sophisticated percutaneous approaches. Eventually, it may be possible to cure atrial fibrillation, much as radiofrequency catheter ablation can now cure supraventricular tachycardias in many and maintain normal sinus rhythm in most. Percutaneous left atrial appendage transcatheter occlusion devices, which are easier to implant, are being evaluated in clinical trials at present. This is an attractive strategy for patients who cannot or will not take warfarin or for patients who have embolic episodes while taking warfarin. Early clinical data suggest that patients with closure devices have lower than expected CVA/TIA rates based on their Congestive heart failure, Hypertension, Age, Diabetes (CHAD) score risk estimates. Randomized data comparing appendage closure devices with warfarin treatment with an INR of 2 to 3 in patients with a high risk for thromboembolism are awaited.

Additional Resources

Fuster V, Ryden LE, Cannom DS, et al: ACC/AHA/ESC 2006 guidelines for the management of patients with atrial fibrillation: A report of the American College of Cardiology/American Heart Association Task Force on practice guidelines and the European Society of Cardiology Committee for Practice Guidelines (Writing Committee to Revise the 2001 guidelines for the management of patients with atrial fibrillation). Developed in collaboration with the European Heart Rhythm Association and the Heart Rhythm Society. Europace 8(9):651-745, 2006.

This paper is a collaborative effort from the ACC, AHA, and ESC to update 2001 guidelines for the diagnosis and management of AF.

EVIDENCE

1. Hsu LF, Jais P, Sanders P, et al: Catheter ablation for atrial fibrillation in congestive heart failure. N Engl J Med 351(23):2373-2383, 2004.

   This study was designed to evaluate whether catheter ablation for atrial fibrillation with restoration of sinus rhythm improves cardiac function, symptoms, exercise capacity and quality of life in patients with CHF. Restoration and maintenance of sinus rhythm by catheter ablation without the use of drugs was effective and improved objective findings of cardiac function.

2. Klein AL, Grimm RA, Murray RD, et al: Use of transesophageal echocardiography to guide cardioversion in patients with atrial fibrillation. N Engl J Med 344(19):1411-1420, 2001.

   A study of 1222 patients tested the hypothesis that cardioversion can be performed safely after only a short period of anticoagulation in patients in whom transesophageal echocardiography reveals no left atrial thrombus. This study found that transesophageal echocardiography-guided management of atrial fibrillation is a feasible option when planning elective cardioversion for the AF patient.

3. Ostermayer SH, Reisman M, Kramer PH, et al: Percutaneous left atrial appendage transcatheter occlusion (PLAATO system) to prevent stroke in high-risk patients with non-rheumatic atrial fibrillation: Results from the international multi-center feasibility trials. J Am Coll Cardiol 46(1):9-14, 2005.

   This article presents the International Multi-Center Feasibility Trials reports on the viability of percutaneous left atrial appendage (LAA) occlusion using the PLAATO system. This study concluded that closing the LAA using the PLAATO system is practical, can be performed with acceptable risk, and should be considered an alternative in patients with AF when long-term anticoagulation treatment is inadvisable.

4. Singer DE, Albers GW, Dalen JE, et al: Antithrombotic therapy in atrial fibrillation: The Seventh ACCP Conference on Antithrombotic and Thrombolytic Therapy. Chest 126(3 Suppl):429S-456S, 2004.

   In this report of the Seventh ACCP Conference on Antithrombotic and Thrombolytic Therapy, grade 1 and 2 recommendations are made for the use of antithrombotic therapy in AF.

5. Wachtell K, Lehto M, Gerdts E, et al: Angiotensin II receptor blockade reduces new-onset atrial fibrillation and subsequent stroke compared to atenolol: The Losartan Intervention for End Point Reduction in Hypertension (LIFE) study. J Am Coll Cardiol 45(5):712-719, 2005.

   The Losartan Intervention for End Point Reduction in Hypertension (LIFE) study compared the effects of losartan and atenolol on new-onset AF. This study concluded that losartan-based antihypertensive therapy (as compared with atenolol-based antihypertensive therapy) significantly reduced new-onset AF and associated stroke.

6. Wyse DG, Waldo AL, DiMarco JP, et al: A comparison of rate control and rhythm control in patients with atrial fibrillation. N Engl J Med 347(23):1825-1833, 2002.

   This study compared the two approaches, rate and rhythm control, in the management of AF. There was no significant difference in survival between the two therapies. Patients randomized to rate control did have a lower risk for adverse drug effects.

William E. Sanders, Jr. ▪ Lukas Jantac

Syncope

Introduction

Derived from the Greek word *synkoptein* meaning "to cut short," syncope was reportedly first described by Hippocrates and is defined as the sudden and transient loss of consciousness and postural tone. Syncope results from cerebral hypoperfusion for 10 or more seconds. The event may be benign or may herald impending sudden death. Even when a benign cause is identified, recurrent syncopal episodes can result in injury and elicit significant patient anxiety. The Framingham Heart Study found that 11% of subjects followed for an average of more than 17 years reported a syncopal episode. Population studies now suggest that about one third of individuals experience a syncopal episode in the course of their lifetime. The incidence increases with age, presenting most commonly in those older than 70 years. In the nonelderly population, 75% of syncope cases occur as isolated events and generally have a benign prognosis. Although men are more likely to experience syncope secondary to a cardiac cause, the overall incidence is equal in men and women. Syncope currently accounts for 3.5% of all emergency room visits and for 1% to 6% of all hospital admissions. The manifestations and consequences of this disorder depend simultaneously on the acute hemodynamics and the underlying cardiac substrate.

Etiology and Pathogenesis

Although the causes of loss of consciousness are numerous, all result in a sudden decrease or brief cessation of cerebral blood flow (Box 38-1). Neurally mediated syncope, including neurocardiogenic and situational types, is most common and is the underlying pathogenesis of more than half of documented cases. A cardiac cause is identified in 18% of patients. Despite the use of modern diagnostic techniques, the etiology remains unexplained in 34% of cases. The most common comorbidity and risk factor associated with this disorder is preexisting cardiovascular disease. Studies have shown that the age-adjusted incidence is almost double in those with cardiovascular disease. Other significant risk factors include systemic hypertension, history of stroke, diabetes mellitus, and excessive use of alcohol. Traditionally, syncope has been categorized into three groups: cardiac, noncardiac, and unknown.

Cardiac Syncope

The rate of sudden cardiac death as well as all cause mortality is significantly higher in patients with syncope and preexisting cardiovascular disease. Cardiovascular causes of syncope are best divided into those caused by arrhythmias (bradycardia and tachycardia) and those caused by structural heart disease.

Arrhythmia

Arrhythmia is the most common cardiogenic cause. In patients with syncope and a history of coronary artery disease, the etiology is ventricular tachycardia unless proven otherwise. Moreover, arrhythmias are the likely cause of most cases of syncope that remain unexplained after a complete diagnostic workup. Associated arrhythmias include bradycardia, ventricular tachycardia, and rarely, supraventricular tachycardia. Typically, bradyarrhythmias are better tolerated than tachyarrhythmias; however, both are equally likely to cause syncope if the onset is abrupt. In addition to heart rate, cerebral blood flow is ultimately influenced by other factors, including ventricular contractile function, body position, and baroreceptor sensitivity.

Structural Heart Disease (Nonarrhythmic)

Reduced cerebral perfusion causing syncope may also occur secondary to transient mechanical obstruction of blood flow. This is observed most frequently in patients

---

Box 38-1 Differential Diagnosis

Cardiac
Tachyarrhythmia
Bradyarrhythmia
Cardiogenic shock
Myocardial infarction
Pericardial tamponade
Hypertrophic cardiomyopathy
Aortic stenosis
Pulmonic stenosis
Congenital heart disease
Atrial myxoma
Prosthetic valve thrombosis

Noncardiac
Vasovagal
Autonomic dysfunction
Hypovolemia or anemia
Carotid hypersensitivity
Drug-induced
Seizure
Hypoxia
Hyperventilation
Hypoglycemia
Adrenal insufficiency
Anxiety
Pulmonary embolism
Primary pulmonary hypertension
Hypertensive encephalopathy
Atherosclerotic disease of carotid or cerebral vessels
Subclavian steal

---

with hypertrophic cardiomyopathy (HCM) and aortic stenosis when outflow from the heart is temporarily reduced or blocked secondary to adverse loading conditions that may occur during tachycardia or hypovolemia. Less commonly, loss of consciousness results from pulmonary embolism, intracardiac tumors, idiopathic pulmonary hypertension, dissecting aortic aneurysm, or cardiac tamponade.

Noncardiac

Noncardiovascular syncopal events are the most common and include neurocardiogenic, orthostatic hypotension, carotid hypersensitivity, cerebrovascular disease, and psychiatric disorders (Box 38-1). Unlike patients with events secondary to a cardiovascular cause, those with noncardiac causes usually have a benign prognosis.

Neurocardiogenic (Vasovagal)

Neurocardiogenic (vasovagal) episodes are the most prevalent of the group of reflex syncopes and are frequently referred to as neurally mediated events. Neurocardiac syncope is characterized by a sudden failure of the autonomic nervous system to sustain adequate blood pressure or heart rate. This pathogenesis accounts for about 20%

of all cases and is slightly more common in women than men. "Situational" syncope may occur after urination, defecation, swallowing, or coughing. Patients presenting with neurocardiogenic syncope are typically young and report a characteristic prodrome consisting of lightheadedness, diaphoresis, and nausea. Episodes may be preceded by long periods of upright posture, noxious emotional or physical stimuli, venipuncture, fear of injury, a warm environment, or vigorous exercise.

Orthostatic Hypotension

Orthostatic hypotension is identified as the cause of syncope in as many as 10% of patients. It is defined as a postural decrease in systolic blood pressure greater than 20 mm Hg or in diastolic blood pressure greater than 10 mm Hg. Symptoms such as lightheadedness or loss of postural tone upon rising from a supine to a sitting or standing position are indicative of orthostatic hypotension. Predisposing factors include reduced intravascular volume, autonomic dysfunction, drugs (primarily vasodilators, diuretics, and tricyclics), and other conditions that impair appropriate vasoconstriction, including significant alcohol use.

Carotid Hypersensitivity and Other Neural Causes

Carotid hypersensitivity is relatively rare and is classified as "situational;" however, recent reports suggest that up to 30% of the unexplained syncopal events in the elderly are due to carotid sinus hypersensitivity. Patients may present with complaints of syncope during shaving or just before crossing a street. Any activity that requires markedly turning one's head to either side can induce a carotid hypersensitive reflex and subsequent loss of consciousness in affected individuals. This is more common in the elderly but should be considered even in younger patients. Carotid hypersensitivity is diagnosed by application of pressure to the carotid sinus and the subsequent observation of marked bradycardia or sinus pauses longer than 3 seconds with associated reproduction of the patient's presenting symptoms.

Cerebrovascular disease rarely results in loss of consciousness because redundant cerebral perfusion usually prevents sudden and significant reduction in blood flow. However, severe multivessel cerebral atherosclerosis and hypoperfusion of the posterior fossa may produce syncope as well as neurologic deficits. Seizures are the primary cause of about 10% of all syncopal events, and this diagnosis may be difficult to establish. An electroencephalogram (EEG) is indicated only in a select group of patients in whom suspicion is high for a neurologic cause.

Unknown Origin

Despite the use of detailed history, physical examination, laboratory work, and advanced diagnostic equipment,

---

Box 38-2   Historical Clues to the Etiology of Syncopal Events

1. Time of occurrence
2. Activity at the time of event
   - Position changes
   - Micturition
   - Defecation
   - Cough
3. Current medications
   - Prescription or over-the-counter
   - Recent changes in doses or medications
4. Alcohol or illicit drug use
5. Concurrent illness
   - Fever
   - Nausea and vomiting
   - Diarrhea
   - Trauma
   - Anemia
6. Family history
   - Arrhythmia
   - Sudden death
7. Episode characteristics
   - Duration
   - Tonic-clonic activity
   - State of consciousness immediately following episode
   - Diaphoresis, pallor, gastrointestinal distress, chest pain, palpitations
   - Inciting visual stimuli (blood, etc.)

---

about one third of syncopal cases are categorized as being of unknown origin.

Clinical Presentation

The reported symptoms and situation associated with an event provide significant clues to the underlying cause (Box 38-2). This history is most important in the ultimate determination of the appropriate diagnosis. Most patients with a benign cause have only a single episode or several episodes that are widely separated over time. Those with syncope secondary to a cardiac cause typically have recurrent events and are more likely to be older and have preexisting cardiac disease.

Symptoms

Patients may present with a wide variety of symptoms. Those with a cardiac cause may complain of preceding chest discomfort or palpitations. Features associated with neurocardiogenic syncope include a prodrome of lightheadedness, nausea, warmth, and diaphoresis. Syncope without preexisting symptoms, especially in the supine position, is usually secondary to bradyarrhythmia or tachyarrhythmia, particularly in patients with known structural heart disease. Situational syncope occurring with coughing, eating, drinking, urinating, or defecating is typically associated with high vagal tone. If loss of conscious-

ness occurs in patients following sudden change in body position, for example, standing up following prolonged sitting, orthostatic hypotension is suspected.

Exertional syncope in older patients may be secondary to ventricular tachycardia and obstructive causes, such as HCM or aortic stenosis. In young patients with exertional syncope, the cause is usually neurocardiogenic; however, long QT syndrome or HCM may also be present in this population. The recovery from an episode may also be helpful in making the correct diagnosis. Persistent diaphoresis and nausea following an event strongly suggests a neurocardiogenic cause rather than a transient arrhythmia, from which recovery is usually fast and complete.

Physical Examination

Careful physical examination is valuable in every syncopal patient, with particular attention given to vital signs and cardiovascular exam. In all patients, blood pressure measurements in the supine, sitting, and standing position are essential to document orthostatic hypotension, and associated symptoms of cerebral hypoperfusion, including lightheadedness, provide further evidence of this diagnosis. The cardiovascular exam should include careful cardiac auscultation and palpation of the peripheral pulses. Auscultation may reveal the characteristic systolic murmur of aortic stenosis or HCM. The murmur of HCM increases after the performance of Valsalva strain or after the patient assumes an upright position. Pulmonary hypertension is suggested by a loud second heart sound. When the history is suspicious for carotid sinus hypersensitivity, carotid sinus massage is indicated, but only with cardiac monitoring and when resuscitative equipment is immediately available. In addition, the examiner should exclude a carotid bruit. Carotid sinus pressure is applied for 3 to 4 seconds during simultaneous recording of the electrocardiogram.

Diagnostic Approach

The cause of a syncopal event can often be elucidated by taking a careful clinical history, performing a thorough physical examination, and reviewing basic laboratory tests as well as an electrocardiogram (ECG). A previous history of heart disease has a high sensitivity for an arrhythmic or cardiac cause of syncope. Laboratory testing, including chemistry profile, complete blood count, and cardiac-specific biomarkers, is helpful in selected patients (Fig. 38-1).

Cardiac Tests

Heart Rhythm Monitoring

ECGs in patients with a cardiac cause of syncope may reveal sinus bradycardia, heart block, prolonged QT

Figure 38-1 Diagnostic Tests Commonly Used to Evaluate a Syncope Patient.

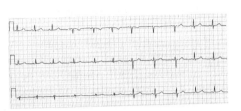

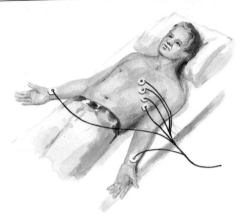

Step 1 ECG

All patients with syncope should undergo electrocardiography. If ECG is abnormal, confirmatory testing and appropriate therapy should be instituted

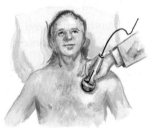

Step 3 Tilt Table Testing

Should be considered if steps 1 and 2 are negative

Step 2 Echocardiography

In most patients without a diagnosis, a structural evaluation with echocardiograph is required

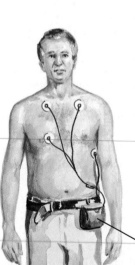

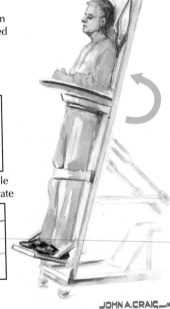

Positive neurocardiogenic tilt-table test shows drop in BP and heart rate

Normal tilt-table test shows maintenance of normal BP and heart rate

Holter monitor

JOHN A. CRAIG—AD
with
D. Mascaro

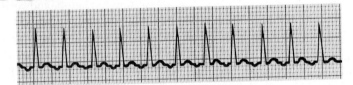

Step 4 Ambulatory Monitoring

Ambulatory monitoring is recommended for patients with negative evaluation. Duration of monitoring is dependent on frequency of episodes. For daily symptoms, 48-hour monitor is adequate

interval, evidence of pre-excitation (Wolfe-Parkinson-White syndrome), prior myocardial infarction, hypertrophy, or Brugada's syndrome. A normal ECG does not exclude a cardiac cause. In patients with frequent (daily) symptoms, 24- to 48-hour ambulatory Holter monitoring may be used for further evaluation. This technique is only diagnostic in 1% to 5% of persons with a history of syncope who experience typical symptoms during the time of the recording. Event or loop recorders are slightly more useful and may be worn for periods of several months; however, they typically require the patient to trigger the recording before the syncopal event, making their utility less practical. Automatic detection algorithms may aid in capturing arrhythmic data, but without the patient triggering the device, the findings may not be readily linked to symptoms. Lastly, an implantable loop recorder warrants consideration in patients who experience recurrent syncope but with a low frequency of events. This device is surgically implanted and automatically stores arrhythmic events according to programmed criteria.

Complementary Cardiac Tests

Transthoracic echocardiograms rarely reveal unsuspected abnormalities, but do provide confirmation of structural heart disease, including prior myocardial infarction, aortic stenosis, and HCM, as well as an assessment of systolic and diastolic function. Such findings alone do not necessarily establish the cause of syncope, and performance of an echocardiogram should not be routine. Exercise testing is useful in patients who experience exercise-induced syncope and in individuals with suspected outflow tract obstruction. In patients who are suspected to have neurocardiogenic syncope based on a suspicious history and the absence of structural heart disease on physical examination, head-up tilt-table testing is particularly valuable in confirming the diagnosis, especially if the exact prodrome and symptoms are reproduced. The addition of isoproterenol or nitroglycerin may be required to elicit a positive response. Signal-averaged ECG has little utility in evaluation of syncope because of its very low positive predictive value. Assessment of T-wave alternans has shown recent promise as a predictor of further arrhythmic events; however, larger studies are required to define its role in this population, and currently the technology is not widely available. The utility of electrophysiologic studies depends on the presence or absence of structural heart disease. In patients with heart disease, about 21% have inducible ventricular tachycardia at electrophysiology study (EPS). In patients with a normal heart, EPS provides minimal useful data.

Neurologic Tests

Imaging of the brain using computed tomography or magnetic resonance imaging is frequently ordered but offers relatively little new information to that obtained by history and physical examination. The use of neurologic testing including EEG and carotid Doppler studies seldom reveals a cause and is generally not recommended.

Management and Therapy

Hospitalization is usually indicated for any case of syncope in which a cardiac source is highly suspected. This is particularly true in elderly patients who have a cardiac cause most frequently and for whom recurrent symptoms can have devastating consequences. Once appropriate testing is performed, however, repeat hospitalizations are usually not enlightening. Correcting any underlying metabolic disturbance is imperative and must be done before any consideration of definitive therapy. This may include removing or substituting medications that may be contributing to the symptoms. The treatment of syncope is then targeted at the suspected cause in the hope of preventing recurrent symptoms and sudden death.

Cardiac: Optimum Treatment

Arrhythmic

Syncope in a patient with a history of coronary artery disease warrants immediate evaluation because it is almost always secondary to ventricular arrhythmia. If sustained ventricular tachycardia is documented on ECG or telemetry without significant coexisting metabolic disturbance, treatment with an implantable cardioverter-defibrillator (ICD) is indicated. If ventricular tachycardia is suspected but not documented, electrophysiologic evaluation may be necessary, and treatment is guided accordingly. Radiofrequency ablation of the arrhythmic focus may be a treatment option but, in the setting of ventricular arrhythmias, is performed only when an ICD is already in place. Pharmacologic therapy alone is not an option when treating malignant ventricular tachycardia or ventricular fibrillation.

Syncope secondary to tachyarrhythmia in patients without coronary artery disease or dilated cardiomyopathy is rare but may be seen in congenital long QT syndrome, Brugada's syndrome, arrhythmogenic right ventricular dysplasia, and catecholaminergic polymorphic ventricular tachycardia. Specific therapy of these particular disorders is beyond the scope of this chapter but is targeted toward preventing symptoms and sudden cardiac death and typically requires ICD placement. Syncope may also occur with rapid atrial fibrillation associated with Wolff-Parkinson-White syndrome. In that instance, radiofrequency catheter ablation of the accessory pathway is curative. Radiofrequency ablation is also the treatment of choice for all supraventricular tachyarrhythmias, particularly those eliciting recurrent symptoms. Both ischemic and nonischemic cardiomyopathy patients with ejection fractions of less than 35% have been shown to have mortality benefit when an ICD is implanted.

In patients with syncope and documented bradycardia secondary to conduction system abnormality, permanent pacemaker placement is the definitive therapy. The complete indications for permanent pacemaker and ICD placement are summarized in recent American College of Cardiology/American Heart Association guidelines.

Structural Heart Disease (Nonarrhythmic)

The two most common structural heart conditions causing obstruction to cerebral blood flow and subsequent syncope are aortic stenosis and HCM. In severe aortic stenosis, aortic valve replacement will alleviate symptoms, including syncope, and will prolong survival. The dynamic outflow obstruction observed in HCM may be treated pharmacologically or surgically. β-blockers, as well as calcium channel blockers, may reduce the outflow tract gradient. Surgical myomectomy and alcohol septal ablation are beneficial in relief of symptoms. Large studies have proven that ventricular pacing is an inadequate treatment for HCM, and it is not recommended.

Noncardiac: Optimum Treatment

Neurocardiogenic (Vasovagal)

Syncope secondary to a neurocardiogenic etiology is common, and treatment options are individualized and often targeted toward specific predisposing environmental exposures. First, patients are advised to avoid trigger situations. Second, because a typical prodrome is usually present, patients are instructed to lie in the supine position with elevated lower extremities if they experience their usual warning symptoms. Other treatment options include lower extremity support stockings and liberal salt intake to expand intravascular volume. Medical therapies including β-blockers, midodrine, fludrocortisone, and selective serotonin reuptake inhibitors have been prescribed, but there are limited data from randomized controlled trials to support their use. Moreover, no drug has been approved by the U.S. Food and Drug Administration for this indication. Studies evaluating implantation of dual-chamber pacemakers in this population have reported no significant reduction in the frequency of syncopal events in the pacemaker-treated groups.

Orthostatic Hypotension

Assessing volume status and appropriately treating hypovolemia with normal saline or other colloid is essential. Appropriate therapy is targeted toward avoiding medications that block sympathetic tone, including β-blockers and some commonly used antidepressants. Wearing lower extremity compression stockings to reduce venous pooling

and rising slowly from a seated position are simple measures that often provide some benefit. Medical therapies employed for orthostatic hypotension resistant to volume expansion have included the use of mineralocorticoids such as fludrocortisone as well as α₁-adrenergic agonists such as midodrine.

Carotid Sinus Hypersensitivity

Therapy for syncope secondary to carotid sinus hypersensitivity is dual-chamber pacemaker placement, although pacing does not always eliminate syncope, especially if the primary underlying mechanism is vasodepression (loss of vascular tone) without cardioinhibition (bradycardia). Avoiding situations in which pressure is placed on the carotid sinus may be helpful. This includes prohibiting extensive movement of the neck and not wearing constricting neckwear, including jewelry or turtleneck sweaters.

Unknown Etiology

No specific therapy is indicated in young patients with unexplained syncope, particularly following the initial hospitalization with negative diagnostic evaluation. Patients with syncope and a history of severe cardiomyopathy of ischemic or nonischemic cause have a 45% 1-year risk of sudden cardiac death. In this population, the use of ICDs has been shown to improve survival.

Avoiding Treatment Errors

A careful clinical history and a thorough physical exam are essential to avoid misdiagnosis in cases of syncope. A previous history of heart disease is extremely sensitive for an arrhythmic or cardiac cause. Judicious selection of ancillary tests should reveal a cause for most of these cases.

Future Directions

Determining the correct cause of syncope may prove difficult with more than one third of patients labeled as having "syncope of unknown etiology" after thorough diagnostic evaluation. It is imperative that the physician use appropriate studies that are directed by a careful clinical history and physical examination. The future development of new, highly sophisticated diagnostic techniques is unlikely to overshadow the importance of obtaining accurate bedside clinical information.

Additional Resource

Heart Rhythm Society. Available at: http://www.hrspatients.org. Accessed October 8, 2007.

The Heart Rhythm Society has an extensive online "Patient and Public Information Center" that provides a guide for the current methods of diagnosis and treatment of cardiac rhythm disorders.

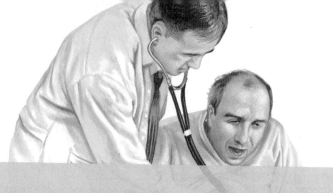

Disorders of Endocrinology and Metabolism

EVIDENCE

1. Gregoratos G, Abrams J, Epstein AE, et al: ACC/AHA/NASPE 2002 Guideline Update for Implantation of Cardiac Pacemakers and Antiarrhythmia Devices—summary article: A report of the American College of Cardiology/American Heart Association Task Force on Practice Guidelines (ACC/AHA/NASPE Committee to Update the 1998 Pacemaker Guidelines). J Am Coll Cardiol 40(9):1703-1719, 2002.

This paper presents guidelines for implantation of devices, pacemakers and defibrillators, used in the treatment of patients with arrhythmic disorders and syncope. The text provides evaluation of data used to support the recommendations.

2. Grubb BP: Clinical practice: Neurocardiogenic syncope. N Engl J Med 352(10):1004-1110, 2005.

The author presents a case review and comprehensive analysis of tests employed to evaluate syncope patients with a presumed neurocardiogenic etiology.

3. Grubb BP: Neurocardiogenic syncope and related disorders of orthostatic intolerance. Circulation 111(22):2997-3006, 2005.

The author details the role of the autonomic nervous system in patients who manifest syncope.

4. Grubb BP, Jorge Sdo C: A review of the classification, diagnosis, and management of autonomic dysfunction syndromes associated with orthostatic intolerance. Arq Bras Cardiol 74(6):537-552, 2000.

The authors propose a classification for autonomic disorders and note the overlap between syndromes.

5. Kapoor WN: Syncope. N Engl J Med 343(25):1856-1862, 2000.

This concise review of all causes of syncope describes clinical features suggestive of specific diagnoses.

6. Shen WK, Decker WW, Smars PA, et al: Syncope evaluation in the emergency department study (SEEDS): A multidisciplinary approach to syncope management. Circulation 110(24):3636-3645, 2004.

This single-center randomized trial demonstrates the value of a designated syncope unit in improving diagnostic yield in the emergency department.

7. Soteriades ES, Evans JC, Larson MG, et al: Incidence and prognosis of syncope. N Engl J Med 347(12):878-885, 2002.

This article discusses the epidemiology and prognosis of syncope among women and men participating in the Framingham Heart Study.

8. Strickberger SA, Benson DW, Biaggioni I, et al: AHA/ACCF scientific statement on the evaluation of syncope. From the American Heart Association Councils on Clinical Cardiology, Cardiovascular Nursing, Cardiovascular Disease in the Young, and Stroke, and the Quality of Care and Outcomes Research Interdisciplinary Working Group; and the American College of Cardiology Foundation in Collaboration with the Heart Rhythm Society. J Am Coll Cardiol 47(2):473-484, 2006.

A consensus statement, which outlines the causes, diagnostic evaluation, and treatment of syncope patients, is presented in this article.

John B. Buse

Diabetes and Prediabetes: Diagnosis and Treatment

Introduction

Diabetes mellitus (DM) affects about 21 million people in the United States and hundreds of millions of people worldwide. Prediabetes, abnormally high glucose levels that are insufficient to meet the diagnostic criteria of diabetes, affects more than 50 million people in the United States. Current estimates for those born in the year 2000 are that one in three will develop diabetes and more than one in two will have prediabetes in their lifetime. This epidemic of DM is driven by increasing obesity and progressively sedentary lifestyles.

DM is a major cause of morbidity and mortality. Premature vascular disease is the eventual cause of death in more than two thirds of people with DM, leading to a loss of more than 10 years of life in those diagnosed at age 40 years. The costs involved in the treatment of people with DM are staggering, accounting by some estimates for one sixth of all health care expenditures in the United States.

We are in the midst of multiple revolutions in DM management. Evidence that lifestyle interventions and patient self-management education are effective has driven improved third-party coverage for these services. Therapeutic targets have been established on the basis of outcomes trials not only for glycemia but also for common comorbidities—hypertension and dyslipidemia. There are new developments in glucose monitoring technology. Multiple new classes of pharmacologic agents are available to treat DM. Together, these advances create the possibility that the early death and disability associated with DM can be avoided.

Etiology and Pathogenesis

Type 1 DM (previously known as insulin-dependent DM) accounts for about 5% to 10% of all cases of diabetes. It can occur at any age but is more common among children and young adults. It is characterized by insulin deficiency generally resulting from autoimmune destruction of insulin-secreting β cells within the pancreatic islets of Langerhans. Other autoimmune endocrine diseases, such as hypothyroidism, ovarian failure, adrenal insufficiency, pernicious anemia, autoimmune hepatitis, and vitiligo, often coexist in patients with type 1 DM. Although classically considered a disease of children, adolescents, and young adults, it is estimated that up to 10% of adults with new-onset DM have a slowly evolving form of type 1 DM. Clinically, these adult-onset patients with type 1 diabetes are essentially indistinguishable from patients with type 2 diabetes except that they tend to be less overweight, to present with weight loss, and to respond poorly to oral antihyperglycemic agents.

The risk for DM is genetically determined and involves several genetic loci, the most important of these being genes within the human leukocyte antigen (HLA) system. However, only 10% of people with type 1 DM exhibit a family history. The risk for future DM in the first-degree relative of a patient with type 1 DM is 2% to 5%. Islet cell antibodies, antibodies to glutamic acid decarboxylase (GAD), antibodies to insulin, and other autoantibodies are often present at diagnosis. There are likely environmental triggers to the development of this autoimmune process, although these are poorly understood.

Type 2 DM (previously known as noninsulin-dependent DM) generally occurs in adulthood, although it can develop at any age. Currently, almost half of children with new-onset diabetes now have type 2 diabetes. Most patients with type 2 DM have a first-degree relative with DM, and most are overweight, generally with a central pattern of obesity. Type 2 DM is more common in all other ethnic groups than in whites of European extraction and tends to occur at an earlier age in these high-risk populations as well as in women. From recent prospective studies, we understand that type 2 DM develops as the result of progressive loss of insulin secretory capacity on the background of insulin resistance. Insulin resistance is defined as an inadequate response of metabolic processes to physiologic insulin concentrations.

A number of clinical phenotypes are associated with insulin resistance and are sometimes discussed together as the metabolic (or dysmetabolic) syndrome. These features include obesity with a central pattern of weight distribution, dyslipidemia, hyperglycemia, hypertension, hypercoagulability, endothelial dysfunction, and accelerated atherosclerosis. The dyslipidemia is characterized by increased triglycerides and decreased high-density lipoprotein (HDL) cholesterol. Although the absolute concentration of low-density lipoprotein (LDL) cholesterol is the same as the population average, the LDL particles are generally small, dense, more numerous, and thus more atherogenic. The pathophysiology of these associations is unknown. Nevertheless, a substantial portion of the increased cardiovascular morbidity in the setting of type 2 DM is likely related to this syndrome and its associated features.

Clinical Presentation

In type 1 DM, clinical deterioration can be quite rapid, and patients can transition from being completely asymptomatic to having rampant polyuria, polydipsia, and polyphagia with weight loss and blurred vision over a matter of days to weeks. Affected individuals generally have fairly widely fluctuating blood sugars. Diabetic ketoacidosis can occur when one or more insulin doses are missed or with physiologic stress. Hypoglycemia is quite common as a complication of insulin therapy in type 1 diabetes.

In type 2 DM, patients may be completely asymptomatic for years. Some present with classic symptoms of microvascular or macrovascular complications. More often, subtle symptoms may be present for years, including fatigue, recurrent cutaneous infections, and intermittent nocturia. If hyperglycemia is allowed to progress unchecked, life-threatening problems, such as diabetic ketoacidosis or hyperosmolar states, can develop.

Differential Diagnosis

Generally, DM is a primary disorder; however, it is worth noting the much less common secondary causes. Among these, pancreatic disorders are the most common, including chronic pancreatitis, cystic fibrosis, and pancreatic cancer. Although for years it was considered that these disorders were the result of destruction of most functioning β cells, the pathophysiology of DM in these cases is more complex, probably involving ill-defined humoral factors. There are iatrogenic causes such as steroid therapy and syndromes associated with hormonal overproduction of glucocorticoids, growth hormone, glucagon, and catecholamines.

Diagnostic Approach

About one third of cases of DM in the United States are undiagnosed. In some studies, 20% to 50% of people with DM have one or more complications of the disease at the time that a diagnosis is made. Estimates suggest that the diagnosis of DM could be made 7 to 12 years earlier with screening than by waiting for symptoms to develop.

Current recommendations suggest screening for DM by measuring a fasting plasma glucose (FPG) starting at age 45 years, with repeat screening every 3 years. Screening should start at an earlier age and be repeated at shorter intervals, particularly in people who are overweight (body mass index [BMI] ≥25 kg/m²) with one or more risk factors (beyond age and weight as above):

- A family history of DM in a first-degree relative
- Belonging to a high-risk ethnic group (essentially all ethnicities except whites of western European extraction)
- Hypertension
- Dyslipidemia (high triglycerides or low HDL)
- Women with a history of gestational diabetes, birth of a child greater than 9 pounds, or ovarian hyperandrogenism
- Prior abnormal fasting glucose or glucose tolerance test
- Acanthosis nigricans
- Known vascular disease

Fasting for the purpose of diabetes screening is defined as nothing by mouth except water for at least 8 hours.

Glucose tolerance testing provides greater sensitivity than FPG but at the expense of greater burden and somewhat less reproducibility. To properly perform an oral glucose tolerance test (OGTT), the patient should be in generally good health without acute or uncontrolled chronic illness and should consume a high-carbohydrate diet (at least 200 g daily) for at least 3 days. The test should be performed in the morning and fasting. Nonpregnant adults should drink an oral solution containing 75 g of dextrose over no more than 3 minutes and should remain seated without smoking for 2 hours. Nausea is a fairly common complication of the OGTT. A single plasma glucose sample is drawn at the 2-hour time point.

Normal levels of glucose are defined as follows:

- Fasting: <100 mg/dL
- 2-hour OGTT: <140 mg/dL

The following levels of glucose are suggestive of diabetes but require confirmation for diagnosis:

- Fasting: ≥126 mg/dL, and/or
- 2-hour OGTT: ≥200 mg/dL
- In patients with symptoms of diabetes (polyuria, polydipsia, weight loss), random glucose measurements: ≥200 mg/dL

Generally, to make the diagnosis, measurements should be made on 2 separate days either repeating the same test or performing another.

Prediabetes is a state of abnormal glucose regulation associated with about twice the risk for developing diabetes and modestly increased risk for developing cardiovascular disease. The diagnosis of prediabetes is suggested by glucose levels as follows:

- Fasting: 100 to 125 mg/dL (i.e., impaired fasting glucose [IFG])
- 2-hr OGTT: 140 to 199 mg/dL (i.e., impaired glucose tolerance [IGT])

Management and Therapy

Optimum Treatment

The American Diabetes Association has recently developed consensus recommendations regarding the management of prediabetes and diabetes, which are summarized in Figure 39-1.

In patients with prediabetes, the development of DM can be prevented or delayed with diet and exercise programs aimed at producing a 5% to 10% loss of body weight, including at least 30 minutes of moderately vigorous physical activity at least 5 days per week.

Because lifestyle therapy is generally well tolerated and associated with broad-based benefits, it is recommended as treatment for both prediabetes and diabetes. To be effective, lifestyle (medical nutrition therapy and physical activity) interventions must be delivered flexibly in a patient-centered approach that both cajoles and seduces patients into a more healthful lifestyle through small steps and frequent follow-up, preferably with the help of a dietitian, diabetes educator, or other qualified lifestyle coach (Fig. 39-2). The major tenets of lifestyle management are to promote consistent moderate carbohydrate intake with an emphasis on whole grains, vegetables, and fruit combined with low saturated and polyunsaturated fat intake and regular aerobic exercise.

Pharmacologic intervention in the setting of prediabetes should be reserved for those at highest risk for developing diabetes and with the best predicted response to therapy: people with both IFG *and* IGT as well as at least one other high-risk feature:

- Age <60 years
- BMI ≥35 kg/m^2
- Family history of diabetes in first-degree relatives
- Elevated triglycerides
- Reduced HDL cholesterol

- Hypertension
- Hemoglobin A1C >6.0%

Based on expense, tolerability, and safety, metformin is the only currently recommended therapy for diabetes prevention. There is evidence that acarbose, orlistat, and rosiglitazone can be effective in preventing or delaying the development of diabetes, but each of these therapies is more expensive and associated with specific adverse effects that make the risk-benefit balance uncertain.

Glycemic control is a central issue for both patients and providers in the management of both type 1 and type 2 DM (see Fig. 39-2); the control of other cardiovascular risk factors is equally important. There are adequate prospective randomized clinical trial data documenting that treatment policies associated with more stringent glycemic targets are associated with decreased rates of retinopathy, nephropathy, and neuropathy. Epidemiologic studies support the potential of intensive glycemic control to reduce cardiovascular risk. For most patients, the following glycemic targets would be associated with a low risk for complications:

- Premeal plasma glucose between 70 and 130 mg/dL
- One- to 2-hour peak postprandial glucose levels less than 180 mg/dL
- Hemoglobin A1C levels below 7%

More stringent control (A1C <6%) is appropriate if the patient tolerates the therapy required. Less stringent treatment goals may be appropriate for patients with limited life expectancies (<6 years). There are no adequately powered clinical trial data available to document the benefit of glycemic control in the setting of advanced complications, in elderly patients (>65 years), and in young children (<13 years). Severe or frequent hypoglycemia is an indication for modification of treatment regimens, including higher premeal and postprandial targets. Self-monitoring of blood glucose, lifestyle modification, and self-management education are integral parts of intensive glucose management strategies associated with a lower risk for complications.

There are inadequate clinical trial data to support dogmatic statements regarding optimal approaches to the management of type 2 DM. Eleven classes of treatments for diabetes are currently available (Table 39-1). In general, long-term clinical trials with metformin, pioglitazone, insulin, and sulfonylureas demonstrate at least trends toward reduction in cardiovascular outcomes. Current recommendations suggest that lifestyle intervention combined with metformin therapy should be initiated at the diagnosis of diabetes. Metformin monotherapy is relatively inexpensive and is not associated with hypoglycemia or weight gain. However, there are a number of contraindications to its use that must be carefully considered.

In patients who do not reach an A1C of less than 7% with lifestyle therapy plus metformin, and particularly in patients with premeal glucose levels of more than 250 mg/

Figure 39-1 Algorithm for Care of People with Prediabetes and Diabetes.
IFG, impaired fasting glucose; IGT, impaired glucoses tolerance; OGTT, oral glucose tolerance test.
Adapted from Nathan DM, Buse JB, Davidson MB, et al: Management of hyperglycemia in type 2 diabetes mellitus: A consensus algorithm for the initiation and adjustment of therapy. Diabetes Care 29(8):1963-1972, 2006; and Nathan DM, Davidson MB, DeFronzo RA, et al: Impaired fasting glucose and impaired glucose tolerance. Diabetes Care 30(3):753-759, 2007.

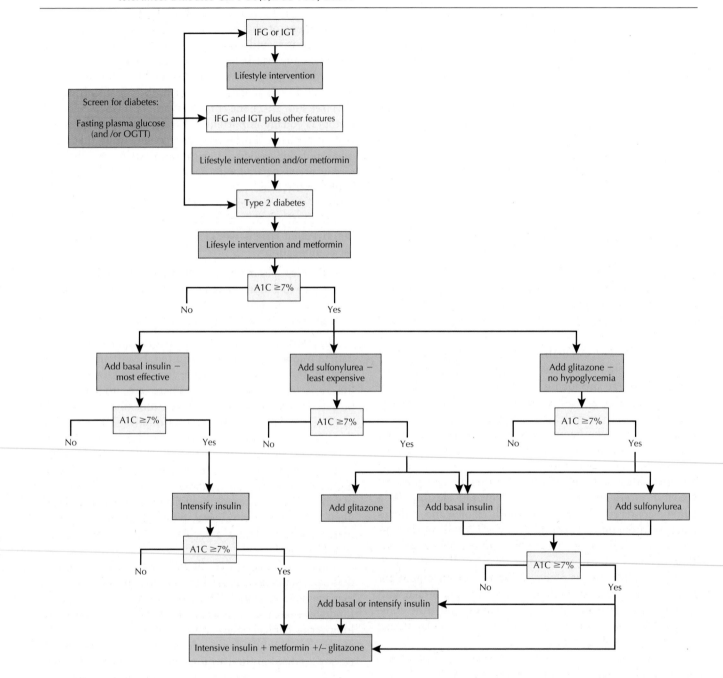

dL, early insulin therapy warrants consideration because it is the most effective antihyperglycemic therapy. Evening doses of long-acting insulin, specifically NPH (neutral protamine Hagedorn) insulin, glargine, or detemir, are highly effective in lowering A1C, although at times doses in excess of 1 U/kg per day are required. Alternative additional therapies in the algorithm include sulfonylureas, which are the least expensive antihyperglycemic treatment,

and thiazolidinediones (rosiglitazone and pioglitazone), which are associated with a low risk for hypoglycemia and progression of β-cell dysfunction. If lifestyle therapy combined with metformin and an additional agent is inadequate to achieve fasting and premeal glucose targets, additional agents should be added sequentially.

There are six additional classes of antihyperglycemic agents that are not included in the algorithm, predomi-

Figure 39-2 Nonpharmacologic Therapy.

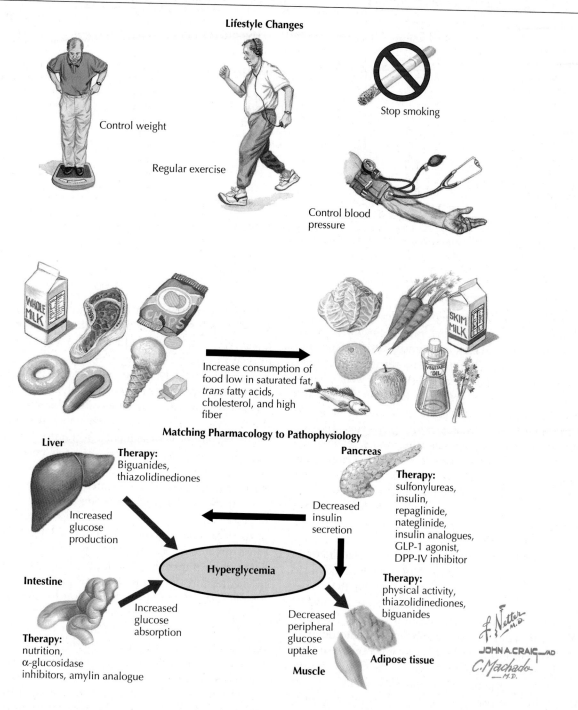

Lifestyle Changes

Control weight

Regular exercise

Stop smoking

Control blood pressure

Increase consumption of food low in saturated fat, *trans* fatty acids, cholesterol, and high fiber

Matching Pharmacology to Pathophysiology

Liver

Therapy: Biguanides, thiazolidinediones

Increased glucose production

Intestine

Therapy: nutrition, α-glucosidase inhibitors, amylin analogue

Increased glucose absorption

Hyperglycemia

Pancreas

Decreased insulin secretion

Therapy: sulfonylureas, insulin, repaglinide, nateglinide, insulin analogues, GLP-1 agonist, DPP-IV inhibitor

Therapy: physical activity, thiazolidinediones, biguanides

Decreased peripheral glucose uptake

Adipose tissue

Muscle

nantly because long-term safety and efficacy studies with these agents have not been completed. The α-glucosidase inhibitors (acarbose and miglitol) lower postprandial glucose by reducing the rate of carbohydrate absorption from the intestinal tract. The major barrier to their use is abdominal complaints. Repaglinide and nateglinide (often lumped together as *glinides*, although technically belonging to two distinct classes of medications) are not sulfonylureas, but their action is mediated through the sulfonylurea receptor; they provide for moderately less risk for hypoglycemia

and some greater postprandial effect than glyburide. Exenatide is a glucagon-like peptide-I (GLP-1) agonist associated with predominantly postprandial glucose lowering, moderate weight loss, and no intrinsic risk for hypoglycemia. Sitagliptin is the first dipeptidyl peptidase (DPP)-IV inhibitor, an oral agent that increases GLP-1 levels modestly, producing glucose lowering without weight gain or hypoglycemia. Pramlintide is an amylin-mimetic approved for use in insulin-treated patients with type 2 diabetes; it reduces postprandial glucose and promotes weight loss.

Table 39-1   Antihyperglycemic Agents in Type 2 Diabetes and Their Characteristics

Class	A1C Reduction	Fasting vs. PPG	Hypoglycemia	Weight Change	Dosing (times/day)
Metformin	1.5	Fasting	No	Neutral	2
Insulin, long acting	1.5-2.5	Fasting	Yes	Gain	1, injected
Insulin, rapid acting	1.5-2.5	PPG	Yes	Gain	1 to 4, injected
Sulfonylureas	1.5	Fasting	Yes	Gain	1
Glitazones	0.5-1.4	Fasting	No	Gain	1
Repaglinide	1-1.5	Both	Yes	Gain	3
Nateglinide	0.5-0.8	PPG	Rare	Gain	3
α-Glucosidase inhibitors	0.5-0.8	PPG	No	Neutral	3
Amylin-mimetics (pramlintide)	0.5-1.0	PPG	No	Loss	3, injected
Incretin agonists (exenatide)	0.5-1.0	PPG	No	Loss	2, injected
DPP-IV inhibitors	0.6-0.8	Both	No	Neutral	1

DPP-IV, dipeptidyl peptidase-IV; PPG, postprandial glucose.
Adapted from Nathan DM, Buse JB, Davidson MB, et al: Management of hyperglycemia in type 2 diabetes mellitus: A consensus algorithm for the initiation and adjustment of therapy. Diabetes Care 29(8):1963-1972, 2006.

Most patients can achieve recommended glucose targets using combinations of agents that improve insulin sensitivity (metformin and thiazolidinediones) with agents that increase insulin levels (sulfonylureas, repaglinide, nateglinide, exenatide, sitagliptin, and insulin) as well as combinations of agents that primarily decrease fasting and premeal glucose levels (metformin, glitazones, sulfonylureas, and long-acting insulins) with agents that decrease postprandial glucose (α-glucosidase inhibitors, repaglinide, nateglinide, rapid-acting insulin, exenatide, sitagliptin, pramlintide). It is even now possible to use combinations of agents that promote weight loss (metformin, exenatide, pramlintide) or are not associated with hypoglycemia (metformin, glitazone, α-glucosidase inhibitor, exenatide, pramlintide, sitagliptin).

Management of type 1 DM requires replacement of insulin in a physiologic fashion. Novel insulin analogues allow this to be achieved to a greater extent than older insulin preparations. In general, most patients with type 1 DM require a multiple daily injection regimen in which they administer a long-acting insulin (i.e., glargine, detemir, NPH human insulin) to control fasting glucose and prevent the rise in glucose between meals. A fast-acting insulin analogue (lispro, aspart, or glulisine) or regular human insulin is administered with each meal in proportion to carbohydrate intake, taking into account planned activity and current levels of glucose. Using this regimen or a continuous subcutaneous insulin infusion (insulin pump) minimizes glycemic excursions. Such intensive regimens generally require substantial commitment on the part of the patient as well as a team of health care providers, including DM educators, dietitians, and physicians, to be effectively implemented. Frequent glucose monitoring (3 to 8 or more times a day) or the use of continuous glucose sensors is necessary to avoid severe hypoglycemia and allow

for rapid adjustments for changes in control. Pramlintide, as an adjunct to rapid-acting insulin, can be used to help lower A1C, postprandial glucose, and weight in the setting of type 1 or type 2 diabetes.

Hypoglycemia is the most common complication of diabetes and the major limitation to tight glycemic control. Particularly in type 1 diabetes, it can be severe, requiring the assistance of another person and even resulting in death, usually as a consequence of trauma. Patients should be asked about hypoglycemia at each encounter—what symptoms they experience and at what level of glucose. Early recognition and treatment of hypoglycemia will prevent more advanced symptoms and may over a period of years delay the development of hypoglycemic unawareness. Occasional glucose levels under 70 mg/dL should not cause great concern unless they occur unexpectedly or without accompanying symptoms. Expectant adjustments in medication, diet, and exercise prescriptions to avoid hypoglycemia are critical. Screening for nocturnal hypoglycemia by home blood glucose monitoring between 1 AM and 4 AM is essential. Temporary but complete avoidance of hypoglycemia (for 3 to 6 months) by raising glycemic goals can reverse hypoglycemic unawareness in many cases. Treatment of hypoglycemia should be measured (15 g carbohydrate, e.g., 4 oz. juice or caloric soda, 3 to 4 glucose tablets), with repeat blood glucose testing after 10 to 15 minutes and additional therapy as necessary. In the case of presumed severe hypoglycemia, intramuscular glucagon can be administered in the field by lay people while awaiting emergency-trained professionals. Certified diabetes educators should always participate in patient education, particularly in regard to hypoglycemia and other complications.

Because more than two thirds of patients with DM die from cardiovascular disease, aggressive management of other cardiovascular risk factors is at least as important as glucose management. Current recommendations suggest that most patients with DM should do the following:

- Take aspirin, 81 mg/d (if older than 40 years or older than 30 years with additional CVD risk factors)
- Reduce blood pressure to less than 130/80 mm Hg with an antihypertensive regimen that generally includes an angiotensin-converting enzyme inhibitor or angiotensin receptor blocker
- Take a statin at a dose adequate to reduce LDL cholesterol by 30% to 40% and to reduce LDL to less than 100 mg/dL (<70 mg/dL in the setting of CVD)
- Reduce triglycerides to less than 150 mg/dL
- Increase HDL cholesterol to more than 40 mg/dL (perhaps 50 mg/dL in women)
- Stop smoking or don't start.

Finally, there are patients who, despite seemingly best efforts, have difficulty achieving adequate control of hyperglycemia and associated cardiovascular risk factors. In those individuals, there is a higher prevalence of depression and other psychological syndromes, sleep-disordered breathing, substance abuse, and physical or emotional abuse that should be screened for and treated if identified.

Avoiding Treatment Errors

The medical regimens required for treatment of diabetes and its comorbidities generally involve several to many pharmacologic agents and are often comanaged by primary care providers, consultants, and diabetes educators. Complicating this situation further is the fact that pharmacy benefit managers often request changes in medications that are not adequately communicated to all providers involved. Patients and providers should take great care in maintaining up-to-date lists of both over-the-counter and prescribed medications. Patients need to have a plan for sick days when oral intake is compromised; generally, they should take their medications as prescribed and monitor glucose more frequently, specifically in the setting of type 1 diabetes. Patients must understand that frequent or severe hypoglycemia is a potentially life-threatening complication of diabetes that must be brought to the attention of health care providers immediately to allow adjustment in therapy.

Future Directions

There is a huge pipeline of drugs in development, including numerous agents that promote weight loss. An exciting possibility for the future is that new islet growth can be fostered. Better glucose monitoring and insulin delivery devices are under development, including approaches that combine these two techniques to create a closed loop or artificial β cell capable of administering insulin based on continuous monitoring of plasma glucose. A number of trials are underway to explore tighter glycemic, blood pressure, and lipid targets and establish their risks and benefits. Increasing efforts are going to focus on diabetes prevention; studies are underway to demonstrate the effectiveness of such approaches to improve outcomes. A broad-based public health approach to deal with the epidemic of obesity and DM is necessary to avoid the almost unimaginable morbidity and expense in managing the metabolic consequences of overnutrition and underactivity.

Additional Resources

American College of Physicians; Diabetes Portal. Available at: http://diabetes.acponline.org.
This website provides both patient and professional information.
American Diabetes Association. Available at: http://www.diabetes.org.
This website provides patient and professional information. Every January, new Clinical Practice Recommendations are published, which can be accessed by clicking on For Health Professionals and Scientists, then Journals, then Diabetes Care, then Clinical Practice Recommendations.
Centers for Disease Control and Prevention. Available at: http://www.cdc.gov/diabetes.
This informative website for patients provides useful information on prevention and therapy with links to useful recent publications and other helpful websites.

EVIDENCE

1. American Diabetes Association: Standards of medical care in diabetes—2007. Diabetes Care 30(Suppl 1):S4-S41, 2007.
   This evidence-based overview of treatment of diabetes is updated annually and is published as the first supplement to Diabetes Care in January each year. The full text is available for free at http://www.diabetes.org.
2. Buse JB, Ginsberg HN, Bakris GL, et al: Primary prevention of cardiovascular diseases in people with diabetes: A joint statement and recommendations from the American Diabetes Association and the American Heart Association. Diabetes Care 30(1):167-172, 2007.
   This evidence-based review describes the techniques of CVD prevention in diabetes. A robust understanding of these principles is critical because about two out of three patients with diabetes die from CVD.
3. Nathan DM, Buse JB, Davidson MB, et al: Management of hyperglycemia in type 2 diabetes mellitus: A consensus algorithm for the initiation and adjustment of therapy. Diabetes Care 29(8):1963-1972, 2006.
   This article provides an algorithm of care for patients with type 2 diabetes and reviews available therapies, including details of insulin titration.
4. Nathan DM, Davidson MB, DeFronzo RA, et al: Impaired fasting glucose and impaired glucose tolerance. Diabetes Care 30(3):753-759, 2007.
   This article presents evidence-based recommendations regarding treatment of prediabetes.

John B. Buse

Prevention and Treatment of Complications of Diabetes

Introduction

Coupled with the current epidemic of diabetes mellitus (DM) is an increasing burden of death and disability. DM is the sixth leading cause of death as reported on death certificates, contributing to more than 200,000 deaths annually. This is likely a gross underestimate of its true burden because only one third of death certificates of those dying with diabetes list diabetes as a contributor despite the fact that more than two thirds succumb to cardiovascular diseases (CVDs) in which diabetes is a clear contributor. DM or prediabetes is present in about two out of three patients with clinical CVD, about two thirds of them are unaware of their diagnosis. The underlying metabolic syndrome of diabetes is clearly a major contributor to CVD, the leading cause of mortality in the Western world.

Microvascular complications of diabetes, namely eye, kidney, and nerve diseases, result in much of the disability associated with diabetes. Diabetes is the leading cause of new cases of blindness among adults with diabetic retinopathy contributing to about 20,000 new cases of blindness each year.

Diabetes is the leading cause of end-stage renal disease, accounting for almost 50% of new cases in the United States. Each year, more than 40,000 people with diabetes begin treatment for end-stage renal disease, and more than 150,000 are maintained on chronic dialysis or with kidney transplantation.

At least 60% of people with diabetes have one or more forms of diabetic neuropathy associated with a wide range of symptoms. Severe peripheral neuropathy is the major contributor to diabetic foot ulcers and amputations. More than 80,000 lower-limb amputations are performed annually among people with diabetes; this is about 60% of nontraumatic amputations in the United States.

Other complications of diabetes are legion. Poor control before conception and during the first trimester of pregnancy causes major birth defects in 5% to 10% of pregnancies and spontaneous abortions in 15% to 20%. Later in pregnancy, poor glycemic control is associated with substantial complications during delivery for both mother and child. Almost one third of people with diabetes have severe periodontal diseases. Musculoskeletal disorders associated with pain and decreased mobility are more common than in the general population. Diabetes is associated with an increased risk for many forms of cancer as well as overall cancer mortality. Particularly in the setting of poorly controlled diabetes, issues such as hypercoagulability and poor immunologic defenses contribute to excess morbidity and mortality across the entire spectrum of human maladies from influenza infections to recovery from surgery.

The costs of diabetes are staggering. In 2002, direct medical costs related to the disease were estimated to be $92 billion, with an additional $40 billion in indirect costs due to disability, work loss, and premature mortality. This estimated $132 billion price tag is an underestimate because it omits costs incurred in the undiagnosed, the cost of care provided by family members and friends, and areas of health care spending unaccounted for in which people with diabetes consume services at higher rates than the general population, including care by optometrists and dentists. Overall health care costs in individuals with diabetes are more than double those in people without diabetes.

Put another way, in the United States, every hour among diagnosed patients with diabetes, the following occur:

- More than $15 million is spent on health care
- Two patients go blind
- Five patients start dialysis
- Six patients suffer stroke
- Nine patients undergo amputation
- Ten patients have a heart attack
- Twenty-six patients die

Etiology and Pathogenesis

Glucose-dependent mechanisms for the development of complications have been described, including the intracellular accumulation of sorbitol, overactivity of protein kinase C, and the development of advanced glycosylation end products. How important these glucose-specific mechanisms are in the generation of complications is unclear. With respect to both CVD and microvascular complications, the contribution of hyperglycemia, increased blood pressure, lipid disorders, hypercoagulability, and smoking is absolutely clear. Finally, as one might expect, patients with any one complication are more likely to suffer others. Primary prevention, screening for early markers of complications, and intensive secondary intervention are critical to provide for optimal outcomes.

Clinical Presentation

With regard to macrovascular disease, the classic presentations of angina, myocardial infarction, stroke, transient ischemic attacks, and claudication are quite common (Figs. 40-1 and 40-2). As is true in nondiabetic individuals, many afflicted with life-threatening vascular disease are asymptomatic. A recent study documented that among patients with type 2 diabetes between the ages of 50 and 75 years who had no history of ischemic heart disease, a normal electrocardiogram, and negative screening questionnaire for anginal symptoms, 22% had silent ischemia by electrocardiograph (ECG)-gated adenosine-stress single-photon emission computed tomography.

Diabetic retinopathy is generally asymptomatic, although, as late manifestations, patients may note a change in their visual field with retinal detachments or may experience blurred vision in the setting of intraocular hemorrhage or macular edema (see Fig. 40-1).

Diabetic nephropathy is also generally asymptomatic until the late stages when patients present with fatigue, edema, symptoms of fluid overload, or a hypertensive crisis (see Fig. 40-1).

Diabetic neuropathy has multiple manifestations as a result of involvement of peripheral motor and sensory nerves, cranial nerves, and the autonomic nervous system. The most common of these is peripheral neuropathy, which can present with numbness or dysesthesias, including burning or tingling (Fig. 40-3; see Fig. 40-2). In general, these symptoms proceed from distal sites proximally and can be associated with motor dysfunction. Mononeuropathies may develop in motor, sensory, or cranial nerves and present with dysfunction of a single nerve. Entrapment neuropathies such as carpal tunnel syndrome are quite common. Autonomic dysfunction can lead to disabling symptoms, including decreased night vision, facial sweating with meals, postprandial bloating, nausea, vomiting, diarrhea, constipation, orthostasis, dyshydrotic skin, urinary retention, and sexual dysfunction (see Fig. 40-2).

Differential Diagnosis

Diabetic retinopathy is pathognomonic of DM, although the retinopathy associated with acromegaly can present in a similar fashion.

Diabetic nephropathy characteristically is associated with increased protein excretion, initially only detected with a very sensitive assay for microalbuminuria, then progressing to the full-blown nephrotic syndrome. In a patient with proteinuria and evidence of retinopathy, the renal disease is most often related to DM. In the absence of retinopathy or significant proteinuria, renal insufficiency is often secondary to other forms of kidney disease, particularly that caused by hypertension.

There is a substantial differential diagnosis for each of the peripheral and autonomic neuropathies. It is prudent to exclude reversible causes, such as vitamin B_{12} deficiency, tertiary syphilis, hypothyroidism, heavy-metal intoxication, and monoclonal gammopathies, by utilizing the history, physical examination, and selected laboratory tests. If physical examination findings are asymmetrical or associated with back pain or other neurologic findings, consideration of spinal or central nervous system pathology is essential. Characteristically, the pain of diabetic neuropathy is worst at rest. Subcritical peripheral vascular disease warrants consideration because it is common and, like neuropathy, is often associated with worse symptoms in the supine position.

Diagnostic Approach

The key to management of the complications of diabetes is screening to detect early manifestations. For CVD, relevant recommendations include the following:

Figure 40-1 Microvascular and Macrovascular Complications.

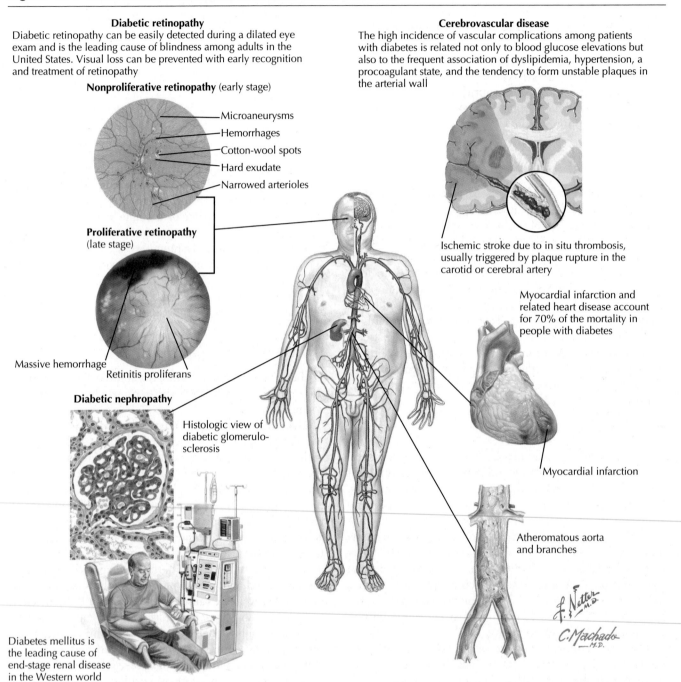

Diabetic retinopathy

Diabetic retinopathy can be easily detected during a dilated eye exam and is the leading cause of blindness among adults in the United States. Visual loss can be prevented with early recognition and treatment of retinopathy

Nonproliferative retinopathy (early stage)

- Microaneurysms
- Hemorrhages
- Cotton-wool spots
- Hard exudate
- Narrowed arterioles

Proliferative retinopathy (late stage)

Massive hemorrhage
Retinitis proliferans

Diabetic nephropathy

Histologic view of diabetic glomerulo-sclerosis

Diabetes mellitus is the leading cause of end-stage renal disease in the Western world

Cerebrovascular disease

The high incidence of vascular complications among patients with diabetes is related not only to blood glucose elevations but also to the frequent association of dyslipidemia, hypertension, a procoagulant state, and the tendency to form unstable plaques in the arterial wall

Ischemic stroke due to in situ thrombosis, usually triggered by plaque rupture in the carotid or cerebral artery

Myocardial infarction and related heart disease account for 70% of the mortality in people with diabetes

Myocardial infarction

Atheromatous aorta and branches

- Blood pressure should be measured at every visit. If the blood pressure is 130 mm Hg or greater systolic, or 80 mm Hg or greater diastolic, the elevation should be confirmed on a separate day.
- A fasting lipid panel should be performed annually. If the patient is not available for testing in the fasting state, a nonfasting non–high-density lipoprotein (non-HDL) cholesterol is a reasonable surrogate for low-density lipoprotein (LDL) cholesterol but may miss even severe disorders of HDL or triglyceride metabolism. If the full

fasting lipid panel is normal, testing may be deferred to every 2 years.
- Patients should be asked about tobacco use at every visit.
- Diagnostic stress testing with imaging procedures should be considered in those with ECG abnormalities, typical or atypical cardiac symptoms, known vascular disease or sedentary lifestyle older than 35 years who are planning to start a vigorous exercise program. Routine stress testing will identify many patients with disease, but it

Figure 40-2 Peripheral Vascular Disease.

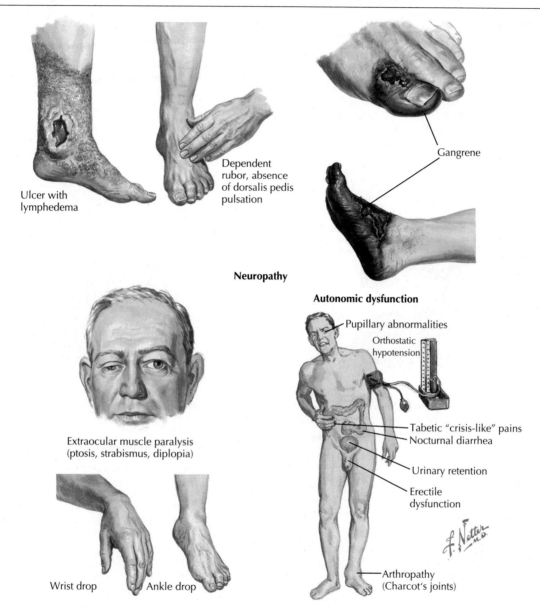

Ulcer with lymphedema

Dependent rubor, absence of dorsalis pedis pulsation

Gangrene

Neuropathy

Extraocular muscle paralysis (ptosis, strabismus, diplopia)

Wrist drop   Ankle drop

Autonomic dysfunction

Pupillary abnormalities

Orthostatic hypotension

Tabetic "crisis-like" pains
Nocturnal diarrhea

Urinary retention

Erectile dysfunction

Arthropathy (Charcot's joints)

remains unclear whether invasive management is associated with improved outcomes in the setting of asymptomatic CVD in diabetes.

To detect other early complications, the following are recommended annually beginning at diagnosis in the setting of type 2 diabetes and within 3 to 5 years in type 1 diabetes:

- Dilated and comprehensive eye exams by an eye care professional
- Spot urine sample for a microalbumin-to-creatinine ratio
  - An albumin excretion ratio of at least 30 µg albumin per mg creatinine suggests diabetic kidney disease.
  - Two out of three measures over a 6-month period are required for diagnosis of albuminuria.

- Serum creatinine for the estimation of glomerular filtration rate (GFR)
- Screen for distal symmetrical polyneuropathy, using simple clinical tests such as vibration perception with a 128-Hz tuning fork and pressure sensation using a 10-g monofilament at the distal plantar aspect of both great toes; electrophysiologic testing is rarely needed.
- Screen for autonomic neuropathy by a general review of systems.
- Identify high-risk foot-related conditions in addition to distal symmetrical polyneuropathy by visual inspection and palpation to identify altered biomechanics, evidence of increased pressure, peripheral vascular disease, or severe nail pathology.
- Semiannual exam and tooth cleaning by oral health professional

Figure 40-3 Neuropathy and Fungal Infection.

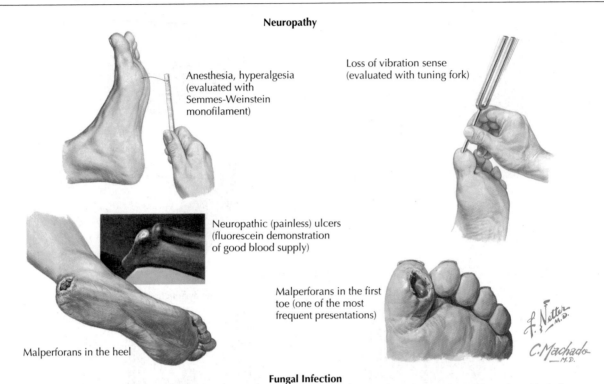

Neuropathy

Anesthesia, hyperalgesia (evaluated with Semmes-Weinstein monofilament)

Loss of vibration sense (evaluated with tuning fork)

Neuropathic (painless) ulcers (fluorescein demonstration of good blood supply)

Malperforans in the first toe (one of the most frequent presentations)

Malperforans in the heel

Fungal Infection

Fungal infections of the nails and skin are common in patients with diabetes. With foot involvement, accompanying minor skin lesions can be the portal of infection and can result in chronic wounds and even amputations. Excellent foot care and antifungal therapy are important preventative measures in the setting of advanced diabetic neuropathy

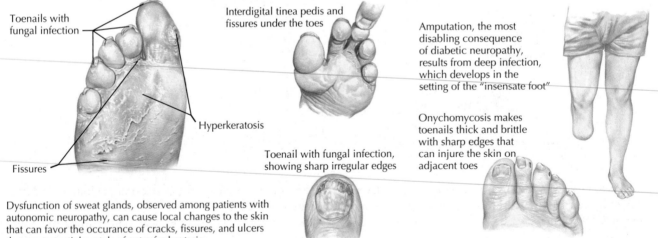

Toenails with fungal infection

Interdigital tinea pedis and fissures under the toes

Amputation, the most disabling consequence of diabetic neuropathy, results from deep infection, which develops in the setting of the "insensate foot"

Onychomycosis makes toenails thick and brittle with sharp edges that can injure the skin on adjacent toes

Hyperkeratosis

Fissures

Toenail with fungal infection, showing sharp irregular edges

Dysfunction of sweat glands, observed among patients with autonomic neuropathy, can cause local changes to the skin that can favor the occurance of cracks, fissures, and ulcers that are potential portals of entry for bacteria

Management and Therapy

Optimum Treatment

Because more than two thirds of patients with DM die from CVD, aggressive management of other cardiovascular risk factors is at least as important as glucose management. Current recommendations suggest that most patients with DM should do the following:

- Take aspirin, 81 mg/d (if older than 40 years or older than 30 years with additional CVD risk factors).

- Reduce blood pressure to less than 130/80 mm Hg with a blood pressure regimen that generally includes an angiotensin-converting enzyme (ACE) inhibitor or angiotensin receptor blocker (ARB).
- Take a statin at a dose adequate to reduce LDL cholesterol by 30% to 40% and to reduce LDL to less than 100 mg/dL (<70 mg/dL in the setting of CVD).
- Reduce triglycerides to less than 150 mg/dL.
- Increase HDL cholesterol to more than 40 mg/dL (perhaps 50 mg/dL in women).
- Stop smoking or don't start.

In addition to glucose management as described in Chapter 39 and control of CVD risk factors as described earlier, there are a number of interventions that have been demonstrated to reduce the risk for developing clinical microvascular complications.

To slow the progression of diabetic kidney disease:

- Blood pressure targets less than 130/80 mg Hg can be considered.
- Prescribe an ACE inhibitor or ARB.
- Reduce dietary protein intake to 0.8 to 1.0 g per kg body weight per day.
- Refer to a physician experienced in the care of diabetic kidney disease when estimated GFR has fallen to less than 60 mL/min per 1.73 m^2.

To minimize the risk for visual loss, refer all patients with macular edema, proliferative retinopathy, or severe nonproliferative diabetic retinopathy to an ophthalmologist expert in the management of diabetic retinopathy.

To minimize the risk for amputation in patients with severe distal symmetrical polyneuropathy or other high-risk foot conditions, provide comprehensive foot self-care education, including the need for daily inspection, nail and skin care, and appropriate footwear. Also consider referral to a foot care specialty center for ongoing preventive care and surveillance.

Only recently have U.S. Food and Drug Administration–approved products for the treatment of painful distal symmetrical polyneuropathy become available: duloxetine and pregabalin. There are a large number of moderately effective therapies for distal polyneuropathy and autonomic neuropathies that can improve symptoms but do not alter the underlying pathophysiology or natural histories of these disorders. Medical providers should discontinue these therapies if relief of symptoms does not occur after titration to an adequate dose.

Avoiding Treatment Errors

The most common errors in the management of diabetic complications are failure to make a timely diagnosis and nonadherence to treatment guidelines once a diagnosis is made, often as a result of oversight. The health care team (both patients and providers) should keep a checklist to ensure that all the listed screening tests are performed at least annually and recommended preventative therapies continued. Nonjudgmental consistent collaboration among the team is the best guarantee that recommendations are adhered to by both patients and providers. In diabetes care, disability results from failure of the team more often than failure of the treatment.

Future Directions

There are a wide variety of treatments that target specific glucose-mediated mechanisms in the development of complications, which although promising, have been somewhat disappointing to date. We have the technology to prevent the development of most complications with glucose control, cardiovascular risk factor management, and screening with referral for specialty care in patients who have early complications. Historically, there has been widespread failure of health care teams to achieve the recommended targets or conduct the recommended screening tests. Recent changes in patient and physician awareness, coupled with potential changes in health care financing, raise the hope that complications of diabetes could be dramatically reduced in the next few decades.

Additional Resources

American Academy of Ophthalmology. Available at: http://www.eyecareamerica.org/eyecare/conditions/diabetic-retinopathy/index.cfm.
This website provides educational materials.
American Podiatric Medical Association. Available at: http://www.apma.org/s_apma/sec.asp?CID=430&DID=17206.
This website provides educational materials.
Centers for Disease Control and Prevention. Available at: http://www.cdc.gov/diabetes. Accessed May 10, 2007.
This informative website for patients provides useful information on prevention and therapy with links to useful recent publications and other helpful websites.
National Kidney Foundation. Available at: http://www.kidney.org/atoz/atozTopic.cfm?topic=2.
This website provides educational materials.

EVIDENCE

1. American Diabetes Association: Standards of medical care in diabetes—2007. Diabetes Care. 30(Suppl 1):S4-S41, 2007.
   This evidence-based overview of treatment of diabetes is updated annually and is published as the first supplement to Diabetes Care in January each year. The full text is available for free at http://www.diabetes.org.
2. Buse JB, Ginsberg HN, Bakris GL, et al: Primary prevention of cardiovascular diseases in people with diabetes: A joint statement and recommendations from the American Diabetes Association and the American Heart Association. Diabetes Care 30(1):167-172, 2007.
   This evidence-based review describes the techniques of CVD prevention in diabetes. A robust understanding of these principles is critical because about two out of three patients with diabetes die from CVD.
3. Centers for Disease Control and Prevention: National diabetes fact sheet, United States 2005. Available at: http://www.cdc.gov/diabetes/pubs/pdf/ndfs_2005.pdf. Accessed February 7, 2007.
   This is an informative website.

Michael J. Thomas ▪ Sue A. Brown

Hypothyroidism

Introduction

Hypothyroidism is a common condition that occurs when the thyroid is unable to produce enough thyroid hormone to meet the body's needs. Onset can occur at any age and is more common in women, with a prevalence of about 2% in some age groups (compared with 0.1% in men). Congenital hypothyroidism is one of the most common endocrine abnormalities present at birth (about 1 in 5000 births).

Etiology and Pathogenesis

Thyroid-stimulating hormone (TSH, or thyrotropin), a glycoprotein produced by pituitary thyrotrophs, stimulates the synthesis and secretion of thyroid hormones by the thyroid. TSH binds to a plasma membrane receptor on thyroid follicular cells and activates adenylate cyclase. It stimulates every facet of thyroid iodine metabolism and promotes thyroid growth. TSH biosynthesis and secretion is inhibited by triiodothyronine (T_3) and thyroxine (T_4), forming a sensitive feedback loop to keep free thyroid hormone concentrations constant. Thyrotropin-releasing hormone (TRH) is a hypothalamic tripeptide that stimulates TSH release. TRH appears to set the level by which the negative feedback loop maintains thyroid hormone levels. Disturbances in the TRH-TSH-thyroid axis can lead to hypothyroidism.

Primary hypothyroidism, the most common cause of thyroid failure, results in low serum thyroid hormone with elevated TSH levels. Loss of functional thyroid tissue and interference of thyroid hormone production are the major causes of primary hypothyroidism (Fig. 41-1).

Loss of functional thyroid tissue is usually due to auto-immune thyroid dysfunction (e.g., Hashimoto's or chronic lymphocytic thyroiditis; see Fig. 41-1). It is sometimes associated with polyglandular autoimmune syndromes and a family history of thyroid dysfunction. High titers of antithyroid antibodies (antithyroid peroxidase and antithyroglobulin antibodies) are common, although titers are sometimes low, particularly in elderly patients. Cell-mediated (T-lymphocyte) destruction of the thyroid probably plays a more significant role in thyroid damage than thyroid antibodies. Pathologic study shows lymphocytic infiltration and fibrosis with destruction of follicles resulting in an atrophic thyroid gland or a firm, nontender diffuse goiter. Gradually, T_4 and T_3 synthesis is impaired, prompting a compensatory rise in TSH and a "subclinical" phase that may precede the onset of frank hypothyroidism. Usually, hypothyroidism is chronic, but transient hypothyroidism as well as hyperthyroidism can occur. Silent ("painless") thyroiditis is a common cause of transient hyperthyroidism, hypothyroidism, or both in the postpartum period (about 5% prevalence). Procedures that remove or destroy functional thyroid tissue, such as surgery or radioactive iodine, can render a person permanently hypothyroid. Finally, congenital agenesis or dysgenesis of the thyroid gland can occur.

Interference with thyroid hormone production is often drug induced. Iodine and lithium inhibit thyroid hormone secretion, particularly in patients with mild autoimmune thyroiditis. Endemic iodine deficiency can lead to goiter, cretinism, and hypothyroidism. Overtreatment with thionamides used for hyperthyroidism can also produce hypothyroidism. Amiodarone, an antiarrhythmic drug containing iodine, can block production of thyroid hormone. Rarely, congenital defects in T_4 biosynthesis or maternal treatment with antithyroid drugs or iodine causes congenital hypothyroidism and goiter.

Secondary hypothyroidism (low TSH or inappropriately normal TSH with low thyroid hormone levels) is usually the result of hypothalamic or pituitary dysfunction due to tumors, trauma, surgery, or irradiation (see Fig. 41-1). TSH deficiency occurs when the anterior pituitary thyrotropes are unable to secrete adequate amounts of TSH to regulate thyroid hormone production. Hypothalamic defects lead to TRH deficiency.

Figure 41-1 Adult Myxedema: Clinical Manifestions and Etiology.

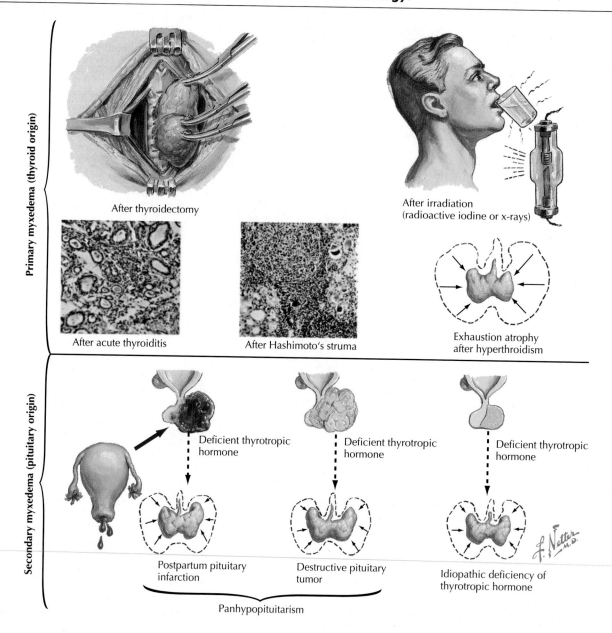

Primary myxedema (thyroid origin)

After thyroidectomy

After acute thyroiditis

After Hashimoto's struma

After irradiation (radioactive iodine or x-rays)

Exhaustion atrophy after hyperthroidism

Secondary myxedema (pituitary origin)

Deficient thyrotropic hormone

Deficient thyrotropic hormone

Deficient thyrotropic hormone

Postpartum pituitary infarction

Destructive pituitary tumor

Idiopathic deficiency of thyrotropic hormone

Panhypopituitarism

Rare familial syndromes exist in which clinical hypothyroidism occurs despite elevated levels of T_4 and T_3 and sometimes an elevated level of TSH. Resistance to thyroid hormone can be due to a mutation in one of the thyroid hormone receptors that binds T_3, rendering the receptor unable to activate target DNA sequences, or the pituitary gland resistant to feedback inhibition of thyroid hormone.

Clinical Presentation

The clinical spectrum of hypothyroidism is broad, ranging from subclinical, with few or no manifestations, to myxedema coma (Fig. 41-2). The onset of symptoms can be insidious and is often overlooked, especially in elderly patients. Cold intolerance is the most specific symptom, and delayed relaxation of deep tendon reflexes is the most specific sign. Some clinical findings are explained by known thyroid hormone effects. Decreased metabolic rates lead to cold intolerance and a tendency to increased weight. The failure to metabolize glycosaminoglycans results in their accumulation in subcutaneous tissue, causing non-pitting edema (myxedema) (Fig. 41-3). A goiter can develop in Hashimoto's thyroiditis or in iodine deficiency, whereas the thyroid gland may be normal size, small, or absent in postprocedural hypothyroidism, congenital thyroid agenesis, or dysgenesis. Mild pituitary gland enlargement occurs in some cases. Laboratory abnormalities often include

Figure 41-2 Hypothyroidism.

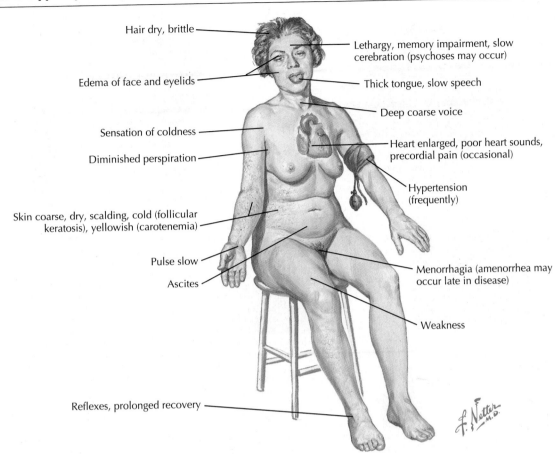

Hair dry, brittle

Edema of face and eyelids

Sensation of coldness

Diminished perspiration

Skin coarse, dry, scalding, cold (follicular keratosis), yellowish (carotenemia)

Pulse slow

Ascites

Reflexes, prolonged recovery

Lethargy, memory impairment, slow cerebration (psychoses may occur)

Thick tongue, slow speech

Deep coarse voice

Heart enlarged, poor heart sounds, precordial pain (occasional)

Hypertension (frequently)

Menorrhagia (amenorrhea may occur late in disease)

Weakness

hypertriglyceridemia, which responds to adequate thyroid hormone replacement (Box 41-1).

Differential Diagnosis

Hypothyroidism is accurately and easily diagnosed with thyroid function tests; however, these tests can be abnormal in sick but apparently euthyroid patients ("nonthyroidal illness" or "euthyroid sick syndrome"). These changes are not believed to indicate abnormal thyroid function because TSH levels are usually normal and other thyroid test abnormalities typically return to normal after the underlying illness resolves. The biologic importance of the euthyroid sick syndromes is not understood, and they may represent an adaptive stress response. The existence of these syndromes emphasizes the importance of exercising sound clinical judgment before ordering diagnostic tests. There are three major patterns of abnormalities in patients with nonthyroidal illness:

1. Low T_3 syndrome with impaired T_4-to-T_3 conversion is seen in most acute and chronic diseases, trauma, surgery, and starvation. T_3 levels are decreased, and reverse T_3 levels are increased, whereas T_4 and TSH concentrations are normal. Although common, this syndrome is seldom a diagnostic problem because T_3 levels are not routinely measured.

2. Low (total) T_4 syndromes, also seen in severe illnesses, often are due to very low levels of plasma-binding proteins. The T_4 index is often low as well, but free T_4 measured by equilibrium dialysis is normal. Normal TSH levels are seen in most patients and provide the best evidence against hypothyroidism.

3. High T_4 syndromes are seen occasionally and may be due to increased plasma-binding proteins. These are usually transient, and normal TSH levels indicate that these patients do not have hypothyroidism.

Diagnostic Approach

An elevated TSH level confirms the diagnosis of primary hypothyroidism. The T_4 level will be low and can be measured directly with a free T_4 assay or estimated by a free thyroxine index (FTI). A decreased serum free T_4 (by equilibrium dialysis) verifies true T_4 deficiency even in the presence of binding protein changes or severe illness and for this reason is generally preferred over the FTI. If the

Figure 41-3 Adult Myxedema: Clinical Manifestations and Etiology.

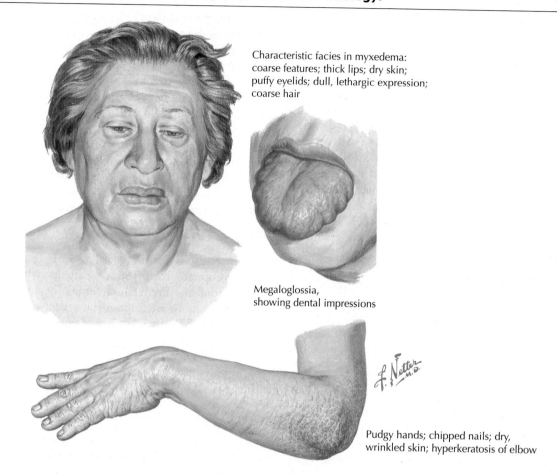

Characteristic facies in myxedema: coarse features; thick lips; dry skin; puffy eyelids; dull, lethargic expression; coarse hair

Megaloglossia, showing dental impressions

Pudgy hands; chipped nails; dry, wrinkled skin; hyperkeratosis of elbow

Box 41-1	Major Clinical Findings of Hypothyroidism

- **Constitutional**: Malaise, cold intolerance, lethargy, fatigue, hoarseness
- **Skin**: Thickened, coarse, dry, cool, nonpitting edema (myxedema), hair loss, decreased sweating
- **Cardiovascular**: Decreased cardiac contractility and rate, cardiac dilation, pericardial and pleural effusions, increased peripheral resistance
- **Gastrointestinal**: Decreased appetite, constipation, mild weight gain
- **Musculoskeletal**: Myalgias, arthralgias
- **Hematologic**: Mild anemia (usually children)
- **Neurologic**: Delayed relaxation phase of deep tendon reflexes, slowing of physical or mental activity, poor memory, somnolence, rarely dementia or anxiety
- **Thyroid gland**: May be large, "normal," or absent
- **Suggestive laboratory abnormalities**: Hypercholesterolemia, increased creatine kinase, hyponatremia, hyperprolactinemia, electrocardiographic changes (prolonged PR interval, low voltage), normochromic anemia, with or without mild increase in mean corpuscular volume
- **Neonatal and pediatric hypothyroidism**: Delayed growth and development, umbilical hernia, prolonged neonatal jaundice, protruding tongue, poor feeding, delayed bone age

FTI is measured, however, it is useful to be aware of a couple of scenarios:

- If the total T_4 is decreased and T_3 uptake is increased, the patient has decreased plasma-binding proteins, not hypothyroidism. The FTI is usually normal, and a normal TSH level confirms that the patient is euthyroid.
- If the total T_4 and the FTI are decreased, but TSH is not elevated, the patient may have secondary hypothyroidism, and evidence of other pituitary hormone deficits should be sought. In most cases, this combination of laboratory findings is due to abnormal plasma hormone binding or the effects of nonthyroidal illness on thyroid tests.

Diagnosis of the distinct cause of hypothyroidism is usually not necessary because most cases are either iatrogenic or due to autoimmune thyroiditis. Antithyroid antibodies, thyroid scans, and uptake measurements are rarely necessary because they do not change the management of the hypothyroidism. If secondary hypothyroidism is suspected, it is more important to assess the function of other pituitary hormones and obtain a magnetic resonance image of the pituitary gland and hypothalamus, than it is to perform a TRH stimulation test.

Management and Therapy

Optimum Therapy

Levothyroxine (L-T$_4$) is the drug of choice. It has supplanted desiccated thyroid extract, which has variable potency and purity. L-T$_4$ is deiodinated and peripherally converted to T$_3$, producing normal plasma levels of both T$_4$ and T$_3$. Therapy begins with average replacement doses of 100 to 125 mg per day (about 1.6 mg/kg/day) and varies depending on age. In elderly patients or those with cardiac disease, therapy should be initiated with smaller doses (25 to 50 mg/day) and increased gradually to avoid precipitating myocardial ischemia or heart failure due to increased metabolic rate and cardiac output. Infants can be treated immediately with full doses (25 to 50 mg/day). The half-life of T$_4$ is about 7 days, so most symptoms gradually resolve within several days to weeks of initiating therapy.

T$_3$ is used infrequently for replacement because of its short half-life and slightly higher cost. Similarly, combination L-T$_4$/T$_3$ preparations offer no pharmacologic advantage because T$_4$ naturally undergoes deiodination in peripheral tissues once absorbed. The role for low supplements of T$_3$ in patients with persistent fatigue, depression, or cognitive problems despite normalization of thyroid function tests is unclear. A recent systematic review did not find evidence supporting its use.

Parenteral L-T$_4$ is indicated for myxedema (see Fig. 41-3) coma or severe life-threatening hypothyroidism, which is rare and occurs most often after an intervening illness. Glucocorticoids are also given in suspected cases because adrenal insufficiency commonly coexists with severe hypothyroidism.

In pregnancy, maternal thyroid requirements increase about 25%, and the increase in total T$_4$ is accompanied by rising levels of thyroid-binding globulin (an effect of increased estrogen). Placental transfer of thyroid hormones is limited, and TSH does not cross the placenta. However, iodine and maternal antibodies readily cross the placenta. Recent studies suggest that maintaining euthyroidism in pregnancy is important for producing a normal intelligence quotient in offspring. Antithyroid drugs cross the placenta in limited amounts but usually do not cause fetal hypothyroidism or goiter unless taken in large doses.

Subclinical hypothyroidism (an increased TSH level with normal T$_4$ levels) is common, occurring in about 7.5% of women and about 3% of men. Treatment is controversial and usually not indicated because of lack of data on relevant clinical outcomes. A recent U.S. Preventive Services Task Force concluded that it is uncertain whether treatment will improve quality of life. A scientific review by Surks and colleagues concluded there was little evidence to support the routine treatment of patients with TSH values between 4.5 and 10.0 mIU/L. However, in individual patients, low doses of thyroid hormone can be given to normalize thyroid function tests and ascertain whether there is an improvement in symptoms.

Avoiding Treatment Errors

The maintenance dose of L-T$_4$ should be adjusted in primary hypothyroidism to normalize the TSH level. Because of the long half-life of T$_4$ and the delayed decrease of chronically elevated TSH levels, dose adjustments are made no more often than every 5 to 6 weeks. It is important to avoid overtreatment because it is associated with accelerated loss of bone mass and a higher prevalence of arrhythmias.

In patients with secondary hypothyroidism, TSH is not regulated normally and cannot be used to adjust the dose. T$_4$ or free T$_4$ levels should be maintained within the normal range. If adrenal insufficiency is present, glucocorticoids should be administered before replacing thyroid hormone to avoid precipitating symptomatic adrenal crisis.

Future Directions

Studies are also underway regarding the long-term outcome and appropriate treatment of patients with subclinical hypothyroidism. Prenatal screening of hypothyroidism will receive more attention given recent evidence of loss of cognitive ability in offspring of untreated mothers.

Additional Resources

Roberts CG, Ladenson PW: Hypothyroidism. Lancet 363(9411):793-803, 2004.
This article provides a recent comprehensive clinical review.

Singer PA, Cooper DS, Levy EG, et al: Treatment guidelines for patients with hyperthyroidism and hypothyroidism. Standards of Care Committee, American Thyroid Association. JAMA 273(10):808-812, 1995.
The authors review the approach by the American Thyroid Association for management of hypothyroidism.

Toft AD: Thyroxine therapy. N Engl J Med 331(3):174-180, 1994.
This paper provides some nuances relating to the administration of thyroxine therapy.

EVIDENCE

1. Escobar-Morreale HF, Botella-Carretero JI, Escobar del Rey F, Morreale de Escobar G: Review: Treatment of hypothyroidism with combinations of levothyroxine plus liothyronine. J Clin Endocrinol Metab 90(8):4946-4954, 2005.
   This is a comprehensive review of the data regarding the controversial use of levothyroxine plus liothyronine.
2. Hak AE, Pols HA, Visser TJ, et al: Subclinical hypothyroidism is an independent risk factor for atherosclerosis and myocardial infarction in elderly women: The Rotterdam Study. Ann Intern Med 132(4):270-278, 2000.
   This large, well-designed epidemiologic study suggests that subclinical hypothyroidism may be a potential risk factor for cardiovascular disease.
3. Helfand M, for the U.S. Preventive Services Task Force: Screening for subclinical thyroid dysfunction in nonpregnant adults: A summary of the evidence for the U.S. Preventive Services Task Force. Ann Intern Med 140(2):128-141, 2004.
   This paper provides a concise summary and grading of the evidence regarding screening patients for subclinical thyroid dysfunction.
4. Surks MI, Ortiz E, Daniels GH, et al: Subclinical thyroid disease: Scientific review and guidelines for diagnosis and management. JAMA 291(2):228-238, 2004.
   The authors present an excellent systematic review of data regarding management of subclinical thyroid disease.

Elizabeth A. Fasy

Thyrotoxicosis

Introduction

Thyrotoxicosis is the constellation of clinical findings that arise when the peripheral tissues are presented with and respond to an excess of thyroid hormone—free thyroxine (T_4) and free triiodothyronine (T_3). Hyperthyroidism refers to sustained increases in thyroid hormone synthesis and secretion by the thyroid gland. The prevalence of hyperthyroidism is estimated at 2% for women and 0.2% for men. About 15% of cases occur in patients older than 60 years.

The most common causes of thyrotoxicosis in Western society are Graves' disease, autonomous single nodules (also known as *toxic hot nodules*), multiple functioning nodules (also called *toxic multinodular goiter*), and thyroiditis. The pathogenesis in each of these conditions is different (Table 42-1). However, the initial therapy is similar and focuses on blocking the peripheral effects of thyroid hormone excess and reducing thyroid hormone overproduction where present.

Etiology and Pathogenesis

Graves' disease is the most common cause of hyperthyroidism in patients younger than 40 years (Fig. 42-1). The pathophysiology represents one of the classic receptor antibody disease states due to thyroid-stimulating hormone (TSH) receptor autoantibodies that continuously stimulate the thyroid gland as TSH agonists. Intrathyroidal lymphocytic infiltrate is the initial abnormality (Fig. 42-2). As in other autoimmune disease states, females are more commonly affected than males. Autonomously functioning thyroid nodules are discrete and function independently of the pituitary-thyroid negative feedback loop. Thyroiditis is characterized by inflammation, with thyroidal damage leading to release of T_4 and T_3 without active formation of T_4 and T_3. Transient hypothyroidism typically follows, with the rare development of permanent hypothyroidism. Other rare causes of hyperthyroidism include (1) TSH-secreting pituitary tumors, (2) struma ovarii, (3) iodine-induced hyperthyroidism (Jod-Basedow), (4) hyperthyroidism mediated by human chorionic gonadotropin, (5) metastatic follicular thyroid cancer, and (6) factitious thyrotoxicosis caused by surreptitious thyroid hormone ingestion.

Clinical Presentation

Common symptoms of thyrotoxicosis include nervousness, emotional lability, fatigability, heat intolerance, weight change (usually weight loss), appetite change (usually increased), myopathic symptoms, increased frequency of bowel movements, sweating, menstrual irregularities (usually oligomenorrhea), and central nervous system disturbance. Common signs include hyperactivity; tachycardia or atrial arrhythmias; systolic hypertension; warm, moist, smooth skin; stare and eyelid retraction; tremor; hyperreflexia; and muscle weakness. Palpitations are a prominent symptom in elderly patients, as is cardiac failure. Generally, elderly patients present with less florid features of thyrotoxicosis and commonly exhibit cardiac symptoms or dementia.

Graves' Disease

A triad of manifestations define the disease: (1) hyperthyroidism and goiter; (2) ophthalmopathy, clinically evident in 10% to 25% of patients, with a higher prevalence in men and in those who smoke; and (3) dermopathy in the form of localized myxedema, which is a skin thickening typically limited to the pretibial area. About 4% of patients

Table 42-1 Disorders Associated with Thyrotoxicosis

Disorder	Pathogenic Mechanism
High Thyroid Radioiodine Uptake	
Graves' disease	Stimulating antibody to TSH receptor
Toxic multinodular goiter	Multiple foci of functional autonomy
Toxic hot nodule	Single focus of functional autonomy
TSH hypersecretion	Thyrotroph adenoma and thyrotroph resistance to T_4
Trophoblastic tumor	Chorionic gonadotropin
Hyperemesis gravidarum	Chorionic gonadotropin
Low Thyroid Radioiodine Uptake	
Silent and subacute thyroiditis	Leakage of stored hormone
Drug-induced thyroiditis (amiodarone, interferon-α)	Leakage of stored hormone
Radiation thyroiditis	Leakage of stored hormone
Infarction of thyroid adenoma	Leakage of stored hormone
Thyrotoxicosis factitia	Hormone ingestion in medication or food
Struma ovarii	Toxic adenoma in a dermoid tumor of ovary
Iodine, iodine-containing drugs, and radiographic contrast agents	Iodine plus thyroid autonomy

T_4, thyroxine; TSH, thyroid-stimulating hormone.

Figure 42-1 Hyperthyroidism with Diffuse Goiter (Graves' Disease).

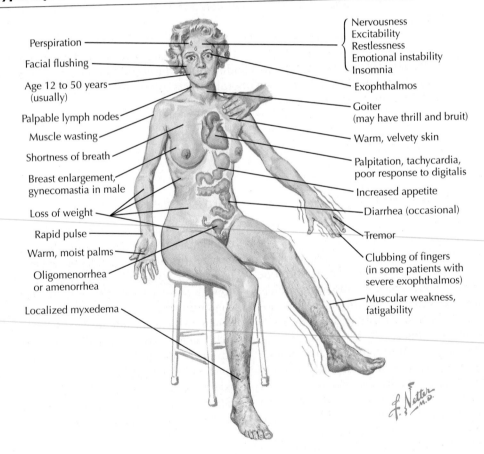

with clinically evident ophthalmopathy have thyroid dermopathy.

The onset of the disease is usually insidious. Some patients may notice the gradual development of goiter and its associated symptoms, including difficulty in fastening the collar button, fullness in the neck, or a choking sensa-tion. Slightly more than one half of the patients experience symptoms of ophthalmopathy (i.e., grittiness and tearing of the eyes, retro-ocular pressure, photophobia, a staring appearance, and the development of diplopia (Fig. 42-3). The thyroid gland is diffusely enlarged and may be firmer, and an audible bruit may be auscultated. Radioactive iodine

Figure 42-2 Thyroid Pathology in Hyperthyroidism with Diffuse Goiter (Graves' Disease).

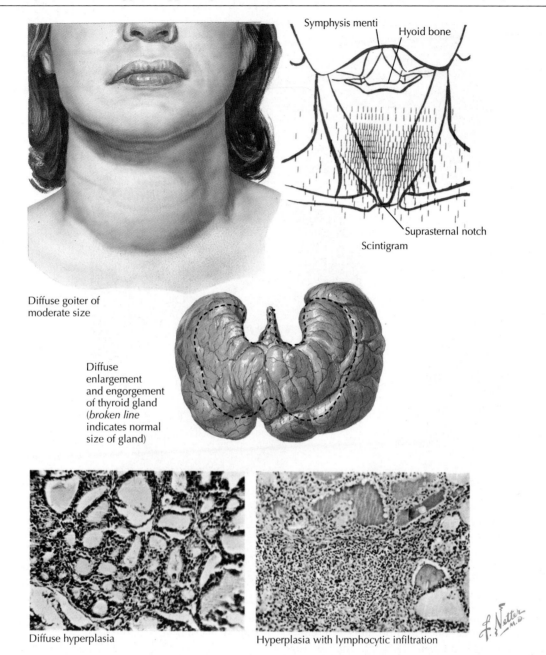

Symphysis menti   Hyoid bone

Suprasternal notch

Scintigram

Diffuse goiter of moderate size

Diffuse enlargement and engorgement of thyroid gland (*broken line* indicates normal size of gland)

Diffuse hyperplasia

Hyperplasia with lymphocytic infiltration

imaging reveals diffuse radioiodine uptake, although this test is not essential to make the diagnosis.

Toxic Multinodular Goiter and Toxic Hot Nodule

Thyroid nodules are the most common cause of thyrotoxicosis in elderly patients. The disease onset is also insidious, and the thyrotoxicosis is usually mild. The goiter may have been diagnosed many years previously. Because these disorders more commonly present in elderly patients, cardiac manifestations, such as tachycardia, atrial fibrillation, precipitation of angina, or cardiac failure, tend to predomi-

nate. On physical exam, toxic solitary nodule presents as a unilateral thyroid mass, and toxic multinodular goiter presents with multiple nodules often not as easily palpated. The nodules appear hyperfunctioning (hot) on radionuclide imaging, concentrating the radioiodide to a greater extent than the surrounding atrophic thyroid tissue (Fig. 42-4).

Thyroiditis

Subacute Thyroiditis

Subacute thyroiditis is also referred to as granulomatous, giant cell, or de Quervain's thyroiditis. Patients present

Figure 42-3 Ophthalmopathy of Graves' Disease.

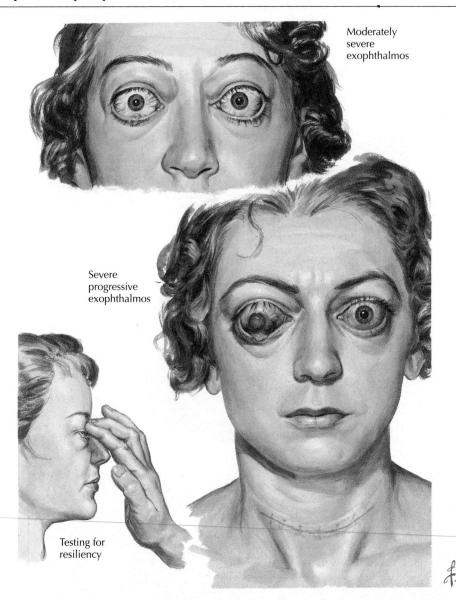

Moderately severe exophthalmos

Severe progressive exophthalmos

Testing for resiliency

with transient symptoms of thyrotoxicosis. Usually, thyroiditis follows a viral-like illness and presents as a tender, enlarged thyroid gland. The pain radiates to the jaw, ears, and occipital area. Episodes are usually self-limiting, although temporary or permanent hypothyroidism can occur. Relapses are common. Because of the lack of active formation of T₃ and T₄, radioiodine thyroid imaging reveals a low thyroid uptake.

Silent Thyroiditis

Silent thyroiditis is thought to be a variant of Hashimoto's thyroiditis with circulating autoantibodies present and lymphocytic infiltration noted in the thyroid gland. The duration of hyperthyroid symptoms is short and has a self-limited course of a few weeks to months, and transient hypothyroidism occurs during recovery. One half of patients have persistent autoantibodies, goiter, and hypothyroidism. Postpartum

thyroiditis is considered a variant of silent thyroiditis, occurring in 5% of postpartum women.

Iodine-Induced Hyperthyroidism

Iodine-induced hyperthyroidism can occur after excess iodine in the diet, exposure to radiographic contrast media, or medications such as amiodarone.

Differential Diagnosis

The differential diagnosis of hyperthyroidism can be categorized by the underlying pathophysiology and broadly divided by radioactive iodine uptake findings. Thyroid disorders that cause excess production and release of thyroid hormone result in increased thyroid radioiodine uptake on thyroid scan and uptake. Autonomous thyroid hormone production characterizes toxic multinodular goiter and

Figure 42-4 Pathophysiology of Hyperfunctioning Thyroid Adenoma.

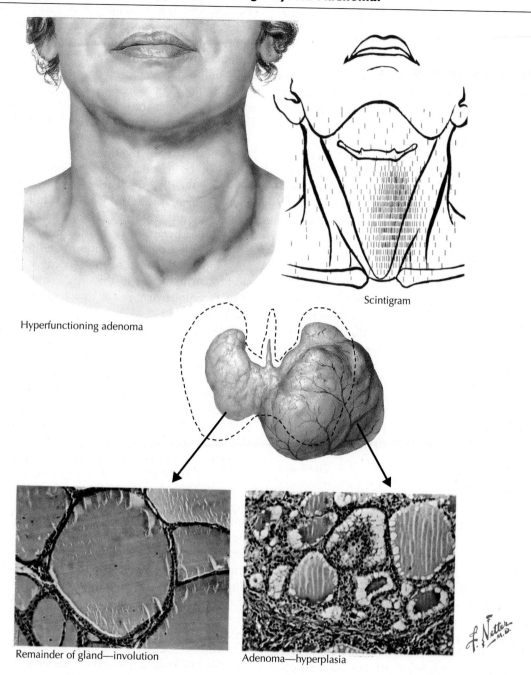

Hyperfunctioning adenoma

Scintigram

Remainder of gland—involution

Adenoma—hyperplasia

toxic hot nodule. Increased stimulation of the thyroid gland by autoantibodies, iodine, and TSH hypersecretion are the cause of Graves' disease, iodine-induced hyperthyroidism, and thyrotroph adenoma, respectively. Human chorionic gonadotropin stimulates the TSH receptor in hyperemesis gravidarum and trophoblastic tumor.

Thyroid disorders that cause release of stored thyroid hormone but no excess production result in low thyroid radioiodine uptake, which is seen in thyroiditis. Excess thyroid hormone not produced by the thyroid gland (thyrotoxicosis factitia, struma ovarii) will also result in a low thyroid radioiodine uptake (see Table 42-1).

Diagnostic Approach

The diagnosis of thyrotoxicosis is established by demonstrating an elevated free thyroxine (FT_4) level accompanied by a suppressed serum TSH level. All patients with thyrotoxicosis have a low or undetectable TSH level (<0.1 μIU/mL), except for TSH-induced thyrotoxicosis. FT_4 levels have generally replaced total T_4 levels, T_3 resin uptake, and corrected measures of FT_4 (e.g., FT_4 index) as the tests for thyrotoxicosis. FT_3 levels are elevated in all patients and are used to monitor response to therapy or in mild states of hyperthyroidism (T_3 toxicosis) where serum FT_4 levels are normal. In Graves' disease and toxic multinodular goiter, T_3 levels typically are higher than T_4 levels (T_3[ng/dL]/T_4[μg/dL] ratio >20).

Thyroid Antibody Testing

Antithyroglobulin and antimicrosomal antibodies are directed toward the detection of cytoplasmic antibodies. These antibodies are usually present in patients with autoimmune thyroid disease, Graves' disease, and Hashimoto's thyroiditis. They are rarely present in patients with other types of thyroiditis. The TSH receptor-binding inhibitory immunoglobulins radioreceptor assay and thyroid-stimulating immunoglobulins bioassay detect antibodies to the TSH receptor, which, if present, are indicative of Graves' thyrotoxicosis.

Imaging

In general, radioisotope imaging of the thyroid is not necessary in all patients with thyrotoxicosis. Scanning may be useful to assess the function of a single nodule in the presence of biochemical evidence of hyperthyroidism, to evaluate the function of nodules in toxic multinodular goiter, to diagnose subacute thyroiditis when other clinical features are absent (i.e., absent uptake in the presence of hyperthyroidism), to confirm the diagnosis of thyrotoxicosis factitia, and to differentiate between silent or postpartum thyroiditis and Graves' disease in the postpartum patient (see Table 42-1).

Management and Therapy

Optimum Treatment

Graves' Disease

Graves' disease is an autoimmune disorder characterized by spontaneous remission and relapse. The three options for managing Graves' disease are antithyroid drugs, radioactive iodine ablation, and surgery. All three options have been shown to be effective, and treatment preferences vary globally. Within the United States, radioiodine ablation is generally preferred as optimal treatment, whereas antithyroid drugs are more popular in Europe and Japan. Antithyroid drugs (e.g., thiourea and β blockers) are the recommended treatment for pregnant women, children, and adolescents and for initial treatment of clinically significant hyperthyroidism. The thionamide antithyroid drugs propylthiouracil (PTU) and methimazole act as competitive inhibitors of thyroid peroxidase to effectively reduce thyroid hormone production. PTU in higher doses may also have the advantage of inhibiting peripheral conversion of T_4 to T_3. These agents may also possess inherent immune-modulating effects that modify the disease pathophysiology. The usual starting doses are PTU, 100 mg every 8 hours, or methimazole, 10 to 30 mg once

daily. For compliance reasons, evidence of increased potency, and lower complication rates, methimazole is preferred. Major side effects develop within the first 3 months of therapy and include agranulocytosis; hepatic dysfunction; a lupus-like syndrome; vasculitis; and, more commonly, skin rash, fever, urticaria, and arthralgia. Patients should be warned about symptoms of fever and sore throat, which are typically seen with agranulocytosis. Follow-up every 4 to 6 weeks is recommended to assess clinical status and thyroid function tests (TSH, T_3 and T_4). The length of treatment is variable, but treatment for about 18 months results in long-term remission in 30% to 40% of cases. Patients with milder disease and small goiters are more likely to fully respond to a course of antithyroid medications and remain in disease remission. Therapy may be discontinued if the patient has been euthyroid for 18 months and the serum TSH is not suppressed. Most relapses occur within the first 6 months. A high dose of thiourea agents plus T_4 replacement technique may result in a higher rate of sustained remission.

For symptomatic relief of hyperthyroidism, β-adrenoceptor antagonists block the peripheral effects of thyroid hormone excess and the peripheral conversion of T_4 to T_3. They are contraindicated in patients with asthma or chronic lung disease. Cardiac failure secondary to thyrotoxicosis is a relative contraindication. The most experience is with propranolol, 40 mg every 8 hours. These agents are given in conjunction with thiourea agents as first-line therapy to provide symptomatic relief of tremor, palpitations, anxiety, and heat intolerance.

For patients with more significant hyperthyroidism and larger goiters, radioactive iodine therapy or surgery is considered (usually subtotal thyroidectomy); radioactive iodine therapy is the preferred treatment in the United States. The decision to proceed to more definitive therapy is governed by the preference of the patient and the treating clinician. Radioactive iodine will provide an effective cure after a single dose of therapy in 70% to 90% of patients. Most centers give a moderate dose of iodine (15 mCi) to ensure adequate ablation of the thyroid gland. The patient is instructed to cease antithyroid therapy 4 to 7 days before the dose of radioactive iodine and then to recommence therapy 2 days after the therapy. Most patients may experience a dry mouth and transient pain in the thyroid and salivary glands during therapy and for a short time afterward and may be rendered hypothyroid 4 to 12 weeks after therapy. The patients must understand that they will become permanently hypothyroid and will require lifelong thyroid hormone replacement. Radioactive iodine is not contraindicated in younger patients or women of childbearing age unless they are pregnant. A pregnancy test is required in women of childbearing age before the administration of therapy.

The effectiveness of radioactive iodine and antithyroid agents has diminished the role of surgery. Thyroidectomy is considered in special circumstances such as patient preference, poor response to antithyroid drugs, nodular or very large goiters, or coexistence of a potentially malignant thyroid nodule.

Second-line agents to treat hyperthyroidism include iodide, iodinated contrast agents, and lithium carbonate.

Autonomous Functioning Nodules

Radioactive iodine is the therapy of choice with a toxic multinodular goiter. Higher doses (in the order of 30 mCi) are usually used to achieve euthyroidism. Radioactive iodine therapy is also successful in patients with a single hot nodule, but repeated doses are often required. An antithyroid drug may be considered to reduce the risk for treatment-induced thyrotoxicosis and to attain euthyroidism faster. Near-total thyroidectomy is also an option. In Europe, percutaneous injection of nodules with ethanol is gaining popularity, but this is rarely used in the United States.

Thyroiditis

Thyroiditis is a self-limited disease in which the hyperthyroidism results from the release of stored thyroid hormone into the circulation. Pain associated with subacute thyroiditis is treated with aspirin or nonsteroidal anti-inflammatory drugs, if mild, or with steroids (prednisone, 30 mg daily, rapidly tapered over a few days) if severe. The hyperthyroidism is treated with β blockers if necessary. Treatment of subsequent hypothyroidism is usually unnecessary, although up to half of patients with silent thyroiditis eventually develop permanent hypothyroidism.

Iodine-Induced Hyperthyroidism

Iodine-induced hyperthyroidism is an extremely difficult condition to treat. Higher doses of thiourea agents are needed to control the hyperthyroidism. If possible, iodine consumption should be reduced, and perchlorate may in addition be useful to block iodine uptake into the gland. Steroid therapy may be useful in amiodarone-induced thyrotoxicosis. Radioactive iodine uptake assessments are useful to determine the degree of uptake before initiation of radioactive iodine (^{131}I) therapy. Early surgery should be considered if no other option is available and the patient is not responding to other therapeutic approaches.

Avoiding Treatment Errors

When following patients on antithyroid drugs, it is recommended to check thyroid function tests (i.e., TSH, T_3, T_4) every 4 to 6 weeks initially until thyroid function is stable. Because thyrotropin levels remain suppressed for weeks to months, it is recommended to follow T_3 and T_4 levels. T_4 levels may normalize more rapidly than T_3 levels, so it is important to follow the T_3 levels to adjust the medication dosage. It is recommended to check the complete blood count before initiation of antithyroid drugs because of the risk for agranulocytosis.

Future Directions

Ongoing research is focused on finding causes of autoimmune hyperthyroidism through genetic and molecular techniques to develop more effective treatments. For example, the molecular diagnosis of hereditary nonautoimmune hyperthyroidism has led to consideration of genetic counseling and primary thyroid ablation in individuals found to have the activated TSH receptor germline mutation.

Additional Resources

American Thyroid Association Website. Available at: http://www.thyroid.org. Accessed October 15, 2006.

The ATA is the professional organization of physicians and scientists dedicated to the research and treatment of thyroid disorders. This website has printable patient handouts in English and Spanish.

Thyroid Disease Manager Website. Available at: http://www.thyroidmanager.org/. Accessed October 15, 2006.

This website is designed to assist physicians caring for patients with thyroid disease with accessible text related to all types of thyroid disease.

EVIDENCE

1. Allahabadia A, Daykin J, Sheppard MC, et al: Radioiodine treatment of hyperthyroidism: Prognostic factors for outcome. J Clin Endocrinol Metab 86(8):3611-3617, 2001.

   This is a retrospective review of high- and low-dose radioactive iodine ablation therapy for patients with Graves' disease.

2. Cooper DS: Hyperthyroidism. Lancet 362(9382):459-468, 2003.

   The author provides an up-to-date clinical review of the etiology and management of hyperthyroidism.

3. Cooper DS: Treatment of thyrotoxicosis. In Braverman LE, Utiger RD (eds): Werner and Ingbar's The Thyroid: A Fundamental and Clinical Text, 8th ed. Philadelphia, Lippincott Williams & Wilkins, 2000, pp 691-715.

   This classic textbook chapter is on the management of hyperthyroidism.

4. Fuhrer D, Warner J, Sequeira M, et al: Novel TSHR germline (Met463Val) masquerading as Graves disease in a large Welsh kindred with hyperthyroidism. Thyroid 10(12):1035-1041, 2000.

   This research paper details nonautoimmune hereditary hyperthyroidism.

5. Reinwein D, Benker G, Lazarus JH, Alexander WD: A prospective randomized trial of antithyroid drug dose in Graves disease therapy. European Multicenter Study Group on Antithyroid Drug Treatment. J Clin Endocrinol Metab 76(6):1516-1521, 1993.

   The authors describe a randomized trial comparing 10 mg versus 40 mg of methimazole in remission rates of Graves' disease in a European iodine-deficient population.

6. Roti E, Gardini E, Minelli R, et al: Sodium ipodate and methimazole in the long-term treatment of hyperthyroid Graves' disease. Metabolism 42(4):403-408, 1993.

   The authors review of the use of antithyroid drugs and sodium ipodate in Graves' disease.

7. Weetman AP: How antithyroid drugs work in Graves disease. Clin Endocrinol (Oxf) 37(4):317-318, 1992.

   The author reviews antithyroid drug pharmacology.

Sue A. Brown

Hyperparathyroidism

Introduction

Hyperparathyroidism is characterized by an elevation in serum parathyroid hormone (PTH) levels. The parathyroid glands synthesize and secrete PTH, which elevates calcium levels to maintain ionized calcium within a narrow physiologic range. PTH stimulates renal conversion of 25-hydroxyvitamin D to 1,25-dihydroxyvitamin D (calcitriol), which increases intestinal calcium absorption. PTH also acts to stimulate bone turnover, thereby releasing calcium and phosphorus from the bone matrix (Fig. 43-1). Appropriate homeostatic increases in PTH can occur from secondary causes; however, this chapter focuses on the inappropriate PTH levels that occur in primary hyperparathyroidism.

Etiology and Pathogenesis

Primary hyperparathyroidism results when the parathyroid glands hypertrophy and secrete excess PTH. Most individuals have four parathyroid glands, located in proximity to the thyroid gland. However, a wide range of variation exists in number and location. Two to eight glands may be found throughout the neck or mediastinum in normal individuals. Most individuals with primary hyperparathyroidism have a solitary parathyroid adenoma (80% to 85%). The remainder have diffuse hyperplasia (12% to 15%), double or triple adenomas (2%), or rarely, parathyroid carcinoma (<1%).

Although most cases are sporadic, there are familial forms of hyperparathyroidism that occur as part of the multiple endocrine neoplasia (MEN) syndromes. About 95% of individuals with MEN 1 have primary hyperparathyroidism along with pituitary and pancreatic tumors. Hyperparathyroidism occurs to a lesser extent in MEN 2a (20% to 30%) in conjunction with pheochromocytomas and medullary thyroid cancer. MEN 2b, which includes neuromas, does not generally have primary hyperparathyroidism as a feature. These familial forms have four-gland hyperplasia and require bilateral neck dissection for therapy.

Clinical Presentation

Primary hyperparathyroidism is usually asymptomatic (75% to 80%) and diagnosed when biochemical screening reveals hypercalcemia. Symptoms vary depending on the level and duration of hypercalcemia (Fig. 43-2). Common symptoms include fatigue, constipation, polyuria, polydipsia, bone pain, and nausea. Neuropsychiatric symptoms (depression, memory loss, headaches) are reported frequently, but their relation to hypercalcemia is less clear because they do not always reverse with its correction. Nephrolithiasis is the most frequent overt complication, occurring in 15% to 20% of individuals. Nephrocalcinosis occurs infrequently. Bone disease is a prominent feature, with osteopenia or osteoporosis and, rarely, osteitis fibrosa cystica. Cortical bone (e.g., the distal radius) is affected more often than cancellous or trabecular bone (e.g., the vertebral column). Thus, bone loss is greater at the distal radius than in the spine. The hip is a mixture of both types of bone and is intermediate in its bone density. Despite decreased bone density, the fracture risk has not been adequately characterized. Cardiovascular manifestations may include hypertension, left ventricular hypertrophy, and myocardial and valvular calcifications. Neuromuscular symptoms occur but are less prominent, and proximal muscle weakness with type II muscle cell atrophy is quite rare. Occasionally, pancreatitis or peptic ulcer disease complicates the clinical course, as do gout and pseudogout.

Differential Diagnosis

The diagnosis is usually made after hypercalcemia is identified. Primary hyperparathyroidism and malignancies

Figure 43-1 Physiology of the Parathyroid Glands.

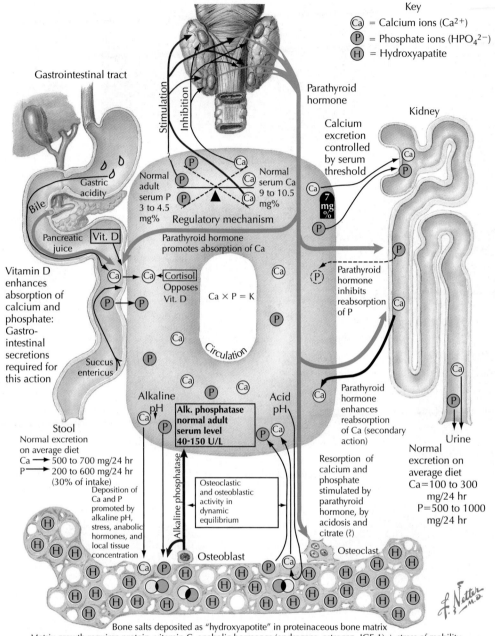

Bone salts deposited as "hydroxyapotite" in proteinaceous bone matrix
Matrix growth requires protein, vitamin C, anabolic hormones (androgens, estrogen, IGF-1) + stress of mobility
Matrix resorption favored by catabolic hormones (11-oxysteroids [cortisol], thyroid), parathyroid hormone + immobilization

account for about 90% of cases of hypercalcemia. Malignancies include multiple myeloma, lymphomas, and prostate, breast, and squamous cell lung carcinomas. Malignant tumors rarely secrete PTH, more often secreting PTH-related peptide, which does not cross-react on the current intact PTH assays. Certain medications cause hypercalcemia and may unmask underlying primary hyperparathyroidism. Thiazide diuretics decrease urinary calcium excretion and may affect the responsiveness of target cells to PTH. Lithium also increases urinary calcium retention

and may directly promote secretion of PTH. Additional causes include other endocrine disorders (hyperthyroidism, primary adrenal insufficiency, and less commonly, hypothyroidism and pheochromocytoma), milk alkali syndrome, excessive vitamin A or D intake, granulomatous disorders (sarcoidosis, tuberculosis), and immobilization. Generally, these conditions have suppressed PTH levels and can be readily distinguished from primary hyperparathyroidism. Benign familial hypocalciuric hypercalcemia is an autosomal dominant condition that causes asymptom-

Figure 43-2 Pathology and Clinical Manifestations of Hyperparathyroidism.

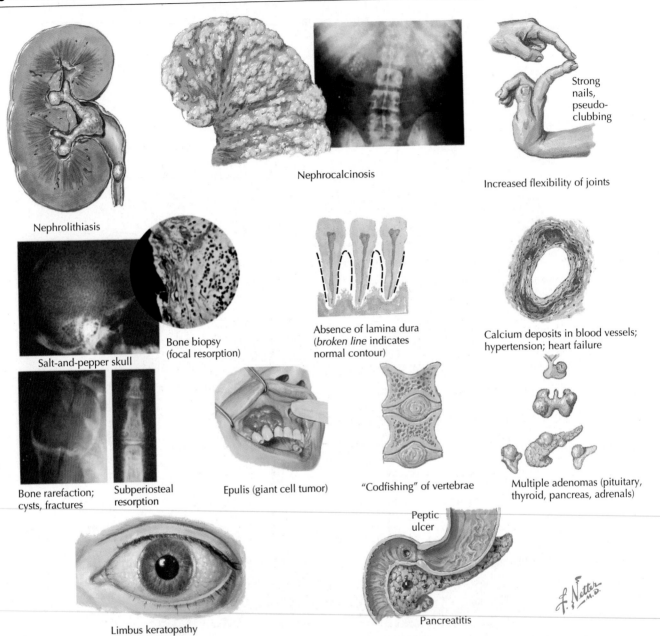

Nephrolithiasis

Nephrocalcinosis

Strong nails, pseudo-clubbing

Increased flexibility of joints

Salt-and-pepper skull

Bone biopsy (focal resorption)

Absence of lamina dura (*broken line* indicates normal contour)

Calcium deposits in blood vessels; hypertension; heart failure

Bone rarefaction; cysts, fractures

Subperiosteal resorption

Epulis (giant cell tumor)

"Codfishing" of vertebrae

Multiple adenomas (pituitary, thyroid, pancreas, adrenals)

Peptic ulcer

Limbus keratopathy

Pancreatitis

atic hypercalcemia with low urinary calcium excretion (<100 mg/day) and usually normal PTH levels. An inactivating mutation of the calcium receptor gene is the common primary underlying abnormality that should be suspected in individuals with a strong family history of hypercalcemia. It is important to diagnose this condition with a 24-hour urinary calcium measurement because these individuals do not require any surgical therapy.

Secondary hyperparathyroidism occurs commonly but is characterized by low or normal serum calcium levels. The elevated PTH often occurs as a physiologic response to conditions that cause hypocalcemia, such as vitamin D deficiency and acute hyperphosphatemia (tumor lysis syn-

drome, acute renal failure, and rhabdomyolysis). It is seen most commonly in renal insufficiency, particularly when renal 1,25-dihydroxyvitamin D production is impaired, with subsequent decreased intestinal calcium absorption. In long-standing renal failure, the parathyroid glands become autonomous, and a condition of tertiary hyperparathyroidism can develop, with PTH levels often greater than 2 to 3 times normal.

Diagnostic Approach

The diagnosis of primary hyperparathyroidism is usually straightforward and only requires the demonstration of elevated PTH levels in the setting of hypercalcemia. The calcium level should be confirmed because venipuncture alone can falsely elevate the serum level. A PTH determination should be performed using the two-site immunoassay. Radiologic studies are not necessary to confirm the diagnosis, but they may be important when considering surgical management. PTH can be in the normal range in some individuals, which is inappropriate for an elevated calcium level. Less commonly, the calcium level remains normal, while the PTH level is elevated. A search for a secondary cause should be considered in these cases, particularly ruling out vitamin D deficiency by measuring 25-hydroxyvitamin D levels. In primary hyperparathyroidism alone, 25-hydroxyvitamin D levels tend to be at the lower end of the normal range, with 1,25-dihydroxyvitamin D levels being normal or even elevated (PTH drives the conversion of 25-hydroxyvitamin D to 1,25-dihydroxyvitamin D).

Although phosphorus is released from bone, there is an increase in urinary phosphorus excretion induced by hyperparathyroidism. Serum phosphorus is, therefore, usually low or at the lower end of normal range. Typically, total urinary calcium excretion is at the upper end of normal, with up to 40% of patients being hypercalciuric (>300 mg/day). Other bone turnover markers (e.g., alkaline phosphatase, urinary *N*-telopeptides, deoxypyridinoline) tend to be elevated, but usually do not aid in the diagnosis or management of primary hyperparathyroidism.

Management and Therapy

Optimum Treatment

Primary hyperparathyroidism can be cured by surgical removal of the parathyroid glands and generally represents the preferred therapy for symptomatic patients. Current accepted surgical indications in symptomatic patients include nephrolithiasis or nephrocalcinosis, osteitis fibrosa cystica, classic neuromuscular disease, or an acute episode of severe hypercalcemia. An experienced surgeon performing a bilateral neck exploration can achieve cure rates of more than 90% (defined as a reduction in serum calcium and PTH levels), with a less than 1% operative mortality rate. Surgical morbidity is low (<5%) but can include bleeding, recurrent laryngeal nerve damage, and rarely, hypoparathyroidism. Many symptoms or signs may improve after parathyroidectomy. There is a significant reduction in recurrent nephrolithiasis after surgery, although no significant improvement in renal insufficiency occurs. Bone mineral density (BMD) also improves consistently by 6% in the first year and up to 10% to 12% after 10 years. Interestingly, BMD gains are usually greatest in cancellous bone and less so in cortical bone. There are conflicting data regarding reduction in fracture risk, with some retrospective studies suggesting a decreased risk and others showing

no change. Classic symptoms of osteitis fibrosa cystica and neuromuscular disease are rare today and can be reversed by surgery. In contrast, cardiac manifestations do not necessarily reverse after surgery, causing some to question their causal association. Specifically, hypertension does not usually improve after parathyroidectomy. Left ventricular hypertrophy may or may not regress after surgery, and cardiac calcifications usually remain unchanged. Neuropsychiatric symptoms also do not improve consistently. The role of surgery in asymptomatic individuals is less clear and continues to be debated. The National Institutes of Health convened a consensus conference in 2002 on the management of asymptomatic primary hyperparathyroidism. The updated recommendations for surgical intervention include the following: total serum calcium levels >1 mg/dL above normal reference ranges, urinary calcium excretion >400 mg/day, reduced creatinine clearance by 30% without other causes, age less than 50 years, and decreased BMD at any site less than 2.5 standard deviations below peak bone density (T score <−2.5).

These recommendations are largely based on expert opinion because few randomized controlled trials exist. One important longitudinal observational study of mild primary hyperparathyroidism enrolled 61 subjects who underwent parathyroidectomy; 60 subjects who did not were followed for 10 years. Surgical management resulted in normalization of biochemical parameters (calcium, PTH, and urinary calcium excretion) that persisted at 10-year follow-up study. There were no recurrences of nephrolithiasis. Subjects had sustained improvements in BMD at the femoral neck and spine throughout the study period (14% and 12% increases over 10 years, respectively). The untreated group also did well overall, with remarkable stability in their disease parameters over 10 years. There was little progression of hypercalcemia or worsening of biochemical profiles. BMD at the spine, hip, and distal radius was unchanged, which was unexpected given that the average age of subjects was 58 years and that more than half of the subjects were postmenopausal women. Subgroup analysis suggested that perimenopausal women did continue to lose bone mass at rates similar to those of normocalcemic healthy women. Additionally, 27% had the development of one or more new indications for parathyroidectomy (calcium >12 mg/dL, increased urinary calcium excretion or distal radius Z score <−2.0). Taken together, these data demonstrate that surgery results in lasting improvements in biochemical parameters and BMD changes, whereas untreated groups overall did not have significant progression. Both sides of the debate have used these data to support their positions. In general, it is thought that additional factors favoring surgical management should include recent fracture in the absence of major trauma; moderate to severe vitamin D deficiency (<15 ng/mL); and perimenopausal women.

The traditional initial surgical approach is bilateral neck dissection. This approach is favored by many experienced surgeons. Because most individuals have a solitary adenoma, surgical techniques for localized exploration (often termed "minimally invasive") have been developed. These are dependent on adequate preoperative or intraoperative localization of the adenoma. Preoperative localization studies include ultrasound, nuclear imaging with technetium-sestamibi scans, computed tomography, magnetic resonance imaging, and selective venous catheterization for PTH measurements. Intraoperative techniques for localization include rapid PTH assays as well as use of sestamibi gamma probes, which allow less extensive and shorter operations. The impact of this approach on surgical cure rates is not proved. Local preferences are important because individual surgeons and institutions have variable expertise in these techniques. For persistent or recurrent disease, there is little debate that bilateral neck dissection is necessary. In this setting, preoperative localization increases the cure rate from about 60% to more than 90%.

Medical therapy should be considered for symptomatic patients awaiting surgery and in those for whom surgery is not an option. Outpatients with mild to moderate hypercalcemia should consume 1 to 1.5 L of fluid per day. Although moderate calcium dietary intake should be maintained, medications such as thiazides, which exacerbate hypercalcemia, should be discontinued. Oral bisphosphonates can be used to decrease bone turnover and improve BMD, but they do not necessarily alter calcium or PTH levels, as reported in a 2-year randomized controlled trial of alendronate. Intermittent intravenous bisphosphonates are another alternative but are rarely used in outpatients except those with severe hypercalcemia awaiting or unable to have surgery (e.g., pamidronate, 30 to 60 mg intravenously every 3 months). Estrogen and progestin therapy has been given to reduce bone resorption, particularly in perimenopausal women, without adversely affecting PTH levels. A calcium-sensing receptor mimetic, cinacalcet, has been studied in mild primary hyperparathyroidism and is effective in lowering calcium at 1 year with a reduction in PTH but no improvement in BMD. Cinacalcet works by mimicking the effect of calcium on the calcium-sensing receptor, which results in lower PTH secretion. However, its use is limited by cost and lack of long-term data. All patients should be encouraged to exercise to maintain bone mass. Calcium levels should be assessed every 4 to 6 months and PTH and creatinine measured at least yearly.

Avoiding Treatment Errors

Furosemide use for outpatient mild hypercalcemia (20 to 40 mg orally once daily) is often not very effective; if used, it is important that adequate hydration be maintained. Patients with primary hyperparathyroidism often have coexistent vitamin D deficiency. Replacement of vitamin D may be necessary, particularly in patients in whom medical rather than surgical therapy will be pursued. Generally, vitamin D, 400 to 800 IU per day, is safe and does not result in significant hypercalcemia. However, more aggressive vitamin D repletion regimens (e.g., 50,000 IU ergocalciferol once a week for 8 weeks) may result in hypercalcemia.

Future Directions

Surgical approaches will continue to be refined, and data will be forthcoming comparing various techniques. Ongoing clinical studies should provide a better understanding of fracture risks and the surgical indications in patients with cardiac and neuropsychiatric manifestations. Future studies should also clarify the role of calcimimetic agents and bisphosphonates in the management of primary hyperparathyroidism.

Additional Resources

Eigelberger MS, Clark OH: Surgical approaches to primary hyperparathyroidism. Endocrinol Metab Clin North Am 29(3):479-502, 2000.
   This paper succinctly outlines an approach to the surgical management of primary hyperparathyroidism.
Silverberg SJ, Bilezikian JP: The diagnosis and management of asymptomatic primary hyperparathyroidism. Nat Clin Pract Endocrinol Metab 2(9):494-503, 2006.
   The authors present a good recent clinical review of the approach to asymptomatic primary hyperparathyroidism.

EVIDENCE

1. Bilezikian JP, Potts JT Jr, Fuleihan Gel-H, et al: Summary statement from a workshop on asymptomatic primary hyperparathyroidism: A perspective for the 21st century. J Clin Endocrinol Metab 87(12):5353-5361, 2002.
   This article summarizes the key recommendation from an expert panel NIH consensus conference on the management of asymptomatic primary hyperparathyroidism.
2. Khan AA, Bilezikian JP, Kung AW, et al: Alendronate in primary hyperparathyroidism: A double-blind, randomized, placebo-controlled trial. J Clin Endocrinol Metab 89(7):3319-3325, 2004.
   These data support the use of alendronate in primary hyperparathyroidism. This is one of the few randomized, placebo-controlled trials on pharmacologic interventions.
3. Peacock M, Bilezikian JP, Klassen PS, et al: Cinacalcet hydrochloride maintains long-term normocalcemia in patients with primary hyperparathyroidism. J Clin Endocrinol Metab 90(1):135-141, 2005.
   This short-term, small study provides information on a novel agent, cinacalcet, when used in maintenance of normocalcemia.
4. Silverberg SJ, Shane E, Jacobs TP, et al: A 10-year prospective study of primary hyperparathyroidism with or without parathyroid surgery. N Engl J Med 341(17):1249-1255, 1999.
   This key study presents the data regarding long-term outcomes in patients who were treated for primary hyperparathyroidism with or without parathyroid surgery.

David A. Ontjes

44

Disorders of the Adrenal Cortex

Introduction

Adrenocorticotropic hormone (ACTH) is the chief determinant of the secretion of cortisol and androgenic steroids by the adrenal cortex. ACTH secretion is controlled by corticotropin-releasing hormone (CRH) from the hypothalamus (Fig. 44-1). At any given moment, ACTH secretion represents a balance between the stimulatory effects of the central nervous system, mediated by CRH, and negative feedback control exerted by circulating glucocorticoids. The secretion of both CRH and ACTH is subject to a diurnal rhythm, reaching a peak at about the time of awakening in the morning, and a nadir in the evening before sleep. Stressful stimuli such as trauma, infection, hemorrhage, or hypoglycemia normally activate CRH and ACTH secretion, causing cortisol levels to rise.

Aldosterone secretion is governed by the renin-angiotensin system (see Fig. 44-1). The chief determinant of aldosterone secretion is angiotensin II, which is generated under the influence of renin. Reduced systemic blood pressure and reduced renal perfusion are responsible for causing the release of renin. In humans, the synthesis of aldosterone is confined to the outer glomerulosa layer of the adrenal cortex; cortisol and androgens are produced by the fasciculata and reticularis layers.

The steroid products of both the adrenal glands and the gonads are derived from a series of biosynthetic steps beginning with cholesterol (Fig. 44-2). The glucocorticoid, cortisol, and the mineralocorticoid, aldosterone, are the most active and important hormones produced by the adrenal cortex. The enzymes involved in steroidogenesis are members of a family of cytochrome P450 oxidases. Each individual enzyme is capable of handling more than one substrate. As a result, a few distinct enzymes are capable of catalyzing transformations leading to more than a dozen steroid products. In the testes, an additional enzyme is present that converts the weak adrenal androgen androstenedione into testosterone. In the ovaries, an aromatase enzyme converts testosterone to estradiol. These terminal steps in the gonads do not occur to an appreciable extent in normal adrenal glands.

ADRENAL INSUFFICIENCY

Adrenal insufficiency arises whenever the quantity of circulating cortisol is insufficient to meet the needs of the body. Under basal conditions, cortisol is needed to maintain normal vascular tone, normal hepatic gluconeogenesis, and normal glycogen stores (hence the name glucocorticoid). Higher concentrations are needed during stress. Lack of adequate cortisol can lead to hypotension, shock, and hypoglycemia. Patients with cortisol deficiency may have variable deficiencies of aldosterone and adrenal androgens as well. Mineralocorticoid deficiency leads to renal wasting of sodium, retention of potassium, and a reduced intravascular volume. Adrenal androgen deficiency leads to a significant reduction of the overall androgen supply in women and can result in a loss of body hair and libido. In men who maintain normal testosterone production from the gonads, loss of adrenal androgens does not lead to an overall androgen deficiency.

Etiology and Pathogenesis

Any disease process causing direct injury to the adrenal cortex can cause primary adrenal insufficiency. Diseases affecting the hypothalamus or pituitary cause secondary adrenal insufficiency by reducing the secretion of ACTH (Box 44-1).

Primary adrenal insufficiency (Addison's disease) is most commonly the result of chronic autoimmune destruction of the adrenal cortex. Lymphocytic infiltration is the usual histologic feature. The adrenal glands are small, and cortical cells are largely absent, although the medulla is preserved. Antibodies to adrenal cortical antigens, including the enzyme 21-hydroxylase, are present early in the disease process. Patients with autoimmune adrenal disease are more likely to have polyglandular autoimmune syndromes causing deficiency of other endocrine glands, including the thyroid, parathyroids, gonads, and pancreatic β cells.

Several other mechanisms can cause primary adrenal insufficiency. Bilateral adrenal hemorrhage occurs in critically ill patients who are taking anticoagulants or who have coagulopathies. The primary antiphospholipid antibody syndrome (lupus anticoagulant) is a common cause of adrenal hemorrhage. The importance of tuberculosis as a cause of adrenal insufficiency has waned in the United States, but not in other parts of the world where it is common. Up to 5% of patients with terminal AIDS may have evidence of adrenal insufficiency, usually due to superinfection with agents such as cytomegalovirus.

The congenital adrenal hyperplasia syndromes are due to inherited defects in specific enzymes involved in the biosynthetic pathway for cortisol production (see Fig. 44-2). The mode of inheritance is usually autosomal recessive. The most common inherited deficiency is of 21-hydroxylase, followed by 11-hydroxylase. These disorders may cause a deficiency of cortisol, aldosterone, or both, and present in infants and children with acute adrenal insufficiency. There is a characteristic overproduction of steroid precursors before the defective enzyme step. In 21-hydroxylase deficiency, these precursors give rise to excessive production of adrenal androgens.

Clinical Presentation

Acute adrenal insufficiency or adrenal crisis should be suspected in patients with unexplained volume depletion and shock, often accompanied by hyperkalemia, acidosis, or hypoglycemia. Chronic insufficiency usually develops more insidiously with symptoms such as weakness, weight loss, anorexia, and postural hypotension. Increased skin pigmentation develops in patients with primary, but not

Figure 44-1 Control of the Secretion of Cortisol and Aldosterone.

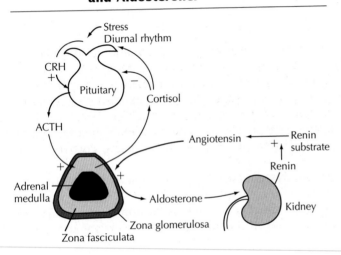

Figure 44-2 Synthetic Pathways for the Adrenal Steroids.

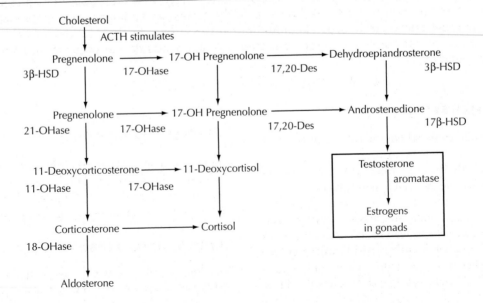

Box 44-1   Causes of Adrenal Insufficiency

Primary Insufficiency

Autoimmune destruction
Infectious diseases (tuberculosis, histoplasmosis, HIV)
Iatrogenic destruction (bilateral adrenalectomy)
Infiltrative diseases (metastatic tumors, amyloidosis, hemochromatosis)
Acute bilateral adrenal hemorrhage
Adrenal leukodystrophy
Congenital adrenal hyperplasias

Secondary Insufficiency

Pituitary or hypothalamic tumors
Iatrogenic ablation (hypophysectomy, radiation therapy)
Pituitary infarction (postpartum necrosis or apoplexy)
Infection (tuberculosis, syphilis)
Sarcoidosis and granulomatous diseases
Idiopathic hypopituitarism
Withdrawal of high dose glucocorticoid therapy

---

secondary, chronic insufficiency due to the melanocyte-stimulating activity of chronically high levels of ACTH and related peptides (Fig. 44-3).

Differential Diagnosis

Volume depletion and vascular collapse can occur with a large number of other conditions causing hypotension, including hemorrhage and sepsis. There are fewer conditions that mimic chronic adrenal insufficiency. Among these are chronic starvation (anorexia nervosa); chronic gastrointestinal disease (inflammation or malignancy); other diseases causing hyperpigmentation (drugs and heavy metals); or fatigue and lassitude (chronic fatigue syndrome). A high level of clinical suspicion is the key to correct diagnosis of both acute and chronic adrenal insufficiency.

Diagnostic Approach

Confirmation of a suspected clinical diagnosis consists of demonstrating inappropriately low cortisol secretion, determining whether the low cortisol level is due to a deficiency of ACTH, and seeking a treatable cause. Baseline measurements of plasma cortisol and ACTH are best obtained in the early morning when levels of both are normally high. A very low morning cortisol level of less than 3 µg/dL strongly suggests adrenal insufficiency, whereas a level of less than 10 µg/dL should arouse suspicion. Administration of synthetic ACTH (cosyntropin) helps in defining adrenal insufficiency in borderline situations and in distinguishing primary from secondary adrenal insufficiency. Normal subjects show a peak cortisol response to greater than 20 µg/dL after cosyntropin, whereas patients with both primary and secondary adrenal insufficiency do not. Primary and secondary insufficiency may then be distinguished by the baseline levels of ACTH, which are high in primary insufficiency only (Fig. 44-4).

Figure 44-3 Chronic Primary Adrenal Cortical Insufficiency (Addison's Disease).

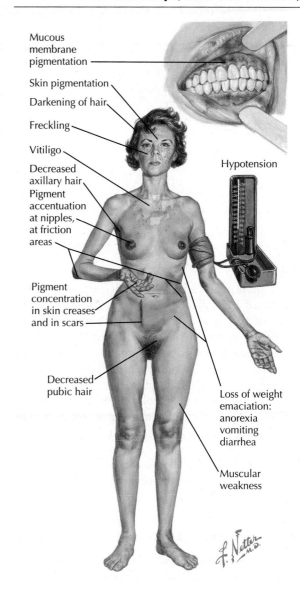

Mucous membrane pigmentation
Skin pigmentation
Darkening of hair
Freckling
Vitiligo
Decreased axillary hair
Pigment accentuation at nipples, at friction areas
Pigment concentration in skin creases and in scars
Decreased pubic hair
Hypotension
Loss of weight emaciation: anorexia vomiting diarrhea
Muscular weakness

In addition, patients with primary insufficiency fail to respond to repeated administration of cosyntropin, whereas patients with secondary insufficiency show an increasing response to repeated testing. In the early stages of primary insufficiency, some patients show evidence of aldosterone deficiency before developing cortisol deficiency. These individuals have low serum levels of aldosterone and high levels of plasma renin activity even before abnormalities in cortisol secretion can be demonstrated.

Patients suspected of having adrenal insufficiency due to congenital adrenal hyperplasia may be diagnosed with the aid of cortisol and ACTH measurements, but further measurement of specific steroid intermediates is essential to identify the specific enzyme defect. For example, in patients with the common form of 21-hydroxylase deficiency, plasma levels of 17-hydroxyprogesterone are markedly elevated (see Fig. 44-2).

Figure 44-4 Outline of Tests for the Differential Diagnosis of Adrenal Insufficiency.

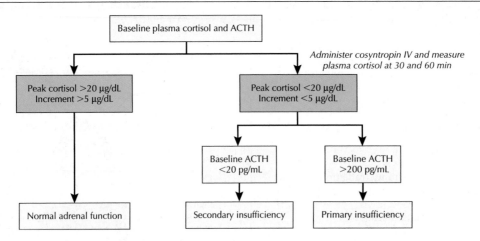

Management and Therapy

Treatment of primary adrenal insufficiency consists of replacement of both glucocorticoids and mineralocorticoids. A combination of hydrocortisone or prednisone, to meet the glucocorticoid requirement, and fludrocortisone, to meet the mineralocorticoid requirement, is usually required. Patients with secondary insufficiency may not require a mineralocorticoid because aldosterone production remains responsive to control by renin and angiotensin. In monitoring therapy, persistent signs and symptoms of adrenal insufficiency should be sought. Periodic laboratory measurement of serum electrolytes, cortisol, and ACTH may also be helpful. Measurement of plasma renin activity is useful in assessing the adequacy of mineralocorticoid replacement.

Avoiding Treatment Errors

During periods of acute illness or stress, the requirement for glucocorticoids typically increases by 2- to 10-fold. To avoid the risk for acute adrenal insufficiency, the dose of glucocorticoid must be increased temporarily until the acute stress is resolved. Patients should carry identification so that unfamiliar caregivers will recognize their need for steroid replacement in case of emergencies. Chronic overtreatment with glucocorticoids can cause insidious side effects, including excessive weight gain, hypertension, glucose intolerance, and osteoporosis. Patients receiving excess glucocorticoid replacement exhibit suppressed early-morning concentrations of serum ACTH.

Optimum Treatment

Patients receiving appropriate replacement therapy for adrenal insufficiency will be well educated about dealing with symptoms of glucocorticoid and mineralocorticoid deficiency during both basal and stress conditions. They will also understand how to avoid the long-term complications of excessive therapy. Optimum therapy for congenital adrenal hyperplasia includes not only providing for basal glucocorticoid and mineralocorticoid requirements but also suppressing the production of excessive steroid byproducts. To suppress excessive androgen production in 21-hydroxylase deficiency, it may be necessary to give high doses of glucocorticoids initially to suppress ACTH and reduce the degree of adrenal hyperplasia. Once control is achieved, the glucocorticoid dose can be reduced for physiologic maintenance.

ADRENOCORTICAL HYPERFUNCTION: CUSHING'S SYNDROME

Chronic glucocorticoid excess leads to a constellation of findings known as Cushing's syndrome. Chronic mineralocorticoid excess leads to a different set of findings, primarily hypertension and hypokalemia.

Etiology and Pathogenesis

Cushing's syndrome is classified as being either ACTH dependent or ACTH independent (Box 44-2).

About 70% of reported cases are due to excess ACTH secretion by a pituitary adenoma (also known as *Cushing's disease*). These adenomas contain basophilic granules and tend to be smaller than adenomas secreting growth hormone or prolactin.

Larger tumors may appear chromophobic on histologic study. ACTH-secreting pituitary tumors usually continue to exhibit feedback suppression by glucocorticoids but require higher than normal levels.

Certain malignant tumors of nonpituitary origin (small cell lung carcinomas, carcinoid tumors, pancreatic islet cell tumors, medullary carcinoma of the thyroid, and pheochromocytomas) have the capacity to secrete ACTH. Ectopic ACTH production accounts for about 10% of all cases of Cushing's syndrome. Typically, these tumors do not exhibit suppression of their production of ACTH,

ACTH Dependent
ACTH-secreting pituitary tumor (Cushing's disease)
ACTH-secreting nonpituitary tumor (ectopic ACTH
    syndrome)
CRH-secreting tumor

ACTH Independent
Cortisol-secreting adrenal tumor; adenoma or carcinoma
Nodular adrenal hyperplasia
Food dependent (GIP-mediated)
Exogenous glucocorticoids (iatrogenic or factitious)

ACTH, adrenocorticotropic hormone; CRH, corticotropin-releasing hormone; GIP, gastric inhibitory peptide.

even at very high glucocorticoid levels. Rarely, a tumor produces ectopic CRH, causing increased ACTH secretion by the normal pituitary gland.

Among the ACTH-independent causes, administration of high doses of exogenous glucocorticoids is by far the most common. Excess production of cortisol by an adrenal tumor is the most common endogenous cause, accounting for about 15% of all spontaneous cases. Food-induced Cushing's syndrome is mediated by gastric inhibitory peptide, which is normally released upon eating and stimulates the adrenal cortex in a few individuals.

Clinical Presentation

Obesity is the most common complaint, occurring in 90% of cases. The distribution of excess fat is typically central, with thin arms and legs (Fig. 44-5). Other features due to chronic glucocorticoid excess include weakening of the connective tissues in the skin (striae, easy bruising), osteoporosis, glucose intolerance, psychiatric disturbances, and increased susceptibility to infections. The manifestations of mineralocorticoid excess include hypertension, edema, hypokalemia, and metabolic alkalosis. Androgen excess in females causes hirsutism, acne, and amenorrhea.

Differential Diagnosis

Most patients with obesity, hypertension, and diabetes mellitus do not have Cushing's syndrome but have exogenous obesity, which is far more common. Most women with obesity, hirsutism, and amenorrhea have the polycystic ovary syndrome, not hypercortisolism. Some patients may have increased secretion of cortisol secondary to another disorder. Examples include patients with primary depression or alcoholism.

Diagnostic Approach

The first step is to demonstrate the presence of inappropriately high cortisol secretion; the second step is to determine the cause of hypercortisolism (Fig. 44-6). The initial step is collection of a 24-hour urine sample for measurement of free cortisol. If this value is normal, the patient is unlikely to have Cushing's syndrome. If the initial cortisol value is elevated, the patient is given a low dose of dexamethasone (2 mg/day for 2 days), and the urine collection is repeated during the second day. If urinary free cortisol is suppressed by more than 50%, the patient is unlikely to have Cushing's syndrome. If low-dose dexamethasone does not suppress the urinary free cortisol by 50%, the suppression test should be repeated with a higher dose of dexamethasone (8 mg/day for 2 days). Patients with an ACTH-producing pituitary tumor usually suppress at the higher dose, whereas patients with adrenal tumors or the ectopic ACTH syndrome do not suppress. The latter two diagnoses may then be distinguished by the baseline ACTH level. In the ectopic ACTH syndrome, ACTH is elevated. In Cushing's syndrome due to functioning adrenal tumors, the ACTH is suppressed.

Magnetic resonance imaging allows visualization of a pituitary tumor in about 80% of cases. If baseline ACTH levels are suppressed, suggesting an adrenal tumor, it is possible to visualize the tumor in 90% of cases with a computed tomography scan of the abdomen.

Management and Therapy

ACTH-secreting pituitary tumors are treated initially by resection, usually through a trans-sphenoidal surgical approach. The cure rate ranges from 60% to 85%. If surgery fails in removing the entire tumor, external pituitary radiation, combined with drug therapy to inhibit cortisol synthesis, induces remissions in most patients. Ketoconazole is the inhibitory drug used most frequently.

Cortisol-secreting adrenal tumors are primarily treated by surgical resection. The cure rate for adenomas is high, but it is much lower for carcinomas because metastases are commonly present at surgery. Second-line therapy for an inoperable tumor involves the use of blockers of cortisol synthesis. Tumors producing ectopic ACTH are almost always malignant. If they are not surgically resectable, they may be controlled with radiation therapy or chemotherapy.

Avoiding Treatment Errors

An accurate diagnosis of the cause of Cushing's syndrome is essential for appropriate therapy. Failure to diagnose an ACTH-secreting pituitary tumor may occur when the tumor is too small to be identified by imaging techniques. Likewise, small nonpituitary tumors producing ACTH ectopically, such as carcinoid tumors of the lung, may be overlooked. In cases in which a tumor is not obvious, direct catheterization of the petrosal sinuses draining the pituitary bed may reveal an ACTH gradient, confirming a pituitary source.

Figure 44-5 Cushing's Syndrome (Clinical Findings).

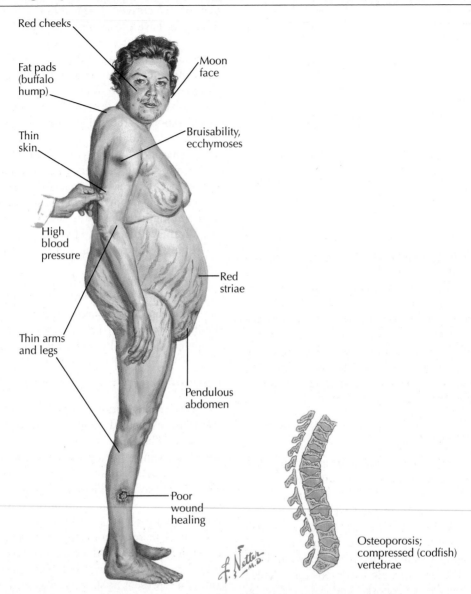

Red cheeks

Fat pads (buffalo hump)

Moon face

Thin skin

Bruisability, ecchymoses

High blood pressure

Red striae

Thin arms and legs

Pendulous abdomen

Poor wound healing

Osteoporosis; compressed (codfish) vertebrae

Figure 44-6 Outline of Tests for the Differential Diagnosis of Cushing's Syndrome.

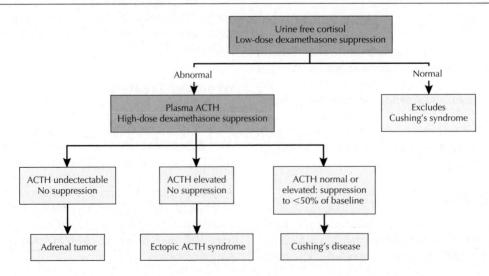

Urine free cortisol
Low-dose dexamethasone suppression

Abnormal

Normal

Plasma ACTH
High-dose dexamethasone suppression

Excludes Cushing's syndrome

ACTH undectectable
No suppression

ACTH elevated
No suppression

ACTH normal or elevated: suppression to <50% of baseline

Adrenal tumor

Ectopic ACTH syndrome

Cushing's disease

Small adrenal cortical tumors are frequently discovered incidentally on computed tomography studies of the abdomen done to investigate an unrelated disease. Although most of these tumors are nonfunctioning, as many as 5% to 10% can produce cortisol and potentially cause Cushing's syndrome. Thus, careful investigation of cortisol secretion is indicated in all patients presenting with adrenal "incidentalomas."

Future Directions

Refinements in the management of adrenal insufficiency are constantly being proposed and tested. The replacement of adrenal androgens, as well as glucocorticoids and mineralocorticoids, may be important in women with adrenal insufficiency. Management of the hyperandrogenism in congenital adrenal hyperplasia continues to be a challenge because the higher doses of glucocorticoids required for full suppression often induce Cushing's syndrome. Drugs capable of blocking androgen receptors may be useful adjuncts in this case. Virilization of the external genitalia in female infants may be reduced by treatment of the mother with dexamethasone during the first trimester of pregnancy.

The accurate diagnosis of ACTH-dependent Cushing syndrome remains difficult in cases in which a pituitary tumor cannot be depicted by current radiologic methods. Improved imaging techniques and petrosal sinus catheterization should identify the correct source of ACTH in all but a few cases.

Additional Resources

Loriaux DL: Adrenal insufficiency. In Becker KL (ed): Principles and Practice of Endocrinology and Metabolism, 3rd ed. Philadelphia, Lippincott Williams & Wilkins, 2001, pp 739-743.
   This reference textbook is available in electronic form through Ovid in participating libraries and institutions.
Schteingart DE: Cushing syndrome. In Becker KL (ed): Principles and Practice of Endocrinology and Metabolism, 3rd ed. Philadelphia, Lippincott Williams & Wilkins, 2001, pp 723-738.
   The author presents a thorough overview of the etiology, diagnosis, and management of Cushing's syndrome.
Speiser PW: Congenital adrenal insufficiency. In Becker KL (ed): Principles and Practice of Endocrinology and Metabolism, 3rd ed. Philadelphia, Lippincott Williams & Wilkins, 2001, pp 743–751.
   This book chapter is a good review of all aspects of congenital adrenal insufficiency, with an emphasis on presentation and management in childhood.

EVIDENCE

1. Bakiri F, Tatai S, Aouali R, et al: Treatment of Cushing's disease by transsphenoidal pituitary microsurgery: Prognosis factors and long-term follow-up. J Endocrinol Invest 19(9):572-580, 1996.
   The authors evaluate long-term results in 50 consecutive patients treated with trans-sphenoidal surgery for ACTH-secreting pituitary tumors.

2. Dittmar M, Kahaly GJ: Polyglandular autoimmune syndromes: Immunogenetics and long-term follow-up. J Clin Endocrinol Metab 88(7):2983-2992, 2003.
   This paper summarizes extensive clinical, epidemiologic, serological and genetic data from 360 patients with polyglandular autoimmune syndrome causing various combinations of type 1 diabetes, autoimmune thyroid disease, Addison's disease, vitiligo, alopecia, hypogonadism and pernicious anemia.

3. Emral R, Uysal AR, Asik M, et al: Prevalence of subclinical Cushing's syndrome in 70 patients with adrenal incidentaloma: Clinical, biochemical and surgical outcomes. Endocr J 50(4):399-408, 2003.
   This evaluation of 70 patients with incidentally discovered adrenal tumors compares the clinical and laboratory features of a subset with subclinical Cushing's syndrome to a larger subset with nonfunctioning tumors.

4. Falorni A, Laureti S, De Bellis A, et al: Italian Addison network study: Update of diagnostic criteria for the etiological classification of primary adrenal insufficiency. J Clin Endocrinol Metab 89(4):1598-1604, 2004.
   This report from the Italian Addison Network on 222 patients with primary adrenal insufficiency documents the value of 21-hydroxylase and adrenal cortex autoantibodies in determining an autoimmune etiology. In this study, 5% of patients had polyglandular autoimmune syndrome, whereas 65% had adrenal autoantibodies without evidence of other autoimmune endocrine diseases.

5. Hammer GD, Tyrrell JB, Lamborn KR, et al: Transsphenoidal microsurgery for Cushing's disease: Initial outcome and long-term results. J Clin Endocrinol Metab 89(12):6348-6357, 2004.
   This retrospective study of 289 patients with Cushing's disease who underwent trans-sphenoidal surgery by a single surgeon for ACTH-secreting pituitary tumors discusses the prognostic factors predicting long-term outcomes.

6. Liu C, Lo JC, Dowd CF, et al: Cavernous and inferior petrosal sinus sampling in the evaluation of ACTH-dependent Cushing syndrome. Clin Endocrinol (Oxf) 61(4):478-486, 2004.
   The authors present a retrospective review of 95 patients undergoing inferior petrosal sinus and cavernous sinus sampling to localize the source of ACTH in ACTH-dependent Cushing's syndrome. These techniques were very accurate in predicting a pituitary source of ACTH, but were not accurate in lateralizing the tumor site within the pituitary.

7. Piedrola G, Casado JL, Lopez E, et al: Clinical features of adrenal insufficiency in patients with acquired immune deficiency syndrome. Clin Endocrinol (Oxf) 45(1):97-101, 1996.
   This retrospective review of 75 AIDS patients with clinical or biochemical manifestations of adrenal insufficiency compares the results of basal and ACTH-stimulated cortisol levels.

8. Yu L, Brewer KW, Gates S, et al: DRB104 and DQ alleles: Expression of 21-hydroxylase autoantibodies and risk of progression to Addison's disease. J Clin Endocrinol Metab 84(1):328-335, 1999.
   An immunogenetic study in 957 patients with type 1 diabetes showed a strong association between the DQ8/DQ2 genotype, the presence of 21-hydroxylase autoantibodies, and the development of Addison's disease.

9. Zelissen PM, Croughs RJ, van Rijk PP, Raymakers JA: Effect of glucocorticoid replacement therapy on bone density in patients with Addison disease. Ann Intern Med 120(3):207-210, 1994.
   In this report on 91 patients with Addison's disease treated with glucocorticoids for a mean of 10.6 years, low bone mineral density was found in 10 of 31 men and 4 of 60 women. In men with low bone mineral density, the mean glucocorticoid dose was significantly higher than in men with normal bone density. There was no correlation between low bone density and glucocorticoid dose in women.

David R. Clemmons

45

Pituitary Diseases

Introduction

The anterior lobe of the pituitary gland produces six polypeptide hormones that regulate the function of other endocrine glands, such as the thyroid and the adrenal glands. The posterior lobe produces hormones that are involved in regulation of salt and water balance. Because of its strategic location, tumors that occur within the sella turcica, the cavernous sinuses, or the hypothalamus can lead to disruption of pituitary hormonal function. From a functional perspective, diseases of the pituitary are grouped into those that destroy or impair hormone function and those that result in increased hormone secretion.

Etiology and Pathogenesis

Normal Pituitary Anatomy and Physiology

The pituitary gland is encased within the sphenoid bone at the base of the brain and is connected directly to the hypothalamus. The hypothalamus contains specific neurons that, following electrochemical stimulation, release peptides termed *releasing factors*. The releasing factors that have been identified include growth hormone–releasing hormone (GHRH); gonadotropin-releasing hormone, which stimulates both luteinizing hormone (LH) and follicle-stimulating hormone (FSH) secretion; thyrotropin-releasing hormone; and corticotropin-releasing factor. Prolactin secretion is negatively regulated by dopamine that is released from hypothalamic neurons. Following direct stimulation, hypothalamic neurons release these polypeptides into the hypophyseal portal vessels where they are transported to the anterior pituitary cells. Each releasing factor stimulates the synthesis and release of the appropriate trophic hormone by a specific pituitary cell type into the general circulation.

Each pituitary hormone acts at specific sites to produce its target effects. Growth hormone (GH) acts upon connective tissue cells to stimulate the synthesis of insulin-like growth factor (IGF)-I. IGF-I in turn stimulates trophic actions related to growth, including protein synthesis, inhibition of protein breakdown, and growth of connective tissue cell types such as bone, muscle, and cartilage. GH is necessary for normal statural growth and for maintenance of normal muscle and bone mass in adults. GH has several important metabolic functions, including stimulation of lipolysis resulting in release of free fatty acids that are used as an energy source; thus, it regulates normal glucose homeostasis and fat stores. GH also stimulates amino acid flux in muscle and contributes to the normal balance between bone formation and absorption. Prolactin acts primarily on the breast to stimulate milk production in the postpartum period. It antagonizes the effects of estrogen, and supraphysiologic concentrations impair normal fertility and estrogen action. Thyroid-stimulating hormone (TSH) acts directly upon the thyroid gland to increase the synthesis and secretion of both T_3 and T_4. Adrenocorticotropic hormone (ACTH) has a similar effect on the adrenal gland, stimulating the conversion of cholesterol to various adrenal steroids, the most important of which is cortisol. LH and FSH act in concert to stimulate gonadal function in males and females. FSH in males is primarily a stimulator of spermatogenesis and Sertoli cell function, and LH functions primarily to stimulate testosterone biosynthesis by the Leydig cells. In females, FSH stimulates follicle maturation, whereas LH is primarily responsible for stimulation of corpus luteal function.

Negative Feedback Regulation

All hormones produced by target cell types are secreted into the general circulation. They provide feedback on the normal pituitary gland and suppress trophic hormone secretion. For example, IGF-I feeds back directly on the somatotropes to inhibit GH release; T_4 inhibits TSH production; cortisol inhibits ACTH secretion; and testosterone in men and estrogen in women inhibit LH and FSH release.

Regulation of posterior pituitary hormone secretion is quite different. The hypothalamus maintains direct neural connections to the posterior pituitary gland through axonal processes. Following their synthesis in the hypothalamic neurons, these small peptides are transported down axonal processes and stored in secretory granules within the posterior pituitary gland. Neural inputs regulate the release of vasopressin, which acts directly on the kidney to control free water clearance. Similarly, under the appropriate stimulus, the brain releases oxytocin, which stimulates uterine contractions. Suckling results in loss of dopaminergic inhibition of prolactin secretion due to a direct reduction in dopamine levels. Lesions that sever the stalk while causing a major loss of stimulation of anterior pituitary hormone synthesis may not cause a complete ablation of posterior pituitary hormone synthesis because these hormones may be released by the severed neurons directly after hypothalamic stimulation. This type of lesion will increase prolactin secretion due to loss of dopamine inhibition.

A number of disease processes—tumors, other destructive lesions, vascular insults—interrupt the delicate balance of the hypothalamic-pituitary axis. A discussion of a selected group of disorders follows.

Clinical Presentation, Differential Diagnosis, Diagnostic Approach, Management, and Therapy

Diseases of the Anterior Pituitary Gland

Most cases of anterior pituitary gland dysfunction are caused by tumors (Fig. 45-1). Usually benign, these tumors disrupt normal pituitary gland function because of their anatomic location. Functionally, tumors are grouped into mass lesions that result in destruction of pituitary hormone secretion and those that result in adenomatous expansion of the specific cell type that produces a single hormone resulting in a hormonal overproduction syndrome.

Mass lesions that can result in pituitary cell destruction and hypofunction include cysts, such as Rathke cleft cyst, arachnoid, and dermoid; and tumors, such as craniopharyngioma, chordoma, glioma, sarcoma, hamartoma, dysgerminoma, metastases, and hormone-secreting or nonfunctional pituitary adenomas. Miscellaneous causes, such as aneurysms, hypophysitis, sarcoidosis, histiocytosis X, Sheehan's syndrome, and traumatic brain injury, can destroy pituitary function.

Usually, tumors destroy multiple cell types. Mass lesions that result in pituitary dysfunction can be divided into three groups: those that arise within the sella turcica; those within the parasellar areas; and those within the hypothalamus. Hypothalamic tumors can cause anterior pituitary dysfunction by destroying hypothalamic-releasing factor production and usually not through expansion within the

sella turcica. Chromophobe adenomas arise within the sella turcica, often secreting only the α subunit of LH or FSH; therefore, they are hormonally silent. These tumors grow slowly and may destroy the entire anterior pituitary gland by pressure necrosis. Extensive proliferation can lead to invasion into the cavernous sinus, or if they extend superiorly, tumors will exert pressure on the optic chiasm, leading to bitemporal hemianopsia.

Other lesions that arise within the pituitary gland include cystic lesions that develop from partial infarction of preexisting pituitary tumors, and granulomatous diseases such as histiocytosis X or sarcoidosis. Hamartomas also occur within the region of the sella turcica, resulting in hypopituitarism. Sheehan's syndrome, a postpartum pituitary infarction due to massive blood loss at delivery that results in panhypopituitarism, is one of the most common circulatory diseases involving the pituitary gland. Carotid artery aneurysms can destroy the pituitary gland. Parasellar and hypothalamic lesions that may produce hormonal dysfunction include meningiomas and craniopharyngiomas. These tumors, which often arise in the hypothalamus, result in disruption of hypothalamic hormone production. Dysgerminomas of the third ventricle can result in hypothalamic dysfunction.

Iatrogenic Causes of Hypopituitarism

Surgery for intrasellar or parasellar lesions can inadvertently result in destruction of the normal pituitary gland by damage to the hypothalamic neurons, stalk section, or direct damage to the anterior pituitary gland. Radiation treatment for pituitary tumors often results in destruction of the normal pituitary gland. Radiation for diseases such as gliomas, central nervous system leukemia or lymphoma, or head and neck tumors can produce sufficient scatter radiation to destroy anterior pituitary gland function.

Consequences of Loss of Hormonal Function

Large mass lesions of the pituitary gland or hypothalamic region can result in complete anterior pituitary hormone destruction (see Fig. 45-1). Generally, the first hormone to be lost is GH, followed by LH and FSH, followed by ACTH and TSH, and lastly, by prolactin. Loss of normal GH secretion in children can result in significant growth failure and hypoglycemia as well as increased body fat and loss of normal muscle mass. In adults, GH deficiency is more likely to lead to changes in body composition with loss of muscle and bone mass. Hypoglycemia in adults is rare. Loss of gonadotrophin secretion in women results in anovulation first followed by amenorrhea and loss of secondary sexual characteristics. In men, loss of gonadotrophin secretion is associated with erectile dysfunction, decreased testicular size, and loss of male secondary sexual characteristics. Loss of TSH secretion results in secondary hypothyroidism. The symptoms—dry skin, constipation, cold intolerance, weight gain, and loss of energy with increased fatigability—are similar to those of primary

Figure 45-1 Pituitary Anterior Lobe Deficiency in the Adult.

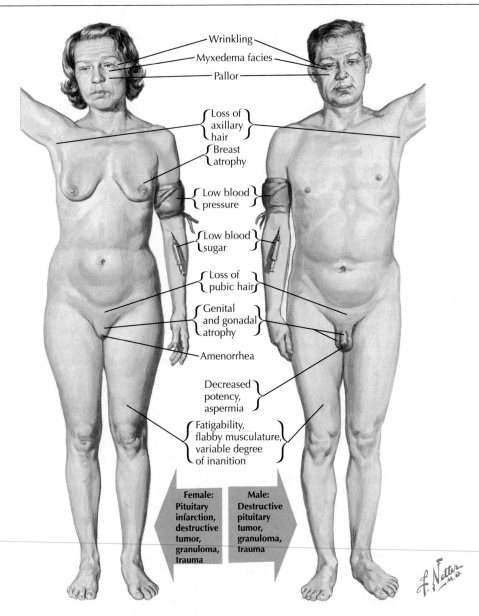

Wrinkling

Myxedema facies

Pallor

Loss of axillary hair

Breast atrophy

Low blood pressure

Low blood sugar

Loss of pubic hair

Genital and gonadal atrophy

Amenorrhea

Decreased potency, aspermia

Fatigability, flabby musculature, variable degree of inanition

Female: Pituitary infarction, destructive tumor, granuloma, trauma

Male: Destructive pituitary tumor, granuloma, trauma

hypothyroidism. Loss of ACTH secretion leads to secondary hypoadrenalism with weight loss, loss of appetite, early satiety, nausea, extreme weakness and lassitude, and inability to mount a normal stress response with resulting circulatory collapse if the deficiency is severe. Unlike primary adrenal insufficiency, mineralocorticoid secretion remains nearly normal; therefore, severe disturbances of sodium and water balance are less common, although hyponatremia results from the loss of direct effect of cortisol on free water clearance.

The loss of prolactin secretion due to diseases such as Sheehan's syndrome results in failure of postpartum lactation. Symptoms of antidiuretic hormone (ADH) deficiency include polyuria, polydipsia, postural hypotension, and hyperosmolarity. Patients with large tumors can present

with symptoms due to the mass lesion, including visual field loss, diplopia, and headaches. The physical signs depend on which hormonal deficits have occurred. Patients with panhypopituitarism often present with dry thin skin, increased truncal fat, decreased muscle mass, loss of pubic and axillary hair, and deep tendon reflexes showing delayed relaxation phase. Ancillary laboratory abnormalities that may occur include anemia, hyponatremia (low cortisol), hypernatremia, hyperosmolarity (ADH deficiency), and hypoglycemia (low GH). Usually the diagnosis of panhypopituitarism or of partial loss of pituitary hormone secretion is confirmed by stimulation tests (Table 45-1). When a hormonal deficit has been confirmed, magnetic resonance imaging of the sella turcica and parasellar region can determine whether a mass lesion is present. Treatment

Table 45-1 Diagnostic Tests Used to Confirm Pituitary Hormone Deficiencies

Hormone	Screening Test	Stimulation Test	Peak Response
GH	IGF-I decreased in 57% of cases	Insulin tolerance test, *or* Arginine infusion plus GHRH	<3 ng/mL <9 ng/ml
FSH/LH*	Testosterone plus LH (men) Estrogen plus FSH and LH (women)	GnRH	<10 IU/mL
TSH*	Free T$_4$ and TSH	TRH	<5 μU/μL
ACTH	Urine cortisol	ACTH stimulation test	Serum cortisol <18 μg/dL
ADH	Polyuria >3 L/24 hr with serum osmolarity >295 mOsm Urine osmolarity <300 mOsm	Water deprivation test	Correction of osmolarity to <298 mOsm after ADH administration

*Usually these deficiencies are confirmed with screening tests, and stimulation testing is usually not required.

ACTH, adrenocorticotropic hormone; ADH, antidiuretic hormone; FSH, follicle-stimulating hormone; GH, growth hormone; GnRH, gonadtropin-releasing hormone; GHRH, growth hormone–releasing hormone; IGF, insulin-like growth factor; LH, luteinizing hormone; TRH, thyrotropin-releasing hormone; TSH, thyroid-stimulating hormone.

usually includes removal of the tumor and institution of hormone replacement therapy. Thyroid hormone and cortisol are replaced orally, and gonadal steroids are replaced either orally (estrogen and progesterone), transdermally, or by injection. GH can be replaced only by injection. ADH is replaced orally or intranasally.

Avoiding Treatment Errors

Hormone replacement in hypopituitarism is challenging because of the inability to use laboratory testing to directly monitor therapy in all cases. For example, ADH replacement is monitored indirectly by measuring urine and serum sodium osmolarity. Thyroid replacement is easily accomplished using direct measurement of free T$_4$. Cortisol replacement is usually monitored using clinical signs (e.g., appetite and weight) as well as electrolyte balance. Cortisol metabolism is decreased with hypothyroidism and GH deficiency; therefore, patients with hypopituitarism often require lower doses than patients with primary adrenal insufficiency.

Pituitary Dysfunction Due to Hypersecretion of Specific Hormones

Adenoma formation with subsequent expansion of somatotropes, thyrotropes, gonadotropes, or lactotropes results in hypersecretion of each of these hormones (Figs. 45-2, 45-3, and 45-4). The most common disorder is prolactin hypersecretion, which accounts for more than half of pituitary adenomas, followed by GH and ACTH hypersecretion. TSH and gonadotropin hypersecretion are rare. The etiology of these tumors in most cases is unknown; however, they represent clonal expansion of a small group of cells. Mutations of oncogenes, such as *PTTG* (pituitary tumor–transforming gene), that are cell growth activators, or mutations of tumor suppressor genes, such as G-protein subunit-α and menin, can result in the formation of pituitary tumors that overproduce hormones. To date, no spe-

cific mutation has been determined in most patients who present with these symptoms. Menin gene mutations result in multiple endocrine neoplasia type 1 syndrome, which is accompanied not only by pituitary mass lesions but also by tumors of the parathyroid gland and pancreas.

Hyperprolactinemia

Overproduction of prolactin leads to different syndromes in men and women. Specifically, modest overproduction of prolactin by very small tumors (<1.0 cm) in women results first in anovulation and then leads to amenorrhea due to direct antagonism of gonadotrophin action in the ovary and attenuation of estrogen action in target tissues such as the endometrium. Severe hyperprolactinemia results in major attenuation of estrogen action, with breast and vaginal atrophy, hot flashes, and development of osteoporosis. Spontaneous lactation occurs in women who are producing sufficient estrogen to stimulate milk production. These patients often present with galactorrhea and amenorrhea. Laboratory diagnosis of hyperprolactinemia is confirmed by serum prolactin measurement greater than 25 ng/mL. Treatment depends on whether a microadenoma or a macroadenoma is present. Almost all prolactin-secreting tumors respond to dopaminergic agonists. Usually, dopaminergic agonist treatment is instituted first, then the decision whether to do surgery or utilize radiation therapy is made, depending on tumor responsiveness. If prolactin values are less than 150 ng/mL, other etiologies, such as medications (e.g., phenothiazines) or hypothyroidism, should be excluded. Prolactin values greater than 150 ng/mL are almost always a result of pituitary tumors. Hypothalamic tumors that result in compression of the pituitary stalk (e.g., craniopharyngiomas) may also cause an increase in prolactin.

Acromegaly

Overproduction of GH leads to gigantism in children and acromegaly in adults (see Figs. 45-2 and 45-3). The physi-

Figure 45-2 Acromegaly.

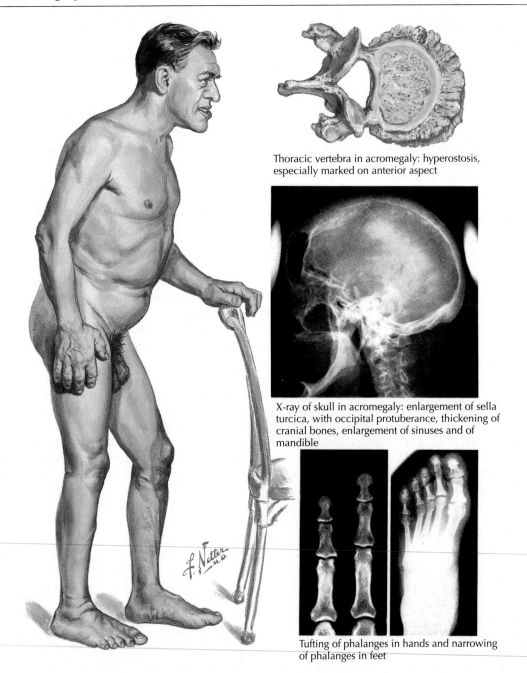

Thoracic vertebra in acromegaly: hyperostosis, especially marked on anterior aspect

X-ray of skull in acromegaly: enlargement of sella turcica, with occipital protuberance, thickening of cranial bones, enlargement of sinuses and of mandible

Tufting of phalanges in hands and narrowing of phalanges in feet

cal features in adults are distinctive and occur because the long bones have undergone epiphyseal fusion but there is overgrowth of the hands and feet, supraorbital ridge, and mandible. Enlargement of soft tissues, including the tongue and skin, and visceromegaly are usually present. Symptoms include sweating, weakness, easy fatigability, and arthralgias. Laboratory abnormalities include fasting hyperglycemia, hyperinsulinemia, and hyperphosphatemia. Treatment includes surgery to remove the primary GH-producing lesion and, sometimes, follow-up radiation therapy. Medical therapy with dopaminergic antagonists, long-acting forms of somatostatin, and GH receptor antagonists is an effective means for reducing the growth-promoting effects of GH. Left untreated, this disease is associated with increased mortality and morbidity, primarily from cardiovascular disease. Because of the increase in mortality, the treatment goals should be normalization of serum IGF-I. The diagnosis of acromegaly is established either

Figure 45-3 Acidophil Adenoma.

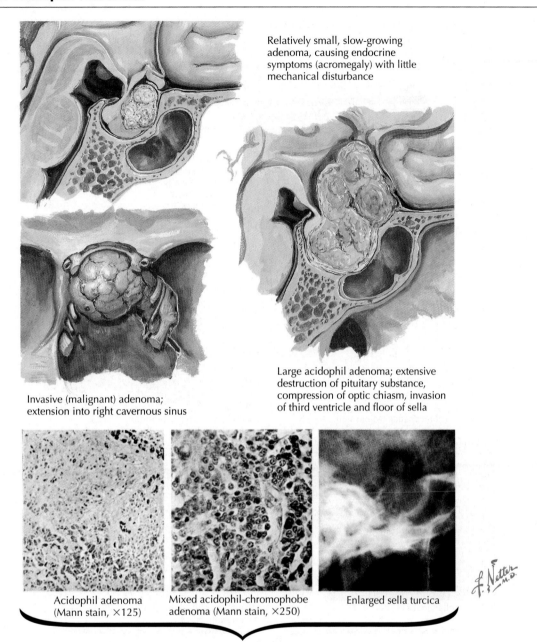

Relatively small, slow-growing adenoma, causing endocrine symptoms (acromegaly) with little mechanical disturbance

Invasive (malignant) adenoma; extension into right cavernous sinus

Large acidophil adenoma; extensive destruction of pituitary substance, compression of optic chiasm, invasion of third ventricle and floor of sella

Acidophil adenoma (Mann stain, ×125)

Mixed acidophil-chromophobe adenoma (Mann stain, ×250)

Enlarged sella turcica

Gigantism, acromegaly (may be asymptomatic if very small)

by obtaining an IGF-I value or by determining that GH cannot be suppressed to less than 0.5 ng/mL after ingestion of 75 g of glucose.

Cushing's Disease

Overproduction of ACTH by the pituitary results in excessive secretion and the development of Cushing's syndrome. This entity presents with a distinct phenotypic appearance, including fat redistribution over the posterior cervical area (buffalo hump), supraclavicular fat pads, and truncal obesity (see Chapter 44, Fig. 44-5). Connective tissue breakdown leads to the distinct appearance of striae over the abdomen, and easy bruisability results from capillary fragility. Other symptoms are hypertension secondary to increased sodium and water retention; hirsutism and amenorrhea (70% of females); weight gain (20 to 30 lb is common); proximal muscle weakness and poor wound healing; and, in most patients, a distinctive facial flush. Laboratory evaluation often reveals hypokalemia, decreased serum urea nitrogen, and decreased bone mineral density. The diagnosis is based

Figure 45-4 Basophil Adenoma.

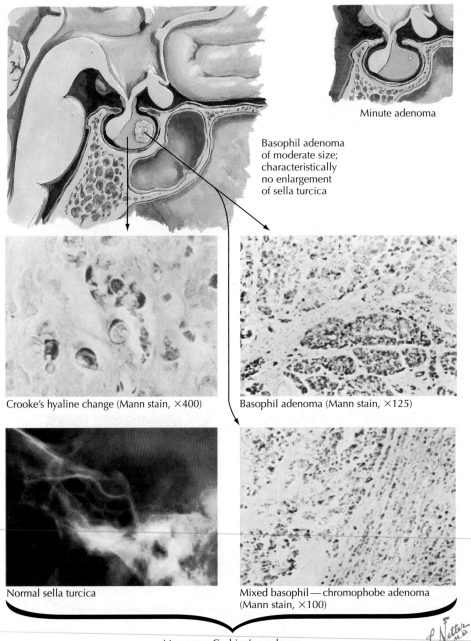

Minute adenoma

Basophil adenoma
of moderate size;
characteristically
no enlargement
of sella turcica

Crooke's hyaline change (Mann stain, ×400)

Basophil adenoma (Mann stain, ×125)

Normal sella turcica

Mixed basophil—chromophobe adenoma
(Mann stain, ×100)

May cause Cushing's syndrome
(may be symptom free)

on an elevated total urinary cortisol excretion over a 24-hour period (>120 μg/day). If this test result is positive, one must distinguish between pituitary tumors and other causes of Cushing's syndrome. This is done by administering dexamethasone, 2.0 mg every 6 hours for 48 hours. Urinary cortisol is suppressed by 50% or greater in patients with ACTH-producing pituitary tumors. Adequate treatment of Cushing's disease requires removal of the ACTH-producing tumor. If a surgical cure is not achieved, radiation treatment and consideration of adrenalectomy are necessary to alleviate the hormonal overproduction. If

left untreated, Cushing's syndrome has a 50% 5-year mortality. Therefore, eliminating the hormonal abnormality is imperative.

Future Directions

Major advances have been made in the past decade in the quality of pituitary imaging and trans-sphenoidal surgery. Progress in these areas is likely to accelerate. Specifically, surgery is now performed endoscopically and in many cases has been extremely successful with much less in-hospital and postoperative morbidity. Improvement in radiation therapy that utilizes techniques that localize radiation to the pituitary mass and limit damage to surrounding structures will continue. Molecular genetics is likely to continue to improve our ability to predict the development of pituitary tumors. Hormonal assays with improved sensitivity and specificity will allow more reliable and rapid diagnostic testing. Whether these tests will be sufficiently precise to obviate stimulation or suppression testing remains uncertain at this time.

Additional Resources

Buchfelder M: Treatment of pituitary tumors: Surgery. Endocrine 28(1):67-75, 2005.

This excellent review of the modern approaches to pituitary surgery covers the most important issues in surgical management.

Cohen LE, Radovick S: Molecular basis of combined pituitary hormone deficiencies. Endocr Rev 23(4):431-442, 2002.

The authors present a succinct review of the molecular defects that result in abnormal pituitary gland development and hormonal deficiencies.

Darzy KH, Shalet SM: Hypopituitarism after cranial irradiation. J Endocrinol Invest 28(5 Suppl):78-87, 2005.

This is an informative review of the most likely clinical syndromes that occur after cranial irradiation.

Gillam MP, Molitch ME, Lombardi G, Colao A: Advances in the treatment of prolactinomas. Endocr Rev 27(5):485-534, 2006.

This review covers all aspects of prolactinoma therapy as well as the mechanisms of pathogenesis. There is an excellent description of the approach to tumors that are relatively resistant to medical therapy.

Hurel SJ, Thompson CJ, Watson MJ, et al: The short Synacthen and insulin stress tests in the assessment of the hypothalamic-pituitary-adrenal axis. Clin Endocrinol (Oxf) 44(2):141-146, 1996.

This well-controlled study reviews the diagnostic sensitivity and specificity of the two best tests for documenting inadequate hypothalamus pituitary adrenal axis function. The authors provide specific guidelines on directing when it is appropriate to use each type of test.

Labeur M, Theodoropoulou M, Sievers C, et al: New aspects in the diagnosis and treatment of Cushing disease. Front Horm Res 35:169-178, 2006.

This article reviews the diagnostic approach to Cushing's disease and provides an algorithm for using combinations of tests to arrive at an accurate diagnosis and to localize the source of excess cortisol secretion. The efficacy of various treatment options are reviewed.

Roelfsema F, Biermasz NR, Romijn JA, Pereira AM: Treatment strategies for acromegaly. Expert Opin Emerg Drugs 10(4):875-890, 2005.

All treatment options for patients with acromegaly are reviewed. Emphasis is placed on individual therapy and the newer treatment options that are available.

EVIDENCE

1. Arafah BM: Medical management of hypopituitarism in patients with pituitary adenomas. Pituitary 5(2):109-117, 2002.

   The author presents a comprehensive review of the essential features of both diagnosis and treatment of hypopituitarism in this category of patients.

2. Burt MG, Ho KK: Newer options in the management of acromegaly. Intern Med J 36(7):437-444, 2006.

   This is an excellent summary of the latest medical treatment options in acromegaly.

3. Ezzat S, Asa SL: Mechanisms of disease: The pathogenesis of pituitary tumors. Nat Clin Pract Endocrinol Metab 2(4):220-230, 2006.

   The authors provide an excellent summary of the modular pathogenesis of pituitary tumors.

4. Freda PU, Wardlaw SL: Clinical review 110: Diagnosis and treatment of pituitary tumors. J Clin Endocrinol Metab 84(11):3859-3866.

   This paper includes a clear outline of the best approaches to diagnosis and management of pituitary tumors.

Hirsutism

Introduction

Hirsutism, which affects about 10% of adult women, is characterized by the presence of terminal hairs that occur in androgen-dependent areas of a woman's body. The prevalence varies according to ethnicity and societal norms. Although most cases are benign, the condition can be extremely distressing to affected patients. The physician must distinguish benign from serious causes and counsel the patient with regard to the efficacy and availability of treatment options.

Etiology and Pathogenesis

Hirsutism results from increased production of androgens by the ovary, adrenal glands, or both, or from increased sensitivity of hair follicles to normal circulating levels of androgens (Fig. 46-1). The latter is frequently caused by increased 5α-reductase activity, which converts testosterone to dihydrotestosterone, a more potent metabolite. Hyperandrogenism, resulting from any of these factors, prolongs the anagen (growth) phase of androgen-sensitive hairs, resulting in their conversion from fine, light, vellus hairs to coarse, dark, terminal hairs.

In women, testosterone is derived mainly from the ovary. About 25% of the total pool is secreted directly by the ovary, and the remainder is produced by peripheral conversion from ovarian and adrenally derived precursors. Androstenedione, a less potent androgen, is produced in equal quantities by both the adrenal gland and ovary. Dehydroepiandrosterone sulfate (DHEAS), also a weak androgen, is secreted almost exclusively by the adrenal gland. Increased testosterone levels indicate ovarian hyperandrogenism; increased DHEAS levels imply adrenal hyperandrogenism. If neither is elevated, and other causes are excluded, increased peripheral conversion is generally assumed.

Circulating androgen levels also affect the concentration of sex hormone–binding globulin (SHBG). SHBG binds testosterone in the circulation. In general, about 80% of testosterone is bound to SHBG, 19% is bound to albumin, and 1% circulates free. Hyperandrogenism and obesity can reduce SHBG concentrations, resulting in a greater percentage of the total testosterone as the free, unbound, active hormone.

Clinical Presentation

The universal feature is an abnormal quantity and quality of sexual hair in the midline body areas. Most commonly, the face, chest, areola, linea alba, buttock, sacrum, inner thigh, and external genitalia are affected (Fig. 46-2). The severity of hirsutism can be quantified based on the Ferriman and Gallwey system, which evaluates nine body areas for absent to severe hirsutism with scores of 0 to 4. A score greater than 7 (of a possible 36) is considered abnormal. Other androgen-dependent symptoms that occur frequently include acne, menstrual irregularity, temporal recession, and frontal alopecia.

Classically, hirsutism is distinguished from virilization, which encompasses more advanced masculinizing features, including increased muscle mass, loss of female body contour, flattening of breasts, deepening of the voice from laryngeal hypertrophy, and clitoral enlargement (greater than 1 cm if measured transversely at base of shaft). This extreme manifestation of hyperandrogenism rarely occurs unless androgen levels are very elevated (>2 to 3 times the upper limit of normal), and if present, suggests ovarian or adrenal neoplasm, or possibly anabolic steroid use.

Hirsutism should also be distinguished from hypertrichosis, which is a diffuse increase in fine, vellus hairs in nonandrogen-dependent areas (often prominent on the cheeks, arms) and can result from glucocorticoid excess,

Figure 46-1 Sources of Hyperandrogenism in Women.

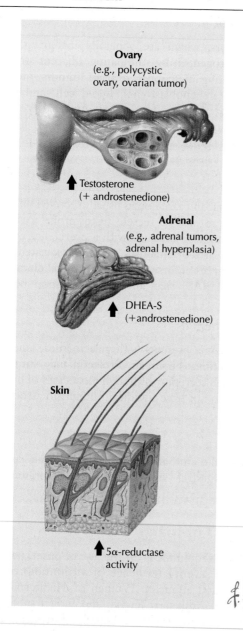

Ovary
(e.g., polycystic ovary, ovarian tumor)

↑ Testosterone (+ androstenedione)

Adrenal
(e.g., adrenal tumors, adrenal hyperplasia)

↑ DHEA-S (+androstenedione)

Skin

↑ 5α-reductase activity

Figure 46-2 Clinical Manifestations of Hyperandrogenism.

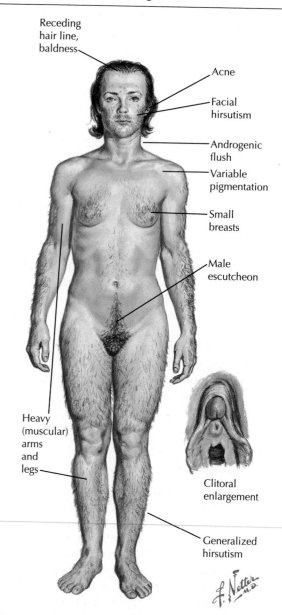

Receding hair line, baldness

Acne

Facial hirsutism

Androgenic flush

Variable pigmentation

Small breasts

Male escutcheon

Heavy (muscular) arms and legs

Clitoral enlargement

Generalized hirsutism

medications (phenytoin, penicillamine, cyclosporine, minoxidil, diazoxide), and systemic disorders (anorexia nervosa, hypothyroidism, porphyrias, dermatomyositis); it can also be familial.

Differential Diagnosis

Most cases of hirsutism in adult women are due to polycystic ovary syndrome (PCOS; about 80%) or idiopathic hirsutism (IH; 15% to 20%). These conditions generally begin in the perimenarcheal or late teen years and progress in a gradual fashion. In contrast, neoplasms of the ovary or adrenal gland present abruptly, progress rapidly, and are

more frequently associated with virilization. More specific characteristics of these disorders, as well as less common etiologies of hirsutism, are presented next.

Common Causes

Polycystic Ovary Syndrome

The criteria for the diagnosis of PCOS were redefined in 2003 to include two of the following three features: (1) *hyperandrogenism*, which may be based on clinical findings such as hirsutism or other androgen-dependent features, or biochemical evidence of increased androgen levels; (2) *oligomenorrhea* (≤8 menses/year); or (3) *polycystic ovaries*

visualized on ultrasound. The diagnosis also requires exclusion of other potentially causative conditions.

Insulin resistance affects ovarian androgen production by dysregulating an ovarian P450 cytochrome-oxidase 17α-dependent pathway involving the conversion of progesterone to androstenedione. Insulin-mediated abnormalities of pituitary luteinizing hormone (LH) secretion may also contribute. Although commonly associated with obesity, cases of PCOS in thin women who are also insulin resistant have been well documented.

In this condition, testosterone is most often mild to moderately elevated, and there may be associated mild elevations in prolactin and DHEAS through mechanisms that are incompletely defined.

Idiopathic Hirsutism

A uniform definition of IH is evolving; a recent review suggests the inclusion of (1) *hirsutism*, (2) *normal androgen levels*, and (3) *regular menses* with normal ovulatory function. Normal ovulatory function can be confirmed by basal body temperature measurement or midluteal phase progesterone measurement. If there is evidence of anovulation despite regular menses, the patient is considered to have PCOS. Pathogenesis of IH involves increased 5α-reductase activity as well as a possible alteration in androgen receptor function, resulting in increased sensitivity of the hair follicle to normal androgen levels.

Rare Causes

Adrenal Hyperplasia

Classic congenital adrenal hyperplasia (21-hydroxylase deficiency) is an autosomal recessive condition diagnosed in infancy because it causes ambiguous genitalia in female infants. A partial form of this condition, nonclassic (late-onset) congenital adrenal hyperplasia (NCAH), may present as a slowly progressive form of hirsutism in adulthood. The pathogenesis involves an enzymatic deficiency in adrenal steroidogenesis, resulting in accumulation of androgen precursors. Clinical features and laboratory findings may be similar to those of PCOS, but can be distinguished by evaluating 17-hydroxyprogesterone levels, which are mild to moderately (>200 ng/dL) elevated at baseline in NCAH and rise to more than 1500 ng/dL after ACTH stimulation. The prevalence of NCAH is less than 3%, although it is known to be particularly common in Ashkenazi Jewish women (prevalence, 1 : 27).

Cushing's Syndrome

Cushing's syndrome presents with hypercortisolemia caused by a cortisol-secreting pituitary adenoma (Cushing's disease), an adrenal adenoma, or an ectopic adrenocorticotropic hormone. It is a rare cause of hirsutism unless induced iatrogenically by glucocorticoid administration. Often, other clinical features predominate (facial plethora, telangiectasias, suboccipital fat pad, violaceous abdominal striae, obesity, hypertrichosis) in this condition.

Ovarian Tumor

Epithelial tumors, which are generally malignant, can cause hyperandrogenism by stimulating adjacent stroma. Androgen-secreting functional ovarian tumors include Sertoli-Leydig (arrhenoblastoma), lipoid cell, and hilus cell tumors. Characteristic features are more severe, and progressive hirsutism and testosterone levels are higher than 150 to 200 ng/dL. Together, these tumors represent less than 1% of causes of hirsutism.

Adrenal Tumor

Adrenal adenomas and carcinomas usually secrete DHEAS, although they can also co-secrete testosterone, cortisol, or both. They are also unusual, with a prevalence of less than 1% of the cases of hirsutism, and are associated with more severe degrees of hirsutism and hormonal elevations (particularly DHEAS) than the more common benign etiologies.

Hyperprolactinemia

Hyperprolactinemia presents with galactorrhea, amenorrhea, and sometimes hirsutism. Prolactin may stimulate adrenal androgen secretion, although most cases of hyperprolactinemia do not have significant hirsutism associated clinically.

Drugs

Danazol, anabolic steroids, glucocorticoids, and certain progestins (norgestrel and levonorgestrel) present in certain oral contraceptive pills can cause hirsutism.

Diagnostic Approach

The evaluation should focus on the age of onset, pattern of progression, severity (evidence of virilization), menstrual history, and ethnicity. Women of Mediterranean, Middle Eastern, Ashkenazi Jewish, and Indian subcontinent origins are more prone to idiopathic hirsutism. The family history of hirsutism is also important. A medication history should be obtained, as well as a history about the extent of mechanical methods (frequency of shaving, tweezing, depilation, or electrolysis) used by the patient to control the condition.

Recommended laboratory tests for all patients are testosterone and DHEAS. Prolactin and thyroid-stimulating hormone should be added if hirsutism is associated with amenorrhea or oligomenorrhea. More extensive laboratory evaluation is seldom indicated because the findings rarely influence treatment. However, additional tests can include 17-hydroxyprogesterone to diagnose NCAH, 3α-androstenediol glucuronide (a metabolite of testosterone used as a marker of 5α-reductase activity), and measurements of free testosterone or SHBG concentrations.

Cortisol (by 24-hour urine collection or overnight 1-mg dexamethasone suppression test) should be assessed if there are clinical features of Cushing's syndrome but otherwise does not need to be part of the routine evaluation for hirsutism.

Management and Therapy

If the laboratory evaluation suggests an ovarian tumor (testosterone levels >150 to 200 ng/dL) or an adrenal gland tumor (DHEAS >700 µg/dL or 2.5 times the upper limit of normal), abdominal and pelvic imaging with ultrasound, computed tomography, or magnetic resonance imaging is indicated, with surgical referral if a mass is detected.

In most other cases, medical therapy is directed at the underlying causative factors. Most agents require 3 to 6 months to achieve a noticeable effect on hirsutism, and patients should be counseled accordingly. Treatment of Cushing's syndrome, a rare cause of hirsutism, is discussed in Chapters 44 and 45.

Suppressing Androgen Production

Combination oral contraceptives decrease ovarian androgen production, and the estrogen component (30 to 35 µg is sufficient) increases the production of SHBG. Agents containing the least androgenic progestins (norgestimate, desogestrel, ethynodiol, drospirenone) are generally recommended, although clinical trial data supporting their superiority over other oral contraceptives in the treatment of hirsutism are lacking. Drospirenone may be particularly useful in light of its structural and antiandrogenic similarities to spironolactone.

Glucocorticoids are indicated for the treatment of NCAH. Dexamethasone, 0.125 to 0.25 mg given at bedtime, suppresses adrenal androgen secretion effectively.

Androgen Receptor Blockers

Spironolactone blocks androgen action peripherally at the level of the hair follicle. The overall response is favorable, with 60% to 70% of patients showing improvement at 6 months. Doses of 50 to 200 mg/daily have been used. The effect is generally dose related, with more than half of patients requiring the maximal dose to benefit. Side effects include a transient initial diuresis and occasional gastrointestinal symptoms. Hyperkalemia occurs but is rare in healthy patients. Spironolactone should be used only in conjunction with adequate contraception because of its potential feminizing effect on a male fetus.

Flutamide at doses of 125 to 250 mg twice daily is similar in efficacy to spironolactone. The potential side effect of liver toxicity and high cost limit its feasibility for routine treatment.

Finasteride, a 5α-reductase inhibitor (at a dose of 5 mg daily), is similar in efficacy to spironolactone and flutamide. It is also costly, and because of its ability to induce ambiguous genitalia in a male fetus, appropriate contraceptive measures are mandatory.

Cyproterone acetate, a progestin with antiandrogenic activity, is used extensively in Europe for the treatment of hirsutism. In several studies in which cyproterone acetate was compared to other drug treatments for hirsutism, no difference in clinical outcome was noted, despite differences produced in hormonal parameters. This drug is not approved for use in the United States because of concerns about it causing cancer in laboratory animals at high doses.

Improving Insulin Sensitivity

Modest weight loss, with resultant improvement in insulin sensitivity, improves the clinical and biochemical features of PCOS. *Pharmacologic insulin sensitizers (metformin and thiazolidinediones)* also improve manifestations of PCOS, although their effects on the hirsutism tend to be milder than those achieved with antiandrogens. Metformin is considered first-line therapy for PCOS, at doses of 500 mg 3 times daily to 1000 mg 2 times a day. Dose titration by 500 mg at weekly intervals to limit gastrointestinal side effects is recommended. Thiazolidinediones (rosiglitazone, pioglitazone) also improve the features of PCOS with results similar to those achieved with metformin. Unlike metformin, however, which is weight neutral and available in a generic formulation, thiazolidinediones are expensive and often associated with modest weight gain, which limits their desirability and feasibility as a long-term treatment option.

Topical and Mechanical Treatments

Eflornithine hydrochloride cream 13.9% became available in 2001 for the treatment of facial hirsutism. Its mechanism of action is to inhibit keratin protein synthesis in the hair follicle, which slows the rate of hair growth. It may reduce the frequency of mechanical treatments, although it will not enhance the conversion of terminal to vellus hair, as will some of the androgen suppression treatments. It is applied twice daily, and effects occur within 4 to 8 weeks; 30% to 60% of patients achieve some degree of clinical improvement. Minor skin irritation, generally infrequent, is the most common side effect.

Electrolysis removes hair permanently by deploying an electrical current through a fine needle to destroy the dermal papilla at the base of the hair. The procedure can be costly and time consuming because only a small number of follicles can be treated in a single session.

Laser treatment has been used recently. Treatment results are roughly equivalent with various types of laser (ruby, alexandrite, diode, which deliver light at a single wavelength) or intense pulsed light (IPL) treatments. Results tend to be best in light-skinned women with dark hair because the contrast improves efficacy. The procedure is generally well tolerated, although it can be very costly

because several treatments are usually necessary to achieve complete and permanent hair removal.

Optimum Treatment

A combination of pharmacologic agents and cosmetic measures are usually required to achieve a satisfactory result.

For PCOS associated with obesity, a brief trial of weight loss achieved through diet and exercise is the initial preferred treatment. If unsuccessful, metformin should be added, with the addition of oral contraceptives, spironolactone, or eflornithine hydrochloride cream as needed. Assessment of glucose and lipid levels should be done in PCOS, given its strong association with these metabolic disturbances.

For IH, if very mild, a trial of eflornithine hydrochloride cream is reasonable, although most cases require a contraceptive for adequate hormonal suppression, and many require the addition of spironolactone for optimal hormonal control.

For both conditions, after a period of hormonal treatment, mechanical measures may then be suggested, and these are often more effective after hormonal therapy has been used to reduce androgen levels or decrease androgen action.

Avoiding Treatment Errors

Patients should be adequately counseled so that their expectations are appropriate. Response to hormonal treatment often requires 6 months, and it is reasonable to wait that long to assess the need for additional agents. Moreover, many women with this condition feel frustrated that the condition is hopeless, having seen minimal effects from mechanical treatments previously tried. The value of controlling the underlying hormonal abnormalities to enhance the effectiveness and permanence of mechanical measures should be appropriately stressed.

Future Directions

Multiple agents are available that exert their effects on hirsutism by different mechanisms. Additional data are needed regarding the most successful and cost-effective treatment combinations. Initial hormonal treatment followed by ever-improving mechanical treatments will likely remain the mainstay of treatment for the near future.

Trials evaluating newer treatment modalities including somatostatin analogues for PCOS are underway. Recognition and treatment of hirsutism diminishes the psychological burden for patients and, for those with PCOS, the potential long-term sequelae of chronic anovulation.

Additional Resources

Azziz R: The evaluation and management of hirsutism. Obstet Gynecol 101(5 Pt 1):995-1007, 2003.
This clinically oriented review is by an expert in the field and includes an extensive bibliography.

Revised 2003 consensus on diagnostic criteria and long-term health risks related to polycystic ovary syndrome (PCOS). Hum Reprod 19(1):41-47, 2004.
This paper summarizes evidence supporting current diagnostic criteria and long-term health implications of PCOS.

Rosenfield RL: Hirsutism. N Engl J Med 353(24):2578-2588, 2005.
The author presents a clinical vignette with discussion of evaluation and treatment recommendations for the hirsute patient.

Wanner M: Laser hair removal. Dermatol Ther 18(3):209-216, 2005.
The author discusses the history, types of lasers, and patient selection recommendations for this treatment modality.

EVIDENCE

1. Dunaif A, Scott D, Finegood D, et al: The insulin-sensitizing agent troglitazone improves metabolic and reproductive abnormalities in the polycystic ovary syndrome. J Clin Endocrinol Metab 81(9):3299-3306, 1996.
   Early evidence of the effect of thiazolidinediones on metabolic and clinical parameters in PCOS is presented.
2. Dunaif A, Segal KR, Futterweit W, Dobrjansky A: Profound peripheral insulin resistance, independent of obesity, in polycystic ovary syndrome. Diabetes 38(9):1165-1174, 1989.
   Evidence is presented that polycystic ovary syndrome occurs in lean as well as obese women.
3. Moghetti P, Tosi F, Tosti A, et al: Comparison of spironolactone, flutamide, and finasteride efficacy in the treatment of hirsutism: A randomized, double blind, placebo-controlled trial. J Clin Endocrinol Metab 85(1):89-100, 2000.
   Comparative efficacy of above regimens in the treatment of hirsutism is discussed.
4. Nestler JE, Jakubowicz DJ, Evans WS, Pasquali R: Effects of metformin on spontaneous and clomiphene-induced ovulation in the polycystic ovary syndrome. N Engl J Med 338(26):1876-1880, 1998.
   Early evidence is provided on the effect of metformin on metabolic and clinical parameters in PCOS.
5. Serafini P, Lobo RA: Increased 5α-reductase activity in idiopathic hirsutism. Fertil Steril 43:74-78, 1985.
   Early evidence is provided of increased 5α-reductase activity in IH.

David A. Ontjes

47

Hypogonadism in the Male

Introduction

Hypogonadism in a male refers to a deficiency of either testosterone production or sperm production, or both. Disorders causing hypogonadism may result from direct damage to the testes (primary hypogonadism) or to the hypothalamus or pituitary (secondary hypogonadism).

The adult male testis consists of two main components: seminiferous tubules, which make up more than 80% of the total testicular mass and contain Sertoli cells and germ cells or sperm; and Leydig or interstitial cells. Sertoli cells, in response to stimulation by pituitary follicle-stimulating hormone (FSH), secrete an androgen-binding protein that increases the concentration of testosterone in the tubular lumen (Fig. 47-1). They also provide an environment necessary for germ cell differentiation into mature sperm. Leydig cells produce testosterone and related steroids in response to stimulation by pituitary luteinizing hormone (LH). Testosterone acts locally on seminiferous tubules to promote sperm formation.

In the adult male, more than 95% of available testosterone is secreted by Leydig cells. In peripheral tissues, a portion of the secreted testosterone is converted into dihydrotestosterone, which is responsible for the androgenic effects of testosterone in some target tissues. Testosterone can also be converted into the potent estrogen, estradiol, in tissues possessing an aromatase enzyme. Adipose tissue and the central nervous system are capable of converting androgens into estrogens by this mechanism.

Most of the activities of the testes, including sperm formation and secretion of testosterone, are controlled by the pituitary gonadotropins, LH and FSH. These hormones are in turn controlled by a peptide hormone produced by the hypothalamus, called gonadotropin-releasing hormone (GnRH). The hormonal control of testicular function is shown in Figure 47-1. GnRH binds to gonadotropin-producing cells in the pituitary and stimulates the secretion of both LH and FSH. Receptors for LH are located on Leydig cells, whereas receptors for FSH are located on Sertoli cells. The testosterone produced by Leydig cells exerts a negative feedback on both the pituitary and the hypothalamus to reduce the release of GnRH, LH, and FSH. Stimulation of Sertoli cells, which have FSH receptors, results in the production of an androgen-binding protein. Under the influence of FSH, the Sertoli cell also secretes proteins called inhibins. These proteins are capable of selectively inhibiting the secretion of FSH by the pituitary. Thus, any process leading to damage of seminiferous tubules will result in a rise of serum FSH, whereas damage to the Leydig cells will result in a rise of both FSH and LH.

Etiology and Pathogenesis

Primary Hypogonadism

Patients have reduced testosterone secretion, reduced sperm production, and increased serum gonadotropins. The disease processes causing primary hypogonadism may damage the seminiferous tubules and Leydig cells to varying degrees, but tend to cause greater damage to sperm production than to testosterone secretion (Box 47-1).

Klinefelter's syndrome, the most common congenital cause of primary hypogonadism in males, is due to the presence of an extra X chromosome. The most common genotype, 47, XXY, is due to nondisjunction of the maternal oocyte, yielding an egg with two X chromosomes. Other chromosomal patterns having extra X chromosome

Figure 47-1 Hypogonadism.

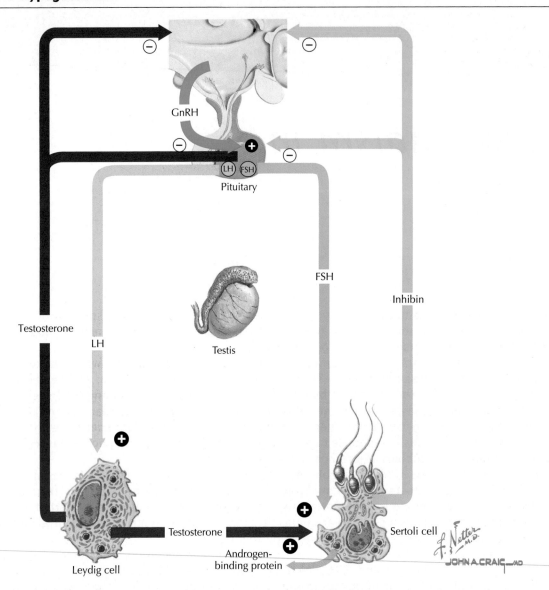

GnRH

Pituitary

LH   FSH

Testosterone

LH

FSH

Inhibin

Testis

Testosterone

Androgen-
binding protein

Leydig cell

Sertoli cell

material may include 48, XXXY; 49, XXXXY; or mosaics such as 46, XY/47, XXY. Klinefelter's syndrome occurs in 1 out of every 1000 live births. Likelihood increases with increasing maternal age. The chromosomal germ cell defect causes severe damage to the seminiferous tubules and variable damage to the Leydig cells. Individuals usually appear normal at birth and may experience normal pubertal development. As adult males, they have small, firm testes, azoospermia, gynecomastia, and usually low testosterone levels. Body proportions are affected, as shown in Figure 47-2. Other abnormalities not directly related to testosterone deficiency occur more frequently, including chronic bronchitis, germ cell tumors, varicose veins, and diabetes mellitus.

Cryptorchidism refers to testes that have not descended from the abdominal cavity into the scrotum by 1 year of age. One or both testes may be involved. About 5% of

males have undescended testes at birth, but in 90%, descent occurs during the first year. The testis may fail to descend because of prenatal androgen deficiency, often due to defective testicular development in utero. In unilateral cryptorchidism, the descended testicle often exhibits abnormalities, including a low sperm count. The undescended testicle may be damaged further because of exposure to higher temperatures inside the abdomen.

Myotonic dystrophy, an autosomal dominant disorder leading to muscle atrophy, is accompanied by hypogonadism that usually develops after puberty. Congenital deficiencies in specific enzymes essential for androgen biosynthesis are rare autosomal recessive disorders that lead to testosterone deficiency during the first trimester of pregnancy, and hence to incomplete virilization of the male infant.

Acquired diseases affecting the testes typically cause greater damage to the seminiferous tubules than to Leydig

Figure 47-2 Testicular Failure: Primary or Hypergonadotropic Hypogonadism, Prepubertal Failure.

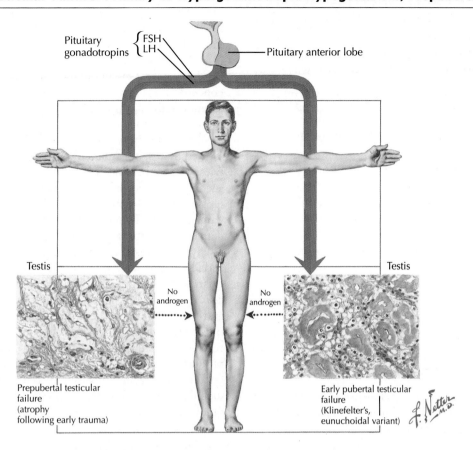

Prepubertal testicular failure (atrophy following early trauma)

Early pubertal testicular failure (Klinefelter's, eunuchoidal variant)

Box 47-1 Causes of Primary Hypogonadism in Males

Congenital Abnormalities

Klinefelter's syndrome and other chromosomal abnormalities
Cryptorchidism
Myotonic dystrophy
Disorders of androgen biosynthesis
Mutation of the follicle-stimulating hormone receptor gene
Spermatic duct obstruction or dysplasia
Varicocele

Acquired Abnormalities

Infections (mumps)
Radiation
Drugs and environmental toxins
Trauma
Autoimmune disease
Acute and chronic systemic diseases
Idiopathic

---

cells. The infection most commonly associated with testicular damage is mumps orchitis. Radiation and certain chemotherapeutic drugs used in the treatment of cancer can cause seminiferous tubule damage proportionate to the exposure. Alkylating agents such as cyclophosphamide and chlorambucil commonly cause oligospermia and elevations in serum FSH. Cisplatin or carboplatin can also decrease the sperm count, but at least partial recovery is usually seen. Many chronic systemic illnesses can cause hypogonadism, both by direct testicular injury and by causing reduced gonadotropin secretion. Cirrhosis, chronic renal failure, and AIDS are all associated with reduced testosterone secretion and variable levels of LH and FSH.

Spermatic Duct Obstruction or Dysplasia

Defects of the epididymis or vas deferens can cause absence of sperm in the semen (azoospermia), whereas spermatogenesis and testosterone secretion by the testes may be normal. Disorders of sperm transport may be either congenital or acquired. Most males with cystic fibrosis have congenital absence of the vas deferens. Acquired obstruction may result from infection (gonorrhea, chlamydia, tuberculosis) or surgical ligation (vasectomy).

Varicoceles are dilations of the venous plexus in the scrotum that exist in 10% to 15% of normal men. Because varicoceles exist in an even higher proportion of infertile men, they have long been proposed as a cause of infertility, perhaps by increasing temperatures within the scrotum. Whether fertility can be improved by ligation of varicoceles remains controversial.

Secondary Hypogonadism

Patients have reduced sperm production, reduced testosterone secretion, and low or normal serum gonadotropins. Sexual differentiation is normal because Leydig cell function during the first trimester, when differentiation occurs, is stimulated by chorionic gonadotropin from the placenta. In contrast, penile growth during the third trimester is dependent on testosterone stimulated by LH from the fetal pituitary (Box 47-2).

Most cases of congenital hypogonadotropic hypogonadism are due to a lack of GnRH, as evidenced by a normal response of serum LH after repetitive administration of synthetic GnRH. In some cases, there are other associated abnormalities, as in the Prader-Willi syndrome, in which hypogonadism is associated with mental retardation and obesity. Kallmann's syndrome is caused by a deletion in a gene on the short arm of the X chromosome that codes for an adhesion molecule, KALIG-1. Lack of this molecule leads to a failure of GnRH-secreting neurons to migrate during embryogenesis from the olfactory placode to the olfactory bulb and arcuate nucleus of the hypothalamus. The consequences are anosmia and hypogonadotropic hypogonadism. Most cases of Kallmann's syndrome are sporadic, but familial inheritance also occurs. Inheritance is usually X linked.

Any acquired disease affecting the hypothalamic-pituitary axis can cause hypogonadotropic hypogonadism. Mass lesions in the pituitary or hypothalamus are more likely to diminish the secretion of gonadotropins than of adrenocorticotropic hormone or thyroid-stimulating hormone. Thus, affected men may have hypogonadism without evidence of adrenal or thyroid deficiency. As a rule, most masses are large enough to cause dysfunction by compressing and damaging surrounding structures in the hypothalamus or pituitary. Prolactin-secreting pituitary adenomas may be an exception. High concentrations of prolactin produced by these tumors can act to inhibit production of GnRH in the hypothalamus. If prolactin concentrations are lowered by appropriate drugs such as bromocriptine, gonadotropin secretion may resume even though the tumor remains.

Meningitis is a rare cause of hypogonadism in the United States, but tuberculous meningitis is seen in countries where tuberculosis is common. Inflammatory diseases such as sarcoidosis and Langerhans cell histiocytosis (eosinophilic granuloma) impair GnRH secretion by damaging the hypothalamus, whereas hemochromatosis damages the pituitary by iron deposition.

Hypogonadism due to pituitary apoplexy occurs with sudden hemorrhage into the pituitary, usually from a preexisting pituitary tumor. Trauma to the base of the skull, as in a basilar skull fracture, can damage the pituitary stalk and impair the movement of GnRH from the hypothalamus to the pituitary. Both apoplexy and basilar skull fracture are usually associated with a deficiency of other pituitary hormones in addition to gonadotropins. Other conditions causing impaired secretion of gonadotropins include severe malnutrition and chronic administration of opioid analgesics.

Clinical Presentation

The clinical manifestations of impaired spermatogenesis are infertility and decreased testicular size. In a normal adult male, both testes should be 4.0 to 7.0 cm in length. The clinical manifestations of testosterone deficiency depend on age at the onset of the deficiency. During embryonic life, testosterone acts to promote differentiation of the external genitalia along male lines. A lack of testosterone in a male infant during early uterine life will result in differentiation along female lines. If the deficiency is complete, the external genitalia may consist of a clitoris and labia, with the vagina ending in a blind pouch. Partial deficiencies lead to incomplete virilization, ranging from posterior labial fusion when the deficiency is more severe to hypospadias when it is mild. Insufficient testosterone late in pregnancy will not prevent normal differentiation of the external genitalia but will result in a very small penis (micropenis).

Lack of testosterone before puberty will result in failure of pubertal development. In the absence of testosterone, the epiphyses of the long bones may fail to close at the usual time, so that linear growth may be prolonged, leading to a eunuchoid body habitus (Fig. 47-3). The lower body segment (floor to pubis) is characteristically more than 2 cm greater than the upper body segment, and arm span is more than 2 cm greater than total height. Testosterone deficiency occurring during adult life results in a loss of

Figure 47-3 Testicular Failure: Seminiferous Tubular Dysgenesis (Klinefelter's Syndrome).

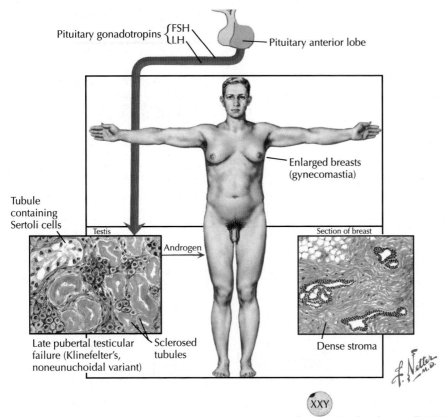

Pituitary gonadotropins {FSH, LH} — Pituitary anterior lobe

Enlarged breasts (gynecomastia)

Tubule containing Sertoli cells

Testis

Androgen

Section of breast

Late pubertal testicular failure (Klinefelter's, noneunuchoidal variant)

Sclerosed tubules

Dense stroma

XXY

Nuclear chromatin often positive (female); usually XXY chromosomal pattern but XXXY, XXXXY, XXYY, and mosaic patterns have been described

libido and overall energy, as well as decreased muscle mass and diminished growth of body hair. Longer-term effects also include a loss of bone mass and development of osteoporosis. Erectile dysfunction, a common problem among adult men, is accompanied by testosterone deficiency in only 5% to 30% of cases. However, testosterone should be measured in men with this complaint because replacement therapy can be helpful when severe deficiency is present.

Differential Diagnosis

Depending on the results of the patient's history and physical examination, measurement of serum testosterone is the most useful test for confirming the presence of hypogonadism in adult males. Semen analysis is indicated when there is a clinical concern regarding fertility. Low testosterone measurements can be difficult to interpret in the teenage boy who is not undergoing pubertal changes at an expected rate, and the differential diagnosis includes constitutionally delayed puberty as well as pathologic causes of secondary hypogonadism. A history of constitutional short stature or delayed dental maturation or a family history of delayed puberty makes a diagnosis of delayed

puberty more likely. A borderline low serum testosterone is also difficult to interpret in the elderly male, in whom the differential diagnosis includes the normal decline in testosterone secretion due to aging. The underlying cause of hypogonadism is often suggested by history and physical examination. For example, a patient with secondary hypogonadism from a large pituitary or hypothalamic mass often has neurologic abnormalities such as visual field defects and evidence of a deficiency of other pituitary hormones. Men with primary hypogonadism are more likely to have breast enlargement (gynecomastia) due to the effects of elevated LH in stimulating testicular aromatase activity.

Diagnostic Approach

Once a low testosterone level is demonstrated, other tests are helpful in arriving at a specific etiologic diagnosis. A simplified scheme for differential diagnosis is shown in Figure 47-4. Semen analysis involves the measurement of the number of sperm in an ejaculated specimen, as well as their motility. Normal men produce more than 20 million sperm per milliliter of ejaculate, or 40 million per total ejaculate, and more than 60% are motile. Serum total

Figure 47-4 Approach to the Differential Diagnosis of Primary and Secondary Hypogonadism.

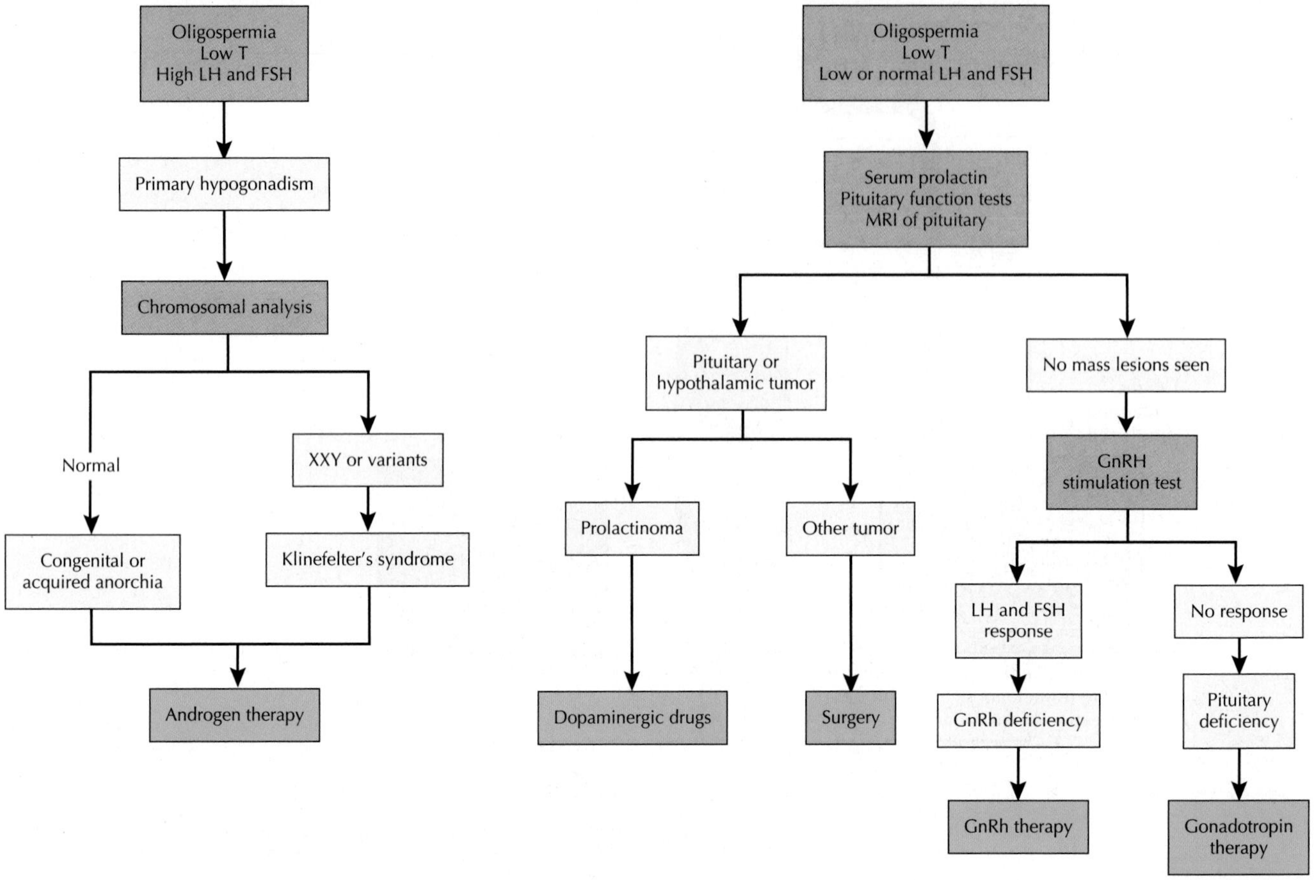

testosterone measurement, which includes free plus protein-bound hormone, is usually the best test for evaluating testosterone secretion. Exceptions occur in obese men, in whom the concentration of sex hormone–binding globulin is frequently low, and in elderly men, in whom it may be high. In such individuals, measurement of the free (unbound) or bioavailable fraction of serum testosterone is a more accurate means of assessment. LH and FSH should also be measured to interpret the significance of a low or borderline testosterone level: elevated gonadotropins confirm the diagnosis of primary hypogonadism even when testosterone is in the low-normal range. Normal gonadotropins in the presence of a low testosterone level indicate secondary hypogonadism.

Management and Therapy

Testosterone replacement is indicated in most adult men with low serum testosterone levels, except in those in whom the underlying cause may be reversible. The preferred testosterone preparations are either testosterone esters for intramuscular injection or special formulations for transdermal administration. Buccal tablets are also available. In the United States, testosterone enanthate and testosterone cypionate are the most frequently used intramuscular forms. Doses of 200 mg every 2 weeks or 300 mg every 3 weeks will maintain serum levels within the normal range throughout most of the dosing interval. Longer dosing cycles result in subnormal serum levels toward the end of the interval. Transdermal formulations are available through skin patches that deliver 5 mg of testosterone every 24 hours and maintain serum testosterone within the normal range. The patch must be changed daily. Testosterone is also available in a hydroalcoholic gel applied in doses of 50 to 100 mg, enough to maintain normal serum levels for 24 hours. Adverse effects can include an increase in acne and aggressive behavior in adolescent boys, and exacerbation of benign prostatic hyperplasia and possibly prostate cancer in older men. Testosterone therapy can also induce erythrocytosis and exacerbate sleep apnea.

Optimum Treatment

Before initiating therapy, a prostate exam should be done, as well as measurements of serum prostate-specific antigen and hematocrit. In older men, bone mineral density should be measured. Serum testosterone should be remeasured after therapy is initiated to ensure that the dose and route of administration are effective in restoring normal serum levels. Within weeks or months, normalization of serum testosterone should lead to improved libido in hypogonadal men and pubertal development in prepubertal boys. Over time, energy, bone mass, and muscle strength should all improve. If no improvement in hypogonadal symptoms is seen after a suitable interval, consider other causes for the symptoms. Monitoring in adults includes repeating the baseline measurements above and inquiring about symptoms of sleep apnea.

Gonadotropin replacement is generally limited to cases of secondary hypogonadism in which fertility is the objective because it is more complex and expensive than testosterone replacement. Some patients are stimulated to produce sufficient sperm for fertilization by injections of human chorionic gonadotropin (hCG), which replicates the effects of LH. Others require combination therapy with hCG and human menopausal gonadotropin, which contains both FSH and LH activity. Monitor effects by repeated semen analysis and measurement of the serum testosterone.

Avoiding Treatment Errors

In younger men, there is no evidence that achieving testosterone levels above the normal range is beneficial. Overtreatment should be avoided in all patients because of the increased risk for side effects. In elderly men with typical age-related declines in serum total and free testosterone, the benefits of testosterone supplements are still unclear, and the risks of untoward effects are higher. Therefore, replacement therapy is not recommended unless there are clear indications of an underlying pituitary or testicular disease.

Future Directions

Improved recognition of the adverse effects of drugs and environmental toxins on testicular function should reduce the incidence of male hypogonadism worldwide. For example, exposure to the nematocide dibromodichloropropane is known to decrease spermatogenesis in farm workers using it in the fields. It is severely restricted in the United States, but it is still exported to and used in other countries. In men undergoing cancer chemotherapy with alkylating agents and other toxic drugs, concurrent suppression of gonadotropins with testosterone or inhibitory analogs of GnRH may protect gonadal function. Further understanding of the benefits and risks of testosterone replacement in aging men will require more data from randomized clinical trials.

Rapid progress in assisted reproductive technology may enable more men with severe oligospermia or low sperm motility to be fertile. Intracytoplasmic sperm injection (ICSI) involves the direct injection of a single spermatozoon into the cytoplasm of an oocyte, previously collected from follicles produced under controlled ovarian stimulation. When there are no sperm in the ejaculate but there are germ cells in the testes, this technique can be performed using spermatozoa isolated from testicular biopsy specimens. ICSI has been successful in some men with Klinefelter's syndrome.

Additional Resources

Handelsman DJ, Zajac JD: Androgen deficiency and replacement therapy in men. Med J Aust 180(10):529-535, 2004.
   This review article for the primary care physician discusses indications for therapy and clinical use of a variety of testosterone products.
Mahmoud A, Comhaire FH: Mechanisms of disease: Late-onset hypogonadism. Nat Clin Pract Urol 3(8):430-438, 2006.
   The authors provide a literature review of the age-related decline in testicular function, focusing on mechanisms.
Margo K, Winn R: Testosterone treatments: Why, when and how? Am Fam Physician 73(9):1591-1598, 2006.
   This review article for the primary care physician deals with the benefits and adverse effects of testosterone therapy in both men and women. It provides an extensive list of testosterone products available in the United States.
Mikhail N: Does testosterone have a role in erectile dysfunction? Am J Med 119(5):373-382, 2005.
   The author presents a review of the literature dealing with the role of testosterone replacement in men with erectile dysfunction.

EVIDENCE

1. Bhasin S, Cunningham GR, Hayes FJ, et al: Testosterone therapy in adult men with androgen deficiency syndromes: An endocrine society clinical practice guideline. J Clin Endocrinol Metab 91(6):1995-2010, 2006.
   The authors provide a set of clinical practice guidelines for testosterone therapy developed by an expert panel of the Endocrine Society. The paper deals extensively with issues of screening, diagnosis, therapy, and applications in patients with sexual dysfunction and in older men.
2. Gruenewald DA, Matsumoto AM: Testosterone supplementation therapy for older men: Potential benefits and risks. J Am Geriatr Soc 51(1):101-115, 2003.
   This structured review of literature relating to the results of testosterone therapy in older men with low-normal or mildly reduced serum testosterone deals with potential positive effects on body composition, muscle strength, bone density, and cognitive and sexual function, as well as potential adverse effects.
3. Tracz MJ, Sideras K, Bolona ER, et al: Testosterone use in men and its effects on bone health. A systematic review and meta-analysis of randomized placebo-controlled trials. J Clin Endocrinol Metab 91(6):2011-2016, 2006.
   The authors describe a meta-analysis of clinical trials on the skeletal effects of testosterone supplementation. Intramuscular testosterone increased lumbar bone density in hypogonadal men, but insufficient information is available to determine whether fracture risk is decreased.

David A. Ontjes

48

Osteoporosis

Introduction

Osteoporosis is the most common bone disease and a major risk factor for fractures. In the United States, there are more than 1.5 million osteoporotic fractures each year, with an annual cost of $15 billion in health care and disability expenses. The average 50-year-old white woman in the United States has a 50% chance of suffering at least one osteoporotic fracture during her remaining lifetime. Because of the aging of our population and the increased occurrence of osteoporosis in elderly people, the incidence of osteoporotic fractures could double over the next 30 years without better methods for prevention and treatment.

Osteoporosis is defined as a low overall bone mass together with a disruption of normal bone architecture, leading to diminished strength and greater risk for fractures after minimal trauma. Histologically, there is an equivalent decrease in both bone mineral (composed of calcium and phosphorus) and bone matrix (composed of collagen and other bone proteins). The normal three-dimensional structure of trabecular bone is altered (Fig. 48-1). In osteoporotic bone, there are fewer connecting bony spicules or "struts," and they are thinner than normal. Thus, both the radiologic density and mechanical strength of osteoporotic bone are diminished. The World Health Organization defines osteoporosis in terms of bone density measurements. Osteoporosis is present when the measured bone density is more than 2.5 standard deviations below the mean for a normal young individual of the same sex and race. This amounts to a loss of 25% to 30% from normal peak bone mass. Osteopenia refers to a lesser degree of bone loss, in which the measured density is between 1.0 and 2.5 standard deviations below normal peak bone mass, amounting to a loss of 10% to 25%.

Bone is a dynamic tissue in which new mineral is constantly being laid down, while previously mineralized sections are being resorbed. This remodeling process is illustrated in Figure 48-2. The cells governing the process are osteoblasts and osteoclasts. Osteoblasts are bone-forming cells derived from connective tissue stem cells that also give rise to fibroblasts. Mature osteoblasts synthesize collagen and other bone matrix proteins such as osteocalcin. They produce the enzyme, alkaline phosphatase, which is believed to play a role in the mineralization process. Osteoclasts are the most important cells involved in bone resorption. They are derived from stem cells in the bone marrow resembling macrophages. Mature osteoclasts are large, multinucleated cells located adjacent to mineralized bone surfaces. These cells contain lysosomes capable of releasing enzymes that can degrade bone matrix proteins.

Etiology and Pathogenesis

A variety of inherited and acquired factors can predispose to low bone mass. Inherited or congenital risk factors include gender (female > male), race (white > African American), body build (thin with small frame), and family history. Acquired risk factors include increasing age, a diet low in calcium and vitamin D, early menopause, a sedentary lifestyle, and cigarette smoking. Osteoporosis results when there is too much bone resorption, too little bone formation, or a combination of both. Estrogen deficiency associated with menopause in normal women is the most common cause of increased bone resorption. Accelerated bone loss continues for about 10 years after menopause, and then the rate of decline decreases to near that of normal aging. Estrogen replacement in the postmenopausal period reduces the rate of resorption and stabilizes bone mass. Men with hypogonadism have accelerated bone loss similar to that of postmenopausal women. Hyperparathyroidism and hyperthyroidism can also cause increased bone resorption.

Age-related bone loss affects both men and women and may be due in part to decreased dietary calcium

Figure 48-1 Structure of Trabecular Bone.

Trabecular bone (schematic)

On cut surfaces (as in sections), trabeculae may appear as discontinuous spicules

Osteoid (hypomineralized matrix)

Active osteoblasts producing osteoid

Inactive osteoblasts (lining cells)

Marrow spaces (containing hematopoietic cells and fat)

Osteocytes

Osteoclasts (in Howship's lacunae)

Trabeculae

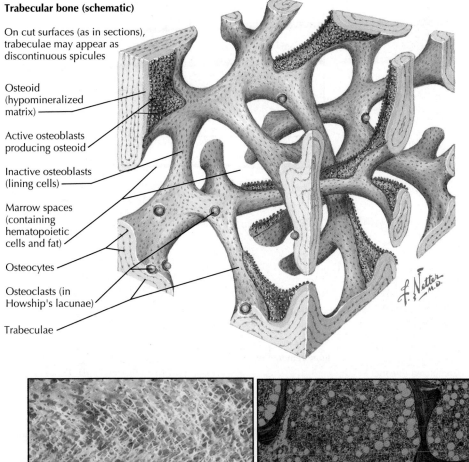

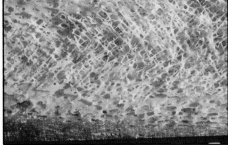

Cross section of cancellous bone (marrow elements removed). Trabecular bone in center; thin cortical bone at bottom

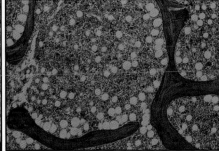

Photomicrograph of decalcified trabecular bone showing relationship of trabeculae to marrow. (H&E stain, ×35)

absorption. In very elderly individuals, the rate of bone formation is often low. Exposure to certain drugs, such as glucocorticoids, and immobilization or lack of mechanical stress on bone itself can cause impaired bone formation.

Heredity undoubtedly plays a major role in determining both the peak bone mass of young adults and the rate of bone loss in older individuals. Multiple genes are likely to influence bone mass and strength. Ongoing research suggests that natural variations (polymorphisms) in a number of genes, including genes for the vitamin D receptor, the estrogen receptor, and type 1 collagen matrix protein, appear to affect bone mass. However, the genes of greatest importance in determining fracture risk are still to be determined.

Clinical Presentation

As bone is lost, there are no symptoms until fractures occur, typically with minimal trauma. Compression fractures of the vertebra are most common, followed by fractures of the proximal femur and the distal radius (Colles's fracture). As a result of vertebral compression with anterior wedging, patients lose height and develop a kyphosis deformity of the spine (Fig. 48-3). Patients who have experienced vertebral compression fractures often have chronic back pain. Proximal femur (hip) fractures are the most disabling, often leading to immobilization and a loss of independent living in elderly men and women. Because the entire skeleton is fragile, fractures are more likely to occur

Figure 48-2 Bone Remodeling.

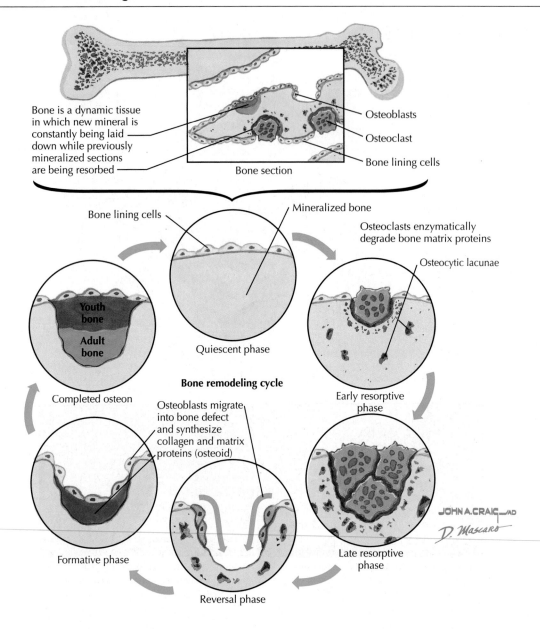

Bone is a dynamic tissue in which new mineral is constantly being laid down while previously mineralized sections are being resorbed

Osteoblasts

Osteoclast

Bone lining cells

Bone section

Bone lining cells

Mineralized bone

Osteoclasts enzymatically degrade bone matrix proteins

Osteocytic lacunae

Quiescent phase

Bone remodeling cycle

Early resorptive phase

Youth bone

Adult bone

Completed osteon

Osteoblasts migrate into bone defect and synthesize collagen and matrix proteins (osteoid)

Late resorptive phase

Formative phase

Reversal phase

JOHN A. CRAIG—AD
D. Mascaro

at other sites as well, including the pelvis, ribs, and long bones.

Differential Diagnosis

Other metabolic bone diseases that can cause structural weakness of bone include osteomalacia and osteitis fibrosis. Osteomalacia occurs when bone mineral fails to be deposited in normally formed bone matrix. Rickets in children is the equivalent of osteomalacia in adults. Osteitis fibrosa is due to high circulating levels of parathyroid hormone (PTH), causing abnormally increased bone resorption.

A number of specific diseases can cause secondary bone loss and should be considered in the differential diagnosis of any patient presenting with low bone mass (Box 48-1).

It is important to identify these conditions because appropriate treatment of the primary problem can often lead to improvement in bone mass as well.

Diagnostic Approach

Plain x-rays of bone can show several types of abnormalities that suggest osteoporosis or another metabolic bone disease. The most common finding is nonspecific osteopenia, or reduced radiographic density. With more advanced disease, deformities or fractures may occur. In early disease, standard x-rays may appear normal. At least 30% of total bone mass must be lost before abnormalities in density are detectable by plain radiographs (Fig. 48-4).

Figure 48-3 Clinical Manifestations of Osteoporosis.

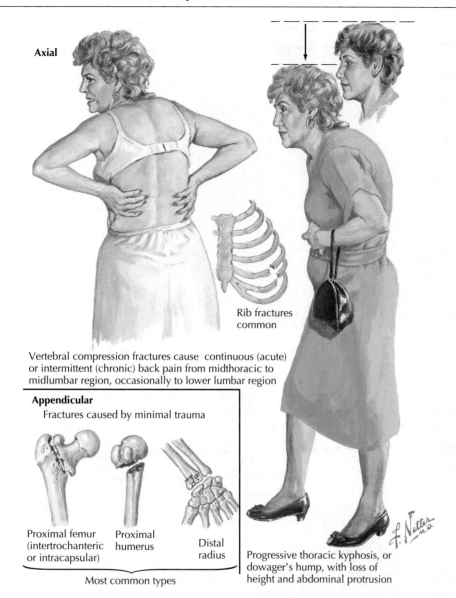

Axial

Rib fractures common

Vertebral compression fractures cause continuous (acute) or intermittent (chronic) back pain from midthoracic to midlumbar region, occasionally to lower lumbar region

Appendicular
Fractures caused by minimal trauma

Proximal femur (intertrochanteric or intracapsular)

Proximal humerus

Distal radius

Most common types

Progressive thoracic kyphosis, or dowager's hump, with loss of height and abdominal protrusion

Quantitative measurement of bone density is the primary means of diagnosing osteoporosis, using World Health Organization standards. The most widely used method for measuring bone mass is dual energy x-ray absorptiometry (DEXA), which uses x-ray beams of two different energy levels. Tissues of differing densities (bone and soft tissue) conduct the beams differently, allowing specific densities to be calculated. Quantitative bone density measurement is used to document the presence of osteopenia or osteoporosis and to predict the risk for fracture. A decline of 1 standard deviation below young normal bone density implies a doubling of fracture risk. The risk doubles again for each standard deviation decline.

Routine laboratory evaluation is limited and used to rule out causes of secondary osteoporosis. Serum creatinine, calcium, phosphorus, alkaline phosphatase, and thyroid-stimulating hormone, as well as complete blood count, should be obtained in most patients. Patients with elevated serum calcium should have a measurement of serum PTH. Those at clinical risk for vitamin D deficiency, especially homebound or institutionalized individuals, should have a measurement of 25-hydroxyvitamin D.

Management and Therapy

Prevention

Osteoporosis is better prevented than cured. The health habits of individuals in early and middle life play a role in their risk for osteoporosis in later life. Adequate dietary intake of calcium and vitamin D, active physical exercise, and avoidance of excessive alcohol, tobacco, and drugs

Figure 48-4 Radiographic Findings in Axial Osteoporosis.

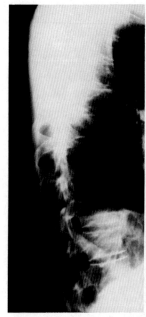

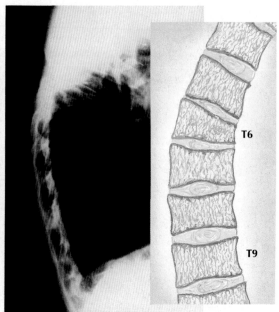

Mild osteopenia in post-
menopausal woman. Vertebrae
appear "washed-out"; no
kyphosis or vertebral collapse

Anterior wedge compression at T6 in same patient 16¹/₂ years later.
Patient has lymphoma, with multiple biconcave ("codfish") vertebral
bodies and kyphosis. Focal lesion at T6 suggests neoplasm

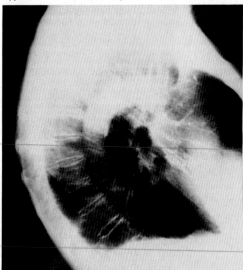

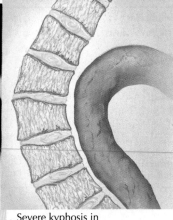

Severe kyphosis in
postmenopausal woman. Mild,
multiple biconcavity and wedging
of vertebrae. Extensive
calcification of aorta

known to cause osteopenia are all useful measures for the prevention of osteoporosis (Table 48-1).

The recommended daily allowance of vitamin D for most healthy individuals is 400 IU, but for the elderly, 800 IU is preferred.

Drug Therapy

The objectives of therapy include prevention of further bone loss, promotion of bone formation, prevention of fractures, reduction or elimination of pain, and restoration of physical function. A growing number of therapeutic agents have been shown to improve bone density and to reduce the incidence of certain fractures in randomized clinical trials. Estrogens, selective estrogen receptor modulators (SERMs), calcitonin, and bisphosphonates are considered to be *antiresorptive agents*, acting primarily to reduce rates of bone resorption by reducing osteoclast activity. PTH analogues, in contrast, are *anabolic agents*, stimulating bone formation through a primary action on osteoblasts.

Ideally the decision to treat with an antiosteoporosis drug should be based on an accurate prediction of the absolute fracture risk in the individual patient. There is currently no generally accepted formula for estimating the probability of future fractures. However, the most powerful predictor is a history of prior fragility fractures. Other key factors known to have independent power to predict fractures include advancing age and low bone mineral density, as measured by DEXA. Thus, antiosteoporosis drug therapy should be strongly considered for both adult women and men with recent fragility fractures, regardless of age. In patients without a history of fractures, drug therapy is usually justified in women and men older than 60 years with bone density measurements more than 2.5 standard deviations below young controls. In younger individuals with low bone density but no history of fractures, drug therapy may be deferred in favor of preventive strategies, with monitoring of bone density every 2 to 3 years.

Estrogen replacement in postmenopausal women prevents the excessive bone loss due to estrogen deficiency. Estrogens should be given together with a progestin in women who have an intact uterus to avoid the increased risk for endometrial cancer. The Women's Health Initiative clinical trial of estrogen replacement in postmenopausal women demonstrated a significant reduction in the risk for hip fracture. Clinical trials have shown that estradiol administered transdermally is also beneficial in postmenopausal osteoporosis. Prolonged administration of estrogens may increase the risk for breast cancer and venous blood clots in susceptible individuals, and estrogens are therefore not the treatment of choice for osteoporosis in many women.

SERMs are synthetic analogues of estrogen that have some of the biologic effects of natural estrogen but lack other effects. Drugs in this class include tamoxifen, a drug used to treat breast cancer, and raloxifene, a drug approved for the treatment of osteoporosis. Raloxifene acts as an estrogen agonist with respect to bone and lipoprotein metabolism. It increases bone density and lowers serum cholesterol when given to postmenopausal women. Clinical trials have demonstrated that raloxifene reduces the risk for vertebral fractures but not hip fractures in postmenopausal women with osteoporosis. Raloxifene does not stimulate the endometrium, and like tamoxifen, it acts as an estrogen antagonist in breast tissue. Thus, raloxifene is a good choice as an antiosteoporosis drug in women at high risk for breast cancer.

Bisphosphonates are a family of compounds that resemble pyrophosphate and are incorporated into the mineral structure of bone. There they inhibit bone resorption and promote increased bone mass. Clinical trials of several bisphosphonates, including etidronate, alendronate, risedronate, and ibandronate, indicate that bone density is increased in postmenopausal women after 2 or more years of treatment. Further trials with orally administered alendronate and risedronate provide strong evidence that these drugs can reduce fracture risk by 40% to 60% at both the spine and the hip, whereas ibandronate reduces fracture risk at the spine. These drugs are effective in men as well as women. Alendronate, risedronate, and ibandronate are currently approved in the United States for treatment of osteoporosis, but other drugs of this class are likely to be approved in the near future.

Calcitonin is a peptide hormone produced in small quantities by the parafollicular cells of the normal thyroid gland. The administration of synthetic human or salmon

---

Box 48-1 Causes of Secondary Osteoporosis

Drugs
Heparin
Ethanol
Glucocorticoids

Endocrine Diseases
Hyperparathyroidism
Thyrotoxicosis
Hypogonadism
Hyperprolactinemia
Glucocorticoid excess (Cushing's syndrome)

Gastrointestinal Diseases
Gastrectomy
Malabsorption syndromes (sprue)
Chronic biliary obstruction

Genetic Abnormalities of Collagen Synthesis
Ehlers-Danlos syndrome
Osteogenesis imperfecta

Malignant Diseases
Myeloma
Leukemia
Lymphoma

Prolonged Immobilization
Bed rest
Cast application to limb

Table 48-1 Calcium Requirements for Optimal Bone Health

Children and Adolescents	Recommended Daily Calcium (mg)
1-3 yr	500
4-8 yr	800
9-18 yr	1300
Adult Women and Men	
19-50 yr	1000
>50 yr	1200
Pregnant and Lactating Women	
15-18 yr	1300
19-50 yr	1000

calcitonin in patients with osteoporosis causes a reduction in bone resorption and a modest increase in bone density. Clinical trials have found that intranasal calcitonin therapy reduces the occurrence of vertebral fractures in postmenopausal women. Large doses of calcitonin may have an analgesic effect through an independent action on the central nervous system.

PTH agonists, including recombinant human PTH 1-34 (teriparatide) and human PTH 1-84, constitute a class of antiosteoporosis drugs whose primary effect is to promote new bone formation. In one clinical trial, teriparatide, given as a daily subcutaneous dose in postmenopausal women, promoted increased bone density and reduced both vertebral and nonvertebral fractures. Teriparatide is also effective in increasing bone mineral density in osteoporotic men. Teriparatide has been approved in the United States for the treatment of osteoporosis. Other drugs of this class are likely to be introduced in the near future.

Optimum Treatment

Osteoporosis is a chronic disease requiring long-term therapy to prevent major complications and morbidity. Effective management requires education of the patient about the risks and benefits of therapy as well as development of an overall therapeutic plan that is acceptable and sustainable. Allied health professionals, including nutritionists and physical therapists, are often helpful in implementing optimal diet and exercise programs. Regular follow-up and monitoring of bone density as well as potential side effects are essential.

Avoiding Treatment Errors

Failure to implement effective strategies for the prevention or treatment of osteoporosis is common. Patients at high risk for developing osteoporosis due to the presence of other diseases or ongoing therapy with agents such as glucocorticoids should be monitored with measurements of bone density and started on antiosteoporosis therapy whenever their bone density is found to be low. Unfortunately, many elderly patients presenting with fragility fractures still receive neither bone density testing nor antiosteoporosis therapy, even though effective treatment is now widely available.

Future Directions

Improved public knowledge about dietary and lifestyle issues affecting risk may offer the greatest promise for avoiding a growing epidemic of osteoporotic fractures. More widely available and affordable screening procedures for low bone density should allow earlier recognition of high-risk individuals. Development of better algorithms

for predicting absolute fracture risk should also enable physicians to select those patients most likely to benefit from long-term therapy with antiosteoporosis drugs. New therapeutic strategies involving both drugs that promote active bone formation and drugs that prevent bone resorption are being studied. The sequential use of bone-forming drugs, such as PTH, followed by antiresorptive drugs, such as bisphosphonates, may provide greater long-term efficacy than the use of either drug alone. Finally, randomized clinical trials allowing head-to-head comparisons of a growing number of antiosteoporosis drugs should eventually lead to improved treatment guidelines and more informed drug selection.

Additional Resources

Häuselmann HJ, Rizzoli R: A comprehensive review of treatments for postmenopausal osteoporosis. Osteoporosis Int 14(1):2-12, 2003.
This is a comprehensive review of randomized, placebo-controlled, double-blind clinical trials of antiosteoporosis drugs registered in Europe and America as of 2002; however, it does not include results of teriparatide or other PTH derivatives.

Miller PD, Bonnick SL, Rosen CJ, et al: Clinical utility of bone mass measurements in adults: Consensus of an international panel. Society for Clinical Densitometry. Semin Arthritis Rheum 25(6):361-372, 1996.
This summary of clinical opinion of an expert panel of the Society of Clinical Densitometry addresses the appropriate use of bone density measurements in determining whom to treat and in following the response to therapy.

Olszynski WP, Shawn Davison K, Adachi JD, et al: Osteoporosis in men: Epidemiology, diagnosis, prevention and treatment. Clin Ther 26(1):15-28, 2004.
This article reviews current information about osteoporosis in men discussing clinical risk factors, pathogenesis, and therapeutic options.

Rosen CJ: Clinical practice. Postmenopausal osteoporosis. N Engl J Med 353(6):595-603, 2005.
This article reviews the clinical management of low bone density and established osteoporosis with an emphasis on both preventive and therapeutic strategies.

Seeman E, Eisman JA: Treatment of osteoporosis: Why, whom, when and how to treat. The single most important consideration is the individual's absolute risk of fracture. Med J Aust 180(6):298-303, 2004.
The authors review the risks and benefits of various therapies for low bone density with guidelines on selection of patients for treatment.

EVIDENCE

1. Black DM, Cummings SR, Karpf DB, et al: Randomised trial of effect of alendronate on risk of fracture in women with existing vertebral fractures. Fracture Intervention Trial Research Group. Lancet 348(9041):1535-1541, 1996.
In this randomized clinical trial of oral alendronate in 2027 postmenopausal women with low bone mineral density and previous vertebral fractures, results showed reduction in fracture risk for both vertebral and nonvertebral fractures, including hip fracture in the treated group.

2. Chapuy MC, Arlot ME, Duboeuf F, et al: Vitamin D3 and calcium to prevent hip fractures in elderly women. N Engl J Med 327(23):1637-1642, 1992.
In a randomized clinical trial in 3270 elderly women with average age of 84 years, supplementation with 1.2 g of calcium and 800 IU of

vitamin D₃ reduced the risk for both vertebral and nonvertebral fractures in the treated group.

3. Chesnut CH 3rd, Silverman S, Andriano K, et al: A randomized trial of nasal spray salmon calcitonin in postmenopausal women with established osteoporosis: The Prevent Recurrence of Osteoporotic Fractures Study. PROOF Study Group. Am J Med 109(4):267-276, 2000.

   In a randomized clinical trial of intranasal salmon calcitonin in 1255 postmenopausal women with established osteoporosis using doses of 100, 200, and 400 IU daily, women receiving 200 IU had fewer new vertebral fractures than the control group.

4. Chesnut CH 3rd, Skag A, Christiansen C, et al: Effects of oral ibandronate administered daily or intermittently on fracture risk in postmenopausal osteoporosis. J Bone Miner Res 19(8):1241-1249, 2004.

   Results of a randomized clinical trial of ibandronate in 2946 osteoporotic women with previous vertebral fractures showed a reduction in risk for new vertebral fractures compared with placebo. Nonvertebral fractures were not significantly reduced except in a higher risk subgroup with bone density T scores of less than 3.0.

5. Cummings SR, Black DM, Thompson DE, et al: Effect of alendronate on risk of fracture in women with low bone density but without vertebral fractures: Results from the Fracture Intervention Trial. JAMA 280(24):2077-2082, 1998.

   In a randomized clinical trial with oral alendronate in 4432 women with low bone density but no previous vertebral fractures, more than 4 years of alendronate reduced fracture risk significantly in a subgroup of women with osteoporosis of the femoral neck (T score ≤−2.5), but there was no significant reduction in women having higher bone density.

6. Ettinger B, Black DM, Mitlak BH, et al: Reduction of vertebral fracture risk in postmenopausal women with osteoporosis treated with raloxifene: Results from a 3-year randomized clinical trial. Multiple Outcomes of Raloxifene Evaluation (MORE) Investigators. JAMA 282(7):637-645, 1999.

   In a randomized clinical trial of raloxifene in 7705 postmenopausal women who had osteoporosis according to World Health Organization Standards, treatment with raloxifene, 60 mg per day, significantly reduced the risk for vertebral but not nonvertebral fractures.

7. Harris ST, Watts NB, Genant HK, et al: Effects of risedronate treatment on vertebral and nonvertebral fractures in women with postmenopausal osteoporosis: A randomized controlled trial. Vertebral Efficacy with Risedronate Therapy (VERT) Study Group. JAMA 282(14):1344-1352, 1999.

   The authors report on a 3-year clinical trial with risedronate in 2458 postmenopausal women who had at least one vertebral fracture treated with oral risedronate or placebo. The treated group had a significant reduction in both vertebral and nonvertebral fractures.

8. Liberman UA, Weiss SR, Broll J, et al: Effect of oral alendronate on bone mineral density and the incidence of fractures in postmenopausal osteoporosis. The Alendronate Phase III Osteoporosis Treatment Study Group. N Engl J Med 333(22):1437-1443, 1995.

   This report on the original trial with alendronate in 994 postmenopausal women with osteoporosis showed that reduction in the risk for new vertebral fractures as well as improvements in bone mineral density of the spine and hip.

9. McClung MR, Geusens P, Miller PD, et al: Effect of risedronate on the risk of hip fracture in elderly women. Hip Intervention Program Study Group. N Engl J Med 344(5):333-340, 2001.

   This clinical trial of oral risedronate in 3886 women at least 80 years old showed reduction in hip fracture risk in a subset who had osteoporosis of the femoral neck (T score ≤3). There was no significant reduction of hip fracture with therapy in a subset who had higher bone mineral density.

10. Neer RM, Arnaud CD, Zanchetta JR, et al: Effect of parathyroid hormone (1-34) on fractures and bone mineral density in postmenopausal osteoporosis. N Engl J Med 344(19):1434-1441, 2001.

    This report of a clinical trial with subcutaneous PTH (1-34) in 1637 postmenopausal women with prior vertebral fractures showed reduction in the risk for both vertebral and nonvertebral fractures in the treated group. The 20-µg dose reduced fractures as much as a 40-µg dose but had fewer side effects.

11. Rossouw JE, Anderson GL, Prentice RL, et al: Risks and benefits of estrogen plus progestin in healthy postmenopausal women: Principal results from the Women's Health Initiative randomized controlled trial. JAMA 288(3):321-333, 2002.

    This article summarizes the overall results of an important clinical trial of estrogen replacement in 16,608 postmenopausal women with an intact uterus. Treatment with 0.6 mg conjugated estrogens plus 2.5 mg medroxyprogesterone daily for 5.2 years significantly reduced hip fractures but not the occurrence of cardiovascular events or all-cause mortality.

Sue A. Brown

49

Paget's Disease of Bone

Introduction

Paget's disease of bone, also known as *osteitis deformans*, is a disorder of accelerated bone turnover. It is characterized by abnormal osteoclast activity that results in increased bone breakdown. Because bone formation and resorption are coupled, there is a concomitant increase in bone formation. However, the new bone that is laid down is abnormal in its organization. Bone biopsy specimens demonstrate loss of the usual lamellar structure that is important for bone strength. As a result, the bone is weakened, with an abnormal bone remodeling surface.

The incidence and prevalence of Paget's disease are difficult to estimate because the disease is largely asymptomatic. Autopsy and radiologic series have found the prevalence to be 3% to 3.7% of patients older than 55 years. Overall, it appears to be a disease of individuals of Anglo-Saxon descent and is much less common in Asian individuals. Nearly all those affected present at a later age, usually older than 40 years. Some series report a male predominance, whereas others suggest that males are equally as affected as females.

Etiology and Pathogenesis

The exact etiology is unknown. Microscopically, osteoclasts are structurally abnormal, of increased size, and found in increased number. They have multinucleated structures with inclusion bodies similar to nucleocapsids found in paramyxoviruses such as measles, respiratory syncytial virus, and canine distemper virus. It has been postulated, but not definitively proved, that Paget's disease results from a viral infection. The involved osteoclasts appear to have an increased sensitivity to substances that alter osteoclast activity, such as 1,25-dihydroxyvitamin D (calcitriol) and RANK-ligand, an important signaling protein secreted by osteoblasts to control osteoclast activity (Fig. 49-1).

Paget's disease may also have a genetic predisposition. It has been reported that 15% to 40% of patients have an affected first-degree relative. Heterozygous mutations of at least two genes have been documented in Paget's disease. A susceptibility gene on the long arm of chromosome 18 has recently been identified in at least one study. This was discovered after an abnormality at a different location on the same chromosome was identified in familial expansile osteolysis, a rare disorder in which osteoclasts also have paramyxovirus-like inclusions. Possibly, viral infection initiates abnormal osteoclast activity and the onset of Paget's disease in individuals with a genetic susceptibility.

Clinical Presentation

Most individuals with Paget's disease of bone are asymptomatic. Often, it is incidentally diagnosed after serum alkaline phosphatase levels are obtained or plain radiographs are performed for unrelated reasons. It predominantly affects the calvarium and axial skeleton, most often involving vertebral bodies, pelvis, and long bones. It can occur in a monostotic form, with a single site affected. However, most patients have polyostotic disease with multiple sites involved (Fig. 49-2). Only 5% of individuals present with bone pain, often described as a dull or persistent ache exacerbated by activity. However, pain is not a good indicator of extent of disease. In one study, only 30% of 863 sites of disease caused symptoms in 170 patients. Bone pain may result from irritation of the periosteum, increased vascularity in affected bone, or mechanical stress with microfractures. There may be warmth at the site of involvement with Paget's disease. Pain in or near a joint may reflect underlying osteoarthritic changes such as osteophyte formation due to the presence of Paget's disease

Figure 49-1 Pathophysiology and Treatment of Paget's Disease of Bone.

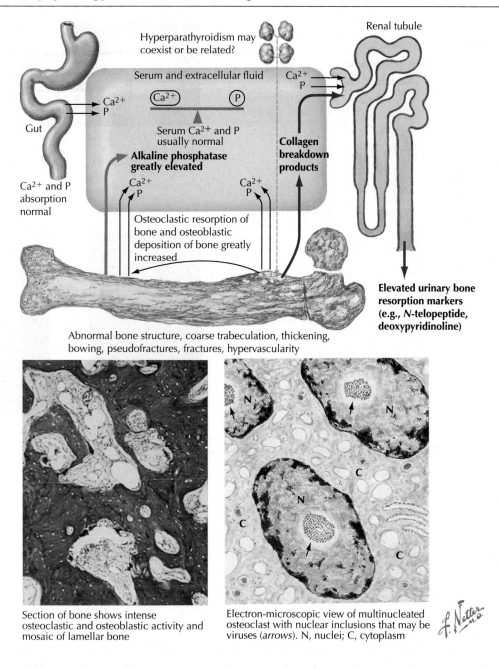

Renal tubule

Hyperparathyroidism may coexist or be related?

Serum and extracellular fluid

Ca^{2+}
P

Ca^{2+} P

Serum Ca^{2+} and P usually normal

Alkaline phosphatase greatly elevated

Gut

Ca^{2+}
P

Collagen breakdown products

Ca^{2+} and P absorption normal

Ca^{2+}
P

Ca^{2+}
P

Osteoclastic resorption of bone and osteoblastic deposition of bone greatly increased

Elevated urinary bone resorption markers (e.g., *N*-telopeptide, deoxypyridinoline)

Abnormal bone structure, coarse trabeculation, thickening, bowing, pseudofractures, fractures, hypervascularity

Section of bone shows intense osteoclastic and osteoblastic activity and mosaic of lamellar bone

Electron-microscopic view of multinucleated osteoclast with nuclear inclusions that may be viruses (*arrows*). N, nuclei; C, cytoplasm

in the adjoining long bone, which may deteriorate cartilage and alter the joint surface. Significant joint deformities can occur with bowing of the lower extremities as well as abnormal facial structures such as frontal bossing. Fractures are a common complication in weight-bearing bones as a result of disorganized bone structure. Neurologic compromise is a concerning complication. Involvement of the vertebral column can result in spinal cord or peripheral nerve root compression. Cranial nerves, particularly ocular and auditory nerves, can be affected as a result of skull deformities. Hearing loss has been reported in up to 37% of individuals and may also be due to acquired bony abnor-

malities in the cochlea. Rarely, hydrocephalus results from deformities at the skull base. With active, widespread disease, high-output congestive heart failure may be caused by increased vascularity of the bone remodeling surface. A rare but dreaded complication is the development of osteosarcoma, which is estimated to occur in less than 1% of patients with long-standing disease.

Differential Diagnosis

Other conditions that can present with bone pain, lytic lesions, and elevated alkaline phosphatase levels include

Figure 49-2 Paget's Disease of Bone.

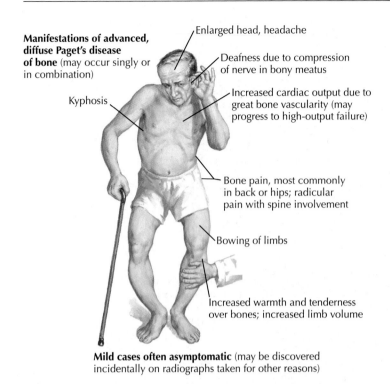

Manifestations of advanced, diffuse Paget's disease of bone (may occur singly or in combination)

Enlarged head, headache

Deafness due to compression of nerve in bony meatus

Increased cardiac output due to great bone vascularity (may progress to high-output failure)

Kyphosis

Bone pain, most commonly in back or hips; radicular pain with spine involvement

Bowing of limbs

Increased warmth and tenderness over bones; increased limb volume

Mild cases often asymptomatic (may be discovered incidentally on radiographs taken for other reasons)

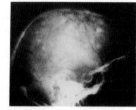

Lateral radiograph shows patchy density of skull, with areas of osteopenia (osteoporosis circumscripta cranii)

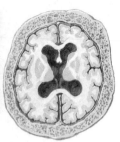

Extremely thickened skull bones, which may encroach on nerve foramina or brainstem and cause hydrocephalus (shown) by compressing cerebral aqueduct

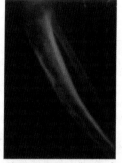

Characteristic radiographic findings in tibia include thickening, bowing, and coarse trabeculation, with advancing radiolucent wedge

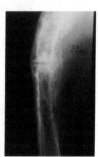

Healing chalk-stick fracture

malignancies, primary or metastatic disease, and infiltrative diseases such as infections and sarcoidosis. With widespread involvement, it can be difficult to distinguish Paget's disease from an underlying malignancy. Usually, the underlying malignancy is more obvious on clinical examination, and the bone metastases are a later complication. Paget's disease is much more likely if previous radiographs demonstrate relative stability of the lesions over time. A distinguishing radiologic feature of Paget's disease is the increase in the diameter of the affected bones, which remains unchanged in infiltrating or metastatic diseases. An isolated pagetic focus in a vertebral body may resemble vertebral hemangiomas or compression fractures. Unfortunately, bone scans do not distinguish among these conditions. Biochemical findings, such as anemia, hypoalbuminemia, or hypercalcemia, may suggest other underlying disorders. Paget's disease may cause hypercalcemia but only with prolonged immobilization or recent fracture. Although characteristic radiographic features exist, the diagnosis of Paget's disease is not always clear, and a search for an underlying malignancy or other disorder may need

to be pursued, including obtaining a bone biopsy specimen in some instances.

Diagnostic Approach

A diagnosis of Paget's disease is often made based on characteristic findings on plain radiographs. Early in the disease, lytic lesions predominate, reflecting increased areas of osteoclast resorption. They are characterized by flame or V-shaped resorption fronts on long bones, or isolated lytic lesions in the skull (also known as *osteoporosis circumscripta*). As the disease progresses, cortical thickening and sclerotic areas result from excessive bone formation from increased osteoblast activity. Bone scans demonstrate increased activity at the involved sites. The extent of the disease varies among individuals. Radiologic identification of sites of involvement is important to document the extent of the disease and to identify asymptomatic lesions located in fracture-prone sites that may require treatment. Although the disease may progress with advancing resorption fronts in a particular bone, there is usually not extensive spread to new bones after the initial diagnosis is made.

On laboratory examination, a significantly elevated alkaline phosphatase level occurs in about 95% of individuals. Baseline values are often greater than 3 times the upper limit of normal. However, monostotic or isolated Paget's disease may have a normal alkaline phosphatase level. The sensitivity of bone-specific alkaline phosphatase is slightly better than that of total alkaline phosphatase. The level of alkaline phosphatase usually correlates with disease activity if followed over time in a single individual. Serum levels of calcium, phosphate, parathyroid hormone, and vitamin D metabolites are usually normal. Hypercalcemia only occurs when the rates of bone formation decrease while the rate of bone resorption remains high, such as during prolonged immobilization or recent fracture. Bone turnover markers or collagen breakdown products, such as urinary N-telopeptides and deoxypyridinoline, are consistently elevated in active, extensive Paget's disease. However, these markers are not specific and have wide intrinsic variability, making their use difficult in treatment of patients. Other markers of osteoblast function, such as osteocalcin, are not helpful in the diagnosis or management of Paget's disease.

Management and Therapy

Optimum Treatment

Treatment of Paget's disease has significantly improved since the availability of potent oral bisphosphonates. Multiple studies have demonstrated an improvement in symptoms, notably bone pain, and a reduction in alkaline phosphatase and other bone turnover markers. Bisphosphonates have been shown to restore normal bone structure on bone biopsy specimens. However, there are no prospective long-term data that demonstrate prevention of future complications after treatment is initiated, and therefore treatment recommendations are often guided by clinical experience or expert consensus panels due to the paucity of randomized long-term clinical trials. Mild disease with isolated involvement in a location unlikely to cause complications, such as the scapula or pelvis, may not need to be treated. Short-term treatment with bisphosphonates or calcitonin may be indicated before orthopedic procedures to prevent excessive blood loss resulting from the hypervascularity of bone. The most common indications for therapy are bone pain, involvement of fracture-prone sites (weight-bearing bones, vertebral bodies), periarticular bone lesions, extensive skull involvement, prior orthopedic procedures, and prolonged immobilization.

Bisphosphonates are pyrophosphate analogs that decrease bone resorption rates by decreasing osteoclast activity and that make the hydroxyapatite structure of the bone matrix less susceptible to resorption. Several preparations are available and are generally given in 3- to 6-month cycles every 1 to 2 years or 1 to 2 months before elective surgery. Etidronate, the initial drug available, is less potent than newer agents and has been associated with osteomalacia when used at higher doses. Tiludronate, alendronate, and risedronate, potent oral bisphosphonates, are also approved by the U.S. Food and Drug Administration (FDA) for the treatment of Paget's disease (400 mg orally once daily, 40 mg orally once daily, and 30 mg orally once daily, respectively). One randomized controlled clinical trial of 89 patients comparing alendronate (40 mg once daily) and etidronate (400 mg once daily) for 6 months demonstrated a normalization of alkaline phosphatase in 63% of patients taking alendronate compared with only 17% taking etidronate. There were significant decreases in urinary bone turnover markers as well as improvements in pain and functional scores on alendronate. A follow-up extension study showed that 52% still had normal alkaline phosphatase levels 25 to 30 months after treatment ended. Radiographic evidence of improvement has varied, with some studies demonstrating regression of bone resorption fronts, but others not showing a significant change. Similar improvements in bone turnover markers are seen with either risedronate or alendronate. Pamidronate is highly effective but must be given in intravenous (IV) form. Dosing has varied from 60 mg given as a single infusion for mild disease to 20 to 60 mg given IV every 3 to 6 months. A randomized controlled study reported that zoledronate (5 mg IV) given as a single infusion reduced bone turnover for the 2-year duration of the trial, which appeared to be more sustained than an oral regimen of risedronate (30 mg once daily for 60 days).

Calcitonin is approved by the FDA in both salmon and human subcutaneous forms for the treatment of Paget's disease. However, bisphosphonates have superior efficacy in inducing and maintaining a remission, which has relegated calcitonin to second-line therapy if bisphosphonates are not tolerated. Calcitonin has a role in perioperative management because it is fast acting and effective for decreasing blood loss during surgery. Other treatment options have included gallium and plicamycin, although they are rarely used today. Often, analgesics and joint replacement surgery need to be considered to treat the associated osteoarthritic changes.

The general goal of treatment is to normalize alkaline phosphatase levels and decrease pain. Serum levels are often measured every 4 to 6 months. An additional treatment course should be considered when the alkaline phosphatase level has increased more than 25% of that achieved after the initial treatment. Bone turnover markers, such as urinary N-telopeptides, may respond earlier than alkaline phosphatase to bisphosphonate therapy. A single 3- to 6-month course of a bisphosphonate can induce a remission for 1 to 2 years or longer. Plain radiographs show changes over time, but they do not always correlate with alkaline phosphatase levels or symptomatic improvement. Bone scans are more reliable for following changes, although radiation exposure and expense limit their use. Although uncontrolled studies suggest there are decreased fracture rates, there is no solid proof that treating individuals will prevent future complications.

Avoiding Treatment Errors

It is important to distinguish radiologic changes associated with Paget's disease from lytic lesions associated with malignant or infiltrating conditions, as discussed under "Differential Diagnosis." An experienced radiologist is instrumental in this regard.

Future Directions

Patients can become less responsive to a single bisphosphonate after successive treatment courses. At least one study suggests, however, that these patients may retain responsiveness when changed to a different bisphosphonate. Combination therapy may prove to be a more effective strategy in the future. Newer, more potent bisphosphonates continue to be developed and may prove even more efficacious for the treatment of Paget's disease of bone. The PRISM (Paget's Disease: A Randomised Trial of Intensive vs. Symptomatic Management) trial is an ongoing United Kingdom multicenter trial comparing treatment strategies for Paget's disease and their impact on clinically relevant outcomes; these forthcoming data may alter management strategies.

Additional Resources

The Paget Foundation. Available at: http://www.paget.org. Accessed February 10, 2007.

The Paget Foundation is a reliable source for patient education.

Siris ES: Goals and treatment for Paget disease of bone. J Bone Miner Res 14(Suppl 2):49-52, 1999.

This concise review outlines the clinical approach to Paget's disease.

Whyte MP: Clinical practice: Paget disease of bone. N Engl J Med 355(6):593-600, 2006.

The author provides an excellent summary of the clinical approach to Paget's disease of bone.

EVIDENCE

1. Hosking D, Lyles K, Brown JP, et al: Long-term control of bone turnover in Paget disease with zoledronic acid and risedronate. J Bone Miner Res 22(1):142-148, 2007.

   This article compared zoledronic acid and risedronate in one of the few long-term clinical studies on the use of bisphosphonates in Paget's disease.

2. Siris E, Weinstein RS, Altman R, et al: Comparative study of alendronate versus etidronate for the treatment of Paget disease of bone. J Clin Endocrinol Metab 81(3):961-967, 1996.

   This paper provides evidence for the efficacy of alendronate compared with etidronate, an earlier-generation bisphosphonate.

3. Gutteridge DH, Ward LC, Stewart GO, et al: Paget disease: Acquired resistance to one aminobisphosphonate with retained response to another. J Bone Miner Res 14(Suppl 2):79-84, 1999.

   This article supports the use of different bisphosphonate preparations in Paget's disease.

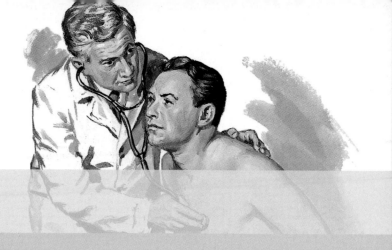
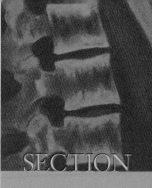

Disorders of the Gastrointestinal Tract

Nicholas J. Shaheen ▪ Ryan D. Madanick

Gastroesophageal Reflux Disease

Introduction

Gastroesophageal reflux disease (GERD) is one of the most common disorders encountered in medical practice. Almost half of Americans suffer heartburn symptoms at least once a month, and greater than 10% experience heartburn weekly. Once considered a nuisance problem, GERD is now associated with several serious conditions, including esophageal strictures, asthma, and esophageal adenocarcinoma. The toll of reflux on quality of life can be substantial. Patients with GERD sometimes rate their quality of life as worse than those with severe chronic diseases such as angina and mild heart failure. For these reasons, clinicians should be aggressive in the management of this disease.

Etiology and Pathogenesis

The pathophysiology of GERD is complex and multifactorial. The body has developed an elegant system of defense mechanisms that allows it to keep gastric acid with a pH of 1 to 2 in proximity to sensitive esophageal tissues. Even minor perturbations of this defense may result in acid injury from reflux.

To a minor degree, reflux occurs in most individuals. However, small amounts of acid refluxate are usually neutralized by salivary secretions and propelled back into the stomach by peristalsis. In GERD, several deficiencies in this defense system are often present. Patients with severe GERD, on average, have decreased lower esophageal sphincter (LES) pressure compared with normal subjects, although there is much overlap between normal subjects and those with reflux. Perhaps more importantly, these subjects have an increased number of transient LES relaxations. Although these short periods of sphincter relaxation occur in normal individuals as well, those with reflux appear to have them more commonly and also have a higher incidence of reflux during the relaxations. Hiatal hernia, or displacement of the stomach through the hiatus so that part of the stomach is in the chest, occurs commonly in those with GERD, impairing the efficiency of the LES. Some patients demonstrate impaired peristalsis, decreasing their ability to propel the refluxate back into the stomach. Other mechanisms, such as differences in the potency and composition of the refluxate, are postulated but are less well understood.

Some manifestations of GERD, including esophagitis, esophageal peptic strictures, and Barrett's esophagus, occur only in those with the most severe disease (Fig. 50-1). Esophagitis is the breakdown of mucosal tissue, so that erosions, exudates, and ulcers replace the normal squamous epithelium. Esophageal peptic stricture, or narrowing of the esophagus secondary to chronic acid exposure, sometimes requires endoscopic dilation and, rarely, surgery. Barrett's esophagus is a metaplastic change of the lining of the esophagus so that it switches from its normal squamous epithelium to a columnar epithelium with goblet cells. It appears that chronic acid exposure is a necessary prerequisite in the pathogenesis. However, because many subjects with severe GERD never develop Barrett's esophagus, other poorly understood host factors must also play a role.

Clinical Presentation

Heartburn, or substernal chest burning, is the most common clinical presentation of GERD (Fig. 50-2). This sensation is often worse when recumbent or after a large meal. Regurgitation of food, water brash (a filling of the

Figure 50-1 Complications of Peptic Reflux (Esophagitis and Stricture).

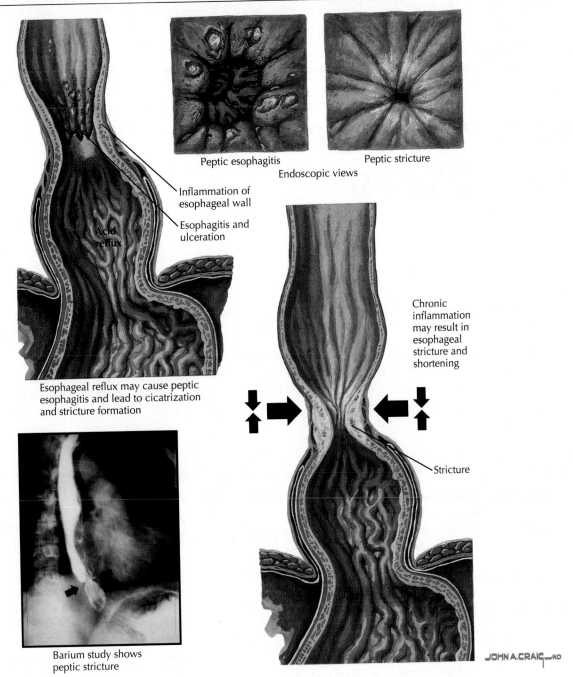

Peptic esophagitis

Peptic stricture

Endoscopic views

Inflammation of esophageal wall

Esophagitis and ulceration

Acid reflux

Esophageal reflux may cause peptic esophagitis and lead to cicatrization and stricture formation

Chronic inflammation may result in esophageal stricture and shortening

Stricture

Barium study shows peptic stricture

JOHN A. CRAIG—AD

mouth with saliva), dysphagia (difficulty swallowing), odynophagia (pain with swallowing), and chest pain are also common.

Recently, there has been an increased appreciation for the extraesophageal manifestations of reflux. GERD may cause a variety of pulmonary and ear, nose, and throat conditions, including asthma, bronchitis, chronic cough, halitosis, hoarseness, pulmonary fibrosis, aspiration pneumonia, and erosion of the dental enamel.

Differential Diagnosis

The presentation of GERD can be similar to many other conditions. Patients with heart disease may describe their chest pain as "burning." Among those complaining of chest pain, it is essential to rule out cardiac disease, especially in high-risk subgroups. Dysphagia is associated with esophageal cancer and esophageal strictures. The extraesophageal symptoms of GERD may be especially

Figure 50-2 Symptoms and Medical Management of GERD.

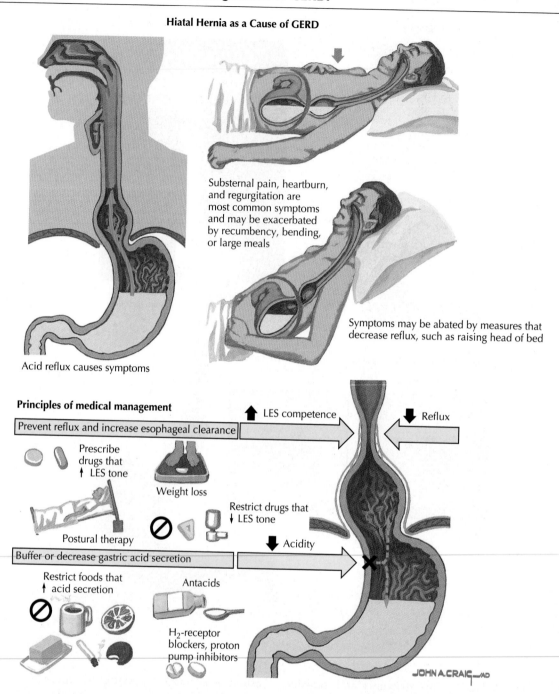

Hiatal Hernia as a Cause of GERD

Substernal pain, heartburn, and regurgitation are most common symptoms and may be exacerbated by recumbency, bending, or large meals

Symptoms may be abated by measures that decrease reflux, such as raising head of bed

Acid reflux causes symptoms

Principles of medical management

Prevent reflux and increase esophageal clearance

Prescribe drugs that ↑ LES tone

Weight loss

Postural therapy

Restrict drugs that ↓ LES tone

↑ LES competence   ↓ Reflux

↓ Acidity

Buffer or decrease gastric acid secretion

Restrict foods that ↑ acid secretion

Antacids

H_2-receptor blockers, proton pump inhibitors

JOHN A. CRAIG—AD

hard to recognize. GERD-induced asthma is a commonly missed diagnosis and should be considered in patients who do not respond as expected to therapies directed at asthma.

Diagnostic Approach

Most individuals with classic reflux symptoms do not require further diagnostic workup beyond a good history and physical examination (see Fig. 50-2). In these patients, an empiric trial of antacid therapy may be used as both a diagnostic and therapeutic measure. Appropriate response to therapy confirms the diagnosis and obviates further workup.

Invasive workup in reflux disease is generally reserved for three categories of patients: those with alarm symptoms (dysphagia, weight loss, bleeding, and anemia); those with uncommon or unclear presentations, in whom the diagnosis is uncertain; and those who do not demonstrate the expected clinical response to therapy.

Several tests are available to evaluate symptoms (Fig. 50-3). Upper endoscopy is a sensitive test for assessing

Figure 50-3 Diagnostic Techniques.

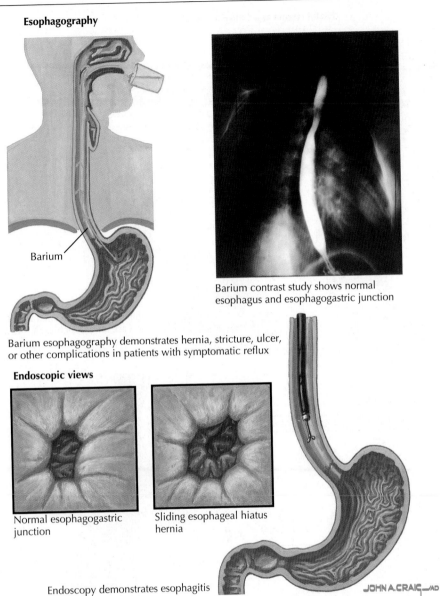

Esophagography

Barium

Barium esophagography demonstrates hernia, stricture, ulcer, or other complications in patients with symptomatic reflux

Barium contrast study shows normal esophagus and esophagogastric junction

Endoscopic views

Normal esophagogastric junction

Sliding esophageal hiatus hernia

Endoscopy demonstrates esophagitis

JOHN A. CRAIG—AD

mucosal damage and detecting strictures and cancers. Normal results of upper endoscopy do not rule out GERD because many patients have nonerosive reflux disease. The 24-hour pH probe is a small tube placed through the nares into the esophagus. It continually monitors and electronically records esophageal acid, allowing the clinician to note the extent of reflux, how high up the esophagus the reflux travels, and the relation of reflux episodes to other symptoms such as coughing or wheezing. Esophageal manometry assesses the contractions of the esophagus and the function of the LES. Because many patients have normal esophageal motility, it is not sensitive for reflux. Barium radiographs are excellent for identifying the presence and extent of esophageal strictures or cancer but are not sensitive or specific for the presence of reflux. Other tests, such as the Bernstein acid perfusion test, scintigraphy, and esophageal impedance studies, either lack specificity or are not commonly available.

Some authorities advocate a once-in-a-lifetime upper endoscopy for those with chronic reflux symptoms, both to screen for adenocarcinoma and to identify those with Barrett's esophagus who might then be enrolled in endoscopic surveillance programs to identify any resultant cancer at an early and potentially curable stage. Neither the efficacy nor cost effectiveness of such a screening endoscopy has been substantiated.

Management and Therapy

Optimum Treatment

The goal of management is complete relief of symptoms and prevention of complications. Given the armamentarium of medical and surgical therapies available, this goal is achievable in most patients. Optimum treatment depends on the severity of the disease and the patient's response to therapy. Generally, therapy commences with conservative measures, is escalated through pharmacologic therapy if necessary, and proceeds to surgical therapy in a small number of severely afflicted patients.

Conservative Therapy

Some GERD patients may respond to simple dietary and lifestyle modifications (see Fig. 50-2). Elevating the head of the bed, preferably on blocks, is a simple measure that is especially effective in those with nighttime symptoms. Weight loss reduces intra-abdominal pressure and may reduce symptoms. Avoidance of late-night meals gives the stomach adequate time to empty before recumbency. Smoking decreases LES pressure, and smoking cessation may improve symptoms. Caffeine, fatty foods, and alcohol may all decrease LES pressure, and limited intake of these items is recommended.

Pharmacologic Therapy

For those with very occasional GERD symptoms precipitated by dietary indiscretion, self-medication with either antacids or over-the-counter H$_2$-receptor antagonists appears to be safe and is widely practiced. Patients with severe or frequent symptoms require more intensive therapy. Both H$_2$-receptor antagonists, such as cimetidine, ranitidine, famotidine, and nizatidine, and proton pump inhibitors, such as omeprazole, pantoprazole, rabeprazole, lansoprazole, and esomeprazole, may provide symptomatic relief. The proton pump inhibitors are more effective at decreasing acid production than the H$_2$-receptor antagonists, but are more expensive. Some authorities have advocated a step-up approach to therapy with these agents; the clinician starts by treating with an H$_2$-receptor antagonist and steps up therapy to a proton pump inhibitor only in patients unresponsive to the H$_2$-receptor antagonist. Others advocate a step-down approach, so that therapy is initiated with a proton pump inhibitor to achieve symptom control, and then the patient is stepped down to the lowest level of acid inhibition that still provides good symptom control. No matter which strategy is adopted, it is important to assess symptom response shortly after the initiation of therapy and to adjust the medication regimen appropriately.

It is rare that patients do not achieve good symptom control with standard doses of proton pump inhibitors. In these situations, the dose of the proton pump inhibitor may be increased to twice a day. If the patient continues to be unresponsive, the clinician should question the diagnosis and consider further workup. If twice-a-day proton pump inhibitors do not control GERD, the addition of a nighttime H$_2$-receptor antagonist to the two doses of proton pump inhibitor or a third dose of proton pump inhibitor may help. Use of a promotility agent in addition to the anti-acid regimen is reasonable. Unfortunately, few agents are available. Use of metoclopramide is limited. Cisapride is also effective, but safety concerns have curtailed its use and availability. Other promotility agents may soon be available. Sucralfate, a mucosal coating agent, may be used either alone or in combination with acid inhibition, but its frequent dosing interval and efficacy make it a less commonly used drug in reflux.

Surgical Therapy

A surgical antireflux procedure for control of symptoms warrants consideration in patients who require chronic pharmacologic therapy, especially high-dose proton pump inhibition. Laparoscopic Nissen fundoplication is the most common antireflux surgical procedure performed in the United States. The recovery time is short, and the procedure is generally well tolerated. Studies indicate that most patients obtain symptom relief and are not taking antireflux medications at 2 years. Long-term outcomes are less clear; data suggest that operator experience and appropriate patient selection are key to improving outcomes.

Multiple endoscopic antireflux devices have been developed to attempt to change the anatomy of the hiatus without a surgical intervention. These include devices that form a plication at the gastroesophageal junction and that apply energy to the submucosal tissue to cause thickening of the area of the LES. The long-term utility of these devices remains unclear.

Avoiding Treatment Errors

Duration of therapy is a commonly overlooked issue in reflux disease. GERD is a chronic condition often requiring chronic therapy. In the subgroup of patients with erosive esophagitis, most of those healed with medication have recurrence of their esophagitis if taken off therapy. In these patients, symptom control after initial treatment may be maintained with less intensive therapy. For instance, a patient initially requiring proton pump inhibitors to heal erosive esophagitis may remain symptom- and disease-free on H$_2$-receptor antagonists. However, healing of erosive esophagitis does not always ensure complete symptom relief, and patients may still require aggressive acid suppression to maintain symptom control.

Future Directions

Several avenues hold promise for improving care of patients with reflux. Several new promotility agents are under development and are likely to be useful in GERD. Endoscopic alterations of the anatomy offer the chance to improve symptoms without subjecting the patient to surgery. Better treatments for the complications of reflux, such as strictures and Barrett's esophagus, may decrease the number of subjects who suffer the most severe manifestations of this disease. Finally, objective analysis of our practices in caring for the reflux patient should allow us to recognize the most cost-effective approaches to therapy.

Additional Resources

International Foundation for Functional Gastrointestinal Disorders Website. Available at: http://www.aboutgerd.org/. Accessed September 22, 2006.

This website is directed at patients with GERD who wish to understand more about their symptoms and how to deal with them.

National Institutes of Health GERD Information Clearinghouse Website. Available at: http://digestive.niddk.nih.gov/ddiseases/pubs/gerd/. Accessed September 22, 2006.

This patient-focused website has detailed information written by GERD experts about both pediatric and adult GERD.

EVIDENCE

1. Dean BB, Gano AD, Knight K, et al: Effectiveness of proton pump inhibitors in nonerosive reflux disease. Clin Gastroenterol Hepatol 2(8):656-664, 2004.

   This systematic review reports that the therapeutic gain of proton pump inhibitors for heartburn resolution is lower in nonerosive reflux disease than in erosive disease.

2. DeVault KR, Castell DO: Updated guidelines for the diagnosis and treatment of gastroesophageal reflux disease. Am J Gastroenterol 100(1):190-200, 2005.

   This excellent guideline critically reviews the level of evidence for various strategies for diagnosis and management of GERD.

3. Fass R, Fennerty MB, Ofman JJ, et al: The clinical and economic value of a short course of omeprazole in patients with noncardiac chest pain. Gastroenterology 115(1):42-49, 1998.

   The empiric "omeprazole test" for noncardiac chest pain is shown to be an accurate noninvasive method for diagnosing GERD in these patients.

4. Spechler SJ, Lee E, Ahnen D, et al: Long-term outcome of medical and surgical therapies for gastroesophageal reflux disease: Follow-up of a randomized controlled trial. JAMA 285(18):2331-2338, 2001.

   This investigation reveals that 62% of patients who underwent open fundoplication for treatment of GERD in a randomized controlled trial had resumed taking antireflux medications after a mean of 9 years.

Douglas R. Morgan ▪ Nicholas J. Shaheen

Peptic Ulcer Disease

Introduction

Peptic ulcers are gastrointestinal mucosal defects that extend through the muscularis mucosa that can be symptomatic or asymptomatic. Peptic ulcer disease (PUD) is associated with significant morbidity and expenditures related to work loss, hospitalizations, and outpatient care (excluding medications) of more than $5 billion per year in the United States. Major advances have been made in the past two decades with the etiologic linkage of *Helicobacter pylori* to PUD and the development of more effective medical therapies. However, despite advances in diagnosis and therapy, the prevalence of PUD remains unaltered, and the cumulative mortality rate in complicated ulcer disease remains significant.

The estimated worldwide lifetime incidence of PUD is 5% to 10%. These estimates double in those harboring *H. pylori* infection. The incidence of PUD increases with age for two major reasons in developed nations. First, the incidence of *H. pylori* infection is decreasing in people younger than 40 years, primarily as a result of improved socioeconomic conditions. Despite this, about 75% of duodenal ulcers and 75% of gastric ulcers not caused by nonsteroidal anti-inflammatory drugs (NSAIDs) are a result of *H. pylori*. The second leading cause of peptic ulcers, the use of NSAIDs, increases with age. NSAID use is an independent predictor of experiencing a gastrointestinal complication such as peptic ulcer disease.

Etiology and Pathogenesis

Although *H. pylori* infection and NSAID use account for most cases of PUD, there are important, less common causes, including hypersecretory states, stress ulcers, neoplasia, and idiopathic ulcers. Cigarette smoking can increase the risk for relapse and delay healing. Corticosteroid use is a risk factor for PUD, but only when used in combination with NSAIDs.

More than half of the world's population is infected with *H. pylori*, most with a mild infection and without clinical manifestations. *H. pylori* infection can result in either or both peptic ulcers and gastric cancer. The interaction between host factors (e.g., genetic), *H. pylori* virulence factors (particularly cytotoxin-associated gene A), and other environmental factors (e.g., diet) drives a subset of patients either to an antral predominant gastritis, the ulcer pathway, or a corpus predominant gastritis, the gastric cancer pathway. In antral gastritis, there is an inhibition of somatostatin and increased gastrin production. These two hormonal alterations cause parietal cells to increase secretion of acid in the gastric body. The increased acid secretion creates an increased duodenal acid load and may contribute to gastric metaplasia in the duodenal bulb, with possible *H. pylori* colonization. This explains, in part, the paradoxical observation that *H. pylori* causes duodenal ulceration but is generally not resident in normal duodenal epithelium.

NSAID use is the second most important etiologic factor in PUD in this country. With the aging of the American population and the ready availability of these agents over the counter, NSAID-induced gastrointestinal toxicity has risen in incidence during the past 3 decades. The U.S. Food and Drug Administration approximates the risk for a clinically significant gastrointestinal event, including perforations, ulcerations, or bleeding, to be 1% to 4% per year for the nonselective class of NSAIDs. The mechanisms by which NSAIDs cause ulceration involve both direct topical injury and systemic effects mediated by endogenous prostaglandins. NSAID use induces changes in the local mucosal blood flow of the stomach and duodenum. These changes impede repair of damaged mucosa. Also, traditional NSAIDs inhibit both the cyclooxygenase (COX-1 and COX-2) isoenzymes. Although inhibition of the COX-2 isoenzyme leads to the anti-inflammatory effects that provide the NSAIDs beneficial effects, inhibition of the COX-1 isoenzyme causes an impaired response

Figure 51-1 Peptic Ulcer Disease: Acute Gastric Ulcers.

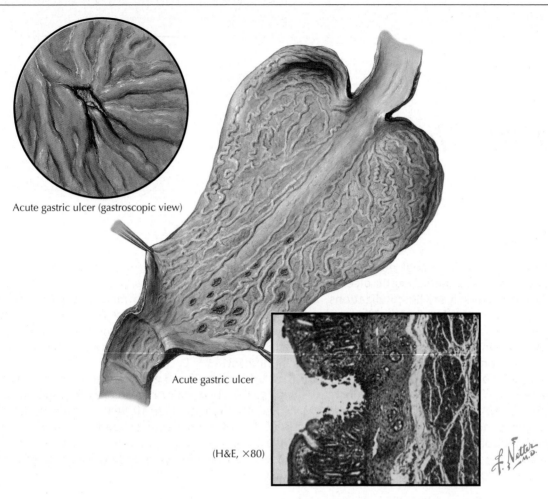

Acute gastric ulcer (gastroscopic view)

Acute gastric ulcer

(H&E, ×80)

to mucosal damage. Because the COX-1 isoenzyme is involved in multiple housekeeping functions, such as hemostasis and protection of the gastric mucosa, inhibition of this enzyme is thought to be responsible for most of the mucosal toxicity of NSAIDs. Nearly 100% of people ingesting NSAIDs have endoscopic evidence of erosions. However, symptoms of clinically important ulcers develop in only a minority of these individuals (Fig. 51-1).

Clinical Presentation

The most common presenting complaint in patients with PUD is dyspepsia. Classic teaching suggests that duodenal ulcers characteristically present with symptoms of burning hunger-type pain that occurs 2 to 3 hours after eating or awakening a patient from sleep and is relieved with antacids. These symptoms lack sensitivity and specificity: the presence of symptoms does not reliably predict ulcers, nor does the absence of symptoms exclude disease (Fig. 51-2). Patients may present with symptoms of a complication of PUD, such as bleeding (hematemesis, melena), perforation with peritonitis, or gastric outlet obstruction from pyloric channel edema (Fig. 51-3). Rarely, patients may present

with syncope or angina secondary to previously undetected blood loss. Some subjects with PUD, especially those taking NSAIDs, may have no symptoms from the disease.

The clinical signs of PUD are often subtle. Vital signs are usually normal unless significant hemorrhage has occurred. Pain on palpation of the mid or right epigastrium is common, but not diagnostic. Stool test results for fecal occult blood may be positive but are neither sensitive nor specific for PUD.

Differential Diagnosis

An accurate history is essential to discriminate between common and uncommon disorders that imitate PUD. With a detailed history and minimal testing, conditions such as gastroesophageal reflux, gastric adenocarcinoma, biliary tract disease, and pancreatic disease can be excluded. Functional or nonulcer dyspepsia is the most common cause of epigastric pain. This poorly understood entity likely represents several different pathophysiologic processes, only some of which are acid peptic in nature. Functional dyspepsia and irritable bowel syndrome are the most common functional gastrointestinal disorders.

Figure 51-2 Peptic Ulcer Disease: Chronic Gastric Ulcers.

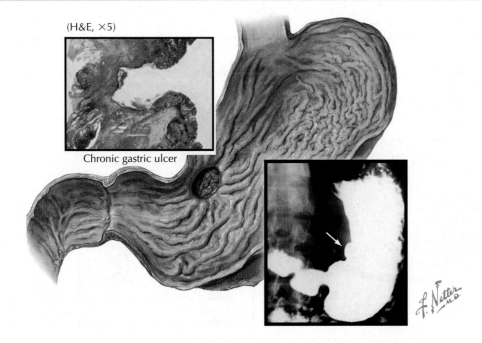

(H&E, ×5)

Chronic gastric ulcer

Diagnostic Approach

Older patients presenting with abdominal pain or any patient with alarm symptoms (early satiety, weight loss, bleeding, anemia) should undergo endoscopy for exclusion of gastric adenocarcinoma. In patients younger than 45 years without alarm symptoms, a test-and-treat strategy may be pursued. To test and treat, one obtains a noninvasive measure of *H. pylori* infection such as a serum or breath test and treats to eradicate the organism if it is present.

Endoscopy is the gold standard for the evaluation of PUD (Fig. 51-4). It allows detection of ulcer disease with accuracy and permits biopsy, to exclude carcinoma as well as confirm infection with *H. pylori* by histology or rapid urease testing (e.g., CLOtest). The margins of all gastric ulcers should be examined and undergo biopsy to exclude malignancy.

Upper gastrointestinal radiography for the diagnosis of PUD is largely of historical interest but is an acceptable substitute in areas where endoscopy is not available. Although certain radiographic features suggest benign or malignant disease, the test has insufficient accuracy to rule out malignancy as a cause of ulceration, especially in the case of gastric ulcers.

Management and Therapy

Optimum Treatment

The goals of treatment are fourfold: relief of symptoms, ulcer healing, prevention of complications, and decreasing the risk for recurrent ulceration. Repeat endoscopy has been advocated for gastric ulcer diseases to document

healing and disprove malignancy; however, it is unclear whether this is necessary in all cases.

Multiple forms of therapy (histamine-2 receptor antagonists, proton pump inhibitors [PPI], or misoprostol) are effective for symptom relief and ulcer healing. For an NSAID-associated ulcer, the agent should be discontinued, if possible. If the patient must remain on the NSAID, PPIs achieve superior healing rates and decrease the risk for relapse. Treatment with COX-2 inhibitors appears to lessen the risk for gastrointestinal side effects in patients requiring chronic NSAID use, but the increased risk for cardiovascular and cerebrovascular events has precluded their use in most cases. Surreptitious or inadvertent NSAID use is the most common reason for recurrent ulcer disease.

The role of *H. pylori* in duodenal and gastric ulcer formation is indisputable. If infection is documented, eradication with a standard regimen of a PPI with two antibiotics for 10 to 14 days is important (see Chapter 52). Successful eradication decreases the recurrence of endoscopically diagnosed duodenal ulcers from about 55% to 19% at 6 months. Follow-up testing is performed 4 weeks or more following therapy to ensure eradication in patients with complicated ulcer disease (e.g., bleeding, perforation).

Although many chronic NSAID users are *H. pylori* positive, the incremental benefit of eradicating the infection for all subjects who are *H. pylori* positive and require chronic NSAIDs remains controversial. Smoking cessation should be encouraged in any form of ulcer disease. Universal dietary modifications are not indicated.

Endoscopic therapy is the initial management step for PUD complicated by bleeding (see Fig. 51-4). At the time

Figure 51-3 Peptic Ulcer Disease: Complications of Gastric and Duodenal Ulcers.

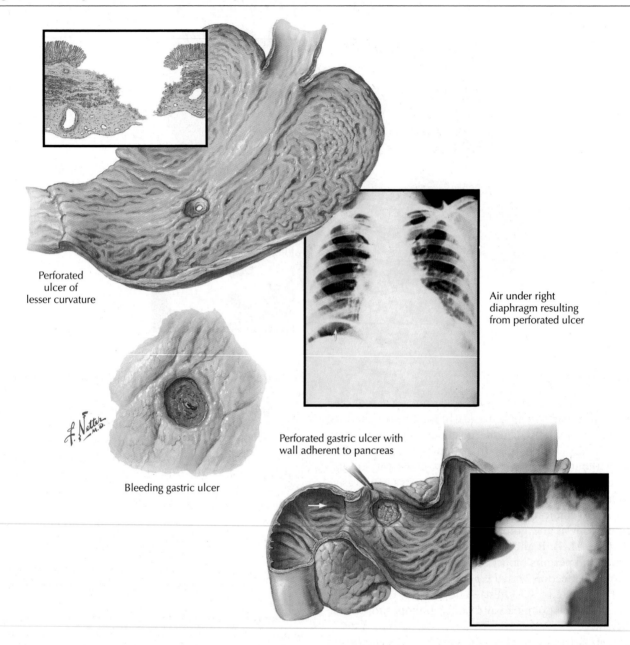

Perforated
ulcer of
lesser curvature

Air under right
diaphragm resulting
from perforated ulcer

Perforated gastric ulcer with
wall adherent to pancreas

Bleeding gastric ulcer

of upper endoscopy, if a visible vessel is seen, either with or without bleeding, treatment can usually be accomplished with various techniques (e.g., cautery, injection, endoclip). Successful endoscopic therapy can also lower the short-term risk for recurrent bleeding as well as the need for surgery. In addition, intravenous PPIs offer the promise of decreasing the acute morbidity and mortality associated with ulcer hemorrhage.

Upper endoscopy can also be useful in gastric outlet obstruction secondary to chronic scarring from PUD because endoscopic balloon dilation may relieve the obstruction, obviating surgery. Generally, ulcers complicated by refractory bleeding may be managed with interventional radiology or surgery. Potent acid suppression

and antimicrobial therapy have lessened the role of surgery in the management of ulcers, and today, surgical intervention is rarely necessary.

Avoiding Treatment Errors

The long-term use of PPI therapy is not indicated for most patients with prior peptic ulcer disease. For *H. pylori*–associated ulcers, antisecretory therapy may be stopped after 3 months. For NSAID-associated ulcers, the patient should be counseled to cease NSAID use, if possible. Lastly, follow-up endoscopy at a 2- to 3-month interval remains warranted for gastric ulcers to exclude malignancy. Definitive studies are needed to facilitate revision of this recommendation.

Figure 51-4 Diagnostic Evaluation.

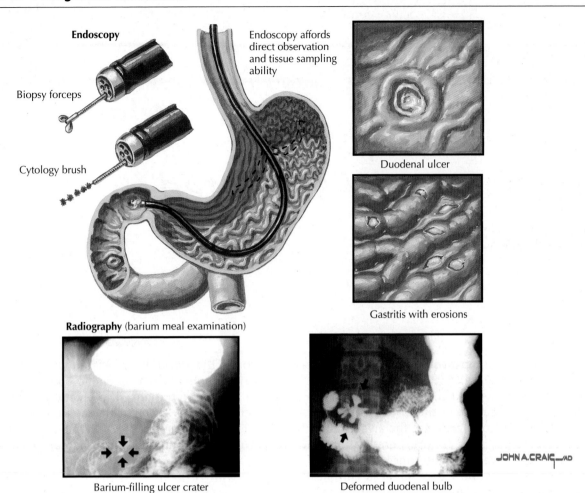

Endoscopy

Biopsy forceps

Cytology brush

Endoscopy affords direct observation and tissue sampling ability

Duodenal ulcer

Gastritis with erosions

Radiography (barium meal examination)

Barium-filling ulcer crater

Deformed duodenal bulb

JOHN A.CRAIG—AD

Future Directions

Although the relative risk for ulcer formation is increased in patients with *H. pylori* infection or NSAID ingestion, the absolute risk is low. Challenges facing investigators include identifying the subsets of these populations who are at higher risk. High-risk patients could be targeted for *H. pylori* testing and eradication. In the case of those requiring chronic NSAID use, prophylactic therapy with PPIs is an option. The epidemiology of PUD is likely to change as the prevalence of *H. pylori* infection in developed nations such as the United States declines; the proportion of *H. pylori*–negative and NSAID-negative ulcers will increase. Thus, investigations aimed at understanding the pathophysiology of ulcer formation and healing will return to center stage.

Additional Resources

Katz PO, Scheiman JM, Barkun AN: Review article: Acid-related disease—what are the unmet clinical needs? Aliment Pharmacol Ther 23(Suppl 2):9-22, 2006.

Despite the revolution in our management of peptic ulcer disease with PPIs and H. pylori therapies, important gaps remain in our understanding and management options.
Yuan Y, Padol IT, Hunt RH: Peptic ulcer disease today. Nat Clin Pract Gastroenterol Hepatol 3(2):80-89, 2006.
The authors present a state-of-the-art review.
Sonnenberg A: Time trends of ulcer mortality in Europe. Gastroenterology 132:2320-2327, 2007.
Time trend analysis of ulcer disease mortality in six European countries over eight decades underscores the importance of H. pylori.

EVIDENCE

1. Ford AC, Delaney BC, Forman D, Moayyedi P: Eradication therapy for peptic ulcer disease in Helicobacter pylori positive patients. Cochrane Database Syst Rev (2):CD003840, 2006.
   This is the Cochrane systematic review of the evidence for the benefit of H. pylori eradication in peptic ulcer disease.
2. Papatheodoridis GV, Sougioultzis S, Archimandritis AJ: Effects of Helicobacter pylori and nonsteroidal anti-inflammatory drugs on peptic ulcer disease: A systematic review. Clin Gastroenterol Hepatol 4(2):130-142, 2006.
   The authors review the roles of NSAIDs and H. pylori infection in peptic ulcer disease.

Douglas R. Morgan

52

Helicobacter pylori Infection and Associated Disorders

Introduction

Helicobacter pylori, the most common chronic bacterial infection in the world, is associated with chronic gastritis, peptic ulcer disease, gastric adenocarcinoma, and gastric lymphoma. Phylogenetic analysis suggests that the organism coevolved with humans, dating to the initial human migrations. The pivotal work by Barry Marshall and Robin Warren in the 1980s confirmed the association of *H. pylori* with gastric disease. Their contributions were recognized with the award of the Nobel Prize in Medicine in 2005. The more recent notion that antibiotic therapy with *H. pylori* eradication may prevent gastric adenocarcinoma and cure gastric lymphoma is of equal potential importance.

Nearly half of the world's population is chronically infected with *H. pylori. H. pylori* is endemic in most of the developing world, affecting about three fourths of adults, compared with about one third of adults in the developed world. Childhood socioeconomic status is the strongest determinant of the likelihood of infection. Related risk factors include inadequate sanitation, crowded living conditions, and sibling infection. In the United States, there are also significant racial and ethnic differences with respect to infection prevalence (Table 52-1).

Person-to-person transmission, specifically gastro-oral, is the postulated mode of infection. Studies suggest that most infections are acquired in childhood before 5 years of age, with familial clustering. Viable organisms have also been isolated from feces and water supplies, suggesting that low-level sporadic transmission may also occur. Adult infection in the developed world is uncommon, with an estimated rate of less than 1% per annum. Importantly, persistent infection following an antibiotic regimen is likely a result of treatment failure (compliance, resistance) rather than new infection.

The decrease in *H. pylori* infection worldwide resulting from improved socioeconomic conditions has several implications. A cohort effect is observed in developed nations, with older individuals more likely to be infected, which reflects childhood socioeconomic status rather than new adult infection. In part, this explains the decrease in incidence in duodenal ulcers and gastric cancer in the developed world. The prevalence of *H. pylori* infection is likely to decrease further owing to our improved understanding of the role of racial and ethnic differences in infection rates and for treatment—underlining the importance of an individualized approach to dyspepsia.

Etiology and Pathogenesis

H. pylori is a gram-negative spiral-shaped gastric organism. The bacteria inhabit the stomach's mucosal surface without invasion. The usual organism burden in the stomach is 1 billion, with a plethora of quasi-species present within each individual. *H. pylori* infection triggers a robust host immune response, resulting in chronic active gastritis in most infections. The organism uses a novel pH-dependent urea channel (UreI) and urease to generate ammonia and create

Table 52-1 *Helicobacter pylori* Seroprevalence in the United States

Race or Ethnicity	Age (yr)			
	All Ages	20-30	50-60	>70
White	27%	8	36	55
African American	51	38	54	73
Hispanic	58	49	63	74
Total	33	17	40	57

Adapted from CDC and NHANES III data; Everhart JE, Kruszon-Moran D, Perez-Perez GI, et al: Seroprevalence and ethnic differences in H. pylori infection among adults in the United States. J Infect Dis 181(4):1359-1363, 2000; and McQuillan GM, Kruszon-Moran D, Kottiri BJ, et al: Racial and ethnic differences in the seroprevalence of 6 infectious diseases in the United States: Data from NHANES III, 1988-1994. Am J Public Health 94(11):1952-1958, 2004.

Box 52-1 *Helicobacter pylori* Infection and Pathways to Gastric Carcinogenesis

Host genetic susceptibility (e.g., cytokine risk genotypes)
Childhood *H. pylori* infection
Proinflammatory cytokine up-regulation by *H. pylori*
Diffuse gastritis with subsequent achlorhydria
Atrophic gastritis
Intestinal metaplasia
Parallel environmental exposures (e.g., dietary, coinfections)
Microniche disequilibrium: additional host genetic and *H. pylori* factors
Gastric dysplasia
Gastric adenocarcinoma

a buffered microenvironment. The urease enzyme is produced at a higher level by *H. pylori* than by other bacteria and serves as the basis for many of the diagnostic tests.

H. pylori infection is a model for understanding gene-environment interactions that can lead to disease through chronic inflammation. The development of ulcer disease or cancer depends on the complex interaction at the gastric microniche level between host genetics, virulence factors, diet, and the environment. Several virulence factors have been described for the organism, the most important of which is the cytotoxin-associated gene A (cagA), which increases the likelihood of both ulcer disease and cancer. Other virulence factors include vacuolization factors (vacA) and adhesion factors (babA). Proinflammatory cytokine genotypes (e.g., polymorphisms of interleukin [IL]-1β, IL-10, tumor necrosis factor-α) are associated with gastric adenocarcinoma in *H. pylori*–infected subjects (Box 52-1).

Three patterns of *H. pylori* infection are associated chronic active gastritis. Most infected persons have a mild gastritis, without clinical manifestations. Second, antral predominant gastritis can be present and is associated with peptic ulcer disease. Third, corpus gastritis is correlated with intestinal metaplasia and gastric adenocarcinoma (Fig. 52-1). Failure to account for the heterogeneity of *H. pylori* infection accounts for much of the discordant literature, particularly in relation to esophageal disease. Lastly, the gene-environment model may vary globally as a result of racial and ethnic differences as well as variance in *H. pylori* virulence factors.

Clinical Presentation

The principal diseases associated with *H. pylori* infection are chronic gastritis, peptic ulcer disease, gastric adenocarcinoma, and low-grade B-cell non-Hodgkin's lymphoma. The *H. pylori*–associated lymphoma is also termed *mucosa-associated lymphoid tissue lymphoma* (MALToma).

Most infected persons have an asymptomatic chronic active gastritis. Dyspepsia is the hallmark of symptomatic infection. Initial infection with acute gastritis is self-limited but may cause discomfort, halitosis, nausea, and vomiting. Transient achlorhydria often develops for 1 to 6 months.

H. pylori is the most important cause of peptic ulcer disease and is implicated in 75% of both duodenal and nonsteroidal anti-inflammatory drug (NSAID)-negative gastric ulcers. The lifetime risk for an ulcer with infection is 5% to 20%. Active ulcer disease may cause epigastric pain, nausea, vomiting, and, if complicated, hemorrhage or obstruction. Eradication of *H. pylori* decreases the risk for ulcer recurrence, but less so than initially postulated. A meta-analysis of trials suggested that the duodenal ulcer recurrence rate with successful eradication is 20% at 6 months, versus 56% in untreated patients. Most commonly, the failure of antibiotic therapy is related to an inadequate course of therapy. Infection testing and treatment are strongly recommended for patients with past or current peptic ulcer disease.

The concept of antibiotic therapy for cancer prevention or cure is intriguing. Patients with *H. pylori*–related gastric cancer or MALToma usually have nonspecific symptoms until large tumors are present. Although the etiology of gastric adenocarcinoma is multifactorial, *H. pylori* infection has a proven role, although it is neither necessary nor sufficient. Epidemiologic studies consistently suggest a relative risk increase of 3 to 9 times, similar to the relation between tobacco and lung cancer. A definitive cancer prevention trial has not been performed and probably will not be because a half-million patient-years would be required to prove efficacy. Thus, treatment recommendations are based on cost-effectiveness analyses, and the current recommendation is to screen for *H. pylori* in high-risk patient populations: family history of gastric cancer and immigrants from high incidence regions (e.g., Asia, Latin America).

Most patients with gastric MALToma also have evidence of infection. A number of studies suggest that nearly 80% of patients with low-grade tumors attain remission

Figure 52-1 Etiology and Pathogenesis of *Helicobacter pylori*.

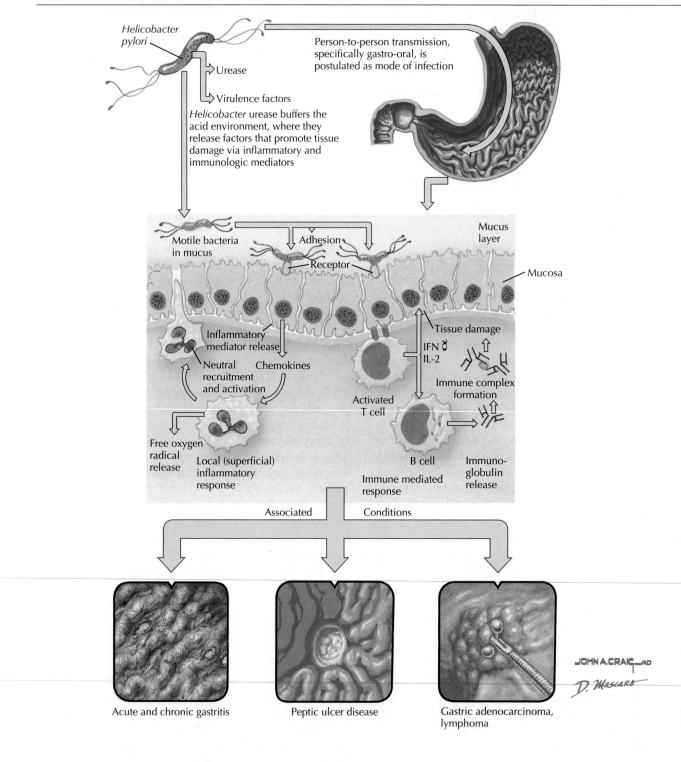

Helicobacter pylori

Urease

Virulence factors

Person-to-person transmission, specifically gastro-oral, is postulated as mode of infection

Helicobacter urease buffers the acid environment, where they release factors that promote tissue damage via inflammatory and immunologic mediators

Motile bacteria in mucus

Adhesion

Receptor

Mucus layer

Mucosa

Inflammatory mediator release

Neutral recruitment and activation

Chemokines

Free oxygen radical release

Local (superficial) inflammatory response

Activated T cell

Tissue damage

IFN ♂
IL-2

Immune complex formation

B cell

Immune mediated response

Immuno-globulin release

Associated   Conditions

Acute and chronic gastritis

Peptic ulcer disease

Gastric adenocarcinoma, lymphoma

JOHN A. CRAIG—AD

D. Mascaro

with antibiotic therapy. It must be noted, however, that half of these patients demonstrate a persistent monoclonal B-cell clone.

A number of entities have been less convincingly associated with *H. pylori* infection. These include functional dyspepsia, gastroesophageal reflux disease (GERD), and synergistic effects with NSAIDs and proton pump inhibi-tors (PPIs). Most randomized controlled trials have shown a borderline benefit of eradication therapy for functional dyspepsia, supporting the notion that it is a functional disease. Some patients may derive benefit from antibiotic therapy, however, suggesting that an individualized approach is appropriate. This has important implications for the approach to uninvestigated dyspepsia.

There may be an additive effect in peptic ulcer disease between *H. pylori* and NSAIDs. The current literature fails to provide a consensus regarding the benefit of testing and eradication before the initiation of chronic NSAID therapy. In the setting of a dual NSAID and *H. pylori* ulcer, eradication is indicated. Continued PPI therapy may be considered if ongoing NSAID use is needed. Subsequent studies have not substantiated the initial report of an increased risk for atrophic gastritis and, by inference, gastric cancer in infected patients treated with chronic PPI therapy. Currently, testing for and treatment of *H. pylori* are not recommended before the initiation of chronic NSAID or PPI therapy.

Postulated extragastric manifestations of disease are tenuous. Studies have yielded discordant results regarding the worsening of GERD and its complications in some patients following *H. pylori* treatment. In the moderate to severe GERD population, the indication for initial testing should be clear, and patients with positive results should be offered treatment. Despite initial reports, there is little evidence for an association with coronary artery disease, iron-deficiency anemia, rosacea, chronic idiopathic urticaria, or growth delay.

Differential Diagnosis

Dyspepsia is broadly defined as the symptom of upper abdominal discomfort and encompasses the clinical entities caused by *H. pylori*. The differential diagnosis for dyspepsia is broad and includes many non–*H. pylori*–related causes: NSAID (and other) peptic ulcer diseases, gastric cancer, esophageal disease and GERD, myocardial ischemia, and hepatobiliary disease. Functional dyspepsia, also known as nonulcer or endoscopy negative dyspepsia, refers to pain in this region without alarm features, laboratory abnormalities, or findings on upper endoscopy. Uninvestigated dyspepsia refers to the initial presentation with epigastric pain or discomfort before clinical evaluation. At upper endoscopy in patients with uninvestigated dyspepsia, about 15% each have ulcer disease, esophageal disease, or gastritis, whereas the remaining 40% to 60% are negative, suggestive of functional or self-limited dyspepsia.

A variety of approaches to uninvestigated dyspepsia have been suggested, including empiric acid suppression, immediate endoscopy, and the test-and-treat and test-and-scope approaches. The latter approaches refer to *H. pylori* testing with either treatment or endoscopy for positive results. The dominant strategy in the United States is test and treat. Patients with new-onset dyspepsia, younger than 45 to 50 years, and without alarm signs or symptoms (vomiting, weight loss, bleeding, anemia) are tested for *H. pylori* infection and treated if results are positive. Persons with persistent symptoms are referred for endoscopy. Recent outcome studies support the efficacy of this approach. The test-and-scope approach is often used in Asia and Latin America where gastric cancer rather than ulcer disease is

the main concern. Some European centers use immediate endoscopy for uninvestigated dyspepsia. Small studies suggest that outcomes and patient satisfaction are slightly better with direct endoscopy. If endoscopy costs in the United States decrease, particularly with the use of unsedated endoscopy, this may become a reasonable approach. Empiric acid suppression for 1 to 2 months has returned to favor with the availability of PPIs. Although the test-and-treat strategy is reasonable for most patients, the approach should be individualized with consideration of test and scope or immediate endoscopy based on symptoms, age, ethnicity, family history, and test availability.

Diagnostic Approach

Testing for *H. pylori* is suggested for those with active or prior peptic ulcer disease, uninvestigated dyspepsia, family history of gastric cancer, moderate-to-severe gastritis diagnosed on upper endoscopy, and gastric cancer or MALToma. All infected patients should be offered treatment.

Diagnostic tests include both noninvasive and invasive approaches (Box 52-2; Fig. 52-2). Serology (enzyme-linked immunosorbent assay detects immunoglobulin G antibodies) can be used to document past or current infection but cannot be used to document successful eradication. The urea breath tests (UBT) and stool antigen assay are active tests, documenting operative infection, and may be used to confirm eradication. For patients undergoing upper endoscopy, gastric biopsy specimens may be submitted for either histology or rapid urease testing (RUT). Histologic studies are the gold standard. Both the UBT and RUT depend on the detection of bacterial urease activity. Culture of *H. pylori* remains difficult and is limited to the research setting.

In low-prevalence populations, such as young whites in the United States, the false-positive rate of serologic testing is unacceptable, and active testing is recommended, particularly for the test-and-treat strategy for uninvestigated dyspepsia. Recent treatment (within 2 to 4 weeks) with any

---

Box 52-2 Diagnostic Tests for *Helicobacter pylori* Infection

Serology
   Immunoglobulin G
   Enzyme-linked immunosorbent assay
Stool antigen test*
Urea breath tests*
   ^{13}C, nonradioactive isotope
   ^{14}C, radioactive isotope
Endoscopy- and biopsy-based tests*
   Histopathology, gold standard
   Rapid urease tests

*Active tests, which may be used to document eradication.

Figure 52-2 Diagnosis and Management of *Helicobacter pylori*.

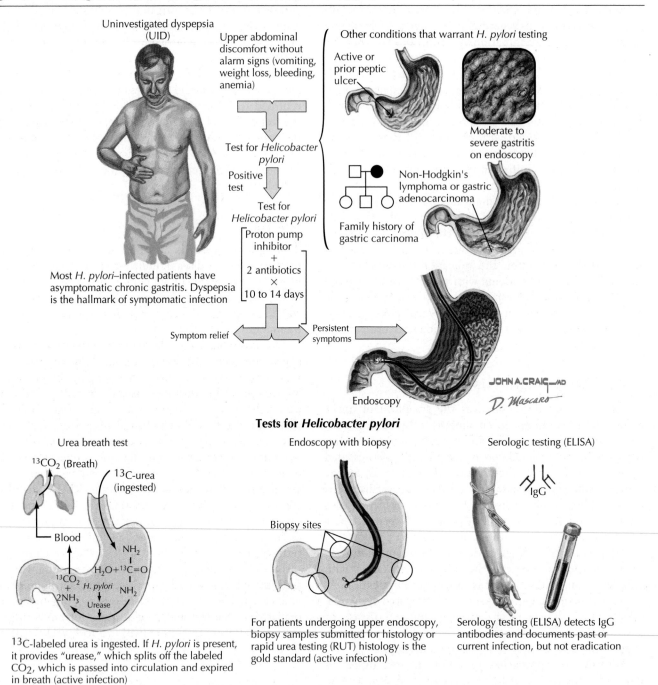

Uninvestigated dyspepsia (UID)

Upper abdominal discomfort without alarm signs (vomiting, weight loss, bleeding, anemia)

Test for *Helicobacter pylori*

Positive test

Test for *Helicobacter pylori*

Proton pump inhibitor
+
2 antibiotics
×
10 to 14 days

Most *H. pylori*–infected patients have asymptomatic chronic gastritis. Dyspepsia is the hallmark of symptomatic infection

Symptom relief

Persistent symptoms

Other conditions that warrant *H. pylori* testing

Active or prior peptic ulcer

Moderate to severe gastritis on endoscopy

Non-Hodgkin's lymphoma or gastric adenocarcinoma

Family history of gastric carcinoma

Endoscopy

JOHN A. CRAIG—MD
D. Mascaro

Tests for *Helicobacter pylori*

Urea breath test

$^{13}CO_2$ (Breath)

^{13}C-urea (ingested)

Blood

NH_2
$H_2O + ^{13}C = O$
$^{13}CO_2$
+
$2NH_3$ *H. pylori* NH_2
Urease

^{13}C-labeled urea is ingested. If *H. pylori* is present, it provides "urease," which splits off the labeled CO_2, which is passed into circulation and expired in breath (active infection)

Endoscopy with biopsy

Biopsy sites

For patients undergoing upper endoscopy, biopsy samples submitted for histology or rapid urea testing (RUT) histology is the gold standard (active infection)

Serologic testing (ELISA)

IgG

Serology testing (ELISA) detects IgG antibodies and documents past or current infection, but not eradication

of the components of *H. pylori* treatment (PPIs, bismuth compounds, and antibiotics) decreases the sensitivity of all nonserologic tests.

In general, documentation of successful eradication is unnecessary. Confirmation of clearance should be considered in patients with complicated peptic ulcer disease, gastric adenocarcinoma, MALToma, or persistent symptoms, and for those requesting such documentation. Active testing or endoscopy is indicated at least 1 month after

treatment to avoid false-negative results in the immediate post-treatment period.

Management and Therapy

Optimum Treatment

Optimal therapy for *H. pylori* infection requires a PPI with two antibiotics for 10 to 14 days (Table 52-2). Treatment

Table 52-2 Standard *H. pylori* Treatment Regimens*

Antibiotic	Proton Pump Inhibitor (PPI)†
PAC, twice daily	PPI, clarithromycin (500 mg), amoxicillin (1 g)
PMC, twice daily	PPI, clarithromycin (250-500 mg), metronidazole (250-500 mg)
PBMT, 4 times daily‡	PPI (twice daily), bismuth (525 mg), metronidazole (250 mg), tetracycline (500 mg)

*Treatment duration is 10-14 days.
†The PPIs (omeprazole, esomeprazole, lansoprazole, pantoprazole, rabeprazole) are equivalent.
‡The PBMT regimen is a 4 times daily regimen, except for twice daily PPI administration.
PAC, a PPI, amoxicillin, and clarithromycin; PBMT, a PPI, bismuth, metronidazole, and tetracycline; PMC, a PPI, metronidazole, and clarithromycin.

should be offered to all patients with positive diagnostic test results. The three principal regimens have similar efficacy of 80% to 85%.

The PAC regimen (a PPI, amoxicillin, and clarithromycin) is the most common combination. The PMC combination (a PPI, metronidazole, and clarithromycin) is appropriate for those individuals who have a penicillin allergy. The use of a PPI with the bismuth-based regimen significantly improves its efficacy. No significant difference has been noted between PPIs, although some physicians have preferences, based on their clinical experience in prescribing these agents. Prepackaged or combination products may improve compliance (e.g., PrevPac, Helidac, Pylera). Of note, the efficacy rates of various regimens and shorter treatment durations have largely been based on studies performed elsewhere and often have not been duplicated in the United States.

Avoiding Treatment Errors

Eradication failure is usually due to patient noncompliance or antibiotic resistance. Patients should be advised that completion of therapy is required and that the choice of a 2-week period without competing factors (e.g., travel) is important. There is no significant resistance to either amoxicillin or tetracycline. Primary resistance rates with clarithromycin and metronidazole are 5% to 10% and 25% to 35%, respectively, with age, sex, racial, and regional differences. Higher resistance rates are noted in elderly, female, and African-American patients. Metronidazole resistance may be an in vitro effect and can be overcome with the use of bismuth or PPI. Clarithromycin resistance

markedly decreases efficacy, and in this case PBMT (a PPI, bismuth, metronidazole, and tetracycline) is the principal retreatment regimen (Fig. 52-2). The use of other antibiotics has been reported in small studies for patients who have failed the PAC and PBMT regimens (e.g., rifabutin, furazolidone, levofloxacin, azithromycin).

Future Directions

H. pylori infection suggests a model for gene-environment interactions leading to disease through chronic inflammation, particularly for gastric cancer. Ongoing research should provide insights into the mode of transmission, childhood infection, and immunology. New antibiotic regimens are expected. A vaccine would provide the most cost-effective manner to prevent gastric cancer in high-incidence regions of the developing world, but development has proved difficult owing to the organism's genetic diversity. Because *H. pylori* has coevolved with humans, continued basic and clinical research will likely offer insights into the organism itself, other bacterial infections, and other human diseases.

Additional Resources

Moayyedi P, Soo S, Deeks J, et al: Eradication of *Helicobacter pylori* for non-ulcer dyspepsia. Cochrane Database Syst Rev 2:CD002096, 2006.
   This article presents the Cochrane systematic review of the evidence regarding the benefit of H. pylori eradication in functional dyspepsia.
Vilaichone RK, Mahachai V, Graham DY: *Helicobacter pylori* diagnosis and management. Gastroenterol Clin North Am 35(2):229-247, 2006.
   This review article is by one of the leaders in the field (Graham).

EVIDENCE

1. Camargo MC, Mera R, Correa P, et al: Interleukin-1beta and interleukin-1 receptor antagonist gene polymorphisms and gastric cancer: A meta-analysis. Cancer Epidemiol Biomarkers Prev 15(9):1674-1687, 2006.
   The role of proinflammatory cytokine polymorphisms in the development of gastric cancer is supported in this study, the first such meta-analysis.
2. El-Omar EM, Carrington M, Chow WH, et al: Interleukin-1 polymorphisms associated with increased risk of gastric cancer. Nature 404(6776):398-402, 2000.
   This seminal paper suggests that proinflammatory cytokine polymorphisms are important cofactors with H. pylori infection for the development of gastric cancer in European populations.
3. Peek RM Jr: Pathogenesis of *Helicobacter pylori* infection. Springer Semin Immunopathol 27(2):197-215, 2005.
   This article provides an overview of important H. pylori risk factors in the development of peptic ulcers and gastric cancer.

Gastrointestinal Bleeding

Introduction

Gastrointestinal (GI) bleeding refers to bleeding from a source in the esophagus, stomach, small intestine, colon, anus, or rarely the liver and pancreas. In 2002, there were 116,724 hospital discharges with a principal diagnosis of GI hemorrhage (ICD-9 code 578.9), which was the 51st among all discharge diagnoses, and 74,717 hospital discharges with a principal diagnosis of diverticulosis with hemorrhage (ICD-9 code 562.12). Various descriptors have been used to categorize GI bleeding including the following: acute, chronic, active, occult, and obscure. In addition, GI bleeding is usually classified as upper versus lower. Upper GI bleeding refers to bleeding from a source from the esophagus to the duodenum at the ligament of Treitz. Lower GI bleeding refers to bleeding from the jejunum to the anus. Because of the breadth of this topic, the focus here is primarily on the causes of GI bleeding and the management strategies for acute bleeding.

Etiology and Pathogenesis

There are many different causes of GI bleeding (Fig. 53-1). Several factors can increase an individual's risk for GI bleeding. These include cirrhosis, coagulopathy, the use of aspirin or nonsteroidal anti-inflammatory drugs, and the use of antiplatelet or anticlotting drugs.

Clinical Presentation

The clinical presentation depends on the rate, source, and volume of blood loss. Upper GI bleeding can present in several ways: hematemesis, vomiting of bright red blood; coffee ground emesis, vomiting of blood that has been digested by gastric acid; and melena, the passage of black tarry stool. Upper GI blood loss can also be occult, with no visible evidence of blood to the naked eye.

Lower GI bleeding can present as hematochezia, the passage of bright red blood per rectum, and less commonly as melena. Lower GI bleeding does stop spontaneously in most cases (about 85%). It can also be occult.

A person who is experiencing a rapid, large-volume GI bleed will manifest hemodynamic instability. Orthostatic blood pressure changes (a decrease in blood pressure of 20 mm Hg systolic or 10 mm Hg diastolic with an associated 20-point rise in heart rate after standing) can be seen with a 15% reduction in blood volume. Hypotension usually occurs with a 20% blood volume reduction.

Slow chronic blood loss can result in a significant reduction in hemoglobin without a change in hemodynamic stability. These patients often present with weakness, fatigue, shortness of breath, or chest pain as a result of anemia.

All patients presenting with GI bleeding should be checked for physical examination findings suggestive of chronic liver disease, including palmar erythema, spider angiomas, splenomegaly, ascites, and scleral icterus. Underlying cirrhosis with portal hypertension is a common cause of upper GI hemorrhage from gastric and esophageal varices.

Some etiologies of GI bleeding are associated with abdominal pain, but many are not. A careful abdominal examination looking for distention, the presence of bowel sounds, and tenderness is a critical step in patient evaluation.

Differential Diagnosis

Numerous lesions can cause upper GI bleeding (Box 53-1) as well as lower GI bleeding (Box 53-2). The following questions yield very important historical information that helps to narrow a very broad differential list of diagnoses:

- Have there been similar prior episodes?
- Did nonbloody emesis precede bloody emesis?
- What medications, both prescription and over the counter, have been taken recently?

Figure 53-1 Gastrointestinal Hemorrhage.

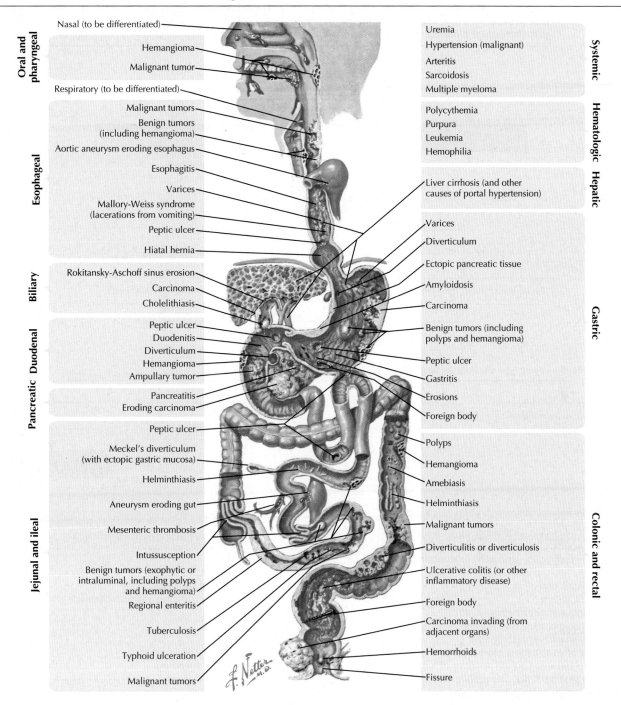

- Is there a history of clotting disorder?
- Is there associated abdominal pain?
- Is there a history of abdominal aortic aneurysm repair?
- Are there risk factors for chronic liver disease?

Diagnostic Approach

When a patient presents with GI bleeding, the urgency of evaluation is highly dependent on an initial assessment of hemodynamic stability and on whether there is significant ongoing bleeding. Monitoring vital signs, obtaining good intravenous access with large-bore intravenous catheters, and ordering a complete blood count, prothrombin time and partial thromboplastin time, and a type and cross-match for blood products should occur early in the evaluation. Hypotension requires aggressive intravenous fluid resuscitation and blood transfusions as indicated. The correction of an underlying coagulopathy is also a key initial therapeutic step. If a patient is having ongoing hacademe-

Figure 53-2A Acute Upper Gastrointestinal Bleeding, Part 1.
AVM, arteriovenous malformation; ED, emergency department; ICU, intensive care unit; UGI, upper gastrointestinal. *From Eisen GM, Dominitz JA, Faigel DO, et al: An annotated algorithmic approach to upper gastrointestinal bleeding. Gastrointest Endosc 53(7):853-858, 2001.*

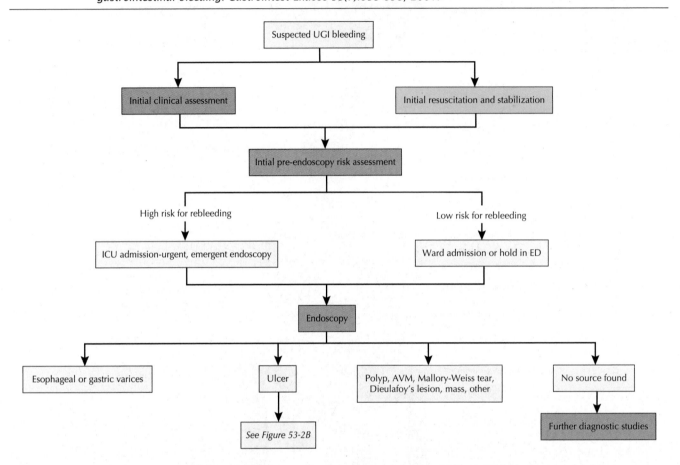

Box 53-1 Differential Diagnoses of Upper Gastrointestinal Bleeding
Ulcers of esophagus, stomach, or duodenum
Varices
Mallory-Weiss tear
Dieulafoy's lesion
Arteriovenous malformation
Esophagitis, gastritis, duodenitis
Portal hypertensive gastropathy
Neoplasia of esophagus, stomach, duodenum
Other rare lesions: Crohn's disease of upper gastrointestinal tract, hemobilia, hemosuccus pancreaticus, aortoenteric fistula

Box 53-2 Differential Diagnoses of Lower Gastrointestinal Bleeding
Diverticulosis
Arteriovenous malformation
Radiation-induced telangiectasias
Colitis (infectious, inflammatory, ischemic)
Neoplasia
Ulcers
Hemorrhoids
Anal fissure
Postpolypectomy bleeding

sis, airway protection may require tracheal intubation. The patient should not receive anything by mouth except essential oral medications.

An experienced endoscopist should see the patient as soon as possible, and the medical care team should ask for a surgical consultation if the patient's hemodynamic state remains unstable with evidence of continuing blood loss. If an upper GI bleed is suspected, the patient should have an urgent upper endoscopy. Endoscopy provides diagnos-

tic and prognostic information and also allows for therapeutic intervention.

If the patient can be stabilized hemodynamically and if it is clear that a lower GI bleed is occurring, a polyethylene glycol purge should be given over 3 to 4 hours.

If the patient presents with evidence of chronic occult GI bleeding and is hemodynamically stable, an outpatient upper and lower endoscopy is a reasonable approach. When there is no definite diagnosis after these studies, the next step is capsule endoscopy of the small bowel or other small bowel imaging modality.

Figure 53-2B Acute Upper Gastrointestinal Bleeding, Part 2.

ICU, intensive care unit; Rx, therapy. *From Eisen GM, Dominitz JA, Faigel DO, et al: An annotated algorithmic approach to upper gastrointestinal bleeding. Gastrointest Endosc 53(7):853-858, 2001.*

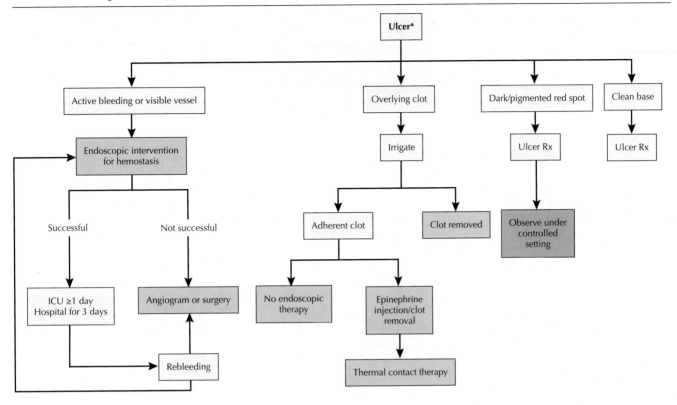

Continued from Figure 53-2A

Management and Therapy

In 2001, the American Society for Gastrointestinal Endoscopy published algorithmic approaches to upper and acute lower GI bleeding (Figs. 53-2 and 53-3). These approaches remain relevant. A 250-mg dose of intravenous erythromycin is often given before upper endoscopy to help empty blood clots from the stomach. Also, most endoscopists now try to remove all adherent clots and provide endoscopic therapy to the lesions found beneath them, if indicated.

In upper GI bleeding, the following are predictors for rebleeding: older age; shock, hemodynamic instability, and orthostasis; comorbid disease states (e.g., coronary artery disease, congestive heart failure, renal and hepatic diseases, cancer); specific endoscopic diagnosis (e.g., GI malignancy); use of anticoagulants and coagulopathy; and presence of a high-risk lesion (e.g., arterial bleeding or nonbleeding, visible vessel).

Optimum Treatment

For upper GI bleeding, optimum treatment involves a combination of endoscopy and medications. The findings on endoscopy identify lesions at risk for rebleeding, which affect the length of hospitalization. Helpful adjunctive medications are available. Proton pump inhibitors, given in high-dose oral or intravenous forms, have decreased rebleeding rates and the need for surgery in patients with peptic ulcer disease. Somatostatin or its synthetic analogue octreotide is used to help control variceal bleeding along with the use of endoscopic therapeutic techniques.

For acute lower GI bleeding, the optimum treatment strategy is shown in the algorithm in Figure 53-3. Stabilization of the patient must be the first priority, followed by evaluation for a specific bleeding source. Some lower GI bleeding lesions are amenable to endoscopic hemostatic therapy, including a culprit diverticulum, arteriovenous malformation, polypectomy sites, and radiation proctitis. Angiography should be reserved for those with massive bleeding that precludes colonoscopy and those in whom colonoscopy was nondiagnostic but bleeding persists. If an extravasation site is identified, arterial embolization is an alternative. Surgery is reserved for those failing endoscopic and angiographic therapy.

Avoiding Treatment Errors

Not paying enough attention to a bleeding patient's hemodynamic stability both at the time of presentation and over

Figure 53-3A Acute Lower Gastrointestinal Bleeding, Part 1.
Coags, coagulation studies including prothrombin time and partial thromboplastin time; CBC, complete blood count; EGD, esophagogastroduodenoscopy; PEG, polyethylene glycol solution; UGIB, upper gastrointestinal bleeding. *From Eisen GM, Dominitz JA, Faigel DO, et al: An annotated algorithmic approach to acute lower gastrointestinal bleeding. Gastrointest Endosc 53(7):859-863, 2001.*

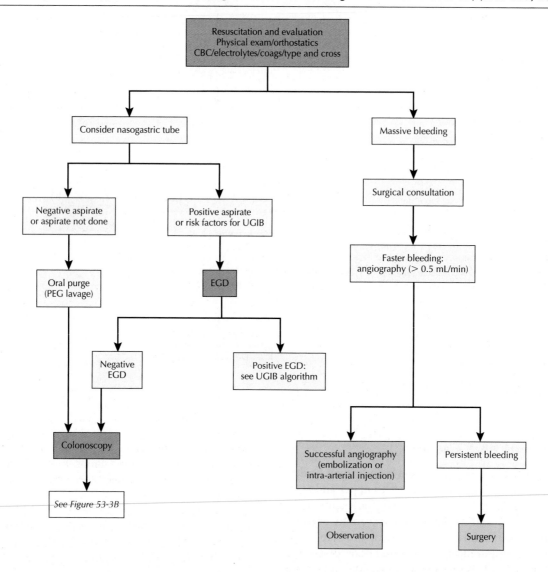

the ensuing hours of hospitalization is the most important treatment error. These patients must have frequent, if not continuous, monitoring of vital signs, cessation or reversal of anticoagulant therapy, ongoing monitoring of hematocrits, adequate intravenous access, fluid support, and blood product support.

Future Directions

Capsule technology will continue to evolve and in the future may have a role in diagnosing lower GI bleeding. Device manufacturers will continue to develop tools to aid the endoscopist in achieving hemostasis. Endoscopic suturing devices are being developed.

Additional Resources

Gastrointestinal bleeding. Gastroenterol Clin North Am 34(4):581-775, 2005.
  Ten chapters of this volume are dedicated to the topic of gastrointestinal bleeding in this quarterly publication.
Tramer MR, Moore RA, Reynolds DJ, et al: Quantitative estimation of rare adverse events which follow a biological progression: a new model applied to chronic NSAID use. Pain 85:169-182, 2000.
  A large review of studies of patients exposed to nonsteroidal anti-inflammatory medications for 2 months found that 1 in 150 developed upper gastrointestinal bleeding.
Triadafilopoulos G: Review article: The role of antisecretory therapy in the management of non-variceal upper gastrointestinal bleeding. Aliment Pharmacol Ther 22(Suppl 3):53-58, 2005.
  The author provides a concise review of nonvariceal upper GI bleeding and the role of proton pump inhibitor therapy.

Figure 53-3B Acute Lower Gastrointestinal Bleeding, Part 2.

AVMs, arteriovenous malformations; EGD, esophagogastroduodenoscopy or UGI endoscopy; h/o, history of; PRBC, packed red blood cells; TRBC, tagged red blood cell scan; UPRBC, units of packed red blood cells. *From Eisen GM, Dominitz JA, Faigel DO, et al: An annotated algorithmic approach to acute lower gastrointestinal bleeding. Gastrointest Endosc 53(7):859-863, 2001.*

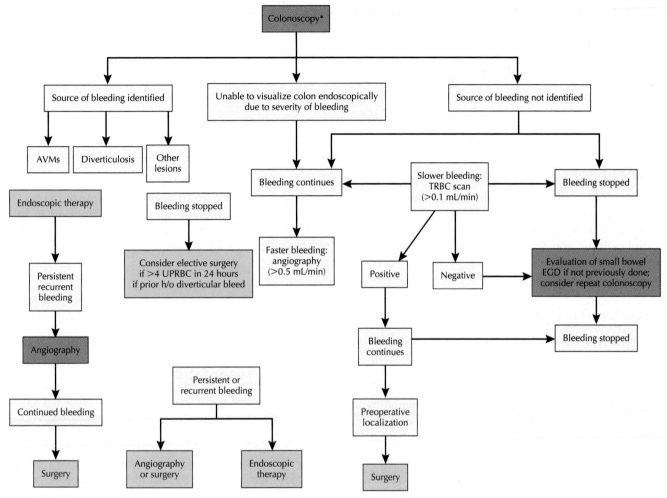

*Continued from Figure 53-3A

EVIDENCE

1. Agency for Healthcare Research and Quality: H-CUPnet Web Site. Available at: http://hcup.ahrq.gov/HCUPNet.asp. Accessed October 7, 2006.

   This website contains hospitalization statistics by year derived from a representative sample of U.S. hospitals.

2. Carbonell N, Pauwels A, Serfaty L, et al: Erythromycin infusion prior to endoscopy for acute upper gastrointestinal bleeding: A randomized, controlled, double-blind trial. Am J Gastroenterol 101(6):1211-1215, 2006.

   A randomized controlled trial of preprocedure erythromycin versus placebo showing improved gastric clearance of blood and quality of endoscopic exam.

3. Corley DA, Cello JP, Adkisson W, et al: Octreotide for acute esophageal variceal bleeding: A meta-analysis. Gastroenterology 120(4):946-954, 2001.

   A meta-analysis of 13 randomized trials shows improved control of acute esophageal variceal hemorrhage with octreotide as compared with all alternative therapies, vasopressin/terlipressin, and no additional intervention/placebo in those who had undergone endoscopic therapy before randomization.

4. Eisen GM, Dominitz JA, Faigel DO, et al. An annotated algorithmic approach to upper gastrointestinal bleeding. Gastrointest Endosc 53(7):853-858, 2001.

   This article contains the American Society of Gastrointestinal Endoscopists' guideline on approach to upper GI bleeding.

5. Farrell JJ, Friedman LS: Review article: The management of lower gastrointestinal bleeding. Aliment Pharmacol Ther 21:1281-1298, 2005.

   The authors present a comprehensive review of all pertinent management strategies for patients with lower GI bleeding.

6. Leontiadis GI, Sharma VK, Howden CW: Systematic review and meta-analysis of proton pump inhibitor therapy in peptic ulcer bleeding. BMJ 330:568, 2005.

   A Cochrane collaboration meta-analysis of 21 trials compares oral or intravenous proton pump inhibitor therapy to placebo.

Cholelithiasis

Introduction

The prevalence of gallstones in the United States increases from about 4% in 20-year-olds to more than 15% in those older than 60 years. Cholecystectomy is the most common abdominal operation performed in this country, with about 750,000 completed each year. The annual cost for the management of gallstones, their complications, and the associated economic losses to society is close to $5 billion.

Etiology and Pathogenesis

Gallstones are classified according to their composition. They vary in shape, number, size, and consistency; however, these characteristics play little role in whether symptoms develop (Fig. 54-1).

Cholesterol gallstones are the most common type. Three factors are necessary for their formation: supersaturation of gallbladder bile with cholesterol, crystal nucleation, and gallbladder hypomotility (Fig. 54-2). The solubility of cholesterol in bile depends on the incorporation of cholesterol in solubilizing bile acid–lecithin micelles. Alterations in the relative concentrations of cholesterol, bile acids, or lecithin can lead to cholesterol supersaturation. Mucin glycoprotein molecules act as nucleating agents to form gallstones. Cholesterol crystals in the mucin gel, coupled with defective emptying of the gallbladder, lead to the growth and development of stones.

Pigmented stones include black or brown varieties. Black pigmented stones are composed of pure calcium bilirubinate or polymer-like complexes of calcium, copper, and large amounts of glycoproteins. These stones are most common in cirrhosis and chronic hemolytic states. Brown pigmented stones are usually associated with infection. Bacteria present in the biliary system hydrolyze glucuronic acid from conjugated bilirubin. Calcium salts of the now unconjugated bilirubin crystallize and form brown stones.

Most epidemiologic series indicate that the prevalence of gallstones in women varies from 5% to 20% between the ages of 20 and 55 years, and from 25% to 30% after age 50 years. The prevalence for men is about half that of women at any age. Other risk factors are listed in Box 54-1.

Clinical Presentation

Gallstones cause symptoms by obstruction of the cystic duct, common bile duct, or erosion into neighboring organs (Fig. 54-3). Seventy-five percent of gallstones do not cause symptoms; 20% cause intermittent pain or biliary colic; 10% result in acute cholecystitis; 5% pass into the common duct, causing bile duct obstruction or pancreatitis; and less than 0.1% are associated with fistulas or gallbladder cancer.

Biliary Colic and Chronic Cholecystitis

About 75% of patients with symptomatic cholelithiasis present with biliary colic. Pain results from the intermittent obstruction of the cystic duct by one or more stones. Inflammation is not present, so there are usually few, if any, systemic signs or symptoms. Biliary colic is a visceral pain that is poorly localized but typically felt in the epigastrium, right upper quadrant, or even left upper quadrant. The pain is steady rather than intermittent and lasts 1 to 6 hours. Describing the pain as "colic" is a misnomer. Pain lasting longer than 6 hours is more commonly associated with the onset of inflammation and hence cholecystitis. Physical examination is typically normal, but mild tenderness in the right upper quadrant may be elicited. Laboratory tests are frequently unrevealing. Seventy percent of patients experience recurrent symptoms within 2 years of

Figure 54-1 Cholelithiasis: Pathologic Features, Choledocholithiasis.

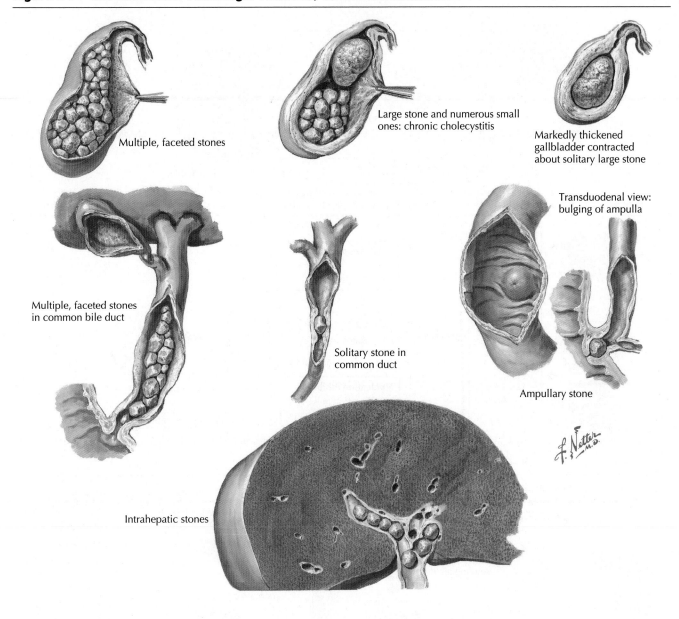

Multiple, faceted stones

Large stone and numerous small ones: chronic cholecystitis

Markedly thickened gallbladder contracted about solitary large stone

Multiple, faceted stones in common bile duct

Solitary stone in common duct

Transduodenal view: bulging of ampulla

Ampullary stone

Intrahepatic stones

Box 54-1   Risk Factors for Gallstone Development

- Older age
- Female
- Obesity
- Weight loss
- Total parenteral nutrition
- Pregnancy
- Genetic predisposition
- Diseases of the terminal ileum
- Hypertriglyceridemia

the initial attack. Recurrent episodes of biliary colic are referred to as *chronic cholecystitis*.

Acute Cholecystitis

Similar to biliary colic, acute cholecystitis is brought on by impaction of a gallstone or stones in the cystic duct or infundibulum (Fig. 54-4). Prolonged obstruction of the cystic duct leads to stasis of bile within the gallbladder, damage to the gallbladder mucosa, and the consequent release of intracellular enzymes and activation of inflammatory mediators. As concentrations of inflammatory mediators rise within the gallbladder, ongoing inflammation produces increased protein and prostaglandin secre-

Figure 54-2 Pathogenesis of Gallstones.

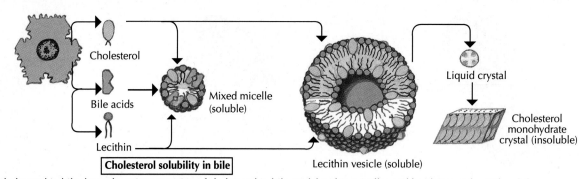

Cholesterol

Bile acids

Lecithin

Mixed micelle (soluble)

Liquid crystal

Cholesterol monohydrate crystal (insoluble)

Cholesterol solubility in bile

Lecithin vesicle (soluble)

Solubility of cholesterol in bile depends on incorporation of cholesterol in bile acid–lecithin micelles and lecithin vesicles. When bile becomes saturated with cholesterol, vesicles fuse to form liposomes, or liquid crystals, from which crystals of cholesterol monohydrate nucleate

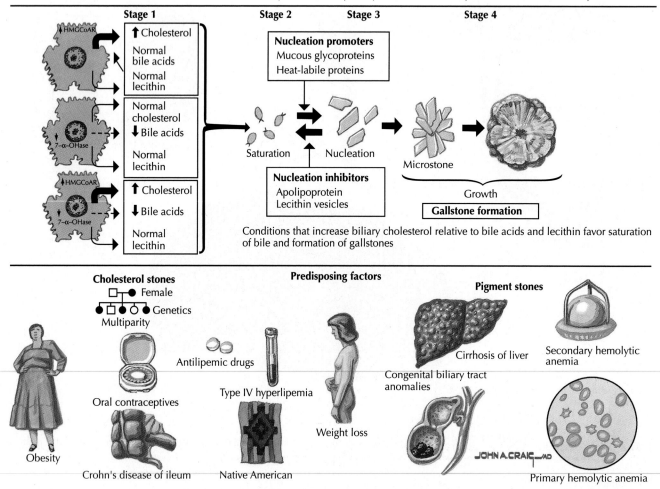

Conditions that increase biliary cholesterol relative to bile acids and lecithin favor saturation of bile and formation of gallstones

tion, decreased water absorption, and white blood cell infiltration. Acute cholecystitis is initially a chemically mediated inflammatory process. Enteric bacteria may be cultured from the bile, but they are not responsible for the onset or activation of acute cholecystitis.

Symptoms persist and usually worsen. Over time, inflammation of the gallbladder ensues, and the pain becomes parietal in nature with localization to the right upper quadrant. Radiation of pain to the back or scapular area is common. Fever is fairly common, but the temperature is usually less than 102° F. Nausea and vomiting may occur. Jaundice may develop in up to 20% of patients, whereas bilirubin levels typically are less than 4 mg/dL. Frequently, white blood cell counts are elevated. Abdominal examination often reveals right subcostal tenderness. A palpable gallbladder occurs in about one third of patients. Murphy's sign, an insensitive but moderately specific finding described as inspiratory arrest during palpation of

Figure 54-3 Cholelithiasis II: Clinical Aspects.

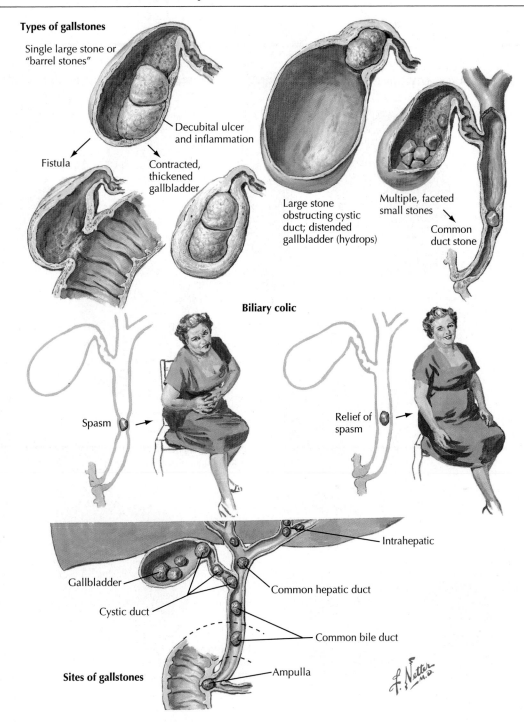

Types of gallstones

Single large stone or "barrel stones"

Fistula

Decubital ulcer and inflammation

Contracted, thickened gallbladder

Large stone obstructing cystic duct; distended gallbladder (hydrops)

Multiple, faceted small stones

Common duct stone

Biliary colic

Spasm

Relief of spasm

Sites of gallstones

Gallbladder

Cystic duct

Intrahepatic

Common hepatic duct

Common bile duct

Ampulla

the right subcostal area during deep inspiration, may be detected.

Choledocholithiasis, Cholangitis, and Gallstone Pancreatitis

Gallstones may pass from the gallbladder into the common bile duct and cause pain, obstructive jaundice, cholangitis, or pancreatitis (Fig. 54-5). Five to 15% of patients with

gallstones also have common duct stones. Stones within the common duct cause pain that is colicky, occurring in the epigastrium with radiation to the back. Jaundice is very common because bilirubin levels rise with the degree of obstruction. Elevations in alkaline phosphatase occur frequently.

Of all the complications of gallstones, cholangitis kills most quickly. The usual clinical presentation consists of

Figure 54-4 Mechanisms of Biliary Pain.

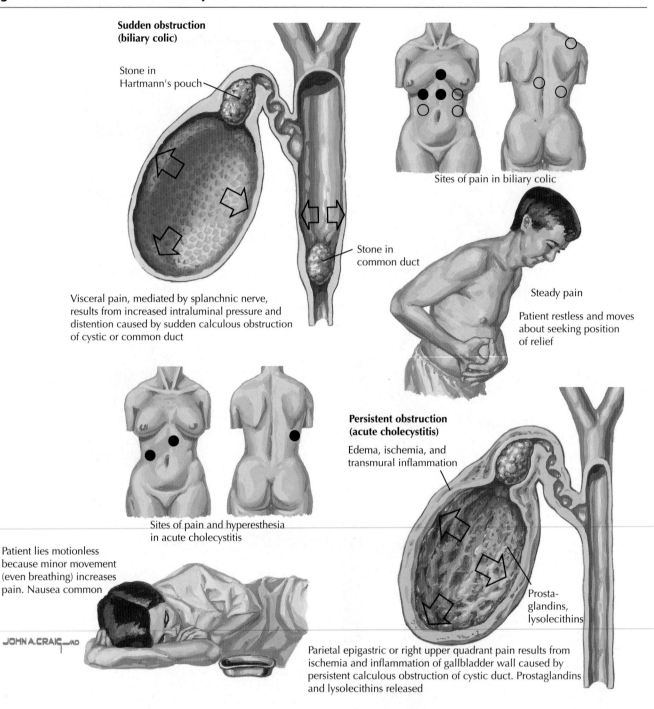

Sudden obstruction (biliary colic)

Stone in Hartmann's pouch

Stone in common duct

Visceral pain, mediated by splanchnic nerve, results from increased intraluminal pressure and distention caused by sudden calculous obstruction of cystic or common duct

Sites of pain in biliary colic

Steady pain

Patient restless and moves about seeking position of relief

Sites of pain and hyperesthesia in acute cholecystitis

Patient lies motionless because minor movement (even breathing) increases pain. Nausea common

JOHN A. CRAIG—AD

Persistent obstruction (acute cholecystitis)

Edema, ischemia, and transmural inflammation

Prosta-glandins, lysolecithins

Parietal epigastric or right upper quadrant pain results from ischemia and inflammation of gallbladder wall caused by persistent calculous obstruction of cystic duct. Prostaglandins and lysolecithins released

pain, jaundice, and chills (i.e., Charcot's triad). Refractory sepsis characterized by altered mentation, hypotension, with Charcot's triad constitutes Reynold's pentad.

Gallstone pancreatitis occurs when a biliary stone causes a transient or sustained blockage of the ampulla of Vater. Most patients experience a mild, self-limited attack that resolves within several days, characterized by abdominal or back pain and elevated serum amylase and lipase levels. Clinical symptoms and abnormal serum biochemistries resolve slowly during this time. Severe pancreatitis devel-

ops in a finite number of patients, manifested by persistent retroperitoneal inflammation, pseudocyst formation, or pancreatic necrosis with or without peripancreatic sepsis.

Uncommon Complications of Gallstone Disease

Emphysematous cholecystitis occurs when gas-forming organisms infect the gallbladder secondary to acute chole-cystitis. Gas pockets present within the gallbladder wall

Figure 54-5 Calculus Obstruction of Common Duct (Choledocholithiasis).

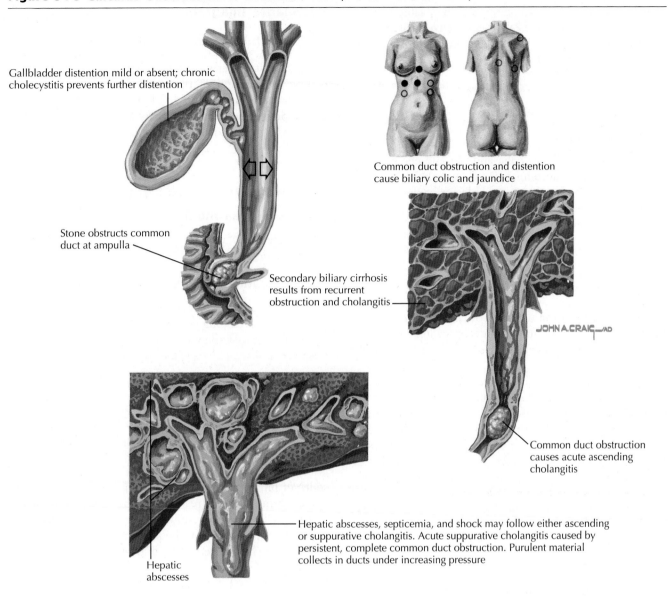

Gallbladder distention mild or absent; chronic cholecystitis prevents further distention

Common duct obstruction and distention cause biliary colic and jaundice

Stone obstructs common duct at ampulla

Secondary biliary cirrhosis results from recurrent obstruction and cholangitis

JOHN A. CRAIG—MD

Common duct obstruction causes acute ascending cholangitis

Hepatic abscesses, septicemia, and shock may follow either ascending or suppurative cholangitis. Acute suppurative cholangitis caused by persistent, complete common duct obstruction. Purulent material collects in ducts under increasing pressure

Hepatic abscesses

can be detected radiographically. Urgent cholecystectomy is recommended. Cholecystoenteric fistulas occur when a stone erodes through the gallbladder wall into an adjacent viscus. The most common sites include the duodenum, the hepatic flexure of the colon, and the stomach.

Differential Diagnosis

Biliary Colic and Chronic Cholecystitis

Colic and chronic cholecystitis mimic episodic upper abdominal symptoms, including gastroesophageal reflux, peptic ulcer disease, pancreatitis, renal colic, diverticulitis, colon cancer, and angina pectoris. Although complaints of gas, bloating, flatulence, and dyspepsia are frequent in patients with gallstones, these symptoms are nonspecific

and should not be considered characteristic clinical manifestations of gallstone disease.

Acute Cholecystitis

The signs and symptoms of acute cholecystitis mimic those of acute appendicitis, acute pancreatitis, right kidney diseases, pneumonia with pleurisy, acute hepatitis, hepatic abscesses, and gonococcal perihepatitis (Fitzhugh-Curtis syndrome).

Choledocholithiasis and Cholangitis

Because the symptoms associated with cystic and common duct obstruction are so similar, biliary colic and acute cholecystitis are always in the differential diagnosis. Malignant obstruction of the common bile duct, acute congestion of the liver associated with congestive heart failure, acute viral hepatitis, and the cholangiopathy of AIDS may also mimic choledocholithiasis.

Diagnostic Approach

Laboratory Tests

In uncomplicated biliary colic and chronic cholecystitis, there are usually no accompanying changes in hematologic and biochemical tests. In acute cholecystitis, leukocytosis is usually observed. Serum aminotransferase, alkaline phosphatase, bilirubin, and amylase levels may also increase.

Sonography

Ultrasonography is the modality of choice for examining the biliary tract. Ultrasound can detect gallbladder stones as small as 2 mm in diameter with sensitivity and specificity rates exceeding 95%.

Sonography is also valuable in the diagnosis of acute cholecystitis. Eliciting a sonographic Murphy's sign (focal gallbladder tenderness under the transducer) has a positive predictive value of more than 90% for diagnosis of acute cholecystitis when stones are seen. The presence of pericholecystic fluid in the absence of ascites and gallbladder wall thickening to more than 4 mm are other nonspecific findings suggestive of acute cholecystitis.

Stones in the common bile duct are seen with sonography in only half of cases. Thus, sonography confirms, but does not exclude, common duct stones.

Hepatobiliary Scintigraphy

Hepatobiliary scintigraphy is most useful in evaluating patients with suspected acute cholecystitis. A normal hepatobiliary scan represents a patent cystic duct and virtually rules out acute cholecystitis in patients who present with abdominal pain. The sensitivity of the test is about 95%, and the specificity is 90%. False-positive results occur primarily in fasting or critically ill patients.

Endoscopic Retrograde Cholangiopancreatography

Endoscopic retrograde cholangiopancreatography (ERCP) is the standard for evaluating common duct stones and pathology. Endoscopic therapeutic applications have revolutionized the treatment of common duct stones and other biliary tract disorders.

Computed Tomography and Magnetic Resonance Imaging

Although not well suited for the evaluation of uncomplicated stones, standard computed tomography (CT) is an excellent test to detect complications such as abscess formation, perforation of the gallbladder or common bile duct, or pancreatitis. Spiral CT and magnetic resonance cholangiography may prove useful as a noninvasive means of excluding common bile duct stones.

Management and Therapy

Optimum Treatment

Cholecystectomy remains the mainstay of treatment of symptomatic gallstones.

Asymptomatic Cholelithiasis

Because up to 80% of all gallstones are asymptomatic and the risk for developing symptoms or complications is low, adult patients with silent or incidental gallstones should be observed and treated expectantly.

Biliary Colic and Chronic Cholecystitis

The natural history of biliary colic is such that recurrent biliary pain occurs in about 38% to 50% of patients per year. The risk for serious biliary complications is relatively low, estimated at 1% to 2% per year. A reasonable approach is to offer cholecystectomy to those with recurring episodes of biliary colic. The laparoscopic approach to gallbladder removal is the treatment of choice for symptomatic gallstones. Laparoscopy, unlike the traditional open operation, allows the surgery to be performed on an outpatient basis with a marked reduction in postoperative pain and a more rapid return to work and usual activities. Conversion to open cholecystectomy is uncommon, averaging less than 3% in most institutions. The incidence of bile duct injury associated with laparoscopic cholecystectomy has decreased to less than 0.5%, and mortality rates are less than 0.1%.

Acute Cholecystitis

If acute cholecystitis is suspected, the patient should be hospitalized for evaluation and treatment. Antibiotics may be withheld in uncomplicated cases but are indicated in toxic-appearing patients or when complications such as perforation or emphysematous cholecystitis are suspected. Definitive therapy is cholecystectomy performed within 24 to 48 hours of the onset of symptoms. Delaying the procedure potentially increases the difficulty in performing surgery, the complication rate, and the need to convert to an open operation. Percutaneous cholecystostomy or transpapillary endoscopic cholecystostomy can be used to drain the inflamed gallbladder for patients deemed to be at high risk for surgery.

Choledocholithiasis

The optimal treatment for common duct stones depends on the level of local expertise in endoscopy and surgery. In general, the presence of obstructive jaundice with a dilated common bile duct should lead promptly to preoperative ERCP with sphincterotomy and stone extraction. Once the bile duct has been cleared, the patient can undergo a routine laparoscopic cholecystectomy within 1 or 2 days.

Cholangitis

The management of sepsis in cholangitis is of paramount importance. Drainage or decompression of the biliary system is definitive. ERCP with stone extraction or at least bile duct decompression with a stent is the treatment of choice. Alternatively, access to the obstructed biliary tract through percutaneous transhepatic cholangiography with drainage catheter placement can temporize by draining the infected obstructed bile duct. Once the patient has recuperated from the infectious insult, elective laparoscopic cholecystectomy can be undertaken.

Gallstone Pancreatitis

For more than three fourths of patients, gallstone pancreatitis is mild, is self-limited, and resolves with conservative management. Cholecystectomy should be performed during the initial admission when the pancreatitis has resolved. Delaying surgery increases the risk for recurrent symptoms and further complications. An evaluation of the biliary system for retained stones should be performed with either a preoperative ERCP or intraoperative cholangiography. For patients with severe biliary pancreatitis, early ERCP with sphincterotomy, if indicated, can be beneficial.

Avoiding Treatment Errors

The widespread use of CT, ultrasound, and nuclear scintigraphy have greatly aided in the diagnosis of cholecystitis and its complications. A team approach in its management is always indicated because coordination of care among primary care physicians, radiologists, gastroenterologists, and surgeons is essential to ensure optimal patient care.

Future Directions

In light of the significant public health impact of gallstones, ongoing research continues to focus on finding the medical means to prevent gallstone formation. Further advances in nonsurgical therapy are expected. Perhaps the most exciting developments will occur in biliary tract imaging techniques with the application of improved resolution ultrasound, endoscopic ultrasound, magnetic resonance imaging, and cholangiography.

Additional Resources

Bellows CF, Berger DH: Management of gallstones. Am Fam Physician 72(4):637-642, 2005.

This concise, complete review article covers the diagnosis and management of gallstones.

Browning JD, Sreenarasimhaiah J: Gallstone disease. In Feldman M, Friedman LS, Sleisenger MH (eds): Sleisenger & Fordtran's Gastrointestinal and Liver Disease, 8th ed. Philadelphia, WB Saunders, 2006.

This is a superb chapter in the hands-down best reference book on gastrointestinal diseases. It is all inclusive—has everything in one source.

NIH Consensus Conference: Gallstones and laparoscopic cholecystectomy. JAMA 269(8):1018-1024, 1993.

This is a great review, "blessing" the introduction of this landmark surgical procedure.

EVIDENCE

1. Gurusamy KS, Samraj K: Early versus delayed laparoscopic cholecystectomy for acute cholecystitis. Cochrane Database Syst Rev 4:CD005440, 2006.

   Clinical trials comparing early versus late cholecystectomy for acute cholecystitis are included in this analysis. Early laparoscopic cholecystectomy during acute cholecystitis seems safe and shortens hospital stay.

2. Keus F, de Jong JA, Gooszen HG, van Laarhoven CJ: Laparoscopic versus open cholecystectomy for patients with symptomatic cholecystolithiasis. Cochrane Database Syst Rev 4:CD006231, 2006.

   Thirty-eight trials randomized 2338 patients. Meta-analysis suggests less overall complications in the laparoscopic group with a shorter hospital stay and convalescence.

3. Urbach DR, Stukel TA: Rate of elective cholecystectomy and the incidence of severe gallstone disease. CMAJ 172:1015-1019, 2005.

   Did the increase in the performance of elective cholecystectomies that occurred after the introduction of laparoscopic cholecystectomy in 1991 result in a reduction in complications of gallstone disease? This study concludes that, as a result of more elective cholecystectomies being performed, there has been an overall reduction in the incidence of severe gallstone disease that is entirely attributable to a reduction in the incidence of acute cholecystitis.

Ian S. Grimm

Pancreatitis

Introduction

Pancreatitis is a general term that encompasses a broad spectrum of pathophysiologic disorders and clinical manifestations. Acute pancreatitis (AP) may range in severity from simple interstitial edema to extensive necrotizing pancreatitis with multisystem organ failure (Fig. 55-1). Most episodes of AP are mild, with an excellent prognosis for complete recovery. However, pancreatic necrosis develops in about 20% of patients, which markedly increases the risk for severe complications and death. The mortality rate for patients with sterile necrosis is 10%, but mortality can exceed 25% in patients with infected pancreatic necrosis. Chronic pancreatitis (CP) refers to irreversible fibrosis and atrophy of the gland, often with a chronic inflammatory cell infiltrate, and progressive loss of exocrine and endocrine function (Fig. 55-2).

Etiology and Pathogenesis

The most common causes of pancreatitis in developed countries are gallstones (45%) and alcohol (35%). About 10% of cases result from miscellaneous causes, whereas another 10% remain unexplained (Box 55-1).

CP can result from recurrent AP; however, it often develops insidiously. Most patients presenting with an initial attack of alcoholic pancreatitis, for instance, already have morphologic changes of CP. Risk factors for CP are listed in Box 55-2.

Clinical Presentation

AP presents with severe epigastric pain of sudden onset, frequently with radiation to the back, nausea, and vomiting (see Fig. 55-1). The pain typically reaches maximal intensity within 30 minutes and persists for hours without relief. Fever, tachycardia, and leukocytosis may be present.

CP may initially present with an attack resembling AP, but it often progresses to a pattern of recurrent inflammatory flares or chronic persistent pain (see Fig. 55-2). Subsequently, malabsorption and diabetes mellitus may develop.

Differential Diagnosis

AP can mimic many causes of an acute abdomen, such as biliary colic, perforated ulcer, mesenteric ischemia or infarction, bowel obstruction, inferior wall myocardial infarction, or ectopic pregnancy. CP can resemble ulcer disease, biliary disorders, gastrointestinal malignancies, malabsorption syndromes, or chronic functional abdominal pain.

Diagnostic Approach

Serum amylase or lipase elevations exceeding 3 times normal are characteristic of acute pancreatitis. Lesser elevations can occur in other conditions. Lipase values are slightly more accurate, especially when the presentation is delayed. An elevation of alanine aminotransferase more than 3 times the upper limit of normal is specific for a gallstone etiology, with a positive predictive value of 95%, in patients without a history of alcohol use. Abdominal computed tomography (CT) detects the presence or absence of pancreatitis in all but the mildest cases and is useful in excluding other conditions having a similar presentation.

The diagnosis of CP requires either evidence of characteristic morphologic abnormalities of the gland or a combination of typical clinical features and abnormal pancreatic functional studies. Pancreatic calcifications on plain radiography or CT represent intraductal stones, which are pathognomonic for CP. Stones may also be seen on transabdominal ultrasonography. Endoscopic retrograde cholangiopancreatography (ERCP) and magnetic resonance

Figure 55-1 Acute Pancreatitis.

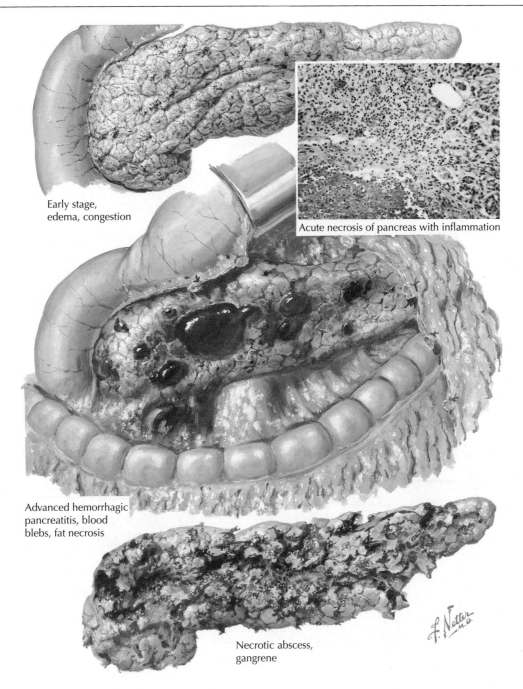

Early stage,
edema, congestion

Acute necrosis of pancreas with inflammation

Advanced hemorrhagic
pancreatitis, blood
blebs, fat necrosis

Necrotic abscess,
gangrene

cholangiopancreatography can provide fine detail of the ductal anatomy, such as irregular dilation of the pancreatic duct, strictures, or ductal filling defects. Endoscopic ultrasonography is the most sensitive means for detecting subtle pancreatic parenchymal changes, although the clinical significance of such findings is uncertain.

The secretin test is the gold standard for documenting pancreatic insufficiency, but it is cumbersome and not widely available. The qualitative fecal fat stain is a simple test to document fat malabsorption, which, in a patient

with suspected CP, implies loss of 90% of exocrine function.

Management and Therapy

Acute Pancreatitis

Optimum Treatment

Management of AP should focus on rapid treatment and early identification of patients at risk for severe AP. All

Figure 55-2 Chronic (Relapsing) Pancreatitis.

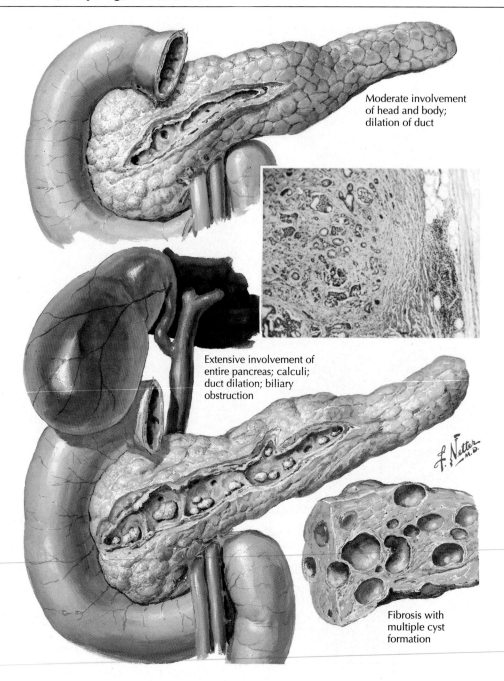

Moderate involvement of head and body; dilation of duct

Extensive involvement of entire pancreas; calculi; duct dilation; biliary obstruction

Fibrosis with multiple cyst formation

patients should receive aggressive fluid replacement, pain management, and careful observation for signs of respiratory insufficiency or significant third-space fluid losses (hemoconcentration, oliguria, hypotension, tachycardia, or azotemia). To promptly identify individuals at risk for severe pancreatitis, the Acute Physiology and Chronic Health Evaluation (APACHE II) score should be calculated on the day of admission. Early predictors of severity include an APACHE II score of 6 or above, obesity (body mass index >30), or pleural effusions. Severe AP is defined as an APACHE II score of 8 or more; a Ranson score of 3 or more; organ failure (shock, pulmonary insufficiency, renal failure, or gastrointestinal bleeding); or local complications, including necrosis, abscess, or pseudocyst. Abdominal ultrasound is indicated to screen for gallstones or biliary ductal dilation. Patients with severe AP and suspected biliary obstruction should undergo urgent ERCP (within 72 hours) to remove bile duct stones. Patients with severe pancreatitis should be transferred to an intensive care setting and undergo dynamic contrast-enhanced CT

Box 55-1 Causes of Acute Pancreatitis and Recurrent Acute Pancreatitis

Common

Gallstones—microlithiasis
Alcohol abuse
Idiopathic causes

Uncommon

Endoscopic retrograde pancreatography
Metabolic: hypertriglyceridemia, hypercalcemia
Obstructive: sphincter of Oddi dysfunction, pancreatic ductal lesions (tumor, stricture)
Duodenal or periampullary lesions: Crohn's disease, blind loop obstruction
Congenital: annular pancreas, pancreas divisum
Trauma
Medications (e.g., azathioprine, 6-mercaptopurine, corticosteroids, dideoxyinosine, estrogens, furosemide, metronidazole, pentamidine, sulfonamides, tetracycline, thiazides, valproic acid)
Toxins
Infections: tuberculosis, cytomegalovirus, mumps, Coxsackie virus, mycoplasma, parasites
Vascular: vasculitis, embolism, hypotension
Autoimmune
Hereditary: hereditary pancreatitis, cystic fibrosis gene mutations

Adapted from Somogyi L, Martin SP, Venkatesan T, Ulrich CD II: Recurrent acute pancreatitis: An algorithmic approach to identification and elimination of inciting factors. Gastroenterology 120(3):708-717, 2001.

Box 55-2 Risk Factors for Chronic Pancreatitis

Alcohol
Tobacco smoking
Chronic renal failure
Hypercalcemia
Hyperlipidemia (possible)
Obstructive
  Pancreas divisum
  Pancreatic ductal stricture
  Duodenal or ampullary lesions
Genetic
  Autosomal dominant hereditary pancreatitis
    Cationic trypsinogen mutations (codons 29, 122)
  Autosomal recessive
    Cystic fibrosis
    Cystic fibrosis gene (*CFTR*) mutations
    Secretory protease inhibitor (*SPINK1*) mutations
    Cationic trypsinogen mutations (codons 16, 22, 23)
Autoimmune
  Primary
  Associated with other diseases: Sjögren's syndrome, inflammatory bowel disease, primary biliary cirrhosis
Recurrent acute pancreatitis
Necrotizing pancreatitis
Postirradiation
Vascular diseases
Idiopathic
  Early onset
  Late onset
  Tropical

Adapted from Etemad B, Whitcomb DC: Chronic pancreatitis: Diagnosis, classification, and new genetic developments. Gastroenterology 120(3):691, 2001.

(ideally after 72 hours) to identify pancreatic necrosis. Oral intake is typically withheld while pain persists. Nasogastric suction is indicated for ileus or for refractory nausea and vomiting. In the absence of ileus, early jejunal feeding is safe and may reduce the risk for complications. Prophylactic antibiotics are widely used in patients with necrotizing pancreatitis (e.g., imipenem-cilastatin for 2 to 4 weeks), although the data and recommendations regarding this practice are conflicting. Patients with necrotizing pancreatitis and clinical deterioration or signs of infection should undergo guided, percutaneous fine-needle aspiration for bacteriology studies. Aggressive surgical débridement is the standard treatment for infected necrosis, which is otherwise uniformly fatal.

Avoiding Treatment Errors

Common errors in the initial management of acute pancreatitis involve the failure to provide adequate fluid resuscitation and the failure to recognize the potential severity of the disease, especially in the first few days of illness. Although most cases of pancreatitis are mild, the full severity of the disease may not be evident in the first several days, during which time patients require close attention for early signs of organ failure. Severity scoring systems, although less than perfect, are valuable clinical tools for predicting complications and mortality, yet they are often not employed in routine practice.

Acute fluid collections are common in acute pancreatitis. Most of these resolve spontaneously with no intervention. They should not be referred to as *pseudocysts* until they have been present for at least 4 weeks because this label tends to invite an unnecessary therapeutic intervention. Percutaneous drainage of acute fluid collections increases the risk for infecting an otherwise sterile environment.

Chronic Pancreatitis

Optimum Treatment

Therapy is directed at managing pain and fat malabsorption primarily. A low-fat diet, non-narcotic analgesics, and abstinence from alcohol are recommended. Narcotics may be required for severe pain. For persistent pain, high protease pancreatic enzyme replacement should be prescribed for at least 8 weeks. Microencapsulated enzyme preparations with high lipase content are useful for treatment of steatorrhea. Treatable problems should be sought, such as pseudocysts or stenosis of the duodenum or intrapancreatic common bile duct. Patients with refractory pain and pancreatic duct strictures or stones may benefit from endoscopic therapy. Those with intractable pain and a dilated

main pancreatic duct often respond to surgical decompression (i.e., lateral pancreaticojejunostomy). Treatments of last resort for pain in patients with nondilated ducts include nerve blocks and pancreatic resection.

Avoiding Treatment Errors

Fluid collections and cystic lesions in the pancreas should be accurately characterized before contemplating a plan of treatment. This may require multiple imaging modalities, including endoscopic ultrasonography. In a patient presenting with a pancreatic cystic lesion in the absence of an antecedent diagnosis of pancreatic disease, the possibility of a cystic neoplasm should be strongly considered. Patients with diffuse dilation of the pancreatic duct are occasionally given an incorrect diagnosis of chronic pancreatitis when the underlying disease is in fact an intraductal mucinous papillary neoplasm. Pancreatic pseudocysts and duct disruptions are increasingly managed by endoscopic means, thereby avoiding prolonged hospitalizations associated with parenteral feeding, percutaneous drainage, or postoperative recovery.

Future Directions

Newer diagnostic tests for pancreatitis (e.g., urinary trypsinogen-2) and biochemical markers of severity (e.g., urinary trypsinogen activation peptide, serum interleukin-6 and -8) may improve current practice. Novel therapies for severe AP will target inhibition of the systemic inflammatory response associated with this disease. The role of genetic factors in the development of pancreatic diseases will remain a major research focus.

Additional Resources

Banks PA: Practice guidelines in acute pancreatitis. Am J Gatroenterol 92(3):377-386, 1997.
   This comprehensive report on management guidelines for acute pancreatitis has stood the test of time.
Baron TH, Moran DE: Acute necrotizing pancreatitis. N Engl J Med 340(18):1412-1417, 1999.
   This is an excellent review on pancreatic necrosis and its complications.

Bradley EL III: A clinically based classification system for acute pancreatitis. Summary of the International Symposium on Acute Pancreatitis, Atlanta, GA, September 11-12, 1992. Arch Surg 128(5):586-590, 1993.
   This report of a consensus conference initially defined standard terms regarding pancreatitis and its complications.
Etemad B, Whitcomb DC: Chronic pancreatitis: Diagnosis, classification, and new genetic developments. Gastroenterology 120(3):682-707, 2001.
   Review on the role of genetics in diagnosis of pancreatitis.
Jacobson BC, Baron TH, Adler DG, et al: ASGE guideline: The role of endoscopy in the diagnosis and management of cystic lesions and inflammatory fluid collections of the pancreas. Gastrointest Endosc 61:363-370, 2005.
   Review of nonsurgical intervention for pancreatic cyst management.
Somogyi L, Martin SP, Venkatesan T, Ulrich CD II: Recurrent acute pancreatitis: An algorithmic approach to identification and elimination of inciting factors. Gastroenterology 120(3):708-717, 2001.
   The authors suggest a diagnostic approach to recurrent pancreatitis.
Uhl W, Warshaw A, Imrie C, et al: IAP guidelines for the surgical management of acute pancreatitis. Pancreatology 2:565-573, 2002.
   The authors provide consensus guidelines on surgical management.
Warshaw AL, Banks PA, Fernandez-Del Castillo C: AGA technical review: Treatment of pain in chronic pancreatitis. Gastroenterology 115(3):765-776, 1998.
   Consensus recommendations are presented on the treatment of pain in chronic pancreatitis.
Whitcomb DC: Acute pancreatitis. N Engl J Med 354:2142-2150, 2006.
   Current clinical practice strategies, evidence, and guidelines are presented.

EVIDENCE

1. Al-Omran M, Groof A, Wilke D: Enteral versus parenteral nutrition for acute pancreatitis. Cochrane Database Syst Rev 1: CD002837, 2003.
   This systematic review concludes that there are insufficient data to recommend one method of feeding over another.
2. Ayub K, Imada R, Slavin J: Endoscopic retrograde cholangiopancreatography in gallstone-associated acute pancreatitis. Cochrane Database Syst Rev 4:CD003630, 2004.
   This systematic review concludes that urgent ERCP is indicated in gallstone pancreatitis that is predicted to be severe.
3. Tenner S, Dubner H, Steinberg W: Predicting gallstone pancreatitis with laboratory parameters: A meta-analysis. Am J Gastroenterol 89:1863-1866, 1994.
   Alanine aminotransferase elevations of more than threefold are highly predictive of a gallstone etiology of acute pancreatitis.

Yolanda V. Scarlett

Diarrhea: Acute and Chronic

Introduction

Diarrhea is defined as increased stool output. The increased fecal output may represent increased stool frequency, increased stool fluidity, or a combination of both. Objectively, diarrhea is defined as a stool weight in excess of 200 g in 24 hours. Diarrhea is classified as acute or chronic, depending on the duration of symptoms. Acute diarrhea lasts no longer than 6 to 8 weeks, with most cases resolving in 2 to 3 weeks. Cases lasting longer than 8 weeks are deemed chronic. Most cases of diarrhea in the United States are acute and self-limited; nevertheless, diarrheal illnesses remain a major cause of morbidity and mortality worldwide.

Etiology and Pathogenesis

Diarrhea occurs because of abnormal fluid and electrolyte transport and altered intestinal motility. The major pathogenic mechanisms include the presence of unusual amounts of poorly absorbable intraluminal solute with associated osmotic diarrhea, abnormal ion absorption or ion secretion that causes secretory diarrhea, inflammatory processes of the mucosa and bowel wall, and abnormal intestinal motility (Fig. 56-1).

In the normal state, in a 24-hour period, about 8 to 10 liters of fluid enters the duodenum from a combination of dietary intake and gut secretions. Two thirds of the fluid is reabsorbed in the duodenum, with one third entering the proximal jejunum. Of the 10 liters of fluid entering the small intestine, only a volume of 1500 mL is presented to the colon. The small intestine has a chloride (Cl^-) and bicarbonate (HCO_3^-) transport mechanism that reduces the concentration of Cl^- and increases the concentration of HCO_3^- such that the concentrations reflect the plasma concentrations. The colon absorbs most of the fluid, excreting only 100 mL in a 24-hour period. The colon's very efficient active transport mechanisms extract sodium (Na^+) and fluid and secrete potassium (K^+). Magnesium (Mg^{2+}) and calcium (Ca^{2+}) are poorly absorbed in the colon. The excreted stool contains 3 millimoles (mmol) of Na^+, 8 mmol of K^+, and 2 mmol of chloride.

Osmotic diarrhea is the result of osmotically active, nonabsorbable solutes accumulating in the gut lumen with resulting intraluminal salt and water retention. A classic feature of osmotic diarrhea is cessation of the symptoms with fasting or after the patient stops ingesting the osmotically active agent. The electrolyte content of the excreted stool is normal in osmotic diarrhea and does not account for the total fecal osmolality. The difference between the measured osmolality and that accounted for by the electrolyte content is termed the *osmotic gap*. The osmotic gap is calculated by doubling the fecal sodium and potassium concentrations and subtracting the value from the stool osmolality or expressed as a formula: osmotic gap = 290 mOsm/L − [2 × (fecal Na^+ + K^+)].

The normal stool osmotic gap is less than 125 and is usually less than 60. A fecal osmotic gap greater than 60 is suggestive of an osmotic diarrhea, a condition in which the osmotic gap is, in fact, usually more than 125. In contrast to osmotic diarrhea, secretory diarrhea does not abate with fasting. There may be a decrease in the stool volume and stool weight, an observation that should not be mistaken for osmotic diarrhea. There is a net luminal secretion of water and electrolytes into the gut, and the osmotic gap is less than 60.

Inflammatory diarrhea is characterized by exudation of blood, mucus, pus, or serum proteins in the stool. This results in increased stool weight and diarrhea.

Figure 56-1 Diarrhea.

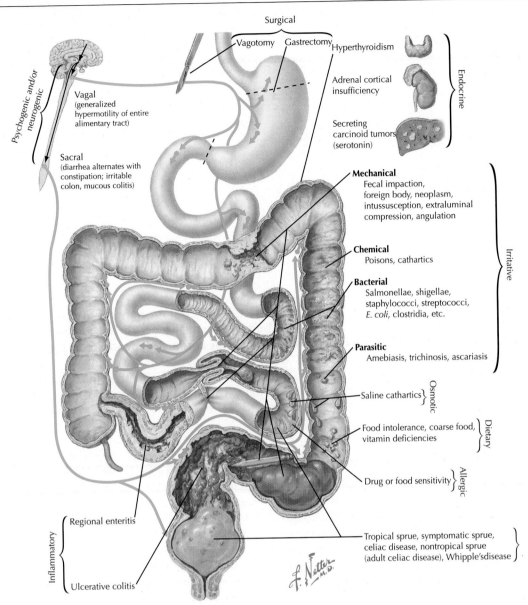

Clinical Presentation

Abnormal intestinal motility may cause diarrhea secondary to rapid intestinal transit or by slow intestinal transit with stasis and resultant bacterial overgrowth.

Clinical Presentation

Individuals who present with diarrhea usually complain of frequent loose, watery stools. Medical attention is often sought because of accompanying dehydration, abdominal discomfort, fever, vomiting, gastrointestinal bleeding, pus in the stool, or chronicity of symptoms. It is crucial to characterize the patient's stool pattern and associated symptoms in order to guide the diagnostic approach.

Differential Diagnosis

The differential diagnoses for both acute and chronic diarrhea is extensive. Either may be caused by infectious agents. Pathogens commonly associated with acute infectious diarrhea include *Salmonella*, *Shigella*, enterohemorrhagic *Escherichia coli*, *Campylobacter*, rotaviruses, and Norwalk agent. *Vibrio cholera* and *Cyclospora* species are less frequent causes of acute diarrhea. Microsporidium and cryptosporidium can cause acute diarrhea and are more likely to affect immunocompromised individuals. *Clostridium difficile* is the agent most frequently associated with nosocomial diarrhea and with antibiotic-associated diarrhea. Common infections associated with chronic

diarrhea include giardiasis, strongyloidiasis, and amebiasis.

Ischemic colitis is a noninfectious cause of acute diarrhea that occurs more frequently in middle-aged and elderly patients with significant peripheral vascular disease or atherosclerotic heart disease. Several medications, including nonsteroidal anti-inflammatory agents, digitalis, vasopressin, and diuretics, have been associated with ischemic colitis.

Osmotic diarrhea with carbohydrate malabsorption from lactase deficiency is seen in lactose intolerance, excessive sorbitol intake, lactulose use, fructose intake, ingestion of magnesium-containing compounds (laxatives, antacids, or supplements), and intestinal mucosal disease such as celiac sprue or gluten intolerance.

A variety of toxin-producing infections cause secretory diarrhea. These include *E. coli* enterotoxin and *V. cholerae* enterotoxin. Senna-containing laxatives, bisacodyl-containing laxatives, vasoactive intestinal peptide, calcitonin, substance P, gastrin, serotonin, and prostaglandins also produce secretory diarrhea. Parasitic infections, including giardiasis, strongyloidosis, and amebiasis, can cause secretory diarrhea. Congenital chloridorrhea is caused by a secretory stimulus from a mucosal ion transport defect. Bile acid malabsorption, microscopic colitis, collagenous colitis, hyperthyroidism, medullary carcinoma of the thyroid, and collagen vascular diseases such as systemic lupus erythematosus and scleroderma are additional causes of secretory diarrhea.

Inflammatory bowel disease secondary to Crohn's disease, ulcerative colitis, and Behçet's disease produces exudative or inflammatory diarrhea. Chemotherapeutic agents, radiation enteritis, microscopic colitis, collagenous colitis, and graft-versus-host disease can also produce inflammatory diarrhea. Parasitic infections, viral agents, and bacterial pathogens may cause inflammatory diarrhea.

Abnormal intestinal motility underlies the functional diarrhea experienced in irritable bowel syndrome (IBS). Constipation may alternate with the diarrhea of IBS. Typically, the diarrhea of IBS is associated with mucus production with absence of inflammatory markers. The nocturnal diarrhea experienced by some patients with advanced diabetes is caused by deranged intestinal motility.

Diagnostic Approach

The initial evaluation of patients with both acute and chronic diarrhea should include a detailed history that includes the duration of symptoms, hydration status, severity of illness, travel history, exposure to potentially contaminated food or water, sick contacts, recent use of antibiotics, medication use, and the immune status of the individual.

A complete physical examination should include careful assessment for evidence of dehydration such as orthostasis, dry mucous membranes, and poor skin turgor. The abdominal exam should include a careful evaluation for peritoneal signs, which are associated with enteroinvasive infectious agents. A rectal exam should include an assessment for fistulas and abscesses.

The diagnostic evaluation of acute diarrhea should include fecal leukocytes and fecal occult blood testing. Routine stool cultures are of little value in healthy individuals who lack fecal leukocytes and fecal occult blood. Also, stool cultures are thought to be of little benefit in cases of nosocomial diarrhea. *C. difficile* is the most likely offending agent and is effectively diagnosed with enzyme-linked immunosorbent assays for toxin A. Stool cultures should be obtained from immunocompromised individuals and from persons with known Crohn's disease or ulcerative colitis. Infectious agents can cause an acute exacerbation of diarrhea in the setting of inflammatory bowel disease. The role of endoscopy is limited. Flexible sigmoidoscopy is helpful if ischemic colitis is suspected. Demonstration of pseudomembranes on endoscopic exam is diagnostic of *C. difficile* colitis and may be beneficial in individuals who are toxic.

Recommended laboratory testing for chronic diarrhea includes a complete blood count to evaluate for inflammation and serum electrolytes for information regarding fluid status. Stool analysis for fecal leukocytes may be helpful in differentiating inflammatory from noninflammatory diarrhea. Calculation of the stool osmotic gap helps to characterize osmotic diarrhea from secretory diarrhea. Fecal occult blood testing is also indicated. Positive fecal occult blood testing is suggestive of an inflammatory process. Stool analysis for excess fecal fat helps to differentiate malabsorption. Stool can be evaluated for fecal fat by a Sudan stain or by quantitatively measuring the fat content of the stool in a 72-hour period. A fecal fat concentration greater than 7 g per 24 hours is consistent with a malabsorptive process. Measuring the stool pH may also be beneficial in differentiating carbohydrate malabsorption—pH usually less than 5.6. Endoscopy has a greater role in chronic diarrhea than in acute diarrhea (Fig. 56-2). Lower endoscopy, flexible sigmoidoscopy, or colonoscopy with biopsies can be helpful with the diagnosis of Crohn's disease, ulcerative colitis, microscopic colitis, and collagenous colitis. Upper endoscopy, esophagogastroduodenoscopy, with biopsy samples taken from the proximal duodenum, is the gold standard for confirming celiac disease or gluten intolerance. In the setting of chronic diarrhea, if the evaluation has been extensive and a diagnosis has not been established, factitious diarrhea should be considered, and the stool should be analyzed for laxative use.

Management and Therapy
Optimum Treatment

The management and therapy of diarrhea depend on the etiology of the disease. Most cases of acute diarrhea are

Figure 56-2 Bacillary Dysentery.

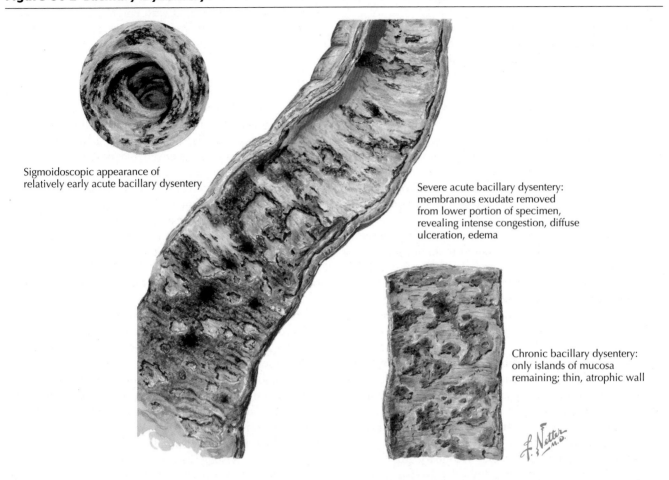

Sigmoidoscopic appearance of relatively early acute bacillary dysentery

Severe acute bacillary dysentery: membranous exudate removed from lower portion of specimen, revealing intense congestion, diffuse ulceration, edema

Chronic bacillary dysentery: only islands of mucosa remaining; thin, atrophic wall

self-limited and do not require therapy beyond supportive care with attention to fluid intake to prevent dehydration. Oral rehydration solutions consisting of sodium chloride, sodium bicarbonate, potassium chloride and sucrose or glucose are designed to use the intestinal sodium-glucose transport system to promote water absorption to decrease the risk for dehydration. Symptomatic therapy with loperamide or diphenoxylate warrants consideration for acute diarrhea if the stool is nonbloody and there is no fever. In general, empiric antibiotic therapy has not been shown to significantly alter the course of acute diarrhea. Empiric antibiotics are generally reserved for patients with bloody diarrhea, fever, and fecal leukocytes who are dehydrated and may require hospitalization and who have been symptomatic for about 1 week. Antibiotic therapy should also be considered in immunocompromised hosts. Probiotics are beneficial in reestablishing the intestinal flora with nonpathogenic microorganisms and in shortening the length of diarrhea in traveler's diarrhea and *C. difficile* infection.

The treatment of chronic diarrhea is guided by the etiology of the disease or disorder and the symptoms. Cases of chronic diarrhea of unknown etiology are often challenging. Long-term use of loperamide is acceptable in

selected cases for symptomatic relief. The long-term use of diphenoxylate, codeine, and tincture of opium requires caution because dependency may develop. Fiber supplementation or bulking agents such as polycarbophil can be beneficial for decreasing the stool fluidity. Alosetron is a highly selective 5-HT$_3$ antagonist that slows transit and reduces stool frequency. Alosetron is approved for use in diarrhea-predominant IBS when prescribed by practitioners knowledgeable of the side-effect profile with close patient monitoring as recommended by the manufacturer. Rifaximin is an antibiotic that inhibits bacterial RNA synthesis by binding DNA-dependent RNA polymerase. It is approved by the U.S. Food and Drug Administration for treatment of travelers' diarrhea caused by noninvasive strains of *E. coli*.

Avoiding Treatment Errors

Treatment of diarrhea, whether acute or chronic, depends on careful evaluation of the stool pattern and associated symptoms. Successful treatment requires proper identification of the underlying cause. A detailed history, including information about travel, dietary intake, and exposure to sick contacts, helps to provide clues about potential infectious agents or dietary factors causing diarrhea. Careful monitoring of fluid and electrolyte status with replacement of both as necessary is essential because dehydration and electrolyte abnormalities are a major source of morbidity and mortality in diarrheal illnesses.

Future Directions

Current research includes the clinical investigation of serotonin 5-HT$_3$ antagonists for the management of diarrhea-predominant IBS. Studies include trials to optimize dosing for alosetron. Ramosetron is a selective 5-HT$_3$ receptor antagonist shown in animal studies to have more potent effects on abnormal colonic function than alosetron. Continued evaluation of ramosetron may provide additional treatment modalities for functional diarrhea. Other investigations include the evaluation of rifaximin in managing the diarrhea associated with small bowel bacterial overgrowth.

Additional Resources

Hirata T, Funatsu T, Keto Y, et al: Pharmacological profile of ramosetron, a novel therapeutic agent for IBS. Inflammopharmacology 15(1):5-9, 2007.

This article provides insight into the research being conducted to develop treatment options for noninfectious diarrhea.

EVIDENCE

1. American Gastroenterological Association: Medical Position Statement: Evaluation and management of chronic diarrhea. Gastroenterology 116:1461-1463, 1999.
   This medical position paper provides a comprehensive guide to the diagnosis and treatment of the most common causes of chronic diarrhea.
2. Camilleri M: Management of the irritable bowel syndrome. Gastroenterology 120:652-658, 2001.
   This practical and concise review of the diagnosis and treatment of irritable bowel syndrome provides a guide to treatment when infectious, inflammatory, or dietary intolerance disorders are not diagnosed.
3. DuPont H: Guidelines on acute infectious diarrhea in adults. The Practice Parameters Committee of the American College of Gastroenterology. Am J Gastroenterol 92:1962-1975, 1997.
   This article provides guidelines for the diagnosis and management of acute infectious diarrhea and is helpful in medical management, including use of antibiotic therapy.
4. Eherer A, Fordtran J: Fecal osmotic gap and pH in experimental diarrhea of various causes. Gastroenterology 103:545, 1992.
   This helpful guide for understanding the physiology of the stool osmotic gap also addresses how it relates to various diarrheal states.

Yolanda V. Scarlett

Constipation

Introduction

Constipation refers to specific symptoms associated with impaired defecation, including abnormal stool frequency, straining with defecation, passage of hard stool, and a sense of incomplete evacuation. It is very common and affects persons of all ages. An individual with constipation may experience one or more of the symptoms. Millions of dollars are spent annually on over-the-counter laxatives, physician visits, and pharmacologic agents to control the symptoms. The true prevalence is not known because many of those affected do not seek medical care. Reported prevalence rates range from 2% to 20%. The Rome III consensus criteria for constipation include two or more of the following: straining during at least 25% of defecations, lumpy or hard stools in at least 25% of defecations, sensation of anorectal obstruction or blockage during at least 25% of defecations, manual maneuvers to facilitate at least 25% of defecations, and fewer than three defecations per week along with rare loose stools and insufficient criteria for diagnosis of irritable bowel syndrome. The symptoms should be present for the past 3 months with onset of symptoms at least 6 months before diagnosis. It is important to define the patient's specific symptoms to determine the most appropriate and cost-effective diagnostic and therapeutic approach.

Etiology and Pathogenesis

Most individuals are toilet trained and able to control defecation by 4 years of age. Successful continent evacuation requires a degree of mental functioning to be able to respond to cues indicating the need to evacuate, normal intestinal motility, proper internal and external anal sphincter function, and coordination of the puborectalis muscle. The rectum is a compliance reservoir with stretch or mechanoreceptors located in the rectal wall. The urge to defecate is experienced once stool is propelled from the distal sigmoid colon into the rectum, activating the mechanoreceptors. Defecation is initiated by sitting and straining to perform a series of maneuvers that increase the intra-abdominal pressure, decrease the resting tone of the internal anal sphincter, straighten the angle of the puborectalis muscle, relax the external anal sphincter, and allow expulsion of the fecal bolus. These maneuvers occur almost simultaneously, and abnormality in any one of the steps can result in constipation.

The causes of constipation are broad and can be divided into metabolic, neurogenic, and idiopathic causes (Fig. 57-1). In addition, numerous drugs are associated with constipation. *Common metabolic or endocrine causes* include hypothyroidism, diabetes mellitus, pregnancy, hypercalcemia, hypokalemia, uremia, glucagonoma, and porphyria. *Neurogenic disorders* include peripheral neuropathy, Hirschsprung's disease, autonomic neuropathy, neurofibromatosis, Chagas' disease, and intestinal pseudo-obstruction. *Central nervous system disorders* include multiple sclerosis, Parkinson's disease, cerebrovascular accident, and spinal cord injury. *Categories of medications* that can cause constipation include narcotic analgesics, anticholinergic drugs, antidepressants, antihypertensives, diuretics, nonsteroidal anti-inflammatory medications, antacids containing aluminum or calcium salts, antihistamines, and antiparkinson agents. *Idiopathic causes* include slow transit-type constipation or colonic inertia, pelvic floor dyssynergia, constipation-predominant irritable bowel syndrome, megacolon, and megarectum.

Clinical Presentation

Individuals who present with complaints of constipation may describe infrequent bowel movements; excessive straining with defecation; inability to evacuate the rectum after experiencing an urge; a desire to have a bowel move-

Figure 57-1 Causes of Constipation.

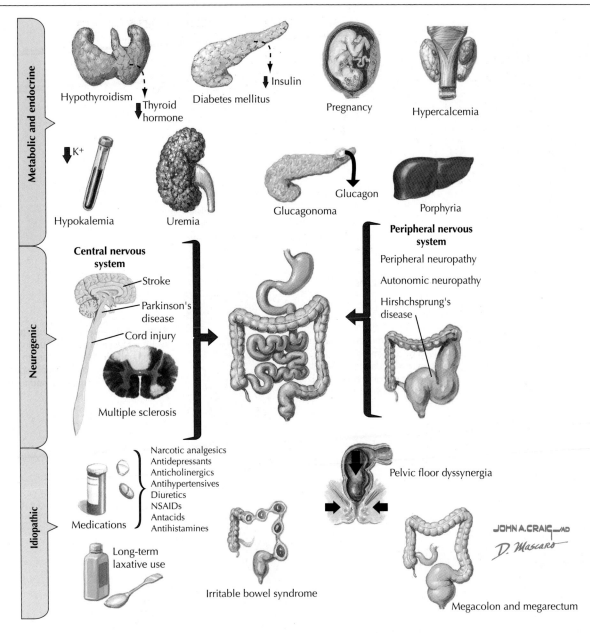

Hypothyroidism
Thyroid hormone

Diabetes mellitus
Insulin

Pregnancy

Hypercalcemia

K+

Hypokalemia

Uremia

Glucagonoma
Glucagon

Porphyria

Central nervous system
Stroke
Parkinson's disease
Cord injury
Multiple sclerosis

Peripheral nervous system
Peripheral neuropathy
Autonomic neuropathy
Hirshchsprung's disease

Medications
Narcotic analgesics
Antidepressants
Anticholinergics
Antihypertensives
Diuretics
NSAIDs
Antacids
Antihistamines

Long-term laxative use

Irritable bowel syndrome

Pelvic floor dyssynergia

Megacolon and megarectum

Metabolic and endocrine

Neurogenic

Idiopathic

JOHN A.CRAIG—AD
D. Mascaro

ment but with lack of an urge to defecate; evacuation of small, hard or dry stools; digital manipulation to achieve evacuation; or a sense of incomplete evacuation. The diagnostic approach depends on what the patient describes as constipation in order to guide the selection of diagnostic tests.

Differential Diagnosis

Most causes of constipation are not life threatening and are of a functional rather than an organic nature. Functional causes of constipation include insufficient fluid and fiber intake as well as physical inactivity. Organic conditions that may cause constipation must be considered.

These include colorectal tumors, hernias, strictures, chronic intermittent volvulus, endometriosis, rectocele, rectal prolapse, and anal stricture.

Diagnostic Approach

Taking a detailed history is the most important factor when evaluating an individual with a complaint of constipation. Information obtained during the history guides selection of appropriate testing. The number of bowel movements in a 7-day period should be documented along with the appearance of the stool. Infrequent stools may reflect slow transit of fecal material through the colon. Small, hard, lumpy stool may reflect inadequate fiber and

Figure 57-2 Diagnosis and Management of Constipation.

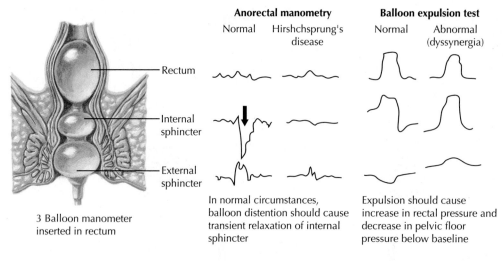

Anorectal manometry

Normal   Hirshchsprung's
                disease

Balloon expulsion test

Normal   Abnormal
                (dyssynergia)

Rectum

Internal
sphincter

External
sphincter

3 Balloon manometer
inserted in rectum

In normal circumstances,
balloon distention should cause
transient relaxation of internal
sphincter

Expulsion should cause
increase in rectal pressure and
decrease in pelvic floor
pressure below baseline

Colonic transit testing

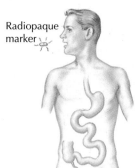

Radiopaque
marker

Patient ingests radiopaque markers
followed by abdominal x-rays
obtained several days after ingestion.
Number of retained markers utilized
to determine colonic transit time

Defecography

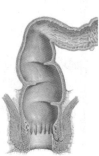

Radiopaque paste introduced into
rectum. Fluoroscopically monitored
imaging provides information on
anorectal angle, pelvic floor descent,
rectocele, intussusception, and rectal
prolapse

General management measures

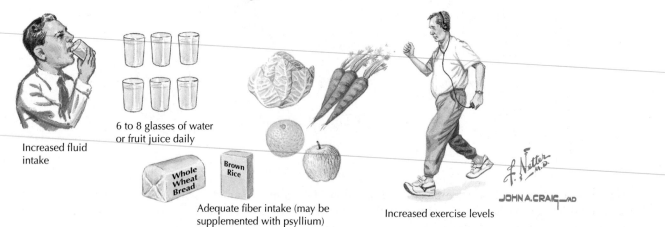

Increased fluid
intake

6 to 8 glasses of water
or fruit juice daily

Whole
Wheat
Bread

Brown
Rice

Adequate fiber intake (may be
supplemented with psyllium)

Increased exercise levels

fluid intake. Long, small-caliber or long, flat stools can be seen with inappropriate relaxation of the puborectalis muscle and external anal sphincter during evacuation. Small-caliber stool can also be associated with tumors, and endoscopic evaluation with colonoscopy should be performed to exclude malignancy.

Standard diagnostic testing includes the balloon expulsion test, colonic transit study, anorectal manometry, and defecography (Fig. 57-2). Other studies such as pelvic floor electromyography, colonic motility testing, and pudendal nerve latency testing are not available at all testing centers; adequate diagnostic information can usually be obtained without these studies.

The *balloon expulsion study* is a simple test that determines whether the patient can evacuate a 50-mL air- or water-filled balloon. Some advocate balloon expulsion testing as a screening study for pelvic floor dysfunction. Inability to expel the balloon may reflect inability to appropriately relax the pelvic floor to allow defecation, as seen with pelvic floor dyssynergia or paradoxical contraction of the pelvic floor in response to straining.

Colonic transit testing evaluates the time required for material to move through the colon. The most cost-effective method to determine the colonic transit time is by ingestion of radiopaque markers in conjunction with having one or more abdominal x-rays obtained several days after ingestion. The number of retained radiopaque markers is used to determine the colonic transit time. There are several protocols for colonic transit marker studies, and the various protocols correlate well with each other. The colonic transit time can also be determined by radionuclide gamma scintigraphic studies. Radionuclide scintigraphic assessment of colon transit is not readily available, but it, too, correlates well with determination of colon transit time when compared with radiopaque markers.

Anorectal manometry testing provides useful information about rectal sensation, internal anal sphincter relaxation, rectal compliance, and pelvic floor responses to straining. Anorectal manometry testing is performed by placing pressure-recording catheters across the anal sphincters. Measurements are obtained by introducing increments of air into a balloon attached to the tip of the catheter. Balloon expulsion testing is often done in conjunction with anorectal manometry. Surface electromyography can be done with skin pads or anal plugs and is often done at the time of anorectal manometry to evaluate for external anal sphincter and puborectalis dysfunction such as paradoxical pelvic floor motions that hinder evacuation. It is very helpful if there is a history of childhood constipation. Screening for Hirschsprung's disease is easily done with manometry. Hirschsprung's disease is excluded by demonstrating appropriate relaxation of the internal anal sphincter in response to balloon distention.

Defecography involves introducing soft barium paste into the rectum and then having the patient evacuate during fluoroscopic exam. It can provide information about the anorectal angle, pelvic floor descent, retentive rectoceles, intussusception, and rectal prolapse.

Management and Therapy

Optimum Treatment

Initial management should include counseling regarding adequate fiber intake, sufficient fluid intake, and physical activity. Most Western diets do not provide the minimum recommended daily requirement of dietary fiber. If the fiber content is deficient, the patient should be instructed to gradually increase the fiber intake to 20 to 35 g daily. Psyllium supplements are effective in increasing fiber intake (Fig. 57-2). Any increase in daily dietary fiber content should occur over a period of days because high dietary fiber is often associated with abdominal bloating and increased flatulence, and individuals with constipation often experience bloating. Fiber should be avoided if there is concern of colonic blockage or stricture because an impaction may develop proximal to the stricture. Patients should drink a minimum of six glasses of fluid, preferably water and fruit juices, daily. Physical limitations often restrict activity, especially in older individuals; nonetheless, the patient should be strongly encouraged to undertake physical activity. Often with attention to fiber, water, and physical activity, the symptoms of constipation improve. If there is still inadequate relief after these initial steps, the history should guide further testing.

Patients with infrequent bowel movements without excessive straining may benefit from stool softening agents such as docusate. Determination of the colonic transit time is indicated if there is inadequate symptom relief despite compliance with basic management. Documented slow colon transit or colonic inertia may be managed with laxatives. If long-term laxative use is required, bulk-forming agents (psyllium), hyperosmolar laxatives (polyethylene glycol, lactulose and sorbitol), and saline laxatives (magnesium sulfate, magnesium citrate, and magnesium phosphate) are preferred to stimulant laxatives. Stimulant laxatives are not recommended for long-term use because they may cause degeneration of the enteric nerve plexus, in turn exacerbating the symptoms of constipation. Common stimulant laxatives include bisacodyl, senna, and cascara. Lubiprostone is a novel type 2 chloride channel activator used to treat chronic constipation by increasing the number of spontaneous bowel movements, improving the stool consistency, and decreasing straining associated with constipation.

Anorectal manometry testing is indicated if there is concern about Hirschsprung's disease and sensory perception or pelvic floor dysfunction. Balloon expulsion testing is often done at the time of anorectal manometry testing. If pelvic floor dysfunction is identified, pelvic floor retraining with biofeedback may be beneficial. Patients are taught to relax, instead of contract, the pelvic floor musculature when attempting to evacuate.

Subtotal colectomy with ileorectal anastomosis is reserved for individuals with constipation that does not respond to conservative measures and to laxative therapy and who do not have pelvic floor dysfunction, including pelvic floor dyssynergia or outlet obstruction. These individuals should have demonstrated normal small bowel neuromuscular function because small bowel neuropathy and small bowel myopathy can contribute to constipation.

Avoiding Treatment Errors

Successful treatment of constipation requires taking a detailed history and tailoring the evaluation to the patient's symptoms. In simple cases, increasing fluid intake along with fiber supplementation and increased activity may provide significant improvement. Diagnostic testing should be reserved for individuals who have failed simple measures, including management of any organic condition that may be contributing to the symptoms.

Future Directions

Tergaserod is a highly selective, partial 5-HT$_4$ receptor agonist with prokinetic properties that increase gastrointestinal transit. Recently, tergaserod was withdrawn from the market under advice from the U.S. Food and Drug Administration secondary to an increased number of cardiovascular events noted in patients taking the drug as part of a treatment study when compared with patients receiving a placebo. In the future, tergaserod may become commercially available for selected patients without significant cardiovascular risks. Recent research includes the clinical investigation of methylnaltrexone for opioid-induced constipation in individuals with advanced illness requiring narcotic analgesics. Methylnaltrexone is derived from naloxone and is a quaternary methyl agent that does not cross the blood-brain barrier. Clinical trials have shown that methylnaltrexone reduces the symptoms of constipation without clinical evidence of loss of analgesia or withdrawal.

This medication may prove useful in narcotic-induced constipation.

Additional Resources

Slatkin N, Karver S, Thomas J, et al: A phase III double blind, placebo controlled trial of every other day dosing of methylnaltrexone for opioid-induced constipation in advanced illness. Gastroenterology 131(3):950, 2006.

The abstract describes a well-designed study addressing the need for additional therapeutic options for constipation in individuals requiring opioids for analgesia.

EVIDENCE

1. Drossman DA, Corazziari E, Delvaux M, et al (eds): Rome III: The Functional Gastrointestinal Disorders, 3rd ed. Mclean, VA, Degnon Associates, 2006, pp 515-523.
This text provides specific diagnostic criteria for functional constipation based on consensus of an international committee of clinicians and scientists.
2. Barnes PR, Lennard-Jones JE: Balloon expulsion from the rectum in constipation of different types. Gut 26:1049-1052, 1985.
This article provides basic information on anorectal physiology and discussion of the mechanics of evacuation.

Mark J. Koruda

Common Anorectal Disorders and Colonic Diseases

Introduction

Anorectal disorders, which often present as pain on defecation, are common and can pose very serious problems for patients. The three most frequent causes of pain on defecation are thrombosed hemorrhoids, fissure in ano, and perirectal abscess. In evaluating these patients, it is important to obtain a thorough history concentrating on the events leading up to the problem and on the aspects of defecation that are troublesome. General physical examination includes an anorectal examination concentrating on external inspection, digital examination, and anoscopy, which allows direct visualization of the anal canal. The pain is often too severe to allow a good anoscopic examination without anesthesia, and some patients may need a general anesthetic to facilitate the diagnosis.

The two most common diseases that afflict the colon relate to the appendix (appendicitis) and diverticuli (diverticulitis). Each presents with somewhat typical signs and symptoms, yet commonly poses challenges in diagnosis and management.

THROMBOSED HEMORRHOIDS

Etiology and Pathogenesis

Hemorrhoids are protrusions of the submucosal veins into the anal canal (Fig. 58-1). External hemorrhoids arise from the inferior hemorrhoidal plexus, occur below the dentate line, and are covered by squamous epithelium. Internal hemorrhoids arise from the superior hemorrhoidal plexus above the dentate line and are covered by rectal mucosa. Mixed hemorrhoids are a combination of both the internal and external varieties. Hemorrhoids are usually caused by constipation with repeated straining to pass hard stool, leading to stretching of the anal mucosa, engorgement, and possible prolapse. If prolapsed hemorrhoids remain out and are not reduced, stasis leads to thrombosis.

Clinical Presentation

The most common symptom of patients with hemorrhoids is bleeding occurring during or after defecation, exacer-bated by straining. Pain usually does not occur unless the hemorrhoid is thrombosed or ulcerated. A prolapsed thrombosed hemorrhoid appears blue or purplish on physical examination. Many patients have edematous tissue around the thrombosed hemorrhoid. The area is usually tender because of stretching of the anoderm.

Differential Diagnosis

Prolapsed hemorrhoids that are not thrombosed, anal condylomata, epidermal inclusion cysts, true rectal prolapse, and sentinel pile (associated with a fissure) deserve consideration. Other causal associations include pregnancy, which can cause increased venous pressure in the hemorrhoidal plexus, or the presence of cirrhosis with portal hypertension.

Diagnostic Approach

Generally, the diagnosis is obvious based on direct physical examination of the external anal canal. Occasionally,

Figure 58-1 Hemorrhoids.

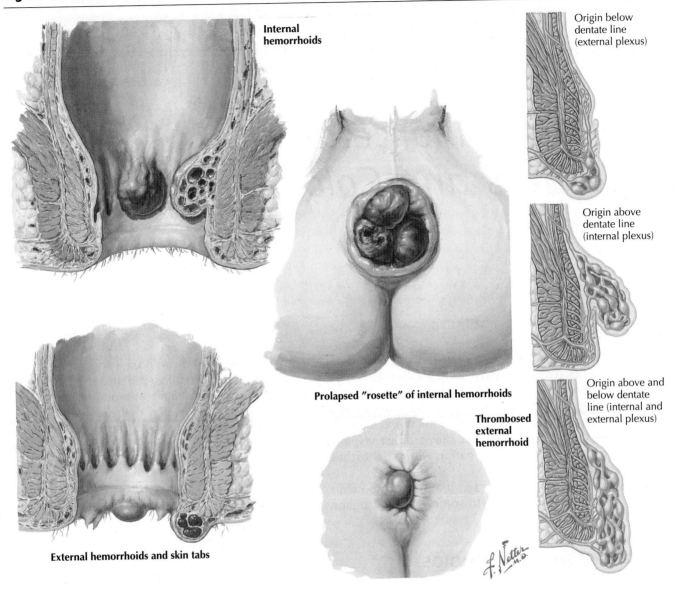

Internal hemorrhoids

Origin below dentate line (external plexus)

Origin above dentate line (internal plexus)

Prolapsed "rosette" of internal hemorrhoids

Origin above and below dentate line (internal and external plexus)

Thrombosed external hemorrhoid

External hemorrhoids and skin tabs

optimal visualization may require examination under local or general anesthesia, especially when the patient is experiencing severe pain. Anoscopy is rarely indicated.

Management and Therapy

Optimum Treatment

Therapy is generally surgical. Incision and drainage of the clot may be adequate, but the excision of the thrombosed hemorrhoid itself is preferable because it allows the tissue to reduce and speeds recovery. Patients can have a local anesthetic with both procedures. Less severe cases can be treated with sitz baths, local steroid creams, and bulk-forming agents. Altering diet, stool consistency, and bowel habits is critical for the long-term treatment of these patients.

Avoiding Treatment Errors

The importance of avoiding errors in diagnosis that lead to a delay in therapy deserves special emphasis. Trials of topical steroids or anesthetics only "prolong the agony" for these patients, whereas timely surgical intervention results in almost immediate relief.

FISSURE IN ANO

Etiology and Pathogenesis

Fissure in ano is a superficial laceration or tear in the anoderm occurring just below the dentate line. The combination of constipation with hard stools and sphincter spasm causes the patient to strain against a spastic sphincter and, as a result, causes the anoderm to give or tear. The skin

in this area is richly innervated by sensory fibers, and the patient is enveloped in a cycle of pain, inflammation, spasm, and more pain. As the patient defecates, the area stretches again, leading to pain that can last several hours. Often, patients will resist having a bowel movement, making the subsequent passage of hard stool even more painful.

Clinical Presentation

The patient presents usually with an acute event or tear causing a cycle of pain and spasm. The physical finding that is pathognomonic in this entity is a sentinel pile or skin tag (Fig. 58-2). This occurs in the posterior midline in 90% of adults. In children, 15% to 20% of lesions can be seen anteriorly. In general, having the patient lie in the lateral decubitus position and spreading the buttocks and asking the patient to strain allows the fissure to be seen. The anoderm will evert out, and the fissure can usually be seen underneath the sentinel pile. Digital examination should be avoided because the area is usually extremely tender. If the diagnosis is suspected and a fissure cannot actually be seen, it may be necessary to perform an examination with the patient under general anesthesia.

Differential Diagnosis

Some patients can sustain tears in this area from physical trauma. Patients with ulcerative colitis commonly have fissures. Various infectious lesions can cause fissures (e.g., amebiasis and tuberculosis), but these are generally quite rare.

Diagnostic Approach

A good history and physical examination are essential to diagnosis. Occasionally, anoscopy with the patient under general anesthesia is necessary.

Management and Therapy

Optimum Treatment

The goal of therapy is to break the spasm of the internal sphincter, so as to reduce pain and improve blood flow to the healing ulcer. Initial therapy for an anal fissure is medical in nature because more than 80% of acute anal fissures resolve without further therapy. First-line therapy includes stool softeners, fiber supplements, and sitz baths for symptomatic relief of pain; they are effective in perhaps 35% of patients.

Nitroglycerin and calcium channel blocker ointments have enjoyed widespread use as second-line therapy. Both serve to relax the internal sphincter muscle and have been met with variable success, 45% to 68% initial healing with up to 35% recurrence rates. Noncompliance with the use of nitroglycerin is common because significant headaches occur in up to 50% of patients.

The injection of botulinum toxin A (BTX) into the internal anal sphincter produces, in effect, a chemical sphincterotomy that lasts up to 3 months. Healing rates up to 90% occur with BTX therapy, with very low recurrence rates.

The gold standard treatment is a lateral anal sphincterotomy, performed by incising the inferior 1 cm of the internal anal sphincter with either an open or closed approach. Complications include bleeding and, rarely, abscess formation and fistula. Incontinence, the most feared complication, occurs when the sphincterotomy performed is too large. This is avoidable with careful surgical technique. Although patients often achieve prompt relief with this procedure, those with chronic fissures may take longer to heal and should be advised accordingly. Comparison of botulinum toxin with lateral internal sphincterotomy showed that at 1 year, more fissures were healed after surgery (94%) than with the injection (75%).

Avoiding Treatment Errors

The timely diagnosis of an anal fissure cannot be overemphasized. Referral to a specialist should not be unduly delayed because therapy results in nearly immediate improvement in a patient's symptoms.

PERIRECTAL ABSCESS
Etiology and Pathogenesis

Almost all anorectal suppurative disease results from infection of the anal glands that extend from the anal crypts, located along the dentate line at the base of the columns of Morgagni. This leads to crypt abscesses, which then penetrate through the wall of the rectum into the perirectal space. Nearly all the anal glands terminate in the intersphincteric plane; therefore, abscesses tend to originate there, and then can travel up, down, or circumferentially around the anus (Fig. 58-3). Perirectal abscesses are classified according to where they are located: perianal, ischiorectal, intersphincteric, or supralevator. Perianal abscesses are the most common, occurring about 50% of the time, whereas the least common type is the supralevator abscess, about 5%.

Clinical Presentation

Patients with perirectal abscesses present with swelling, throbbing, and continuous pain. The onset of pain is usually slower than a fissure and can be more diffuse. On physical examination, there may be edema, induration, or erythema overlying the abscess. Because of the thick fascial bands around the anus, fluctuance is a relatively late sign. Digital examination may be rather painful. If the patient is able to tolerate it, the digital examination can show bogginess.

Figure 58-2 Anal Fissure.

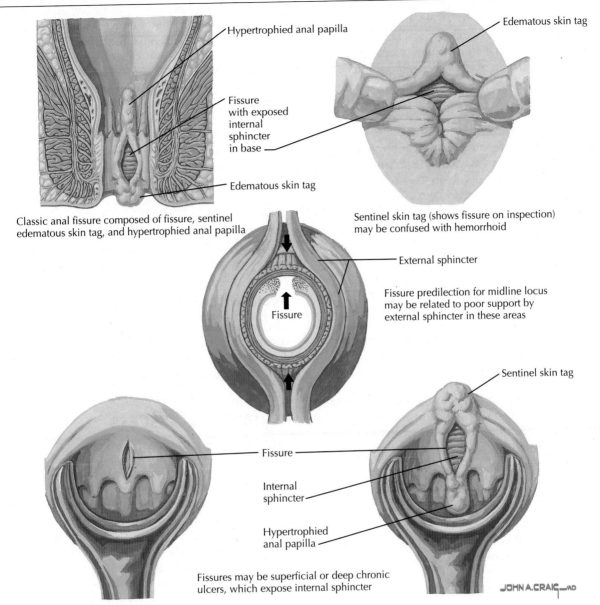

Hypertrophied anal papilla

Fissure with exposed internal sphincter in base

Edematous skin tag

Edematous skin tag

Classic anal fissure composed of fissure, sentinel edematous skin tag, and hypertrophied anal papilla

Sentinel skin tag (shows fissure on inspection) may be confused with hemorrhoid

External sphincter

Fissure predilection for midline locus may be related to poor support by external sphincter in these areas

Fissure

Sentinel skin tag

Fissure

Internal sphincter

Hypertrophied anal papilla

Fissures may be superficial or deep chronic ulcers, which expose internal sphincter

JOHN A.CRAIG—MD

Differential Diagnosis

Very few entities are included in the differential diagnosis of perirectal abscess. Chronic perirectal abscesses with fistula formation are well-known complications of Crohn's disease. Rarely, patients with tuberculosis and actinomycosis present with abscesses in the perirectal area. A localized soft tissue infection from chronic bedsores, as seen in paraplegic patients, can lead to diagnostic confusion.

Diagnostic Approach

The diagnosis is usually made by careful physical examination, looking for induration and occasionally bogginess on the rectal examination. Some clinicians have advocated a computed tomography (CT) scan in difficult patients.

Examination with the patient under anesthesia, with aspiration of the suspected area, may be necessary. Where the perirectal abscess should be drained is obvious in many cases. Newer adjuncts, such as endorectal ultrasound, are helpful in selected patients but generally are not necessary.

Management and Therapy

Optimum Treatment

The critical approach to perirectal abscess is incision and drainage. Antibiotics are also important but are not adequate alone. Localized perianal abscesses can be drained under local anesthesia. Patients with more complicated abscesses require examination in the operating room under

Figure 58-3 Surgical Management of Anorectal Abscess.

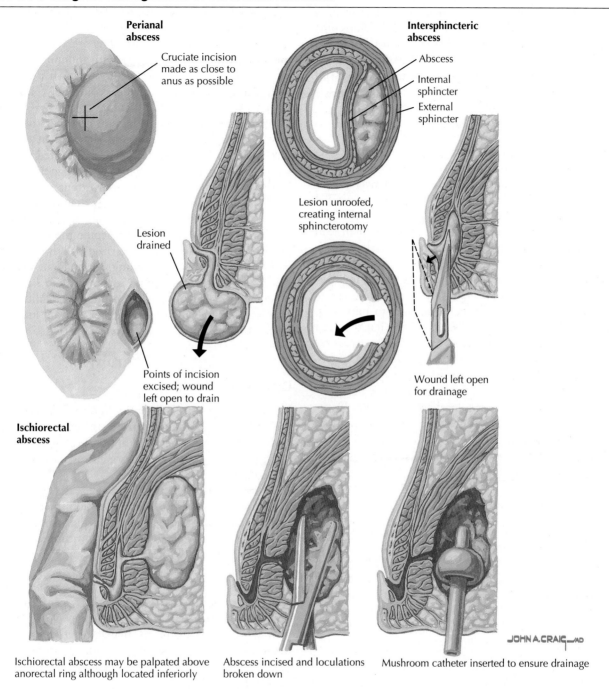

Perianal abscess

Cruciate incision made as close to anus as possible

Lesion drained

Points of incision excised; wound left open to drain

Intersphincteric abscess

Abscess

Internal sphincter

External sphincter

Lesion unroofed, creating internal sphincterotomy

Wound left open for drainage

Ischiorectal abscess

Ischiorectal abscess may be palpated above anorectal ring although located inferiorly

Abscess incised and loculations broken down

Mushroom catheter inserted to ensure drainage

JOHN A. CRAIG—AD

anesthesia. A circumanal incision in the inner sphincteric groove is the safest incision to avoid damage to the sphincters (see Fig. 58-3). If the offending crypt can be identified, then a radial incision can be used to connect it in a submucosal fashion to allow better drainage. Fistula in ano occurs in about 10% to 15% of cases, and these usually drain into the rectum into an area in which the offending crypt has not been identified. Patients with fistula in ano should be referred to a surgeon because of the complexity of management.

Avoiding Treatment Errors

The most common pitfall in the management of perirectal abscesses is over-reliance on antibiotics. Perirectal abscess is a surgical disease, and timely operative intervention is imperative.

DIVERTICULAR DISEASE

Diverticular disease, which includes diverticulosis and diverticulitis, is very common in Western populations.

Some estimates place the incidence of diverticular disease at 10% per decade of life. Most patients with diverticulosis remain symptom free; however, 10% to 30% develop complications, with diverticulitis being the most common. Diverticulitis accounts for more than 200,000 hospitalizations annually and health care costs of more than $300 million (Fig. 58-4).

Etiology and Pathogenesis

Colonic diverticula are actually pseudodiverticula, outpouching of the mucosa through weak areas of the muscularis where blood vessels penetrate. The relatively lower fiber content of Western diets leads to firmer, less bulky stools that require higher intramural pressures within the colon to propel them. The increased pressures then lead to the formation of diverticula at the areas of relative weakness within the colonic wall. Diverticula occur mainly in the left colon, with up to 90% of patients having involvement of the sigmoid colon and only 15% having right-sided disease. They can number from one to hundreds, with the typical size being less than 10 mm, but they can also be as large 2 cm in diameter.

Diverticulitis is characterized as inflammation, infection, or both associated with diverticula. It occurs as the result of perforation of a single diverticulum. Uncomplicated diverticulitis results in a localized phlegmon. Complicated diverticulitis is associated with abscess formation, free perforation with peritonitis, fistula to adjacent viscera, or obstruction. Lower gastrointestinal bleeding may also occur with diverticulosis.

Clinical Presentation

Abdominal pain, typically in the left lower quadrant, is the most common presenting symptom of diverticulitis. The pain may be intermittent or constant. It is frequently associated with a change in bowel habits, either diarrhea or constipation. Anorexia, nausea, and vomiting also may occur, as well as fever. Dysuria and urinary frequency can result from bladder irritation by the adjacent inflamed sigmoid colon.

Differential Diagnosis

The differential diagnosis for diverticulitis is vast. Acute appendicitis is perhaps the most common misdiagnosis that is made. Other diagnoses to be considered are inflammatory bowel disease, ischemic or infectious colitis, peptic ulcer disease, colorectal cancer, and gynecologic abnormalities.

Diagnostic Approach

The diagnosis of acute diverticulitis is commonly made on clinical grounds based on the patient's history, signs, and symptoms and physical exam. Radiologic imaging is the most common modality used not only to confirm the diagnosis but also to assess its severity and the presence of complications.

Plain abdominal and chest films are typically done in the initial evaluation of patients with abdominal pain. Free intraperitoneal air is detected in about 10% of patients with acute diverticulitis. More commonly, nonspecific findings such as ileus are apparent.

Contrast studies such as barium or water-soluble contrast enemas had been the gold standard in diagnosing diverticulitis. These have been supplanted by cross-sectional imaging studies such as CT, magnetic resonance imaging, and ultrasound to a lesser extent.

CT scanning has a sensitivity approaching 98% in diagnosing diverticulitis. It also provides imaging of adjacent structures and the ability to determine the severity of the disease. Mild disease is characterized by bowel wall thickening and pericolic fat stranding. In moderate diverticulitis, the bowel wall thickening is greater than 3 mm with a phlegmon or small abscess. In severe diverticulitis, there is an abscess greater than 5 cm with or without local or free perforation with free intraperitoneal air (Fig. 58-5).

Management and Therapy

Optimum Treatment

Patients with mild diverticulitis (no peritoneal signs and the ability to take fluids) can be treated as an outpatient with close follow-up. Oral antibiotics directed toward gram-negative and anaerobic organisms should be administered for 7 to 10 days.

Patients with moderate to severe disease, complications, or comorbidities require hospitalization. Broad-spectrum antibiotics should be started with the expectation that clinical improvement should occur within 2 to 3 days. About 75% of these patients respond, and the remaining patients come to surgical intervention.

Patients with small, localized, pericolic abscesses can be managed medically with antibiotics. Larger abscesses are best treated with CT-guided drainage, which has been proved very successful in managing these collections because it allows the patient to undergo an elective, less risky surgical resection at a later date after the localized sepsis has resolved.

Indications for immediate surgical intervention include pneumoperitoneum, peritonitis, sepsis, inability to drain the abscess percutaneously, and failure of medical management. The indications for elective surgery are not as well defined. The risk for developing recurrent diverticulitis after an initial episode that responded to medical treatment is about 30%. After a second episode, the chance of a third episode is more than 50%. Because recurrent episodes are less likely to respond to medical management, surgical resection of the involved area should be considered for the second episode of documented uncomplicated diverticulitis.

Figure 58-4 Diverticular Disease.

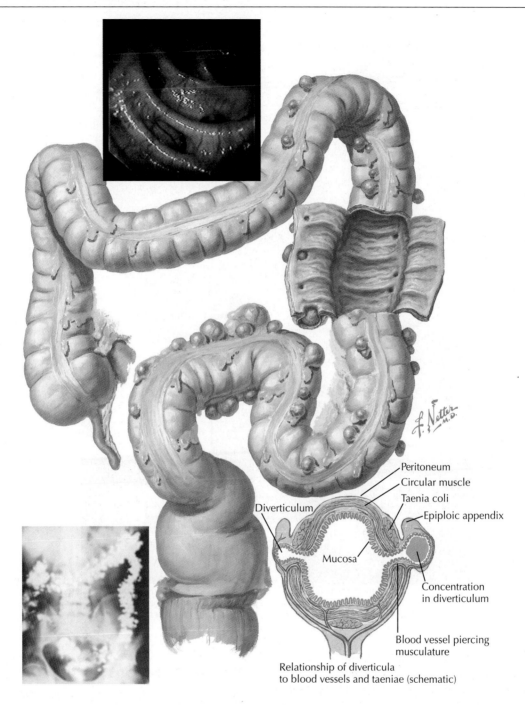

Diverticulum

Peritoneum
Circular muscle
Taenia coli
Epiploic appendix

Mucosa

Concentration
in diverticulum

Blood vessel piercing
musculature

Relationship of diverticula
to blood vessels and taeniae (schematic)

The surgical options that are available in the management of diverticulitis traditionally differ for emergent versus nonemergent, elective operations. In the emergency setting where free perforation with fecal contamination, peritonitis with abscess formation, or systemic sepsis is present, there is a significant risk for anastomotic dehiscence and its associated morbidity if a resection with primary anastomosis is performed. Hence, in these instances, the strategy is to manage the patient in a two-stage manner. At the time of the initial operation, the affected bowel, usually the sigmoid colon, is resected. A colostomy is created of the proximal colon and the site of distal transection (distal sigmoid-proximal rectum) is left within the pelvis as a closed off stump. It is estimated that 50,000 colostomies are created in this country per year under this circumstance. After the patient has recuperated from this initial procedure, the option exists for the second stage, namely takedown of the colostomy with reanastomosis. About 60% of these patients do elect to have their colostomy reversed.

Figure 58-5 Diverticular Disease, with Computed Tomography Scans Showing a Thickened Wall and Diverticula.

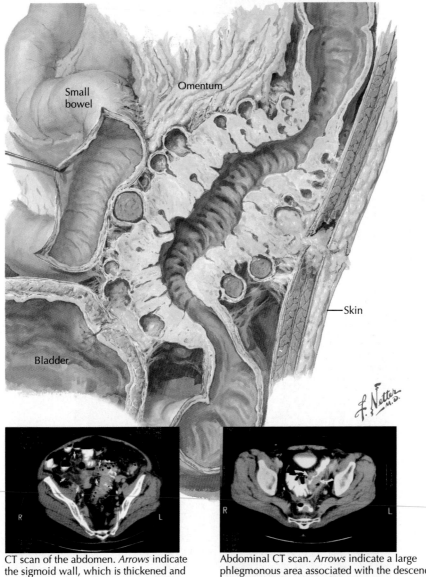

Small bowel

Omentum

Skin

Bladder

CT scan of the abdomen. *Arrows* indicate the sigmoid wall, which is thickened and associated with diverticula.

Abdominal CT scan. *Arrows* indicate a large phlegmonous area associated with the descending colon, which has numerous diverticula.

In the elective setting when the patient is otherwise healthy and local inflammation and infection have resolved, primary resection of the involved bowel with immediate anastomosis is the procedure of choice.

Avoiding Treatment Errors

The widespread use of CT and magnetic resonance imaging have greatly aided in the diagnosis of diverticulitis and its complications. A team approach in its management is frequently indicated because coordination of care among primary care physicians, radiologists, gastroenterologists, and surgeons is essential to ensure optimal patient outcomes.

Future Directions

Whether the far-reaching beneficial effects of increasing the amount of fiber in Western diets will have an effect on the future incidence of diverticular disease and its complications remains in question.

The application of laparoscopic surgery in the management of diverticular disease is becoming more the norm than the exception. It has a low complication rate (<10%) and has shortened hospital stays (2 to 5 days) in most series.

Although the two-stage surgical approach in the management of patients with complications of diverticulitis had been considered the safest alternative, the second stage

Figure 58-6 Progressive Inflammation of the Appendix with Fecaliths.

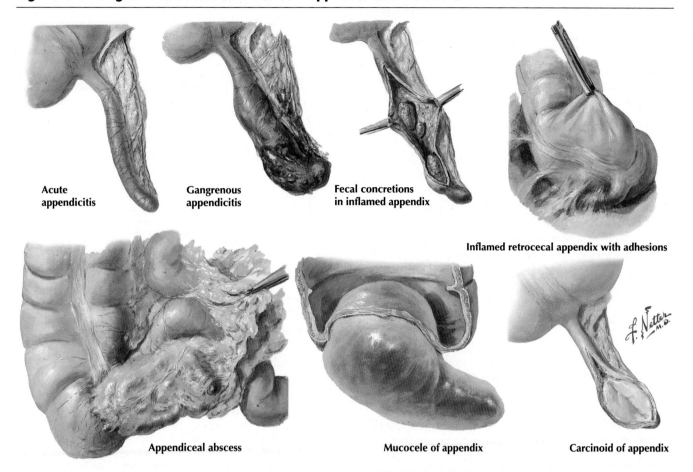

Acute appendicitis

Gangrenous appendicitis

Fecal concretions in inflamed appendix

Inflamed retrocecal appendix with adhesions

Appendiceal abscess

Mucocele of appendix

Carcinoid of appendix

of the procedure, colostomy takedown, is not without morbidity. Anastomotic dehiscence rates for this operation average 4%; wound infections are 4%; and mortality approaches 1%. In light of these complication rates, there are recent reports that even in the presence of abscesses or localized sepsis, resection with primary anastomosis can be performed with satisfactory results.

The traditional acceptance of surgery after two episodes of uncomplicated diverticulitis has been brought into question. Recent analysis supports performing colectomy after the fourth rather than the second episode in patients older than 50 years. This practice resulted in 0.5% fewer deaths, 0.7% fewer colostomies, and saved $1,035 per patient.

APPENDICITIS

Leonardo da Vinci was the first to make anatomic mention of the appendix in the 15th century, and the German surgeon Lorentz Heister first recognized appendicitis in a case report in 1711. The lifetime risk for developing appendicitis is about 8%. Appendectomy is the most common emergency operation performed in the world, with more than 250,000 procedures performed in the United States per year.

Etiology and Pathogenesis

Appendicitis occurs when the appendiceal lumen becomes obstructed (Fig. 58-6). The cause of obstruction can be a fecalith, tumor, foreign body, or hypertrophied lymphatic tissue. Luminal obstruction then produces an increase in intraluminal pressure, which in turn results in venous hypertension, ischemia of the appendiceal wall, and subsequent bacterial invasion of the appendix with necrosis and perforation.

Clinical Presentation

Early on in the progression of appendicitis, distention of the appendiceal lumen typically results in dull, poorly characterized viscerally mediated pain located in the periumbilical area. As the inflammatory process progresses to involve the serosal surface, parietal irritation localizes pain to the right lower quadrant, associated with the location of the appendix. Further progression may then lead to perforation with potential abscess formation. Many patients report anorexia and low-grade temperatures.

Differential Diagnosis

Many, if not most, abdominal pathologic processes may mimic appendicitis. These include bacterial or viral enteritis, mesenteric adenitis, pyelonephritis, renal colic, acute pancreatitis, Crohn's disease, cecal or sigmoid diverticulitis, small bowel obstruction, ectopic pregnancy, ruptured ovarian cyst, ovarian torsion, and acute salpingitis or tubo-ovarian abscess.

Diagnostic Approach

Appendicitis can be a diagnostic challenge because there is no single symptom, finding, or laboratory test that is completely sensitive or specific for the diagnosis. A detailed history and physical exam are the cornerstones in making the diagnosis. Patients with early appendicitis typically appear slightly ill and may manifest low-grade temperature. Localized peritoneal irritation can be detected with localized tenderness in the right lower quadrant as well as the presence of guarding, cough tenderness, or associated Rovsing, psoas, or obturator signs. Elevated white blood cell counts commonly are in the 11,000 to 17,000/mm³. Abdominal CT scans are considered the imaging study of choice in nonclassic cases of appendicitis but are increasingly used in more routine cases.

Management and Therapy

Optimum Treatment

Since its introduction in 1894 by McBurney, appendectomy is the treatment of choice for acute appendicitis, and the technique has remained nearly unchanged. Appendectomies are now commonly performed by the laparoscopic approach. The advantage of laparoscopy over open appendectomy relates to quicker and less painful recovery, fewer complications, and better cosmesis.

Avoiding Treatment Errors

As with most surgical diseases, making the correct diagnosis is key. Conventional wisdom has taught that a negative appendectomy rate (no appendicitis at the time of surgery) should be on the order of 10%. Delaying surgery until the diagnosis is more certain may lead to an increased rate of perforation and other potential complications.

Future Directions

In many instances, the diagnosis of appendicitis can be made on clinical grounds alone. With the development of rapid helical and multidetector CT scanners, CT imaging increasingly is used as the first test to evaluate patients with acute abdominal pain. Clearly, many CT scans are performed unnecessarily in the evaluation of the patient with appendicitis. The proper role of imaging in diagnosing appendicitis has yet to be determined.

Additional Resources

Dominguez EP, Sweeney JF, Choi YU: Diagnosis and management of diverticulitis and appendicitis. Gastroenterol Clin North Am 35(2):367-391, 2006.

This is an excellent review article.

Fox JM, Stollman NH: Diverticular disease of the colon. In Feldman M, Friedman LS, Sleisenger MH (eds): Sleisenger & Fordtran's Gastrointestinal and Liver Disease, 8th ed. Philadelphia, WB Saunders, 2006, pp 2613-2625.

This is a superb chapter in the hands-down best reference book on gastrointestinal disease.

Kaidar-Person O, Person B, Wexner SD: Hemorrhoidal disease: A comprehensive review . J Am Coll Surg 204(1):102-117, 2007.

As the title indicates, this is perhaps the most comprehensive review available. With 15 pages and 166 references, this article covers anatomy, pathogenesis, and all treatment modalities.

Metcalf A: Anorectal disorders. Five common causes of pain, itching, and bleeding. Postgrad Med 98(5):81-84, 87-89, 92-94, 1995.

This older review article is a good source for pathophysiology, diagnosis, and treatment of common anorectal diseases.

EVIDENCE

1. Brisinda G, Cadeddu F, Brandara F, et al: Randomized clinical trial comparing botulinum toxin injections with 0.2 percent nitroglycerin ointment for chronic anal fissure. Br J Surg 94:162-167, 2007.

   One hundred patients were randomized to receive either nitroglycerin or BTX for chronic anal fissure. Although treatment with either agent is effective as an alternative to surgery, Botox is the more effective agent.

2. Lan P, Wu X, Zhou X, et al: The safety and efficacy of stapled hemorrhoidectomy in the treatment of hemorrhoids: A systematic review and meta-analysis of ten randomized control trials. Int J Colorectal Dis 21:172-178, 2006.

   A meta-analysis includes 10 randomized controlled studies that evaluated the safety and efficacy of PPH compared with open hemorrhoidectomy. Stapled hemorrhoidectomy may be as safe as traditional open hemorrhoidectomy.

3. Mentes BB, Irkorucu O, Akin M, et al: Comparison of botulinum toxin injection and lateral internal sphincterotomy for the treatment of chronic anal fissure. Dis Colon Rectum 46(2):232-237, 2003.

   The healing rate of chronic anal fissure is high with Botox; the procedure allows an earlier recovery and fewer complications when compared with sphincterotomy. It occasionally requires repeat injection, and the healing rate is lower in this circumstance.

4. Salem L, Veenstra DL, Sullivan SD, Flum DR: The timing of elective colectomy in diverticulitis: A decision analysis. J Am Coll Surg 199(6):904-912, 2004.

   Decision and cost analysis simulated clinical and economic outcomes after recovery from diverticulitis. This study suggested that the expectant management is associated with lower rates of death and colostomy and is cost-saving for both younger and older patients.

5. Sauerland S, Lefering R, Neugebauer EA: Laparoscopic versus open surgery for suspected appendicitis (review). Cochrane Database Syst Rev 4:CD001546, 2004.

   Fifty-four studies that compared open versus laparoscopic appendectomies were reviewed. Recommendations are to use laparoscopy and laparoscopic appendectomy in patients with suspected appendicitis unless laparoscopy is contraindicated or not feasible. Especially young, female, obese and employed patients appear to benefit.

Yehuda Ringel ▪ Douglas A. Drossman

Irritable Bowel Syndrome

Introduction

Irritable bowel syndrome (IBS), the most common functional gastrointestinal (GI) disorder, is defined as a combination of chronic or recurrent gastrointestinal symptoms not explained by structural or biochemical abnormalities. Studies show that 8% to 23% of adults in the Western world have IBS of varying severity. It accounts for 12% of primary care and 28% of gastroenterologic practice visits yearly.

IBS affects both genders and all ages and demographic groups. Prevalence is higher in females (female-to-male ratio, 2 : 1 in the community setting) and decreases with age. Patients with IBS report lower health-related quality of life as compared with patients who have other chronic GI and non-GI disorders, or healthy controls. IBS poses a considerable socioeconomic burden in terms of health care utilization and costs. On average, patients with IBS miss 3 times more workdays and have significantly more health care and physician visits annually than people without bowel symptoms. The cost of health services for patients with IBS is significantly higher than that for controls. The estimated annual direct cost in the United States is more than $2 billion, and the calculated indirect costs are as high as $20 billion.

Etiology and Pathogenesis

There is no unique pathophysiologic mechanism that explains the symptoms of IBS. It is best understood as an integration of several contributing features. Patients may have exaggerated intestinal motor activity in response to intrinsic (e.g., meals, intraluminal balloon distention) or environmental (e.g., psychological stress) stimuli. However, although certain motility abnormalities have been described, they are not unique or well correlated with pain or with the discomfort that characterize IBS. Patients can also exhibit lower pain thresholds to intestinal or rectal distention (i.e., visceral hypersensitivity and altered pain perception).

The pathophysiologic mechanisms by which visceral hypersensitivity and altered perception are induced or modulated are incompletely understood. Recent studies show that the autonomic nervous system, the neuroendocrine system, and the central nervous system (CNS) have a major role in processing and modulating afferent visceral information from the gut and influencing the conscious experience of visceral sensations and pain through activation of 5-HT afferent receptors (Fig. 59-1). Thus, the experience of IBS symptoms can result from dysfunction at the level of the gut (i.e., abnormal intestinal motor or sensory function) or from dysfunction at any level of neural control of the gut, including the autonomic nervous system, spinal pathways, and CNS (i.e., the brain-gut axis). Figure 59-2 describes the physiologic interactions between brain and gut as well as the visceral pain modulation system.

Considerable attention has been given to potential links between IBS and several predisposing genetic and environmental factors. Recent genetic studies have shown that IBS is twice as prevalent in monozygotic as in dizygotic twins and suggested an association between IBS and several possible gene pleomorphisms (e.g., serotonin reuptake transporter, interleukin-10, and GNb3 protein). The role of intestinal inflammation and activation of the mucosal immune system in the pathophysiology of IBS, as well as in the mechanisms responsible for intestinal dysmotility and visceral hypersensitivity, has also been investigated. Epidemiologic studies have shown that IBS can occur in up to 30% of patients recovering from acute bacterial gastroenteritis, leading to identifying acute GI infections as the greatest single risk factor for IBS. Other studies reported a clinical association between IBS and inflammatory conditions (e.g., inflammatory bowel diseases) and

Figure 59-1 Irritable Bowel Syndrome: Serotonin (5-HT) Receptors on Sensory Afferent Nerves.

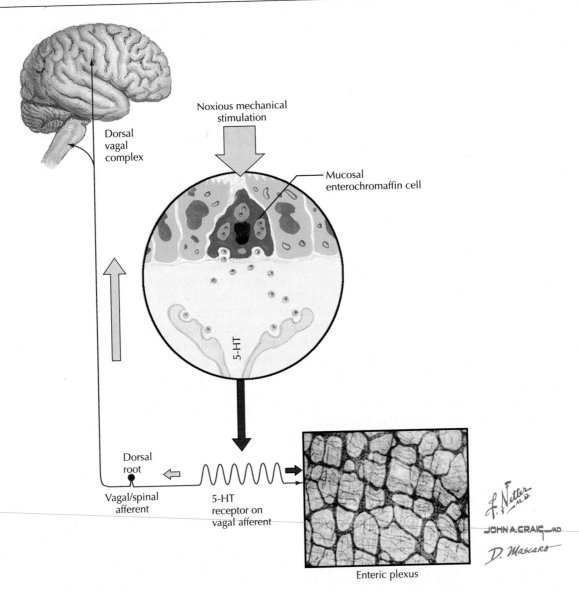

Dorsal vagal complex

Noxious mechanical stimulation

Mucosal enterochromaffin cell

5-HT

Dorsal root

Vagal/spinal afferent

5-HT receptor on vagal afferent

Enteric plexus

documented increased infiltration of chronic inflammatory and activated immunocompetent cells (e.g., intraepithelial lymphocytes and mast cells) in the intestinal mucosa of patients with IBS, suggesting a possible etiologic role for structural or functional changes following acute inflammation or low-grade subclinical inflammation in the pathophysiology of the disorder.

Psychological factors, through their effects on the CNS (e.g., brain cognitive and affective centers) or through autonomic nervous system and neuroendocrine (e.g., hypothalamic-pituitary-adrenal axis) pathways, also influence symptom perception as well as behavioral and emotional responses. Psychological distress affects intestinal motor function and reduces the intestinal sensation threshold, leading to increased gastrointestinal perception.

Because both physiologic and psychological factors contribute to the patient's symptoms and illness, a biopsychosocial model of illness and disease is used for IBS (Fig. 59-3). The biopsychosocial model of illness and disease integrates the physiologic, psychological, behavioral, and environmental factors that contribute to clinical presentation and outcome. Consistent with this model, all these factors interact simultaneously at multiple levels to define illness experience and outcome. The relative contribution and importance of each factor vary among patients and in an individual patient over time. Thus, the clinical presentation, the severity of the symptoms, and the outcome are determined by interaction of all these factors. This complexity carries important implications for establishing a comprehensive and effective diagnosis and treatment plan for patients with IBS.

Figure 59-2 Irritable Bowel Syndrome: Brain-Gut Axis.

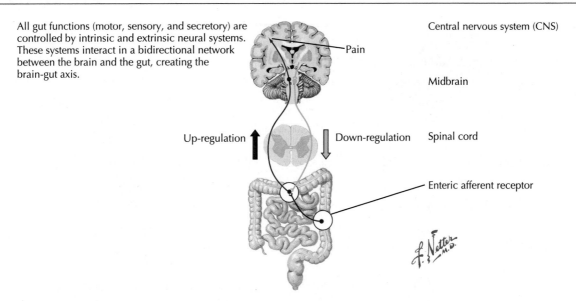

All gut functions (motor, sensory, and secretory) are controlled by intrinsic and extrinsic neural systems. These systems interact in a bidirectional network between the brain and the gut, creating the brain-gut axis.

Central nervous system (CNS)

Pain

Midbrain

Up-regulation   Down-regulation   Spinal cord

Enteric afferent receptor

Figure 59-3 Conceptual (Biopsychosocial) Model for Irritable Bowel Syndrome.

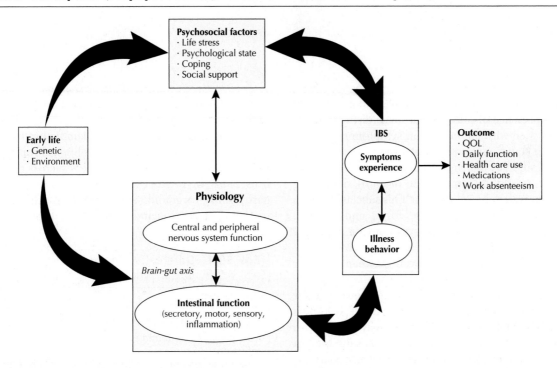

Clinical Presentation

Abdominal pain or discomfort is the most frequently reported symptom in IBS (Fig. 59-4). It is often poorly localized, variable in nature, and usually relieved with defecation. Pain or discomfort is also associated with altered bowel habits (e.g., diarrhea, constipation, or combination of both at times) and with a change in the consistency or frequency of stools. Associated symptoms include bloating, urgency, and a feeling of incomplete evacuation. Although

symptoms tend to occur in clusters, individual symptoms may also occur sequentially and may vary in type, location, and severity over time. In addition, some patients may complain about other (i.e., noncolonic) GI symptoms, such as heartburn and dyspepsia including nausea and early satiety; or non-GI (i.e., extraintestinal) symptoms, including musculoskeletal symptoms (e.g., fibromyalgia), headache, genitourinary symptoms, sexual dysfunction, sleep disturbances, and chronic fatigue. In addition, patients with more severe IBS are more likely to have an increased

Figure 59-4 Irritable Bowel Syndrome.

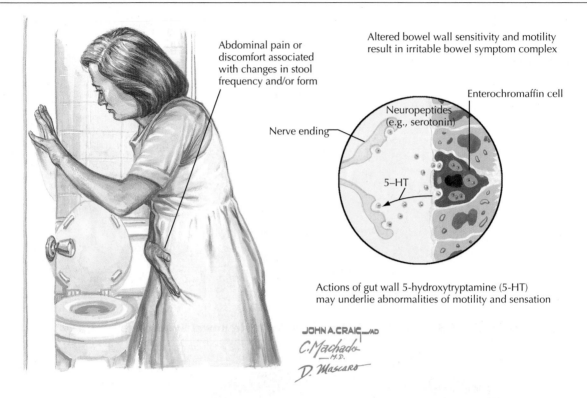

Abdominal pain or discomfort associated with changes in stool frequency and/or form

Altered bowel wall sensitivity and motility result in irritable bowel symptom complex

Enterochromaffin cell

Neuropeptides (e.g., serotonin)

Nerve ending

5–HT

Actions of gut wall 5-hydroxytryptamine (5-HT) may underlie abnormalities of motility and sensation

JOHN A. CRAIG—AD
C. Machado
—M.D.
D. Mascaro

prevalence of comorbid psychosocial disturbances (e.g., anxiety, depression, life stressors, trauma, and a history of abuse). The presence of these psychosocial disturbances is usually associated with an increase in symptom reporting, poorer health status, and poorer outcome.

IBS is classified as diarrhea predominant, constipation predominant, or mixed (combination of both), depending on the most prevalent bowel pattern. This subclassification is determined by stool frequency, form, and passage. However, because the predominant symptom often changes over time, it is not uncommon for a patient to alternate between these IBS subgroups or even between different functional disorders such as IBS and dyspepsia.

As noted, IBS symptoms are heterogeneous in their expression, may overlap other functional GI disorders (e.g., dyspepsia, functional heartburn), or may coexist with other disorders (e.g., ulcerative colitis, Crohn's disease). In these patients, treatment of both disorders is necessary for symptom control and prevention of long-term adverse outcomes. Although symptoms may help direct diagnostic and treatment approaches, they are not sufficient to make a diagnosis.

Differential Diagnosis

The differential diagnosis is broad for IBS (Box 59-1). It includes lactase deficiency; bacterial overgrowth; GI malignancy (e.g., colon or rectal cancer); drugs such as laxative-cathartics or antacids containing magnesium; infection due

to *Salmonella* species, *Campylobacter jejuni, Yersinia enterocolitica, Clostridium difficile, Giardia lamblia, Entamoeba histolytica*; and opportunistic infections in an immunocompromised host. IBS can mimic inflammatory bowel disease (i.e., Crohn's disease, ulcerative colitis); chronic pancreatitis; celiac sprue; metabolic disorders such as diabetes mellitus and thyrotoxicosis; endocrine tumors such as gastrinoma, carcinoid, and vipoma; psychiatric illnesses including depression and somatization disorders; intestinal

---

Box 59-1   Differential Diagnosis of Irritable Bowel Syndrome

Lactase deficiency
Drugs
  Laxative-cathartics
  Magnesium-containing antacids
Infection
  Bacterial infection: *Salmonella* species, *Campylobacter jejuni, Yersinia enterocolitica, Clostridium difficile*
  Parasitic infection: *Giardia lamblia, Entamoeba histolytica*
  Opportunistic infections in immunocompromised host
Inflammatory bowel disease
  Crohn's disease
  Ulcerative colitis
Malabsorption
  Chronic pancreatitis
  Celiac sprue
Metabolic disorders
  Diabetes mellitus

pseudo-obstruction due to primary visceral myopathy and neuropathy or secondary myopathy and neuropathy (e.g., scleroderma, diabetes mellitus). Other colonic diseases in the differential diagnosis include microscopic and collagenous colitis and villous adenoma.

Diagnostic Approach

Because there are no biologic markers for IBS, it is diagnosed by identifying a cluster of clinical symptoms that are consistent with the disorder, excluding other conditions by looking for clinical alert signs (Box 59-2), and performing limited diagnostic testing.

The use of symptom-based diagnostic criteria is standard for IBS. A widely accepted set of diagnostic criteria was developed by multinational working teams known as the Rome Committees. By using the clinical diagnostic criteria, the physician can make a positive diagnosis of IBS, thereby reducing the need for excess diagnostic tests to exclude other conditions.

To meet the Rome III criteria, patients must have abdominal pain or discomfort associated with bowel symptoms. These may include improvement with defecation, changes in bowel frequency, or changes in stool form. The Rome III Committees suggest subtyping of IBS by the predominant stool pattern (hard or lumpy, loose/mushy or watery). Abnormal stool passage (straining, urgency, or feeling of incomplete evacuation), passage of mucus, and bloating or abdominal distention are not essential, but when present, they increase diagnostic confidence and may be used to identify additional subgroups of IBS.

Obtaining the history of the patient's symptoms involves a careful inquiry about the pain or discomfort and its relation to bowel habits and stool characteristics. To meet the IBS criteria, the pain or discomfort must have begun at least 6 months earlier and meet the following criteria for at least 3 days per month for the last 3 months: associated with at least two of the three criteria linking pain to a change in bowel habit (Box 59-3). Initial screening should include blood tests (blood cell count, sedimentation rate, chemistries), stool tests (for ova, parasites, and blood), and sigmoidoscopy to rule out other potential diagnoses. Other studies such as colonoscopy, barium enema, ultrasound, or CT depend on the presence of alarm signs such as symp-

toms that awaken the patient from sleep, initial presentation at an older (>50 years) age; evidence for GI bleeding, weight loss, fever, or a family history of colon cancer or IBD; an abnormal finding on physical examination; or abnormal initial laboratory tests. In addition, specific studies to exclude other conditions such as lactose intolerance, small intestine bacterial overgrowth, thyroid malfunction, or celiac sprue should be considered depending on features in the history or from screening studies that point to other diagnoses. If the initial screening is normal, further diagnostic studies may be withheld, and treatment can be started with a follow-up visit within 4 to 6 weeks. Any changes in the clinical status may lead to further investigation.

Because physiologic and psychological factors influence the presentation of IBS, it is important to consider both in planning the diagnostic approach. Clinicians should evaluate patients for comorbid disorders (e.g., anxiety, panic disorders, depressive disorders, post-traumatic stress disorder, and somatization disorders), personality disturbances, a history of sexual or physical abuse, recent stressful life events, early life experiences, family dysfunction, and maladaptive coping strategies. Understanding the patient's psychosocial status helps to determine an appropriate diagnostic plan while minimizing investigative studies.

Management and Therapy

Optimum Treatment

An effective physician-patient relationship is essential to any treatment plan. This includes appropriate reassurance and education about the condition, its natural history, and its consequences. The patient's understanding of the relevance of physiologic and psychosocial factors to the symptoms, and the acceptance of the need to address both in diagnosis and treatment, is desired but not always achieved.

Given limited understanding and the complexity of the pathophysiologic determinants, the current treatment primarily targets the patient's symptoms and overall well-

being rather than a specific underlying etiologic mechanism. The treatment approach depends on the type of the symptoms, severity of the disorder, presence of other aggravating conditions (e.g., obstructed defecation, fecal incontinence, hemorrhoids), and impact of symptoms on the patient's overall well-being and psychological status. Treatment for symptoms is determined by whether pain, diarrhea, or constipation is predominant. The severity of the symptoms is determined by their intensity and constancy, the degree of psychosocial difficulties, and the frequency of health care utilization. Most patients with IBS symptoms do not see physicians for their symptoms and are usually referred to as *IBS nonpatients*; most patients (about 70%) who do see physicians have mild and infrequent symptoms associated with little disability. These patients usually require only reassurance, education, recommendations for dietary and lifestyle changes, and encouragement for health-promoting behaviors. Short-term medication treatment can be prescribed during exacerbations. Another 25% of patients have moderate symptoms that occasionally interfere with daily activities (e.g., missing school, work, or social functions). These patients may require additional pharmacologic or behavioral treatments. Only a small proportion of patients with IBS (about 5%) have severe symptoms that considerably affect their daily activities and quality of life. These patients usually require psychopharmacologic (e.g., antidepressants) or psychological (e.g., cognitive-behavioral) treatments. In rare cases, referral to tertiary care centers may be needed.

Drug Therapy

Medications directed at the gut can be used to relieve specific GI symptoms. Examples are anticholinergic agents for pain and diarrhea; loperamide for diarrhea; and laxatives such as sorbitol or polyethylene glycol (PEG) solution for constipation. Some new serotonin-receptor acting agents have been recently introduced for use in patients with IBS. These serotonergic medications are directed to reduce gut sensitivity and improve bowel dysfunction. Alosetron, a 5-hydroxytryptamine-3 ($5HT_3$) antagonist, is suggested for female patients with severe diarrhea-predominant IBS who do not respond to other treatments, and a $5HT_3$ agonist (tegaserod) is suggested for female patients with constipation-predominant IBS. Both of these serotonergic medications are currently under restricted use in the United States due to serious adverse events (ischemic colitis and severe constipation with alosetron and cardiovascular effects with tegaserod). Other medications (e.g., κ-opioid active agents for pain) are currently in clinical trials.

Medications with central or psychotropic effects (e.g., antidepressants) can be used to treat comorbid affective or psychiatric disorders (e.g., depression, anxiety). However, low doses of antidepressants also have analgesic properties that are independent of their psychotropic effects. Tricyclic agents such as desipramine (50 to 150 mg) or amitriptyline (25 to 100 mg) appear to be effective in controlling IBS symptoms. Serotonin reuptake inhibitors are used primarily for reduction of associated anxiety and depression but are not as effective for pain control. Newer serotonin norepinephrine reuptake inhibitors such as duloxetine can provide pain relief without the side effects of the tricyclic agents. Consistent with the biopsychosocial model, it is important to view medication therapy as part of a more comprehensive management plan. More recently, there is increasing interest in the use of probiotics because they appear to reduce inflammation in the gut, which may in part be responsible for the visceral hypersensitivity.

Psychological Treatments

Several psychological treatments are used for IBS, including cognitive-behavioral therapy, dynamic or interpersonal therapy, and more passive treatments (e.g., progressive muscle relaxation, hypnosis). Psychological treatments appear superior to conventional medical treatment in reducing psychological distress, improving coping, and reducing some bowel symptoms. However, no one specific treatment is found to be superior. Psychological treatments are recommended for patients with frequent or disabling symptoms, associated psychiatric disorders, history of abuse with maladjustment to the current illness, and somatization with multiple consultations across specialties.

Avoiding Treatment Errors

Chronic use of opioid pain medications should be avoided in patients with IBS. The beneficial effects of these agents are usually short lived, and patients often develop tolerance and sometimes addiction. Chronic use of opioid medications also alter intestinal function and may lead to worsening of constipation and bloating and produce nausea and vomiting. In addition, there is the potential for the development of narcotic bowel syndrome when the chronic use of narcotics prescribed for pain paradoxically produces increased pain, which may lead to escalating dosages in an effort to reduce the pain. Treatment of this condition requires withdrawal of the narcotics. Prescribing of anticholinergic-antispasmodic agents (e.g., hyoscyamine, dicyclomine) or medications with anticholinergic effects (e.g., tricyclic antidepressants) should be done with caution and consideration of bowel habits pattern because these agents decrease intestinal motility and their use may result in worsening of constipation. Similar consideration should be taken with serotonin reuptake inhibitors because many of them have diarrhea as a side effect and therefore may worsen symptoms in patients with diarrhea.

Future Directions

Significant advances in our understanding of functional gastrointestinal disorders and IBS have occurred during the past decade; however, the diagnosis and management of these difficult yet common disorders are still a challenge in clinical practice. Hopefully, the growing interest and recent advances in the multidisciplinary research of these disorders will contribute to the development of novel and more effective diagnostic and treatment approaches.

Additional Resources

Andresen V, Camilleri M: Irritable bowel syndrome: Recent and novel therapeutic approaches. Drugs 66(8):1073-1088, 2006.

The authors provide a recent update that focuses on pharmacologic treatments targeted toward IBS and its clinical subsets.

Longstreth GF, Thompson WG, Chey WD, et al: Functional bowel disorders. In Drossman DA, Corazziari E, Delvaux M, et al (eds): Rome III: The Functional Gastrointestinal Disorders, 3rd ed. McLean, VA, Degnon Associates, 2006.

This chapter reviews the pathophysiology of functional GI disorders with regard to normal and pathologic mechanisms relating to motility, visceral hypersensitivity, bacterial flora, and secretion and provides the basis for pharmacologic treatments targeted to these sites.

Tack J, Fried M, Houghton LA, et al: Systematic review: The efficacy of treatments for irritable bowel syndrome—a European perspective. Aliment Pharmacol Ther 24(2):183-205, 2006.

This review addresses some treatments for IBS not available in the United States.

EVIDENCE

1. American Gastroenterological Association: The burden of gastrointestinal diseases. 2001. Available at: http://www.gastro.org/wmspage.cfm?parm1=3234. Accessed February 26, 2007.

This is a good resource on the health care burden of various GI diseases, including functional GI disorders.

2. Drossman DA, Camilleri M, Mayer EA, Whitehead WE: AGA technical review on irritable bowel syndrome. Gastroenterology 123(6):2108-2131, 2002.

The authors present a detailed and comprehensive review on the etiology, pathophysiology, and management of IBS.

3. Halvorson HA, Schlett CD, Riddle MS: Postinfectious irritable bowel syndrome: A meta-analysis. Am J Gastroenterol 101:1894-1899, 2006.

This meta-analysis provides supporting evidence for the existence of postinfectious IBS as a sequela of intestinal infection and shows a sevenfold increase in the odds of developing IBS following acute infectious gastroenteritis.

4. Hungin AP, Whorwell PJ, Tack J, Mearin F: The prevalence, patterns and impact of irritable bowel syndrome: An international survey of 40,000 subjects. Aliment Pharmacol Ther 17:643-650, 2003.

This large epidemiologic study investigates the prevalence, symptom pattern, and impact of IBS across eight European countries.

5. Levy RL, Olden KW, Naliboff BD, et al: Psychosocial aspects of the functional gastrointestinal disorders. Gastroenterology 130(5):1447-1458, 2006.

The authors provide a detailed and comprehensive review on the importance and approach to the management of psychosocial factors in IBS.

6. Longstreth GF, Thompson WG, Chey WD, et al: Functional bowel disorders. Gastroenterology 130:1480-1491, 2006.

The authors present a detailed and comprehensive review on the etiology, pathophysiology, and management of IBS.

7. Palsson OS, Drossman DA: Psychiatric and psychological dysfunction in irritable bowel syndrome and the role of psychological treatments. Gastroenterol Clin North Am 34(2):281-303, 2005.

This review of the important role of psychosocial factors in IBS provides guidance on how to achieve satisfactory clinical outcomes as well as addressing these factors in clinical work.

8. Ringel Y, Drossman DA: Irritable bowel syndrome: Classification and conceptualization. J Clin Gastroenterol 35(1 Suppl):S7-S10, 2002.

This article summarizes the current understanding of IBS as a multidetermined biopsychosocial disorder in which physiologic, psychological, behavioral, and environmental factors contribute to the clinical presentation of the disorder.

9. Saito YA, Petersen GM, Locke GR 3rd, Talley NJ: The genetics of irritable bowel syndrome. Clin Gastroenterol Hepatol 3(11):1057-1065, 2005.

Genetic basis may relate to the etiology of IBS or its response to therapy. This paper includes reviews of the current literature on genetic factors that might explain the familial clustering of IBS.

10. Saito YA, Schoenfeld P, Locke GR 3rd: The epidemiology of irritable bowel syndrome in North America: A systematic review. Am J Gastroenterol 97(8):1910-1915, 2002.

This is a systematic review of the published literature on the prevalence, incidence, and natural history of IBS in North America.

Kim L. Isaacs

Inflammatory Diseases of the Gastrointestinal Tract

Introduction

Inflammation of the gastrointestinal (GI) tract may occur as a result of infection, physical damage (radiation exposure and ischemia), or an idiopathic, chronic relapsing process commonly referred to as inflammatory bowel disease (IBD). IBD includes Crohn's disease and ulcerative colitis. The pathogenesis, clinical features, and treatments overlap. *Clostridium difficile* colitis is an important nosocomial infection of the colon that is increasingly complicating the course of the hospitalized patient. This chapter reviews the pathogenesis, clinical presentation, diagnostic testing, and treatment for Crohn's disease, ulcerative colitis, and *C. difficile* colitis.

Inflammatory Bowel Disease

Both ulcerative colitis and Crohn's disease are more common in individuals of Northern European origin, with incidence rates from 5 to 12 per 100,000. The incidence of ulcerative colitis has remained fairly constant over the past 50 years. In contrast, the incidence of Crohn's disease is increasing globally, with the most marked changes from 1960 to 1987, followed by a recent plateau. The sex distribution is equal in ulcerative colitis; there is a slight female predominance in Crohn's disease. These diseases are more common in white, and Jewish, populations than in other groups. Both diseases show increased incidence in families, with 6% to 20% of patients having a positive family history of IBD. There is a high concordance of disease among monozygotic twins. As compared with a nondiseased population, patients with Crohn's disease have a higher prevalence of smokers, whereas those with ulcerative colitis are more likely to be nonsmokers. Environmental factors such as infections, toxin or drug exposure, and diet may play a permissive role in the development of disease. Specific agents such as nonsteroidal anti-inflammatory drugs and oral contraceptives have been implicated in Crohn's disease.

Etiology and Pathogenesis

The etiology of ulcerative colitis and Crohn's disease is unknown. Studies indicate an interaction between genetic susceptibility, the host's immune response, and environmental influences. Once inflammation is initiated, there is a failure to down-regulate the immune response. Disordered immunoregulation is thought to occur in part through T-cell responses. Bacteria and bacterial cell products have been implicated in pathogenesis. Genetic variants involving the innate immune system and response to bacteria such as the *NOD2* mutation and toll-like receptor 4 (*TLR4*) have been described in association with Crohn's disease. Certain disease phenotypes have higher associations with these mutations such as early-onset, small bowel disease with the *NOD2* variant in Crohn's disease. Currently, there is an intense effort to identify genes that may play a role in both ulcerative colitis and Crohn's disease, as well as phenotypic associations.

Ulcerative colitis is a mucosal disease limited to the colon. It begins in the rectum and is contiguous throughout the bowel. There may be a sharp cutoff of normal and abnormal mucosa in the distal bowel, or the entire colon may be involved (pancolitis). The ileum is involved in 10% of patients with pancolitis (backwash ileitis). There are no skip lesions, although occasionally there will be a patch of inflammation in the cecum in patients with left-sided ulcerative colitis. Histologically, there is a neutrophilic infiltration with crypt abscess formation and crypt distortion. The inflammation is limited to the mucosal surface. There is foreshortening of the intestine and the development of pseudopolyps with healing.

Figure 60-1 Regional Enteritis (Crohn's Disease).

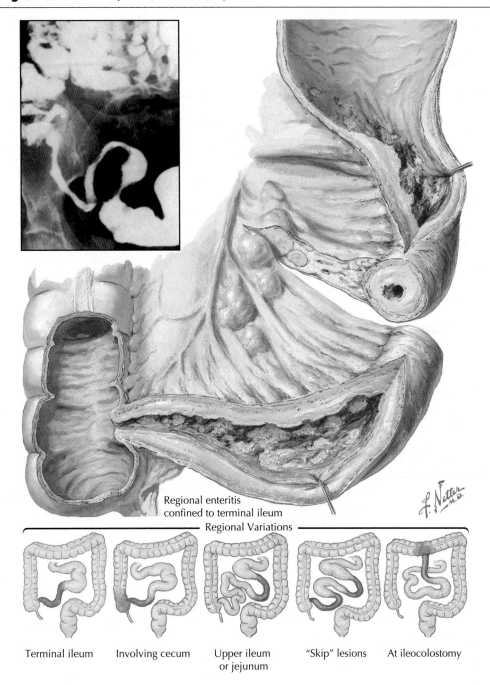

Regional enteritis
confined to terminal ileum

Regional Variations

Terminal ileum   Involving cecum   Upper ileum
or jejunum   "Skip" lesions   At ileocolostomy

In Crohn's disease, the inflammatory process may involve any part of the luminal GI tract from the mouth to the anus (Fig. 60-1). The terminal ileum is affected in 70% to 80% of patients, either alone or in combination with colonic involvement. The inflammation is transmural and characterized by infiltration of the bowel wall with neutrophils, followed by mononuclear-type cells and fibrous tissue. With chronicity, there is architectural dis-tortion. In 60% of cases, noncaseating granulomas may be seen. Small aphthous ulcerations evolve into deep linear ulcerations and fissuring. Mucosal and submucosal fibrosis may lead to stricture formation. The disease is character-ized by skip lesions with normal intervening mucosa. The serosa and mesentery exhibit reactive changes with thick-ening and fibrosis. Grossly, "creeping fat" is noted along the serosal surface. The transmural nature of the disease, along with the deep ulcerations and fissures, leads to the complications of abscess, fistula formation, and obstruction.

Clinical Presentation

Ulcerative Colitis

Patients typically present with bloody diarrhea and tenesmus. With rectal involvement, presenting complaints include bleeding and constipation. Systemic symptoms are not infrequent and include anorexia, weight loss, and fever; localized abdominal cramping may occur with bowel movements. Steady constant pain in the absence of bowel movements suggests severe disease. In toxic dilation, there are decreased bowel sounds and abdominal distention. Long-standing disease may present with a colonic malignancy. After 10 years of pancolonic disease, the incidence of colon cancer increases by about 0.5% to 1% per year.

Crohn's Disease

The presentation of Crohn's disease depends on the affected location. Gastroduodenal disease presents with signs and symptoms that mimic peptic ulcer disease, including midepigastric pain and nausea. In small bowel disease, pain is common; narrowing of the small bowel lumen may lead to obstructive symptoms such as nausea, vomiting, abdominal distention, and pain. In ileal disease, nonbloody diarrhea occurs; patients with substantial ileal disease may have vitamin B_{12} deficiency or bile salt diarrhea. Weight loss and nutrient malabsorption are common. Systemic symptoms such as weight loss and fever and laboratory abnormalities such as anemia and thrombocytosis are more common than in ulcerative colitis. Growth retardation in children may be the presenting complaint.

Complications include abscess formation, enterocutaneous fistulas, and obstruction. Extraintestinal manifestations include axial or central and peripheral arthritis, pyoderma gangrenosum, erythema nodosum, iritis, episcleritis, sclerosing cholangitis, aphthous stomatitis, amyloidosis, gallstones, and kidney stones (Figs. 60-2 and 60-3). The extraintestinal manifestations are seen both in Crohn's disease and ulcerative colitis.

Differential Diagnosis

The differential diagnosis (Box 60-1) of ulcerative colitis covers a wide range of bacterial and parasitic infections of the colon as well as direct damage to the bowel from radiation or ischemia. The patient's history is very important in narrowing the diagnostic list. Potential pathogen exposure, vascular risk factors, a history of radiation exposure, and medication history are important components of the history. If a patient presents with only lower GI bleeding, hemorrhoids, colonic polyps, arteriovenous malformation, and malignancy are in the differential diagnosis.

Box 60-1   Differential Diagnosis of Inflammatory Bowel Disease

Colitis
Inflammatory bowel disease
  Ulcerative colitis
  Crohn's colitis
  Indeterminate colitis
Infection
  Salmonella species
  Campylobacter species
  Shigella species
  Clostridium difficile colitis
  Toxogenic *Escherichia coli*
  Entamoeba histolytica
Other
  Radiation colitis
  Medication-induced colitis
  Ischemic colitis
  Diverticulitis

Enteritis
Inflammatory bowel disease
  Crohn's disease
Infection
  Tuberculosis
  Yersinia enterocolitica
Malignancy
  Lymphoma
Other
  Ulcerative jejunoileitis
  Appendicitis
  Behçet's syndrome
  Chronic granulomatous disease
  Sarcoidosis
  Tubo-ovarian abscess
  Endometriosis

The differential diagnosis for Crohn's disease of the colon is similar to that of ulcerative colitis. In patients who present with small bowel symptoms, disease processes that affect the small bowel must be considered. These include infections, inflammatory processes of other intra-abdominal organs, and other idiopathic inflammatory diseases of the small bowel (see Box 60-1).

Diagnostic Approach

The clinical presentation dictates the types and timing of diagnostic testing. A stool specimen should be examined in patients presenting with a diarrheal illness. White blood cells and blood are seen in ulcerative colitis and infectious colitis. Stool culture for bacterial pathogens, *C. difficile* toxin, and stool prep for parasites will help rule out infectious etiologies. Of note, *C. difficile* infection has been shown to precipitate flares of ulcerative colitis. Compre-

Figure 60-2 Regional Enteritis (Crohn's Disease).

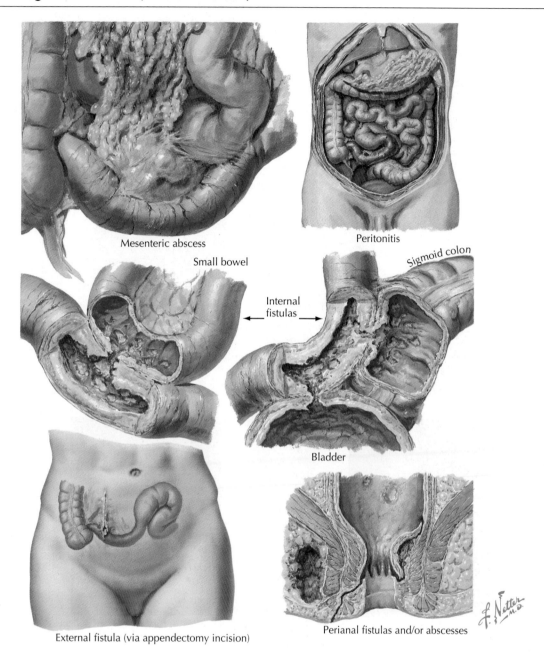

Mesenteric abscess

Peritonitis

Small bowel

Sigmoid colon

Internal fistulas

Bladder

External fistula (via appendectomy incision)

Perianal fistulas and/or abscesses

hensive parasitic screening tests are required in anyone with a travel history or potential parasitic exposure. A qualitative stool fat helps to identify a malabsorptive diarrhea.

Hematologic studies should include hemoglobin, white blood cell count, erythrocyte sedimentation rate, C-reactive protein, and albumin to help define the severity of disease. Serologic testing for antineutrophilic cytoplasmic antibody and anti–*Saccharomyces cerevisiae* antibody has limited diagnostic usefulness. Other serologic markers, such as the antiglycan antibodies laminaribioside and chitobioside, may have a higher specificity

for Crohn's disease but primarily remain research tools at this time.

Sigmoidoscopy, colonoscopy, or both are useful in the diagnosis of colitis (Fig. 60-4). Endoscopic evaluation can help determine the extent and severity of disease. Small bowel radiologic studies help with the diagnosis of small intestinal Crohn's disease demonstrating such findings as luminal narrowing, mucosal irregularity, and internal fistulous disease. They also document the extent of small bowel involvement. In colitis, barium studies of the colon may show a shortened contracted bowel with a loss of bowel wall markings.

Figure 60-3 Extraintestinal Manifestations of Inflammatory Bowel Disease.

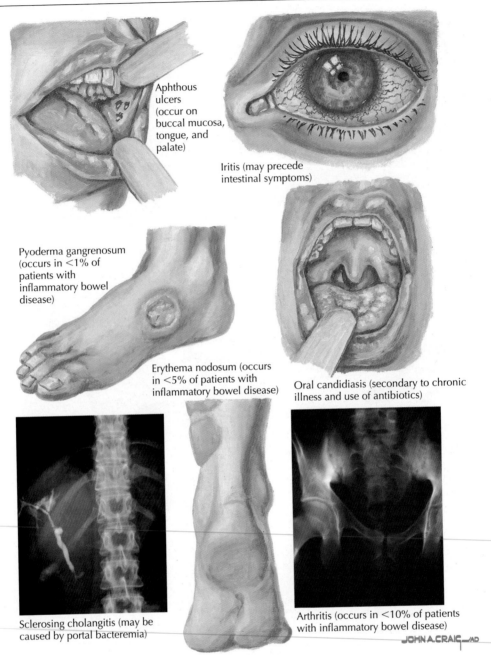

Aphthous ulcers (occur on buccal mucosa, tongue, and palate)

Iritis (may precede intestinal symptoms)

Pyoderma gangrenosum (occurs in <1% of patients with inflammatory bowel disease)

Erythema nodosum (occurs in <5% of patients with inflammatory bowel disease)

Oral candidiasis (secondary to chronic illness and use of antibiotics)

Sclerosing cholangitis (may be caused by portal bacteremia)

Arthritis (occurs in <10% of patients with inflammatory bowel disease)

JOHN A. CRAIG—MD

Management and Therapy

Principles of Therapy

The treatment of ulcerative colitis or Crohn's disease depends on disease location, extent of disease, and severity. Severe disease exacerbations may require inpatient hospitalization. Symptomatic and supportive treatment includes antidiarrheal agents, antispasmodic drugs, hydration, and nutritional support. The history and physical examination should determine whether there are signs and symptoms of toxicity or development of complications, such as toxic dilation, perforation, or abscess formation.

Optimum Treatment

The goals of drug therapy are to use the least toxic drugs first, to reduce long-term steroid use, and to induce remission. Over the past several years, alternative strategies have been proposed that include aggressive, immune active therapy at disease diagnosis in attempts to prevent the

Figure 60-4 Inflammatory Bowel Disease: Colitis.

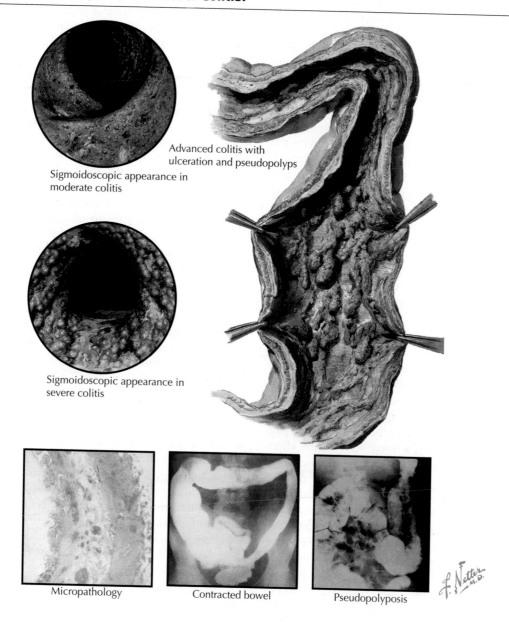

Sigmoidoscopic appearance in
moderate colitis

Advanced colitis with
ulceration and pseudopolyps

Sigmoidoscopic appearance in
severe colitis

Micropathology

Contracted bowel

Pseudopolyposis

long-term development of disease complications. This has been called the top-down approach. It is not clear whether either approach is beneficial for all patients, and attempts are being made to identify the patients who should receive more aggressive initial therapy.

5-Aminosalicylates (5-ASAs) are the first-line therapy in ulcerative colitis. There is controversy about the effectiveness of this class of drugs in Crohn's disease. There are few consistent controlled data to suggest benefit in induction and maintenance of remission with 5-ASAs in Crohn's disease. 5-ASAs are useful in the maintenance of remission in ulcerative colitis. The 5-ASAs differ in the site and mechanism of release. Their activity is dose dependent, and dosage escalation may enhance response.

Sulfasalazine is a 5-ASA bound to sulfapyridine by a diazo bond. Sulfapyridine is a carrier that prevents small bowel absorption. The diazo bond is broken down by bacteria in the colon, releasing 5-ASA and sulfapyridine. Side effects include nausea, vomiting, malaise, sun sensitivity, and rash, which may be caused by the sulfa component. Patients can be desensitized to some of these side effects. Male patients may experience a reduction in sperm count with decreased fertility. Agranulocytosis has also been described. Despite these potential problems, sulfasalazine is a very useful drug and may have benefit for arthritis in patients with both bowel disease and arthritis.

Olsalazine is a 5-ASA dimer in which the 5-ASAs are linked by a diazo bond, which is broken down by bacteria in the colon releasing the 5-ASAs. Up to 20% of patients may experience a secretory diarrhea, which limits its usefulness in treating colitis.

Balsalazide is a 5-ASA with a diazo bond to an inert carrier, 4-aminobenzoyl-beta-alanine. Delivery to the colon is similar to that of sulfasalazine but without the sulfa side effects. Standard dosing is 6.75 g/day.

Oral mesalamine is available in a pH-dependent release form and a delayed release form. The delayed release form is delivered into the terminal ileum and colon. When the capsule opens in the ileum or colon, the drug is released. Standard dosing ranges from 2.4 to 4.8 g/day. The pH-dependent form relies on diffusion of water into an ethyl cellulose granule and displacement of the drug out of the granule. The drug is released in the duodenum. It can be used for disease involving the small bowel or the colon. Standard dosing is 4 g/day.

Topical mesalamine is available in enema and suppository forms. The suppositories (500 and 1,000 mg) are useful for the topical therapy of rectal disease. The enema form, dosed at 4 g, can be used for colonic disease to the splenic flexure; it does not require release from a carrier as with the oral agents.

Steroids are used for more severe ulcerative colitis or Crohn's disease. Corticosteroids can be used topically, orally, or intravenously. Prednisone is the most commonly used oral steroid. Budesonide is available in an ileal release preparation. It has the advantage of a rapid first-pass metabolism and, theoretically, a lower steroid side-effect profile. Orally, the prednisone dosage range is typically 40 to 60 mg/day for 3 weeks, with a variable slow taper if there is a response; there is no benefit to using doses higher than this. Intravenous steroids may be given as a bolus or a continuous infusion. There are anecdotal reports suggesting that continuous corticosteroid infusion is better than bolus infusion. Budesonide is available in 3-mg capsules. Standard therapy starts at 9 mg/day and is tapered by 3 mg/day at varying intervals. Short-term side effects of systemic steroids include glucose intolerance, acne, mood swings, sleep disturbances, and weight gain. Long-term side effects include osteoporosis and cataracts. These agents have no maintenance benefit and should be used for acute disease therapy. Topical steroids are available in suppository, foam, and enema preparations. Foam and suppositories are used in rectal disease. Enemas may be used for left-sided colonic disease. All patients on steroids should be followed closely for the development of steroid-induced osteopenia. Calcium and vitamin D supplementation are important. The development of osteopenia or osteoporosis requires more aggressive management of bone health.

Antibiotics have been shown to have a role in colonic disease, perineal disease, small bowel bacterial overgrowth, and infectious complications such as abscess formation and pouchitis. Metronidazole at 10 to 20 mg/kg is the first-line antibiotic. Unfortunately, it is poorly tolerated by many patients because of nausea and taste disturbances. Peripheral neuropathy may occur with long-term use, and paresthesias are often an early sign of this side effect. Metronidazole should be discontinued if any paresthesias occur because neuropathy is progressive and can be irreversible. Other antibiotics that have been used with some success are ciprofloxacin and clarithromycin. Rifaximin, a nonsystemically absorbed antibiotic, has the theoretical advantage that its activity is limited to the intraluminal GI tract. It is currently in trial in Crohn's disease.

Immunosuppressive agents such as azathioprine and 6-mercaptopurine are used for medically refractory bowel disease, steroid-dependent disease, and perineal disease. These agents are most commonly used in Crohn's disease, but are increasingly used in ulcerative colitis. The white blood cell count should be carefully monitored for evidence of bone marrow suppression. Measurement of metabolites may play a role in determining therapeutic efficacy and potential for toxicity. These agents have a delayed onset of action and should be used for 3 to 6 months before making decisions on lack of efficacy. Other side effects include pancreatitis and cholestasis. Long-term neoplasia risk is not clear.

Parenteral methotrexate has been shown to be of benefit in active Crohn's disease as well as for maintenance therapy. Dosages range from 15 to 25 mg intramuscularly or subcutaneously once per week. Signs of toxicity include liver abnormalities and pulmonary fibrosis. It is absolutely contraindicated in pregnancy, and caution should be used in women of childbearing age.

Cyclosporine is used in severe, acute colitis. It has a limited role in the treatment of Crohn's disease. In fulminant colitis, intravenous dosing has been shown to prevent or delay colectomy. Cyclosporine has a narrow therapeutic window; side effects include renal toxicity, hypertension, hirsutism, and seizures. A surgeon should be closely involved and follow the patient's course, helping to observe for signs and symptoms that indicate the need for an urgent colectomy. Despite the encouraging short-term success of cyclosporine, over the long-term, many patients who were initial responders have a relapse that leads to colectomy.

Infliximab, a chimeric antibody to tumor necrosis factor-α is used to treat Crohn's fistulous disease as well as to induce remission and decrease steroid requirements in patients with luminal disease. It has also been approved for use in the induction and maintenance of remission in ulcerative colitis. The drug is given as a 5 mg/kg IV infusion over 2 hours. The average duration of response is 8 weeks. An induction course of therapy at 0, 2, and 6 weeks is commonly employed with subsequent maintenance dosing every 8 weeks. Potential side effects include infusion reactions, infections, arthritis or arthralgias, and malignancy. Development of antibodies to infliximab may lead to increased infusion reactions and decreased efficacy of drug therapy. Premedication with intravenous hydrocortisone and concomitant alternative immunosuppression with antimetabolites or methotrexate are strategies that have been employed in attempts to decrease antibody formation. Adalimumab and certolizumab are alternative anti–tumor necrosis factor agents that may be used in patients who have developed antibodies to infliximab.

Avoiding Treatment Errors

In the therapy of inflammatory bowel disease, there are multiple potential treatment errors that can be predicted and avoided. Both Crohn's disease and ulcerative colitis are characterized by disease exacerbations and remissions. With the treatment of an exacerbation, it is important to make sure that the symptoms are due to recurrent IBD. Enteric infections, bowel ischemia, and functional bowel disease can mimic the symptoms of active inflammatory bowel disease. Escalation of disease therapy for IBD may be harmful if the bowel symptoms are not due to worsening of the IBD. With each change in IBD therapy, reconsider the differential diagnosis with physical examination, endoscopic evaluation, stool examination, and laboratory testing as indicated.

All the therapies used in the treatment of IBD have potential side effects that require vigilance to allow for early detection of complications. The clinician should be familiar with the common side effects of these medications and institute appropriate monitoring procedures.

This is especially important with the immune active agents because complications such as infection from profound immunosuppression may occur. Suggested monitoring for 6-mercaptopurine and azathioprine includes a complete blood count (CBC), aspartate transaminase (AST), alanine transaminase (ALT), alkaline phosphatase, total bilirubin, and when appropriate, lipase and amylase. Before starting 6-mercaptopurine and azathioprine, check the patient's thiopurine methyl transferase (TPMT) phenotype and genotype to detect patients with low enzyme activity. Individuals with low TPMT activity are susceptible to profound early immunosuppression and should be started on lower initial 6-mercaptopurine and azathioprine doses with more frequent initial monitoring.

Suggested monitoring for methotrexate includes CBC, AST, ALT, alkaline phosphatase, total bilirubin, and monitoring of respiratory function. For cyclosporine, monitoring includes CBC, creatinine, AST, ALT, alkaline phosphatase, total bilirubin, and monitoring of blood pressure.

Future Directions

There has been an explosion of knowledge regarding important factors in the pathophysiology of inflammatory bowel disease. This is reflected in how we consider and treat Crohn's disease and ulcerative colitis. As we move forward into a new era of treatment, clinical and genetic phenotyping of disease may allow for more specific thera-

peutic regimens. Advances are being made in the use of biologics in the treatment of IBD, and we are likely to see drug regimens that include growth factors, antibodies to different components of immune active cells, and drugs that stimulate certain classes of white blood cells. The recognition that gut bacterial flora may play a role in disease activity will likely lead to increased manipulation of the gut flora with both probiotics and antibiotics. With these new therapies, attempts will be made to develop therapeutic regimens to avoid steroid exposure and allow for early intervention that may change the disease course.

Clostridium difficile Colitis

C. difficile was first shown to play a causative role in the development of pseudomembranous colitis associated with antibiotic usage in 1978. It has become a more and more important nosocomial pathogen, complicating hospital stays, precipitating inflammatory bowel disease, and causing significant morbidity and increasing mortality in affected patients. The asymptomatic colonization rate of hospitalized patients with *C. difficile* is as high as 20%, compared with a less than 5% colonization rate in the community. In approximately one third of patients colonized, a toxin is produced that leads to diarrhea.

Etiology and Pathogenesis

C. difficile is an anaerobic, gram-positive, spore-forming bacterium. It is spread by the fecal-oral route, often by spores that are left on surfaces. Handwashing helps prevent spread. In colonized patients who receive antibiotics, *C. difficile*, which is resistant to many antibiotics, proliferates in the environment of decreased normal colonic flora. *C. difficile* produces toxins that cause diarrhea in affected patients. If the organism carries the gene for toxin production, disease develops. There are two major toxins: the A and B toxins. Toxin B is more cytotoxic than toxin A. The toxin binds to a receptor on the colonocyte and is incorporated into the cell, which then leads to a loss of polarity of the cell and ultimately cell death. This process leads to a colitis and often pseudomembrane formation. A particularly virulent strain of *C. difficile*—the NAP1/027 strain—has been recently associated with widespread outbreaks in Canada and the United States. This strain produces much larger quantities of toxin than strains previously isolated.

Clinical Presentation

Patients typically present with diarrhea during or immediately after antibiotic exposure. Factors that increase the risk for infection include increasing age, severe comorbid disease, patients on an antisecretory medicine such as proton pump inhibitors, multiple antibiotics, hospitalization (particularly in the intensive care unit), patients with nasogastric tubes, and patients who have a long duration of antibiotic therapy. Stools are typically watery and liquid in consistency. Occasionally, the stool is bloody. Patients may have abdominal pain. In more severe cases, patients have systemic symptoms of fever, malaise, dehydration, and delirium.

Differential Diagnosis and Diagnostic Approach

The approach to diagnosis is similar in all patients presenting with diarrhea. The historical information of prior antibiotic exposure should place *C. difficile* infection high in the differential diagnosis. The differential diagnosis for *C. difficile* colitis is nearly the same as that for ulcerative colitis (see Box 60-1). Diagnostic studies include stool culture and stool testing for *C. difficile* toxin. Complete blood count and albumin measurements help with assessment of severity of the ongoing infection. Endoscopic evaluation with a sigmoidoscopy and biopsy may identify pseudomembranes (Fig. 60-5).

Management and Therapy

Optimum Treatment

First-line therapy for *C. difficile* colitis is metronidazole, 500 mg three times daily, based on cost and efficacy. In early studies, up to 90% of patients were cured of infection with metronidazole; however, the response rate appears to be decreasing, with a recent study demonstrating only a 50% relapse-free response rate. Intravenous metronida-

Figure 60-5 Pseudomembranous Colitis.

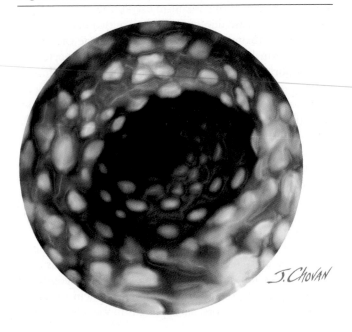

J. CHOVAN

zole is excreted in the bile and may be used for treatment in patients who cannot tolerate oral medication. Oral vancomycin is also effective for treatment of *C. difficile* colitis, with an initial dose of 125 mg four times a day, increasing to 250 mg four times a day for more severe disease. A vancomycin taper is used in relapsing disease. Intravenous vancomycin is not excreted into the lumen of the GI tract and is ineffective for treatment. Nitazoxanide at 500 mg twice a day for 7 days appears to be as effective as metronidazole in the treatment of this disease entity. Repopulating the colon with nonpathogenic bacteria (probiotics) is one proposed therapeutic option in *C. difficile* colitis. *Saccharomyces boulardii* does appear to play a role in decreasing recurrent *C. difficile* colitis. The standard dosage is one 500 mg capsule twice a day for 4 weeks. For symptomatic control of diarrhea, cholestyramine has been used to bind the toxin produced by *C. difficile*. If a patient becomes increasingly toxic despite medical therapy, colectomy should be considered.

Prevention should also be considered as an important therapeutic maneuver in colitis related to *C. difficile* infection. Hospitalized patients with *C. difficile* infections should be placed on contact precautions with handwashing, gloves, and gowns during contact with the patient. The patient should have a dedicated stethoscope and thermometer available in the room. There should be monitoring and surveillance activity by infection control on the hospital floor units and intensive care units.

Avoiding Treatment Errors

In treating *C. difficile* colitis, it is important to recognize that the antibiotics must reach the lumen of the gastrointestinal tract to be effective. Oral vancomycin is effective, whereas intravenous vancomycin is not effective. Both intravenous and oral metronidazole can be used for therapy. *C. difficile* can complicate other forms of inflammatory bowel disease. If a patient is not responding to therapy, it is important to reassess the disease process and treat coexistent disease appropriately.

Future Directions

There are multiple newer antibiotics that are thought to have a role in the treatment of *C. difficile* colitis. In addition to nitazoxanide as mentioned, other antibiotics include ramoplanin, rifaximin, rifalazil, and OPT-80. Both passive and active immunization strategies are being assessed for disease prevention. The vaccines in trial include those directed against the A and B toxin (active immunization) and MDX-066, which is a monoclonal antibody to toxin A.

Additional Resources

Carter MJ, Lobo AJ, Travis SP; IBD Section, British Society of Gastroenterology: Guidelines for the management of inflammatory bowel disease in adults. Gut 53(Suppl 5):V1-V16, 2004.

This paper summarizes current management guidelines for patients with ulcerative colitis and Crohn's disease.

Crohn's and Colitis Foundation of America. Available at: http://www.ccfa.org. Accessed November 21, 2006.

This website provides comprehensive information on Crohn's disease and ulcerative colitis for patients. Patient education brochures are also available through this site.

Crohn's and Colitis Foundation of Canada. Available at: http://www.ccfc.ca. Accessed November 21, 2006.

This website has information about Crohn's disease and ulcerative colitis, as well as ongoing programs, events, and research in Canada.

Itzkowitz SH, Present DH; Crohn's and Colitis Foundation of America Colon Cancer in IBD Study Group. Consensus conference: Colorectal cancer screening and surveillance in inflammatory bowel disease. Inflamm Bowel Dis 11(3):314-321, 2005.

Practice guidelines are presented regarding current recommendations for colorectal cancer screening in patients with inflammatory bowel disease.

Kornbluth A, Sachar DB; Practice Parameters Committee of the American College of Gastroenterology: Ulcerative colitis practice guidelines in adults (update): American College of Gastroenterology, Practice Parameters Committee. Am J Gastroenterol 99(7):1371-1385, 2004.

The authors present practice guidelines for the management of patients with ulcerative colitis.

Lichtenstein GR, Abreu MT, Cohen R, Tremaine W: American Gastroenterological Association Institute Medical Position Statement on Corticosteroids, Immunomodulators, and Infliximab in Inflammatory Bowel Disease. Gastroenterology 130(3)935-939, 2006.

In this summary of the current treatment options for IBD, monitoring practices are recommended, and the level of evidence that supports those recommendations is discussed.

Thorpe CM, Gorbach SL: Update on Clostridium difficile. Curr Treat Options Gastroenterol 9(3):265-271, 2006.

The authors provide a summary of the diagnosis and treatment of Clostridium difficile colitis.

EVIDENCE

1. Akobeng AK, Zachos M: Tumor necrosis factor-alpha antibody for induction of remission in Crohn's disease. Cochrane Database Syst Rev 1:CD003574, 2004.

   This review and summary of all the available clinical trial data looks at the use of TNF-α antagonists for the induction of remission in Crohn's disease.

2. Lawson MM, Thomas AG, Akobeng AK: Tumour necrosis factor alpha blocking agents for induction of remission in ulcerative colitis. Cochrane Database Syst Rev 3:CD005112, 2006.

   This review and summary of all the available clinical trial data looks at the use of TNF-α antagonists for the induction of remission in ulcerative colitis.

3. Lemann M, Mary JY, Colombel JF, et al: A randomized, double-blind, controlled withdrawal trial in Crohn's disease patients in long-term remission on azathioprine. Gastroenterology 128(7):1812-1818, 2005.

   This trial addresses the question of the effectiveness of maintenance therapy with azathioprine in patients with Crohn's disease.

4. Sutherland L, MacDonald JK: Oral 5-aminosalicylic acid for induction of remission in ulcerative colitis. Cochrane Database Syst Rev 2:CD000543, 2006.

   This is a review and summary of all the available clinical trials that look at the use of 5-aminosalicylates for the induction of remission in ulcerative colitis.

Ryan D. Madanick ▪ Nicholas J. Shaheen

Esophageal Disorders: Dysphagia

Introduction

Dysphagia, or difficulty swallowing, is among the most common gastrointestinal symptoms experienced by the general population. More than one fourth of elderly patients experience dysphagia at least intermittently. The causes of this symptom are diverse, ranging from the benign to dreaded malignancies such as esophageal cancer. This chapter reviews the etiologies, presentation, diagnostic workup, and treatment of this condition.

Etiology and Pathogenesis

Dysphagia has a myriad of causes that require careful assessment. To understand the etiology and pathogenesis, it is helpful to use the anatomic location of the sensation of dysphagia. Patients who complain of difficulty initiating swallowing, with frequent sensations of choking or suffocation, are said to have *transfer dysphagia*, or difficulty transferring the food bolus from the oropharynx into the upper esophagus. Subjects localizing the sensation of dysphagia to the neck area have *cervical dysphagia*, whereas those who experience lodging of food, pills, or fluid in the chest have *thoracic dysphagia*.

The etiology of dysphagia differs based on the localization of symptoms (Box 61-1). Subjects who complain of transfer dysphagia may have underlying neurologic damage secondary to a cerebrovascular accident (CVA) or multiple sclerosis. Oropharyngeal malignancies also warrant consideration. In patients with cervical dysphagia, cervical spine osteophytes, esophageal webs, squamous cell carcinoma of the esophagus, and esophageal strictures predominate. In subjects with thoracic dysphagia, gastroesophageal reflux disease (GERD), esophageal stricture (Fig. 61-1), Schatzki's ring (a benign ring at the gastroesophageal junction), motility disorders such as achalasia, and esophageal cancer of either squamous or adenomatous histology (Fig. 61-2) are common diagnoses. Extrinsic compression of the esophagus by any structure in the neck or thorax may lead to symptoms referable to the location of the compression.

The pathogenesis of aerodigestive malignancies commonly causing dysphagia differs by location and histology. The main risk factors for cancers of the tongue, pharynx, and larynx, as well as squamous cell cancers of the esophagus, are tobacco use, alcohol consumption, and African American race. Conversely, the pathogenesis of esophageal adenocarcinoma appears to involve chronic inflammation of the distal esophagus by acid reflux (see Chapter 50). This cancer occurs in increased frequency in white males.

Clinical Presentation

The defining characteristic of dysphagia is the sensation of blockage to the passage of solid or liquid contents, or both. Subjects may describe a gradual course, with escalating symptoms initially to only bulky solids such as meats or breads, progressing to dysphagia to substances of a pudding-like consistency, and culminating in complete intolerance to solids. Such a crescendo pattern of symptoms is suggestive of a worsening mechanical obstruction, such as esophageal cancer, or a tightening esophageal peptic stricture. Alternatively, the patient may describe dysphagia to liquids and solids equally, with no crescendo pattern. Such a history is more suggestive of a motor abnormality, such as achalasia or diffuse esophageal spasm. The latter is especially suggested when substances of an especially hot or cold temperature precipitate symptoms. Long-term, nonprogressive problems with intermittent dysphagia to bulky solids is suggestive of the presence of Schatzki's ring (Fig. 61-3).

Box 61-1   Etiology of Dysphagia

Transfer Dysphagia
Neuromuscular disorders
  Cerebrovascular accident
  Parkinson's disease
  Multiple sclerosis
  Head trauma
  Amyotrophic lateral sclerosis
  Peripheral neuropathy
  CNS tumors
  Myasthenia gravis
  Inflammatory myopathy (polymyositis)
Oropharyngeal malignancies
Xerostomia
Depression
 	
Cervical Dysphagia
UES dysfunction
  Cricopharyngeal bar
  Cricopharyngeal spasm
Proximal esophageal stricture
  Radiation
  Caustic ingestion
Esophageal web
Squamous cell carcinoma of larynx/proximal esophagus
Zenker's diverticulum
Cervical osteophyte
Extrinsic compression (goiter)
 	
Thoracic Dysphagia
Motility disorders
  Achalasia
  Diffuse esophageal spasm
  Ineffective esophageal motility
  Systemic sclerosis
Esophageal malignancy
  Adenocarcinoma
  Squamous cell carcinoma
Distal esophageal stricture
  Peptic/GERD
  Pill-induced
  Radiation
  Caustic ingestion
Schatzki's rings
Eosinophilic esophagitis
Aberrant subclavian artery (dysphagia lusoria)

CNS, central nervous system; GERD, gastroesophageal reflux disease; UES, upper esophageal sphincter.

Profound weight loss may be seen with almost all the causes of dysphagia listed in Box 61-1; however, in elderly patients, this alarm feature is especially concerning for esophageal cancer. Close examination of the patient with dysphagia may yield additional clues as to the pathogenesis of the symptoms. For instance, patients with motility disorders secondary to systemic sclerosis may manifest characteristic changes of the skin of the fingers (sclerodactyly) (see Chapter 154). Those with CREST (calcinosis, Raynaud's phenomenon, esophageal dysfunction, sclerodactyly, and telangiectasia) syndrome may demonstrate several of the cutaneous manifestations of the disorder, so a thorough dermatologic evaluation should be performed.

Differential Diagnosis

As noted in Box 61-1, the differential diagnosis of the symptom of dysphagia is broad. It is important to clarify the patient's symptom complex. Patients may complain of trouble swallowing when they are really experiencing odynophagia, or pain on swallowing. Additionally, severe erosive esophagitis may have a degree of dysphagia as a component of its presentation due to edema of the esophageal wall from inflammation.

Diagnostic Approach

Because of the specter of possible malignancy, as well as the progressive and destructive nature of many of the etiologies of the symptom, dysphagia generally demands immediate attention and a prompt workup. Dysphagia is one of the alarm symptoms of GERD, and dysphagia in the setting of heartburn mandates diagnostic testing.

The diagnostic measures of choice depend on the character of the dysphagia. Subjects with transfer dysphagia should have a good examination of the oropharynx and neck. Depending on the patient profile, if this examination fails to demonstrate an etiology of the symptoms, further testing with either modified barium swallow (contrast radiography concentrating on the swallowing mechanism and the proximal esophagus) or a fiberoptic endoscopic evaluation of swallowing (FEES) study may be indicated. In a FEES study, the subject is asked to ingest foods of varying consistency while a speech pathologist observes the swallowing mechanism through a fiberoptic scope passed through the nose and positioned in the nasopharynx above the vocal cords. Both the barium study and the FEES study allow evaluation of bolus formation, movement of the epiglottis, and detection of aspiration of even minute amounts of material. The choice between the two modalities may depend on local expertise and availability. Further workup, such as brain imaging studies to assess for multiple sclerosis or CVA, depends on the patient profile and findings of the initial evaluation.

The workup of true cervical dysphagia is similar to that of transfer dysphagia. However, the absence of an obvious risk factor such as a stroke is an indication for cross-sectional imaging of the neck to rule out an extrinsic lesion compressing the cervical esophagus. If the evaluation of the transfer mechanism and proximal esophagus is negative, the patient should have an evaluation for distal esophageal pathology. The sensation of food sticking may be referred to the sternal notch or above in these thoracic esophageal conditions.

Several modalities exist to evaluate thoracic dysphagia. A barium esophagram is helpful in assessing the gross anatomic structure of the esophagus, including evaluation for intrinsic lesions and extrinsic compression. It may also be helpful in the diagnosis of achalasia. Frequently, a dilated esophagus without peristaltic contractions will be seen, with a contrast-filled esophagus and a narrow tapered

Figure 61-1 Two Types of Benign Esophageal Strictures.

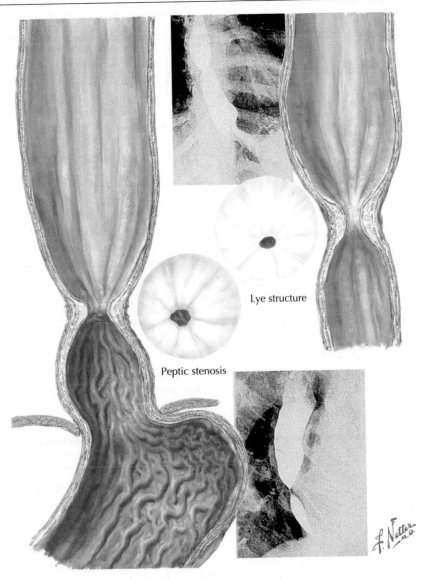

Lye structure

Peptic stenosis

gastroesophageal junction, the so-called bird's beak appearance. When the location of dysphagia is uncertain, a tablet esophagram can help to further localize the pathologic region. Ultimately, many patients will require an upper endoscopy for thoracic dysphagia. Endoscopy allows the physician to assess the esophageal mucosa for esophagitis, to perform biopsies of masses, to dilate strictured regions, and to rule out subtle lesions that may have been missed on barium swallow. Additionally, in patients with suspected achalasia, upper endoscopy allows the exclusion of secondary achalasia, or pseudoachalasia, in which a tumor at the gastric cardia mimics the presentation of achalasia. In the absence of obvious structural abnormalities on upper endoscopy, esophageal biopsies are recommended to rule out eosinophilic esophagitis. If the structural studies do not reveal an obvious etiology for the problem, esophageal manometry is then warranted to rule out esophageal motor disorders.

Management and Therapy

Optimum Treatment

Management of the patient with dysphagia ultimately depends on the type of dysphagia (Table 61-1). For patients with oropharyngeal dysphagia, therapy is directed at improving bolus transfer and nutritional intake, reducing pulmonary aspiration, and ameliorating the quality of life. If structural issues such as webs or strictures exist, they should be addressed initially, usually by endoscopic dilation. However, for most underlying causes of oropharyngeal dysphagia, the largest component of care for patients with oropharyngeal dysphagia is swallowing therapy by a

Figure 61-2 Malignant Tumors of Midportion and Distal Portion of Esophagus.

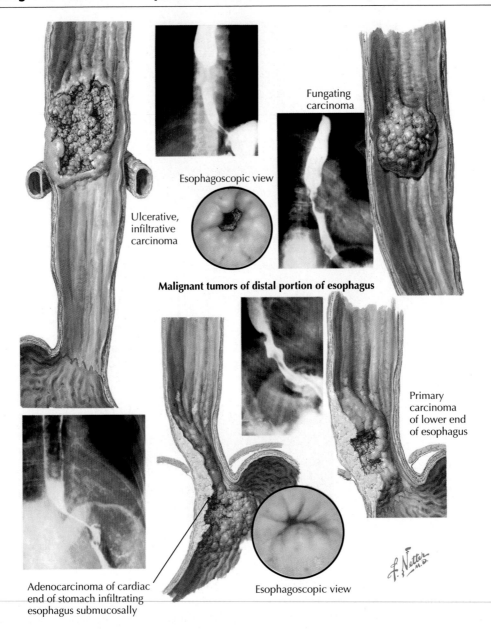

Fungating carcinoma

Esophagoscopic view

Ulcerative, infiltrative carcinoma

Malignant tumors of distal portion of esophagus

Primary carcinoma of lower end of esophagus

Adenocarcinoma of cardiac end of stomach infiltrating esophagus submucosally

Esophagoscopic view

speech pathologist. Various maneuvers are taught that focus on increasing propulsion of the bolus from the mouth to the pharynx and subsequently through the upper esophageal sphincter, such as tucking the chin or tilting the head to the stronger side. Increasing bolus consistency with thickening products is valuable because thin liquids often cause the greatest problems. In highly selected patients, primarily those whose dysfunction is isolated to hypertension or impaired relaxation of the cricopharyngeus muscle, consideration may be given to surgical myotomy. Ultimately, if patients cannot support their nutritional needs through the oral route, or if there is significant pulmonary aspiration, enteral alimentation through gastrostomy or jejunostomy is required.

The management of esophageal dysphagia is tailored much more toward the underlying pathology. Achalasia can be managed with surgical myotomy or endoscopic pneumatic balloon dilation, depending on local expertise and patient preference. In patients with achalasia who are not candidates for surgical intervention, injection of botulinum toxin A into the lower esophageal sphincter is a useful but temporary treatment. The management of esophageal stenoses is directed at increasing the luminal diameter by endoscopic means. Benign strictures can be dilated with various types of dilating balloons or *bougies*, which are thin, flexible, tapered rods that gently widen the narrowed segment within the esophagus. The choice of dilating device used depends on the length and character

Figure 61-3 Inferior Esophageal (Schatzki's) Ring.

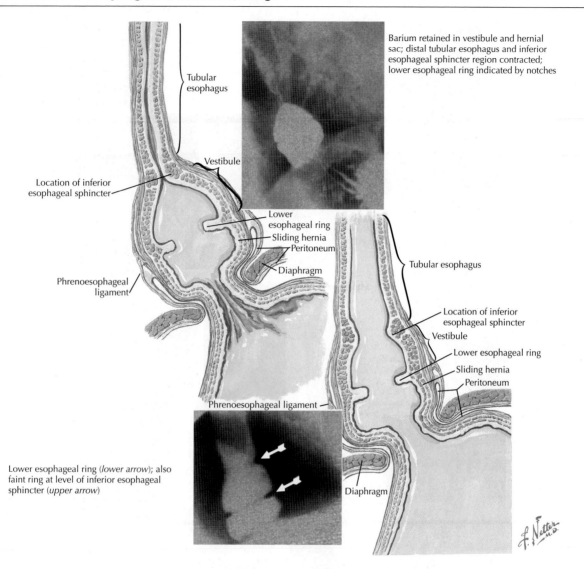

Tubular esophagus

Barium retained in vestibule and hernial sac; distal tubular esophagus and inferior esophageal sphincter region contracted; lower esophageal ring indicated by notches

Vestibule

Location of inferior esophageal sphincter

Lower esophageal ring

Sliding hernia

Peritoneum

Diaphragm

Phrenoesophageal ligament

Tubular esophagus

Location of inferior esophageal sphincter

Vestibule

Lower esophageal ring

Sliding hernia

Peritoneum

Phrenoesophageal ligament

Lower esophageal ring (*lower arrow*); also faint ring at level of inferior esophageal sphincter (*upper arrow*)

Diaphragm

of stricture, the underlying etiology, and the preference of the endoscopist. Many mild stenoses, as well as Schatzki's rings, can be treated with just a single dilation. However, if the stricture is very tight upon presentation, or results from insults such as radiation, lye ingestion, or long-standing GERD, several sessions may be required over months to years to achieve optimal success. If the pathology is malignant in etiology, then curative resection should be attempted if possible. When the tumor is unresectable or the patient is inoperable, palliative care can be achieved with serial dilations, placement of endoscopic stents, or endoluminal ablative therapy.

For patients with esophageal motility disorders other than achalasia, management can be much more difficult. There is a dearth of well-designed randomized controlled trials for these disorders, especially since manometric criteria for diagnosing them are continually evolving. Aggressive control of GERD with proton pump inhibitors may improve esophageal motility or the dysphagia symptoms

to some degree, although it is unlikely to result in complete resolution. For patients whose symptoms are associated with diffuse esophageal spasm, smooth muscle relaxants, such as calcium channel blockers or long-acting nitrates, are frequently prescribed. Antidepressants, especially the tricyclics, can be tried as well to improve symptoms secondary to the central effects of these agents.

Avoiding Treatment Errors

The first major principle in evaluating dysphagia is to recognize that its presence is an alarm sign that warrants further evaluation, not an empiric trial of therapy for GERD or dyspepsia. Once a neoplastic etiology has been ruled out, further treatment strategies can be directed at the results of diagnostic testing. Second, because eosinophilic esophagitis has been increasingly recognized only within the past few years, a heightened level of suspicion should be maintained in patients who have dysphagia,

Table 61-1   Management of Dysphagia

Disorder	Management Options
Oropharyngeal dysphagia	Swallowing therapy
	Gastrostomy/jejunostomy
	Cricopharyngeal myotomy/botulinum toxin injection*
Cervical or esophageal stricture/ring/web	Endoscopic dilation
	Acid suppression (PPI)
Unresectable esophageal tumor	Serial endoscopic dilation
	Endoluminal ablation
	Endoscopic stenting
Achalasia	Surgical (Heller) myotomy
	Endoscopic pneumatic dilation
	Botulinum toxin injection
	Smooth-muscle relaxants (isosorbide dinitrate, nifedipine)
Other esophageal motility disorders	Acid suppression (PPI)
	Smooth muscle relaxants
	Tricyclic antidepressants
Eosinophilic esophagitis	Swallowed aerosolized fluticasone
	Systemic corticosteroids
	Cromolyn sodium
	Endoscopic dilation (judicious)

PPI, proton pump inhibitor.
*For selected patients with isolated upper esophageal sphincter dysfunction.

especially with recurrent food obstructions, but no obvious pathology on endoscopic, radiologic, or manometric investigation. If no structural lesions are encountered, random esophageal biopsies should be considered. Treatment of eosinophilic esophagitis is principally with swallowed aerosolized fluticasone, cromolyn sodium, or systemic steroids and endoscopic dilation must only be undertaken judiciously with appropriate informed consent.

Future Directions

The diagnosis and classification of esophageal motility disorders have been an active matter of research in motility labs, and new technology called multichannel intraluminal impedance (MII) has been developed recently. MII complements standard esophageal manometry by adding a formal assessment of bolus transit to quantify the function of the esophagus in dysphagia patients. It remains to be seen exactly how this new technology will affect patient care, and current research will hopefully clarify its utility. The basis of therapy for oropharyngeal and esophageal dysphagia will not likely change in the near future; however, injection of botulinum toxin A has been used to treat cricopharyngeal disorders and other nonachalasia esophageal motility disorders with some degree of success. Finally the ongoing development of gastrointestinal promotility agents will hopefully lead to improved therapy for patients with esophageal motor dysfunction in the coming years.

Additional Resources

Cook IJ, Kahrilas PJ: AGA technical review on management of oropharyngeal dysphagia. Gastroenterology 116(2):455-478, 1999.

This comprehensive literature-based review examines the evaluation and management of patients with oropharyngeal dysphagia.

Ferguson DD: Evaluation and management of benign esophageal strictures. Dis Esophagus 18(6):359-364, 2005.

This review focuses on the options available for managing patients with benign strictures, from simple dilation techniques to more complex issues for refractory strictures.

Richter JE: Oesophageal motility disorders. Lancet 358(9284):823-828, 2001.

The author discusses the manometric diagnosis of recognized esophageal motility disorders and the management options available for these conditions.

EVIDENCE

1. Lopushinsky SR, Urbach DR: Pneumatic dilatation and surgical myotomy for achalasia. JAMA 296(18):2227-2233, 2006.

   This retrospective study found that patients with achalasia who had undergone either pneumatic dilation or surgical myotomy often required subsequent intervention (surgical or endoscopic) when followed for many years after their first treatment. The risk for requiring a subsequent intervention was higher in the pneumatic dilation group.

2. Remedios M, Campbell C, Jones DM, Kerlin P: Eosinophilic esophagitis in adults: Clinical, endoscopic, histologic findings, and response to treatment with fluticasone propionate. Gastrointest Endosc 63(1):3-12, 2006.

   The authors reported that all patients in their series who were treated with swallowed aerosolized fluticasone improved clinically and histologically, but many had recurrent symptoms after completing the course of treatment.

3. Tutuian R, Castell DO: Combined multichannel intraluminal impedance and manometry clarifies esophageal function abnormalities: Study in 350 patients. Am J Gastroenterol 99(6):1011-1019, 2004.

   This investigation highlighted the utility of multichannel intraluminal impedance to show normal and abnormal bolus transit in several esophageal motility disorders.

Mark Russo ▪ Steven Zacks

Diseases of the Liver— Abnormal Liver Function Tests, Nonalcoholic Fatty Liver Disease, and Drug- Induced Liver Injury

Introduction

Abnormal liver tests occur in 1% to 4% of the population. There are many causes for test abnormalities. Non-alcoholic liver disease (NAFLD) and drug-induced liver injury (DILI) are among the most common etiologies. More than 30% of the population meets criteria for obesity, and many of these individuals have underlying NAFLD. Clinicians are likely to encounter patients who have abnormal liver tests from NAFLD. The clinical picture is often complicated further by medications like statins used to treat the complications of obesity and associated with medication-induced liver function test abnormalities.

ABNORMAL LIVER CHEMISTRY TESTS

Etiology and Pathogenesis

Serum liver chemistry testing is often done during periodic health maintenance, in screening before blood donation, as part of insurance and employment physicals, and during hospitalizations. Proper interpretation of abnormalities in liver chemistries within the context of a patient's risk factors and medical history guide further evaluation and management. Because normal laboratory values are defined as the mean distribution and 2 standard deviations above or below the normal population, 2.5% of the population, by definition, will have one or more liver tests that are either below or above normal. Normal values for liver tests may vary by age, race, and gender.

Alanine aminotransferase (ALT), aspartate aminotransferase (AST), alkaline phosphatase, and total bilirubin constitute the most common blood tests typically included in a liver panel. γ-Glutamyltransferase (GGT) and 5′-nucleo-tidase are typically used to confirm the liver, rather than bone, as the source of alkaline phosphatase elevation. The above tests are erroneously labeled as liver "function" tests because ALT, AST, GGT, and alkaline phosphatase are enzymes and not markers of synthetic function. Albumin and prothrombin are proteins synthesized by the liver that can provide an estimate of liver synthetic function.

AST and ALT are abundant hepatic enzymes that catalyze the transfer of amino groups to form the hepatic metabolites pyruvate and oxalate. ALT is found in the hepatocyte cytosol, and AST is found in hepatocyte cytosol and mitochondria. Both are released into the blood when there is hepatocellular injury or death. AST is also found in heart, skeletal muscle, and blood. Bilirubin is a product of hemoglobin degradation. It is insoluble and requires conjugation, glucuronidation, before it can be secreted. Bilirubin uridine diphosphate-glucuronyl transferase conjugates bilirubin so that it can be secreted into the bile canaliculus. Alkaline phosphatase is an enzyme found in many tissues, including liver, bone, intestine, and placenta. Elevations in alkaline phosphatase may be seen during pregnancy.

Clinical Presentation

Elevations in liver chemistries are usually detected during routine physical exams or during blood donation in asymptomatic patients. Patients with elevated liver tests from acute viral hepatitis or obstructive jaundice can manifest malaise, nausea, vomiting, or abdominal pain as presenting symptoms. Liver tests are not 100% sensitive for the presence of liver disease, and patients with chronic viral hepatitis B or C, or even cirrhosis, may have normal liver tests.

Differential Diagnosis

The differential diagnosis of elevated liver tests is broad (Box 62-1). A systematic approach to evaluation can help minimize testing and reduce costs initiated. In patients presenting with symptoms of jaundice, acute viral hepatitis, and gallstone disease, alcoholic hepatitis and drug-induced liver injury are in the differential. In asymptomatic patients who have elevations in liver tests, chronic viral hepatitis, fatty liver disease, and hemochromatosis warrant consideration.

Diagnostic Approach

Abnormal liver tests should be repeated with patients fasting and abstaining from alcohol and off of nonessential medications, including over-the-counter medicines and complementary or alternative medicines. Elevations in liver chemistries documented on two or more occasions require further evaluation.

The evaluation of patients with elevated liver tests should take into consideration the most common causes of chronic liver disease: alcohol use, medications, hemochromatosis,

Box 62-1	Differential Diagnosis of Elevated Liver Tests

Common
Alcohol
Medications
Fatty liver disease
Gallstone disease
Hemochromatosis
Chronic hepatitis B or C

Rare
Autoimmune liver disease
Primary sclerosing cholangitis
Primary biliary cirrhosis
α_1-Antitrypsin deficiency

Very Rare
Wilson's disease
Budd-Chiari syndrome

chronic hepatitis C, and nonalcoholic fatty liver disease. Hepatitis B is relatively rare in the United States, having become less common after the implementation of universal immunization. Other liver disorders are relatively rare and should not be included in the initial evaluation unless a risk factor or predisposing condition is present. An abdominal ultrasound is useful for detecting gallstones, although it may miss common bile duct stones and fatty infiltration of the liver. Liver biopsy seldom identifies an etiology of liver disease that is not detected on blood testing but may be useful to stage the amount of liver fibrosis.

The pattern of liver test elevation may be useful for determining the underlying disease. Elevations in total bilirubin or alkaline phosphatase suggest cholestatic liver disease or obstruction, such as primary sclerosing cholangitis, primary biliary cirrhosis, pancreatic head mass or choledocholithiasis. Elevations in AST and ALT suggest hepatocellular disease. The pattern of elevation may be mixed with elevations of AST, ALT, alkaline phosphatase, and total bilirubin in drug-induced liver injury. Nonalcoholic fatty liver disease and drug-induced liver injury, two common causes of elevations in liver tests, are discussed in this chapter.

NONALCOHOLIC FATTY LIVER DISEASE

Etiology and Pathogenesis

NAFLD was first described by Ludwig in patients who presented with elevations in liver tests and hepatic steatosis on liver biopsy without a significant history of alcohol use. The current hypothesis is that two insults or "hits" cause liver injury in NAFLD. In the first hit, insulin resistance leads to the retention of lipids, particularly triglycerides, within hepatocytes. The underlying mechanism is decreased fatty acid disposal due to impaired mitochondrial β oxidation. Macrovesicular steatosis within hepatocytes arises from the first hit and produces a chicken-wire appearance on liver biopsy (Fig. 62-1). The second hit, oxidative stress, causes peroxidation of hepatocyte membrane lipids and cytokine production. The oxidative stress may be responsible for the progression from steatosis to steatohepatitis with or without fibrosis or cirrhosis (see Fig. 62-1). Adipokines, cytokines elaborated in fat cells, also play a role. Increased serum leptin and decreased adiponectin may promote hepatic steatosis and steatohepatitis.

The common etiologic factors for NAFLD are visceral obesity, type II diabetes mellitus, low high-density lipoprotein cholesterol, and hypertriglyceridemia. Mitochondrial dysfunction is linked to insulin resistance and hepatic steatosis. However, emerging evidence suggests a significant proportion of NAFLD patients lack these risk factors. Increasing age is associated with worse fibrosis, possibly because of increased NAFLD duration or increased hepatocyte mitochondria dysfunction in elderly people.

Figure 62-1 Nutritional Liver Diseases—Nonalcoholic Fatty Liver Disease.

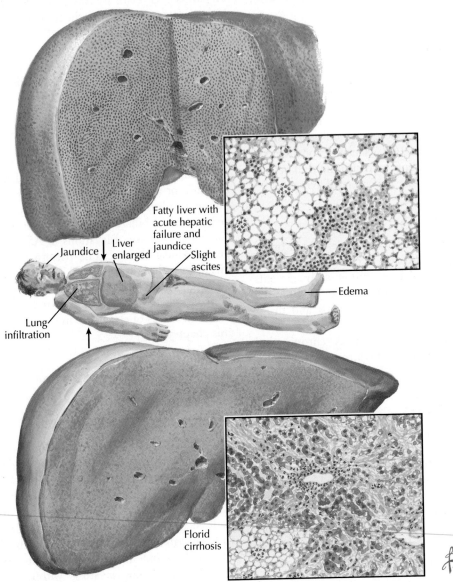

Secondary hepatic steatosis or steatohepatitis is seen with inborn errors of metabolism and medications. Amiodarone, methotrexate, tamoxifen, glucocorticoids, nucleoside analogues, calcium channel blockers, nonsteroidal anti-inflammatory drugs, and the tetracycline antibiotics have been associated with hepatic steatosis. Secondary fatty liver disease has also been associated with weight loss surgeries creating extensive small bowel diversion, total parenteral nutrition, and jejunal diverticulosis with bacterial overgrowth.

Clinical Presentation

The clinical presentation of NAFLD is variable. The most common presentation is asymptomatic elevation of aminotransferases, usually up to fivefold elevated, with ALT usually greater than AST. NAFLD is usually suspected in patients with abnormal liver chemistries after the exclusion of other liver diseases and the presence of fatty infiltration of the liver on imaging studies or unexplained hepatomegaly. The liver enzymes may fluctuate and may decrease with weight loss. NAFLD can be detected by ultrasonography, often done for unrelated reasons, such as investigation of right upper quadrant pain. Some patients can present with cryptogenic cirrhosis. Indeed, NAFLD may be the most common cause of cryptogenic cirrhosis.

The most common signs of NAFLD are visceral obesity and hepatomegaly. When presenting with cirrhosis, patients may have splenomegaly, spider angiomas, and palmar erythema. Mild to moderate elevation of ALT and AST is the most common and often the only laboratory abnormality. The ALT/AST ratio is usually greater than 1, but decreases as cirrhosis develops. There is no correlation between the degree of AST or ALT elevation and histologic severity. Hypoalbuminemia, hyperbilirubinemia, and prolonged prothrombin time are seen in decompensated cirrhosis. Serum ferritin is frequently elevated, and in 6% to 11%, the transferrin saturation is elevated.

The diagnosis of NAFLD is suggested by the presence of NAFLD etiologic factors. As previously noted, imaging studies may reveal features that suggest fatty infiltration. Liver biopsy is the gold standard to confirm a diagnosis of NAFLD and to distinguish steatohepatitis from simple steatosis. Moreover, a liver biopsy will assess the extent of fibrosis in steatohepatitis and provide prognostic information. The steatohepatitis variant of NAFLD is characterized by histologic features, including steatosis, hepatocyte ballooning degeneration, lobular inflammation with polymorphonuclear leukocytes, lobular necrosis, Mallory bodies, and perisinusoidal fibrosis.

Differential Diagnosis and Diagnostic Approach

To diagnose NAFLD, secondary causes of hepatic fat must be excluded. Hepatitis C and alcoholic liver disease are particularly important because of the high prevalence of these two disorders. It is generally believed that a fatty liver does not develop with alcohol consumption levels of less than 20 g/day in females and less than 30 g/day in males.

Ultrasonography, computed tomography, and magnetic resonance imaging can identify hepatic steatosis and have been advocated as diagnostic tests for NAFLD. None is sufficiently sensitive to detect hepatic inflammation, fibrosis, or cirrhosis. With the inability to distinguish simple steatosis from steatohepatitis and to stage the severity of injury, liver biopsy remains the best diagnostic test for steatohepatitis. However, the lack of effective medical therapy for NAFLD and the risks associated with biopsy require careful consideration before making the decision to proceed.

Management and Therapy

Optimum Treatment

There is no currently established treatment for NAFLD. In the absence of proven therapies, the emphasis is to correct NAFLD etiologic factors. Sustained, gradual, and moderate (10% or less) weight loss through exercise and diet may improve liver enzymes and histology. The proximal gastric bypass operation may be superior to the vertical-banded gastroplasty for weight loss and may be beneficial in NAFLD, provided the weight loss is gradual and maintained. Insulin sensitizers that decrease hepatic steatosis and fibrosis are being investigated. In pilot studies using rosiglitazone and pioglitazone for 48 weeks, NAFLD patients had improvement in insulin sensitivity, liver his-

tology, and liver enzymes. In a small study, metformin for 4 months was associated with liver enzyme improvement. Subjects also lost a significant amount of weight. Therefore, it is uncertain whether the improvement was secondary to weight loss or to the metformin. Vitamin E at 400 to 1200 IU per day was associated with improvement in ALTs in children with NAFLD, but biopsy data were not collected as part of the trial. Betaine, a precursor of the hepatoprotective factor S-adenosyl methionine, has shown promise. However, NAFLD can recur and rapidly progress. The results of small trials using fibrates for hypertriglyceridemia are mixed, with the most rigorously designed showing no histologic benefit. There are currently no data on the use of 3-hydroxy-3-methylglutaryl–coenzyme A reductase inhibitors (i.e., the statins) for the treatment of NAFLD. Liver transplantation is offered to NAFLD patients with decompensated cirrhosis.

Avoiding Treatment Errors

A misconception in treating patients with NAFLD is that certain classes of medications should be avoided that have been associated with elevating aminotransferases. For example, statins are associated with elevations in aminotransferases. Clinicians are reluctant to prescribe statins in patients with NAFLD and hyperlipidemia. Patients with NAFLD who have indications for statins, especially hypertriglyceridemia, should be prescribed these and other agents for hyperlipidemia because there is no evidence suggesting an increased risk for severe liver injury in NAFLD patients treated with statins. The same line of reasoning holds true for patients with NAFLD and diabetes. NAFLD patients with diabetes who have indications for metformin or glitazones should be prescribed these medications.

Future Directions

Because NAFLD is prevalent, larger, well-designed clinical trials with liver histology as an outcome are needed. The most promising drugs are the thiazolidinediones and statins. Studies of disease pathogenesis will help identify patients at greatest risk for progression and need of treatment. The nonalcoholic steatohepatitis clinical research network funded by the National Institutes of Health (NIH) is poised to answer many questions about the natural history and treatment of NAFLD.

DRUG-INDUCED LIVER INJURY

Etiology and Pathogenesis

Drug-induced liver injury (DILI) is typically classified as dose dependent or idiosyncratic. Most drugs are associated with idiosyncratic injury, defined as unpredictable elevations in liver tests that occur at any dose or duration of use (Fig. 62-2). Acetaminophen is an example of a dose-

Figure 62-2 Drug-Induced Hepatic Injuries.

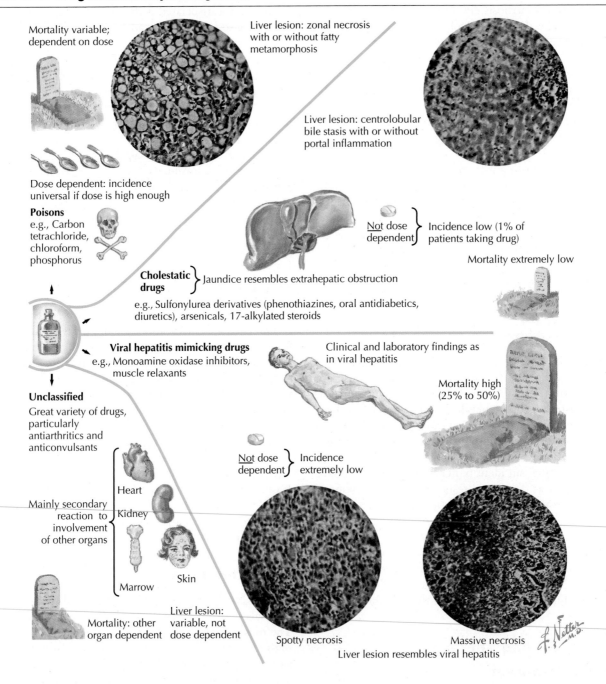

Mortality variable; dependent on dose

Liver lesion: zonal necrosis with or without fatty metamorphosis

Liver lesion: centrolobular bile stasis with or without portal inflammation

Dose dependent: incidence universal if dose is high enough

Poisons
e.g., Carbon tetrachloride, chloroform, phosphorus

Not dose dependent } Incidence low (1% of patients taking drug)

Mortality extremely low

Cholestatic drugs } Jaundice resembles extrahepatic obstruction

e.g., Sulfonylurea derivatives (phenothiazines, oral antidiabetics, diuretics), arsenicals, 17-alkylated steroids

Viral hepatitis mimicking drugs
e.g., Monoamine oxidase inhibitors, muscle relaxants

Clinical and laboratory findings as in viral hepatitis

Mortality high (25% to 50%)

Unclassified
Great variety of drugs, particularly antiarthritics and anticonvulsants

Not dose dependent } Incidence extremely low

Mainly secondary reaction to involvement of other organs

Heart

Kidney

Skin

Marrow

Mortality: other organ dependent

Liver lesion: variable, not dose dependent

Spotty necrosis

Massive necrosis

Liver lesion resembles viral hepatitis

dependent hepatotoxin; most individuals develop elevations in AST or ALT with a single dose of more than 10 g.

Hepatotoxicity from most drugs is believed to occur through a reactive metabolite. The metabolite may covalently bond to proteins that disrupt protein function, resulting in cell necrosis and death. Metabolites may act as haptens, and cell injury may occur through immune-mediated injury. On liver biopsy, drugs may produce characteristic patterns of injury, including spotty or massive necrosis, cholestasis, chronic hepatitis, or microvesicular or macrovesicular steatosis (see Fig. 62-2). Less common histologic patterns of DILI include fibrosis,

veno-occlusive disease, phospholipidosis, and peliosis hepatitis.

The factors that render an individual susceptible to developing DILI are largely unknown. Studies have described differences in genetic sequences of drug metabolism or human leukocyte antigen (HLA) haplotypes between individuals who did and did not develop DILI from a specific drug. Polymorphisms in glutathione S-transferase have been associated with DILI from tacrine and troglitazone. Polymorphisms in the HLA-DR haplotype are associated with cholestatic liver injury from amoxicillin-clavulanic acid. Genetic testing may eventually prove to be useful for identifying individuals at increased risk for DILI from a specific drug.

Clinical Presentation

Fatigue, mild abdominal pain, and jaundice are among the most common symptoms reported by patients with DILI. Most patients may not experience any symptoms, and the first sign of a drug reaction is detected by a friend or clinician who notices scleral icterus. Medications associated with hypersensitivity reactions may be accompanied by a skin rash or peripheral eosinophilia. Generalized pruritus with or without a skin rash is characteristic of cholestatic reactions. Physical exam is typically unremarkable, but mild right upper quadrant tenderness to palpation is a frequent finding. Hepatosplenomegaly is not a common sign in DILI.

Differential Diagnosis

The differential diagnosis for DILI is broad, but most commonly acute viral hepatitis, gallstone disease, and autoimmune liver disease require exclusion (Box 62-2). DILI can be difficult to diagnose because there is no diagnostic test that can definitively implicate a drug as a cause for hepatotoxicity. The closest gold standard is a rechallenge in which the patient is re-exposed to a drug and redevelops hepatotoxicity. Rechallenge only occurs inadvertently; thus, there are few cases that meet this gold standard.

Diagnostic Approach

The temporal association between elevations in liver tests and the initiation of a drug and the exclusion of other causes of increased liver tests are important components in the diagnosis. Hepatitis A immunoglobulin M (IgM) should be obtained to exclude acute hepatitis A, and hepatitis B surface antigen and core IgM should be obtained to exclude acute hepatitis B. Abdominal imaging is necessary in patients who present with elevations in total bilirubin or alkaline phosphatase to exclude cholangitis or choledocholithiasis. DILI may be difficult to distinguish from autoimmune liver disease. Both can present with hepatocellular, mixed, or cholestatic patterns of liver injury. Autoantibodies are not pathognomic for autoimmune liver

disease, and patients with DILI may develop antinuclear antibodies. A liver biopsy can be helpful. The characteristic finding in DILI is the presence of eosinophils. Instruments have been developed to provide a quantitative score used to assign a probability that the implicated drug is the cause of the liver test abnormalities, but they are cumbersome and not used in clinical practice.

Drug reactions can be classified as hepatocellular, cholestatic, or mixed (Box 62-3). A hepatocellular reaction is defined as an ALT/alkaline phosphatase ratio greater than 5, a cholestatic reaction as an ALT/alkaline phosphatase ratio less than 2, and a mixed reaction as values between hepatocellular and cholestatic reactions. Cholestatic reactions typically take longer to resolve than hepatocellular reactions.

Management and Therapy

Optimum Treatment

Management of DILI should be directed at early recognition of hepatotoxicity and prompt discontinuation of the potential offending agent. With the exception of N-acetylcysteine for acetaminophen hepatotoxicity and deferoxamine for iron overdose, there are no antidotes for DILI. N-acetylcysteine should be administered if hepatotoxicity from acetaminophen is suspected, even if the acetaminophen level is undetectable. Although prescribing corticosteroids for DILI is frequently contemplated, there is no evidence supporting their use.

Box 62-2   Differential Diagnosis of DILI

Acute hepatitis A
Acute hepatitis B
Epstein-Barr virus hepatitis
Cytomegalovirus hepatitis
Autoimmune liver disease
Cholangitis or choledocholithiasis
Vascular insult (ischemic or thrombotic)
Alcoholic hepatitis

Box 62-3   Pattern of Liver Injury from Selected Drugs, Classes of Drugs, and Complementary Alternative Medicines

Hepatocellular
Isoniazid
Statins
Acetaminophen
Halothane
Methyldopa
Amanita mushrooms
Chaparral

Cholestatic
Amoxicillin-clavulanate
Azathioprine
Barbiturates
Erythromycin
Methyltestosterone
Celandine

Mixed
Phenytoin
Trimethoprim-sulfamethoxazole
Ketoconazole
Allopurinol
Valerian
Germander
Kava

Most patients with DILI recover without significant sequelae. However, if jaundice develops (total bilirubin >3 mg/dL), patients need to be followed more closely. Mortality rate is estimated at 10% in patients who develop jaundice following a hepatocellular injury (hepatocellular jaundice) from a drug reaction.

Prescribing Medications in Patients with Elevated Liver Tests

A common clinical scenario that arises is whether to prescribe a medication known to be associated with elevations in liver tests, such as statins, in patients with abnormal liver tests. Under most circumstances, the indication and benefit of the drug far outweigh the rare risk for DILI. Statins have not been associated with an increased risk for DILI in patients with elevated liver tests and can be prescribed for hypercholesterolemia in patients with NAFLD. Liver tests should be obtained before starting a medication associated with elevations in liver tests so that a new drug is not incorrectly implicated as a cause for liver test elevations in a patient who has underlying chronic liver disease. One approach is to continue patients on the drug as long as AST or ALT does not exceed 3 times the baseline value and the bilirubin does not exceed the upper limit of normal range.

Avoiding Treatment Errors

Recognizing DILI early, stopping the offending agent, and avoiding re-exposure are the mainstays of therapy. In a patient who typically does not complain of symptoms and presents with abdominal discomfort or nausea after starting a new medication, particularly a known hepatotoxin, such as isoniazid, it is reasonable to stop the medication and check liver tests. Steroids may be prescribed in certain situations, such as a hypersensitivity reaction, although there is no evidence to support the use of steroids in DILI.

Future Directions

Because DILI is among the most common reasons for regulatory action against a drug, there is much interest in developing accurate preclinical testing for identifying drugs that are potentially hepatotoxic. Hepatocyte cell culture systems and identification of genetic polymorphisms associated with DILI are among the most actively investigated areas. The Drug Induced Liver Injury Network is prospectively collecting DILI cases for potential genetic association studies.

Additional Resources

Drug Induced Liver Injury Network. Available at: http://dilin.dcri.duke.edu/index.html. Accessed August 29, 2006.

This website provides information about the multicenter drug-induced liver injury study sponsored by the NIH. It is a useful resource for references and medications that have been associated with severe hepatotoxicity.

Green RM, Flamm S: AGA technical review on the evaluation of liver chemistry tests. Gastroenterology. 2002;123:1367-1384.

This guideline provides a structured approach for evaluating patients with elevated liver tests.

Farrell GC, Larter CZ: Nonalcoholic fatty liver disease: From steatosis to cirrhosis. Hepatology 43(2 Suppl 1):S99-S112, 2006.

This comprehensive review on the pathogenesis and management of fatty liver disease provides a perspective on potential therapeutics.

Novak D, Lewis JH: Drug-induced liver disease. Curr Opin Gastroenterol 3:203-215, 2003.

This review is a useful clinical resource because it describes the clinical presentation of specific medications associated with drug-induced liver injury. The article includes information on herbal hepatotoxicity.

Sanyal AJ; American Gastrointestinal Association: AGA technical review on nonalcoholic fatty liver disease. Gastroenterology 123(5):1705-1725, 2002.

This article provides a detailed review on the natural history, pathogenesis, and management for fatty liver disease.

EVIDENCE

1. Andrade RJ, Jucena ML, Fernandez MC, et al: Drug induced liver injury: An analysis of 461 incidences submitted to the Spanish registry over a 10-year period. Gastroenterology 129:512-521, 2005.

   The authors describe one of the largest series of patients with drug-induced liver injury and provide a description of clinical and laboratory data as well as a list of drugs that cause DILI.

2. Belfort R, Harrison SA, Brown K, et al: A placebo-controlled trial of pioglitazone in subjects with nonalcoholic steatohepatitis. N Engl J Med 255:2297-2307, 2006.

   This key randomized clinical trial demonstrated biochemical and histologic improvement in patients with nonalcoholic steatohepatitis (NASH) treated with pioglitazone compared with placebo.

3. Matteoni CA, Younossi ZM, Gramlich T, et al: Nonalcoholic fatty liver disease: A spectrum of clinical and pathological severity. Gastroenterology 116(6):1413-1419, 1999.

   The authors provide a complete series of pathologic findings in patients with fatty liver disease. The study is particularly useful because the specific pathologic findings associated with fibrosis are provided.

4. Neuschwander-Tetri BA, Brunt EM, Wehmeier KR, et al: Improved nonalcoholic steatohepatitis after 48 weeks of treatment with the PPAR-gamma ligand rosiglitazone. Hepatology 38(4):1008-1017, 2003.

   The authors describe one of the first trials demonstrating histologic improvement on liver biopsy with medication. The data from this study supported the development of larger studies of glitazones in patients with NASH.

5. Sanyal AJ, Mofrad PS, Contos MJ, et al: A pilot study of vitamin E versus vitamin E and pioglitazone for the treatment of nonalcoholic steatohepatitis. Clin Gastroenterol Hepatol 2(12):1107-1115, 2004.

   This small randomized trial of 20 patients demonstrated that vitamin E only resulted in a biochemical response with no benefit seen in liver histology. The combination of vitamin E and pioglitazone resulted in a biochemical, histologic, and metabolic response.

6. Ueno T, Sugawara H, Sujaku K, et al: Therapeutic effects of restricted diet and exercise in obese patients with fatty liver. J Hepatol 27(1):103-107, 1997.

   Data from this study demonstrated that patients with fatty liver disease benefited from weight loss and exercise, supporting the clinicians' recommendation that changes in lifestyle can lead to improvement in liver disease.

A. Sidney Barritt ▪ Michael W. Fried

Viral Hepatitis: Acute and Chronic Disease

Introduction

Acute viral hepatitis and chronic viral hepatitis are major sources of morbidity and mortality worldwide. There are an estimated 1.5 million new cases of hepatitis A each year. More than 2 billion people worldwide have been exposed to hepatitis B at some point during their lives, and 350 million of these remain chronically infected. Nearly 3% of the world's population is infected with hepatitis C, totaling about 170 million people.

Infection with one of the hepatotropic viruses (hepatitis A, B, C, D, E) (Table 63-1) can cause an acute, chronic, or acute and chronic illness. The clinical manifestations of these infections range from a viral prodrome to fulminant hepatic failure to chronic liver disease and cirrhosis. Other viruses, such as cytomegalovirus, Epstein-Barr virus, herpesvirus, and varicella-zoster virus, may also cause an acute hepatitis, but usually in the context of a systemic illness. In such cases, the liver is not the primary target of infection.

HEPATITIS A

Etiology and Pathogenesis

Hepatitis A is caused by the hepatitis A virus (HAV) and is transmitted in a fecal-oral manner. The most common method of transmission is through contaminated food or water. The infection is endemic in developing areas. There is an incubation period of anywhere from 1 to 6 weeks before the onset of symptoms (Fig. 63-1). HAV manifests as an acute illness, with exposure granting lifelong immunity. There is no chronic phase to HAV infection.

Clinical Presentation

The symptoms of HAV infection are nonspecific and can resemble a flu-like illness. Commonly, infected persons suffer from malaise, fatigue, nausea, and vomiting as well as low-grade fever and mild right upper quadrant pain. Diarrhea can also occur and facilitate transmission of HAV. As the illness progresses to the icteric phase of acute hepatitis, dark or tea-colored urine and jaundice are noted. The physical exam is often notable for icteric sclerae, jaundice and occasionally, a tender palpable liver. Like the symptoms, however, physical exam signs are not specific for HAV.

Differential Diagnosis

Acute hepatitis caused by any of the hepatotropic viruses, acute systemic viral infection, drug hepatotoxicity, and cholangitis, among other etiologies, should all be considered in the differential diagnosis of acute hepatitis A.

Diagnostic Approach

Laboratory analysis of the patient with HAV demonstrates liver enzyme abnormalities with a pattern of acute hepatocellular injury. Initially, the serum transaminases (alanine aminotransferase [ALT] and aspartate aminotransferase [AST]) can rise to greater than 10 times the upper limit of normal. Serum bilirubin becomes elevated as well, usually below 10 mg/dL, and is slower to rise and fall than the serum transaminases. In endemic areas, subclinical infection is common in children, and the likelihood of symptomatic acute icteric infection rises with the patient's age at acquisition. The definitive laboratory test for acute

Table 63-1   Hepatotropic Viruses

	Mode of Transmission	Approximate Incubation	Endemic Areas	Potential for Chronicity
Hepatitis A	Fecal-oral Food-and water-borne outbreaks	1-6 wk	Developing countries	No
Hepatitis E	Fecal-oral Food- and water-borne outbreaks	1-6 wk	Mexico, SE Asia	No
Hepatitis B	Parenteral, sexual, perinatal	1-6 mo	Asia, Africa	Yes
Hepatitis D	Parenteral, sexual	1-6 mo	Mediterranean	Yes
Hepatitis C	Parenteral	1-6 mo	Egypt	Yes

Figure 63-1 Viral Hepatitis: Acute Form.

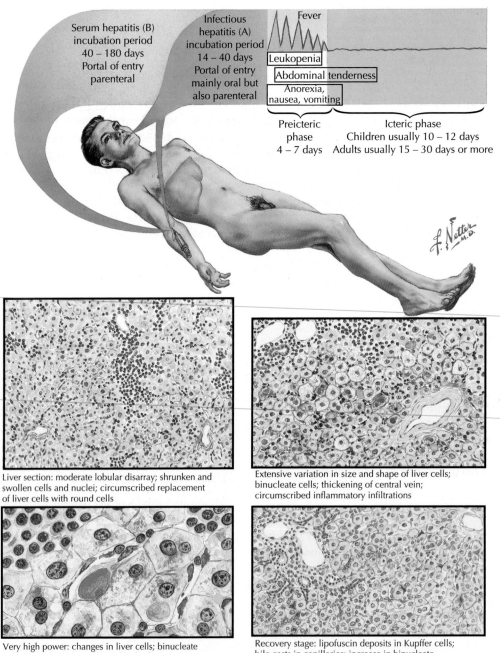

Liver section: moderate lobular disarray; shrunken and swollen cells and nuclei; circumscribed replacement of liver cells with round cells

Extensive variation in size and shape of liver cells; binucleate cells; thickening of central vein; circumscribed inflammatory infiltrations

Very high power: changes in liver cells; binucleate cells, infiltration, councilman-like body

Recovery stage: lipofuscin deposits in Kupffer cells; bile casts in capillaries; increase in binucleate cells; occasional trinucleate cells

Figure 63-2 Viral Hepatitis: Fulminant Form (Acute Massive Necrosis).

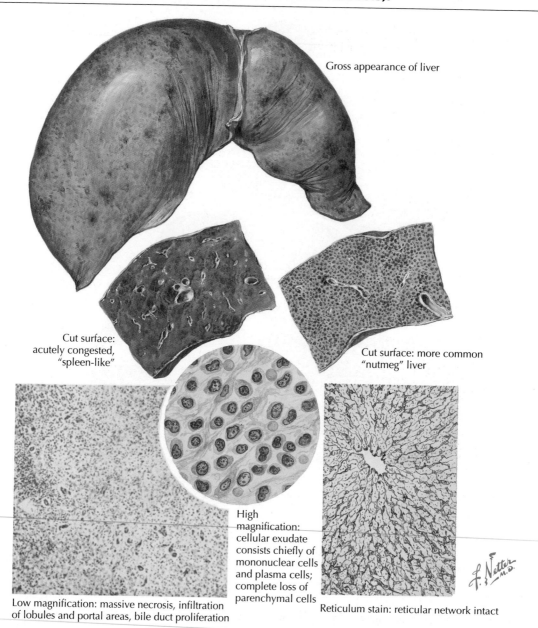

Gross appearance of liver

Cut surface: acutely congested, "spleen-like"

Cut surface: more common "nutmeg" liver

High magnification: cellular exudate consists chiefly of mononuclear cells and plasma cells; complete loss of parenchymal cells

Low magnification: massive necrosis, infiltration of lobules and portal areas, bile duct proliferation

Reticulum stain: reticular network intact

hepatitis A is serum HAV IgM. Prior exposure or vaccination, and thus immunity, is confirmed by a reactive HAV total IgG.

Management and Therapy

Optimum Treatment

There are no specific interventions for treatment except for supportive care and monitoring for the development of fulminant liver failure, a rare complication of HAV infection (Figs. 63-2 and 63-3). The urgency of evaluation of hepatitis and considerations for hospital admission or referral to a liver specialist are based on the functional status of the patient, the tempo of changes in liver enzyme levels, and the presence of hepatic synthetic dysfunction. Patients with social support to monitor their status, who are sufficiently reliable to keep follow-up appointments, and who are able to maintain their oral intake may convalesce as outpatients. Those with evidence of progressive hepatic synthetic dysfunction (prolonged prothrombin time, altered mental status) should be hospitalized until clinical improvement is noted or referred for evaluation for liver transplantation if progressive liver failure develops.

Acute HAV infection must be reported to public health officials so that they can watch for clustering of cases and perhaps identify a common link to an outbreak. The index

Figure 63-3 Viral Hepatitis: Subacute Fatal Form.

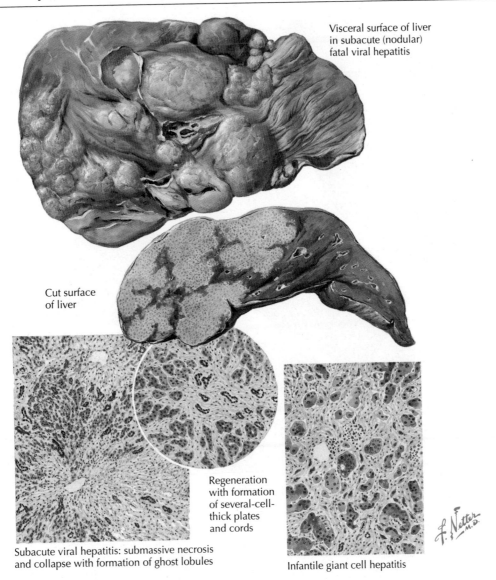

Visceral surface of liver
in subacute (nodular)
fatal viral hepatitis

Cut surface
of liver

Regeneration
with formation
of several-cell-
thick plates
and cords

Subacute viral hepatitis: submassive necrosis
and collapse with formation of ghost lobules

Infantile giant cell hepatitis

case in HAV outbreaks is most infectious before the icteric phase of the illness. Fecal shedding of the HAV is at its peak while the patient suffers from nonspecific flu-like symptoms of malaise, nausea, and diarrhea. Close personal and household contacts are at risk for acquiring HAV from the index case. Close contacts of an index case should receive hepatitis A immune globulin within 2 weeks of exposure, which offers the best chance of preventing infection.

Most recent recommendations advise all children to receive the hepatitis A vaccine at age 1 year as part of routine childhood vaccinations. Catch-up vaccination of unvaccinated children between ages 2 and 18 years should also be considered. Susceptible adults, especially those at increased risk for HAV infection, such as travelers to developing countries where HAV is endemic, men who have sex with men, intravenous drug users, residents and employees of institutionalized living facilities, and day care workers, should also be vaccinated for HAV. Patients with a chronic liver disease require HAV vaccination given their higher risk for hepatic decompensation if they acquire the virus.

HEPATITIS E

The hepatitis E virus (HEV) is another hepatotropic virus that is spread by the fecal-oral route. It is endemic to developing countries, especially in Central America and South and Southeast Asia. Like HAV, its incubation period is 1 to 6 weeks. HEV has no potential for inducing chronic liver disease. Pregnant women seem particularly at risk for development of fulminant liver failure; however, the overall rate of severe hepatitis is low. Serologic testing for anti-HEV is now available and should be considered if travel

Table 63-2 Serologic Profile of Hepatitis B

	Serum ALT	HBsAg	Anti-HBs	HBcAb	HBeAg	Anti-HBe	HBV DNA
Acute	++++	+	–	+ IgM	+/–	+/–	+/–
Resolved	Normal	–	+	+ (Total)	–	+	–
Chronic (wild type)	++	+	–	+	+	–	>20,000 IU/mL
Chronic (pre-core mutant)	++	+	–	+	–	+	>2000 IU/mL
Inactive carrier	Normal	+	–	+	–	+	<20,000 IU/mL
Vaccinated	Normal	–	+	–	–	–	–

ALT, alanine aminotransferase; Anti-HBe, hepatitis B envelope antibody; Anti-HBs, hepatitis B surface antibody; HBcAb, hepatitis B core antibody; HBeAG, hepatitis B envelope antigen; HBsAg, hepatitis B surface antigen; HBV, hepatitis B virus; Ig, immunoglobulin; IU, international units.

to an endemic region occurred before the onset of acute hepatitis. Like hepatitis A, supportive care is the hallmark of treatment for hepatitis E. Most cases resolve spontaneously; however, the advent of encephalopathy or coagulopathy should prompt referral to a transplantation center.

HEPATITIS B

Etiology and Pathogenesis

The hepatitis B virus (HBV) has the potential to cause both acute and chronic hepatitis. Acute infection can range from a flu-like icteric illness to fulminant hepatic failure. Chronic HBV infection may remain asymptomatic or lead to cirrhosis, portal hypertension, hepatocellular carcinoma, and end-stage liver disease (Fig. 63-4). This DNA virus is transmitted sexually, parenterally, or perinatally. Nearly half of the world's population lives in areas where HBV is endemic, particularly parts of Asia and Africa (Fig. 63-5).

Clinical Presentation

Acute infection manifests with fever, anorexia, nausea, vomiting, and abdominal tenderness, followed by an icteric phase that, in adults, can last for more than a month. Nearly 95% of adults recover and develop natural immunity after acute infection. About 5% develop chronic HBV infection, whereas less than 1% develop fulminant hepatic failure. Newborns that acquire HBV from their mothers by vertical transmission have a 90% risk of developing chronic HBV.

Extrahepatic manifestations of HBV include urticaria, polyarteritis nodosa, and chronic kidney disease through membranous and membranoproliferative glomerulonephritis.

Diagnostic Approach

Acute hepatitis B produces liver enzyme abnormalities consistent with hepatocellular injury, with marked elevations of serum ALT and AST activities. In general, the ALT and AST will rise rapidly, often to levels greater than 10 to 15 times the upper limits of normal, followed by a more gradual and sustained elevation of the serum bilirubin. Serologic confirmation of infection is essential, as is the correct identification of acute disease versus chronic carriers, vaccinated patients, and those with resolved infection and immunity. These various clinical scenarios are defined in Table 63-2. A patient may traverse several of these clinical stages during the natural course of their HBV infection (Fig. 63-4).

Management and Therapy

Acute Hepatitis B: Optimum Treatment

Like HAV infection, the mainstay of acute HBV infection is supportive care and surveillance for the signs and symptoms of hepatic dysfunction. The development of encephalopathy or coagulopathy is ominous, and patients should be immediately referred for transplantation evaluation. There appears to be no role for direct antiviral therapy in patients with acute hepatitis B, although the use of this therapy in severe acute hepatitis B remains controversial. People with acute HBV should have repeat serologic testing 6 months after the initial infection to confirm clearance of hepatitis B surface antigen (HBsAg) and immunity versus chronic infection.

Patients with acute HBV infection should be reported to local public health authorities. Susceptible persons who have had sexual contact with the index case within 2 weeks of presentation should receive hepatitis B immune globulin and the hepatitis B vaccine.

Chronic Hepatitis B: Optimum Treatment

Chronic HBV infection can progress to cirrhosis, portal hypertension, end-stage liver disease, and hepatocellular carcinoma. Some of these patients may be candidates for antiviral therapy if they have evidence of active HBV DNA replication in their serum. Several agents, including immunomodulators such as interferon and peginterferon and direct antivirals such as lamivudine, adefovir, entecavir, and telbivudine have demonstrated efficacy for the treatment of chronic hepatitis B. Decisions regarding treatment for chronic HBV and monitoring are complex, and patients may benefit from specialty evaluation. Patients with chronic

Figure 63-4 Natural History of HBV Infection.
HBeAg, hepatitis B envelope antigen.

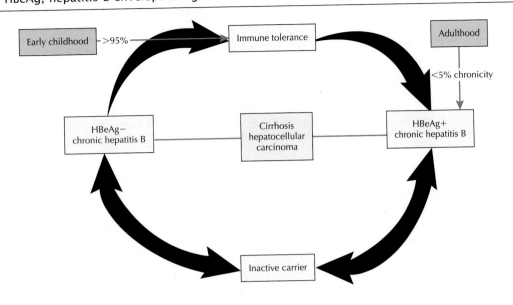

Figure 63-5 Acute Hepatitis B: Risk Factors 1991-1996.
IVDA, intravenous drug abuse. *Adapted from Epidemiology and Prevention of Viral Hepatitis. Centers for Disease Control and Prevention. Available at: http://www.cdc.gov.*

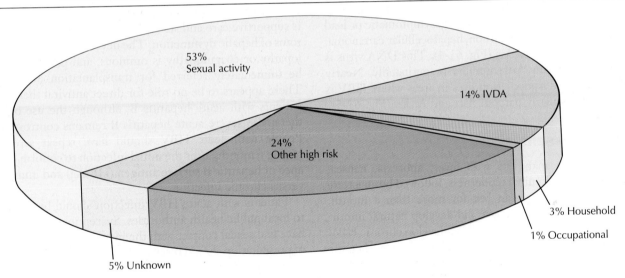

HBV should receive the hepatitis A vaccine. Because of the high incidence of hepatocellular carcinoma in patients with chronic hepatitis B, those at highest risk (cirrhotic patients, Asian men >40 years and women >50 years, African patients >20 years, and individuals with family history of hepatocellular carcinoma, among others) should be screened for liver cancer with hepatic ultrasound at 6- to 12-month intervals.

Prevention

Prevention is the key to decreasing the incidence of HBV infection. The hepatitis B vaccine is highly immunogenic and induces protective antibodies in most people who receive the vaccine. Those who are immunosuppressed or already have advanced liver disease are the exceptions to this rule. Currently, vaccination against HBV is recommended for all newborns, health care workers, and patients with another liver disease. In the United States, thanks to newborn vaccinations and catch-up vaccination programs for older children, the incidence and prevalence of HBV infection should dramatically decrease within a generation. In other countries where HBV is endemic, newborn vaccinations have reduced the rates of vertical transmission, chronic HBV, and hepatocellular carcinoma.

HEPATITIS D

Hepatitis D virus (HDV) is a defective ribonucleic acid (RNA) virus that requires the hepatitis B surface antigen for replication. Thus, only people with acute HBV infection (coinfection) or chronic carriers of HBV (superinfection) are at risk for HDV infection. Also known as the *delta virus*, HDV is endemic to countries surrounding the Mediterranean Sea, particularly Italy and Turkey. This diagnosis should be considered in acute HBV patients who have a difficult clinical course or in chronic HBV patients who have a flare of their disease. Laboratory confirmation requires a positive serum HBsAg as well as the presence of hepatitis delta antibody. Therapy entails treatment of the underlying hepatitis B, if applicable, and continued supportive care.

HEPATITIS C

Etiology and Pathogenesis

Hepatitis C virus (HCV) infects nearly 2% of the population in the United States and 3% of the population worldwide. HCV differs from the other heterotropic viruses because it is much more likely to induce a chronic hepatitis. HCV can progress to hepatocellular carcinoma or cirrhosis and end-stage liver disease and, as a result, is a major public health problem. HCV is the leading cause of death from liver disease in the United States. An acute form of HCV does exist, but it is rarely encountered because nearly 75% of cases are asymptomatic.

Hepatitis C is a heterogeneous single-stranded RNA virus with six major genotypes. Genotype 1 is the most common type found in the United States, 70% of cases, with genotypes 2 and 3 accounting for the remainder. Genotype 4 is endemic to Egypt and the Middle East. Genotypes 5 and 6 are rarely encountered outside of southern Africa. Although the genotype does not impact severity of disease, genotype 1 is more often refractory to therapy.

The natural history of HCV infection is in dispute. Some patients will have stable, mild disease, whereas others will have disease progression over decades and develop cirrhosis. Factors associated with rapid disease progression include alcohol use, male gender, coinfection with HIV, and hepatic steatosis.

Clinical Presentation

Often, HCV is diagnosed after routine liver function tests, drawn for an alternative indication, are found to be abnormal. Most acute infections are asymptomatic; those with chronic infection have fatigue, malaise, and other nonspecific symptoms. Some patients' initial symptoms are those of chronic liver disease: jaundice, ascites, and confusion, often after they have unknowingly harbored the virus for decades.

Risk factors for infection include intravenous drug use (70%), blood transfusion before 1992 (6%), and occupational exposures (3%). Transmission by sexual exposure is possible, but the rate of transmission is low. Risks associated with tattoos, body piercing, and intranasal cocaine use are not well defined. Nearly 10% of HCV-infected people do not have an identifiable risk factor.

Extrahepatic manifestations of HCV infection include cryoglobulinemia, glomerulonephritis, porphyria cutanea tarda, and thyroid disease. There are associations among HCV, diabetes mellitus, lichen planus, and B-cell lymphoma.

Diagnostic Approach

Because chronic HCV is usually asymptomatic, screening with anti-HCV antibody for hepatitis C is recommended for all patients with an abnormal ALT, any history of intravenous drug use, blood transfusions or organ transplantation before 1992, hemophilia, or hemodialysis. Health care workers with documented exposure to HCV-infected blood and children born to HCV-infected mothers should also be screened.

In the setting of a risk factor or elevated ALT, the presence of anti-HCV is virtually diagnostic of HCV infection. Before consideration of therapy for HCV, the presence of HCV as a measure of active viremia and the genotype of HCV should be determined. Viral levels do not indicate the severity of infection but are useful in following response to therapy.

Management and Therapy

Optimum Treatment

If identified early, as in the case of an occupational exposure, acute HCV infection is amenable to treatment with interferon. Chronicity can be prevented in 98% of patients if treatment begins within 3 to 6 months after infection.

Patients with chronic HCV infection require the same health maintenance as any other patient with a chronic liver disease; hepatitis A and B immunizations and hepatocellular cancer screening in the presence of cirrhosis.

Liver biopsy is a generally safe and useful, although not a mandatory, tool in staging hepatitis C infection. Therapy is usually recommended for those with evidence of some degree of hepatic fibrosis, although all patients with chronic hepatitis C may be considered for antiviral therapy provided they have no contraindications.

The current regimen for HCV treatment is once-weekly subcutaneous injections of peginterferon administered with twice-daily ribavirin for 6 months to 1 year.

Successful HCV therapy is defined as an undetectable HCV RNA in serum 6 months after completion of therapy. This is called a *sustained virologic response* (SVR) and is synonymous with a "cure." Patients with genotype 1 HCV achieve SVR 40% to 50% of the time. Genotype 2 and 3 patients achieve SVR 75% to 80% of the time. Patients should be carefully screened before therapy. Interferon can exacerbate psychiatric illness and thus is contraindicated for patients with poorly controlled depression or bipolar disorder. Other side effects of therapy include neutropenia, hemolytic anemia, thrombocytopenia, and thyroid dysfunction. Treatment is also contraindicated for patients with significant cardiac disease or decompensated cirrhosis.

Patients should be counseled that there is no risk for transmission of hepatitis C through casual contact, sharing food, utensils, kissing, or hugging. Care should be taken to avoid sharing items that may be exposed to blood, like razors or toothbrushes. As above, the risk for sexual transmission is low, but measurable; sexual partners should undergo screening for HCV, but mandatory barrier protection is not routinely recommended in monogamous relationships. The risk for vertical transmission is also low. Currently, there are no recommendations for changing birthing practices or breast-feeding in HCV-positive women.

Avoiding Treatment Errors

The most common treatment error with the entire series of hepatotropic viruses is one of correct diagnosis and determination of chronicity. Care should be taken in interpreting the HAV serologies; if misread, an alternative diagnosis and thus expeditious treatment may be delayed. HAV IgM is indicative of acute disease, whereas a reactive HAV total antibody confirms immunity. The HBV serologies can be more confusing because there are subtle differences in the serologic profiles for acute disease, resolved infection, chronic active disease, chronic inactive carriers, and vaccinated individuals (see Table 63-2). Additionally, the period between 2 weeks and 4 months after infection, when the HBsAg has disappeared, but the hepatitis B surface antibody is not yet detectable, can make diagnosis more difficult. In individuals in whom the suspicion of acute infection is high, checking the hepatitis B core IgM titer can resolve this issue.

Treating HCV is fraught with possible complications, mostly due to the side effects of peginterferon and ribavirin. Anemia, leukopenia, thyroid dysfunction, and psychiatric problems can complicate therapy. Thus, referral to a subspecialist should be considered. The primary physician can play a large role in screening for hepatitis C patients with risk factors for infection, counseling newly diagnosed individuals, and assisting with the identification of candidates for antiviral therapy who will be jointly managed with the subspecialist.

FUTURE DIRECTIONS

Hepatitis B therapy is rapidly changing thanks to innovations made with nucleoside analogues used for HIV infection. Like HIV treatment, combination therapy with interferons, lamivudine, entecavir, adefovir, and telbivudine will receive a new emphasis in coming years. The goal of combination therapy will be to prevent resistance and to improve eradiation of HBV.

Understanding virus and host characteristics that influence progression of disease, and response to therapy, will be the key to advancing treatment for hepatitis C. Direct antivirals that inhibit key enzymes in HCV replication are under development.

Although therapy for chronic hepatitis B and hepatitis C will continue to evolve, prevention of viral hepatitis remains crucial. Although an HCV vaccine is not likely in the near future, extensive use of vaccinations for HAV and HBV has the potential to reduce, if not eliminate, these infections within a few generations as well as to significantly reduce the incidence of cirrhosis and hepatocellular carcinoma.

Additional Resources

Up-To-Date. Available at: http://www.uptodate.com.
> This website has continuously updated reviews of a variety of internal medicine, obstetric-gynecologic, and pediatric topics, including the acute and chronic hepatotropic viruses as well as the sequelae of infection.

Centers for Disease Control and Prevention. Available at: http://www.cdc.gov.
> The CDC website has information about immunization practices, the epidemiology of disease, and disease prevention.

EVIDENCE

1. Fiore AE, Wasley A, Bell BP: Prevention of hepatitis A through active or passive immunization: Recommendations of the advisory committee on immunization practices (ACIP). MMWR Recomm Rep 55:1-23, 2006.
   > This article advocates universal immunization against hepatitis A in an effort to eradicate the disease.
2. Keeffe EB, Dieterich DT, Han SH, et al: A treatment algorithm for the management of chronic hepatitis B virus infection in the United States: An update. Clin Gastroenterol Hepatol 4:926-962, 2006.
   > Keeffe and colleagues have updated an algorithm for managing chronic hepatitis B.
3. Lok AS, McMahon BJ: Chronic hepatitis B. Hepatology 45:507-539, 2007.
   > This article includes the American Association for the Study of Liver Disease (AASLD) guidelines on chronic hepatitis B.
4. Mast EE, Weinbaum CM, Fiore AE, et al: A comprehensive immunization strategy to eliminate transmission of hepatitis B virus infection in the United States: Recommendations of the Advisory Committee on Immunization Practices (ACIP). Part II: Immunization of adults. MMWR Recomm Rep 55:1-33, 2006.
   > Mast and associates discuss catch-up immunizations in adults and the effects of universal immunizations in children as well as the natural history of hepatitis B.
5. Strader DB, Wright T, Thomas DL, Seeff LB; the Practice Guidelines Committee, American Association for the Study of Liver Diseases: Diagnosis, management and treatment of hepatitis C. Hepatology 39;1147-1171, 2004.
   > This article includes the American Association for the Study of Liver Disease (AASLD) guidelines for management of hepatitis C.

Roshan Shrestha

Cirrhosis

Introduction

Cirrhosis and its complications comprise one of the top 10 causes of mortality in this country. Cirrhosis of the liver is an irreversible alteration of hepatic architecture, characterized by diffuse fibrosis and areas of nodular regeneration. These nodules can be micronodular (<3 mm) or macronodular (>3 mm). Features of both micronodular and macronodular cirrhosis are frequently present in the same liver. Determining the etiology is often not possible based on the gross and microscopic appearance of the cirrhotic liver and requires careful utilization of the history, physical examination, biochemical and serologic tests, and histochemical stains.

Etiology and Pathogenesis

The relationship between alcohol abuse and cirrhosis is well established. Ethanol is a hepatotoxin that leads to the development of fatty liver, alcoholic hepatitis, and ultimately, cirrhosis (Fig. 64-1). The pathogenesis may differ depending on the underlying causes of the liver disease. In general, there is ongoing chronic inflammation either due to toxins (alcohol and drugs), infections (hepatitis virus, parasites), autoimmune phenomenon (chronic active hepatitis, primary biliary cirrhosis), or biliary obstruction (common bile duct stone, primary sclerosing cholangitis [PSC]), and recently well-recognized chronic inflammation caused by nonalcoholic fatty liver disease (NAFLD) with the subsequent development of diffuse fibrosis and cirrhosis (Box 64-1).

Clinical Presentation

Patients may be entirely asymptomatic or may present with nonspecific constitutional symptoms, or symptoms of liver failure, complications of portal hypertension, or both.

Nonspecific symptoms include weakness, lethargy, anorexia, weight loss, abdominal pain, loss of libido, altered sleep-wake pattern, and nausea or vomiting. Specific symptoms due to hepatic synthetic dysfunction and portal hypertension include jaundice, pruritus, coagulopathy leading to easy bruising, fluid retention with ankle edema, ascites, gastroesophageal variceal bleeding leading to hematemesis or melena, and symptoms of hepatic encephalopathy ranging from mild confusion to coma.

On physical examination, patients may have stigmata of chronic liver disease such as Dupuytren's contractures, palmar erythema, spider angiomas, parotid enlargement, and bruising. Palpation of the abdomen may reveal an enlarged or shrunken liver, splenomegaly, ascites, or dilated superficial anterior abdominal wall veins. Male patients may show signs of feminization (gynecomastia), testicular atrophy, and loss of body hair. Patients with hepatic encephalopathy may present with a "flapping tremor" or asterixis.

Differential Diagnosis

The new onset of ascites presenting with no history and stigmata of chronic liver disease may not be secondary to cirrhosis and portal hypertension. Other causes include portal vein occlusion, nephrotic syndrome, protein-losing enteropathy, severe malnutrition, myxedema, ovarian diseases (Meig's syndrome, struma ovarii), pancreatic ascites, chylous ascites, nephrogenic ascites, tuberculous peritonitis, or secondary malignancy.

The differential diagnosis for hematemesis and melena includes duodenal ulcer, gastric ulcer, esophagitis, gastritis, Mallory-Weiss tear, hematobilia, anastomotic ulcer, and Ménétrier's disease.

Diagnostic Approach

After a thorough history and physical examination, complete laboratory data, radiologic examination, and histologic studies may be necessary to establish the diagnosis and the most likely cause of cirrhosis.

Figure 64-1 Septal Cirrhosis.

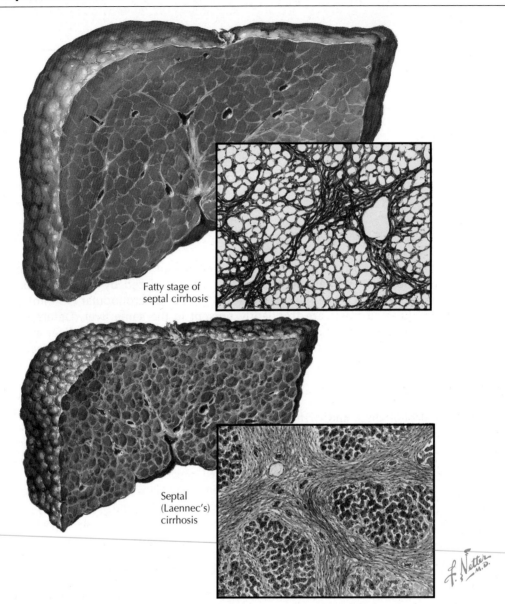

Fatty stage of
septal cirrhosis

Septal
(Laennec's)
cirrhosis

The complete blood cell count may show anemia, leukopenia, or thrombocytopenia. Hypersplenism causes both leukopenia and thrombocytopenia. Chronic blood loss and vitamin deficiency can cause anemia. Prolongation of the prothrombin time occurs secondary to vitamin K deficiency or impaired clotting factor synthesis.

Serum biochemistry often demonstrates an elevated bilirubin level and a low albumin level. Some patients with established cirrhosis may have normal aspartate aminotransferase (AST) and alanine aminotransferase (ALT) levels. Elevated AST and ALT levels are found in patients with autoimmune hepatitis, viral hepatitis, alcoholic hepatitis, and drug-induced liver injury. Patients with cholestatic liver disease usually have elevated alkaline phosphatase, γ-glutamyltransferase, and conjugated bilirubin levels.

Several other serologic tests are necessary to establish cause: viral serology for hepatitis B (HBsAg), C (anti-HCV Ab), and quantitative DNA and RNA levels, respectively, to define the activity status; iron studies and *HFE* gene analysis for hereditary hemochromatosis; serum and 24-hour urine copper, ceruloplasmin level for Wilson's disease; α_1-antitrypsin level and genotype for α_1-antitrypsin deficiency. Serum autoantibodies (antinuclear antibody, anti–smooth muscle antibody, antimitochondrial antibody and anti-liver-kidney microsomal antibody) and quantitative serum immunoglobulins levels may help to diagnose autoimmune liver disease. Periodic evaluation of tumor markers is indicated to detect complicating primary hepatocellular carcinoma; these include alpha fetoprotein and the combination of carcinoembryonic antigen and CA 19-9. Moni-

> **Box 64-1   Causes of Cirrhosis**
>
> **Infections:** Hepatitis B, hepatitis C, possibly other viruses, schistosomiasis
>
> **Drugs and toxins:** Alcohol, methyldopa, methotrexate, isoniazid, amiodarone
>
> **Biliary obstruction:** Primary and secondary sclerosing cholangitis, cystic fibrosis, biliary atresia, common bile duct stones
>
> **Metabolic disorders:** Hereditary hemochromatosis, Wilson's disease, α_1-antitrypsin deficiency, cystic fibrosis, glycogen storage disease
>
> **Autoimmune diseases:** Chronic active hepatitis, primary biliary cirrhosis
>
> **Cardiovascular:** Chronic right heart failure, Budd-Chiari syndrome, veno-occlusive disease
>
> **Miscellaneous:** Nonalcoholic fatty liver disease, sarcoidosis, jejunoileal bypass, neonatal hepatitis
>
> **Cryptogenic:** Unknown cause

toring for cholangiocarcinoma is recommended in patients with cirrhosis from PSC.

Radiologic studies (ultrasound with or without Doppler, computed tomography, or magnetic resonance imaging) provide additional diagnostic information. Although these studies are not always necessary, they are useful in screening for primary hepatocellular carcinoma and cholangiocarcinoma. They provide information in addition to serum tumor markers, which are commonly associated with cirrhosis of various causes.

Histologic examination of the liver biopsy specimen is often key for diagnosis. Micronodules, fatty infiltration, and Mallory's hyaline usually accompany alcoholic cirrhosis. Primary biliary cirrhosis, primary and secondary sclerosing cholangitis, and autoimmune hepatitis have typical histologic findings. Special stains such as Prussian blue for iron and periodic acid–Schiff diastase for α_1-antitrypsin globules can confirm the diagnosis. Liver biopsy is necessary to stage the disease, to help determine the prognosis, and to guide optimum therapy. There are various noninvasive measurements of liver fibrosis in the serum and liver by measuring markers of connective tissue and liver stiffness. The sensitivity and specificity of serum markers (hyaluronic acid, type III procollagen peptide, etc.) for detection of extensive fibrosis are not acceptable. The measurement of liver stiffness with transient elastography and its correlation to fibrosis have been validated in viral hepatitis and cholestatic liver diseases. The results provide a promising simple and reliable noninvasive means to assess liver fibrosis; however, in clinical practice, its use to replace the liver biopsy is yet to be determined.

Management and Therapy

In general, management of cirrhosis includes the following:

- Withdrawal of the causative agent (e.g., alcohol, drugs)
- Treatment of the specific underlying cause (e.g., antiviral therapy for viral hepatitis, prednisone or azathioprine for autoimmune hepatitis, phlebotomy for hemochromatosis, D-penicillamine or trientine for Wilson's disease)
- Treatment of underlying risks for NAFLD (obesity, diabetes, hyperlipidemia, drugs)
- Treatment of decompensated cirrhosis: ascites, infection, gastrointestinal hemorrhage, hepatic encephalopathy, and hepatorenal syndrome
- Orthotopic liver transplantation for decompensated cirrhosis if the patient is a suitable candidate

Ascites

Patients with cirrhosis in whom ascites develops need a diagnostic (10 to 20 mL) abdominal paracentesis. Indications include new-onset ascites, clinical deterioration with fever, abdominal pain, and change in mental status. The factors producing ascites in cirrhosis are a low serum albumin level, hepatic outflow block with overproduction of lymph, and portal venous hypertension. Ascites can be mild, moderate, or severe on the basis of the amount of fluid in the peritoneal cavity (Figs. 64-2 and 64-3).

Optimum Treatment

The initial treatment includes restriction of dietary sodium intake and the use of oral diuretics. Approximately 20% of patients respond to sodium restriction alone. Sodium is usually limited to 2 g (90 mEq) per day. Diuretics include spironolactone and furosemide. More than 90% of patients respond to this combination therapy. The maximum spironolactone dose is 400 mg/day, and for furosemide, 160 mg/day. Amiloride, 10 to 20 mg/day, is an alternative to spironolactone if there are side effects such as tender gynecomastia.

Approximately 10% of patients with cirrhosis will develop ascites refractory to routine medical treatment with sodium restriction and diuretic therapy. Large-volume paracentesis (LVP) can be used before alternative therapies such as transjugular intrahepatic portosystemic shunt (TIPS) or peritoneovenous shunt. TIPS is a relatively safe nonsurgical procedure that is effective in reducing portal hypertension. TIPS placement is indicated in cirrhotic patients with refractory ascites who require LVP more than 2 or 3 times per month. Compared with serial LVP, placement of an uncovered TIPS stent is more effective at preventing ascites from recurring; however, an increased incidence of hepatic encephalopathy and shunt dysfunction rates after TIPS placement are complications that increase its cost. The development of a newer polytetrafluoroethylene-covered stent may provide better results in shunt dysfunction rates and patient survival. The TIPS procedure has gained wide popularity and provides a bridge to liver transplantation in patients with advanced cirrhosis.

Figure 64-2 Ascites.

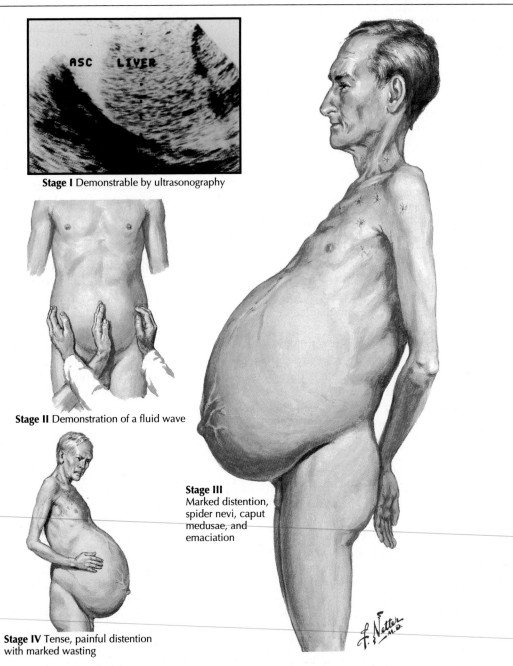

Stage I Demonstrable by ultrasonography

Stage II Demonstration of a fluid wave

Stage III
Marked distention, spider nevi, caput medusae, and emaciation

Stage IV Tense, painful distention with marked wasting

Peritoneovenous shunt (LeVeen/Denver) can be used if the placement of a TIPS is contraindicated.

Avoiding Treatment Errors

Making an appropriate diagnosis before initiating treatment is critical. Diuretic therapy should be used cautiously and in a stepwise fashion to avoid potential severe electrolyte and fluid imbalance and renal dysfunction. For patients with refractory ascites, the risks and benefits of placement of a peritoneovenous shunt or TIPS should be evaluated thoroughly for a successful outcome.

Gastrointestinal Hemorrhage

Gastroesophageal variceal bleeding is the most ominous complication of cirrhosis (see Fig. 64-4).

Optimum Treatment

Initial management of suspected variceal bleeding requires immediate hospitalization, volume resuscitation, and airway protection for massive bleeding. If the diagnosis is reasonably certain, pharmacologic therapy with somatostatin or its analogue octreotide can be initiated. If

Figure 64-3 Pathophysiology of Ascites Formation.

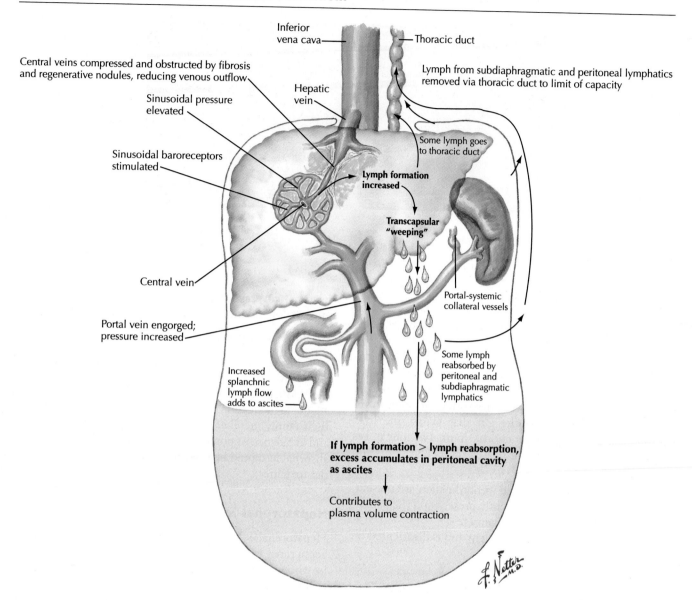

Inferior vena cava

Thoracic duct

Central veins compressed and obstructed by fibrosis and regenerative nodules, reducing venous outflow

Lymph from subdiaphragmatic and peritoneal lymphatics removed via thoracic duct to limit of capacity

Hepatic vein

Sinusoidal pressure elevated

Some lymph goes to thoracic duct

Sinusoidal baroreceptors stimulated

Lymph formation increased

Transcapsular "weeping"

Central vein

Portal-systemic collateral vessels

Portal vein engorged; pressure increased

Some lymph reabsorbed by peritoneal and subdiaphragmatic lymphatics

Increased splanchnic lymph flow adds to ascites

If lymph formation > lymph reabsorption, excess accumulates in peritoneal cavity as ascites

Contributes to plasma volume contraction

endoscopy confirms esophageal varices, endoscopic therapy with either variceal ligation or sclerotherapy is indicated. Endoscopic therapy controls acute variceal bleeding in 80% to 95% of patients, a success rate superior to pharmacologic agents or balloon tamponade. There is a 50% to 80% risk for recurrent variceal bleeding. Options to prevent recurrent variceal bleeding include endoscopic ligation or sclerotherapy, nonselective β-blockers (propranolol, nadolol), surgical shunts, TIPS, and liver transplantation.

TIPS is one of the most promising therapies for the control of acute variceal bleeding. The goal of TIPS is to achieve a hepatic venous gradient of less than 12 mm Hg and a reduction or loss of contrast opacification of varices.

TIPS is reserved for those patients who are refractory to endoscopic therapy along with pharmacotherapy or who have acute, severe bleeding from gastric varices. The technical success rate and control of acute variceal bleeding is more than 90% (Fig. 64-4).

Avoiding Treatment Errors

Gastroesophageal hemorrhage carries a high morbidity and mortality; timely aggressive resuscitation and therapeutic interventions are important in the management of these critically ill patients. Airway protection by ventilator support should be done to avoid aspiration pneumonia in patients with agitation and massive bleeding.

Figure 64-4 Endoscopic Appearance of Esophageal Varices with Evidence of Recent Hemorrhage.

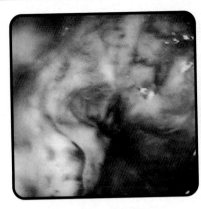 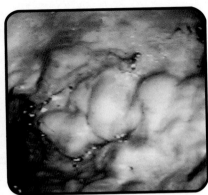

Hepatic Encephalopathy

Hepatic encephalopathy represents a constellation of reversible neurologic signs and symptoms accompanying advanced, decompensated liver disease or extensive porto-systemic shunting. The pathogenesis of hepatic encephalopathy remains unclear. It is partially attributable to toxic compounds that are derived from the metabolism of nitrogenous substrates in the gut that bypass the liver through an anatomic and functional shunt. The four stages of hepatic encephalopathy are based on mental status and neurologic findings:

Stage 1: Mild confusion and incoordination are present.
Stage 2: Asterixis is consistently present and the patient has obvious personality changes.
Stage 3: The patient is somnolent and is disoriented on arousal.
Stage 4: The patient is comatose.

Common precipitating factors include deterioration in hepatic function, gastrointestinal hemorrhage, excess protein intake, alcohol, sedatives or hypnotics, surgery, hepatoma, infection, dehydration, electrolyte imbalance (hypokalemia), constipation, and placement of a surgical shunt or TIPS.

Optimum Treatment

Management includes identification and correction of any precipitating factor, restriction of dietary protein to 40 g/day, and administration of lactulose. Antibiotics to decontaminate the gut, such as neomycin, metronidazole, amoxicillin, and rifaximin, can be added if there is no response to dietary manipulation and lactulose or if there is intolerance to lactulose. Rifaximin, a nonaminoglycoside antibiotic derived from rifamycin, has gained popularity because it is not absorbed from the gut, thereby eliminating potential toxicities of other antibiotics (renal failure, ototoxicity, and peripheral neuropathy) and has broad-spectrum anti-

bacterial coverage. Patients with severe refractory hepatic encephalopathy need urgent liver transplantation.

Avoiding Treatment Errors

Identification of precipitating factors correctly is the key in the management of hepatic encephalopathy. Ensuring the optimal use and effectiveness of lactulose requires the adequate education and understanding of patients and their family members. The result is improved compliance and avoidance of potential side effects. Antibiotics that are absorbable should be used cautiously to avoid their potential toxicities.

Hepatorenal Syndrome

Hepatorenal syndrome is a distinct type of progressive acute renal failure that develops in a patient with cirrhosis in whom all other causes of renal dysfunction have been excluded. It is a functional type of renal failure. If the liver disease improves, normal renal function returns. The pathogenesis of the hepatorenal syndrome is unknown. The probability of hepatorenal syndrome in cirrhosis is about 20% in 1 year and 40% in 5 years. Hyponatremia and azotemia are characteristic. The urinary sodium concentration is less than 10 mEq/L. The urinary sediment is unremarkable. Other important chemical findings include a urine-to-plasma creatinine ratio of more than 30 and a urine-to-plasma osmolality ratio of more than 1.

Optimum Treatment

In the management of hepatorenal syndrome, specific causes for renal failure should be excluded (i.e., acute tubular necrosis, prerenal azotemia from intravascular volume depletion, drug-induced nephrotoxicity, or pre-existing chronic renal disease). Renal replacement therapy should be considered for patients who are potential candidates for liver transplantation. Experimental forms of therapy include prostaglandin E₁, dopamine, terlipressin, peritoneovenous shunt, and TIPS.

Avoiding Treatment Errors

The hepatorenal syndrome carries a high mortality, and liver transplantation can reverse the syndrome. Therefore, timely and comprehensive evaluation of patients to determine their candidacy for liver transplantation is important in their management.

Liver Transplantation

Optimum Treatment

Liver transplantation is no longer experimental and is considered the standard of care for patients with advanced cirrhosis. With improved surgical technique and better immunosuppressive drugs, it has become a successful therapy for end-stage liver disease with long-term survival rates approaching 90% and excellent quality of life. Unfortunately, the gap between the numbers of deceased donors and recipients continues to widen.

Living donor liver transplantation (LDLT) is used by many transplantation centers worldwide. First used in a child in 1989, LDLT has become a viable alternative for pediatric recipients. Over the past decade, LDLT has been used successfully in adult recipients with patient and graft survivals similar to those with deceased donor liver transplantation. The rate-limiting factor is the availability of suitable donors for this procedure. With appropriate donor and recipient selection, further refinement in surgical technique, and increasing experience, LDLT may give superior results. About 5% to 10% of liver transplantations in the United States have involved the use of living donors.

Avoiding Treatment Errors

Liver transplantation is the only definitive therapy in decompensated cirrhosis. About 18,000 patients in the United States are on the United Network of Organ Sharing waiting list, and the number increases 25% per year. Only about 5000 to 6000 deceased donor liver transplantations are performed each year in the United States. Because there is an excess of potential recipients, careful identification and evaluation of transplant recipients is critical.

Future Directions

Major improvements in diagnostic techniques now allow the diagnosis of chronic liver diseases earlier in their course. Improvement in pharmacologic agents that include antiviral drugs (hepatitis B and C) will help to prevent progression to cirrhosis.

Liver transplantation is a highly effective option in the management of advanced cirrhosis. Hepatocyte, stem cell, and xenotransplantation may provide additional therapeutic options in the management of end-stage liver disease.

Additional Resources

Rossle M, Haag K, Ochs A, et al: The transjugular intrahepatic portosystemic stent-shunt procedure for variceal bleeding. N Engl J Med 330:165-171, 1994.

One of the original articles published using TIPS in the management of variceal bleeding, this paper describes the technique and success of the procedure.

Runyon BA: Care of patients with ascites. N Engl J Med 330:337-342, 1994.

The author provides a comprehensive discussion in the management of patients with ascites.

Starzl TE, Demetris AJ, Van Thiel D: Liver transplantation (1). N Engl J Med 321:1014-1022, 1989.

Starzl TE, Demetris AJ, Van Thiel D: Liver transplantation (2). N Engl J Med 321:1092-1099, 1989.

Both of these articles provide the original documentation of the overall success of liver transplantation for patients with end-stage liver disease.

Stiegmann GV, Goff JS, Michaletz-Onody PA, et al: Endoscopic sclerotherapy as compared with endoscopic ligation for bleeding esophageal varices. N Engl J Med 326:1527-1532, 1992.

This is one of the leading articles describing two different endoscopic techniques in the management of esophageal variceal hemorrhage. The authors demonstrate the superiority of endoscopic band ligation in the management of bleeding esophageal varices and in decreasing the potential complications of endoscopic therapy.

EVIDENCE

1. Garcia-Tsao G: The transjugular intrahepatic portosystemic shunt for the management of cirrhotic refractory ascites. Nat Clin Pract Gastroenterol Hepatol 3:380-389, 2006.

   This review article outlines the pathophysiology and utility of TIPS in patients with refractory ascites. It encompasses all relevant clinical studies to date in the literature.

2. Rector WG Jr: Complications of Liver Disease. St Louis, Mosby-Year, 1992.

   This book outlines all potential complications of liver disease and is simple to follow.

3. The Organ Procurement and Transplantation Network Web site. Available at: http://www.optn.org. Accessed August 14, 2006.

   This site provides information on all activities related to transplantation, including data from specific transplant centers, regions, and the entire country.

William D. Heizer

Celiac Disease

Introduction

Celiac disease occurs throughout the world and has prevalence estimates ranging from 1 in 500 to 1 in 67, except in Japan, where the prevalence is very low. A large study demonstrated a prevalence in the United States of 1 in 133 for those with no risk factors, 1 in 56 among individuals with gastrointestinal symptoms associated with the disease, 1 in 39 in second-degree relatives of celiac disease patients, and 1 in 22 in first-degree relatives. Therefore, about 3 million people in the United States have the disease. However, it is estimated that fewer than 5% of affected individuals have been diagnosed.

Celiac disease is one of a number of diseases of the small intestine that can cause malabsorption syndrome. Others include Whipple's disease, diffuse mucosal malignancies, bacterial overgrowth syndrome, and short bowel (Fig. 65-1).

Etiology and Pathogenesis

Celiac disease results from an immune response to peptides present in gluten, a protein found in wheat, and similar proteins found in rye and barley. The toxic peptides are resistant to intraluminal and brush border proteolytic activity, enter the submucosa either through or between epithelial cells, and are transformed to more antigenic forms by the enzyme tissue transglutaminase. The immune response stimulates a T-lymphocyte attack on small bowel mucosa, resulting in an epithelial stress response and death of enterocytes—an autoimmune process. Only genetically susceptible individuals develop the disease, and multiple genes are involved. The presence of one of the human major histocompatibility molecules, HLA-DQ2 or HLA-DQ8, is almost essential and occurs in about 98% of cases. In addition to dietary gluten exposure and genetic susceptibility, some triggering event may be necessary to initiate the disease. Damage to the small intestinal mucosa is manifested histologically by a progression of changes, which include migration of lymphocytes to intraepithelial locations, crypt hyperplasia, shortening and thickening of the villi, and shortening of the columnar epithelial cells. Tissue transglutaminase promotes the immune response by converting glutamine side chains of the toxic peptides to glutamate and also cross-linking these residues to lysine in other proteins, including in the enzyme itself. Serum antibodies against tissue transglutaminase (TTGA) are useful diagnostically and are the same as endomysial antibodies (EMA), although characteristics of the two tests for the antibody are such that they may occasionally give different results.

Clinical Presentation

Symptoms and signs leading to diagnosis may be intestinal (e.g., diarrhea) or nonintestinal (e.g., anemia or bone loss). Relatives of celiac disease patients and individuals with conditions associated with celiac disease are increasingly being diagnosed with screening blood tests or endoscopic duodenal biopsies despite having no symptoms attributable to the disease. The mode of presentation has changed over time with the advent of serologic tests, endoscopic duodenal biopsies, and greater awareness of the disease. Features leading to the diagnosis at a major medical center between 2000 and 2004 were diarrhea in 37% of cases, anemia in 13%, screening in 12%, bone disease in 8%, incidental in 5%, and other features in 26%. The incidental diagnosis was usually the result of unexpected discovery of an abnormal duodenal mucosa during upper endoscopy for reflux or dyspepsia symptoms. The other features leading to diagnosis included abdominal pain, constipation, weight loss, neurologic symptoms (peripheral neuropathy, seizures, ataxia), dermatitis herpetiformis, macroamylasemia, hypoproteinemia, elevated sedimentation rate, need for

Figure 65-1 Malabsorption Syndrome: Small Intestinal Causes.

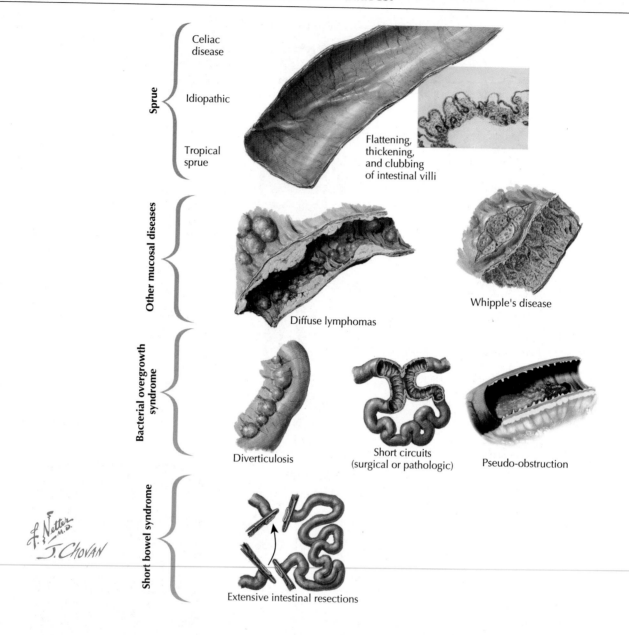

Sprue
- Celiac disease
- Idiopathic
- Tropical sprue

Flattening, thickening, and clubbing of intestinal villi

Other mucosal diseases

Diffuse lymphomas

Whipple's disease

Bacterial overgrowth syndrome

Diverticulosis

Short circuits (surgical or pathologic)

Pseudo-obstruction

Short bowel syndrome

Extensive intestinal resections

increased amounts of oral medication, and liver test abnormalities. Additional presenting signs and symptoms reported by others include irritable bowel syndrome, nausea, vomiting, dyspepsia, bloating, abdominal distention, glossitis, muscle cramps, bleeding, miscarriage, infertility, growth retardation, paresthesias, weakness, lassitude, hyposplenism, and small bowel intussusception. The diagnosis is most frequently made in 40- to 60-year-olds, although prevalence of the disease appears to be equal in children and adults. Females are three times more frequently affected than males. The disease is diagnosed in obese and even morbidly obese individuals. The mean delay from onset of symptoms to diagnosis is 4 to 5 years.

The classic presentation of celiac disease, dominated by signs and symptoms of malabsorption, is now very rare in developed countries but can occur. Advanced malabsorption syndrome is characterized by diarrhea; weight loss or poor weight gain; and bulky, greasy, and unusually foul-smelling stools (Fig. 65-2). Signs of vitamin or mineral deficiencies may include glossitis from B vitamins and iron deficiency, osteomalacia from vitamin D and calcium deficiency, tetany from calcium and magnesium deficiency, and ecchymoses from vitamin K deficiency. Edema may result from hypoalbuminemia caused by decreased protein absorption, decreased hepatic synthesis of albumin, and protein-losing enteropathy. Medications and nutrients are poorly absorbed. Anemia may be macrocytic, due to folic

Figure 65-2 Advanced Malabsorption Syndrome.

Physical findings

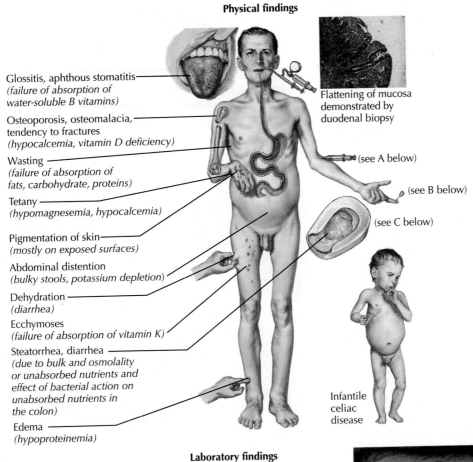

Glossitis, aphthous stomatitis
(failure of absorption of water-soluble B vitamins)

Flattening of mucosa demonstrated by duodenal biopsy

Osteoporosis, osteomalacia, tendency to fractures
(hypocalcemia, vitamin D deficiency)

(see A below)

Wasting
(failure of absorption of fats, carbohydrate, proteins)

(see B below)

Tetany
(hypomagnesemia, hypocalcemia)

(see C below)

Pigmentation of skin
(mostly on exposed surfaces)

Abdominal distention
(bulky stools, potassium depletion)

Dehydration
(diarrhea)

Ecchymoses
(failure of absorption of vitamin K)

Steatorrhea, diarrhea
(due to bulk and osmolality or unabsorbed nutrients and effect of bacterial action on unabsorbed nutrients in the colon)

Edema
(hypoproteinemia)

Infantile celiac disease

Laboratory findings

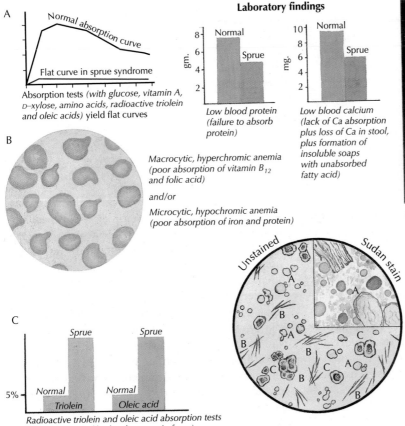

A

Normal absorption curve

Flat curve in sprue syndrome

Absorption tests *(with glucose, vitamin A, D–xylose, amino acids, radioactive triolein and oleic acids)* yield flat curves

B

Macrocytic, hyperchromic anemia *(poor absorption of vitamin B_{12} and folic acid)*

and/or

Microcytic, hypochromic anemia *(poor absorption of iron and protein)*

Normal / Sprue (gm.)

Low blood protein *(failure to absorb protein)*

Normal / Sprue (mg.)

Low blood calcium *(lack of Ca absorption plus loss of Ca in stool, plus formation of insoluble soaps with unabsorbed fatty acid)*

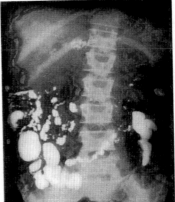

X-ray – typical "deficiency" pattern with breaking up and flocculation of barium column

C

Sprue / Sprue

Normal / Normal

5%

Triolein / Oleic acid

Radioactive triolein and oleic acid absorption tests *(increased loss of both substances in feces)*

Unstained / Sudan stain

Stool examination reveals abundance of:
A – neutral fats
B – fatty acid crystals
C – soaps

acid and occasionally vitamin B$_{12}$ malabsorption, microcytic, due to iron and protein malabsorption, or mixed.

Several malignancies are associated with celiac disease, including non-Hodgkin's lymphoma, small intestinal adenocarcinoma, and squamous carcinoma of the esophagus and head and neck. They may be discovered before, at, or after the diagnosis of celiac disease, but the incidence of malignancies, with the possible exception of lymphoma, decreases over several years after beginning a gluten-free diet.

Differential Diagnosis

The great variety of ways that celiac disease can present results in a broad differential diagnosis. For those presenting with diarrhea, the differential includes irritable bowel syndrome, lactase deficiency, inflammatory bowel disease, giardiasis, small bowel bacterial overgrowth, pancreatic insufficiency, human immunodeficiency virus enteropathy, radiation enteropathy, and food allergy. Celiac patients are often lactose intolerant because of lactase deficiency resulting from decreased lactase activity in the damaged mucosa. This secondary lactase deficiency must not be mistaken for primary acquired lactase deficiency. In the differential for anemia, one must consider colon or gastric neoplasm or pernicious anemia; possible causes for decreased bone mineral density include age-related osteoporosis, hypogonadism, thyroid disease, and primary or metastatic bone neoplasm.

Diagnostic Approach

A high level of clinical suspicion is important, recognizing the many ways the disease can present. The availability of a noninvasive and highly sensitive and specific diagnostic test, namely detection of antibodies to tissue transglutaminase, has been a major advance. The diagnosis should be confirmed, in almost all instances, by upper endoscopy and small bowel mucosal biopsy. Final confirmation requires an unequivocal response of clinical signs or symptoms or mucosal histology to gluten withdrawal.

Serum antibodies, immunoglobulin G (IgG) and immunoglobulin A (IgA), against tissue transglutaminase can be detected as either EMA or TTGA. The IgA antibodies are more sensitive and specific than IgG antibodies. However, about 2% of celiac disease patients are IgA deficient; therefore, a serum IgA level may be needed to properly interpret the serologic test. The cost-effectiveness of ordering a serum IgA level when celiac disease serology is ordered is not known. It is probably more cost effective to order an IgA level only if the EMA-IgA or TTGA-IgA is weakly positive or the EMA-IgG or TTGA-IgG is elevated. In the EMA test, antibody is detected by its attachment to connective tissue in monkey esophagus or human umbilical cord using immunofluorescence, although an enzyme-linked immunoassay has been reported. Sensitivity of 90% to 97% and specificity of 98% to 99% for EMA-IgA have been reported. The TTGA-IgA test is an enzyme-linked immunoassay. When it is done using recombinant or purified human tissue transglutaminase, as opposed to earlier tests using guinea pig antigen, sensitivity is 94% to 95% and specificity is 95% to 97%. Sensitivity of both tests is lower in celiac disease with milder mucosal changes, and can be negative when mucosal changes are minimal. Antibody levels decrease and may disappear after 6 to 12 months of gluten withdrawal. Either test is more specific than antigliadin and antireticulin tests, which should no longer be used to diagnose celiac disease. Although some believe the antigliadin and antireticulin tests help identify celiac disease patients with minimal histologic changes who benefit symptomatically from a gluten-restricted diet, the apparent benefit may be a placebo response. Other investigators report that the antigliadin test is more sensitive than EMA or TTGA for diagnosing gluten-associated neurologic disease.

As a general rule, mucosal biopsy should be done in all patients before initiating diet therapy. Exceptions can include patients with biopsy-proven dermatitis herpetiformis and those with high-titer TTGA or EMA who have classic symptoms or a relative with celiac disease. The mucosal changes have been thought to begin in the duodenum and progress slowly distally, very seldom reaching the terminal ileum. However, studies have revealed some patients with patchy changes and some with positive biopsy results only in the distal duodenum or jejunum, although this observation was not supported by other studies. To minimize the chance of missing a mucosal abnormality, at least two biopsy specimens should be obtained from the second, third, and fourth parts of the duodenum each, if possible. An experienced surgical pathologist should report the histologic abnormalities and classify them as Marsh type I (increased intraepithelial lymphocytes, IELs), II (increased IELs and crypt hyperplasia), IIIa (partial villous atrophy), IIIb (subtotal villous atrophy), or IIIc (total villous atrophy). Studies show that celiac disease is eventually confirmed in 95% of patients with Marsh III lesions, in most with Marsh II, but only in 10% with Marsh I.

Almost all celiac disease patients have one or both of the HLA antigens, DQ2 and DQ8. Therefore, their absence essentially excludes the diagnosis with a negative predictive value of 99.9%. However, the antigens are present in 30% to 40% of the general population, so the presence of one or both of these antigens has a positive predictive value of only 1.7%. Situations in which testing may be useful include individuals with weakly positive serology and equivocal biopsies, individuals who have placed themselves on dietary restriction months earlier and insist on knowing if they have the disease but do not want to go off the diet for a prolonged time, and children of individuals with diagnosed celiac disease who hope to avoid periodic serologic testing in future years.

Small bowel radiographs, stool fat assay, and the D-xylose absorption test are neither sensitive nor specific enough to be useful for diagnosing celiac disease. The utility of capsule endoscopy is promising but has not been adequately studied.

A therapeutic trial of a gluten-free diet is not appropriate for several reasons. The diet is difficult and lifelong for celiac disease and should not be started without a confirmed diagnosis. Individuals who do not have the disease may experience some improvement of symptoms on the diet, leading to a false-positive diagnosis. The diet may not be followed well and, even if it is, up to 30% of celiac disease patients will require longer than a month to respond, and up to 5% will take longer than 6 months. Therefore, patients may not follow the diet well or long enough, leading to a false-negative diagnosis. Finally, once on the diet, patients often seek medical help to make a definitive diagnosis in order to decide if they should stay on a strict diet or their relatives should be considered at increased risk. Because both the serologic test and biopsy may normalize with time on the diet, diagnostic tests should not be done until the patient has been on a gluten-containing diet for at least 6 weeks, and preferably 3 months.

Individuals with any of the many features listed under "Clinical Presentation" for which there is no other reasonable explanation should be considered for testing. Testing the large number of individuals who meet Rome criteria for irritable bowel syndrome or those who have a documented decrease in bone mineral density remains controversial. The reported incidence of celiac disease among individuals with reduced bone mineral density compared with controls who have normal bone density ranges from the same to a 10-fold increased incidence.

An increased prevalence of celiac disease has been documented in a number of conditions. The conditions and reported prevalence, compared with a prevalence of 0.5% to 1% in the general population, include dermatitis herpetiformis (100%), type I diabetes mellitus (2.5% to 10%), Sjögren's syndrome (10%), Addison's disease (8%), autoimmune thyroid disease (1% to 5%), inflammatory bowel disease (2% to 18%), Down syndrome (1% to 10%), autoimmune hepatitis (6%), primary biliary cirrhosis (5% to 10%), autoimmune myocarditis (4%), IgA deficiency (2%), and microscopic colitis. Routinely screening all patients with these conditions for celiac disease is not recommended because current data do not indicate a clear outcome benefit for early detection and treatment of asymptomatic individuals. Instead, physicians taking care of patients with any of these conditions should be aware of the association and maintain a low threshold for testing those with symptoms that could be a result of celiac disease. Because abnormal small bowel mucosa, often patchy and mild, is present in 100% of biopsy-proven dermatitis herpetiformis patients, and the skin lesion improves on a gluten-restricted diet independent of the severity of the mucosal lesion, small bowel biopsy is not mandatory in this condition.

In practice, the diagnosis of celiac disease often presents a dilemma. A substantial number of patients present with serology, histology, symptoms, or response to gluten withdrawal that are not consistent with each other. Because there is not complete agreement among experts about the designation or management of such individuals, a brief opinion, if not quite a consensus, is in order.

The diagnosis of *celiac disease* requires a compatible histologic abnormality of the small intestinal mucosa that improves on a gluten-restricted diet. However, if the patient also has symptoms compatible with celiac disease that respond to the diet, the symptomatic response can be accepted as adequate indirect evidence of histologic improvement so that a repeat mucosal biopsy is not required to establish the diagnosis.

Patients with positive serology and positive histology but no significant symptoms are designated as having *silent* or *asymptomatic celiac disease*. There is disagreement about whether these patients should be placed on a gluten-restricted diet. This should be decided after thorough discussion with the patient of the risks and benefits of therapy.

Patients with positive serology but mucosal histology that is normal or shows only increased IELs (Marsh I) are designated as having *latent* or *potential celiac disease*, assuming a false-positive serologic test can be reasonably excluded. The same designation is used for patients with previously diagnosed celiac disease who maintain normal histology when gluten is later reintroduced. On long-term follow-up, some patients with latent celiac disease go on to develop full-blown celiac disease, and some maintain or revert to normal serology and histology. Diet therapy is optional.

Patients with negative serology and mucosal histology showing only increased IELs (Marsh I) may have latent or even symptomatic celiac disease, but most do not. Many other conditions cause this histology, including bacterial overgrowth syndrome, food allergies, enteric parasites, inflammatory bowel disease, drugs including nonsteroidal anti-inflammatory agents and proton pump inhibitors, and gastric *Helicobacter* species infection. Details of the number, distribution, and type of IELs in various conditions are still being investigated. Diet therapy is not recommended.

Patients with flat intestinal mucosa and positive serology, who do not improve symptomatically or histologically after a year on an adequate gluten-restricted diet, or patients who responded initially and then stopped responding, are designated as having *refractory celiac disease* (RCD). They usually respond to a combination of immunosuppressant and gluten restriction. Other patients with flat mucosa and usually negative serology, who are not gluten sensitive, are designated as having *idiopathic sprue*. The etiology of this condition is unknown, although some of these patients improve on restriction of dietary

proteins other than gluten, and some respond to immunosuppression.

In contrast to patients who have the mucosal abnormalities of celiac disease, there are patients, with or without positive serology, who have normal mucosal histology but have symptoms that respond to gluten withdrawal, for example, ataxia, peripheral neuropathy, aphthous stomatitis, or diarrhea. The pathophysiology and nomenclature for these conditions are unsettled. Some of these patients may actually have a mucosal abnormality that is missed because it is patchy or because it is submicroscopic, seen only by electron microscopy. Others are best designated as having *gluten sensitivity* or *gluten sensitivity syndrome*. Gluten sensitivity has been defined as a systemic disease caused by heightened immunologic responsiveness to ingested gluten in genetically susceptible individuals that may primarily attack one or more organs such as the intestine (celiac disease), skin (dermatitis herpetiformis), central nervous system (gluten ataxia, seizures), peripheral nerves (peripheral neuropathy), muscles, or other tissues. Deposition of TTGA-IgA or other types of IgA has been found in the histologically normal intestinal mucosa and in other tissues, including brain, in some of these cases. The prevalence of gluten sensitivity in the absence of celiac disease is unknown.

Management and Therapy

Optimum Treatment

The mainstay of treatment is elimination of gluten from the diet, which is far from easy. Gluten or a similar toxic protein is present in wheat, rye, and barley. The average daily U.S. diet contains 9000 to 15,000 mg of gluten, and a slice of bread contains 1500 to 2000 mg. The minimum toxic dose of gluten for celiac disease patients is unclear and is probably not the same for all patients. A daily amount of 100 mg of gluten, the amount in about 1/20 slice of bread, was shown to produce histologic changes in a group of patients with the disease, so ideally, the diet should be restricted to less than that, probably 10 to 50 mg daily. One well-studied patient was sensitive to 1 mg of gluten per day. However, in practice, many patients on a gluten-restricted diet are ingesting 1000 mg or more of gluten daily. It is possible, but by no means certain, that many celiac patients can tolerate 200 to 1000 mg daily with minimal symptoms or risk. Pure oats are safe, but commercial oat products are usually contaminated with other grains, so oat products should also be avoided at least until the patient is free of the presenting celiac symptoms and then only if the oat product is thought to be pure. Most patients report experiencing symptoms within 24 hours after accidentally ingesting gluten, but absence of such immediate symptoms is not an indication that the diet is gluten free.

Initially, the dietary restrictions may seem overwhelming. Counseling by a dietitian experienced in treating celiac disease is essential. Many helpful resources are available on the Internet (see "Additional Resources"). Talking with someone who has had celiac disease for several years and is doing well can be a great help to the newly diagnosed patient.

A multivitamin and multimineral supplement providing about the recommended daily amounts should be given twice daily for the first 6 months of dietary therapy and once daily thereafter. Any anemia should be characterized. Iron or folic acid deficiency should be treated with appropriate oral supplements. Determine a serum 25-hydroxy vitamin D level for any newly diagnosed patient. If it is below normal, give 50,000 IU of vitamin D_2, or preferably vitamin D_3, orally 1 to 7 times weekly, depending on the level, and redetermine the serum level in 1 to 3 months. Adjust the dose to keep the serum 25-hydroxy vitamin D level in the high-normal range. Determine bone mineral density, and if it is low, repeat after 1 year of diet and vitamin therapy. If it has not improved, consider bisphosphonate or calcitonin therapy.

Clinic visits, in conjunction with seeing a dietitian, should be at 1- to 2-month intervals initially to ensure that the patient understands and is following the diet, and every 6 to 12 months thereafter. Each visit should include a review of the patient's diet, symptoms, and mood. Serum folic acid, carotene, 25-hydroxy vitamin D, and ferritin levels should be checked periodically if they were initially low. Monitoring the serum TTGA level yearly is recommended. It usually decreases and becomes negative after 6 to 12 months of appropriate diet therapy. An increase in titer is presumptive evidence of inadequate dietary compliance. Routine follow-up duodenal biopsies are not recommended. The occurrence of abdominal pain, weight loss, bleeding, or reoccurrence of diarrhea should be investigated with a careful history, and, if indicated, small bowel and colon biopsy, abdominal and pelvic computed tomography scan, or capsule endoscopy.

Symptomatic response to treatment often takes more than a month and may take up to 1 year. In a group of 161 patients with diarrhea as the major symptom, the cumulative response (cessation of diarrhea) after starting the diet was 3% in 1 day, 32% in 1 week, 69% in 1 month, and 87% in 6 months.

Reasons for lack of symptomatic response to dietary therapy (approximate percentages) are accidental or deliberate gluten ingestion (47%); incorrect diagnosis (10%); complication of celiac disease such as lymphoma, small bowel cancer, or ulcerative jejunitis (10%); coexisting disease such as small bowel bacterial overgrowth, lymphocytic colitis, collagenous colitis, pancreatic insufficiency, giardiasis, lactase deficiency, or irritable bowel syndrome (17%); and RCD (16%).

The definition of RCD is evolving. By strict definition, it is an enteropathy that is histologically consistent with celiac disease that either responds initially to a gluten-restricted diet but stops responding or has not responded histologically or symptomatically after 12 months of diet therapy but responds with addition of immunosuppressive therapy. Two forms of RCD are distinguished. Patients with RCD I have a normal IEL population, respond well to diet and immunosuppression, and have a good prognosis. Patients with RCD II have an abnormal (immature) IEL population, do not respond well to diet and immunosuppression, and have a generally poor outcome, many dying of disseminated enteropathy-associated T-cell lymphoma within 1 year of starting treatment. Immunosuppressant therapy for RCD has included oral corticosteroids or azathioprine and intravenous anti–tumor necrosis factor-α antibodies (infliximab). Some patients with RCD have a thickened subepithelial band of collagen, termed *collagenous celiac disease*.

Avoiding Treatment Errors

Few physicians are knowledgeable about the details of a gluten-free diet. However, the physician can and should provide the knowledge, encouragement, and resources to help the patient become committed to the diet and expert in following it. The patient must be willing to read labels even on products known previously to be free of gluten, contact pharmaceutical companies to ensure that prescription and nonprescription medications being taken are gluten free, read printed or online material written by knowledgeable individuals, plan ahead and talk with the chef when eating out, and join a support group, if available. Wheat strains and products that are forbidden and that a patient may not recognize as wheat include durham, kamut, spelt, einkorn, emmer, farro, semolina, couscous, farina, orzo, bulgar, graham flour, and triticale. Products that may contain gluten unanticipated by the patient include medications, malt, modified food starch, rice syrup, soy sauce, hydrolyzed plant protein, hydrolyzed vegetable protein, extracts, spices, ice cream, canned fruit, canned soups, many candies, imitation seafood, flavored coffees, root beer, beer and many other alcoholic drinks, envelope adhesive, lipstick, and lip balm. Wheat starch contains trace amounts of gluten and is excluded from the diet, at least in the United States.

Products that are gluten free if not contaminated include rice, corn, millet, sorghum, potato, chestnut, almond, soy, amaranth, arrowroot, buckwheat, quinoa, sweet potato, and teff. Flours from these products are usually deficient in B vitamins and iron, so patients on a gluten-free diet should be supplemented.

Occasionally a patient, because of misinformation or a compulsive nature, becomes overly cautious. So long as normal dishwashing and sanitation are practiced, it is not necessary for the patient to maintain a separate set of kitchenware, for a spouse to wash the face and brush the teeth before kissing the patient, or for the patient to avoid use of shampoos and body lotions containing gluten. Gluten peptides are too large to be absorbed through intact skin. On the other hand, significant gluten may be ingested from butter, peanut butter, or other spread contaminated with bread by a previous user or from toasting gluten-free bread in a toaster oven that is not thoroughly cleaned after being used to toast gluten-containing bread. With time and appropriate resources, the patient can become educated and careful without being excessively compulsive.

Future Directions

At a clinical level, it will be important to document the risk for asymptomatic celiac disease, the benefit and burden of treating the asymptomatic patient, and the related issue of who, if anyone, should be screened for the disease. Better documentation of the minimum toxic dose of gluten is needed. Less intrusive therapy will certainly be welcomed, including a very achievable goal of more, and more clearly labeled, gluten-free foods and drugs, and a more challenging goal of reducing or eliminating dietary restrictions. This might be accomplished by developing wheat and other grains genetically engineered to eliminate the toxic peptides, bacterial endopeptidases that digest the toxic peptides when taken orally with gluten-containing foods, and drugs that prevent the toxic peptides from entering the mucosa or activating the immune system.

Additional Resources

Celiac.com. Available at: http://www.celiac.com. Accessed October 7, 2006.
> *This site contains lists of ingredients, foods, and alcoholic beverages that are gluten-free and a list of food items forbidden on a gluten-free diet.*

Celiac Disease Awareness Campaign. Available at: http://www.celiac.nih.gov. Accessed October 7, 2006.
> *This is an NIH website for physicians and patients to increase awareness and provide up-to-date information about celiac disease.*

Celiac Disease Foundation. Available at: http://www.celiac.org. Accessed October 7, 2006.
> *This site is maintained by the Celiac Disease Foundation.*

Celiac Sprue Association. Available at: http://www.csaceliacs.org. Accessed October 7, 2006.
> *This site is maintained by the Celiac Sprue Association/USA, Inc.*

Clan Thompson's Celiac Site. Available at http://www.clanthompson.com/index.php3. Accessed October 7, 2006.
> *Clan Thompson's "Smartlist" contains gluten-free and vegetarian status on hundreds of items and is constantly updated.*

Gluten-Free Restaurant Program. Available at: http://www.glutenfreerestaurants.org. Accessed October 7, 2006.
> *This site lists restaurants that have gluten-free menu items but includes only some restaurants in some states.*

Gluten Intolerance Group. Available at: http://www.gluten.net. Accessed October 7, 2006.
> *This site is maintained by the Gluten Intolerance Group of North America. Patients who join this nonprofit organization for a yearly membership fee receive an informative quarterly newsletter and a card that can be used when eating out to help the chef identify what foods on the menu are gluten free.*

Lowell JP: The Gluten-Free Bible. New York, Henry Holt, 2005.
> *This is a comprehensive and entertaining guide.*

EVIDENCE

1. Fasano A, Berti I, Gerarduzzi T, et al: Prevalence of celiac disease in at-risk and not-at-risk groups in the United States: A large multicenter study. Arch Intern Med 163(3):286-292, 2003.

    The authors present results of a screening study of more than 13,000 U.S. subjects that established the prevalence of celiac disease among various not-at-risk and at-risk groups.

2. Abdulkarim AS, Burgart LJ, See J, Murray JA: Etiology of non-responsive celiac disease: Results of a systematic approach. Am J Gastroenterol 97(8):2016-2021, 2002.

    This study establishes the cause of clinical nonresponsiveness to gluten-free diet among 55 patients diagnosed with celiac disease.

3. Goerres MS, Meijer JW, Wahab PJ, et al: Azathioprine and prednisone combination therapy in refractory coeliac disease. Aliment Pharmacol Ther 18(5):487-494, 2003.

    This article presents the outcomes of 18 refractory celiac disease patients treated with prednisone and azathioprine, including 10 with RCD I and 8 with RCD II.

4. Green PH, Fleischauer AT, Bhagat G, et al: Risk of malignancy in patients with celiac disease. Am J Med 115(3):191-195, 2003.

    This study presents the incidence of malignancy among 381 celiac disease patients from 1981 to 2000.

5. Green PH, Jabri B: Celiac disease. Annu Rev Med 57:207-221, 2006.

    This is a current summary by one of the leaders in the field.

6. Murray JA, Watson T, Clearman B, Mitros F: Effect of a gluten-free diet on gastrointestinal symptoms in celiac disease. Am J Clin Nutr 79(4):669-673, 2004.

    This study establishes the rate of cessation of diarrhea in celiac disease patients after beginning a gluten-free diet.

7. National Institutes of Health Consensus Development Panel: National Institutes of Health Consensus Development Conference Statement on Celiac Disease, June 28-30, 2004. Gastroenterology 128(4):S1-S9, 2005.

    This statement and the remainder of the supplement summarize the available information on pathogenesis, diagnosis, and therapy as of mid-2004.

8. Marsh MN: Gluten, major histocompatibility complex, and the small intestine. A molecular and immunobiologic approach to the spectrum of gluten sensitivity (celiac sprue). Gastroenterology 102:330-354, 1992.

    The author presents a widely accepted classification of the histologic changes seen in the intestinal mucosa in celiac disease.

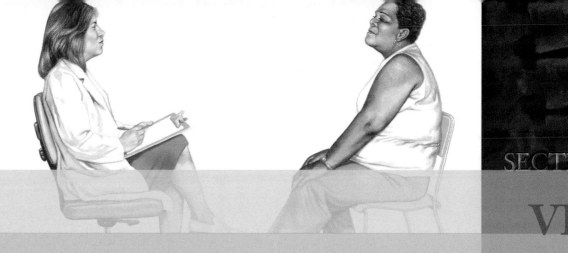

Disorders of Coagulation and Thrombosis

Stephan Moll

Hypercoagulable States

Introduction

Hypercoagulable states are conditions that predispose to thrombosis. They can be inherited or acquired. Thrombophilia is the tendency to develop thromboses. Formerly, idiopathic thrombosis characterized a thrombosis in which an underlying hypercoagulable state could not be identified. The term is best avoided because many cases of so-called idiopathic thrombosis can now be attributed to one or more of the known thrombophilias and, thus, are not truly unexplained any more. Thromboses can be separated into those associated with transient risk factors and those not associated with transient risk factors.

Etiology and Pathogenesis

Overview

In hypercoagulable states, an imbalance between the procoagulant and fibrinolytic mechanisms may lead to thrombosis. Several known disturbances of plasmatic coagulation result predominantly in venous thromboembolism (Box 66-1). Relatively little is known about disturbances in blood vessel wall and platelet function that lead to hypercoagulability. About half of patients with venous thromboembolism without transient risk factors have an inherited or acquired thrombophilia (Table 66-1). Patients with arterial thromboembolism do not usually have an identifiable hypercoagulable abnormality (Box 66-2). Thrombosis is a multifactorial process, with environmental and lifestyle factors, as well as inherited and acquired thrombophilias.

The Individual Thrombophilias

Factor V Leiden

Factor V Leiden is a point mutation in the coagulation factor V gene, discovered in 1994 and named for the city of Leiden, the Netherlands. It is the most common known inherited risk factor for venous thromboembolism. The mutation results in a factor V protein (Arg506Gln) that cannot be normally inactivated by its physiologic inactivator, activated protein C (APC), thus causing APC resistance. It is the most common inherited risk factor for venous thromboembolism (Fig. 66-1). The heterozygous state is a mild risk factor for venous thrombosis (risk increased 3-fold); the homozygous state is associated with a higher risk (increased 18-fold). Factor V Leiden is not a risk factor for arterial events, except in young women who smoke tobacco. Found primarily in whites, the mutation does not occur in native Africans or Asians. About 5% of the general U.S. population and, due to mixture of races, 1.2% of the African American population is heterozygous for factor V Leiden.

Prothrombin 20210 Mutation

The prothrombin 20210 mutation, a point mutation in the noncoding sequence of the prothrombin gene (G20210A), is associated with elevated prothrombin (factor II) levels. Discovered in 1996, it is the second most common inherited risk factor for venous thromboembolism (see Table 66-1). It is a mild risk factor for venous thromboembolism (risk in heterozygotes increased 2-fold to 4.8-fold compared with individuals without this mutation), but is not a risk factor for arterial thrombosis. The mutation is found in the same population as the factor V Leiden mutation; 2.3% of the overall U.S. population and 0.5% of the African American population is heterozygous for the mutation.

Protein C Deficiency

Protein C deficiency, a moderate risk factor for venous thromboembolism (risk is 7 to 15 times increased compared with a control population), is caused by a multitude of mutations. However, clinical penetrance is variable, and selected families are at greater risk. Arterial thrombosis is less common in individuals with protein C deficiency than venous events.

Protein S Deficiency

Protein S deficiency is a mild risk factor for venous thromboembolism and increases the risk for venous thromboembolism about twofold. However, the clinical picture is variable among families. Arterial thrombosis is less common in individuals with protein S deficiency than venous events. It is caused by a large number of different mutations.

Antithrombin

Antithrombin deficiency is associated with venous thromboembolism, less commonly with arterial events, and has variable clinical penetrance. Selected families are at high risk, and half of individuals in these families have thromboses before the age of 30 years. Overall, antithrombin deficiency appears to be a moderate to strong risk factor for venous thromboembolic disease, but accurate risk estimates are not available because the disorder is uncommon. A variety of different mutations lead to the deficiency.

Homocystinuria and Homocystinemia

Homocystinuria is a rare homocysteine metabolism disturbance in children, leading to extremely high serum homocysteine levels. Fifty percent of these patients have arterial or venous thromboses before the age of 30 years. Homocystinemia is a disorder of mildly to moderately increased

---

Box 66-1 Hypercoagulable States Predisposing to Venous Thromboembolism

Acquired

Surgery, trauma, prolonged immobilization
Older age
Obesity, smoking
Hormones (oral contraceptives, pregnancy, hormone replacement therapy)
Malignancy, chemotherapy
Previous venous thromboembolism
Inflammatory disorders (Crohn's disease, ulcerative colitis)
Myeloproliferative disorders
Hyperhomocysteinemia (inherited or acquired)
Antiphospholipid antibodies (see Fig. 66-2)
    Anticardiolipin antibodies
    Lupus anticoagulant
    Anti-β_2-glycoprotein I antibodies
Paroxysmal nocturnal hemoglobinuria

Inherited

Factor V Leiden (G1691A mutation)
Prothrombin G20210A mutation
Protein C deficiency
Protein S deficiency
Antithrombin deficiency
Rare causes (e.g., dysfibrinogenemia, elevated PAI1 levels)
Elevated levels of factor VIII, factor IX, factor XI, or fibrinogen (inherited or acquired)
Factor XIII Val34 Leu polymorphism (protective against venous thromboembolism)

Box 66-2 Hypercoagulable States Predisposing to Arterial Thromboembolism

Acquired

Arteriosclerosis
Vasculitis
Heparin-induced thrombocytopenia
Thrombotic thrombocytopenic purpura (acquired or inherited)
Hemolytic-uremic syndrome (usually acquired)
Hyperhomocysteinemia (acquired or inherited)
Antiphospholipid antibodies (see Fig. 66-2)
    Lupus anticoagulant
    Anticardiolipin antibodies
    Anti-β_2-glycoprotein I antibodies

Inherited

Deficiency of protein C, protein S, antithrombin
Rare causes (dysfibrinogenemia)
Elevated levels of fibrinogen, factor VIII, and von Willebrand factor (inherited or acquired)
Factor XIII Val34 Leu polymorphism (protective effect against arterial thromboembolism)

Table 66-1 Prevalence of Hypercoagulable States in Venous Thromboembolism

Hypercoagulable State	Prevalence in Unselected Patients with Venous Thromboembolism (%)	Prevalence in Patients with Venous Thromboembolism without Transient* Risk Factors (%)
Protein C deficiency	3	1-9
Protein S deficiency	1-2	1-13
Antithrombin III deficiency	1	0.5-7
Factor V Leiden	12-21	52
Prothrombin 20210 mutation	6	16-19
Hyperhomocysteinemia	10-14	18.8
Antiphospholipid antibodies	8.5-14	No reliable studies available

* Transient risk factors: surgery, trauma, and immobilization.

Figure 66-1 Factor V Leiden and Prothrombin 20210 Mutations.

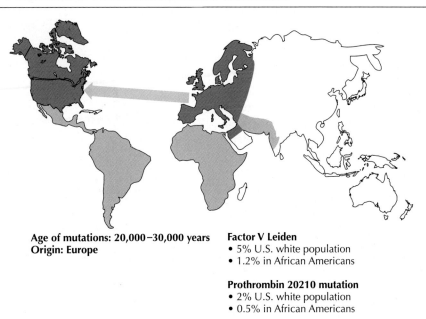

Age of mutations: 20,000–30,000 years
Origin: Europe

Factor V Leiden
• 5% U.S. white population
• 1.2% in African Americans

Prothrombin 20210 mutation
• 2% U.S. white population
• 0.5% in African Americans

serum homocysteine levels, associated with an increased risk for venous thromboembolism, arteriosclerosis, and arterial thromboembolism. Elevated levels may also be found in patients with a homozygous mutation in the methylene-tetrahydrofolate reductase gene (thermolabile C677T MTHFR) and individuals double heterozygous for the C677T MTHFR and A1298C MTHFR polymorphisms; however, these mutations are not risk factors for thromboembolic disease by themselves if homocysteine levels are normal. Elevated homocysteine levels can be decreased in many individuals with folic acid, or a combination of folic acid, vitamin B_6, and vitamin B_{12}. However, lowering of the homocysteine level does not lead to a decreased risk for arterial or venous thrombosis.

Antiphospholipid Antibody Syndrome

Antiphospholipid antibody (APLA) syndrome is defined as the occurrence of thrombosis (arterial or venous) or recurrent pregnancy loss in patients with repeatedly positive APLA tests (see Fig. 66-2). It occurs as the primary APLA syndrome not associated with any other diseases, or as the secondary APLA syndrome, associated with autoimmune diseases, malignancy, or drugs (see Chapter 152).

Diagnostic Approach

Opinions vary about what constitutes an appropriate workup and who requires testing. If testing is done, then appropriate timing of testing and correct interpretation of test results are essential, as is education of the patient and family about thrombophilia in the case of an inherited disorder.

In venous thromboembolism not associated with surgery, trauma, or prolonged immobilization, the following tests may be helpful: factor V Leiden, prothrombin 20210 mutation, protein C activity, protein S activity, antithrombin activity, homocysteine level, and antiphospholipid antibodies (lupus anticoagulant, anticardiolipin immunoglobulin G [IgG] and immunoglobulin M [IgM] antibodies, anti-β_2-glycoprotein I antibodies). Malignancy as an underlying contributor to the thromboembolism warrants consideration and evaluation using a thorough medical history, physical examination, and appropriate screening tests.

In unexplained arterial thromboembolic events, thrombophilia tests may include protein C activity, protein S activity, antithrombin activity, homocysteine, and antiphospholipid antibodies (lupus anticoagulant, anticardiolipin IgG and IgM antibodies, anti-β_2-glycoprotein I antibodies). A lipid profile (low-density lipoprotein, cholesterol, triglycerides, lipoprotein-a) may also be appropriate to assess for risk factors of premature arteriosclerosis. Furthermore, a thorough evaluation of all causes of arterial thromboembolism (e.g., arteriosclerosis, intracardiac thrombus, atrial fibrillation, patent foramen ovale) is important.

The diagnosis of factor V Leiden is made by either genetic (polymerase chain reaction) or coagulation (APC resistance) testing. APC resistance and factor V Leiden are not synonyms; 5% to 10% of patients with APC resistance do not have factor V Leiden, but another abnormality, such as a lupus anticoagulant, that interferes with the APC-resistance assay. An abnormal APC resistance test should be followed by the genetic test for factor V Leiden.

A normal APC resistance test excludes the presence of factor V Leiden and does not need to be followed by a genetic test.

The diagnosis of prothrombin 20210 mutation is made by genetic testing (polymerase chain reaction). Factor II activity levels are not helpful.

The evaluation of protein C deficiency requires measurement of protein C activity levels, also referred to as *functional protein C*. Obtaining only a protein C antigen level will miss the occasional functional protein C deficiency that is caused by a dysfunctional protein. Protein C activity levels are low in patients taking vitamin K antagonists (e.g., warfarin, phenprocoumon). Levels normalize up to 2 weeks after discontinuation of warfarin. They are also low in liver disease.

Protein S circulates in the plasma in two forms: bound to the transport protein C4b–binding protein, and unbound, as free protein S. Only the free protein is enzymatically active. Tests include protein S activity (*functional protein S*), free protein S antigen, and total protein S antigen. Obtaining only free or total protein S antigen levels is insufficient to exclude protein S deficiency, because a patient may have normal protein S antigen levels, but a functional deficiency caused by a dysfunctional protein S molecule. Low protein S activity levels occur in patients taking oral contraceptives or hormone replacement therapy, during pregnancy, during oral anticoagulant treatment, in the setting of liver synthetic dysfunction, and at the time of an acute thrombotic event. Congenital protein S deficiency cannot be diagnosed under these circumstances. Levels normalize up to 3 weeks after discontinuation of oral anticoagulants.

Antithrombin activity can be low in the acute setting of a thromboembolism, during heparin therapy, in patients with liver synthetic dysfunction, and in nephrotic syndrome. Low levels in these circumstances do not necessarily indicate congenital antithrombin deficiency.

Plasma homocysteine levels increase after a protein-rich diet, but the change is typically less than 10% from baseline, an elevation that, for practical purposes outside of clinical studies, is not relevant. Because the MTHFR polymorphisms do not appear to be associated with arterial or venous thromboembolism, nor with pregnancy complications, there is no clinical indication to test for them if homocysteine levels are normal.

APLAs are a heterogeneous group of antibodies (Fig. 66-2) that can be detected in the laboratory by either functional coagulation assays (*lupus anticoagulant*) or enzyme-linked immunosorbent assay (e.g., anticardiolipin and anti-β₂-glycoprotein I antibodies). These tests are discussed in detail elsewhere (see Chapter 152).

Testing for rare causes of thrombophilia, such as dysfibrinogenemia, plasminogen deficiency, paroxysmal nocturnal hemoglobinemia, and myeloproliferative disorders is preferably done after consultation with a thrombophilia specialist.

Figure 66-2 Antiphospholipid Antibodies.

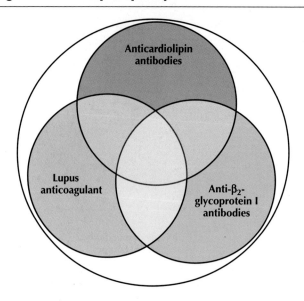

Management and Therapy

Optimum Treatment

The presence or absence of certain thrombophilic risk factors may have bearing on the length of anticoagulant treatment after venous thromboembolism and on the accuracy of anticoagulation monitoring (in the case of the presence of antiphospholipid antibodies), and may have implications for other family members. Management and therapy of various arterial and venous thromboembolic problems are discussed in the other chapters of this book (see Chapters 29, 31, 67, and 125). Referral for evaluation in a specialized thrombophilia center deserves careful consideration for patients with spontaneous or unusual thrombotic events and for asymptomatic individuals with known thrombophilia. The opportunity to perform thrombophilia testing brings the responsibility to counsel patients and their families about the implications of positive or negative test results and to educate them about their thrombophilia. Some patient education tools are available on the Internet.

Avoiding Treatment Errors

Knowledge of the factors that cause false-positive and false-negative test results (Table 66-2; Box 66-3) is important to avoid labeling a patient with a thrombophilia that the patient does not have, or missing the presence of a thrombophilia.

Future Directions

Significant developments in thrombophilia include the identification of new genetic polymorphisms and haplotypes that predispose carriers to venous or arterial thromboembolism, and the performance of clinical studies that

Table 66-2 Influence of Acute Thrombosis, Heparin, and Warfarin on Thrombophilia Test Results

Test	Acute Thrombosis	Unfractionated Heparin	Low Molecular Weight Heparin	Vitamin K Antagonists
Factor V Leiden genetic test	Reliable	Reliable	Reliable	Reliable
Activated protein C resistance assay	Reliable[1]	Caveat[2]	Caveat[2]	Reliable[1]
Prothrombin 20210 genetic test	Reliable	Reliable	Reliable	Reliable
Protein C activity or antigen	Caveat[3]	Reliable	Reliable	Low
Protein S activity or antigen	May be low	Reliable	Reliable	Low
Antithrombin activity	May be low	May be low	May be low	May be elevated
Lupus anticoagulant	Reliable[4]	Caveat[5]	Caveat[5]	Caveat[5]
Anticardiolipin antibodies	Reliable[4]	Reliable	Reliable	Reliable
Homocysteine	Reliable	Reliable	Reliable	Reliable
Factor VIII antigen or activity	High[6]	Reliable	Reliable	Reliable
Factor IX antigen or activity	Reliable[6]	Reliable	Reliable	Low
Factor XI antigen or activity	Reliable[6]	Reliable	Reliable	Reliable

[1] Reliable if the assay is performed with factor V–depleted plasma; thus, the clinician needs to inquire how the individual laboratory performs the assay.
[2] Depending on the way the assay is performed, results may be unreliable; the health care provider needs to contact the laboratory and ask how the specific test performs on heparin.
[3] Probably reliable, but limited data in literature.
[4] Test often positive or elevated at time of acute thrombosis, but subsequently negative. *Data from Paramthosy K: Prevalence of antiphospholipid antibodies in idiopathic venous thromboembolism. Blood 104:153a, 2004.*
[5] Although many test kits used for lupus anticoagulant testing contain a heparin neutralizer that inactivates unfractionated heparin (UF) and possibly low molecular weight heparin (LMWH), thus making these tests reliable on UF and LMWH, clinicians need to inquire with their laboratory how their individual test kit performs in samples with UF and LMWH.
[6] No indication for testing in the acute setting.
From Moll S. Thrombophilias: Practical implications and testing caveats. J Thromb Thrombolysis 21(1):7-15, 2006.

Box 66-3 Conditions Leading to Acquired Coagulation Factor Deficiencies

- Liver disease: decreased protein C, protein S, and antithrombin
- Warfarin therapy: decreased protein C and protein S
- Estrogens (oral contraceptives, pregnancy, postpartum state, hormone replacement therapy): decreased protein S
- Inflammatory diseases: decreased protein S
- Acute thrombosis: decreased antithrombin and protein S
- Heparin therapy: decreased antithrombin

From Moll S. Thrombophilias: Practical implications and testing caveats. J Thromb Thrombolysis 21(1):7-15, 2006.

assess the risk for recurrent thrombosis in patients with various thrombophilias. These studies should also help determine the optimal length and intensity of oral anticoagulant treatment. Patients will also benefit from the formation of comprehensive thrombophilia treatment centers and an active national patient advocacy group, such as the National Alliance for Thrombosis and Thrombophilia.

Additional Resources

National Alliance for Thrombosis and Thrombophilia (NATT). Available at: http://www.nattinfo.org. Accessed May 22, 2007.
The NATT website is primarily for patients and public, but also has a section for health care providers that allows them to print peer-reviewed educational materials on topics surrounding diagnosis and management of thrombosis and thrombophilia, to be used as handout materials in hospitals and clinics.

Thrombophilia Support Page. Available at: http://www.fvleiden.org/. Accessed May 22, 2007.
This education website is primarily for patients with thrombosis or thrombophilia, but also provides information suitable for health care providers. It provides a question-and-answer section, which discusses clinically relevant topics.

EVIDENCE

1. Gris JC, Lissalde-Lavigne G, Quere I, et al: Prophylaxis and treatment of thrombophilia in pregnancy. Curr Opin Hematol 13(5):376-381, 2006.
   This article provides a useful summary of the data on pregnancy complications related to thrombophilia and the use of anticoagulants to prevent or treat them.
2. Moll S: Thrombophilias: Practical implications and testing caveats. J Thromb Thrombolysis 21(1):7-15, 2006.
   This clinically oriented summary includes the most common thrombophilias, their clinical relevance, and practical aspects pertaining to testing, such as when and what to test and causes of false-positive and false-negative test results.
3. Varga E: Inherited thrombophilia: Key points for genetic counseling. J Genet Couns 16(3):261-277, 2007.
   This detailed and clinically useful review educates the genetic counselor on risk assessment and genetic counseling for hereditary thrombophilia.
4. Wu O, Robertson L, Twaddle S, et al: Screening for thrombophilia in high-risk situations: Systematic review and cost-effectiveness analysis. The Thrombosis Risk and Economic Assessment of Thrombophilia Screening (TREATS) study. Health Technol Assess 10(11):1-110, 2006.
   This is an exhaustive presentation of published data on thrombophilic risk associated with the various thrombophilias, including assessments and conclusions on populations to screen.

Darren A. DeWalt ▪ Marschall S. Runge

67

Deep Venous Thrombosis and Pulmonary Embolism

Introduction

Deep venous thrombosis (DVT) and pulmonary embolism (PE) are the two most important clinical events that occur in individuals with venous thrombosis. Approximately 0.1% of the population will experience a DVT, and PE is the third leading cause of cardiovascular mortality. Early diagnosis and treatment of DVT and PE substantially reduce mortality and morbidity, but autopsy series consistently find that DVT and PE are still underdiagnosed. The numerous publications of algorithms aimed at improving diagnostic accuracy and optimizing treatment illustrate the frequency with which both DVT and PE elude diagnosis. In this chapter, we review the various presentations of these syndromes and provide an overview of the most promising modalities for early diagnosis and treatment.

Etiology and Pathogenesis

Deep venous thromboses may occur anywhere in the venous system, but most begin in the lower extremities between the lower leg and the pelvis. Virchow's classic triad of vessel wall injury, stasis, and hypercoagulability is as relevant today as when proposed for understanding the pathogenesis and risk factors for thrombosis. Both stasis and vessel wall injury can lead to platelet aggregation, which triggers the clotting cascade, including cellular and protein components. This can result in an imbalance in the naturally occurring procoagulant and anticoagulant proteins, and formation of an intravascular thrombus. Chapter 66 describes this complex system in more detail.

Although pulmonary emboli usually result from embolization of thrombi in the venous system of the lower extremities or pelvis, one must also consider the inferior vena cava (IVC), renal or upper extremity veins, and even the right side of the heart as potential sources of pulmonary emboli (Fig. 67-1). Thrombi can also form in smaller veins below the popliteal vein, but these thrombi rarely embolize, and thus present a low risk.

Many of the classic risk factors for DVT or PE affect one aspect of Virchow's triad (Fig. 67-2). Immobility from surgery, trauma, or paralysis can lead to stasis because venous flow in the lower extremities is partially dependent on muscular contraction. By entirely different mechanisms, surgery, trauma, or infection can cause vessel wall injury. Additionally, most malignancies are accompanied by some degree of hypercoagulability, a complication particularly well documented in mucinous adenocarcinomas and referred to as *Trousseau's syndrome*.

Another common cause of DVT involves pregnancy; the combination of a hypercoagulable state, local venous stasis (from the uterus compressing the IVC), and immobility (e.g., with travel) is a common setting for DVT in individuals who have none of the above risk factors. Indeed, other identified hypercoagulable states are increasing in number and are discussed in Chapter 66. Understanding the settings in which DVT and PE occur may offer the clinician a clue toward diagnosis. However, it is important to consider the clinical findings (Tables 67-1 and 67-2), particularly for patients with no known precipitants.

Clinical Presentation

Patients with DVT or PE present with a spectrum of symptoms ranging from mild tenderness or swelling in the calf to acute dyspnea and syncope. A careful history may reveal one or more of the predisposing risk factors listed

Figure 67-1 Deep Venous Thrombosis.

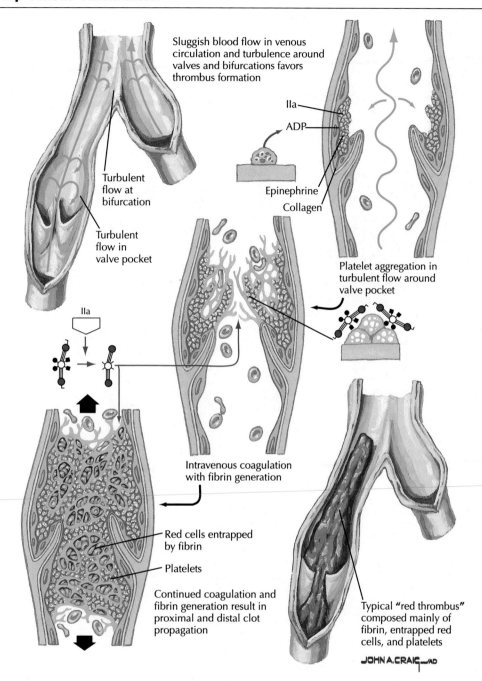

Sluggish blood flow in venous circulation and turbulence around valves and bifurcations favors thrombus formation

IIa

ADP

Epinephrine

Collagen

Turbulent flow at bifurcation

Turbulent flow in valve pocket

Platelet aggregation in turbulent flow around valve pocket

IIa

Intravenous coagulation with fibrin generation

Red cells entrapped by fibrin

Platelets

Continued coagulation and fibrin generation result in proximal and distal clot propagation

Typical "red thrombus" composed mainly of fibrin, entrapped red cells, and platelets

JOHN A. CRAIG—AD

in Tables 67-1 and 67-2. The classic constellation of symptoms for an isolated DVT includes unilateral leg symptoms of swelling, tenderness, and dilated collateral veins. As previously noted, most patients do not present with this complete set of findings, making early diagnosis more challenging. It is important to remember, however, that about 40% of patients with isolated DVT will have asymptomatic PEs on ventilation-perfusion ($\dot{V}/\dot{Q}$) scans. For this reason, patients with either DVT or PE should be considered to have both until proved otherwise.

The more ominous presentation of PE may (but does not invariably) include the symptoms of DVT and also reflects the effect of acute cessation of perfusion to parts of the lung. The sudden onset of dyspnea and tachycardia may be the initial clue (Fig. 67-3). Other common symptoms and signs include chest pain (pleuritic or nonpleuritic), hemoptysis, pleural rub, hypoxemia, or fever (less than 38.9°C). A patient who also has syncope, hypotension, or signs of new-onset right-sided heart failure falls into the category of severe PE. At highest risk are those patients

Figure 67-2 Predisposing Factors for Pulmonary Embolism.

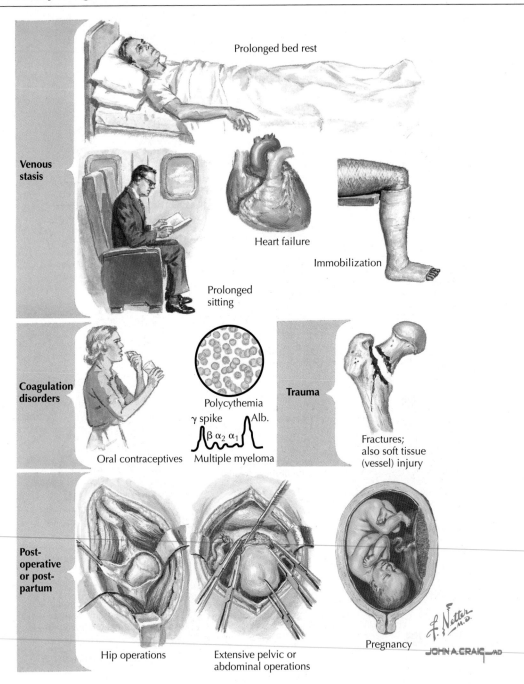

Prolonged bed rest

Venous stasis

Heart failure

Immobilization

Prolonged sitting

Coagulation disorders

Polycythemia

γ spike   Alb.

β α₂ α₁

Oral contraceptives   Multiple myeloma

Trauma

Fractures; also soft tissue (vessel) injury

Post-operative or post-partum

Pregnancy

Hip operations   Extensive pelvic or abdominal operations

with PE who present with hemodynamic compromise. One should always include PE in the differential diagnosis for patients presenting in cardiogenic shock until another cause is proved.

Differential Diagnosis

Many processes can masquerade as a DVT or PE and, thus, should be kept in mind while proceeding through diagnostic algorithms. One of the most important factors in determining the probability of DVT or PE is the likelihood of a competing diagnosis. For DVT, the most common competing diagnoses are muscle strain or leg injury, venous insufficiency, lymphatic obstruction, popliteal cyst, drug-induced edema, and cellulitis. The differential diagnosis of dyspnea and tachycardia is also quite long and includes pneumonia, congestive heart failure, myocardial infarction, chronic obstructive pulmonary disease, pulmonary hemorrhage, and aspiration pneumonitis. One of the first steps in the diagnosis of DVT or PE is to assess the likelihood that one of the competing diag-

Table 67-1 Clinical Model for Predicting Pretest Probability for Deep Venous Thrombosis

Clinical Feature	Score
Active cancer (treatment ongoing or within previous 6 months or palliative)	1
Paralysis, paresis, or recent plaster immobilization of the lower extremities	1
Recently bedridden for >3 days or major surgery within 4 weeks	1
Localized tenderness along the distribution of the deep venous system	1
Entire leg swollen	1
Increased calf swelling (>3 cm in circumference comparing affected vs asymptomatic side; measured 10 cm below tibial tuberosity)	1
Pitting edema confined to the symptomatic leg	1
Collateral superficial veins (nonvaricose)	1
Alternative diagnosis as likely or greater than that of DVT	−2

DVT, deep vein thrombosis. In patients with symptoms in both legs, the more symptomatic leg is used. Pretest probability calculated as the total score: high ≥3; moderate 1 or 2; low ≤0. *Adapted from Wells PS, Anderson DR, Bormanis J, et al: Value of assessment of pretest probability of deep-vein thrombosis in clinical management. Lancet 350(9094):1795-1798, 1997.*

Table 67-2 Algorithm to Determine Pretest Probability of Pulmonary Embolism

Clinical Feature	Score
Clinical symptoms of DVT	3
Heart rate >100 beats/min	1.5
Immobilization or surgery in the previous 4 weeks	1.5
Previous objectively diagnosed DVT or PE	1.5
Hemoptysis	1
Malignancy	1
PE as likely as or more likely than an alternative diagnosis	3

DVT, deep vein thrombosis; PE, pulmonary embolism. Probability: high >6 pts, moderate 2 to 6 pts, low <2 pts. *Adapted from Wells PS, Anderson DR, Rodger M, et al: Excluding pulmonary embolism at the bedside without diagnostic imaging: Management of patients with suspected pulmonary embolism presenting to the emergency department by using a simple clinical model and D-dimer. Ann Intern Med 135(2):98-107, 2001.*

noses accounts for the symptoms and physical examination findings.

Diagnostic Approach

The most accurate and cost-effective approach to the diagnosis of DVT and PE remains an active area of research and a challenge for clinicians. Currently, most authors recommend algorithms that combine the pretest probability with careful selection of diagnostic tests. Because DVT and PE are commonly missed, these diagnoses must be kept in mind until proved otherwise. This does not mandate comprehensive testing for a given patient, but the pretest probability for DVT and PE increases in circumstances when other leading diagnoses are excluded in the course of the initial assessment.

Deep Venous Thrombosis

The diagnostic evaluation for suspected DVT should begin with an assessment of the pretest probability. Countless models have been proposed. The most widely used model was developed by Wells and associates (see Table 67-1). Unfortunately, because of varied presentations, the clinical diagnosis of DVT is very inaccurate, leading to difficulty establishing an accurate pretest probability. This issue is presented in greater detail in Chapter 3. Pretest probability is extremely important, however, in interpreting the results of noninvasive tests for DVT (as in other clinical syndromes), as described later.

The options for objective testing include D-dimer, compression venous ultrasonography, impedance plethysmography, and contrast venography. Contrast venography remains the gold standard for the diagnosis of DVT, and compression venous ultrasonography has largely replaced impedance plethysmography as the noninvasive diagnostic test of choice. The accuracy of compression venous ultrasonography has greatly reduced the need for contrast venography.

The D-dimer assays measure a degradation product of cross-linked fibrin and are commonly used in assessment of DVT. Theoretically, any patient with active coagulation should have an elevated D-dimer, suggesting the usefulness of a negative result to rule out DVT. Clinically, the D-dimer can sufficiently lower the probability of DVT in the low-risk group to avoid proceeding with ultrasound. In the moderate- and high-risk groups, the false-negative rate of the D-dimer is too high to render it useful. For patients in the moderate- or high-risk group, clinicians should proceed directly to ultrasound. Additionally, a positive result on a D-dimer test is woefully nonspecific and cannot be used to diagnose DVT. Certain patient groups are known to have especially high rates of false-positive results, including hospitalized patients and those who have had recent surgery or malignancy.

Compression venous ultrasonography leads the list of noninvasive tests for the diagnosis of DVT. A positive test result occurs when the femoral or popliteal veins are noncompressible under ultrasound visualization. The ability to perform this test in a timely manner is the most difficult barrier because most studies must be done during normal working hours. The sensitivity and specificity of this test have been reported to be as high as 95% and 96%, respectively, for symptomatic, proximal DVT, although this clearly depends on the skill and experience of the technolo-

Figure 67-3 Embolism of Lesser Degree without Infarction.

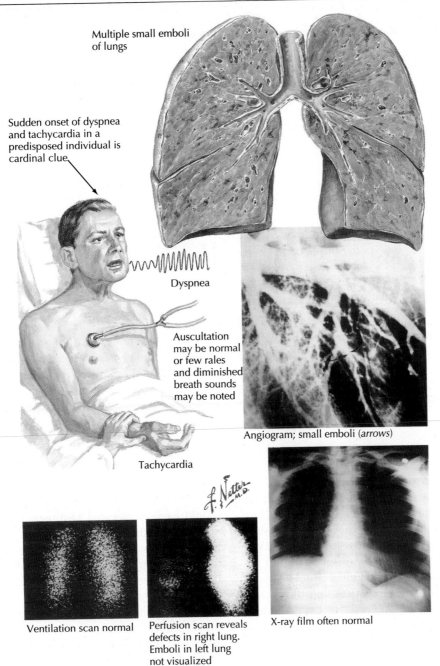

Multiple small emboli of lungs

Sudden onset of dyspnea and tachycardia in a predisposed individual is cardinal clue

Dyspnea

Auscultation may be normal or few rales and diminished breath sounds may be noted

Tachycardia

Angiogram; small emboli (*arrows*)

Ventilation scan normal

Perfusion scan reveals defects in right lung. Emboli in left lung not visualized

X-ray film often normal

gist and interpreting physician. For the diagnosis of isolated thrombosis in the calf vein, sensitivity and specificities are 60% to 70%, but as previously described, patients with only distal thromboses are at very low risk. When the ultrasound result confirms the clinical suspicion, one can stop further testing and proceed with therapy. Another test is required only if there is discord between the clinical suspicion and the ultrasound result.

Contrast venography is occasionally needed as the arbiter of discordant results between the clinical predictor model and the initial ultrasound. If a patient is thought to be at low risk, but has a positive ultrasound, venography is used to confirm the result. A negative venogram will abrogate long-term anticoagulation. Alternatively, if clinical suspicion is high but the ultrasound result is negative, most clinicians will consider venography to be certain that the ultrasound did not yield a false-negative result. The use of serial ultrasound examinations instead of venography has been proposed, but expert opinion varies on the efficacy of this approach, and head-to-head comparisons are limited. Certainly, this approach is preferable in individuals at risk for contrast dye nephropathy or with known dye allergy.

Figure 67-4 Massive Embolization.

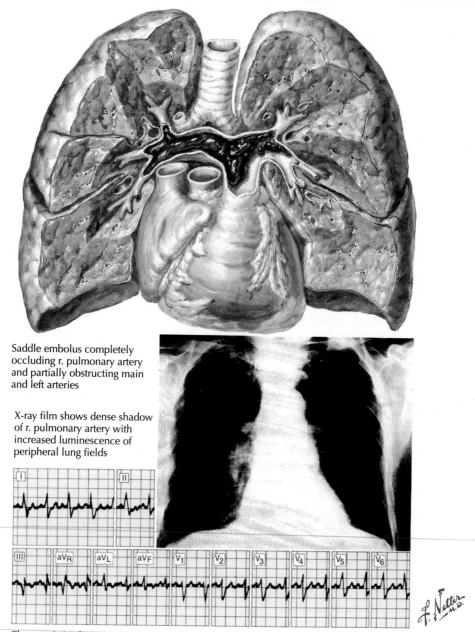

Saddle embolus completely occluding r. pulmonary artery and partially obstructing main and left arteries

X-ray film shows dense shadow of r. pulmonary artery with increased luminescence of peripheral lung fields

Characteristic electrocardiographic findings in acute pulmonary embolism. Deep S_1; prominent Q_3 with inversion of T_3; depression of S-T segment in lead II (often also in lead I) with staircase ascent of S-T_2; T_2 diphasic or inverted; r. axis deviation; tachycardia

Serial duplex examinations should be considered 7 days after the initial workup.

Pulmonary Embolism

The diagnosis of PE begins in the same manner—with an assessment of the clinical probability of disease (see Fig. 67-3). Table 67-2 is a useful set of clinical criteria to determine pretest probability of PE. The last item is determined by the physician based on all available clinical data, includ-ing history, physical examination, electrocardiography (ECG), and chest radiography. In the initial study of this tool, patients in the high-risk group had an incidence of 41%; the moderate-risk group, 16%; and the low-risk group, 1.3%.

The ECG does not reliably diagnose PE, but it may offer clues to its presence. The classic ECG finding of S1Q3T3 is infrequently present, and nonspecific ST- or T-wave changes appear more commonly (Fig. 67-4). Evidence of new right ventricular strain or right-axis deviation

can be an early marker for massive PE. The ECG can also help determine whether other differential diagnoses, particularly myocardial infarction, are present.

The chest radiograph is mainly helpful in identifying other diagnoses and lessening the likelihood that the presentation is caused by PE. The classic findings of pulmonary infarct that have been described (Hampton's hump or a dilated proximal pulmonary artery) are rarely seen.

The D-dimer test occupies the same place in the workup of PE as it does for DVT. In a patient in the lowest risk group, a negative D-dimer makes the presence of a PE unlikely. In any other group of patients, the D-dimer is not useful.

The imaging procedures for the determination of PE are computed tomography (CT) scan, $\dot{V}/\dot{Q}$ scan, and pulmonary angiography.

The contrast-enhanced CT scan has gained rapid acceptance in the diagnosis of PE and has decreased the use of $\dot{V}/\dot{Q}$ scanning for most groups of patients. The CT has a high specificity and sensitivity for emboli in the proximal pulmonary arteries and the large branches, and is constantly improving in the diagnosis of subsegmental defects. A recent meta-analysis suggests that the CT scan is sufficiently sensitive and specific to use in diagnosis of PE. For patients with a high clinical suspicion of PE, a negative CT result should be followed with additional testing such as lower extremity ultrasound or pulmonary angiogram. The CT can be used in settings where underlying lung pathology makes $\dot{V}/\dot{Q}$ scanning difficult to interpret and can be helpful for evaluating other suspected diagnoses. One important limitation of CT scanning is that it requires the administration of venous contrast material, which may be contraindicated in some groups of patients. The CT scan has largely replaced the $\dot{V}/\dot{Q}$ scan in clinical practice.

The $\dot{V}/\dot{Q}$ scan remains a reliable noninvasive test for diagnosis of PE. The possible test results include normal, low probability, intermediate probability, and high probability. A normal $\dot{V}/\dot{Q}$ scan will eliminate the possibility of PE, and a high probability scan will diagnose PE. Low or intermediate probability scans lack the accuracy to either dismiss the diagnosis of PE entirely or to begin therapy, and, depending on the clinical setting, may mandate further testing. Many other illnesses can complicate interpretation of the test, including neoplasm, infection, and heart failure. A normal baseline radiograph increases the chances that the $\dot{V}/\dot{Q}$ scan will yield useful results. In our institution, many of our complicated patients, for whom knowing a diagnosis is essential, will be placed in the low or intermediate category and require further testing.

As for DVT, angiography remains the gold standard for the diagnosis of PE. This invasive procedure requires passage of a catheter into the pulmonary arteries and injection of contrast under fluoroscopy. The mortality risk of pulmonary angiography is less than 0.5% in skilled hands, and thus is far less than the complications of misdiagnosis of PE. Delaying anticoagulation in patients with thrombus can be disastrous, and chronic unnecessary anticoagulation should be avoided. Thus, any patient with a high clinical suspicion of PE but an ambiguous diagnosis should undergo pulmonary angiography.

In the stable patient, an often reasonable alternative is to perform lower-extremity venous ultrasonography. Although not all PEs result from DVT, the presence of DVT offers confirmatory evidence that, in the presence of appropriate symptoms, the patient has had a PE.

Management and Therapy

Optimum Treatment

The recommendations for therapy for DVT and PE are currently the same, except for very large PEs, or PEs in the presence of hemodynamic compromise. The efficacy of anticoagulation is clear, but controversies remain over the acute management of DVT and PE and the necessary length of long-term anticoagulation. Both of these are addressed in the American College of Chest Physicians (ACCP) guidelines in more detail.

Acute management of DVT and PE requires administration of heparin. Multiple studies have evaluated the effectiveness of continuous-infusion unfractionated heparin (UH) and low-molecular-weight heparin (LMWH), both of which are indirect thrombin inhibitors (requiring the presence of antithrombin III). Most authorities consider both therapies effective for DVT and hemodynamically stable PE. Many hospitals have developed standard protocols for the administration of UH, and we strongly support this approach. At our hospital, UH is started with a bolus dose of 80 IU/kg and a continuous infusion of 18 IU/kg/hr. The activated partial thromboplastin time (aPTT) should be checked 6 hours after initiation and the dose of heparin adjusted to reach an aPTT of 1.5 to 2.3 times normal. Studies have demonstrated that subcutaneous UH can be administered twice daily as an alternative to intravenous UH. Most guidelines (including the ACCP guidelines) recommend giving a 5000-unit intravenous bolus followed by 17,500 units subcutaneously twice daily.

Many physicians prefer LMWH because of its ease of administration (subcutaneously once or twice daily) and because therapeutic monitoring is not usually required. Several studies indicate that LMWH is at least as effective as UH for the treatment of DVT and PE. Because LMWH is subject to renal clearance, it is not recommended for patients with renal failure. In stable patients, LMWH can be given on an outpatient basis. Note that different preparations of LMWH vary in their relative antithrombin and anti-Xa activities, and they may not be readily interchangeable. Altogether, however, the only reason that LMWH is not the clear treatment of choice for patients with DVT and PE is its cost, which is much higher than that of UH.

Table 67-3 Duration of Anticoagulation for Deep Venous Thrombosis and Pulmonary Embolism

3 months	First event with reversible or time-limited risk factor
≥6 months	First episode of DVT/PE with documented deficiency of protein C or protein S, or the factor V Leiden or prothrombin 20210 gene mutation, homocystinemia, or high factor VIII levels
12 months or lifetime	First event with: ■ Cancer (therapy with LMWH for first 3-6 months is safer and more effective) ■ Antiphospholipid antibody ■ Two or more thrombophilic conditions (e.g., combined factor V Leiden and prothrombin 20210 gene mutations) ■ Idiopathic Recurrent event

DVT, deep vein thrombosis; LMWH, low-molecular-weight heparin; PE, pulmonary embolism. *From Buller HR, Agnelli G, Hull RD, et al: Antithrombotic therapy for venous thromboembolic disease. Chest 126(3 Suppl):401S, 2004.*

Fondaparinux is a newer antithrombotic agent that may be of use for the acute treatment of DVT or PE. Initial data suggest it is a reasonable alternative to UH or LMWH. At our center, fondaparinux is considered if a patient develops heparin-induced thrombocytopenia. Fondaparinux is contraindicated for patients with creatinine clearance of less than 30 mL/min.

Long-term anticoagulation is recommended for any patient with either DVT or PE, and at this time, warfarin is the mainstay of this therapy. Warfarin exerts its effect by inhibiting the formation of vitamin K–dependent proteins, and thus does not achieve therapeutic anticoagulation until it has been administered for several days. It is currently recommended to start warfarin concurrently with heparin therapy and continue administration of heparin until the International Normalized Ratio reaches the therapeutic range of 2.0 to 3.0.

The duration of anticoagulation depends on the underlying cause of the thrombosis and is still a subject of much debate and research. The current ACCP guidelines are reasonable (Table 67-3), but these recommendations may change as we learn more about the causes of idiopathic venous thromboembolism.

Most patients can be treated according to the previous guidelines. However, patients with very large PEs or with PE and hemodynamic compromise may require a more aggressive approach. Thrombolytic therapy has been studied in patients with massive PE but has not uniformly proved to decrease mortality, probably because of the comorbidities present in patients with massive PE. However, most experts agree that hemodynamically unstable patients should be considered for thrombolytic therapy. If thrombolytic therapy is considered, the potential for bleeding (particularly from an underlying malignancy) must be carefully weighed. Surgical embolectomy should be considered for patients with massive PE and hemodynamic compromise with contraindications to thrombolytic therapy or who fail thrombolysis.

Another subset of patients who require special consideration includes those with contraindications to anticoagulation or with repetitive DVT or PE. In individuals with contraindications to anticoagulation, an IVC filter may be inserted to lessen the chance of further pulmonary emboli. Temporary filters that can be removed after the situation is resolved are now available. Occasionally, long-term IVC filters are used as a last option in patients with a contraindication to anticoagulation, although in this circumstance, complications can arise from local thrombosis at the site of the filter.

Avoiding Treatment Errors

To avoid treatment errors, the treating clinician should carefully review the patient's creatinine clearance (in case of consideration of LMWH) and any previous allergies to heparin, including heparin-induced thrombocytopenia. In patients with renal insufficiency, UH is a better choice than LMWH. For patients with a history of heparin-induced thrombocytopenia, clinicians should consider fondaparinux and consultation with a coagulation specialist.

Prophylaxis

Prevention of DVT and PE has been well studied and proved effective in several instances. Patients at high risk for DVT and PE include (in order of descending risk) those undergoing surgical procedures (especially orthopedic and neurosurgical); after ischemic stroke; and medical patients with cancer, heart failure, severe lung disease, or myocardial infarction. Those at highest risk clearly benefit from more aggressive measures to prevent thrombus formation. Therapy with LMWH or fondaparinux is recommended for patients undergoing hip or knee replacements. For patients at lower risk (medical patients), the best therapy remains unclear. Current guidelines recommend subcutaneous UH or LMWH as reasonable choices for prophylaxis of DVT and PE among medical patients. Ultimately, DVT and PE prophylaxis should be instituted for any patients at risk. A detailed analysis of the vast research in this area can be found in the ACCP guidelines on prevention of venous thromboembolism.

Future Directions

The diagnostic algorithms of DVT and PE will benefit from further refinement of the imaging modalities, but the most exciting developments will be in anticoagulants with fewer side effects and a broader therapeutic window.

Additional Resources

Buller HR, Agnelli G, Hull RD, et al: Antithrombotic therapy for venous thromboembolic disease: The Seventh ACCP Conference on Antithrombotic and Thrombolytic Therapy. Chest 126(3 Suppl):401S-428S, 2004.

This review is the product of a consensus conference and represents an international consensus on therapy for VTE.

Geerts WH, Pineo GF, Heit JA, et al: Prevention of venous thromboembolism: The Seventh ACCP Conference on Antithrombotic and Thrombolytic Therapy. Chest 126(3 Suppl):338S-400S, 2004.

This review is the product of a consensus conference and represents an international consensus on prevention VTE.

Piazza G, Goldhaber SZ: Acute pulmonary embolism, part I: Epidemiology and diagnosis. Circulation 114(2):e28-e32, 2006.

This concise, case-based review of acute PE provides practical information for the diagnostic workup of PE.

EVIDENCE

1. Quiroz R, Kucher N, Zou KH, et al: Clinical validity of a negative computed tomography scan in patients with suspected pulmonary embolism: A systematic review. JAMA 293(16):2012-2017, 2005.

    This thorough systematic review includes several studies on the validity of CT scanning for the diagnosis of PE.

2. Stein PD, Hull RD, Patel KC, et al: D-dimer for the exclusion of acute venous thrombosis and pulmonary embolism: A systematic review. Ann Intern Med 140(8):589-602, 2004.

    This systematic review summarizes the numerous studies on the role of D-dimer in the diagnosis of VTE.

3. Wells PS, Anderson DR, Bormanis J, et al: Value of assessment of pretest probability of deep-vein thrombosis in clinical management. Lancet 350(9094):1795-1798, 1997.

    This prospective cohort study used pretest probability and ultrasound in the workup of patients with suspected DVT.

4. Wells PS, Anderson DR, Rodger M, et al: Excluding pulmonary embolism at the bedside without diagnostic imaging: Management of patients with suspected pulmonary embolism presenting to the emergency department by using a simple clinical model and D-dimer. Ann Intern Med 135(2):98-107, 2001.

    This prospective cohort study demonstrates the safety and usefulness of using pretest probability to manage the workup of patients with suspected PE.

Disseminated Intravascular Coagulation

Introduction

Disseminated intravascular coagulation (DIC) is a complex coagulation disorder that is characterized by widespread activation of the clotting and fibrinolytic systems, with resultant thrombotic and hemorrhagic complications. DIC is not a disease, but rather a clinicopathologic syndrome resulting from various inciting conditions (Box 68-1).

Etiology and Pathogenesis

DIC is the result of inappropriate and excessive activation of the hemostatic process. The pathologic activators of this process are only partially understood. One or more mechanisms are likely, including the de novo synthesis or release of tissue factor into the systemic circulation following endothelial injury (in extensive trauma, abruptio placentae, or retained dead fetus); production of tissue factor-like substances by circulating malignant tumor cells or amniotic fluid; and vessel wall disruption leading to platelet activation, followed by activation of the hemostatic system (in sepsis, extensive burns, hypothermia, hypoxemia and acidosis, and extensive carcinomatosis).

Unchecked activation of the coagulation system leads to excessive thrombin generation, with subsequent fibrin formation. Fibrin is widely deposited throughout the vasculature, particularly in small-caliber vessels, resulting in end-organ dysfunction. Natural regulatory proteins, such as antithrombin III (AT) and protein C, are consumed in the process. Additionally, secondary activation of the fibrinolytic system typically occurs, resulting in the generation of fibrin and fibrinogen split products. However, in many forms of DIC, such as in sepsis, the excessive synthesis and release of plasminogen activator inhibitor by endothelial cells is counterproductive and results in insufficient fibrinolysis to remove the ubiquitous deposited fibrin.

In DIC, procoagulant, anticoagulant, and fibrinolytic factors are consumed (Fig. 68-1). Circulating thrombin also leads to platelet activation, which further enhances the prothrombotic state. Consumption of platelets leads to thrombocytopenia. When procoagulant activity dominates (such as in cancer and sepsis), thrombi formed in the microvasculature produce multiorgan failure. However, if fibrinolytic activation or the consumption of procoagulant factors and platelets dominate, bleeding may ensue. The latter outcome may be seen, for example, in acute promyelocytic leukemia owing to synthesis of plasminogen activators by the leukemic cells and in DIC associated with surgery or obstetric disasters. Microangiopathic hemolytic anemia (MAHA) occurs when thrombi narrow the lumen of the microvasculature, and erythrocytes, in their attempt to pass through, become fragmented. In this circumstance, hemolysis occurs, with the circulation of fragmented red blood cells (helmet cells or schistocytes).

Clinical Presentation

The clinical presentation of DIC is highly variable and is determined to a large extent by the underlying etiology (Box 68-1). In many cases, clinical complications may be subtle or even absent. Although vaso-occlusive manifestations are significantly more prevalent overall, certain subtypes of DIC may be associated with bleeding, usually in the form of widespread microvascular oozing from mucocutaneous surfaces. Manifestations of this microvascular oozing can include easy bruising, microscopic or macroscopic hematuria, or bleeding from venipuncture or intra-

Figure 68-1 Disseminated Intravascular Coagulation (DIC).

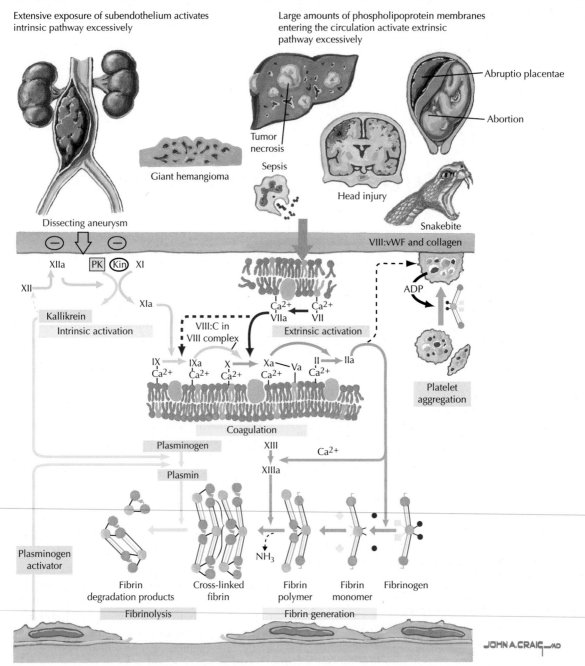

Extensive exposure of subendothelium activates intrinsic pathway excessively

Large amounts of phospholipoprotein membranes entering the circulation activate extrinsic pathway excessively

Abruptio placentae

Abortion

Tumor necrosis

Sepsis

Giant hemangioma

Head injury

Dissecting aneurysm

Snakebite

VIII:vWF and collagen

XIIa   PK Kin XI

XII

ADP

Kallikrein

XIa

Ca2+   Ca2+
VIIa   VII

Intrinsic activation

VIII:C in VIII complex

Extrinsic activation

IX   IXa   X   Xa — Va   II — IIa
Ca2+   Ca2+   Ca2+   Ca2+   Ca2+

Platelet aggregation

Coagulation

Plasminogen

XIII

Ca2+

Plasmin

XIIIa

Plasminogen activator

NH3

Fibrin degradation products

Cross-linked fibrin

Fibrin polymer

Fibrin monomer

Fibrinogen

Fibrinolysis

Fibrin generation

JOHN A. CRAIG—MD

Physiology and molecular events leading to DIC

venous catheter sites, surgical wounds, or endotracheal tubes. At the most extreme end of the spectrum is fulminant DIC, for example as seen in severe sepsis, presenting as massive and diffuse bleeding, unmanageable by blood product transfusions (Fig. 68-2). As outlined previously, bleeding is more frequently encountered in hyperacute forms of DIC, in which there is rapid and decompensated consumption of clotting factors and platelets as a result of hyperfibrinolysis. Low-grade DIC is found most frequently in patients with sepsis or malignant tumors and, rarely, in

the obstetric patient with a retained dead fetus. Because liver synthetic function is able to replace the consumed coagulation proteins and a steady state is reached, patients may be asymptomatic, and the diagnosis of DIC is made only by laboratory testing.

DIC in the obstetric patient can be particularly challenging to diagnose and manage because of the high risk to both the mother and fetus and, in part, because DIC can present in any of several different ways. Amniotic fluid embolism occurs in 1 : 20,000 to 1 : 30,000 deliveries,

Box 68-1 Clinical Conditions Associated with Disseminated Intravascular Coagulation

- Sepsis and severe infection
- Trauma (e.g., polytrauma, neurotrauma, fat embolism)
- Organ destruction (e.g., severe pancreatitis)
- Malignancy
  - Solid tumors
  - Myeloproliferative or lymphoproliferative malignancies
- Obstetric calamities
  - Amniotic fluid embolism
  - Abruptio placentae
  - Preeclampsia, eclampsia, HELLP syndrome (hemolysis, elevated liver enzymes, low platelet count)
  - Retained dead fetus
- Vascular disorders
  - Large aneurysms
  - Kasabach-Merritt syndrome
- Severe hepatic failure
- Severe toxic or immunologic reactions
  - Snake bites
  - Recreational drugs
  - Transfusion reactions
  - Transplant rejection
- Therapy with prothrombin complex concentrates

carries a 26% to 86% maternal mortality rate, and is responsible for about 10% of maternal deaths. Amniotic fluid embolism can occur during labor, during cesarean birth, or within 30 minutes postpartum. Fulminant, diffuse hemorrhage develops because of the consumption of coagulation factors. Acute hypotension, hypoxemia, and cardiopulmonary arrest may occur as a result of widespread microthrombi. Previous pregnancy, carriage of a male fetus, and a history of allergies and atopy are risk factors, but prolonged labor and the use of oxytocin are not. A less severe DIC, ranging from mild vaginal bleeding to maternal hemorrhagic shock, may occur in abruptio placentae. The extent of DIC in septic abortion, intra-amniotic infection, and postpartum endometritis is variable.

Diagnostic Approach

The diagnosis of DIC should only be contemplated when an associated underlying cause has been identified. There is no single laboratory test for the diagnosis of DIC, but a typical DIC laboratory panel includes a prothrombin time (PT), activated partial thromboplastin time (aPTT), fibrinogen activity assay, platelet count, and a D-dimer or fibrin degradation product (FDP) level. A diagnostic scoring algorithm utilizing these widely available coagulation tests was proposed by the International Society of Thrombosis and Haemostasis in 2001. The design of this scoring system has a pathophysiologic basis, incorporating the concepts of nonovert and overt DIC as distinct entities, each with its own scoring system (Table 68-1). Overt DIC can be defined as a state in which the vascular endothelium

and blood and its components have lost the ability to compensate and restore homeostasis in response to injury. The result is a progressively decompensating state with thrombotic multiorgan dysfunction, bleeding, or both. Nonovert DIC may be defined as a clinical vascular injury state that results in stress to the hemostatic system, the response to which, for the moment, is sufficient to forestall further rampant inflammatory and hemostatic activation. The nonovert DIC score emphasizes repeat assessments because the overall trend is an important facet for both diagnosis and prognosis. To some extent, these subsets reflect different points in the continuum, although it is clear that nonovert DIC may be associated with adverse outcomes in critically ill patients independently of progression to overt DIC.

Both scoring systems have been validated in prospective studies, generally in the intensive care unit setting. In overt DIC, a score of 5 or more is considered to be diagnostic, as it is in nonovert DIC (see Table 68-1). It should be noted that the term *fibrin-related products* can include direct assays for the presence of fibrin (e.g., soluble fibrin monomers) and indirect assays of fibrin generation (such as D-dimer, FDPs). Of these, D-dimers are now the most frequently used assay in North America. The scoring system for the diagnosis of nonovert DIC (see Box 68-1) includes, in addition to the previously mentioned global studies, more specific (but less widely available) tests, such as plasma antithrombin and protein C levels.

It should be especially noted that a low plasma fibrinogen level is not a sensitive marker of DIC, nor is it considered necessary for the diagnosis. In fact, high plasma fibrinogen levels are much more frequently encountered. In addition, even though a review of the peripheral blood smear should be performed, MAHA in DIC is neither invariably present, nor required to make the diagnosis.

Differential Diagnosis

Often the clinical and laboratory presentation is such that DIC cannot be diagnosed with absolute certainty. Many of the patients in whom the diagnosis of DIC is entertained are in the intensive care unit and have multiple medical problems. The coagulopathy and thrombocytopenia in these patients are often multifactorial. The differential diagnosis includes coagulopathy resulting in liver synthetic dysfunction in chronic or acute liver failure; thrombocytopenia caused by hypersplenism; vitamin K deficiency in the postsurgical or intensive care unit patient; dilutional coagulopathy and thrombocytopenia after multiple red blood cell transfusions; heparin- or other drug-induced thrombocytopenia; thrombotic thrombocytopenic purpura (TTP); hemolytic-uremic syndrome (HUS); other MAHA; immune-mediated thrombocytopenia triggered by infection; or infective endocarditis. Measurement of factor VIII activity can be used to differentiate between severe DIC and severe liver synthetic dysfunction. Although factor

Figure 68-2 Disseminated Intravascular Coagulation (DIC) in Fulminant Bacterial Sepsis

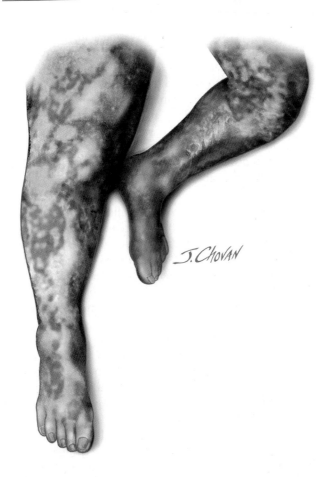

J. CHOVAN

Table 68-1	Scoring System for Disseminated Intravascular Coagulation of the International Society of Thrombosis and Haemostasis

1. **Risk assessment:** Does the patient have an underlying disorder known to be associated with overt DIC?
   If no: Do not use this algorithm.
   If yes, order global coagulation tests: platelet count, prothrombin time, fibrinogen, and soluble fibrin monomers or fibrin degradations products (such as D-dimer)

2. **Score global coagulation test results and calculate total score:**

Test Result	Score
Platelet Count >100 = 0 <100 = 1 <50 = 2	☐
Prolonged Prothrombin Time <3 sec = 0 >3 sec and <6 sec = 1 >6 sec = 2	☐
Fibrinogen Level >100 mg/dL = 0 <100 mg/dL = 1	☐
Elevated Fibrin-Related Markers No increase = 0 Moderate increase = 2 Strong increase = 3	☐
Total:	☐

3. Evaluate total score:
   If total score ≥5: compatible with overt DIC; repeat scoring daily
   If total score <5: suggestive (not affirmative) for nonovert DIC; repeat in the next 1 to 2 days

DIC, disseminated intravascular coagulation.

VIII is low in severe DIC, it is normal or elevated in most instances of severe liver synthetic dysfunction. The activity of the vitamin K–dependent factors (II, VII, IX, X) can be compared with that of non–vitamin K–dependent factors (fibrinogen, AT, V, VIII, XI, XII) to differentiate between vitamin K deficiency and DIC. In the pregnant or postpartum patient, the differential diagnosis includes preeclampsia, eclampsia, HELLP syndrome (hemolysis, elevated liver enzymes, low platelet count), and TTP/HUS.

Management and Therapy

Optimum Treatment

Management of DIC should focus on the treatment of the underlying disorder, blood product support in the bleeding patient, and consideration of the use of heparin, AT concentrate, or activated protein C concentrate (drotrecogin alfa [Xigris]). In the handful of small prospective randomized clinical trials that have been performed, no clear benefit of heparin has been demonstrated in DIC. However, heparin anticoagulation is appropriate for those patients with a documented thromboembolic event, acral ischemia, or purpura fulminans. There remains a range of opinion on the most appropriate dosing protocol for heparin.

The patient with DIC who is bleeding clearly needs blood product support. In the nonbleeding patient with DIC who is at increased risk for bleeding (e.g., postsurgical, postpartum, intubated), blood products may also be indicated. In other nonbleeding patients with DIC, blood product transfusions are probably not routinely indicated. It has been proposed that blood product transfusions, such as plasma and platelets, may worsen DIC, but this theory has neither been proved nor disproved. However, avoidance of transfusion products in DIC patients not at risk for bleeding appears prudent. In the absence of any randomized trials (or even consensus guidelines) on the use of blood products in DIC, reasonable transfusion goals in the DIC patient who is bleeding or is being prepared for an invasive procedure are a platelet count higher than

$50 \times 10^9/L$, fibrinogen more than 100 mg/dL, and maintenance of PT and aPTT as close to the normal range as possible.

The various blood product and drug therapies used in DIC are as follows.

Fresh Frozen Plasma

Fresh frozen plasma (FFP) contains all coagulation factors, but none in concentrated form. Thus, a bleeding patient with severe DIC might require such large volumes of FFP to achieve the previously mentioned targets that the potential for fluid overload would be a real limitation. To avoid a dilutional coagulopathy in the patient who receives multiple packed red blood cell (PRBC) transfusions, a patient should receive one bag of FFP for every 4 units of PRBCs.

Cryoprecipitate

Cryoprecipitate contains mainly fibrinogen, factor VIII, von Willebrand factor, and fibronectin. In some countries, not including the United States, purified fibrinogen products are available. In the United States, cryoprecipitate is the product of choice for hypofibrinogenemia. One dose of cryoprecipitate (derived from 10 donors) increases the fibrinogen plasma level by about 100 mg/dL in a non-DIC patient, but generally less in a patient with ongoing consumption due to DIC.

Platelet and Red Blood Cell Transfusions

One bag of apheresis platelets from a single donor, or 5 to 6 pooled units from whole blood collection, typically leads to an anticipated increase in platelet count of 30,000 to 60,000/μL in the non-DIC patient, and less in the DIC patient. PRBCs should be transfused as needed, although it is not known what the optimal hemoglobin level is in patients with DIC.

Drotrecogin Alfa

Drotrecogin alfa (recombinant human activated protein C concentrate) was shown to decrease mortality in adult patients with severe sepsis and has been approved by the U.S. Food and Drug Administration (FDA) since 2001. Drotrecogin alfa is an intravenous anticoagulant that proteolytically inactivates coagulation factors Va and VIIIa. In addition, it may possess anti-inflammatory, profibrinolytic, and antiapoptotic activities in vivo. A recent post hoc analysis of the Pivotal Recombinant Human Protein C Worldwide Evaluation in Severe Sepsis (PROWESS) study demonstrated that (1) overt DIC, as defined by the International Society on Thrombosis and Haemostasis scoring system and representing about 30% of the total cohort, is a strong predictor of mortality in severe sepsis; and (2) patients with overt DIC are the most likely to benefit from the use of activated protein C concentrate. The benefit of the drug in noninfectious DIC has not been examined to date.

Antithrombin (III) Concentrate

Antithrombin III (AT) concentrate indications are not clear-cut. In a large phase III prospective randomized study on the use of AT concentrate in severe sepsis, no significant reduction in 90-day mortality could be shown compared with placebo. However, post hoc analyses have suggested that benefit might have been observed had the use of concomitant heparin been excluded, and if randomization had been limited to patients with DIC at baseline. Although this suggests that AT concentrates may yet be shown to have some benefit in DIC, the level of evidence at this time is insufficient to recommend its routine use.

Avoiding Treatment Errors

When considering the use of blood products and anticoagulant drugs in DIC, the indications should be carefully assessed, as should the potential bleeding complications of heparin, antithrombin, and drotrecogin alfa.

Future Directions

It is clear that the role of established and new anticoagulants in the treatment of DIC should be further examined. In particular, the demonstrated proinflammatory and procoagulant activities of thrombin make it an attractive therapeutic target, if excessive bleeding can be avoided. The role of drotrecogin alfa in severe sepsis has recently been questioned by several prospective clinical trials. It may be that the agent is of most benefit in a subset of patients with more life-threatening disease associated with DIC. Despite this, it would be of interest to examine the efficacy and safety of drotrecogin alfa in nonsepsis-related DIC, and recombinant thrombomodulin or other new anticoagulants in phase II and III studies. FDA approval of fibrinogen concentrate for bleeding patients with DIC is desirable, as is a clinical study of recombinant factor VIIa.

Additional Resource

Levi M, Ten Cate H: Disseminated intravascular coagulation. N Engl J Med 341(8):586-592, 1999.
This is a review article on pathogenesis and management of DIC.

EVIDENCE

1. Bakhtiari K, Meijers JC, de Jonge E, Levi M: Prospective validation of the International Society of Thrombosis and Haemostasis scoring system for disseminated intravascular coagulation. *Crit Care Med* 32(12):2416-2421, 2004.
   This prospective study shows the accuracy of the simple ISTH scoring system for DIC to diagnose or reject a diagnosis of DIC in intensive care unit patients with clinical suspicion of DIC.
2. Bernard GR, Vincent JL, Laterre PF, et al: Efficacy and safety of recombinant human activated protein C for severe sepsis. *N Engl J Med* 344(10):699-709, 2001.

This is the sentinel clinical study on the use of drotrecogin alfa in sepsis.

3. Dhainaut JF, Yan SB, Joyce DE, et al: Treatment effects of drotrecogin alfa (activated) in patients with severe sepsis with or without overt disseminated intravascular coagulation. J Thromb Haemost 2(11):1924-1933, 2004.

   This retrospective analysis of the PROWESS trial demonstrates that a modified ISTH overt DIC scoring system may be useful as an independent assessment for identifying severe sepsis patients at high risk for death with a favorable risk-to-benefit profile for drotrecogin alfa treatment.

4. Feinstein DI: Diagnosis and management of disseminated intravascular coagulation: The role of heparin therapy. Blood 60(2):284-287, 1982.

   This review of clinical publications addressing the use of heparin in DIC concludes that the majority of studies suggest that heparin is not helpful.

5. Kienast J, Juers M, Wiedermann CJ, et al: Treatment effects of high-dose antithrombin without concomitant heparin in patients with severe sepsis with or without disseminated intravascular coagulation. J Thromb Haemost 4(1):90-97, 2006.

   This retrospective analysis of a large phase III antithrombin sepsis trial demonstrates that an adapted ISTH DIC score may identify patients with severe sepsis who potentially benefit from high-dose antithrombin treatment.

6. Taylor FB Jr, Toh CH, Hoots WK, et al: Scientific Subcommittee on Disseminated Intravascular Coagulation (DIC) of the International Society on Thrombosis and Haemostasis (ISTH): Towards definition, clinical and laboratory criteria, and a scoring system for disseminated intravascular coagulation. Thromb Haemost 86(5):1327-1330, 2001.

   The authors describe the clinically useful ISTH scoring system for DIC.

7. Toh CH, Downey C: Performance and prognostic importance of a new clinical and laboratory scoring system for identifying non-overt disseminated intravascular coagulation. Blood Coagul Fibrinolysis 16(1):69-74, 2005.

   This prospective study validates the clinical usefulness of the ISTH scoring system by demonstrating its prognostic relevance.

8. Warren BL, Eid A, Singer P, et al: Caring for the critically ill patient. High-dose antithrombin III in severe sepsis: A randomized controlled trial. JAMA 286(15):1869-1878, 2001.

   This prospective clinical trial demonstrates that high-dose antithrombin therapy had no effect on 28-day all-cause mortality in adult patients with severe sepsis and septic shock when administered within 6 hours after the onset, but that there was some evidence to suggest a treatment benefit of antithrombin in the subgroup of patients not receiving concomitant heparin.

Stephan Moll

69

Anticoagulation Management

Introduction

Several anticoagulants are in clinical use, and additional agents are in development (Table 69-1). Although anticoagulants can be very effective in preventing thrombotic events, they can also lead to devastating bleeding complications (Fig. 69-1). Thus, detailed knowledge of their optimal dosing and monitoring, their clearance mechanisms and drug interactions, and the management of supratherapeutic levels and bleeding complications is essential to minimize risk and optimize efficacy.

Unfractionated Heparin, Low-Molecular-Weight Heparin, and Fondaparinux

Heparins are a mixture of different lengths of polysaccharides. *Unfractionated heparins* have a mean length of 40 monosaccharide units. They inactivate thrombin, and, to a much lesser degree, factor Xa (Fig. 69-2). Low-molecular-weight heparins (LMWHs) are derived from unfractionated heparin through chemical and physical fractionation processes. In contrast to unfractionated heparins, LMWHs have a mean length of 15 monosaccharide units and preferentially inhibit factor Xa and, to a lesser degree, thrombin. *Fondaparinux* (Arixtra) is a synthetic pentasaccharide of the antithrombin-binding region of heparin and can be considered an extremely low-molecular-weight heparin. It has specific anti-Xa inhibitory activity, without any activity against thrombin.

Dosing and Monitoring

Heparin

Unfractionated heparin at therapeutic doses typically needs to be monitored with the activated partial thromboplastin time (aPTT; see Fig. 69-2). The therapeutic aPTT range depends on the heparin sensitivity of the aPTT reagent and the instrument used by a laboratory. There is no standardization of the aPTT for heparin therapy, as there is for the prothrombin time (PT) through the International Normalized Ratio (INR) for vitamin K antagonist therapy. Optimally, a coagulation laboratory should provide the clinicians with the therapeutic heparin aPTT range for the reagent-instrument combination used in that laboratory, and clinicians should use a nomogram for heparin dosing. If a laboratory-specific therapeutic aPTT range has not been established, then an aPTT ratio of 2.0:2.5 of the mean aPTT of the normal range can be used as an approximation. It should be noted, however, that this range is subtherapeutic with some aPTT reagents, and heparin underdosing may occur.

Heparin is mostly cleared by the reticuloendothelial system and, to a smaller degree, by the kidney; patients with renal failure may require less heparin for therapeutic aPTTs to be achieved. The plasma half-life of heparin depends on the dose given: the half-life of unfractionated heparin is about 60 minutes after a 100 U/kg intravenous (IV) bolus. A patient taking therapeutic doses of continuous-infusion IV unfractionated heparin will likely have a return to baseline aPTT within 3 to 4 hours after discontinuation of heparin. A loading dose of 80 U/kg heparin IV followed by a continuous infusion of 18 U/kg/hr is usually an appropriate starting dose for patients at average risk for bleeding. For patients at increased risk for bleeding, such as those receiving concomitant thrombolytics or with thrombocytopenia, this dosing may have to be modified. The aPTT should be determined 6 hours after initiation of heparin and each dose change, and once daily after a therapeutic aPTT has been achieved.

Table 69-1   Anticoagulants in Clinical Use and Selected Agents in Development

Generic	Brand Name*	Dosing†
Heparin		
Unfractionated heparin	Various names	Various nomograms; aPTT adjusted
Dalteparin	Fragmin	*Prophylaxis:* various doses
		Full-dose: 100 U/kg every 12 hr SC or 200 U/kg every day SC
Enoxaparin	Lovenox	*Prophylaxis:* various doses
	Clexane	*Full-dose:* 1.0 mg/kg every 12 hr or 1.5 mg/kg every day SC
Tinzaparin	Innohep	*Prophylaxis:* various doses
		Full-dose: 175 U/kg every day SC
Certoparin	Monoembolex	*Prophylaxis:* various doses
Nadroparin	Fraxiparin	Not approved for full-dose anticoagulant treatment
Reviparin	Clivarin	
Anti-Xa Inhibitors		
Pentasaccharides		
Fondaparinux	Arixtra	*Prophylaxis:* 2.5 mg every day SC
		Full-dose: 7.5 mg every day SC
Idraparinux‡	None yet	In development
Apixaban‡	None yet	In development
Rivaroxaban‡	Xarelto	In development
Thrombin Inhibitors		
Argatroban	Acova	No bolus; continuous infusion: 2 µg/kg/min IV; aPTT adjusted
	Novastan	
Bivalirudin	Angiomax	*In percutaneous coronary interventions:*
		▪ Bolus: 0.75 mg/kg IV
		▪ Continuous infusion: 1.75 mg/kg/hr IV until 4 hrs after intervention; then 0.2 mg/kg/hr for up to 20 hours
Desirudin	Iprivask Revasc	15 mg every 12 hr SC
Lepirudin	Refludan	*Bolus:* 0.4 mg/kg IV
		Continuous infusion: 0.15 mg/kg/hr IV; aPTT adjusted
Danaparoid	Orgaran	*Prophylaxis:* 750 U SC every 12 hr or every 8 hr
		Full-dose: Bolus 2500 U IV, then continuous infusion 150-400 U/hr; anti-Xa level adjusted
Ximelagatran	Exanta	Withdrawn from market
Dabigatran‡	Rendix	In development
Vitamin K Antagonists		
Coumarins		
Warfarin	Coumadin	
	Jantoven	
Phenprocoumon	Marcumar	
	Falithrom	Interindividual variability; dosing is INR adjusted
	Phenpro	
Acenocoumarol	Sinthrome	
Tioclomarol	Apegmone	
Indandiones		
Anisindione	Miradon	
Fluindione	Previscan	Interindividual variability; dosing is INR adjusted
Phenindione	Dindevan	
	Pindione	

* Other products may exist.
† Dosing regimens may vary depending on indication, country of use, presence or absence of renal or liver dysfunction, and concomitant use of antiplatelet drugs or anticoagulants.
‡ Agents printed in *italics* are investigational.
aPTT, activated partial thromboplastin time; INR, International Normalized Ratio; SC, subcutaneous.

Low-Molecular-Weight Heparins

The various LMWHs (see Table 69-1) differ in their chemical composition; therefore, dose recommendations for prophylaxis and treatment indications differ for the various drugs. The lack of significant plasma protein binding of LMWHs gives them a more predictable anticoagulant effect than unfractionated heparin. As a result, fixed or weight-adjusted dosing is possible. For this reason, laboratory monitoring of their anticoagulant effect is unnecessary except in unusual circumstances. Peak plasma levels are reached 3 to 4 hours after injection. The half-

Figure 69-1 Intracranial Hemorrhage in a Patient Taking a Vitamin K Antagonist.

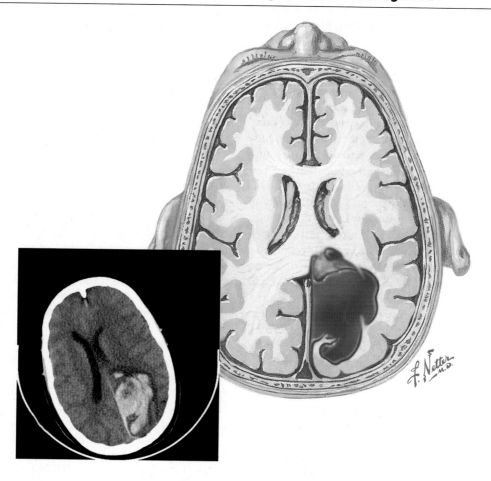

Figure 69-2 Coagulation Cascade.

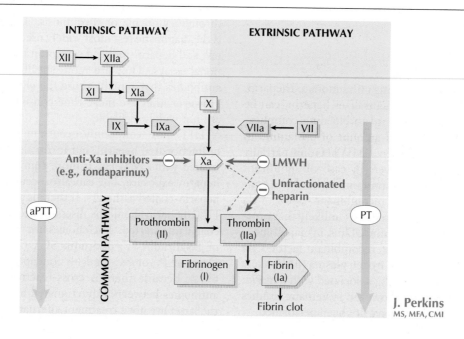

lives of the various agents differ, ranging between 3 to 7 hours. Once- or twice-daily dosing regimens are available for the different LMWHs. In special patient populations, for whom monitoring of LMWH becomes necessary, an anti-Xa level (also called quantitative heparin level) should be obtained. The aPTT is typically only slightly prolonged in patients treated with LMWH and is not a useful parameter to measure the anticoagulation status of that patient. Because the LMWHs are cleared by the kidney, dose reduction and anti-Xa monitoring are needed in patients with creatinine clearances of less than 30 mL/min. LMWHs should be avoided and unfractionated heparin used instead in patients with severe renal impairment or dialysis dependence. In obese patients, LMWH dosing should be based on actual body weight, but in the patient with a body mass index of 40 kg/m^2 or more, anti-Xa level determination should be considered to avoid overanticoagulation. Therapeutic anti-Xa levels are in the order of 1.0 to 2.0 U/mL for once-daily dosing, and 0.6 to 1.2 U/mL for twice-daily dosing, obtained 3 to 4 hours after subcutaneous (SC) injection. Anti-Xa levels should always be obtained if a patient taking LMWH has a recurrent thrombotic event or a significant bleed, to determine whether the patient was subtherapeutically or supratherapeutically anticoagulated.

Fondaparinux

Fondaparinux (Arixtra) is given subcutaneously and reaches its peak plasma level at 2 hours. It has a half-life of 17 to 21 hours and is dosed once daily. Because it does not significantly bind to plasma proteins, it can be given as a fixed dose, either in prophylactic or therapeutic doses (see Table 69-1). Fondaparinux, like the LMWHs, is excreted by the kidney and should not be used in patients with renal failure. Fondaparinux does not appear to cause the clinical syndrome of heparin-induced thrombocytopenia (HIT) and can be considered as an alternative anticoagulant in patients with established HIT.

Bleeding

If bleeding occurs in a patient taking unfractionated heparin, intravenous protamine, which neutralizes heparin, can be given. Because protamine can lead to bleeding complications if overdosed, the minimal amount of protamine to neutralize heparin should be given. LMWH is only partially reversed by protamine. However, in case of significant bleeding while taking LMWH, protamine should be considered. For major bleeding, recombinant factor VIIa (NovoSeven) should be considered. It is unlikely that protamine has any effect on fondaparinux. Thus, in major bleeding associated with fondaparinux, recombinant factor VIIa is the treatment of choice. Fresh frozen plasma (FFP) likely has little, if any, effect on bleeding associated with heparin, LMWH, and fondaparinux, however systematic studies assessing its effect and efficacy have not been performed.

Heparin-Induced Thrombocytopenia

HIT is an incompletely understood immunologic phenomenon in which antibodies to the heparin–platelet factor 4 complex form. It is defined as the occurrence of thrombocytopenia in a patient treated with heparin and the presence of a positive test for heparin-associated antibodies. Although in some patients these antibodies are clinically irrelevant, in others they lead to thrombocytopenia and, in about one third of such patients, to thrombotic events. These can be arterial or venous and most commonly occur in large to mid-sized vessels, causing deep venous thrombosis, pulmonary embolism, or arterial occlusion resulting in myocardial infarction, stroke, or gangrene of extremities or digits (Fig. 69-3). Strict classification criteria for HIT require a platelet count decrease to less than 100,000/μL or a decrease in platelet count of more than 50% from baseline. A less strict definition for HIT is a platelet count decrease to less than 150,000/μL or a decrease of more than 30% from baseline. The clinical picture of HIT (thrombosis plus demonstration of heparin-associated antibodies) occasionally occurs even in patients who do not have a decrease in their platelet count. A high suspicion for HIT is needed in any patient who develops a decreasing platelet count while taking heparin or a patient with a new thrombotic event that has occurred during heparin therapy.

Tests that can be used for diagnostic purposes include (1) heparin–platelet factor 4 antibody enzyme-linked immunosorbent assay (HIT-PF4 ELISA), (2) heparin-induced platelet aggregation (HIPA) study, and (3) heparin-induced serotonin release assay. The HIT-PF4 ELISA is the most sensitive assay to detect HIT antibodies, but the least specific for clinically relevant antibodies. Many patients exposed to high doses of heparin, such as patients with cardiopulmonary bypass surgery, develop heparin–platelet factor 4 antibodies, which often do not lead to thrombocytopenia or thrombosis. The HIT-PF4 ELISA is the diagnostic test most widely used for HIT. The HIPA test and heparin-induced serotonin release assay are functional assays. They are more specific for the pathogenic antibodies that actually cause the clinical picture of HIT. However, they are more time consuming to perform and are not widely available.

HIT most commonly occurs in patients treated with unfractionated heparin, but it can also develop in patients treated with LMWHs. It more commonly occurs with IV heparin exposure, but can also occur with SC dosing or heparin-coated catheters. If there is a clinical suspicion for HIT, heparin should be discontinued and alternative anticoagulants started. The choices are (1) hirudins (lepirudin or bivalirudin IV; desirudin SC), (2) argatroban IV, (3) Orgaran IV or SC, and (4) fondaparinux SC (see Table 69-1). Because there is cross-reactivity of the HIT-PF4 antibodies between unfractionated heparin and LMWHs, the latter are not a treatment alternative when HIT caused

Figure 69-3 Digital Ischemia in a Patient with Heparin-Induced Thrombocytopenia.

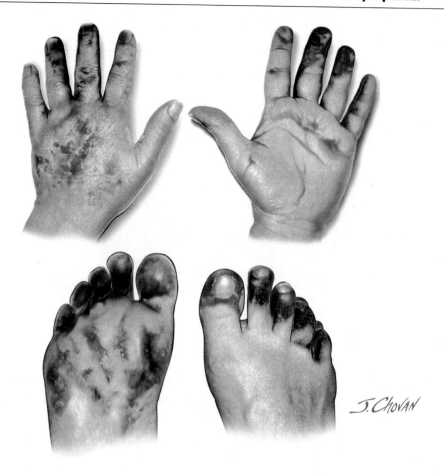

J. CHOVAN

by unfractionated heparin has occurred. HIT-PF4 antibodies do not appear to cross-react with fondaparinux to cause HIT, and fondaparinux has, therefore, in recent years become an attractive treatment option. To date, however, large treatment trials using fondaparinux in HIT have not been performed. Initiation of warfarin should be delayed until the platelet count has increased to 100,000/μL, preferably to 150,000/μL. Vitamin K antagonists should not be started without a patient receiving one of the alternate anticoagulants, and administration of both anticoagulants should be overlapped for at least 5 days and until the warfarin therapy has resulted in an INR greater than 2.0. Detailed recommendations for platelet count monitoring in patients taking heparin, as well as for the diagnosis and treatment of HIT, are available in the guidelines of the American College of Chest Physicians (ACCP).

Oral Anticoagulants

Coagulation factors are synthesized in the liver. The factors II, VII, IX, and X (see Fig. 69-2) require the presence of vitamin K to become fully functional. The available oral anticoagulants (see Table 69-1) are all vitamin K antagonists. Because the half-lives of some of these factors are quite long (50 hours for factor II), the full antithrombotic effect of vitamin K antagonists is not reached for several days after starting these drugs.

An important issue in the use of oral anticoagulants is the short half-life of protein C, an endogenous anticoagulant with a half-life of about 8 hours. Protein C levels can decrease early after initiation of vitamin K antagonist drug therapy, thus rendering the patient hypercoagulable during the first few days of treatment, before factor II has decreased sufficiently to protect the patient from thrombosis. Thus, vitamin K antagonists create a prothrombotic state in the first 5 days, before they have a full anticoagulant effect. This puts the patient at risk for vitamin K antagonist–induced skin necrosis (Fig. 69-4) or progression of thrombosis, unless a parenteral anticoagulant is given overlapping with the vitamin K antagonist for at least 5 days and until the INR is above 2.0. Such overlap is not needed in the patient initiated on vitamin K antagonists who does not have an acute thrombotic event, such as a patient with newly discovered atrial fibrillation without transient ischemic attack or stroke.

Figure 69-4 Vitamin K Antagonist–Induced Skin Necrosis.

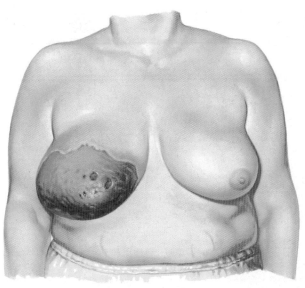

Dosing and Monitoring

The anticoagulant effect of vitamin K antagonists is determined by measuring the PT (see Fig. 69-2), expressed as the standardized INR. The typical loading dose of warfarin in a hospitalized patient is 5 mg daily on day 1 and 2, with subsequent dosing based on the INR measurement after the first two doses. A frail or elderly patient, one who has been treated with prolonged antibiotics, has liver disease, or has undergone intestinal resection, will need a lower dose in the first few days. Some clinicians prefer using higher loading doses of 7.5 mg or 10 mg, particularly in an outpatient with normal nutritional status. For maintenance dosing, the highest dose requirements for keeping a patient in the therapeutic range are in men younger than 50 years (median dose, 6.4 mg/day), the lowest in women older than 70 years (median dose, 3.1 mg/day). Occasional patients need doses as high as 20 or 30 mg per day.

The effectiveness of coordinated anticoagulation clinics in improving anticoagulation control, reducing bleeding and thromboembolic event rates, and decreasing health care cost by reducing hospitalizations and emergency department visits has been shown. The use of so-called point-of-care instruments or near-patient-testing devices in clinics, using a blood drop from a fingerstick for whole blood PT testing, allows immediate reporting of the result to the patient and dose adjustment. Patients can also use these devices at home for self-monitoring and, if trained well and encouraged by the health care system in which they live, for self-management. If patients are carefully selected and trained, the use of point-of-care testing can improve anticoagulation control, decrease in thrombo-embolic and bleeding complications, and achieve higher patient satisfaction.

Supratherapeutic INRs, Bleeding

The management of elevated INRs and bleeding that occurs in patients taking vitamin K antagonists depends on the degree of INR elevation and the presence or absence of risk factors for bleeding and whether active bleeding is present or not. Management options have been published as recommendations from the ACCP (Table 69-2) and include omitting the next anticoagulant dose and giving vitamin K. Too much vitamin K should be avoided if there is no major bleeding, because it may lower the INR dramatically and, as a result, make re-anticoagulation of the patient more difficult. FFP can lower the INR to some degree but not markedly. FFP does not reverse overanticoagulation completely because the short half-life of coagulation factor VII of 4 to 6 hours would require huge doses of FFP to be given for full reversal. If complete and immediate INR reversal is needed, such as when treating a major bleeding or life-threatening event in a patient on vitamin K antagonists, a prothrombin complex concentrate (e.g., Bebulin, Profilnine) or recombinant factor VIIa (NovoSeven) should be given.

Fluctuating INRs

Some patients treated with vitamin K antagonists may, at times, have unexpected and seemingly unexplained high or low INRs, or may have significant INR fluctuations over

Table 69-2 Recommendations for Management of Elevated INRs in Patients Taking Vitamin K Antagonists

INR	Bleeding	Risk Factor for Bleeding	Intervention
<5.0	No	No/yes	Omit next VKA dose and reduce dose
5.0-9.0	No	No	Omit next VKA doses and reduce dose
5.0-9.0	No	Yes	Vitamin K, <5 mg by mouth
>9.0	No	No/yes	Vitamin K, 5-10 mg by mouth
Serious bleed at any INR	Yes	No/yes	Vitamin K, 10 mg IV + FFP or PCCs
Life-threatening bleed	Yes	No/yes	Vitamin K, 10 mg IV + PCCs. Consider recombinant VIIa

FFP, fresh frozen plasma; PCCs, prothrombin complex concentrates, VKA, vitamin K antagonist. *Modified from Ansell J, Hirsh J, Poller L, et al: The pharmacology and management of the vitamin K antagonists: The Seventh ACCP Conference on Antithrombotic and Thrombolytic Therapy. Chest 126(3 Suppl):204S-233S, 2004.*

time. In these situations, the following reasons for aberrant or fluctuating INRs should be considered: (1) Was the out-of-line INR a lab error? Lab errors are more common when there was significant trouble at the time of blood draw with tissue trauma or when the blood tube was not filled appropriately. (2) Has any new prescription medication that could affect protein binding or the half-life of warfarin been started or has any one been discontinued? (3) Is the patient taking any new over-the-counter medications, vitamins, herbs, homeopathic medications, or weight control pills, which may have a similar effect? (4) Is the patient taking his or her various medications at the same times as usual? (5) Have there been dietary changes that would change the patient's vitamin K intake? (6) Has the patient recently had an infection or diarrhea? (7) Is the patient noncompliant with taking the oral anticoagulant or confused about the prescribed dose to take? (8) Was the package of the oral anticoagulant outdated? (9) Does the patient have a lupus anticoagulant? (10) Has there been an unusual amount of stress, sleep deprivation, or physical activity in the days preceding the INR test? If no reason for widely fluctuating INRs can be determined, daily supplementation with low-dose vitamin K, for instance, at a dose of 150 µg/day, can lead to better INR control in some patients.

Side Effects

Bleeding is the main side effect of oral anticoagulant therapy. The risk for bleeding is highest in elderly individuals; in persons who have not had stable anticoagulant control and have a tendency to supratherapeutic INRs; in patients with comorbidities that increase the bleeding risk, such as malignancy, uncontrolled hypertension, or a preexisting bleeding disorder; and in the first few months of anticoagulant initiation. A striking, yet rare side effect of oral and parenteral anticoagulants is that of purple toe syndrome (Fig. 69-5), a violaceous painful discoloration of the feet and sometimes the hands. The etiology is thought to be formation of cholesterol emboli, released from atherosclerotic lesions as a result of plaque rupture or as a

Figure 69-5 Purple Toe Syndrome Associated with Vitamin K Antagonist Therapy.

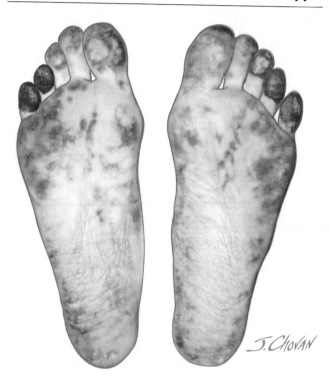

J. CHOVAN

result of weakening of the fibrin mesh overlying atheromatous lesions. Evidence of cholesterol embolization in other skin areas can also be present, leading to livedo reticularis and renal impairment.

Periprocedural Bridging Therapy

Whether there is a need to stop oral anticoagulant therapy before a surgical or radiologic procedure depends on the bleeding risk associated with the procedure. How soon before the procedure the drug should be stopped depends on the INR that the patient has when the drug is stopped and the half-life of the drug being used. Warfarin, when

Table 69-3 Recommendations When Interrupting Warfarin Therapy for Invasive Procedures*

Risk for Clot	Preoperative	Postoperative
Low	Stop warfarin about 4 days before surgery	Prophylactic dose LMWH/UFH (if intervention causes thrombotic risk)
	No LMWH/UFH	Restart warfarin
Intermediate	Stop warfarin about 4 days before surgery	Prophylactic dose LMWH/UFH
	Prophylactic dose LMWH/UFH	Restart warfarin
High	Stop warfarin about 4 days before surgery	LMWH/UFH (no dose recommendation given)
	Full-dose LMWH/UFH 2 days before surgery	Restart warfarin

* These recommendations are all so-called grade C recommendations, i.e., very weak recommendations, where treatment alternatives may be equally reasonable.
LMWH, low-molecular-weight heparin; UFH, unfractionated heparin. *Modified from Ansell J, Hirsh J, Poller L, et al: The pharmacology and management of the vitamin K antagonists: The Seventh ACCP Conference on Antithrombotic and Thrombolytic Therapy. Chest 126(3 Suppl):204S-233S, 2004.*

targeted to keep the INR between 2 and 3, can typically be stopped 5 days before a procedure for which an INR of about 1 is required. The need for bridging therapy with a subcutaneous or intravenous anticoagulant before and after the procedure depends on the thromboembolic risk of the patient. How soon an anticoagulant can be restarted after surgery depends on the bleeding risk associated with the surgery. Some guidelines have been created by the American College of Chest Physicians (Table 69-3), but individual risk assessment of a patient and good communication between the health care provider managing the patient's anticoagulants and the surgeon is typically needed for optimal periprocedural anticoagulation planning.

Pregnancy and Anticoagulants

Prophylactic or full-therapeutic doses of anticoagulants may be indicated in the pregnant woman with (1) a strong thrombophilia but no previous thromboembolism, (2) previous thromboembolism or a mechanical heart valve, or (3) a history of recurrent early pregnancy losses or one or more late pregnancy losses as a result of thrombophilia. Warfarin can be teratogenic when taken during pregnancy weeks 6 to 12, but this risk is low; coumarin embryopathy occurs in only 0.6% of pregnancies in which women received oral vitamin K antagonists between weeks 6 and 12. However, warfarin taken at any time during pregnancy may lead to bleeding complications in the fetus. Discontinuation of warfarin and institution of LMWH or unfractionated heparin is, therefore, the anticoagulant management strategy of choice during pregnancy. The heparin can either be started as soon as pregnancy is confirmed and before week 6 of pregnancy, or before conception.

Warfarin is not detectable in the breast milk of mothers who take warfarin, but only a limited number of women taking warfarin have been studied. These data cannot exclude the passage of small amounts of warfarin into breast milk, but such doses are unlikely to cause bleeding in the newborn. It, therefore, appears safe for the woman taking warfarin to breast-feed. There are very limited data in the medical literature on other coumarin drugs (see Table 69-1), and it is, therefore, not known, whether they are also safe. Phenindione and anisindione (see Table 69-1) do appear in breast milk. Unfractionated heparin and LMWH are not secreted in breast milk and can be safely administered to nursing mothers.

Patient Education

Treatment with anticoagulants and antiplatelet agents is associated with a significant risk for bleeding, and lack of appropriate treatment with these drugs can lead to significant morbidity and mortality. The therapy recommended and prescribed by health care providers may be optimized by having an educated patient. Patients can find information about anticoagulant drugs, as well as the diseases treated with these drugs, at websites listed in the "Additional Resources" section of this chapter.

Avoiding Treatment Errors

Of premier importance for the optimization of safety and efficacy of anticoagulant and antiplatelet agents is an accurate assessment in each patient about the indication or lack thereof for the use of anticoagulants, based on established treatment guidelines as well as the patient's individual risk factors for thromboembolism and bleeding. Treatment algorithms should be used for unfractionated heparin and oral anticoagulant management whenever possible. Patients taking oral anticoagulants should be followed by a specialized anticoagulation service or, at least, through a systematic management approach. Awareness of a patient's renal status and weight is important to avoid inappropriate LMWH and fondaparinux dosing. HIT should be considered in any patient who develops thrombocytopenia or a new thrombotic event while being treated with a heparin product.

Future Directions

More efficacious, safer, and easier to use anticoagulant agents are under development. Several promising oral agents that may not require monitoring of their anticoagulant effect and will, therefore, be less cumbersome to use and are presently being tested in phase 2 and 3 clinical trials (e.g., dabigatran, rivaroxaban, apixaban). Local delivery of anticoagulants or genes modulating anticoagulant control at sites of increased thrombogenicity, such as in diseased arteries, is a promising treatment modality that may decrease systemic bleeding problems. Much about the initiating pathophysiologic events leading to venous thrombotic disease needs to be elucidated before such local therapy can be tested in the venous vasculature. While waiting for better anticoagulants to become clinically available, patient management with the existing drugs needs to be improved by instituting coordinated anticoagulation services, promoting patient self-monitoring and self-management, and improving patient and health care provider education on the use of anticoagulant drugs.

Additional Resources

American College of Cardiology. Available at: http://www.acc.org/media/patient/index.htm. Accessed May 22, 2007.

This educational website of the American College of Cardiology provides a wealth of clinical and practical information regarding anticoagulant issues surrounding atrial fibrillation, mechanical heart valves, coronary artery disease, and other disorders in which anticoagulants and antiplatelet agents are used. Several treatment guidelines are included. The site is suitable for health care providers, with some information materials suitable for patients.

American Heart Association. Available at: http://www.americanheart.org. Accessed May 22, 2007.

This website of the American Heart Association includes extensive clinical and practical information regarding anticoagulant issues surrounding atrial fibrillation, mechanical heart valves, coronary artery disease, and other disorders in which anticoagulants and antiplatelet agents are used. Several treatment guidelines of interest for clinicians are included. Some information is also suitable for patients.

American Stroke Association. Available at: http://www.strokeassociation.org. Accessed May 22, 2007.

This website of the American Stroke Association contains extensive clinically relevant information on anticoagulant and antiplatelet use for primary and secondary stroke prevention, including important treatment guidelines. Some information is also suitable for patients.

ClotCare Online Resources. Available at: http://www.clotcare.com. Accessed May 22, 2007.

This multispecialty education website covers anticoagulant issues for health care providers and patients.

National Alliance for Thrombosis and Thrombophilia (NATT). Available at: http://www.nattinfo.org. Accessed May 22, 2007.

This website is primarily for patients and public, but also has a section for health care providers that allows them to print peer-reviewed educational materials on topics surrounding diagnosis and management of thrombosis and thrombophilia to be used as handout materials in hospitals and clinics.

Thrombophilia Support Page. Available at: http://www.fvleiden.org. Accessed May 22, 2007.

This educational website is primarily for patients with thrombosis or thrombophilias, but also includes information suitable for health care providers. A question-and-answer section provides a discussion of clinically relevant topics.

Vascular Disease Foundation. Available at: http://www.vdf.org. Accessed May 22, 2007.

This website contains information material on venous and arterial disease, mostly for patients.

EVIDENCE

1. Ansell J, Hirsh J, Poller L, et al: The pharmacology and management of the vitamin K antagonists: The Seventh ACCP Conference on Antithrombotic and Thrombolytic Therapy. Chest 126(3 Suppl):204S-233S, 2004.

   This article provides a comprehensive discussion of clinically relevant aspects of oral anticoagulant management, with weighing of clinical evidence and specific management recommendations based on published clinical trials. The article contains a multitude of relevant references. Updated guidelines are schedule to be published in Chest in 2008.

2. Bates S, Greer IA, Hirsh J, Ginsberg JS: Use of antithrombotic agents during pregnancy: The Seventh ACCP Conference on Antithrombotic and Thrombolytic Therapy. Chest 126(3 Suppl): 627S-644S, 2004.

   This clinically relevant discussion of anticoagulant management during pregnancy weighs the clinical evidence and specific management recommendations based on published clinical trials. Updated guidelines are scheduled to be published in Chest in 2008.

3. Hirsh J, Raschke R: Heparin and low-molecular weight heparin: The Seventh ACCP Conference on Antithrombotic and Thrombolytic Therapy. Chest 126(3 Suppl);188S-203S, 2004.

   This comprehensive discussion of clinically relevant aspects of parenteral anticoagulant management weighs the clinical evidence and specific management recommendations based on published clinical trials. Updated guidelines are scheduled to be published in Chest in 2008.

4. Warkentin T, Greinacher A: Heparin-induced thrombocytopenia: Recognition, treatment, and prevention: The Seventh ACCP Conference on Antithrombotic and Thrombolytic Therapy. Chest 26(3 Suppl):311S-337S, 2004.

   This clinically relevant discussion of heparin-induced thrombocytopenia weighs the clinical evidence and specific management recommendations, based on published clinical trials. Updated guidelines are scheduled to be published in Chest in 2008.

Lee R. Berkowitz

Bleeding Disorders

Introduction

The coagulation system is based on an intricate set of checks and balances between procoagulant and anticoagulant proteins, all interacting with platelets and the vascular endothelium. The end result is protection from bleeding and inhibition of excessive thrombosis. A great deal is known about many of the proteins in this system as well as the structure and function of platelets. This knowledge enables the internist to approach bleeding disorders with diagnostic and therapeutic sophistication.

Etiology and Pathogenesis

Congenital Bleeding Disorders

Von Willebrand's Disease

Von Willebrand's Disease (vWD) is a common congenital bleeding diathesis. Both quantitative and qualitative abnormalities have been described in the von Willebrand protein, which allows platelet adherence to the endothelium and provides factor VIII stability. The most common variant of vWD is type I, which is autosomal dominant in inheritance. Patients have a quantitative decrease in vWD protein to 30% to 50% of normal. Type II variants are defined by qualitative differences in the multimeric structure of the von Willebrand protein. At least eight different type II variants have been described. They are labeled alphabetically as types IIa to IIh. Inheritance is either autosomal dominant or recessive.

Hemophilia A

Hemophilia A is the most common inherited bleeding disorder. The inheritance is X linked, so this disorder is seen almost exclusively in males. Affected individuals have reduced factor VIII levels. Patients with severe hemophilia have no detectable factor VIII activity. Those with mild hemophilia have 1% to 5% factor VIII activity (Fig. 70-1).

Acquired Bleeding Disorders

Disseminated intravascular coagulation (DIC) is a multisystem process resulting in bleeding and thrombosis in the microvasculature. DIC occurs in the setting of life-threatening disorders, including sepsis and massive trauma, that overwhelm the clotting cascade, leading to excessive amounts of activated thrombin. This, in turn, causes fibrin deposition with activation of the lytic system and depletion of clotting factors (see Chapter 68, Fig. 68-1).

Immune thrombocytopenic purpura (ITP) is an autoimmune process in which patients generate antibodies directed to surface proteins on platelets. The antibody-coated platelets are then prematurely destroyed in the reticuloendothelial system. ITP occurs spontaneously or as a manifestation of an autoimmune disease or B-cell neoplasm.

Thrombotic thrombocytopenic purpura (TTP) is characterized by platelet clumping in the microcirculation. This results in thrombocytopenia, microangiopathic hemolytic anemia, and varying degrees of organ dysfunction, particularly in the brain and kidney.

Qualitative Disorders of Platelets

Platelets follow a multistep sequence to form a platelet plug over a site of damaged vascular endothelium. The sequence begins with platelet adherence, followed by platelet aggregation and activation. Activation is dependent in part on cyclooxygenase-induced release of intracellular granules. Once the platelet plug is formed, coagulation factors are then activated, resulting in fibrin deposition and hemostasis. Both congenital and acquired qualitative platelet disorders have been recognized. Glanzmann's thrombasthenia is a congenital disorder in which the platelets have a defect in the glycoprotein IIb/IIIa complex, altering platelet aggregation. A number of congenital storage granule disorders have been described. The most common

Figure 70-1 Hemophilia A and B.

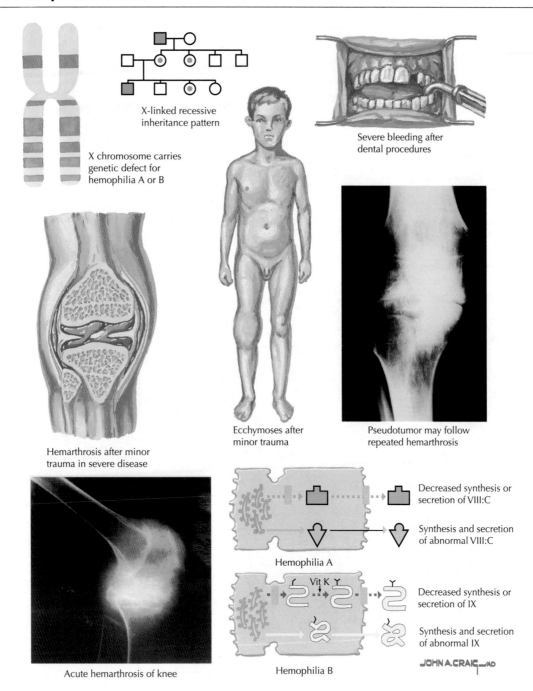

X-linked recessive
inheritance pattern

X chromosome carries
genetic defect for
hemophilia A or B

Severe bleeding after
dental procedures

Hemarthrosis after minor
trauma in severe disease

Ecchymoses after
minor trauma

Pseudotumor may follow
repeated hemarthrosis

Acute hemarthrosis of knee

Decreased synthesis or
secretion of VIII:C

Synthesis and secretion
of abnormal VIII:C

Hemophilia A

Vit K

Decreased synthesis or
secretion of IX

Synthesis and secretion
of abnormal IX

Hemophilia B

JOHN A. CRAIG—AD

acquired defects are seen with the use of aspirin and non-steroidal anti-inflammatory drugs (NSAIDs). Both inhibit cyclooxygenase; aspirin's effect is irreversible, whereas NSAIDs cause reversible inhibition.

Liver Disease

The liver is the site of synthesis of most clotting proteins. In addition, activated factors are cleared from the circulation by the liver. Any disease that causes impaired liver function will lead to decreased synthesis of clotting factors

and a DIC-type picture because of the prolonged half-life of activated thrombin. The liver is also the site of vitamin K–dependent modulation of factors II, VII, IX, and X, a process that is also impaired with significant liver disease and results in decreased factor activity.

Clinical Presentation and Differential Diagnosis

Congenital bleeding disorders may present in childhood or in adults (Fig. 70-2). Patients with hemophilia A have

Figure 70-2 Clinical Presentation of Patients with Bleeding Disorders.

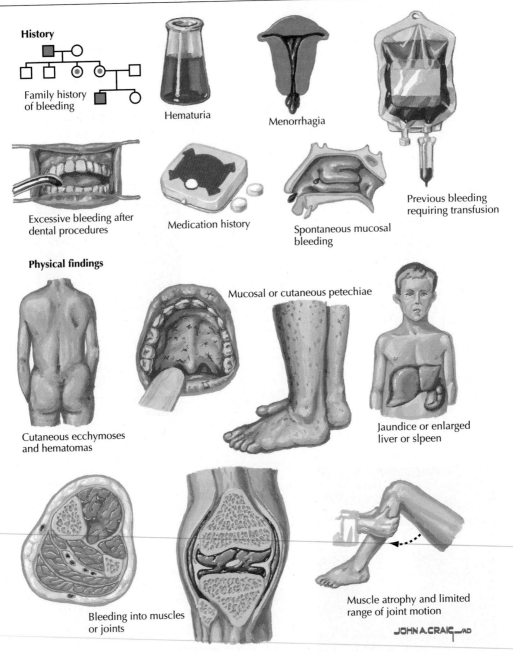

History

Family history of bleeding

Hematuria

Menorrhagia

Previous bleeding requiring transfusion

Excessive bleeding after dental procedures

Medication history

Spontaneous mucosal bleeding

Physical findings

Mucosal or cutaneous petechiae

Cutaneous ecchymoses and hematomas

Jaundice or enlarged liver or slpeen

Bleeding into muscles or joints

Muscle atrophy and limited range of joint motion

JOHN A. CRAIG—MD

bleeding beginning in infancy. As these patients mature, spontaneous hemarthroses are common. Any trauma will result in localized hemorrhage. Patients with von Willebrand's disease (vWD) usually present later in life, and most often with easy bruisability, heavy menses, or significant bleeding secondary to dental work or surgery. Hemarthroses are rare.

With acquired bleeding disorders, there are several key findings. Patients with ITP or thrombocytopenia associated with DIC usually have petechiae on the lower extremities. The lesions are small parafollicular erythematous macules and are seen at platelet counts less than 50,000/µL. Oozing from any puncture site, such as from intravenous sites, blood-drawing sites, and surgical scars, is common. TTP has been described in patients with *Escherichia coli* sepsis and in patients taking certain drugs (quinine, mitomycin C, cisplatin, gemcitabine, clopidogrel). These patients also have neurologic findings, evidence of a hemolytic anemia, and renal abnormalities. Patients with qualitative platelet disorders or liver disease generally have an increased tendency to bruise.

Figure 70-3 Hemostasis Tests.

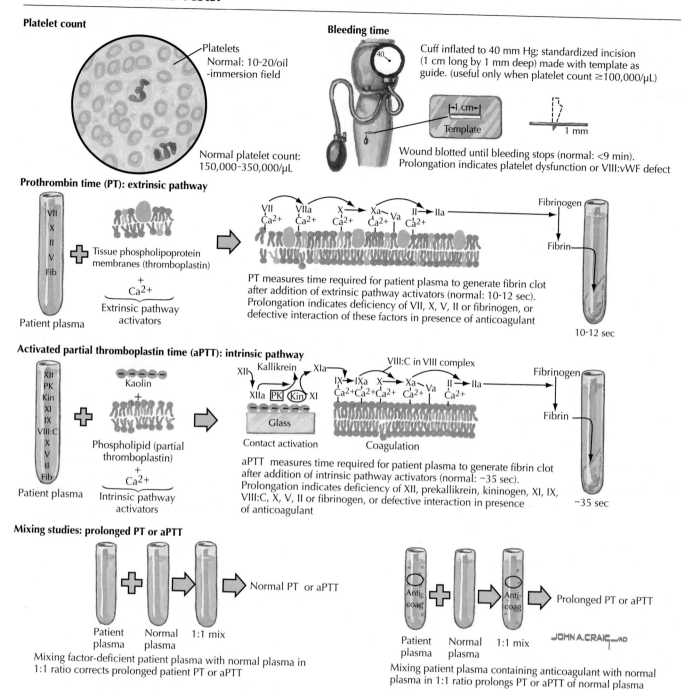

Platelet count

Platelets
Normal: 10-20/oil
-immersion field

Normal platelet count:
150,000-350,000/µL

Bleeding time

Cuff inflated to 40 mm Hg; standardized incision
(1 cm long by 1 mm deep) made with template as
guide. (useful only when platelet count ≥100,000/µL)

Template

1 cm

1 mm

Wound blotted until bleeding stops (normal: <9 min).
Prolongation indicates platelet dysfunction or VIII:vWF defect

Prothrombin time (PT): extrinsic pathway

VII
X
II
V
Fib

Patient plasma

Tissue phospholipoprotein
membranes (thromboplastin)
+
Ca²⁺
Extrinsic pathway
activators

VII   VIIa   X → Xa   II → IIa
Ca²⁺   Ca²⁺   Ca²⁺   Va   Ca²⁺

Fibrinogen

Fibrin

PT measures time required for patient plasma to generate fibrin clot
after addition of extrinsic pathway activators (normal: 10-12 sec).
Prolongation indicates deficiency of VII, X, V, II or fibrinogen, or
defective interaction of these factors in presence of anticoagulant

10-12 sec

Activated partial thromboplastin time (aPTT): intrinsic pathway

XII
PK
Kin
XI
IX
VIII:C
X
V
II
Fib

Patient plasma

Kaolin
+
Phospholipid (partial
thromboplastin)
+
Ca²⁺
Intrinsic pathway
activators

XII   Kallikrein   XIa
XIIa   PK   Kin   XI
Glass
Contact activation

VIII:C in VIII complex

IX → IXa   X → Xa   II → IIa
Ca²⁺ Ca²⁺ Ca²⁺   Ca²⁺   Va   Ca²⁺
Coagulation

Fibrinogen

Fibrin

aPTT measures time required for patient plasma to generate fibrin clot
after addition of intrinsic pathway activators (normal: ~35 sec).
Prolongation indicates deficiency of XII, prekallikrein, kininogen, XI, IX,
VIII:C, X, V, II or fibrinogen, or defective interaction in presence
of anticoagulant

~35 sec

Mixing studies: prolonged PT or aPTT

Normal PT or aPTT

Patient
plasma

Normal
plasma

1:1 mix

Mixing factor-deficient patient plasma with normal plasma in
1:1 ratio corrects prolonged patient PT or aPTT

Anti-
coag

Anti-
coag

Prolonged PT or aPTT

Patient
plasma

Normal
plasma

1:1 mix

Mixing patient plasma containing anticoagulant with normal
plasma in 1:1 ratio prolongs PT or aPTT of normal plasma

JOHN A. CRAIG—AD

With all bleeding problems, there is a great deal of overlap in findings, and none is pathognomonic for a particular disease process. With any of the above findings, the physician should have a low threshold to evaluate the coagulation system.

Diagnostic Approach

Several tests are readily available and will significantly narrow the diagnostic possibilities (Fig. 70-3). The prothrombin time (PT) and activated partial thromboplastin time (aPTT) measure the activities of all clotting factors. Prolongations indicate significant factor deficiency, which is seen in hemophilia, vWD, DIC, and the coagulopathy of liver disease. The platelet count detects quantitative platelet problems (alterations in platelet number), and the bleeding time detects qualitative platelet problems (alterations in platelet function). Table 70-1 shows specific differences in these tests for the common coagulopathies.

Following the results of screening tests, more specific assays can be done. Tests are available for factor VIII and von Willebrand protein. Measurement of other factors and

Table 70-1   Diagnostic Studies in Common Coagulations

Disorder	PT	aPTT	Platelet Count	Bleeding Time
Hemophilia A	Normal	Prolonged	Normal	Normal
vWD	Normal	Prolonged	Normal	Prolonged
DIC	Prolonged	Prolonged	Decreased or normal	Normal
ITP	Normal	Normal	Decreased	Normal
TTP	Normal	Normal	Decreased	Normal
Qualitative platelet disorders	Normal	Normal	Normal	Prolonged
Liver disease	Prolonged	Prolonged	Normal	Normal

aPTT, activated partial thromboplastin time; DIC, disseminated intravascular coagulation; ITP, immune thrombocytopenic purpura; PT, prothrombin time; TTP, thrombotic thrombocytopenic purpura; vWD, von Willebrand's disease.

Box 70-1   The Pentad of TTP

1. Microangiopathic hemolytic anemia
2. Thrombocytopenia
3. Renal insufficiency
4. Fluctuating neurologic abnormalities
5. Fever

fibrinogen can be helpful for the diagnosis of DIC. The D-dimer assay, which measures lytic system activity, is often used in DIC. The diagnosis of ITP is usually a diagnosis of exclusion. Assays for platelet antibodies are available but have poor specificity (see Fig. 70-3). The diagnosis of TTP is dependent on a pentad of findings shown in Box 70-1.

Management and Therapy

Congenital Bleeding Disorders: Optimum Treatment

von Willebrand's Disease

Type I disease can be treated with desmopressin (DDAVP) for mild bleeding and preoperative prophylaxis. The drug can be administered intravenously or subcutaneously and will increase levels of von Willebrand protein in several hours. For more significant bleeding, purified concentrates containing von Willebrand protein should be administered intravenously. Type II disease is treated similarly, except the IIb variant, in which DDAVP is contraindicated.

Hemophilia A

The treatment of choice for significant bleeding is administration of recombinant factor VIII intravenously. The target factor VIII level depends on the severity of bleeding. For isolated hemarthroses, in which the target level is 30% to 50%, patients can be taught to self-administer factor VIII.

With treatment, inhibitors to factor VIII develop in 10% to 15% of patients. A variety of approaches can be used in this situation, depending on the severity of the bleeding and the level of the inhibitor.

Acquired Bleeding Disorders: Optimum Treatment

Disseminated Intravascular Coagulation

In patients with DIC, the primary focus should be to treat the underlying condition causing the coagulopathy. Until this is done, there will be no substantial improvement. This usually takes hours to several days. In the interim, fresh frozen plasma and cryoprecipitate can be given to replace clotting factors and fibrinogen. Platelets are also given if the platelet count is less than 50,000/μL with active bleeding. If there is no bleeding related to a surgical procedure, a lower platelet count can be tolerated without transfusion. The use of heparin is controversial because of its bleeding risk. In general, it is given if treatment of the underlying condition and replacement therapy do not appear to be working.

Immune Thrombocytopenic Purpura

At presentation, most patients are treated with prednisone (1 mg/kg body weight per day), which will normalize the platelet count in 3 to 7 days. The process is chronic, and an attempt at tapering steroids will often result in a decrease in the platelet count. Patients then must undergo splenectomy, which produces a complete response in 70% to 80% of cases. Intravenous immunoglobulin (IVIG) is an alternative to prednisone that improves the platelet count in days. Whether there is any advantage to IVIG compared with prednisone is not clear, nor is it clear that the combination of prednisone and immunoglobulin is superior to either alone. For patients who continue with significant thrombocytopenia after splenectomy, there are a number of options, including chemotherapy, high-dose pulse steroids, or chronic daily steroids. Responses are quite individualized.

Thrombotic Thrombocytopenic Purpura

TTP is a life-threatening emergency with a mortality rate of greater than 90%, if not treated. The mainstay of treatment is exchange of the patient's entire plasma volume with normal donor plasma. Corticosteroids are also used in doses similar to the treatment of ITP.

Liver Disease: Optimum Treatment

Because many patients have irreversible liver pathology, the coagulopathy is usually a chronic process. Repeated doses of vitamin K may be helpful. Otherwise, patients are treated for acute bleeding with fresh frozen plasma, which will transiently raise factor levels.

Avoiding Treatment Errors

Patients with type IIb vWD should not receive DDAVP. This may cause aggregation of platelets and thrombocytopenia. Platelet transfusions are contraindicated in TTP. There are case reports of acute worsening and even death after platelets were given to these patients.

Future Directions

Patients with newly diagnosed ITP may respond to rituximab. In TTP, deficiency of a metalloproteinase that cleaves von Willebrand factor has been observed in patients with recurrent TTP. Protein C infusions have been shown to be effective in the purpura fulminans variant of DIC.

Additional Resources

United States National Institutes of Health Web Site. Available at: http://clinicaltrials.gov. Accessed October 7, 2006.

This site is updated frequently for both patients and health care providers. It includes links to the National Library of Medicine.

EVIDENCE

1. American Society of Hematology Web Site. Available at: http://www.hematology.org. Accessed October 7, 2006.

    This site provides an annual review of many important subjects in hematology.
2. National Hemophilia Foundation Web Site. Available at: http://www.hemophilia.org. Accessed October 7, 2006.

    This site provides materials for both patients and health care providers.

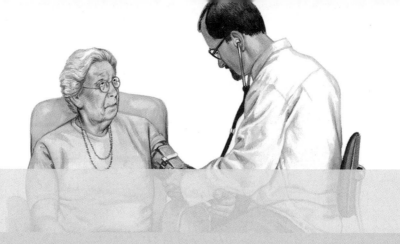

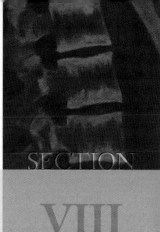

Hematologic Disorders

Lee R. Berkowitz

Anemias

Introduction

Anemia, a hemoglobin concentration below the normal range for a standard complete blood count (CBC), is a common finding in internal medicine patients. Most anemias have a specific etiology. Defining the cause is critical for determining therapy and for uncovering other significant associated disease processes. Although these anemias are familiar to most clinicians, understanding them continues to be a dynamic process because new information is always emerging.

Etiology and Pathogenesis, Differential Diagnosis

Iron Deficiency

This common anemia should be considered in any patient presenting with a microcytic anemia and a low or normal reticulocyte count. Because adults have several grams of iron in circulating red blood cells and another gram in storage iron, the diagnosis of iron deficiency requires searching for a source of blood loss. The sequence of findings in iron deficiency is loss of storage iron, followed by development of anemia, and finally by development of microcytosis.

Thalassemia

This disorder is a common anemia in certain areas of the world, including the Mediterranean, India, Southeast Asia, and Africa. A high prevalence has also been observed in Western countries in individuals descended from those regions where thalassemia is common. At a molecular level, there are hundreds of globin abnormalities leading to either α-chain underproduction (α-thalassemia) or β-chain underproduction (β-thalassemia). The phenotype is similar. The underproduction of either α or β chains results in a microcytic red blood cell. There is also hemolysis because the imbalance results in excess globin chains, which are oxidized and precipitate on the surface of the red blood cell, resulting in premature red blood cell removal in the spleen. The bone marrow partially compensates by increasing the number of reticulocytes.

Vitamin B$_{12}$ and Folate Deficiency

The folate metabolic pathway is responsible for thymidine synthesis. Thymidine is then incorporated into DNA. Vitamin B$_{12}$ is a cofactor in this pathway. Vegetables and fruits are rich in folates, but vitamin B$_{12}$ is only found in foods from animals. The absorption of folate occurs in a straightforward pathway in the jejunum. Vitamin B$_{12}$ absorption is more complex, requiring intrinsic factor production in the stomach, pancreatic secretion, and then passage through the mucosa of the terminal ileum.

The hematologic findings in folate and vitamin B$_{12}$ deficiency are identical. Because nuclear maturation is arrested, red blood cells are macrocytic. Reticulocytes are low or normal. The folate–vitamin B$_{12}$ pathway is also present in neutrophils and platelets, so deficiencies can result in reductions in all three cell lines. Neutrophils are often hypersegmented.

Vitamin B$_{12}$ deficiency can also lead to neurologic findings as a consequence of demyelination. These include peripheral neuropathy with decreased proprioception, optic atrophy, and dementia. These abnormalities may precede hematologic changes and may not improve after B$_{12}$ replacement when recognized late in the disease course.

Anemia of Chronic Disease

A normocytic anemia with a suboptimal reticulocyte response may develop in patients with a variety of chronic inflammatory diseases, infections, or neoplastic diseases. Because a precise cause has not been found, this anemia is called the *anemia of chronic disease* and is the most common cause of anemia in hospitalized patients. One theory is that elevated levels of cytokines induce blockage of the release of storage iron into circulating iron. Another theory is that elevated levels of cytokines result in decreased endogenous erythropoietin levels. There are no specific diagnostic tests, so the diagnosis is made by careful clinical observation and by excluding other causes of anemia.

Sickle Cell Anemia

Sickle cell anemia is an inherited hemoglobinopathy secondary to a single amino acid substitution in the β-globin chain. In the homozygous state, sickle hemoglobin becomes insoluble when deoxygenated. This results in a loss of red cell deformity, which in turn causes vaso-occlusion in the microcirculation and a shortened life span of these erythrocytes. The prevalence for the gene that encodes hemoglobin S is 8% in the African American population. There are about 50,000 patients with sickle cell anemia in the United States. There are also sickle variants that combine hemoglobin S with another abnormal hemoglobin such as sickle thalassemia (hemoglobin S-β-thalassemia) or hemoglobin C (hemoglobin SC disease). These variants have a similar phenotype to sickle cell anemia but are less severe.

Clinical Presentation

Patients with anemia may or may not be symptomatic (Fig. 71-1). Key factors include the degree of anemia and how

Figure 71-1 Anemia.
Hgb, hemoglobin; HCT, hematocrit; RBC, red blood cell; MCV, mean corpuscular volume.

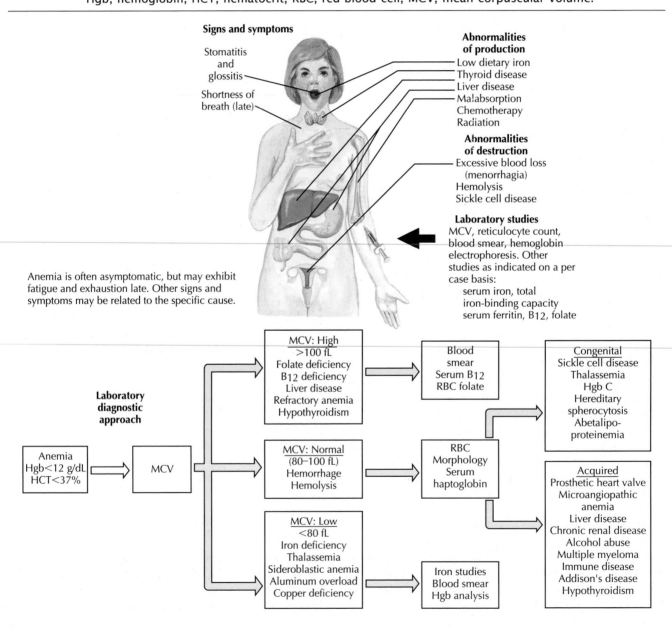

Box 71-1 Crises in Sickle Cell Anemia

Vaso-occlusive
Aplastic
Splenic sequestration
Hyperhemolytic

Box 71-2 Complications of Sickle Cell Anemia

Cholelithiasis
Acute chest syndrome
Hematuria
Priapism
Osteomyelitis
Stroke
Pulmonary hypertension
Spontaneous abortion

---

rapidly it develops. In general, symptoms develop at a hemoglobin level of 8.0 to 9.0 g/dL, when the anemia develops over hours to a few days. A slower evolving process will allow the patient to compensate hemodynamically, so patients with hemoglobin values below 7.0 g/dL may have few symptoms. All patients will have symptoms at a hemoglobin level of 5.0 to 6.0 g/dL.

Early symptoms of anemia include fatigue and dyspnea on exertion. As the anemia worsens, patients will experience organ ischemia, often presenting with angina pectoris or focal neurologic findings. Shock is common with acute blood loss. In the setting of ischemic symptoms or shock, patients should undergo an emergency transfusion before a cause for the anemia is investigated.

Almost all sickle cell patients are diagnosed in childhood. In adult patients, the recognition of acute and chronic complications is the major challenge for the internist. An acute vaso-occlusive crisis is the most common acute presentation. Patients present with pain in the back and extremities, anywhere the small-sized arterioles become occluded. The average number of crises per year per patient is two, and the average duration of each crisis is 7 days. Hypoplastic or aplastic crises are the next most common presentation. Patients present with signs and symptoms of worsening anemia. This is due to parvovirus B19 infection of red cell precursors, which causes reticulocytopenia. Other types of crises are listed in Box 71-1.

Sickle cell patients have an average hemoglobin level of 7 to 8 g/dL. This degree of anemia plus chronic vaso-occlusion leads to widespread organ damage. A dilated cardiomyopathy is found in 50% of adults. Pulmonary hypertension occurs in 30% and carries a mortality rate of 50%. All adult patients are asplenic, resulting in susceptibility to infection with encapsulated organisms. Pregnancy complications occur more frequently than in the general population, and cholelithiasis with cholecystitis is common. Additional complications are listed in Box 71-2.

Diagnostic Approach

Because there are many causes of anemia, a selective diagnostic approach is recommended. A prudent place to begin is to categorize the anemia based on the mean corpuscular volume (MCV) of the patient's red blood cells and the reticulocyte count (see Figs. 71-1 and 71-2). Dividing the red blood cells into microcytic (MCV <80 μL), normocytic (80 to 100 μL), or macrocytic (>100 μL) will greatly narrow the diagnostic possibilities. The reticulocyte count gives additional information regarding the status of the bone marrow. If the bone marrow's red blood cell productive mechanism is intact, anemia will result in an increased production of reticulocytes. A low or even normal reticulocyte count in the anemic patient (3% or less) indicates that the marrow is not responding appropriately, and a search for a marrow abnormality will define the cause of the anemia. A word of caution about interpreting reticulocyte counts is warranted. They are usually reported as a percentage of the red blood cells, a relative value. To convert this to an absolute value, the patient's percentage of reticulocytes should be multiplied by the ratio of the patient's hematocrit and a normal hematocrit value (ratio = the patient's hematocrit divided by a normal hematocrit value).

Figure 71-2 illustrates how the MCV and reticulocyte count can be used to categorize anemias. After the anemia has been categorized by MCV and the reticulocyte count, more specific tests can be done.

Iron Deficiency

A number of diagnostic tests are useful for diagnosing iron deficiency. Serum markers include serum iron, total iron binding capacity, and ferritin. A low serum ferritin (<18 μg/L) has a positive likelihood ratio over 40, and a serum ferritin of 19 to 45 μg/L has a positive likelihood ratio of about 3. A transferrin saturation (Fe/total iron binding capacity) of 0.05 has a positive likelihood ratio of 16.5. However, a transferrin saturation of 0.06 to 0.08 only has a positive likelihood ratio of 1.43. The gold standard for iron deficiency is a Prussian blue stain of the bone marrow, indicating the presence or absence of iron. Because bone marrow aspiration is an invasive procedure, the morbidity must be considered on an individual basis. When the diagnosis remains unclear, a trial of iron can be diagnostic. The response will take weeks, and patient compliance is necessary. The diagnostic approach, whether serologic markers, bone marrow aspiration, or a trial of iron, depends on the severity of illness.

Thalassemia

Because the erythrocytes underproduce hemoglobin in individuals with thalassemia, microcytosis is universally

Figure 71-2 Categorizing Anemia Based on Reticulocyte Count.
MCV, mean corpuscular volume.

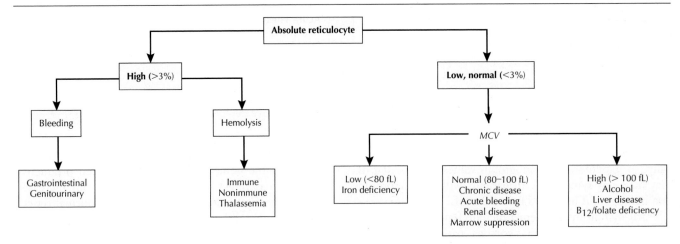

present. This underproduction also results in hemolysis. The combination of microcytosis and increased reticulocytes seen in thalassemia is unique and thus can be used to make the diagnosis. Further information can be obtained from a hemoglobin electrophoresis, which in β-thalassemia shows increased hemoglobin A_2 and increased hemoglobin F.

Vitamin B_{12} and Folate Deficiency

The diagnosis of folate deficiency is made when there is a macrocytic anemia with or without pancytopenia in clinical settings that could lead to folate deficiency. These settings include pregnancy, poor nutrition, hemolysis, and malabsorption. A serum folate assay may be helpful, but it should be noted that levels increase quickly with proper diet. A red blood cell folate assay that does not change with refeeding can confirm the diagnosis. The diagnosis of vitamin B_{12} deficiency is usually made by measuring serum vitamin B_{12}. Current assays have high sensitivity but are only moderately specific. Assays of homocysteine and methylmalonic acid are helpful in that they both increase with vitamin B_{12} deficiency. The Schilling test, in which a patient ingests radiolabeled vitamin B_{12} with or without intrinsic factor, is rarely done because of the difficulty in obtaining an adequate urine collection and the reduced sensitivity of the test in early vitamin B_{12} deficiency.

Sickle Cell Anemia

The findings of a normochromic, normocytic anemia with reticulocytosis and sickle forms on peripheral smear is diagnostic of sickle cell disease. Microcytosis suggests sickle thalassemia. A person with sickle cell trait has no abnormalities on physical examination or of the CBC. The gold standard for diagnosis is hemoglobin electrophoresis. Unless there is suspicion of a variant phenotype, electrophoresis is not necessary.

Management and Therapy

Optimum Treatment

Iron Deficiency

Patients need sufficient iron to restore erythrocyte as well as storage iron. The standard treatment is ferrous sulfate, 325 mg orally 3 times a day for 6 months. Other iron preparations are also available and equally efficacious, with the exception of enteric-coated products. These reduce gastrointestinal toxicity but have poor absorption. Iron can also be given intravenously if a patient cannot tolerate oral iron. A single total replacement dose is given. This carries a small risk for anaphylaxis. Transfusions also provide intravenous iron, 250 mg per unit of packed red blood cells.

Thalassemia

Patients with heterozygous α- or β-thalassemia have a mild hemolytic anemia. Folic acid daily (1 mg orally) will more than meet the increased demands resulting from the increased red blood cell turnover. A severe anemia develops in patients with homozygous thalassemia, which requires transfusions, usually beginning in childhood.

Vitamin B_{12} and Folate Deficiency

The most common cause of vitamin B_{12} deficiency is pernicious anemia, in which loss of intrinsic factor does not allow vitamin B_{12} absorption; vitamin B_{12} must be given intramuscularly. At diagnosis, 1 mg of vitamin B_{12} is given weekly for 4 weeks followed by monthly injections. The same treatment is applicable for other causes of vitamin B_{12} deficiency such as gastric achlorhydria from protein pump inhibitors and diseases of the terminal ileum. The treatment of all causes of folate deficiency is daily oral folate, 1 mg. If the patient cannot take oral folate, it can be given intravenously.

Anemia of Chronic Disease

If improvement of the underlying condition occurs, an improvement in the anemia will follow. This is not always the case in conditions that are chronic. Measurement of the endogenous erythropoietin level is recommended. If the level is less than 500 mU/mL, patients are candidates for recombinant human erythropoietin, given weekly by subcutaneous injection. An increase in the hemoglobin is usually seen in 4 to 8 weeks. Administration is maintained as long as the chronic condition is present.

Sickle Cell Anemia

The management of an acute vaso-occlusive crisis includes pain relief, hydration, and treatment of any precipitating infection. Narcotics are often required for pain control. Management of chronic complications such as pulmonary hypertension and cardiomyopathy are the same for the sickle cell patient and any other patient with these medical problems. Adult patients are given hydroxyurea daily, which reduces sickling by increasing hemoglobin F. There is no role for ongoing transfusions in sickle cell patients. Exchange transfusions are done for life-threatening complications such as acute chest syndrome, stroke, and acute hepatic failure.

Avoiding Treatment Errors

A diagnosis of iron deficiency in an adult requires that a source of blood loss be found. In premenopausal females, menstruation is the most likely cause. In postmenopausal females and men, a bleeding site in the gastrointestinal tract should be thoroughly evaluated. For all causes of vitamin B_{12} deficiency the treatment must be lifelong because storage B_{12} will only suffice for several months.

Future Directions

Vasodilators and antiproliferative agents have been tried in sickle cell patients with pulmonary hypertension. Recent studies have shown that sildenafil can reduce pulmonary arterial pressure and improve exercise tolerance. Two oral iron chelators, deferiprone and deferasirox, have been used in patients with sickle cell anemia, β-thalassemia, and the anemia of chronic disease. These agents appear to have similar efficacy and toxicity to deferoxamine. Further trials are ongoing.

Additional Resources

Cooley's Anemia Foundation Web site. Available at: http://www.thalassemia.org. Accessed October 10, 2006.
> Historical as well as current issues in thalassemia are reviewed.

Medline Plus Web site. Available at: http://www.nlm.nih.gov/medlineplus. Accessed October 10, 2006.
> This website can be used by both patients and health care providers.

EVIDENCE

1. American Society of Hematology Education Program Book. Available at: http://www.asheducationbook.org. Accessed October 10, 2006.
> This book is an excellent annual update of many topics in hematology.
2. Goldman L, Ausiello C: Cecil Textbook of Medicine, 22nd ed. Philadelphia, WB Saunders, 2004.
> The authors present a definitive review of the causes and treatments of anemia.

Bone Marrow Failure States

Anne W. Beaven ▪ Maria Q. Baggstrom ▪ Thomas C. Shea

Introduction

Bone marrow failure refers to any condition in which peripheral blood cell counts are low because of failure of the marrow to produce adequate numbers of circulating cells. Marrow failure is due to many different causes but is broadly classified as aplastic anemia (fatty bone marrow), myelodysplasia (disordered hematopoiesis), and agnogenic myeloid metaplasia and myelofibrosis (fibrosis).

Despite different etiologies, the signs and symptoms of all bone marrow failure syndromes are similar (Fig. 72-1). Patients with anemia may present with fatigue, dyspnea, or pallor. Thrombocytopenia can lead to petechiae, bruising, or bleeding. Infections are the hallmark of neutropenia. Most deaths are due to complications of bleeding, infection, transfusion-associated complications such as iron overload, or progression to acute leukemia.

Aplastic Anemias

Etiology and Pathogenesis

Aplastic anemia is an acquired or inherited disorder with multiple- or single-lineage cytopenia. Although adults are more likely to have acquired aplastic anemia, some congenital forms (Fanconi's anemia, dyskeratosis congenita) may not be diagnosed until adulthood because up to half of affected people may not have typical physical anomalies.

Most cases of aplastic anemia are idiopathic, but it can also occur secondary to exposure to radiation, chemicals, drugs, infections, or immunologic diseases (Box 72-1).

Clinical Presentation

Patients usually present with a history of infection, bleeding, or symptomatic anemia. There is a bimodal age distribution with peaks at 20 years of age and again in the fifth decade.

Differential Diagnosis

The differential diagnosis for cytopenia is very broad. During initial workup, it is important to rule out reversible causes (drugs, infection, and thymoma). Testing for acquired causes such as paroxysmal nocturnal hemoglobinuria (PNH) is also important because of a higher risk for progression to acute leukemia and the possible need to change treatment decisions. If clinically indicated, diseases such as cirrhosis, cancer, systemic lupus erythematosus, and tuberculosis should be considered.

Diagnostic Approach

Examination of the peripheral blood smear and bone marrow biopsy specimens is required to diagnose aplastic anemia. The blood smear shows few abnormalities except a decrease in the numbers of white blood cells, red blood cells, and platelets. Examination of the bone marrow specimen reveals a hypocellular marrow that is replaced by variable amounts of fat. Other diagnostic tests include cytogenetic analysis, which is usually normal; flow cytometry to look for the coexpression of the CD55/59 antigens (diagnostic of PNH); and testing for antibodies for parvovirus. A chest x-ray should be performed to screen for thymoma, and a subsequent computed tomography scan of the neck and chest is performed if indicated.

Figure 72-1 Bone Marrow Failure: Clinical Presentation.

Symptoms of anemia (pallor, dyspnea, and tiredness) are common to **aplastic anemias**, **myelodysplasia** (when it affects the red cell line), **agnogenic myeloid metaplasia,** and **myelofibrosis**

Patients with **agnogenic myeloid metaplasia** present with night sweats; low-grade fever; digestive symptoms such as early satiety and diarrhea; marked splenomegaly

Examination of peripheral blood smear:
Aplastic anemia: Decrease in overall number of platelets, white and red cells

Myelodysplasia: Anisocytosis is common with both microcytic and macrocytic red blood cells present in most cases

Agnogenic myeloid metaplasia and **myelofibrosis:** Immature granulocytes, nucleated red cells, and teardrop-shaped red cells

Ecchymoses and petechiae are common findings in those conditions that affect platelet production, such as **aplastic anemia,** and **myelodysplasia**

Hepatomegaly routinely present in the **agnogenic myeloid metaplasia syndromes**

Examination of the bone marrow smear:
Myelodysplasia: Most marrow biopsies are hypercellular, and abnormal cytogenetics are important prognostic markers found in 50% of these patients
Agnogenic myeloid metaplasia and **myelofibrosis:** Fibroblasts, reactive myelofibrosis, dysplastic-megakaryocyte hyperplasia, osteosclerosis, and dilation of marrow sinusoids with intravascular hematopoiesis

Replacement of the bone marrow by fatty tissue is seen in **aplastic anemia**. **Myelofibrosis** is characterized by the presence of diffuse fibrotic tissue replacing the bone marrow

Peripheral edema is another sign seen in patients with **agnogenic myeloid metaplasia** and **myelofibrosis**

Histopathology of normal and abnormal marrow states

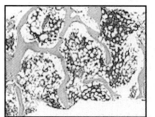
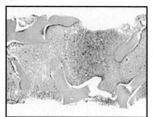
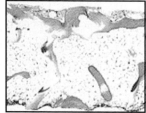
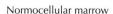

| Normocellular marrow | Hypercellular marrow | Hypocellular marrow |

Management and Therapy

Management involves a combination of supportive care and immunosuppressive therapy and, for selected individuals, bone marrow transplantation (BMT). Patients commonly need medical support with antibiotics and blood transfusions. Blood products should be depleted of white blood cells before infusion to reduce the risk for alloimmunization. Cytokines such as granulocyte colony-stimulating factor (G-CSF), granulocyte-macrophage colony-stimulat-ing factor, and erythropoietin may be helpful in patients with recurrent infections or profound anemia.

Immunosuppressive therapy with cyclosporine and antithymocyte globulin (ATG) is frequently used and has an overall response rate of about 70%. Response to immu-nosuppressive therapy is correlated with long-term sur-vival (Box 72-2). However, partial responses with late relapses of disease or development of secondary malignan-cies, including myelodysplasia and acute leukemia, are frequent.

Box 72-1 Classification of Aplastic Anemias and Single Cytopenias

Causes of Aplastic Anemia

Acquired

Radiation

Drugs and chemicals
Cytotoxic agents, benzene
Idiosyncratic reactions: chloramphenicol, nonsteroidal anti-inflammatory drugs, antiepileptic drugs, gold, other drugs and chemicals

Viruses

Epstein-Barr virus (infectious mononucleosis)
Hepatitis (non-A, non-B, non-C hepatitis)
Human immunodeficiency virus (HIV)
Parvovirus

Immune Diseases

Eosinophilic fasciitis
Hypoimmunoglobulinemia
Thymoma and thymic carcinoma
Graft-versus-host disease after transplantation or blood transfusion
Paroxysmal nocturnal hemoglobinuria
Pregnancy
Idiopathic—the most frequent diagnosis

Inherited

Fanconi's anemia
Dyskeratosis congenita
Schwachman-Diamond syndrome
Reticular dysgenesis
Amegakaryocytic thrombocytopenia
Familial aplastic anemias
Nonhematologic syndromes (Down's, Dubovitz's, Seckel's)

Causes of Cytopenias

Acquired

Anemias
Pure red blood cell aplasia
Idiopathic
Thymoma
Transient erythroblastopenia of childhood
Neutropenia
Idiopathic
Drugs, toxins
Thrombocytopenia
Drugs, toxins
Inherited

Inherited

Anemias
Congenital pure red blood cell aplasia
Neutropenia
Kostmann's syndrome
Schwachman-Diamond syndrome
Reticular dysgenesis
Thrombocytopenia
Thrombocytopenia with absence of radii
Idiopathic amegakaryocytic thrombocytopenia

Modified from Young NS, Maciejewski JP: Aplastic Anemia. In Hoffman R, Benz EJ Jr, Shattil SJ, et al (eds): Hematology: Basic Principles and Practice. Philadelphia, Churchill Livingstone, 2000, p 298; with permission from Elsevier.

Box 72-2 Aplastic Anemia and Therapies

Antithymocyte Globulin and Cyclosporine

Response rate: 60%-74%
Relapse rate of responders: 20%-38%
Overall survival: Up to 55% 7 years after treatment

Bone Marrow Transplantation

Overall response rate with sustained engraftment: 83%-97%
Graft-versus-host disease: 31%-33%
Overall survival: 78%-94% after 5 years

Data from Frickhofen N, Heimpel H, Kaltwasser JP, Schrezenmeier H: Blood 101:1236-1242, 2003; Marsh J, Schrezenmeier H, Marin P, et al: Blood 93:2191-2195, 1999; Rosenfeld S, Follmann D, Nunez O, Young NS: JAMA 289:1130-1135, 2003; Locatelli F, Bruno B, Zecca M, et al: Blood 96:1690-1697, 2000; and Ahn MJ, Choi JH, Lee YY, et al: Int J Hematol 78:133-138, 2003.

Allogeneic transplantation is generally used as initial therapy for patients younger than 40 years who have a matched sibling donor or for other patients after failure of immunosuppressive therapy. Transplant-related mortality and morbidity are significant, however, and increase dramatically in patients older than 40 years, those with an unrelated donor, and those with multiple prior transfusions. Despite these risks, allogeneic transplantation offers a benefit over immunosuppressive therapy because the risk for disease relapse or progression to acute leukemia or PNH is much smaller in this group. These clonal diseases develop in 15% to 20% of patients within 10 years after immunosuppressive therapy but are rare after allogeneic transplantation.

Optimum Treatment

Treatment decisions are influenced by severity of disease and patient age. Patients with severe (absolute neutrophil count [ANC] = 0.2-0.5×10^9/L) and very severe (ANC $<0.2 \times 10^9$/L) aplastic anemia should be considered for immunosuppressive therapy or, if they are younger than 40 years with a matched sibling donor, for BMT. Patients with nonsevere aplastic anemia (ANC $>0.5 \times 10^9$/L), those older than 40 years, and those lacking a matched related sibling donor should be treated with supportive care (growth factors, transfusions) and immunosuppression.

Myelodysplasia

Etiology and Pathogenesis

Myelodysplasia is a clonal disorder of hematopoietic progenitor cells, which results in ineffective hematopoiesis. The marrow is usually hypercellular, but stem cells are unable to differentiate into mature cells that leave the marrow cavity and function normally in the peripheral blood. Myelodysplastic syndromes are classified into five categories (Table 72-1). Myelodysplasia is generally an

Table 72-1 World Health Organization Criteria for Myelodysplastic Syndromes

Syndrome	Cytopenia	Dysplasia in Bone Marrow	Ringed Sideroblasts	Blasts Peripheral Blood	Blasts Bone Marrow	Auer Rods
Refractory anemia	Anemia	Erythroid	<15%	No	<5%	No
Refractory anemia with ringed sideroblasts	Anemia	Erythroid	≥15%	No	<5%	No
Refractory cytopenia with multilineage dysplasia	Bi- or pancytopenia; monocytes <1000/μL	≥10% in two or more myeloid cell lines	<15%	Rare	<5%	No
Refractory cytopenia with multilineage dysplasia and ringed sideroblasts	Bi- or pancytopenia; monocytes <1000/μL	≥10% in two or more cell lines	≥15%	Rare	<5%	No
Refractory anemia with excess blasts-1	Cytopenia; monocytes <1000/μL	Single- or multiple-lineage dysplasia		<5%	5%-9%	No
Refractory anemia with excess blasts-2	Cytopenia; monocytes <1000/μL	Single- or multiple-lineage dysplasia		5%-19%	10%-19%	±
Myelodysplastic syndrome (MDS), unclassified	Cytopenia	Dysplasia in granulocytes or megakaryocytes		Rare	<5%	No
MDS with 5q deletion (5q-syndrome)	Anemia; normal or increased platelets	Megakaryocytes normal or increased with hypolobated nuclei		<5%	<5%	No

idiopathic acquired process, but it has been associated with exposure to chemicals (solvents, pesticides), chemotherapy, and radiation therapy.

Clinical Presentation

As with all bone marrow failure syndromes, presentation depends on which cell line is primarily affected (see Fig. 72-1). Patients can present with fatigue, dyspnea, bleeding, petechiae, or recurrent infection; asymptomatic patients may be diagnosed after routine blood work. Although initial cytopenia may be mild, progressive pancytopenia usually occurs over several years.

Differential Diagnosis

The differential diagnosis of pancytopenia in myelodysplastic syndrome (MDS) patients includes hypersplenism, aplastic anemia, congenital causes, PNH, viral marrow suppression, marrow infiltration, and anemia of chronic disease. Dysplastic changes in the bone marrow can also be caused by vitamin deficiency (B_{12}, folate), drugs (antibiotics, diphenylhydantoin, and chemotherapy), ethanol, benzene, lead, and viral infections (HIV).

Diagnostic Approach

Diagnosis requires examination of the peripheral blood smear and the bone marrow biopsy specimen. The peripheral blood smear may show macrocytic red blood cells, hypogranular neutrophils (pseudo–Pelger-Huët anomaly), and giant platelets. Bone marrow evaluation shows normal or increased cellularity, megaloblastic red blood cell precursors, ringed sideroblasts, and immature myeloid cells, often with an increase in myeloblasts.

Cytogenetic analysis is important for determining the biology and prognosis of the disease. Half of all cases of myelodysplasia include a cytogenetic abnormality. Complex abnormalities are associated with an aggressive course and rapid progression to acute leukemia. However, those with an isolated deletion of chromosome 5 (5q-syndrome) have a more benign course that includes a tendency to develop an isolated anemia without other cell lines being involved; the median survival of patients with 5q-syndrome is longer than 5 years, and only 25% experience progression to acute leukemia (Tables 72-2 and 72-3).

Management and Therapy

Supportive care includes the administration of hematopoietic cytokines and growth factors, especially the

Table 72-2 International Prognostic Scoring System for Myelodysplastic Syndromes

Prognostic variables	0	0.5	1.0	1.5	2.0
		Survival and Acute Myeloid Leukemia Evolution Score Value			
Marrow blasts (%)	<5	5-10	—	11-20	21-30
Karyotype	Good	Intermediate	Poor	—	—
Cytopenia	0-1	2-3	—	—	—

Karyotypes: good = normal, -Y, del(5q), del(20q); poor = complex (>3 abnormalities) or chromosome 7 anomalies; intermediate = other abnormalities. Cytopenias: neutrophils <1800/μL, platelets <100,000/μL, hemoglobin <10 g/dL.

Modified from Greenberg P: Aplastic anemia. In Hoffman R, Benz EJ Jr, Shattil SJ, et al (eds): Hematology: Basic Principles and Practice, 3rd ed. New York, Churchill Livingstone, 2000, p 298.

Table 72-3 Survival by International Prognostic Scoring System

Risk Category	Combined Score	Median Survival (yr)
Low	0	5.7
Intermediate		
1	0.5-1.0	3.5
2	1.5-2.0	1.2
High	≥2.5	0.4

Note: Median age at diagnosis is the seventh decade, with a 3 : 2 proportion favoring men. Many patients progress to acute myeloid leukemia (AML). This can range from 5% transformation in refractory anemia with ringed sideroblasts (median survival, 73 months) to 40% to 50% in refractory anemia with excess blasts (median survival, 12 months) and refractory anemia with excess blasts in transformation (median survival, 5 months), respectively. AML following evolution of myelodysplastic syndrome (MDS) is an especially aggressive form of leukemia that is difficult to treat and is fatal in 90% of the one third to one half of MDS patients in whom it develops. *Reprinted with permission from Heaney ML, Golde DW: Myelodysplasia. N Engl J Med 340:1651, 1999.*

combination of erythropoietin and G-CSF. Patients with less than 20% blasts in their marrow can be given a trial of 5-azacytidine or decitabine to induce differentiation and maturation of the abnormal cells. Lenalidomide warrants consideration in patients with a 5q deletion because complete cytogenetic responses with decreased splenomegaly and transfusion requirements have been seen with this therapy. Other management options include chemotherapy and stem cell transplantation. Immunomodulation may be promising. In a pilot study of 25 patients, 11 patients, most of whom had the HLA-DR15 haplotype, became transfusion independent after treatment with ATG (Table 72-4).

Patients who develop blast counts greater than 20% are frequently treated with standard induction regimens for acute leukemia. Results have been disappointing, with a remission rate of 50% to 60% and a relapse rate of 90% for anthracycline-cytarabine combinations. Although BMT is the only curative therapy for such patients and should be undertaken when feasible, patients often fare poorly because of their advanced age and resistant disease.

Optimum Treatment

Care of patients with myelodysplasia is directed at symptom control with growth factor support including G-CSF and erythropoietin plus blood transfusions when necessary. Lenalidomide is the recommended therapy in patients with 5q-syndrome; azacitidine or decitabine can be used in other MDS patients. If a patient progresses to acute leukemia, standard leukemia chemotherapy regimens are implemented. For younger patients, BMT should be considered as the only potentially curative option; the optimal timeframe for BMT is when the disease is progressing but before leukemic transformation has occurred.

Agnogenic Myeloid Metaplasia and Myelofibrosis

Etiology and Pathogenesis

Fibrosis of the bone marrow (myelofibrosis) is divided into primary (idiopathic) and secondary processes. Myelofibrosis can be caused by infiltration of the bone marrow by a neoplastic process, granulomatous infections, and metabolic abnormalities.

Malignant disorders associated with myelofibrosis include agnogenic myeloid metaplasia, polycythemia vera, chronic myeloid leukemia, essential thrombocytosis, acute myelofibrosis, acute myeloid leukemia, hairy cell leukemia, acute myelodysplasia with myelofibrosis, multiple myeloma, non-Hodgkin's lymphoma, and metastatic carcinoma.

Nonmalignant conditions associated with myelofibrosis include tuberculosis, histoplasmosis, renal osteodystrophy, vitamin D deficiency, hypoparathyroidism, hyperparathyroidism, gray platelet syndrome, systemic lupus erythematosus, scleroderma, radiation exposure, osteopetrosis, Paget's disease, benzene exposure, thorotrast exposure, and Gaucher's disease.

Table 72-4 Myelodysplasia and Therapies

	(G-CSF) + Epo vs. Epo Alone	Azacitidine vs. Best Supportive Care	Decitabine vs. Best Supportive Care	Lenalidomide
Overall response rate	73.3% vs. 40% (erythroid response)	60% vs. 5% (response in at least one blood cell line)	17% vs. 0% (all cell lines improved, and a 50% decrease in bone marrow blasts)	56% Overall; 83% 5q-syndrome; 57% normal cytogenetics; 12% abnormal cytogenetics (erythroid response)
Median time to event (AML or death)	Not available	21 mo vs. 12 mo (*P* = 0.007)	12 m vs. 6.8 m (*P* = 0.03) (in the subgroup of patients with IPSS Int-2/high-risk MDS)	Not available
Overall survival	Not available	20 mo vs. 14 mo (*P* = 0.10)	Not available	Not available

AML, acute myeloid leukemia; G-CSF, granulocyte colony stimulating factor; Epo, erythropoietin; IPSS, International Prognostic Scoring System; MDS, myelodysplastic syndrome. *Data from Balleari E, Rossi E, Clavio M, et al: Ann Hematol 85:174-180, 2006; Kantarjian H, Issa JPJ, Rosenfeld CS, et al: Cancer 106:1794-1880, 2006; List A, Kurtin S, Roe DJ, et al: N Engl J Med 352:549-557, 2005; and Silverman LR, Demakos EP, Peterson BL, et al: J Clin Oncol 20:2429-2440, 2002.*

Clinical Presentation

Patients present with marked splenomegaly, progressive anemia, and constitutional symptoms including fatigue, weight loss, night sweats, fever, early satiety, diarrhea, and peripheral edema. Upon examination, they have pancytopenia, leftward shift in the granulocyte count, and increased levels of lactate dehydrogenase as a result of extramedullary hematopoiesis and accelerated marrow cell turnover. Complications can include portal hypertension or splenic infarction, as well as symptoms from extramedullary hematopoiesis associated with lymphadenopathy, ascites, pleural effusions, pneumonia, hematuria, or compression of the spinal cord and nerve roots. Median age at diagnosis is 65 years, with no definitive gender distribution.

Differential Diagnosis

The differential diagnosis includes other hematologic malignancies such as chronic myelogenous leukemia, lymphoma, multiple myeloma, Hodgkin's disease, hairy cell leukemia, and myelodysplastic syndromes. Solid tumors such as metastatic breast, prostate, or lung cancer can also cause this syndrome.

Diagnostic Approach

The diagnosis is made through examination of the peripheral blood smear and the bone marrow. The peripheral blood smear shows immature granulocytes, nucleated red cells (leukoerythroblastosis), and teardrop-shaped red blood cells. Biopsy of the bone marrow shows fibroblasts in the marrow space with reactive myelofibrosis along with dysplastic-megakaryocyte hyperplasia. Cytogenetic studies

are most useful for excluding chronic myelogenous leukemia and identifying those patients at risk for rapid transformation to acute leukemia.

The diagnosis of myelofibrosis with myeloid metaplasia is based on the following combinations: two necessary criteria plus any two optional criteria when splenomegaly is present, or two necessary criteria plus any four optional criteria when splenomegaly is absent.

> *Necessary criteria:* (1) diffuse bone marrow fibrosis, and (2) absence of Philadelphia chromosome or *BCR-ABL* rearrangement in peripheral blood cells
>
> *Optional criteria:* splenomegaly, anisopoikilocytosis with teardrop erythrocytes, circulating immature myeloid cells, circulating erythroblasts, clusters of megakaryoblasts and dysplastic megakaryocytes in bone marrow sections, myeloid metaplasia

Management and Therapy

Median survival is 3 to 6 years (Table 72-5). Death is usually due to complications of thrombocytopenia (bleeding) or neutropenia (infection). Transformation to acute leukemia is uncommon, occurring in less than 5% of cases. Prognostic factors associated with shortened survival include advanced age, anemia, hypercatabolic symptoms, leukocytosis, leukopenia, circulating blasts, increased numbers of granulocyte precursors, thrombocytopenia, and abnormalities in karyotype.

Management and therapy of myelofibrosis are largely palliative. Androgen preparations and corticosteroids are used to alleviate anemia. Hydroxyurea or thalidomide can be used to control leukocytosis, thrombocytosis, and organomegaly. Alternative treatments include interferon-

Table 72-5 Lille Scoring System for Predicting Survival in Myelofibrosis with Myeloid Metaplasia

No. of Adverse Prognostic Factors	Risk Group	Median Survival (mo)
0	Low	93
1	Intermediate	26
2	High	13

Note: Adverse prognostic factors were hemoglobin count less than 10 g/dL and white blood cell count less than 4 or greater than 30 × 10⁹/L. *Data from Barosi G: Myelofibrosis with myeloid metaplasia: Diagnostic definition and prognostic classification for clinical studies and treatment guidelines. J Clin Oncol 17(9):2961, 1999.*

α and cladribine. In anemic patients with low serum erythropoietin levels, darbepoetin or epoetin alfa injections may be helpful.

Splenectomy is recommended for patients with hydroxyurea-resistant symptomatic splenomegaly, overt portal hypertension, and progressive anemia requiring transfusion. For patients with contraindications to surgery, splenic irradiation can be effective. Allogeneic stem cell transplantation is an option in young patients and is the only potentially curative therapy.

Optimum Treatment

The goal of therapy is to minimize symptoms while avoiding treatment-related toxicities. Therefore, patients with mild cytopenia and minimal symptoms do not require treatment. As the disease progresses, stem cell transplantation is a good option in young patients. Otherwise, treatment with either hydroxyurea or thalidomide is an acceptable option, with responses seen in up to half of patients. For patients with massive symptomatic splenomegaly, splenectomy or splenic irradiation should be considered.

Avoiding Treatment Errors

All patients with marrow failure syndromes should be referred to a hematologist. Before subjecting patients to intensive therapy or BMT, easily reversible causes of disease must be ruled out. For any patients who have the potential for proceeding to BMT, blood transfusions should be minimized because a history of multiple blood transfusions is associated with worse outcomes after transplantation. Additionally, patients who have received multiple blood transfusions (>20 to 30 units) should be monitored for iron overload, with possible initiation of iron chelation to prevent long-term complications. Every patient, even those who obtain a complete response to therapy, must be closely monitored for relapse or progression of disease and transformation to acute leukemia or, in patients with aplastic anemia, to PNH.

Future Directions

Aplastic Anemias

Future directions for the therapy of aplastic anemia include nonablative BMT, growth factors (megakaryocyte growth factors, stem cell–stimulating factors, and other cytokines), high-dose cyclophosphamide, recombinant humanized anti–interleukin-2 receptor antibody–directed therapy, and gene therapy for identifiable lesions such as Fanconi's anemia.

Myelodysplasia

Future directions include nonablative BMT, immunomodulation, and molecular genetic approaches. Thalidomide and arsenic trioxide have also shown some benefit in treating patients with MDS, but more data are needed. Long-term outcomes with methylation-altering agents such as 5-azacytidine and decitabine or immunomodulating agents like lenalidomide remain to be determined.

Agnogenic Myeloid Metaplasia and Myelofibrosis

Future directions for therapy include lenalidomide, antifibrotic therapy, cytokine-directed approaches, and safer, more effective methods of allogeneic transplantation.

Additional Resources

Aplastic Anemias

Aplastic Anemia & MDS International Foundation, Inc. Available at: http://www.aamds.org/aplastic/. Accessed October 8, 2006.
   This website for patients provides details about diseases, clinical trials, and support networks.
Bagby GC, Lipton JM, Sloand EM, Schiffer CA: Marrow failure. Hematology Am Soc Hematol Educ Prog; 318-336, 2004.
   This paper provides a broad review of marrow failure syndromes.
Young NS, Calado RT, Scheinberg P: Current concepts in the pathophysiology and treatment of aplastic anemia. Blood 108:2509-2519, 2006.
   This is an excellent review of the pathophysiology and treatment of aplastic anemia.

Myelodysplasia

Aplastic Anemia & MDS International Foundation, Inc. Available at: http://www.aamds.org/aplastic/. Accessed October 8, 2006.
   This website for patients provides details about aplastic anemia and MDS treatment, clinical trials, and support networks.
The National Comprehensive Cancer Network (NCCN) Clinical Practice Guidelines in Oncology. Available at http://www.nccn.org/professionals/physician_gls/f_guidelines.asp. Accessed October 8, 2006.
   The NCCN website has guidelines for the treatment of myelodysplastic syndromes.

Agnogenic Myeloid Metaplasia and Myelofibrosis

Barosi G: Myelofibrosis with myeloid metaplasia: Diagnostic definition and prognostic classification for clinical studies and treatment guidelines. J Clin Oncol 17:2954-2970, 1999.

The author reviews the pathophysiology and diagnosis of myelofibrosis with myeloid metaplasia.

Tefferi A: Pathogenesis of myelofibrosis with myeloid metaplasia. J Clin Oncol 23:8520-8530, 2005.

This is an excellent, detailed review of pathogenetic causes of myelofibrosis and their therapeutic implications.

EVIDENCE

Aplastic Anemias

1. Di Bona E, Rodeghiero F, Bruno B, et al: Rabbit antithymocyte globulin (r-ATG) plus cyclosporine and granulocyte colony stimulating factor is an effective treatment for aplastic anaemia patients unresponsive to a first course of intensive immunosuppressive therapy. Br J Haematol 107:330-334, 1999.

   Up to 77% of patients unresponsive to first-line immunosuppressive therapy respond to treatment with rabbit-ATG, cyclosporine, and G-CSF.

2. Frickhofen N, Heimpel H, Kaltwasser JP, et al: Antithymocyte globulin with or without cyclosporin A: 11-Year follow-up of a randomized trial comparing treatments of aplastic anemia. Blood 101:1236-1242, 2003.

   Results are reported from a randomized trial comparing ATG/methylprednisolone with or without cyclosporine in 84 patients after a median follow-up of 11 years. Cyclosporine improved disease-free survival and overall response rate but not overall survival.

3. Kojima S, Frickhofen N, Deeg HJ, et al: Aplastic anemia. Int J Hematol 82:408-411, 2005.

   The authors present recommendations of a 2004 international consensus panel on the treatment of severe aplastic anemia.

4. Marsh J, Schrezenmeier H, Marin P, et al. Prospective randomized multicenter study comparing cyclosporin alone versus the combination of antithymocyte globulin and cyclosporin for treatment of patients with nonsevere aplastic anemia: A report from the European Blood and Marrow Transplant (EBMT) Severe Aplastic Anaemia Working Party. Blood 93(7):2191-2195, 1999.

   This study concluded that cyclosporine plus ATG has a higher overall response rate than cyclosporine alone.

5. Rosenfeld S, Follmann D, Nunez O, Young NS: Antithymocyte globulin and cyclosporine for severe aplastic anemia: Association between hematologic response and long-term outcome. JAMA 289:1130-1135, 2003.

   Long-term outcomes of aplastic anemia patients treated with ATG and cyclosporine showed durable responses in half of patients.

Myelodysplasia

1. Balleari E, Rossi E, Clavio M, et al: Erythropoietin plus granulocyte colony-stimulating factor is better than erythropoietin alone to treat anemia in low-risk myelodysplastic syndromes: Results from a randomized single-centre study. Ann Hematol 85:174-180, 2006.

   Results showed a higher erythroid response rate with G-CSF plus erythropoietin than with erythropoietin alone.

2. Kaminskas E, Farrell A, Abraham S, et al: Approval summary: Azacitidine for treatment of myelodysplastic syndrome subtypes. Clin Cancer Res 11:3604-3608, 2005.

   This is a summary of the data used by the U.S. Food and Drug Administration to approve azacitidine for treatment of MDS.

3. Kantarjian H, Issa JPJ, Rosenfeld CS, et al: Decitabine improves patient outcomes in myelodysplastic syndromes: Results of a phase III randomized study. Cancer 106:1794-1880, 2006.

   Results showed a longer time to progression to AML or death in high-risk patients treated with decitabine than in patients treated with best supportive care.

4. List A, Kurtin S, Roe DJ, et al: Efficacy of lenalidomide in myelodysplastic syndromes. N Engl J Med 352:549-557, 2005.

   Lenalidomide decreases erythroid transfusion requirements and induces some cytogenetic remissions. The highest response rates were seen in patients with 5q deletions.

5. Silverman LR, Demakos EP, Peterson BL, et al: Randomized controlled trial of azacitidine in patients with the myelodysplastic syndrome: A study of the cancer and leukemia group B. J Clin Oncol 20:2429-2440, 2002.

   Higher response rates, decreased leukemic transformation, and improved survival were seen with azacitidine therapy compared with best supportive care.

Agnogenic Myeloid Metaplasia and Myelofibrosis

1. Deeg HJ, Gooley TA, Flowers MED, et al: Allogeneic hematopoietic stem cell transplantation for myelofibrosis. Blood 102:3912-3918, 2003.

   Allogeneic transplantation can lead to long-term relapse-free survival.

2. Marchetti M, Barosi G, Balestri F, et al: Low-dose thalidomide ameliorates cytopenias and splenomegaly in myelofibrosis with myeloid metaplasia: A phase II trial. J Clin Oncol 22:424-431, 2004.

   Thalidomide therapy can lead to decreased splenomegaly, cytopenia, and fatigue.

Mark E. Brecher

Blood Component Therapy

Introduction

The transfusion of blood was the first successful transplantation of living tissue in humans. Today, transfusion of blood components is so common and safe that it is rarely thought of as a transplantation. In 2001, for allogeneic transfusions within the United States alone, it is estimated that 13,898,000 units of whole blood/red blood cells, 2,614,000 units of whole blood–derived platelets, 1,264,000 units of apheresis platelets, and 3,926,000 units of plasma were administered. For red blood cell–containing products alone, this equates to 1 unit transfused every 2.3 seconds. A basic understanding of compatibility, indications, and the risks of blood component therapy are essential both for optimal patient care and for providing patients with information for a truly informed decision.

Basic Immunohematology

Pretransfusion testing confirms compatibility between the blood component and the recipient and detects unexpected but clinically significant antibodies that might harm the recipient or compromise the survival of the transfused cells. Red blood cell serologic testing depends on in vitro hemolysis or agglutination resulting from red blood cell antigen-antibody interaction. ABO typing involves testing of the recipient's red blood cells with potent anti-A and anti-B typing reagent (forward typing) and reaction of the recipient's plasma or serum with A1 (the major subtype of group A) and B red blood cells (reverse typing). Typically, ABO antibodies are immunoglobulin M antibodies and are reactive at room temperature. Rh typing tests the recipient's red blood cells with a chemically modified immunoglobulin G anti-D antibody that is reactive at room temperature.

Antibody screening for unexpected red blood cell antibodies requires testing of serum or plasma with group O reagent red blood cells selected to express all commonly occurring clinically significant antigens. Clinically significant antibodies present in serum or plasma are detected after 37° C incubation or after the addition of antihuman globulin (an indirect antihuman globulin test or indirect Coombs' test). If an unexpected antibody is detected, further serologic testing to identify the antigen specificity of the antigen is performed. A nonreactive antibody screen allows for the rapid selection of red blood cells that require only a confirmation of ABO compatibility. The presence of unexpected antibodies requires the more time-consuming identification of antigen-negative units and a full crossmatch. A full crossmatch requires testing the recipient's serum or plasma with red cells from the units to be transfused, incubation at 37° C, and testing with antihuman globulin.

With the exception of infants, the lack of expression of either the A or B antigen results in the formation of anti-B or anti-A, respectively. A group O individual lacks both the A and the B antigens and thus forms both anti-A and anti-B. The ABO antigens, their antibodies, and compatibility of red blood cell and plasma components are summarized in Table 73-1.

Platelets can be thought of as bags of plasma, and ideally one would transfuse platelets with the compatibility of plasma. However, because of the short shelf life of platelets (5 days, or 7 days for some apheresis products), platelets are frequently transfused across ABO compatibility barriers. Cryoprecipitate due to the limited volume transfused is also frequently transfused across ABO plasma compatibility barriers. Group O is a universal red blood cell unit. Group AB is a universal plasma unit.

Table 73-1 ABO Types and Compatibility of Red Cells and Plasma

ABO Type (Antigens Expressed)	Percentage of Population	ABO Red Blood Cell Compatibility	Plasma Compatibility
O	45	O	O, A, B, AB
A	40	A, O	A, AB
B	11	B, O	B, AB
AB	4	AB, A, B, O	AB

Rh-negative (D-negative) red blood cells and platelets (which account for only 15% of the donor base) are reserved principally for female recipients of childbearing potential, and thus at risk for hemolytic disease of the newborn with pregnancy. To preserve an inventory of Rh-negative units, trauma cases involving males, in which the type is not initially known, are frequently transfused with Rh-positive red blood cells.

Blood Components and Indications for Transfusion

Individual institutions must have guidelines for the transfusion of blood components. These guidelines are based on the scientific literature and local practice and serve as the basis for the focused review of transfusion practices. Although guidelines represent institution consensus, they cannot substitute for clinical judgment and the need for flexibility in practice, and should not be considered a mandate to transfuse or not to transfuse.

Before the administration of blood or blood components, the indications, risks, and benefits of a blood transfusion and possible alternatives must be discussed with the patient and documented in the medical record. Transfusions should be documented in the patient's record, including both indications and outcome. Specific notations should be made when exceptions to the institutional guidelines exist.

Red Blood Cells

The purpose of red blood cell transfusion is to provide oxygen-carrying capacity and to maintain tissue oxygenation when the intravascular volume and cardiac function are adequate for perfusion. One unit of red blood cells should increase the patient's hemoglobin (Hgb) level by 1 g/dL or the hematocrit by 3% in a 70-kg recipient. Red blood cell transfusion should only be used when time or underlying pathophysiology precludes other management (e.g., iron, erythropoietin, and folate).

Criteria are as follows: (1) Hgb <8 g/dL in an otherwise healthy patient; (2) Hgb <11 g/dL in cases of increased risk for ischemia (e.g., pulmonary disease, coronary artery disease, cerebral vascular disease); (3) acute blood loss resulting in blood loss >15% of total blood volume (750 mL in 70-kg male) or with evidence of inadequate oxygen delivery (e.g., electrocardiographic signs of cardiac ischemia, tachycardia, cyanosis); (4) symptomatic anemia in a normovolemic patient (e.g., tachycardia, mental status changes, electrocardiographic signs of cardiac ischemia, angina, shortness of breath, lightheadedness or dizziness with mild exertion); or (5) regular predetermined therapeutic program for severe hypoplastic or aplastic anemia or for bone marrow suppression for hemoglobinopathies. The post-transfusion Hgb should not exceed 11.5 g/dL (12.5 g/dL in those cases of increased risk for organ/tissue ischemia).

It is not acceptable to use red blood cell transfusions to increase wound healing or merely to take advantage of readily available predonated autologous blood without an acceptable medical indication.

Platelets

Platelets are used for patients suffering from or at significant risk for hemorrhage due to thrombocytopenia or platelet dysfunction. One unit of whole blood–derived platelets (a random unit) should increase the platelet count by 7 to 10×10^9/L in a 70-kg recipient. Dosing is generally a pool of 4 to 6 U. A single donor apheresis platelet transfusion should increase the platelet count by 40 to 60×10^9/L in a 70-kg recipient. In the United States, the use of apheresis platelets has been increasing annually. In 2004, it was estimated that 77% of all therapeutic doses of platelets transfused were apheresis platelets.

Criteria are as follows: (1) platelet count $\leq 10 \times 10^9$/L (for prophylaxis in stable, nonfebrile patients), or $<20 \times 10^9$/L for prophylaxis with fever or instability; (2) platelet count $\leq 50 \times 10^9$/L in a patient with documented hemorrhage or rapidly decreasing platelet count or planned invasive or surgical procedure; (3) diffuse microvascular bleeding in a patient with disseminated intravascular coagulation or following a massive blood loss (>1 blood volume) with a platelet count not yet available; or (4) bleeding in a patient with platelet dysfunction.

Unacceptable indications for platelet transfusion include patients with the following syndromes, but no evidence of bleeding or coagulopathy: thrombotic thrombocytopenic purpura (TTP), hemolytic-uremic syndrome (HUS), or idiopathic thrombocytopenic purpura; empiric use during massive transfusion in which the patient does not exhibit a clinical coagulopathy; and extrinsic platelet dysfunction, such as in renal failure, hyperproteinemia, or von Willebrand's disease.

Plasma

This component contains adequate levels of all soluble coagulation factors. Plasma is available as fresh frozen plasma (FFP), plasma frozen within 24 hours, and thawed plasma. These products are indicated for the correction of multiple or specific coagulation factor deficiencies, or for the empiric treatment of TTP or HUS. One unit contains about 220 mL, and the usual starting dose is 5 to 15 mL/kg (2 to 4 U in a 70-kg recipient).

Criteria for transfusion include treatment or prophylaxis of multiple or specific coagulation factor deficiencies (prothrombin time [PT] or partial thromboplastin time [PTT] >1.5 times the mean normal value). Congenital deficiencies (antithrombin III; factors II, V, VII, IX, X, XI; plasminogen; or antiplasmin) or acquired deficiencies related to warfarin therapy, vitamin K deficiency, liver disease, massive transfusion (>1 blood volume in 24 hours), and disseminated intravascular coagulation are acceptable indications for the transfusion of plasma. Plasma is also indicated in patients with a suspected coagulation deficiency (PT/PTT pending) who are bleeding, or at risk for bleeding, from an invasive procedure. Unacceptable criteria are empiric use during massive transfusion in which the patient does not exhibit clinical coagulopathy, nutritional supplementation, or volume replacement.

Cryoprecipitate

Cryoprecipitate is a cold insoluble fraction of FFP; each bag contains about 80 to 100 U of factor VIII and 250 mg of fibrinogen. It also contains factor XIII and von Willebrand's factor. The usual starting dose is one concentrate per 7 to 10 kg. In a 70-kg male, 10 U would be expected to raise the fibrinogen 40 mg/dL. Cryoprecipitate may also be applied topically, with an equal volume of bovine thrombin, taking advantage of its adhesive, hemostatic, and sealant properties. Single units are appropriate as a fibrin sealant or glue.

Appropriate indications for cryoprecipitate use include treatment or prevention of bleeding associated with certain known or suspected clotting factor deficiencies (factor VIII, von Willebrand's factor, factor XIII, or factor I) and of a prolonged bleeding time or fibrinogen of less than 150 mg/dL or other specific coagulation factor assay-documented deficiency. Cryoprecipitate may also be used for the treatment of surface oozing and the maintenance of tissues in tight apposition to each other or the sealing of leaking spaces (fibrin glue). The use of desmopressin acetate may frequently be a preferred or acceptable alternative to use of cryoprecipitate for patients with type I von

Willebrand's disease, mild hemophilia A (factor VIII deficiency), or certain platelet dysfunctional disorders.

Other Blood-Derived Products

Other blood-derived products, such as intravenous immunoglobulin preparations, normal serum albumin, and coagulation factor concentrates, are beyond the scope of this chapter. Their use is covered in other relevant chapters.

Risks of Blood Products

Infectious Disease

Although blood products today are considered safer than ever, a truly zero-risk blood supply is probably unattainable. Currently, blood donations in developed countries are screened for HIV types 1 and 2, hepatitis C, hepatitis B, and syphilis. Recently, many countries have begun testing for hepatitis C and HIV with nucleic amplification testing (NAT). Knowledge of the current risk for disease transmission (summarized later) is a prerequisite for proper informed consent for transfusion (Table 73-2).

Table 73-2 Risk for Infectious Disease	
Infectious Agent	**Estimated Risk/Unit (with Nucleic Amplification Testing)**
Virus	
HIV types 1 and 2	1 : 400,000-1 : 2,400,000
Human T-cell lymphotrophic virus types I and II	1 : 256,000-1 : 2,000,000
Hepatitis B	1 : 58,000-1 : 147,000
Hepatitis C	1 : 872,000-1 : 700,000
West Nile virus	<1 : 2,000,000 but in flux, with regional, temporal, and testing variation
Bacteria	
Red blood cells	1 : 1000 (contaminated) <1 : 1,000,000 (fatal)
Platelets screened with Gram stain, pH, or glucose concentration	1 : 2000-1 : 4000 >40% result in clinical sequelae
Platelets screened with aerobic culture	<1 : 10,000
Syphilis	<1 : 10,000,000
Parasites	
Malaria, *Babesia* species	<1 : 1,000,000

Note: The high risk for bacterial contamination of platelets is due to the required storage at 20° C to 24° C; 1 : 2500 per pool of 6 or 1 : 13,400 single donor apheresis platelets result in clinical sepsis (without a bacterial detection screen). The related mortality is about 1 : 17,000 for random donor pools and 1 : 16,000 for single donor apheresis platelets (nonscreened for bacteria).
Modified from Brecher ME (ed): Technical Manual, 15th ed. Bethesda, MD, American Association of Blood Banks, 2005, p 700.

Table 73-3 Noninfectious Complications of Transfusion

Type	Rate
Acute (≤24 Hours of Transfusion)	
Immunologic	
Hemolytic	1 : 38,000-1 : 70,000
Nonhemolytic (febrile, chills)	1 : 100-1 : 200
Transfusion-related acute lung injury	1 : 5000-1 : 190,000
Allergic (mild)	1 : 33-1 : 100
Anaphylactic	1 : 20,000-1 : 50,000
Angiotensin-converting enzyme inhibitor—mediated hypotension	Dependent on clinical setting
Nonimmunologic	
Fluid overload	<1%
Air embolism	Rare
Citrate toxicity (hypocalcemia)	Dependent on clinical setting
Pseudohemolytic	Unknown
Delayed (>24 Hours after Transfusion)	
Immunologic	
Delayed hemolytic	1 : 5000-1 : 11,000
Graft-versus-host disease	Rare
Post-transfusion purpura	Rare
Nonimmunologic	
Iron overload	After >100 units of red blood cells

Modified from Brecher ME (ed): Technical Manual, 15th ed. Bethesda, MD, American Association of Blood Banks, 2005, pp 634-638.

Noninfectious Disease

The greatest risk of transfusion involves noninfectious complications. The most common noninfectious cause for death is the transfusion of ABO-incompatible allogeneic red blood cells (with the administration of ABO-incompatible red blood cells at a rate of 1 : 38,000 units and a fatality rate of 1 : 1,300,000 units transfused). These events are invariably due to human error, classically, the misidentification of a patient or sample. It is because of the recognition of this avoidable source of error that blood banks and transfusion services have very stringent policies regarding patient and sample identification. Noninfectious complications of transfusion can be divided into acute (≤24 hours of transfusion) and delayed (>24 hours after transfusion) (Table 73-3).

Future Directions

Future directions for blood component therapy include additional initiatives to reduce the risk for infectious disease such as wider application of NAT testing, use of viral and bacterial inactivation technologies, or both. Currently, the use of bacterial culture of apheresis platelets is allowing a transition to a 7-day extended storage. Red blood cell "substitutes" made from polymerized Hgb are currently in clinical trials. Such products with a prolonged shelf life will not require compatibility testing and may provide transient (24 to 48 hours) oxygen-carrying capacity in patients for whom transfusion of red blood cells is not an option (e.g., trauma patients in the field) or allow extensive acute normovolemic hemodilution in the operative setting.

Additional Resources

Goodnough LT, Brecher ME, Kanter MH, AuBuchon JP: Transfusion medicine. Second of two parts—blood conservation. N Engl J Med 340(7):525-533, 1999.
  This is the second part of a review article on the current state of transfusion medicine, with emphasis on blood conservation.

EVIDENCE

1. Brecher ME (ed): Technical Manual, 15th ed. Bethesda, MD, American Association of Blood Banks, 2005.
    This is one of the most referenced sources of information in blood banking and transfusion medicine.
2. Goodnough LT, Brecher ME, Kanter MH, AuBuchon JP: Transfusion medicine. First of two parts—blood transfusion. N Engl J Med 340(6):438-447, 1999.
    This review article provides an overview of the current state of transfusion medicine.
3. Goodnough LT, Shander A, Brecher ME: Transfusion medicine: Looking to the future. Lancet 361(9352):161-169, 2003.
    This review article looks to the future of transfusion medicine.
4. Stehling L, Luban NL, Anderson KC, et al: Guidelines for blood utilization review. Transfusion 34(5):438-448, 1994.
    This is the American Association of Blood Banks example of guidelines and indications for transfusion.

Peter M. Voorhees ▪ Robert Z. Orlowski

Malignant Lymphomas

Introduction

Lymphomas arise from a malignant transformation of lymphoid cells (B-, T-, or natural killer cells) and are classified as Hodgkin's disease (HD) or non-Hodgkin's lymphoma (NHL). HD is divided into five subtypes that share many characteristics, while NHL comprises a heterogeneous group of more than 20 malignancies that are distinct not only from HD, but in many cases from one another (Box 74-1). NHL can be divided broadly into low-, intermediate-, and high-grade malignancies based on their clinical aggressiveness. Low-grade NHL is associated with long survival but, in most instances, is not curable. In contrast, although the median survival for intermediate- and high-grade NHL is shorter, they often can be cured. With current therapy, HD is curable in most patients.

In developed areas, the incidence of HD is about 3 of 100,000 persons. A bimodal age distribution is seen, with a first peak occurring in the third decade and a second peak after the age of 50 years. NHL is more common than HD, representing 4% of all new cancer diagnoses in the United States. In 2006, it is estimated that there will be 58,700 new cases of NHL diagnosed in the United States, in contrast to 7800 new cases of HD. The 5-year survival rates for HD and NHL during the period from 1974 to 1976 were 71% and 47%, respectively, but have since increased to 85% and 60% during the period from 1995 to 2001, which is testimony to the significant advances made in the therapy for these diseases.

Etiology and Pathogenesis

Several factors support a possible role for Epstein-Barr virus (EBV) in the pathogenesis of HD as evidenced by the fact that patients with a history of infectious mononucleosis have a twofold to threefold increased risk for developing HD, and that EBV is found in the tumor cells of about half of cases. Patients with HIV are at increased risk for the development of HD. Furthermore, there appears to be a slight genetic predisposition to the development of HD, in that about 1% of patients have a family history of HD, with first-degree relatives and monozygotic (compared with dizygotic) twins being at increased risk.

Whereas HD is typically cytogenetically normal, in NHL nonrandom chromosomal translocations are frequently encountered and play important pathogenic roles. Notable examples include translocations involving chromosome 8q24, which lead to overexpression of *c-Myc* in Burkitt's lymphoma (BL); t(14;18), which leads to overexpression of the B-cell survival factor, *Bcl-2*, in follicular lymphoma; and t(11;14), which results in up-regulation of the cell cycle regulator, cyclin D1, in mantle cell lymphoma.

Several risk factors for NHL have been identified, including primary immunodeficiency syndromes (e.g., ataxia-telangiectasia, Wiskott-Aldrich syndrome) and secondary immunodeficiency from pharmacologic immunosuppression of organ transplant recipients or HIV infection. Other infectious agents associated with an increased risk for NHL include hepatitis C virus (splenic marginal zone lymphoma), human T-cell leukemia virus type I (adult T-cell leukemia and lymphoma), EBV (primary central nervous system [CNS] lymphomas and BL), human herpesvirus-8 (primary effusion lymphoma), *Helicobacter pylori* (gastric mucosa-associated lymphoid tissue [MALT] lymphomas), and *Chlamydia psittaci* (ocular adnexal MALT lymphomas). Autoimmune and chronic inflammatory disorders associated with an increased risk for NHL include celiac sprue (enteropathy-type intestinal T-cell lymphomas), rheumatoid arthritis (large granular lymphocytic leukemia), Sjögren's disease (extranodal marginal zone lymphomas), autoimmune thyroid disease (thyroid lymphomas), and inflammatory bowel diseases. Finally, exposure to pesticides and radiation has been associated with an increased risk for NHL.

Non-Hodgkin's Lymphomas and Leukemias

B-Cell Tumors

Immature B-cell tumors
  Precursor B-cell lymphoblastic lymphoma
Mature B-cell tumors
  Follicular lymphoma
  Chronic lymphocytic leukemia, small lymphocytic lymphoma
  Prolymphocytic leukemia
  Lymphoplasmacytic lymphoma, Waldenström's macroglobulinemia
  Mantle cell lymphoma
  Marginal zone lymphoma of mucosa-associated lymphoid tissue (MALT) type
  Nodal marginal zone lymphoma
  Splenic marginal zone lymphoma
  Hairy cell leukemia
  Diffuse large cell lymphoma
  Mediastinal large B-cell lymphoma, primary CNS lymphoma, primary effusion lymphoma, intravascular large B-cell lymphoma
  Burkitt's lymphoma

T-Cell and Natural Killer (NK) Cell Tumors

Immature T-cell tumors
  Precursor T-cell lymphoblastic lymphoma
Mature T-cell tumors
  Prolymphocytic leukemia
  Large granular lymphocytic leukemia
  NK cell leukemia
  Extranodal NK and T-cell lymphoma, nasal type
  Mycosis fungoides
  Sézary's syndrome
  Angioimmunoblastic T-cell lymphoma
  Peripheral T-cell lymphoma
  Adult T-cell leukemia and lymphoma
  Systemic anaplastic large cell lymphoma
  Primary cutaneous anaplastic large-cell lymphoma
  Subcutaneous panniculitis-like T-cell lymphoma
  Enteropathy-type intestinal T-cell lymphoma
  Hepatosplenic T-cell lymphoma

Hodgkin's Lymphoma

Nodular lymphocyte predominant Hodgkin's lymphoma
Classic Hodgkin's lymphoma
  Nodular sclerosis
  Lymphocyte-rich type
  Mixed cellularity
  Lymphocyte depleted

involvement. Mediastinal involvement is common in HD, but may be seen in NHL as well, particularly primary mediastinal large cell and lymphoblastic lymphomas, and is commonly heralded by symptoms of chest pain, cough, and dyspnea. Constitutional symptoms in HD and NHL are common and can include fever, night sweats, weight loss, fatigue, and pruritus. In HD, rare manifestations include pain in affected nodes after drinking alcohol and Pel-Ebstein fever, which builds to a peak over several days, lasts several weeks, wanes, and then begins anew. Patients with low-grade NHL may have several years of waxing-waning adenopathy before seeking medical attention and tend not to have systemic symptoms or extranodal involvement until disease is more advanced. Low-grade NHL can transform into intermediate- or high-grade NHL, which declares itself as a disproportionately increasing nodal mass or the rapid acceleration of symptoms. With intermediate- and high-grade NHL, symptoms develop over weeks to months, and extranodal involvement, such as of the gastrointestinal tract, bone marrow, or CNS, can occur even in early-stage disease. CNS involvement may manifest as spinal cord compression from epidural lesions, focal neurologic deficits from intraparenchymal brain lesions, or headaches, mental status changes, neck pain and stiffness, cranial neuropathies, or radicular symptoms from leptomeningeal involvement.

Hematologic abnormalities most commonly include anemia, although leukopenia and thrombocytopenia can be seen, especially with bone marrow involvement or hypersplenism from splenic infiltration. Liver test abnormalities can be seen with hepatic involvement, and an increased creatinine might be seen in patients with bilateral ureteral obstruction from bulky retroperitoneal lymphadenopathy. Lactate dehydrogenase (LDH) is frequently elevated in patients with advanced HD and NHL and is reflective of significant tumor burden. Hypercalcemia can be seen in the presence of bony involvement or through the increased conversion of 25-hydroxy-vitamin D to 1,25-hydroxy-vitamin D. Tumor lysis syndrome (hyperuricemia, hyperkalemia, hyperphosphatemia, hypocalcemia, and renal failure) may occur in high-grade NHL, most notably BL and lymphoblastic lymphoma, and occasionally in intermediate-grade NHL, even before the initiation of treatment, but is rare in HD.

Clinical Presentation

Patients with HD and NHL typically have adenopathy that is firm, nontender, and mobile. Contiguous spread of disease to adjacent lymph node chains is the rule in HD, and supradiaphragmatic presentations involving the neck, supraclavicular fossa, or axilla are most common, whereas sites of involvement are more varied in NHL because of its predilection for early hematogenous spread. Disease limited to areas below the diaphragm is less frequent in HD, as is epitrochlear, Waldeyer ring, or extranodal

Differential Diagnosis

The differential diagnosis for adenopathy is broad and should prompt consideration of infectious etiologies, autoimmune processes, hypersensitivity reactions, and other malignancies (Table 74-1).

Diagnostic Approach

For patients with adenopathy and no constitutional symptoms, a period of close observation for a few weeks, possi-

Table 74-1 Differential Diagnosis of Lymphadenopathy

Infectious	
Bacterial	Streptococcal infections, secondary syphilis, Lyme disease, cat-scratch disease, tularemia
Viral	Infectious mononucleosis, cytomegalovirus, HIV, hepatitis B
Fungal	Cryptococcosis, histoplasmosis, coccidioidomycosis
Mycobacterial	Tuberculosis, atypical mycobacterial infections
Protozoal	Toxoplasmosis
Malignancy	Solid tumors (e.g., lung, breast, head and neck)
Endocrine	Thyroid disease, Addison's disease
Autoimmune	Rheumatoid arthritis, systemic lupus erythematosus, Wegener's granulomatosis, Still's disease, Churg-Strauss syndrome, dermatomyositis
Immunologic	Serum sickness, other hypersensitivity reactions (e.g., phenytoin)
Other	Sarcoidosis, Kikuchi's disease, Rosai-Dorfman disease, amyloidosis, Castleman's disease, the histiocytoses, Kawasaki's disease, Whipple's disease

bly with a course of antibiotics, is usually reasonable, provided that the involved area is not growing at a rapid rate. Empiric use of steroids should be avoided because steroids are lympholytic and can make interpretation of a future lymph node biopsy difficult. Regression of adenopathy does not rule out a malignant process because nodes may wax and wane. Patients with persistent or progressive adenopathy, especially in the presence of unexplained constitutional symptoms; abnormal screening laboratory studies including anemia; elevations of the erythrocyte sedimentation rate, liver function tests, or LDH; abnormal chest radiographs, or those at high HIV risk, should be considered for prompt referral for biopsy.

An incisional or excisional biopsy is usually required to diagnose lymphoma, and the most accessible node is targeted. If there is concern for transformation of a low-grade lymphoma, the most symptomatic or suspicious node should be removed. Standard hematoxylin and eosin staining is supplemented with flow cytometry, immunohistochemistry, cytogenetic analysis, or DNA testing (e.g., immunoglobulin or T-cell receptor gene rearrangement studies) to establish the diagnosis of lymphoma and the correct subtype. Needle aspiration is not adequate in most cases because the neoplastic Reed-Sternberg cells in HD can make up 1% or less of the total cell population, and the nodal architecture used in histologic classification of lymphomas is lost.

Staging of Hodgkin's Disease and Non-Hodgkin's Lymphoma

In addition to a careful history and physical examination, management of HD and NHL depends on accurate staging (Fig. 74-1). Staging is typically accomplished with the use of computed tomography (CT) of the neck, chest, abdomen, and pelvis. [^{18}F]-2-fluoro-2-deoxy-D-glucose positron emission tomography (FDG-PET), particularly when combined with CT, is a highly sensitive technique for detecting metabolically active lymphoma. Bone marrow aspiration and biopsy remain an essential part of staging given the limitations of CT and FDG-PET in the detection

of marrow involvement. The staging laparotomy, once commonly used in the workup of HD, is infrequently performed today, but might be considered in favorable-prognosis, stage I and II HD if a negative result would dictate the use of radiation therapy without chemotherapy. Certain subtypes of NHL (BL, lymphoblastic lymphoma, or diffuse large B-cell NHL with bone marrow involvement, extensive extranodal involvement, or in HIV patients) have a predilection for spreading to the CNS, and a lumbar puncture at diagnosis is warranted to exclude CNS involvement. Patients are staged according to the Ann Arbor classification system (see Fig. 74-1). However, clinical factors other than stage play an important role in determining prognosis from HD and NHL. To better determine long-term outcomes and treatment, scoring systems have been devised for HD and NHL (Table 74-2).

Management of Hodgkin's Disease

Optimum Treatment

Favorable-prognosis, stage I, and II classic HD: Patients with supradiaphragmatic, laparotomy-staged disease may receive primary radiation therapy, and enjoy a 75% to 85% relapse-free survival rate and a 90% 20-year survival rate because many relapsed patients are successfully salvaged with chemotherapy. Patients with clinical stage I or II disease with favorable prognostic factors may receive extended-field radiation therapy that includes para-aortic and splenic fields, but are more commonly treated with combined-modality chemotherapy and radiation therapy. Patients with unfavorable prognostic factors are also treated with combined-modality therapy, which includes the use of four to six chemotherapy cycles, followed by involved-field radiation therapy (IFRT) at lower doses than those used when primary radiation therapy is employed.

Advanced, stage III, and IV classic HD: Most stage III and IV patients receive six to eight cycles of combination chemotherapy. Radiation is used in select instances, such as for patients with bulky masses at presentation,

Figure 74-1 Malignant Lymphomas—Staging.
CBC, complete blood count; ESR, erythrocyte sedimentation rate; HD, Hodgkin's disease; HIV, human immunodeficiency virus; LDH, lactate dehydrogenase; NHL, non-Hodgkin's lymphoma.

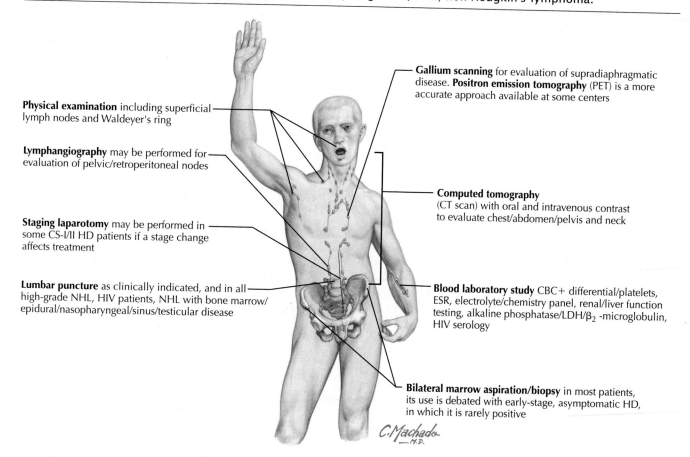

Gallium scanning for evaluation of supradiaphragmatic disease. **Positron emission tomography** (PET) is a more accurate approach available at some centers

Physical examination including superficial lymph nodes and Waldeyer's ring

Lymphangiography may be performed for evaluation of pelvic/retroperitoneal nodes

Computed tomography (CT scan) with oral and intravenous contrast to evaluate chest/abdomen/pelvis and neck

Staging laparotomy may be performed in some CS-I/II HD patients if a stage change affects treatment

Lumbar puncture as clinically indicated, and in all high-grade NHL, HIV patients, NHL with bone marrow/epidural/nasopharyngeal/sinus/testicular disease

Blood laboratory study CBC+ differential/platelets, ESR, electrolyte/chemistry panel, renal/liver function testing, alkaline phosphatase/LDH/β_2 -microglobulin, HIV serology

Bilateral marrow aspiration/biopsy in most patients, its use is debated with early-stage, asymptomatic HD, in which it is rarely positive

Ann Arbor Classification

Stage I
Involvement of a single lymph node region (I) or of a single extralymphatic organ or site (IE)

Stage II
Involvement of two or more lymph node regions on the same side of the diaphragm (II) or localized involvement of extralymphatic organ or site and of one or more lymph node regions on the same side of the diaphragm (IIE)

Stage III
Involvement of lymph node regions on both sides of the diaphragm (III), which may also be accompanied by localized involvement of extralymphatic organ or site (IIIE) or by involvement of the spleen (IIIS) or both (IIISE)

Stage IV
Diffuse or disseminated involvement of one or more extralymphatic organs or tissues with or without associated lymph node enlargement

Certain symptoms are commonly associated with lymphoma:
* Night sweats
* Temperature > 38.5°C
* Weight loss > 10%
These are called "B" symptoms and are included in the stage designated to a patient. For instance, a patient with involved lymph nodes in the neck and under the arms only, and without any of the "B" symptoms, has stage IIA disease. The same patient with night sweats has stage IIB disease.

Table 74-2 Prognostic Scoring Systems for Malignant Lymphomas

A. The International Prognostic Index for Diffuse Large Cell Lymphoma

Score	Risk Group	Complete Response Rate	5-Year Overall Survival
0 to 1	Low	87%	73%
2	Low-intermediate	67%	51%
3	High-intermediate	55%	43%
4 to 5	High	44%	26%

1 point is assigned for each of the following clinical parameters: age >60 years, serum lactate dehydrogenase (LDH) > the normal range, an Eastern Cooperative Oncology Group (ECOG) performance status of ≥2, Ann Arbor stage III or IV disease, and >1 extranodal site of disease.

B. The Follicular Lymphoma International Prognostic Index

Score	Risk Group	5-Year Overall Survival	10-Year Overall Survival
0 to 1	Low	90.6%	70.7%
2	Intermediate	77.6%	50.9%
≥3	High	52.5%	35.5%

1 point is assigned for each of the following clinical parameters: age >60 years, serum LDH > the normal range, Ann Arbor stage III or IV disease, number of nodal sites >4, hemoglobin <12 mg/dL.

or for those whose disease has not completely regressed radiographically after chemotherapy. Freedom from relapse in stage IIIB and IV disease can occur in up to 70% of cases, with an overall survival rate of more than 80%. The most common regimens include ABVD (Adriamycin, bleomycin, vinblastine, and dacarbazine) or MOPP (mechlorethamine, oncovin, procarbazine, and prednisone). ABVD is generally preferred because it is associated with a decreased risk for myelodysplasia or secondary leukemia, is better tolerated, and improves the chance of preserving fertility.

Nodular lymphocyte-predominant HD: Most patients present with early-stage disease, and radiation therapy, sometimes with more limited fields, is a consideration given their good prognosis.

Relapsed HD: Relapsed HD is curable in many instances. Most patients who received radiation as initial treatment undergo combination chemotherapy. For those who underwent chemotherapy initially and had a long remission (>1 year), repeat chemotherapy, often combined with radiation therapy for those with limited disease at relapse, is reasonable; but after a brief or no remission, patients should be considered for salvage chemotherapy followed by autologous stem cell transplantation.

Late toxicities of radiation therapy vary, in part, with the radiation field used, but may include hypothyroidism, accelerated atherosclerosis, solid tumors (lung, breast, gastrointestinal, thyroid, soft tissue, and skin), and hematologic malignancies, including myelodysplasia, acute myeloid leukemia, and NHL. Chemotherapy (especially alkylating agents and topoisomerase II inhibitors) further increases the risk for myelodysplasia and acute myeloid leukemia. Congestive heart failure can occur as a result of anthracycline exposure, especially in those who have received a higher cumulative dose, are older, or have received prior radiation therapy to the chest. Bleomycin can cause an acute hypersensitivity pneumonitis or, more commonly, a subacute or chronic fibrosing alveolitis, which is more likely in those who have received chest radiation.

Management of Non-Hodgkin's Lymphoma

The histologic type and stage are taken into account in making treatment recommendations. General guidelines for follicular and diffuse large cell lymphomas, the most common NHLs, are presented next.

Low-Grade, Follicular Lymphomas

Optimum Treatment

Low-grade, follicular lymphomas are incurable with standard chemotherapy, and there is no evidence that early treatment prolongs survival. A watchful waiting approach is reasonable for asymptomatic patients. For many with systemic symptoms, chemotherapy can effectively decrease tumor burden and symptoms, often for long periods of time, although relapse is inevitable.

Early, stage I, and II disease: Although stage I or limited stage II disease at presentation is uncommon, these patients are candidates for radiation therapy, which may be curative in some. Whether this approach is better than observation alone for patients with early-stage, asymptomatic disease is debatable.

Advanced, stage III, and IV disease: Watchful waiting is still appropriate for most asymptomatic patients, whereas symptomatic patients are candidates for systemic chemotherapy. Options for cytotoxic chemotherapy include chlorambucil or cyclophosphamide, alone or with prednisone (these are oral regimens but expose patients to alkylating agents, which confer a risk for myelodysplasia and secondary leukemia); fludarabine-based chemotherapy (higher response rates, but more immunosuppressive); or the combination regimen CHOP (cyclophosphamide, doxorubicin, oncovin, and prednisone) or CVP (cyclophosphamide, oncovin, and prednisone). Rituximab is a monoclonal antibody directed against the CD20 antigen on B cells and has significant activity against low-grade B-cell lymphomas. In combination with cytotoxic chemotherapy regimens and as maintenance therapy after completion of chemotherapy, rituximab has been shown to improve remission durations for patients with follicular lymphoma. Rituximab can also be used as single-agent therapy, especially for those who are medically unfit to receive conventional chemotherapy. More recently, radioisotope-conjugated anti-CD20 antibodies have emerged for the treatment of follicular lymphoma and have demonstrated impressive response rates in newly diagnosed and relapsed disease.

Relapsed disease: When patients experience relapse, they can usually be treated with another of the many available chemotherapeutic modalities. Autologous and allogeneic transplantation remains investigational.

Diffuse Large B-Cell Lymphomas

Optimum Treatment

Early, stage I, and II disease: Three cycles of CHOP chemotherapy followed by IFRT is associated with a 70% to 80% progression-free and overall survival rate at 5 years. Rituximab is typically given with chemotherapy and will likely improve survival further, given its successful use in more advanced disease.

Advanced, stage III, and IV disease: Six to eight cycles of CHOP produces complete response rates in up to 60% of cases, but therapy is curative in less than 50%. The addition of rituximab to CHOP has improved the overall survival from this disease and is now routinely incorporated into therapy. Autologous stem cell transplantation is sometimes used for patients with high-risk disease as defined by the International Prognostic Index score (see Table 74-2), which has been shown to improve disease-free survival but has not led to a consistent improvement in overall survival compared with chemotherapy alone.

Relapsed disease: Relapsed disease is treated with salvage chemotherapy, followed in most cases by autologous stem cell transplantation, with intent to cure. Patients who are not eligible for transplantation are treated with non-cross-resistant chemotherapy regimens, palliative radiation therapy, or both, and are rarely cured.

Avoiding Treatment Errors

Decisions regarding the use of radiation therapy, chemotherapy, or a combination of the two, and the choice of chemotherapy agents used critically depend on a thorough staging evaluation and accurate pathologic diagnosis for both Hodgkin's and non-Hodgkin's lymphoma. Furthermore, aggressive supportive care is crucial to the successful outcome of a chosen therapy, requires a thorough understanding of the toxicity profiles of the therapeutics used, and may include the use of hematopoietic growth factors (e.g., erythropoietin for malignancy-related anemia, granulocyte colony-stimulating factor for prevention of febrile neutropenia), antiemetics for acute and delayed chemo-therapy-induced nausea and vomiting, and prophylactic antibiotics for specific infections (e.g., *Pneumocystis carinii* pneumonia prophylaxis for patients receiving fludarabine-based chemotherapy).

Future Directions

Ongoing studies in HD and NHL will determine whether more extended chemotherapy can effectively replace radiation therapy in the management of early-stage HD, thereby decreasing long-term radiation-associated morbidity and mortality. Fueled by the success in NHL, current and future studies in HD will incorporate antibody-based treatment strategies into current standards of care (e.g., anti-CD30 antibodies). Ongoing and future studies in NHL will clarify the efficacy and role of immunotherapy (anti-idiotype vaccine strategies, novel antibody-based therapies, radioimmunotherapy). Finally, our increased understanding of the molecular pathogenesis of lymphomas has paved the way for the development and incorporation of targeted pharmacologic agents into current management strategies for these diseases.

Additional Resources

National Cancer Institute: Cancer topics. Available at: http://cancer.gov/cancerinformation. Accessed December 13, 2006.

> *The National Cancer Institute provides up-to-date information regarding lymphoma management for the health care professional as well as patients and is an invaluable resource for information regarding clinical trials in lymphoma.*

The National Comprehensive Cancer Network (NCCN). Available at: http://www.nccn.org. Accessed December 13, 2006.

> *The NCCN is a consortium of cancer programs across the United States that has drafted up-to-date, evidence-based clinical practice guidelines for the treatment of a variety of malignancies, including the lymphomas, as well as patient-directed guidelines for lymphoma management and appropriate oncologic supportive care.*

EVIDENCE

A predictive model for aggressive non-Hodgkin's lymphoma. The International Non-Hodgkin's Lymphoma Prognostic Factors Project. N Engl J Med 329(14):987-994; 1993.

> *This study helped identify clinical parameters that on multivariate analysis predicted survival outcomes for patients with aggressive NHL and remains the most commonly used prognostication tool.*

Canellos GP, Anderson JR, Propert KJ, et al: Chemotherapy of advanced Hodgkin's disease with MOPP, ABVD, or MOPP alternating with ABVD. N Engl J Med 327(21):1478-1484, 1992.

> *This phase 3 study established ABVD as the standard of care chemotherapy regimen for patients with advanced HD, and the ABVD regimen remains in use today.*

Coiffier B, Lepage E, Briere J, et al: CHOP chemotherapy plus rituximab compared with CHOP alone in elderly patients with diffuse large-B-cell lymphoma. N Engl J Med 346(4):235-242, 2002.

> *This phase 3 study demonstrated an improvement in overall survival for elderly patients with diffuse large B-cell lymphoma who received the anti-CD20 monoclonal antibody, rituximab, with their CHOP chemotherapy, and defined the current standard of care for this disease.*

Hanna K. Sanoff ▪ Beverly S. Mitchell

Leukemias

Introduction

The leukemias are a group of disorders characterized by neoplastic transformation of hematopoietic cells, with resultant accumulation of these cells in the bone marrow and commonly, although not universally, in the peripheral blood. Leukemias may arise from lymphoid or from myeloid cells and are generally classified as acute if the cells are arrested early in differentiation (blasts or early progenitors), or as chronic if the cells are mature. Most leukemias are characterized by chromosomal or cytogenetic abnormalities that contribute to the assessment of overall prognosis. Risk factors for leukemia include exposure to ionizing radiation, previous chemotherapy, and increasing age.

Acute Myeloid Leukemia

Etiology and Pathogenesis

Acute myeloid leukemia (AML) arises in a stem cell capable of giving rise to granulocytes, monocytes, red blood cells, and platelets. Malignant transformation occurs at different stages of differentiation, giving rise to subtypes that can be distinguished by morphology, histochemistry, and specific surface markers using a panel of monoclonal antibodies (flow cytometry). The subtypes of AML have been codified in a French-American-British classification system that divides the leukemias into eight groups (M0-7) based on the myeloid phenotype. Because cells accumulate at a very immature stage of development, they replace the bone marrow and cause anemia and thrombocytopenia. Many cytogenetic abnormalities have been described that lead to the production of specific proteins that cause the leukemias. Of these, the translocation of a portion of chromosome 17 onto the long arm of chromosome 15 in acute progranulocytic or M3 leukemia is the best understood. The resulting aberrant gene product contains a portion of the nuclear retinoic acid receptor, and clinical remissions in this disorder can be achieved with pharmacologic doses of all-*trans*-retinoic acid. This vitamin A derivative binds to the receptor and overcomes the block in differentiation, allowing maturation of the leukemic cells into neutrophils.

Clinical Presentation

Patients present with symptoms related to anemia (fatigue, pallor, and dyspnea), neutropenia (infection), or thrombocytopenia (petechiae, bleeding). Different subtypes may have specific manifestations. Acute progranulocytic leukemia (M3) may present with disseminated intravascular coagulation and bleeding or purpura. Leukemias derived from monocytes (M4 and M5) may present with skin, gum, or lung infiltration. AML may also develop from preexisting myelodysplasia that is characterized by a period of low blood counts, frequently requiring blood product support.

Differential Diagnosis

Patients presenting with high white blood counts consisting predominantly of blasts are easily diagnosed based on examination of the peripheral blood smear (Fig. 75-1). Patients with pancytopenia may have acute leukemia on the basis of blasts in the bone marrow only. The differential diagnosis includes aplastic anemia, myelodysplasia, marrow infiltration with fibrosis or tumor, or, rarely, hypersplenism.

Diagnostic Approach

Examination of the peripheral blood smear is always warranted. A bone marrow aspiration and biopsy should be

Figure 75-1 Leukemias: Clinical Presentation of Leukemias.

AML, acute myeloid leukemia; ALL, acute lymphoblastic leukemia; CML, chronic myelogenous leukemia; CLL, chronic lymphocytic leukemia.

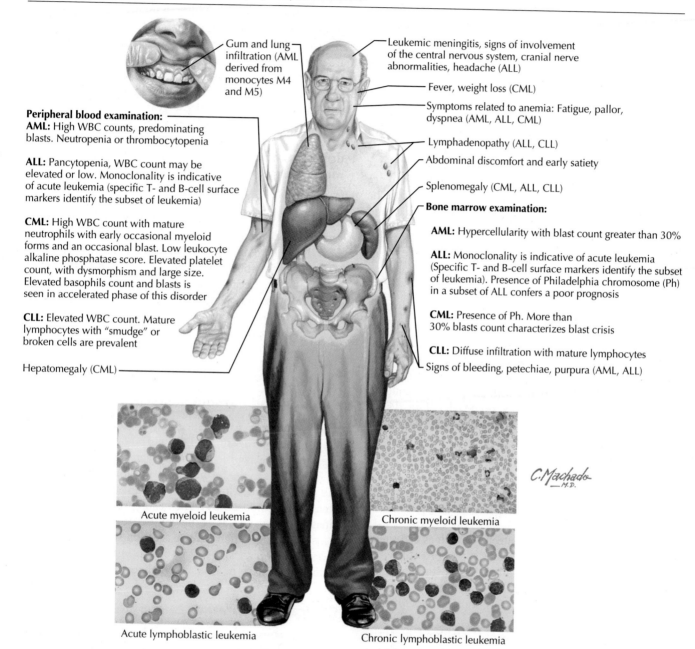

Gum and lung infiltration (AML derived from monocytes M4 and M5)

Leukemic meningitis, signs of involvement of the central nervous system, cranial nerve abnormalities, headache (ALL)

Fever, weight loss (CML)

Symptoms related to anemia: Fatigue, pallor, dyspnea (AML, ALL, CML)

Lymphadenopathy (ALL, CLL)

Abdominal discomfort and early satiety

Splenomegaly (CML, ALL, CLL)

Peripheral blood examination:
AML: High WBC counts, predominating blasts. Neutropenia or thrombocytopenia

ALL: Pancytopenia, WBC count may be elevated or low. Monoclonality is indicative of acute leukemia (specific T- and B-cell surface markers identify the subset of leukemia)

CML: High WBC count with mature neutrophils with early occasional myeloid forms and an occasional blast. Low leukocyte alkaline phosphatase score. Elevated platelet count, with dysmorphism and large size. Elevated basophils count and blasts is seen in accelerated phase of this disorder

CLL: Elevated WBC count. Mature lymphocytes with "smudge" or broken cells are prevalent

Hepatomegaly (CML)

Bone marrow examination:

AML: Hypercellularity with blast count greater than 30%

ALL: Monoclonality is indicative of acute leukemia (Specific T- and B-cell surface markers identify the subset of leukemia). Presence of Philadelphia chromosom (Ph) in a subset of ALL confers a poor prognosis

CML: Presence of Ph. More than 30% blasts count characterizes blast crisis

CLL: Diffuse infiltration with mature lymphocytes

Signs of bleeding, petechiae, purpura (AML, ALL)

Acute myeloid leukemia

Chronic myeloid leukemia

Acute lymphoblastic leukemia

Chronic lymphoblastic leukemia

performed with requests for flow cytometry and cytogenetics. Bone marrow specimens are generally hypercellular, and a blast count of greater than 30% is diagnostic of acute leukemia.

Management and Therapy

Optimum Treatment

Patients with AML are treated with combination chemotherapy in an attempt to empty the bone marrow of malignant cells and allow normal progenitors to repopulate the marrow. Patients are generally hospitalized for 3 to 4 weeks and require intensive blood product and antibiotic support. Following the induction of remission (less than 5% blasts in the marrow), patients are treated with several cycles of high-dose chemotherapy as consolidation of the remission. Patients with cytogenetic abnormalities portending a poor prognosis or who relapse are candidates for bone marrow transplantation. The overall survival rate is 30% to 40% at 3 to 5 years, with most deaths due to relapse of the disease.

Avoiding Treatment Errors

Because treatment regimens are markedly different for AML and acute lymphoblastic leukemia (ALL), it is critical to definitively classify the leukemic blasts as either myeloid or lymphoid before initiating therapy.

Acute Lymphoblastic Leukemia

Etiology and Pathogenesis

ALLs are associated with cytogenetic abnormalities and translocations. Most frequently they occur in immunoglobulin or T-cell receptor loci that undergo recombination in the normal course of lymphoid maturation and are regions of active transcription. These diseases may also be subcategorized as of pre-T-, T-, pre-B-, or B-cell origin based on their surface markers. The presence of a Philadelphia chromosome (a translocation between chromosomes 9 and 22) occurs in some patients with ALL and has a poor prognosis.

Clinical Presentation

As with AML, ALL presents with anemia and thrombocytopenia (see Fig. 75-1). The white blood cell count may be elevated or low, and blasts have a lymphoid morphology. In contrast to AML, patients with ALL more frequently have lymphadenopathy and splenomegaly. The disease may also involve the central nervous system and present with cranial nerve abnormalities and headache. Lumbar puncture is indicated to make a diagnosis of leukemic meningitis in such cases.

Differential Diagnosis

Toxoplasmosis or acute viral infections such as cytomegalovirus and infectious mononucleosis may present with a reactive lymphocytosis that is difficult to distinguish from an acute leukemia. Appropriate antibody titers in conjunction with suspicion of an infectious etiology should establish the appropriate diagnosis. The leukemic phase of certain lymphomas and the occasional lymphoid blast crisis of chronic myelogenous leukemia are also in the differential diagnosis.

Diagnostic Approach

Examination of the peripheral blood and bone marrow by morphology, cytogenetics, and flow cytometry should establish the diagnosis. Specific T- and B-cell surface markers identify the subset of leukemia. Monoclonality is indicative of an acute leukemia, as opposed to a reactive lymphocytosis, and can be determined by finding identical rearrangements of the immunoglobulin or T-cell receptor loci in all cells.

Management and Therapy

Optimum Therapy

The treatment of ALL consists of intensive induction chemotherapy with multiple drugs and consolidation treatment that is carried out over 1 to 2 years. The regimens are very intensive and include prophylactic intrathecal administration of chemotherapy drugs such as methotrexate and cytosine arabinoside. Although most patients enter remission, patients may relapse years after treatment, and the overall cure rate with chemotherapy alone in adults is roughly 20%, with a worse prognosis for individuals older than 50 years. Childhood ALL has a far better prognosis, with an overall cure rate of more than 80%.

Avoiding Treatment Errors

The management of patients with both AML and ALL requires meticulous supportive care and clinical familiarity with the many complications of therapy; therefore, if possible, patients should be referred to a tertiary care center for treatment. Because patients with acute leukemia can experience a rapid decline in their clinical status, prompt attention to any new or worsening signs or symptoms, such as fever or dyspnea, is warranted.

Chronic Myelogenous Leukemia

Etiology and Pathogenesis

The hallmark of chronic myelogenous leukemia (CML) is the presence of the Philadelphia chromosome (Ph), involving a reciprocal translocation between chromosomes 9 and 22. This leads to the formation of a fusion protein between the bcr region of chromosome 22 and the c-abl tyrosine kinase on chromosome 9. The fusion protein has increased kinase activity and is sufficient to cause the disease in transgenic mice. The disease frequently undergoes progression to a blast crisis form by a progression of genetic changes that have not been well characterized.

Clinical Presentation

CML presents with a high white blood count that may be detected on routine complete blood cell count and splenomegaly in 90% of cases. Patients may complain of generalized fatigue or abdominal discomfort and early satiety. Occasionally, patients present with hypermetabolic symptoms of fever and weight loss. Hepatomegaly is also common. The peripheral blood smear shows mature neutrophils with occasional earlier myeloid forms and an occasional blast (see Fig. 75-1). The platelet count is frequently elevated, and platelets may appear somewhat large and dysmorphic on peripheral smear. An accelerated phase of the disorder is a harbinger of blast crisis and is characterized by progressive splenomegaly and elevation of the white blood cell (WBC) count with basophils and an increasing percentage of blasts. Blast crisis occurs in untreated patients at a mean of 3 to 4 years from diagnosis and is characterized by more than 30% blasts in the bone marrow of either myeloid or lymphoid type.

Differential Diagnosis

Reactive leukocytosis, resulting most commonly from infection, malignancy, or drug reaction, is the most common entity to be differentiated from CML. Other myeloproliferative disorders, including polycythemia vera and myelofibrosis, also present with elevated WBC counts and splenomegaly. The blast crisis of CML must be distinguished from de novo forms of AML and ALL.

Diagnostic Approach

The Ph, as ascertained from cytogenetic analysis of the peripheral blood or bone marrow, definitively distinguishes CML from both infectious causes of a high WBC count and from other myeloproliferative diseases. ALL may also be associated with a Ph. A leukocyte alkaline phosphatase score may be obtained on peripheral WBCs and is generally high in reactive leukocytosis and low in CML.

Management and Therapy

Optimum Therapy

Patients presenting with a very high WBC count may require initial therapy with hydroxyurea, which controls the blood counts but does not prolong overall survival.

A drug that specifically inhibits the tyrosine kinase activity of the bcr-abl fusion protein (imatinib) is highly effective in inducing hematologic remissions with normalization of blood counts in more than 90% of patients. Unfortunately, many patients develop resistance to imatinib over time. A second bcr-abl tyrosine kinase inhibitor (dasatinib) has recently been approved for patients who are either intolerant of, or have disease resistance to, imatinib. In this setting, dasatinib produces hematologic remissions in about 60% of patients. Because the long-term efficacy of these new tyrosine kinase inhibitors is unknown, the optimum strategy for integrating tyrosine kinase inhibitors and bone marrow transplantation is evolving; however, imatinib and dasatinib offer the least toxicity and highest response rate of any therapy developed to date.

Avoiding Treatment Errors

Imatinib and dasatinib have markedly improved the outlook and quality of life of patients with CML. However, they have also made treatment of young patients with CML increasingly complex. Because the optimal way to integrate these advances into clinical practice is somewhat uncertain, consultation with a physician specializing in malignant hematology is now warranted.

Chronic Lymphocytic Leukemia

Etiology and Pathogenesis

Chronic lymphocytic leukemia (CLL) is the most common type of leukemia, frequently occurring in patients older than 50 years. This disorder involves the accumulation of slowly dividing mature B, or rarely T, lymphocytes in the peripheral blood and bone marrow. The molecular basis for this disorder remains obscure, although a number of different cytogenetic abnormalities have been described. It appears to be associated with an increase in the anti-apoptotic or anti–cell death proteins, such as bcl-2, that characterize the indolent lymphomas.

Clinical Presentation

Patients most commonly present with an elevated WBC count on routine complete blood count (CBC). Most cells are mature lymphocytes (see Fig. 75-1). Other less common presentations include lymph node enlargement, recurrent infections because of the associated hypogammaglobulinemia, or immune-mediated hemolytic anemia or thrombocytopenia. A simple Rai staging classification, which has prognostic import, defines the stage of the disease (Table 75-1).

The anemia and thrombocytopenia in CLL result from decreased production due to bone marrow involvement. In addition to clinical stage, the intracellular tyrosine kinase ZAP-70 has been shown to be useful in further defining the prognosis of CLL. Patients with ZAP-70 expression require treatment an average of 6 years earlier than those with ZAP-70-negative CLL. Whether early treatment in ZAP-70-positive patients alters their accelerated clinical course is not yet known.

Differential Diagnosis

Viral infections, the leukemic phase of non-Hodgkin's lymphoma, and hairy cell leukemia, an unusual lymphoproliferative disease characterized by pancytopenia,

Table 75-1	Rai Staging Classification for Chronic Lymphocytic Leukemia	
Stage	Features	Median Survival (yr)
0	Lymphocytosis only (>5 × 10⁹/L)	>15
I	Lymphocytosis and lymphadenopathy	8
II	Lymphocytosis and splenomegaly	6
III	Lymphocytosis and anemia (hemoglobin ≈1 g/dL)	3
IV	Lymphocytosis and thrombocytopenia (platelets <100 × 10⁹/L)	2

splenomegaly, and a distinctive surface marker phenotype, are in the differential diagnosis.

Diagnostic Approach

Examination of the peripheral blood reveals mature lymphocytes, frequently with "smudge" or broken cells characteristic of lymphoproliferative diseases. Bone marrow transplantation may be indicated in patients presenting with cytopenia. Flow cytometry is a useful diagnostic tool in difficult cases. A serum protein electrophoresis and Coombs' test with reticulocyte count are indicated in patients with recurrent infections and anemia, respectively.

Management and Therapy

Optimum Treatment

Patients with stage 0, I, or II disease can be observed at 3- to 6-month intervals with physical examination and CBC to assess disease progression. Patients with stable disease can be observed annually. Initial therapy for patients with stage III or IV disease is either intermittent treatment with an alkylating agent and prednisone or therapy with fludarabine, a nucleoside analogue. Although fludarabine results in a higher remission rate and longer disease-free intervals, overall survival is similar with the two regimens. Fludarabine results in prolonged immunosuppression, and patients should be monitored for opportunistic infections. Patients with more aggressive CLL or who have failed primary therapy are candidates for combination chemotherapy. Monoclonal antibodies against B-lymphocyte antigens CD20 (rituximab) and CD52 (alemtuzumab) also have activity against CLL, and alemtuzumab has been approved for use in refractory CLL.

Richter's syndrome represents a transformation of the disease into a more aggressive lymphoma and confers a poor prognosis. Patients with recurrent infections and hypogammaglobulinemia should receive intravenous immunoglobulin. Immune-mediated hemolysis or thrombocytopenia requires treatment of the underlying disease for a good response.

Avoiding Treatment Errors

Consultation with an experienced hematopathologist is critical to ensure the correct diagnosis of CLL, which can be difficult to distinguish from other chronic lymphoproliferative disorders such as hairy cell leukemia. Although ZAP-70 shows promise as a way to select patients who might benefit from more intense therapy early in their disease course, current best evidence still supports watchful waiting until the onset of disease progression or symptoms.

Future Directions

Progress in treating the acute leukemias has been slow. New approaches include the combined use of monoclonal antibodies with chemotherapeutic drugs and stimulation of the host immune system to leukemia-associated antigens. As new molecular mechanisms of oncogenesis are discovered, they will be become subjects for specific targeting by pharmacologic agents. CML has opened a new era of tumor-specific therapies that should revolutionize the current approaches to leukemia treatment.

Additional Resources

The American Cancer Society Web site. Available at: http://www.cancer.org. Accessed October 15, 2006.
  The American Cancer Society offers teaching materials, clinical trials information, and survivor support. The website and materials are all available in Spanish. This is an excellent resource for physicians and patients.
The Leukemia and Lymphoma Society Web site. Available at: http://www.leukemia-lymphoma.org. Accessed October 15, 2006.
  The Leukemia and Lymphoma Society website offers teaching materials and clinical trials search engines for patients. Information booklets are available from the Society in Spanish and French.
The National Comprehensive Cancer Network Web site. Available at: http://www.nccn.org. Accessed October 15, 2006.
  The National Comprehensive Cancer Network's treatment guidelines include recommendations from a panel of experts on the treatment on AML, CML, and CLL.

EVIDENCE

1. Druker BJ, Talpaz M, Resta DJ, et al: Efficacy and safety of a specific inhibitor of the BCR-ABL tyrosine kinase in chronic myeloid leukemia. N Engl J Med 344(14):1031-1037, 2001.
    This sentinel paper describes imatinib response in patients with chronic-phase CML resistant to interferon therapy.
2. Hoelzer D, Gokbuget N: New approaches to acute lymphoblastic leukemia in adults: Where do we go? Semin Oncol 27(5):540-559, 2000.
    The authors review the state-of-the-art treatment options for ALL in adults.
3. Keating MJ, O'Brien S, Lerner S, et al: Long-term follow-up of patients with chronic lymphocytic leukemia (CLL) receiving fludarabine regimens as initial therapy. Blood 92(4):1165-1171, 1998.
    The authors present evidence for the efficacy of fludarabine as first-line treatment of CLL.
4. Pui CH, Evans WE: Treatment of acute lymphoblastic leukemia. N Engl J Med 354(2):166-178, 2006.
    This article reviews current treatment of ALL with a focus on emerging therapeutic options.
5. Rassenti LZ, Huynh L, Toy TL, et al: ZAP-70 compared with immunoglobulin heavy-chain gene mutation status as a predictor of disease progression in chronic lymphocytic leukemia. N Engl J Med 351(9):893-901, 2004.
    This paper presents evidence for ZAP-70 as a prognostic marker of CLL disease course.
6. Tallman MS, Gilliland G, Rowe JM: Drug therapy for acute myeloid leukemia. Blood 106(7):1154-1163, 2005.
    The authors review the prognostic features and treatment options of AML.

Robert Z. Orlowski • Don A. Gabriel

Multiple Myeloma

Introduction

Multiple myeloma is a malignant clonal disorder of plasma cells typically found in the bone marrow. About 15,000 new cases are diagnosed yearly in the United States, with a prevalence of approximately 50,000 patients, making myeloma the second most common hematologic malignancy. The peak incidence occurs in the sixth decade of life, but this disease can also be found in older and younger patients. Certain exposures, such as to radiation or to some chemicals, may modestly increase the risk for developing myeloma, but most patients have no such exposure history. In most patients, multiple myeloma is sporadic, but its incidence in African Americans is twofold higher than in whites, suggesting the possibility of an influence from genetic factors.

Presentation and Evaluation

Patients with multiple myeloma have varied presentations, but common manifestations include bony pain, anemia, renal dysfunction, hypercalcemia, recurring infections, and peripheral neuropathy. Evaluation of any patient begins with a careful history and physical examination (Box 76-1). Bone pain develops secondary to lytic bony lesions or pathologic fractures, including vertebral compression fractures. Fatigue and dyspnea are consequences of anemia caused by marrow involvement, anemia of chronic disease, or in a few cases, high paraprotein levels causing hyperviscosity. Elevation of serum viscosity may also induce mental status changes, congestive heart failure, coagulopathy, and changes on examination of the optic fundus. Serum viscosity measurements aid in the diagnosis of this syndrome, which is a clinical emergency that can be rapidly reversed by plasmapheresis and exchange. Renal insufficiency of varying degrees is seen in up to 40%, and hypercalcemia can occur as a result of osteoclast activation by the myeloma cell and its microenvironment. Recurring infections, especially of the sinopulmonary tract, present as complications of functional hypogammaglobulinemia, as well as granulocytopenia and impaired cell-mediated immunity. Peripheral neuropathies may develop as a result of compression fractures or localized masses of plasma cells, known as *plasmacytomas*, which can induce nerve root impingement. Some patients may present with amyloidosis, which can also cause peripheral neuropathy and other clinical problems, including nephrotic syndrome, congestive cardiomyopathy, hepatomegaly, macroglossia, carpal tunnel syndrome, periorbital purpura, and malabsorption. Of note, 20% of patients are asymptomatic and come to medical attention because of an abnormality in a laboratory or radiographic evaluation performed for another indication.

The diagnosis of myeloma is ultimately based on laboratory findings, with the hallmark being identification of a monoclonal paraprotein on electrophoresis or immunofixation of the serum or urine (Box 76-2). Most commonly, patients have immunoglobulin G (IgG), IgA, or light chain disease, but IgM, IgD, and IgE myelomas are also seen, as is oligosecretory or nonsecretory disease. This last category means that even patients without a monoclonal protein can have myeloma, and they are diagnosed with a bone marrow aspiration and biopsy. Marrow sampling is important to evaluate the extent of involvement and for cytogenetic studies, including routine karyotyping and fluorescence in situ hybridization. Patients with at least 10% clonal marrow plasmacytosis, a serum or urine paraprotein, and signs of end-organ damage have symptomatic multiple myeloma. Those patients who have no disease-related symptoms have asymptomatic myeloma. Finally, patients with a lower-level paraprotein, lesser marrow involvement, and no symptoms have monoclonal gammopathy of undetermined significance (MGUS). If amyloidosis is suspected, Congo red staining of the marrow can be performed but has a sensitivity of only 50%. More reliable diagnostic tests include biopsies of the kidney, rectum, or gingiva and abdominal fat pad aspirates.

Box 76-1   Diagnostic Evaluation of a Plasma Cell Dyscrasia

Complete history and physical exam
Complete blood cell count with differential and platelets
Examination of peripheral blood smear for rouleaux formation
Creatinine, blood urea nitrogen, and electrolytes
Calcium and albumin; obtain ionized calcium in the setting of hypercalcemia
Quantitative immunoglobulins
Serum protein electrophoresis and immunofixation, with monoclonal protein quantitation
Random urine collection for protein electrophoresis and immunofixation
Twenty-four-hour urine collection for total protein, light chain quantitation, and creatinine clearance
Myeloma skeletal survey, including evaluation of the spine, pelvis, skull, humeri, and femurs; in some patients, magnetic resonance imaging and/or positron emission tomography may be appropriate
Unilateral bone marrow aspirate and biopsy, with cytogenetics both by routine karyotyping and fluorescence in situ hybridization for characteristic myeloma-associated abnormalities, immunophenotyping, and plasma cell labeling index, if available; bilateral marrow sampling may be of benefit in patients suspected of having oligosecretory or nonsecretory disease
β_2-microglobulin, C-reactive protein, and lactate dehydrogenase
Serum viscosity, if clinically indicated

Box 76-2   Diagnostic Criteria for Plasma Cell Dyscrasias

Monoclonal gammopathy of undetermined significance
■ Monoclonal protein in the serum <3.0 g/dL
■ Clonal marrow plasmacytosis <10%, if a marrow is done
■ No related organ or tissue impairment (see below)
■ No signs of another malignancy associated with a monoclonal protein

Asymptomatic multiple myeloma
■ Monoclonal protein in the serum ≥3.0 g/dL
■ Clonal marrow plasmacytosis, usually ≥10%
■ No related organ or tissue impairment (see below)

Symptomatic multiple myeloma
■ Monoclonal protein in the serum and/or urine
■ Clonal marrow plasmacytosis, usually ≥10% *and/or,*
■ Documented clonal plasmacytoma
■ Related organ or tissue impairment, including at least one of the following:
   Hypercalcemia (>11.5 mg/dL; >2.65 mmol/L)
   Renal insufficiency (serum creatinine >2 mg/dL; ≥177 µmol/L
   Anemia (hemoglobin <10 g/dL, or 2 g/dL below lower limit of normal)
   Bone disease (lytic lesions or osteopenia with compression fracture)
   Symptomatic hyperviscosity
   Amyloidosis
   Frequent bacterial infections (>2 in previous 12 months)

Differential Diagnosis

Although one of the hallmarks of multiple myeloma is the presence of a monoclonal protein in the serum or urine, most patients with a paraprotein do not have myeloma. Other malignant entities to consider include Waldenström's macroglobulinemia, amyloidosis, indolent non-Hodgkin's lymphoma, mantle cell lymphoma, and chronic lymphocytic leukemia. Even more common is MGUS, which is generally a benign condition, although it does carry a 1.0% to 1.5% per year risk of progression to one of the hematologic malignancies described earlier. MGUS is also associated with an increased risk for developing solid tumors. Patients with adult T-cell leukemia and lymphoma can present with bony lesions and hypercalcemia reminiscent of myeloma, but often have abnormal circulating lymphocytes and generally do not have a monoclonal protein. Polyclonal increases in immunoglobulins without a paraprotein are often a result of chronic immune stimulation, such as from HIV or hepatitis C virus infection. A variety of autoimmune disorders can also produce a polyclonal increase in immunoglobulins and in some cases may be associated with a low-level monoclonal protein.

Staging and Risk Stratification

Several different staging systems have been used to stratify patients into different risk groups to better predict outcome and guide therapy. The International Staging System, which is based on serum levels of albumin and β_2-microglobulin (Table 76-1), is superior in its ability to predict overall survival (OS) compared with older approaches. In the future, this may be modified or replaced with systems that incorporate the results of cytogenetics because chromosomal abnormalities can affect the response to, and durability of, both standard and high-dose therapies. DNA ploidy has an impact, in that patients with hypodiploid disease have a shorter survival, whereas hyperdiploid patients have an improved prognosis. Many patients with myeloma are found to have one of several recurring, nonrandom genetic lesions. Loss of a portion of, or an entire copy of, chromosome 13 is frequently reported and may induce cell cycle dysregulation through loss of the retinoblastoma protein. This genetic abnormality confers an inferior prognosis. Translocations in which one partner is the immunoglobulin heavy-chain locus, such as t(11;14), t(4;14) or t(14;16), and t(6;14), are also frequent, and may affect cell cycle control in part by dysregulation of *cyclin D1*,

Table 76-1 The International Staging System for Multiple Myeloma

Stage	Criteria	Median Overall Survival
I	Serum β_2-microglobulin <3.5 mg/L *and* Serum albumin ≥3.5 g/dL	62 mo
II	Neither stage I nor stage III	44 mo
III	Serum β_2-microglobulin ≥5.5 mg/L	29 mo

cyclin D2, or *cyclin D3*, respectively. Interestingly, t(11;14) is associated with a neutral or good prognosis, whereas t(4;14) and t(14;16) confer a poor risk. Other genetic lesions that are found include mutations of the p53 locus at 17p13, *c-myc*, *ras*, and 1q21 lesions that may involve *CKS1B*.

Management and Therapy

Optimum Initial Treatment

Patients with symptomatic multiple myeloma require treatment to reduce tumor burden, ameliorate symptoms, reduce the risk for complications, improve quality of life, and prolong survival. The choice of initial induction regimens is often guided by a decision about whether or not the patient is a candidate for high-dose chemotherapy with autologous peripheral blood stem cell transplantation (PBSCT). Factors that are weighed in this decision include the age and performance status of the patient and the presence of comorbid medical conditions and vital organ compromise. Those patients who are candidates for autologous PBSCT typically undergo initial therapy with regimens that avoid alkylating agents because these drugs damage stem cells and impair their collection in adequate numbers.

For patients who are older or who for another reason are not candidates for PBSCT, initial therapy has in the past consisted of a combination of the alkylator melphalan (Alkeran) and prednisone (MP; Fig. 76-1). Recent studies have added novel agents to the MP backbone, and results with the MPT regimen, incorporating the immunomodulatory and antiangiogenic agent thalidomide (Thalomid), have been encouraging. Two randomized trials have shown that MPT induced a higher overall and complete response rate, as well as a superior time to progression (TTP) and OS, suggesting MPT should be the standard of care for this population. Unfortunately, MPT carries with it a higher risk for toxicities, including thromboembolic and infectious complications, with the former indicating the need for concurrent prophylactic anticoagulation. MP is still, therefore, acceptable in patients of very advanced age or poor performance status and organ function. Current studies are investigating the utility of adding other agents,

such as lenalidomide (Revlimid) or the proteasome inhibitor bortezomib (Velcade), to the MP regimen. In some cases, it may also be appropriate to utilize an induction therapy more typically used in younger, transplant-eligible patients. Barring toxicity or disease progression, treatment is continued until either a complete remission is achieved or patients enter a plateau phase, with 3 months of stable disease despite continued therapy. Induction is then stopped in favor of watchful waiting, or patients may receive maintenance therapy.

In patients who are eligible for PBSCT, induction therapy with four to six cycles is pursued to reduce the disease burden before stem cell mobilization. One regimen used commonly combines infusional doxorubicin (adriamycin) and vincristine with oral dexamethasone, or a similar combination except using pegylated liposomal doxorubicin (Doxil; DVd). An oral combination of thalidomide with dexamethasone (thal/dex) appears to provide a higher overall response rate of 60% to 70% and may result in a prolonged TTP and OS in patients who do not proceed to transplantation. Lenalidomide with dexamethasone seems to improve upon these benefits further and may be less toxic than thal/dex, although both require prophylactic anticoagulation because of the risk for thromboembolic complications. Studies with hybrid regimens, such as DVd with thalidomide, have shown response rates approaching or exceeding 90%, with a high proportion of complete responses. However, these regimens are more toxic, and long-term follow-up is needed to determine whether the higher response rates will translate into a benefit after PBSCT. Bortezomib is also being actively investigated in combination with some of the agents described earlier in the front-line setting.

Supportive care is an important aspect of the multidisciplinary approach to multiple myeloma. Bisphosphonates, such as pamidronate (Aredia) and zoledronate (Zometa), reduce the risk for pathologic bony fractures in patients with lytic lesions or osteoporosis and compression fractures and may also affect survival. Their risks include acute flu-like infusion-related reactions, renal insufficiency, and jaw osteonecrosis with extended use. Erythropoietic agents (Aranesp, Epogen, or Procrit) affect disease- and treatment-related anemia and improve quality of life while reducing transfusion requirements, although care should be taken to not exceed a hemoglobin value of 12.0 g/dL with their use. Kyphoplasty or vertebroplasty in patients with acute vertebral compression fractures and pain can provide significant relief of pain and reduce the need for analgesics. Local radiation therapy can also be of benefit in pain control and is helpful for patients with solitary plasmacytomas as well.

Transplantation Options

High-dose chemotherapy for myeloma is employed in an attempt to extend both the event-free survival and the OS.

Figure 76-1 A Current Treatment Algorithm for Multiple Myeloma.
A current treatment algorithm for patients who are or are not suitable candidates for stem cell transplantation is presented. Further detail is provided in the text. Dex, dexamethasone; DVd, pegylated liposomal doxorubicin with vincristine and oral dexamethasone; DVd-T, DVd with thalidomide; MP, melphalan and prednisone; MPT, melphalan and prednisone with thalidomide; PAD, bortezomib with infusional doxorubicin and dexamethasone; PBSCT, peripheral blood stem cell transplantation; SCT, stem cell transplantation; VAD, infusional doxorubicin and vincristine with oral dexamethasone.

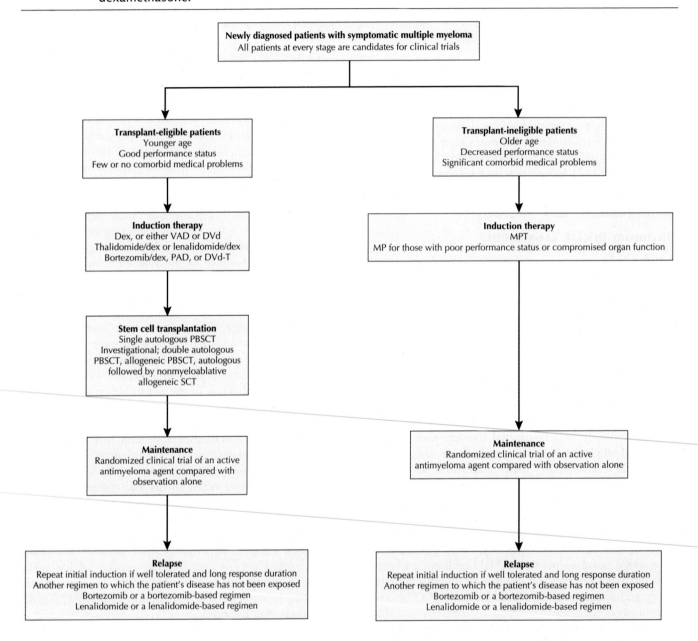

Several randomized studies comparing single autologous PBSCT after induction chemotherapy with a chemotherapy-only approach have shown an advantage for transplantation. Complete remissions can be achieved in up to 40% or more of patients, and median OS of up to 5 years or more can be seen, with a 100-day transplant-related mortality (TRM) rate of less than 2% to 3%. Some studies suggest that a tandem approach, in which two auto-PBSCTs are performed, with the second shortly following the first, may be superior to a single transplantation. Unfortunately, most patients ultimately relapse, probably because of residual myeloma present in the patient despite conditioning with high-dose melphalan, or contamination of the stem cell product with plasma cells, or both. As a result, there has been interest in following a single auto-PBSCT with a reduced-intensity, nonmyeloablative approach, using stem cells from a matched allogeneic donor that would not be contaminated with myeloma and would induce a graft-versus-myeloma effect. In younger patients, a fully ablative allogeneic transplant may be an option as well, but these approaches are complicated by graft-versus-host disease, and the latter is plagued by a high TRM.

Maintenance Therapy

Because front-line myeloma therapy is not curative, a maintenance approach with a lower dose of an active anti-myeloma agent is an attractive strategy to prolong the response duration. For patients treated with conventional dose regimens, no studies have shown a benefit in OS for any currently available drug when compared with observation alone. In patients who have received high-dose therapy with stem cell support, interferon was shown to improve survival by about 6 months, but its use was complicated by significant toxicities. Recently, thalidomide has been shown to improve post-transplantation event-free survival by more than 10 months, and also to improve overall survival. Lenalidomide, as well as other agents such as bortezomib, continue to be studied in this setting.

Treatment of Relapsed and Refractory Disease

Despite the use of induction chemotherapy, and even of autologous PBSCT, multiple myeloma will relapse and become symptomatic again in most patients, who then need additional therapy. In some cases, it may be appropriate to repeat whatever regimen was used previously, especially if it induced a remission of 6 to 12 months or more. Responding patients treated with such an approach typically have a remission duration one half the length of that seen previously. More commonly, patients are treated with a single-agent or combination regimen to which their disease has not been previously exposed. Bortezomib was the first new drug recently approved for therapy of relapsed and refractory disease, and in a randomized study induced a superior response rate, TTP, and OS compared with dexamethasone alone. Combination regimens based on bortezomib have even greater activity, and bortezomib with pegylated, liposomal doxorubicin has been shown to be superior to bortezomib alone. A second, newly approved agent is the novel immunomodulatory drug lenalidomide, which in combination with dexamethasone, was shown to be superior to dexamethasone alone and to improve TTP and OS.

Avoiding Treatment Errors

It is important to perform a full initial evaluation because patients with asymptomatic multiple myeloma do not benefit from early initiation of therapy, whereas those with symptomatic disease should generally be started promptly on treatment. Careful assessment of renal function and correction of abnormalities, when possible, is important before the initiation of therapy because several of the commonly used agents, including melphalan and lenalidomide, may need to be dose-adjusted in patients with renal insufficiency. Also, cytogenetic studies and fluorescence in situ hybridization probing for myeloma-associated chromosomal abnormalities are becoming increasingly important both prognostically and in deciding on optimal therapeutic strategies. For example, patients with t(4;14) have a poor outcome after autologous stem cell transplantation and may be candidates for novel chemotherapeutic approaches or allogeneic transplantation, whereas patients with deletion 13 may respond especially well to bortezomib-containing regimens.

Future Directions

Even though multiple myeloma remains an incurable disease, recent advances that have been incorporated into the current treatment algorithm (see Fig. 76-1) have produced a significant trend toward an improving OS. Many novel agents being studied in the relapsed and refractory disease population are showing promising results, including heat shock protein 90 inhibitors and monoclonal antibodies to interleukin-6, among others. Therefore, all patients should be considered candidates for clinical trials, which offer access to new, promising drugs that usually have been extensively validated in increasingly physiologically relevant preclinical models. It is likely that our expanding knowledge of the molecular pathogenesis of multiple myeloma will lead, in the near future, to a risk-adapted and cytogenetically adapted treatment strategy that will personalize therapy for patients and bring us closer to a cure for this disease.

Additional Resources

The International Myeloma Foundation. Available at: http://www. myeloma.org/. Accessed December 2, 2006.
  The International Myeloma Foundation is an important patient advocacy group that provides resources for multiple myeloma patients, as well as their caregivers and health care providers, including information about clinical trials.
The Leukemia and Lymphoma Society. Available at: http://www. leukemia.org/hm_lls. Accessed December 2, 2006.
  The Leukemia & Lymphoma Society is an important patient advocacy group that provides resources for multiple myeloma patients, as well as their caregivers and health care providers, including information about clinical trials.
The Multiple Myeloma Research Foundation. Available at: http://www. multiplemyeloma.org. Accessed December 2, 2006.
  The Multiple Myeloma Research Foundation is an important patient advocacy group that provides resources for multiple myeloma patients, as well as their caregivers and health care providers, including information about clinical trials.

The National Cancer Institute. Available at: http://www.clinicaltrials. gov/. Accessed December 2, 2006.

This National Cancer Institute website provides resources for multiple myeloma patients, as well as their caregivers and health care providers, including information about clinical trials.

EVIDENCE

1. Attal M, Harousseau JL, Facon T, et al: Single versus double autologous stem-cell transplantation for multiple myeloma. N Engl J Med 349(26):2495-2502, 2003.

   This was the first prospective, randomized clinical trial showing that patients receiving induction chemotherapy followed by two autologous peripheral blood stem cell transplants had an improved time to progression and overall survival compared with patients receiving chemotherapy and only a single transplantation for multiple myeloma.

2. Attal M, Harousseau JL, Stoppa AM, et al: A prospective, randomized trial of autologous bone marrow transplantation and chemotherapy in multiple myeloma. InterGroupe Français du Myélome. N Engl J Med 335(2):91-97, 1996.

   This was the first prospective, randomized clinical trial showing that patients receiving induction chemotherapy followed by autologous peripheral blood stem cell transplantation had an improved response rate, time to progression, and overall survival compared with patients receiving chemotherapy alone for multiple myeloma.

3. The International Myeloma Working Group: Criteria for the classification of monoclonal gammopathies, multiple myeloma and related disorders: A report of the International Working Group. Br J Haematol 121(5):749-757, 2003.

   This report presents the currently accepted criteria for diagnosis of plasma cell dyscrasias as formulated by the International Myeloma Working Group.

4. Greipp PR, San Miguel J, Durie BG, et al: International staging system for multiple myeloma. J Clin Oncol 23(15):3412-3420, 2005.

   The authors discuss the derivation and validation of the most accurate prognostic system for multiple myeloma, which relies on the results of serum studies of albumin and β_2-microglobulin.

5. Palumbo A, Bringhen S, Caravita T, et al: Oral melphalan and prednisone chemotherapy plus thalidomide compared with melphalan and prednisone alone in elderly patients with multiple myeloma: Randomised controlled trial. Lancet 367(9513):825-831, 2006.

   This phase III, randomized, international trial demonstrated that melphalan, prednisone, and thalidomide induced a higher response rate, response quality, and improved overall survival compared with melphalan and prednisone alone, making the three-drug regimen the standard of care for myeloma patients not eligible for stem cell transplantation.

6. Rajkumar SV, Blood E, Vesole D, et al: Phase III clinical trial of thalidomide plus dexamethasone compared with dexamethasone alone in newly diagnosed multiple myeloma: A clinical trial coordinated by the Eastern Cooperative Oncology Group. J Clin Oncol 24(3):431-436, 2006.

   This phase III, randomized trial demonstrated that thalidomide and dexamethasone induced a higher response rate and response quality compared with dexamethasone alone as an initial therapy for patients with myeloma requiring chemotherapy.

7. Rajkumar SV, Hayman SR, Lacy MQ, et al: Combination therapy with lenalidomide plus dexamethasone (Rev/Dex) for newly diagnosed myeloma. Blood 106(13):4050-4053, 2005.

   This phase II study demonstrated promising activity of the novel thalidomide analogue lenalidomide, in combination with dexamethasone, as an initial induction regimen for patients with multiple myeloma.

8. Richardson PG, Sonneveld P, Schuster MW, et al: Bortezomib or high-dose dexamethasone for relapsed multiple myeloma. N Engl J Med 352(24):2487-2498, 2005.

   This phase III, randomized, international trial demonstrated that bortezomib induced a higher response rate, response quality, and improved time to progression and overall survival compared with dexamethasone for patients with relapsed myeloma.

9. Stewart AK, Fonseca R: Prognostic and therapeutic significance of myeloma genetics and gene expression profiling. J Clin Oncol 23(15):6339-6344, 2005.

   The authors review some of the important cytogenetic findings commonly seen in multiple myeloma, their biology, and how they affect prognosis and therapy.

James M. Coghill ▪ Thomas C. Shea

Hematopoietic Stem Cell Transplantation

Introduction

During the past three decades, hematopoietic stem cell transplantation (HSCT) has been established as curative therapy for hematopoietic malignancies, marrow failure syndromes, primary immunodeficiencies, and genetic disorders. Current efforts are improving the efficacy of this therapy and expanding its role in the treatment of other disorders such as the hemoglobinopathies and autoimmune diseases. Underlying the use of HSCT is the principle of dose response in regard to tumor cell kill (i.e., increasing dose overcomes drug resistance and eradicates more malignant cells). The ensuing pancytopenia following marrow-ablative therapy is abrogated by the infusion of stem cells from either an autologous or allogeneic (histocompatible donor) source (Fig. 77-1). In the autologous setting, tumors that are still responsive to standard doses of chemotherapy (chemosensitive disease) respond even better to the dose escalation used in transplantation. Additional benefits of allogeneic transplantation include the infusion of a tumor-free stem cell graft and the graft-versus-tumor (GVT) immune effect mediated by donor cells against residual host cancer cells. This concept has recently led to treatments that use lower doses of chemotherapy or irradiation, so called nonmyeloablative or reduced intensity transplantations, which focus on establishing a stable donor graft to allow for GVT with less emphasis on direct cytotoxicity from the conditioning regimen itself. Advances in the fields of immunology, infectious disease, and transfusion medicine have all contributed to the encouraging results listed in Table 77-1.

Management and Therapy

The decisions regarding application and initiation of transplantation are complex and best addressed by early referral to centers with experience in a full-range of options regarding the use of autologous versus allogeneic transplants as well as the different types of donor cells available. Maintaining good communication with the transplantation center is critical to the successful long-term management of patients after they are discharged and reintegrated into their local health care system. This is particularly important in managing allogeneic transplant recipients who may develop opportunistic infections or graft-versus-host disease (GVHD) requiring the long-term use of immunosuppressive medications.

Autologous Transplantations

Prospective trials have identified a disease-free survival and overall survival benefit for autologous transplantations over conventional therapy in relapsed Hodgkin's and non-Hodgkin's lymphoma and multiple myeloma. Numerous phase II trials also attest to the value of autologous transplantation in patients with acute myelogenous leukemia (AML) in second complete remission. Although autologous transplantation is better tolerated than allogeneic transplantation, it is not feasible in patients with significant residual disease in the marrow and is generally unsuccessful in disease that is resistant to conventional doses of chemotherapy. Although conceptually attractive, the value of removing contaminating tumor

Figure 77-1 Hematopoietic Stem Cell Transplantation.
BK, a polyomavirus; CMV, cytomegalovirus; GU, genitourinary; GI, gastrointestinal.

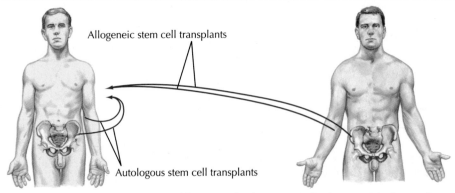

Allogeneic stem cell transplants

Autologous stem cell transplants

In autologous transplantation, the patient is the source of the stem cells (the patient is the donor and the host at the same time). When the stem cells come from another person who is a histocompatible donor, this is called allogeneic transplantation

Sources of hematopoietic stem cells

Peripheral blood

Umbilical cord blood (used primarly for children)

Bone marrow (preferable from iliac crest)

Placenta

Transplant complications

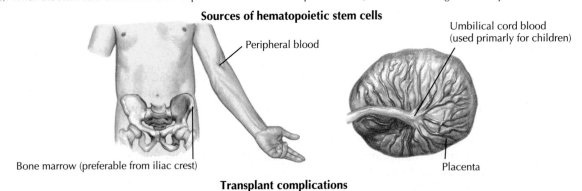

Graft-versus-host disease (graft rejection)

Persistent immune reaction against the skin

Persistent immune reaction against liver and GI tract

Polyomavirus

Reactivation of varicella zoster

Invasive pulmonary infections—
Fungi: nocardiosis, aspergillosis, pneumocystis
Gram+: staphylococcal, pneumococcal infections
Gram−: *E. coli, Klebsiella, Pseudomonas aeruginosa*
Viral: CMV, herpes simplex, influenza infections

Bacteremias and catheter infections: staphylococcal, streptococcal, gram-negative infections

Hepatic infections—
fungal: aspergillosis
Viral: CMV

Infections

Encephalitis: viruses: herpes simplex
Protozoa: toxoplasmosis
Fungi: aspergillosis

Sinus infections— fungal: mucormycosis

GU tract infections: adenoviruses CMV, BK

GI tract infections: CMV and adenoviral infections

cells from reinfused products, so-called purging, remains unproved.

Allogeneic Transplantations

The decision to undergo an allogeneic transplantation depends on the underlying disease, the existing age and comorbidities of the patient, and the availability of a suitable donor. The decreased leukemia relapse rate after allo-geneic transplantations compared with that after identical twin (syngeneic) or autologous transplantations exemplifies the advantage of a GVT response. Mild chronic GVHD enhances GVT in diseases such as chronic myelogenous leukemia (CML) and is associated with a decreased relapse rate. This immune effect is also the basis for treating recurrent disease after transplantation with infusions of lymphocytes collected from the donor (donor lymphocyte infusions). Usually, allogeneic transplantation is pref-

Table 77-1 Diseases Responsive to Hematopoietic Stem Cell Transplantation

Disease	Type of Transplantation	Timing	Clinical Results
AML	Allogeneic	CR 2 or high-risk CR 1	OS 30%-60%
	Autologous	CR 1 or CR 2 if no donor available	OS 30%-40%
ALL (children)	Allogeneic	Second CR	OS 40%-65%
ALL (high risk)	Allogeneic	First CR	OS 50%
CML	Allogeneic	Tyrosine kinase (imatinib) resistant	OS 50%-60%
Myelodysplastic syndrome	Allogeneic	Age <65 yr	OS 40%
Aplastic anemia	Allogeneic	Individualized	OS 70%-90%
CLL	Allogeneic or autologous	Participation in clinical trial	Small series of patients with durable CR. Nonablative transplantation under investigation
Intermediate-grade NHL	Autologous	Chemosensitive relapse	OS 40%-50%
High-risk NHL	Autologous	First CR	OS 50%-60%
Low-grade NHL	Allogeneic or autologous relapse	Chemosensitive	DFS 25%-50% at 5 yr
Mantle cell lymphoma	Allogeneic or autologous	First CR	Small series with autologous durable CR rates of 25%-50%
Hodgkin's disease	Autologous	Chemosensitive relapse	15%-25% DFS
Multiple myeloma	Autologous	Chemosensitive relapse or first remission	5-yr OS 50%; DFS of 20%
Thalassemia	Allogeneic	Clinical trial	OS 75% for patients without cirrhosis
Sickle cell anemia	Allogeneic	Clinical trial	OS 75%
Autoimmune disorders	Allogeneic or autologous	Clinical trial	Small series of remissions

CR, complete response; DFS, disease-free survival; OS, overall survival; AML, acute myelogenous leukemia; CLL, chronic lymphocytic leukemia; CML, chronic myelogenous leukemia; ALL, acute lymphocytic leukemia; NHL, non-Hodgkin's lymphoma.

erable for relapsed leukemias and patients with refractory lymphomas because of the immune effect of the donor cells against residual tumor and the lack of contaminating tumor cells in the infusion product. Early identification and transplantation in patients with high-risk features who are destined to do poorly with standard therapies optimize the chance for cure in such settings.

Histocompatibility

Major histocompatibility class I (human leukocyte antigens [HLA]-A, -B, -C) and class II (HLA-D, -DR, -DQ, -DO, -DN, -DP) antigens are the HLA used to determine patient-donor compatibility. Six alleles from three HLA antigens (A, B, and DR) are used for routine typing of siblings. A six-for-six match is considered to be an HLA identical full match. Additional alleles can be evaluated for unrelated donor transplantations.

Donor Availability

Matched sibling donors are available for about 30% of patients and have historically been preferred over partially matched or unrelated donors because of the decreased risk for graft rejection and GVHD. The National Marrow Donor Program includes a registry with more than 5.5 million volunteer donors that can provide a match for

about 80% of patients overall, with the probability of finding a donor varying by the patient's racial and ethnic background. Transplantations using umbilical cord blood cells or cells from donors who are mismatched at more than one allele are available for certain patients at a limited number of centers. Virtually all patients have a haplotype or three-antigen-matched donor, provided they have a living first-degree relative. The infusion of large numbers of stem cells, depletion of T cells from the donor product, and aggressive immunosuppression may overcome the high risk for acute graft rejection and severe GVHD in these transplant recipients.

Sources of Hematopoietic Stem Cells

Bone Marrow

Marrow harvesting usually requires general anesthesia and multiple aspirations from the iliac crest. Typically, 15 to 20 mL/kg recipient body weight, yielding a minimum of 2×10^8 nucleated cells/kg, is adequate for engraftment. Donors usually go home the same day and seldom require more than oral analgesics for 1 to 2 days postoperatively.

Peripheral Blood

Low numbers of stem cells expressing the CD34 surface antigen exist in the peripheral blood under normal circumstances. This number can be markedly increased, allowing for collection by a process called *apheresis*, following treatment with granulocyte colony-stimulating factor (G-CSF) alone, or, for autologous transplant recipients, G-CSF plus chemotherapy. Advantages over bone marrow infusions include more rapid hematopoietic recovery and decreased transplantation-related mortality. This process does, however, result in the infusion of 10 times more donor T cells in allogeneic transplants, leading to an increased risk for GVHD. This complication is offset by earlier graft recovery and a lower risk for both infection and relapse and has led to peripheral blood becoming the most common stem cell source for both related and unrelated adult allogeneic transplantations. In children, however, especially in the treatment of nonmalignant diseases such as aplastic anemia, related donor marrow may be preferred to stem cells because of the decreased risk for GVHD.

Umbilical Cord Blood

Hematopoietic stem cells are present in umbilical cord blood and can be collected from the placenta after delivery. Because neonatal lymphocytes remain immunologically naive, they are less likely to result in GVHD and permit the use of partially matched patient-donor pairs. The ability to undertake transplantation with mismatched donors and the rapid availability of frozen and stored cord blood products are the major advantages of this approach. Disadvantages include delayed engraftment and an increased risk for infection. Currently, umbilical cord transplantations are used primarily for children, but research on in vitro stem cell expansion and use of multiple cord blood products may allow for the more widespread use of this approach in adult patients.

Transplantation-Related Therapy

Conditioning Regimens

Preparative regimens given before allogeneic stem cell or bone marrow infusion are designed to eradicate the underlying disease and permit engraftment of donor stem cells without rejection. Full myeloablation of the hematopoietic system may be accomplished by total-body irradiation (TBI) or high-dose busulfan. In addition to marrow aplasia and infection, major toxicities include infertility, lung and liver toxicity, and severe mucositis. Each of these treatments is generally administered with other agents to augment both the immunosuppressive and antitumor effect of the treatment. In the autologous setting, a variety of combination regimens have been used including TBI-cyclophosphamide-etoposide and carmustine-etoposide-cytarabine-melphalan (BEAM).

There has also been interest in the integration of radioimmunotherapy (RIT) into both autologous and allogeneic transplantation conditioning regimens. RIT involves coupling radioactive isotopes to monoclonal antibodies directed at molecular targets found on the surfaces of malignant cells. Such a therapeutic strategy permits the targeting of high levels of radiation directly to a tumor, thereby minimizing damage to adjacent, normal tissues. Iodine-131 tositumomab and yttrium-90 ibritumomab are currently approved at nonmyeloablative doses for the management of non-Hodgkin's lymphoma. In the allogeneic setting, protocols incorporating immunoconjugates directed against CD33, CD45, and CD66 are currently underway to augment therapy for patients with leukemia, myelodysplastic syndrome, and lymphoma. The toxicity of such approaches does not appear greater than with chemotherapy alone, and efficacy may be improved compared with historical controls.

Nonmyeloablative regimens consisting of immunosuppressive drugs such as fludarabine and cyclophosphamide, low-dose TBI, and most recently RIT have been used to establish a mixed-chimera hematopoietic state (both donor and host cells). In less aggressive tumors such as the chronic leukemias or indolent lymphomas, the advantages of this strategy include less toxicity and a shorter duration of pancytopenia while maintaining a GVT effect. Early efficacy data using this approach has been encouraging, with complete remission rates approaching 85% in CML, chronic lymphocytic leukemia (CLL), and the low-grade lymphomas. Also, because of the reduced acute toxicity of the nonmyeloablative conditioning regimens, stem cell transplantation is becoming a viable treatment alternative for increasing numbers of older patients. Since 1984, the number of transplantations performed for those older than 50 years has risen more than in any other age group, with such patients currently receiving nearly 20% of all allogeneic transplantations for AML, acute lymphocytic leukemia, and CML.

Immunosuppression

The main factor allowing allogeneic transplantation is the use of medications that dampen the T-cell response. Agents such as methotrexate, corticosteroids, and cyclosporine or tacrolimus are used to prevent graft rejection and GVHD during the initial period after transplantation. Additional agents such as antithymocyte globulin and alemtuzumab have also been used both before and immediately after transplantation in an effort to prevent GVHD. Both agents are clearly effective in reducing the incidence and severity of acute and chronic GVHD, but they may increase the risk for infectious complications, graft rejection, and disease relapse, depending on the particular dosing regimen used. Newer anti-inflammatory medications such as infliximab, etanercept, rituximab, and daclizumab have been successfully used in the management of established acute or chronic GVHD but also may increase the risk for infectious complications.

Transfusion Therapy

Transfusions for immunosuppressed patients require removal of leukocytes from infused blood products to

Table 77-2 Comparison of Complications between Autologous, Allogeneic, and Nonmyeloablative Transplantations

Complication	Autologous	Allogeneic	Nonablative
Bacterial infection	3+	4+	2+
Viral infections	1+	4+	4+
Fungal infections	1+	4+	4+
Graft vs. host	—	3+	2+
Graft rejection	Slow recovery 1+	2%-5%	5%-10%
Graft vs. tumor	—	2+	3+
Veno-occlusive disease	1%-3%	5%	Rare
Relapse	4+	2+	3+
Secondary myelodysplastic syndrome or acute myelogenous leukemia	5%-15%	—	—
Treatment-related mortality	5%	20%-40%	15%-25%

lower the risk for alloimmunization and cytomegalovirus (CMV) transmission. Blood products must also be irradiated after transplantation to reduce the risk for transfusion-associated GVHD. These measures should be continued as long as patients are receiving immunosuppressive medication or have evidence of GVHD.

Transplant Complications

Treatment-Related Morbidity and Mortality

Weighing the risk for disease relapse and the potential for cure with transplantation against the likelihood of treatment-related effects on quality of life are paramount considerations for both the transplantation team and patient (Table 77-2). Overall mortality rates with allogeneic transplants range from 15% to 50% in the first 1 to 2 years, depending on patient age, organ function, and quality of the patient-donor match. Early toxicity for nonmyeloablative transplant regimens is generally low, although delayed GVHD remains a significant risk, and long-term treatment-related mortality (TRM) may be similar to fully ablative regimens. TRM rates vary from 2% to 10% for autologous transplants, depending primarily on the type and stage of malignancy, age and physiologic status of the patient, and conditioning regimen used. Although complications are more common following allogeneic transplantation than autologous transplantation, the risk for relapse is substantially higher for most autologous transplant recipients. These variables lead to complex decisions that are best made by an informed patient at an experienced center where multiple options are available.

Graft-versus-Host Disease

The degree of HLA disparity is directly associated with the incidence and severity of GVHD. More severe GVHD has historically been observed with matched unrelated or mismatched donor transplants, although outcomes comparable to those of matched related donor transplants are now being reported as a result of recent advances in immunosuppression and HLA typing. Acute GVHD by definition occurs before day 100 and develops in 10% to 70% of matched sibling transplant recipients. Chronic GVHD occurs beyond day 100 and manifests as a persistent autoimmune reaction against the host's skin, gut, and liver. Although mild GVHD is associated with a decreased relapse rate, severe GVHD conveys a poor quality of life and higher risk for TRM. The incidence of acute and possibly chronic GVHD appears to be reduced with the use of nonmyeloablative conditioning regimens compared with fully ablative protocols.

Infection

Bacterial infections occur early after transplantation during the period of neutropenia and mucosal injury. Infection with CMV and other viral pathogens, such as adenovirus, usually occurs 30 to 100 days after transplantation. The risk for bacterial, fungal, and viral infection continues with prolonged immunosuppression and can present months to years later as unexplained fevers (see Fig. 77-1). Patients requiring prolonged immunosuppression for GVHD are at risk for rapidly fatal bacterial infections with encapsulated organisms such as streptococcus and pneumococcus. Fevers in these patients must be treated aggressively with broad-spectrum antibiotics while the underlying cause is being investigated. Reactivation of varicella zoster occurs in 30% to 40% of patients, typically within 12 months of transplantation. Life-threatening dissemination may occur if not recognized and treated early with medications such as acyclovir. Fungal infections with invasive organisms such as aspergillosis or mucormycosis can also be seen in patients on long-term immunosuppressive therapy. Amphotericin B has been the mainstay of management for presumed and documented invasive fungal infections in transplant recipients but is now being replaced by newer agents such as liposomal amphotericin B, voriconazole, and caspofungin. These agents have less renal and infusional toxicity than amphotericin, with comparable or improved efficacy in most situations.

Avoiding Treatment Errors

Most HSCT recipients are closely monitored at an experienced center after transplantation. Such patients, however, do occasionally present to local physicians and emergency departments with urgent complications. It is important to realize that such patients, in particular those undergoing allogeneic procedures, may continue to demonstrate qualitative immune system dysfunction for months or even years after the recovery of their blood counts, and that this increases their risk for serious opportunistic infectious complications. Findings such as fever, cough, skin rash, and pain should be aggressively worked up because HSCT patients can rapidly decompensate. When questions do arise, local physicians are encouraged to directly contact the patient's transplantation center for additional advice.

Future Directions

Continued improvements in supportive care and expansion of the donor transplant pool through the use of cord blood cells, mismatched, and matched unrelated donors will continue to increase the number of transplantation candidates in upcoming years. Combining vaccines and other immunotherapy approaches with either autologous or allogeneic transplantation will be used to eliminate tumor cells and the risk for relapse in the future, and approaches using regulatory T-cell infusions, total lymphoid irradiation, and new immunosuppressant agents are being investigated for the prevention and treatment of GVHD.

Additional Resources

Blume KG, Forman SJ, Appelbaum FR (eds): Thomas's Hematopoietic Cell Transplantation, 3rd ed. Malden, MA, Blackwell Science, 2004.
   This excellent textbook is devoted exclusively to stem cell transplantation for those wishing to study HSCT in greater detail.
The National Marrow Donor Program Web site. Available at http://www.marrow.org. Accessed November 21, 2006.
   The official website of the National Marrow Donor Program is an excellent source of information on practically every aspect of stem cell transplantation, including up-to-date survival statistics by disease type.

EVIDENCE

1. Alyea EP, Kim HT, Ho V, et al: Comparative outcome of non-myeloablative and myeloablative allogeneic hematopoietic cell transplantation for patients older than 50 years of age. Blood 105(4):1810-1814, 2005.
   This retrospective analysis from a single transplantation center in the United States demonstrates improved overall survival and a reduced
incidence of GVHD in patients older than 50 years undergoing nonmyeloablative conditioning versus standard ablative regimens.
2. Aoudjhane M, Labopin M, Gorin NC, et al: Comparative outcome of reduced intensity and myeloablative conditioning regimen in HLA identical sibling allogeneic haematopoietic stem cell transplantation for patients older than 50 years of age with acute myeloblastic leukaemia: A retrospective survey from the Acute Leukemia Working Party (ALWP) of the European group for Blood and Marrow Transplantation (EBMT). Leukemia 19:2304-2312, 2005.
   This large retrospective series from Europe demonstrates comparable overall survival and reduced transplant-related toxicity in leukemia patients older than 50 years treated with nonmyeloablative conditioning regimens compared with those undergoing traditional, myeloablative procedures.
3. Child JA, Morgan GJ, Davies FE, et al: High-dose chemotherapy with hematopoietic stem-cell rescue for multiple myeloma. N Engl J Med 348(19):1875-1883, 2003.
   This landmark study demonstrates improved progression-free and overall survival in multiple myeloma patients treated with autologous HSCT compared with traditional chemotherapy.
4. Laughlin MJ, Eapen M, Rubinstein P, et al. Outcomes after transplantation of cord blood or bone marrow from unrelated donors in adults with leukemia. N Engl J Med 351: 2265-2275, 2004.
   This retrospective analysis from the United States demonstrates similar long-term outcomes between leukemia patients receiving mismatched umbilical cord stem cells and those receiving bone marrow from mismatched, unrelated, adult donors.
5. Philip T, Guglielmi C, Hagenbeek A, et al: Autologous bone marrow transplantation as compared with salvage chemotherapy in relapses of chemotherapy-sensitive non-Hodgkin's lymphoma. N Engl J Med 333(23):1540-1545, 1995.
   This important study, also known as the Parma trial, demonstrates improved event-free and overall survival in patients with relapsed non-Hodgkin's lymphoma treated with autologous stem-cell transplantation versus traditional, salvage chemotherapy.
6. Press OW, Eary JF, Gooley T, et al: A phase I/II trial of iodine-131-tositumomab (anti-CD20), etoposide, cyclophosphamide, and autologous stem cell transplantation for relapsed B-cell lymphomas. Blood 96(9):2934-2942, 2000.
   This important early study demonstrates the feasibility of combining radioimmunotherapy with traditional cytotoxic agents in the autologous HSCT setting for relapsed non-Hodgkin's lymphoma.
7. Tallman MS, Gray R, Robert NJ, et al: Conventional adjuvant chemotherapy with or without high-dose chemotherapy and autologous stem-cell transplantation in high-risk breast cancer. N Engl J Med 349(1):17-26, 2003.
   This landmark trial demonstrates a lack of benefit for HSCT compared with traditional chemotherapy for high-risk breast cancer.
8. Tauro S, Craddock C, Peggs K, et al: Allogeneic stem-cell transplantation using a reduced-intensity conditioning regimen has the capacity to produce durable remissions and long-term disease-free survival in patients with high-risk acute myeloid leukemia and myelodysplasia. J Clin Oncol 23(36):9387-9393, 2005.
   This study demonstrates that reduced-intensity transplantations are effective in producing long-term remissions of both acute leukemia and myelodysplasia, despite their reduced toxicity compared to traditional allogeneic HSCT regimens.

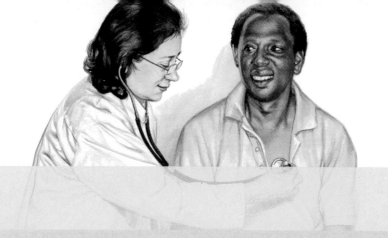
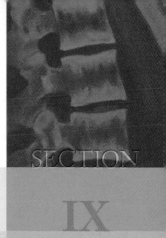

Oncologic Disorders

Mark A. Socinski

Lung Cancer

Introduction

Lung cancer is diagnosed in about 170,000 people annually in the United States. It is the second most common cancer in men (behind prostate) and in women (behind breast), accounting for 14% of all cancers in men and 13% in women. It is the most common cause of cancer-related death, with about 160,000 deaths annually. In men, the number of lung cancer deaths has been decreasing since the late 1980s, but it still accounts for 31% of all cancer deaths. In women, lung cancer deaths surpassed breast cancer deaths in 1986 and now account for 25% of all cancer deaths. The number of deaths from lung cancer exceeds deaths from colon, breast, prostate, and pancreatic cancer combined (Fig. 78-1).

Etiology and Pathogenesis

Smoking is the major risk factor for lung cancer. Although 85% to 90% of all patients have a history of direct exposure to tobacco, it is likely that the cause of lung cancer is multifactorial. Susceptibility clearly plays a role because most lifetime smokers do not develop lung cancer. A dose-response relationship exists between the number of cigarettes smoked and lung cancer risk. Once smoking cessation occurs, risk decreases but remains above the risk of lifetime nonsmokers for at least 18 years. More than half of all lung cancers are diagnosed in current nonsmokers. Other risk factors are shown in Box 78-1.

Lung cancer is classified into two major categories (Table 78-1): small cell lung cancer (SCLC) and nonsmall cell lung cancer (NSCLC). Each category and subtype of lung cancer has variations in the histology and degree of differentiation. About 1% to 4% of lung cancers have mixed histology consisting of both small cell and nonsmall cell. The differentiation by pathologists between SCLC and NSCLC is good (>90%). However, it is not 100%, and careful attention to the clinical presentation is necessary.

Clinical Presentation

The clinical presentation of lung cancer (Table 78-2) is generally related to symptoms referable to the disease in the chest or to disease at sites of metastasis. The most common chest symptoms are cough, dyspnea, chest pain, and hemoptysis. Other symptoms resulting from invasion into or obstruction of vital thoracic structures may include superior vena cava syndrome, pleural or pericardial effusion, postobstructive pneumonia, and Pancoast's syndrome.

Metastatic disease may occur anywhere, but the most common sites include the liver, adrenals, bone, brain, and lymph nodes. Patients often present with symptoms referable to sites of metastases including bone pain, seizures, hemiplegia, or hepatomegaly. Generalized symptoms such as weight loss, fatigue, malaise, and anorexia are very common and occur more often with advanced disease.

Several paraneoplastic syndromes are associated with lung cancers, including the syndrome of inappropriate antidiuretic hormone, hypercalcemia, gynecomastia, and Cushing's syndrome, and several neurologic syndromes, including Eaton-Lambert syndrome, cerebellar degeneration, peripheral neuropathy, and dementia.

Screening

The role of screening remains controversial. Table 78-3 shows trials published to date in which chest radiograph with or without sputum cytology were performed. No clear benefit was demonstrated when lung cancer mortality was the end point. These trials involved men only and really addressed less intense versus more intense screening strategies. The message is that screening has not been adequately addressed, rather than ineffective. Recent efforts have focused on the role of spiral computed

Figure 78-1 Annual Mortality Rate (in Thousands).

From Detterbeck FC, Rivera MP, Socinski MA, Rosenman JG (eds): Diagnosis and Treatment of Lung Cancer: An Evidence-Based Guide for the Practicing Clinician. Philadelphia, WB Saunders, 2001.

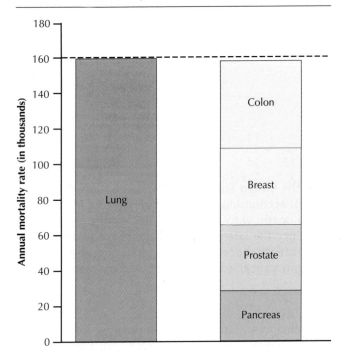

Table 78-2 Clinical Presentation of Lung Cancer

Symptom	Percentage of Patients
Cough	46
Weight loss	32
Dyspnea	30
Chest pain	30
Hemoptysis	27
Fever	28
Asymptomatic	15

From Detterbeck FC, Rivera MP, Socinski MA, Rosenman JG (eds): Diagnosis and Treatment of Lung Cancer: An Evidence-Based Guide for the Practicing Clinician. Philadelphia, WB Saunders, 2001.

Table 78-1 Histologic Classification of Lung Cancer*

Cancer Type	Age-Adjusted Incidence Rate[†]
Small cell	9.4
Nonsmall cell	
▪ Large cell	9.6
▪ Squamous cell carcinoma	15.3
▪ Adenocarcinoma	15.3
▪ Bronchioloalveolar carcinoma	1.4
▪ Adenosquamous carcinoma	0.8
Other	
▪ Bronchial gland carcinoma	0.6
▪ Adenoid cystic carcinoma	
▪ Mucoepidermoid tumor (MET)	
▪ Carcinoid tumor	0.5
▪ Typical	
▪ Atypical	
▪ Sarcoma	0.1
▪ Carcinosarcoma	

* Based on the World Health Organization system classification.
† Age-adjusted incidence rates per 100,000 population according to Surveillance, Epidemiology, and End Results (SEER) registry statistics, 1983-1987.
From Detterbeck FC, Rivera MP, Socinski MA, Rosenman JG (eds): Diagnosis and Treatment of Lung Cancer: An Evidence-Based Guide for the Practicing Clinician. Philadelphia, WB Saunders, 2001.

tomography (CT) scans for screening. Preliminary studies suggest that lung cancer can be found at an earlier stage, but the impact of this approach on survival remains uncertain. The results of several ongoing randomized trials are awaited and will help clarify the role of screening. The National Lung Cancer Screening Trial in the United Sates has randomized about 50,000 people to either plain chest x-ray or spiral CT scan. Until these results, as well as results from other similar trials, become available, routine screening cannot be recommended.

Diagnostic Approach

Histologic or cytologic confirmation is required to make the diagnosis of lung cancer. All patients should have multidisciplinary input into the optimal approach to making the diagnosis using the chest CT scan and positron emission tomography (PET) scan for direction. Options include sputum cytology, bronchoscopy, transthoracic fine-needle aspiration (TTFNA), endoscopic esophageal or bronchial ultrasound-guided fine-needle aspiration, cervical mediastinoscopy or anterior mediastinotomy, and biopsy or fine-needle aspiration of a metastatic site.

Sputum Cytology

This method is the least invasive, but accuracy depends on rigorous sample collection and optimal preservation. The

Table 78-3 Screening for Lung Cancer

Study*	N	Accrual Years	Intervention Frequency (mo) Control	Intervention Frequency (mo) Screen	Study Duration (yr)	Lung cancer Detection Rate in Population Control	Lung cancer Detection Rate in Population Screen	Percentage of Resectable Patients with Lung Cancer Control	Percentage of Resectable Patients with Lung Cancer Screen	Five-Year Survival of Patients with Cancer (%) Control	Five-Year Survival of Patients with Cancer (%) Screen	Lung cancer Mortality in Population[a] Control	Lung cancer Mortality in Population[a] Screen
Erfurt[b]	143,880	1972-1977			6	0.65	0.95	19	28	8	14	0.8	0.6
North London[b]	55,034	1960-1963	CXR q36	CXR q6	3	0.38	0.44	29[c]	44[c]	6	15	0.8	0.7
Hopkins	10,387	1973-1978	CXR q12 / —	CXR q12 / Sp q4	5-7	5.5	4.8	44	47	20[d]	20[d]	4.6	3.6
Memorial Sloan-Kettering Cancer Center	10,040	1974-1978	CXR q12 / —	CXR q12 / Sp q4	5-8	3.8	3.7	51	53	33	37	2.7	2.7
Mayo Clinic	9,211	1971-1976	CXR q12[e] / Sp q12[e]	CXR q4 / Sp q4	6	3.5	4.5	32	46	15	33	3.0	3.2
Czechoslovakia[f]	6,346	1976-1977	CXR q36[g] / —	CXR q6[g] / Sp[h] q6[g]	3	2.0	3.9	16	25	0	26	1.5	1.7

* Inclusion criteria: randomized trials of a screening intervention for lung cancer.
[a] Per 1000 patients/year.
[b] Groups of patients randomized rather than individual patients.
[c] $P < 0.05$.
[d] Eight-year survival.
[e] Yearly studies advised with about 50% compliance.
[f] Based on data from 3-year study period.
[g] Annual CXR during 3-year follow-up period.
[h] Single sputum specimen.
CXR, chest radiograph; Screen, screened arm; Sp, sputum (three samples).

sensitivity is about 65% and highly dependent on tumor size and location (large central tumors have the highest sensitivity rates). There is a 2% false-positive rate and a 10% false-negative rate.

Bronchoscopy

The overall sensitivity of bronchoscopy is 80% to 85% in central tumors and 60% to 65% in more peripheral lesions. In tumors smaller than 2 cm, the sensitivity is less than 33%.

Transthoracic Fine-Needle Aspiration

The overall sensitivity of TTFNA is 88%, specificity is 97%, and a false-positive rate is 1%. It carries a 27% false-negative rate, so lesions highly suspicious for lung cancer should still be considered malignant even with a negative TTFNA.

Endoscopic Esophageal or Bronchial Ultrasound-Guided Fine-Needle Aspiration

Newer approaches using endoscopic transesophageal or transbronchial techniques are currently available that may be the optimal approach depending on the findings on chest CT scan. The transesophageal approach is complementary to mediastinoscopy. With careful selection of patients, the overall sensitivity is 80% or greater with rates of specificity approaching 100%.

Cervical Mediastinoscopy or Anterior Mediastinotomy

Mediastinal lymph node sampling is often the method of diagnosing lung cancer. A cervical mediastinoscopy involves an incision in the sternal notch and sampling lymph nodes with the mediastinoscope in the paratracheal and subcarinal spaces. Important stations for sampling are shown in bold in figure 78-2. A station designates a specific anatomic location of an intrathoracic lymph node as defined by the American Joint Committee on Cancer [Fig. 78-2]. In tumors arising in the left upper lobe, it is necessary to sample nodes in the aortopulmonary window through an anterior mediastinotomy. This procedure involves an incision in the left second intercostal space and direct visualization of the anteroposterior window (station 10).

Biopsy or Fine-Needle Aspiration of a Metastatic Site

Biopsy of extrathoracic sites is a strategy that can accomplish both diagnosis and staging. For example, biopsies of the liver, bones, adrenal gland, or a brain lesion will provide the diagnosis and the stage (IV in the case of brain metastasis).

Differential Diagnosis and Staging

Lung cancer should be suspected when the appropriate signs and symptoms suggest this diagnosis, particularly in a patient with a history of smoking (Table 78-4). Radiographic abnormalities often suggest the diagnosis, but new abnormalities need to be differentiated from benign pulmonary lesions including infectious, inflammatory, granulomatous, vascular abnormalities, hamartomas, and metastatic lesions.

Staging is the most important determinant of a patient's treatment plan and prognosis. All patients must be carefully staged at the time of initial presentation. Staging is done using the tumor, mode, metastasis (TNM) system briefly summarized in Table 78-5.

Clinical staging relies on physical examination and radiographic studies (Table 78-6). Pathologic staging confirms the findings of radiographic studies with biopsies of suspected areas of pathologic involvement. In general, pathologic staging is more accurate than clinical staging in defining the presence of cancer.

All patients require a complete history and physical exam, chest x-ray, and a staging chest CT (a chest CT extending all the way through the liver and adrenals). Additional testing may include a head CT or magnetic resonance imaging, radionuclide bone scan, and a PET scan. Pathologic staging may include mediastinoscopy, thoracoscopy, or biopsy of suspected metastatic lesions.

Although the TNM system should also be used for SCLC, a more simplified system has historically been limited- or extensive-stage disease. Limited-stage disease is defined as disease limited to a reasonable thoracic radiation port. This typically includes the primary tumor and N1-3 nodes. Areas of controversy include the contralateral hilar and supraclavicular nodes. Disease beyond this definition is classified as extensive-stage SCLC and includes patients with malignant pleural or pericardial effusions.

Intrathoracic Staging

Figure 78-2 shows the regional lymph node stations for lung cancer staging. The initial evaluation of the mediastinal lymph nodes should be a chest CT scan. However, the sensitivity of CT is about 65%, with a specificity of 75%. False-negative rates are 10% to 15%, with false-positive rates of 30% to 40%. PET scanning increases the sensitivity (about 84%) and specificity (93%) but still has false-positive and false-negative rates of about 7% and 16%, respectively. CT and PET should be used together in selected cases. Mediastinoscopy remains the gold standard for mediastinal evaluation. The overall sensitivity of mediastinoscopy is similar to PET (about 84%), but its specificity is 100%. It does carry a 9% false-negative rate because all the mediastinal nodal stations are not accessible by mediastinoscopy. Obviously, its false-positive rate is 0%.

Figure 78-2 Regional Lymph Node Stations for Lung Cancer Staging.
Adapted from Mountain CF, Dresler CM: Regional lymph node classification for lung cancer staging.
Chest 1997; 111:1718-1723.

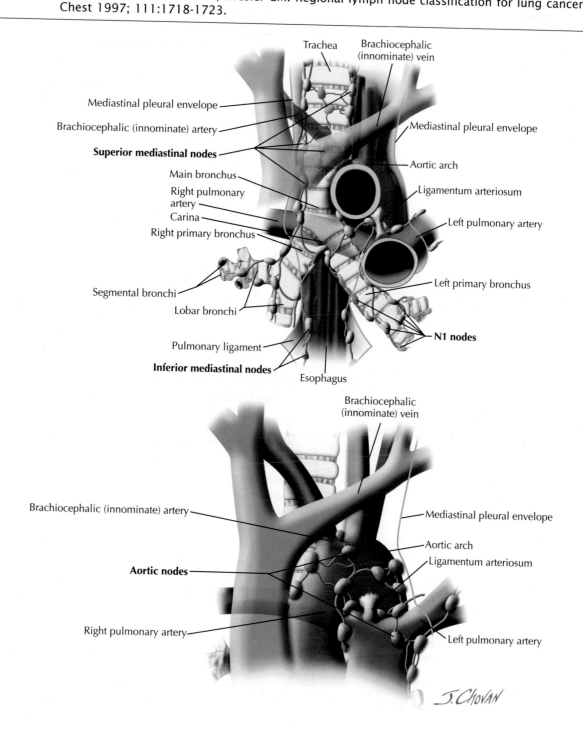

Extrathoracic Staging

Judicious use of noninvasive staging tests should be the standard for the evaluation of extrathoracic metastases. The intrathoracic clinical stage and overall signs and symptoms obtained by the history and physical examination should guide the use of such tests. The most common sites of metastases are the brain, bones, liver, adrenal gland, and contralateral lung. Directed testing including bone scans, brain CT or magnetic resonance imaging, and CT and PET scan should be done on an individualized basis. Once stage IV disease is documented, testing can stop unless patients are having organ-specific symptoms, which need therapeutic attention (particularly brain or bone metastases).

Table 78-4 Differential Diagnosis of a Pulmonary Mass or Abnormality

Diagnostic Category	Helpful Clinical Factors
Primary lung cancer	Age, risk factors
Metastatic cancer	Medical history, number of lesions
Chronic benign lesion	
Granuloma, scar	Prior chest x-ray, diffuse calcification
Hamartoma	Prior chest x-ray, fat on fine cut computed tomography
Acute benign lesion	
Rounded atelectasis	Radiographic appearance, resolution
Pseudotumor (fluid in fissure)	Radiographic appearance, resolution
Foreign body, obstruction	Clinical history
Lung abscess	Clinical history
Bacterial pneumonia	Clinical history
Tuberculosis, atypical acid-fast bacillus	Clinical history, purified protein derivative skin test
Fungal infection	Clinical history
Pulmonary embolus	Clinical history, resolution
Vasculitis	Clinical history

Table 78-5 TNM Staging System

T Status

T0	Primary cannot be defined
Tis	In situ carcinoma
T1	Lesions less than 3 cm and surrounded by lung
T2	Lesions greater than 3 cm or invading the visceral pleura
T3	Lesions in a structure that can potentially be resected (chest wall or pericardium)
T4	A lesion in a vital structure that cannot be resected (aorta or heart) or a malignant pleural or pericardial effusion

N Status

N0	No lymph nodes involved
N1	Lymph nodes within the lung only (peribronchial or hilar)
N2	Ipsilateral mediastinal nodes
N3	Contralateral mediastinal or supraclavicular nodes

M Status

M0	No metastatic disease
M1	Metastatic disease

Stage Groupings

Stage	T	N	M	Approximate Percentage of Cases
IA	1	0	0	Stage I: 36%
IB	2	0	0	
IIA	1	1	0	Stage II: 7%
IIB	2	1	0	
	3	0	0	
IIIA	1-3	2	0	Stage IIIA: 10%
IIIB	1-4	3	0	Stage IIIB: 20%
	4	0-3	0	
IV	Any	Any	1	Stage IV: 27%

Detterbeck FC, Rivera MP, Socinski MA, Rosenman JG (eds): Diagnosis and Treatment of Lung Cancer: An Evidence-Based Guide for the Practicing Clinician. Philadelphia, WB Saunders, 2001.

Management and Therapy

Accurate staging is essential because treatment depends on histology and stage of the disease.

Optimum Treatment of Nonsmall Cell Lung Cancer

Stage I

The standard of care is complete surgical resection through lobectomy or a more extensive procedure if needed. Systematic sampling or complete mediastinal node dissection is performed on all patients at the time of resection. The expected cure rates or 5-year survival rates range from 70% to 80% for stage IA to 50% to 65% for stage IB. The role of postoperative adjuvant chemotherapy remains controversial in stage IB but is probably justified in tumors 4 cm or greater in size. The role of adjuvant chemotherapy in stage IA remains investigational.

Stage II

Complete surgical resection by lobectomy or more if needed is standard. Systematic sampling or complete mediastinal node dissection is performed on all patients at the time of resection. The expected cure rates or 5-year survival rates range from 30% to 50% in stage II NSCLC. If a complete surgical resection is accomplished, postoperative chemotherapy is indicated. Three to four cycles of cisplatin-based chemotherapy is considered the standard of care. There is no defined role for adjuvant radiotherapy in completely resected patients.

Stage IIIA/B

Stage IIIA includes two groups: those with bulky mediastinal disease and those with nonbulky mediastinal disease. In patients with nonbulky disease, surgical resection may

Table 78-6 Types of Staging Assessments

Prefix	Concept	Definition
c	Clinical	Before initiation of any treatment, using any and all information available (including mediastinoscopy)
p	Pathologic	After resection, based on pathologic assessment
y	Restaging	After part or all of the treatment has been given
r	Recurrence	Stage at time of a recurrence
a	Autopsy	Stage as determined by autopsy

be entertained. Survival with surgery alone is poor (9% to 30% 5-year survival rate). Several small phase III studies suggest that preoperative chemotherapy improves 5-year survival rates. In resected stage IIIA patients, postoperative thoracic radiation therapy reduces local recurrences but does not improve survival. These patients have a 5-year survival rate of about 20% to 35%. Like stage II patients, they should receive adjuvant cisplatin-based chemotherapy.

In patients with unresectable stage IIIA/B NSCLC with a good performance status (PS), combined chemotherapy and thoracic radiation therapy are the standard of care. When concurrent approaches have been directly compared with sequential therapy in phase III trials, concurrent chemoradiotherapy has yielded superior survival. The 5-year survival rate is about 10% to 20%.

Stage IV

Combination platinum-based chemotherapy improves survival and palliates disease-related symptoms in most with a good pathologic stage. Studies comparing platinum-based chemotherapy versus best supportive care (BSC) show improvement in survival as a result of the chemotherapy. The 1-year survival with BSC alone is about 10%. With platinum-based chemotherapy, the 1-year survival is about 20% to 25%. Recently developed cytotoxic agents (paclitaxel, docetaxel, gemcitabine, vinorelbine, irinotecan) used with the platinums have improved the survival outcomes in stage IV NSCLC. These new agents are associated with a 1-year survival rate of 30% to 40%. Recently, the addition of bevacizumab (a monoclonal antibody to vascular endothelial growth factor [VEGF]) improved survival in combination with chemotherapy compared with chemotherapy alone in selected patients (nonsquamous histology and lack of brain metastases and hemoptysis) with advanced disease. Because stage IV disease is not curable, all patients will eventually progress. Treatment options for these patients include docetaxel, pemetrexed, and erlotinib, all of which have the potential to improve survival and palliate symptoms in patients at the time of progression.

BSC is the standard for patients with a poor pathologic stage. These patients suffer more treatment-related morbidity and mortality and show no improvement in survival as a result of treatment.

Optimum Treatment of Small Cell Lung Cancer

Limited-Stage Small Cell Lung Cancer

LS SCLC constitutes one third of all cases of SCLC. The optimal therapeutic approach is combined chemoradiotherapy. Cisplatin-etoposide is the standard regimen, and radiotherapy is given concurrently with chemotherapy early in the course. Because brain relapse is so common in patients achieving remission, prophylactic cranial irradiation is recommended to improve survival rates.

Extensive-Stage Small Cell Lung Cancer

This is a treatable but incurable disease. Although response rates to combination chemotherapy range from 60% to 80%, the 2-year survival rate is less than 10%. The median survival is 8 to 12 months. The standard regimen is either cisplatin or carboplatin in combination with etoposide.

Avoiding Treatment Errors

Because staging is the most important determinant of a patient's treatment and prognosis, errors in the staging process are the most likely to lead to errors in treatment. The presentation of each patient's clinical database to a combined team composed of a medical oncologist, a radiation oncologist, a pulmonologist, and a thoracic surgeon is the most effective mechanism to avoid treatment errors and to ensure the selection of an optimal therapeutic plan. The utilization of a team of experts takes advantage of the perspective of each of these specialists and, in the process, also leads to more efficiency in the selection of diagnostic tests. Optimal diagnostic testing increases the likelihood of accurate staging.

Future Directions

Two major growth pathways (the VEGF and epidermal growth factor pathways) have been validated as important targets in lung cancer. Several new targeted agents are being tested in advanced NSCLC. These new drugs are targeted at novel pathways, including angiogenesis, signal transduction, and apoptosis. They will likely lead to further

improvements in survival and be incorporated into treatment in earlier stages of NSCLC. New radiotherapy technologies, including three-dimensional treatment planning, intensity-modulated approaches, stereotactic radiotherapy, and the use of protective agents to ameliorate the toxicity of radiation, will likely improve the therapeutic index of radiation therapy. Chemopreventive strategies in early-stage disease are under study and may lead to a reduction in the risk for second primary tumors. Rapid spiral CT scanning has brought about a resurgence of interest in screening for lung cancer although the role of screening remains controversial. Lastly, reduction in the number of smokers would dramatically decrease the incidence of lung cancer. Strategies directed at smoking prevention and more effective smoking cessation therapies should be high priorities.

Additional Resource

Centers for Disease Control and Prevention. Available at: http://www.cdc.gov/cancer/lung. Accessed June 24, 2007.
   The CDC's website provides helpful information about all aspects of lung cancer for patients and their families.

EVIDENCE

1. Detterbeck FC, Rivera MP, Socinski MA, Rosenman JG (eds): Diagnosis and Treatment of Lung Cancer: An Evidence-Based Guide for the Practicing Clinician. Philadelphia, WB Saunders, 2001.
   This very helpful overview of lung cancer provides a practical guide to diagnosis and treatment.

2. Lee CB, Morris DE, Fried DB, Socinski MA: Current and evolving treatment options for limited stage small cell lung cancer. Curr Opin Oncol 18:162-172, 2006.
   This article provides an analysis and review of the modern treatment approach to this disease process, including possible new therapies.

3. Mountain CF: Revisions in the International System for Staging Lung Cancer. Chest 111:1710-1717, 1997.
   The author presents a useful review of changes in the lung cancer staging system.

4. Socinski MA: Adjuvant therapy for resected non-small cell lung cancer. Clin Lung Cancer 6:162-169, 2004.
   The author addresses the role of adjuvant therapy following resection of non-small cell lung carcinoma.

5. Socinski MA, Morris DE, Masters GA, Lilenbaum R; American College of Chest Physicians. Chemotherapeutic management of stage IV non-small cell lung cancer. Chest 123:226S-243S, 2003.
   This article reviews the options available in the management of stage IV lung cancer.

6. Stinchcombe TE, Fried D, Morris DE, Socinski MA: Combined modality for stage III non-small cell lung cancer. Oncologist 11:809-823, 2006.
   This article reviews the rapidly evolving concept of combined radiation and chemotherapy therapy for the treatment of stage III NSCLC.

Robert S. Wehbie ▪ Bert H. O'Neil ▪ Richard M. Goldberg

79

Colorectal Cancer

Introduction

Deaths due to colorectal cancer (CRC) are second only to lung cancer in site-specific mortality and constitute about 11% of the cancer-related deaths in the United States. During the past decade, advances have been made in our understanding of CRC genetics, screening, surgical techniques, adjuvant therapies, and treatment of the patient with metastatic disease. Despite these advances, the etiology of most CRCs remains ill defined, metastatic disease develops in a number of patients with localized disease at diagnosis despite adjuvant therapy, and metastatic CRC, with a few exceptions, remains fatal.

Etiology and Pathogenesis

Usually, CRC is a disease of elderly people, with incidence not rising appreciably until the fifth decade of life (Fig. 79-1). Incidence varies around the world, with rates higher in Western industrialized nations. Migrating populations tend to assume the CRC risk of the region into which they move; thus, environmental factors have long been suspected to play a role in CRC development. Epidemiologic data suggest an association between dietary constituents such as fats and risk; however, identification of the specific dietary or other environmental factors involved in CRC development has been elusive.

A family history of CRC is a strong predictor of development, with up to 20% of patients reporting a family history of the disease. Having an affected first-degree relative increases the lifetime risk to about 10%. However, defined genetic syndromes account for about 5% of CRC cases.

The sequence of molecular events leading to carcinogenesis is better described for CRC than for any other solid tumor. This is partly due to insights offered by the known inherited CRC syndromes: familial adenomatous polyposis (FAP) and hereditary nonpolyposis colorectal cancer (HNPCC).

FAP accounts for less than 1% of CRCs. It is caused by an inherited defect in one of two adenomatous polyposis coli (*APC*) genes. Affected individuals lose their only functional APC copy in certain somatic cells (such as colonocytes) through random deletion and develop hundreds to thousands of colorectal adenomas during adolescence.

CRC develops in nearly all these patients by 40 years of age. Spontaneous loss of both APC copies is thought to be a key event in the development of colorectal adenomas in most patients with sporadic CRC.

HNPCC (or Lynch's syndrome) accounts for 2% to 4% of CRC. It is due to an inherited defect in one of a family of DNA mismatch repair (*MMR*) genes and leads to an accumulation of genetic errors. CRC develops in more than 60% of affected individuals by age 50 years. About 15% of sporadic CRCs have acquired rather than inherited microsatellite instability, the genetic manifestation of *MMR* mutation.

It is believed that almost all CRC develops from adenomatous polyps. The current hypothesis of colorectal carcinogenesis suggests that CRC is caused by an accumulation of mutations. Although there is probably an order to these defects, it is the overall accumulation of abnormalities that is most important. More than 90% of cancers have two or more defects. In general, genetic changes accumulate with an initial mutation in the 5q chromosome (*APC* gene mutations) noted in polyps and followed by changes in chromosome 12 (*K-ras* oncogene) as the polyps become more dysplastic. Deletions are then noted in a chromosome 18 gene (deleted in colon cancer). Finally, *p53* (chromosome 17p) mutations appear and mark the transition from benign adenoma to malignant carcinoma.

Chronic inflammatory bowel diseases such as ulcerative colitis and Crohn's disease may lead to CRC development in up to 10% of affected individuals. Other conditions associated with an increased risk include Gardner's syndrome, Turcot's syndrome, and juvenile polyposis.

Figure 79-1 Clinical Manifestations of Colorectal Cancer.

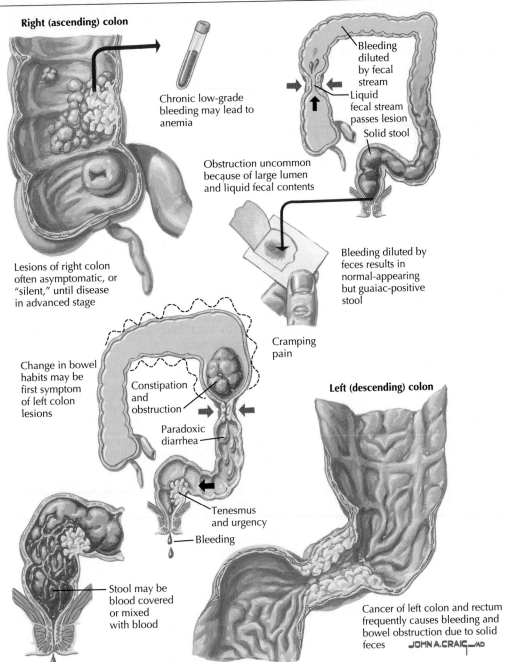

Right (ascending) colon

Chronic low-grade bleeding may lead to anemia

Bleeding diluted by fecal stream

Liquid fecal stream passes lesion

Solid stool

Obstruction uncommon because of large lumen and liquid fecal contents

Lesions of right colon often asymptomatic, or "silent," until disease in advanced stage

Bleeding diluted by feces results in normal-appearing but guaiac-positive stool

Cramping pain

Left (descending) colon

Change in bowel habits may be first symptom of left colon lesions

Constipation and obstruction

Paradoxic diarrhea

Tenesmus and urgency

Bleeding

Stool may be blood covered or mixed with blood

Cancer of left colon and rectum frequently causes bleeding and bowel obstruction due to solid feces

JOHN A. CRAIG—MD

Together, these conditions account for about 1% of CRC cases.

Clinical Presentation

It is important to remember that even advanced CRC is most often asymptomatic. When symptoms occur, they depend on the size and location of the tumor (Fig. 79-2). Typical presenting symptoms include abdominal pain, changes in bowel habits, and rectal bleeding. Colon cancers on the right side tend to be large and present with occult bleeding resulting in anemia (fatigue, heart failure). Left-sided cancers tend to present with symptoms of bowel obstruction (e.g., cramping, change in bowel habits or stool caliber). Blood mixed with the stool is the most frequent symptom of rectal cancer. Other symptoms include mucous discharge, unsatisfied defecation, rectal discomfort, abdominal pain, and the symptoms (or signs) of anemia. Not uncommonly, patients present with signs or symptoms of metastatic disease. The liver is the most common site of CRC metastasis, but other sites can be involved.

Figure 79-2 Screening Techniques.

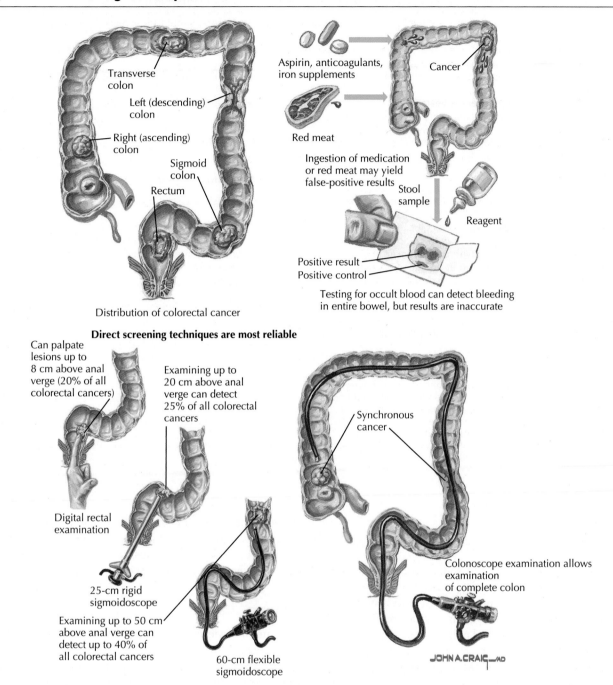

Transverse colon

Left (descending) colon

Right (ascending) colon

Sigmoid colon

Rectum

Distribution of colorectal cancer

Aspirin, anticoagulants, iron supplements

Cancer

Red meat

Ingestion of medication or red meat may yield false-positive results

Stool sample

Reagent

Positive result
Positive control

Testing for occult blood can detect bleeding in entire bowel, but results are inaccurate

Direct screening techniques are most reliable

Can palpate lesions up to 8 cm above anal verge (20% of all colorectal cancers)

Examining up to 20 cm above anal verge can detect 25% of all colorectal cancers

Synchronous cancer

Digital rectal examination

25-cm rigid sigmoidoscope

Examining up to 50 cm above anal verge can detect up to 40% of all colorectal cancers

60-cm flexible sigmoidoscope

Colonoscope examination allows examination of complete colon

JOHN A.CRAIG—AD

Differential Diagnosis

Most CRCs are adenocarcinomas; other histologic varieties account for less than 5% of cases and include carcinoid tumors, sarcomas, lymphomas, melanomas, and in patients with HIV, Kaposi's sarcoma. Locally advanced tumors from other pelvic structures can involve the rectum and present with rectal cancer symptoms. Because symptoms of CRC are nonspecific, malignancy should be included in the differential diagnosis of nearly any chronic gastrointestinal or abdominal illness and should always be considered in the differential diagnosis of iron-deficiency anemia. Never dismiss the possibility of CRC because of a patient's age; although the incidence of CRC in the young has not increased over time, the percentage of CRC patients younger than 50 years is gradually increasing (as older patients who are screened are prevented from getting the disease).

Table 79-1 American Gastroenterological Association Screening Recommendations

- Average- or standard-risk patients, defined as the absence of any high-risk factors, should be screened annually beginning at age 50 years
- Starting at age 50 years, both men and women should have one of the following after discussion of relative merits and risks:
  - Yearly fecal occult blood test (without sample rehydration) and flexible sigmoidoscopy every 5 years; or
  - FOBT yearly; or
  - Flexible sigmoidoscopy every 5 years; or
  - Double contrast barium enema every 5 years; or
  - Colonoscopy every 10 years
  - High-risk patients should begin colorectal cancer screening earlier and more often (see Fig. 79-3)
- Screening recommendations for high-risk groups are as follows:

Familial Risk Category	Screening Recommendation
First-degree relative affected with colorectal cancer or an adenomatous polyp at age ≥60 years, or 2 second-degree relatives affected with colorectal cancer	Same as average risk but starting at age 40 years
Two or more first-degree relatives[a] with colon cancer, or a single first-degree relative with colon cancer or adenomatous polyps diagnosed at an age <60 years	Colonoscopy every 5 years, beginning at age 40 years or 10 years younger than the earliest diagnosis in the family, whichever comes first
One second-degree or any third-degree relative[b,c] with colorectal cancer	Same as average risk
Gene carrier or at risk for familial adenomatous polyposis[d]	Sigmoidoscopy annually, beginning at age 10-12 years[e]
Gene carrier or at risk for hereditary nonpolyposis colorectal cancer	Colonoscopy, every 1-2 years, beginning at age 20-25 years or 10 years younger than the earliest case in the family, whichever comes first

[a]First-degree relatives include parents, siblings, and children.
[b]Second-degree relatives include grandparents, aunts, and uncles.
[c]Third-degree relatives include great-grandparents and cousins.
[d]Includes the subcategories of familial adenomatous polyposis, Gardner's syndrome, some Turcot's syndrome families, and antibiotic-associated pseudomembranous colitis (AAPC).
[e]In AAPC, colonoscopy should be used instead of sigmoidoscopy because of the preponderance of proximal colonic adenomas. Colonoscopy screening in AAPC should probably begin in the late teens or early 20s.

Diagnostic Approach

Screening and Diagnosis

Fecal occult blood testing and sigmoidoscopy screening have been shown to decrease CRC-related mortality (Table 79-1). The concept that most cases of CRC follow the adenoma-to-carcinoma pathway has led to the important application of colonoscopy and polypectomy because more than 90% of polyps can be removed by colonoscopy. Adenoma removal has been shown to decrease the incidence of CRC by 70% to 90%. With increasing use of screening technologies, more CRCs are asymptomatic. Most cancers that present today are symptomatic because screening is still not uniformly practiced (Fig. 79-3).

Endoscopy

A rigid sigmoidoscope facilitates reliable examination of the rectum, but frequently the rectosigmoid junction cannot be negotiated; therefore, the sigmoid colon may not be visualized. Flexible sigmoidoscopy allows visualization of only the distal third of the colon. Colonoscopy provides a view of the entire colon and is more sensitive for both early CRC and colorectal adenomas than double-contrast barium enema. Synchronous lesions are present in up to 15% of patients; thus, the entire colon should be assessed whenever possible (see Fig. 79-3).

Staging

The tumor-node-metastasis classification for rectal cancer has replaced the Dukes staging system (Table 79-2). Tumor stage, determined by the depth of tumor penetration into the bowel wall, the number of regional lymph nodes involved, and the presence or absence of distant metastases, is the most important prognostic indicator of survival.

CT scanning of the chest and abdomen are commonly employed in initial staging, although intraoperative examination of the abdomen may be adequate in select cases. Transrectal ultrasound or, more recently, specialized magnetic resonance imaging scans can determine the depth of tumor invasion and the presence of pelvic lymph node metastases. It is an important rectal cancer staging tool at many institutions, particularly those where preoperative chemoradiation therapy is employed.

Figure 79-3 Algorithm for Colorectal Cancer Screening.
See Table 79-1. FAP, familial adenomatous polyposis; HNPCC, hereditary nonpolyposis colorectal cancer. *Reprinted with permission from Winawer S, Fletcher R, Rex D, et al; U.S. Multisociety Task Force on Colorectal Cancer: Colorectal cancer screening and surveillance: Clinical guidelines and rationale. Update based on new evidence. Gastroenterology 124(2):544-560, 2003.*

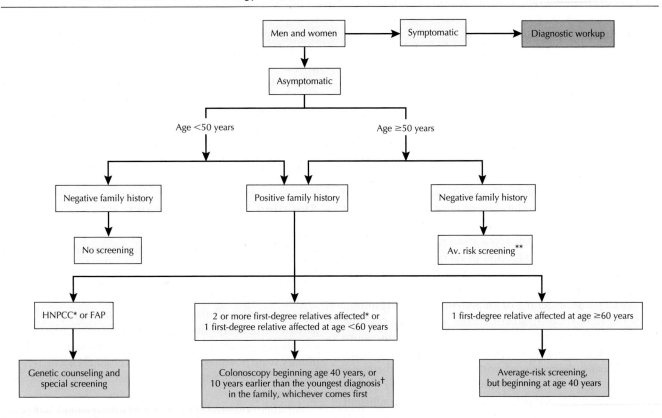

†Either colorectal cancer or adenomatous polyp.
*HNPCC, hereditary nonpolyposis colorectal cancer and FAP, familial adenomatous polyposis.
**See Table 79-1.

Table 79-2	AJCC/UICC Stage Grouping		
Stage 0	Tis*	N0	M0
Stage I	T1	N0	M0
	T2	N0	M0
Stage IIa	T3	N0	M0
IIb	T4	N0	M0
Stage IIIa	T1-2	N1	M0
IIIb	T3-4	N1	M0
IIIc	Any T	N2†	M0
Stage IV	Any T	Any N	M1

*Carcinoma in situ.
†Metastasis in four or more regional nodes.
AJCC, American Joint Committee on Cancer; UICC, International Union Against Cancer. *From American Joint Committee on Cancer: AJCC Cancer Staging Manual, 6th ed. Philadelphia, Lippincott-Raven, 2002.*

Routine preoperative laboratory studies, including a complete blood cell count and blood chemistry studies with liver-related tests, usually suffice. A preoperative carcinoembryonic antigen (CEA) test may be helpful in the postoperative follow-up of patients but should not be used as a screening or diagnostic test.

Management and Therapy

Optimum Treatment

Surgery

Tumor resection is the cornerstone of CRC management. The goal of surgery is the removal of all macroscopic tumor with clear surgical margins, plus areas of draining lymphatics. Most colon cancers can be treated with a one-stage resection and anastomosis. The rectum is divided into equal thirds. Tumors arising in the upper third are handled most satisfactorily by low anterior resection. A proportion of low rectal cancers and cancers of the anal canal are best managed by abdominoperineal resection of the rectum together with the anal canal and subsequent permanent colostomy. Some low mobile cancers, especially in poor operative candidates, may be best treated by transanal local excision.

Adjuvant and Neoadjuvant Therapy

Adjuvant chemotherapy with 5-fluorouracil (5-FU), leucovorin (LV), and oxiliplatin for 6 months improves survival for patients with node-positive CRC. There is increasing evidence that there may also be a survival advantage with adjuvant chemotherapy in patients with T3, N0, M0 (stage II) disease, but the absolute magnitude of this benefit is relatively small, on the order of 2% to 5%. Calculators of chemotherapy benefit are now available on the Internet and can be very useful in educating patients for decision making about therapy.

Rectal cancers (tumors arising below the peritoneal reflection) present an additional challenge. A substantial fraction of patients will have local recurrence if the tumor extends through the bowel wall (T3 disease) or if there are positive lymph nodes. Postoperative adjuvant pelvic radiation therapy is effective in controlling these local recurrences. Standard practice is to augment radiation therapy with the protracted infusion of 5-FU. It is notable also that recent advances in surgery such as sharp dissection of the entire mesorectum (total mesorectal excision or TME) may decrease the risk for local recurrence in select patients without need for radiotherapy. TME is now considered the standard operation for rectal cancer.

There has been an evolution in rectal cancer management to the delivery of chemoradiation therapy preoperatively. Benefits of this strategy include lower volume of irradiated tissue, lessening of long-term ill effects resulting from the removal of irradiated tissue at surgery, and the potential that tumor down-staging will permit more sphincter-sparing surgeries. Because a number of cases are pathologically down-staged with preoperative chemoradiation therapy, all patients treated in this manner should be considered for completion of their 6-month adjuvant chemotherapy course with additional chemotherapy postoperatively, regardless of the pathologic stage at surgery.

Follow-up includes colonoscopy 12 months postoperatively and then at 2- to 3-year intervals. Patients should be seen every 6 to 12 months for 5 years. CEA monitoring can be useful for the early discovery of disease recurrence. There is also some evidence to support routine imaging studies in the follow-up period, and American Society of Clinical Oncology guidelines now support routine imaging during surveillance.

Management of Metastatic Disease

Recurrent CRC is frequently localized to resectable organs (Fig. 79-4). The most common organ is the liver; the lung is the second most common. When confined to a resectable segment of either liver or lung, long-term survival is 25% to 40%. In select patients, liver lesions may be directly ablated by percutaneous or laparoscopic radiofrequency thermal ablation.

Patients with unresectable or widespread metastatic disease may benefit from systemic chemotherapy. Combination chemotherapy regimens are more effective than the core regimen of 5-FU/LV. The past several years have seen the addition of irinotecan (a topoisomerase I inhibi-

tor) and oxiliplatin (a DNA cross-linker) to 5-FU/LV regimens with enhanced survival, albeit with increased toxicities. Roughly half of patients respond to first-line chemotherapy.

More recently, several therapeutic antibodies have entered clinical practice, with targets that were discovered through genetic research. Of particular promise has been an antibody against the proangiogenic vascular endothelial growth factor known as bevacizumab. This antibody appears to enhance the effect of chemotherapy on survival, with limited side effects when compared with classic chemotherapeutic agents. Antibodies against the epidermal growth factor receptor have also been approved for use in colon cancer and also appear to augment the effectiveness of chemotherapy on colorectal cancers.

Avoiding Treatment Errors

Management of colorectal cancer has become increasingly complex in recent years, particularly the management of rectal cancer, which often involves multiple subspecialists. For example, sequencing of therapies can be of substantial importance. To avoid potential complications and maximize outcomes, all patients with rectal cancer and many patients with colon cancer (particularly metastatic colorectal cancer) should be managed by an organized multidisciplinary team composed of gastroenterologists, experienced surgeons, radiologists, radiation oncologists, and medical oncologists.

Another potential error in initial management is missing a second primary cancer because initial colonoscopy was incomplete (often due to an obstructing distal lesion). All patients should undergo a complete colonoscopy after appropriate recovery from surgery if the initial endoscopy was suboptimal.

Future Directions

The future for advances in all aspects of CRC management is bright. Increasing knowledge of CRC molecular biology and genetics is pivotal in these developments. Identification of molecular targets and lesions will allow the rational design of strategies for CRC prevention, screening, and treatment.

Better identification of environmental and dietary factors will have obvious ramifications for CRC prevention. Preventive therapies remain a hot area of research, although use of the most promising class of drugs, the cyclooxygenase-2 inhibitors, has been clouded by concerns about increased cardiovascular risk. The use of aspirin, calcium supplementation, and exercise has been linked to reduced incidence of polyps and colorectal cancers. New screening modalities promise both increased sensitivity and specificity by analyzing for genetic anomalies linked to CRC (such as *K-ras* mutations) in stool

Figure 79-4 Metastasis in Colorectal Cancer.
CEA, carcinoembryonic antigen; CT, computed tomography.

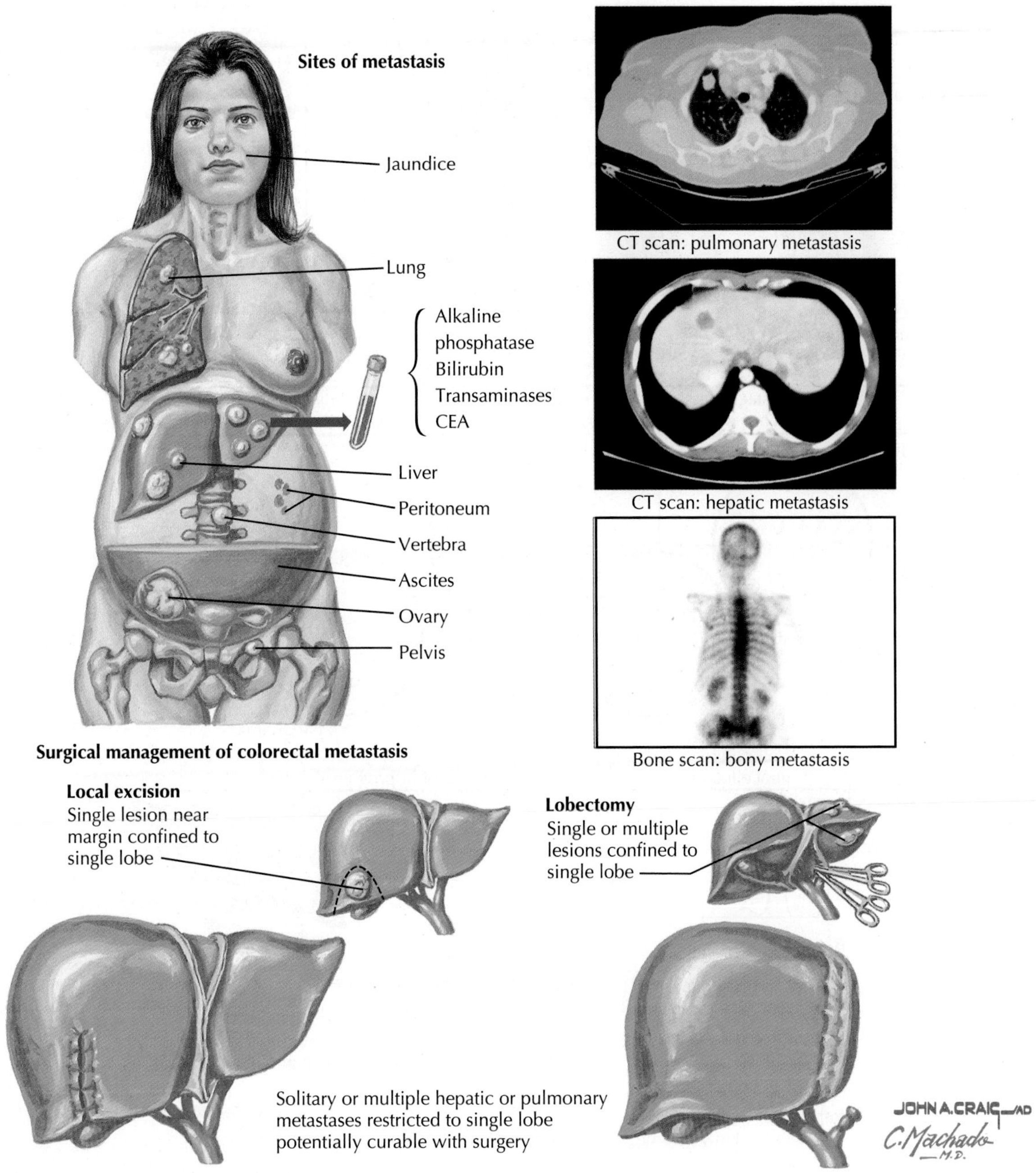

Sites of metastasis

- Jaundice
- Lung
- Alkaline phosphatase
- Bilirubin
- Transaminases
- CEA
- Liver
- Peritoneum
- Vertebra
- Ascites
- Ovary
- Pelvis

CT scan: pulmonary metastasis

CT scan: hepatic metastasis

Bone scan: bony metastasis

Surgical management of colorectal metastasis

Local excision
Single lesion near margin confined to single lobe

Lobectomy
Single or multiple lesions confined to single lobe

Solitary or multiple hepatic or pulmonary metastases restricted to single lobe potentially curable with surgery

JOHN A. CRAIG—AD
C. Machado—M.D.

samples. New imaging techniques such as CT virtual colonoscopy may provide noninvasive means of detecting polyps and CRC.

Advances in adjuvant therapies will consist of both more effective regimens and improved patient selection for these treatments. Targeted therapies such as bevacizumab and cetuximab are already being studied for their potential benefits in the adjuvant setting.

Our ever-increasing understanding of CRC biology and markers of treatment responses, plus a rapidly expanding armamentarium of effective agents, will likely permit a more patient-directed approach to treatment (Fig. 79-5). As a current example, CRC with high-level thymidylate synthase (an important target of 5-FU) expression may have a poorer response to 5-FU. A host of other molecular markers may have prognostic and predictive importance.

Figure 79-5 Prognostic Indicators in Colorectal Cancer.

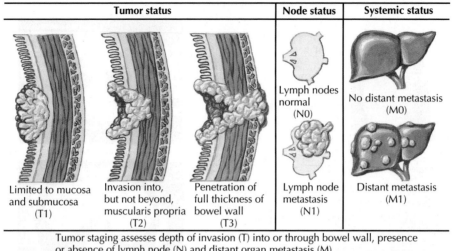

Tumor staging assesses depth of invasion (T) into or through bowel wall, presence or absence of lymph node (N) and distant organ metastasis (M)

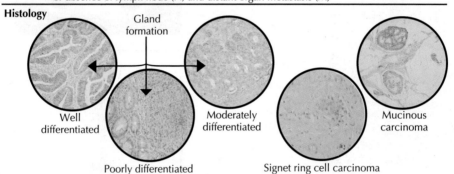

Well-differentiated tumors have better outcome than poorly differentiated tumors; intracellular or extracellular mucin indicates poor prognosis

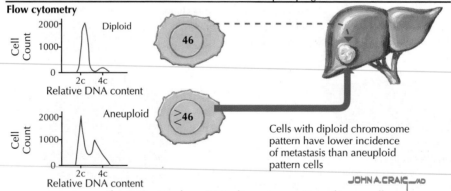

Flow cytometry shows DNA chromosome pattern of tumor cells

Additional Resources

Mayo Clinic Adjuvant Systemic Therapy Calculator. Available at: http://www.mayoclinic.com/calcs/. Accessed November 4, 2006; and Adjuvant! Online. Available at: http://www.adjuvantonline.com. Accessed November 4, 2006.

These websites include the two available risk calculators that are valuable for discussion of risks of recurrence with or without various chemotherapy treatments for patients with colon cancer.

Winawer S, Fletcher R, Rex D, et al: Gastrointestinal Consortium Panel: Colorectal cancer screening and surveillance: Clinical guidelines and rationale. Update based on new evidence. Gastroenterology 124(2):544-560, 2003.

The authors present the authoritative consensus guidelines for screening of standard and high-risk patients for CRC.

EVIDENCE

1. American Cancer Society: Cancer Facts and Figures. New York, American Cancer Society, 2004.

This book provides annually updated cancer statistics for the United States.

2. Beaven AW, Goldberg RM: Adjuvant therapy for colorectal cancer: Yesterday, today, and tomorrow. Oncology (Williston Park) 20(5): 461-9; discussion 469-70, 473-5, 2006.

This review compares today's standard of care for adjuvant colorectal carcinoma to that practiced 20 years ago. The authors examine key questions asked about adjuvant therapy and the answers that ultimately changed clinical practice standards and improved overall survival for patients.

3. Desch CE, Benson AB III, Somerfield MR, et al: Colorectal cancer surveillance: 2005 Update of an American Society of Clinical Oncology Practice Guideline 10.1200/JCO.2005.04.0063. J Clin Oncol 23(33):8512-8519, 2005.

This update of the 2000 American Society of Clinical Oncology guideline on colorectal cancer surveillance adds a recommendation for annual surveillance CT scans of the chest, abdomen, and in certain circumstances, pelvis, for patients eligible for further potentially curative surgery.

4. Itzkowitz SH, Present DH: Consensus conference: Colorectal cancer screening and surveillance in inflammatory bowel disease (IBD). Inflamm Bowel Dis 11(3):314-321, 2005.

No standardized guidelines have yet been set forth to guide the gastroenterologist in performing surveillance in patients with IBD. A panel of international experts was assembled to develop consensus recommendations for the performance of surveillance. The findings are presented herein.

5. Kaz AM, Brentnall TA: Genetic testing for colon cancer. Nat Clin Pract Gastroenterol Hepatol 3(12):670-679, 2006.

Colon cancer remains the third leading cause of death due to cancer in the United States, where it affected more than 145,000 individuals in 2005. Up to 30% of these cases exhibit familial clustering, which means that tens of thousands of individuals have a disease with a potentially definable genetic component. About 3% to 5% of colon cancers are associated with high-risk, inherited colon cancer syndromes. Identification of the genes that cause these colon cancer syndromes, coupled with additional insights into their clinical course, has led to the development of specific management guidelines—and genetic tests—that can diagnose these familial disorders. These guidelines can be life saving, not only for the affected patient, but also for their family members.

6. O'Neil BH, Goldberg RM: Chemotherapy for advanced colorectal cancer: Let's not forget how we got here (until we really can). Semin Oncol 32(1):35-42, 2005.

Physicians and patients alike have been heartened by the recent advances in the treatment of colorectal cancer. The emergence of novel agents active in the treatment of this devastating disease, such as cetuximab and bevacizumab, has been particularly notable. However, even before these recent events, a substantial change in prognosis for patients with metastatic colorectal cancer had occurred as a result of advances in traditional chemotherapeutic agents. Refinements in dose, schedule, and sequence continue to be made that could lead to further improvements in outcomes. Additionally, new chemotherapeutic agents with promise for activity in colorectal cancer are being studied. Chemotherapy is likely to remain a central element of the treatment strategy. Our understanding of its current role is discussed in this article.

7. Ransohoff DF: Colon cancer screening in 2005: Status and challenges. Gastroenterology 128(6):1685-1695, 2005.

This is an authoritative review on screening from a well-respected epidemiologist in the field.

8. Sandler RS. Epidemiology and risk factors for colorectal cancer. Gastroenterol Clin North Am 25(4):717-735, 1996.

This is an authoritative review on CRC epidemiology from a renowned epidemiologist in the field.

Lisa A. Carey

Breast Cancer

Introduction

Breast cancer will be diagnosed in nearly 178,480 U.S. women and 2,030 U.S. men in the year 2007, making it the most common malignancy in women. The lifetime risk for the development of breast cancer for an American woman is about 1 in 10, with advancing age as the strongest risk factor. Two thirds of cases occur in postmenopausal women; the disease is extremely rare in women younger than 30 years. Incidence has recently been stable, whereas breast cancer mortality within the entire population decreased about 25% during the past 10 to 20 years. About half of that improvement in mortality comes from successful screening, and the other half from improved adjuvant therapy.

Etiology and Pathogenesis

Age is the strongest risk factor for noninherited breast cancer. Women older than 65 years have a risk several-fold higher than that of 40-year-old women. At any age, a history of breast or ovarian cancer increases the risk for subsequent breast cancer. Family history is an important, but smaller, contributor to risk (about twofold to fivefold increased risk for first-degree relatives), except in those families with an inherited form of breast cancer, in whom the risk is highest. Inherited breast cancer is responsible for 5% to 10% of all breast cancers and is primarily due to mutations in the *BRCA1* or *BRCA2* gene, which are inherited in an autosomal dominant fashion. *BRCA1* or *BRCA2* mutation carriers have a 60% to 80% lifetime risk for breast cancer and an increased risk for premenopausal and bilateral disease. Identification of families with inherited breast cancer patterns is crucial because genetic testing can identify carriers of a mutation, and there are effective prevention strategies.

Hormonal risk factors may be broadly grouped as factors that increase the number of normal menstrual cycles in a lifetime, especially if the cycles occur before a first full-term pregnancy. They include early age of menarche, late menopause, and nulliparity or age at first pregnancy older than 30 years. Several other variables have been associated with breast cancer risk, possibly by increasing hormone levels. For example, obesity, a high-fat diet, and alcohol can all cause higher circulating estrogen levels. Certain benign breast diseases confer increased risk for breast cancer. Atypical hyperplasia is associated with an up to 1% yearly risk of invasive breast cancer. Despite the name, lobular carcinoma in situ is not a neoplastic or preneoplastic lesion, but is a marker of increased breast cancer risk in any quadrant of either breast. This risk can approach 1.5% per year for invasive breast cancer.

Clinical Presentation

There are two major forms of primary breast cancer: invasive and noninvasive. Noninvasive breast cancer includes ductal carcinoma in situ (DCIS), which is truly a preneoplastic lesion in that up to 30% of inadequately treated DCIS cases recur or progress to invasive cancer. Most DCIS cases are detected by mammography; only 10% are palpable. Paget's disease is a rare variant of DCIS that can occur alone or at the same time as invasive disease. It appears as eczematous changes of the nipple that represent extension of the DCIS component of the cancer into the main ducts.

Invasive breast cancer usually presents as a painless mass or mammographically detected calcifications, architectural distortion, or asymmetrical density. Clinical or breast self-examination may also detect a tumor by overlying dimpling or retraction of the skin or asymmetry of the breasts (Fig. 80-1). Occasionally, breast cancer will be associated with nipple inversion or discharge. Suspicion of malignancy should be higher if the discharge is heme positive. Rarely, breast cancers present with inflammatory

Figure 80-1 Palpation of the Breasts.

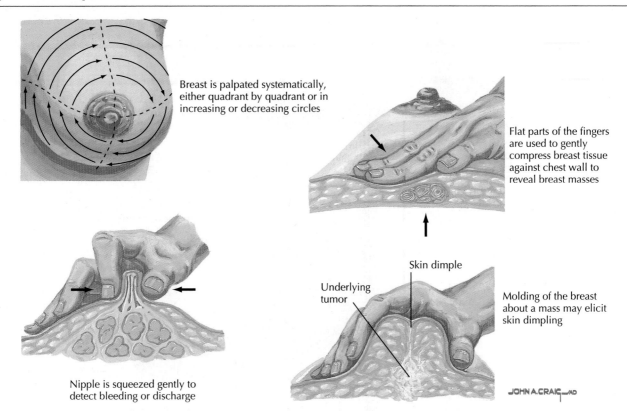

Breast is palpated systematically, either quadrant by quadrant or in increasing or decreasing circles

Flat parts of the fingers are used to gently compress breast tissue against chest wall to reveal breast masses

Skin dimple

Underlying tumor

Molding of the breast about a mass may elicit skin dimpling

Nipple is squeezed gently to detect bleeding or discharge

JOHN A. CRAIG—AD

changes in the skin of the breast. Since the advent of screening, more breast cancers present at an early curable stage, with disease limited to the breast only or breast and local lymph nodes. Fewer than 10% of patients with breast cancer present with distant metastases.

Most invasive primary breast cancers are adenocarcinomas of ductal, lobular, or a mixed pattern. Less than 5% are pure tubular, colloid, mucinous, or atypical medullary type, which are considered to have a better prognosis. Clinical oncologists use several features of the patient and the tumor to gauge likelihood of recurrence. The American Joint Commission on Cancer tumor, node, metastasis (TNM) system, although imperfect, is used most commonly. *T* refers to tumor size or fixation to local structures, with larger sizes or fixed status conferring worse prognosis. *N* refers to regional lymph node metastasis; the presence of involved axillary, mammary, supraclavicular or infraclavicular lymph nodes connotes a poorer prognosis. *M* refers to distant metastasis, which is generally considered incurable. There are several prognostically relevant features of the patient or the tumor that are not included in the TNM system. Some studies suggest that high-grade tumors carry a worse prognosis. Recent research has focused on the biologic heterogeneity of breast cancer. A molecular profiling using gene expression array suggests that breast cancer actually represents several biologically distinct diseases. Although these breast cancer subtypes can only accurately be distinguished using microarray technology

that is not currently clinically available, they do differ in some easily identifiable ways using clinical assays that are routinely performed on breast cancers for the estrogen receptor (ER), progesterone receptor (PR), and receptor tyrosine kinase HER2. The presence of ER or PR identifies the luminal subtypes, which make up about 70% of breast cancers, are considered sensitive to endocrine therapies, and carry a slightly better prognosis and later recurrence. The hormone receptor–negative subtypes, which constitute about 30% of breast cancers, are about equally made up of the basal-like and HER2+/ER– subtypes, which clinically can be crudely identified as negative for all three markers (basal-like) or negative for ER and PR but positive for HER2 (HER2+/ER–). Both these subtypes are typically highly proliferative and carry a poor prognosis and a higher risk for early relapse, although the use of HER2-targeted therapy in the HER2+/ER– is altering the natural history of that subtype. Overexpression of the cell surface receptor tyrosine kinase HER2 is found not only in the HER2+/ER– subtype but also in some luminal breast cancers. As with the ER and targeted hormonal agents such as tamoxifen, HER2 predicts success of treatment with targeted anti-HER2 drugs such as the monoclonal antibody trastuzumab.

Most patients present with early-stage nonmetastatic breast cancer, at a time when prompt multimodality therapy can reduce breast cancer recurrence and death. Breast cancer recurrence as metastatic disease can occur at

Figure 80-2 Pathways of Tumor Dissemination.

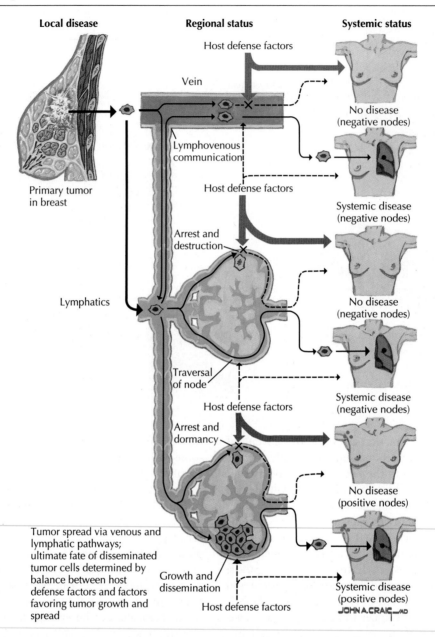

Local disease

Primary tumor
in breast

Lymphatics

Tumor spread via venous and
lymphatic pathways;
ultimate fate of disseminated
tumor cells determined by
balance between host
defense factors and factors
favoring tumor growth and
spread

Regional status

Host defense factors

Vein

Lymphovenous
communication

Host defense factors

Arrest and
destruction

Traversal
of node

Host defense factors

Arrest and
dormancy

Growth and
dissemination

Host defense factors

Systemic status

No disease
(negative nodes)

Systemic disease
(negative nodes)

No disease
(negative nodes)

Systemic disease
(negative nodes)

No disease
(positive nodes)

Systemic disease
(positive nodes)

JOHN A. CRAIG_MD

any time; however, the risk is highest within the first 5 to 10 years after diagnosis. There are multiple tumor and host factors that affect a tumor's ability to exit the breast, survive in the blood and lymphatics, arrest and extravasate in a new site, and finally survive and grow in that site to become clinically evident metastatic disease (Fig. 80-2). The most common sites of recurrence are local (including conserved breast or chest wall), bone, lymph nodes, lung, and liver. Central nervous system (CNS) recurrences, rare before the era of aggressive systemic therapy, appear to be increasing, probably because the drugs used to prevent systemic relapse do not penetrate the CNS adequately. Local recurrence, particularly in a conserved breast, is curable with surgery and radiation therapy; however, it is a poor prognostic factor. Metastatic breast cancer is considered incur-

able, although a small percentage of patients live longer than 10 years, and the prognosis after metastic diagnosis is improving.

Differential Diagnosis

Several nonmalignant conditions can mimic breast cancer. Cysts and fibroadenomas often present with palpable masses. These may be distinguished from malignancy on clinical or radiographic grounds, such as the tenderness, cyclic changes, and sonographic appearance of cysts, and the characteristic mammographic density and circumscribed feel and appearance of fibroadenomas. Papillomas or mammary duct ectasia can produce nipple discharge. Mastitis or cellulitis of the breast is very difficult to distin-

Figure 80-3 Mammograms.
Left: Mammogram depicting a partially lobulated, partially indistinct mass that proved to be infiltrating ductal carcinoma. *Right:* Mammogram depicting branching, casting, and pleomorphic calcifications that proved to be ductal carcinoma in situ. *Courtesy of Etta Pisano, MD.*

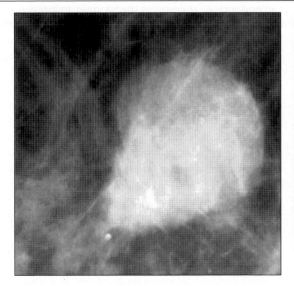
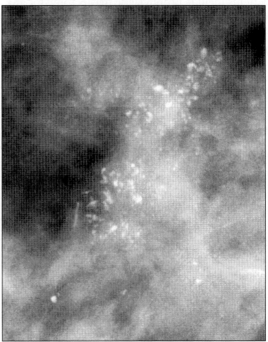

guish clinically from inflammatory breast cancer. Breast malignancies other than primary breast cancer are rare. These include sarcomas (cystosarcoma phyllodes among others), lymphomas, and chloromas as well as metastases from melanomas or other carcinomas. Breast cancer metastasis to the contralateral breast is rare. A woman with a history of breast cancer is at increased risk for developing breast cancer in the contralateral breast. In general, these represent second primary tumors.

Diagnostic Approach

About 20% to 30% of invasive and 80% of noninvasive breast cancers are not palpable; 10% of invasive cancers are not visible on mammograms. For this reason, physical examination and radiology are considered complementary (Fig. 80-3). Ultrasound may provide valuable information in evaluating palpable masses. The American Cancer Society guidelines for breast cancer screening are that women older than 20 years should perform breast self-examination every month; women should have clinical breast examination by a health professional every 3 years from ages 20 to 39 years, and yearly thereafter; and women 40 years and older should undergo annual mammography. Mammography in women between 40 and 50 years of age has been controversial, although emerging data suggest a smaller but real benefit in this age group. The benefit is smaller in younger women because breast cancer is less prevalent and mammograms are technically limited in more glandular and dense premenopausal breasts. Recent studies suggest that screening in women at high risk or with dense breasts may be improved with digital mammography or breast magnetic resonance imaging.

Diagnosis of a palpable lesion can be made by fine-needle aspiration, core needle biopsy, or open surgical biopsy. Lesions seen by mammography or ultrasound only can be biopsied by stereotactic core needle biopsy, by ultrasound-guided needle biopsy, or by needle-localized open biopsy. A complete history and physical examination is the best screening test for systemic spread of cancer. Chest radiography, complete blood cell count, and screening liver chemistries are often performed to screen for metastatic disease; however, these tests are unlikely to be abnormal in early stage tumors. More aggressive evaluations such as bone scans and CT scans are generally reserved for symptomatic patients and those with more locally advanced or metastatic disease.

Management and Therapy

Prevention

There are both medical and surgical strategies for breast cancer prevention. In women at moderate to high risk, the selective ER modulators tamoxifen or raloxifene have been shown to reduce the risk for noninvasive and invasive breast cancer by more than 40%. Tamoxifen decreases the incidence of ER-positive breast cancer and does not appear to affect the development of ER-negative breast cancer.

Toxicity includes increased endometrial cancer risk (seen primarily with tamoxifen not raloxifene), venous thrombosis, menopausal symptoms, and a small increase in cataract progression. Surgical strategies used primarily in very-high-risk patients include prophylactic mastectomy for any woman and prophylactic oophorectomy for premenopausal women. Prophylactic mastectomy reduces the risk for breast cancer by at least 90% in high-risk patients treated by skilled surgeons. Prophylactic oophorectomy has been evaluated in *BRCA* mutation carriers, in whom it reduces breast cancer by about 50%.

Optimum Treatment

Local and Regional Therapy

Surgical options include breast conservation, which is local excision of the tumor with dissection of the level I and II axillary lymph nodes followed by radiation therapy to the breast. Breast conservation is standard of care and offers comparable 5-year survival to modified radical mastectomy. Some tumors are too large or poorly placed for conservation; for those patients, mastectomy is standard. Dissection of the ipsilateral axillary lymph nodes allows tumor debulking and prognostication. Sentinel lymphadenectomy allows surgeons to selectively identify the first draining lymph node or nodes (the "sentinel" node) from a tumor region using vital blue dye or radiolabeled colloid. In experienced hands, if this first draining lymph node does not contain tumor, the remainder of the axilla is also likely to be free of tumor and does not require dissection. Radiation therapy is required for patients who have breast conservation; otherwise, the local recurrence rate may exceed 30% with long-term follow-up. Local recurrence in conserved and radiated breasts is less than 10%. Radiation is also given to the chest wall and local lymph node groups remaining after surgery for large tumors or for some tumors with involved axillary lymph nodes.

Systemic Therapy

Systemic therapy refers to chemotherapy, hormone therapy, bisphosphonates, or biotherapy given to patients to prevent or treat metastatic disease throughout the body. Adjuvant therapy is given as an adjunct to local therapy to decrease the chance of recurrence. Neoadjuvant, or preoperative, therapy is a newer approach that involves the same drugs as in adjuvant therapy given before the surgery to decrease the tumor size, allow breast conservation and provide important data to researchers regarding the effect of drugs and combinations of drugs in the primary breast cancer. The use of adjuvant therapy, primarily chemotherapy, hormone therapy, or biologic therapy is determined by the patient's general health, age, ER status of the tumor, and the probability of recurrence based on stage and other prognostic variables. Accurately predicting risk for recurrence has previously involved mathematic models that include these clinical variables; newer genomic models based on gene expression patterns in the tumor promise to improve this accuracy. Chemotherapy includes several non–cross-resistant drugs, called *polychemotherapy*. Overall, adjuvant chemotherapy decreases the risk of recurrence by 23% and the risk of death by 17%. Hormone, also known as endocrine, therapy is useful only in preventing recurrence of tumors that express the ER; it is not effective in ER-negative cancer. Among hormone receptor-positive breast cancers, the selective ER modulator tamoxifen decreases the risk of recurrence by 41% and risk of death by 34%. Although there are fewer long-term data, in postmenopausal women aromatase inhibitors have better relapse-free survival than tamoxifen alone and should be considered instead of or subsequent to tamoxifen. In premenopausal patients with ER-positive tumors, oophorectomy may be a useful adjunct to tamoxifen, particularly in high-risk patients who cannot or will not take chemotherapy. Giving both chemotherapy and subsequent endocrine therapy is more effective than either strategy alone. For the 20% to 30% of patients with HER2-positive breast cancer, HER2-targeted therapy with the monoclonal antibody trastuzumab added to certain chemotherapy and after chemotherapy improves both relapse-free and overall survival compared with chemotherapy alone.

Metastatic therapy is given to women with systemic relapse. The goals of metastatic therapy are to palliate symptoms and prolong life; however, given the incurable nature of the disease at this stage, quality-of-life considerations become very important in choosing therapy. This therapy may include chemotherapy—either with one of the many single agents with documented effectiveness or polychemotherapy; hormone therapy (if hormone receptor positive—with tamoxifen or other antiestrogens; aromatase inhibitors [if postmenopausal] or ovarian ablation [if premenopausal]); bisphosphonates therapy for lytic bone metastases or targeted biotherapy such as HER2-targeted agents such as trastuzumab or lapatinib for appropriate patients. Antiangiogenics such as VEGF inhibitors improve outcome, although patient selection is a challenge. Surgery and radiation are also sometimes used for treatment of local complications. A number of clinical trials are evaluating the best combinations of chemotherapy and other drugs for adjuvant treatment and newer drugs and compounds for metastatic therapy.

Avoiding Treatment Errors

The most common errors in treating breast cancer are failures to diagnose this disease and failures to manage the disease at the time of diagnosis optimally with multimodality assessment and therapy. Failure to diagnose breast cancer can occur through ineffective screening, which often represents problems with access to health care, or poorly performed screening. Screening mammography should be performed using machinery that has met quality standards, and by experienced personnel. Therapeutic decision-making is optimized when surgical decisions are made with direct consultation with radiologists and pathologists and adjuvant therapy decisions are made in the setting of multidisciplinary tumor boards.

Future Directions

Since 1990, breast cancer mortality in the United States has markedly decreased, largely because of aggressive efforts to detect and treat the disease at early stages. A significant additional strategy has been to develop effective preventive treatments for those at high risk. Certain groups, such as medically underserved populations in the United States and many populations in undeveloped countries, have not seen these improvements in outcome. An important accomplishment will be to provide better screening and prevention efforts to these groups. Given the improvement in outcome with mammographic screening, better imaging techniques may provide additional benefits. New strategies are at hand to determine the metastatic potential of the tumor and to refine selection of adjuvant therapy. These include examination of bone marrow or blood for evidence of micrometastases, definition of individual tumor biology through tumor markers, and classification of tumor subtypes using sophisticated molecular techniques analysis. Bisphosphonates, new hormonal approaches, and new targeted therapies are being tested in the adjuvant setting to try to improve the cure rate in early breast cancer. The success and low toxicity of tamoxifen and trastuzumab suggest that the future of breast cancer therapy is likely to involve other targeted therapies, with treatment determined by the molecular profile of the particular tumor.

Additional Resources

National Cancer Institute. The Breast Cancer Risk Assessment Tool. Available at: http://www.cancer.gov/bcrisktool. Accessed February 25, 2007.

This tool estimates a woman's risk for developing breast cancer for two time periods: over the next five years and over her lifetime.

Adjuvant Online. Breast cancer recurrence risk and impact of adjuvant therapy mathematical estimates. Available at: www.adjuvantonline.com. Accessed December 3, 2006.

This web-based program uses several clinical variables for estimating the risk of recurrence and the benefit of adjuvant therapy in nonmetastatic breast cancer.

EVIDENCE

1. American Cancer Society: Cancer facts and figures 2006. Available at: http://www.cancer.org/downloads/STT/CAFF2006PW Secured.pdf. Accessed February 25, 2007.

    This website provides regularly updated statistics on cancer incidence and mortality.

2. Barrett-Connor E, Mosca L, Collins P, et al: Effects of raloxifene on cardiovascular events and breast cancer in postmenopausal women. N Engl J Med 355(2):125-137, 2006.

    This randomized, placebo-controlled evaluation of the selective estrogen receptor modulator raloxifene addresses several important end points, including breast cancer prevention.

3. Berry DA, Cronin KA, Plevritis SK, et al: Effect of screening and adjuvant therapy on mortality from breast cancer. N Engl J Med 353(17):1784-1792, 2005.

    This mathematic model-based evaluation addresses the relative contributions of improvements in screening and treatment on mortality from breast cancer.

4. Early Breast Cancer Trialists' Collaborative Group: Effects of chemotherapy and hormonal therapy for early breast cancer on recurrence and 15-year survival: An overview of the randomised trials. Lancet 365(9472):1687-1717, 2005.

    This paper presents a meta-analysis of the impact of adjuvant endocrine therapy and chemotherapy on reducing the risk of recurrence in nonmetastatic breast cancer.

5. Eifel P, Axelson JA, Costa J, et al: National Institutes of Health Consensus Development Conference Statement: Adjuvant therapy for breast cancer, November 1-3, 2000. J Natl Cancer Inst 93(13):979-989, 2001.

    This report of a consensus conference reviews the impact of various forms of adjuvant therapy in reducing the risk for recurrence in nonmetastatic breast cancer.

6. Fisher B, Anderson S, Bryant J, et al. Twenty-year follow-up of a randomized trial comparing total mastectomy, lumpectomy, and lumpectomy plus irradiation for the treatment of invasive breast cancer. N Engl J Med 347(16):1233-1241, 2002.

    This article discusses the long-term impact of breast conservation versus mastectomy in local and systemic control of breast cancer.

7. Fisher B, Costantino JP, Wickerham DL, et al: Tamoxifen for the prevention of breast cancer: Current status of the National Surgical Adjuvant Breast and Bowel Project P-1 study. J Natl Cancer Inst 97(22):1652-1662, 2005.

    The authors present results of a randomized, placebo-controlled trial on the selective estrogen receptor modulator tamoxifen in breast cancer prevention.

8. Greene F, Page D, Fleming I, et al (eds): AJCC Cancer Staging Handbook, 6th ed. Philadelphia, Lippincott-Raven, 2002.

    The AJCC provides a comprehensive description of TNM staging.

9. Hartmann LC, Schaid DJ, Woods JE, et al: Efficacy of bilateral prophylactic mastectomy in women with a family history of breast cancer. N Engl J Med 340(2):77-84, 1999.

    This article reports on an observational study of the long-term impact of prophylactic mastectomy in women with a family history of breast cancer.

10. Newman EA, Guest AB, Helvie MA, et al: Changes in surgical management resulting from case review at a breast cancer multidisciplinary tumor board. Cancer 107(10):2346-2351, 2006.

    The authors present results of an observational study of the changes in treatment plan due to multidisciplinary review.

11. Perou CM, Sorlie T, Eisen MB, et al: Molecular portraits of human breast tumours. Nature 406(6797):747-752, 2000.

    This is the first of many publications examining gene expression array–identified subtypes of breast cancer.

12. Smith RA, Saslow D, Sawyer KA, et al: American Cancer Society guidelines for breast cancer screening: Update 2003. CA Cancer J Clin 53(3):141-169, 2003.

    This article provides the guidelines for screening for breast cancer from the American Cancer Society.

13. Sorlie T, Perou CM, Tibshirani R, et al: Gene expression patterns of breast carcinomas distinguish tumor subclasses with clinical implications. Proc Natl Acad Sci USA 98(19):10869-10874, 2001.

    This is the first description of the clinical and prognostic implications of molecular subtypes of breast cancer.

14. U.S. Preventive Services Taskforce. Screening for breast cancer: Recommendations and rationale. Ann Intern Med 137(5 Part 1):344-346, 2002.

    This paper presents a comprehensive review of the evidence for and against various screening modalities in breast cancer.

William Y. Kim ▪ Paul A. Godley ▪ Young E. Whang

Prostate Cancer

Introduction

Prostate cancer constitutes 33% of noncutaneous malignancies diagnosed in males, making it the most commonly diagnosed malignancy in men. An estimated 234,000 new cases are anticipated in the United States in 2006. These figures represent a sharp decline from the 1997 estimates of 334,500 new cases, a trend consistent with an effect from the recent adoption of prostate-specific antigen (PSA) screening for prostate cancer. Prostate cancer is the third leading cause of male cancer deaths, with 27,350 deaths anticipated in 2006. Mortality rates from prostate cancer as well as several other cancers have been decreasing since the early 1990s, although a relationship of this decrease to current screening efforts has not been established.

The incidence and mortality rates among African-American men surpass those of other racial and ethnic groups and are twice as high as those of white Americans. Risk increases sharply as men age, and men with a strong family history of prostate cancer may have several times the risk for prostate cancer as men without such a history.

Etiology and Pathogenesis

Research on men who migrate from areas of low prostate cancer mortality to areas of high mortality provides compelling evidence for unidentified environmental causes. Japanese males aged 65 to 74 years who migrated to the United States had age-specific prostate cancer mortality rates (40.2/100,000/year) intermediate between the high rate of U.S. whites (92.6/100,000/year) and Japan's lower rate (11.2/100,000/year). These studies imply that immigrants are exposed to environmental or lifestyle factors that place them at higher risk for prostate cancer. Systematic review of prostate cancer risk factors has not demonstrated consistent environmental, behavioral, or dietary risk factors amenable to primary prevention, although some studies have suggested that dietary saturated fat consumption may increase risk.

Several prostate cancer prevention strategies are under investigation. SELECT, a large randomized, controlled trial of selenium and vitamin E as nutritional cancer prevention agents, began in 2002. The Prostate Cancer Prevention Trial examined the chemoprevention of prostate cancer using finasteride, an inhibitor of 5α-reductase (the intracellular enzyme that converts testosterone to its active metabolite dihydrotestosterone). Finasteride appears to decrease the development of prostate cancer by 25% but may increase the risk for high-grade cancer and cause sexual side effects.

Clinical Presentation

Early-stage prostate cancer is usually asymptomatic. Symptoms referable to the prostate gland are often due to benign prostatic hyperplasia, which is not related to nor a risk factor for prostate cancer. Locally advanced prostate cancer may present with symptoms of bladder outlet obstruction or hematuria, and patients with metastatic disease may present with bone pain and, less commonly, spinal cord compression or obstructive uropathy (Fig. 81-1).

Differential Diagnosis

In addition to prostate cancer, prostatitis and benign prostatic hypertrophy are associated with an elevated serum PSA level. A course of antibiotics may lead to normalization of elevated PSA in patients with prostatitis. PSA levels in prostate cancer and benign prostatic hypertrophy overlap significantly, and currently a biopsy is the only test that can distinguish these two conditions.

Figure 81-1 Prostate Cancer.

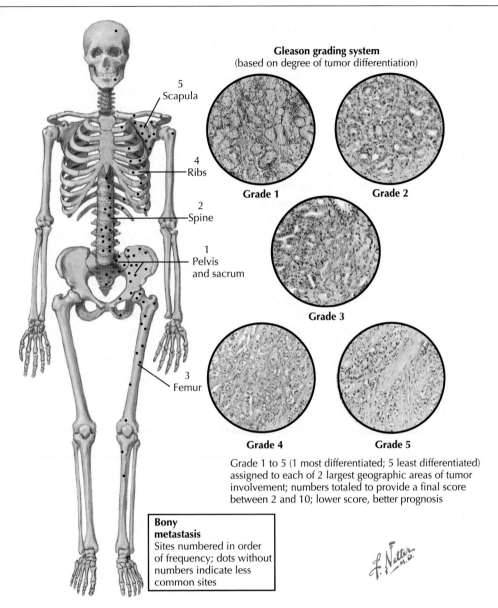

Gleason grading system
(based on degree of tumor differentiation)

Grade 1

Grade 2

Grade 3

Grade 4

Grade 5

Grade 1 to 5 (1 most differentiated; 5 least differentiated) assigned to each of 2 largest geographic areas of tumor involvement; numbers totaled to provide a final score between 2 and 10; lower score, better prognosis

5
Scapula

4
Ribs

2
Spine

1
Pelvis
and sacrum

3
Femur

Bony metastasis
Sites numbered in order of frequency; dots without numbers indicate less common sites

Diagnostic Approach

Screening remains a controversial issue. The lack of consensus on PSA screening is reflected in the diversity of recommendations from public health and physician organizations. The American Cancer Society, the American Urological Association, and others recommend annual screening with PSA and digital rectal examination (DRE) starting at age 50 years. These same groups recommend initiating screening at age 45 years for high-risk patients—men of African-American descent or with a family history of prostate cancer, defined as a first-degree relative diagnosed before the age of 65 years. The National Cancer Institute, the U.S. Preventive Services Task Force, the Canadian Task Force on the Periodic Health Exam, the Office of Technology Assessment, and the American College of Physicians have either not made a recommendation, recommended that screening be discussed with patients, or recommended explicitly against screening.

Of the screening tests for early prostate cancer, only the PSA assay stands out as both convenient to administer and potentially sensitive enough to detect cancer while it is localized to the prostate gland. DRE alone is not a reliable screening test, having failed to demonstrate effectiveness in preventing metastatic prostate cancer or death from prostate cancer in a case-control study and a quasi-cohort study. DRE, however, does detect some prostate cancers that are missed by PSA testing. Uncertainty about the natural history of prostate cancer and the wisdom of detecting and treating asymptomatic patients is reflected in the extraordinarily high prevalence of prostate cancer detected at autopsy in men without a previous clinical diagnosis of prostate cancer. These studies from various countries consistently document that 20% to 30% of men die with unsuspected carcinoma of the prostate.

Pathology and Staging and Risk Stratification

Tissues obtained from transurethral resection of the prostate may be incidentally found to be involved with cancer. Patients with an elevated PSA level or a palpable nodule on DRE should undergo a needle biopsy of the prostate gland. Almost all prostate carcinomas are adenocarcinomas. In the Gleason grading system, the glandular differentiation patterns of the primary (largest) and secondary tumors are each scored from 1 (well differentiated) to 5 (poorly differentiated) and then added together to give a number from 2 to 10 (see Fig. 81-1).

Staging using the tumor-node-metastasis (TNM) system classifies T1 as not palpable and T2 as palpable tumors confined to the prostate gland. T1c describes nonpalpable tumors detected by random prostate biopsies performed because of an elevated PSA test. T3 tumors extend beyond the gland, and T4 tumors invade adjacent organs. N1 and M1 denote the presence of positive lymph nodes and metastatic disease, respectively.

Patients can be divided into well-defined prognostic groups based on the clinical characteristics of T stage on DRE, PSA level, and Gleason grade. Low-risk patients are defined as clinical stage T1c or T2a (tumor involving one half of one lobe), PSA <10, and Gleason score ≤6. Intermediate-risk patients have clinical stage T2b (tumor involving more than one half of one lobe but not both lobes), PSA of 10 to 20, or Gleason score of 7. High-risk patients have a clinical stage T2c (tumor involving both lobes) or higher, PSA >20, or a Gleason score of 8 or higher. Risk category is prognostic. After definitive local therapy, low-, intermediate-, and high-risk patients have been shown to have approximate likelihoods of 15%, 50%, and 70%, respectively, of having biochemical recurrence (detectable and rising PSA) at 5 years.

Management and Therapy

Localized Disease

Patients with clinically localized disease have several treatment options, including radical prostatectomy, external-beam radiation therapy, brachytherapy, and watchful waiting. Although radical prostatectomy has been shown to decrease disease-specific and overall mortality at 10 years when compared with watchful waiting, there are no randomized trials comparing surgery to radiation therapy.

Thus, treatment of localized prostate cancer remains controversial. Radical prostatectomy is the most frequently chosen treatment in patients younger than 70 years (Fig. 81-2). With a retropubic approach, the procedure is frequently preceded by a regional pelvic lymph node dissection. More than one third of patients with clinically localized disease are upstaged with capsular penetration, positive surgical margins, or involvement of the seminal vesicles or lymph nodes. The risk of finding positive lymph nodes increases with the T stage, Gleason grade, and PSA. A frozen section can be obtained intraoperatively and the prostatectomy aborted if the results are positive for metastatic nodal disease. The major side effects associated with radical prostatectomy include erectile dysfunction and urinary incontinence.

Radiation therapy can be delivered by external beam or by brachytherapy using iodine or palladium prostatic interstitial implants. External-beam radiation is given to a dose of about 70 to 78 Gy in daily fractions over 7 to 8 weeks. Seed implants permanently placed during an outpatient procedure may be used alone or in combination with external-beam radiation. Temporary high-dose-rate brachytherapy devices, inserted into the prostate gland for less than an hour and removed, remain investigational. Radiation therapy is associated with erectile dysfunction and rectal damage (radiation proctitis) and less commonly with urinary incontinence. Urinary retention secondary to prostate inflammation is a common but transient side effect of brachytherapy.

The third option is no treatment, also variously termed watchful waiting, expectant management, active surveillance, or observation. It involves deferring treatment until signs of progression or development of symptoms, but not initially attempting to eradicate the disease. The advantage is the lack of early complications associated with aggressive therapy but at the cost of potential late complications from locally advanced or metastatic prostate cancer, and death from prostate cancer, a possibility also faced by men who choose more aggressive treatment. Watchful waiting may be recommended to patients with low-grade disease, or a life expectancy of less than 10 years.

The treatment of locally advanced disease (T3 or T4) may consist of radiation and androgen deprivation. Addition of androgen deprivation therapy to radiation for patients with intermediate- or high-risk disease has been demonstrated to increase survival and should be strongly considered in these patients.

Relapsed Disease

Many men (up to 30% by some estimates) who were treated with curative intent for presumed organ-confined prostate cancer will have recurrence of their disease, first detected as a consistent rise in PSA level but without radiologic evidence of disease or symptoms. This scenario is termed *biochemical* or *PSA-only relapse*. Therapy for patients

Figure 81-2 Radical Prostatectomy.

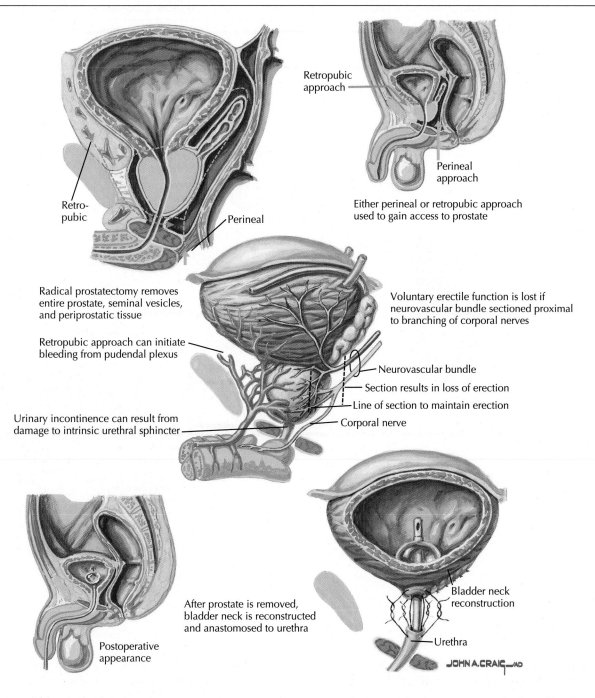

Retropubic
approach

Perineal
approach

Either perineal or retropubic approach
used to gain access to prostate

Radical prostatectomy removes
entire prostate, seminal vesicles,
and periprostatic tissue

Retropubic approach can initiate
bleeding from pudendal plexus

Urinary incontinence can result from
damage to intrinsic urethral sphincter

Retro-
pubic

Perineal

Voluntary erectile function is lost if
neurovascular bundle sectioned proximal
to branching of corporal nerves

Neurovascular bundle

Section results in loss of erection

Line of section to maintain erection

Corporal nerve

Postoperative
appearance

After prostate is removed,
bladder neck is reconstructed
and anastomosed to urethra

Bladder neck
reconstruction

Urethra

JOHN A.CRAIG_AD

with PSA-only relapse hinges on whether the relapse is thought to represent systemic disease or local recurrence of the tumor. Factors suggestive of systemic recurrence include both attributes of the original tumor (Gleason score 8 or greater, seminal vesicle invasion, or lymph node metastases) and characteristics at the time of recurrence (PSA recurrence-free survival <2 to 3 years and fast PSA doubling time, i.e., <9 months). Patients with presumed local recurrence of tumor can be offered treatment with salvage local therapy. Patients first treated with prostatec-

tomy can be administered salvage radiotherapy, whereas patients originally treated with radiation therapy can be salvaged with prostatectomy. Men with biochemical relapse thought to represent systemic disease often receive androgen deprivation therapy (ADT). However, when to institute ADT, immediately or delayed until clinical metastatic disease develops, remains controversial. Patients with biochemical recurrence have a varied prognosis, and many patients may develop clinical progression and death from prostate cancer over a period of 10 to 15 years, during

Figure 81-3 Androgen Deprivation in Metastatic Disease.
DHT, dihydrotestosterone; LH, luteinizing hormone; LHRH, luteinizing hormone–releasing hormone.

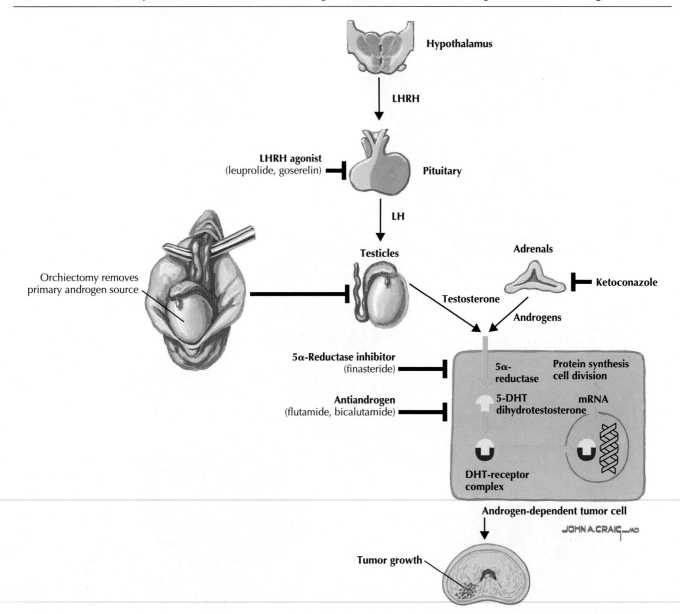

which time they are also at risk for dying from other conditions. Although there is some evidence that early ADT may delay disease progression and result in prolonged survival, the data are indirect and not consistent. Additionally, these studies do not take into account side effects of ADT, such as impotence, osteoporosis, and other quality-of-life parameters. Thus, the optimal timing of ADT for these patients is undefined and will need to be individualized.

Metastatic Disease

Metastatic prostate cancer is incurable. Patients are treated palliatively with ADT because prostate cancer cells initially require circulating testosterone for viability and prolifera-

tion (Fig. 81-3). Advantages of surgical castration with bilateral orchiectomy include immediate efficacy, compliance, and low cost. Medical castration using the long-acting preparations of a luteinizing hormone–releasing hormone (LHRH) agonist (leuprolide or goserelin) is used more commonly because of the psychological trauma associated with orchiectomy. LHRH is normally secreted from the hypothalamus in a pulsatile fashion; however, continuous stimulation of the LHRH receptor by the LHRH agonists leads to its down-regulation on the pituitary cells. LHRH agonists initially cause a transient surge in the testosterone level due to the stimulation of the pituitary LHRH receptor (flare phenomenon) and are therefore contraindicated in men with impending spinal cord compression or urinary obstruction from prostate cancer. Short-term use of an antiandrogen agent such as flutamide or bicalutamide, which acts as a competitive inhibitor of the androgen receptor, is indicated for the first several weeks after administration of the LHRH agonist. The major common side effects of ADT (both surgical and medical) include loss of libido, erectile dysfunction, gynecomastia, hot flashes, loss of muscle mass, osteoporosis, anemia, and fatigue. Osteoporosis induced by ADT increases the rate of skeletal fractures; bisphosphonates prevent this treatment-related osteoporosis.

ADT is effective only temporarily because progressive disease will develop again after a median of 18 to 24 months. In this setting, second-line endocrine manipulations involving antiandrogens, low-dose steroids, or ketoconazole are often attempted. For patients who have been on long-term antiandrogen therapy, its discontinuation leads to reduction in PSA in 15% to 20% of cases; however, responses to second-line hormonal treatment tend to be infrequent and short lived.

The traditional view of prostate cancer as resistant to chemotherapy is changing. The combination of mitoxantrone and prednisone does not prolong the survival of hormone-refractory metastatic prostate cancer patients but does improve pain control and quality of life. Furthermore, docetaxel-based combination chemotherapy has been shown in randomized studies to impart a 2- to 3-month improvement in median survival over mitoxantrone and prednisone. Docetaxel represents the current standard of care for patients with metastatic hormone-refractory prostate cancer.

Zoledronic acid, a new potent bisphosphonate, decreases skeletal complications such as bone pain, fracture, and spinal cord compression in patients with hormone-refractory prostate cancer and bone metastases and is currently indicated as adjunct therapy. In addition to chemotherapy, palliation of pain associated with bone metastases may be achieved by external-beam radiation or systemic administration of bone-seeking radioactive isotopes (strontium-89 or samarium-153).

Medical Emergencies in Prostate Cancer Management

Prostate cancer frequently metastasizes to the bones and lymph nodes of the pelvis and retroperitoneum. It is one of the most common causes of spinal cord compression, an oncologic emergency that arises from epidural metastasis in the vertebral bodies and usually presents with midline accelerating back pain. Loss of ambulation due to weakness, and bowel and bladder incontinence are late symptoms that are usually irreversible despite treatment. The diagnosis can be made with computed tomography myelography or noninvasively with magnetic resonance imaging. Treatment consists of corticosteroids and radiation therapy or, in selected patients, surgical intervention. Initiation of

the LHRH agonist by itself in noncastrated patients is not recommended in this setting because of concerns about the flare phenomenon.

Obstructive uropathy may result from primary prostate cancer locally invading into the urethra and the bladder or extrinsic compressive obstruction of ureters by soft tissue nodal masses in the pelvis or retroperitoneum. It may progress to complete renal failure. Renal function can be preserved by relief of obstruction through percutaneous nephrostomy tube or internal stent placement.

Avoiding Treatment Errors

Optimal treatment of localized prostate cancer is currently undefined. Decisions should take into account the clinical risk factors for relapse, the life expectancy and comorbid illnesses of the patient, side-effect profile of the therapy, and patient preference. Primary care physicians should help patients understand the range of available options and the benefits and side effects of each option considered and avoid overly aggressive treatment in some cases. Recent surveys indicate that the use of androgen deprivation therapy as primary therapy for low-risk localized disease has been increasing in the United States recently, and this trend raises concerns about overtreatment of elderly patients with indolent disease.

Future Directions

Availability of the human genome sequence and advances in molecular profiling of tumors hold great promise for developing better prognostic and predictive markers and therapeutic agents specifically targeting cancer cells (e.g., drugs inhibiting kinases). Approaches to improve the treatment outcome of those patients unlikely to be cured by local treatment alone (e.g., high-risk group) will be explored. Treatment approaches to hormone-refractory prostate cancer will continue to be refined with available chemotherapeutic agents and novel molecularly targeted agents.

Additionally, technologic improvements in the treatment of early-stage prostate cancer are gaining popularity. The use of laparoscopic prostatectomy and, more recently, robotic prostatectomy is becoming more widespread because of their less invasive nature and faster patient recovery time. However, surgical and oncologic outcomes of these procedures will require additional long-term follow-up studies.

Additional Resources

American Cancer Society Website. Available at: http://www.cancer.org. Accessed October 9, 2006.
  The American Cancer Society site provides extensive resources for education and treatment decisions.
National Cancer Institute Website. Available at: http://www.cancer.gov/ cancertopics/types/prostate. Accessed October 9, 2006.

The National Cancer Institute provides extensive information on common cancer types.

People Living with Cancer Website. Available at: http://www.plwc.org. Accessed October 9, 2006.

The People Living with Cancer website provides patient-oriented information approved by the American Society of Clinical Oncology.

Stanford JL, Stephenson RA, Coyle LM, et al: Prostate Cancer Trends 1973-1995, SEER Program, National Cancer Institute. NIH Pub. No. 99-4543. Bethesda, MD, 1999. Available at: http://seer.cancer.gov/publications/prostate/. Accessed October 9, 2006.

This is the most comprehensive available analysis of population-based trends in prostate cancer.

EVIDENCE

1. Albertsen PC, Hanley JA, Fine J: 20-Year outcomes following conservative management of clinically localized prostate cancer. JAMA 293(17):2095-2101, 2005.
   The indolent natural history of low-grade prostate cancer supports watchful waiting for some patients.
2. Bill-Axelson A, Holmberg L, Ruutu M, et al: Radical prostatectomy versus watchful waiting in early prostate cancer. N Engl J Med 352(19):1977-1984, 2005.
   There is long-term benefit of radical prostatectomy.
3. Bolla M, Gonzalez D, Warde P, et al: Improved survival in patients with locally advanced prostate cancer treated with radiotherapy and goserelin. N Engl J Med 337(5):295-300, 1997.
   This trial supports the addition of androgen deprivation to radiation therapy in intermediate- and high-risk prostate cancer.
4. D'Amico AV, Manola J, Loffredo M, et al: 6-Month androgen suppression plus radiation therapy vs radiation therapy alone for patients with clinically localized prostate cancer: A randomized controlled trial. JAMA 292(7):821-827, 2004.
   This trial supports the addition of androgen deprivation to radiation therapy in intermediate- and high-risk prostate cancer.
5. Freedland SJ, Humphreys EB, Mangold LA, et al: Risk of prostate cancer-specific mortality following biochemical recurrence after radical prostatectomy. JAMA 294(4):433-439, 2005.
   This article provides estimates of death from prostate cancer using clinical risk factors in patients with biochemical relapse.
6. Johansson JE, Andren O, Andersson SO, et al: Natural history of early, localized prostate cancer. JAMA 291(22):2713-2719, 2004.
   This study supports early radical treatment, especially in patients with a life expectancy of more than 15 years.
7. Petrylak DP, Tangen CM, Hussain MH, et al: Docetaxel and estramustine compared with mitoxantrone and prednisone for advanced refractory prostate cancer. N Engl J Med 351(15):1513-1520, 2004.
   This article establishes docetaxel chemotherapy for advanced prostate cancer.
8. Saad F, Gleason DM, Murray R, et al: A randomized, placebo-controlled trial of zoledronic acid in patients with hormone-refractory metastatic prostate carcinoma. J Natl Cancer Inst 94(19):1458-1468, 2002.
   Zoledronic acid decreases skeletal-related morbidity in advanced prostate cancer.
9. Tannock IF, de Wit R, Berry WR, et al: Docetaxel plus prednisone or mitoxantrone plus prednisone for advanced prostate cancer. N Engl J Med 351(15):1502-1512, 2004.
   This article establishes docetaxel chemotherapy for advanced prostate cancer.

Mark Taylor ▪ Bert H. O'Neil

82

Upper Gastrointestinal Cancers

Introduction

Cancers of the upper gastrointestinal (GI) tract, including those of the pancreas, esophagus, stomach, liver, and biliary system, in order of U.S. prevalence, are together the most common cancer killers worldwide. Several of these tumors continue to have rising incidence in the United States, particularly esophageal cancer and hepatocellular (liver cell) carcinoma (HCC). Pancreatic cancer, despite being relatively uncommon, is the fourth leading cancer killer in the United States because of a nearly 1:1 ratio of cases and deaths. There has been a decline in proximal squamous cell carcinoma (SCC) of the esophagus and distal adenocarcinoma of the stomach, whereas the incidence of distal esophageal adenocarcinoma and proximal gastric carcinoma has increased. Upper GI cancers are 2 to 3 times more common in men than in women. SCC of the esophagus is 4 to 5 times more common in African Americans; adenocarcinoma is more prevalent in the white population. Cancer of the stomach is second only to lung carcinoma in incidence, with more than 750,000 new cases diagnosed worldwide each year. Incidence is highest in the Russian Federation and Japan. In the United States, there were an estimated 21,900 new cases and 13,500 deaths in 1999. This represents a dramatic decline in the past seven decades.

Pancreatic Cancer

Etiology and Pathogenesis

Tobacco use is the most well-established risk factor for pancreatic cancer, accounting for about 25% of cases. Known genetic syndromes and chronic pancreatitis account for only a small percentage of cases. At this point, most cases of pancreatic cancer are of unknown cause. Onset of diabetes has been shown to occur 1 to 3 years before diagnosis of pancreatic cancer in many cases.

Clinical Presentation

The most common presenting symptom of pancreatic cancer is abdominal pain, which is nonspecific in nature. Radiation of pain to the back is one distinguishing feature that also has ominous implications. Cancer of the head of the pancreas should always be considered in the differential diagnosis of painless jaundice. Venous thrombosis is exceedingly common in patients with pancreatic malignancies.

Differential Diagnosis

The differential diagnosis for a patient with epigastric pain and abnormalities of the pancreas on computed tomography (CT) includes pancreatitis (which can mimic tumors), cysts of the pancreas, cystadenocarcinomas (a relatively indolent form of tumor), and neuroendocrine tumors of the pancreas (Fig. 82-1).

Diagnostic Approach

Diagnosis of pancreatic cancer can occasionally be difficult because of the presence of significant amounts of scarring and inflammatory tissue in an apparent pancreatic mass. Not infrequently, patients with masses in the pancreatic head are taken to surgery without prior tissue confirmation of malignancy. CA19-9 is a carbohydrate antigen that can be a useful adjunct to diagnosis, but is not a specific marker. Staging of pancreatic cancer consists of imaging of the abdomen and chest, usually by CT. High-quality imaging is required to determine the relationship between the

Figure 82-1 Malignant Tumors—Cystadenocarcinoma, Islet Cell Carcinoma, and Chronic Relapsing Pancreatitis.

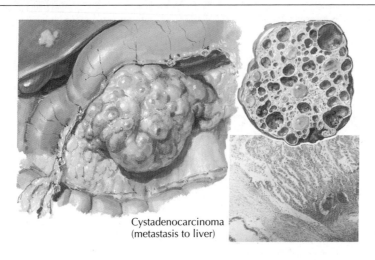

Cystadenocarcinoma
(metastasis to liver)

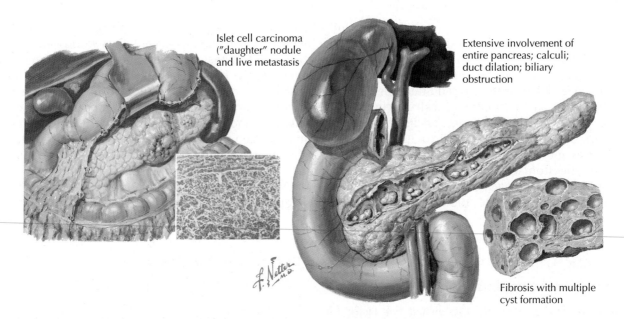

Islet cell carcinoma
("daughter" nodule
and live metastasis

Extensive involvement of
entire pancreas; calculi;
duct dilation; biliary
obstruction

Fibrosis with multiple
cyst formation

cancer and the local vasculature, which determines whether surgical resection is possible.

Management and Therapy

Optimum Treatment

LOCALIZED DISEASE. About 20% of patients present with disease that is amenable to surgical resection, a procedure that results in roughly a 20% chance of long-term survival. Pancreatic head tumors are treated surgically with a Whipple procedure, whereas more distal tumors are treated with partial pancreatectomy (Fig. 82-2). Adjuvant therapy is controversial; patients have been treated with a combination of 5-fluorouracil and radiation therapy based on a small randomized study, but subsequent data have not confirmed this early result. Very recently, a German group showed that chemotherapy using gemcitabine can improve recurrence-free survival after surgery, a result that should prompt a study of chemotherapy alone versus chemoradiotherapy after surgical resection. Some centers routinely treat patients with chemoradiotherapy preoperatively, but to date, no randomized data support this practice. One advantage of preoperative therapy is that the patients with the worst prognosis often progress systemically during radiation and are thereby spared major surgery.

ADVANCED DISEASE. Advanced disease is generally palliated with either chemoradiotherapy in the case of non-metastatic but unresectable disease, or chemotherapy (again, gemcitabine based) in the case of metastatic disease. New therapies are desperately needed for patients with this disease.

Figure 82-2 Carcinoma of the Pancreas.

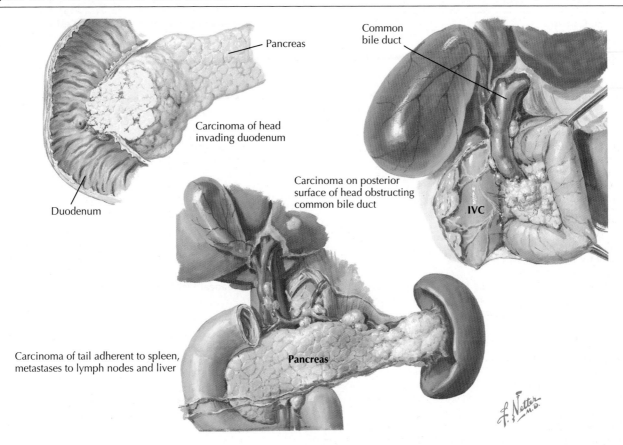

Pancreas

Carcinoma of head invading duodenum

Duodenum

Common bile duct

Carcinoma on posterior surface of head obstructing common bile duct

IVC

Carcinoma of tail adherent to spleen, metastases to lymph nodes and liver

Pancreas

Avoiding Treatment Errors

Although a detailed discussion of treatment errors surrounding chemotherapy is beyond the scope of this book, it is important that patients with possible pancreatic tumors be managed by an experienced multidisciplinary team for optimal treatment planning before initiation of any treatment plan.

Stomach Cancer

Etiology and Pathogenesis

Environmental and genetic factors both play a role in development (Table 82-1). Migrants from high-risk areas who move to low-risk areas have an intermediate risk for development of cancer, as do their subsequent generations. *Helicobacter pylori* infection is associated with a threefold to sixfold increase in the risk for developing distal intestinal-type adenocarcinoma. The incidence of proximal gastric cancer has increased in parallel with distal esophageal cancer (see next section).

Clinical Presentation

Gastric carcinoma is asymptomatic in its early stages, or presents with vague abdominal symptoms (anorexia, abdominal discomfort, nausea and vomiting, melena, and

weakness) that are not clearly attributable to carcinoma; therefore, most gastric cancers are not diagnosed until the disease is advanced. Early satiety is a symptom associated with diffusely infiltrating carcinoma (Fig. 82-3). Weight loss, seen in more than 80% of patients, is associated with poorer survival. Symptoms attributable to metastatic disease include jaundice (from biliary obstruction), ascites, and abdominal pain.

Differential Diagnosis

Both the presentation and endoscopic appearance of gastric cancer can mimic benign gastric ulcers. Other malignancies that can mimic stomach cancer are GI stromal tumors (with a much better prognosis than adenocarcinomas), lymphomas, and other rare variants of carcinoma and sarcoma.

Diagnostic Approach

Many patients are diagnosed by endoscopy performed for symptomatic reasons or anemia. Upper endoscopy should always follow a negative colonoscopy in a patient with iron-deficiency anemia. Staging of gastric cancer is generally done by CT of the chest and abdomen. The main sites of spread of gastric cancer are liver, intra-abdominal lymph nodes, peritoneum, and lung. Peritoneal metastasis is often

Table 82-1 Risk Factors

Gastric Cancer	Esophageal Cancer (Squamous Cell Carcinoma)
Nutritional Factors	
High salt consumption	Alcohol
High nitrate consumption	
Low dietary vitamin A and C	
Lack of refrigeration	
Exposure	
Rubber workers	Smoking
Coal workers	Lye ingestion
Helicobacter pylori infection	Human papillomavirus infection
Epstein-Barr virus infection	
Radiation exposure	
Prior gastric surgery for benign disease	
Genetic Factors	
Type A blood	Tylosis
Pernicious anemia	Autosomal dominant condition manifest by
Hereditary nonpolyposis colon cancer	hyperkeratosis of palms and soles
Li-Fraumeni syndrome	Plummer-Vinson syndrome
Autosomal dominant syndrome involving *p53* tumor suppressor gene mutation associated with soft tissue sarcoma, breast cancer, osteosarcoma, brain tumors, adrenal cortical tumors, acute leukemia	Esophageal webs and iron-deficiency anemia
Family history	
Preexisting Conditions	
Adenomatous gastric polyps	Achalasia
Chronic atrophic gastritis	Celiac sprue
Dysplasia	Other aerodigestive cancer
Intestinal metaplasia	Barrett's esophagus (adenocarcinoma)
Ménétrier's disease	
Poorly outlined disease, diagnosed in patients with giant gastric folds, dyspeptic symptoms, and hypoalbuminemia due to GI protein loss; the etiology is unknown	
Gastric ulcers	

Adapted from Karpeh M, Kelsen DP, Tepper JE: Cancer of the stomach. In DeVita VT, Hellman S, Rosenberg SA (eds): Cancer Principles and Practice of Oncology, 6th ed. Philadelphia, Lippincott, Williams & Wilkins, 2001, pp 1092-1126.

missed by conventional imaging studies, so laparoscopy is often performed before open surgery to avoid unnecessary laparotomy. Mediastinal lymph node spread is also common, and supraclavicular adenopathy (Sister Mary Joseph node) can also be found.

Prognosis

Depth of invasion and number of involved lymph nodes significantly alter prognosis. Additional adverse prognostic factors include advancing age, linitis plastica type, aneuploidy, and tumors of the gastric cardia or the gastro-esophageal junction. The median survival time for metastatic cancer is less than 1 year even with therapy.

Management and Therapy

Optimum Treatment

LOCALIZED DISEASE. Localized gastric cancer is treated with partial or total gastrectomy depending on site, along with partial esophagectomy for gastroesophageal junction

tumors. There is controversy as to the extent of lymph node dissection required at the time of surgery. In Japan, a more extensive nodal dissection is performed, with reports of better overall survival rates. In the United States and Europe, a more limited dissection is performed because it is thought that more extensive operations only add to morbidity. Two randomized studies of Western versus Japanese lymph node dissection revealed no differences in outcome. The difference in outcomes has been attributed to more accurate staging (the so-called Will Rogers phenomenon) with the Japanese procedure. The operative mortality rate is about 5%, and long-term sequelae include dumping, heartburn, and reduced appetite. Gastric cancer can recur at the site of the initial tumor, local lymph nodes, in the peritoneal cavity, or distantly (usually the liver or lungs). Adjuvant therapy for stomach cancer currently includes concomitant chemotherapy and radiotherapy with further chemotherapy.

ADVANCED DISEASE. Advanced or metastatic stomach cancer may be treated with surgery for palliation, with

Figure 82-3 Carcinoma of the Stomach: Polypoid Adenocarcinoma and Scirrhous Carcinoma.

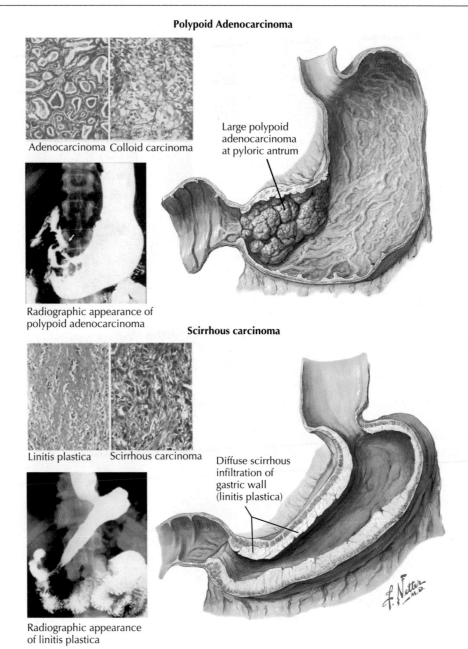

Polypoid Adenocarcinoma

Adenocarcinoma Colloid carcinoma

Radiographic appearance of polypoid adenocarcinoma

Large polypoid adenocarcinoma at pyloric antrum

Scirrhous carcinoma

Linitis plastica   Scirrhous carcinoma

Diffuse scirrhous infiltration of gastric wall (linitis plastica)

Radiographic appearance of linitis plastica

radiation often a reasonable alternative to palliate bleeding or symptoms related to eating. Chemotherapy can palliate symptoms, but effects are on average short-lived, and prolongation of survival by chemotherapy is on the order of 2 to 3 months.

Avoiding Treatment Errors

Although a detailed discussion of treatment errors surrounding surgery and chemotherapy is beyond the scope of this book, it is important that patients with stomach cancer be managed by an experienced multidisciplinary team for optimal treatment planning before initiation of any treatment plan.

Esophageal Cancer

Etiology and Pathogenesis

For squamous cell cancer of the esophagus, the most significant risk factors are alcohol consumption and tobacco use, which act both independently and synergistically. Patients with upper aerodigestive tract tumors have a 4% to 7% risk per year of esophageal cancer, suggesting a field effect of the aforementioned agents. The major known risk factor for adenocarcinoma is presence of Barrett's esophagus, which is associated with a 30- to 40-fold increase in risk (Fig. 82-4).

Figure 82-4 Malignant Tumors of Midportion and Distal Portion of Esophagus.

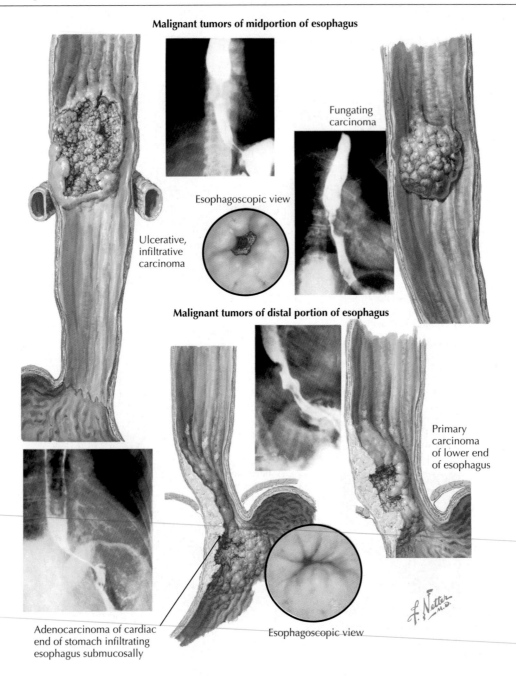

Malignant tumors of midportion of esophagus

Fungating carcinoma

Esophagoscopic view

Ulcerative, infiltrative carcinoma

Malignant tumors of distal portion of esophagus

Primary carcinoma of lower end of esophagus

Adenocarcinoma of cardiac end of stomach infiltrating esophagus submucosally

Esophagoscopic view

Clinical Presentation

Progressive dysphagia is present in 90% of patients. Dysphagia for solids precedes that for liquids. Typically, patients give a history of symptoms for 3 to 6 months before seeking medical attention. Weight loss is common, and symptoms can include cough or pneumonia from tracheoesophageal fistulas, chest pain from invasion of mediastinal structures, hoarseness from recurrent laryngeal nerve palsy, odynophagia, and hematemesis from tumor bleeding.

Differential Diagnosis

The differential diagnosis of esophageal dysphagia is given in Box 82-1.

Diagnostic Approach

The diagnosis of esophageal cancer is made endoscopically. Staging of the disease always involves CT scanning and often involves endoscopic ultrasound and positron emission tomography scanning (to look for occult meta-

From Castell DO: Approach to the patient with dysphagia. In Yamada T (ed): Textbook of Gastroenterology, 2nd ed. Philadelphia, Lippincott Williams & Wilkins, 1995.

static disease). Bronchoscopy is used in cases in which CT is suggestive of possible tracheal involvement (a finding that would denote surgical nonresectability).

Management and Therapy

Optimum Treatment

SURGERY. Surgery should be considered in localized or loco-regional disease that has not invaded essential structures. Patients must be fit enough to withstand a thoracotomy. Even with lymphatic spread, prolonged local control and relief of symptoms are best achieved if surgery is included in the therapy. The decision on surgical approach is based on location of the tumor and the surgeon's preference. Right thoracoabdominal (Ivor-Lewis) procedure), left thoracoabdominal, and transhiatal approaches are most common; morbidity and mortality rates are similar. Prognosis is related to tumor stage, not type of procedure performed. The long-term survival rate after surgical resection ranges from 10% to 30% in most series. Most recurrences are at the site of the initial tumor, but metastatic recurrence is seen most commonly in the liver and lungs.

RADIATION THERAPY AND CHEMOTHERAPY. As primary therapy, chemoradiation is approximately equivalent to surgical resection in terms of rate of cure, but is inferior in local disease control. Chemotherapy and radiation therapy given before (neoadjuvant) surgery is considered standard at many centers based on weight of phase II data but is still somewhat controversial.

Recent consideration has been given for treating carcinomas of the cardia of the stomach as well as tumors of the gastroesophageal junction similarly to adenocarcinoma of the esophagus. The rationale is the similarity in epidemiology, genetic abnormalities, prognosis of these malignancies, and the frequency at which gastric carcinoma invades submucosally into the distal esophagus.

Avoiding Treatment Errors

As in the case of other cancers discussed in this chapter, the importance of a multidisciplinary team in initial patient evaluation and therapeutic decision making cannot be stressed enough. The key is to involve multiple specialty perspectives.

Hepatocellular Carcinoma

Etiology and Pathogenesis

Most HCCs arise in a background of chronic liver disease (Fig. 82-5). Worldwide, the most common cause is hepatitis B infection, which can lead to HCC before the development of cirrhosis. In the Western world and Japan, hepatitis C virus infection has become the most common cause of HCC. In this setting, significant cirrhosis is usually (>70% of cases) present at the time of cancer diagnosis. Alcohol use can be a major contributor to the development of HCC in patients with chronic hepatitis, but alcoholic cirrhosis alone induces cancer development with far lower frequency. Other less common causes of chronic liver disease, such as hemochromatosis, Wilson's disease, and α_1-antitrypsin deficiency, can also predispose to HCC.

Clinical Presentation

Tumors in the liver are largely asymptomatic. Occasionally, HCCs can present with pain, but other symptoms are nonspecific and include anorexia, weight loss, worsening ascites, and encephalopathy. Occasionally HCC can present dramatically with peritoneal hemorrhage or with the signs and symptoms of metastatic disease. Screening is recommended for patients with known chronic hepatitis or end-stage liver disease, generally with serum alpha fetoprotein (AFP) measurements and ultrasound or magnetic resonance imaging (MRI) depending on the patient's risk.

Differential Diagnosis

The signs and symptoms of developing HCC overlap with those of progressive end-stage liver disease, thus worsening liver function in such a patient should warrant consideration of imaging studies and measurement of serum

Figure 82-5 Primary Hepatic Carcinoma.

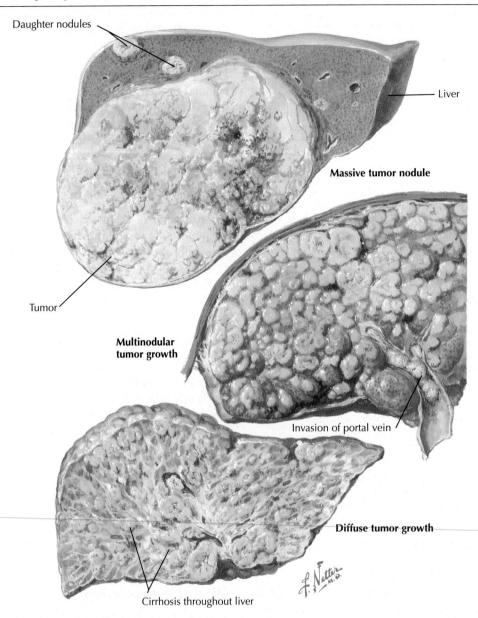

Daughter nodules

Liver

Massive tumor nodule

Tumor

Multinodular
tumor growth

Invasion of portal vein

Diffuse tumor growth

Cirrhosis throughout liver

AFP. The pathologic differential diagnosis of HCC includes metastatic tumors from other sites and intrahepatic bile duct tumors (cholangiocarcinomas). Most metastatic cancers in the liver are adenocarcinomas and are generally distinguishable from HCC morphologically or by immunohistochemistry.

Diagnostic Approach

Imaging of HCC is difficult because of the background of chronic liver disease. CT scans have a propensity to underestimate disease, whereas MRI often shows lesions that are difficult to interpret as cancer or noncancerous processes such as inflammation or liver regeneration. Because HCC remains confined to the liver in most cases, extensive extra-

hepatic imaging is not necessary except in the case of symptoms that require investigation. Prognosis and treatment options are strongly influenced by the presence of portal vein thrombosis, so attention should be paid to this on imaging studies.

Management and Therapy

Optimum Treatment

When possible, transplantation or resection is the treatment of choice. Unfortunately, a minority of patients are eligible for these therapies. Small tumors detected by screening can be effectively managed by radiofrequency ablation. Because the criteria for listing of patients for liver transplantation is often in flux, patients with end-stage liver disease should be managed by a multidisciplinary team of gastroenterologists, surgeons, radiologists, and medical oncologists. HCC that is not amenable to surgery or ablation is very difficult to manage; the disease is resistant to most chemotherapy agents, and the liver is intolerant of external-beam radiotherapy. One potentially palliative therapy with controversial efficacy is embolization (or chemoembolization) through the hepatic artery using particulate matter such as Gelfoam or beads composed of various soluble polymers.

Avoiding Treatment Errors

Patients with hepatobiliary cancers are complicated, particularly given the possibility of transplantation as a treatment, and should for the most part be managed at a tertiary care center by an experienced multidisciplinary team.

Future Directions

Despite improvements in survival during the past few decades, the prognosis of upper GI tract malignancies remains poor. Because of the relative rarity of most of these conditions in Western countries, research progress has been slow. Pancreatic cancer remains perhaps the most difficult of all cancers, with rapid progression and few effective therapies. Recently erlotinib, an agent targeting the epidermal growth factor receptor, has shown promise in a well-conducted randomized trial; but gains in survival were on the order of only weeks. In the coming years, newer agents studied in more common conditions such as lung cancer and colon cancer will be studied in the upper GI cancers, with hope that improvements in prognosis will follow. For the moment, advances in predictive capabilities, particularly for patients known to be at risk for esophageal cancer (Barrett's esophagus patients) and HCC, will be important in discovering these diseases at curable stages.

Additional Resources

Wong R, Malthaner R: Combined chemotherapy and radiotherapy (without surgery) compared with radiotherapy alone in localized carcinoma of the esophagus. Cochrane Database Syst Rev 25(1): CD002092, 2006.

This systematic review of available evidence addresses the controversial subject of the appropriate therapy for esophageal cancer.

EVIDENCE

1. American Cancer Society: Cancer facts and figures. New York, American Cancer Society, 2004.
   The American Cancer Society provides annually updated cancer statistics for the United States.
2. Blackstock AW, Cox AD, Tepper JE: Treatment of pancreatic cancer: Current limitations, future possibilities. Oncology 10(3):301-307; discussion, 308-323, 1996.
   This is an excellent state-of-the-art review on pancreatic cancer treatment.
3. Blot WJ, Devesa SS, Kneller RW, Fraumeni JF Jr: Rising incidence of adenocarcinoma of the esophagus and gastric cardia. JAMA 265(10):1287-1289, 1991.
   This is a very widely cited and important article on the epidemiology of distal esophageal adenocarcinoma.
4. Bonenkamp JJ, Hermans J, Sasako M, et al: Extended lymph-node dissection for gastric cancer. N Engl J Med 340(12):908-914, 1999.
   This well-conducted European trial demonstrated the lack of apparent survival benefit of the Japanese extended lymphadenectomy in a Western population with stomach cancer.
5. Bosch FX, Ribes J, Cleries R, Diaz M: Epidemiology of hepatocellular carcinoma. Clin Liver Dis 9(2):191-211, 2005.
   The authors present an interesting review of HCC epidemiology.
6. Braga L, Guller U, Semelka RC: Modern hepatic imaging. Surg Clin North Am 84(2):375-400, 2004.
   This is a good review of commonly employed diagnostic imaging techniques (US, CT, MRI, PET) in the evaluation of liver metastatic lesions and HCC.
7. Devesa SS, Blot WJ, Fraumeni JF Jr: Changing patterns in the incidence of esophageal and gastric carcinoma in the United States. Cancer 83(10):2049-2053, 1998.
   The authors provide a follow-up article to their seminal work.
8. El-Seraq HB, Davila JA, Petersen NJ, McGlynn KA: The continuing increase in the incidence of hepatocellular carcinoma in the United States: An update. Ann Intern Med 139(10):817-823, 2003.
   This article confirmed a significant rise in hepatocellular carcinoma incidence in the United States.
9. Konner J, O'Reilly E: Pancreatic cancer: Epidemiology, genetics, and approaches to screening. Oncology 16(12):1615-1622, 1631-1632; discussion, 1632-1633, 1637-1638, 2002.
10. Macdonald JS, Smalley SR, Benedetti J, et al: Chemoradiotherapy after surgery compared with surgery alone for adenocarcinoma of the stomach or gastroesophageal junction. N Engl J Med 345(10):725-730, 2001.
    This study defined current standard-of-care therapy for resectable stomach cancer in the United States.
11. Neuhaus P, Oettle H, Post S, et al: A randomised, prospective, multicenter, phase III trial of adjuvant chemotherapy with gemcitabine vs. observation in patients with resected pancreatic cancer. ASCO Meeting Abstracts 23:LBA4013, 2005.
12. Nomura A, Stemmermann GN, Chyou PH, et al: Helicobacter pylori infection and gastric carcinoma among Japanese Americans in Hawaii. N Engl J Med 325(16):1132-1136, 1991.
    This is one of two simultaneous articles documenting this important epidemiologic association.
13. Oettle H: Adjuvant chemotherapy with gemcitabine vs observation in patients undergoing curative-intent resection of pancreatic cancer: a randomized controlled trial. JAMA 297(3):267-277, 2005.
    This study utilized chemotherapy alone as adjuvant therapy for pancreatic cancer and defines the European standard of care.
14. Parsonnet J, Friedman GD, Vandersteen DP, et al: Helicobacter pylori infection and the risk of gastric carcinoma. N Engl J Med 325(16):1127-1131, 1991.
    This is one of two simultaneous articles documenting this important epidemiologic association.
15. Shaheen NJ: Advances in Barrett's esophagus and esophageal adenocarcinoma. Gastroenterology 128(6):1554-1566, 2005.
    The author presents an up-to-date expert review of the pathogenesis and controversies surrounding management of Barrett's esophagus.

Skin Cancer

Introduction

Skin cancer is a major health problem in the United States with 1.3 million new nonmelanoma skin cancers and 51,000 new melanomas diagnosed annually. Nonmelanoma and melanoma skin cancers together account for 40% of all malignancies. The annual cost to treat nonmelanoma skin cancers in the United States approaches $650 million. The incidence of both nonmelanoma and melanoma skin cancers has been steadily increasing. This increase is most likely due to increased sunlight exposure, increased longevity of the population, and increased surveillance. Early detection and treatment can have a significant impact on morbidity and mortality.

BASAL CELL CARCINOMA

Etiology and Pathogenesis

Basal cell carcinoma (BCC) is the most common skin cancer, accounting for more than 75% of all nonmelanoma skin cancers. There are 750,000 to 900,000 new cases in the United States each year. The ultraviolet radiation of sunlight is the most important causative factor, with both sunburns and cumulative dose over years being important. Thus, most of these cancers are located on sun-exposed areas, 85% of them on the head and neck. Incidence increases with age; it is uncommon in those younger than 50 years and rare in young adults. Persons with light skin, blue eyes, and blonde hair are at greater risk because of their relative lack of natural photoprotection with melanin pigment.

Clinical Presentation

The patient is often unaware of these painless tumors because of their very slow growth rate. Frequently slight bleeding after minor trauma (e.g., face washing) brings the patient to the physician. The most common clinical appearance of a BCC is a discrete, smooth, pink papule or nodule with a translucent or pearly sheen, telangiectasias, and a rolled border. A central erosion or ulceration is often evident; however, the appearance may vary considerably. Superficial BCC may present as a thin, scaly, red plaque easily confused with eczema or tinea. Morpheaform BCC may appear similar to a yellow-white scar. Pigmented BCCs most often have a blue-black stippling or may have sufficient melanin to appear as a black nodule.

Differential Diagnosis

The common, nodular type of BCC has a distinctive appearance that is seldom missed because of its pearly sheen and central dell or ulceration (Fig. 83-1). At times, nodular BCC may resemble sebaceous adenoma or other appendage tumors. Superficial BCC is often mistaken for actinic keratosis, tinea, or eczema. Morpheaform BCC may resemble scar tissue, morphea, or chronic radiodermatitis. Pigmented BCC is infrequently confused with melanoma.

Diagnostic Approach

The diagnosis is not difficult to make clinically, but the skin biopsy provides confirmation.

Management and Therapy

Optimum Treatment

Basal cell carcinomas are slow-growing tumors, and treatment is usually not urgent. Metastasis is rare, but the tumor is capable of unrestricted growth causing local destruction; hence, complete ablation of the tumor is indicated. BCCs with morpheaform, infiltrating, or

Figure 83-1 Nodular Basal Cell Carcinoma.

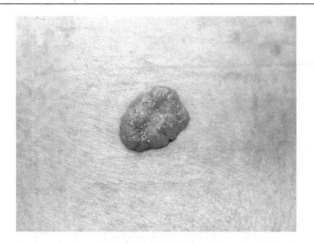

micronodular histopathologic patterns are more difficult to cure. Tumors in certain facial sites are more resistant to ablation regardless of the method used. High-risk areas include the medial canthus, nasolabial fold, alar crease, postauricular sulcus, and concha. The selection of the type of treatment requires consideration of several factors: the size and location of the tumor, its histologic subtype, ready access to and cost of the treatment, time frame available for treatment, skill of the physician, patient age, and intervening medical conditions. Guidelines for use of different modalities are as follows:

Curettage and electrofulguration: small tumors (<1 cm), sites not prone to high recurrence rates, nonaggressive histologic patterns, speed and ease of treatment, when secondary intention healing is adequate, to minimize cost

Cryosurgery: indications similar to those for curettage and electrofulguration

Radiation therapy: larger tumors, older patients, tissue conservation, to avoid disfiguring scars

Topical chemotherapy (5-fluorouracil): for superficial tumors only (in the epidermis and at the dermal-epidermal junction), to avoid or minimize scarring

Surgical excision: any size tumor, any location or histopathologic pattern, rapid healing, planned scar placement

Mohs chemosurgery (micrographic surgery): any size tumor, aggressive histopathologic patterns, sites prone to high recurrence rates, recurrent tumors, tissue conservation relative to traditional surgical excision

The prognosis for BCC is excellent. Overall, the 5-year cure rate for small, primary (i.e., previously untreated) BCCs is about 95%, regardless of the treatment used. Larger tumors, tumors in select sites, and tumors with certain histopathologic patterns will not have as high a cure rate.

Avoiding Treatment Errors

The simple expedient of performing a biopsy before definitive treatment will prevent most cases of undertreatment and overtreatment. The pathology report should comment on whether or not the tumor has a histopathologic pattern that warrants a particular treatment. For example, by obtaining a biopsy report that confirms an infiltrating pattern in the BCC, the physician will know to use a more aggressive treatment, such as scalpel excision or Mohs chemosurgery, and to avoid undertreatment with curettage and electrofulguration.

Another avoidable treatment error is selecting an appropriate treatment based on the location and size of the malignancy.

Future Directions

Newer treatment modalities for BCC include topical imiquimod, photodynamic therapy, and systemic retinoids. A greater impact will be felt from prevention programs: public education to limit sun exposure, use of topical sunscreens and protective clothing, increased skin cancer screening by physicians, patient awareness and self-screening, and cessation of tanning bed use.

SQUAMOUS CELL CARCINOMA
Etiology and Pathogenesis

Squamous cell carcinoma (SCC) is the second most common cutaneous malignancy with an incidence of 7 to 12 per 100,000 in the white population of the United States. It is a sun-associated tumor; acute sunburns and cumulative dose are both important in causation. Hence, these cancers are more likely to develop in those with blue eyes, blonde hair, and fair skin. Persons with outdoor occupations, those with heavy recreational sun exposure, and those living in semitropical or tropical regions are at greatest risk. Most SCCs probably arise from an antecedent lesion, the actinic keratosis, a premalignant focus of intraepidermal dysplasia brought about by chronic sun exposure. It is an erythematous, scaly lesion from a few millimeters to several centimeters in size. The scale may be so thick as to form a cutaneous horn. SCC in situ is referred to as Bowen's disease (Fig. 83-2).

Factors other than sunlight that can play a significant role in the pathogenesis include certain strains of human papillomavirus, especially in the periungual and genital regions, topical agents (tar, creosote, nitrogen mustard), and some ingested chemicals (arsenic). Any chronic inflammatory focus on the skin can lead to SCC, but usually the inflammation is present for years before the cancer forms; chronic discoid lupus erythematosus lesions and vascular ulcers are examples of cancer-inciting lesions. Old thermal burn scars and sites of therapeutic x-ray exposure are well

Figure 83-2 Bowen's Disease.

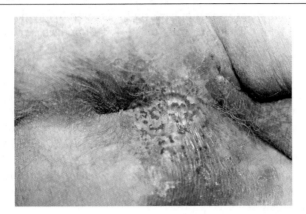

known to cause SCC decades after the initial injury or treatment.

Clinical Presentation

SCC presents as papules, nodules, or plaques, which are erythematous and hyperkeratotic (Fig. 83-3). Bowen's disease is a thin, pink, scaly plaque, which may mimic a superficial fungal infection or dermatitis; the scale may be thin or compact, yellow, and thick. Although the tumor begins in the epidermis and may remain superficial for a long time, ultimately it invades into the dermis, and even subcutaneous tissues, forming a deep nodular mass. Erosion of the epidermis or deeper ulceration may occur early or late. The growth rate is variable. It may grow slowly or may double in size in a matter of weeks. In an early, superficial phase, it may be indistinguishable from an actinic keratosis or eczema. Later, its malignant nature is more obvious when a deeper, ulcerated nodule develops. The clinical appearance of even the advanced SCC may not be sufficiently distinct from other, less common cutaneous malignancies; however, its localization in an area of sun-damaged skin or in an area of old burn injury or radiation dermatitis leads one to suspect the diagnosis.

Differential Diagnosis

SCC that is in situ can resemble actinic keratosis, eczema, dermatophytosis, or in the perineum, extramammary Paget's disease. Invasive SCC must be differentiated from actinic keratosis, keratoacanthoma, granulomas, and a wide variety of benign and malignant, primary and metastatic, cutaneous tumors.

Diagnostic Approach

A definitive diagnosis can seldom be made on the basis of clinical examination alone. Skin biopsy should always be done.

Figure 83-3 Squamous Cell Carcinoma.

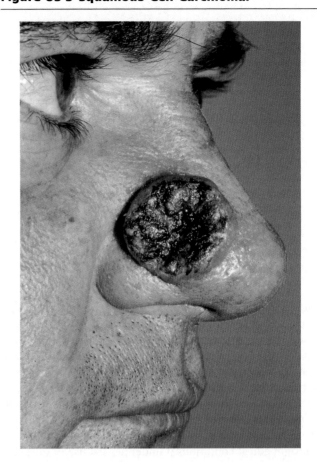

Management and Therapy

Optimum Treatment

The modalities and the criteria for selection used in the treatment of BCC are also used for SCC. The prognosis for SCC of the skin is good. Five-year cures are greater than 90% overall, although rates for larger and more deeply invasive tumors are lower. Metastases are not rare, approaching 3% to 4%. Tumors on the ears and lips and those that develop in thermal burn or radiation treatment sites are particularly likely to metastasize.

Avoiding Treatment Errors

Obtaining a definitive biopsy diagnosis is important before undertaking tumor ablation. The physician must also recognize that the treatment technique needs to be customized for the size and location of the carcinoma.

Future Directions

As in the case of BCC, prevention programs will have the greatest impact on this disease. Pathogenesis-based therapies under investigation include cyclooxygenase inhibitors, topical immunomodulators, and inhibitors of hedgehog signaling.

MELANOMAS

Etiology and Pathogenesis

Melanomas develop in fair-skinned people most frequently; they are unusual in dark-skinned people. In 1% to 6% of cases, there is a familial history. Patients with large numbers of nevocellular nevi may have an increased risk, especially if some of those nevi are dysplastic. Melanomas develop in normal-appearing skin most often but may evolve from a preexisting nevus of either the congenital or acquired type. History of perceptible change in any pigmented lesion is of paramount importance. Although there is an association between melanomas and sun exposure, it is quite common for melanomas to develop on relatively sun-protected sites; head and neck, torso, and upper and lower extremities are all common sites. Usually, they first appear as nonpalpable, pigmented lesions. Their innocuous appearance and small size cause them to be overlooked or thought of as a "mole" or "age spot." They expand laterally at the dermal-epidermal junction, and increasing diameter or perimeter irregularities prompt the patient or the physician to be suspicious. Eventually they change from macular, nonpalpable, lesions to nodular lesions.

The rate of melanoma diagnosis has doubled since 1986. Yet there is no change in the melanoma death rate, nor is there a change in the incidence of advanced disease. Some authors contend that there is not an epidemic of melanomas but an epidemic of biopsies and diagnoses.

Clinical Presentation

On examination, one usually sees a pigmented lesion with color that may vary from light brown to black, but areas of red or white are not rare (Fig. 83-4). The size of the lesion can vary from a few millimeters to several centimeters, and borders are usually irregular and indistinct. Ulceration is a late change. The natural variation in the appearance of benign, nevocellular nevi makes the diagnosis difficult.

Differential Diagnosis

Melanoma most often must be differentiated from benign, congenital, or dysplastic nevi; seborrheic keratosis; tattoo; foreign body; or in the case of amelanotic melanoma, pyogenic granuloma.

Diagnostic Approach

Several tools have been developed recently to more precisely define melanomas. Epiluminescence is the use of an illuminated magnifying lens to examine lesions for subtle variations in pigment pattern, which might indicate malignancy. Digital epiluminescence microscopy is available to store and compare images of suspicious lesions. Ultimately, the diagnosis is made histopathologically after a biopsy specimen is taken. Incisional biopsy of a portion of a melanoma does not predispose to metastasis or worsen prognosis; however, it is important to get a representative specimen to make a diagnosis and aid in prognosis. A shave biopsy should not be done because it may not provide the opportunity to assess the depth of invasion of the melanoma. The dermatopathologist will make the diagnosis of melanoma and assess a level of invasion. A number of subclassifications exist, with corresponding histopathologic and clinical features: lentigo maligna melanoma, nodular melanoma, superficial spreading melanoma, acral lentiginous melanoma, and desmoplastic melanoma. These classifications are less important than the level of invasion in planning treatment and assessing prognosis.

Management and Therapy

Optimal Treatment

The treatment of melanomas is surgical. The extent of surgery depends on the location, size, and depth of invasion of the melanoma. A microstaging is done at biopsy to determine the histopathologic level of invasion, measured in millimeters (Breslow levels). The Breslow level is the single most important predictor of survival for patients with melanoma. Patients with tumors less than 0.76 mm thick have a 96% 5-year survival rate, whereas patients with tumors greater than 4 mm have a 47% chance of 5-year survival. Larger melanomas, deeper melanomas, and melanomas on the head, neck, hands, and feet require wider margins of excision. The Breslow level determines the margin of excision: in general, in situ melanomas are excised with 0.5- to 1.0-cm margins, tumors with levels less than 1 mm are excised with 1.0-cm margins of clinically normal skin; tumors with levels of 1 to 2 mm are

Figure 83-4 Melanoma.

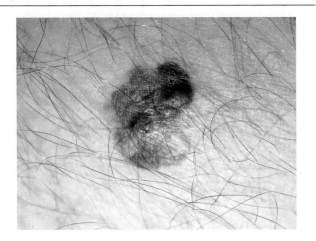

excised with 1- to 2-cm margins, and tumors with levels greater than 2 mm get 2- to 2.5-cm margins.

Additional Treatment

Elective lymph node dissection for patients with melanoma confined to the skin has not been shown to improve survival. It may improve survival if there are clinically involved regional lymph nodes. Sentinel lymph node biopsy uses lymphoscintigraphy to determine the first ("sentinel") node in a regional basin with subsequent biopsy of that node to search for metastatic foci. This is a useful staging procedure but imparts no survival benefit for the patient and is not the standard of care. Interferon-α_{2b} for patients with metastatic disease has been approved by the U.S. Food and Drug Administration, although no statistically significant benefit has been demonstrated in prospective trials. Numerous tumor vaccine therapy trials are ongoing, but no systemic adjuvant therapy provides survival benefit yet.

Avoiding Treatment Errors

The most common error in the treatment of pigmented lesions is failure to accurately diagnose the lesion. Melanomas can clinically mimic several different benign pigmented lesions, and vice versa. Skin biopsy is essential before treatment. Further error can be avoided if the biopsy removes the entire lesion, thereby eliminating the chance of sampling error wherein a nonrepresentative portion of the lesion only is examined.

Follow-Up Care

Patients who have had a BCC or a SCC should be observed for 5 years with routine skin examinations and palpation for lymph nodes to check for recurrence of the tumors as well as surveillance for the development of new, primary cutaneous malignancies. About 30% to 50% of patients with skin cancer experience another, separate skin cancer within a few years. The frequency of the follow-up examinations varies depending on the character of the initial tumor, the level of sun damage, and precancerous change.

Patients who have had a melanoma should undergo lifelong follow-up to check for recurrence or the development of second primary melanomas, which may occur in as many as 8% of patients. Initially, check-up visits should be no longer than every 6 months, extending to 12 months in later postoperative years. Patients with a family history of melanoma and dysplastic nevi should be observed more closely. Screening for occult metastases from early melanomas is generally not warranted, although chest x-rays are often obtained in patients with thicker melanomas.

All patients should be educated about the risks of sun exposure and need to use sunscreens that have sun protection factor of 15 or higher and provide ultraviolet A and B protection. Instruction in self-examination should also be a routine part of follow-up care.

FUTURE DIRECTIONS

Although the principal treatment for all skin cancers remains surgical ablation, several new treatment modalities are under investigation. Photodynamic therapy uses a systemic or topical application of a photosensitizing chemical followed by intense or laser light to the area to bring about a more or less selective destruction of the tumor tissue with relative sparing of adjacent tissue. Immunomodulators are currently under investigation. Imiquimod, a heterocyclic amine, has shown potent antiviral and antitumor action both experimentally and in recent clinical trials. The role of radiation therapy is being revisited because some melanomas have been shown to be radiosensitive.

Additional Resources

Giblin AV, Thomas JM: Incidence, mortality and survival in cutaneous melanoma. J Plast Reconstr Aesthet Surg 60(1):32-40, 2007; Epub July 7, 2006.
  This literature-based review also addresses etiology and public awareness issues.
Gloster HM Jr, Neal K: Skin cancer in skin of color. J Am Acad Dermatol 55(5):741-760, 2006.
  Although far more common in whites, skin cancer in dark-skinned people is not rare and may have greater morbidity and mortality.
Lewis KG, Jellinek N, Robinson-Bostom L: Skin cancer after transplantation: A guide for the general surgeon. Surg Clin North Am 86(5):1257-1276, viii, 2006.
  This review addresses the difficult management issues for skin cancer in the transplant population.

EVIDENCE

1. Balch CM, Soong SJ, Bartolucci AA, et al: Efficacy of an elective regional lymph node dissection of 1 to 4 mm thick melanomas for patients 60 years of age and younger. Ann Surg 224:255-266, 1996.
  This article documents that overall 5-year survival is not any better after elective node dissection, but some advantage is shown in a subset of patients younger than 60 years.
2. Buzaid AC, Ross MI, Balch CM, et al: Critical analysis of the current American Joint Committee on Cancer staging system for cutaneous melanoma and proposal of a new staging system. J Clin Oncol 15:1039-1051, 1997.
  This article demonstrates that tumor thickness and ulceration remain the most important factors in prognosis.
4. Johnson TM, Sondak VK, Bichakjian CK, et al: The role of sentinel node biopsy for melanoma: Evidence assessment. J Am Acad Dermatol 54:19-27, 2006.
  The author notes that "no conclusive or high-level evidence exists that a positive sentinel lymph node biopsy (SLNB) followed by immediate complete lymph node dissection (CLND) improves overall survival in patients with melanoma."
5. Kanzler MH, Mraz-Gernhard S: Treatment of primary cutaneous melanoma. JAMA 285:1819-1821, 2001.
  This article presents a succinct summary of the current surgical options in the treatment of melanoma.

6. Martinez JC, Otley CC: The management of melanoma and nonmelanoma skin cancer: A review for the primary care physician. Mayo Clin Proc 76:1253-1265, 2001.

The authors address reasonable approaches for the primary care physician.

7. MEDLINEplus Health Information: Skin cancer. 2002. Available at: http://www.nlm.nih.gov/medlineplus/skincancer.html. Accessed December 14, 2002.

This website contains a wealth of information regarding all types of skin cancer suitable for the physician and for patients.

8. Morton DL, Thompson JF, Cochran AJ, et al: Sentinel-node biopsy or nodal observation in melanoma. N Engl J Med 355:1307-1317, 2006.

The authors show that the melanoma-specific survival rates were similar in the two groups.

9. National Institutes of Health Consensus Development Conference Statement on Diagnosis and Treatment of Early Melanoma. January 27-29, 1992. Am J Dermatopathol 15:34-43, 1993.

This article represents a good summary of expert opinion.

10. Randle HW: Basal cell carcinoma. Identification and treatment of the high-risk patient. Dermatol Surg 22:255-261, 1996.

The author identifies basal cell carcinomas that have features putting the patient at greater risk for recurrence and those that should lead the clinician to more aggressive treatment and follow-up.

11. Skin Cancer Foundation. Available at: http://www.skincancer. org. Accessed December 15, 2002.

This website is a valuable source of information for patients concerning all types of skin cancer, including their prevention and treatment.

12. Szepietowski JC, Salomon J: Typical and atypical locations of basal-cell carcinoma: Relationship with clinical and histological types. Skin Cancer 15(4):193-200, 2000.

This is a reasonable guide to the subtypes of basal cell carcinoma and their management.

13. Welch, HG, Woloshin S, Schwartz LM: Skin biopsy rates and incidence of melanoma: Population-based ecological study. BMJ 331(7515):481, 2005.

The authors conclude: "increased incidence [of melanoma] being largely the result of increased diagnostic scrutiny and not an increase in the incidence of disease."

14. Verma, S, Quirt I, McCready D, et al: Systematic review of systemic adjuvant therapy for patients at high risk for recurrent melanoma. Cancer 106(7):1431-1442, 2006.

These authors suggest that high-dose interferon can give a reduction in 2-year mortality but stop short of claiming any benefit in sentinel lymph node–positive patients.

Allen F. Marshall ▪ William W. Shockley

84

Cancer of the Oral Cavity and Oropharynx

Introduction

The oral cavity and oropharynx are among the most common sites of head and neck cancer. In the United States, there are 30,000 new cases of cancer arising in these sites, accounting for 8000 deaths per year. In developing nations, these numbers are much higher, with oral cavity cancer being the third most common malignancy after cervical and gastric cancers. Squamous cell carcinoma (SCC) accounts for greater than 90% of oral cavity and oropharyngeal malignancies followed by minor salivary gland malignancies in the oral cavity and lymphoma in the oropharynx. Discussion in this chapter is limited to SCC of the oral cavity and oropharynx.

Etiology and Pathogenesis

The oral cavity is defined as the region beginning at the vermilion border of the lip extending posteriorly to the end of the hard palate superiorly, the circumvallate papillae inferiorly, and the anterior tonsillar pillars laterally. Subsites of the oral cavity are the lips, buccal mucosa, gingiva and alveolar ridge, hard palate, floor of the mouth, retromolar trigone, and anterior two thirds of the tongue. The oropharynx begins at the posterior border of the oral cavity and extends posteriorly to the posterior pharyngeal wall, inferiorly to the epiglottis, and superiorly to the soft palate. Subsites of the oropharynx are the base of the tongue (posterior one third), lateral and posterior pharyngeal walls, tonsillar area (including pharyngeal tonsils, tonsillar pillars, and tonsillar fossae), and soft palate. Together, the oral cavity and oropharynx have important roles in airway protection, deglutition, and communication. Loss or compromise of these functions increases with tumor extent, and preservation of these functions is an important principle in treatment.

Alcohol consumption and cigarette use are the primary risk factors in the development of SCC of the head and neck. In fact, 75% of oral cancers are associated with alcohol and tobacco use. Smoking confers a 1.9-fold risk to males and a 3.0-fold risk to females for developing head and neck cancer. The risk is proportional to pack-years and drinks per day. Other forms of tobacco use, including cigar smoking, pipe smoking, and smokeless tobacco, are also associated with these lesions. Although alcohol consumption and tobacco use are accepted independent risk factors for SCC, their concurrent use results in a synergistic effect with an even greater propensity for malignancy. Induction of *p53* mutations in the oropharyngeal mucosa has been described in patients with an alcohol and tobacco history. Popular in India and Southeast Asia, the long-term use of betel nut quid, a mixture of cured tobacco and the product of *Areca catechu* tree, is also a known risk factor. Additionally, multiple studies have shown an association between human papillomavirus and a subset of SCC. Although it is included in discussion of oral cavity carcinoma, SCC of the lip differs from other oral cavity SCCs in that ultraviolet radiation exposure is the primary risk factor. Other associations include long-term immunosuppression and tertiary syphilis.

Clinical Presentation

SCC of the oral cavity and oropharynx can present in a variety of ways. The patient may experience seemingly innocuous persistent mouth or throat symptoms. Some patients may notice a new mouth or throat lesion. With clinical suspicion, careful attention is placed on the history. The presence of bleeding, halitosis, dysphagia, odynophagia, dysarthria, paresthesias, oral-dental pain, otalgia, poor fitting dentures, trismus, or weight loss is noted. A history of cigarette smoking or alcohol use should alert the clinician that the patient is at high risk for SCC of the oral cavity and oropharynx.

Thorough physical examination should incorporate the use of a headlight and dental mirrors to facilitate examination of all mucosal surfaces in the oral cavity and oropharynx. Lesions of the retromolar trigone and anterior floor of mouth are missed most often during cursory examination because of their location behind the teeth. A tongue blade is instrumental in examining these "hidden" lesions. After examination of all mucosal surfaces, palpation of the floor of the mouth, tongue, base of the tongue, and tonsillar region should be performed. Palpable masses, areas of induration, ulceration, and tenderness should alert the clinician to the possibility of malignancy. Upon palpation, the extent of fixation to underlying periosteum should be noted, indicating mandibular or maxillary involvement. Cranial nerve function should be documented with particular attention to the hypoglossal nerve as well as the mandibular and lingual branches of the trigeminal nerve. Trismus may indicate invasion of the muscles of mastication. Examination of the neck for lymphadenopathy should always be performed.

Oral Cavity

Oral cavity SCC most commonly arises in the tongue (30% to 40%), lips (25% to 30%), and floor of mouth (15%). Within the oral cavity, SCC is likely to present as a nonhealing ulcer, an exophytic lesion, or an indurated infiltrating mass. Of primary tongue lesions, posterolateral oral tongue (75%) and anterolateral tongue (20%) are most common (Fig. 84-1). These tumors are often asymptomatic until advanced stages, when they present with pain, bleeding, dysphagia, loose teeth, or difficulty with articulation.

SCC of the lip (see Fig. 84-1) presents as a nonhealing, crusting, ulcerative lesion or a scaly, hyperkeratotic lesion of the vermilion; about 90% occur on the lower lip as a result of increased sun exposure. The most common age range for patients with SCC of the lip is 50 to 70 years.

Primary malignancy of the maxillary and mandibular gingival ridges represents 10% of all oral cavity cancers, with a mean age of 66.7 years. Invasion of tumor into bone at presentation is not uncommon because the gingiva closely approximates it.

A palpable neck mass representative of metastasis to a cervical lymph node is present on initial evaluation in 15% to 30% of patients with oral cavity SCC (Fig. 84-2). However, neck metastases are less frequent (10%) with SCC of the lower lip. Submental and submandibular lymph nodes are the first-echelon drainage for most of the oral cavity, and these regions are most likely to be involved when metastasis is present. The upper deep jugular lymph nodes are also often involved. Because of the rich lymphatic drainage and near midline position of many oral cavity cancers, bilateral or contralateral cervical metastases are relatively common.

Oropharynx

Oropharyngeal tumors typically appear as ulcerative or infiltrating mucosal lesions. SCC of the base of the tongue (see Fig. 84-2) is often not visible during routine physical examination and is noticeable only on palpation. The most common sites for oropharyngeal SCC are the tonsil and the anterior tonsillar pillar. To a greater extent than its counterpart in the oral cavity, SCC of the oropharynx remains asymptomatic until the disease is advanced. The most common presenting symptoms are pain and dysphagia. In more advanced cases, these symptoms can be accompanied by dysarthria, referred otalgia, weight loss, hemoptysis, hoarseness, and stridor. Cervical metastases are identifiable upon presentation in up to 60% of patients and are most commonly seen in the deep jugular nodes.

Differential Diagnosis

Differential diagnosis includes inflammatory processes and benign lesions (see Chapter 11), salivary gland neoplasms (adenoid cystic carcinoma, mucoepidermoid carcinoma, and adenocarcinoma), lymphoma (primarily with tonsillar involvement), and sinonasal malignancies, which may erode into the oral cavity and oropharynx.

The concept of *field cancerization*, where widespread epithelial dysplasia occurs in high-risk individuals, applies to SCC of the upper aerodigestive tract. The incidence of synchronous primary SCC for the upper aerodigestive is reported between 3% and 15%.

Premalignant lesions should be recognized and followed closely because early identification of asymptomatic lesions is associated with much lower morbidity and mortality. Erythroplakia is the most important premalignant lesion of the oral cavity and oropharynx. Generally seen as a red, slightly raised lesion or a smooth, atrophic red lesion, erythroplakia is associated with a 90% chance of representing dysplasia, carcinoma in situ, or SCC at the time of presentation. Erythroplakia may also represent an inflammatory lesion of the mucosa, and management includes removal of irritating factors and treatment of infection, with follow-up in 10 to 14 days. If the lesion has not resolved, incisional biopsy of the periphery of the lesion is recommended to rule out carcinoma.

Leukoplakia (Fig. 84-3), defined as a white patch of mucosa not associated with any other disease, is associated with less than 5% malignant transformation. Management of leukoplakia involves serial examination by the clinician. Biopsy is necessary only for lesions that undergo rapid growth, become symptomatic, or are otherwise clinically suspicious. Lichen planus (LP) is associated with malignancy rarely (3% to 5%), and observation or symptomatic treatment is adequate for most cases. Erosive LP occasionally merits biopsy for diagnosis because this subtype is more likely to be associated with oral cancer. Like leukoplakia, all suspicious areas of LP should undergo biopsy. ▪

Figure 84-1 Malignant Tumors of Oral Cavity.

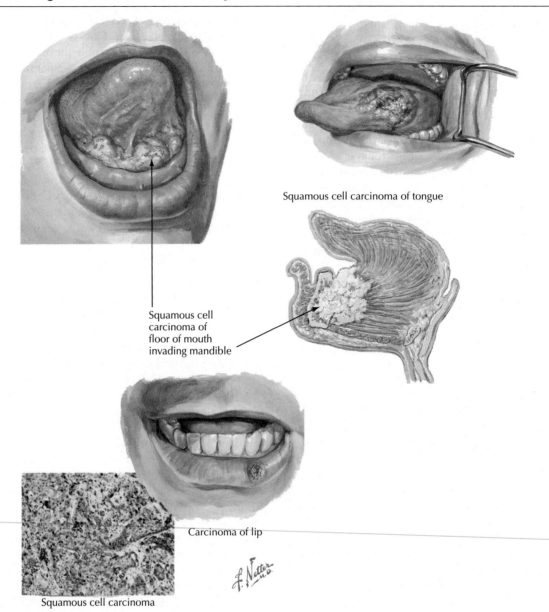

Squamous cell carcinoma of tongue

Squamous cell carcinoma of floor of mouth invading mandible

Carcinoma of lip

Squamous cell carcinoma

Diagnostic Approach

A thorough history and physical examination is the most important step in diagnosis of lesions of the oral cavity and oropharynx. Early diagnosis is of paramount importance because small, asymptomatic lesions may be treated with a high rate of cure, with minimal morbidity. Once lesions become symptomatic, the cure rate drops, and the morbidity of treatment modalities increases dramatically.

After treatment for 10 to 14 days and removal of irritants, the lesion should be reevaluated. If substantial improvement has not occurred, biopsy is indicated. Sore throat unresponsive to medical treatment, otalgia without evidence of ear disease, and unexplained dysphagia should receive further workup. Biopsy of suspicious lesions may be performed under local anesthesia if the lesion is easily accessible. Biopsy should not be excisional and should include a section of the lesion as well as a small portion of adjacent normal-appearing mucosa. Biopsy of oropharyngeal lesions may be difficult to perform without general anesthesia.

Management and Therapy

Management

If the lesion is a superficial early SCC of the oral cavity, excision without extended workup may be appropriate. Otherwise, once the diagnosis is confirmed or strongly suspected, the patient should undergo panendoscopy (laryngoscopy, bronchoscopy, and esophagoscopy) to rule out a second primary SCC of the upper aerodigestive tract. A second primary will occur in as many as 15% of patients with SCC of the oral cavity or oropharynx. Preoperative

Figure 84-2 Malignant Tumors of Oropharynx.

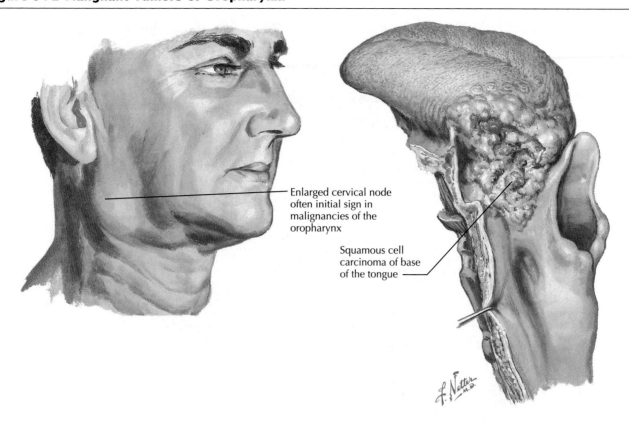

Enlarged cervical node often initial sign in malignancies of the oropharynx

Squamous cell carcinoma of base of the tongue

studies include a chest radiograph and liver function tests to rule out distant metastasis or synchronous lung cancer. Radiographic evaluation of the mandible with a dental x-ray is indicated in some oral cavity cancers. Computed tomography (CT) or magnetic resonance imaging (MRI) may be indicated to better define the location and extent of the tumor and cervical metastases. Generally, contrast-enhanced CT of the neck (from skull base to clavicles) is most useful and expedient. Exceptions include cancer at the base of the tongue or suspicion of perineural invasion, when tissue planes are better imaged with MRI. On occasion, these imaging studies identify pathologic lymph nodes not palpable on physical examination.

Tumor staging is the most reliable predictor of prognosis. Staging using the tumor-node-metastasis (TNM) system is performed according to the guidelines of the American Joint Committee on Cancer (Table 84-1). T1 and early T2 lesions have an associated 60% to 95% 5-year survival rate when no cervical metastases are present. The presence of cervical metastasis results in a worse prognosis, with only 25% to 40% 5-year survival rate. More advanced disease (T3 and T4 lesions) carries 5-year survival rates of 11% to 40%. In general, oropharyngeal cancers have a worse prognosis than oral cavity tumors.

Other considerations in prognosis include tumor thickness and patient age. Tumor thickness has recently been shown to affect prognosis of oral cavity SCCs, with lesions more than 5 mm thick associated with significantly lower 5-year survival rates. Presence of SCC in young patients (<35 years old) is generally a poor prognostic indicator, with most of these tumors representing aggressive disease.

Optimum Treatment

Precise staging is essential to developing an appropriate treatment plan. Treatment is comprised of surgical excision, radiation therapy, and combined modalities. Chemotherapy alone has not been shown to have curative potential in SCC of the head and neck but does have a role in palliation of advanced disease.

Early lesions (T1 and early T2) are generally amenable to single-modality treatment. Surgical resection with a wide margin (1 to 2 cm) of excision is the treatment of choice for most of these lesions. Radiation provides an alternative for patients in poor health or in whom surgical morbidity is deemed too great. Advanced lesions (infiltrative T2, and all T3 and T4) require combined modality treatment. In the oral cavity, resection is accompanied by postoperative radiation treatment. Advanced oropharyngeal SCC is treated with combined chemotherapy and radiation or resection and adjuvant radiation therapy. Tonsillar and base of tongue tumors appear to be particularly amenable to combined chemoradiation as the primary treatment.

Treatment depends on the size of the primary tumor and the presence of nodal disease. Patients with early lesions and no clinical evidence of lymphatic spread may be followed closely without specific therapy directed to the

Figure 84-3 Leukoplakia.

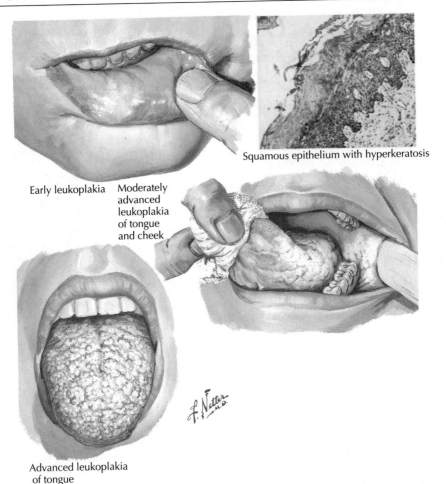

Squamous epithelium with hyperkeratosis

Early leukoplakia   Moderately advanced leukoplakia of tongue and cheek

Advanced leukoplakia of tongue

cervical lymph nodes. For more advanced disease, neck dissection with removal of lymph nodes at risk or radiation of the neck is required, even in the absence of clinically evident cervical metastasis. Presence of enlarged cervical lymph nodes requires neck dissection and adjuvant radiation treatment.

Treatment for advanced cancer of the oral cavity and oropharynx often results in functional loss. Primary radiation, or organ preservation therapy, followed by surgical excision of residual disease may result in decreased long-term morbidity. Despite continued improvement in treatment modalities and reconstructive techniques, dysphagia, dysarthria, and aspiration may occur after treatment. Patients often require tracheostomy and feeding tubes in the immediate postoperative period, and some require one or both for an extended period. Xerostomia, mucositis, fibrosis, lymphedema, and dysphagia are common side effects of radiation treatment.

Avoiding Treatment Errors

Early recognition of the signs and symptoms of oral cavity and oropharyngeal carcinoma is critical to optimum treatment. Referral to an otolaryngologist in a timely manner will assist proper diagnosis and management. A neck mass should not be excised without a thorough head and neck exam to establish a primary site. A complete head and neck exam includes performing an office flexible fiber-optic laryngoscopy to assess extent of tumor and possible presence of second primary. Fine-needle aspirate of a neck mass with unknown primary will also aid in the diagnosis and management before surgical excision.

Future Directions

Several new chemotherapeutic agents such as epidermal growth factor receptor inhibitors show promise as adjuvant therapies for head and neck cancer. Other areas of promise include the use of intraoperative radiation. Gene micro-array analysis has a promising role in identification of tissue biomarkers used to identify patients who are at risk for head and neck SCC or those who might benefit from certain treatment modalities. In the surgical realm, sentinel node biopsy is being evaluated as an alternative to neck dissection in patients with larger primary lesions and no evidence of nodal spread.

Although many new therapeutic options may soon be available, the role of tobacco and alcohol use in the devel-

Table 84-1 AJCC Staging of Oral Cavity and Oropharyngeal Cancer

Primary Tumor (T)	Oropharyngeal Cancer
TX: Primary tumor cannot be assessed	T1: Tumor diameter <2 cm in greatest dimension
T0: No evidence of primary tumor	T2: Tumor diameter >2 cm, but not >4 cm
Tis: Carcinoma in situ	T3: Tumor diameter >4 cm
T1: 2 cm or less	T4a: Tumor invades the larynx, deep or extrinsic muscle of tongue, medial pterygoid, hard palate, or mandible
T2: Tumor more than 2 cm but not more than 4 cm	
T3: More than 4 cm	T4b: Tumor invades lateral pterygoid muscle, pterygoid plates, lateral nasopharynx, or skull base or encases carotid artery
T4 (lip): Tumor invades adjacent structures (e.g., through cortical bone, inferior alveolar nerve, floor of mouth, skin of face)	
T4a (oral cavity): Tumor invades adjacent structures (e.g., through cortical bone, into deep (extrinsic) muscle of tongue, maxillary sinus, skin	
T4b (oral cavity): Tumor invades masticator space, pterygoid plates, or skull base or encases the internal carotid artery	

Regional Lymph Nodes (N)	Distant Metastases (M)
NX: Regional lymph nodes cannot be assessed	MX: Distant metastasis cannot be assessed
N0: No regional lymph node metastasis	M0: No distant metastases
N1: Metastasis in a single ipsilateral lymph node, <3 cm in greatest dimension	M1: Distant metastases present
N2: Metastasis in a single ipsilateral lymph node, >3 cm but not >6 cm in greatest dimension; or in multiple ipsilateral lymph nodes, none >6 cm in greatest dimension; or in bilateral or contralateral lymph nodes, none more than 6 cm in greatest dimension	
N2a: Metastasis in a single ipsilateral lymph node, >3 cm but not >6 cm in greatest dimension	
N2b: Metastasis in multiple ipsilateral lymph nodes, none >6 cm in greatest dimension	
N2c: Metastasis in bilateral or contralateral lymph nodes, none >6 cm in greatest dimension	
N3: Metastasis in a lymph node, >6 cm in greatest dimension	

AJCC, American Joint Committee on Cancer.
From the American Joint Committee on Cancer: AJCC Cancer Staging Manual, 6th ed. New York, Springer-Verlag, 2002.

opment of oral and oropharyngeal cancer cannot be over-emphasized. Avoidance of these risk factors is the most effective measure in reducing the incidence of head and neck cancer, and the clinician should take the responsibility of patient education as seriously as diagnosis and treatment.

Additional Resources

Spiegel JH, Jalisi S: Contemporary diagnosis and management of head and neck cancer. Otolaryngol Clin North Am 38(1): xiii-xiv, 2005.
This collection of papers focuses on the newest and latest algorithms for diagnosis and treatment of head and neck cancer.

Warner GC, Reis PP, Makitie AA, et al: Current applications of microarrays in head and neck cancer research. Laryngoscope 114(2):241-248, 2004.
This article provides an introduction to microarray technology and how it is currently being applied to head and neck cancer research.

EVIDENCE

1. Gassner HG, Sabri AN, Olsen KD: Oropharyngeal malignancy. In Cummings CW, Haughey BH, Thomas JR, et al (eds): Cum-

mings Otolaryngology Head and Neck Surgery, 4th ed. Philadelphia, Elsevier Mosby, 2005 pp 1717-1757.
This chapter in a core otolaryngology text is an in-depth review of the diagnosis and management of oropharyngeal cancer.

2. Mashberg A, Samit A: Early diagnosis of asymptomatic oral and oropharyngeal squamous cancers. CA Cancer J Clin 45(6):328-351, 1995.
This important paper addresses diagnosing oral and oropharyngeal SCC in the asymptomatic patient by assessing risk factors and performing a thorough directed physical exam. Management of precancerous lesions and the use of toluidine blue staining are discussed.

3. Prince S, Bailey BM: Squamous carcinoma of the tongue: Review. Br J Oral Maxillofac Surg 37(3):164-174, 1999.
The authors present a good review of cancer confined to the tongue with a focus on prognosis and outcomes.

4. Summerlin DJ: Precancerous and cancerous lesions of the oral cavity. Dermatol Clin 14(2):205-223, 1996.
This paper guides the reader to a greater understanding of the clinicopathologic appearance of oral cavity cancers and precancers.

5. Wein RO, Weber RS: Malignant neoplasms of the oral cavity. In Cummings CW, Haughey BH, Thomas JR, et al (eds): Cummings Otolaryngology Head and Neck Surgery, 4th ed. Philadelphia, Elsevier Mosby, 2005, pp 1579-1617.
This chapter in a core otolaryngology text is an in-depth review of the diagnosis and management of oral cavity cancer.

John F. Boggess ▪ Victoria Lin Bae-Jump

Cervical Neoplasia

Introduction

Since its adoption in the United States in the 1940s, universal screening using the Papanicolaou (Pap) test has decreased death from cervical cancer by more than 70%. Cervical cancer screening is the most successful cancer screening program in history.

Although the Pap smear has reduced cervical cancer deaths in the United States, many challenges remain. The most significant barrier is lack of compliance with screening recommendations, particularly in older women, the uninsured, ethnic minorities, and women in rural areas. In the United States, 50% to 70% of cervical cancer cases occur among women who have never been screened or who have not been screened within the past 5 years. Significant racial disparity exists in both incidence and death from cervical cancer, with the highest-risk ethnic group being Vietnamese women. Although cervical cancer accounts for only 2% of all cancer deaths in women, it ranks second among women aged 20 to 39 years.

Prevention of cervical cancer and cervical cancer mortality is feasible because (1) progression from early cellular abnormalities, termed low-grade dysplasia (LGSIL), through more severe dysplasia (high-grade dysplasia [HGSIL]), to carcinoma in situ (CIS) and invasive cancer is generally slow, allowing time for detection; (2) associated cellular abnormalities can be identified; and (3) effective treatment is available for premalignant lesions. Although screening has been successful in reducing squamous cancer incidence and mortality, the incidence of glandular or adenocarcinoma is increasing.

Etiology and Pathogenesis

Most cervical cancer develops within the cervical transformation zone, the region where the epithelial cells of the cervix and vagina undergo metaplastic transformation to the columnar epithelium that lines the endocervical glands. Figure 85-1 demonstrates the findings in this area, visualized during colposcopy. The susceptibility of women to squamous cancer is due to the fragility of this tissue in combination with its direct exposure to environmental carcinogens, the most important being the human papilloma virus (HPV).

HPV plays a central role in the development of cervical cancer. Ninety-five percent to 99% of squamous cell cervical cancers and 75% to 95% of high-grade CIN lesions have detectable HPV DNA. HPV is transmitted primarily by sexual intercourse and can persist in vulvar, vaginal, and cervical tissue throughout a woman's lifetime. As a group of more than 100 viral types, HPV viruses cause a diverse spectrum of diseases. HPV types 6 and 11 cause warts, and types 16 and 18 cause cancer. Among women without cervical cytology abnormalities at baseline, those with high-risk HPV types have a relative risk for developing high-grade cervical lesions that is 58- to 71-fold higher than those without detectable HPV.

HPV DNA must integrate into the host genomic DNA to promote the changes that lead to cervical cancer. This event appears to be rare, but it is essential for cancer progression. In the absence of viral integration, the normal viral life cycle produces morphologic changes in the cervical epithelium characteristic of LGSIL. With viral integration, cellular changes characteristic of HGSIL and ultimately cancer are observed (Fig. 85-2). Interrelated host factors such as age, nutritional status, immune function, smoking, and possibly silent genetic polymorphisms modulate incorporation of viral DNA. It is estimated that nearly 100% of CIS and cancer lesions have integrated HPV DNA compared with a small minority of low-grade dysplastic lesions. The transition time from simple viral infection to integration of DNA and oncogenesis is unknown and may be influenced by the patient's risk profile. Natural history studies confirm that, in most cases,

Figure 85-1 Colposcopy.

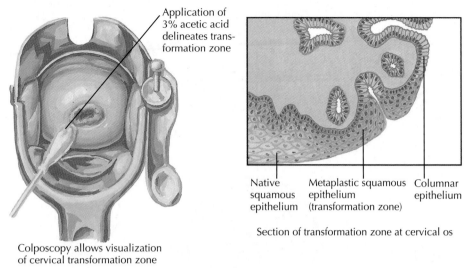

Application of 3% acetic acid delineates transformation zone

Colposcopy allows visualization of cervical transformation zone

Native squamous epithelium | Metaplastic squamous epithelium (transformation zone) | Columnar epithelium

Section of transformation zone at cervical os

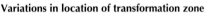

Variations in location of transformation zone

Prepubertal | Reproductive | Postmenopausal

Exocervical | Exocervical | Endocervical

Features of normal transformation zone

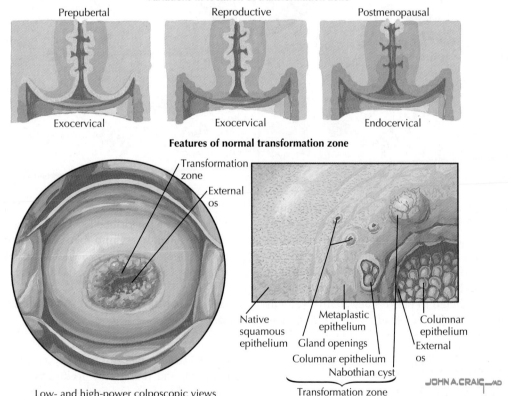

Transformation zone

External os

Low- and high-power colposcopic views of normal transformation zone

Native squamous epithelium | Metaplastic epithelium | Gland openings | Columnar epithelium | Nabothian cyst | Columnar epithelium | External os

Transformation zone

JOHN A. CRAIG—AD

the course of infection and cervical abnormalities progress in an orderly fashion from less to more severe lesions. Thus, the sequence of changes associated with HPV infection and the development of cervical cancer parallel the cytologic changes observed and are amenable to surveillance with Pap tests.

In the United States, peak incidence and prevalence of HPV infection occurs among women younger than 25 years; however, more than 30% of postmenopausal women have detectable HPV DNA using polymerase chain reac-

tion detection methods. Because most cervical cancers are associated with HPV infection, independent of age of cancer incidence, screening for epithelial changes caused by the virus is indicated in all age groups.

Clinical Presentation

Cervical cancer develops a clinically visible lesion when invasive, and, when deeply invasive, it spreads by local extension, through lymphatics or the bloodstream (Fig.

Figure 85-2 Cervical Cell Pathology in Squamous Tissue.

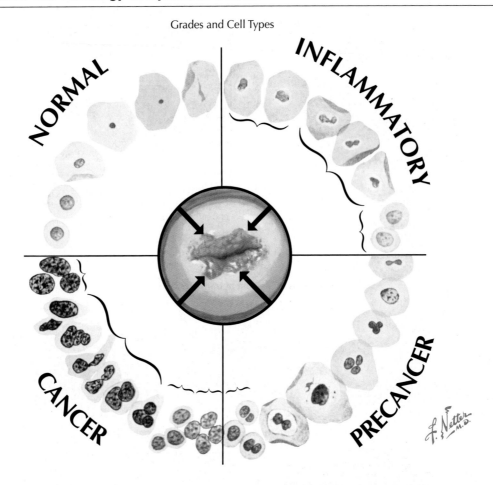

Grades and Cell Types

NORMAL

INFLAMMATORY

CANCER

PRECANCER

85-3). Preinvasive cervical neoplasias are rarely associated with symptoms. With progression to invasive cervical cancer, women are more likely to complain of abnormal vaginal discharge and intermenstrual bleeding, specifically after douching or coitus. Pain, loss of appetite, and weight loss are all late manifestations. Back pain may indicate ureteral obstruction related to pelvic sidewall involvement by tumor. Involvement of the bladder or rectum may present with bleeding as well as fistula formation.

Differential Diagnosis

Many cervical conditions, including genital tract infection, can influence Pap test interpretation and may result in false-positive findings. Certain benign conditions such as leiomyomas, primary herpes infection, endometriosis, and cervical polyps can cause a palpable or visible cervical mass. Uterine cancer can extend to the cervix and vagina and needs to be considered in the differential diagnosis.

Management and Therapy

Screening

Pap test screening is recommended in women who are sexually active or age 18 or older. After three or more

consecutive annual examinations with normal findings, the Pap test may be performed less frequently at the discretion of the physician. In asymptomatic women who have undergone hysterectomy and who do not have a history of genital dysplasia or cancer, Pap tests are not necessary.

Conventional Triage of Abnormal Pap Tests

Treatment and management of screening cytologic abnormalities begins with referral to a specialist trained in colposcopy and therapy of preinvasive cervical dysplasia. Documented cases of invasive cervical cancer should be referred to a gynecologic oncologist. Understanding the triage of abnormal Pap tests requires an understanding of the current Bethesda classification of Pap test abnormalities (Box 85-1). Women with two atypical squamous cells of undetermined significance (ASCUS) or LGSIL Pap tests should undergo colposcopy and directed biopsy. A single HGSIL or cancer Pap test should prompt immediate referral for colposcopic evaluation. Whenever a clinically suspicious lesion or ulceration of the cervix is observed, referral for examination with colposcopy and biopsy should occur, irrespective of the Pap test result. Colposcopy includes magnified examination of the cervix

Figure 85-3 Cancer of Cervix.

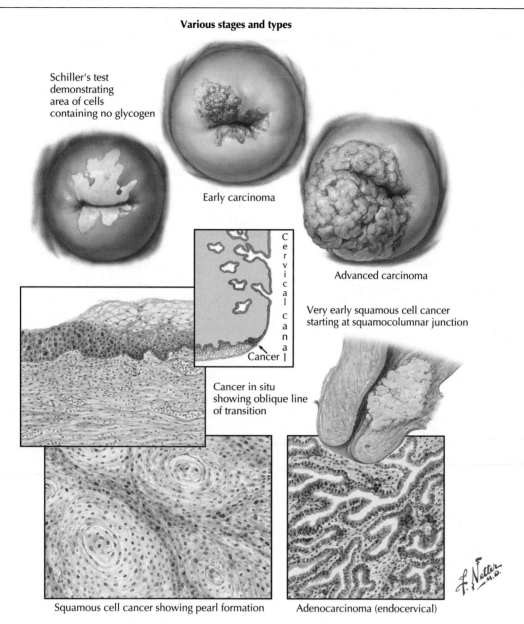

Various stages and types

Schiller's test demonstrating area of cells containing no glycogen

Early carcinoma

Advanced carcinoma

Cervical canal

Cancer

Cancer in situ showing oblique line of transition

Very early squamous cell cancer starting at squamocolumnar junction

Squamous cell cancer showing pearl formation

Adenocarcinoma (endocervical)

after the application of dilute acetic acid, which accentuates dysplastic epithelium by turning it white. Directed punch biopsies of the cervix of all acetowhite lesions and any ulcerative areas showing atypical vascular patterns are performed to determine which patients require treatment and which require routine or close follow-up (Fig. 85-4).

Curettage of the endocervix is performed when the entire transformation zone cannot be visualized or when a visible lesion extends within the cervical canal. In most cases, histologically proven LGSIL is benign, and Pap test screening at frequent intervals is acceptable for compliant patients. HGSIL lesions are much more likely to develop into invasive cancer and therefore are treated. If the whole

lesion is visible on colposcopy, removal of all abnormal epithelium together with the whole transformation zone is performed by cryotherapy, laser ablation, or loop electrical excision. If the lesion is not totally visible or if it is large, cold knife conization is preferred.

Follow-up of patients with LGSIL lesions or who have undergone definitive treatment includes Pap test assessment every 3 to 6 months until three normal Pap tests are obtained. Yearly screening should be continued thereafter. Cytologic abnormalities detected on follow-up screening should be reevaluated with colposcopy.

Hysterectomy may be appropriate for certain women who have completed childbearing and desire definitive

Box 85-1 2001 Bethesda System (Abridged)
Specimen Adequacy
■ Satisfactory for evaluation (note presence/absence of endocervical/transformation zone component)
■ Unsatisfactory for evaluation (specify reason)
■ Specimen rejected/not processed (specify reason)
■ Specimen processed and examined, but unsatisfactory for evaluation of epithelial abnormality because of (specify reason)
General Categorization (Optional)
■ Negative for intraepithelial lesion or malignancy
■ Epithelial cell abnormality
■ Other
Interpretation/Result
■ Negative for intraepithelial lesion or malignancy
■ Organisms
■ *Trichomonas vaginalis*
■ Fungal organisms morphologically consistent with *Candida* species
■ Shift in flora suggestive of bacterial vaginosis
■ Bacteria morphologically consistent with *Actinomyces* species
■ Cellular changes consistent with herpes simplex virus
■ Other non-neoplastic findings (optional to report; list not comprehensive)
■ Reactive cellular changes associated with
■ Inflammation (includes typical repair)
■ Radiation
■ Intrauterine contraceptive device
■ Glandular cells status after hysterectomy
■ Atrophy
■ Epithelial cell abnormalities
■ Squamous cell
■ Atypical squamous cells (ASCs)
■ Of undetermined significance (ASC-US)
■ Cannot exclude HSIL (ASC-H)
■ Low-grade squamous intraepithelial lesion (LSIL) encompassing: human papillomavirus/mild dysplasia/cervical intraepithelial neoplasia (CIN) 1
■ High-grade squamous intraepithelial lesion (HSIL) encompassing: moderate and severe dysplasia, carcinoma in situ; CIN 2 and CIN 3
■ Squamous cell carcinoma
■ Glandular cell
■ Atypical glandular cells (AGCs) (specify endocervical, endometrial, or not otherwise specified)
■ Atypical glandular cells (AGCs), favor neoplastic (specify endocervical, or not otherwise specified)
■ Endocervical adenocarcinoma in situ (AIS)
■ Adenocarcinoma
■ Other (list not comprehensive)
■ Endometrial cells in a woman older than 40 years
Automated Review and Ancillary Testing (Include as Appropriate)
Educational Notes and Suggestions (Optional)

Adapted from Solomon D, Davey D, Kurman R, et al: The 2001 Bethesda System: Terminology for reporting results of cervical cytology. JAMA 287(16):2116, 2002. Copyright © 2002, American Medical Association.

treatment. Care must be taken to exclude invasive disease.

Optimum Treatment of Invasive Lesions

The current staging system of the International Federation of Gynecology and Obstetrics is presented in Box 85-2. Early-stage disease is amenable to both surgical and radiation therapy. The choice of method is based on many social and clinical factors. For tumors stage II and greater, radiation is the mainstay of therapy, with chemotherapy added to potentiate the efficacy of the radiation.

Radiation therapy can be used in all stages of disease, but surgery alone is limited to patients with stage I and IIa disease. The 5-year survival rate for stage I cancer of the cervix is about 85% with either radiation therapy or radical hysterectomy. The advantage of surgical management is evident in younger women in whom conservation of ovarian function is important.

The governing principle behind treating invasive cervical lesions surgically is based on the observation that cervical cancer typically spreads locally and to regional lymph nodes in a stepwise and predictable manner. En bloc resection of the primary tumor with margins requires radical dissection of both parametrial tissues and excision of a 2- to 3-cm vaginal margin. The degree of resection is tailored to the primary lesion size. If significant extracervical disease is demonstrated in the parametrial tissues or lymph nodes, hysterectomy is abandoned in favor of radiation therapy. Postoperative assessment of the hysterectomy specimen and lymph nodes for occult lymph node metastasis, parametrial involvement, or extensive lymphatic space invasion is critical in selecting which patients would benefit from adjuvant radiation therapy.

Radiation therapy can be administered by external beam to a total pelvic dose of 5000 cGy and as brachytherapy applied transvaginally to the cervix, and vaginal and parametrial tissues to boost the total dose to the tumor to 7500 cGy. In selected patients with large tumors or known pelvic lymph node involvement, the radiation fields are extended to include the para-aortic lymph nodes.

Recent reports of increasing the efficacy of radiation therapy with the infusion of low-dose platinum chemotherapy have led to this regimen becoming the standard of care for extracervical disease.

Local-regional cervical cancer recurrences can often be salvaged, with some long-term survivors. After primary surgical management, pelvic recurrences can be treated with radiation therapy with curative intent if no distant metastatic disease is present. Isolated lung metastasis can be treated with surgical excision with good results in patients without other sites of recurrence. Chemotherapy for advanced or recurrent disease yields short-lived responses of 30%.

Figure 85-4 Colposcopic Views of Abnormal Cervical Changes.

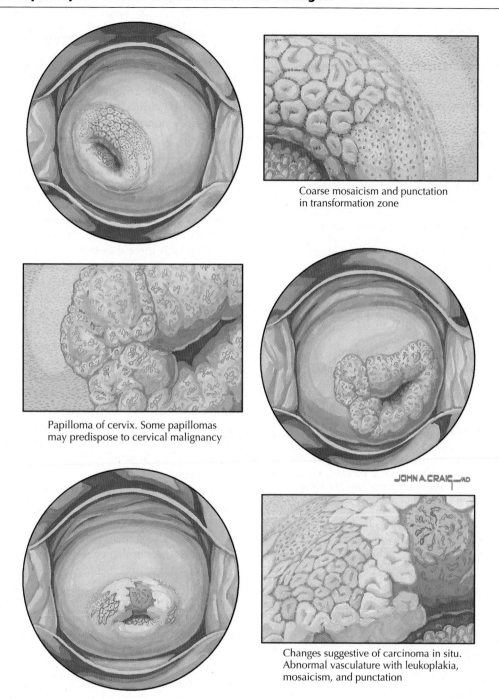

Coarse mosaicism and punctation
in transformation zone

Papilloma of cervix. Some papillomas
may predispose to cervical malignancy

JOHN A.CRAIG⏤MD

Changes suggestive of carcinoma in situ.
Abnormal vasculature with leukoplakia,
mosaicism, and punctation

Avoiding Treatment Errors

Although screening algorithms for preventing cervical cancer have been successful, errors occur and represent one of the most common reasons for litigation. Most errors occur for two reasons: failure of the cytopathologist to detect an abnormality due to human error or limitations in sensitivity of the Pap test, or inadequate triage and follow-up Pap abnormalities. Many technologic innovations, such as liquid-based cytology and computer-assisted screening, have improved incrementally the sensitivity of the Pap test for detecting high-grade lesions. In addition, incorporating HPV testing can improve sensitivity of testing at the expense of specificity.

All clinical offices that perform Pap smear screening need to have well-documented processes in place for following patients and communicating all abnormal results to them. Documentation of such communication is critical to ensure compliance. Several computer software systems are available to automate communication and provide prompts

Box 85-2   Staging of Cervical Cancer

Stage I

The carcinoma is strictly confined to the cervix (extension to the corpus should be disregarded).

Stage IA: Invasive cancer identified only microscopically. All gross lesions even with superficial invasion are stage IB cancers. Invasion is limited to measured stromal invasion with maximum depth of 5.0 mm and no wider than 7.0 mm.

Stage IA1: Measured invasion of stroma no greater than 3.0 mm in depth and no wider than 7.0 mm

Stage IA2: Measured invasion of stroma greater than 3.0 mm and no greater than 5.0 mm and no wider than 7.0 mm. The depth of invasion should not be more than 5.0 mm taken from the base of the epithelium, either surface or glandular, from which it originates. Preformed space involvement (vascular or lymphatic) should not alter the staging but should be specifically recorded so as to determine whether it should affect treatment decisions in the future.

Stage IB: Clinical lesions confined to the cervix or preclinical lesions greater than IA

Stage IB1: Clinical lesions no greater than 4.0 cm in size

Stage IB2: Clinical lesions greater than 4.0 cm in size

Stage II

The carcinoma extends beyond the cervix but has not extended to the pelvic wall. The carcinoma involves the vagina but not as far as the lower third.

Stage IIA: No obvious parametrial involvement

Stage IIB: Obvious parametrial involvement

Stage III

The carcinoma has extended to the pelvic wall. On rectal examination, there is no cancer-free space between the tumor and the pelvic wall. The tumor involves the lower third of the vagina. All cases with a hydronephrosis or nonfunctioning kidney are included unless they are known to be due to other causes.

Stage IIIA: No extension to the pelvic wall

Stage IIIB: Extension to the pelvic wall and/or hydronephrosis or nonfunctioning kidney

Stage IV

The carcinoma has extended beyond the true pelvis or has clinically involved the mucosa of the bladder or rectum. A bullous edema as such does not permit a case to be allotted to stage IV.

Stage IVA: Spread of the growth to adjacent organs

Stage IVB: Spread to distant organs

Adapted from Modifications in the staging for stage I vulvar and stage I cervical cancer. Report of the FIGO Committee on Gynecologic Oncology. International Federation of Gynecology and Obstetrics. Int J Gynaecol Obstet 50(2):215-216, 1995.

for unresolved abnormal testing and may be helpful at reducing such errors.

Future Directions

Given the pathogenetic role of HPV in cervical cancer and the virus prevalence among sexually active women, much research has focused on the development of an HPV vaccine. Two prophylactic HPV vaccines have emerged, Gardasil (Merck & Co.) and Cervarix (Glaxo-Smith-Kline). Both are composed of noninfectious, recombinant HPV viral-like particles from HPV 16 and 18, which account for about 70% of all cervical cancers. Gardasil also offers protection from HPV 6 and 11, associated with genital warts. The results from large-scale randomized phase II and III clinical trials of these vaccines have been impressive, demonstrating almost 100% short-term protection from cervical dysplasia. Persistent protective effects have been seen beyond 2 years for each of these vaccines.

The quadrivalent Gardasil vaccine is approved by the U.S. Food and Drug Administration for use in women and adolescents aged 9 to 26 years. In June 2006, the Federal Advisory Committee on Immunization Practices (ACIP) recommended routine vaccination of females 11 to 12 years of age with three doses of this vaccine. This vaccination series can be started as early as 9 years of age. The ACIP also endorsed vaccination for all females 13 to 26 years of age, regardless of prior sexual activity.

Although these highly effective and well-tolerated vaccines have great potential in the reduction of cervical dysplasia and cervical cancer, many questions remain both in the implementation of routine vaccination and the durability of immunity. It is also unclear whether these vaccines may offer cross-protection against other HPV types or if these vaccines may also be efficacious in men. Challenges also exist in the future for the much needed distribution of these vaccines to economically disadvantaged women worldwide in the hope of reducing the global burden of cervical disease.

Although HPV vaccination and newer screening technologies offer great promise, the major failure in preventing cervical cancer death in the United States remains lack of compliance with screening. Studies show that the strongest influence on compliance is whether physicians emphasize the importance of screening. Racial disparity still exists in outcomes of treatment. Finally, the National Cancer Institute (NCI) has recognized that the identification of biomarkers, which might better identify those cytologic abnormalities that are clinically significant, would dramatically improve the cost-effectiveness of current screening algorithms. A consequence of the improved sensitivity of current screening methods is a loss of specificity. The number of women with an abnormal Pap test has increased significantly since the Bethesda system was adopted in 1988. Screening techniques, like liquid-based cytology and computer-assisted analysis, have greater sensitivity, but their cost is prohibitive for many patients.

Based on a recent study of minimally abnormal Pap tests, the NCI has concluded that women with ASCUS tests who do not have high-risk HPV may be screened yearly. The results of this study are significant given that ASCUS is the most common Pap test abnormality but correlates with biopsy-proven dysplasia in fewer than half of women with the finding.

Cervical cancer prevention will require a look forward to new technology while continuing to look back and fully implement what has been to date the most successful cancer prevention strategy adopted.

Additional Resource

Centers for Disease Control and Prevention. Available at: http://www.cdc.gov/cancer/cervical. Accessed June 23, 2007.

The CDC provides a very useful, well-organized, patient-friendly website that reviews risk factors, screening, and clinical presentation.

EVIDENCE

1. Berek JS, Hacker NF (eds): Practical Gynecologic Oncology, 3rd ed. Philadelphia, Lippincott Williams & Wilkins, 2000.

    This excellent resource text covers screening, epidemiology, and treatment of cervical cancer.

2. National Cancer Institute. Available at: http://www.cancer.gov. Accessed May 8, 2007.

    This website provides up-to-date information for both patients and clinicians on the latest recommendations regarding screening and treatment of cervical cancer.

3. Rock JA, Thompson JD (eds): Te Linde's Operative Gynecology, 8th ed. Philadelphia, Lippincott-Raven, 1997.

    This excellent text provides an atlas of gynecologic operative procedures with an emphasis on history and technique.

4. Schiller JT, Lowy DR: Prospects for cervical cancer prevention by human papillomavirus vaccination. Cancer Res 66(21):10229-10232, 2006.

    The authors provide an excellent review of recent innovations in cervical cancer screening.

5. U.S. Preventive Services Task Force: Guide to Clinical Preventive Services, 2nd ed. Washington, DC, U.S. Dept of Health and Human Services, 1996.

    This is a meta-analysis of all available published literature related to cervical cancer screening.

W. Kimryn Rathmell ▪ Paul A. Godley

Testicular Cancer

Introduction

Testicular cancer is the leading cancer among men ages 15 to 35 years, although it is responsible for less than 1% of all human tumors. Up to 95% of tumors presenting in the testes in this age group are germ cell tumors, with the remainder primarily accounted for by lymphomas and some gonadal stromal tumors. Testicular germ cell tumors are primarily of pure seminoma or nonseminoma (embryonal, yolk sac, teratoma, choriocarcinoma) histology.

In 2006, about 8250 new cases of testicular germ cell tumor were diagnosed in the United States. With the implementation of effective chemotherapeutic strategies, fewer than 5% of affected patients will succumb to the illness. The incidence of testicular cancer has continued to rise over the past several decades. Although the cause of this trend remains unknown, the disease is much more prevalent in white males when compared with their African American counterparts, and the rising incidence appears to be limited to whites. The incidence of testicular cancer in African American males is about one fourth of that observed for white males.

Etiology and Pathogenesis

Several risk factors are associated with the development of this cancer; however, most patients will not display any of the known risk factors. The increased risk associated with cryptorchidism is especially notable, and patients with an undescended testicle that is not repaired by age 5 years pose a particularly high risk for the development of carcinoma in *either* testicle. About 10% of testicular tumors are associated with cryptorchidism; 25% of these tumors occur in the contralateral, normally descended testicle. The reported rate of malignant transformation of the cryptorchid testis varies from 3- to 14-fold that of a normal testis. Other risk factors include infertility or subfertility, HIV infection, and family history of testicular cancer.

Clinical Presentation

Testicular germ cell tumors most commonly present as a painless nodule on the testis, although about 30% of patients report dull pain in the testicle. Roughly 10% of patients present with acute testicular pain, and another 10% have symptoms or signs of metastatic disease (Fig. 86-1). Any concerning lesion or symptom requires expeditious evaluation with a testicular ultrasound, a highly sensitive test in the diagnosis of testicular cancer. The general ultrasound appearance of testicular germ cell tumors is that of parenchymal irregularities in an otherwise smooth and homogeneous-appearing testis (Fig. 86-2).

Germ cell tumors sometimes arise outside of the testicle, generally along the midline of the body in developmental rest areas of germinal tissue. Another presentation is that of metastatic disease without evidence of a primary testicular tumor. In this case, the primary lesion has "burned out." These clinical scenarios require a high index of suspicion in the absence of a testicular mass when there is midline lymphadenopathy and other signs compatible with underlying testicular cancer. Finally, paraneoplastic phenomena such as gynecomastia or other signs or symptoms of widespread disease can add to the diagnostic challenge.

Differential Diagnosis

The differential diagnosis of testicular cancer includes alternate causes of testicular nodularity, pain, or swelling. Testicular torsion, epididymitis, and hydrocele lead the differential diagnostic list. Additional diagnoses to consider include orchitis, trauma or hematoma, hernia, and gumma associated with syphilis.

Figure 86-1 Scrotum and Contents.

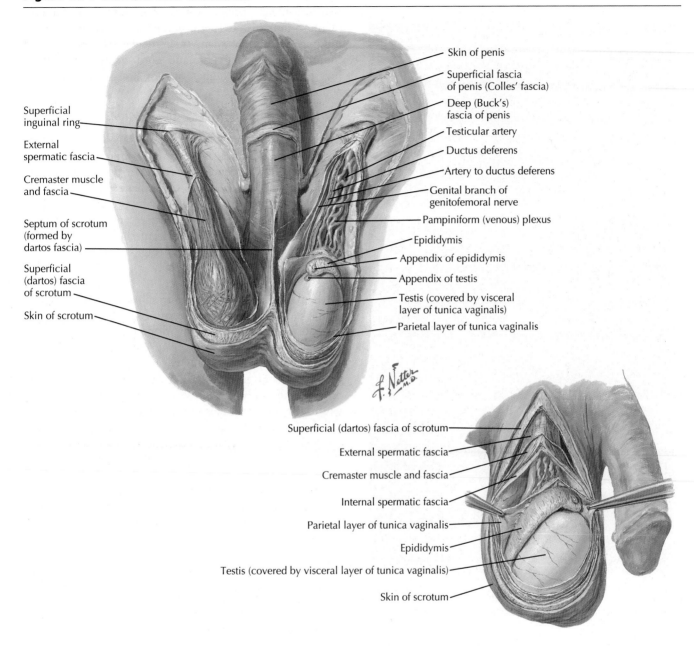

Diagnostic Approach

Biology of Testicular Neoplasm

Tumors of the testis often secrete biologic markers that are detectable in the peripheral blood. The availability of reliable serum tumor markers has greatly improved the screening and identification of tumors of germ cell origin. Alpha fetoprotein (AFP), human chorionic gonadotropin (β-HCG), and lactate dehydrogenase (LDH) provide rapid and quantitative measures of testicular germ cell tumor activity in many cases. Additional utilization of tumor markers in staging, surveillance, and prognosis is discussed later in this chapter. These markers should be obtained as a priority in the evaluation of a testicular nodule.

AFP is commonly secreted by embryonal cells of non-seminomatous germ cell tumors. This protein is not produced by pure seminoma cells and always marks the presence of nonseminomatous germ cells either in the primary tumor or in a metastatic site, even when the tumor histology favors a pure seminoma diagnosis. The 6-day serum half-life of AFP may lead to confusion in the interpretation of samples drawn soon after orchiectomy.

β-HCG is secreted by syncytiotrophoblast giant cells, which may be a component of choriocarcinoma, embryo-

Figure 86-2 Ultrasound Findings in the Testicle.

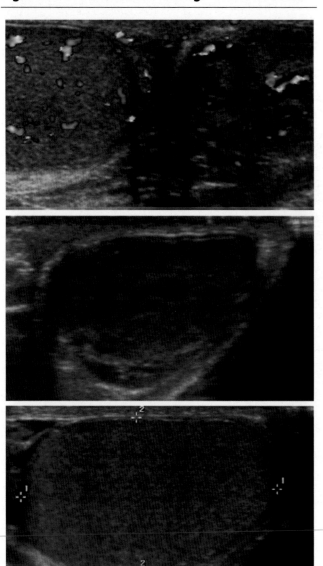

A, Side by side vascular flow evaluations of the normal testicle (left) and diseased testicle (right). **B,** Standard ultrasound findings in the testicle, with hypoechoic lesions in a homogeneous background. **C,** Homogeneous bland appearance on ultrasound of a normal testis.

nal carcinoma, and pure seminoma. As a functional hormone, β-HCG may induce paraneoplastic phenomena such as gynecomastia by enhancing secretion of estrogen by the testis.

Several cytogenetic markers are associated with testicular germ cell tumors. In particular, isochrome 12p (i12p) is a frequent cytogenetic abnormality that can be identified with each of the germ cell tumor histologies. It is associated with a poorer prognosis.

Pathologic Classification

The classification of testicular germ cell neoplasms includes two main subdivisions: seminoma and nonseminomatous germ cell tumor (NSGCT). The incidence of each of these two histologic types is roughly equivalent. Key elements of the tumor histology are uniquely important in determining a treatment plan. In particular, the presence of tumor cells in the spermatic cord or lymphovascular invasion portends a higher risk for disease spread to the abdomen.

Nonseminomatous Germ Cell Tumor

Because testicular cancer is derived from cells with pluripotency, the NSGCT is generally composed of a mixed histology, although one or more tumor types may be predominant among the others. Cells that resemble yolk sac, embryonal, or teratoma tissue may be present mixed with cells derived from seminoma. These tumors can produce all or some of the classic tumor markers and classically produce both AFP and β-HCG (Fig. 86-3).

Seminoma

Testicular seminoma is a unique subtype of the testicular neoplasms. Although the pattern of spread for both types of testicular neoplasm is identical, the susceptibility to chemotherapy, and in particular radiation, of the pure seminoma makes this distinction critical to treatment, follow-up, and prognosis. The diagnosis of seminoma requires not only the presence of abundant seminoma within the tumor, but also the *exclusion* of other malignant cellular features. The presence of even a small contribution by an alternate cell type is sufficient for diagnosis of mixed NSGCT. Typically, seminoma does not secrete any measurable tumor markers, but this tumor can occasionally result in positive β-HCG tests. In contrast, the presence of measurable serum levels of AFP or LDH should alert the physician to the presence of unsampled NSGCT.

Gonadal Stromal Tumors

Tumors arising from the gonadal stroma, although uncommon, constitute a distinct subset of tumors. These neoplasms are classified as Leydig, Sertoli, or gonadoblastoma tumors and together account for less than 5% of all tumors of testicular origin.

Staging

The staging of testicular germ cell neoplasms is dependent on the following: tumor invasiveness within the contents of the scrotal sac, the presence of retroperitoneal lymphadenopathy, tumor marker level, and the presence of metastatic disease (excluding pulmonary metastatic disease). When evaluating a patient with a testicular nodule, the clinician should keep in mind that the primary lymphatic drainage of the testis follows the pattern of embryonic descent of the testicle from the ipsilateral region of the renal hilum (Fig. 86-4). Once staged using the conventional TNM staging algorithm, patients are assigned to one of three risk group categories: good risk, intermediate

Figure 86-3 Testicular Tumors I: Seminoma, Embryonal Carcinoma.

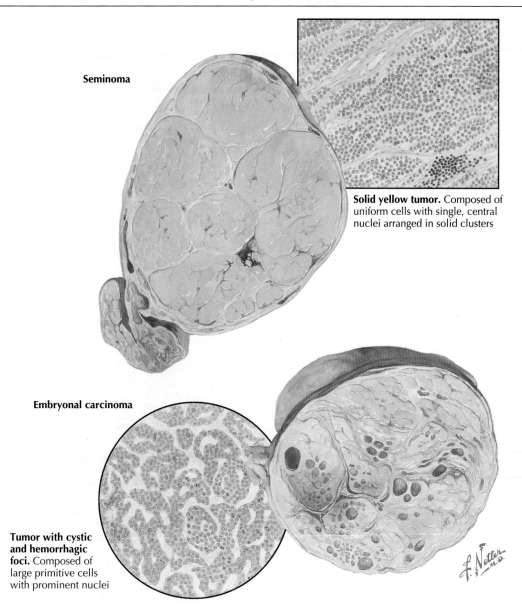

Seminoma

Solid yellow tumor. Composed of uniform cells with single, central nuclei arranged in solid clusters

Embryonal carcinoma

Tumor with cystic and hemorrhagic foci. Composed of large primitive cells with prominent nuclei

risk, and poor risk. The central purpose is to predict long-term disease-free survival and cure. Risk stratification is also a critical determinant in the choice of chemotherapy. Tables for TNM staging and inclusion criteria for risk categories stratification are provided (Tables 86-1, 86-2, 86-3, and 86-4).

Management and Therapy

Optimum Treatment of Seminoma

Stage I

The treatment of stage I seminoma remains an area of active controversy because 15% to 20% of patients who undergo surveillance will relapse in the retroperitoneum. Seminomas are radiosensitive neoplasms, and radiation to the infradiaphragmatic region including para-aortic lymph nodes with 20 to 30 Gy has become the standard of care for most individuals. The emerging use of adjuvant single-agent cisplatin or carboplatin for one or two cycles has been increasingly considered an appropriate alternative to radiation therapy. However, 85% or more of stage I patients will achieve a long-term disease-free outcome with no further therapy after orchiectomy. Therefore, for selected patients who are committed to a strict regimen of surveillance (Table 86-5), or for whom a relative contra-indication to radiation therapy or chemotherapy exists, orchiectomy alone is a reasonable option. With radiation

Figure 86-4 Testis Descent through the Deep Body Wall.

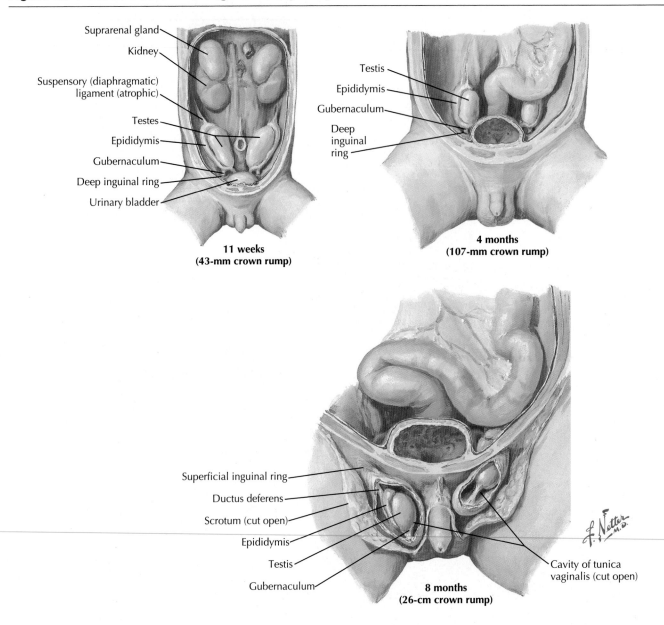

Suprarenal gland
Kidney
Suspensory (diaphragmatic) ligament (atrophic)
Testes
Epididymis
Gubernaculum
Deep inguinal ring
Urinary bladder

**11 weeks
(43-mm crown rump)**

Testis
Epididymis
Gubernaculum
Deep inguinal ring

**4 months
(107-mm crown rump)**

Superficial inguinal ring
Ductus deferens
Scrotum (cut open)
Epididymis
Testis
Gubernaculum

Cavity of tunica vaginalis (cut open)

**8 months
(26-cm crown rump)**

or chemotherapy, the rate of recurrence in these individuals following adjuvant treatment is less than 5%.

Stage II

Stage II seminoma is treated as stage II nonseminomatous germ cell tumor with conventional chemotherapy [see Principles of Chemotherapy].

Treatment of Nonseminoma

Principles of Chemotherapy

Cisplatin is the single most effective chemotherapeutic agent in the management of testicular germ cell tumors; carboplatin is not an alternative except in the case of adju-

vant therapy for pure seminoma. Since the advent of cisplatin-containing multidrug combinations, testicular germ cell tumors have become highly curable cancers, even in advanced stages. The focus of recent advances in the treatment of testicular germ cell tumors has been to limit the intensity of therapy with the goal of reducing the severity of both short-term and long-term sequelae of chemotherapy treatment without compromising efficacy. The standard three-drug regimen for testicular germ cell tumor is BEP, comprising bleomycin, etoposide, and cisplatin given in 3-week cycles. Long-term side effects associated with chemotherapy include premature ischemic heart disease, kidney disease, and hypertension. Another late effect that must be considered in patients who receive chemotherapy is the potential negative impact on fertility.

Table 86-1   Risk Stratification of Seminoma and Nonseminoma

Risk	Seminoma	Nonseminoma
Good	Any primary, any markers, no nonpulmonary visceral mets	Testicle or retroperitoneum primary, *and* No nonpulmonary visceral mets, *and* Good markers (all): AFP <1000; β-HCG <5000; LDH <1.5× ULN
Intermediate	Any primary, any markers, nonpulmonary visceral mets	Testicle or retroperitoneum primary, *and* No nonpulmonary visceral mets, *and* Int. markers (any): AFP, 1000-10,000; β-HCG, 5000-50,000, LDH 1.5× to 10× ULN
Poor		Mediastinum primary tumor, *or* Nonpulmonary visceral mets, *or* Poor markers (any): AFP >10,000; β-HCG >50,000; LDH >10× ULN

AFP, alpha fetoprotein; β-HCG, human chorionic gonadotropin; LDH, lactate dehydrogenase; ULN, upper limit of normal.

Table 86-2   TNM and Serum Marker Stages

T Stage	Tumor Status	M Stage	Metastatic Involvement
pTx	Primary tumor cannot be assessed	Mx	Distant metastasis cannot be assessed
pT0	No evidence of primary tumor	M0	No metastatic disease
pTis	Intratubular germ cell neoplasia	M1	Distant metastasis
pT1	Limited to the testis and epididymis, no lymphatic/vascular invasion; tumor may invade into the tunica albuginea but not the tunica vaginalis	M1a	Nonregional nodal or pulmonary metastasis
pT2	Tumor limited to the testis and epididymis with vascular/lymphatic invasion, or tumor extending through the tunica albuginea with involvement of the tunica vaginalis	M1b	Distant metastasis other than to nonregional lymph nodes and lungs
pT3	Invades the spermatic cord	**S Stage**	**Serum Markers**
pT4	Invades the scrotum	Sx	Marker studies not available or not performed
N Stage	**Nodal Status**	S0	All marker studies within normal limits
Nx	Regional lymph nodes cannot be assessed	S1	LDH, <1.5× ULN; AFP <1000; β-HCG <5000
N0	No involved regional lymph nodes	S2	LDH, 1.5× to 10× ULN; AFP, 1000-10,000; β-HCG, 5000-50,000
N1	Total lymph node mass ≤2 cm	S3	LDH >10× ULN; AFP >10,000; β-HCG >50,000
N2	Total lymph node mass 2-5 cm		
N3	Total lymph node mass >5 cm		

AFP, alpha fetoprotein; β-HCG, human chorionic gonadotropin; LDH, lactate dehydrogenase; ULN, upper limit of normal.

Although these individuals often have primary sperm defects in count or viability on analysis, every patient considering chemotherapy should receive counseling about the likelihood of infertility and be given the option of expeditious sperm banking.

Stage I Optimum Treatment

Nonseminomatous germ cell tumors are less radiosensitive than pure seminomas, and therefore adjuvant therapy with radiation is not considered a part of the algorithm for stage I disease (Fig. 86-5). These patients also have a risk for relapse between 25% and 35%, but with a rate of cure that approaches 95% after salvage therapy. Three appropriate management options are available: (1) surgical retroperitoneal lymph node dissection, (2) adjuvant chemotherapy, or (3) surveillance (see Table 86-5).

Surgical management of these tumors requires the involvement of a skilled urologic surgeon. Although laparoscopic approaches are an exciting and potentially highly valuable addition to management, an open ipsilateral tem-

Figure 86-5 Treatment Algorithm: Stage 1 Nonseminoma.
BEP, bleomycin, etoposide, and cisplatin; F/U, follow-up; RPLND, retroperitoneal lymph node dissection.

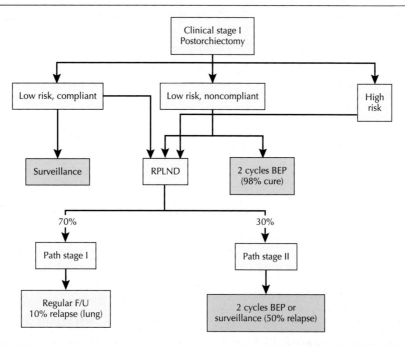

Table 86-3 Definition of Stages

Stage	Definition
I	Limited to the testis
Ia	T1, N0, M0, S0
Ib	T2-T4, N0, M0, S0
Is	Any T, N0, M0, S1-3
II	Spread to regional nodes
IIa	Any T, N1, M0, S0-1
IIb	Any T, N2, M0, S0-1
IIc	Any T, N3, M0, S0-1
III	Metastatic disease
IIIa	Any T, any N, M1a, S0-1
IIIb	Any T, N1-3, M0, S2
	Any T, any N, M1a, S2
IIIc	Any T, N1-3, M0, S3
	Any T, any N, M1a, S3
	Any T, any N, M1b, any S

Table 86-4 Five-Year Disease-Free Survival Estimates for Each Stage of Testicular Cancer

Stage	Seminoma	Nonseminoma	Overall
Stage I	99%	98%	98%
Stage II	95%	95%	95%
Stage III	90%	76%	78%
All stages			96%

Table 86-5 Follow-up Care Schedules

Year	Exam	Markers	Imaging
1	Monthly	Monthly	Every 2 mo
2	Every 2 mo	Every 2 mo	Every 4 mo
3-5	Every 3 mo	Every 3 mo	Every 6 mo
>5	Annually	As needed	As needed

plate retroperitoneal lymph node dissection (RPLND) remains the standard of care. The advantage of surgical management is that it provides both diagnostic material and local control. When the RPLND specimen is pathologically negative, the risk for development of recurrence in the abdomen is essentially nil. These patients, however, maintain an overall risk for recurrence of about 10% with the primary site of relapse in the lung. They should undergo routine annual follow-up for disease recurrence. When the RPLND specimen reveals viable germ cell tumor, the risk for recurrence in the abdomen is significantly lessened. However, the possibility of recurrence inside or outside the abdomen is still significant, about 50%. These indi-

viduals must continue to undergo intensive surveillance, including imaging and tumor marker studies, for at least 5 years, or they should consider adjuvant chemotherapy. The potential late effects of RPLND include retrograde ejaculation as a result of nerve damage along the node template. Because of this risk, an experienced urologic surgeon should have specific training in nerve-sparing approaches. With these newer approaches, the risk for retrograde ejaculation is less than 5% to 10%; however, the risk for both minor and major complications of RPLND is greater when performed after chemotherapy.

Adjuvant chemotherapy (conventionally two cycles of BEP) will reduce the risk for recurrence to less than 5%.

Finally, compliant patients who are good candidates for close follow-up due to lower risk features of their primary tumor can consider surveillance as a reasonable alternative to both RPLND and adjuvant chemotherapy.

Stage II Optimum Treatment

Surgery and chemotherapy are the mainstays of treatment in stage II patients. RPLND is considered a standard of care when markers are negative after orchiectomy. Additional chemotherapy is considered based on the identification of viable tumor and the extent of involvement. Chemotherapy for good-risk disease consists of either four cycles of EP or three cycles of BEP. Both regimens are equivalent based on randomized clinical trials. Alternatively, the use of primary chemotherapy is an appropriate course of action. Residual masses in the retroperitoneum should be resected to prevent the malignant degeneration of what may represent mature teratoma. Observation only is also acceptable if indicated by the clinical situation. Patients who meet criteria for intermediate or poor-risk disease despite of the apparent staging should be treated with additional chemotherapy or early consideration for enrollment in a clinical trial.

Clinicians must recognize the not uncommon development of retroperitoneal or other masses during the course of chemotherapy. This occurrence may herald primary refractory disease but more commonly represents the growth of a teratoma component of these masses despite chemotherapeutic efficacy for the remaining germ cell tissue.

Stage III Optimum Treatment

The management of stage III disease virtually parallels that of stage II disease. Standard chemotherapy followed by resection of residual masses in the absence of persistent marker elevation is appropriate for good-risk disease. In intermediate- or poor-risk disease, the more intensive four cycles of BEP or consideration of clinical trial therapy remains the mainstay of treatment decision making.

Management of Relapsed or Refractory Disease

Numerous regimens have been developed as salvage treatment for those situations in which primary chemotherapy is ineffective. Most still depend on the use of cisplatin as the single most active chemotherapeutic drug. Multiagent chemotherapy regimens incorporate ifosfamide and vinblastine or paclitaxel, with cisplatin, and have reasonable rates of response and even benefits to survival. Additionally, the use of ablative chemotherapy followed by autologous stem cell transplant has been used successfully in specialty centers. In patients with a long time to disease recurrence, reexposure to EP or BEP may be feasible and effective.

Avoiding Treatment Errors

The most significant treatment errors in testicular cancer involve dosing errors of the chemotherapeutic agents that comprise the BEP regimen. Severe pulmonary toxicity, fever and neutropenia, and renal failure may develop in these cases. Standardized, and preferably computerized, chemotherapy order sheets and a redundant system of checking chemotherapy dose calculations can help minimize the possibility of medication errors.

Future Directions

When treating a generally young population with curative intent, the importance of considering the long-lasting effects of therapeutic interventions requires special emphasis. Although the high cure rate of testicular cancer is a therapeutic triumph, new research efforts must now focus on identifying the late effects of treatment, including premature coronary artery disease, neuropathy, and renal impairment, as patients treated in their late teens and early 20s reach retirement age and beyond. Finally, the importance of educating patients about the problems to anticipate in the months and years following treatment warrants special emphasis. This will require the development of an effective system of care that provides long-term support and follow-up.

Additional Resources

American Cancer Society. Available at: http://www.cancer.org. Accessed September 29, 2006.
> The American Cancer Society website provides extensive resources for education and treatment decisions.

Lance Armstrong Foundation Survivor Care. Available at: http://www.laf.org. Accessed September 29, 2006.
> This informative website is oriented toward cancer survivors.

National Cancer Institute: Testicular Cancer Home Page. Available at: http://www.cancer.gov/cancertopics/types/testicular/. Accessed September 29, 2006.
> The National Cancer Institute provides extensive information on common cancer types.

NCCN Guidelines for the Management of Testicular Cancer, vol. 1, 2006. Available at: http://www.nccn.org. Accessed September 29, 2006.
> The NCCN provides frequently updated treatment algorithms for the management of common cancer types.

People Living with Cancer. Available at: http://www.plwc.org. Accessed September 29, 2006.
> This website provides patient-oriented information approved by the American Society of Clinical Oncology.

EVIDENCE

> Chemotherapy regimens for stage II and III nonsemitomatous germ cell tumors are supported by randomized phase III clinical trials. The U.S. Preventive Services Task Force Rating of the quality of the evidence is good, and the strength of the chemotherapy treatment recommendations is A–.

1. Bosl GJ, Motzer RJ: Testicular germ cell cancer. N Engl J Med 337(4):242-253, 1997.

   The authors present an elegantly written and authoritative review of testicular cancer.

2. Huddart RA, Norman A, Shahidi M, et al: Cardiovascular disease as a long-term complication of treatment for testicular cancer. J Clin Oncol 21(8):1513-1523, 2003.

   Late effects of chemotherapy can be significant in treating a youthful population. This manuscript describes a concerning late sequelae of chemotherapy.

3. International Germ Cell Collaborative Group: International germ cell consensus classification: A prognostic factor-based staging system for metastatic germ cell cancers. J Clin Oncol 15(2):594-603, 1997.

   This authoritative assessment of the tumor and patient-specific factors that affect the prognosis for testicular cancers establishes the currently utilized classification system.

4. McGlynn KA, Devesa SS, Sigurdson AJ, et al: Trends in the incidence of testicular germ cell tumors in the United States. Cancer 97(1):63-70, 2003.

   This article examines the trends in incidence of germ cell tumors over the previous 30 years.

5. Read G, Stenning SP, Cullen MH, et al: Medical research council prospective study of surveillance for stage I testicular teratoma. Medical Research Council Testicular Tumors Working Party. J Clin Oncol 10:1762-1768, 1992.

   This article examines the utilization of surveillance for disease recurrence in patients with stage I tumors as an alternative to adjuvant surgical or chemotherapy.

6. Saxman SB, Finch D, Gonin R, Einhorn LH: Long-term follow-up of a phase III study of three versus four courses of bleomycin, etoposide, and cisplatin in favorable-prognosis germ-cell tumors: The Indiana University experience. J Clin Oncol 16(2):702-706, 1998.

   Three cycles of chemotherapy were established here as the new standard of care for good-risk germ cell tumors, thus significantly reducing the short- and long-term toxicities of the exposure to chemotherapy.

7. Toner GC, Stockler MR, Boyer MJ, et al: Comparison of two standard chemotherapy regimens for good-prognosis germ cell tumours. Lancet 357:739-745, 2001.

   This study established the superiority of the standard BEP regimen over similar variations. The impact of this paper is to document the necessity of full-dose-intensity chemotherapy to maximize patient survival outcomes.

8. Williams SD, Birch R, Einhorn LH, et al: Treatment of disseminated germ cell tumors with cisplatin, bleomycin and either vinblastine or etoposide. N Engl J Med 316:1435-1440, 1987.

   This seminal manuscript established BEP chemotherapy as the standard of care for treatment of testicular cancer.

Thyroid Cancer

Introduction

Thyroid cancer is a relatively rare malignancy. It is estimated that in the United States in 2006 there will be about 30,000 new cases and 1500 deaths related to thyroid cancer. A frequent presentation of thyroid cancer is as a thyroid nodule, and the prevalence of thyroid nodules is high. It is estimated that in the United States about 275,000 new thyroid nodules will be detected each year and about 5% of all adults have a palpable thyroid nodule. However, only 5% of palpable nodules are malignant. Thus, despite the relative rarity of thyroid cancer, many patients will undergo an evaluation for thyroid cancer.

Clinical Presentation

The clinical history may provide insight into the diagnosis. A very rapid enlargement over hours suggests hemorrhage into an existing thyroid nodule. Most hemorrhagic nodules are benign; however, up to 10% may be malignant. A rapid growth over weeks is suggestive of malignancy. Thyroid nodules that are larger (>3 cm) and develop in a short period of time (<2 months) are concerning for anaplastic thyroid cancer, lymphoma, or metastasis to the thyroid. However, the absolute size of the thyroid nodule is not predictive of malignancy. A change in size of an existing nodule or rapid growth during thyroid replacement therapy is suggestive of malignancy.

The patient's gender, age, environmental exposure, and family history may provide additional value information and help estimate the risk for malignancy. The risk of a thyroid nodule being malignant is twice as high in men as in women. The risk for malignancy increases with younger age, and about 20% of solitary nodules in patients younger than 20 years are malignant. A history of radiation exposure to the neck increases the risk for developing benign and malignant thyroid masses. Therapeutic radiation to the neck for skin infections, enlarged tonsils, adenoids, and thymus was common practice in the 1950s and 1960s. The Chernobyl nuclear accident spread radiation throughout Europe, with short-lived iodine isotopes being deposited in Russia, Ukraine, and Belarus. Thyroid cancer incidence in these regions has increased 12- to 34-fold, especially among children who were exposed. A careful history of radiation exposure is particularly important for immigrants from these regions.

A prior history of malignancy, the presence of tumor syndrome, and other clinical syndromes should raise clinical suspicion of thyroid cancer as well. The syndrome of multiple endocrine neoplasia (MEN) types IIA and IIB raises the suspicion for medullary thyroid cancer (MTC). MEN IIA consists of MTC cancer (all cases), pheochromocytoma, and hyperparathyroidism, whereas MEN IIB consists of MTC, mucosal neuromas, and pheochromocytomas, and patients tend to have a marfanoid body habitus. A family history of non–MTC is important as well because about 5% to 10% of patients with papillary thyroid cancer may have a family history of thyroid cancer. Gardner's syndrome and Cowden's disease (multiple hamartomas) are associated with well-differentiated thyroid cancer.

Differential Diagnosis and Diagnostic Approach

The differential diagnosis of thyroid nodule is extensive (Box 87-1). A through physical examination of the head and neck should be the initial step in the evaluation. The size, number, and consistency of any nodules should be noted. The thyroid gland and thyroid nodules will move with swallowing, whereas mass external to thyroid will not. A careful palpation of the neck for any lymphadenopathy should be performed. Large, multiple, or fixed lymph nodes are suggestive of malignant involvement. The next

Box 87-1 Differential Diagnosis of Thyroid Nodule
Malignant Causes
Thyroid carcinoma
Thyroid metastases
Thyroid lymphoma
Nonmalignant Causes
Nontoxic nodular goiter
Hashimoto's thyroiditis
Benign adenoma
Cyst
Hemorrhagic nodule
Pyogenic thyroiditis
Subacute (de Quervain) thyroiditis
Riedel's thyroiditis
Hyperplastic nodule

step in the evaluation is a fine-needle aspiration (FNA). This test is accurate and has limited morbidity, and the results are generally available in several days. The sensitivity and specificity are about 90% and 70%, respectively. The results of an FNA are generally reported as benign, malignant, suspicious, and nondiagnostic. A nondiagnostic biopsy, generally as a result of insufficient cells for evaluation, should not be considered evidence of a benign process. The level of clinical suspicion is used in guiding the workup when a definitive diagnosis cannot be made cytologically. The negative predictive value has been reported to be 97%; however, a biopsy negative for malignancy when there is a high clinical suspicion for malignancy should be further evaluated with a surgical or ultrasound-guided biopsy. If the fine-needle biopsy is suggestive of lymphoma, an excisional biopsy should be pursued.

Several laboratory tests are frequently included in the initial evaluation. A thyroid-stimulating hormone (TSH) level may be useful in determining whether the patient is euthyroid, hypothyroid, or hyperthyroid, and is helpful if a benign disorder such as Hashimoto's thyroiditis is being considered in the differential diagnosis. Patients with an elevated TSH should have a complete thyroid function panel performed. If a patient has a personal or family history of MTC or if the FNA is suggestive of MTC, a serum calcitonin and a screening for the *RET* proto-oncogene should be included in the initial evaluation. The disease phenotype is correlated with the position and type of *RET* proto-oncogene mutation. Thyroglobulin levels are useful for monitoring for recurrence of well-differentiated thyroid cancer after complete thyroidectomy; however, they should not be part of the initial evaluation. The use of radioactive iodine or technetium-99m to evaluate the thyroid nodule is of limited utility and does not help to discriminate between benign and malignant nodules. The initial imaging modality of choice is a thyroid ultrasound. This can be used to detect nonpalpable nodules, evaluate neck lymph nodes for malignant involvement, and serially follow nodules. Certain characteristics seen on ultrasound are suggestive of malignancy; however, ultrasound characteristics cannot accurately distinguish between malignant and benign lesions. Ultrasound-guided FNA may increase the sensitivity of the biopsy by reducing the chances of missing the nodule in question.

Management and Therapy

Surgical Management

Thyroid cancer is frequently divided into three general categories: well differentiated, poorly differentiated, and medullary, and the histology directly affects the surgical management. The primary management of thyroid cancer is surgical resection. A fiberoptic evaluation of the larynx to assess for vocal cord paralysis should be performed on all patients undergoing thyroid surgery. This is required because assessment for vocal cord paralysis based on symptoms and clinical history is insensitive, and vocal paralysis may indicate invasion of the recurrent laryngeal nerve or the airway. The use of computed tomography (CT) scans results in a delay radioactive iodine scanning and treatment of about 6 to 8 weeks. Thus, the use of CT scanning should be limited to select patients whose surgical resection may be improved with the additional information obtained by the CT scan. Patients with lymphadenopathy on physical exam or ultrasound and patients with diagnosis of papillary thyroid cancer, which has a higher rate of nodal involvement, should undergo preoperative CT scanning. A thorough assessment of the nodal involvement preoperatively will facilitate a more complete and directed nodal dissection at the time of surgery. In this situation improvement in surgical resection is probably of greater benefit than earlier postoperative treatment with radioiodine.

Well-Differentiated Thyroid Cancers

The well-differentiated category generally consists of papillary thyroid cancer, follicular thyroid cancer, and Hürthle cell carcinoma. Papillary thyroid cancer is associated with the microscopic feature of psammoma bodies that can be calcified and can appear as microcalcifications on ultrasound (Fig. 87-1). One feature of papillary thyroid cancer is its tendency for being multifocal, and about one third of patients will have lymph node involvement at the time of diagnosis. Of the well-differentiated thyroid cancers, papillary thyroid cancer has the lowest rate of distant metastases. Follicular thyroid cancer is pathologically characterized by capsular or vascular invasion. Follicular thyroid cancer tends to present as solitary tumors and has a more aggressive clinical course and a higher rate of distant metastases than papillary thyroid cancer. At the time of diagnosis, about 10% to 15% of patients will have metastatic disease. Hürthle cell carcinoma is characterized

Figure 87-1 Papillary Carcinoma of the Thyroid.

Clinical characteristics of papillary carcinoma of the thyroid.

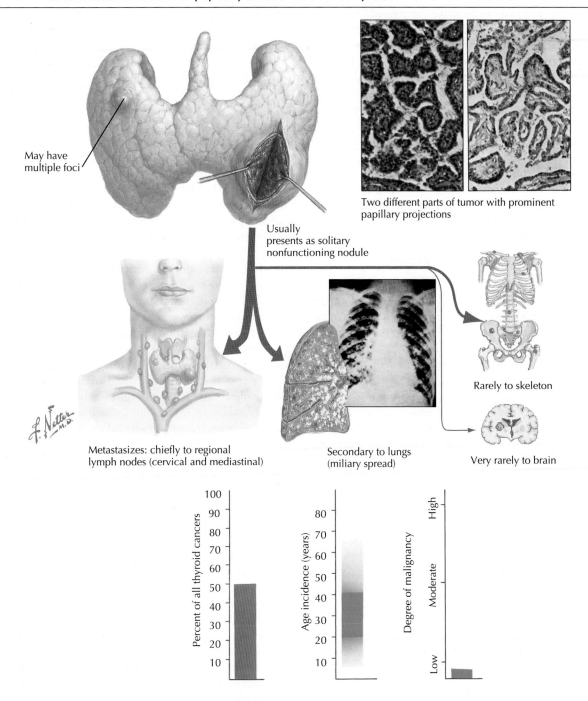

May have multiple foci

Two different parts of tumor with prominent papillary projections

Usually presents as solitary nonfunctioning nodule

Rarely to skeleton

Metastasizes: chiefly to regional lymph nodes (cervical and mediastinal)

Secondary to lungs (miliary spread)

Very rarely to brain

by the presence of oncocytes rich in mitochondria (Hürthle cells), and vascular and capsular invasion. The diagnosis of Hürthle cell cancer and follicular thyroid cancer can only be made on a surgical specimen because evidence of capsular or vascular invasion is required for the diagnosis.

The primary principle of the surgical management of well-differentiated thyroid cancer is that there should be complete resection of all gross disease in the thyroid and involved lymph nodes. The extent of surgery, partial thy-roidectomy versus total thyroidectomy, is a debated issue. Most of the studies are retrospective and do not defini-tively support one procedure over the other. There are several risk stratification systems to better estimate the chances of recurrence, and many physicians select the sur-gical procedure on the potential for recurrence. However, many of these risk stratification systems use factors that are not known preoperatively, which limits the application of these systems in selecting the surgical procedure. Patients without evidence of nodules in the contralateral lobe, no evidence of lymph node involvement, and thought to be at low risk for recurrence can probably be treated effectively with resection of the involved lobe and the isthmus. It is recommended that patients who are thought to be at high risk for recurrence undergo total thyroidectomy. Most surgeons in the United States perform a total thyroidectomy. Potential advantages of performing a total thyroidectomy are the removal of occult microscopic disease in the contralateral lobe, allowing the monitoring for disease recurrence with serial thyroglobulin levels, and allowing the use of radioiodine to ablate any remaining thyroid tissue. Patients with no clinical evidence of lymph node involvement do not require an elective neck dissection, and patients with clinically evident disease preoperatively should have the involved lymph nodes removed, but do not require a formal neck dissection.

Poorly Differentiated Thyroid Cancers

Anaplastic thyroid cancer and the rare types of thyroid cancer, insular and large cell, are often included in the category of poorly differentiated thyroid cancers. Anaplastic thyroid cancer represents the most aggressive form and accounts for about 1% to 2% of all thyroid cancers. This is a very aggressive malignancy with a median survival in most studies of 3 to 6 months. Most patients present with locally advanced disease with symptoms consisting of stridor, dysphagia, dyspnea, neck pain, and tenderness. Regional lymph node metastases, vocal cord paralysis, and direct invasion into the surrounding tissues are common. Many patients will have metastatic disease at presentation, with the most frequent sites of metastases being the bone, lung, and brain. Pathologically, anaplastic thyroid cancer can be confused with lymphoma and MTC; however, MTCs stain positive for calcitonin, and lymphoma cells are positive for leukocyte common antigen. Frequently, securing a safe airway to prevent death from asphyxiation can be a critical component of palliating patients. If the patient develops an emergent airway obstruction, securing the airway requires a tracheostomy. In nonemergent circumstances, an elective tracheostomy and radiotherapy are treatment options. Radiotherapy can achieve local control in about 80% of the cases, but does not provide long-term control of this disease.

Medullary Thyroid Cancer

The surgical management of MTC differs. The current guidelines recommend that surgical treatment should include a total thyroidectomy and a modified radical neck dissection. The chances of biochemical cure, defined as normalization of basal and stimulated calcitonin levels, is dependent on the presence or absence of lymph node involvement.

Patients should have calcitonin levels checked before surgery. If the calcitonin level remains elevated postoperatively, residual disease in the neck is unlikely, and serum

calcitonin scan of the chest and abdomen or MRI is indicated to detect distant metastases. In persistent or recurrent MTC, the chance of biochemical cure with surgical resection is about 20% at experienced centers. Patients who are determined to have a MEN syndrome who have a high risk for developing thyroid cancer may undergo a prophylactic thyroidectomy.

Postoperative Management

The three components of the postoperative care consist of thyroid ablation with radioiodine, TSH suppression, and surveillance for recurrence. There is significant variability and debate about which groups of patients should receive radioiodine thyroid ablation. It is generally not offered to patients with tumors smaller than 1 cm because the risk for recurrence of these cancers is thought to be low. Some clinicians offer radioiodine to patients with tumors larger than 1.5 or 2.0 cm regardless of risk factors, whereas other physicians use it only in patients with tumors larger than 2.0 cm or those with other risks factors. Treatment with radioiodine in high-risk tumors has been shown to reduce the rate of recurrence and cancer-specific mortality.

A common method of delivering radioiodine is for patients to withdraw thyroid hormone until the TSH is elevated to 30 µIU/mL. This can take about 4 to 6 weeks. Two weeks before therapy, the patient is placed on a low iodine diet and then undergoes a low-dose radioiodine whole-body scan, which can assist in choosing the appropriate treatment dose of radioiodine. Radioiodine ablation is usually performed after the whole-body scan, and a post-treatment whole-body scan is performed. Patients who have had an iodinated contrast CT scan in the previous 6 to 9 months should have a low 24-hour urinary iodine clearance measured. The urinary iodine clearance should be less than 200 µg/d per gram of creatinine before radioiodine ablation. The administration of radioactive iodine should be delayed until this level is reached.

Thyroid hormone is initiated after radioiodine treatment, and the dose is titrated to suppress TSH. Some studies indicate a lower rate of tumor recurrences with lifelong TSH suppression, and the optimal level of TSH suppression may vary with the risk for recurrence. The surveillance for recurrence should consist of periodic physical exams, TSH, and thyroglobulin levels, and antithyroglobulin antibodies every 6 to 12 months. Antithyroglobulin antibodies should be checked with thyroglobulin because antibodies make thyroglobulin measurements unreliable. Because of problems of laboratory variability, the thyroglobulin levels should ideally be performed at the same laboratory. Patients with distant metastases or soft tissue invasion on initial staging or a detectable thyroglobulin level should undergo periodic neck scans and diagnostic radioiodine scans every 12 months. A recombinant TSH-stimulated thyroglobulin test is appropriate in low-risk patients. Thyroglobulin and diagnostic radioiodine tests cannot be used in patients who underwent a subtotal thyroidectomy. When patients have elevated thyroglobulin levels, a workup for metastatic disease should be initiated. The initial workup frequently includes an ultrasound to evaluate for a local recurrence and radioiodine scans. If the tumor produces thyroglobulin, but is not radioiodine-avid, an 18-fluorodeoxyglucose positron emission tomography scan may provide valuable information. CT scans and bone scans are also frequently used.

Recurrent or Metastatic Disease

About one third of patients will experience a tumor recurrence, and most will recur within the first 10 years after diagnosis. The rate of metastases varies with histology, and about 10% of patients with papillary thyroid cancer, 25% with follicular thyroid cancer, and 35% with Hürthle cell cancer will develop distant metastases. The prognosis is better for patients with radioiodine-avid lung metastases, and worse for skeletal and non–radioiodine-avid metastases. If a patient is suspected of having a local recurrence, the diagnosis should be confirmed on FNA biopsy given the risks of additional surgery in the neck. Surgical resection of the local recurrence is the preferred treatment, and it is generally followed by radioiodine ablation. External-beam radiotherapy may be used for recurrent cancers that are not amendable to surgical resection and not responsive to radioiodine. The fibrosis that develops after external-beam radiotherapy complicates or prevents any further surgical interventions; therefore, this treatment should only be used after consultation with surgical colleagues.

When patients have nonresectable metastases or distant metastatic disease, the primary treatment is radioiodine. This can be a very effective therapy. However, about one third of patients will undergo dedifferentiation, which consists of the loss of the ability to produce thyroglobulin and the ability to concentrate radioiodine. This creates difficulty in monitoring the disease burden and renders radioiodine ineffective. Chemotherapy is generally the standard therapy for metastatic malignancies. In metastatic thyroid cancer, several chemotherapeutic agents have been explored; however, there is no established chemotherapy for well-differentiated thyroid cancer. For anaplastic thyroid cancer, agents such as doxorubicin and paclitaxel have demonstrated activity with a response rate of about 20%. The treatment of metastatic MTC is surgical resection if recurrence is localized. If the recurrence is diffuse, chemotherapy has a limited role in the treatment of metastatic disease. Given the lack of proven effective therapies for metastatic thyroid cancer of all subtypes, the enrollment of patients in clinical trials is critical to develop new therapeutic options.

Avoiding Treatment Errors

One potential clinical decision-making error is interpreting a nondiagnostic or suspicious biopsy result as negative for malignancy. If the clinical suspicion for malignancy is high, nondiagnostic results should lead to an ultrasound-guided FNA or surgical biopsy. In the preoperative workup, one potential error is the indiscriminate use of CT scanning, which can also limit the ability of the patient to receive radioactive iodine after the surgical resection. Only carefully selected patients should undergo preoperative CT scans. In the postoperative surveillance period, two potential errors are inadequate thyroid suppression and biochemical monitoring for recurrence. Anaplastic thyroid cancer is a rare and very aggressive malignancy, and a delay in a referral for airway management can result in airway compromise and the need for emergent tracheostomy.

Future Directions

Given the modest activity of current agents in the treatment of recurrent and metastatic disease, there is increasing interest in the development of novel therapeutic agents. During the past several years, there has been greater understanding of the proto-oncogenes and pathways responsible for the development of malignancy, and agents that specifically target these pathways are entering clinical trials. The *RET* oncogene and RAF kinases are frequently mutated in papillary thyroid cancer, and there is interest in exploring the multitargeted tyrosine kinase inhibitors, ZD6474 and AZD6244, which target this pathway. These agents are currently entering phase II trials. Other targeted therapies are currently in development and will soon enter clinical trials.

Additional Resources

Lansford CD, Teknos TN: Evaluation of the thyroid nodule. Cancer Control 13(2):89-98, 2006.
    This is an up-to-date, concise, well-written article about the valuation of a thyroid nodule.
Patel KN, Shaha AR: Poorly differentiated and anaplastic thyroid cancer. Cancer Control 13:119-128, 2006.
    This is an excellent review of a rare and very difficult disease to manage and treat.
Sherman SI, Angelos P, Ball DW, et al: Thyroid carcinoma. J Natl Compr Canc Netw 3(3):404-457, 2005.
    This article provides clear-cut guidelines and algorithms for the evaluation and management of thyroid cancer.
Slough CM, Randolph GW: Workup of well-differentiated thyroid carcinoma. Cancer Control 13(2):99-105, 2006.
    This excellent review article is about the preoperative workup for thyroid cancer.
Sturgeon C, Angelos P: Identification and treatment of aggressive thyroid cancers. Part 1: Subtypes. Oncology 20(3):253-260, 2006.
    This excellent review article is about thyroid cancer.
Sturgeon C, Angelos P: Identification and treatment of aggressive thyroid cancers. Part 2: Risk assessment and treatment. Oncology 20(4):397-408, 2006.
    This excellent review article is about thyroid cancer.

EVIDENCE

1. Ain KB, Egorin MJ, DeSimone PA: Treatment of anaplastic thyroid carcinoma with paclitaxel: Phase 2 trial using ninety-six-hour infusion. Collaborative Anaplastic Thyroid Cancer Health Intervention Trials (CATCHIT) Group. Thyroid 10(7):587-594, 2000.

   This study demonstrated the activity of paclitaxel in anaplastic thyroid cancer.

2. Belfiore A, Garofalo MR, Giuffrida D, et al: Increased aggressiveness of thyroid cancer in patients with Graves' disease. J Clin Endocrinol Metab 70(4):830-835, 1990.

   This paper evaluates thyroid cancers associated with Grave's disease.

3. Bitton RN, Sachmechi I, Tabriz MS, et al: Papillary carcinoma of the thyroid with manifestations resembling Graves' disease. Endocr Pract 7(2):106-109, 2001.

   This article describes the risks factors for thyroid cancer.

4. Bouvet M, Feldman JI, Gill GN, et al: Surgical management of the thyroid nodule: Patient selection based on the results of fine-needle aspiration cytology. Laryngoscope 102(12 Pt 1):1353-1356, 1992.

   This article describes the role of fine-needle aspirate in evaluation of a thyroid nodule.

5. Castro MR, Gharib H: Thyroid nodules and cancer. When to wait and watch, when to refer. Postgrad Med 107(1):113-116, 119-120, 123-124, 2000.

   This review article helps with the management of a common clinical problem.

6. Eng C: Familial papillary thyroid cancer—many syndromes, too many genes? J Clin Endocrinol Metab 85(5):1755-1757, 2000.

   The author describes familial thyroid cancers.

7. Frank-Raue K, Hoppner W, Frilling A, et al: Mutations of the ret proto-oncogene in German multiple endocrine neoplasia families: Relation between genotype and phenotype. German Medullary Thyroid Carcinoma Study Group. J Clin Endocrinol Metab 81(5):1780-1783, 1996.

   This paper reviews the important relationship between the RET proto-oncogene and the phenotype.

8. Gilliland FD, Hunt WC, Morris DM, Key CR: Prognostic factors for thyroid carcinoma. Cancer 79(3):564-573, 1997.

   The authors provide a classification of the current prognostic factors for thyroid cancer and cancer recurrence.

9. Haigh PI, Urbach DR, Rotstein LE: AMES prognostic index and extent of thyroidectomy for well-differentiated thyroid cancer in the United States. Surgery 136(3):609-616, 2004.

   This paper includes a prognostic index that helps estimate the chance of recurrence and the extent of surgery.

10. Hegedus L: Clinical practice. The thyroid nodule. N Engl J Med 351:1764-1771, 2004.

    This is an excellent review article of this common clinical problem.

11. Jemal A, Siegel R, Ward E, et al: Cancer statistics, 2006. CA Cancer J Clin 56(2):106-130, 2006.

    This is a review of the epidemiology of thyroid cancer with the expected rates and deaths for 2006.

12. King AD, Ahuja AT, King W, et al: The role of ultrasound in the diagnosis of a large, rapidly growing, thyroid mass. Postgrad Med J 73(861):412-414, 1997.

    This review article describes the role of ultrasound.

13. Lansford CD, Teknos TN: Evaluation of the thyroid nodule. Cancer Control 13(2):89-98, 2006.

    This comprehensive and useful review article is highly recommended.

14. Leonard N, Melcher DH: To operate or not to operate? The value of fine needle aspiration cytology in the assessment of thyroid swellings. J Clin Pathol 50(11):941-943, 1997.

   The authors provide an assessment of the role of FNA in the evaluation.

15. Machens A, Gimm O, Hinze R, et al: Genotype-phenotype correlations in hereditary medullary thyroid carcinoma: Oncological features and biochemical properties. J Clin Endocrinol Metab 86(3):1104-1109, 2001.

    This article describes the genotype and phenotype.

16. Maxon HR, Thomas SR, Saenger EL, et al: Ionizing irradiation and the induction of clinically significant disease in the human thyroid gland. Am J Med 63(6):967-978, 1977.

    This paper describes the risk for prior radiation therapy in the development of thyroid cancer.

17. Mazzaferri EL: Management of a solitary thyroid nodule. N Engl J Med 328(8):553-559, 1993.

    This is an excellent review article on the management of a solitary thyroid nodule.

18. Mazzaferri EL: Thyroid cancer in thyroid nodules: Finding a needle in the haystack. Am J Med 93(4):359-362, 1992.

    The authors address management of a thyroid nodule.

19. Mazzaferri EL, Jhiang SM: Long-term impact of initial surgical and medical therapy on papillary and follicular thyroid cancer. Am J Med 97(5):418-428, 1994.

    This article presents a valuable follow-up of patients treated with surgical resection.

20. McHenry CR, Slusarczyk SJ, Khiyami A: Recommendations for management of cystic thyroid disease. Surgery 126(6):1167-1172, 1999.

    This paper provides guidelines and recommendation for management of cystic thyroid disease.

21. Nel CJ, van Heerden JA, Goellner JR, et al: Anaplastic carcinoma of the thyroid: A clinicopathologic study of 82 cases. Mayo Clin Proc 60(1)51-58, 1985.

    This paper presents the pathologic characteristics of anaplastic thyroid cancer.

22. Pasieka JL: Anaplastic thyroid cancer. Curr Opin Oncol 15(1):78-83, 2003.

    The author describes treatment options for anaplastic thyroid cancer.

23. Patel KN, Shaha AR: Poorly differentiated and anaplastic thyroid cancer. Cancer Control 13(2):119-128, 2006.

    The authors present an excellent review of a rare and very difficult disease to manage and treat.

24. Raab SS, Silverman JF, Elsheikh TM, et al: Pediatric thyroid nodules: Disease demographics and clinical management as determined by fine needle aspiration biopsy. Pediatrics 95(1):46-49, 1995.

    This article describes thyroid nodules in the pediatric population.

25. Rojeski MT, Gharib H: Nodular thyroid disease. Evaluation and management. N Engl J Med 313(7):428-436, 1985.

    This is a review article on nodular thyroid disease.

26. Ruegemer JJ, Hay ID, Bergstralh EJ, et al: Distant metastases in differentiated thyroid carcinoma: A multivariate analysis of prognostic variables. J Clin Endocrinol Metab 67(3):501-508, 1988.

    This paper provides prognostic variables in the metastatic setting.

27. Samaan NA, Schultz PN, Haynie TP, Ordonez NG: Pulmonary metastasis of differentiated thyroid carcinoma: Treatment results in 101 patients. J Clin Endocrinol Metab 60(2):376-380, 1985.

    This article reflects the distribution of metastases and the response to therapy.

28. Shaha AR: Controversies in the management of thyroid nodule. Laryngoscope 110(2 Pt 1):183-193, 2000.

    The author addresses management of a thyroid nodule.

29. Sherman SI, Angelos P, Ball DW, et al: Thyroid carcinoma. J Natl Compr Canc Netw 3(3):404-457, 2005.

This article provides clear-cut guidelines and algorithms for the evaluation and management of thyroid cancer.

30. Shimaoka K, Schoenfeld DA, DeWys WD, et al: A randomized trial of doxorubicin versus doxorubicin plus cisplatin in patients with advanced thyroid carcinoma. Cancer 56(9):2155-2160, 1985.

    This trial demonstrates the activity of doxorubicin in the treatment of advanced thyroid cancer.

31. Singer PA, Cooper DS, Daniels GH, et al: Treatment guidelines for patients with thyroid nodules and well-differentiated thyroid cancer. American Thyroid Association. Arch Intern Med 156(19):2165-2172, 1996.

    The authors present guidelines for the management of thyroid cancer.

32. Slough CM, Randolph GW: Workup of well-differentiated thyroid carcinoma. Cancer Control 13(2):99-105, 2006.

This is an excellent review article about the management of well-differentiated thyroid cancer.

33. Sturgeon C, Angelos P: Identification and treatment of aggressive thyroid cancers. Part 1: Subtypes. Oncology 20(3):253-260, 2006.

    This is an excellent review article about thyroid cancer.

34. Sturgeon C, Angelos P: Identification and treatment of aggressive thyroid cancers. Part 2: Risk assessment and treatment. Oncology 20(4):397-408, 2006.

    This is an excellent review article about thyroid cancer.

35. Weber T, Schilling T, Buchler MW: Thyroid carcinoma. Curr Opin Oncol 18(1):30-35, 2006.

    The authors provide a current update about the therapeutic options for thyroid cancer.

Stephen A. Bernard ▪ Thomas E. Stinchcombe

Palliative Care for Patients with Advanced Cancer

Introduction

Palliative care refers to care at the end of life. Palliative medicine is now increasingly recognized as a distinct area of medicine, and the principles of symptom management are being incorporated into surgery, pediatrics, family medicine, and internal medicine. The goals of the interventions are to relieve symptoms and suffering in individuals with advanced disease. Although these goals are often addressed in patients with cancer, similar goals are now acknowledged as important in end-stage heart and lung disease and in neurodegenerative conditions such as Alzheimer's disease and amyotrophic lateral sclerosis. Although simple medical management of a symptom such as pain does not require this type of specialized approach, the broader context within which the symptom of pain may be seen often benefits from psychological counseling and from addressing social, existential, spiritual, and other dimensions of the symptom. It is the use of a multidisciplinary approach that recognizes and utilizes the numerous facets of care at end of life that distinguishes palliative care from other disciplines.

Approach to the Patient

The approach to a cancer patient at the end of life must address the futility of additional active, disease-oriented treatments. In the United States, this has been particularly difficult because of the environment in which cancer is treated. This environment has lead to a continued reduction in the number of days that the patient is on hospice in the United States (a surrogate marker for stopping active treatment).

A recent review by Okon and Gomez describes an approach that acknowledges the multidimensional nature of end-of-life care. Pain should be addressed in the context of the totality of depression, impact on function, and social support. Several tools and approaches are discussed by the authors to evaluate the role of autonomy, communication, closure of life affairs, economic burden, and transcendental and existential issues on symptoms at the end of life.

Pain

Pain that is seen at the end of life in cancer patients is often a combination of disease and treatment effects. Surveys of this population throughout the world have shown that 70% to 80% of patients with cancer will have pain and that in at least one third of those patients, the pain will interfere with function. Points that are important in the history are location, character, and severity. The role of movement (incidental pain) is also important. The perception of pain is commonly altered by other symptoms (e.g., fatigue, weakness, nausea, constipation, dyspnea, coughing); or psychological factors (e.g., depression, anxiety, and feelings of hopelessness or anger). The impact that the pain has on a patient's daily activities and psychosocial functioning varies greatly. Pain and the context within which it is viewed may change frequently, and reassessments should be done at intervals that account for the rate of change.

Pathophysiology of Pain

The afferent pathways for pain in the nervous system begin with nociceptors, specialized receptors that respond to noxious physical or chemical stimuli widely distributed throughout the body except in the brain. Pain afferent fibers enter the spinal cord through the dorsal root and synapse in the dorsal horn and then ascend through the spinothalamic and spinoreticular paths to the thalamus and the reticular system, respectively. The efferent pathways, which modulate nociceptive transmission, originate in the central nervous system and travel down the lateral posterior column into the peripheral nerves. The efferent pathways are activated by endogenous endorphins and can be activated centrally by opioids that mimic the activity of endogenous endorphins. The neurotransmitter serotonin is also believed to be important in some of these descending pathways, and this may account for the action of antidepressants in the treatment of pain.

Classification of Pain

Nociceptive pain arises from direct stimulation of the nociceptors by physical or chemical stimulation of the nerve endings due to tissue damage; it is often divided into somatic and visceral pain. Somatic pain is described as aching pain that is often well localized. Visceral pain is poorly localized and described as squeezing or a pressure sensation; it may be referred to distant cutaneous sites. It is caused by infiltration, compression, or distention of thoracic or abdominal viscera that are innervated by the sympathetic nervous system. Neuropathic pain is burning or tingling with intermittent lancinating pain that results from tumor infiltration or compression of a peripheral nerve or the spinal cord. This type of pain is also seen in diabetic neuropathy or postherpetic neuralgia.

Optimum Treatment of Pain

If the disease is responsive, treatment of the underlying condition can provide significant pain relief. However, for most patients during their disease course, symptom management will also be needed. The management of cancer pain has employed the World Health Organization (WHO) Analgesic Ladder that was developed 20 years ago. A review of the history of this three-step ladder by Foley emphasizes the multidimensional nature of pain that is addressed in this document. For many patients with cancer, treatment begins with the strong opioids described in WHO step 3. Most of these patients' pain will not be controlled with drugs that are used at steps 1 and 2. The step 3 drugs include morphine, hydromorphone, and methadone. Analgesia may have been used at the beginning of the illness, but with progression of the disease or inability to relieve the pain with disease-focused therapy, symptom management with stronger opioids and other measures become more important. Radiation of a painful bone lesion may still play a role in this population, and many of the short-course schedules used outside of the United States are now being used in this country with excellent results. Stabilization of the spine by external bracing may diminish incident pain. Use of bisphosphonates for selected tumors—breast and prostate cancer and myeloma—may relieve the pain of bony metastases. Although the WHO Analgesic Ladder is not ideal, it remains the best known effort to adopt principles of cancer pain management throughout the world. There are now more than 30 guidelines from more than 12 countries. Worldwide, access to pain medications remains a major issue.

Avoiding Treatment Errors

An extensive review is beyond the scope of this chapter; several topics are briefly discussed. Balancing the need to relieve pain with the side effects of the analgesics used occurs with the management of almost all patients. Several of these agents have unique issues associated with them. For example, the use of drugs such as fentanyl, given in micrograms, with a patient-controlled analgesia pump requires attention to the programming of the pump. Drugs that have a long half-life in the body, such as methadone, have the potential for cumulative effects that may not be immediately seen. Recently, the U.S. Food and Drug Administration has published a warning for this drug and the potential for cardiac arrhythmias. Many of the opioids are cleared by drug-metabolizing enzymes in the liver (the cytochrome P-450 system), and there is the potential for clinically apparent drug interactions, such as phenocopying, that could occur with codeine and other drugs that affect the CYP 2D6 isozyme.

Conversions of all the opioids, especially methadone, need to take into account the issue of incomplete cross-tolerance for the new drug leading to overdosing if a reduction in starting dose is not done.

Anorexia and Cachexia

Cancer cachexia refers to the weight loss and particularly loss of muscle mass and adipose tissue commonly associated with advanced cancer. The syndrome of loss of appetite and weight loss is as common in the advanced cancer patient as that of pain. Although other conditions such as AIDS have similar loss of weight, the alteration of metabolism is more profound in cancer. In contrast to starvation, there is an increase in energy expenditure and much greater proteolysis. Although originally thought to be a form of starvation of the host as a result of the consumption of calories by a highly metabolic tumor creating a calorie deficit for the body, recent work has shown a more complex picture. Substances produced by the tumor such as proteolysis-inducing factor promote breakdown of protein. In response to the tumor, the patient (host) may make such

factors as tumor necrosis factor (TNF), interleukin-6, and interleukin-1. These host-derived cytokines further accelerate the loss of weight. There may be derangements in the autonomic nervous system such as decreased emptying of the stomach or slowing of transit time in bowel emptying.

Anorexia is defined as the decline in food intake to the point that caloric intake does not provide enough energy for the amount of caloric expenditure. In advanced cancer, this symptom is due to several causes. These include alteration in taste thresholds to bitter and sweet; changes in the oropharyngeal environment due to treatment with damage to the mucosa, and loss of salivary function. The degree of symptoms may vary by the type of tumor and its treatment. The two syndromes often occur simultaneously, and symptoms can be very disturbing to the patient's family or caretakers; however, they do not always cause the patient discomfort. Patient and family education is very important.

Optimum Treatment

The initial treatment involves encouraging increased oral intake or the use of high calorie nutritional supplements; however, as the patient becomes more ill, these measures may not be sufficient. The use of total parenteral nutrition has not been shown to be beneficial in affecting survival in a variety of cancers, both adult and pediatric. Treating symptoms that may be contributing to the syndrome is an important aspect of managing anorexia and cachexia.

Pharmacologic approaches may result in an increased appetite or sense of well-being; less frequently, they result in improvement in objective parameters such as weight gain or lean muscle mass. Potential adverse effects must be balanced against the relatively modest benefits. Often, decisions are made based on the patient's and the family's preferences and the level of anxiety and discomfort created by the anorexia and cachexia.

Corticosteroids, usually dexamethasone or methylprednisolone, are used most often. Trials have shown an improvement in appetite and performance status, but they have been associated with adverse events such as gastrointestinal hemorrhage, cushingoid body features, and myopathy. These relatively inexpensive medications are also beneficial in the treatment of chronic nausea and pain and may be beneficial in the treatment of cancer-associated fatigue. The proper dose and duration of treatment have not yet been definitively determined.

The progestational agent, megestrol acetate, is often used in this situation. Several studies have documented its effectiveness in increasing appetite and food intake in a significant percentage of patients. The dose used has varied from 480 to 1600 mg daily. Side effects include fluid retention, edema, and erectile dysfunction in men. There is some concern about a possible increased risk for deep venous thrombosis. The high cost of megestrol acetate, especially in comparison to corticosteroids, must be considered with the use of this agent.

Emerging Therapies

Dronabinol, a derivative of marijuana, has shown some activity as an appetite stimulant and in the treatment of chronic nausea, benefits that have increased interest in its use in the treatment of cancer cachexia and anorexia. As expected, there are associated mood effects, somnolence, and confusion. Thalidomide is believed to alter levels of TNF, a cytokine that may be responsible for anorexia and cachexia. A preliminary study revealed some therapeutic efficacy. Thalidomide may be of benefit in the treatment of coexisting insomnia also. It is a teratogen and has been associated with adverse events such as dry mouth, somnolence, and peripheral neuropathy. Melatonin is believed to alter TNF levels and is relatively well tolerated. A preliminary study revealed some efficacy in preventing weight loss in patients with metastatic cancer. Anabolic steroids have been considered as a possible treatment for these symptoms, although a recent randomized controlled trial showed that they were inferior to dexamethasone or megestrol acetate. Recently, attention has focused on the use of ghrelin, a peptide that stimulates food intake.

Hydration

Often patients with advanced cancer have a decline in their oral intake due to cancer fatigue, persistent nausea and vomiting, and cancer anorexia and cachexia. Family members and members of the medical staff will often raise the issue of the palliative benefits of intravenous hydration. Many family members have concerns that if intravenous fluids (IVF) are not initiated, the patient will "die of thirst," and this fear is often compounded if the patient has dry mucous membranes or the appearance of dehydration. The family may perceive the decision to discontinue intravenous hydration as letting him or her die, and they must be educated before any discussion or decision to forego or discontinue hydration.

The risks and benefits of IVF are debated in the palliative care community because many studies evaluating its use have been done in very heterogeneous patient populations. The symptoms, clinical outcomes evaluated, and evaluation methods used have varied among studies, making direct comparison difficult. The argument in favor of the use of IVF is that the patient may have less delirium related to dehydration and a lower frequency of adverse events from altered drug metabolism due to renal insufficiency. There is no evidence that the use of IVF in this setting prolongs life to any significant degree. Arguments against the use of IVF focus on the risk for fluid overload and possible benefits such as decreased pulmonary and gastrointestinal secretions with less nausea and vomiting; decreased urine production with fewer episodes of incontinence; and diminished need for use of urinary catheters.

Many patients complain of thirst or dry mouth while in the terminal phases of their illness, and this can cause significant discomfort for the patient and the patient's family. A study by McCann and colleagues found that 66% of patients admitted to a palliative care unit complained of thirst or dry mouth on admission, but with the use of small amounts of oral fluids, ice chips, and routine mouth care, these symptoms were relieved for several hours in most patients. This study supports the use of these simple measures initially to address a patient's complaint of thirst or dry mouth before considering the initiation of IVF.

Avoiding Treatment Errors

Given the relative paucity of data on the risks and benefits of intravenous hydration and the relative risks and benefits of fluid deficiency in the palliative setting, it is impossible to give definitive recommendations on this subject. Often the decision will have to be made based on the condition and wishes of the individual patient and his or her family and on the opinion of the physician and medical staff caring for the patient. Careful attention to the volume of fluid may avoid the possibility of rapidly worsening renal function and the potential for opioid-induced neurotoxicity, but at the same time not overhydrate the individual to cause a worsening of dyspnea.

Future Directions

Worldwide, there are increasing numbers of palliative care specialists both in developed and developing countries. In the United States, the development of a separate boarded specialty is underway. The development of such programs in the United States requires resolution of reimbursement issues; however, demand for such services continues to increase.

Additional Resources

The Cochrane Collection Website. Reviews of evidence-based palliative care. http://www.cochrane.org/reviews/en/topics/85.html. Accessed November 4, 2006.

Okun T, Gomez C: Patient evaluation in palliative care. Available at: http://www.uptodateonline.com.libproxy.lib.unc.edu. Accessed August 26, 2006.

This is one of several topics on this website dealing with palliative care.

Walker P, Bruera E (eds): Palliative care. Hematol Oncol Clin North Am 16(3):511-762, 2002.

The entire June 2002 issue is devoted to topics in palliative care.

EVIDENCE

1. Bernard S, Bruera E: Drug interactions in palliative care. J Clin Oncol 18(8):1780-1799, 2000.
   The authors review drug interactions seen with the common classes of drugs used in palliative care.
2. Bruera E, Neumann CM, Pituskin E, et al: Thalidomide in patients with cachexia due to terminal cancer: Preliminary report. Ann Oncol 10:857-859, 1999.
   A trial of thalidomide for relief of symptoms that included appetite and caloric intake as outcome variables showed a positive result in this study; however, only 28 patients were evaluated.
3. Cleary J: Putting evidence about cancer pain into practice: The role of clinical guidelines. Cancer Pain Release 18:1-12, 2005.
   An interview with one of the individuals responsible for developing the revision of the American Pain Society 2005 guidelines addresses the goals, current views of guidelines, and their limitations.
4. Foley K: Appraisal of the WHO Analgesic Ladder on its 20th anniversary. Cancer Pain Release 19:1-8, 2006.
   In this interview with one of the key individuals who developed the WHO Ladder, the rationale, limitations, and future use are discussed.
5. U.S. Food and Drug Administration, Center for Drug Evaluation and Research: Methadone hydrochloride information. Available at: http://www.fda.gov/cder/drug/infopage/methadone/default.htm. Accessed January 19, 2007.
6. Caraceni A, Portenoy RK: An international survey of cancer pain characteristics and syndromes. IASP Task Force on Cancer Pain. International Association for the Study of Pain. Pain 82:263-274, 1999.
   Fifty-one clinicians in 24 countries and 1095 patients were surveyed to provide an overview of cancer-related pain. A multivariate model suggested that the presence of breakthrough pain, somatic pain, and lower performance status were the most important predictors of intense pain.
7. Clark D, Centeno C: Palliative care in Europe: An emerging approach to comparative analysis. Clin Med 6:197-201, 2006.
   The article discusses the variation in palliative care in European countries. Future directions to better integrate palliative care in health care delivery are discussed.
8. Cleeland CS, Gonin R, Hatfield AK, et al: Pain and its treatment in outpatients with metastatic cancer. N Engl J Med 330:592-596, 1994.
   A survey of a group of 1308 outpatients seen at Eastern Oncology Group institutions showed that 67% had pain, and 36% had pain severe enough to interfere with function. In 42%, the pain was not adequately treated.
9. Fainsinger R, Bruera E: When to treat dehydration in a terminally ill patient? Support Care Cancer 5(3):205-211, 1997.
   This article reviews the issues in hydration and dehydration in the terminally ill patient, suggesting that hydration may have some advantages. The advantages and disadvantages of each side in this controversy are addressed.
10. Loprinzi CL, Kuglet JW, Sloan JA, et al: Randomized comparison of megestrol acetate versus dexamethasone versus fluoxymesterone for the treatment of cancer anorexia/cachexia. J Clin Oncol 17:3299-3306, 1999.
    This randomized, double-blind trial showed equivalency of megestrol acetate to dexamethasone in improvement in appetite in a population with cancer anorexia and cachexia.
11. McCann RM, Hall WJ, Groth-Juncker A: Comfort care for terminally ill patients. The appropriate use of nutrition and hydration. JAMA 272:1263-1266, 1994.
    The authors report on a prospective observational and interventional trial of patients admitted to a palliative care unit. Thirst was either not experienced or experienced only initially. The symptom could be alleviated with small amounts of oral fluid, suggesting that more aggressive hydration is not appropriate.
12. Pereira J, Lawlor P, Vigano A, et al: Equianalgesic dose ratios for opioids: A critical review and proposals for long-term dosing. J Pain Symptom Manag 22(2): 672-687, 2001.
    The authors provide a review of the literature on equianalgesic dosing that includes articles on methadone. Discrepancies in this literature are discussed.

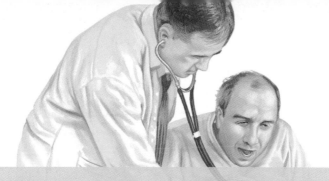
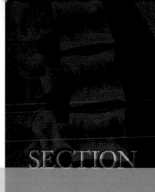

Infectious Diseases

William C. Miller ▪ Cynthia Gay

89

Fever of Unknown Origin

Introduction

Fever is common with many acute illnesses. The fever usually resolves spontaneously. However, certain patients develop prolonged fever without clear cause, posing a diagnostic challenge for their physicians.

Petersdorf and Beeson established the classic definition of fever of unknown origin (FUO) in 1961. They defined FUO as (1) illness of more than 3 weeks' duration, (2) temperature of 38.3° C (101° F) on several occasions, and (3) uncertain diagnosis after 1 week of study in hospital. Although this definition of FUO has been very useful, changes in the practice of medicine have significantly altered the approach to patients with persistent fever. In 1991, Durack and Street proposed revisions to the definition, including the substitution of three outpatient visits or 3 hospital days for the third criterion. Alternatively, the third criterion can be replaced with uncertain diagnosis after 1 week of evaluation. In addition, Durack and Street proposed distinguishing classic FUO from nosocomial, neutropenic, or HIV-associated FUO, given differences in etiologies and underlying conditions.

Etiology and Pathogenesis

More than 200 diseases have been linked to FUO. The five primary categories of FUO are infection, malignancy, noninfectious inflammatory diseases, miscellaneous, and undiagnosed (Fig. 89-1). Infections represent about 30% to 50% of cases; malignancies, 20% to 30%; noninfectious inflammatory diseases, 10% to 30%; miscellaneous, 15% to 25%; and undiagnosed, 5% to 15%. Most case series on FUO report infections as the most common diagnosis; however, some studies have shown an increase in cases due to noninfectious inflammatory diseases. The prevalence of febrile illnesses varies geographically, with infections being more common in developing countries and tropical regions. Causes also vary according to host factors such as underlying immunosuppression and hospital and health service exposures.

The most commonly identified infections are abscesses, tuberculosis, and viral infections. Abscesses, predominantly intra-abdominal, have remained a leading cause of FUO over the past three decades. Hepatic, subhepatic, and subdiaphragmatic abscesses are common. Other locations include the retroperitoneal, splenic, appendiceal, pericolonic, perinephric, and pelvic areas. Underlying conditions such as diabetes mellitus, immunosuppressive medications,

prior surgery, and cirrhosis have been associated with the development of occult abscesses.

Tuberculosis is the most common source of FUO in most case series and often presents with miliary or extrapulmonary involvement. Viral infections have been increasingly recognized because of the availability of tests for cytomegalovirus (CMV) and Epstein-Barr virus (EBV). HIV infection, either with acute or previously undiagnosed established infection with concurrent opportunistic infection, also may cause FUO. Acute HIV infection as a cause of fever is frequently not considered but should be included in the differential diagnosis of individuals presenting with a mononucleosis-like illness, particularly with high-risk sexual or injection drug use exposure. Acute HIV infection is also among the most common causes of FUO among returned travelers in addition to malaria and typhoid fever. Many other infections have been associated with FUO, including cat-scratch disease (*Bartonella* species infection), brucellosis, histoplasmosis, leishmaniasis, malaria, psittacosis, relapsing fever, and leptospirosis.

Subacute bacterial endocarditis (SBE), osteomyelitis, sinusitis, and urinary tract infections also cause FUO. SBE is a less common cause than in the past because of improvements in blood culture methods and echocardiography. However, true culture-negative cases (without antibiotic

Figure 89-1 Potential Causes of Fever of Unknown Origin.

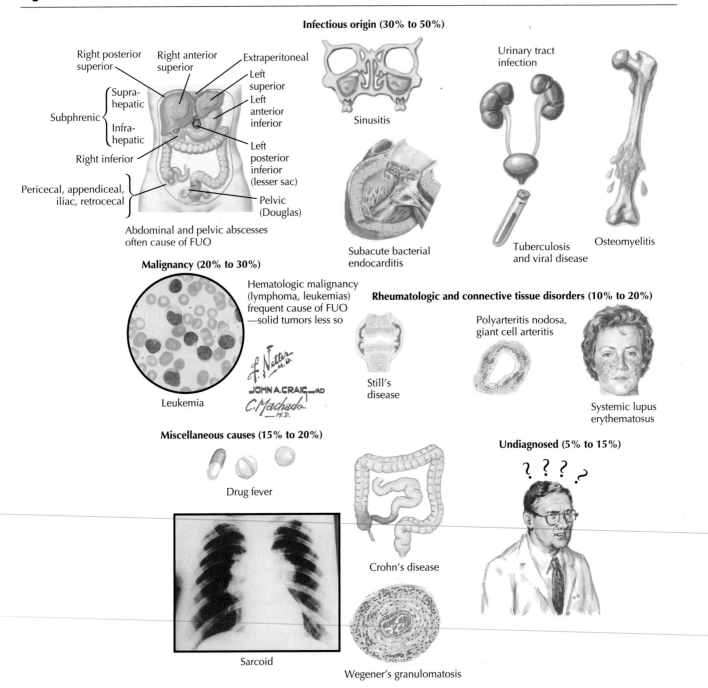

Infectious origin (30% to 50%)

Right posterior superior / Right anterior superior / Extraperitoneal / Left superior / Left anterior inferior / Left posterior inferior (lesser sac)

Suprahepatic / Infrahepatic — Subphrenic

Right inferior

Pericecal, appendiceal, iliac, retrocecal

Pelvic (Douglas)

Abdominal and pelvic abscesses often cause of FUO

Sinusitis

Urinary tract infection

Subacute bacterial endocarditis

Tuberculosis and viral disease

Osteomyelitis

Malignancy (20% to 30%)

Hematologic malignancy (lymphoma, leukemias) frequent cause of FUO —solid tumors less so

Leukemia

Rheumatologic and connective tissue disorders (10% to 20%)

Still's disease

Polyarteritis nodosa, giant cell arteritis

Systemic lupus erythematosus

Miscellaneous causes (15% to 20%)

Drug fever

Crohn's disease

Sarcoid

Wegener's granulomatosis

Undiagnosed (5% to 15%)

administration before obtaining blood culture specimens) still constitute 3% to 5% of large series. Culture-negative endocarditis is more common with infections due to *Coxiella burnetii* (Q fever); *Tropheryma whippelii; Brucella, Mycoplasma, Chlamydia, Histoplasma, Legionella,* and *Bartonella* species infection; and the HACEK group, including *Haemophilus, Actinobacillus, Cardiobacterium, Eikenella,* and *Kingella* species. Fastidious organisms may be missed in routine culture.

Several neoplastic diseases may cause fever and may present as FUO. Hematologic malignancies are most common, including Hodgkin's and non-Hodgkin's lymphoma. Leukemia also may cause FUO, but less commonly. Solid tumors cause FUO less commonly than lymphomas and leukemias. Renal cell carcinoma may cause fever and FUO, although only 2.5% of cases present with FUO. Carcinoma of the colon may cause persistent fever. Other solid tumors occasionally associated with FUO include hepatocellular carcinoma, gastric carcinoma, pancreatic carcinoma, mesothelioma and leiomyosarcoma.

The two most common rheumatologic diseases associated with FUO are Still's disease (juvenile rheumatoid arthritis) and giant cell arteritis. Still's disease occurs in young adults and is associated with episodic fever, arthralgias, arthritis, and commonly, a rash. Fever may precede the onset of joint symptoms, but the diagnosis cannot be made until arthritis develops. Giant cell arteritis is an important cause of FUO in patients older than 50 years with a high erythrocyte sedimentation rate (ESR). FUO in elderly patients is more frequently due to noninfectious inflammatory diseases and, in developed countries, exceeds infection as the most common cause. Polyarteritis nodosa is a rare but important cause of FUO. Other rheumatologic diseases causing FUO include systemic lupus erythematosus (SLE), polymyositis, rheumatoid arthritis, Takayasu's arteritis, and mixed cryoglobulinemia.

Many other disorders fall under the miscellaneous category. Drug fever is another common cause. Drug fever may be caused by allergic reactions, idiosyncratic reactions, or altered thermoregulation. Drug fever is more common in hospitalized patients and in patients with AIDS. Drug fever can occur without other symptoms or signs but is suggested by simultaneous rash or peripheral eosinophilia.

Factitious fever, which is most often identified in young people who are associated in some way with the medical profession, is surprisingly common. Several granulomatous diseases are associated with FUO, including Crohn's disease, Wegener's granulomatosis, sarcoidosis, and granulomatous hepatitis. Alcoholic hepatitis can be associated with persistent fever and appears to be common in the community setting. Other conditions associated with FUO include recurrent pulmonary emboli, thyroid disease, hematoma, atrial myxoma, and familial Mediterranean fever. Fever can also result from hypothalamic dysfunction related to massive strokes and anoxic brain injury.

Despite adequate diagnostic evaluation, a significant proportion of patients with FUO will remain without a confirmed diagnosis. Many of these patients will recover spontaneously without sequelae. Other patients will develop manifestations of their underlying illness over time, eventually leading to a definitive diagnosis.

Clinical Presentation

By definition, the clinical presentation of FUO includes fever. The fever may be high or low and relatively constant or intermittent. Generally, the more prolonged the fever, the less likely that an infection is the cause. Other symptoms and signs may or may not be present. If present, these can provide crucial clues to the diagnosis. Relatively minor findings should not be overlooked or dismissed.

Differential Diagnosis

As discussed, a wide variety of diseases can cause FUO. In approaching the patient meeting criteria for FUO, one should first consider if they have classic, nosocomial, neutropenic, or HIV-associated FUO. Classic FUO occurs in immunocompetent hosts, with onset as an outpatient and fever documented on at least three outpatient visits or persistent for at least 3 weeks. Nosocomial FUO represents all patients with fever onset after admission to the hospital, and persisting for at least 3 days with no diagnosis after initial workup. Differential diagnosis of nosocomial FUO includes drug-resistant bacteria, drug fever, deep venous thrombosis secondary to immobility, *Clostridium difficile* colitis, noninfectious postoperative fever due to inflammatory responses, and increased risk for infections secondary to surgical procedures, urinary and respiratory instrumentation, and intravascular devices. In addition, endotracheal intubation and gastric and enteral feeding tubes increase the risk for nosocomial sinusitis, which can present as FUO in intensive care units.

Immunosuppressed patients have the highest incidence of FUO among all patient groups and frequently do not manifest signs or symptoms of inflammation. FUO in either the neutropenic or HIV-infected patient significantly alters and broadens the differential diagnosis. Diagnostic workup for neutropenic or immune-suppressed patients should consider reactivation of latent viral infections such as herpesviruses, fungal infections including *Candida* and *Aspergillus* species, drug fever, and graft-versus-host disease. The differential diagnosis for infectious etiologies in HIV-infected patients broadens to include opportunistic infections such as toxoplasmosis, disseminated *Mycobacterium avium* complex infection, *Pneumocystis jiroveci* pneumonia, and CMV, and can be guided by CD4 cell count.

Because infections are the most common etiology of fever, travel history is crucial to assess the risks for tropical illness from travel abroad and infections associated with particular geographic areas, such as Rocky Mountain spotted fever in the southeast and midwestern United States and malaria and leishmaniasis in endemic regions. A history of animal and insect exposure should be obtained to assess the risk for infections related to arthropods, particularly during seasons when mosquitoes and ticks are most active.

Evidence of particular organ system involvement should lead to a narrowing of the differential diagnosis. For example, lymph node involvement may suggest lymphoma, CMV, EBV, tuberculosis, toxoplasmosis, or *Bartonella* species infection (cat-scratch disease), among others.

Diagnostic Approach

A critical step in the evaluation of FUO, although commonly overlooked, is the documentation of fever. If fever

Figure 89-2 Diagnostic Considerations in Fever of Unknown Origin.
TB, tuberculosis; ETOH, alcohol; AST, asparate aminotransferase; ALT, alanine aminotransferase.

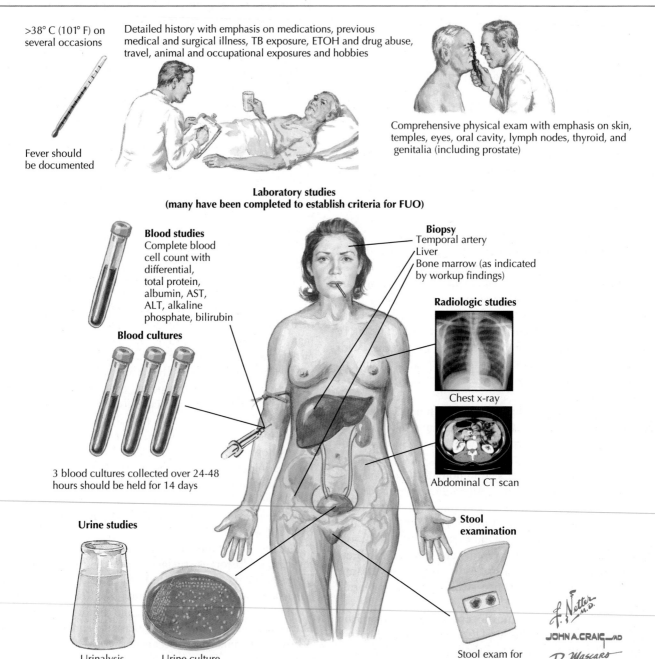

>38° C (101° F) on several occasions

Fever should be documented

Detailed history with emphasis on medications, previous medical and surgical illness, TB exposure, ETOH and drug abuse, travel, animal and occupational exposures and hobbies

Comprehensive physical exam with emphasis on skin, temples, eyes, oral cavity, lymph nodes, thyroid, and genitalia (including prostate)

Laboratory studies
(many have been completed to establish criteria for FUO)

Blood studies
Complete blood cell count with differential, total protein, albumin, AST, ALT, alkaline phosphate, bilirubin

Blood cultures

3 blood cultures collected over 24-48 hours should be held for 14 days

Biopsy
Temporal artery
Liver
Bone marrow (as indicated by workup findings)

Radiologic studies

Chest x-ray

Abdominal CT scan

Urine studies

Urinalysis   Urine culture

Stool examination

Stool exam for occult blood

is not demonstrated during the evaluation, the patient should document the fever with a reliable thermometer. Documentation and evaluation of fever patterns, however, rarely lead to the diagnosis.

An extremely thorough history and physical examination is essential (Fig. 89-2). Frequently, the clues to appropriate next steps in the evaluation are found within the history and physical examination. The history should include detailed questions about medications, previous medical illnesses, previous surgical illnesses, tuberculosis exposure, prior evaluations with purified protein derivative

(PPD), alcohol and illicit drug use, domestic and foreign travel, animal exposures, occupational exposures, sexual history, sick contacts, and hobbies. Careful questioning about all body systems is essential to detect relatively minor symptoms that might provide important clues to the diagnosis. The presence of immunosuppression expands the breadth of initial laboratory and radiographic studies and the pace of diagnostic pursuit given the potential for rapid deterioration.

Special attention should be given to examination of the skin, temples, eyes, oral cavity, lymph nodes, thyroid, and genitalia as part of a comprehensive examination. In men, the prostate should be examined and a careful pelvic examination is essential in women to evaluate for pelvic inflammatory disease. Positive physical findings should lead to a targeted investigation and early diagnosis. However, subtle physical findings may be overlooked, especially in older patients. Findings may also change over time, necessitating repeated, careful examinations.

Many common laboratory tests are likely to have been completed before a patient satisfies the criteria for FUO. Initial laboratory studies should include routine studies, such as complete blood count with differential, total protein, albumin, aspartate aminotransferase, alanine aminotransferase, alkaline phosphatase, and bilirubin. Urinalysis and urine culture should be performed. A pregnancy test should be obtained to rule out the possibility of ectopic pregnancy as the cause of fever, particularly in the presence of abdominal discomfort in women.

Typically, three blood cultures spaced over a 24- to 48-hour period are sufficient. False-negative blood cultures can occur in the face of antibiotic therapy, which may necessitate repeat cultures if empirical therapy was initiated before collection of the cultures. With the satisfaction of FUO criteria, blood cultures for rare pathogens should be performed. Blood cultures should be held for up to 14 days. A culture using alternative techniques, such as lysis centrifugation procedure, should be considered to enhance detection of fastidious organisms. Direct communication with the microbiology laboratory is encouraged to identify preferred procedures for isolating rare or fastidious organisms in a given laboratory.

A chest x-ray should be obtained. A tuberculin skin test should be placed early in the evaluation, but a negative PPD alone does not rule out tuberculosis. The sensitivity of PPD in extrapulmonary tuberculosis is often relatively low, and immunosuppressed patients may be anergic. Biopsy of involved lymph nodes, bone marrow, or the liver is often required because the yield of sputum acid-fast bacillus stain and culture is decreased for miliary tuberculosis. Stool should be examined for occult blood at least three times to provide clues to underlying gastrointestinal diseases, such as Crohn's disease or carcinoma of the colon.

An antibody test for HIV should be performed to rule out chronic HIV infection, or a viral detection assay should be used if acute HIV infection is suspected. The erythrocyte sedimentation rate (ESR) may provide useful information. In most cases, an ESR greater than 100 mL/hour suggests the presence of a major systemic disease, such as giant cell arteritis or tuberculosis. Unfortunately, slightly or moderately elevated ESR (20 to 40 mm/hr) is common in FUO and can be difficult to interpret, especially in elderly patients. A normal ESR argues against connective tissue diseases.

CT scan of the abdomen and pelvis should be obtained early in the evaluation. Occult abscesses, which can often be readily identified by CT, are one of the most common causes of FUO. Detection of an abnormality by CT may be followed by a CT-guided biopsy to establish the definitive diagnosis. CT of the chest occasionally provides evidence of lung disease not readily apparent by chest radiography. MRI or angiogram should be obtained if vasculitis is suspected.

Several radionuclide scanning techniques have been used in the evaluation of FUO. The most commonly used tests are gallium-67 scans and indium-labeled leukocyte scans. Bone scans are sometimes useful in the diagnosis of occult osteomyelitis or metastatic neoplastic disease. Positron emission tomography with ^{18}F-fluorodeoxyglucose has also been used. Generally, these tests do not provide a specific diagnosis, but on occasion, they may yield a focus for further evaluation. Nuclear medicine tests should generally be used as second-line imaging tests in the absence of clinical diagnostic clues or when clinical clues are confusing. Physicians should not rely heavily on these tests and should interpret results cautiously.

In younger patients, serologic studies can play a role in the diagnostic evaluation. Generally, serum samples should be obtained and frozen for later testing during the initial evaluation of the patient with persistent fever. Generally, indiscriminate use of serologic studies is not cost effective. Given the low prevalence of many of the diseases that cause FUO, the pretest probability of serologic tests is low, and they may lead to false-positive results. A classic example is serologic tests for Lyme disease, which is not associated with FUO but may have false-positive serology. Serologic tests should generally be selected only in response to diagnostic clues in the history, physical examination, and routine laboratory tests. However, routine serology for certain pathogens may be warranted in endemic areas, such as for *Brucella* and *Leishmania* species and Q fever in Mediterranean countries and the Middle East. Another important exception is serologic tests for SLE, for which antinuclear antibody and anti–double-stranded DNA should be performed in most younger patients with persistent fever.

Patients with lymphadenopathy and persistent fever may be evaluated with serologic titers for CMV, EBV, and HIV. Antibody titers for CMV and EBV must be interpreted cautiously. Serologic tests for HIV should be repeated after 2 to 3 months to identify seroconversion. Polymerase chain reaction (PCR) testing allows more rapid diagnosis of several infections and is available for EBV, CMV, tuberculosis, HIV, and human herpesvirus 6 and 7.

Biopsy procedures, particularly of the bone marrow and liver, can be important diagnostic tools in the evaluation of FUO. Bone marrow biopsy may be helpful in identifying hematologic malignancies and miliary tuberculosis. Cultures for mycobacteria, as well as bacteria and fungi, should be performed on all biopsy specimens. Bone marrow aspiration alone is probably not adequate in the evaluation of FUO. Liver biopsy can yield the diagnosis, but only if abnormalities are detected on routine studies of liver function.

Temporal artery biopsy is indicated early in the evaluation of the elderly patient with FUO and elevated ESR. Signs and symptoms of giant cell arteritis may be minimal or limited to persistent fever alone. A generous length (2 to 3 cm) of temporal artery should be obtained at biopsy. Bilateral specimens may be necessary.

In older patients, colonoscopy to search for colon carcinoma is reasonable. Echocardiography, both transthoracic and transesophageal, may also be considered to look for valvular lesions consistent with endocarditis, especially if blood cultures may have been obscured by prior antibiotic therapy.

Laparoscopy is occasionally necessary when other evaluations have failed to yield a diagnosis. Most intra-abdominal processes can be identified with CT, and biopsies can be performed percutaneously with CT guidance. Generally, if the imaging studies are negative, invasive exploration of the abdomen is not indicated.

Many patients with FUO will have no diagnosis at the end of an intensive evaluation. If no diagnosis has been established after a thorough investigation and the patient is stable, a period of observation is indicated if the patient's general condition is not compromised. The period of observation may lead to new findings that lead to the diagnosis or the symptoms may resolve spontaneously.

Management and Therapy

The appropriate management of FUO depends primarily on the identification of the underlying etiology. However, certain general rules of management should be considered.

Early in the evaluation of FUO, especially in older patients, all nonessential medications should be discontinued, including medications that have been used for a lengthy period of time. Drug fevers can be caused by long-standing medications. A costly investigation may be avoided if fever resolves after discontinuation of medications.

Empirical therapeutic trials should be avoided whenever possible, particularly in the setting of immunocompetent hosts with classic FUO. Given the frequent spontaneous resolution of the FUO, cure cannot be ascribed to the treatment with certainty. Furthermore, use of therapeutic agents, especially antibiotics, can obscure findings or tests that might lead to a definitive diagnosis.

In contrast, prompt empirical antibiotics, and sometimes antifungals, are the cornerstone of management for patients with neutropenic FUO. These patients are routinely taking antibiotics and antifungals as prophylaxis before the onset of fever and necessitate consideration of broader antimicrobial coverage while the diagnostic workup is underway. Fever often resolves following the recovery of neutrophil counts, with no clear diagnosis. Empirical antibiotics also may be warranted in the case of nosocomial or HIV-associated FUO, depending on clinical severity and likely infectious causes.

Optimum Therapy

The treatment of FUO is specific to the cause of fever, and prognosis is determined by both the cause and the presence of underlying immunosuppression or comorbidities.

Avoiding Treatment Errors

Failure to obtain a thorough medical history and to perform a comprehensive physical examination is likely the most critical error in identifying possible causes of FUO. Empirical therapeutic trials should be avoided except for cases in which all diagnostic approaches have failed and the clinical condition of the patient does not allow for careful observation. If empirical antimicrobial therapy is initiated, cultures should be obtained before administration if possible, to allow subsequent targeted and optimized therapy to cultured pathogens.

Future Directions

FUO will remain an important diagnostic challenge despite advances in imaging and diagnostic tests allowing rapid diagnoses of many causes of persistent fever. The availability and the number of pathogens detectable by rapid antigen and PCR testing will likely continue to expand in the next decade. New molecular genetic tools are being investigated for difficult-to-diagnose disorders such as familial Mediterranean fever and Muckle-Wells syndrome, and such genetic analysis may prove useful in the future for selective diseases. Those cases that remain undiagnosed present a substantial challenge to the physician.

Additional Resources

Erten N, Saka B, Ozturk G, et al: Fever of unknown origin: a report of 57 cases. Int J Clin Pract 59:958-960, 2005.

Knockaert DC: Fever of unknown origin in adults. Clin Infect Dis 24:291-302, 1997.

Mourad O, Palda V, Detsky A: A comprehensive evidence-based approach to fever of unknown origin. Arch Intern Med 163:545-551, 2003.

Sørensen HT, Mellemkjaer L, Skriver MV, et al: Fever of unknown origin and cancer: A population-based study. Lancet 6:851-855, 2005.

EVIDENCE

1. Durack DT, Street AC: Fever of unknown origin reexamined and redefined. Curr Clin Top Infect Dis 11:35-51, 1991.
   The authors revisit FUO and provide a new framework for thinking about FUO in an era where evaluations occur more commonly in the outpatient context. The authors also consider FUO in special populations, such as nosocomial FUO.

2. Gaeta GB, Fusco FM, Nardiello S: Fever of unknown origin: A systematic review of the literature for 1995-2004. Nucl Med Commun 27(3):205-211, 2006.

 A systematic review of the published literature, including reports from developing countries, on classical FUO from 1995 to 2004. Case series were reviewed to evaluate the use of tests in determining the cause of FUO, and failed to reveal a standardized diagnostic approach for all cases of FUO.

3. Hirschmann JV: Fever of unknown origin in adults. Clin Infect Dis 24(3):291-302, 1997.

 The author provides an overview of FUO including common causes and approach to diagnosis.

4. Knockaert DC, Vanderschueren S, Blockmans D: Fever of unknown origin in adults: 40 Years on. J Intern Med 253(3):263-275, 2003.

 The authors report on a systematic search of published literature of FUO from 1990 to 2002, focusing on changes in FUO during this time period and compared with a prior review of literature published from 1961 to 1990 by the same author.

5. Mackowiak PA, Durack DT: Fever of unknown origin. In Mandell GL, Bennett JE, Dolin R (eds): Principles and Practice of Infectious Diseases, 6th ed. Philadelphia: Churchill Livingstone, 2005, pp 718-727.

 The authors present a comprehensive review of FUO with specific attention given to classic FUO, nosocomial FUO, immune-deficient FUO, and HIV-related FUO, in addition to FUO in return travelers. They present a thorough differential diagnosis for each category and provide historical, diagnostic, and imaging recommendations for the evaluation of FUO.

6. Petersdorf RG, Beeson PB: Fever of unexplained origin: Report of 100 cases. Medicine 40:1-30, 1961.

 In this landmark paper, Petersdorf and Beeson developed criteria for the definition of FUO that remained the medically accepted definition in the clinical evaluation and studies of FUO until changes to the original definition were proposed in 1991.

7. Vanderschueren S, Knockaert D, Adriaenssens T, et al: From prolonged febrile illness to fever of unknown origin. Arch Intern Med 163(9):1033-1041, 2003.

 A prospective study of FUO among only immunocompetent patients between 1900 and 1999 reported on the time period until diagnosis, the final diagnoses, and the percentage of cases that remained undiagnosed.

Joseph J. Eron ▪ Cynthia Gay

Septicemia

Introduction

The clinical condition characterized by fever, tachycardia, hypotension, and metabolic acidosis in the presence of demonstrated or suspected infection has been labeled with various terms such as septicemia, sepsis, sepsis syndrome, and septic shock. These terms are used interchangeably by some clinicians, but experts have developed more precise definitions to provide clinicians and clinical research scientists with a common basis for their observations and treatments. However, there is clinical evidence and utility in the recognition that patients may progress along a continuum from sepsis to septic shock.

Sepsis is defined as a systemic response to presumed or confirmed infection (organisms in a normally sterile site) with clinical evidence of abnormal body temperature (>38° C or <36° C); tachycardia; metabolic acidosis, usually accompanied by compensatory respiratory alkalosis and tachypnea; and an elevated or depressed white blood cell count. Severe sepsis implies evidence of organ hypoperfusion such as decreased renal function, hypoxemia, or altered mental status. Septic shock applies to the presence of hypotension and organ hypoperfusion despite adequate fluid resuscitation (Table 90-1).

Sepsis and septic shock are common clinical conditions that are extremely challenging to manage successfully. Often, the microbiologic diagnosis is obscured because of antimicrobial therapy given before the patients arrive at the treating facility or during acute resuscitation before diagnostic cultures are obtained. Frequently, patients have underlying severe illness such as immune suppression, hematologic or other malignancies, or disruption of host defenses such as severe burns. Patients may present with altered mental status so that medical history is unobtainable or unreliable. The rapid progression to multiorgan failure may make identification of the initial pathogenic process (e.g., pneumonia, pyelonephritis, or intra-abdominal infection) difficult.

Sepsis is the 10th leading cause of death in the United States and the leading cause of death in critically ill patients. However, sepsis may be the immediate cause of death in other common, independently categorized causes of mortality such as cancer and pneumonia. About 80% of severe sepsis cases in intensive care units in the United States and Europe during the 1990s occurred after admissions for unrelated causes. The incidence of sepsis increased almost fourfold from 1979 to 2000, to an estimated 660,000 cases (240 cases per 100,000 population) of sepsis or septic shock per year in the United States. Mortality due to sepsis remains high despite recent trends showing a decline in some settings.

Etiology and Pathogenesis

For consistency in this chapter, sepsis and septic shock will be considered to be caused by a microbiologic organism with or without documented bloodstream infection. Other conditions can cause clinical syndromes indistinguishable from sepsis-related infection, although the exact mechanisms leading to the clinical presentation in those conditions are less clearly defined.

In the past, gram-negative bacilli were most commonly associated with bacteremia and sepsis in the United States.

During the past 15 to 20 years, gram-positive cocci such as *Staphylococcus aureus*, coagulase-negative staphylococci, and enterococci have become more common, especially as causes of nosocomial bloodstream infections. Recent trends also show an increase in cases of severe sepsis caused by fungi, in particular *Candida* species. However, almost any overwhelming microbiologic infection can lead to sepsis syndrome and septic shock. Possible etiologic agents include rickettsia and rickettsia-like organisms; fungi, such as *Candida*, *Aspergillus*, and *Cryptococcus* species; parasites such as those that cause malaria; acute toxoplasmosis in the

Table 90-1 Diagnostic Criteria for Sepsis

Syndrome	Criteria	Comment

Sepsis	Confirmed or suspected infection in normally sterile site
	Temperature >38° C or <36° C
	Heart rate >90 beats/minute
	Respiratory rate >20 breaths/minute or $PaCO_2$ <32 mm Hg
	WBC >12,000 cells/mm³ or <4000 cells/mm³, or >10%
	    immature forms
	Systolic blood pressure of <90 mm Hg, MAP <70 mm Hg,
	    or a reduction of >40 mm Hg from baseline
		Sepsis-related hypotension must have no
		    other cause.

Severe sepsis	Lactic acidosis
	Oliguria
	Altered mental status
	Acute lung injury
		Implies sepsis-associated organ dysfunction
		    distant from the site of infection.
		Hypotension can be reversed by fluid
		    resuscitation.

Septic shock	Requires administration of pressor therapy to maintain
	    blood pressure
		Hypotension persists despite adequate fluid
		    resuscitation.

MAP, mean arterial pressure; $PaCO_2$, arterial carbon dioxide partial pressure, WBC, white blood cell.

immunocompromised host; and even some viral infections. The lung, abdomen, and urinary tract are the most common sites of infection, but the source of infection remains unidentified in up to one third of cases. Blood culture specimen results are positive in only about 30% of cases. Culture of other sites such as sputum, urine, cerebrospinal fluid, or pleural fluid may reveal a specific etiology, but areas of localized infection that trigger the process may not be accessible to culture.

Infectious agents activate both proinflammatory and anti-inflammatory responses, which are mediated, in part, by monocytes, macrophages, and neutrophils. These activated cells interact with endothelial receptors leading to the release of cytokines such as tumor necrosis factor (TNF), interleukin (IL), proteases, leukotrienes, reactive oxygen species, nitric oxide, arachidonic acid, and platelet-activating factor. Microvascular injury, thrombosis, and capillary leak result from the multiple interactions at the vascular endothelium and are further affected by dysregulation of the coagulation and complement cascades. Diffuse endothelial disruption leads to tissue hypoxia and associated organ dysfunction.

The exact pathogenesis underlying the development of severe sepsis and septic shock remains elusive, likely related to the heterogeneity of patients, infectious agents, and events that initiate inflammatory mechanisms. The previous prevailing theory that septic shock represents an exaggerated, uncontrolled inflammatory response to bacteremia, endotoxemia, fungemia, or more localized severe infection (Fig. 90-1) was based primarily on animal studies in which high levels of circulating cytokines such as TNF-α were found. However, the levels of TNF-α and IL-1, which are the major proinflammatory cytokines, were exponentially higher in these animals than in septic patients. Notably, high levels of TNF-α have been associated with sepsis due to meningococcemia in humans, and

are correlated with mortality. However, additional research in humans revealed that the presence of an exaggerated systemic inflammatory response, as measured by levels of TNF, TNF-α, or IL-1β, was much less frequent than expected.

The precise role of TNF-α and IL-1 in the pathophysiology of sepsis remains to be determined. These cytokines produce leukocyte-endothelial adhesion followed by the release of platelet-activating factor, IL-8, arachidonic acid metabolites, and clotting factors, all of which contribute to the generation of fever, tachycardia, tachypnea, ventilation-perfusion abnormalities, lactic acidosis, and disseminated intravascular coagulation. However, more recent work has revealed that septic patients demonstrate features of immunosuppression, including increased susceptibility to nosocomial infections, loss of delayed hypersensitivity, and failure to clear pathogens. A newer theory proposes that early sepsis may involve increases in inflammatory mediators, but then progresses toward an immunosuppressive state in which anti-inflammatory responses predominate.

Clinical Presentation

The initial presentation of sepsis may be subtle, but the rapid progression of this syndrome usually makes the general diagnosis obvious, although the specific infectious agent may remain obscure. Minor mental status changes or confusion may be very early signs of sepsis. Hyperventilation has been noted as an early sign in closely monitored patients who are found subsequently to be septic. Most patients are either hyperthermic or hypothermic and complain of chills or have rigors. Some debilitated and elderly patients may have minimal symptoms other than confusion, and negligible signs other than orthostasis or

Figure 90-1 Septicemia.

PAI-1, plasminogen activator inhibitor-1; TAFI, thrombin activatable fibrinolysis inhibitor.

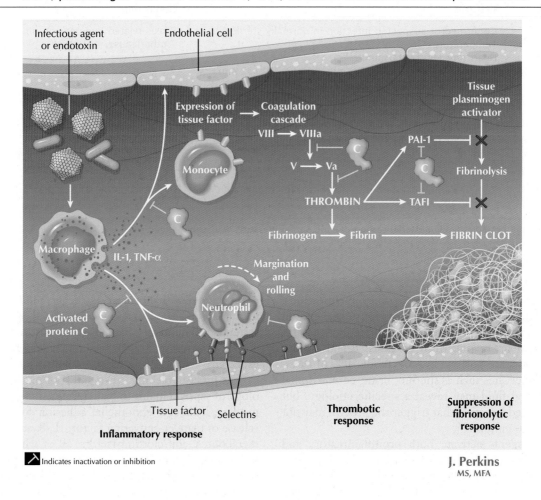

⚒ Indicates inactivation or inhibition

J. Perkins
MS, MFA

frank hypotension. Neutrophil counts may be high, but neutropenia is also a common manifestation.

Although the line between primary clinical manifestations and subsequent complications is arbitrary, the complications of sepsis, including organ hypoperfusion, coagulopathy, and endothelial damage, represent a continuum from sepsis syndrome to septic shock. Patients frequently present with evidence of organ hypoperfusion such as hypotension, oliguria, hypoxemia, acidosis, and liver function abnormalities. Patients may also have signs of a consumptive coagulopathy with thrombocytopenia and bleeding, and depressed myocardial function with elevated heart rate and cardiac output. Adult respiratory distress syndrome (ARDS) or diffuse pulmonary capillary leak syndrome may be a somewhat later finding. Because of the very rapid progression of sepsis, some patients may present with evidence of ARDS.

Differential Diagnosis

Other processes or stimuli may cause systemic inflammatory responses resulting in a clinical syndrome that is indistinguishable from sepsis. Burns and pancreatitis are the most common noninfectious causes, as well as adrenal insufficiency, pulmonary embolism, myocardial infarction, cardiac tamponade, dissecting or ruptured aortic aneurysm, occult hemorrhage, and drug overdose. Other causes of severe tissue injury such as trauma may also result in a sepsis-like appearance.

Diagnostic Approach

Diagnostic signs of septic shock syndrome may be subtle during the very early manifestations, but they are usually obvious once the process has evolved. Determining the source of the infection and the specific microbial agent is the main issue in diagnosis. Medical history, including predisposing disorders, recent antimicrobial therapy, diet, travel, and exposure information is important. If possible, one should obtain a history of symptoms from the patient to help localize the source of infection. Cultures of blood, urine, and sputum (cerebrospinal fluid, wounds, and peritoneal fluid when indicated) are essential. If possible, the appropriate diagnostic studies should be obtained before antibiotic administration to increase the diagnostic yield. Most retrospective studies evaluating the effect of antibi-

Table 90-2 Evidence-Based Recommendations for Treatment of Sepsis

Treatment Modality	Recommendation	Grade of Evidence
Antimicrobials	Intravenous antibiotics should be initiated within one hour of suspected sepsis	E
Bicarbonate	Not indicated for lactic acidosis with pH ≥7.15 due to hypoperfusion	C
Cultures	Cultures from appropriate sites should be obtained before antimicrobial administration	D
Deep venous thrombosis prophylaxis	Low-dose unfractionated heparin or low-molecular-weight with heparin or mechanical device if heparin use is contraindicated	A
Fluid resuscitation	Natural or artificial colloids or crystalloids are appropriate because data do not support superiority of either type	C
Glucose control	Maintenance of blood glucose <150 mg/dL (8.3 mmol/L) Continuous insulin and glucose infusion with glucose monitoring every 30-60 minutes to achieve above	D
Initial resuscitation within first 6 hours	Resuscitation goals in first 6 hours: ▪ Central venous pressure: 8-12 mm Hg ▪ Mean arterial pressure ≥65 mm Hg ▪ Urine output ≥0.5 mL/kg/hr ▪ Central venous or mixed venous oxygen saturation ≥70%	B
Mechanical ventilation	Low tidal volumes of 6 mL/kg of predicted body weight while maintaining end-inspiratory plateau pressures <30 cm H_2O for ALI/ARDS	B
Recombinant human activated protein C	Indicated for APACHE II ≥25, multiple organ failure, or ARDS due to sepsis, septic shock, and no absolute contraindication related to bleeding risk or relative contraindication for which risk exceeds benefit	B
Blood transfusion	Red blood cell transfusion if central venous or mixed venous oxygen of 70% not achieved after first 6 hours Red blood cell transfusion only for hemoglobin <7.0 g/dL (<70 g/L) after hypoperfusion resolved, in the absence of coronary artery disease or lactic acidosis during initial resuscitation	B
Steroids	IV corticosteroids (hydrocortisone 200-300 mg/day, for 7 days in 3-4 divided doses or by continuous infusion) with septic shock unresponsive to fluid replacement	C
	Corticosteroid doses of >300 mg of hydrocortisone daily should not be used as treatment for severe sepsis or septic shock	A
Stress ulcer prophylaxis	H_2 receptor inhibitors for all patients with severe sepsis	A

ALI, acute lung injury; APACHE, Acute Physiology and Chronic Health Evaluation; ARDS, adult respiratory distress syndrome.
Grade of recommendations: A, supported by at least two level I investigations; B, supported by one level I investigation; C, supported by level II investigations only; D, supported by at least one level III investigation; E, supported by level IV or V evidence.
  Grade of evidence: I, large, randomized trials with clear-cut results; II, small, randomized trials with uncertain results; III, nonrandomized, contemporaneous controls; IV, nonrandomized, historical controls and expert opinion; V, case series, uncontrolled studies, and expert opinion. *Adapted from Dellinger RP, Carlet JM, Masur H, et al: Surviving Sepsis Campaign guidelines for management of severe sepsis and septic shock. Crit Care Med 32(3):858-873, 2004.*

otic initiation in bacteremic patients found a decrease in mortality when "appropriate" empirical antimicrobials were started within 48 hours of collecting blood cultures. Stool culture and screening for *Clostridium difficile* toxin are sometimes overlooked.

Management and Therapy

Therapy is divided into several categories including hemodynamic support, antimicrobials, tissue oxygenation goal-directed therapy, and specific interruption of the inflammatory cascade. Despite advances in antimicrobial therapy during the past half century, dramatic improvements in mortality from severe sepsis syndrome have not occurred. Imbalance between oxygen demand and supply results in total tissue and organ hypoxia due to the physiologic hallmarks of sepsis and septic shock, including peripheral vasodilation, decreased cardiac function, intravascular volume loss due to endothelial dysfunction, and increased metabolic demand. Recent therapeutic advances for sepsis include recombinant human activated protein C for severe sepsis, corticosteroids in septic shock, prompt goal-directed therapy to improve tissue hypoperfusion, and intensive insulin therapy (see later). In 2003, an expert panel reconvened to update key recommendations for the management of severe sepsis and septic shock based on available data (Table 90-2), and key recommendations are discussed next.

Table 90-3 Empiric Antibiotic Therapy	
Clinical Setting	**Possible Therapies**
Outpatient admission	Third-generation cephalosporin (e.g., ceftriaxone, cefotaxime) or piperacillin/tazobactam, or imipenem (or meropenem or ertapenem) each with an aminoglycoside; plus vancomycin
Intra-abdominal	Piperacillin/tazobactam or imipenem (or meropenem or ertapenem), each with an aminoglycoside; tigecycline is an alternative when *Pseudomonas* coverage is not thought to be indicated; plus vancomycin
Hospitalized patient*	Imipenem (or meropenem or ertapenem) or piperacillin/tazobactam (at doses to cover *Pseudomonas aeruginosa*) plus aminoglycoside; ceftazidime, cefepime, and ciprofloxacin are alternatives; plus vancomycin
Neutropenic patient	Imipenem (or meropenem or ertapenem), cefepime, ceftazidime alone or with an aminoglycoside; piperacillin/tazobactam (at doses to cover *Pseudomonas aeruginosa*) is an alternative; plus vancomycin plus fluconazole (caspofungin is an alternative)
Possible methicillin-resistant *Staphylococcus aureus*	Linezolid and daptomycin are possible alternatives to vancomycin depending on the site of infection. (Daptomycin should not be used in the case of pneumonia, and there is limited experience with linezolid for certain syndromes such as endocarditis and meningitis)
Possible tick exposure	Add doxycycline

* Local epidemiology of nosocomial infection and antibiotic resistance patterns should be used to guide therapy.

Optimum Treatment

Diagnostic cultures should be obtained before antibiotic administration, and antibiotic therapy should ideally be directed at specific pathogens. However, early in the course of septic shock, the precise pathogen is usually not known and may remain obscure after extensive investigation. In general, the severity of the illness dictates broad antimicrobial coverage unless there is a high degree of certainty as to the likely pathogen, and should be initiated within 1 hour of the suspicion or recognition of severe sepsis. Table 90-3 presents suggested empiric antibiotic therapy for patients with sepsis or septic shock in a variety of settings.

Early goal-oriented therapy focuses on optimization of tissue oxygen delivery as measured by mixed venous oxygen saturation, pH, or arterial lactate levels. This approach has demonstrated improved survival compared with standard fluid resuscitation and maintenance of blood pressure. Physiologic goals during the first 6 hours of resuscitation include the following: (1) central venous pressure 8 to 12 mm Hg, (2) mean arterial pressure ≥65 mm Hg, (3) central venous oxygen saturation ≥70%, and (4) urine output ≥0.5 mL/kg/hr (using transfusion, inotropic agents, and supplemental oxygen with or without mechanical ventilation).

Recombinant human activated protein C (drotrecogin alfa), which promotes fibrinolysis and inhibits thrombosis and inflammation, reduced mortality in patients with severe sepsis from 30.8% to 24.7% in a randomized, controlled trial. Not surprisingly, the drug was associated with

a small but statistically significant increase in the incidence of severe bleeding, including intracranial hemorrhage. A second trial was conducted to evaluate the benefit of drotrecogin alfa in adults with severe sepsis and a low risk for death, defined as an Acute Physiology and Chronic Health Evaluation (APACHE) II score of less than 25 and no more than single organ failure. The study revealed no beneficial treatment effects for this patient group, but an increased incidence of serious bleeding complications. Drotrecogin alfa (activated) is currently approved by the U.S. Food and Drug Administration only for the treatment of severe sepsis in patients with more than one organ dysfunction or an APACHE II score of greater than 25.

During the past decade, multiple trials of mediator-based therapy designed to disrupt the inflammatory cascade involved in the pathogenesis of sepsis have been disappointing. Agents including antiendotoxin antibodies, TNF antagonists, IL receptor antagonists, and other agents have not demonstrated significant benefit. However, several randomized, controlled trials of glucocorticoid therapy for septic shock demonstrated a significant benefit in shock reversal. Current guidelines recommend intravenous corticosteroids (hydrocortisone, 200 to 300 mg/day in 3 or 4 divided doses for 7 days) for septic shock unresponsive to fluid resuscitation.

Intensive glycemic control emerged as an important management strategy following a large trial that demonstrated decreased mortality in patients with severe sepsis and blood glucose kept between 80 and 110 mg/dL (4.4 to 6.1 mmol/L) on continuous insulin and glucose infusion. Intensive insulin therapy for bacteremic patients was associated with a lower mortality rate than conventional therapy (12.5% vs. 29.5%) and reduced the frequency of sepsis episodes by 46%. The beneficial effect of intensive insulin therapy on mortality persisted regardless of a prior history of diabetes. Current guidelines suggest keeping blood glucose less than 150 mg/dL (8.3 mmol/L) or between 100 and 140 mg/dL. Frequent monitoring is critical to avoid hypoglycemic brain injury.

Although catheter-related infections (CRIs) have decreased with improved sterilization techniques and equipment, they remain the leading cause of bloodstream infections. Several randomized controlled trials evaluating the prevention of CRI through the use of catheters coated with heparin, chlorhexidine-sulfadiazine, and antibiotics showed a reduction in catheter colonization but not in bloodstream infections.

Avoiding Treatment Errors

The most serious errors associated with sepsis syndrome are likely to be diagnostic rather than therapeutic. Noninfectious causes of systemic inflammatory response syndrome (e.g., pancreatitis) should always be considered, as should mimics of the sepsis syndrome such as large pulmonary emboli and adrenal insufficiency. More unusual pathogens that may not yield positive blood cultures, such as malaria, tuberculosis, or histoplasmosis, should also be considered.

Future Directions

Sepsis is an increasingly common clinical syndrome with a high mortality rate despite modern interventions. The failure of anti-inflammatory agents to improve the outcome of sepsis has prompted investigators to rethink the pathophysiology underlying sepsis and septic shock, and to consider whether sepsis syndrome results from both proinflammatory and immune suppressive responses. In the past decade, new treatment strategies for sepsis have emerged, including drotrecogin alfa (activated), glucocorticoid treatment for septic shock, intensive insulin therapy, and goal-directed resuscitation. More refined supportive care, including the elucidation of target physiologic parameters and specific interventions most effective at achieving them, should result in wider implementation and increased survival. Interventions directed at the inflammatory and coagulation cascade continue in development and need to be further studied. Newer strategies targeting anti-inflammatory mediators and their role in causing immune suppression in sepsis need to be explored. Given the increasing number of elderly and immune-suppressed patients and the increasing prevalence of antibiotic resistance, antibiotic therapy alone is unlikely to improve mortality from sepsis. Accordingly, the substantial utilization of health care resources associated with severe sepsis and septic shock will likely increase.

Additional Resources

Annane D, Sebille V, Charpentier C, et al: Effect of treatment with low doses of hydrocortisone and fludrocortisones on mortality in patients with septic shock. JAMA 288(7):862-871, 2002.

The paper reports findings from a randomized, placebo-controlled, double-blind trial of hydrocortisone and fludrocortisone versus matching placebos in 300 patients with septic shock. The authors concluded that a 7-day treatment course of low-dose hydrocortisone and fludrocortisone reduced mortality in patients with septic shock and relative adrenal insufficiency.

Matthay MA: Severe sepsis—new treatment with both anticoagulant and antiinflammatory properties. N Engl J Med 344(10):759-762, 2001.

This editorial accompanied the publication by Bernard and colleagues (below) on findings from the randomized controlled trial of activated protein C for the treatment of severe sepsis. The editorial discusses potential theories regarding drug efficacy and provides a critique of the study.

Nguyen HB, Rivers EP, Abrahamian FM, et al: Severe sepsis and septic shock: Review of the literature and emergency department management guidelines. Ann Emerg Med 48(1):28-54, 2006.

Nguyen and colleagues present a comprehensive review of sepsis and septic shock with a focus on the early management of sepsis in the emergency department.

EVIDENCE

1. American College of Chest Physicians/Society of Critical Care Medicine Consensus Conference Committee: Definitions for sepsis and organ failure and guidelines for the use of innovative therapies in sepsis. Crit Care Med 20(6):864-874, 1992.

   This report by the ACCP/SCCM Consensus Conference Committee presents the consensus definitions for sepsis and related syndromes developed by the committee.
2. Andrews P, Azoulay E. Antonelli M, et al: Year in review in intensive care medicine, 2004. I. Respiratory failure, infection, and sepsis. Intensive Care Med 31(1):28-40, 2005.

   Andrews and colleagues present a review of research published on respiratory failure, infection, and sepsis. In regard to sepsis, a summary of findings from studies of catheter-related infection and endocarditis, nosocomial infections and antimicrobial use, and sepsis in HIV-infected patients is presented.
3. Angus DC, Linde-Zwirble WT, Lidicker J, et al: Epidemiology of severe sepsis in the United States: Analysis of incidence, outcome, and associated costs of care. Crit Care Med 29(7):1303-1310, 2001.

   The authors report on an observational cohort study of the incidence, cost, and outcomes of severe sepsis in the United States in the year 1995.
4. Bernard GR, Vincent JL, Laterre PF, et al: Efficacy and safety of recombinant human activated protein C for severe sepsis. N Engl J Med 344(10):699-709, 2001.

   Bernard and colleagues present findings from their randomized, double-blind, placebo-controlled trial of recombinant human activated protein C for the treatment of severe sepsis.
5. Dellinger RP, Carlet JM, Masur H, et al: Surviving Sepsis Campaign guidelines for management of severe sepsis and septic shock. Crit Care Med 32(3):858-873, 2004.

   The Surviving Sepsis Campaign Management Guidelines Committee published a systematic review of the literature on sepsis. Treatment and diagnostic recommendations are summarized and graded by the level of recommendation and class of evidence to support the recommendation.
6. Hotchkiss RS, Karl IE: The pathophysiology and treatment of sepsis. N Engl J Med 348(2):138-150, 2003.

   Hotchkiss and colleagues published a review of sepsis focusing on advances in the understanding of the pathogenesis of sepsis and therapeutic strategies.

7. Martin GS, Mannino DM, Eaton S, Moss M: The epidemiology of sepsis in the United States from 1979 to 2000. N Engl J Med 348(16):1546-1554, 2003.

A retrospective study of sepsis that analyzed discharge records from hospitals participating in the National Hospital Discharge Survey, providing a nationally representative sample. The authors report on temporal changes in incidence, sepsis outcomes, and risk factors for sepsis.

8. Munford R: Sepsis, severe sepsis, and septic shock. In Mandell GL, Bennett JE, Dolin R (eds): Mandell, Douglas, and Bennett's Principles and Practice of Infectious Diseases, 6th ed. Philadelphia, Churchill Livingstone, 2005, pp 906-922.

Munford and colleagues provide a comprehensive review of sepsis, severe sepsis, and septic shock encompassing the epidemiology, clinical manifestations, diagnostic approach, and therapy of sepsis and associated syndromes. They present an in-depth review of the current evidence on the pathogenesis of sepsis and related syndromes.

9. Rivers E, Nguyen B, Havstad S, et al: Early goal-directed therapy in the treatment of severe sepsis and septic shock. N Engl J Med 345(19):1368-1377, 2001.

The authors report on findings from a randomized study of 6 hours of early goal-directed therapy versus standard therapy for sepsis or septic shock in the emergency department.

10. Wheeler AP, Bernard GR: Treating patients with severe sepsis. N Engl J Med 340(3):207-214, 1999.

Wheeler and Bernard published a review of severe sepsis with a particular focus on the pathophysiology and treatment of specific organ system involvement.

Mary C. Bowman ▪ David A. Wohl ▪ Andrew H. Kaplan

91

Staphylococcal Infections

Introduction

Within the genus *Staphylococcus*, a single species, *Staphylococcus aureus,* and a group of species known as coagulase-negative staphylococci (CoNS) cause significant human disease. *S. aureus* is the most virulent of all staphylococcus species and is one of the most important of all human bacterial pathogens. It is a major cause of serious nosocomial as well as community-acquired infections that include skin and soft tissue infections (SSTIs), septicemia, endovascular infections, and infections of indwelling catheters or implanted prosthetic devices. Infections due to methicillin-resistant *S. aureus* (MRSA) have emerged as "super bugs" and are associated with excess morbidity, mortality, and increasing health care costs. Once relatively isolated to health care environments, MRSA is increasingly being acquired and spread within the community. CoNS, of which *Staphylococcus epidermidis* constitutes the major pathogen, are the most common bacteria isolated from blood cultures. Although most often a contaminant, *S. epidermidis* has emerged as a true cause of infection in hospitalized patients with implanted foreign bodies and in immunocompromised hosts. Resistance of staphylococcal organisms to many of the available classes of antibiotics is widespread and represents a serious challenge for clinicians. The mainstays of treatment are the appropriate choice and length of antibiotic treatment, removal of infected tissues or foreign objects, and surgical drainage of infected fluid collections.

Epidemiology

S. aureus is a human commensal organism most commonly recovered from the anterior nares. Studies show that asymptomatic carriers of *S. aureus* are relatively common, representing between 20% and 40% of adults, and suggest that 50% of adults will be colonized at some time during their life. Cross-sectional studies in high-risk populations, including those with diabetes mellitus or chronic exfoliative skin conditions and those receiving chronic hemodialysis, have demonstrated carriage rates as high as 90%. Health care workers and users of intravenous drugs are also at greater risk for colonization. The clinical relevance of asymptomatic carriage is underlined by several studies that have demonstrated both an increased risk for infection in colonized patients and for the transfer of strains from colonized health care workers to patients.

The nosocomial spread of *S. aureus* has significant impact on both clinical outcomes and health care costs. *S. aureus* is the most commonly reported cause of hospital-acquired infection and is estimated to cause clinical disease in 2% of all patients that are admitted. Patients with nosocomial *S. aureus* infection have about twice the length of

hospital stay and are at an increased risk for dying during the hospitalization. The widespread transmission of strains resistant to β-lactam antibiotics is of particular concern. Virtually all the isolates recovered from both hospital and community-acquired infections are resistant to penicillin, and recent reports indicate that 55% to 59% of isolates from hospitals and long-term care facilities are resistant to methicillin. Risk factors associated with hospital-acquired MRSA include prolonged hospitalization (often greater than 14 days), preceding antimicrobial therapy (especially with cephalosporins or fluoroquinolones), presence in an intensive care unit or burn unit, hemodialysis, having a surgical site infection, and proximity to a patient colonized or infected with MRSA.

In the community, *S. aureus* represents the most common cause of SSTIs, and community-acquired methicillin-resistant *S. aureus* (CA-MRSA) infections are becoming more common. Studies performed between 1997 and 2001 demonstrate that 12% to 22% of all staphylococcal isolates in patients presenting from community settings were methicillin resistant. In a study performed in 2004, 59% of staphylococcal isolates obtained strictly from SSTIs were characterized as CA-MRSA. Risk factors that have been associated with CA-MRSA infection include African American race, HIV infection, recent antibiotic therapy within the past 6 months, and skin trauma. That the infection appears to spread in circumstances that involve close contact between people and their sharing of equipment is supported by the frequency with which CA-MRSA outbreaks have been reported among incarcerated individuals, military personnel, football players, and family members.

CoNS are found among the normal flora of human skin and mucous membranes. Historically, the isolation of CoNS in blood cultures has been viewed as a contaminant occurring through percutaneous venous blood sampling. Reports show that up to 50% of positive blood culture isolates are CoNS. However, in recent years, paralleling advances in medicine, CoNS have emerged as true pathogens. Risk factors associated with infection are indwelling central venous catheters, implanted prosthetic devices, and immunocompromised hosts, most frequently patients with hematologic malignancies. Misinterpretation of a positive blood culture has important implications. CoNS are virtually resistant to penicillin and the antistaphylococcal penicillins, so positive blood cultures necessitate therapy with vancomycin most frequently. An important study by Tokars helped to clarify which cultures are likely contaminants versus true pathogens in patients without obvious signs and symptoms of sepsis and is dependent on number of cultures drawn, the site of phlebotomy, and length of time to positivity.

Pathogenesis

S. aureus is a very robust organism, able to persist on surfaces at wide ranges of temperature, pH, and salt concentrations. Several bacterial products are associated with the ability of the organism to persist in the environment and cause disease. These are grouped into substances that allow the organism to persist on surfaces in vivo and toxins and enzymes that appear to be important in tissue invasion and destruction.

A hallmark of *S. aureus* infection is its ability to colonize and persist on both implanted and indwelling foreign bodies such as intravenous catheters or prosthetic joints. The organism is also commonly found on disrupted native endovascular epithelium such as abnormal cardiac valves or thrombosed blood vessels. Attachment of the organism is mediated by a number of bacterial products, including teichoic acid. Once the organism adheres to a surface, its persistence at that site is supported by several factors that interfere with immune clearance. These include factors that inhibit neutrophil access to the organisms (coagulase), limit phagocytosis (capsule or slime layer), inhibit opsonization (clumping factor and protein A), and interfere with intracellular killing (catalase).

After adherence, a group of enzymes and toxins allow the organism to destroy involved tissue. These include several extracellular enzymes that are directly involved in

tissue destruction through a disruptive effect on cellular membranes.

Secreted toxins that act at a distance and are responsible for many of the clinical manifestations of *S. aureus* infection are particularly important. These toxins are grouped into those that produce tissue destruction directly (A-, B-, C-, and D-toxins) and those that act by producing immune dysregulation (toxic shock syndrome [TSS] toxins, enterotoxins, and exfoliative toxins). Many of the staphylococcal toxins act as superantigens. These bacterial proteins interact with major histocompatibility class II receptors outside of the antigen-binding groove. This high-affinity binding activates a large number of T lymphocytes, which in turn produce large amounts of cytokines. Elaboration of these cytokines plays a critical role in the pathogenesis of many of the clinical manifestations of *S. aureus* infection, including TSS, scalded skin syndrome, and staphylococcal food poisoning syndrome.

A prominent feature of the genome is the presence of mobile genetic elements that can carry genes involved in pathogenicity and drug resistance. These have typically been called *pathogenicity islands* and are able to move between bacteria. Of current interest are the SCC*mec* cassettes that carry methicillin resistance as well as a virulence factor, the Panton-Valentine leukocidin toxin. Sequence-specific types of SCC*mec* cassettes (types I to IV) have been instrumental in epidemiologic tracking of hospital-versus community-acquired MRSA.

Clinical Presentation

The clinical manifestations of *S. aureus* infection are protean and reflect the interaction between host and bacterial factors. Host factors predispose a patient to infection as well as influence the course of the disease and its presentation. Quantitative and qualitative defects in phagocytic function and conditions that disrupt the integrity of the skin increase the risk for infection. Among patients with phagocytic defects, those with deficiencies in neutrophil chemotaxis (e.g., Job's syndrome and Chediak-Higashi syndrome) and intracellular killing (e.g., chronic granulomatous disease) are at greatest risk. Patients with poorly controlled diabetes mellitus are also at increased risk for serious infection.

Skin and Soft Tissue Infections

Staphylococcal infection of the skin and soft tissues presents with a range of syndromes. Most characteristic is the tendency of the organism to form abscesses. Infections may progress from superficial, relatively benign infections of the hair follicle (folliculitis) to invasion of the tissue surrounding the follicle (furuncles). These small abscesses may coalesce and form larger collections of pus (carbuncles). Uncommonly, the underlying muscle and fascia become involved (pyomyositis and necrotizing fasciitis).

Patients experiencing these deep-seated syndromes are generally febrile, complain of pain in the involved area, and appear ill. They require surgical intervention as well as appropriate antibiotic therapy. Staphylococcal wound infections associated with the presence of a foreign body such as a suture or surgical drain are of particular concern. The milder manifestations may be treated conservatively with oral antibiotics. Myositis and necrotizing fasciitis require aggressive surgical intervention for drainage and removal of infected tissue. Although there is a trend to greater incidence of MRSA SSTIs in the community, there is no difference in clinical outcomes compared with sensitive organisms when there is appropriate intervention.

Staphylococcal Scalded Skin Syndrome

A bullous disease seen almost exclusively in children, staphylococcal scalded skin syndrome is associated with infection with an exfoliative toxin-producing *S. aureus*. Pathologically, the disease is associated with splitting of the granular layer of the epidermis. Generally, infected children are younger than 5 years of age and present with fever and irritability. Sloughing of apparently uninvolved skin (Nikolsky's sign) is characteristic. Upon rupture of the fluid-filled bullae, large areas of epidermis may be disrupted, producing potentially serious volume and electrolyte losses, particularly in very young children. Therapy includes antibiotics and supportive care for electrolyte and volume loss.

Staphylococcal Toxic Shock Syndrome

This toxin-mediated syndrome was initially described in menstruating women using tampons (Fig. 91-1). Staphylococcal TSS has since been recognized in men and in women who are not menstruating. TSS initially presents as rash, fever, myalgias, diarrhea, and a depressed level of consciousness. Renal failure, hepatitis, and shock may rapidly follow these initial signs and symptoms within 24 to 48 hours. The shock may be severe and produce digital necrosis. TSS is often accompanied by the appearance of a desquamative rash, commonly on the hands and feet.

Unlike menses-associated TSS seen most commonly in young women, nonmenstrual TSS is often associated with surgical procedures and may occur in the absence of frank evidence of active infection. A high level of suspicion for TSS must be maintained for patients with a sunburn-appearing rash and a rapidly evolving shock picture following a surgical intervention. Patients with TSS should receive antibiotics active against *S. aureus* as well as supportive care for shock and organ failure. For life-threatening disease, intravenous immunoglobulin is often given in concert with standard therapy. Any potential site of ongoing bacterial replication and toxin production (i.e., infected surgical suture, tampon) should be removed.

Staphylococcal Food Poisoning

S. aureus is associated with about 10% to 20% of the reported outbreaks of food-borne disease in the United States. The syndrome results from ingestion of any of the several heat-stable bacterial exotoxins. Because the preformed toxin is present in the food and does not require ongoing bacterial replication, rapid onset and resolution of symptoms mark the illness. Nausea and vomiting usually occur within 6 hours of ingesting the contaminated food, and symptoms generally resolve within 12 hours. Patients are not febrile, but may appear quite ill from the hypovolemia associated with often explosive diarrhea and vomiting. Outbreaks are usually associated with the ingestion of partially cooked food (e.g., potato salad). Therapy is supportive; antibiotics are not required.

Pneumonia

S. aureus is an important cause of purulent pneumonia (Fig. 91-2). The organism gains access to the lungs either through aspiration of nasopharyngeal contents colonized with staphylococci or hematogenous spread (e.g., metastatic spread from bacteremia or septic emboli from right-sided endocarditis). Staphylococcal pneumonia tends to be fulminant and is often associated with infiltrative lesions that progress to cavitation as well as to pleural empyemas. *S. aureus* is also a common cause of secondary bacterial pneumonia following infection with influenza virus. Antistaphylococcal antibiotics are usually effective in clearing the infection; however, surgical drainage may be required in cases of pleural empyema.

Endocarditis

S. aureus, the second most common etiologic agent in infective endocarditis, is responsible for between 20% and 30% of the cases (Fig. 91-3). Although the aortic and mitral valves are most likely to be involved, there is an increased prevalence of tricuspid valve involvement among intravenous drug users. As is the case for other organisms, *S. aureus* is more likely to infect heart valves with underlying abnormalities (e.g., degenerative valvular disease, rheumatic heart disease, or congenital abnormalities). However, the valves may be normal in as many as one third of all cases. Staphylococcal endocarditis is also associated with the use of indwelling vascular catheters.

In comparison with endocarditis due to the viridans streptococci, staphylococcal endocarditis tends to be more aggressive and has an acute presentation. Myocardial abscesses are more frequent in the setting of *S. aureus* endocarditis, as are valve ring abscesses, which often require surgical repair. Emboli to large organs occur in nearly half of all cases.

Treatment includes appropriate antibiotics active against the organism. Surgical replacement of the infected valve may be required because of serious conduction dis-

Figure 91-1 Toxic Shock Syndrome.

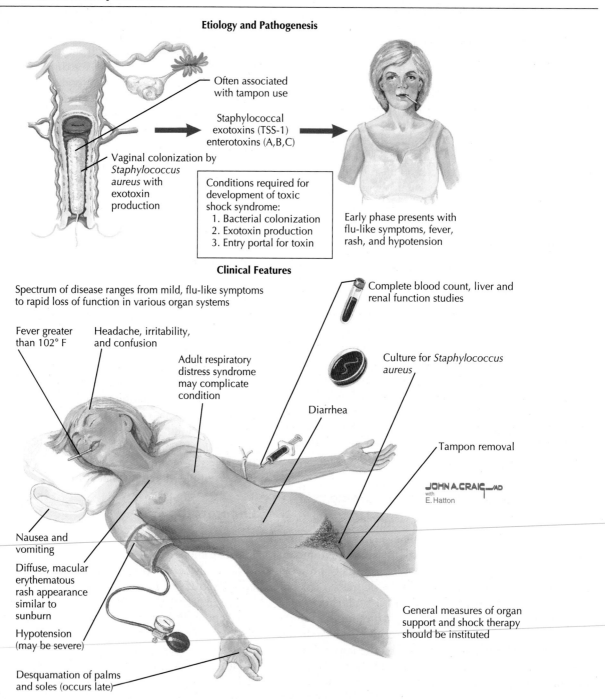

Etiology and Pathogenesis

Often associated with tampon use

Staphylococcal exotoxins (TSS-1) enterotoxins (A,B,C)

Vaginal colonization by *Staphylococcus aureus* with exotoxin production

Conditions required for development of toxic shock syndrome:
1. Bacterial colonization
2. Exotoxin production
3. Entry portal for toxin

Early phase presents with flu-like symptoms, fever, rash, and hypotension

Clinical Features

Spectrum of disease ranges from mild, flu-like symptoms to rapid loss of function in various organ systems

Complete blood count, liver and renal function studies

Fever greater than 102° F

Headache, irritability, and confusion

Adult respiratory distress syndrome may complicate condition

Culture for *Staphylococcus aureus*

Diarrhea

Tampon removal

JOHN A. CRAIG—AD
with
E. Hatton

Nausea and vomiting

Diffuse, macular erythematous rash appearance similar to sunburn

Hypotension (may be severe)

General measures of organ support and shock therapy should be instituted

Desquamation of palms and soles (occurs late)

turbances, myocardial abscesses, evidence of valvular instability, multiple large organ emboli, ongoing bacteremia despite appropriate antibiotic therapy, and refractory congestive heart failure.

Differential Diagnosis/ Diagnostic Approach

Infection with *S. aureus* may be indistinguishable from other bacterial infections. Culture of the organism from infected tissue or blood is the basis of diagnosis. Given the

aggressive nature of many staphylococcal infections, however, a high level of suspicion should be maintained in the presence of predisposing conditions such as defects in phagocytic function and in patients with diabetes mellitus.

Management and Therapy

Optimum Treatment

Drainage of infected material and antibiotics are the mainstays of therapy. Organisms resistant to many of the

Figure 91-2 Staphylococcal Pneumonia.

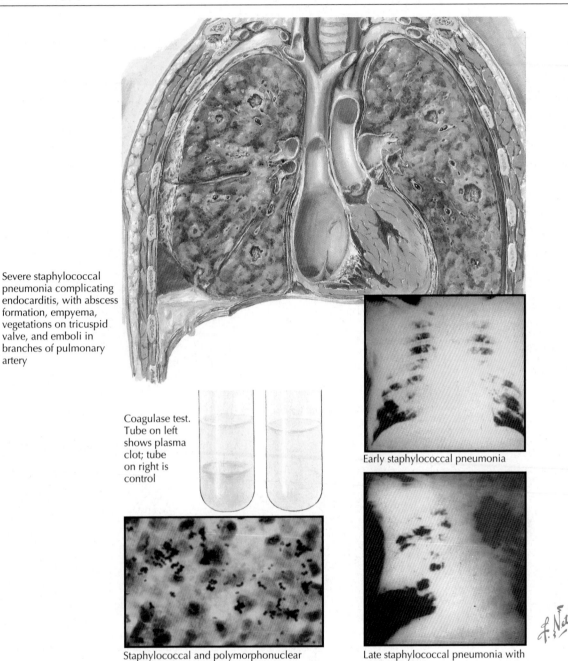

Severe staphylococcal pneumonia complicating endocarditis, with abscess formation, empyema, vegetations on tricuspid valve, and emboli in branches of pulmonary artery

Coagulase test. Tube on left shows plasma clot; tube on right is control

Early staphylococcal pneumonia

Staphylococcal and polymorphonuclear leukocytes in sputum (Gram stain)

Late staphylococcal pneumonia with abscesses and pneumothorax

available antimicrobial agents are routinely recovered in the hospital as well as in the community setting.

Resistance may be due to either elaboration of β-lactamase or alterations in one of the penicillin-binding proteins (PBPs). The β-lactamase enzyme is secreted extracellularly and acts by cleaving the β-lactam ring, thereby inactivating the compound. Organisms using this mode of resistance may be treated with β-lactamase stable antibiotics such as nafcillin or oxacillin. In organisms with altered PBPs, represented by methicillin-resistant strains, penicillins and cephalosporins are ineffective. These β-

lactam antibiotics directly target the PBPs to interfere with cell wall integrity. In the methicillin-resistant strains, there are different drug susceptibility profiles that are seen in hospital- versus community-acquired isolates. There is also a difference in patterns of drug resistance depending on geography. It is therefore important to tailor treatment according to regional antibiotic susceptibility patterns.

The appearance of strains of *S. aureus* that have reduced susceptibility to the glycopeptide antibiotics (e.g., vanco-mycin) is a particular concern. Several such isolates have been reported from Japan and the United States. Thus far,

Figure 91-3 Bacterial Endocarditis.

Early lesions

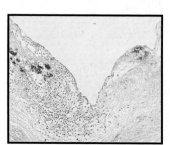

Deposit of platelets and organisms (stained dark), edema, and leukocytic infiltration in very early bacterial endocarditis of aortic valve

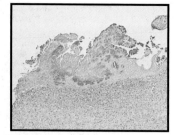

Development of vegetations containing clumps of bacteria on tricuspid valve

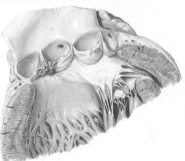

Early vegetations of bacterial endocarditis on bicuspid aortic valve

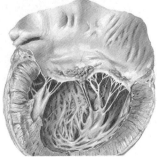

Early vegetations of bacterial endocarditis at contact line of mitral valve

Advanced lesions

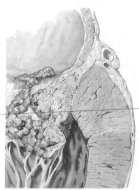

Vegetations of bacterial endocarditis on under-aspect as well as on atrial surface of mitral valve

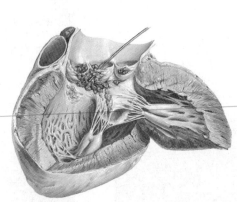

Advanced bacterial endocarditis of aortic valve: perforation of cusp; extension to anterior cusp of mitral valve and chordae tendineae: "jet lesion" on septal wall

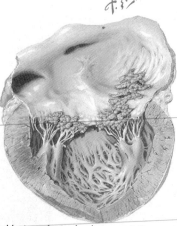

Advanced lesion of mitral valve: vegetations extending onto chordae tendineae with rupture of two chordae; also extension to atrial wall and contact lesion on opposite cusp

these organisms show only intermediate levels of resistance to vancomycin and retain susceptibility to the newer classes of antistaphylococcal antibiotics, the oxazolidinones, quinupristin-dalfopristin, the cyclic lipopeptide daptomycin, and the glycylcycline tigecycline.

Newer approaches to therapy involve decolonization to prevent person-to-person transmission and to break the cycle of recurrent outbreaks of MRSA SSTIs in a single individual. Currently no clear consensus guidelines exist, and evidence from controlled trials is limited. However,

general measures include intranasal mupirocin, topical antiseptic washes (i.e., chlorhexidine gluconate) during daily showers and weekly chlorine baths (about 1 tsp per gallon of bath water with a 10-minute soak). Personal hygiene measures include keeping nails trimmed short and scrubbed daily with soap, single use only of bath towels and garments, and washing clothes in hot water. If a single patient has recurrent MRSA outbreaks, then oral antibiotics are often used in conjunction. Also, all members of the household should be treated with the general decoloniza-

tion measures. A recent study was the first to show that a combination of intranasal mupirocin, chlorhexidine gluconate washes, and rifampin and doxycycline treatment for 7 days was effective in the eradication of MRSA colonization in hospitalized patients for at least 3 months.

Avoiding Treatment Errors

Appropriate management of every infectious disease involves early recognition of the presence of infection, inclusion of the causative organism in the differential diagnosis, and when possible, treatment with antimicrobials active against the infecting organisms for a sufficient duration to achieve the desired outcome. Because most serious infections caused by staphylococci are not subtle, pitfalls in the management of these infections typically involve the failure to consider staphylococci as the infectious agent and lack of consideration for the drug-resistance potential of this organism. Cultures of material (e.g., wound drainage, sputum, blood) are essential for the establishment of the diagnosis and the determination of drug susceptibilities to guide therapeutic management.

A common error in the management of endovascular infections caused by *S. aureus* is the assumption that detection of this organism in the urine indicates only a urinary tract infection. Isolation of *S. aureus* in the urine should prompt evaluation for the presence of endocarditis or other endovascular infection because this organism commonly enters the genitourinary system hematogenously.

Future Directions

Future studies are likely to yield a more thorough understanding of the pathogenetic mechanisms of staphylococcal disease. Of special interest are insights that should arise from studies of whole bacterial genomes, with an emphasis placed on the further elucidation of the mobile genetic elements.

Epidemiologic studies of drug resistance will also be of continued importance. Although the newer classes of antibiotics have enhanced the ability to treat resistant strains of *S. aureus*, and resistance to these agents appears to be uncommon, it is anticipated that resistant organisms will become prevalent as the use of these antibiotics becomes widespread. Therefore, prevention of infection is of paramount importance. Strategies involving decolonization regimens of chronic carriers need further investigation but are showing promise. Vaccine development and targeted antiadhesion strategies are areas of ongoing study.

Additional Resources

Crossley KB, Archer GL: The Staphylococci in Human Disease. New York, Churchill Livingstone, 1997.

This book provides a more in-depth discussion of the disease processes associated with staphylococci that are beyond the scope of discussion in this chapter.

Lewis JS, Jorgensen JH: Inducible clindamycin resistance in staphylococci: Should clinicians and microbiologists be concerned? Clin Infect Dis 40:280-285, 2005.

This article reviews the clinical importance of inducible clindamycin resistance in Staphylococcus aureus. Patients with life-threatening infections due to CA-MRSA should not be treated with clindamycin alone because of this concern.

Liu C, Chambers HF: *Staphylococcus aureus* with heterogeneous resistance to vancomycin: Epidemiology, clinical significance, and critical assessment of diagnostic methods. Antimicrob Agents Chemother 47:3040-3045, 2003.

This article provides an excellent overview of staphylococcal resistance and intermediate resistance to vancomycin that may aid general practitioners in understanding appropriate therapeutic use of vancomycin.

Mandell GL, Bennett JE, Dolin R (eds): Principles and Practice of Infectious Diseases, 6th ed. Philadelphia, Churchill Livingstone, 2004.

This text provides a more in-depth discussion of the disease processes associated with staphylococci that are beyond the scope of discussion in this chapter. It is the primary general reference source of infectious disease practitioners.

EVIDENCE

1. Foster TJ: The Staphylococcus aureus "superbug." J Clin Invest 114:1693-1696, 2004.

   This article reviews the factors contributing to Staphylococcus aureus virulence. These include its altered PBP, adhesion molecules present on its surface, and ability to produce exotoxins that are capable of promoting inflammation and cellular injury.

2. Miller LG, Quan C, Shay A, et al: A prospective investigation of outcomes after hospital discharge for endemic, community-acquired methicillin-resistant and -susceptible *Staphylococcus aureus* skin infection. Clin Infect Dis 44(4):483-492, 2007.

   The authors report on a prospective trial comparing the 30-day outcome of CA-MRSA vs. CA-MSSA skin and soft tissue infections. They found no significant differences between the groups when appropriate incision and drainage of abscesses was performed. However, there was a trend noted toward close contacts of persons with CA-MRSA developing an infection.

3. Moran GJ, Krishnadasan A, Gorwitz RJ, et al: Methicillin-resistant *S. aureus* infections among patients in the emergency department. N Engl J Med 355(7):666-674, 2006.

   This paper reports the prevalence of MRSA as a cause of skin infections among adult patients presenting to emergency departments in several geographically diverse, metropolitan areas in the United States. It also presents data on antimicrobial-resistant patterns and strain genotypes.

4. Simor A, Phillips E, McGeer A, et al: Randomized controlled trial of chlorhexidine gluconate for washing, intranasal mupirocin, and rifampin and doxycycline versus no treatment for the eradication of methicillin-resistant *Staphylococcus aureus* colonization. Clin Infect Dis 44:178-185, 2007.

   This is the second randomized controlled trial performed to assess the efficacy of eradication of MRSA colonization. Such therapies are often offered to patients with recurrent infections despite the lack of evidence. The results of this study, using a combination of topical and oral systemic antimicrobial agents, indicate that MRSA decolonization in hospitalized patients may be achieved for prolonged periods of time and that such treatment is generally well tolerated without significant adverse effects.

5. Tokars JI: Predictive value of blood cultures positive for coagulase-negative staphylococci: Implications for patient care and health care quality assurance. Clin Infect Dis 39(3):333-341, 2004.

   The author presents a mathematical model for the interpretation of whether blood cultures positive for CoNS are likely to represent true bacteremia vs. contamination and thus necessitate antimicrobial therapy. These clinical guidelines are very useful in daily practice.

David J. Weber ▪ Amanda Peppercorn ▪ William A. Rutala

Cellulitis

Introduction

Cellulitis is an infection of the skin that may extend into the subcutaneous tissues. Despite being a common clinical entity, the incidence and epidemiology have not been well delineated. Cellulitis accounted for 2.2% of office visits in an analysis of a large health care plan.

Etiology and Pathogenesis

Cellulitis represents a subset of skin and soft tissue infections (Fig. 92-1). The epidemiology, pathogenesis, clinical manifestations, pathogens, and treatment differ by the depth of infection. Cellulitis is an acute, spreading infection of the dermis that may involve the subcutaneous tissues. Erysipelas is a distinct form of superficial cellulitis that is associated with marked swelling of the skin and does not involve subcutaneous tissues. The margins of involved and normal tissues are sharply demarcated, particularly at bony prominences, in contrast to cellulitis, in which the margins are generally not distinct. Cellulitis is distinct from primary pyodermas such as impetigo (a superficial vesiculopustular skin infection), folliculitis (infection of the hair follicles), furuncles (inflammatory nodule of the hair follicles), and carbuncles (abscesses of the subcutaneous tissue that drain through hair follicles). These infections differ from cellulitis in that they are usually caused by *Staphylococcus aureus* as opposed to streptococci, often respond to local measures (topical agents and drainage), and rarely require hospitalization. Infections deeper in the soft tissues include fasciitis (infection between the subcutaneous tissue and muscle) and myositis (infection in the muscle).

Cellulitis generally results from a breach in the skin due to trauma (e.g., cut), underlying disorders of the skin (e.g., psoriasis, eczema), ulcers (e.g., diabetic or decubitus ulcers), or superficial dermal infections (dermatoses, particularly tinea pedis). Major predisposing factors include venous (e.g., venous insufficiency, prior saphenectomy) or lymphatic compromise (e.g., prior pelvic radiation, filariasis, radical mastectomy). Previous cellulitis is also a predisposing factor. Recurrent bouts of cellulitis are common in patients with impaired lymphatic drainage following radical mastectomy or associated with morbid obesity.

Erysipelas is almost always caused by group A β-hemolytic streptococcus. Less commonly, erysipelas may develop secondary to group C and G streptococcal infection, especially in patients with underlying venous or lymphatic compromise. Rarely, *Staphylococcus aureus* (including methicillin-resistant strains), *Streptococcus pneumoniae*, enterococci, or aerobic gram-negative bacilli may cause erysipelas. Group A β-hemolytic streptococcus is the most common causative organism in cellulitis. Other streptococci, including groups B, C, and G, are also common causes. After streptococci, *Staphylococcus aureus* is the most common pathogen in cellulitis. However, there are a variety of other pathogens (Table 92-1).

Clinical Presentation

Cellulitis is generally an easily recognized clinical syndrome. Typical local findings include macular erythema that is generally confluent and blanching with associated swelling, warmth, and tenderness of the involved area. Lymphangitis with tender regional lymphadenopathy is common. Cellulitis most commonly occurs in the lower extremities, followed by the upper extremities and then head and neck. Systemic findings are common, especially fever and chills. Patients may complain of myalgias and fatigue.

In general, the onset is subacute with enlargement of the erythematous area over several days. Progression is generally proximal. In some patients, the onset of symptoms may be abrupt with high fever and pronounced rigors. Disorientation or an altered mental status may occur, especially in elderly patients.

Figure 92-1 Cross-Section of the Skin Showing Layer and Types of Infections.

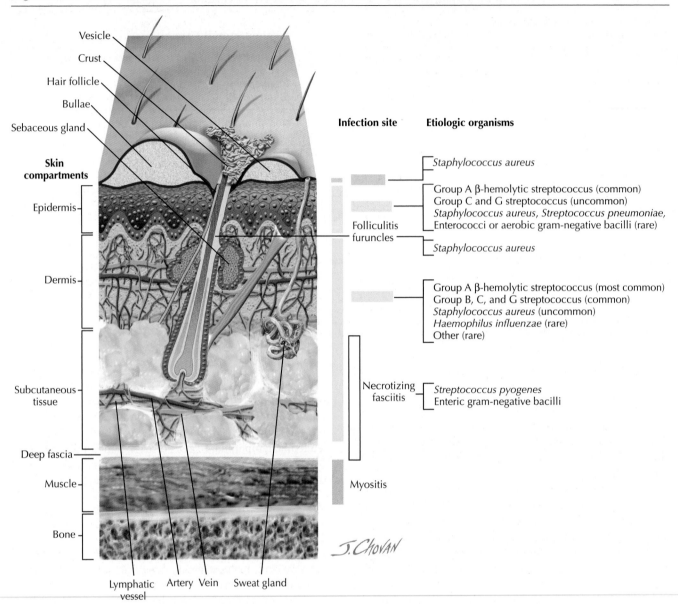

Table 92-1	Uncommon Pathogens Causing Cellulitis and Their Risk Factors
Pathogen	**Risk Factors**
Aeromonas hydrophilia	Swimming in fresh or brackish waters: trauma in the water or contamination of open wounds. Use of medicinal leaches
Community-associated MRSA	Participant in contact sports (e.g., football), inmate of a correctional institute, injection drug use, recipient of a tattoo (failure to use aseptic technique), household member with *S. aureus* colonization or infection, and poor personal hygiene. Recent studies have noted that community-associated MRSA may occur in the absence of identifiable risk factors
Erysipelothrix rhusiopathiae	Wound with occupational exposure to infected animals including swine, sheep, horses, cattle, chickens, crabs, fish, dogs, and cats
Pasteurella multocida	Cat scratches or bites, dog bites
Pseudomonas aeruginosa	Puncture wounds on plantar surfaces of foot; water exposure
Vibrio vulnificus	Swimming in brackish or marine waters: trauma in the water or contamination of open wounds

MRSA, methicillin-resistant *Staphylococcus aureus*.

Table 92-2 Specific Anatomic Variants of Cellulitis and Causes of Predisposition

Anatomic Variant of Cause of Predisposition	Location	Likely Bacterial Cause
Periorbital cellulitis	Periorbital (origin may be sinuses or dental)	*Staphylococcus aureus*, pneumococcus, group A streptococcus
Buccal cellulitis	Cheek	*Haemophilus influenzae*
Cellulitis complicating body piercing	Ear, nose, umbilicus	*S. aureus*, CA-MRSA, group A streptococcus
Mastectomy (with axillary node dissection) for breast cancer	Ipsilateral arm	Non–group A hemolytic streptococcus
Lumpectomy with radiation (with limited axillary node dissection) for breast cancer	Ipsilateral arm	Non–group A hemolytic streptococcus
Harvest of saphenous vein for coronary artery bypass	Ipsilateral leg	Group A or non–group A hemolytic streptococcus
Liposuction	Thigh, abdominal wall	Group A streptococcus, peptostreptococcus
Postoperative (very early) wound infection	Abdomen, chest, hip	Group A streptococcus
Injection drug use ("skin popping")	Extremities, neck	*S. aureus*, CA-MRSA, streptococci (groups A, C, F, G)
Perianal cellulitis	Perineum	Group A streptococcus, enteric gram-negative bacilli
Crepitant cellulitis	Trunk, extremities	*Clostridium* species, mixed infections (anaerobes and gram-negative bacilli)

CA-MRSA, community-associated methicillin-resistant *Staphylococcus aureus*.
Adapted from Swartz MN: Clinical practice: Cellulitis. N Engl J Med 350:904-912, 2004.

Differential Diagnosis

The distinctive appearance of cellulitis usually leads to an accurate clinical diagnosis. Occasionally, the rash of erythema migrans in Lyme disease leads to diagnostic confusion.

Severe pain in a limb, frank necrosis, blebs, or crepitus should suggest gangrenous cellulitis or fasciitis. Necrotizing fasciitis is a medical emergency that requires emergent surgical débridement and intravenous antibiotics. Type I fasciitis is an acute, rapidly developing infection of deep fascia, characterized by severe pain, tenderness, swelling, bullae, and necrosis of the skin. It is often accompanied by crepitus in a mixed infection caused by anaerobes plus facultative species such as streptococci or enteric gram-negative bacilli. A clinical pearl worth committing to memory is that necrotizing fasciitis should remain high on the differential in any patient with pain out of proportion to the clinical findings on physical examination.

Type II fasciitis is an acute infection, often accompanied by toxic shock syndrome. Physical examination reveals rapid progression of marked edema to violaceous bullae and necrosis of subcutaneous tissue without associated crepitus. Type II fasciitis is generally caused by group A streptococci.

Deep venous thrombosis (DVT) in the lower extremities may mimic cellulitis because patients with DVT often present with erythema overlying the involved veins with associated tenderness and swelling. Fever may also accompany DVT. Other noninfectious syndromes that may lead to diagnostic confusion include contact dermatitis, insect bites or stings, drug reactions, venous stasis, and foreign body reactions. Less common syndromes may also mimic cellulitis: cutaneous larva migrans, pyoderma gangrenosa, leukemia, lymphoma, Paget's disease, panniculitis, sarcoidosis, Sweet's syndrome (acute febrile neutrophilic dermatosis), systemic lupus erythematosus, and urticaria.

Diagnostic Approach

The diagnosis of cellulitis depends on the appearance of the skin and, in most cases, does not require an attempt to establish a microbial etiology. Moreover, attempts to establish an etiologic or microbiologic diagnosis by culturing blood, skin aspirates, or skin biopsy samples are rarely successful. In one study of more than 500 patients with cellulitis, blood cultures were positive in only 2% of cases. In patients with environmental exposures, it may be useful to try to isolate the causative pathogen by blood cultures or skin biopsy (Table 92-2). Skin biopsy and blood cultures are indicated for cellulitis in patients who are highly immunocompromised (e.g., neutropenia associated with therapy for malignancies). In such patients, fungal and other systemic infections (e.g., candidiasis, histoplasmosis, and blastomycosis) may present with cellulitis.

Physical examination should focus on determining the extent of disease. It is mandatory to completely undress the patient to allow maximal visualization of all skin areas. The examiner should delineate the area of cellulitis with a marking pen to allow assessment of the extent of spread after the initiation of therapy. The observation of blebs,

necrosis, decreased sensation, or crepitus should suggest fasciitis or myositis. Such infections are medical emergencies and require prompt institution of therapy, evaluation of the extent of disease using computed tomography or magnetic resonance imaging, and prompt assessment for emergent surgery to achieve drainage and removal of necrotic material. For cellulitis involving an extremity, the distal web spaces should be examined for superficial bacterial or fungal infection such as tinea pedis. Treatment of these superficial infections reduces the risk for recurrent cellulitis. Documentation of both venous and arterial blood flow in the involved limb is especially important given the association of venous or arterial insufficiency as a risk factor both for infection and failure to respond to antibacterial therapy. Structures adjacent to the area of cellulitis such as joints and bones should be evaluated for septic involvement. In patients with facial cellulitis, evaluation for sinusitis or dental infection is important given the association of these infections with cellulitis.

The only laboratory test generally useful is a white blood cell count with differential. If the antibiotic chosen is appropriate, the patient's fever and white blood cell count should respond.

Management and Therapy

Optimum Treatment

In most patients with cellulitis, outpatient therapy with oral antibiotics is adequate. A complicating abscess requires drainage with Gram stain and culture of the aspirated contents. Patients who have the following risk factors require consideration for inpatient admission and therapy: failure to respond to oral therapy within 72 hours, inability to take oral medication, and severe underlying diseases such a chronic renal or liver failure or insulin-dependent diabetes. Signs and symptoms of systemic toxicity (e.g., tachycardia [heart rate >100 beats/min], hypotension [systolic blood pressure <90 mm Hg or 20 mm Hg below baseline] are also indications for admission. Patients who require hospitalization should have the following laboratory tests: two blood cultures, complete cell count with differential, blood urea nitrogen and creatinine, bicarbonate, and creatinine phosphokinase.

Clues to potentially severe, deep, soft tissue infection include pain disproportionate to the physical findings; violaceous bullae, cutaneous hemorrhage; skin sloughing or necrosis; hypesthesia of the involved skin; rapid progression; and the presence of gas in the tissues. These patients should have an emergent surgical consultation. Computed tomography or magnetic resonance imaging is often useful to determine the extent of infection if myositis or necrotizing fasciitis is suspected; however, prompt surgery should not be delayed to obtain scans unless the diagnosis is in doubt. In patients with staphylococcal or streptococcal toxic shock, clindamycin rapidly turns off toxin production and is ordered in conjunction with other antibiotics used to treat streptococcal (e.g., penicillin) or staphylococcal (e.g., oxacillin or vancomycin) infections.

Topical mupirocin is effective for mild erysipelas. Bacitracin and neomycin are considered less effective therapy. Patients who have numerous lesions or who are not responding to topical agents should receive an oral antibiotic active against both *Streptococcus pyogenes* and *S. aureus*. Such agents include dicloxacillin (adult dose, 250 mg 4 times per day orally), cephalexin (adult dose, 250 mg 4 times per day orally), clindamycin (adult dose, 300 to 450 mg 3 times per day orally), or amoxicillin-clavulanate (adult dose, 875/125 mg 2 times per day orally). Therapy should be continued for 7 days. Penicillin is the drug of choice in patients who require hospitalization.

Cellulitis that is associated with furuncles, carbuncles, or abscesses is usually caused by *S. aureus*. In such patients, the abscess requires drainage, and the aspirate should be sent for Gram stain and bacterial culture. Community-associated methicillin-resistant *S. aureus* (CA-MRSA) should be strongly considered in these patients. Initial outpatient therapy should include an agent likely effective against CA-MRSA such as trimethoprim-sulfamethoxazole (adult, 2 double-strength tablets 2 times per day orally) or clindamycin (adult dose, 300 to 450 mg 3 times per day orally). The culture results should provide a guide for optimal antibiotic selection. For inpatients, initial therapy should include a drug with activity against MRSA such as vancomycin, daptomycin, linezolid, or tigecycline.

Cellulitis that is diffuse or unassociated with a defined portal is most commonly caused by streptococcal species. Treatment with dicloxacillin (adult dose, 250 mg 4 times per day orally) or cephalexin (adult dose, 250 mg 4 times per day orally) is usually effective in these patients. For penicillin-allergic patients, clindamycin (adult dose, 300 to 450 mg 3 times per day orally) is the recommended alternative. Important clinical clues to other causes of cellulitis include physical activity, trauma, water contact, animal bites, insect bites, and human bites. In such patients, antibiotics with a wider spectrum or multiple antibiotics may be required. Treatment with intravenous cefazolin or oxacillin is reasonable in patients who require hospitalization; however, the possibility of MRSA infection warrants consideration of initial therapy with vancomycin, daptomycin, linezolid, or tigecycline. The length of therapy is 7 to 10 days, depending on the response. However, conversion to oral therapy is possible when the cellulitis is stable (not progressing) and the patient is clinically responding, as evidenced by decrease in pain, resolution of fever, and shrinkage of the area of cellulitis (it helps to demarcate the extent of initial involvement with a marking pen, as previously noted). An important adjuvant in therapy is to elevate the involved limb to reduce swelling and to promote healing.

Avoiding Treatment Errors

Patients with simple cellulitis managed as outpatients require close follow-up. Failure to respond within 72 hours, progressive spread of infection, or development of systemic signs requires hospitalization. Cellulitis associated with bite wounds (antibiotic depends on biting species), intravenous drug use, infection associated with injury in water, and postoperative surgical wound infections requires a broader spectrum of therapy or different agents. Initial hospitalization and broad-spectrum antibiotics are usually required for patients who have cellulitis and are immunocompromised; demonstrate evidence of systemic toxicity; have suspected necrotizing cellulitis, fasciitis, or myositis; have arterial or venous insufficiency in the infected limb; or have underlying disorders such as insulin-dependent diabetes, renal failure, or liver failure.

Future Directions

The epidemiology of CA-MRSA has not been completely defined. It is likely that the increasing prevalence of CA-MRSA will require alterations in the standard empiric therapy for cellulitis. Management of these patients, once their initial infection has resolved, from the standpoint of personal hygiene and potential decolonization is still evolving. At present, there is no recommendation to attempt to decolonize such patients after a single bout of CA-MRSA skin infection.

New drugs active against MRSA have recently been introduced, including linezolid, daptomycin, and tigecycline. Although all are approved by the U.S. Food and Drug Administration for the therapy of skin and soft tissue infections, when to use these newer agents is incompletely defined. Additional agents with activity against MRSA are likely to be available in the near future.

Rapid tests (e.g., polymerase chain reaction) to detect MRSA are becoming clinically available. Such tests have been used primarily to detect colonization in newly hospitalized patients to determine whether contact precautions are indicated. Whether such tests will have a role in aiding in the choice of therapy for treating skin infections has not been evaluated.

Attempts to develop a vaccine to prevent *S. aureus* infections continue. To date, such vaccines have not been effective.

Additional Resources

Hanson, PG, Standridge, J, Jarrett, F, Maki, DG: Freshwater wound infection due to *Aeromonas hydrophila*. JAMA 238:1053-1054, 1977.
   This brief paper describes freshwater wound infections due to Aeromonas hydrophila.
Noonburg GE: Management of extremity trauma and related infections occurring in the aquatic environment. J Am Acad Orthop Surg 13:243-253, 2005.
   The author presents an excellent review of infections related to the aquatic environment, including those due to Vibrio species, Aeromonas hydrophila, Erysipelothrix rhusiopathiae, and Mycobacterium marinum. Also covered is the management of noninfectious aquatic injuries such as boating accidents, propeller injuries, Morey eel and barracuda bites, and envenomation injuries (e.g., stingrays).
Ulusaraac O, Carter E: Varied clinical presentation of *Vibrio vulnificus* infections: A report of four unusual cases and review of the literature. South Med J 97:163-168, 2004.
   The authors present four cases of Vibrio vulnificus infections and review the literature on this important pathogen.

EVIDENCE

1. Falagas ME, Vergidis PI: Narrative review: Diseases that masquerade as infectious cellulitis. Ann Intern Med 142:47-55, 2005.
   This is an excellent review of noninfectious diseases that masquerade as infectious cellulitis, such as vascular disorders, primary dermatologic disorders, rheumatic disorders, immunologic-idiopathic disorders, malignant diseases, familial syndromes, and foreign-body reactions.
2. Perl B, Gottehrer NP, Raveh D, et al: Cost-effectiveness of blood cultures for adult patients with cellulitis. Clin Infect Dis 29:1483-1488, 1999.
   This important paper demonstrates that blood cultures are rarely positive in patients with cellulitis.
3. Stevens DL, Bisno AL, Chambers HF, et al: Practice guidelines for the diagnosis and management of skin and soft-tissue infections. Clin Infect Dis 41:373-406, 2005.
   This comprehensive guideline focuses on appropriate antibiotic therapy for skin and soft tissue infections.
4. Stulberg DL, Penrod MA, Blatny RA: Common bacterial skin infections. Am Fam Physician 66:119-124, 2002.
   This good review of the common bacterial skin infections includes cellulitis, erysipelas, impetigo, folliculitis, furuncles, and carbuncles.
5. Swartz MN: Clinical practice: Cellulitis. N Engl J Med 350:904-912, 2004.
   A comprehensive, concisely written review of cellulitis, including specific anatomic variants, important processes that should be distinguished from cellulitis, and initial treatment recommendations.

Kristine B. Patterson ▪ Cam Patterson

93

Infective Endocarditis

Introduction

Infective endocarditis (IE) is an infection of the endocardial surface of the heart and implies the presence of microorganisms in the lesion. Despite advances in medical and surgical interventions, IE continues to be associated with high morbidity and mortality, especially given the evolution of antimicrobial resistance. Early diagnosis, prompt and appropriate antimicrobial therapy, echocardiographic evaluation, and timely surgical intervention are cornerstones of successful management.

Etiology and Pathogenesis

The three main bacterial causes of IE are streptococci, staphylococci, and enterococci. *Staphylococcus aureus* has now replaced viridans group streptococci as the leading cause owing to an increased frequency of oxacillin-resistant *S. aureus* in tertiary centers and community-acquired infections. IE typically occurs in the setting of a previously damaged valve surface. This provides a suitable site for bacterial colonization and adherence, allowing replication to a critical mass and the formation of mature, infected vegetation.

Clinical Presentation

Any organ system can be involved in patients with IE, and thus the clinical presentation is highly variable. Four processes contribute to the clinical manifestations of IE: (1) the infectious process on the valve causing local intracardiac complications (e.g., perivalvular abscess, incompetent valve, conduction disturbances, congestive heart failure [CHF]) (Fig. 93-1); (2) vascular phenomena (e.g., septic pulmonary or arterial emboli, mycotic aneurysm, intracranial hemorrhage); (3) bacteremic seeding of remote sites (e.g., osteomyelitis, psoas or perirenal abscess) (Fig. 93-2); and (4) immunologic phenomena (e.g., glomerulonephritis, Osler's nodes, Roth spots, positive rheumatoid factor, and antinuclear antibodies).

The presentation of IE is straightforward when the classic signs and symptoms are present: fever, bacteremia or fungemia, valvular incompetence, peripheral emboli, and immune-mediated vasculitis as is seen in subacute IE.

However, acute IE may evolve too quickly for immunologic phenomena to develop, and patients may present only with fever or severe manifestations such as those related to valve incompetency. In both acute and subacute IE, fever is the most common presenting symptom.

Frequently, the diagnosis can be made clinically if a careful physical examination is performed. Attention should be given to the conjunctiva (petechial hemorrhages), dilated funduscopic exam (Roth spots), complete cardiovascular exam (new or changing murmur, especially aortic, mitral or tricuspid regurgitation, and signs of CHF), splenomegaly, and extremities (splinter hemorrhages, septic emboli, Janeway's or Osler's nodes) (Fig. 93-3). The comprehensive physical examination can be complemented by several nonspecific yet suggestive laboratory findings including (but not limited to) anemia, thrombocytopenia, leukocytosis, an active urinary sediment, an elevated sedimentation rate, hypergammaglobulinemia, positive rheumatoid factor, antinuclear antibodies, hypocomplementemia, and false-positive Venereal Disease Research Laboratory and Lyme disease serology.

Differential Diagnosis

Almost any disseminated severe bacterial, fungal, mycobacterial, viral, parasitic, or spirochete infection can manifest some of the features of IE. Several connective tissue or autoimmune diseases and hematologic malignancies can also mimic IE. By using the expertise of the microbiologist and the cardiologist early in the process, a definitive positive diagnosis will alert the clinician to any potential

Figure 93-1 Bacterial Endocarditis.

Early lesions

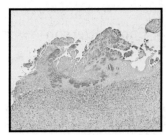

Deposit of platelets and organisms (stained dark), edema, and leukocytic infiltration in very early bacterial endocarditis of aortic valve

Development of vegetations containing clumps of bacteria on tricuspid valve

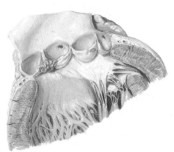

Early vegetations of bacterial endocarditis on bicuspid aortic valve

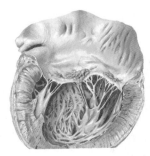

Early vegetations of bacterial endocarditis at contact line of mitral valve

Advanced lesions

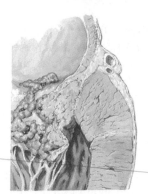

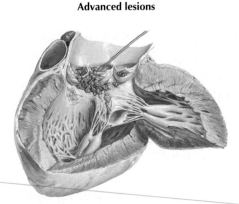

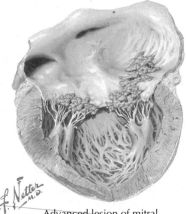

Vegetations of bacterial endocarditis on under-aspect as well as on atrial surface of mitral valve

Advanced bacterial endocarditis of aortic valve: perforation of cusp; extension to anterior cusp of mitral valve and chordae tendineae: "jet lesion" on septal wall

Advanced lesion of mitral valve: vegetations extending onto chordae tendineae with rupture of two chordae; also extension to atrial wall and contact lesion on opposite cusp

complications and therapeutic interventions. Conversely, a negative echocardiogram will allow alternative diagnoses to be explored more rapidly.

Diagnostic Approach

Since 1994, the Duke criteria have been the diagnostic strategy most consistently used in stratifying patients suspected of IE into definite, possible, or rejected categories. Most recently, these criteria have been modified to include newer diagnostic methods. Although the modified Duke criteria can provide a primary diagnostic schema, they should not replace clinical judgment.

Microbiology

The first definitive test obtained should be at least three sets of routine blood cultures during the first 24 hours of observation. More cultures may be necessary if the patient has received antibiotics in the preceding weeks. Almost 50% of culture-negative IE can be attributed to antibiotic use before obtaining cultures. Organisms, such as the HACEK group (*Haemophilus* species, *Actinobacillus*

Figure 93-2 Bacterial Endocarditis: Remote Embolic Effects.

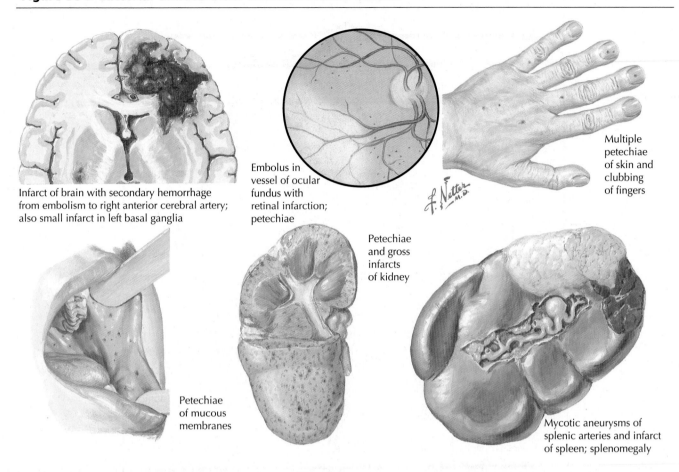

Infarct of brain with secondary hemorrhage from embolism to right anterior cerebral artery; also small infarct in left basal ganglia

Embolus in vessel of ocular fundus with retinal infarction; petechiae

Multiple petechiae of skin and clubbing of fingers

Petechiae and gross infarcts of kidney

Petechiae of mucous membranes

Mycotic aneurysms of splenic arteries and infarct of spleen; splenomegaly

actinomycetemcomitans, *Cardiobacterium hominis*, *Eikenella corrodens*, and *Kingella* species) and *Brucella* species are slow growing and require extended incubation of cultures (4 weeks). Special culture techniques or media may be required for some organisms (e.g., *Legionella* species). Blood culture results are negative in more than 50% of fungal endocarditis cases. Serologic studies are frequently necessary to diagnose Q fever, brucellosis, legionellosis, and psittacosis and are now included as a surrogate marker in lieu of positive blood cultures for diagnosis.

Specific Pathogens

Staphylococcal Endocarditis

Staphylococci are now the most common cause of IE, especially *S. aureus* native valve IE. Increasing rates of methicillin-resistant *S. aureus* are being reported. The course of *S. aureus* is typically fulminant with myocardial and valve-ring abscesses and widespread metastatic infection common. Thirty percent of patients experience neurologic manifestations. IE caused by oxacillin-resistant *S. aureus* is particularly common in injection drug users (IDUs) or patients with nosocomial infection. Coagulase-negative staphylococci are an important cause of prosthetic

valve endocarditis (PVE). Right-sided IE is more commonly seen in IDUs and may be either oxacillin sensitive or resistant.

Streptococcal Endocarditis

Streptococci are now the second most common causative agents of IE, with the viridans streptococci the most common subgroup. The cure rate exceeds 90%, but complications are seen in about 30% of cases.

Streptococcus pneumoniae IE is rare and usually involves the aortic valve. It frequently has a fulminant course and is often associated with perivalvular abscess, pericarditis, and concurrent meningitis. Penicillin resistance is increasing. Valve replacement may be beneficial in preventing early death.

S. anginosus has a predilection to disseminate and form abscesses and may require a longer course of therapy compared with other α-hemolytic streptococci. *S. bovis* IE should prompt a colon malignancy evaluation.

IE due to nutritionally variant streptococci typically is indolent in onset and associated with previous heart disease. Special media are required for microbiologic identification. Therapy is difficult because of systemic embolization and frequent relapse.

Figure 93-3 Common Portals of Bacterial Entry in Bacterial Endocarditis.

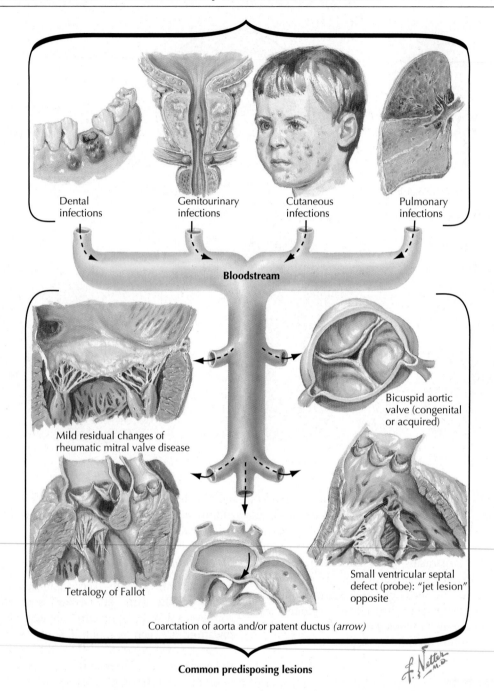

Dental infections

Genitourinary infections

Cutaneous infections

Pulmonary infections

Bloodstream

Mild residual changes of rheumatic mitral valve disease

Bicuspid aortic valve (congenital or acquired)

Tetralogy of Fallot

Small ventricular septal defect (probe): "jet lesion" opposite

Coarctation of aorta and/or patent ductus *(arrow)*

Common predisposing lesions

Enterococcal Endocarditis

Enterococcus faecalis and *Enterococcus faecium* IE usually affect older men after genitourinary tract manipulation or younger women after an obstetric procedure. Classic peripheral manifestations are uncommon. There is a rapidly increasing rate of penicillin-resistant enterococcus in tertiary care centers.

Gram-Negative Endocarditis

Persons using injection drugs, prosthetic valve recipients, and patients with cirrhosis are at increased risk for gram-negative endocarditis. CHF is common.

Salmonella species IE usually involves abnormal valves and is associated with significant valvular destruction, atrial thrombi, myocarditis, and pericarditis. Valve replacement after 7 to 10 days of antimicrobial therapy is typically required.

Pseudomonas species IE is almost exclusively seen in IDUs and often affects normal valves. Embolic phenomena, inability to sterilize valves, neurologic complications, ring and annular abscesses, splenic abscesses, bacteremic relapses, and progressive heart failure are common. Early surgical intervention is recommended for left-sided involvement.

Neisseria gonorrhoeae rarely causes IE and typically follows an indolent course, with aortic valve involvement, large vegetations, valve-ring abscesses, CHF, and nephritis.

HACEK Endocarditis

The gram-negative bacilli of the HACEK group account for 5% to 10% of cases of native valve IE. All are fastidious and may require 3 weeks or more for primary isolation. HACEK endocarditis is more common in patients who have dental infections or in IDUs who contaminate the injection with saliva.

Fungal Endocarditis

Candida and *Aspergillus* species are the most common cause of fungal IE. *Candida* species are more common in persons with central venous catheters or parenteral nutrition. Both can be seen following prosthetic valves. Other *Candida* species, *C. parapsilosis* and *C. tropicalis*, predominate in IDUs. Blood culture results are usually negative in *Aspergillus* species IE. Surgical intervention is almost always required, especially with prosthetic valves, following a course of antifungal agents. Lifelong antifungal suppressive therapy is frequently considered.

Culture-Negative Endocarditis

Culture-negative IE is common. Causes include recent administration of antimicrobial agents; slow growth of fastidious organisms, such as the HACEK group; fungal endocarditis; *Coxiella* species; intracellular parasites, such as *Bartonella* or *Chlamydia* species; and noninfectious endocarditis.

Prosthetic Valve Endocarditis

PVE occurs in up to 10% of patients during the lifetime of the prosthesis. Early PVE (within 60 days after implantation) usually results from valve contamination during the perioperative period. Late PVE (after 60 days) results from transient bacteremia. Clinical manifestations are similar to those of native valve IE; however, new or changing murmurs are more common. Persistently positive blood culture results and valvular dysfunction by echocardiography are the hallmarks. Transesophageal echocardiography (TEE) is recommended for diagnosis and assessment of complications such as perivalvular abscess, regurgitation, and so forth. Coagulase-negative staphylococci are the dominant cause of PVE in the first year. After 1 year, the causative organisms are similar to those of native valve IE. Therapy is, by necessity, aggressive. Rifampin and gentamicin can be added to nafcillin for methicillin-sensitive *S. aureus* or to vancomycin for methicillin-resistant *S. aureus*. For culture-negative PVE, vancomycin and gentamicin should be used to provide broad bactericidal coverage.

Echocardiography

Echocardiography is an essential tool in the diagnosis and management of patients with IE and should be performed in all patients with suspected and confirmed IE (Fig. 93-4). An oscillating vegetation or mass, annular abscess, prosthetic valve dehiscence, and new regurgitation are all major Duke criteria and, as such, confirm IE. Transthoracic echocardiography (TTE) is rapid, noninvasive, and has excellent specificity for vegetations (98%); however, sensitivity is less than 60%. TTE should be performed initially when the suspicion is low. TEE allows imaging of very small vegetations and is the procedure of choice for assessing the pulmonic valve, prosthetic valves, and perivalvular areas for abscesses. TEE has a substantially higher sensitivity (76% to 100%) and specificity (94%) than TTE for perivalvular extension of infection. TEE should be obtained initially when clinical suspicion is high, especially when PVE is suspected or when images obtained by TTE will be poor (i.e., severe pulmonary disease or obesity). If clinical suspicion of IE persists after an initially negative TEE, a repeat study is warranted within 7 to 10 days. The combination of a negative TEE and a negative TTE confers a 95% negative predictive value.

Management and Therapy

Optimum Treatment

Antimicrobial Therapy

After initial empiric therapy, antimicrobial agents should be selected based on susceptibility testing of the isolated causative microbe (Table 93-1). Prolonged administration of antimicrobial agents is required, almost always through the parenteral route. Bactericidal agents or antibiotic combinations that produce synergistic, rapidly bactericidal effects are the agents of choice. Serum concentrations must be closely monitored when using aminoglycosides. Blood culture specimens should be obtained early in therapy to ensure eradication of the bacteremia and throughout therapy when persistent or recurrent fever is present. Patients with IE complicated by cardiac arrhythmias and CHF require close observation in an intensive care unit. Anticoagulation is contraindicated in patients with native valve IE.

Many of the newer antimicrobial agents may not have been specifically evaluated in IE patients. Daptomycin, a cyclic lipopeptide antibiotic, is bactericidal in vitro against most gram-positive bacteria, especially oxacillin-sensitive

Figure 93-4 Echocardiography in the Diagnosis and Management of Infective Endocarditis.
IE, infective endocarditis; Rx, antibiotic treatment for endocarditis; TEE, transesophageal echocardiography; TTE, transthoracic echocardiography. *Modified with permission from Bayer AS, Bolger AF, Taubert KA, et al: Diagnosis and management of infective endocarditis and its complications. Circulation 98(25):2936-2948, 1998.*

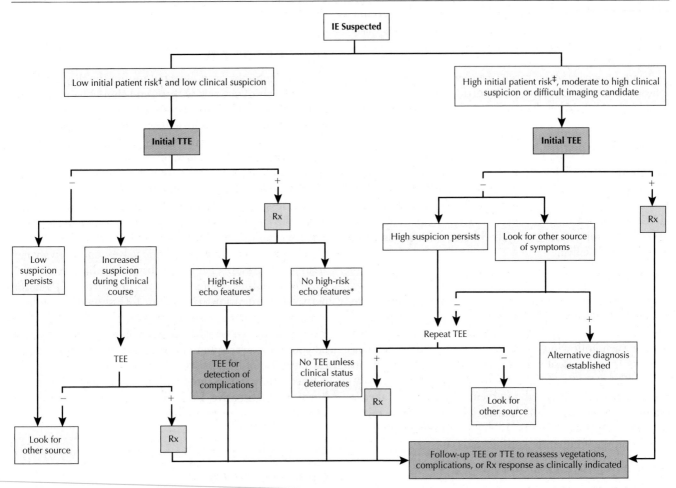

*High-risk echocardiographic features include large and/or mobile vegetations, valvular insufficiency, suggestion of perivalvular extension, or secondary ventricular dysfunction.
†For example, a patient with fever and a previously known heart murmur and no other stigmata of IE.
‡High initial patient risks include prosthetic heart valves, many congenital heart diseases, previous endocarditis, new murmur, heart failure, or other stigmata of endocarditis.
Rx indicates antibiotic treatment for endocarditis.

and oxacillin-resistant *S. aureus*. Recently, daptomycin was shown to be noninferior to standard therapy for bacteremia and right-sided IE. There were too few subjects with left-sided IE to demonstrate noninferiority.

Echocardiography

After the initial diagnosis, echocardiography is useful in management, identifying those patients at high risk for complications, and assessing the need for surgery. Findings that indicate increased risk for complications or need for surgical intervention include the following:

- Persistent vegetation after embolization
- Vegetations larger than 10 mm, especially those on the anterior mitral leaflet (greater risk for embolization)
- Large vegetations
- Vegetations that increase in size while on therapy

- Acute aortic or mitral insufficiency with CHF
- CHF unresponsive to therapy
- Valve perforation or rupture
- Large abscess or abscess unresponsive to therapy
- New heart block
- Valvular dehiscence

Cardiac Surgery

Appropriate, timely surgical intervention can reduce morbidity and mortality substantially. Relatively substantiated indications for surgical intervention include the following:

- Refractory CHF
- More than one serious systemic embolic episode
- Fungal IE, especially involving prosthetic valve
- IE with antibiotic-resistant bacteria or ineffective antimicrobial therapy

Table 93-1 Antimicrobial Therapy for Infective Endocarditis*

Etiology	Antimicrobial Therapy
Viridans streptococci and *S. bovis* penicillin-susceptible (MIC <0.2 μg/mL)	Penicillin G, 12-18 million U/24 hr IV in 6 doses[†] for 4 wk *or* Ceftriaxone, 2 g IV once daily for 4 wk, *or* Penicillin G, 12-18 million U/24 hr IV in 6 doses[†] for 2 wk *with* gentamicin, 3 mg/kg IV every day for 2 wk *or* Vancomycin, 30 mg/kg/24 hr IV in two divided doses for 4 wk (recommended only for patients allergic to β-lactams)
Viridans streptococci and *S. bovis* relatively resistant to penicillin (MIC, 0.1-0.5 μg/mL)	Penicillin G, 24 million U/24 hr IV continuously or 6 doses for 4 wk *with* gentamicin, 3 mg/kg IV every day for 2 wk (first-generation cephalosporins may be substituted for penicillin in patients with penicillin hypersensitivity not of the immediate type), *or* Vancomycin, 30 mg/kg/24 hr IV in two divided doses for 4 wk (only recommended for patients allergic to β-lactams)
Enterococci (and viridans streptococci with penicillin MIC >0.5 μg/mL, nutrient variant viridans streptococci)	Penicillin G, 18-30 million U/24 hr IV in 6 doses *with* gentamicin, 1 mg/kg IV every 8 hr for 4-6 wk, *or* Ampicillin, 12 g/24 hr in six doses *with* gentamicin, 1 mg/kg IV every 8 hr for 4-6 wk, *or* Vancomycin, 30 mg/kg/24 hr IV in two divided doses for 4-6 wk *with* gentamicin, 1 mg/kg IV every 8 hr for 4-6 wk (only recommended for patients allergic to β-lactams; cephalosporins are not acceptable alternatives for patients allergic to penicillins)
Staphylococci (penicillin-susceptible)	Penicillin G, 20 million U/24 hr IV in six doses for 6 wk[†]
Staphylococci (methicillin-susceptible, penicillin-resistant)	Nafcillin (or oxacillin), 2 g IV every 4 hr[†] for 6 wk *with* gentamicin, 1 mg/kg IV every 8 hr for 3-5 days,[†] *or* Cefazolin (or other first-generation cephalosporin), 2 g IV every 8 hr for 6 wk *with* gentamicin, 1 mg/kg IV every 8 hr[†] for 3-5 days
Staphylococci (methicillin-resistant)	Vancomycin, 30 mg/kg/24 hr IV in two divided doses for 6 wk
HACEK microorganisms	Ceftriaxone, 2 g once daily IV for 4 wk, *or* Ampicillin-sulbactam, 12 g/24 hr IV in 4 doses for 4 wk
Culture-negative (native valve)	Ampicillin-sulbactam, 12 g/24 hr IV in 4 doses for 4-6 wk *with* gentamicin, 3 mg/kg each day for 4-6 wk, *or* Vancomycin, 30 mg/kg in 2 doses for 4-6 wk *plus* gentamicin, 1 mg/kg in 3 doses for 4-6 wk *with* ciprofloxacin, 1000 mg/24 hr PO or 800 mg/24 hr in 2 doses IV for 4-6 wk
Prosthetic valve endocarditis	Refer to 2005 American Heart Association endocarditis guidelines

MIC, minimum inhibitory concentration.

* Antibiotic dosages for adult patients with normal renal and hepatic function. Test infecting strain of *Enterococcus* for resistance to aminoglycosides. High-level resistance means loss of synergy, and thus aminoglycosides should not be used in these instances. Therapy should be prolonged to 8-12 wk.

[†] Dosing of penicillin, nafcillin, and oxacillin is frequent and often problematic for home therapy patients. Because these drugs are stable for 24 hr at room temperature, they may be given through a pump that remains with the patient, requiring adjustment only once every 24 hr. Aminoglycosides are used for synergy in gram-positive infections. Requires continuous therapy.

Adapted from Wilson WR, Karchmer AW, Dajani AS, et al: Antibiotic treatment of adults with infective endocarditis due to streptococci, enterococci, staphylococci, and HACEK microorganisms. American Heart Association. JAMA 274:1706-1713, 1995. Copyrighted 1995 American Medical Association.

- Persistent positive blood cultures following 1 week of antibiotic therapy
- Left-sided IE with *Pseudomonas* or *Salmonella* species
- Prosthetic valve IE of 12 months' or less duration after initial replacement
- Echocardiographic findings listed earlier

Avoiding Treatment Errors

Effective treatment of IE requires a multidisciplinary approach with input from infectious disease specialists, cardiology, and cardiothoracic surgery. Although guide-lines and criteria such as the Duke criteria have been established, treatment should be individualized based on clinical judgment.

After a person is put on appropriate antimicrobial therapy, it is imperative to ensure that repeat blood cultures are negative. If not, one should reevaluate therapy and look for complications. Blood cultures should be repeated near the end of antimicrobial therapy and shortly after completing therapy to ensure resolution, and a new baseline echocardiogram should be obtained. It is imperative to educate patients regarding signs of symptoms of IE. Often overlooked are the need for thorough dental evaluation and treatment for substance abuse.

Prophylaxis

Antimicrobial prophylaxis is recommended for patients with increased risk of endocarditis due to underlying cardiac conditions undergoing invasive procedures likely to generate bacteremia. Detailed prophylaxis recommendations are available on the American Heart Association website.

Future Directions

Some clinicians believe that the size of the vegetation and other echocardiographic characteristics predict who is at risk for poor outcome and needs early surgery. At the present time, specific echocardiographic criteria have not been demonstrated. Future studies will help to determine whether echocardiographic findings other than perivalvular or myocardial abscesses are added to the current list of indications for surgery.

Additional Resources

American Heart Association Website. Available at: http://www.americanheart.org.

The AHA website provides guidance in the management of other cardiac-related diseases.

European Society of Cardiology: 2004 European Society for Cardiologist guidelines for infective endocarditis. Available at: http://www.escardio.org/knowledge/guidelines/Guidelines_list.htm. Accessed November 25, 2006.

The European guidelines, which differ from the IDSA and AHA guidelines, are reviewed.

Schlant RC, Alexander RW, O'Rourke RA, et al (eds): Hurst's The Heart, 10th ed. New York, McGraw-Hill, 2001.

The management of IE from a cardiologist's perspective is comprehensively reviewed in this textbook.

EVIDENCE

1. Infectious Diseases Society of America: 2005 American Heart Association infective endocarditis guidelines. Available at: http://www.idsociety.org/. Accessed November 25, 2006.

   The IDSA publishes updated guidelines for the management of IE and serves as an essential tool in managing these complicated patients.

2. Mandell GL, Bennett JE, Dolin R (eds): Mandell, Douglas, and Bennett's Principles and Practice of Infectious Diseases, 5th ed. New York, Churchill Livingstone, 2000.

   This chapter provides more specific guidance in the diagnosis and treatment of suspected or confirmed IE. Less common pathogens and complicated IE are comprehensively reviewed.

3. Fowler VG Jr, Boucher HW, Corey GR, et al: Daptomycin versus standard therapy for bacteremia and endocarditis caused by *Staphylococcus aureus*. N Engl J Med 355(7):653-665, 2006.

   The authors describe the use of a newer-generation antibiotic in resistant bacterial infections.

Shannon Galvin

Meningitis

Introduction

Meningitis is an inflammation of the meninges, characterized by cellular pleocytosis in the cerebrospinal fluid (CSF). It manifests as headache, fever, meningismus (painful stiff neck), seizures, focal neurologic deficits, and disturbances of consciousness. Meningitis is an infectious disease emergency, requiring prompt evaluation and treatment. Because many bacterial and nonbacterial pathogens can cause meningitis, early broad-spectrum treatment and diagnostic testing are of great importance.

Etiology and Pathogenesis

Patients with meningitis can present acutely or chronically, the distinction helping determine likely etiologies. The most common acute presentations result from bacterial and aseptic meningitis. Aseptic meningitis may occur in patients with viral infections or in association with an adverse drug reaction. A subacute picture, in which CSF pleocytosis persists for longer than 4 weeks, is more likely to be associated with fungal or vasculitic meningitis.

Acute Bacterial Meningitis

The most common causes of bacterial meningitis in most case series are *Streptococcus pneumoniae*, which accounts for about 50% to 60% of community-acquired cases, and *Neisseria meningitides*, which accounts for 14% to 37% of reported community-acquired cases, based on numerous studies on the etiology of bacterial meningitis. Other frequent causes are *Haemophilus influenzae* (3% to 4%) and *Listeria monocytogenes* (4% to 11%). Rarely, bacterial meningitis is associated with other bacteria, including gram-negative bacilli, other streptococci, *Staphylococcus aureus*, anaerobes, and diphtheroids. Elderly or immuno-compromised patients are more likely than others to develop infection due to *Listeria* and gram-negative bacilli. Patients with prior neurosurgery are more likely to develop infection with skin organisms such as *Staphylococcus aureus* and *Staphylococcus epidermis*, and somewhat less commonly, *Pseudomonas aeruginosa* and other gram-negative bacilli.

Acute Viral Meningitis

Viral meningitis is most commonly caused by Coxsackie virus and echoviruses. West Nile virus, HIV, arboviruses, herpes simplex virus types 1 and 2, adenovirus, cytomegalovirus, varicella-zoster virus, Epstein-Barr virus, lymphocytic choriomeningitis virus, and influenza virus are other causes.

Other Causes of Acute and Chronic Meningitis

Other infectious causes of meningitis include cryptococcosis, tuberculosis, leptospirosis, syphilis, Lyme disease, other fungi, and amebic meningoencephalitis. With the exception of amebic meningoencephalitis, subacute or chronic presentations are more common with these etiologies.

Aseptic meningitis can be caused by a number of drugs and can also be a manifestation of certain rheumatologic or other systemic disorders (Box 94-1). Carcinomatous meningitis is frequently seen in hematologic malignancies and in some adenocarcinomas.

Clinical Presentation

Signs and Symptoms

Headache, fever, and neck stiffness are the hallmarks of meningitis. The headache is usually severe and frontal and can be accompanied by photophobia and vomiting. More severe and acute symptoms suggest a bacterial cause, although the ability of the patient to mount immune

Box 94-1 Etiology of Aseptic Meningitis
Viral
Echovirus, coxsackievirus, arboviruses, herpes simplex type 2, HIV, lymphocytic choriomeningitis, adenovirus, mumps, influenza, parainfluenza, cytomegalovirus, Epstein-Barr virus, varicella-zoster virus, West Nile virus, others
Drugs
Nonsteroidal anti-inflammatory drugs, trimethoprim-sulfamethoxazole, isoniazid, penicillin, ciprofloxacin, OKT3, azathioprine, immunoglobulin, carbamazepine, cytosine arabinoside, others
Systemic
Sarcoidosis, Behçet's syndrome, systemic lupus erythematosus, central nervous system vasculitis, Vogt-Koyanagi-Harada syndrome, Wegener's granulomatosis, carcinomatous meningitis, others
Other Infectious Syndromes in which Cerebrospinal Fluid Cultures Can Be Negative
Rocky Mountain spotted fever, typhus, human ehrlichiosis, endocarditis, amebiasis, others

responses must be kept in mind when assessing severity of symptoms. Immunocompromised patients may have a more subtle presentation, yet these patients are at very high risk for poor outcome. In bacterial meningitis, the temperature usually exceeds 37.7° C. Low-grade fever is more often present in viral meningitis. Fever may be entirely absent in immunocompromised patients. Neck stiffness is a specific sign and has a sensitivity of about 70%. Mental status changes occur in bacterial meningitis in 44% of cases but are found in only 3% of viral meningitis cases. Seizures occur in the range of 20% to 25% of patients with bacterial meningitis, and focal findings such as cranial nerve deficits are even somewhat more common, occurring in 25% to 30% of these patients. Unfortunately, the classic triad of fever, neck stiffness, and mental status changes occurs in less than half of patients even in bacterial meningitis. However, in one series, 95% had at least two of the four symptoms of headache, fever, neck stiffness, and mental status changes. In *Neisseria* meningitis especially, symptoms can progress from onset to death in a matter of hours, with sepsis symptoms preceding meningeal symptoms.

The clinical presentation and course of viral meningitis are often less severe than in bacterial meningitis. In viral meningitis, examination of the CSF often shows a lymphocytic pleocytosis, and the illness most commonly has a self-limited course of 5 to 7 days. Some less common causes of viral meningitis, such as West Nile virus in particular, can cause a mixed meningoencephalitic picture and present with profound changes in mentation.

A thorough history may elicit clues to more unusual causes of meningitis. The meningitis of leptospirosis often occurs in patients with a history of exposure to rodent, dog, or livestock urine, and these patients often have associated jaundice and renal dysfunction. Both syphilis and Lyme disease present with the clinical picture of aseptic meningitis during their secondary phases and are almost always associated with relevant exposures when a complete history can be obtained. Amebic disease secondary to *Naegleria fowleri* and *Acanthamoeba* species is fulminant and usually occurs in persons with exposure to fresh-water lakes.

Physical Examination

Meningeal signs, most commonly meningismus, are present in about 88% of cases of bacterial meningitis. Other classic signs are Kernig and Brudzinski signs (Fig. 94-1). The Kernig sign is pain in the back upon passive extension of one leg at the knee and the thigh. The Brudzinski sign is flexion of the legs at the thighs when the patient's neck is flexed. Jolt accentuation of headache is a very sensitive finding for meningitis. This is elicited by having the patient turn the head rapidly horizontally a number of times per second to assess for worsening of the headache.

A thorough neurologic examination should be performed, with attention given to accurate assessment of the level of consciousness, presence or absence of cranial nerve deficits, assessment for papilledema, and documentation of any focal motor or sensory defects. The skin should be carefully examined for lesions. Purpura strongly suggests meningococcal disease. Petechiae are almost as frequently seen as purpura in meningococcal meningitis and can occur in rickettsial diseases and sometimes in pneumococcal meningitis. Embolic phenomena such as splinter hemorrhages, Janeway's lesions, and Roth's spots suggest endocarditis, both a cause and a mimic of meningitis. A note should be made of CSF shunts, prior neurosurgical procedures, or head trauma because all predispose to meningitis.

Patients can also present with evidence of potentially contiguous infections associated with bacterial meningitis, such as sinusitis, otitis media, and mastoiditis, and with complications of meningitis, such as cavernous sinus thrombosis and thrombophlebitis of the cranial sinuses (Fig. 94-2).

Differential Diagnosis

The differential diagnosis for patients presenting with fever, headache, and altered mental status includes encephalitis, focal brain lesion, and systemic infections, including endocarditis and rickettsial infections. Encephalitis is classically distinguished from meningitis by the absence of meningeal symptoms and the presence of diffuse neurologic deficits such as altered mentation, confusion, and seizures. Brain lesions (infectious or malignant) are more likely to present with focal neurologic complaints and can

Figure 94-1 Kernig's Sign and Brudzinski's Neck Sign.

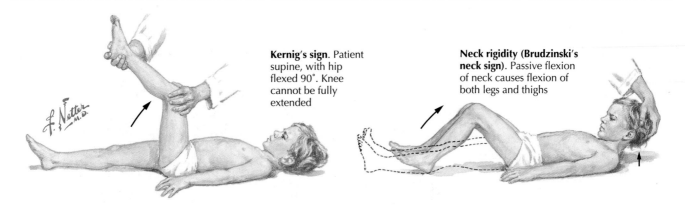

Kernig's sign. Patient supine, with hip flexed 90°. Knee cannot be fully extended

Neck rigidity (Brudzinski's neck sign). Passive flexion of neck causes flexion of both legs and thighs

Figure 94-2 Bacterial Meningitis.

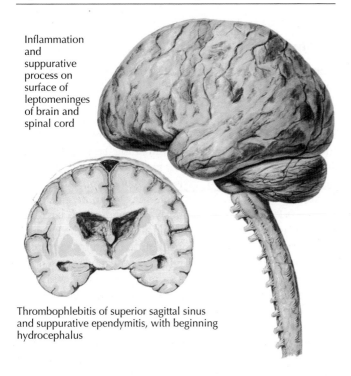

Inflammation and suppurative process on surface of leptomeninges of brain and spinal cord

Thrombophlebitis of superior sagittal sinus and suppurative ependymitis, with beginning hydrocephalus

be detected by computed tomography (CT) imaging. Blood culture to detect systemic bacteremia and consideration of rickettsial diseases is always warranted. In tropical countries, cerebral malaria must also be excluded.

Diagnostic Approach

The diagnosis of meningitis is made by lumbar puncture (Figs. 94-3 and 94-4). It is important to document the opening pressure and appearance of the CSF. CSF should be sent for cell count and differential, glucose, protein, Gram stain, and culture in all cases (Table 94-1). The addition of a Venereal Diseases Research Laboratory (VDRL) and a cryptococcal antigen is helpful when an

immunocompromised state is possible or in a subacute presentation. Other important tests include viral polymerase chain reaction (PCR) for herpes family viruses and enteroviruses; examination for acid-fast organisms and tuberculosis PCR; and CSF cell cytology. Cytology and mycobacterial culture usually require 10 mL of fluid. Table 94-1 shows typical results for the various type of meningitis using CSF results immediately available.

Some confusion surrounds the appropriate use of imaging studies and the timing of antibiotics. Meningitis, and suspected meningitis, should be considered an infectious emergency. If the lumbar puncture is to be delayed at all, empiric antibiotics should be started immediately. CSF cultures are often sterile for bacterial pathogens if taken after antibiotics have been given. CSF cell count and makeup are not affected to any great degree if taken within the first 24 hours of treatment. The risk for causing herniation in a patient by performing a lumbar puncture is no more than 6% and probably only happens when the intracranial pressure is not evenly distributed because of mass effect. The current recommendation is to obtain a CT scan before doing lumbar puncture on all comatose patients, those with focal deficits or papilledema, those with prior central nervous system (CNS) disease or new-onset seizures, and HIV-positive patients.

Culture is the gold standard for making a diagnosis of bacterial meningitis. Latex agglutination tests for bacterial pathogens can be considered; however, because the sensitivity of these tests is only about 70%, a negative test does not rule out a bacterial cause. False-positive agglutination tests have also been reported.

CSF PCR for enteroviruses such as Coxsackie virus and echoviruses and the herpes viruses (herpes simplex virus, varicella-zoster virus, cytomegalovirus) are available and are useful in cases of suspected viral meningitis. CSF PCR and serologic studies for West Nile virus and arboviruses, such as Venezuelan equine encephalitis and Eastern equine encephalitis, should be considered during the summer and fall or given the possibility of mosquito exposure.

Figure 94-3 Bacterial Meningitis.

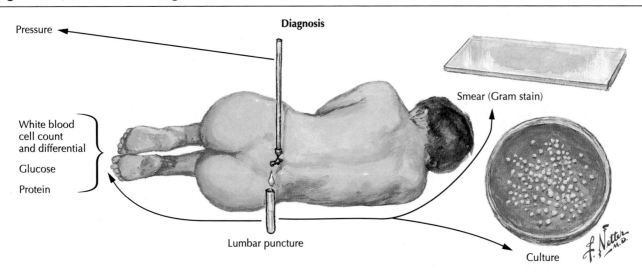

Figure 94-4 Diagnostic Algorithm.
CT, computed tomography; PCR, polymerase chain reaction; LP, lumbar puncture; VDRL, Venereal Diseases Research Laboratory. *Modified from Tunkel AR, Hartman BJ, Kaplan SL, et al: Practice guidelines for the management of bacterial meningitis. Clin Infect Dis 39(9):1267-1284, 2004.*

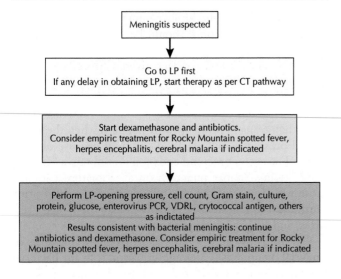

Neurosyphilis is associated with a mild CSF pleocytosis, and the CSF VDRL test result is positive in only 60% of cases. The diagnosis of leptospirosis is made by serology. CSF and serum serologies can be ordered for suspected Lyme disease with CNS involvement, but are best ordered in the setting of an appropriate clinical picture and the results must be interpreted with care as both false-positive and false-negative are common. The diagnosis of amebic disease requires CSF examination for motile amebas.

Management and Therapy

Optimum Treatment

Treatment is directed toward covering likely pathogens until bacterial meningitis has been ruled out (Tables 94-2 and 94-3). The current recommendation is to use a third-generation cephalosporin such as ceftriaxone, 2 g given intravenously every 12 hours, plus vancomycin, 1 g given intravenously twice a day (maintaining trough levels of 15-20 µg/mL) plus dexamethasone. Dexamethasone has been shown to reduce adverse outcomes in adults with bacterial meningitis. Dexamethasone should be given in a dose of 0.15 mg/kg intravenously every 6 hours if bacterial meningitis is suspected; it should be given before or concomitant with first dose of antibiotics. It can be continued for 4 days if bacterial meningitis is confirmed.

Listeria monocytogenes is not optimally treated with ceftriaxone. At-risk patients such as those older than 50 years or with immune compromise and any ill patient with meningitis not responding to therapy should receive ampicillin, 2 g intravenously every 4 hours, in addition to empiric therapy while awaiting cultures. Doxycycline, 100 mg twice daily, should be added to the treatment regimen in any patient with meningitis and an illness consistent with Rocky Mountain spotted fever in an endemic area. Often empiric treatment with intravenous acyclovir to cover for herpes encephalitis is begun because the presentation may be similar to meningitis. Treatment with an agent active against *Pseudomonas* species such as ceftazidime or cefepime in place of ceftriaxone, along with vancomycin, can be given as empiric therapy for neurosurgical or head trauma patients. All empiric treatment should be modified as appropriate cultures and antibiotic sensitivities become available. Tuberculous meningitis is treated with four drugs and the consideration of adding steroids. Cryptococcal meningitis requires amphotericin B therapy, usually along with 5-fluorocytosine (5FC).

The duration of therapy for bacterial meningitis depends on the isolated pathogen as well the patient's response. At a minimum, intravenous antibiotics should be administered for at least 7 days and extended to 14 days for pneumococcus, less common bacteria such as gram-negative rods, and *S. aureus* and to at least 21 days for *Listeria* species. In low resource settings, single-dose ceftriaxone has been shown to be effective in outbreaks of meningococcal disease.

Prevention

Vaccination against three organisms that cause meningitis has been shown to be an effective means toward preventing meningitis. Vaccination against *H. influenzae* type B should be part of the routine immunization schedule for children. Vaccination with pneumococcal polysaccharide vaccine protects against invasive disease and is helpful in reducing cases of pneumococcal meningitis in at-risk populations. It

Table 94-1 Typical Cerebrospinal Fluid Findings in Meningitis

	Normal	Bacterial	Viral	Fungal	Tuberculosis	Other
WBC count	0-5/mm^3	100-10,000/mm^3	5-3000/mm^3	5-500/mm^3	5-500/mm^3	—
WBC makeup	—	>50% polymorphonuclear leukocytes	>50% lymphocytes	>50% lymphocytes	>50% lymphocytes	Carcinomatous can have monoclonal population and cellular atypia
Protein	50-80 mg/dL	>200 mg/dL	Normal or slightly high	Normal or slightly high	Elevated	Protein can be elevated in any illness that disrupts blood-brain barrier
Glucose	70-80 mg/dL or >60% of serum glucose	<40 mg/dL or <60% of serum glucose	Normal	Normal	<40 mg/dL may be normal in 20% of cases	Can be low in carcinomatous meningitis
Gram stain	Negative	60% positive	Negative	India ink positive 50% for *Cryptococcus* species	Acid-fast stain positive in 25%-37%	—
Pressure	75-200 mm Hg	Elevated	Normal	Elevated	Normal or elevated	—

Note: Exceptions to these values can occur, and clinical findings should be taken into account when making a diagnosis.

Table 94-2 Recommendations for Specific Antimicrobial Therapy in Bacterial Meningitis Based on Isolated Pathogen and Susceptibility

Microorganism, Susceptibility	Standard Therapy	Alternative Therapies
Streptococcus pneumoniae		
Penicillin MIC		
<0.1 µg/mL	Penicillin G or ampicillin	Third-generation cephalosporin,[a] chloramphenicol
0.1-1.0 µg/mL[b]	Third-generation cephalosporin[a]	Cefepime (B-II), meropenem (B-II)
≥2.0 µg/mL	Vancomycin plus a third-generation cephalosporin[a,c]	Fluoroquinolone[d] (B-II)
Cefotaxime or ceftriaxone MIC ≥1.0 µg/mL	Vancomycin plus a third-generation cephalosporin[a,c]	Fluoroquinolone[d] (B-II)
Neisseria meningitidis		
Penicillin MIC		
<0.1 µg/mL	Penicillin G or ampicillin	Third-generation cephalosporin,[a] chloramphenicol
0.1-1.0 µg/mL	Third-generation cephalosporin[a]	Chloramphenicol, fluoroquinolone, meropenem
Listeria monocytogenes	Ampicillin or penicillin G[e]	Trimethoprim-sulfamethoxazole, meropenem (B-III)
Streptococcus agalactiae	Ampicillin or penicillin G[e]	Third-generation cephalosporin[a] (B-III)
Escherichia coli and Other Enterobacteriaceae[g]	Third-generation cephalosporin (A-II)	Aztreonam, fluoroquinolone, meropenem, trimethoprim-sulfamethoxazole, ampicillin
Pseudomonas aeruginosa[g]	Cefepime[e] or ceftazidime[e] (A-II)	Aztreonam,[e] ciprofloxacin,[e] meropenem[e]

continued

Table 94-2 Recommendations for Specific Antimicrobial Therapy in Bacterial Meningitis Based on Isolated Pathogen and Susceptibility—cont'd

Microorganism, Susceptibility	Standard Therapy	Alternative Therapies
Haemophilus influenzae		
β-Lactamase negative	Ampicillin	Third-generation cephalosporin,[a] cefepime, chloramphenicol, fluoroquinolone
β-Lactamase positive	Third-generation cephalosporin (A-I)	Cefepime (A-I), chloramphenicol, fluoroquinolone
Staphylococcus aureus		
Methicillin susceptible	Nafcillin or oxacillin	Vancomycin, meropenem (B-III)
Methicillin resistant	Vancomycin[f]	Trimethoprim-sulfamethoxazole, linezolid (B-III)
Staphylococcus epidermidis	Vancomycin[f]	Linezolid (B-III)
Enterococcus Species		
Ampicillin susceptible	Ampicillin plus gentamicin	
Ampicillin resistant	Vancomycin plus gentamicin	
Ampicillin and vancomycin resistant	Linezolid (B-III)	

Note: All recommendations are A-III, unless otherwise indicated.
[a] Ceftriaxone or cefotaxime.
[b] Ceftriaxone- or cefotaxime-susceptible isolates.
[c] Consider addition of rifampin if the MIC of ceftriaxone is >2 µg/mL.
[d] Gatifloxacin or moxifloxacin.
[e] Addition of an aminoglycoside should be considered.
[f] Consider addition of rifampin.
[g] Choice of a specific antimicrobial agent must be guided by in vitro susceptibility test results.
From Tunkel AR, Hartman BJ, Kaplan SL, et al: Practice guidelines for the management of bacterial meningitis. Clin Infect Dis 39(9):1267-1284, 2004.

Table 94-3 Recommended Dosages of Antimicrobial Therapy in Patients with Bacterial Meningitis (A-III)

Total Daily Dose (Dosing Interval in Hours)

Antimicrobial Agent	Neonates, Age in Days 0-7[a]	8-28[a]	Infants and Children	Adults
Amikacin[b]	15-20 mg/kg (12)	30 mg/kg (8)	20-30 mg/kg (8)	15 mg/kg (8)
Ampicillin	150 mg/kg (8)	200 mg/kg (6-8)	300 mg/kg (6)	12 g (4)
Aztreonam	—	—	—	6-8 g (6-8)
Cefepime	—	—	150 mg/kg (8)	6 g (8)
Cefotaxime	100-150 mg/kg (8-12)	150-200 mg/kg (6-8)	225-300 mg/kg (6-8)	8-12 g (4-6)
Ceftazidime	100-150 mg/kg (8-12)	150 mg/kg (8)	150 mg/kg (8)	6 g (8)
Ceftriaxone	—	—	80-100 mg/kg (12-24)	4 g (12-24)
Chloramphenicol	25 mg/kg (24)	50 mg/kg (12-24)	75-100 mg/kg (6)	4-6 g (6)[c]
Ciprofloxacin	—	—	—	800-1200 mg (8-12)
Gatifloxacin	—	—	—	400 mg (24)[d]
Gentamicin[b]	5 mg/kg (12)	7.5 mg/kg (8)	7.5 mg/kg (8)	5 mg/kg (8)
Meropenem	—	—	120 mg/kg (8)	6 g (8)
Moxifloxacin	—	—	—	400 mg (24)[d]
Nafcillin	75 mg/kg (8-12)	100-150 mg/kg (6-8)	200 mg/kg (6)	9-12 g (4)
Oxacillin	75 mg/kg (8-12)	150-200 mg/kg (6-8)	200 mg/kg (6)	9-12 g (4)
Penicillin G	0.15 mU/kg (8-12)	0.2 mU/kg (6-8)	0.3 mU/kg (4-6)	24 mU (4)
Rifampin	—	10-20 mg/kg (12)	10-20 mg/kg (12-24)[e]	600 mg (24)
Tobramycin[b]	5 mg/kg (12)	7.5 mg/kg (8)	7.5 mg/kg (8)	5 mg/kg (8)
TMP-SMZ[f]	—	—	10-20 mg/kg (6-12)	10-20 mg/kg (6-12)
Vancomycin[g]	20-30 mg/kg (8-12)	30-45 mg/kg (6-8)	60 mg/kg (6)	30-45 mg/kg (8-12)

[a] Small doses and longer intervals of administration may be advisable for very-low-birth-weight neonates (<2000 g).
[b] Need to monitor peak and through serum concentrations.
[c] Higher dose recommended for patients with pneumococcal meningitis.
[d] No data on optimal dosage needed in patients with bacterial meningitis.
[e] Maximun daily dose of 600 mg.
[f] Dosage based on trimethoprim component.
[g] Maintain serum trough concentrations of 15-20 µg/mL.
TMP-SMZ, trimethoprim-sulfamethoxazole.
From Tunkel AR, Hartman BJ, Kaplan SL, et al: Practice guidelines for the management of bacterial meningitis. Clin Infect Dis 39(9):1267-1284, 2004.

should be given to all adults older than 65 years, persons with chronic diseases, and those with asplenia. The heptavalent pneumococcal polysaccharide protein conjugate vaccine is given to children as part of the routine childhood immunization schedule.

A polysaccharide vaccine against *Neisseria meningitidis* serogroup A, C, Y, and W-135 is available and is currently recommended for use in 11 to 12 year olds, in disease outbreaks, and in persons with complement deficiencies and functional asplenia. This vaccine should also be offered to matriculating college freshmen, military recruits, and travelers to endemic areas of sub-Saharan Africa.

Prophylaxis

Close contacts of persons with meningococcal meningitis should receive one dose of ciprofloxacin, 500 mg orally, or four doses of rifampin, 600 mg orally every 12 hours, to eradicate colonization of the pharynx. *Close contacts* are those who live in the same household or have other significant or prolonged contact.

Avoiding Treatment Errors

The most common and devastating treatment error is delay in initiating appropriate antibiotics. If meningitis is suspected, treatment and evaluation must begin immediately. Initial broad coverage is wise and can then be narrowed based on diagnostic results. Early consideration of an immunocompromised state that would necessitate treatment for *Listeria* or fungal etiologies is crucial. Patients with bacterial meningitis need close and frequent neurologic assessment, especially of cranial nerves; any changes should prompt evaluation for herniation, cavernous sinus thrombosis, or other catastrophic sequelae.

Future Directions

The prevalence of pneumococcal meningitis may begin to change now that children are being routinely vaccinated using the conjugate vaccine. The use of magnetic resonance imaging in diagnosing meningitis is under further study but will probably not supplant the need for lumbar puncture. The usefulness of such tests as C-reactive protein and procalcitonin in differentiating between bacterial and viral meningitis is being explored.

Additional Resources

Gilbert DN, Moellering RC Jr, Eliopolous GM, Sande MA: The Sanford Guide to Antimicrobial Therapy, 36th ed. Sperryville, VA, Antimicrobial Therapy, 2006.

Splendiani A, Puglielli E, De Amicis R, et al: Contrast-enhanced FLAIR in the early diagnosis of infectious meningitis. Neuroradiology 47(8):591-598, 2005.

Thwaites GE, Nguyen DB, Nguyen HD, et al: Dexamethasone for the treatment of tuberculous meningitis in adolescents and adults. N Engl J Med 351(17):1741-1751, 2004.

Tyler KL, Pape J, Goody RJ, et al: CSF findings in 250 patients with serologically confirmed West Nile virus meningitis and encephalitis. Neurology 14;66(3):361-365, 2006.

EVIDENCE

1. Archer BD: Computed tomography before lumbar puncture in acute meningitis: A review of the risks and benefits. CMAJ 148(6):961-965, 1993.
   The author provides a general discussion of the timing of CT when planning a lumbar puncture.
2. Attia J, Hatala R, Cook DJ, Wong JG: The rational clinical examination. Does this adult patient have acute meningitis? JAMA 282(2):175-181, 1999.
   The authors present a very useful discussion of findings that suggest the diagnosis of meningitis.
3. de Gans J, van de Beek D: Dexamethasone in adults with bacterial meningitis. N Engl J Med 347(20):1549-1556, 2002.
   This trial has led to the use of dexamethasone along with antibiotics in adults with suspected bacterial meningitis.
4. Durand ML, Calderwood SB, Weber DJ, et al: Acute bacterial meningitis in adults. A review of 493 episodes. N Engl J Med 328(1):21-28, 1993.
   This article describes the etiologies, presentations, and outcomes of a large case series of meningitis patients.
5. Nathan N, Borel T, Djibo A, et al: Ceftriaxone is effective as long-acting chloramphenicol in short-course treatment of meningococcal meningitis during epidemics: A randomised non-inferiority study. Lancet 366(9482):308-313, 2005.
   A single dose of ceftriaxone had efficacy in epidemics of meningococcal disease.
6. Tunkel AR, Hartman BJ, Kaplan SL, et al: Practice guidelines for the management of bacterial meningitis. Clin Infect Dis 39(9):1267-1284, 2004.
   The authors provide complete guidelines for the treatment of bacterial meningitis.
7. van de Beek D, de Gans J, Spanjaard L, et al: Clinical features and prognostic factors in adults with bacterial meningitis. N Engl J Med 351(18):1849-1859, 2004.
   This excellent paper describes the clinical presentation and outcomes in patients with bacterial meningitis.

Septic Arthritis

Introduction

Septic arthritis is a bacterial infection of the synovial space that can occur in both native and prosthetic joints. It usually presents with monoarticular involvement but can be polyarticular. Septic arthritis deserves prompt attention to prevent morbidity and mortality. Although the focus of this chapter is septic arthritis, viruses and other systemic infections can also cause arthritis, usually of the polyarticular type and occurring as part of a syndromic presentation. These illnesses are discussed in relation to the differential diagnosis of suspected septic arthritis.

Etiology

Risk factors for septic arthritis include specific characteristics of a joint that increase its susceptibility to infection when seeded by bacteria and specific host factors that increase the risk for infection. Preexisting joint disease is a major risk factor. Rheumatoid arthritis (RA) and prosthetic joints pose the highest risks, but diseases like osteoarthritis also carry elevated risk. Host factors that increase risk include diabetes mellitus, chronic renal failure, age greater than 80 years, and immunocompromised states.

The leading cause of all cases of septic arthritis is *Staphylococcus aureus*—about 40% to 60% of cases. *S. aureus* is the main cause in RA patients and in those with polyarticular septic arthritis. Streptococci are the second in frequency at 14% to 18%, including group A, as well as groups B, C, and G, and less commonly *Streptococcus pneumoniae*. Gram-negative organisms account for about 7% to 12% of cases. *Haemophilus influenzae* was a leading cause in the past, especially in children, but the incidence has declined dramatically in countries with the *H. influenzae* vaccine. *Neisseria gonorrhoeae* can account for about 5% of cases. Other important pathogens include *Kingella* and *Brucella* species and tuberculosis. Fungal joint infections occasionally occur and include coccidiomycosis, blastomycosis, and those secondary to other soil fungi.

Certain conditions lead to an elevated risk for particular pathogens. Diabetic and elderly patients are more likely to have arthritis due to gram-negative organisms. Immunocompromised hosts can develop septic arthritis due to mycobacteria and fungi and other unusual organisms like *Listeria* species.

Certain exposures also confer risk for particular pathogens. *N. gonorrhoeae* is the most likely etiology of septic arthritis in sexually active young adults in the United States. Intravenous drug users and persons with indwelling catheters can have septic arthritis from hematogenous spread of organisms such as *S. aureus*. Exposure to soil organisms from trauma can lead to fungal arthritis.

Prosthetic joint infections are caused by, in decreasing order of frequency, *Staphylococcus epidermidis* and other coagulase-negative staphylococci, *S. aureus*, streptococci, gram-negative rods, enterococci, and anaerobes. In about 10% of cases of prosthetic joint infections, multiple organisms are isolated.

Clinical Presentation

Joint pain is the most common presenting symptom. In the classic scenario, patients present with the recent onset of pain and associated swelling in one joint. Less than half of all patients have fever. The knee is the most commonly affected joint, followed by the hip. Other joints may be involved, and a polyarticular presentation is not unusual, especially in bacteremic patients and those with RA.

RA patients may experience a more insidious onset, and a high index of suspicion is needed to distinguish septic arthritis from a RA flare. New pain in a previously unaffected joint, pain in one joint out of proportion to others, and the new onset of joint disease in two or more joints are clues to septic arthritis in these patients. A chronic presentation with less acute, more insidious symptoms is also more common in septic arthritis caused by tuberculous or fungal infection.

The physical exam usually demonstrates a warm, erythematous joint with effusion and a limited range of motion. The examination of all other joints is key to excluding polyarticular involvement. The skin should be examined for rashes; disseminated gonorrhea is associated with pustular or papular lesions that can be few and easy to miss. The examiner should carefully observe for conjunctivitis, uveitis, and enthesopathies that are characteristic of a viral or reactive arthritis syndrome. Cardiac examination and search for embolic phenomena should be done carefully to eliminate endocarditis as a cause of the septic arthritis.

Many patients have a leukocytosis. C-reactive protein (CRP) is almost always elevated, and the erythrocyte sedimentation rate (ESR) is usually but not invariably high. Plain films usually do not show any changes in native joints, but they may show prosthesis loosening in prosthetic joints. Magnetic resonance imaging (MRI) is not diagnostic but can suggest the diagnosis when synovial enhancement is seen. Joint effusions are seen by MRI in about 70% of cases.

Prosthetic infection presentations can be classified as early, occurring less than 3 months from surgery, or late. Prosthetic joint infections that occur early typically present with more inflammation and are more likely to be secondary to highly virulent pathogens like *S. aureus*. Later presentations of prosthetic joint infections may have a more insidious onset of pain and swelling or simply instability of the joint and be due to less virulent organisms. A draining sinus tract may be the first presentation.

Differential Diagnosis

The differential diagnosis of acute arthritis includes crystal-induced arthritis such as gout and pseudogout, lupus erythematosus, RA, seronegative arthritis syndromes such as psoriatic arthritis, Reiter's syndrome, and other reactive arthritis such as that occurring in poststreptococcal infection. Other noninfectious causes of arthritis include sarcoidosis, but this is typically more insidious and polyarticular. Other infectious causes that predominantly cause polyarticular disease but should be considered are viral infections, Lyme disease, and mycoplasmal infection. Viral causes of arthritis include hepatitis A, hepatitis B, hepatitis C, parvovirus, and mumps. Globally, the mosquito-borne viruses that cause febrile arthritis syndromes are important and include the alphaviruses-Ross River, chikungunya, o'nyong-nyong, and Sindbis viruses. Common viruses that uncommonly cause arthritis are adenovirus, Coxsackie virus, echovirus, and Epstein-Barr virus. Acute HIV infection can also present with arthritis.

Diagnostic Approach

The diagnosis of septic arthritis is made from synovial fluid analysis (Fig. 95-1). Synovial fluid should be sent for cell

Figure 95-1 Septic Joint Aspiration.

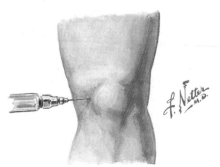

Sample of joint fluid aspirated for culture

count, Gram stain and culture, and crystal examination. Usually, synovial white blood cells exceed 50,000 cells/mm³; often, frank pus is aspirated. Crystal examination is important to exclude gout or pseudogout, which can present identically to septic arthritis. The Gram stain is critical to guiding initial antibiotic therapy.

Blood cultures are frequently positive in septic arthritis (about 50% of all patients) and should always be obtained. Other routine blood work has limited utility for diagnosing or excluding septic arthritis. Leukocytosis is found in only about 40% of cases. An elevated ESR is usually found but is nonspecific, and the sedimentation rate can occasionally be normal. Reported sensitivities for elevation of CRP routinely seem to be about 100%; however, the test has poor specificity because it can also be elevated in other types of inflammatory arthritis. One study found that serum procalcitonin levels higher than 0.5 ng/mL had a 55% sensitivity but a 94% specificity for septic arthritis compared with crystal-induced arthritis or RA, but current clinical application of this test remains limited. Arthrocentesis is mandatory to diagnose and guide treatment in suspected cases of septic arthritis.

Certain etiologies require specific diagnostic considerations. Gonococcal arthritis can be culture negative from the joint fluid, but urethral, cervical, rectal, and pharyngeal swabs cultured on Thayer-Martin media are often positive and yield the diagnosis. Brucellosis warrants consideration in persons with sacroiliitis and a history of occupational animal exposure; the diagnosis often requires holding cultures for up to 35 days and sending for brucella serologies. Fungal arthritis should be considered in cases of soil exposure secondary to penetrating trauma and in immunocompromised hosts. The diagnosis should also be considered in areas endemic for coccidiomycosis and blastomycosis. Mycobacterial arthritis can be caused by tuberculosis and by atypical mycobacteria, including *Mycobacterium marinum*. In *M. marinum* infection, the patient often gives a history of fish or water contact. Likewise, fungal or mycobacterial arthritis should be considered in any patient not responding to antibiotics. Joint fluid should be sent for fungal and mycobacterial culture in these cases.

Serologies for hepatitis A, B, and C, parvovirus serologies, and serum parvovirus DNA polymerase chain reaction can be ordered in patients with polyarticular arthritis. These patients should also have an evaluation for rheumatologic diseases beginning with rheumatoid factor and antinuclear antibodies and other subsequent evaluations as appropriate. Lyme disease is a complex diagnosis that requires a positive Western blot in the appropriate clinical setting. Mycoplasma can often be diagnosed by serology.

Prosthetic joint infections are strictly diagnosed using one of the following criteria: growth of a pathogen from synovial fluid, growth of a low-virulence organism from two synovial fluid or surgical specimens, purulent synovial fluid, inflammation on histopathologic examination of periprosthetic tissue, or presence of a sinus tract. However, many joint infections exist that do not meet these criteria, and a symptomatic patient may warrant treatment.

Management

Optimum Treatment

Empiric antibiotic therapy is guided by classifying the patient into three different groups: sexually active adults, non–sexually active adults, and persons with prosthetic joints.

Sexually active adults should have initial therapy directed at gonorrhea and gram-positive organisms with ceftriaxone; vancomycin should be added for better gram-positive coverage if the Gram stain reveals gram-positive cocci. Persons at low risk for gonorrhea should start vancomycin and either a third-generation cephalosporin or a quinolone to cover staphylococci and streptococci species, as well as gram-negative organisms. Persons with prosthetic joints should have therapy directed also at staphylococcal and streptococcal species with vancomycin; however, in prosthetic infections in particular, therapy should ideally be started after cultures are obtained. Once culture results are available, therapy should be modified as needed based on speciation and sensitivity data.

Parenteral antibiotic therapy that is tailored to the specific organism should continue for at least 2 and possibly 4 weeks.

If gonococcal arthritis is diagnosed, ceftriaxone may be switched to oral quinolones to complete 7 days of treatment. As with any sexually transmitted disease, testing for HIV and syphilis and treatment for chlamydia should also be provided.

Antibiotic treatment of prosthetic joints may include the addition of rifampin to vancomycin for staphylococcal infections to improve penetration into biofilms. Any patient receiving rifampin needs monitoring of liver function tests and a complete blood count periodically, as well as attention to the multidrug interactions of rifampin.

In native joints, repeated arthrocentesis to drain the joint effusion is often advisable, especially in purulent infections. In joints such as the hip and sometimes the shoulder, this usually requires arthroscopic or open procedures. The role of routine surgery for native joints is debated. There has been no randomized trial examining this question. Although some series have pointed to increased morbidity in joints treated surgically, this may correlate only with more aggressive disease.

Conversely, septic arthritis in a prosthetic joint requires surgical removal of the prosthesis for cure. The prosthesis is removed, and parenteral antibiotics are administered for about 6 weeks guided by culture. Reimplantation can be scheduled after cure of the infection is confirmed. A single-stage procedure has been advocated by some authors in settings where the pathogen is of low virulence, such as coagulase-negative staphylococci; the prosthesis is well seated; and the surrounding tissue is intact. This one-stage strategy may work better for hip prostheses than knee joints. The known difficulties of eradicating infection in the presence of foreign materials and the subsequent higher risk for treatment failure and its consequences suggest that a two-stage removal would usually be optimal; however, this must be balanced with other surgical considerations, such as the technical feasibility of and the patient's ability to tolerate repeated surgeries.

The treatment of other infectious causes of arthritis obviously depends on the particular diagnosis. Lyme arthritis is treated with doxycycline, 100 mg by mouth twice daily for 30 days. Treatment of fungal or mycobacterial arthritis is directed at the specific pathogen. Symptomatic treatment is given for reactive or viral arthritis.

Avoiding Treatment Errors

Making the correct diagnosis is the first step in avoiding treatment errors. This means maintaining a high index of suspicion for septic arthritis and obtaining joint fluid for analysis and culture. Treatment should be directed at the most common pathogens but must be tailored to the culture results. Optimal antibiotic dosing must be given so that adequate synovial and bone drug levels are achieved; this usually requires at least 2 weeks of parenteral therapy. The patient's clinical and microbiologic response should always guide the duration of therapy because longer courses may be required. If no organism has been identified and the patient is not responding, therapy may need to be broadened or an alternative diagnosis reconsidered. Prosthetic joint infections usually require surgical removal of the prosthesis because any other strategy results in lower cure rates. Although early and appropriate use of antibiotics can be life saving, clinicians must always be familiar with the patient's allergy history and the known side effects of antibiotics and monitor appropriately to avoid adverse events.

Future Directions

Further studies may refine the use of serologic and radiographic tests that distinguish septic from other causes of arthritis; however, joint fluid culture will probably not be abandoned in the near future. Evolving patterns of resistance should be monitored to guide initial treatment, especially in gram-positive organisms and gonococci.

Additional Resources

Goldenberg DL: Septic arthritis. Lancet 351(9097):197-202, 1998.
The author presents an excellent review of the topic.
Zimmerli W, Trampuz A, Ochsner PE: Prosthetic joint infections. N Engl J Med 351(16):1645-1654, 2004.
The authors provide a complete discussion of the medical and surgical management of prosthetic joint infections.

EVIDENCE

1. Eder L, Zisman D, Rozenbaum M, Rosner I: Clinical features and aetiology of septic arthritis in northern Israel. Rheumatology (Oxford) 44(12):1559-1563, 2005.
The authors present a case series that describes the presentation and etiology.
2. Gupta MN, Sturrock RD, Field M: A prospective 2-year study of 75 patients with adult-onset septic arthritis. Rheumatology (Oxford) 40(1):24-30, 2001.
The authors report on a prospective study of the presentation, etiology, and outcome in patients with septic arthritis.
3. Karchevsky M, Schweitzer ME, Morrison WB, Parellada JA: MRI findings of septic arthritis and associated osteomyelitis in adults. AJR Am J Roentgenol 182(1):119-122, 2004.
This article discusses the utility of MRI in septic arthritis.
4. Li SF, Henderson J, Dickman E, Darzynkiewicz R: Laboratory tests in adults with monoarticular arthritis: Can they rule out a septic joint? Acad Emerg Med 11(3):276-280, 2004.
This useful article examines which tests can be used to exclude or confirm septic arthritis from other causes of arthritis.
5. Martinot M, Sordet C, Soubrier M, et al: Diagnostic value of serum and synovial procalcitonin in acute arthritis: A prospective study of 42 patients. Clin Exp Rheumatol 23(3):303-310, 2005.
The authors describe a new test in the evaluation of acute arthritis.
6. Weston VC, Jones AC, Bradbury N, et al: Clinical features and outcome of septic arthritis in a single UK Health District, 1982-1991. Ann Rheum Dis 58(4):214-219, 1999.
This case series describes the management and outcome of septic arthritis.

Osteomyelitis

Introduction

Bone infection is associated with significant morbidity and is often not effectively treated solely with antibiotics. Infected bone regenerates slowly and can represent an ischemic compartment that is poorly penetrated by antibiotics or the immune system. The incidence of osteomyelitis is likely to increase as a result of changing health care practices, an aging population, and evolving pathogens. Trends such as the increasing use of prosthetic joint implantation and an increased use of central venous catheters (with the attendant risk for bacteremia) may translate to higher rates of osteomyelitis. There is evidence that the development of community-acquired methicillin-resistant *Staphylococcus aureus* (MRSA) as a pathogen may increase the rates of bone and joint infections.

Osteomyelitis can be secondary to hematogenous seeding, a contiguous focus of infection, open fractures, or vascular insufficiency of an extremity. Chronic osteomyelitis is associated with retained, avascular bone and is ineffectively treated with antibiotic therapy alone. The spectrum of bone infections is so vast that no rule of thumb applies to treatment. Medical therapy alone is sometimes sufficient, but surgical therapy is often necessary, and the treatment team may involve the primary care physician, orthopedic surgeon, plastic surgeon, infectious diseases specialist, and vascular surgeon.

Etiology and Pathogenesis

The disease state of osteomyelitis is due to both an infecting microorganism and an associated host inflammatory response. An infecting organism can reach the bone through direct inoculation (such as a penetrating injury), a hematogenous route, or contiguous spread from infection in adjacent tissue. In the case of acute hematogenous osteomyelitis of the long bones, the initial infection is endosteal, with subsequent extension to cortical bone and the periosteum, whereas other forms of osteomyelitis may first affect cortical bone. As acute osteomyelitis progresses to chronic osteomyelitis (generally over months to years), there is retained dead bone and frequently extension through cortical bone with sinus tracts draining to the skin (Fig. 96-1).

The Waldvogel system is most commonly used to classify osteomyelitis and describes three categories based on the underlying etiology of bone infection. The first is hematogenous osteomyelitis, a type that occurs in both adults and children. In adults, the vertebrae are more often involved; in contrast, the long bones are more often involved in children. The hematogenous source of infection may be due to overt septicemia but often is secondary to subclinical bacteremia related to a remote site of infection (Fig. 96-2). A second category is osteomyelitis secondary to a contiguous focus of infection. This includes osteomyelitis secondary to trauma, implanted hardware (prosthetic joints, external or internal fixation), adjacent soft tissue infection, dental infection, and pressure ulcers (Fig. 96-3). The last category is osteomyelitis secondary to vascular insufficiency, which is most often associated with soft tissue infection. This is exacerbated by poor tissue perfusion due to large or small vessel disease. Most patients in this category have diabetes mellitus, and the bones of the feet (especially the phalanges and metatarsals) are most often involved.

The Cierny-Mader system is also used to classify osteomyelitis and is more anatomic in description; it is composed of four stages. Stage 1 is medullary osteomyelitis; examples include acute hematogenous endosteal infections or infections associated with intramedullary rods. Stage 2 is superficial osteomyelitis, such as contiguous infection involving the cortical surface of bone. Stage 3 is full-thickness involvement of the bone that can be debrided without compromising bone. Stage 4 is diffuse osteomy-

Figure 96-1 Chronic Osteomyelitis Involving the Metaphysis of the Tibia.

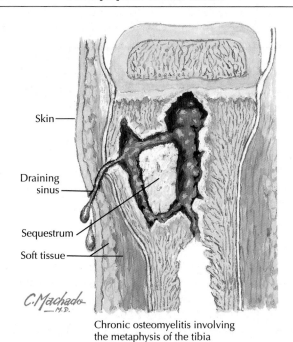

Skin
Draining sinus
Sequestrum
Soft tissue

Chronic osteomyelitis involving the metaphysis of the tibia

Figure 96-2 Hematogenous Osteomyelitis.

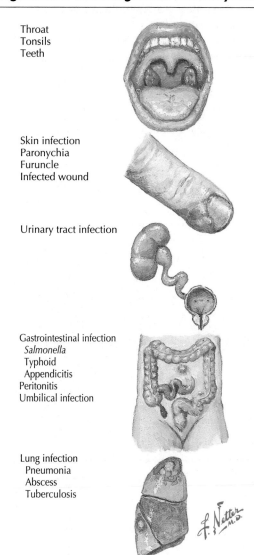

Throat
Tonsils
Teeth

Skin infection
Paronychia
Furuncle
Infected wound

Urinary tract infection

Gastrointestinal infection
Salmonella
Typhoid
Appendicitis
Peritonitis
Umbilical infection

Lung infection
Pneumonia
Abscess
Tuberculosis

Hematogenous osteomyelitis may be secondary to subclinical bacteremia associated with numerous infections, including tonsillitis, cellulitis, pyelonephritis, intra-abdominal infections, and pneumonia

elitis that either will result in bony instability after debridement or has through-and-through involvement that requires transection of a bone segment.

The pathogens that most often cause osteomyelitis are aerobic gram-positive cocci and various gram-negative bacteria. *S. aureus* is the most common pathogen and is seen in all types of osteomyelitis. Enterobacteriaceae and *Pseudomonas* species are commonly encountered gram-negative pathogens. Anaerobic bacteria can also infect bone and may do so alone or as part of a mixed infection. Fungi—most often *Candida albicans*, but less commonly endemic mycoses, *Cryptococcus* species, or filamentous fungi—can also cause osteomyelitis. In adults, *Mycobacterium tuberculosis* is well known to cause disease in the axial (rarely the appendicular) skeleton. In the final analysis, any microorganism that can cause invasive disease is capable of causing osteomyelitis, and the literature contains many case reports of osteomyelitis due to less commonly encountered pathogens. This breadth of potential pathogens speaks to the importance of establishing a culture diagnosis whenever possible. Unique associations are listed in Table 96-1.

Clinical Presentation

The clinical presentation varies based on the etiology of disease. In many cases, the patient does not present with sepsis, and the degree of fever and leukocytosis is mild. Pain is almost always present unless masked by neuropathy or obtundation, and this can be an important clue. Statisti-cally, most patients with symptoms of focal limb, joint, or back pain do not have bone infection, and therefore it is not surprising that in cases of hematogenous or other forms of osteomyelitis, pain may initially be attributed to other more common causes.

Hematogenous osteomyelitis in adults can affect the long bones but more often affects the vertebrae. The lumbar spine is involved more often than the thoracic spine, and cervical spine disease (rarely the dens) is seen in a small minority of cases. Patients always have associated pain, and this can range from mild to severe. In the absence of systemic symptoms, it is difficult to differentiate early vertebral osteomyelitis from benign lumbago. Fever may be present, and in cases of advanced disease or associated epidural abscess, neurologic deficits may develop. One

Figure 96-3 Examples of Contiguous Infections That May Be Associated with Osteomyelitis.

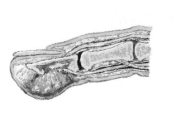

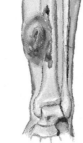

Felon (or other hand infection) that involves bones

Abscess or infected wound adjacent to bone

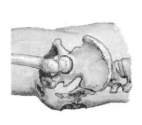

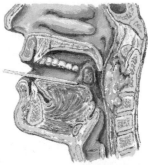

Pressure ulcers that extend to sacrum, pelvis, or spine

Retropharyngeal abscess that spreads to cervical vertebrae

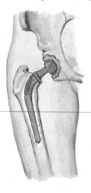

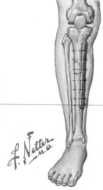

Total joint replacement (loosening of prosthesis usually occurs but does not necessarily indicate infection)

Internal fixation of fractures

should consider this diagnosis in patients with new-onset back pain that steadily worsens or does not improve.

Osteomyelitis associated with vascular insufficiency presents with concurrent soft tissue infection in most cases. Detecting the subset of diabetic foot ulcers with accompanying osteomyelitis can be challenging. Patients may note fever, erythema, and draining ulcers overlying involved bone. Most patients have few systemic symptoms, and many do not complain of pain. In patients who neglect early symptoms, secondary sepsis and bacteremia may result with overt rigors and fever. In advanced cases, bone may be visible in the bed of the wound.

Prosthetic joint infections represent a form of osteomyelitis secondary to a contiguous infection. These patients uncommonly have fever or systemic symptoms. The primary clinical finding is pain, especially with weight bearing. It is common to encounter patients with worsening pain over an extended period of time (months) who are ultimately diagnosed with a prosthesis infection. Delay in diagnosis may be related to initial neglect of pain and to the similarity of symptoms to those experienced in aseptic loosening or mechanical dysfunction.

Chronic osteomyelitis often presents with overlying pain and erythema. Draining sinus tracts can be found adjacent to the infected bone. Most such patients describe chronic pain and drainage and have a known history of osteomyelitis.

Differential Diagnosis

The differential diagnosis of osteomyelitis is not broad but can be challenging to establish. The degree of diagnostic difficulty depends on the form of osteomyelitis being considered. Issues in diagnosing bone infection range from failing to consider the diagnosis (as in early hematogenous osteomyelitis) to being uncertain how to confirm a suspected case (as in the setting of an infected soft tissue ulcer in close proximity to bone). Differentiating between Charcot's foot (neuropathic osteoarthropathy) and osteomyelitis in the diabetic foot often presents a special challenge. In addition, osteomyelitis in patients with sickle cell disease can be difficult to differentiate from bone infarction.

The diagnosis of vertebral osteomyelitis requires a high index of suspicion. Herniated intervertebral disks, vertebral compression fractures, muscular strain, and arthritis can all present with similar pain.

Osteomyelitis of the diabetic foot ranges from a subtle to obvious diagnosis; this depends on the degree of soft tissue infection and bone destruction. The differential diagnosis may include diabetic foot ulcer (with no underlying bone infection), Charcot's foot, crystal arthropathy, degenerative joint disease, and bone fracture.

In the setting of prosthetic joint infection, the differential diagnosis is narrow. Diagnostic considerations include aseptic loosening, mechanical dysfunction (such as patellofemoral instability), infection, and rarely, secondary sarcoma.

Diagnostic Approach

Given the various clinical presentations of osteomyelitis, there is no commonly accepted algorithm to guide diagnosis. A careful initial history and physical examination is key. The diagnosis may be further substantiated by laboratory studies, pathology, culture, and radiologic imaging. Ultimately, it is the clinician's thoughtful synthesis of this material that leads to a diagnosis of confirmed or probable osteomyelitis.

Table 96-1 Common Osteomyelitis Pathogens and Clinical Associations

Clinical Setting	Pathogen	Comments
Hematogenous osteomyelitis	*Staphylococcus aureus*, Enterobacteriacae, *Pseudomonas aeruginosa*	A single pathogen is most often isolated
Prosthetic joint–associated osteomyelitis	Coagulase-negative staphylococci, *S. aureus*, Enterobacteriaceae	Blood cultures are rarely positive; joint aspirates and multiple operative cultures can aid diagnosis
Vertebral osteomyelitis	See "Hematogenous osteomyelitis"; *Mycobacterium tuberculosis*	Tuberculosis should be considered, although it is responsible for a small minority of cases
Osteomyelitis associated with diabetic foot infections	*S. aureus*, *Streptococcus agalactiae* and other streptococci, Enterobacteriaceae, anaerobes, *Pseudomonas* and *Enterococcus* species, coagulase-negative staphylococci	Almost always a polymicrobial infection
Osteomyelitis associated with sickle cell disease	*Salmonella* species, Enterobacteriaceae, *S. aureus*	Hematogenous source
Unique endemic pathogens	*Brucella* species, endemic mycoses (*Blastomyces*, *Coccidioides*, and *Histoplasma* species), melioidosis (*Burkholderia pseudomallei*)	Osteomyelitis occurs in a small subset of infections due to these pathogens

Certain elements of the history and physical exam are useful in diagnosing osteomyelitis. Pain at the involved site is frequently seen. When accompanied by fever, the clinician's index of suspicion should increase. When bone is visible in the bed of an infected ulcer, or if encountered by gentle probing of the wound, osteomyelitis, as a rule, is diagnosed. Draining fistulas often accompany chronic osteomyelitis, and most such patients carry a previous diagnosis of osteomyelitis.

The white blood cell count (WBC) is often elevated (with neutrophilic predominance), but a normal WBC count should never be used to exclude the diagnosis. In cases of chronic osteomyelitis and late prosthetic joint infections, a normal WBC is especially common. The erythrocyte sedimentation rate is high in most cases of bone infection but is slow to change over time, and it can also be elevated with other disease states. C-reactive protein (CRP) changes more quickly with response to therapy, but a normalized CRP does not equate with cure.

Culturing an etiologic pathogen is often diagnostic and, along with antibiotic susceptibility testing, is important in guiding treatment decisions. Samples for culture can include blood, bone, joint aspirates, or deep samples of soft tissue adjacent to a focus of osteomyelitis. In cases of hematogenous osteomyelitis, positive blood cultures can provide a diagnosis and obviate the need for biopsy. The importance of holding antibiotic therapy until cultures are obtained warrants emphasis. A single blood culture positive for a pathogen that might represent a skin contaminant (e.g., coagulase-negative staphylococci, *Propionibacterium acnes*, or corynebacteria) is not diagnostic. Cultures from draining sinus tracts can be misleading, although the growth of *S. aureus* is usually dependable. Surface swab cultures from an ulcer contiguous to osteo-

myelitis are also often misleading. Bone biopsy cultures obtained by surgical or computed tomography (CT)-guided biopsy are the most specific. All samples should be sent for aerobic and anaerobic culture, and in certain circumstances (prior negative cultures, suggestive pathology, or a compatible clinical scenario), samples should be sent for mycobacterial and fungal culture. In vertebral osteomyelitis with negative blood cultures, CT-guided biopsy is often used for diagnosis. If the biopsy culture is negative, undertaking repeat CT-guided biopsy or open biopsy, or in certain cases, proceeding to empiric treatment, is indicated. In the setting of prosthetic joint infection, multiple samples from periprosthetic bone and soft tissue (up to five) should be sent for culture. Some orthopedic surgeons rely on intraoperative frozen section pathology during joint revision surgery to suggest persistent infection (>10 neutrophils per high-power field).

Plain radiographs should routinely be done when there is clinical suspicion of osteomyelitis. Although plain radiography has poor sensitivity, it often can help support the diagnosis and is also useful for future comparison. Plain films may show narrowing of the joint space, periosteal elevation, and osteopenia or lytic changes. In acute osteomyelitis, it takes several weeks or more for any visible abnormalities to be visible on plain films, and it is not uncommon to diagnose osteomyelitis despite unremarkable plain radiographs.

CT and magnetic resonance imaging (MRI) can provide better delineation of bony anatomy and are useful in making the diagnosis. CT provides excellent imaging of cortical bone and adjacent soft tissue and, in chronic osteomyelitis, adequately detects sequestra. When there are implanted metal devices in the viewing field, scatter artifact seriously limits the quality of imaging. Implants may also interfere with MRI interpretation. MRI is superior in detecting acute osteomyelitis because of its ability to detect marrow edema (which appears white on T2-weighted sequences and black on T1). In cases of vertebral osteomyelitis, MRI is also useful in the diagnosis of epidural abscess. Charcot's osteoarthropathy and marrow changes secondary to sickle cell anemia are difficult to separate from osteomyelitis on MRI. MRI is also less useful in following response to therapy because marrow changes often persist after the infection has been successfully treated.

Three-phase bone scans are done using technetium-99m bound to phosphate, an isotope that accumulates in areas of new bone formation. This scanning technique is useful in suspected cases of osteomyelitis with normal plain films. False-positive findings can occur in the setting of post-traumatic injury, noninfectious inflammatory bone disease, and healed osteomyelitis. Radionuclide-labeled WBC scans are less sensitive and uncommonly used in diagnosing osteomyelitis.

Management and Therapy

The treatment of osteomyelitis should take into account the host status, etiologic pathogens, and extent of bone involvement. Optimal care often requires multidisciplinary input. Although medical therapy alone is appropriate in many circumstances, there are numerous situations that require surgical intervention.

Certain principles should be kept in mind. First, when treating bone infection in association with implanted hardware, osteomyelitis is seldom cured without removal of the hardware (plate and screw fixation, intramedullary nails, prosthetic joints). Early prosthetic joint infection treated with débridement and prosthesis retention may be an exception, but this, too, may cause persistent infection without hardware removal. Second, debridement is most often indicated in diabetic foot infection with contiguous osteomyelitis; dogma has generally been that diseased bone should be debrided to healthy, bleeding bone, although some suggest that limited debridement or antibiotic treatment alone can be successful. Third, chronic osteomyelitis is a surgical disease that is not cured with antibiotic therapy. Antibiotics may be used in conjunction with surgical treatment or as short-course therapy to effect symptomatic improvement. Fourth, when amputation is carried out well above the level of infection (i.e., below the knee amputation to treat a refractory diabetic foot infection), antibiotic therapy should be discontinued in the absence of disseminated infection. Fifth, in patients with arterial insufficiency and osteomyelitis in an extremity, consideration should be given to revascularization.

The appropriate length of antibiotic treatment remains an area of some uncertainty. For cases of acute hematogenous osteomyelitis, most physicians treat with a 6-week course of antibiotics. This is based on time for bone regeneration and on the body of clinical experience in treating osteomyelitis. There are scenarios in which a shorter or longer course of antibiotics is appropriate. In diabetic foot infections with associated osteomyelitis, a shorter course of antibiotics is often effective, about 4 weeks, if there has been aggressive debridement of soft tissue and resection of osteomyelitic bone. In contrast, some patients with vertebral osteomyelitis due to difficult pathogens, such as MRSA, are treated with longer courses of antibiotics; this is especially the case in patients with complicated infections involving epidural or paravertebral abscesses. In such cases, some physicians treat with an extended course of parenteral antibiotics (8 to 12 weeks), and others attempt a switch to extended oral antibiotics after an initial 6- to 8-week course of parenteral antibiotics.

Whether to give intravenous or oral antibiotics is also a common question. In most cases, treatment is with parenteral antibiotics. There are, however, situations in which oral therapy is appropriate. Fluoroquinolones have excellent bioavailability and bone penetration, and in infections due to susceptible gram-negative rods (*Pseudomonas* species excluded), monotherapy with an oral fluoroquinolone is appropriate. Although patients with *S. aureus* osteomyelitis have been successfully treated using a combination oral regimen of rifampin and a fluoroquinolone, this approach has not become the standard of care. Clindamycin can be used to treat *S. aureus* infections that have no evidence of constitutive or inducible resistance. It offers excellent bioavailability and good bone penetration and is appropriate to use orally or parenterally. In treating adults with *S. aureus* osteomyelitis, oral clindamycin can be used to de-escalate from initial treatment with a parenteral antibiotic. Linezolid is a newer antibiotic that is highly bioavailable and has good gram-positive activity and good bone penetration; extended use can be associated with neuropathy and more commonly with cytopenia, and these complications have tempered its utility in treating osteomyelitis.

Antibiotic regimens appropriate for common pathogens are listed in Table 96-2. When indicated based on drug metabolism and excretion, renal or hepatic insufficiency requires dose adjustments. In cases of enterococcal infections, an aminoglycoside dosed for synergy can be used through all or part of the treatment course. Oral rifampin can be added as an adjunctive agent in treating *Staphylococcus* osteomyelitis associated with hardware. Dual antibiotic therapy for *Pseudomonas* osteomyelitis is often used for part or all of treatment.

Optimum Treatment

In vertebral osteomyelitis, medical therapy is the standard. Culture and antibiotic susceptibility testing should always guide the selection of antibiotics. In the unusual circumstance when cultures are negative, concern about fastidious pathogens, fungi, and mycobacteria should increase. Empiric treatment in these cases is most often with a regimen that covers gram-positive and gram-negative

Table 96-2 Accepted Antibiotic Treatment Options for Selected Osteomyelitis Pathogens

Pathogen	Antibiotics of Choice	Alternative Treatment
Methicillin-sensitive *Staphylococcus aureus*	Oxacillin or nafcillin (2 g IV every 4-6 hr)	Cefazolin (1-2 g IV every 8 hr) Clindamycin[a] (600-900 mg IV every 8 hr; 300-450 mg by mouth every 6 hr) Vancomycin (1 g IV every 12 hr) Rifampin[b] (600 mg by mouth every day or 300 mg by mouth twice a day)
Methicillin-resistant *S. aureus*	Vancomycin (1g IV every 12 hr)	Teicoplanin (400 mg IV every 12 hr for 1 day, then every 24 hr) Rifampin[b] (600 mg by mouth every day or 300 mg by mouth twice a day)
Streptococci (groups A, B, C, F, G)	Penicillin G (12-20 mU IV daily in six doses or as continuous infusion)	Clindamycin[a] (600-900 mg IV every 8 hr; 300-450 mg by mouth every 6 hr) Vancomycin (1g IV every 12 hr)
Enterococcus species	Ampicillin (2 g IV every 4 hr), *or* Penicillin G (as above)	Gentamicin[c] (1 mg/kg IV every 8 hr) Vancomycin (1 g IV every 12 hr)
Enterobacteriacae[d]	Fluoroquinolone (i.e., ciprofloxacin [400 mg IV every 12 hr; 750 mg by mouth twice a day]), *or* Third-generation cephalosporin (i.e., ceftriaxone [2 g IV every 24 hr])	Cefepime (2 g IV every 12 hr) Imipenem[e] (500 mg IV every 6 hr)
Pseudomonas aeruginosa	Piperacillin (2-4 g IV every 4-6 hours), or piperacillin-tazobactam (3.375-4.5 g IV every 6 hr), or ceftazidime (2 g IV every 8 hr) and gentamicin (once daily dosing)[f], or ciprofloxacin (400 mg IV every 12 hr; 750 mg by mouth twice a day)	Cefepime (2 g IV every 8-12 hr), *or* Imipenem (500 mg IV every 6 hr), *and* Ciprofloxacin, *or* Gentamicin (once-daily dosing)

[a]If no evidence of constitutive or inducible resistance.
[b]Not to be used as a single agent.
[c]Consider using ampicillin, penicillin, or vancomycin *and* an aminoglycoside dosed for synergy during part or all of treatment.
[d]Cephalosporin monotherapy should be used with caution in *Enterobacter* or *Serratia* species infections.
[e]For use in resistant isolates.
[f]Gentamicin may be discontinued after several weeks to decrease the risk of vestibular, oto- or nephrotoxicity.

pathogens. Treatment duration is for a minimum of 6 weeks. In patients with spinal instability, associated neurologic symptoms, a large paravertebral infection not responding to medical treatment, or extensive epidural abscess, surgical intervention may be necessary. Surgery usually involves a two stage procedure: initial anterior debridement followed by delayed posterior instrumented fusion.

In osteomyelitis associated with diabetic foot infection, large vessel disease is often an underlying problem that requires revascularization to maximize the chances for treatment success. In patients who present with sepsis and an advanced, neglected foot infection, immediate amputation may offer the only alternative to decrease morbidity. Fortunately, most patients can be treated with debridement of soft tissue and infected bone. After debridement, wound management is critical and may involve negative-pressure dressings and skin grafting. Such infections are almost always polymicrobial, and surface-swab cultures are inadequate guides to therapy.

For most patients with prosthetic joint infections, the standard of care is a two-stage procedure. The first stage consists of removal of the infected prosthesis, debridement, and placement of a spacer containing antibiotic

impregnated cement; many orthopedic surgeons will use an articulating spacer that allows the patient to bear weight and maintain limited joint mobility. Parenteral antibiotics are administered for 6 or more weeks and then discontinued. Subsequently, a new arthroplasty is implanted unless there are findings to suggest persistent infection.

Chronic osteomyelitis requires surgical treatment for patient recovery. Patients who are not acceptable operative candidates may be treated with intermittent antibiotics for symptomatic flares. Surgical treatment is complicated, especially for through-and-through infection of bone. Management of dead space after resection of sequestrum is a primary issue in treatment and often requires multiple-stage procedures. Management by both orthopedic and plastic surgery may be required, and local or free flap repair is sometimes used to manage dead space. Adjunctive antibiotic treatment is indicated and should be guided by bone culture.

Avoiding Treatment Errors

In making therapeutic decisions for patients with osteomyelitis, the physician must carefully consider the patient's ability to tolerate ideal therapy. When osteomyelitis is associated with adjacent decubitus ulcers, depending on the level of patient debility, it may be appropriate to treat associated sepsis with minor debridement and a short course of antibiotics but not seek to treat curatively. In patients with late prosthetic joint infections, often there is the temptation to treat with debridement but to retain the prosthesis. This approach may be appropriate in frail patients, but in general, retention of the prosthesis leads to chronic infection, even with aggressive parenteral antibiotic treatment. The treating physician should always realize the limitations of antibiotic therapy; in patients with osteomyelitis associated with a contiguous infection, an extended course of antibiotics is inappropriate if critical ischemia is not addressed or if necrotic, devitalized tissue is not debrided.

Future Directions

S. aureus is the single-most important bacterial pathogen causing osteomyelitis, and MRSA has steadily become more predominant. Clinical anecdotes have suggested a poor response to vancomycin in some cases. Rarely, treatment failure has been due to frank vancomycin resistance or to intermediate resistance related to increased cell wall thickness. Some have described "hetero-resistant" MRSA as a cause of vancomycin treatment failure, and others have suggested that dysfunction in the *S. aureus* accessory gene regulator (*agr*) may be associated with vancomycin treatment failure. At the moment, vancomycin continues to be first-line treatment for significant disease due to MRSA; future research should focus on developing techniques to predict MRSA isolates that respond poorly to vancomycin and explore alternate antibiotic therapy for such infections.

EVIDENCE

1. Calhoun JH, Manring MM: Adult osteomyelitis. Infect Dis Clin North Am 19(4):765-786, 2005.
   The authors provide a comprehensive review of osteomyelitis in adults.
2. Jeffcoate WJ, Lipsky BA: Controversies in diagnosing and managing osteomyelitis of the foot in diabetes. Clin Infect Dis 39(Suppl 2):S115-S122, 2004.
   This is a good discussion of the pitfalls in diagnosis and treatment of osteomyelitis associated with diabetic foot infection.
3. Lew DP, Waldvogel FA: Osteomyelitis. Lancet 364(9431):369-379, 2004.
   The authors provide a comprehensive review of osteomyelitis, including its pathogenesis.
4. Mader JT, Calhoun JC: Osteomyelitis. In Mandell GL, Bennett JE, Dolin R (eds): Mandell, Douglas, and Bennett's Principles and Practice of Infectious Diseases, 5th ed. Philadelphia, Churchill Livingstone, 2000, pp 1182-1195.
   This chapter presents a comprehensive review of osteomyelitis.
5. Parsons B, Strauss E: Surgical management of chronic osteomyelitis. Am J Surg 188(1A Suppl):57-66, 2004.
   The authors present a discussion of staged surgical procedures used to treat chronic osteomyelitis.

David J. Weber ▪ Vickie Brown ▪ Emily E. Sickbert-Bennett ▪
William A. Rutala

97

Intravascular Catheter Infections

Introduction

The Centers for Disease Control and Prevention (CDC) estimates that health care–associated infections account for 2 million infections, 90,000 deaths, and $4.5 billion in excess health care costs annually. Hospital-acquired bloodstream infections have been estimated at 250,000 infections per year with 26,250 associated deaths—the eighth leading cause of death in the United States. A prospective analysis of data from 49 hospitals evaluated 24,179 nosocomial bloodstream infections between 1995 and 2002 and found an incidence of 60 cases per 10,000 hospital admissions. About 51% of cases occurred in the intensive care unit. Intravascular devices were the most common predisposing factor; a central venous catheter (CVC) was in place in 72%, a peripheral intravenous catheter in 35%, and an arterial catheter in 16%.

This chapter addresses the prevention and management of intravascular catheter-related infections.

Types of Intravascular Catheters and Their Use

Intravascular catheters are widely used in medicine to provide fluid replacement, allow hemodynamic monitoring, and administer medication (Table 97-1). CVCs are intravascular catheters whose tip lies within a great vessel such as the vena cava (Fig. 97-1).

Intravascular Catheter-Related Complications

Complications associated with peripheral venous catheters include phlebitis, bleeding, infiltration, and infection. Of these, sterile phlebitis is the most common. Generally, removal of the catheter and warm soaks is sufficient to bring relief. Complications of CVCs differ depending on the type and location of the central catheter but include thrombosis, air embolism, catheter misplacement, vein laceration, and local and systemic infection. Pneumothorax and hemothorax are risks with subclavian and to a lesser extent with internal jugular placement. Subclavian artery puncture may occur with subclavian vein placement. Complications of pulmonary artery placement include cardiac arrhythmias and pulmonary infarction. Rarely, during

manipulation, a piece of a CVC may shear off, resulting in catheter embolization.

Etiology and Pathogenesis of Catheter-Related Infections

All intravascular catheters represent an infection risk because the skin must be breached during insertion and use. Catheter-related infections develop by several mechanisms (Fig. 97-2). Migration of skin organisms at the insertion site into the cutaneous catheter tract with colonization of the catheter tip is the most common route of infection for percutaneously inserted, short-term catheters. Contamination of the catheter hub with bacterial invasion through the lumen (i.e., colonization of the internal surface of the catheter) contributes substantially to colonization of CVCs. Occasionally, catheters might become hematogenously seeded from another focus of infection. Rarely, intrinsic (i.e., from the manufacturer) or extrinsic (i.e., during manipulation at the health care facility) contamination of the infusate leads to catheter-related bloodstream infection. Safdar and Maki assessed the mechanism of catheter-related bloodstream infections with noncuffed short-term CVCs and reported that 45% of infections were extraluminally acquired, 26% were intraluminally

Table 97-1   Types of Intravascular Devices and Comments on Their Use

Type of Intravascular Device	Comments
Peripheral venous catheter	Usually inserted into veins of the forearm or the hand; most commonly used short-term intravascular device; rarely associated with bloodstream infection
Peripheral arterial catheter	For short-term use; commonly used to monitor hemodynamic status and to determine blood gas levels of critically ill patients; risk for bloodstream infections may approach that of central venous catheters (CVCs)
Midline catheter	Peripheral catheter (size, 7.6-20.3 cm) is inserted via the antecubital fossa into the proximal basilic or cephalic veins, but it does not enter central veins; it is associated with lower rates of phlebitis and infections than are CVCs
Nontunneled CVC	Most commonly used CVC; accounts for an estimated 90% of all catheter-related bloodstream infection; increased risk for infection with internal jugular or femoral vein site of infection
Pressure-monitoring system	Used in conjunction with arterial catheter; associated with both epidemic and endemic nosocomial bloodstream infections; source is often fluid column in the tubing between the patient's intravascular catheter and the pressure-monitoring apparatus, contaminated infusate, or nondisposable transducers
Peripherally inserted CVC (PICC)	Provides an alternative to subclavian or jugular vein catheterization; is inserted via the peripheral vein into the superior vena cava, usually by way of the basilar or cephalic veins; is easier to maintain; and is associated with fewer mechanical complications (e.g., hemothorax) than are nontunneled CVCs. However, PICC-associated venous thrombosis is noted in about 2.5% of inserted lines
Pulmonary artery catheter	Inserted through a Teflon introducer (e.g., Cordis) and typically remains in place for an average duration of only 3 days; most catheters are heparin bonded to reduce catheter thrombosis and microbial adherence to the catheter
Tunneled CVC	Surgically implanted CVC (e.g., Hickman, Broviac, Groshong, or Quinton catheter) with the tunneled portion exiting the skin and a Dacron cuff just inside the exit site; the cuff inhibits migration of organisms into the catheter tract by stimulating growth of surrounding tissue, thus sealing the catheter tract; used to provide vascular access to patients who require prolonged intravenous chemotherapy, home-infusion therapy, or hemodialysis
Totally implantable catheter	A subcutaneous port or reservoir with self-sealing septum is tunneled beneath the skin and is accessed by a needle through intact skin; low rates of infection
Intra-aortic balloon pump (IABP)	An IABP is a catheter with a balloon position in the descending thoracic aorta that is used to provide temporary support of cardiac function
Phoresis catheter, Vas-Cath, PermCath	These are larger and sturdier catheters used for high flow blood withdrawals for apheresis or dialysis
Powercath	This is a central catheter that allows high flow rate and pressure for rapid injection of contrast media

Adapted from O'Grady NP, Alexander M, Dellinger EP, et al: Guidelines for the prevention of intravascular catheter-related infections. Centers for Disease Control and Prevention. MMWR Recomm Rep 51(RR-10):1-29, 2002.

acquired through the ports, and the mechanism of infection was indeterminate in 29%.

Biofilm formation on the surfaces of indwelling catheters is central to the pathogenesis of infection in indwelling catheters. The distinguishing feature of biofilms is the presence of extracellular polymeric substances, primarily polysaccharides, surrounding and encasing the microbes. Virtually all percutaneous CVCs are colonized by microorganisms embedded in a biofilm matrix. The organisms most commonly isolated from catheter biofilms are coagulase negative staphylococci, *Staphylococcus aureus*, *Klebsiella pneumoniae*, *Pseudomonas aeruginosa*, and *Candida albicans*. Although biofilm formation on CVCs is universal, the extent and location of biofilm formation depend on duration of catheterization: short-term catheters (<10 days) have greater biofilm formation on the external surfaces; long-term catheters (30 days) have greater biofilm forma-

tion on the catheter inner surfaces. Pathogens contained within biofilms exhibit increased resistance to antimicrobial therapy.

Epidemiology and Microbiology of Catheter-Related Infections

The prevalence of bloodstream infections has been described in a prevalence study of 10,038 patients in 1447 European intensive care units; on the date of the study, 247 patients (2.5%) were being treated for a hospital-acquired bloodstream infection. Risk factors for infection included pulmonary artery catheters (odds ratio, 1.2) and CVCs (odds ratio, 1.35). The incidence of catheter-related bloodstream infections occurring in intensive care units is available from the Center for Disease Control and Prevention (CDC) National Nosocomial Infection Surveillance

Figure 97-1 Catheter Placement.

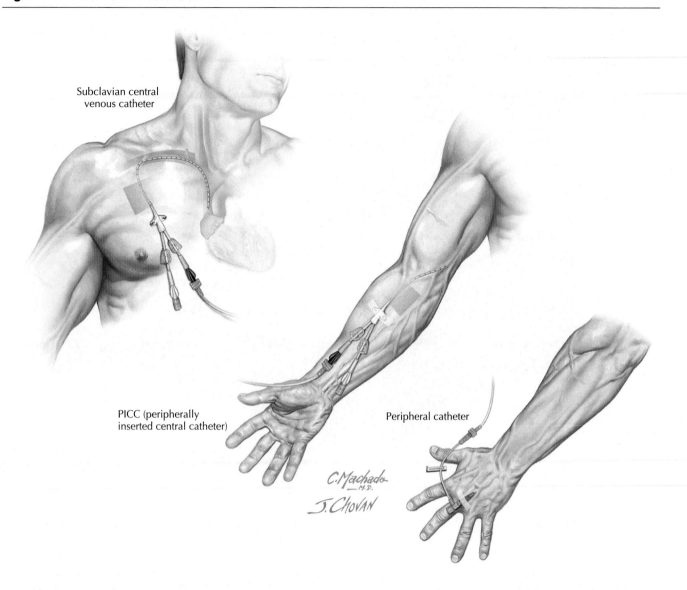

Subclavian central
venous catheter

PICC (peripherally
inserted central catheter)

Peripheral catheter

C. Machado
_M.D._

J. Chovan

(NNIS). The incidence of infections (per 1000 catheter-days), June 2002 through June 2004, ranged from 2.7 to 7.4 depending on the type of intensive care unit. A meta-analysis has reported the rates of catheter-related bloodstream infections by type of catheter (Table 97-2).

The microbiology of CVC-related bloodstream infections has been reported. The most common pathogens are coagulase-negative staphylococci, *S. aureus*, *Enterococcus* species, enteric gram-negative bacilli (*Escherichia coli*, *K. pneumoniae*, *Enterobacter* species), *Pseudomonas aeruginosa*, and *Candida* species (Table 97-3).

The incidence of catheter-related bloodstream infections varies considerably by type of catheter, frequency of catheter manipulation, and patient-related factors (e.g., underlying disease and acuity of illness). Duration of catheterization is the most important risk factor. Risk factors

associated with a higher incidence of peripheral venous catheter–related infections are placement in lower extremity (lowest risk with placement into hand veins), failure to rotate the site every 72 to 96 hours, and use of steel needles. Risk factors associated with a higher incidence of CVC-related bloodstream infection include the following:

- Hospital characteristics
  - Teaching hospital versus nonteaching hospital
  - Larger hospitals
- Patient characteristics
  - Severity of underlying disease
  - Active infection at other site
  - Care in an intensive care unit
  - Immunosuppression (e.g., HIV, organ transplant)
  - Surgery patient

Figure 97-2 Pathogenesis of Infection.

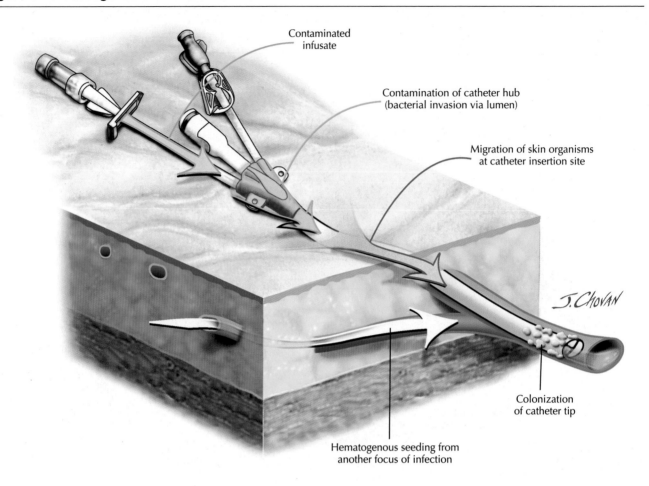

Contaminated
infusate

Contamination of catheter hub
(bacterial invasion via lumen)

Migration of skin organisms
at catheter insertion site

J. CHOVAN

Colonization
of catheter tip

Hematogenous seeding from
another focus of infection

- Features of insertion
  - ~~Emergent placement~~
  - Location of insertion (femoral site > internal jugular site > subclavian site)
  - Multilumen catheters
  - Failure to use maximal barrier precautions (sterile drape that covers entire body; sterile gloves and gown, and mask for physician)
  - Nontunneled catheters
- Features of maintenance
  - Duration of catheterization
  - Colonization of catheter hub
  - Parenteral nutrition
  - Inappropriate catheter use

Prevention of Intravascular Catheter-Related Infections

Key measures to prevent intravascular catheter-related infections include strict adherence to aseptic insertion and maintenance, preparation of the insertion site with an antiseptic, and prompt removal when the catheter is no longer medically necessary. There is no evidence that prophylactic antibiotics are successful in preventing catheter-related infections. Antiseptic and antibiotic impregnated CVCs have been demonstrated to reduce the incidence of catheter colonization and catheter-related bloodstream infections. Their use should be considered for prolonged catheterization. Implantable CVCs warrant consideration if central venous access is required for more than 30 days. Peripherally inserted central catheter (PICC) lines are useful for prolonged venous access when central venous access through the subclavian or internal jugular sites is not required. Based on currently available data, central venous or PICC catheters do not require changes at set intervals. Recommendations for the prevention of intravascular catheter-related infections have been published (Box 97-1).

Clinical Presentation

Catheter-related infections include both local and systemic infections. Exit-site infections, tunnel infections, and pocket infections constitute the local infection group. Erythema, induration, and tenderness within 2 cm of the catheter exit site are the usual manifestations of exit-site

Table 97-2 Risk for Catheter-Related Bloodstream Infections by Type of Catheter

	CR-BSI Pooled Mean (95% CI) per 100 Catheters	CR-BSI Pooled Mean (95% CI) per 1000 Catheter-Days
Peripheral venous catheters		
Plastic catheters	0.1 (0.1-0.2)	0.5 (0.2-0.7)
Steel needles	2.0 (0.0-4.3)	8.6 (0.0-18.2)
Venous cutdown	3.7 (0.0-10.8)	9.0 (0.0-26.6)
Midline catheters	0.4 (0.0-0.9)	0.2 (0.0-0.5)
Arterial catheters for hemodynamic monitoring	0.8 (0.6-1.1)	1.7 (1.2-2.3)
Peripherally inserted central catheters		
Inpatient and outpatient	3.1 (2.6-3.7)	1.1 (0.9-1.3)
Inpatient	2.4 (1.2-3.6)	2.1 (1.0-3.2)
Outpatient	3.5 (2.8-4.1)	1.0 (0.8-1.2)
Short-term noncuffed central venous catheters		
■ Nonmedicated		2.7 (2.6-2.9)
Nontunneled	4.4 (4.1-4.6)	1.7 (1.2-2.3)
Tunneled	4.7 (3.2-6.2)	1.6 (1.3-2.0)
■ Medicated		1.2 (0.3-2.1)
Chlorhexidine-silver-sulfadiazine	2.6 (2.1-3.2)	4.7 (1.5-8.0)
Minocycline-rifampin	1.0 (0.3-1.8)	3.3 (1.7-5.0)
Silver impregnated	5.2 (1.7-8.7)	4.8 (2.1-7.5)
Silver iontophoretic	4.0 (2.1-6.0)	3.7 (2.4-5.0)
Benzalkonium chloride	4.3 (1.9-6.7)	
Pulmonary artery catheters	1.5 (0.9-2.0)	
Hemodialysis catheters		
Temporary, noncuffed	8.0 (7.0-9.0)	4.8 (4.2-5.3)
Long-term, cuffed and tunneled	21.2 (19.7-22.8)	1.6 (1.5-1.7)
Cuffed and tunneled central venous catheters	22.5 (21.2-23.7)	1.6 (1.5-1.7)
Subcutaneous venous ports		
Central	3.6 (2.9-4.3)	0.1 (0.0-0.1)
Peripheral	4.0 (2.4-5.6)	0.1 (0.1-0.2)
Intra-aortic balloon pumps	3.0 (0.0-6.3)	7.3 (0.0-15.4)
Left ventricular assist devices	26.1 (19.2-33.0)	2.1 (1.5-2.7)

CI, confidence interval; CR-BSI, catheter-related bloodstream infection.
Adapted from Maki DG, Kluger DM, Crnich C: The risk of bloodstream infection in adults with different intravascular devices: A systematic review of 200 published prospective trials. Mayo Clin Proc 81(9):1159-1171, 2006.

Table 97-3 Pathogens Isolated from Central Venous Catheter-Associated Bloodstream Infections

Pathogen	1986-1989	1992-1999
Gram-Positive Cocci		
Coagulase-negative staphylococci	27%	37%
Staphylococcus aureus	16%	13%
Enterococcus species	8%	13%
Gram-Negative Bacilli		
Escherichia coli	19%	14%
Klebsiella pneumoniae	4%	3%
Enterobacter species	5%	5%
Pseudomonas aeruginosa	4%	4%
Fungi		
Candida species	8%	8%
Miscellaneous	9%	3%

Adapted from O'Grady NP, Alexander M, Dellinger EP, et al: Guidelines for the prevention of intravascular catheter-related infections. Centers for Disease Control and Prevention. MMWR Recomm Rep 51(RR-10):1-29, 2002.

infections. Other associated signs and symptoms of infection include fever or pus emerging from the exit site. Tunnel infections are characterized by tenderness, erythema, and induration more than 2 cm from the catheter exit site, along the subcutaneous tract of a tunneled catheter (e.g., Hickman or Broviac catheter). Pocket infections are defined as infected exudate in the subcutaneous pocket of a totally implanted intravascular device. They are often associated with tenderness, erythema, and induration over the pocket. Spontaneous rupture and drainage, or necrosis of the overlying skin, may also occur. Local infections may be associated with concomitant bloodstream infection. Systemic signs are common and may be categorized as constitutional (fever, rigors, hypotension, shock), respiratory (hyperventilation, respiratory failure), gastrointestinal (abdominal pain, vomiting, diarrhea), and neurologic (confusion, seizures).

Clinical findings are unreliable for establishing a diagnosis of intravascular catheter-related infection, because of their poor sensitivity and specificity. Symptoms and signs suggestive of intravascular catheter-related sepsis include

---

Box 97-1   Selected Recommendations for Placement of Intravascular Catheters in Adults and Children

Hand Hygiene

A. Perform hand hygiene procedures by washing hands with conventional antiseptic-containing soap and water or with waterless alcohol-based gels or foams. Observe hand hygiene before and after palpating catheter insertion sites, as well as before and after inserting, replacing, accessing, repairing, or dressing an intravascular catheter. Palpation of the insertion site should not be performed after the application of antiseptic, unless aseptic technique is maintained (IA).

Aseptic Technique during Catheter Insertion and Care

A. Maintain aseptic technique for the insertion and care of intravascular catheters (IA).

B. Wear clean or sterile gloves when inserting an intravascular catheter as required by OSHA (IC). Wearing clean gloves rather than sterile gloves is acceptable for the insertion of peripheral intravascular catheters if the access site is not touched after the application of skin antisepsis. Sterile gloves should be worn for the insertion of arterial and central catheters (IA).

C. Wear clean or sterile gloves when changing the dressing on intravascular catheters (IC).

Catheter Insertion

A. Do not routinely use arterial or venous cutdown procedures as a method to insert catheters (IA).

Selection and Placement of Intravascular Catheters

A. Select the catheter, insertion technique, and insertion site with the lowest risk for complications (infectious and noninfectious) for the anticipated type and duration of intravenous therapy (IA).

B. Promptly remove any intravascular catheter that is no longer essential (IA).

C. Do not routinely replace central venous or arterial catheters solely for the purpose of reducing the incidence of infection (IB).

D. Replace peripheral venous catheters at least every 72 to 96 hours in adults to prevent phlebitis. Leave peripheral venous catheters in place in children until intravenous therapy is completed, unless complications (e.g., phlebitis and infiltration) occur (IB).

E. When adherence to aseptic technique cannot be ensured (i.e., when catheters are inserted during a medical emergency), replace all catheters as soon as possible and after no longer than 48 hours (II).

F. Use clinical judgment to determine when to replace a catheter that could be source of infection (e.g., do not routinely replace catheters in patients whose only indication is fever. Do not routinely replace venous catheters in patients who are bacteremic or fungemic if the source of infection is unlikely to be the catheter (II).

G. Replace any short-term central venous catheter if purulence is observed at the insertion site, which indicates infection (IB).

H. Replace all central venous catheters if the patient is hemodynamically unstable and a catheter-related bloodstream infection is suspected (II).

I. Do not use guidewire techniques to replace catheters in patients suspected of having catheter-related infection (IB).

Prophylactic Antibiotics

A. Do not administer intranasal or systemic antimicrobial prophylaxis routinely before insertion or during use of an intravascular catheter to prevent catheter-related colonization or bloodstream infection (IA).

Peripheral Venous Catheters
Selection of Peripheral Venous Catheters

A. Select catheters on the basis of the intended purpose and duration of use, known complications (e.g., phlebitis and infiltration), and experience of individual catheter operators (IB).

B. Avoid the use of steel needles for the administration of fluids and medications that might cause tissue necrosis if extravasation occurs (IA).

C. Use a midline or PICC when the duration of intravenous therapy will likely exceed 6 days (IB).

Selection of Peripheral Catheter Insertion Site

A. In adults, use an upper instead of lower extremity site for catheter insertion (IA).

B. In pediatric patients, the hand, the dorsum of the foot, or scalp can be used as the catheter insertion site (II).

Central Venous Catheters
General Principles

A. Use a central venous catheter with the minimum number of ports or lumens essential for the management of the patient (IB).

B. Use totally implantable access devices for patients who require long-term, intermittent vascular access. For patients requiring frequent or continuous access, a PICC or tunneled central venous catheter is preferable (II).

Selection of Catheter Insertion Site

A. Weigh the risks and benefits of placing a device at a recommended site to reduce infectious complications against the risk for mechanical complications (e.g., pneumothorax, subclavian artery puncture, subclavian vein thrombosis, hemothorax, thrombosis, air embolism, and catheter misplacement) (IA).

B. Use a subclavian site (rather than a jugular or a femoral site) in adult patients to minimize infection risk for nontunneled central venous catheter placement (IA).

PICC, peripherally inserted central catheter.

IA. Strongly recommended for implementation and strongly supported by well-designed experimental, clinical, or epidemiologic studies.

IB. Strongly recommended for implementation and supported by some experimental, clinical, or epidemiologic studies, and a strong theoretical rationale.

IC. Required by state or federal regulations, rules, or standards.

II. Suggested for implementation and supported by suggestive, clinical, or epidemiologic studies or a theoretical rationale.

Adapted from O'Grady NP, Alexander M, Dellinger EP, et al. Guidelines for the prevention of intravascular catheter-related infections. Centers for Disease Control and Prevention. MMWR Recomm Rep 51(RR-10):1-29, 2002.

the following: inflammation or purulence at the catheter insertion site; signs of sepsis without an identifiable local infection (e.g., pneumonia, skin or soft tissue infection, urinary tract infection); abrupt onset of shock; signs or symptoms of sepsis plus catheter malfunction; evidence of septic thrombophlebitis of the great veins associated with a CVC; bloodstream infection caused by staphylococci (especially coagulase-negative staphylococci) or *Corynebacterium*, *Candida*, or *Bacillus* species; high-grade bacteremia or candidemia (multiple positive blood cultures); and sepsis refractory to appropriate antimicrobial therapy.

Diagnostic Approach

All patients who develop a fever or other signs of infection and have a vascular catheter in place require evaluation for catheter-related infection. The area around the catheter exit site should be evaluated for erythema, tenderness, and purulence. Examination of the tunnel track is also important. Patients with suspected intravascular catheter-related infection should have at least two sets of blood samples drawn for culture, with at least one set drawn percutaneously. Catheter-related bloodstream infections are defined as bacteremia or fungemia in a patient who has an intravascular device in place and more than one positive blood culture obtained from a peripheral vein, clinical manifestations of infection (e.g., fever, chills, hypotension), and no apparent source for bloodstream infection other than the catheter. They may be detected by use of semiquantitative (≥15 colony forming units [cfu] per catheter segment) or quantitative (≥10² cfu per catheter segment) cultures of a subcutaneous segment of the catheter where the isolate from the catheter cultures and blood cultures is identical. Other diagnostic criteria include simultaneous quantitative cultures of blood obtained from the catheter and peripherally with a ratio of at least 5 : 1 (CVC versus peripheral) and a differential time to a positive blood culture (i.e., a positive result of culture from a CVC is obtained at least 2 hours earlier than is a positive result of culture from peripheral blood). In a meta-analysis that evaluated the accuracy of diagnostic tests for diagnosing intravascular catheter-related bloodstream infections, the most accurate test was paired (i.e., one culture drawn through the catheter and a second drawn from a peripheral vein) quantitative blood cultures followed by paired qualitative blood culture. The most accurate diagnostic method that requires removal of the catheter was the catheter segment culture test (segment from the removed catheter is immersed in broth media and incubated for 24 to 72 hours) followed by semiquantitative culture (5 cm segment of catheter is rolled 4 times across a blood agar plate and incubated). Although paired quantitative blood cultures were the most accurate test for diagnosis of catheter-related bloodstream infection, other methods studied showed acceptable sensitivity and specificity (both >0.75) and negative predictive value (>99%). Importantly, catheters should not be removed and

cultured routinely but rather only if catheter-related bloodstream infection is suspected clinically.

Management and Therapy

Optimum Treatment

The choice of initial antibiotic therapy will depend on the severity of the patient's disease, the risk factors for infection, and the likely pathogens associated with the specific intravascular device. In general, therapy will consist of an antibiotic active against staphylococci, especially methicillin-resistant strains, such as vancomycin or daptomycin, and an antibiotic active against gram-negative bacilli, especially *P. aeruginosa*, such as ceftazidime, cefepime, piperacillin-tazobactam, or a carbapenem (i.e., imipenem or meropenem). Initial antimicrobial therapy should be administered intravenously and should be adjusted once culture data are available. The duration of therapy ranges from 10 to 14 days to 4 to 6 weeks and depends on the patient's underlying diseases (e.g., immunosuppression), promptness of response to therapy, and presence of complicated infections (e.g., septic thrombosis, endocarditis, osteomyelitis, or other metastatic seeding). Algorithms are available to aid in the diagnosis and management. Indications for catheter-removal include the following:

- Tunnel or pocket site infection
- Infection with multiple bacteria, *S. aureus* or *Candida*, *Bacillus*, *Corynebacterium* species
- Unexplained sepsis
- Septic thrombophlebitis
- Endocarditis
- Refractory or progressive exit site infection
- Continued bacteremia (i.e., blood cultures remain positive for more than 3 days)

Avoiding Treatment Errors

The determination of the specific pathogen is critical. Patients with suspected intravenous catheter-related infections should have two sets of blood samples drawn for culture, with at least one set drawn percutaneously. For indwelling catheters, patients with evidence of a tunnel infection should have the exudates sent for culture and Gram stain. Antibiotic susceptibility testing of isolated pathogens is especially critical. The Infectious Diseases Society of America (IDSA) Guideline for the Management of Intravascular Catheter-Related Infections provides pathogen-based recommendations for correct antimicrobial therapy.

Patients who have a complicated bloodstream infection (i.e., septic thrombosis, endocarditis, osteomyelitis) with a removable CVC should have the CVC removed and be treated with systemic antibiotics for 4 to 6 weeks (6 to 8 weeks for osteomyelitis). Failure to remove the catheter or to treat for the proper duration is often associated with ongoing sepsis, development of metastatic infection, and serious morbidity or death. Catheter removal is also required for infections due to *S. aureus*, gram-negative bacilli, and *Candida* species.

Patients with a complicated infection (tunnel infection, port abscess, septic thrombosis, endocarditis, osteomyelitis) who have a tunneled CVC or implantable device-related bacteremia require removal of the catheter or device. In general, as with removal of tunneled CVCs, removal of nontunneled catheters is recommended with infections due to *S. aureus*, gram-negative bacilli, or *Candida* species. However, salvage therapy may be attempted for infections due to *S. aureus* or gram-negative bacilli using systemic antibiotics and antibiotic lock therapy for 14 days. The CVC or intravascular device should be removed if there is clinical deterioration, persisting or relapsing bacteremia, or no response to therapy.

As with all patients on antibiotic therapy, appropriate laboratory tests should be routinely performed to assess for adverse events. These minimally include a complete blood count and platelet count every week and weekly assessment of renal function.

Future Directions

The development of a culture of safety, ongoing surveillance by trained infection control personnel, a supportive education program, and adoption of a five-component intervention have recently been shown by Pronovost and colleagues to lead to a 66% reduction in CVC-related infections in the intensive care unit. The five components of intervention include appropriate hand hygiene, use of chlorhexidine for skin preparation, use of full-barrier precautions during insertion of CVCs, use of the subclavian vein as preferred site for insertion of the catheter, and removal of unnecessary CVCs. Widespread adoption of this intervention could potentially save more than 10,000 lives per year in the United States.

In addition to implementing current CDC recommendations, development of catheters with new materials that inhibit biofilm formation and bacterial adhesion could likely lead to reduced rates of catheter-related infections.

EVIDENCE

1. Maki DG, Kluger DM, Crnich C: The risk of bloodstream infection in adults with different intravascular devices: A systematic review of 200 published prospective trials. Mayo Clin Proc 81(9):1159-1171, 2006.
   This is an impressive meta-analysis of all published studies that report infectious complications associated with intravascular catheters.

2. Mermel LA, Farr BM, Sherertz RJ, et al: Guidelines for the management of intravascular catheter-related infections. Clin Infect Dis 32(9):1249-1272, 2001.
   This article presents the IDSA Guideline for management of intravascular catheter-related infection.

3. National Nosocomial Infection Surveillance (NNIS) System Report: Data summary from January 1992 through June 2004, issued October 2004. Am J Infect Control 32(8):470-485, 2004.
   This article includes the most recent surveillance data from CDC of health care–associated device-related infections.

4. O'Grady NP, Alexander M, Dellinger EP, et al: Guidelines for the prevention of intravascular catheter-related infections. Centers for Disease Control and Prevention. MMWR Recomm Rep 51(RR-10):1-29, 2002.
   This CDC guideline for the prevention of intravascular catheter-related infection is key reading for persons inserting or caring for catheters.

5. Pronovost P, Needham D, Berenholtz S, et al: An intervention to decrease catheter-related bloodstream infections in the ICU. N Engl J Med 355:2725-2735, 2006.
   This recent paper details a five-component intervention that reduced catheter-related infections by more than 50%.

6. Safdar N, Fine JP, Maki DG: Meta-analysis: Methods for diagnosing intravascular device-related bloodstream infection. Ann Intern Med 142(6):451-466, 2005.
   The authors provide an excellent analysis of methods used to diagnose catheter-related bloodstream infections.

7. Safdar N, Maki DG: The pathogenesis of catheter-related bloodstream infection with noncuffed short-term central venous catheters. Intensive Care Med 30(1):62-67, 2004.
   This article represents an excellent and concise review.

8. Trautner BW, Darouiche RO: Catheter-associated infections: Pathogenesis affects prevention. Arch Intern Med 164(8):842-850, 2004.
   The authors present an important discussion of the pathogenesis of catheter-related infections.

9. Vincent J-L, Bihari DJ, Suter PM, et al: The prevalence of nosocomial infections in intensive care units in Europe. Results of the European Prevalence of Infections in Intensive Care (EPIC) Study. JAMA 274(8):639-644, 1995.
   This is the best prevalence study of health care–associated infections.

10. Weber DJ, Rutala WA, Sickbert-Bennett E: Efficacy of antibiotic or antiseptic impregnated devices in preventing nosocomial infections. In Rutala WA (ed): Disinfection, Sterilization and Antisepsis: Principles, Practices, Challenges, and New Research. Washington, DC, Association for Professionals in Infection Control and Epidemiology, 2006.
    The authors provide a concise review of efficacy and safety of antibiotic or antiseptic impregnated intravascular catheters.

11. Wenzel RP, Edmond MB: The impact of hospital-acquired bloodstream infections. Emerg Infect Dis 7(2):174-177, 2001.
    This excellent analysis addresses the overall impact of hospital-acquired bloodstream infections in the United States.

12. Wisplinghoff H, Bischoff T, Tallent SM, et al: Nosocomial bloodstream infections in US hospitals: Analysis of 24,179 cases from a prospective nationwide surveillance study. Clin Infect Dis 39(3):309-317, 2004.
    The authors review a very large data set of nosocomial bloodstream infections.

Influenza

Adaora A. Adimora ▪ David J. Weber

Introduction

Influenza is an acute respiratory illness characterized by fever, cough, myalgias, and malaise due to influenza type A or B virus that occurs in epidemics each winter. Influenza's public health importance is largely due to the magnitude of its annual global epidemics and associated morbidity and mortality. Recently, infection with the avian influenza H5N1 virus strain has become endemic among birds in Eurasia; sporadic transmission to humans has generated concern that efficient person-to-person transmission could emerge and become a major public health threat.

Etiology and Pathogenesis

Influenza viruses are ribonucleic acid viruses classified as type A, B, or C on the basis of antigenic differences. All belong to the family Orthomyxoviridae. Influenza C causes only mild illness and does not occur in epidemics, so its public health importance is substantially less than that of types A and B. Influenza A viruses are further subtyped based on two structural proteins: hemagglutinin and neuraminidase. Hemagglutinin binds the virus to cell receptors; neuraminidase promotes release of virus from infected cells following replication as well as spread of virus in the respiratory tract (Fig. 98-1). At least 9 neuraminidases and 15 hemagglutinins have been identified in influenza A viruses. Currently, circulating influenza A viruses include H1N1 and H3N2 strains. Antibodies to these antigens are important determinants of the immune response to influenza virus. The ability of influenza A to cause epidemics is largely due to the propensity of its hemagglutinin and neuraminidase antigens to undergo major antigenic variation, known as *antigenic shifts*, and minor variations, known as *antigenic drifts*. Influenza B only undergoes antigenic drift. As a result of these periodic antigenic variations in circulating influenza virus strains, a large proportion of the population lacks immunity and is left vulnerable to infection.

Transmission occurs predominantly through droplet transmission produced by coughs and sneezes and by other mechanisms, such as hand-to-hand contact. Human influenza A H5N1 transmission has resulted from close contact with infected birds; its transmission from human to human has been rare. Influenza virus infects the respiratory epithelium, where it replicates within infected cells, causes degenerative changes and cell death, and is then released to infect other cells. Illness severity appears to be related to the amount of viral replication and host defenses. Extrapulmonary viral infection is uncommon. The host immune response is complex and involves an array of defenses, including cell-mediated immunity, local and systemic antibody, and interferon production. Constitutional symptoms, such as myalgias, fever, and headache, may be due to cytokine production because viremia is rare. The increased clinical severity of human influenza H5N1 infection may be partly due to its unusually high levels of serum cytokine induction with resultant increased stimulation of proinflammatory responses.

Clinical Presentation

The illness usually begins abruptly after an incubation period of 24 to 72 hours. Fever, chills, headache, malaise, and myalgias are the predominant symptoms. Respiratory symptoms, such as cough, clear nasal discharge, and sore throat, are typically present but less prominent than the systemic manifestations. The presentation varies widely, from the classic presentation described previously to minimal or no symptoms. Elderly patients may present with only fever, confusion, and weakness. Typically, the physical examination is notable for a toxic-appearing patient with pharyngeal erythema but no exudate and tender cervical lymphadenopathy. Fever and systemic

Figure 98-1 Influenza Virus and Its Epidemiology.
From Kilbourne ED: The molecular epidemiology of influenza. J Infect Dis 127:478-487, 1973.

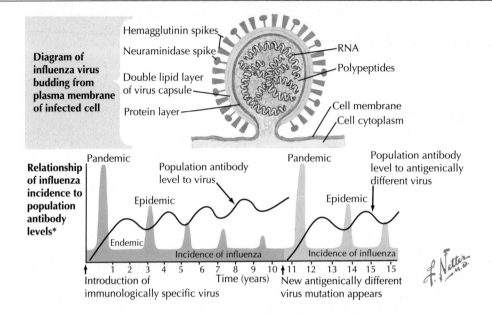

Differential Diagnosis

Because a variety of infectious diseases are associated with abrupt onset of fever, headache, malaise, and myalgias, the differential diagnosis is generally based on epidemiologic evidence of an illness characteristic of influenza occurring during a confirmed outbreak. The differential diagnosis includes adenoviruses, respiratory syncytial virus, parainfluenza, *Mycoplasma pneumoniae*, *Legionella* species, and *Chlamydia psittaci*.

The diagnosis of avian H5N1 virus infection should be considered for patients with pneumonia or severe respiratory distress syndrome whose cause has not been determined if they have traveled to a country with H5N1 infection in poultry or humans within 10 days of the onset of symptoms. The differential diagnosis of avian influenza includes the pathogens listed earlier and potentially may include severe acute respiratory syndrome.

Diagnostic Approach

The most useful laboratory techniques for diagnosis of infection due to human influenza virus in the setting of acute illness involve either virus isolation or detection of viral antigen in respiratory secretions. Nasal swabs or washes, throat swabs, or sputum samples provide acceptable specimens. Virus can be detected in culture within 3 to 7 days by cytopathic effect or hemadsorption. The time for diagnosis can be decreased to 1 or 2 days by centrifuging specimens onto cells in shell vials and using either immunofluorescence or enzyme-linked immunosorbent assay to detect antigen. Some assays yield results within a few hours with comparable sensitivity and specificity to culture results. In contrast, the diagnosis of avian influenza

symptoms usually last about 3 days, but convalescence is often marked by malaise and weakness. Complete recovery may require several weeks.

A variety of respiratory tract conditions can complicate influenza, such as tracheobronchitis, croup, and exacerbation of chronic pulmonary disease. Primary influenza viral pneumonia is associated with fever, cough, dyspnea, and respiratory compromise with minimal evidence of bacteria on sputum Gram stain (Fig. 98-2). Sputum culture specimens show growth of only normal oral flora. A common complication, secondary bacterial pneumonia, is usually due to *Streptococcus pneumoniae*, *Haemophilus influenzae*, or less commonly *Staphylococcus aureus*, and is usually seen among elderly patients and those with chronic lung, heart, or renal disease or diabetes mellitus. It tends to occur about 7 days after onset of influenza, usually after the patient appears to be recovering. Recently, community-associated methicillin-resistant *S. aureus* (CA-MRSA) has been reported to follow influenza. Such infections have been characterized by high fever, hemoptysis, shock, multiple pulmonary cavities, and empyema.

Nonpulmonary complications are relatively uncommon but include myositis, myocarditis, pericarditis, Guillain-Barré syndrome, encephalopathy, and toxic shock syndrome from secondary staphylococcal or streptococcal infection. Reye's syndrome is now a rare complication of influenza because of recognition of aspirin as a risk factor in children and recommendations to avoid aspirin use in children with influenza.

The H5N1 strain has caused particularly severe clinical disease with high mortality rates. Common features include fever, pneumonia and respiratory symptoms, and gastrointestinal symptoms. Laboratory studies have revealed pancytopenia and increased serum aminotransferase levels.

Figure 98-2 Influenza Pneumonia.

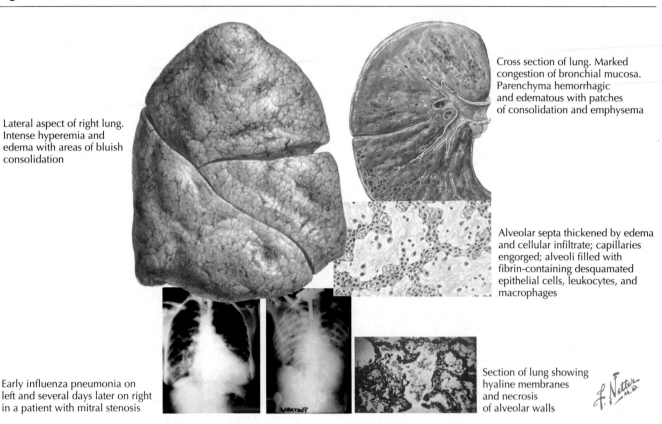

Lateral aspect of right lung. Intense hyperemia and edema with areas of bluish consolidation

Cross section of lung. Marked congestion of bronchial mucosa. Parenchyma hemorrhagic and edematous with patches of consolidation and emphysema

Alveolar septa thickened by edema and cellular infiltrate; capillaries engorged; alveoli filled with fibrin-containing desquamated epithelial cells, leukocytes, and macrophages

Early influenza pneumonia on left and several days later on right in a patient with mitral stenosis

Section of lung showing hyaline membranes and necrosis of alveolar walls

H5N1 can be made by viral culture or polymerase chain reaction assay for influenza H5N1. When this diagnosis is suspected, clinicians should alert laboratory personnel so that appropriate biosafety measures can be used to process specimens.

Serologic testing of acute and convalescent sera by complement fixation or hemagglutination assays is sensitive and specific but is not useful in treating acute illness.

Management and Therapy

Uncomplicated cases of influenza usually require only supportive care and therapy for relief of symptoms. Appropriate recommendations include rest, maintenance of adequate hydration, and if needed, use of acetaminophen for relief of fever and headache. Children should not receive aspirin because of its association with Reye's syndrome.

Optimum Therapy

Antiviral therapy is available for treatment of influenza. The neuraminidase inhibitors, zanamivir and oseltamivir, have activity against both influenza A and B. Amantadine and rimantadine are active against influenza A. Because of the marked increase in resistance to amantadine and riman-

tadine among influenza A isolates obtained during the 2005-2006 influenza season in the United States, the Centers for Disease Control and Prevention has recommended that these drugs not be used for treatment of influenza in the United States; oseltamivir or zanamivir is recommended instead. Oseltamivir is recommended for treatment of influenza H5N1 because isolates from Southeast Asia had amino acid substitutions that rendered them resistant to amantadine and rimantadine.

When given to otherwise healthy adults within 2 days of the start of illness, zanamivir and oseltamivir can decrease the duration of uncomplicated influenza A or B by about 24 hours. Zanamivir is given as an inhaled powder at doses of 10 mg twice daily for 5 days. Because zanamivir inhalation can exacerbate bronchospasm among patients with asthma or chronic obstructive pulmonary disease, it is not recommended for persons with underlying airway disease. Oseltamivir is given in doses of 75 mg orally twice daily for 5 days. Its most common adverse effects are nausea and vomiting, which may be reduced by taking the drug with food. Evidence now suggests that treatment of viral influenza may decrease the risk for hospitalization and secondary bacterial pneumonia; thus, oseltamivir administration should be considered for influenza patients with underlying diseases.

Avoiding Treatment Errors

Failure to consider the diagnosis of influenza is probably the most common treatment error. Given the very limited number of treatment options and the need to begin therapy early in the disease course, the importance of considering influenza as the underlying pathogen in patients presenting with toxic upper respiratory illness cannot be overemphasized. The presence of other documented cases of influenza in the community often helps the clinician to make the correct diagnosis. To be effective, therapy must be initiated within 2 days of the start of illness.

Prevention

The primary method for preventing influenza is annual administration of influenza vaccine. Influenza vaccine is prepared from influenza A and B strains isolated during the previous influenza season and therefore likely to circulate in the United States in the upcoming winter. Immunization is recommended for people at high risk for complications from influenza infection, including children aged 6 to 59 months; persons older than 50 years; and those of any age who have chronic diseases of the heart, lung, or kidneys; diabetes mellitus; immunosuppression; or hemoglobinopathies. Also recommended for vaccination are residents of nursing homes and other facilities that house persons with chronic medical conditions; children and teenagers who receive chronic aspirin therapy and might therefore be at risk for Reye's syndrome; and women who will be pregnant during influenza season. Vaccination of health care workers and household members of persons in high-risk groups is also strongly recommended to decrease risk for influenza transmission. People known to have anaphylactic hypersensitivity to eggs or other vaccine components should not receive influenza vaccine. The optimal time for vaccine administration in the United States is from the beginning of October through mid-November.

Influenza vaccine efficacy depends on the vaccine recipient's age and immunocompetence as well as the degree of similarity between the vaccine virus strains and strains in circulation during influenza season. When vaccine and circulating virus strains are well matched, efficacy in healthy adults younger than 65 years is 70% to 90%. Although the vaccine is less effective among elderly persons living in nursing homes (30% to 40%), its efficacy is about 50% to 60% in preventing pneumonia and 80% in preventing death.

Two influenza vaccine preparations are licensed in the United States: an injectable inactivated vaccine and a live-attenuated vaccine that is administered intranasally. The intranasal live-attenuated vaccine is licensed for use in healthy individuals between the ages of 5 and 49 years but not for immunocompromised patients, pregnant women, persons with a history of Guillain-Barré syndrome, or those with chronic metabolic, renal, pulmonary, or cardiovascular diseases.

Although the primary method of influenza prevention is vaccination, antiviral agents are important adjuncts. Oseltamivir (75 mg once daily for persons >13 years of age) can be used for chemoprophylaxis of influenza. However, chemoprophylaxis is not a substitute for vaccination. During influenza outbreaks, clinicians should consider antiviral prophylaxis for several target populations: (1) people at high risk for complications of influenza who receive the vaccine after the onset of an influenza outbreak in their community; (2) unvaccinated health care workers, or health care workers, regardless of vaccine status, in an outbreak that is due to a strain that might not be controlled by the vaccine; (3) people who have immune deficiencies; and (4) people at high risk for influenza complications who should not be vaccinated and others who wish to avoid influenza illness. Prophylaxis should be provided for 6 weeks because this would cover the duration of most seasonal influenza outbreaks. When determining the timing and duration for administering influenza antiviral medications for chemoprophylaxis, factors related to cost, compliance, and potential side effects should be considered.

Future Directions

Influenza remains one of the most common and important infectious diseases. Recent threats of potentially more virulent strains in Asia have galvanized efforts to develop effective vaccine and treatment strategies. New therapies directed against influenza are expected to play an important role in both endemic and epidemic situations.

Additional Resources

Advisory Committee on Immunization Practices; Smith NM, Bresee JS, et al: Prevention and control of influenza: Recommendations of the Advisory Committee on Immunization Practices (ACIP). MMWR Recomm Rep 55(RR-10):1-42, 2006.
  This paper presents a useful general review of prevention and control measures.
Centers for Disease Control and Prevention: Influenza (flu). Available at: http://www.cdc.gov/flu/. Accessed November 28, 2006.
  This article contains information for clinicians and patients.
Dolin R: Influenza. In Braunwald E, Fauci AS, Kasper DL, et al (eds): Harrison's Principles of Internal Medicine, 16th ed. New York, McGraw-Hill, 2004.
  This chapter on influenza provides a helpful general textbook overview.
Francis JS, Doherty MC, Lopatin U, et al: Severe community-onset pneumonia in healthy adults caused by methicillin-resistant *Staphylococcus aureus* carrying the Panton-Valentine leukocidin genes. Clin Infect Dis 40(1):100-107, 2005.
  The authors document the increasing impact of MRSA infections in the community.
Gubareva LV, Kaiser L, Hayden FG: Influenza virus neuraminidase inhibitors. Lancet 355(9206):827-835, 2000.
  This article presents a useful review of the agents currently used in influenza prevention and therapy.
Smith C: Influenza viruses. In Gorbach SL, Bartlett JG, Blacklow NR (eds): Infectious Diseases, 2nd ed. Philadelphia, WB Saunders, 1998, pp 2120-2124.

The author presents a useful general textbook review of the influenza viruses.

Treanor J: Influenza virus. In Mandell GL, Bennett JE, Dolin R (eds): Mandell, Douglas, and Bennett's Principles and Practice of Infectious Diseases, 5th ed. Philadelphia, Churchill Livingstone, 2000, pp 1823-1849.

The author presents a useful overview of influenza infection.

UpToDate. Available at: http://www.uptodateonline.com. Accessed November 28, 2006.

This website contains information for clinicians and patients.

EVIDENCE

1. Hayden FG, Atmar RL, Schilling M, et al: Use of the selective oral neuraminidase inhibitor oseltamivir to prevent influenza. N Engl J Med 341(18):1336-1343, 1999.

   In this randomized placebo-controlled trial of oseltamivir (75 mg, 150 mg, or placebo) for influenza prophylaxis, protective efficacy of the two active-treatment groups combined was 74%.

2. Hayden FG, Osterhaus AD, Treanor JJ, et al: Efficacy and safety of the neuraminidase inhibitor zanamivir in the treatment of influenza virus infections. N Engl J Med 337(13):874-880, 1997.

   In randomized double-blind studies of adults with influenza in Europe and North America, zanamivir decreased the duration of illness compared with placebo.

3. Nicholson KG, Aoki FY, Osterhaus AD, et al: Efficacy and safety of oseltamivir in treatment of acute influenza: A randomised controlled trial. Neuraminidase Inhibitor Flu Treatment Investigator Group. Lancet 355(9218):1845-1850, 2000.

   The authors conducted a randomized, controlled trial of influenza treatment with oseltamivir among 726 healthy adults. Oseltamivir use shortened the duration of illness by about 1 day.

4. Randomised trial of efficacy and safety of inhaled zanamivir in treatment of influenza A and B virus infections. The MIST (Management of Influenza in the Southern Hemisphere Trialists) Study Group. Lancet 352(9144):1877-1881, 1998.

   Zanamivir reduced the duration and severity of illness in this randomized double-blind placebo-controlled trial.

5. Treanor JJ, Hayden FG, Vrooman PS, et al: Efficacy and safety of the oral neuraminidase inhibitor oseltamivir in treating acute influenza: a randomized controlled trial. US Oral Neuraminidase Study Group. JAMA 283(8):1016-1024, 2000.

   In this randomized, double-blind placebo-controlled trial, oseltamivir treatment reduced the duration of fever, and oseltamivir recipients were able to return to their usual activities 2 to 3 days earlier than those who received placebo.

Infectious Mononucleosis

Introduction

Infectious mononucleosis (IM) is the typical clinical presentation of primary Epstein-Barr virus (EBV), defined by the clinical triad of fever, pharyngitis, and cervical lymphadenopathy, in conjunction with increased circulating atypical lymphocytes. About 95% of all adult populations worldwide will have experienced prior EBV infection. Transmission normally occurs through saliva, and EBV has been called "the kissing disease," although transmission probably can also occur sexually. Initial infection occurs more commonly during childhood in the developing world and in persons of low socioeconomic status, with more than 80% of such children being seropositive by age 4 years, a much higher rate than in the United States and United Kingdom, where the rate of seropositivity at age 5 years is only 50%. The incidence of primary infection peaks during adolescence and young adulthood in developed countries. Infections in childhood often do not present to medical providers, being subclinical or asymptomatic events, whereas the rare persons who experience primary infection beyond their 30s are more likely to present atypically, but with substantial morbidity. Diagnostic testing is key in distinguishing EBV infection, which is usually a self-limited disease, from other more serious illnesses that may present in a similar manner.

Etiology and Pathogenesis

EBV is a human gamma herpesvirus, which normally is restricted to infecting the pharynx and B cells. Primary EBV infection occurs when an uninfected subject is exposed to EBV virions, usually transmitted in saliva from a persistently infected host to the oropharynx of the susceptible person. Sexual transmission of EBV does also occur, but is less frequent. Viral infection occurs first at the mucosal layer, and quickly infects the circulating B cells present locally. EBV within epithelial and B cells can follow a virally encoded program of lytic replication, producing many lytic viral proteins that are both highly immunogenic and required for generating free virions. Acute infection is followed by viremia and circulating infected B cells. A subset of infected B cells adopt an alternative viral life cycle called *latent replication*, characterized by expression of latent (less immunogenic) viral genes that promote persistence of the host cell, replication of latent virus during mitosis of the host cell, and evasion of immune surveillance. Soon after primary infection, a vigorous cellular-mediated immune response is generated, and the subsequent diffuse immune response occurs. Many of the clinical manifestations of EBV infection occur as a result of immune mechanisms, targeting infected circulating B cells. Large numbers of activated CD8+ T cells are produced, which over several weeks eradicate lytically infected cells. The atypical lymphocytes seen on peripheral blood smears are actually these CD8+ cytotoxic T cells. As seen with many other viral infections, symptoms, physical findings, and laboratory abnormalities (such as elevated liver function tests) arise during the CD8+ T-cell response and resolve as the infection is controlled. Thus, by the time patients show symptoms, they have already generated an initial humoral and cellular response. This pattern of illness is helpful in diagnosis of EBV infection, as discussed later. It is important to note that the latent reservoir is never eradicated. Periodically, the lytic viral genes are reactivated at mucosal surfaces to allow shedding of new virions that may infect a new host. Reactivation is asymptomatic. A great deal has been published regarding the role of latent EBV in a variety of malignancies, including African and spontaneous Burkitt's lymphoma, B-cell lymphomas in patients with compromised T-cell immunity, and nasopharyngeal carcinoma. In contrast, acute EBV infection is rarely associated with the development of cancer (discussed later).

Figure 99-1 Infectious Mononucleosis.

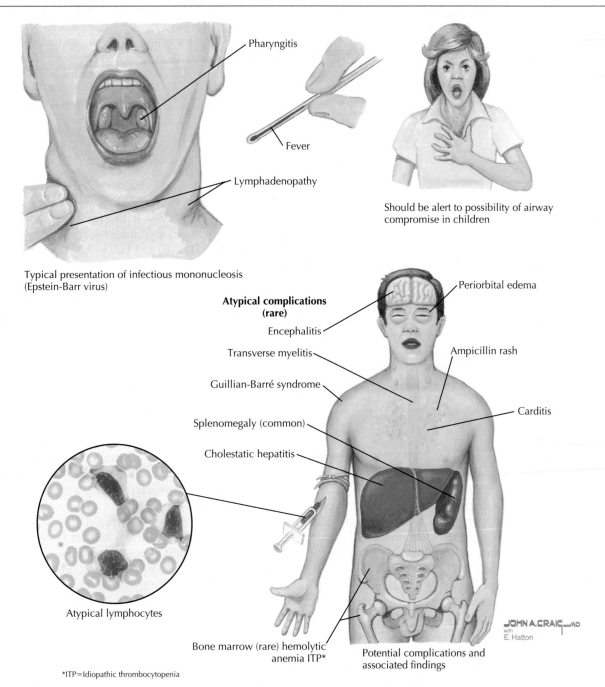

Typical presentation of infectious mononucleosis
(Epstein-Barr virus)

Pharyngitis

Fever

Lymphadenopathy

Should be alert to possibility of airway
compromise in children

**Atypical complications
(rare)**

Encephalitis

Transverse myelitis

Guillian-Barré syndrome

Splenomegaly (common)

Cholestatic hepatitis

Periorbital edema

Ampicillin rash

Carditis

Atypical lymphocytes

Bone marrow (rare) hemolytic
anemia ITP*

Potential complications and
associated findings

*ITP=Idiopathic thrombocytopenia

JOHN A. CRAIG—AD
with
E. Hatton

Clinical Presentation

Most often, primary EBV infection is asymptomatic or
subclinical, but among cases that present to the clinician,
the triad of fever, pharyngitis, and cervical lymphadenopathy is typical. These classic findings, coupled with reactive
atypical lymphocytes and an absolute lymphocytosis, define
IM syndrome (Fig. 99-1). Primary EBV infection in adolescents and young adults predominantly manifests this
way, usually with malaise, and often with inflammation of

vascular reticuloendothelial organs producing mild hepatitis (with abdominal pain, nausea, vomiting, or elevated
transaminases) and splenomegaly. Symptoms and laboratory abnormalities usually resolve spontaneously within 4
to 6 weeks of onset, although evidence of EBV infection
may last for several months. Significant rashes and other
skin findings are not associated with EBV infection alone.
However, treatment with antibiotics during acute EBV
infection often results in a diffuse maculopapular rash. β-
Lactam antibiotics, especially ampicillin and amoxicillin,

are strongly associated with the development of such a rash, but dermatologic reactions have been described with many other antibiotics, including cephalosporins and fluoroquinolones.

Atypical clinical manifestations can occur at any age and involve almost any organ system; cholestatic hepatitis and splenic rupture (following trauma) are among the more severe manifestations seen in clinical practice. Rarely, other complications can occur. These include meningitis or encephalitis, transverse myelitis, Guillain-Barré syndrome, myocarditis, hemophagocytic syndrome, hemolytic anemia, thrombocytopenia, and aplastic anemia (Box 99-1). In middle-aged or older patients, the typical features of fever, pharyngitis, or lymphadenopathy are often absent, whereas more severe complications are more common. Infection generally does not occur in infants until after 8 months of age, perhaps because of protective maternal antibodies. Infection in infants and young children may have a milder presentation, although any of the above syndromes may occur. In addition, severe peritonsilar edema can occur in young children and infrequently results in airway obstruction. Although malignancy is not associated with acute infection in normal hosts, those rare individuals with familial X-linked lymphoproliferative syndrome do not have an effective immune response to EBV and usually succumb to either fulminant IM or develop acute B-cell lymphoma. In extremely rare cases, a chronic active EBV (CAEBV) infection occurs, associated with chronic IM, multiple organ system disease, progressive illness, and high mortality. CAEBV has been more commonly reported in Japanese populations for unknown reasons. There is a popular misconception that chronic fatigue syndrome (CFS) is related to prior EBV infection, but there is no evidence to support this contention, and CFS is clearly distinguished from CAEBV by fever and objective evidence of organ involvement seen in the latter.

Differential Diagnosis

Many disseminated infections in their acute phase, especially viruses, can produce a clinical syndrome that overlaps with IM. Still, EBV is the most common cause of IM-like syndromes. Cytomegalovirus (CMV), human herpesvirus-6 (HHV-6) and HHV-7 are similar clinically, although in immunocompetent subjects, most atypical sequelae with HHV-6 and HHV-7 are rarely described. HHV-6 causes roseola and is commonly associated with febrile seizures in children. HIV can closely mimic acute EBV infection, sometimes presenting with fever, pharyngitis, lymphadenopathy, or reactive lymphocytes (although often the absolute lymphocyte count may be depressed transiently). Acute HIV may also occasionally produce a mild exanthem, aseptic meningitis, or mild hepatitis. In susceptible or unvaccinated, immunosuppressed women of childbearing age, HIV, CMV, measles, mumps, rubella, and toxoplasmosis should be considered in particular because of the potential ramifications regarding fetal infection and development. In some patients, measles may cause atypical lymphocytes with fever and lymphadenopathy, but frequently a cough is present, and the enanthem (Koplik's spots) and extensive exanthem toward the end of symptoms can be helpful in distinguishing measles from other infections. Similarly, mumps may produce atypical lymphocytes but can be differentiated by parotitis or orchitis. Parvovirus produces slapped-cheek erythema in children and may cause small-joint arthralgias or arthritis in adults. Adenoviral infection can produce upper respiratory infection with atypical lymphocytes. Rubella has few pathognomonic associations in childhood or adult disease. Acute toxoplasmosis may be clinically indistinguishable from EBV infection. When a history of cat exposure can be elicited, acute toxoplasmosis should be strongly considered. Of the hepatitis viruses, transaminase levels in the thousands of units per liter generally distinguish hepatitis A and hepatitis B from acute EBV infection. In hepatitis C, transaminase elevation is often less than 10-fold normal values, similar to EBV. Serologic evaluation can help distinguish the two. In children, Kawasaki's disease must be considered in the differential diagnosis of patients presenting with an IM-like syndrome. Group A streptococcal pharyngitis may also acutely masquerade as IM. In a patient with persistent or progressive fever or lymphadenopathy, exclusion of various malignancies or rheumatologic disease may be indicated.

Finally, some drugs, including dapsone and phenytoin, have been associated not only with fever and elevated liver function tests but also with reactive atypical lymphocytes.

Diagnostic Approach

With EBV being almost universally experienced in children and adolescents, it frequently is diagnosed (nondefinitively) from clinical presentation and reactive lymphocytosis alone. Because the differential diagnosis is largely made up of self-limited diseases, this is reasonable in mild cases. A streptococcal test (rapid streptococcal antigen or culture) is usually indicated because treatment of streptococcal pharyngitis is important, but avoidance of amoxicillin with a negative test may spare the patient an EBV-related β-lactam rash. One of the more important viral illnesses to rule out is acute HIV infection, which may present with nonspecific findings. Correct identification of cases is critical to the individual patient and for public health reasons. The clinician needs to maintain a low threshold for initial baseline HIV serology (which may be negative for weeks following acute HIV infection) and follow-up testing. If a patient is deemed at high risk for HIV (recent unprotected sex or unsafe needle use), HIV viral load testing may occasionally be appropriate. As suggested in the prior section, women of childbearing age should have a vaccine and exposure history taken, with possible further testing done.

In atypical or more severe cases of IM, such as evaluation of a fever of unknown origin, a specific identification of acute EBV infection (in addition to HIV exclusion) may be useful in limiting the evaluation. Several blood or serum assays are available.

Heterophile Antibodies (Monospot)

The production of heterophile antibodies is an incompletely understood epiphenomenon of EBV infection of B cells in the acute phase. Polyclonal, nonspecific, nonadaptive antibodies are generated, and these often include antibody species capable of agglutinating erythrocytes of horses and sheep. This phenomenon is common in adolescents with acute EBV infection, with a sensitivity of 90%. However, the specificity and sensitivity are significantly decreased in both children and adults older than 35 years. Thus, the monospot is not an effective means for EBV screening of these populations.

Specific Epstein-Barr Virus Serology

Serologic testing is highly sensitive and specific and is the gold standard for evaluating EBV exposure. There are two immunogenic lytic viral proteins (viral capsid antigen [VCA] and early antigen-D [EA-D]) and one latent viral protein of low immunogenicity (Epstein-Barr nuclear antigen-1 [EBNA-1]) that are routinely assayed in com-

Table 99-1	Interpretation of Epstein-Barr Virus–Specific Serology		
Serology	**No Prior EBV Infection**	**Acute IM**	**Past Infection**
VCA IgM	−	+	−
VCA IgG	−	+/−	+
EBNA-1 IgG	−	−	+

EBNA-1, Epstein-Barr nuclear antigen-1; Ig, immunoglobulin; VCA, viral capsid antigen.

mercially available kits. By the time a patient is symptomatic, immunoglobulin M (IgM) to VCA is almost always present, whereas the IgG response develops within the first few weeks and will persist for the life of the subject. EA-D antibodies appear quickly but do not add much to the evaluation. The IgG response to EBNA-1 usually takes several weeks to months to develop, but then is maintained for life, marking persistent infection. Thus, serum taken during the acute phase of an illness can be used to rule out EBV infection, to diagnose early initial infection, or to diagnose prior infection (Table 99-1). Most adults have serologic evidence of prior infection (EBNA-1 IgG antibodies); this is in no way suggestive of CAEBV (described earlier). Because persistent infection and viral reactivation are asymptomatic, disease in a patient with EBNA-1 IgG antibodies is virtually never explained by EBV IM and may require further evaluation.

Epstein-Barr Virus Quantitative Polymerase Chain Reaction (Viral Load)

Quantitative polymerase chain reaction techniques have been evaluated in a variety of EBV-related conditions. Persons who have not been exposed to EBV will have undetectable viral loads. Immunocompetent persons with resolved previous infection will similarly have very low to undetectable levels of EBV DNA circulating in the blood. A markedly elevated level is consistent with acute EBV IM, although the assays commonly available will not distinguish acute infection from other EBV-associated conditions, malignancies in particular. The test is relatively expensive and, thus, appropriate for the investigation of IM only in complicated or difficult to discern circumstances.

Management and Therapy

Patients should be counseled to avoid contact sports or similar activities with risk for trauma because splenic rupture has been frequently reported and is one of the few causes of mortality associated with EBV. Rarely, small children with significant oropharyngeal obstruction may require emergent intubation for protection of the airway. Otherwise, because acute IM is generally self-limited, supportive care is sufficient.

Optimum Treatment

Medical therapy for acute EBV infection has been disappointing. Although acyclovir, a generally well-tolerated antiviral that is active against lytic EBV, is capable of suppressing oropharyngeal shedding of EBV, it is not indicated for treatment of acute EBV infection except under exceptional circumstances. This is based on a number of small randomized studies that have failed to show efficacy. Similarly, because many of the atypical EBV-associated syndromes are thought to result from the exuberant CD8+ T-cell response, treatment with high-dose steroids has been advocated but not proved useful. It is important to note that the studies reported to date have been small and were not powered to detect subtle effects. Additionally, randomized trials have not focused on patients with more severe or atypical disease. Thus, for patients with uncomplicated IM, no specific intervention is indicated. For patients with severe or life-threatening complications, low toxicity regimens such as acyclovir with or without steroids are reasonable to consider.

Avoiding Treatment Errors

Treatment with β-lactam antibiotics should be avoided in IM.

Future Directions

Various novel medical agents have been explored in preclinical investigations for treatment of IM, but because symptoms normally resolve without intervention, prospective, appropriately powered, randomized trials are needed to document both efficacy and lack of significant toxicity. Interventions to target atypical EBV disease, with its higher morbidity, are still needed as well. Because of the scarcity of such severe cases, no such trials are currently underway. A vaccine against EBV is an attractive approach, whether for vaccination of only high-risk individuals or larger groups, and such an approach is currently being tested in clinical trials.

Additional Resources

Epstein-Barr Virus and Infectious Mononucleosis. Available at: http://www.cdc.gov/ncidod/diseases/ebv.htm. Accessed December 3, 2006.

This website provides useful information about the disease and diagnosis of EBV in a format appropriate for both patients and physicians.

EVIDENCE

1. Auwaerter PG: Infectious mononucleosis in middle age. JAMA 281(5):454-459, 1999.

    This case report and literature review addresses atypical features of EBV in middle-aged and older adults.

2. Chan KH, Tam JS, Peiris JS, et al: Epstein-Barr virus (EBV) infection in infancy. J Clin Virol 21(1):57-62, 2001.

    The authors report on a prospective longitudinal survey of EBV seroconversion in infants up to 2 years old in Hong Kong.

3. Crawford DH, Macsween KF, Higgins CD, et al: A cohort study among university students: Identification of risk factors for Epstein-Barr virus seroconversion and infectious mononucleosis. Clin Infect Dis 43(3);276-282, 2006.

    A prospective cohort of university students showed an association between sexual intercourse and EBV acquisition.

4. Jenson HB: Acute complications of Epstein-Barr virus infectious mononucleosis. Curr Opin Pediatr 12(3):263-268, 2000.

    The author provides a literature review of common and atypical complications in pediatric cases.

5. Linde A: Diagnosis of Epstein-Barr virus-related diseases. Scand J Infect Dis Suppl 100:83-88, 1996.

    Viral capsid antigen antibody, in the absence of EBNA antibodies, defines acute EBV seroconversion.

6. Ohga S, Nomura A, Takada H, et al: Epstein-Barr virus (EBV) load and cytokine gene expression in activated T cells of chronic and active EBV infection. J Infect Dis 183(1):1-7, 2001.

    One of numerous studies showing the ability of EBV viral load to discriminate between active EBV-related disease, prior infection, and uninfected patients.

7. Rea TD, Russo JE, Katon W, et al: Prospective study of the natural history of infectious mononucleosis caused by Epstein-Barr virus. J Am Board Fam Pract 14(4):234-242, 2001.

    This prospective observational case series describes 150 subjects, 16 to 46 years old, with acute primary infection with EBV. Most clinical findings resolved within 1 month, although a minority of cases resolved more slowly.

8. Torre D, Tambini R: Acyclovir for treatment of infectious mononucleosis: A meta-analysis. Scand J Infect Dis 31(6):543-547, 1999.

    The authors report on a meta-analysis of five randomized controlled trials of acyclovir used for treating IM. A trend toward efficacy did not achieve statistical significance.

Peter A. Leone

100

Herpes Simplex Virus Infections

Introduction

Genital and oral infections due to herpes simplex virus (HSV) are endemic in the United States. Genital herpes infection is caused by HSV-2 and less frequently by HSV-1. Genital HSV infection causes vesicular and ulcerative disease in adults and severe systemic disease in neonates and immunocompromised individuals.

HSV-2 transmission is almost always sexual, whereas HSV-1 is usually transmitted through nonsexual human contact. The incidence of new HSV-2 infections is estimated at greater than 1.5 million cases annually. HSV-2 seroprevalence, which is extremely rare before 12 years of age, rises sharply with the onset of sexual activity and peaks by the early 40s. The seroprevalence of HSV-2 infection rose 30% between 1978 and 1991 to 21.7%. The national seroprevalence estimates in 1999 to 2004 decreased to 17%. The decrease was primarily seen in persons 14 to 18 years of age. Most individuals with genital HSV infection have undiagnosed initial infections and unrecognized recurrent outbreaks. Orolabial HSV-2 infection is rare and is almost always associated with genital infection.

HSV-1 infection frequently occurs in childhood, with seropositivity in about 20% of children younger than 5 years. The seroprevalence of HSV-1 rises almost linearly with increasing age to about 50%. HSV-1 is increasingly common, with an estimated 50% of incident genital infection attributable to it.

Etiology and Pathogenesis

Primary HSV infection occurs at the mucosal site of inoculation with retrograde infection of sensory nerve ganglia. Following resolution of primary infection, HSV enters a latent state in the sensory nerve ganglia and can reactivate to cause active infection at any mucosal site innervated by the infected ganglia.

During primary HSV infection, natural killer (NK) cells are important effectors of immunity. NK-cell activation depends on the production of several cytokines that have direct and indirect effects important in limiting viral replication. As the immune response matures, clearance of HSV from infected tissues is T-cell mediated and involves cytokine-mediated effector mechanisms and direct cytolysis of virus-infected cells. Both CD4+ and CD8+ T cells are important in resolution of infection.

The efficiency of the immune response appears to influence the quantity of virus-established latency in the ganglia. The elements that contribute to this control are not com-pletely known, but interferon-γ is likely to be important. Initial evidence suggests that immune response may play a supplemental role in maintaining latency of HSV, but this remains to be confirmed.

Clinical Presentation

Genital infection with HSV is classified into five categories.

The primary first episode refers to infection with either HSV-1 or HSV-2 in an individual who has never been infected with a herpes simplex virus. In immunocompetent hosts, this event usually goes unrecognized. After an incubation period of 1 to 14 days (average, 4 days), a papule appears that evolves into a vesicle within 24 hours (Fig. 100-1). These vesicles can be clear or pustular and rapidly evolve into shallow, nonindurated, painful ulcers. Clinical associations include dysuria, inguinal lymphadenitis, vaginal discharge, and cervicitis. Systemic symptoms,

Figure 100-1 Lesions of Herpes Simplex.

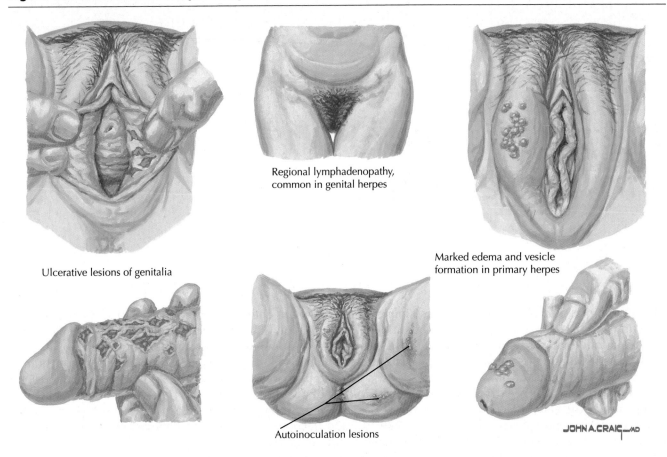

Ulcerative lesions of genitalia

Regional lymphadenopathy, common in genital herpes

Marked edema and vesicle formation in primary herpes

Autoinoculation lesions

JOHN A.CRAIG—AD

including myalgias, malaise, fever, and other flu-like symptoms, may also develop. Crops of lesions occur over 1 to 2 weeks. Crusting and healing require an additional 1 to 2 weeks.

A nonprimary first episode is an infection in an individual who has had a previous infection with either HSV type, typically a previous orolabial infection with HSV-1, in whom a genital HSV-2 infection develops. Generally, it is less severe than the primary first episode because of a partial humoral and cellular immune response. There are fewer lesions, less pain, fewer systemic symptoms, and more rapid resolution of lesions (usually 5 to 7 days). This episode is clinically similar to that of recurrent disease and can be mistaken for recurrent infection.

A first recognized episode is an initial infection, whether it is a first episode or recurrent infection.

A recurrent episode is the second or subsequent episode of genital herpes with the same virus type. HSV-2 accounts for more than 90% of recurrent genital herpes. The median number of recurrences is four, with 38% of individuals having six or more recurrences annually. Recurrent outbreaks are usually not associated with systemic symptoms, are fairly mild, and often go unrecognized, but they may be preceded by a prodrome of paresthesia or dysesthesia.

A cluster of localized vesiculopustular or ulcerative lesions develops and tends to lateralize to one side of the midline. Atypical lesions are common and may be mistaken for excoriation or irritation. Predominant locations of lesions are the glans or shaft of the penis in men, the vaginal introitus or labia in women, and the buttocks and anal area in both sexes. A neuropathic prodrome may occur 6 to 24 hours before the appearance of lesions.

Subclinical shedding refers to the detection of virus in the absence of visible lesions. Our understanding of genital herpes has shifted from that of intermittent outbreaks to one of low-grade continuous shedding of virus that can be detected by viral culture of the genitals and anus 5% to 7% of days and 15% to 20% of days by polymerase chain reaction (PCR). The frequency of subclinical shedding is greatest the first 6 to 12 months after acquiring genital herpes. It is less common in HSV-1. In HSV-2, subclinical shedding occurs in virtually all individuals but is more common in women and diminishes in frequency over time. Many episodes are temporally associated around clinically recognized outbreaks, with virus detected 1 day to several days preceding or following resolution of lesions. The development of symptoms or lesions appears to be most related to duration of viral shedding and not to the host immune response. Patients who are counseled about the mild signs and symptoms of recurrent outbreaks may learn to recognize some periods when they are at risk for transmitting HSV to partners. Unfortunately, because up to 70% of transmission is attributable to asymptomatic viral shedding, patients are potentially infectious to all sexual partners regardless of signs or symptoms.

Differential Diagnosis

Discrete genital or anal ulcers in sexually active young adults have a relatively narrow differential diagnosis. Chancroid is rare in the United States, and syphilis is at a historical low and highly concentrated in certain geographic areas.

The differential diagnosis should include the following infectious etiologies: genital herpes, syphilis, chancroid, primary HIV, lymphogranuloma venereum, and donovanosis.

Primary syphilis may be distinguished from other ulcers by the presence of a nontender, indurated, nonpurulent ulcer. Other ulcer characteristics are not helpful in distinguishing infectious etiologies but are more likely to be due to herpes. Diagnostic testing is critical to prevent a missed diagnosis of genital herpes for any genital ulcer.

Diagnostic Approach

Viral culture has, until recently, been the gold standard for the diagnosis. It is now known that PCR for HSV DNA is 3 to 4 times more sensitive than viral culture and can increase viral detection from genital lesions by 11% to 70% compared with cell culture. Although PCR is offered by many reference laboratories, it is not commercially available. Viral detection methods, whether culture or PCR, allow the etiologic diagnosis of a genital ulcer. They also permit distinction of HSV-1 from HSV-2, an important consideration for prognosis and counseling. Cultures are most sensitive while lesions are in the vesicular-pustular stage. Sensitivity rapidly declines as lesions ulcerate and crust. Direct immunofluorescent antibody testing is more rapid (4 to 6 hours) than culture, but does not differentiate HSV-1 and HSV-2.

Enzyme-linked immunosorbent assay (ELISA) testing for HSV antigens in clinical specimens is a rapid alternative to culture (results in 3 to 4 hours), but its use is generally confined to large laboratories and teaching institutions. Microscopy of Papanicolaou smears or Giemsa staining (Tzanck test) is insensitive and nonspecific and not recommended for the diagnosis of genital herpes. A type-specific antibody test based on HSV glycoprotein G is the most important and reliable diagnostic tool for HSV infection. Antibody tests based on complement fixation, indirect immunofluorescence, or neutralization technologies do not distinguish antibodies to HSV-1 from HSV-2. A nega-

tive antibody test result is reassuring in that it excludes the diagnosis in a patient who has symptoms suggestive of recurrent herpes. A positive test result that is not HSV glycoprotein G–based is of little diagnostic value because it does not distinguish reliably between type 1 and type 2 infections. Because more then half of U.S. adults are HSV-1 seropositive, a positive test result is not useful in the evaluation of genital ulcer disease. Immunoglobulin M (IgM) antibody is often present with recurrent HSV outbreaks and does not indicate recent infection. IgM antibodies are only indicated for the evaluation and diagnosis of neonatal herpes infection.

New type-specific serologic assays have specificities of more than 98% for the detection of HSV-2 antibody and sensitivities of more than 90%, depending on the population studied. A rapid, office-based assay that can be run on serum or fingerstick analyses and provide results in less than 10 minutes is also available. It is imperative to specify a glycoprotein G–based test when ordering an HSV serologic test.

The following are the current U.S. Food and Drug Administration–approved, type-specific assays: Western immunoblot, HerpeSelect HSV-1 and HSV-2 ELISA (Focus Diagnostics, Cypress, CA), HerpeSelect HSV-1 and HSV-2 immunoblot (Focus Diagnostics, Cypress, CA), BioKit HSV-2 Rapid Assay (Biokit USA, Lexington, MA), and Captia HSV-1 and HSV-2 (Trinity Biotech, Wicklow, Ireland).

Management and Therapy

There is an undeserved stigma attached to genital herpes, and most patients require reassurance and appropriate counseling. This can be given only if one has full access to the facts and myths surrounding this condition.

Pharmacologic and Other Treatment

Antiviral therapy for initial genital herpes prevents new lesion formation and rapidly reduces viral shedding, infectivity, and the risk for autoinfection. However, it has no effect on preventing subsequent recurrences. When taken continuously, it effectively suppresses HSV recurrences and reduces subclinical shedding and the risk for transmission of HSV by about 50%. Episodic treatment shortens the course of recurrences. The current recommended antiviral regimens for genital herpes cause few adverse effects, but serum levels can become elevated when renal function is impaired (requiring a reduction in dosage) (Table 100-1). Acyclovir, famciclovir, and valacyclovir are not approved for use during pregnancy. Some experts recommend the use of suppressive acyclovir therapy during the last month of pregnancy for women with symptomatic recurrent herpes to prevent unnecessary cesarean births by reducing the likelihood of an outbreak near term.

Table 100-1   Drug and Dose for a Specific Type of HSV-2 Infection

Type of Infection or Therapy	Acyclovir	Famciclovir	Valacyclovir
Initial	400 mg tid for 10 days	250 mg PO tid for 10 days	1 g PO bid for 10 days
Recurrent	800 mg PO tid, for 2 days	1000 mg PO bid for 1 day	500 mg PO bid for 3 days
Suppressive	400 mg PO bid	250 mg PO bid	500 mg PO qd (<10 outbreaks/year) *or* 1000 mg PO qd (≥10 outbreaks/yr)

Topical lidocaine jelly 2% is a useful adjunct to oral antiviral drugs in managing severe first episodes in women. It should be applied frequently, and especially before voiding, but for no longer than 24 to 36 hours. There is a theoretical risk of sensitization, but this is very rarely seen in practice. Antifungal or antibacterial agents may be needed to treat secondary infections.

There is no evidence that salt baths, topical antiseptics, lysine, vitamins, or other nonmainstream remedies are more effective than placebo in the treatment or prevention of genital herpes.

Optimum Treatments

First Episodes

After diagnosis, assess the need for further immediate tests if there is clinical suspicion of syphilis, chancroid, primary HIV, or other infection. Tests include darkfield examination, serum for rapid plasma reagin, HIV p24 antigen or serum HIV RNA, or antibody testing.

Use of an oral antiviral for 7 to 10 days should be considered. Symptoms usually resolve in 3 to 4 days. If this is not the case, consider the possibility of secondary infection. Lesions persisting for longer than 14 days should prompt consideration of HIV coinfection, and one should consider repeat serologic testing for syphilis and examination for other genital infections after 2 to 4 weeks. If the initial HSV virologic test results were negative, HSV type-specific serology should be obtained 6 weeks and again 3 months after presentation. HIV testing is recommended for all individuals diagnosed with genital herpes.

Recurrent Episodes

Virologic specimens should be obtained from active lesions if the diagnosis has not yet been confirmed. Consider obtaining type-specific serology in patients with atypical lesions, negative virologic tests, or lesions that cannot be tested for the presence of HSV.

HIV testing should be strongly encouraged for those who have not been recently tested.

Other important considerations include episodic treatment with oral antiviral agents and counseling patients on treatment options, including continued episodic therapy that may be started at the first signs or symptoms of an outbreak, or suppressive therapy to prevent recurrences.

COUNSELING. First and most importantly, accurate information about all aspects of the disease should be provided. New diagnoses of genital herpes can be emotionally devastating and may make comprehension and retention of information difficult. Important information to cover at the first visit includes the following:

- The availability of effective therapy for primary infection
- The availability of effective therapy for recurrences
- Recurrent episodes tend to be milder than the initial episode
- Transmission of herpes usually occurs from a partner who was not aware of his or her infection or did not believe he or she was infectious when exposure occurred
- Daily suppressive therapy can reduce the risk for transmission by 50%
- Condom use more than 25% of the time can reduce transmission of HSV by 50%

Time should be taken at follow-up visits to address the patient's concerns and to provide appropriate counseling. Patients may be given written information and referred to Internet websites and telephone hotlines.

Prevention

The majority of patients once educated on the mild signs and symptoms of outbreaks will recognize symptomatic outbreaks. The following steps can help prevent the acquisition and transmission of genital herpes:

- Disclosure of HSV status to sexual partners
- Abstinence during outbreaks
- Condoms can reduce transmission, especially during the first 6 to 12 months after initial infection
- Choosing partners with like serologic status
- Daily suppressive therapy has been shown to reduce the risk for HSV transmission to an uninfected partner by about 50%

Avoiding Treatment Errors

Major issues in patients with HSV infections include (1) failure to actively investigate whether other sexually transmitted infections are present in the same individual and (2) failure to counsel infected patients on treatment options. It is also important to understand the need to treat HSV infection more aggressively in immunocompromised individuals.

Future Directions

Preventive and therapeutic vaccines are currently in phase 2 and 3 clinical trials. Clinical efficacy data on these vaccines will be available in 4 years. Even with an effective vaccine, questions concerning the acceptability of a sexually transmitted infection vaccine for the general public and whether the target population should be preteens or young adults will need to be addressed. The development of vaginal microbicides will offer women protection against HSV and a broad array of other sexually transmitted infections.

Additional Resources

American College of Obstetricians and Gynecologists. Available at: http://www.acog.com.
  This website provides the latest recommendations for ACOG guidelines on HSV and HSV management.
American Social Health Association. Available at: http://www.ashastd.org.
  This is one of the best sites for patients looking for the latest information on STDs in an easily understood yet complete manner.
ASHA National Herpes Hotline: (919) 361-8488.
  This hotline is the best immediate resource for herpes information.
Ebel C, Wald A: Managing Herpes: How to Live and Love with a Chronic STD. Research Triangle Park, NC, American Social Health Association, 2002.

This is one of the best overviews of genital herpes for patients. It provides important insights on the impact of diagnosis on patients and gives clear guidance for counseling.
Handsfield HH: Genital Herpes. New York, McGraw-Hill, 2001.
  This book provides a one-stop resource for clinicians and patients.
CDC Division of Sexually Transmitted Diseases. Available at: http://www.cdc.gov\std.
  The CDC provides the best public health site and the website for the STD Treatment Guidelines.
CDC National STD Hotline: English: (800) 227-8922, (800) 342-2437; Spanish: (800) 344-7432.
  This hotline is bilingual and offers an excellent service.
WebMD. Available at: http://www.webMD.com.
  This excellent site for patients and clinicians provides information on counseling patients concerning HSV.

EVIDENCE

1. Ashley RL, Wald A: Genital herpes: Review of the epidemic and potential use of type-specific serology. Clin Microbiol Rev 12:1-8, 1999.
    This excellent overview of the HSV epidemic addresses the utility of type-specific serology for diagnosis and counseling of genital herpes.
2. Corey L, Wald A, Patel R, et al: Once-daily valacyclovir to reduce the risk of genital herpes. N Engl J Med 350:11-20, 2004.
    The authors present pivotal data on the benefit of suppressive therapy to reduce the transmission risk of genital HSV-2.
3. Wald A: New therapies and prevention strategies for genital herpes. Clin Infect Dis 28(Suppl 1):S4-S13, 1999.
    This paper provides a summary for approach to treatment of this disease.
4. Workowski KA, Berman SM: Centers for Disease Control and Prevention: Sexually transmitted diseases treatment guidelines, 2006. MMWR Recomm Rep 55(RR-11):1-94, 2006.
    This article provides the latest and best expert guidance for treatment of genital herpes.
5. Xu F, Sternberg MR, Kottri BJ, et al: Trends in herpes simplex virus type 1 and type 2 seroprevalence in the United States. JAMA 296(8):964-973, 2006.
    The authors report on the latest population-based survey for the prevalence of HSV-1 and HSV-2 in the United States.

Adaora A. Adimora ▪ David J. Weber

101

Varicella-Zoster Infections

Introduction

Varicella-zoster virus (VZV), a large DNA virus, belongs to the family Herpesviridae and, like all herpesviruses, induces lifelong latent infection. VZV causes two clinical syndromes: varicella (chickenpox), a highly contagious childhood rash illness due to primary infection with VZV; and herpes zoster (shingles), usually a dermatomal vesicular rash caused by reactivation of latent VZV infection. Varicella is usually benign in immunocompetent children but causes substantially greater morbidity and mortality in adults, pregnant women, and immuno-compromised hosts. Herpes zoster can cause severe and prolonged pain and, like varicella, is sometimes much more severe in compromised hosts. Introduction of the varicella vaccine in the mid-1990s dramatically decreased the incidence of chickenpox in the United States, as well as hospitalizations and deaths due to vari-cella and its complications among children and adults.

Etiology and Pathogenesis

Primary infection occurs through airborne transmission of infectious droplets from vesicular skin lesions or respiratory secretions resulting in infection of the upper respiratory tract, followed by viral replication in regional lymph nodes, viremia, and subsequent infection of endo-thelial cells of the skin and the epidermis. The rash of varicella-zoster infection is characterized initially by clear vesicles that contain infectious virus. Vesicles become pus-tular with migration of polymorphonuclear cells and sub-sequently either rupture or resorb.

After primary VZV infection, the virus becomes latent in dorsal root ganglia. The factors that promote reactiva-tion and subsequent development of clinical herpes zoster are poorly understood.

Clinical Presentation

Varicella is extremely contagious; the reported attack rate among persons without previous infection exceeds 90%. Before the vaccination era, children aged 5 through 9 years were affected most commonly. About 10% of the U.S. population older than 15 years is susceptible to VZV infec-tion. Illness, characterized by rash, malaise, and fever, appears 8 to 21 days after infection. The rash, varicella's hallmark, begins as a vesicular eruption that occurs in crops of lesions over several days and spreads from the head to the trunk and finally to the extremities (Fig. 101-1). The skin lesions undergo a characteristic series of changes as vesicles umbilicate and then evolve into pus-tules and finally crusted papules. Varicella is contagious 1 or 2 days before the onset of rash and until all lesions have formed crusts.

Chickenpox in a previously immunized person (break-through varicella) is usually a mild illness, and the rash often differs from typical varicella. Patients with break-through infection have fewer lesions, and their rash tends to be papulovesicular or papular instead of vesicular. They can transmit varicella to others but do so less often than individuals with typical varicella.

Varicella is usually a benign illness in immunocompe-tent children; however, it is generally more severe in older adolescents and adults. In the neonate, it is associated with high mortality risk when maternal disease develops within 5 days before or 2 days after delivery. Disease may be severe in immunocompromised hosts of all ages. Varicella may cause fetal malformations (about 4% of infected mothers) if the mother develops disease, especially in the first trimester.

Complications include secondary skin infections, usually due to *Staphylococcus aureus* or *Streptococcus pyogenes*, which occur as a result of scratching the pruritic lesions. Pneu-monia is uncommon in children but complicates about 16% to 20% of adult infections, usually about 3 to 5 days after the onset of illness (see Fig. 101-1). Pneumonia is

Figure 101-1 Varicella Pneumonia.

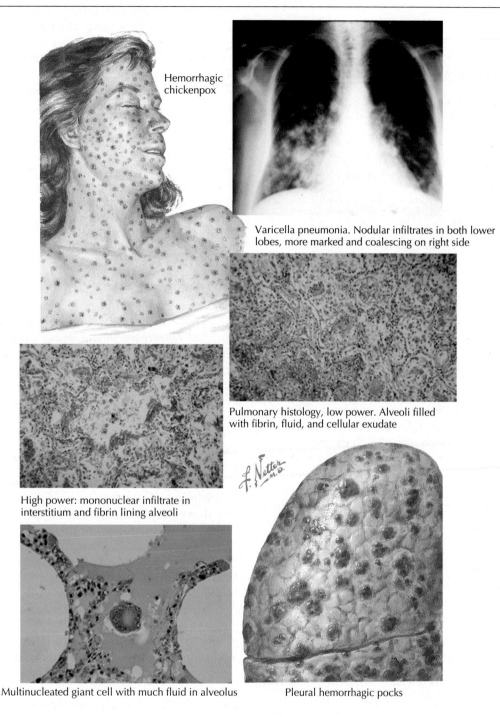

Hemorrhagic chickenpox

Varicella pneumonia. Nodular infiltrates in both lower lobes, more marked and coalescing on right side

Pulmonary histology, low power. Alveoli filled with fibrin, fluid, and cellular exudate

High power: mononuclear infiltrate in interstitium and fibrin lining alveoli

Multinucleated giant cell with much fluid in alveolus

Pleural hemorrhagic pocks

often associated with dyspnea, cough, and fever, but radiographic evidence of pneumonitis may develop in the absence of respiratory symptoms. Common radiographic findings include interstitial and nodular infiltrates. Morbidity is especially severe in pregnant women with varicella and pneumonia. Central nervous system complications include cerebellar ataxia, aseptic meningitis, encephalitis, Guillain-Barré syndrome, Reye's syndrome, and transverse myelitis. Myocarditis, hepatitis, nephritis, and arthritis are other complications.

Herpes zoster occurs at all ages, but incidence rises with old age and the waning of cell-mediated immunity. The first symptom is pain, followed within 48 to 72 hours by eruption of a unilateral maculopapular rash in a dermatomal distribution that subsequently becomes vesicular. The thoracic and lumbar dermatomes are most frequently

Figure 101-2 Herpes Zoster with Probable Keratitis.

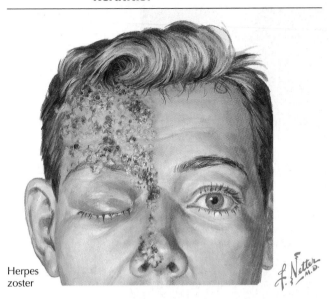

Herpes zoster

involved. Lesions usually persist for 10 to 15 days, but skin may not become completely normal for several weeks. Involvement of the trigeminal nerve may cause eye involvement (herpes zoster ophthalmicus), a potentially sight-threatening condition (Fig. 101-2). Zoster-associated pain and postherpetic neuralgia are the most troublesome symptoms and may be incapacitating, especially in persons older than 50 years. Pain is especially severe in the areas overlying the site of previous blisters. Risk factors for postherpetic neuralgia include increased age, sensory loss, and severity of pain. Prompt treatment with antiviral agents appears to decrease the risk for postherpetic neuralgia. Central nervous system involvement may present as meningoencephalitis or encephalitis. Herpes zoster is more severe in immunocompromised hosts than in normal hosts. Patients with lymphoma, for example, are at increased risk for cutaneous dissemination and visceral involvement.

Differential Diagnosis

Diagnostic considerations include disseminated herpes simplex virus, Coxsackie virus, echovirus, and atypical measles, but these infections more often cause a morbilliform rash than vesicular lesions. Appearance of impetigo can be similar to varicella, but unroofing of impetigo lesions should reveal gram-positive cocci due to *S. aureus* or *S. pyogenes*.

Diagnostic Approach

History and physical examination are usually sufficient for diagnosis. A characteristic skin rash in multiple stages of development should raise suspicion of varicella, especially in a person with a history of exposure. A dermatomally distributed vesicular rash should always raise the possibility of herpes zoster. Laboratory testing can help to define the diagnosis in equivocal cases. Vesicular skin lesions are scraped to obtain material for viral culture or performance of direct fluorescent antibody staining. Antibody testing with immune adherence hemagglutination assay, fluorescent antibody to membrane antigen assay, and enzyme-linked immunosorbent assay are occasionally helpful in demonstrating seroconversion or diagnostic rises in titer. Tzanck smears of lesions may reveal characteristic multinucleated giant cells, but sensitivity is only 60%. Such smears do not distinguish herpes simplex virus from VZV. Polymerase chain reaction assays to detect VZV DNA in cerebrospinal fluid are helpful in the diagnosis of central nervous system involvement.

Management and Therapy

Maintenance of good hygiene with bathing is important to decrease the risk for complications in patients with varicella. Fingernails should be cut closely to reduce risk for secondary infection. Dressings and antipruritic drugs can decrease itching. Oral acyclovir (800 mg 4 times daily by mouth for 5 to 7 days) or other similar drugs (i.e., valacyclovir, famciclovir) decrease the duration and number of lesions and reduce fever when given within 24 hours of onset and should be prescribed for adults and adolescents. Children at high risk for complications should also be treated.

In patients with varicella zoster, antiviral therapy with famciclovir (500 mg thrice daily for 7 days), valacyclovir (1 g thrice daily for 7 days), or acyclovir (800 mg 5 times daily for 7 to 10 days) speeds resolution of lesions and pain but is most efficacious when given within 3 days of onset of rash. Valacyclovir results in faster resolution of pain than acyclovir. The addition of prednisone to acyclovir improved pain and other quality-of-life measurements in one study; however, it should be used with caution in patients with diabetes mellitus and others at risk for complications of corticosteroid use. It is unknown whether administration of prednisone with valacyclovir or famciclovir provides additional benefit because these antivirals are more potent than acyclovir. Amitriptyline, desipramine, and gabapentin may be useful in decreasing postherpetic neuralgia.

Avoiding Treatment Errors

The most critical step in avoiding treatment errors is to make an accurate diagnosis as early during the clinical course of varicella-zoster infection as possible. Treatment efficacy is clearly dependent on the early initiation of antiviral therapy. As previously noted, varicella skin lesions are occasionally misdiagnosed as impetigo. This is one example of an error that could delay the use of antivirals and, in turn, lead to preventable complications, including a greater likelihood of postherpetic neuralgia.

Prevention

Varicella vaccine, a live attenuated virus vaccine, has at least a 95% to 99% efficacy and is approved for use in healthy children at least 12 months old and for susceptible adolescents and adults. All children should be routinely vaccinated between 12 and 18 months, and susceptible children should be vaccinated before their 13th birthday. Varicella-zoster immune globulin (VZIG) can be given after exposure to persons at high risk for complications (e.g., immunocompromised persons, pregnant women, premature infants [born at less than 28 weeks' gestation or birth weight of less than 1000 g]). Varicella immune globulin should be given within 96 hours of exposure. However, VZIG is no longer manufactured in the United States. It may be obtained from Canadian manufacturers but requires administration with informed consent and a research protocol. Although not approved by the U.S. Food and Drug Administration (FDA), antivirals administered at standard doses from postexposure days 8 through 21 have been successful in preventing varicella in immunocompromised persons.

A new vaccine, ZOSTAVAX, was recently approved by the FDA for prevention of VZV among people aged 60 years and older. This vaccine reduced the incidence of both zoster and postherpetic neuralgia in participants in a large clinical trial. Recommendations for use by the Advisory Committee on Immunization Practices are pending.

Future Directions

Introduction and widespread use of the varicella vaccine has changed the epidemiology of varicella infection. Long-term follow-up is essential to definitively determine whether revaccination is necessary and if there are new or different clinical manifestations in people whose waning vaccine immunity allows illness. Varicella may present different clinical manifestations as a result of the vaccine and new types of immunosuppressive therapy. Use of the newly approved zoster vaccine may dramatically decrease the incidence of zoster and postherpetic neuralgia in the future.

Additional Resources

Grose C, Zaia J: Varicella-zoster virus. In Gorbach SL, Bartlett JG, Blacklow NR (eds): Infectious Diseases, 2nd ed. Philadelphia, WB Saunders, 1998, pp 2120-2125.
This chapter provides a good general reference.

Nguyen HQ, Jumaan AO, Seward JF: Decline in mortality due to varicella after implementation of varicella vaccination in the United States. N Engl J Med 352(5):450-458, 2005.
The authors review the population impact of the varicella vaccine.

UpToDate. Available at: http://www.uptodateonline.com. Accessed November 29, 2006.
This website contains information for clinicians and patients.

Vazquez M, Shapiro ED: Varicella vaccine and infection with varicella-zoster virus. N Engl J Med 352(5):439-440, 2005.
This article provides additional perspective on the varicella vaccine.

Whitley R: Varicella-zoster virus. In Mandell GL, Bennett JE, Dolin R (eds): Mandell, Douglas, and Bennett's Principles and Practice of Infectious Diseases, 5th ed. Philadelphia, Churchill Livingstone, 2000, pp 1580-1586.
This chapter provides a good general review.

Whitley R: Varicella-zoster virus infections. In Braunwald E, Fauci AS, Kasper DL, et al (eds): Harrison's Principles of Internal Medicine, 15th ed. New York, McGraw-Hill, 2001.
This chapter provides a good general review.

EVIDENCE

1. Beutner KR, Friedman DJ, Forszpaniak C, et al: Valaciclovir compared with acyclovir for improved therapy for herpes zoster in immunocompetent adults. Antimicrob Agents Chemother 39(7):1546-1553, 1995.
   Valacyclovir administration to immunocompetent adults with herpes zoster older than 50 years resulted in faster resolution of pain than acyclovir in this randomized double-blind study.
2. Nyerges G, Meszner Z, Gyarmati E, Kerpel-Fronius S: Acyclovir prevents dissemination of varicella in immunocompromised children. J Infect Dis 157(2):309-313, 1988.
   In this randomized double-blind study of immunocompromised children with varicella and no signs of dissemination, acyclovir decreased time to full crusting of lesions.
3. Oxman MN, Levin MJ, Johnson GR, et al: A vaccine to prevent herpes zoster and postherpetic neuralgia in older adults. N Engl J Med 352(22):2271-2284, 2005.
   This large randomized placebo-controlled trial of the zoster vaccine demonstrates efficacy in preventing both zoster and postherpetic neuralgia in persons 60 years and older.
4. Wallace MR, Bowler WA, Murray NB, et al: Treatment of adult varicella with oral acyclovir. A randomized, placebo-controlled trial. Ann Intern Med 117(5):358-363, 1992.
   This randomized placebo-controlled trial demonstrates that early treatment (within 24 hours of rash onset) of adults with acyclovir decreased the time to healing of cutaneous varicella as well as duration of fever.

Cynthia Gay ▪ Joseph J. Eron

Encephalitis

Introduction

The term *encephalitis* refers to inflammation in the brain parenchyma caused by a broad range of infectious and noninfectious etiologies. This chapter primarily focuses on infectious encephalitis. Infectious encephalitis is considered a medical emergency because prompt initiation of treatment for specific pathogens, such as herpes simplex virus (HSV) and Rocky Mountain spotted fever (RMSF), can substantially decrease associated morbidity and mortality. Acute encephalitis, the most common form of fatal sporadic encephalitis in developed countries, is a frightening and potentially devastating manifestation of HSV infection.

Etiology and Pathogenesis

Encephalitis and meningitis share many features including a clinical presentation dominated by fever and headache. The presence of abnormal brain function in the case of pure encephalitis helps to distinguish the two syndromes; however, this distinction may be blurred when patients present with both parenchymal and meningeal involvement. Separating the two entities is important because the etiologies for meningitis and encephalitis vary considerably. The altered consciousness seen with infectious encephalitis reflects diffuse involvement of the cerebral cortex by an infectious pathogen or inflammation produced in response to infection. HSV-1, varicella-zoster virus (VZV), mumps, measles, and enteroviruses are the most common viral causes in immunocompetent hosts. HSV encephalitis has an estimated incidence of between 2 and 4 cases per million individuals per year, and accounts for about 10% to 20% of cases of viral encephalitis. Many arboviruses can cause encephalitis such as Japanese encephalitis and West Nile virus encephalitis. *Listeria monocytogenes* and *Rickettsia rickettsii* (the causative agent of RMSF) are bacterial causes of encephalitis. Important nonviral causes of encephalitis also include African trypanosomiasis in endemic regions and toxoplasmosis in immune-compromised individuals.

Central nervous system (CNS) invasion can occur through hematogenous spread from a primary site such as the respiratory tract (i.e., measles, mumps) or subcutaneous tissues (Eastern and Western equine virus). CNS infection can also result from retrograde transport from peripheral nerves, as in the case of rabies, or from retrograde transport from skin or mucous membranes into sensory ganglia, as occurs with HSV and VZV infection.

In the case of HSV, the virus enters through mucosal or cutaneous surfaces with initial local, sometimes subclinical, infection, which then leads to infection of autonomic or sensory nerve endings with subsequent transport to the nerve cell bodies in the ganglia. Most HSV encephalitis is caused by HSV-1. In initial infection, HSV replication occurs in the ganglia and surrounding neural tissue before the establishment of latency. In children and some young adults, HSV encephalitis may result from oral or labial infection and neurotropic extension through the olfactory bulb. In many adults, the presence of serologic or historical evidence of HSV-1 infection at the time of HSV encephalitis presentation suggests that the encephalitis is a manifestation of reactivation of latent infection in the ganglion with extension to the CNS. HSV DNA has also been identified with polymerase chain reaction (PCR) in brain tissue from individuals dying of non-neurologic causes; therefore, reactivation of latent infection within the CNS itself may be possible. Thus, HSV infection of the CNS can occur through three routes: (1) immediate CNS invasion through the trigeminal nerve following primary oropharyngeal HSV-1 infection; (2) HSV-1 reactivation followed by CNS invasion; and (3) in situ reactivation of HSV-1 within the CNS.

The temporal lobe is the characteristic site of infection early in the course of HSV encephalitis. This suggests a common mode of entry into the CNS, for example, from reactivation in the trigeminal ganglia and entry into the brain through the rami meningeals of the trigeminal nerve. In some cases, the HSV-1 variant associated with encephalitis differs from the variant isolated from a patient's oropharynx, suggesting that encephalitis may result from a second HSV infection. The encephalitis is caused by lytic HSV infection of neuronal and astroglial cells with associated necrosis of brain tissue. The infection may extend from the temporal lobe to other areas of the brain.

The differences in the clinical presentation of encephalitis due to various infectious agents may reflect differences in the types of cells infected in the CNS. Infection of neurons can cause focal or generalized seizures. Isolated demyelination, as can be seen by magnetic resonance imaging (MRI), may result from oligodendroglia involvement and cause stroke-like symptoms. Cortical infection or reactive parenchymal swelling can manifest as altered consciousness, and infection of brainstem neurons can cause coma or respiratory failure.

Histopathologic changes vary according to the infectious etiology, host immune response, and the stage of infection but generally show parenchymal damage, reactive gliosis, and the infiltration of inflammatory cells. Meningeal and perivascular mononuclear inflammation predominate in fatal viral encephalitis, although polymorphonuclear cells can be seen. Histologic changes also show degenerating neural cells and phagocytosis of neurons. The characteristic intranuclear inclusions associated with adenovirus, measles, and herpesvirus infections of other tissues are also seen in encephalitis, and Negri bodies are found in the brain tissue with rabies encephalitis. Vasculitis is prominent in encephalitis due to rickettsia.

Viral encephalitis can result from primary viral invasion of the CNS with neuronal involvement, or can be categorized as postinfectious encephalitis. In primary viral infection, neurons are affected, and the pathogen can be recovered. In postinfectious encephalitis, virus cannot be detected or recovered. Histopathologic changes in postinfectious encephalitis show perivascular mononuclear inflammation and perivenous demyelination with sparing of neurons. Histologic findings and the fact that the clinical onset usually begins as the primary infection is resolving or following subclinical illness suggest the syndrome is immune mediated. The clinical distinction between the two disorders is difficult, and some viruses, such as measles, have been associated with both.

Clinical Presentation

Infectious encephalitis is generally an uncommon manifestation of common infections and is most common in young children, adults older than 65 years, and the immunocompromised. Infection with the viruses associated with encephalitis usually does not result in clinically evident disease, with about 1% of St. Louis and West Nile infections causing symptoms of encephalitis. Eastern equine virus is an exception; infection with this virus frequently produces symptomatic encephalitis in all age groups.

Patients with encephalitis usually present with the acute onset of fever, headache, altered level of consciousness, and brain dysfunction. Altered consciousness can vary from mild lethargy to coma. Abnormal brain function encompasses behavioral and cognitive changes as well as focal neurologic signs and seizures. Clinical manifestations can range from agitation and acute memory disturbances to psychosis and unresponsiveness. Autonomic and hypothalamic disturbances, diabetes insipidus, and the syndrome of inappropriate antidiuretic hormone secretion can also complicate the clinical course. Focal neurologic findings usually develop during the course of encephalitis regardless of the pathogen, and focal and generalized seizures are common. Various other neurologic abnormalities may occur, including hemiparesis, hemianopsia, cranial nerve palsies, abnormal movements, and altered deep tendon reflexes. Meningitis presents similarly with fever, headache, and nuchal rigidity but is generally not associated with abnormal brain function, especially earlier in the disease process, and vomiting and photophobia may also be prominent.

The clinical presentation of encephalitis is usually nonspecific, although certain features can provide clues to specific causes. Parotitis is highly suggestive of mumps, and gastrointestinal symptoms increase the likelihood of enteroviral infection. A parkinsonian tremor has been associated with Japanese encephalitis. Flaccid paralysis in an immunocompromised host with possible mosquito exposure should prompt consideration of West Nile virus. Rabies encephalitis may be preceded by local paresthesias at the site of an animal bite and later evolve to pharyngeal spasms, hydrophobia, and aerophobia (Fig. 102-1). The presence of a rash may lend support to certain diagnoses: rash on the palms and soles with RMSF, the bull's eye lesion of Lyme disease, and the dermatomal, vesicular eruption characteristic of VZV. Focal neurologic findings such as personality change, seizure, hallucinations, and aphasia suggest localization to the temporal lobe and should raise suspicion for HSV encephalitis (Fig. 102-2). Behaviors may be bizarre with HSV encephalitis and include Kluver-Bucy syndrome—visual agnosia, excessive oral tendencies, placidity, altered sexual behavior, and changes in dietary habits. Other presentations include amnesia and hypomanic symptoms such as elevated mood, decreased need for sleep, and hypersexuality. In addition, dysphasia may present as a localizing finding with HSV encephalitis.

Encephalitis related to bacterial and viral pathogens is usually acute in onset; however, Lyme disease, as well as enteroviral, adenoviral, and toxoplasma encephalitis in immunocompromised patients, may present as a subacute process. Subacute presentation of neurologic symptoms with persistent fever is more common with parameningeal infections such as brain abscesses or tuberculous

Figure 102-1 Rabies.

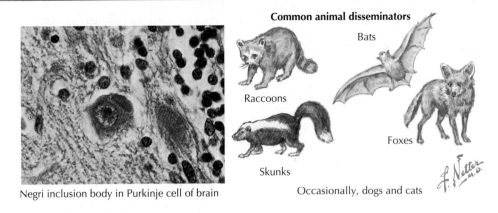

Negri inclusion body in Purkinje cell of brain

Common animal disseminators

Raccoons

Bats

Skunks

Foxes

Occasionally, dogs and cats

Figure 102-2 Herpes Simple Virus—Encephalitis.

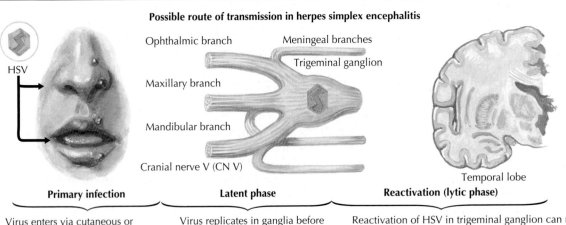

Possible route of transmission in herpes simplex encephalitis

HSV

Ophthalmic branch

Maxillary branch

Mandibular branch

Cranial nerve V (CN V)

Meningeal branches

Trigeminal ganglion

Temporal lobe

Primary infection

Virus enters via cutaneous or mucosal surfaces to infect sensory or autonomic nerve endings with transport to cell bodies in ganglia

Latent phase

Virus replicates in ganglia before establishing latent phase

Reactivation (lytic phase)

Reactivation of HSV in trigeminal ganglion can result in spread to brain (temporal lobe) via meningeal branches of CN V

Clinical features of HSV encephalitis

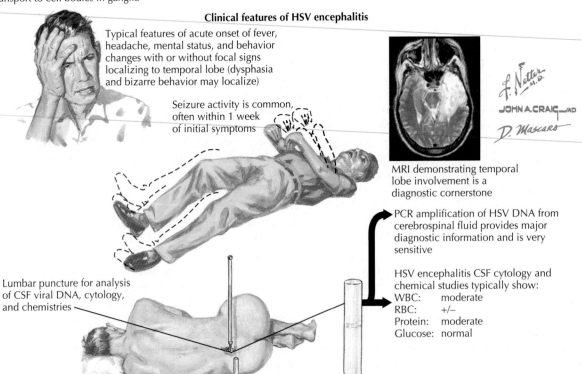

Typical features of acute onset of fever, headache, mental status, and behavior changes with or without focal signs localizing to temporal lobe (dysphasia and bizarre behavior may localize)

Seizure activity is common, often within 1 week of initial symptoms

MRI demonstrating temporal lobe involvement is a diagnostic cornerstone

PCR amplification of HSV DNA from cerebrospinal fluid provides major diagnostic information and is very sensitive

Lumbar puncture for analysis of CSF viral DNA, cytology, and chemistries

HSV encephalitis CSF cytology and chemical studies typically show:
WBC: moderate
RBC: +/−
Protein: moderate
Glucose: normal

Box 102-1   Differential Diagnosis of Encephalitis, Excluding Viral Pathogens

Noninfectious

Acute disseminated encephalomyelitis
Adrenal leukodystrophy
Drug-induced meningitis (NSAIDs, sulfa drugs,
  antithymocyte globulin, intravenous immune globulin)
Dural venous sinus thrombosis
Migrainous syndromes with pleocytosis
Neuro-Behçet's disease
Neuroleptic malignant syndrome
Primary and secondary tumors (meningeal or parenchymal)
Reye's syndrome
Sarcoidosis
Subdural hematoma
Systemic lupus erythematosus
Thyrotoxicosis
Toxic encephalopathy
Cerebral vasculitis

Infectious

Amebic infection
Bartonella henselae, disseminated
Brucella species infection
Cerebral malaria
Coxiella burnetii infection
Echinococcus granulosus infection
Fungal CNS infection (cryptococcosis, coccidioidomycosis,
  histoplasmosis, North American blastomycosis,
  candidiasis)
Legionella species infection
Listeria monocytogenes meningitis
Mycoplasma pneumoniae infection
Naegleria fowleri infection
Partially treated bacterial meningitis
Rickettsial (*R. rickettsii, R. typhi, R. prowazekii, Ehrlichia
  chaffeensis*) infection
Parameningeal infection (brain abscess, epidural or subdural
  abscess)
Prion disease
Salmonella typhi infection
Schistosomiasis
Spirochetal infection (syphilis, Lyme disease, leptospirosis)
Mycobacterium tuberculosis infection
Toxoplasmosis
Trypanosomiasis
Tuberculosis
Whipple's Disease (*Tropheryma whippelii*)

CNS, central nervous system; NSAIDs, nonsteroidal anti-inflammatory drugs.

meningitis. The onset of neurologic symptoms with postinfectious encephalitis is usually acute and occurs 2 to 12 days after symptom onset related to the primary infection.

Differential Diagnosis

There is a broad range of infectious and noninfectious syndromes that can cause encephalitis or present with similar clinical characteristics (Box 102-1). Bacterial meningitides, brain abscesses, and meningoencephalitis (e.g., *Listeria* species) should be excluded and may require empiric therapy until the appropriate diagnostic tests have been completed. Encephalopathy, due to intoxications and malaria, should be considered. Noninfectious causes include intracranial hemorrhage, CNS autoimmune diseases with or without systemic manifestations such as systemic lupus erythematosus, Wegener's granulomatosis, or primary CNS vasculitis. Thyrotoxicosis, neuroleptic malignant syndrome, and exposure to certain toxins or drugs also warrant consideration. Distinguishing encephalitis from meningitis narrows the differential and is critical in the case of HSV. HSV encephalitis can be fatal and cause significant morbidity, but HSV meningitis is usually a self-limited syndrome, typically caused by HSV-2 and associated with the primary episode. Other infectious causes of encephalitis include syphilis, tuberculosis, and opportunis-

tic CNS pathogens such as *Cryptococcus neoformans* or *Toxoplasma gondii* in undiagnosed or advanced HIV infection.

Common causes of viral encephalitis vary worldwide. Rabies is a common cause in India and Mexico; measles is the leading cause in Africa; and Japanese B encephalitis accounts for a large number of cases in China and Southeast Asia. Many viruses can cause encephalitis, and several have clinical features or a seasonal or geographic predilection that suggest their diagnosis (Table 102-1).

As previously noted, HSV encephalitis commonly presents with clinical deficits suggestive of temporal lobe necrosis, including personality changes, dysphasia, and seizures. Other herpesviruses can present similarly, including cytomegalovirus (CMV), VZV, and Epstein-Barr virus (EBV). Additional viral infections include enteroviral and vector-borne viral encephalitides (Eastern equine, St. Louis, and West Nile encephalitis, among others). Less common sporadic viral encephalitides, such as those related directly or indirectly to adenoviruses, influenza, mumps, measles, and acute HIV infection, should be considered (see Table 102-1).

Infectious causes are often suggested by seasonal variation, medical or travel history, or physical, laboratory, or radiologic examinations. HSV encephalitis occurs sporadically throughout the year and in patients of all ages,

Table 102-1   Viral Causes of Encephalitis

Viral Family	Virus	Location
Adenoviridae	Adenovirus	Worldwide
Bunyaviruses	California encephalitis	Midwest and Northeast United States, Southern Canada
	La Crosse	Northern United States
	Rift Valley	Sub-Saharan Africa
	Toscana	Europe
Enteroviruses	Coxsackie virus	Worldwide
	Echovirus	Worldwide
	Hepatitis A	Worldwide
	Poliovirus	—
Flaviviridae	Dengue	Central and South America, Caribbean, Southeast Asia, Africa
	Murray valley	Australia, New Guinea
	Japanese encephalitis virus	East and Southeast Asia, India
	St. Louis encephalitis	South and Central United States, Canada, Caribbean
	West Nile virus	United States, Israel, Mideast
Human herpesvirus (HHV)	Cytomegalovirus	Worldwide
	Epstein-Barr virus	Worldwide
	HHV-6 and HHV-7	Worldwide
	Herpes simple virus-1	Worldwide
	Herpes simplex virus-2	Worldwide
	Varicella-zoster virus	Worldwide
Orthomyxoviridae	Influenza A	Worldwide outbreaks, epidemics
Arenaviridae	Lymphocytic choriomeningitis virus	Europe and North and South America
	Junin	Argentina
	Lassa	Western Africa
	Machupo	Bolivia
Paramyxoviridae	Hendra	Australia
	Measles virus	Worldwide
	Mumps	Worldwide
	Nipah	Malaysia, Singapore, Bangladesh
Polyomavirus	JC virus	Worldwide
Rhabdoviridae	Rabies	Worldwide
	Lyssavirus	Australia
Reoviridae	Colorado tick fever	Rocky Mountains of United States
Retroviruses	HIV	Worldwide
Rubivirus	Rubella	Worldwide
Togaviruses	Eastern equine encephalitis	Eastern and Gulf coasts of United States, Caribbean, South America
	Venezuelan equine encephalitis	South and Central America, Florida, Southwest United States
	Western equine	Western United States and Canada

although it may be more common in adolescents and young adults and in individuals older than 50 years. In contrast, viral encephalitides due to arboviruses occur when mosquitoes and ticks are active in respective locales. In temperate regions, mosquito-borne encephalitis tends to peak in late summer, and tick-borne encephalitides occur primarily in late spring and summer. Most arboviruses also have specific geographic distributions (see Table 102-1) related to their animal hosts and vectors. Eastern equine virus occurs predominantly in coastal marshlands of the Atlantic and Gulf coasts of North and South America, whereas St. Louis encephalitis virus infection occurs most commonly in the Midwest and Southern region of the United States. Enterovirus causes encephalitis predominately in the late summer and fall. Viruses associated with

postinfectious encephalitis include mumps, measles, VZV, EBV, rubella, and influenza.

Travel and outdoor exposure to locales with prevalent tick populations also raise the possibility of nonviral etiologies such as RMSF, Lyme disease, or Colorado tick fever. Lyme disease should be considered with exposure in areas where *Borrelia* species are endemic, such as the Northeastern United States and Europe. Additional animal exposures and geography can further broaden the differential. Nipah virus was first identified following an outbreak of encephalitis among pig farm workers in Malaysia and was subsequently also found in Singapore and Bangladesh. Nipah virus is one of several emerging infections that cause encephalitis and mandates consideration of evolving epidemiologic patterns, particularly with arboviruses. The

West Nile virus was first discovered in North America during an epidemic in 1999 and has since demonstrated substantial geographic expansion attributed to bird migration. Japanese encephalitis was initially focused in China and southeastern Asia but has expanded into India, Pakistan, Russia, the Philippines, and Australia. Other previously unknown pathogens that were responsible for recent outbreaks of encephalitis include hendra virus isolated from horses and humans in Australia, and Australian bat Lyssavirus, which causes a rabies-like disease.

Patients with immune deficiency can also present with subacute or chronic encephalitis due to toxoplasmosis or enteroviruses. Additional causes of encephalitis in individuals who are immunosuppressed due to AIDS or medications include CNS infection with *Histoplasma* species, CMV, JC virus (progressive multifocal leukoencephalopathy), and less commonly *Cryptococcus* species infection, which typically causes meningitis.

HSV-1 encephalitis does not occur more commonly in immune-suppressed patients despite an increased frequency and severity of mucocutaneous HSV-1 infections in this population. Accordingly, it has been postulated that much of the pathophysiology of CNS HSV-1 infection is immune mediated and may explain the subacute presentation and mild histopathologic changes on biopsy specimens that can occur in immunosuppressed patients with HSV encephalitis.

Diagnostic Approach

Diagnostic tests should be guided by medical history, with careful attention to geography, recent travel history, occupation, season, animal and insect exposures, and the immune status of the patient. History should be sought from relatives or other contacts if the patient cannot provide this information because of altered neurologic status. Peripheral blood tests are rarely useful but may show a lymphocytosis common with viral encephalitis. They may also detect malaria or atypical lymphocytes associated with EBV infection. MRI of the brain is the preferred imaging technique because it more sensitive than computed tomography (CT) for the detection of edema and inflammation seen early in encephalitis. Brain imaging by CT or MRI is preferable in patients presenting with mental status changes before lumbar puncture, to evaluate for space-occupying lesions and brain abscesses, and to determine the risk for herniation. Lumbar puncture should be delayed for evidence of elevated intracranial pressure on imaging, for status epilepticus, and immediately after generalized seizure, coagulopathy, or severe thrombocytopenia.

Timely cerebrospinal fluid (CSF) examination is critical and should include opening pressure measurement, cellular analysis, protein, glucose, viral culture, and appropriate PCR and serologic testing, as dictated by history and probable infectious causes. Bacterial and fungal stains and cultures should be obtained given the overlap in clinical presentation between meningitis, meningoencephalitis, and parameningeal infections. Acid-fast bacillus stain and culture should be performed on immunocompromised hosts and considered in immunocompetent hosts at high risk for tuberculous meningitis.

The initial CSF examination may not distinguish aseptic or bacterial meningitis from viral encephalitis. However, the absence of a pleocytosis suggests a noninfectious cause, unless the patient is severely immunosuppressed and unable to mount an inflammatory response. CSF findings characteristic of viral infectious encephalitis include a predominantly mononuclear pleocytosis, ranging from 10 to 2000 cells/mm^3, but usually less than 250 cells/mm^3. Early in the course, a neutrophil predominance can occur, and a repeat lumbar puncture 8 to 24 hours later is often useful to evaluate for cellular evolution. CSF protein is usually normal or mildly elevated. A significant decrease in CSF glucose is unusual in viral encephalitis, in contrast to a characteristic decrease with tuberculous, bacterial, fungal, and amebic infections. CSF findings of a lymphocytic pleocytosis with a reduced glucose are strongly associated with tuberculous meningoencephalitis. An increased number of red blood cells in the absence of a traumatic tap suggests HSV and hemorrhagic encephalitis, or listerial and primary amebic meningoencephalitis. In contrast, CSF examination with bacterial meningitis characteristically shows a more significant pleocytosis of more than 2000 cells/mm^3 with a neutrophil predominance, a protein concentration of more than 200 mg/dL, and hypoglycorrhachia.

Viral culture has been the gold standard for diagnosis of viral encephalitis, but specific PCR for viral DNA amplification technique has advanced diagnostic testing considerably and is currently available for HSV-1, HSV-2, VZV, human herpesvirus-6 and -7, CMV, EBV, enteroviruses, respiratory viruses, HIV, and *Chlamydia pneumoniae* and *Mycobacterium tuberculosis* on CSF. Advantages of this technique include excellent sensitivity and specificity and rapid response times on a small amount of CSF fluid. PCR detection of HSV DNA is the gold standard diagnostic test and has 98% sensitivity and 94% to 100% specificity, and is positive early in the course. Diagnostic yield is highest in the first week of illness and decreases substantially and sequentially in the second and third weeks following symptom onset. Diagnostic workup for encephalitis should generally include PCR for HSV, enteroviruses, and West Nile virus. Additional PCR and serologic testing work will vary according to travel and exposure history and immune status. In some cases, testing for rabies, mumps, EBV, and HIV should be considered. All immunocompromised individuals should have a cryptococcal antigen test and PCR for CMV performed on CSF.

PCR tests have largely replaced serum and CSF antibody tests because they are more rapid and because interpretation of antibody tests can be more difficult. Elevated viral antibody titers may be nonspecific and reflect polyclonal activation due to infection, previous infection, or reactivation rather than primary infection. However, the detection of specific immunoglobulin M in the CSF does suggest CNS infection. Many viral causes require acute and convalescent serologies for diagnosis, and serum during the acute phase should be tested or saved for later testing, as indicated by the history.

Chest radiography should be obtained in consideration of mycoplasma, legionella, or tuberculosis. MRI of the brain can be useful in diagnosing HSV encephalitis showing abnormalities ranging from localized edema with increased signal on T2-weighted images to large areas with radiographic evidence of frank necrosis and hemorrhage. However, only minimal abnormalities may be seen early in the disease (see Fig. 102-2). MRI of the brain is the preferred imaging method because CT of the brain has only about 50% sensitivity for detecting temporal lobe abnormalities early in the disease. Electroencephalogram is rarely diagnostic except in the case of HSV encephalitis. However, it is sensitive in demonstrating early cerebral involvement and in distinguishing encephalopathy from infectious encephalitis.

Management and Therapy

There are many treatable, nonviral infections that can present similarly and for which diagnosis should be aggressively sought (see Box 102-1). Treatment of bacterial, fungal, and parasitic causes of encephalitis is pathogen specific and will not be covered here. Most viral encephalitis cases remain undiagnosed, but studies have shown VZV and HSV-1 to be commonly involved pathogens. Specific therapy for viral encephalitides is limited. Therefore, supportive care is paramount and may include airway intubation, sedation, and mechanical ventilation when mental status is significantly compromised. The potential for rapid deterioration requires that even patients with minimal alteration in sensorium be carefully observed.

HSV is the most important viral cause of encephalitis to consider because it can be fatal, can cause serious morbidity, and is treatable. The therapy of choice for HSV encephalitis is intravenous acyclovir. Acyclovir administration should not be delayed for diagnostic certainty, but initiated as soon as the diagnosis is entertained and while awaiting results of HSV PCR testing. Acyclovir has poor oral bioavailability and must be given at high doses (10 to 15 mg/kg) intravenously every 8 hours for 14 to 21 days to ensure adequate levels in the CNS and prevent relapse. In the initial comparative study with vidarabine, acyclovir reduced mortality by 50% (from 54% to 28%). Therefore, despite the fact that HSV-1 is very sensitive to inhibition by acyclovir, death or serious sequelae related to HSV encephalitis remain common, especially if therapy is initiated when the patient is near coma or comatose. Even with acyclovir therapy, only 38% of patients with confirmed HSV encephalitis were considered to be functioning normally 6 months after infection, although only 9% were considered to have moderate debility. Long-term cognitive and memory impairments are not uncommon.

Acyclovir is also indicated for VZV encephalitis at the same doses and duration. If PCR testing for HSV and VZV is negative, acyclovir should, in most cases, be discontinued. Most recommendations include acyclovir for herpes B encephalitis transmitted from infected macaques monkeys given a high fatality rate; however, supportive data are limited. Combination therapy with ganciclovir (5 mg/kg intravenously twice daily) and foscarnet (60 mg/kg every 8 hours or 90 mg/kg every 12 hours) is the preferred treatment for CMV encephalitis. Antiretroviral therapy should be continued or initiated in AIDS patients with CMV encephalitis.

Corticosteroid use for encephalitis remains controversial and is generally advised only for vasculitis due to severe VZV encephalitis or severe and progressive vasogenic edema with a short course (3 to 5 days) of high-dose dexamethasone or methylprednisolone. Supportive and symptomatic management remains crucial, particularly for most viral causes without specific therapy. Brain biopsy is generally considered only if the cause remains unknown and the patient fails to improve, or if surgical decompression is indicated for refractory increased intracranial pressure. Prognosis is dependent on the specific pathogen, the immune status of the host, and timely initiation of appropriate treatment. Isolation precautions are not indicated for community-acquired infective encephalitis, unless rabies or contagious, viral hemorrhagic fever is suspected. Vaccines are available for hepatitis A, influenza, Japanese encephalitis, measles, mumps, polio, and rabies.

Avoiding Treatment Errors

Failure to consider encephalitis and its causes in the differential diagnosis of a patient who presents with fever and headache is a common error that delays diagnosis and initiation of appropriate therapy for treatable causes of encephalitis, such as HSV, *Listeria* species infection, and RMSF. If fever and headache are more prominent than subtle cognitive abnormalities, clinicians may focus more on the diagnosis and treatment of meningitis and may not collect historical clues needed to construct and unravel the differential diagnosis of encephalitis. Broader initial therapy, including acyclovir, doxycycline, ampicillin, or a combination, may avoid sequelae of encephalitis such as persistent neurologic deficits or death.

A delay in performing a lumbar puncture, indicated in almost all patients presenting with fever, headache, nuchal rigidity, or altered mental status, may also impede diagnosis and administration of effective therapy. Not uncommonly, HSV PCR is not performed on the initial CSF sample, which can delay diagnosis and treatment and necessitate repeat lumbar puncture for additional diagnostic studies. Neither a negative MRI nor CT of the brain can definitively rule out encephalitis because both can be normal early in the disease. Administration of antibiotics before lumbar puncture frequently complicates the interpretation of CSF findings and may make distinguishing between partially treated bacterial meningitis and viral encephalitis of unknown etiology difficult, necessitating a prolonged course of intravenous antibiotics for the former. A careful and thorough history, including travel, occupation, and exposures, is critical in generating a full differential diagnosis because historical information could point to specific etiologies not otherwise considered such as intoxication or tuberculosis.

Future Directions

Advances in PCR testing have provided newer and more rapid diagnostic tests for encephalitis. Currently available PCR tests can be expected to become more widely available, and newer tests for additional etiologies are likely. Multiplex PCR tests in which individual PCR tests are combined into microarrays are a promising new technique for the detection and genotyping of microbes. Microarray-based detection could become a rapid and efficient standard diagnostic technique in the future if the sensitivity improves and the cost is not prohibitive. The past decade has witnessed encephalitis outbreaks due to the expansion of known arboviruses into new geographic distributions and the appearance of encephalitides due to previously unknown pathogens. These trends are likely to continue. New drugs for the treatment of common causes of encephalitis, particularly viral pathogens, are urgently needed. The mortality rate of patients with untreated HSV encephalitis approaches 70%, and most survivors have serious neurologic sequelae. Thus, the wider availability of HSV PCR testing, as well as PCR tests for other etiologies, will allow more rapid diagnosis and initiation of indicated treatment.

Additional Resources

Bellini WJ, Harcourt BH, Bowden N, et al: Nipah virus: An emergent paramyxovirus causing severe encephalitis in humans. J Neurovirol 11:481-487, 2005.

A review of henipaviruses includes their virology and epidemiology and the clinical presentation of Nipah virus infection.

Hayes EB, Gubler DJ: West Nile virus: Epidemiology and clinical features of an emerging epidemic in the United States. Annu Rev Med 57:181-194, 2006.

A comprehensive review of West Nile Virus, including updated data on epidemiology and clinical manifestations with symptomatic infection.

Koskiniemi M, Rantalaiho T, Piiparinen H, et al: Infections of the central nervous system of suspected viral origin: A collaborative study from Finland. J Neurovirol 7(5):400-408, 2001.

This article reviews the causes of acute central nervous system symptoms in 3231 patients suspected of related viral infection; 46% of cases were due to viral infection, with varicella-zoster virus the most common cause, followed by herpes simplex virus and enteroviruses.

Koskiniemi M, Piiparinen H, Rantalaiho T, et al: Acute central nervous system complications in varicella zoster virus infections. J Clin Virol 25(3):293-301, 2002.

This study of 174 patients with CNS infection due to varicella-zoster infection defined the best diagnostic approach.

Mackenzie JS: Emerging zoonotic encephalitis viruses: Lessons from Southeast Asia and Oceania. J Neurovirol 11:434-440, 2005.

The author presents an updated review of emerging viral infections with a focus on Japanese encephalitis virus, tick-borne encephalitis virus, Nipah virus, hendra virus, and Australian bat Lyssavirus.

EVIDENCE

1. Chaudhuri A, Kennedy PG: Diagnosis and treatment of viral encephalitis. Postgrad Med J 78(924):575-583, 2002.

   This comprehensive review of the diagnostic investigations and treatment of viral encephalitis gives special attention to distinguishing between viral encephalitis and encephalopathy. The authors provide clear recommendations for the diagnostic approach to infectious encephalitis and a more detailed discussion of encephalitis due to HSV, CMV, and Nipah virus.

2. Corey L: Herpes simplex virus. In Mandell GL, Bennett JE, Dolin R (eds): Mandell, Douglas, and Bennett's Principles and Practice of Infectious Diseases, 6th ed. Philadelphia, Churchill Livingstone, 2005, pp 1762-1780.

   The author has written a comprehensive review of herpes simplex virus including pathogenesis, clinical presentations, and treatment recommendations.

3. Griffin DE: Encephalitis, myelitis, and neuritis. In Mandell GL, Bennett JE, Dolin R (eds): Mandell, Douglas, and Bennett's Principles and Practice of Infectious Diseases, 6th ed. Philadelphia, Churchill Livingstone, 2005, pp 1143-1147.

   This comprehensive review of encephalitis and myelitis due to infectious and noninfectious causes encompasses the distinctive pathogenesis and pathologic findings of encephalitis, as well as the clinical, laboratory, neuroimaging, and epidemiologic characteristics. It includes an in-depth discussion of the lumbar puncture procedure and CSF evaluation.

4. Jääskeläinen AJ, Piiparinen H, Lappalainen, et al: Multiplex-PCR and oligonucleotide microarray for detection of eight different herpes viruses from clinical specimens. J Clin Virol 37(2):83-90, 2006.

   This paper documents findings from an evaluation of multiplex PCRs and microarray for the detection of eight herpesviruses compared with conventional PCR tests on CSF, whole blood, plasma, and serum. Microarray detected 94% (214 of 227) of herpes viruses positive by conventional PCR testing.

5. Klein RS: Herpes simplex virus type 1 encephalitis. UpToDate. Last updated September 27, 2005. Available at: http://www.uptodateonline.com.

   The author provides a thorough review of the pathogenesis, clinical manifestations, diagnosis, treatment, and outcomes of encephalitis due to HSV-1.

6. Lakeman FD, Whitley RJ: Diagnosis of herpes simplex encephalitis: Application of polymerase chain reaction to cerebrospinal fluid from brain-biopsied patients and correlation with disease. National Institute of Allergy and Infectious Diseases Collaborative Antiviral Study Group. J Infect Dis 171(4):857-863, 1995.

   The authors review the findings of a study evaluating the sensitivity of PCR detection of HSV in CSF as compared with isolation of HSV from tissue from brain biopsy.

7. Schmutzhard E: Viral infections of the CNS with special emphasis on herpes simplex infections. J Neurol 248:469-477, 2001

   The author reviews CNS infections due to herpes simplex and herpes zoster. This article includes an extensive compilation of viruses causing CNS infection and a thorough differential diagnosis for HSV encephalitis.

8. Steiner I, Budka H, Chaudhuri A, et al: Viral encephalitis: A review of diagnostic methods and guidelines for management. Eur J Neurol 12(5):331-343, 2005.

    The European Federation of Neurological Societies (EFNS) task force published a systematic review of the literature from 1966 to May of 2004 and present an up-to-date comparison of diagnostic investigations including neuroimaging, viral culture, PCR testing, serological testing, antigen detection and histopathology, and a review of the management of viral encephalitis.

9. Whitley RJ, Cobbs CG, Alford CA Jr, et al: Diseases that mimic herpes simplex encephalitis. Diagnosis, presentation, and outcome. NIAD Collaborative Antiviral Study Group. JAMA 262:234-239, 1989.

    This report is on diagnoses following brain biopsy in a study of patients suspected of having herpes simplex encephalitis.

10. Whitley RJ, Gnann JW: Viral encephalitis: Familiar infections and emerging pathogens. Lancet 359(9305):507-513, 2002.

    The authors review the pathogenesis, clinical manifestations, and diagnosis of viral encephalitis. The epidemiology, clinical presentation, diagnosis, and treatment of viral encephalitis due to HSV, B virus, rabies, enterovirus, and several arthropod-borne viruses are reviewed in more detail.

11. Zunt JR, Marra CM: Cerebrospinal fluid testing for the diagnosis of central nervous system infection. Neurol Clin 17:675-689, 1999.

    The authors review CSF testing for the diagnosis of CNS infection due to bacteria, virus, fungi, and prion disease.

David J. Weber ▪ Peter A. Leone ▪ William A. Rutala

103

Pulmonary Tuberculosis

Introduction

Tuberculosis remains a major scourge of humankind, with an estimated one third of the world's population currently infected. Worldwide, more than 8 million persons develop active tuberculosis each year, leading to an estimated 1.9 million deaths. Worldwide, coinfection with HIV and tuberculosis represents a public health crisis because it is the leading cause of HIV-related morbidity and mortality in developing countries. In the United States, 14,097 (4.8 cases per 100,000 population) were reported in 2005, the lowest rate ever recorded. Overall, an estimated 15 million Americans are infected with *Mycobacterium tuberculosis*. The incidence of tuberculosis in the United States varies independently by age and gender, with higher rates reported among older persons and men. In 2005, disparities in tuberculosis rates persisted among members of racial and ethic minority populations. In descending order, the highest rates per 100,000 population were reported among Asians (29.6), Native Hawaiians or other Pacific Islanders (16.1), non-Hispanic blacks (11.7), Hispanics (10.3), American Indians or Alaska Natives (8.2), and non-Hispanic whites (1.4). Foreign-born persons accounted for 54.3% of all tuberculosis cases. The percentage of foreign-born persons among all persons with tuberculosis has risen steadily since 1993, when foreign-born persons accounted for 29% of U.S. cases.

Etiology and Pathogenesis

Human tuberculosis is caused by three closely related mycobacteria grouped in the *Mycobacterium tuberculosis* complex: *M. tuberculosis*, *M. bovis*, and *M. africanum*. They are aerobic, non–spore-forming, nonmotile, slightly curved or straight bacilli, 0.2 to 0.6 μm × 1.0 to 10 μm in size. Their cell walls have a high lipid content that render them impermeable to Gram staining (termed *acid-fastness*). Most laboratories use a fluorochrome stain that allows visualization of the mycobacteria using a fluorescent microscope (Fig. 103-1).

In the United States, *M. tuberculosis* is the only important human pathogen in the *M. tuberculosis* complex. It is found worldwide, and humans are the only known reservoir. *M. bovis*, an important pathogen in developing countries, is most commonly acquired from cattle by ingestion of contaminated milk. The disease produced in humans by *M. bovis* is virtually indistinguishable from that caused by *M. tuberculosis* and is treated similarly. Bacille Calmette-Guérin (BCG), an attenuated strain of *M. bovis*, is used in many parts of the world as a vaccine to prevent tuberculosis. Although there is evidence that BCG vaccine protects against disseminated tuberculosis and meningitis in children, the efficacy of BCG to protect against pulmonary disease has not been proved.

Tuberculosis is spread from person to person through the air by droplet nuclei, particles 1 to 5 μm in diameter that contain *M. tuberculosis* (Fig. 103-2). Droplet nuclei are produced when persons with pulmonary or laryngeal tuberculosis cough, sneeze, speak, or sing. *M. tuberculosis* infection occurs if, after inhalation of infective droplet nuclei, viable bacilli survive the initial host defenses. The organisms grow for 2 to 10 weeks, at which time they elicit a cellular immune response that can be detected by a reaction to the tuberculin skin test (TST). Before development of cellular immunity, tubercle bacilli spread through the lymphatics to the hilar lymph nodes and then through the bloodstream to distant sites. Tuberculous disease (tuberculosis) will develop at some time in about 10% of individuals who acquire tuberculous infection and are not provided preventive therapy.

The interaction between HIV and tuberculosis is synergistic, each increasing the pathogenicity of the other. Unlike many of the pathogens associated with HIV that lead to disease only in the later stages of HIV infection

Figure 103-1 Tuberculosis: Sputum Examination (Stained Smear).

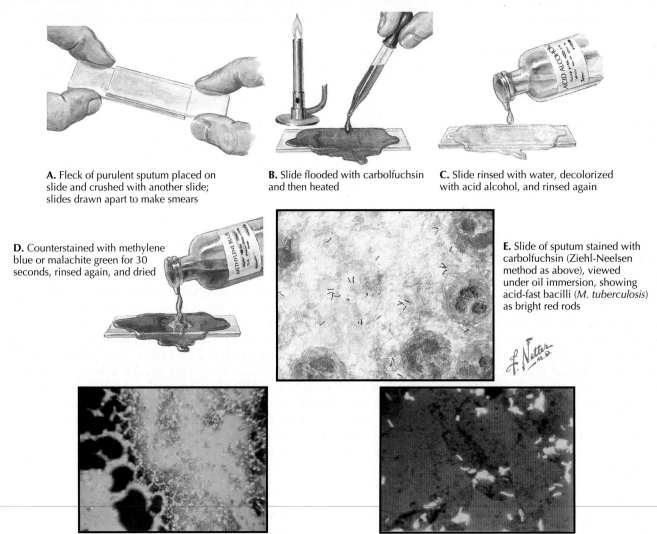

A. Fleck of purulent sputum placed on slide and crushed with another slide; slides drawn apart to make smears

B. Slide flooded with carbolfuchsin and then heated

C. Slide rinsed with water, decolorized with acid alcohol, and rinsed again

D. Counterstained with methylene blue or malachite green for 30 seconds, rinsed again, and dried

E. Slide of sputum stained with carbolfuchsin (Ziehl-Neelsen method as above), viewed under oil immersion, showing acid-fast bacilli (*M. tuberculosis*) as bright red rods

F. *M. tuberculosis* stained with auramine O, which causes acid-fast bacilli to fluoresce (×200)

G. Auramine O stain of *M. kansasii* (acid-fast "atypical" mycobacteria), which are much larger than *M. tuberculosis* (×200)

(e.g., *Pneumocystis carinii*, *Toxoplasma* species, cytomegalovirus), *M. tuberculosis* causes disease at any stage of HIV infection.

Clinical Presentation

Primary tuberculosis is generally a self-limited, mild pneumonic illness that often goes undiagnosed. Primary infection may result in granulomas visible on chest radiography. Most pulmonary tuberculosis infections are inapparent radiographically. Thus, the only indication that infection has occurred is a positive TST or whole blood interferon-γ (IFN-γ) assay.

The symptoms of tuberculosis are protean and nonspecific and can be classified as either systemic or organ spe-

cific. Classic systemic symptoms include fever (present in about 35% to 85%), night sweats, unexplained weight loss, anorexia, and fatigue. Laboratory findings may include an increased peripheral blood leukocyte count (about 10%), anemia (about 10%), and occasionally, an increased monocyte or eosinophil count. The lung is the most common site involved, accounting for 80% of cases reported to the Centers for Disease Control and Prevention (CDC; Fig. 103-3). Organ-specific symptoms in pulmonary tuberculosis include cough, pleuritic chest pain, and hemoptysis. In primary tuberculosis, chest radiographs often show infiltrates in the middle or lower lung zones, with ipsilateral hilar adenopathy (see Fig. 103-3). In reactivation tuberculosis, classic radiographic findings include upper lobe infiltrates, frequently with cavitation. In patients infected with HIV with less than 200 CD4 cells/mm^3, the radiographic

Figure 103-2 Dissemination of Tuberculosis.

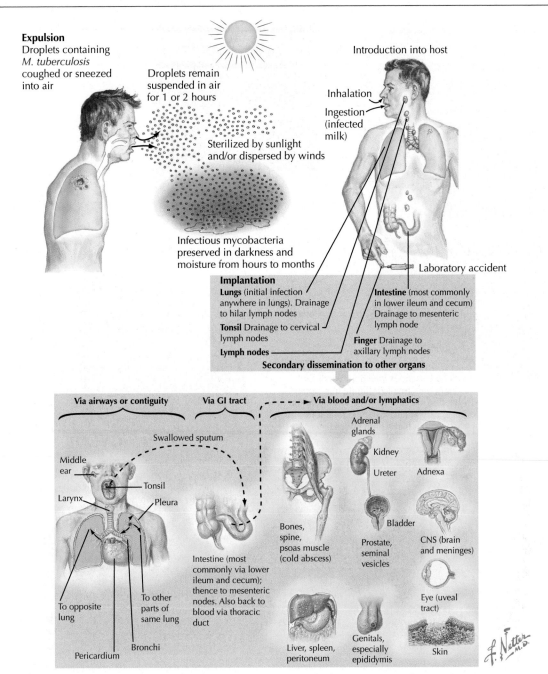

Expulsion
Droplets containing *M. tuberculosis* coughed or sneezed into air

Droplets remain suspended in air for 1 or 2 hours

Sterilized by sunlight and/or dispersed by winds

Infectious mycobacteria preserved in darkness and moisture from hours to months

Introduction into host

Inhalation

Ingestion (infected milk)

Laboratory accident

Implantation
Lungs (initial infection anywhere in lungs). Drainage to hilar lymph nodes

Tonsil Drainage to cervical lymph nodes

Lymph nodes

Intestine (most commonly in lower ileum and cecum) Drainage to mesenteric lymph node

Finger Drainage to axillary lymph nodes

Secondary dissemination to other organs

Via airways or contiguity   **Via GI tract**   **Via blood and/or lymphatics**

Swallowed sputum

Middle ear
Tonsil
Larynx
Pleura
To opposite lung
To other parts of same lung
Pericardium
Bronchi

Intestine (most commonly via lower ileum and cecum); thence to mesenteric nodes. Also back to blood via thoracic duct

Adrenal glands
Kidney
Ureter
Adnexa
Bladder
Bones, spine, psoas muscle (cold abscess)
Prostate, seminal vesicles
CNS (brain and meninges)
Eye (uveal tract)
Liver, spleen, peritoneum
Genitals, especially epididymis
Skin

findings frequently are atypical: cavitation is uncommon; lower lung zone or diffuse infiltrates and mediastinal adenopathy are frequent; and extrapulmonary disease occurs in about half of cases.

Extrapulmonary tuberculosis may involve the pleura, lymphatics, bone or joints, genitourinary system, meninges, peritoneal cavity, or other sites. It often presents a diagnostic challenge with varied symptoms and signs depending on the organ system involved. Signs and symptoms of disseminated tuberculosis are generally nonspe-

cific and include fever, weight loss, night sweats, anorexia, and weakness. A productive cough is common because most patients with disseminated disease also have pulmonary tuberculosis. Physical findings are variable but often include fever, wasting, hepatomegaly, pulmonary findings, lymphadenopathy, and splenomegaly. Small, 1- to 2-mm granulomas are visible on chest radiography in about 85% of patients. These lesions that look like millet seeds have led to disseminated disease being termed *miliary tuberculosis*.

Figure 103-3 Initial (Primary) Tuberculous Complex.

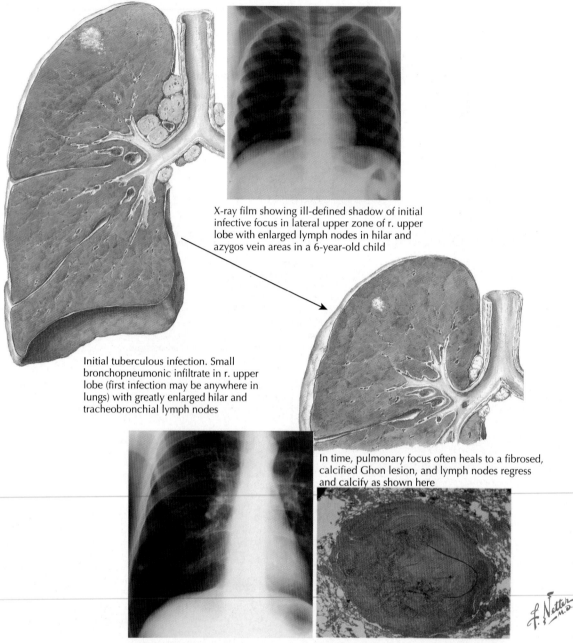

X-ray film showing ill-defined shadow of initial infective focus in lateral upper zone of r. upper lobe with enlarged lymph nodes in hilar and azygos vein areas in a 6-year-old child

Initial tuberculous infection. Small bronchopneumonic infiltrate in r. upper lobe (first infection may be anywhere in lungs) with greatly enlarged hilar and tracheobronchial lymph nodes

In time, pulmonary focus often heals to a fibrosed, calcified Ghon lesion, and lymph nodes regress and calcify as shown here

Calcified Ghon lesion in lateral portion of r. lower lobe

Section of a very inspissated, dried-out focus with fibrous capsule

Differential Diagnosis

Patients with pulmonary tuberculosis may present with acute or chronic disease. The differential diagnosis of acute infection includes the common viral and bacterial causes of pneumonia such as *Streptococcus pneumoniae, Haemophilus influenzae, Mycoplasma* species, and respiratory viruses. Chronic infection may be confused with noninfectious causes of pulmonary disease, including sarcoidosis, collagen vascular diseases, autoimmune diseases, and cancer. It may also be confused with other causes of chronic pulmonary infection, especially endemic fungi (blastomycosis, cryptococcosis, histoplasmosis, coccidioidomycosis) and nontuberculous mycobacteria. Guidelines for when to consider pulmonary tuberculosis have been published (Box 103-1).

Tuberculosis must be considered in the diagnosis of fever of unknown origin. Mycobacterial cultures of blood, bone marrow, and liver may sometimes establish the diagnosis. Biopsy specimens of organs with evidence of dys-

Box 103-1 Guidelines for the Evaluation of Pulmonary Tuberculosis

Any patient with a cough ≥2 to 3 weeks' duration, with a least one additional symptom, including fever, night sweats, weight loss, or hemoptysis

Any patient at high risk for TB* with an unexplained illness, including respiratory symptoms of ≥2 to 3 weeks' duration

Any patient with HIV infection and unexplained cough and fever

Any patient at high risk for TB with a diagnosis of community-acquired pneumonia who has not improved after 7 days of therapy

Any patient at high risk for TB with incidental findings on chest radiograph suggestive of TB even if symptoms are minimal or absent

TB, tuberculosis.

*Patients with one of the following characteristics: recent exposure to a case of infectious TB; history of a positive test result for *Mycobacterium tuberculosis* infection; HIV infection; injection or noninjection drug use; foreign birth and immigration ≤5 years from a region in which incidence is high; residents and employees of high-risk congregate settings; membership in a medically underserved, low-income population; or a medical risk factor for TB (i.e., diabetes mellitus, conditions requiring prolonged corticosteroids and other immunosuppressive therapy; chronic renal failure; certain hematologic malignancies and carcinomas, weigh >10% below ideal body weight, silicosis, gastrectomy, or jejunoileal bypass).

Adapted from Taylor Z, Nolan CM, Blumberg HM; American Thoracic Society; Centers for Disease Control and Prevention; Infectious Diseases Society of America: Controlling Tuberculosis in the United States. Recommendations from the American Thoracic Society, CDC, and the Infectious Diseases Society of America. MMWR Recomm Rep 54(RR-12):1-81, 2005.

function or abnormalities on radiographic scans should also include culture testing for mycobacteria.

Consideration of mycobacterial infection is important in chronic organ system disorders including meningitis, peritonitis, epididymitis, pericarditis, pleuritis, and osteomyelitis. The finding of granulomas on biopsy should always raise the suspicion of tuberculosis, although they may also be found in histoplasmosis, coccidioidomycosis, blastomycosis, and sarcoidosis.

Recently, tuberculosis has been associated with the use of tumor necrosis factor-α (TNF-α) antagonists. These drugs (infliximab, etanercept, adalimumab) are effective in the management of rheumatoid arthritis and active Crohn's disease. They have been used to treat Behçet's disease, psoriasis, uveitis, pyoderma gangrenosum, Still's disease, sarcoidosis, and Sjögren's syndrome. Most cases of tuberculosis have been reported with infliximab, but etanercept and adalimumab may also be associated with an increased risk. Potential recipients of these drugs should be screened with a TST or QuantiFERON tuberculosis Gold test (QFT-G, see later), detailed questionnaire about recent travel and potential tuberculosis exposures, assessment for symptoms such as cough and weight loss, and chest radi-

ography to minimize their risk for acquiring or reactivating tuberculosis. Patients with latent tuberculosis should receive therapy before initiation of therapy with TNF-α antagonists.

Diagnostic Approach

Until recently, latent tuberculosis infection (LTBI) could only be detected by a TST using purified protein derivative (PPD) (Fig. 103-4). This test is subject to both false-positive and false-negative results (Table 103-1) that can be minimized by careful attention to proper placement and interpretation of the test. In most persons, TST sensitivity persists throughout life; however, the size of the skin test may decrease and disappear over time. If PPD is administered to infected persons whose skin tests have waned, an initial test may be small or absent, but a subsequent test (2 to 4 weeks later) may demonstrate an accentuated response. This booster effect should not be misinterpreted as skin test conversion, but rather the second test should be considered as reflecting the individual's true exposure to *M. tuberculosis*. Two-step testing is recommended in people who are likely to undergo repeated tuberculin testing (i.e., health care workers) or for whom immunity is likely to have waned (i.e., elderly people), and who have not had a TST within the previous 12 months. The criteria used for classifying a TST result as positive are based on the size of induration and epidemiologic and clinical characteristics of the patient (Table 103-2). The sensitivity of the TST to detect active tuberculosis is in the range of 75% to 80% but may be lower in some groups such as elderly and HIV-infected persons. The specificity of the TST is about 99% in populations that have no other mycobacterial exposure or BCG vaccination, but decreases to about 95% in populations in which cross-reactivity with other mycobacteria is common (e.g., Southeast United States). Routine testing is recommended only for high-prevalence and high-risk groups (see Table 103-1). Prior receipt of BCG vaccination does not alter the interpretation of TST reactivity. Pregnancy is not a contraindication to TST.

More recently, a blood test, the QFT-G, has become available for diagnosing latent tuberculous infection. The QFT-G test includes a mixture of synthetic peptides representing two *M. tuberculosis* proteins, ESAT-6 and CFP-10. If the patient is infected with *M. tuberculosis*, white blood cells will release IFN-γ in response to contact with these antigens. In the QFT-G test, the patient's blood is incubated with the test antigens for 16 to 24 hours and the amount of IFN-γ is measured. QFT-G can be used in all circumstances in which the TST is currently used, including contact investigations, evaluation of recent immigrants who have had BCG vaccination, and tuberculosis screening of health care workers. Potential advantages of the QFT-G include convenience; avoidance of subjectivity inherent in measurements of cutaneous induration produced by the TST; the need for only one patient visit; and

Figure 103-4 Tuberculin Testing.

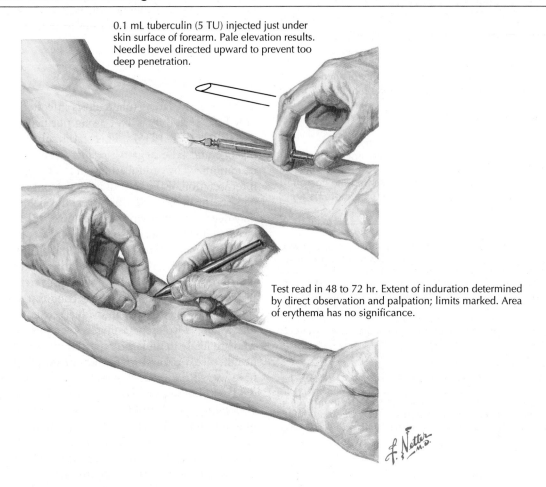

0.1 mL tuberculin (5 TU) injected just under skin surface of forearm. Pale elevation results. Needle bevel directed upward to prevent too deep penetration.

Test read in 48 to 72 hr. Extent of induration determined by direct observation and palpation; limits marked. Area of erythema has no significance.

Table 103-1 Potential Causes of False-Positive and False-Negative Tuberculin Reactions

Causes of False-Positive Reactions	Causes of False-Negative Reactions
Mistaking erythema for induration	Anergy due to overwhelming tuberculous infection
Infection with nontuberculous mycobacteria	Recent infection with *M. tuberculosis* (<10 weeks)
Receipt of BCG vaccine	Drugs (steroids, immunosuppressive agents)
Early reading of skin test with reaction due to immunoglobulins rather than cell-mediated immunity	Metabolic derangements (e.g., chronic liver or renal disease)
Use of incorrect strength of PPD (i.e., 250 TU)	Immune suppressive diseases (e.g., HIV, hematologic malignancies, or lymphoma)
Poorly standardized antigen	Malnourishment
	Recent receipt of live virus vaccine (e.g., measles)
	Newborns, elderly population
	Improper storage or dilution of PPD
	Inappropriate administration (e.g., too little antigen, or subcutaneous administration)
	Errors in reading or recording TST

BCG, bacillus of Calmette-Guerin; PPD, purified protein derivative; TST, tuberculin skin test; TU, tuberculin unit.
Adapted from Diagnostic Standards and Classification of Tuberculosis in Adults and Children. Am J Respir Crit Care Med 161(4 Pt 1): 1390, 2000.

Table 103-2 Criteria for Tuberculin Positivity, by Risk Group

Induration ≥5 mm	Induration ≥10 mm	Induration ≥15 mm
HIV-positive persons	Recent arrivals (<5 years) from high-prevalence countries*	Persons with no known risk factors for tuberculosis
Recent contacts of tuberculosis cases*	Injection drug users	
Fibrotic changes on chest radiograph consistent with prior tuberculosis	Mycobacterial laboratory personnel*	
Patients with organ transplants and other immunosuppressed patients (receiving the equivalent of >15 mg/day prednisone for ≥1 month)‡	Residents and employees of high-risk congregate settings: prisons and jails, nursing homes and other health care facilities, residential facilities for AIDS patients, and homeless shelters*	
	Persons with clinical conditions that make them high risk*,†	
	Children <4 years of age or infants, children, and adolescents exposed to adults in high-risk categories*	

TST, tuberculin skin test.

*Epidemiologic criteria used in classifying the TST skin reaction.

†High-risk medical conditions include silicosis, diabetes mellitus, chronic renal failure, leukemia, Hodgkin's disease, immunosuppressive therapy, and malnutrition.

‡Clinical conditions used in classifying the TST skin reaction.

From Targeted tuberculin testing and treatment of latent tuberculosis infection. A joint statement of the American Thoracic Society (ATS) and the Centers for Disease Control and Prevention (CDC). Am J Respir Crit Care Med 161(4 Pt 2):S221-S247, 2000. Also adapted from Screening for tuberculosis and tuberculosis infection in high-risk populations. Recommendations of the Advisory Council for the Elimination of TB. MMWR Recomm Rep 44(RR-11):19-34, 1995.

the ability to perform repeated testing without boosting the response, as may occur with serial tuberculin testing. However, caution should be used when testing certain populations because of limited data in the use of QFT-G, including immunocompromised persons, patients with extrapulmonary tuberculosis, children, and populations in high-incidence countries. In addition, there are limited data on the long-term reproducibility of this assay, particularly in serial testing situation (e.g., health care workers). Before the QFT-G is conducted, arrangements should be made with a qualified laboratory and courier service, if needed, to ensure prompt and proper processing of blood.

For suspected active tuberculosis, all patients should be evaluated with a TST. A careful history should attempt to elicit the nonspecific symptoms of tuberculosis and organ-specific symptoms, especially of pulmonary disease. Physical examination is of limited utility in the diagnosis but may aid in detecting specific organ infection requiring further investigation. All patients with a positive TST or QFT-G result or symptoms of tuberculosis should have a chest radiograph to aid in the diagnosis of pulmonary tuberculosis and to determine the extent of disease.

A presumptive diagnosis of pulmonary tuberculosis can often be made using the chest radiograph. For suspected cases of pulmonary tuberculosis, mycobacteria may be demonstrated in sputum by acid-fast staining (Ziehl-Neelsen or Kinyoun method) or a fluorochrome procedure using auramine-O or auramine-rhodamine dyes. Smear positivity indicates greater infectiousness. For smear-

positive pulmonary cases, a nucleic acid amplification assay (NAA) can be used to rapidly detect M. tuberculosis, with a sensitivity of about 95% and specificity approaching 100%. The U.S. Food and Drug Administration advises against the use of NAA in smear-negative samples because of low sensitivity.

Isolation of M. tuberculosis from specimens of sputum and other tissues is essential for confirmation of the identity of the organism and for subsequent drug susceptibility testing, which is recommended for initial isolates for each patient. Cultures also remain the cornerstone for the diagnosis of tuberculosis in smear-negative pulmonary and extrapulmonary cases and, along with sputum smears for acid-fast bacillus, provide the basis for monitoring a patient's response to treatment, for release from isolation, and for diagnosing treatment failure and relapse. Sputum may be obtained every 8 to 12 hours. Induction of sputum with hypertonic saline may increase the yield of obtaining adequate sputum specimens, especially in HIV-infected patients. Detection of mycobacterial growth on conventional Löwenstein-Jensen or Middlebrook 7H10 medium requires 4 to 8 weeks. Assays that detect either the production of carbon dioxide or the consumption of small amounts of oxygen by microorganisms in culture may be used to detect mycobacterial grown in 14 to 21 days. The precise time required for detection of mycobacteria by these metabolic assays is largely dependent on the number of organisms in the inoculum. A computed tomography scan may provide valuable information in assessing whether an abnormal chest radiograph is consistent with tuberculosis.

Table 103-3 Recommended Therapy for Latent Tuberculous Infection

Drug	Duration (mo)	Interval	Rating* (Evidence)† HIV Negative	Rating* (Evidence)† HIV Positive
Isoniazid	9	Daily	A (II)	A (II)
		Twice weekly	B (II)	B (II)
Isoniazid	6	Daily	B (I)	C (I)
		Twice weekly	B (II)	C (I)
Rifampin	4	Daily	B (II)	B (III)

*A, preferred; B, acceptable alternative; C, offer when A and B cannot be given.
†I, Randomized clinical trial data; II, data from clinical trials that are not randomized or were conducted in other populations; III, expert opinion. *From Targeted tuberculin testing and treatment of latent tuberculosis infection. A joint statement of the American Thoracic Society (ATS) and the Centers for Disease Control and Prevention (CDC). Am J Respir Crit Care Med 161(4 Pt 2):S221-S247, 2000.*

Aspiration of gastric fluid for culture is often helpful in young children unable to produce sputum. Fiberoptic bronchoscopy is a useful diagnostic test to obtain specimens from the respiratory tract in patients unable to produce sputum.

The diagnosis of extrapulmonary tuberculosis usually requires an invasive procedure to obtain fluid (e.g., cerebrospinal fluid [CSF]) for smear or culture, and biopsy to obtain tissue for culture. A first morning-voided midstream urine specimen should be cultured to establish the diagnosis of genitourinary tuberculosis. Blood for mycobacterial culture should be anticoagulated with heparin and processed by a lysis-centrifugation system or inoculated into broth media designed for mycobacterial blood cultures. The diagnosis of central nervous system tuberculosis is established by culture of the CSF; a minimum of 5 mL of fluid should be submitted to the laboratory in a sterile container for culture. Invasive procedures to obtain specimens from the lung, pericardium, lymph nodes, bones and joints, bowel, salpinges, and epididymis warrant consideration when noninvasive techniques do not provide a diagnosis. Antimicrobial susceptibility testing is essential on all cultures that yield *M. tuberculosis*.

Management and Therapy

Optimum Treatment

All patients with known or suspected tuberculosis should be placed on airborne precautions (>6 to 12 air exchanges per hour, negative pressure, and air directly exhausted to the outside) when receiving care within a health care facility. Health care personnel should don an N95 respirator before entering the room of a patient with potentially communicable tuberculosis. Patients should remain on airborne isolation until they have received at least 2 to 3 weeks of standard multidrug antituberculosis therapy, demonstrated clinical improvement (i.e., reduction in the frequency of cough), and have three consecutive negative sputum smears cultured 8 to 24 hours apart with at least one sputum being an early morning specimen. Patients with known or suspected multidrug-resistant *M. tuberculosis* should remain isolated until culture results are negative. Close contacts of persons with active pulmonary tuberculosis require evaluation for tuberculosis because active disease is already present in 2% to 3% and latent infection in 5% to 15%.

All persons with a reactive TST (see Table 103-1) or positive QFT-G should have therapy of LTBI recommended (Table 103-3) after excluding active tuberculosis with history, physical examination, chest radiography, and bacteriologic studies (when indicated). Ideally, patients should receive follow-up evaluations at least monthly. Follow-up evaluations should include questioning about adverse drug reactions and a brief physical assessment for signs of hepatitis. Baseline testing of liver function (i.e., alanine transaminase/aspartate transaminase and bilirubin) is recommended only for persons at high risk for liver dysfunction, including patients with HIV infection, persons with a history of chronic liver disease (e.g., hepatitis C), pregnant women, postpartum women within 3 months of delivery, and persons who use alcohol regularly. Active hepatitis and end-stage liver disease are relative contraindications to the use of isoniazid or pyrazinamide. Routine monitoring during treatment of LTBI is indicated for persons whose baseline liver function test results are abnormal and persons at risk for hepatic disease. Such tests should also be performed on persons with signs or symptoms of hepatitis. Isoniazid therapy should be stopped if transaminase levels exceed three times the upper limit of normal if associated with symptoms, and five times the upper limit of normal if the patient is asymptomatic.

Patients with active tuberculosis require therapy with multiple drugs to prevent the development of resistance, enhance tuberculocidal therapy, and properly treat if their strain of *M. tuberculosis* is resistant to one or more drugs. The preferred regimen for patients with fully susceptible bacilli is a 6-month course initially consisting of isoniazid, rifampin, ethambutol (use streptomycin in children too young to be monitored for visual acuity), and pyrazinamide, given for 2 months, followed by isoniazid and rifampin for 4 months. If there is evidence of a slow or suboptimal response, therapy should be given for a total of 9 months, or for 4 months after culture results become negative. All patients should be treated using enhanced, directly observed therapy (DOT) to ensure compliance. Extrapulmonary tuberculosis in adults should be managed in a manner similar to that for pulmonary tuberculosis (i.e., 6 months of therapy), except for meningitis for which a 9- to 12-month regimen is recommended. Children who have miliary tuberculosis, bone and joint tuberculosis, or tuberculous meningitis, should receive a minimum of 12 months of therapy. Expert consultation is usually needed when treating tuberculosis in HIV-infected persons because treatment is more difficult because of the possibility of malabsorption of antituberculous medications and because of drug interactions between rifampin and protease inhibitors.

Physicians should be familiar with the administration, adverse reactions, and contraindications of the first-line antituberculous medications. In pulmonary tuberculosis, the response to therapy is monitored by obtaining follow-up sputa for culture. Reevaluation of therapy is necessary if sputum culture results have not become negative after 2 months. In this case, repeat drug susceptibility testing is essential, and DOT therapy should be continued or initiated. Patient education with regard to compliance, symptoms of drug toxicity, and drug interactions is critical to ensure proper therapy.

Treating persons dually infected with HIV and *M. tuberculosis* is challenging because of potential overlapping toxicities, drug interactions, and paradoxical reactions. For example, many antiretrovirals interact with antituberculous medications, especially the rifamycins. In HIV treatment-naïve patients, the timing of initiating highly active antiretroviral therapy (HAART) is complex. Consultation with an infectious disease specialist is recommended. Multidrug resistance (MDR), defined as resistance to at least isoniazid and rifampin, is a growing problem worldwide. In the United States, MDR tuberculosis is more common in persons who are foreign born, who remain culture positive, or whose symptoms do not resolve after 3 months of therapy. All patients with MDR tuberculosis should receive DOT and be managed by persons familiar with use of second-line medications such as aminoglycosides (e.g., streptomycin), polypeptides, fluoroquinolones (e.g., ciprofloxacin), thioamides, cycloserine, and para-aminosalicylic acid. Use of second-line drugs is less effective, more toxic, and costlier than use of first-line isoniazid- and rifampin-based regimens. Recently, extensively drug-resistant (XDR) tuberculosis has emerged as a worldwide problem. The CDC and World Health Organization define XDR tuberculosis as the occurrence of tuberculosis in persons whose *M. tuberculosis* isolates are resistant to isoniazid and rifampin and also to any fluoroquinolone and at least one of three injectable second-line

drugs (i.e., amikacin, kanamycin, or capreomycin). Between 2000 and 2006, about 1% of culture-confirmed cases (N = 922) in the United States were due to MDR TB strains; of these MDR TB strains, about 2% (N = 17) were due to XDR TB strains. Although XDR TB is uncommon in the United States, it is more common in South Korea (15% of all MDR tuberculosis isolates) and the countries of eastern Europe and western Asia (14% of all MDR tuberculosis isolates).

Avoiding Treatment Errors

The most common error in detecting tuberculosis is failure to consider the diagnosis in a patient as it often presents with protean manifestations including low-grade fever, gradual weight loss, cough, night sweats, and fatigue. An appropriate evaluation with a chest radiograph and three sputum collections for smear plus culture will usually allow detection of pulmonary tuberculosis. Diagnosis of extrapulmonary disease is more difficult because it usually requires an invasive procedure. Tissue is the preferred source for material for smears and cultures to detect extrapulmonary tuberculosis rather than fluids (e.g., peritoneal biopsy rather than ascites fluid, pericardial tissue rather than pericardial fluid). A bone marrow aspirate or biopsy is often useful to detect disseminated tuberculosis (laboratory should be notified ahead of time to expect the specimen).

To prevent possible nosocomial transmission, all patients with known or *suspected* tuberculosis should immediately be placed on airborne precautions. Health care personnel should be properly trained in the use of an N95 respirator.

Patients with LTBI should be carefully counseled regarding the need to properly take their medications and to complete the entire course of therapy. Patients with active tuberculosis should ideally be treated with DOT. Failure to properly take medications or complete a full course of antituberculous therapy is the main reason for the development of drug resistance.

Future Directions

The major challenges of tuberculosis are the increasing proportion of multidrug-resistant strains and the prevention and treatment of tuberculosis in HIV-infected persons. Progress against tuberculosis is being made on several fronts. New diagnostic tests are being developed for the rapid detection of *M. tuberculosis* (e.g., polymerase chain reaction) in sputum or tissue samples, and for the rapid identification of drug-resistant strains. New drugs are being studied for the therapy of tuberculosis, including the quinolone moxifloxacin, nitroimidazopyrans (e.g., PA-824), macrolides (e.g., azithromycin, clarithromycin), oxazolidinones (e.g., linezolid, PNU-100480), diamines (e.g., SQ109), and ring-substituted imidazoles. Finally, a major research effort is being directed toward developing new tuberculosis vaccines. Several candidate vaccines should be ready for human testing within a few years.

Additional Resources

Campbell IA, Bah-Sow O: Pulmonary tuberculosis: Diagnosis and treatment. BMJ 332(7551):1194-1197, 2006.

The authors provide an excellent, concise review of current advances in the diagnosis and treatment of pulmonary tuberculosis.

de Jong BC, Israelski DM, Corbett EL, Small PM: Clinical management of tuberculosis in the context of HIV infection. Annu Rev Med 55:283-301, 2004.

This superb paper reviews the management of patients dually infected with HIV and M. tuberculosis.

Diagnostic Standards and Classification of Tuberculosis in Adults and Children. Official statement of the American Thoracic Society and the Centers for Disease Control and Prevention. Am J Respir Crit Care Med 161(4 Pt 1):1376-1395, 2000.

This official guideline describes methods of detecting tuberculosis.

Nahid P, Pai M, Hopewell PC: Advances in the diagnosis and treatment of tuberculosis. Proc Am Thorac Soc 3(1):103-110, 2006.

The authors provide a brief review of new methods for the diagnosis and treatment of tuberculosis.

Rychly DJ, DiPiro JT: Infections associated with tumor necrosis factor-alpha antagonists. Pharmacotherapy 25(9):1181-1192, 2005.

This important paper reviews the evidence that tumor necrosis factor-α antagonists are a risk factor for reactivation of tuberculosis.

Screening for tuberculosis and tuberculosis infection in high-risk populations. Recommendations of the Advisory Council for the Elimination of Tuberculosis. MMWR Recomm Rep 44(RR-11):19-34, 1995.

This important guideline describes the standards for tuberculosis screening.

Taylor Z, Nolan CM, Blumberg HM; American Thoracic Society; Centers for Disease Control and Prevention; Infectious Diseases Society of America. Controlling Tuberculosis in the United States. Recommendations from the American Thoracic Society, CDC, and the Infectious Diseases Society of America. MMWR Recomm Rep 54(RR-12):1-81, 2005.

This important statement describes public health measures for controlling tuberculosis in the United States.

Winthrop KL, Siegel JN, Jereb J, et al: Tuberculosis associated with therapy against tumor necrosis factor alpha. Arthritis Rheum 52(10):2968-2974, 2005.

The authors provide an excellent review of tumor necrosis factor-α antagonists associated with reactivation of tuberculosis.

Winthrop KL: Risk and prevention of tuberculosis and other serious opportunistic infections associated with the inhibition of tumor necrosis factor. Nat Clin Pract Rheumatol 2:602-610, 2006.

This is the most recent review of tumor necrosis factor-α antagonists associated with reactivation of tuberculosis.

EVIDENCE

1. American Thoracic Society; CDC; Infectious Disease Society of America: Treatment of tuberculosis. MMWR Recomm Rep 52(RR-11):1-77, 2003.

   This excellent guideline provides detailed recommendations for the treatment of tuberculosis.

2. Blumberg HM, Leonard MK Jr, Jasmer RM: Update on the treatment of tuberculosis and latent tuberculous infection. JAMA 293(22):2776-2784, 2005.

   This excellent, concise review describes current therapy guidelines for the treatment of tuberculosis.

3. Furin JJ, Johnson JL: Recent advances in the diagnosis and management of tuberculosis. Curr Opin Pulmon Med 11(3):189-194, 2005.

   This short paper provides an excellent review of new methods for the diagnosis and management of tuberculosis.

4. Small PM, Fujiwara PI: Management of tuberculosis in the United States. N Engl J Med 345(3):189-200, 2001.

   This older paper provides a comprehensive review of the treatment of tuberculosis.

5. Targeted tuberculin testing and treatment of latent tuberculosis infection. A joint statement of the American Thoracic Society and the Centers for Disease Control and Prevention. Am J Respir Crit Care Med 161(4 Pt 2):S221-S247, 2000.

   This important guideline describes the detection and treatment of latent tuberculosis infection.

Amanda Peppercorn ▪ Jonathan S. Serody

104

Fungal Infections

Introduction

The incidence of medically significant fungal infections has dramatically increased over the past two decades and strongly correlates with the rise in the number of immunocompromised patients. The AIDS epidemic, the expansion of stem cell and solid organ transplantation, and the ever-increasing use of chemotherapy and immunosuppressive agents have placed more hosts at risk for invasive fungal disease and have broadened the range of fungi capable of causing significant disease in humans (Box 104-1). During the past decade, significant advances have occurred in the diagnosis and treatment of these infections as several new antifungal drugs have become available. However, given the complexity of the population of patients who remain at highest risk for these infections (Box 104-2), substantial challenges in, and opportunities for, early diagnosis and management remain. Mortality remains high in certain settings and can be as high as 90% for invasive mold infections in hematopoietic stem cell transplant recipients.

Fungi can exist as yeast or molds (also spelled "moulds"). Yeast-like fungi generally are round, unicellular organisms that reproduce by budding and form flat smooth colonies. Molds are composed of longitudinal tubular structures called hyphae, grow by extension, and have a fuzzy appearance on a growth plate. Although most fungi exist as either yeast or molds, the dimorphic fungi, which include the agents of histoplasmosis, blastomycosis, sporotrichosis, coccidioidomycosis, paracoccidioidomycosis, and chromoblastosis, grow in the host as a yeast but exist in the environment as a mold. Mycoses are infections caused by fungi. With rare exception, mycoses are generally not transmissible from one person to another.

The fungal cell wall is a rigid barrier composed of glucans and chitin. Some fungi, such as *Cryptococcus* species, have a polysaccharide capsule that acts as an added layer of protection and aids in evasion from the immune system. Inside the cell wall is the cytoplasmic membrane that contains ergosterols. Antifungal agents such as azoles and polyene antifungal agents target ergosterols. The new echinocandin class of antifungals targets the production of β-D-glucan in the cell wall (Table 104-1).

Current diagnostic testing includes culture of the affected site, histologic examination of tissue with the use of special staining techniques (Gomori methenamine-silver, periodic acid–Schiff, and calcofluor stain), use of antigen studies (the galactomannan, β-1,3-D-glucan, cryptococcal and histoplasmic antigen assays) and paired acute and convalescent antibody titers. There are limitations to the utility of antibody-based studies. Cross-reactivity and high false-negative rates, particularly in immunocompromised hosts who cannot mount a forceful humoral immune response, can limit the accuracy of this approach. Thus, the current standard for diagnosis of invasive fungal infections relies primarily on clinical suspicion, culture, and histopathologic diagnosis.

HIV-Related Immunodeficiency

Many mycoses are caused by important pathogens in those with immunosuppression caused by HIV, including candidiasis, cryptococcosis, histoplasmosis, and pneumocystosis. Histoplasmosis is discussed in the section on endemic fungi. Mucocutaneous candidiasis is extremely common in people with AIDS and can be a clue to the diagnosis of immune system dysfunction in the setting of HIV/AIDS. Its presence in a previously healthy patient should prompt an evaluation for an underlying immunologic problem such as malignancy or AIDS. (See "Candidiasis.")

Box 104-1   Important Causes of Fungal Infections in Humans

Candida Species
- *C. albicans, C. glabrata, C. guilliermondii, C. kefyr, C. krusei, C. lusitaniae, C. parapsilosis, C. rugosa, C. tropicalis*

Other Yeasts
- *Cryptococcus neoformans*
- *Malassezia* species
- *Rhodotorula* species
- *Saccharomyces* species
- *Trichosporon* species

Zygomycetes
- *Absidia* species
- *Cunninghamella* species
- *Mucor* species
- *Rhizomucor* species
- *Rhizopus* species
- *Saksenaea* species

Other Molds
- *Acremonium* species
- *Aspergillus* species (*A. fumigatus, A. niger, A. flavus, A. terreus, A. versicolor*)
- *Emmonsia* species
- *Fusarium* species
- *Scedosporium* species
- *Trichoderma* species

Dematiaceous Molds
- *Alternaria* species
- *Bipolaris* species
- *Curvularia* species
- *Cladophialophora* species
- *Dactylaria* species
- *Exophiala* species
- *Phialophora* species
- *Ramichloridium* species
- *Wangiella* species

Dimorphic Fungi
- *Blastomyces dermatitidis*
- *Coccidioides immitis*
- *Histoplasma capsulatum*
- *Paracoccidioides brasiliensis*
- *Penicillium marneffei*
- *Sporothrix schenckii*

Other
- *Pneumocystis jiroveci*

Box 104-2   People at Risk for Invasive Fungal Infections

Transplant recipients (solid organ and bone marrow transplantations)
Patients with hematologic malignancies (leukemias, lymphomas)
Injection drug users
People with HIV/AIDS and low CD4 counts/advanced immunosuppression
Immunosuppressive drug therapy (chemotherapy, corticosteroids, tumor necrosis factor inhibitors, cyclosporine, azathioprine, CellCept, sirolimus, anakinra)
Preterm infants (<26 weeks' gestation or <1000 g)
Hospitalized patients with:
- Prolonged length of stay
- Intensive care unit
- Broad-spectrum antibiotics
- High acuity
- Diabetes mellitus
- Renal failure and hemodialysis
- Parenteral nutrition
- Cancer and chemotherapy
- Severe pancreatitis
- Major surgery
- Invasive devices (urinary catheters, central venous catheters)

Cryptococcosis

Cryptococcus neoformans is an encapsulated yeast-like organism that can cause disease in both immunocompetent and immunocompromised hosts but has been an important cause of morbidity and mortality in people with AIDS (Fig. 104-1). *Cryptococcus* is found in soil contaminated with pigeon droppings. Infection occurs after inhalation of the organism with dissemination to other organs through the bloodstream. Although the organism can remain in the bloodstream and cause disease in the lungs, urinary tract, skin, joints, and bones, the most common sites of disease are the brain and the meninges. Before the advent of combination antiretroviral therapy, 5% to 10% of people with HIV developed cryptococcal meningitis.

The clinical course can be subacute or acute, with the typical signs and symptoms of meningitis, including fever, nuchal rigidity, photophobia, lethargy, and confusion. Diagnosis can be made by fungal stain and culture of the cerebrospinal fluid (including India ink stain). The cryptococcal antigen assay can also detect the presence of the organism in serum and cerebrospinal fluid. Poor prognostic features include altered mental status at the time of presentation, high opening pressure on lumbar puncture, and a low cerebrospinal fluid white blood cell count, which suggests more advanced immunosuppression. If left untreated, the mortality rate is virtually 100%.

For patients with HIV and meningeal disease, treatment guidelines recommend induction therapy with amphotericin B (or a lipid formulation) at 0.7 to 1 mg/kg/day plus flucytosine (100 mg/kg/day) for 2 weeks followed by a minimum of 10 weeks of oral fluconazole (400 mg/day), followed by lifelong suppression with fluconazole, 200 mg/day. Recent data support discontinuation of maintenance fluconazole in patients with immune reconstitution after the institution of highly active antiretroviral therapy.

Table 104-1 Antifungal Agents and Properties

Agent	Route of Administration	Mechanism of Action	Spectrum of Activity
Polyenes ■ Amphotericin B ■ Lipid-based formulations ■ Amphotericin B lipid complex ■ Amphotericin B colloidal dispersion ■ Liposomal amphotericin B	Intravenous	Binds to ergosterol in fungal cell membrane, increasing permeability	Broad spectrum, includes *Candida* species, dimorphic and filamentous fungi
Azoles ■ Ketoconazole (K) ■ Fluconazole (F) ■ Itraconazole (I) ■ Voriconazole (V) ■ Posaconazole—approval pending (P) ■ Ravuconazole—approval pending (R)	Intravenous (F, I, V) and oral (all azoles)	Inhibition of enzyme required for biosynthesis of cell membrane structural component ergosterol	*Candida albicans*, voriconazole active against *Aspergillus*, posaconazole active against Zygomycetes
Echinocandins ■ Caspofungin ■ Micafungin ■ Anidulafungin	Intravenous	Inhibition of β-D-glucan synthesis, required for fungal cell wall integrity	All *Candida* species, *Aspergillus* species

Pneumocystosis

Pneumocystis jiroveci is the etiologic agent of pneumocystis pneumonia (PCP). It is an unusual organism that was originally classified as a protozoan but recently was reclassified based on ribosomal ribonucleic acid analysis as a unicellular fungi. It lacks ergosterol in its cellular membrane, however, and is thus unresponsive to treatment with azole and polyene antifungal agents. *Pneumocystis* was recognized as a rare cause of pneumonia in immunocompromised hosts before the AIDS epidemic. There was a dramatic rise in the incidence and mortality related to this pathogen in patients with AIDS in the 1980s and 1990s (Fig. 104-2). Although the advent of highly active antiretroviral therapy caused a significant decrease in the incidence of PCP in the late 1990s, there are still about 16,000 cases per year in the United States, and it remains the most common AIDS-related opportunistic infection, often occurring in people who are unaware of their HIV diagnosis. There is now increasing recognition of the importance of this pathogen as a cause of pneumonia in developing countries of Africa and Asia in the setting of the AIDS pandemic.

Pneumocystis jiroveci can cause a subacute or acute pneumonia that can deteriorate rapidly to respiratory failure. Chest x-ray findings can include honeycombing (which gave rise to the name pneumo*cyst*is), interstitial infiltrates, or minimal abnormalities, but these findings usually are not associated with pleural effusions. The serum lactate dehydrogenase level may be elevated, and generally there is a widened alveolar-arterial oxygen gradient. Diagnosis is made using high clinical index of suspicion, symptoms of dyspnea on exertion, fever, chest pain, and progressive shortness of breath paired with imaging findings and visu-

alization of trophozoites or cysts on special staining of deep (induced) sputum or specimens obtained by bronchoscopy. The organism cannot be cultured. Treatment includes high-dose trimethoprim-sulfamethoxazole (15 mg/kg/day divided in three doses given intravenously or orally) for 21 days followed by chemoprophylaxis; if the partial pressure of oxygen is less than 70 mm Hg or the alveolar-arterial gradient is more than 35 mm Hg, a course of corticosteroids is recommended at the start of therapy to decrease the inflammatory response and subsequent lung damage during treatment.

Candidiasis

Etiology and Pathogenesis

About 154 species of the yeast *Candida* have been described. *Candida* exists as part of the normal human flora of the genitourinary and gastrointestinal tracts and heavily colonizes the skin. It remains the most common cause of fungal infections worldwide and is of particular significance in the hospital setting. Fungal infections make up about 8% of all nosocomial infections, and of these, 80% are attributable to *Candida* species. Historically, *Candida albicans* was the primary candidal pathogen in humans. However, a recent epidemiologic shift has been documented with a rise in the proportion of non-*albicans* species such as *C. glabrata*, *C. parapsilosis*, *C. tropicalis*, and *C. krusei*. This is particularly significant because these species can be resistant to fluconazole, which is commonly used in prevention and as first-line therapy.

Candida of most species form biofilms, which are a matrix-enclosed population that adheres to a surface. These form on catheters and are difficult to eradicate,

Figure 104-1 Cryptococcosis and Torulosis.

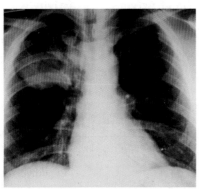

Pulmonary cryptococcosis presenting as a large mass-like lesion, easily mistaken for carcinoma

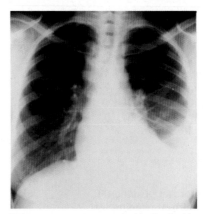

Pulmonary cryptococcosis. Mediastinal lymph nodes enlarged and pleural effusion on left

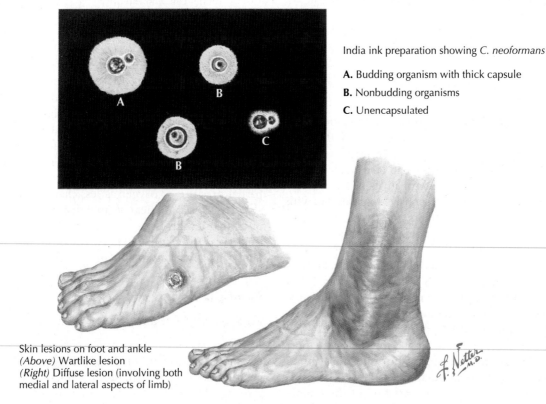

India ink preparation showing *C. neoformans*

A. Budding organism with thick capsule

B. Nonbudding organisms

C. Unencapsulated

Skin lesions on foot and ankle
(Above) Wartlike lesion
(Right) Diffuse lesion (involving both medial and lateral aspects of limb)

allowing persistence in sterile sites through instrumentation such as bladder catheters, abdominal drains, and central venous lines. *Candida* species represent the fourth most common bloodstream isolate, and mortality rates range from 30% to 60%. Candidemia also accounts for about a 10-day increase in hospital length of stay. Candidiasis is more common in patients who have undergone stem cell or solid organ transplantation or prolonged care in an intensive care unit and those who have a history of intravenous drug use, a prolonged course of antibiotics, parenteral nutrition, frequent major surgeries, or AIDS.

Clinical Presentation and Diagnostic Approach

Candida species infection causes a wide spectrum of disease, ranging from vulvovaginitis to oropharyngeal ("thrush") and esophageal candidiasis, cheilitis, bloodstream infections, endocarditis, surgical abdominal infections, urinary tract infections, and deep-seated organ infection. The type of infection is strongly influenced by the host's immune status. Vulvovaginal candidiasis is most commonly observed in immunocompetent women, particularly in the setting of antibiotic usage with alterations in the normal flora. Hema-

Figure 104-2 *Pneumocystis carinii* **Pneumonia.**

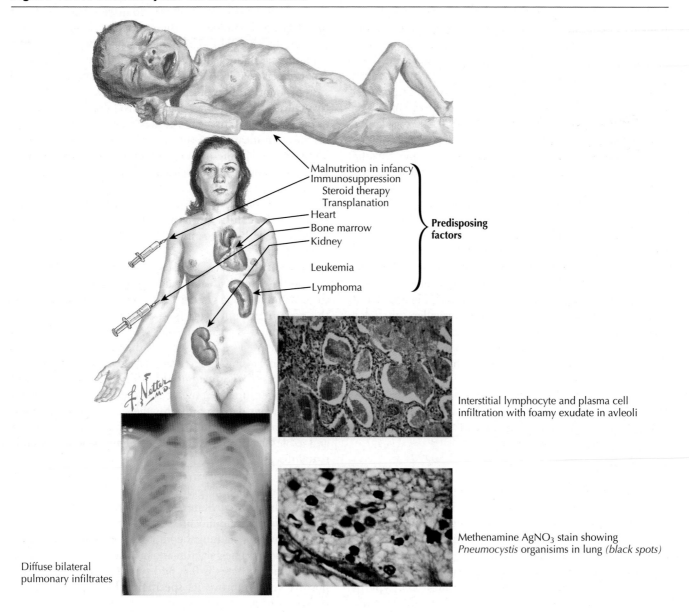

Malnutrition in infancy
Immunosuppression
Steroid therapy
Transplanation
Heart
Bone marrow
Kidney

Leukemia

Lymphoma

Predisposing factors

Interstitial lymphocyte and plasma cell infiltration with foamy exudate in avleoli

Methenamine AgNO₃ stain showing *Pneumocystis* organisims in lung *(black spots)*

Diffuse bilateral pulmonary infiltrates

togenous disseminated candidal infection is more commonly found after stem cell transplantation and in the setting of prolonged neutropenia. Mucocutaneous candidiasis is commonly seen in individuals with cell-mediated immune dysfunction, such as those with chronic steroid use or AIDS. Invasive candidiasis often presents with nonspecific clinical manifestations such as fever and signs and symptoms of sepsis. However, chorioretinitis, nodular skin lesions that can be excised for biopsy, and hepatosplenic abscesses can be specific clues to its diagnosis.

Culture is the mainstay of diagnosis but can take several days, and often treatment must begin empirically. *Candida* that can be grown from a sterile site such as the peritoneum or the bloodstream provides definite evidence of infection. However, positive cultures from pulmonary specimens and urinary specimens in patients who have a bladder catheter in place may indicate colonization rather than active infection. These cultures must be interpreted in the context of the immune status of the host and other clinical signs and symptoms. The β-1,3-D-glucan assay is under investigation as an antigen-based diagnostic technique to rapidly detect invasive candidiasis and, thus, could be useful in selecting candidates who need aggressive therapy.

Management and Therapy

Candida species are susceptible to all three antifungal classes of drugs, and all are used in different settings to prevent and treat infection. However, certain non-*albicans* species such as *C. glabrata* can be resistant to fluconazole, and this resistance does, in some cases, cross over to other azoles. *C. krusei* is inherently resistant to fluconazole but remains susceptible to voriconazole. Susceptibility testing has recently become available in many academic and research settings for different candidal species, and these patterns of susceptibility differ by geography and medical setting. For treatment of mucocutaneous disease, topical treatments can be used initially. If extensive thrush or esophagitis is present, fluconazole (100 to 200 mg/day) is initiated for a short course. In those with severe immunosuppression who relapse at the end of therapy, chronic suppression with fluconazole is recommended. In the setting of candidemia, the central venous line must be removed expediently and an evaluation undertaken to exclude endocarditis. For initial treatment, amphotericin B (or a lipid formulation, based on side-effect profile) or an echinocandin offers full susceptibility, although there are in vitro data to suggest decreased activity of *C. parapsilosis* to echinocandins. The clinical importance of these data remains unclear. Once the organism is identified and susceptibility data are complete, the provider can tailor therapy accordingly. Invasive disease from *Candida* species is generally treated for a prolonged course depending on the site involved and the level of immunosuppression of the patient.

Infections in Oncology, Transplantation, and Severely Immunocompromised Hosts

Aspergillus

Aspergilli are filamentous molds that generate conidia, the spore formed at the side or tip of the hyphae. There are multiple different strains of aspergillus, although most infections are due to *Aspergillus fumigatus, Aspergillus flavus, Aspergillus niger,* and *Aspergillus terreus* (Fig. 104-3). Aspergillus organisms are ubiquitous, and significant numbers are found in soil, dust, and possibly water. The type of infection caused by aspergillus differs based on the immune state of the individual (Table 104-2). Most commonly, individuals acquire infection with aspergillus species by inhalation.

The diagnosis of aspergillosis has been extensively reviewed and a system generated to discern the likelihood of infection. Radiologic findings include nodular lesions, cavities, or the halo sign, which represents edema surrounding a pulmonary nodule. A definite diagnosis of aspergillosis requires culture of the organism from sterile sites or identification of the organism in tissue with a positive culture. Probable aspergillosis requires identification of the organism in tissue in the absence of a positive culture or the identification of the organism in bronchoalveolar lavage sample in the presence of an abnormal radiograph. For transplant recipients who have a higher probability of infection, the criteria for "definite" disease is not generally required to consider therapy. Radiographic evidence in the presence of a culture from bronchoalveolar lavage and the absence of other organisms supports the diagnosis of aspergillosis.

Mortality associated with aspergillosis in the immunocompromised individual is quite high and approaches 60% to 95% in allogeneic stem cell transplant recipients. For this reason, prompt diagnosis is critical. Neutropenia and prolonged use of corticosteroids are significant risk factors for infection. The mainstay of therapy at this time is voriconazole (4 mg/kg intravenously given twice a day preceded by a 6 mg/kg loading dose for two doses) followed by prolonged oral therapy at 200 mg twice a day. There are no current data to indicate whether surgical resection or combination antifungal therapy using an echinocandin and azole or polyene is indicated for invasive or disseminated disease.

Several new noninvasive tests have become available for the diagnosis of aspergillosis. The test most commonly used in the United States is the Platelia galactomannan enzyme-linked immunosorbent assay that detects galactomannan, which is a fungal component present in serum of infected hosts. The galactomannan assay cutoff for positive in the United States is 0.5, and typically two consecutive positive tests improve its specificity. False-positive reactions can occur in patients infected with other molds, in neonates, and in individuals receiving antibiotics generated from fungal products such as piperacillin-tazobactam. False-negative tests are seen in individuals on fungal

Table 104-2 Clinical Manifestations of *Aspergillus* Infections

Type	Immune Status of Host	Clinical Manifestations	Treatment
Allergic bronchopulmonary aspergillosis	Immune competent	Asthma	Steroids, voriconazole
Aspergilloma	Immune competent	Often asymptomatic, cough, malaise, weight loss, hemoptysis	Surgical resection, voriconazole
Invasive pulmonary	Immune compromised	Fever, chest pain, cough, shortness of breath; radiographic findings	Voriconazole
Disseminated invasive	Immune compromised	Organ system dependent	Voriconazole with or without echinocandin
Sino-orbital	Immune competent and immune compromised	Acute form: fever, headache, facial pain; chronic form: headache, congestion	Voriconazole

Figure 104-3 Aspergillosis.

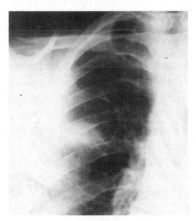

Film showing an aspergilloma within a cavity in right lung

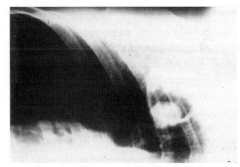

Film of same patient as shown at *left*, in I. lateral decubitus position demonstrating shift of fungus ball to dependent portion of cavity

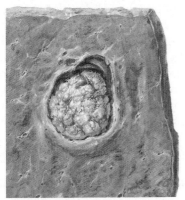

Gross appearance of an aspergilloma in a chronic lung cavity

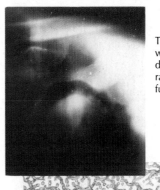

Tomogram of an aspergilloma within a cavity in I. upper lobe, demonstrating characteristic radiolucent crescent above fungus ball

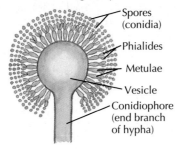

Spores (conidia)

Phialides

Metulae

Vesicle

Conidiophore (end branch of hypha)

Structure of fruiting form of *Aspergillus niger*. Other species of *Aspergillus* vary in configuration, but their general structure is similar

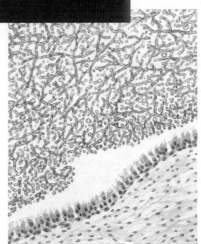

Microscopic structure of an aspergilloma composed of a tangled mass of hyphae within a dilated broncus. No evidence of tissue invasion

prophylaxis. Other tests that can be used are assays for detecting circulating β-1,3-D-glucan and real-time polymerase chain reaction techniques. The galactomannan assay is helpful in monitoring response to therapy because this test should rapidly normalize in adequately treated patients.

Zygomycetes

Zygomycetes are a group of fungi predominantly found in soil that cause infections primarily in immunocompro-

mised hosts. There are multiple different species of fungi in the zygomycete family (see Box 104-1). Zygomycete infections are typically acquired from aerosol exposure to the fungus in a susceptible host. Thus, the most common sites of zygomycete infection are rhinocerebral and pulmonary, with less common sites of infection being the gastrointestinal tract, skin, kidney, and central nervous system. The most common risk factors for zygomycete infection are diabetes mellitus, neutropenia, allogeneic stem cell and solid organ transplantation, and individuals chronically treated with corticosteroids. Because the organism requires iron for growth and can utilize chelated iron, treatment with the iron chelation agent deferoxamine is a risk factor for invasive zygomycete infection.

Rhinocerebral zygomycete infection should be suspected in susceptible patients who present with fever, headache, nasal congestion, and nasal discharge. Patients with poorly controlled diabetes mellitus and ketoacidosis are particularly at risk. Typical black eschars due to local tissue invasion and necrosis may be apparent on the nasal mucosa. Direct extension to overlying skin, orbit, cavernous sinus, and central nervous system occur commonly and are often devastating. Pulmonary zygomycete infection is typically found in individuals with neutropenia, stem cell transplantation, or chronic steroid treatment. Presenting signs include fever, cough, and hemoptysis. X-rays demonstrate multiple nodular lesions, and the lesions are often confused with aspergillosis. Gastrointestinal disease involving the stomach or colon often presents as diarrhea with abdominal pain.

Treatment of zygomycete infection requires therapy with amphotericin B or lipid products for a prolonged course. Posaconazole, an oral azole, has been used effectively in the treatment of zygomycete infections; however, neither voriconazole nor the echinocandins are active as treatment. Aggressive surgical débridement is critical for patients with rhinocerebral zygomycete infection. The overall mortality rate for zygomycete infection ranges from 25% to 50% for sinus disease to 80% or greater for pulmonary and cerebral disease.

Endemic Mycoses

Multiple different fungi exist in the soil specific to particular geographic areas and are largely responsible for the primary endemic mycoses in the United States: blastomycosis, histoplasmosis, coccidioidomycosis, and sporotri-

chosis. For most of these organisms, the clinical symptoms and signs depend on the route of acquisition and the immune status of the host.

In the United States, *Blastomyces dermatitidis* is typically found in the Ohio and Mississippi river valleys and the Midwestern states and areas along the Great Lakes and St. Lawrence River. Infection with *B. dermatitidis* has been found in individuals who spend time outdoors either through work or recreation and has been associated with exposure to excavation and water. Infection occurs most commonly due to inhalation of conidia. Thus, the most common clinical presentation of blastomycosis is acute or subacute respiratory infection. Based on surveys from endemic areas in Wisconsin and Minnesota, it is estimated that most infected patients are either asymptomatic or develop a mild flu-like illness. However, an acute process that appears similar to bacterial pneumonia with fever, cough, shortness of breath, and consolidation on chest x-ray can occur. Or, the presentation can consist of subacute respiratory symptoms. Dissemination to the skin, bone, genitourinary tract, central nervous system, and other sites have also been described. The disease is diagnosed by the presence of organisms cultured from an involved area or detected microscopically. X-ray findings for blastomycosis are nonspecific and include lobar and interstitial infiltrates, nodular lesions, and pleural effusions.

Unlike many of the endemic mycoses, immunocompromised patients do not appear to be at greater risk for infection with *B. dermatitidis*. Infection in the immunocompromised host is associated with a higher mortality rate, poorer response rate to therapy, and increased risk for recurrence. Therapeutic approaches for the endemic mycoses are shown in Table 104-3.

In the United States, *Histoplasma capsulatum* is found commonly in the Ohio River and the St. Lawrence River valleys. The organism is found in the droppings of birds

Table 104-3	Therapy for Endemic Mycoses			
Mycosis	**Acute**	**Disseminated**	**Chronic**	**Immunocompromised***
Blastomyces dermatitidis	Itraconazole, 200 mg/day	Amphotericin B or lipid complex followed by itraconazole		Amphotericin B or lipid derivatives followed by long-term itraconazole
Histoplasma capsulatum	Itraconazole	Amphotericin B followed by azole therapy	Amphotericin B followed by prolonged azole therapy	Amphotericin B followed by prolonged azole therapy
Coccidioides immitis	Either no treatment, itraconazole, or fluconazole	Itraconazole or fluconazole; meningitis: high-dose fluconazole		High-dose prolonged azole therapy (itraconazole, fluconazole) or amphotericin B then azole therapy
Sporothrix schenckii	Fluconazole, itraconazole	Amphotericin B or lipid product	Bone or joint involvement treated with itraconazole	Amphotericin B or lipid product or itraconazole

* For these infections, prolonged (>2 years) or lifelong therapy for the immunocompromised individual is required.

Figure 104-4 Histoplasmosis.

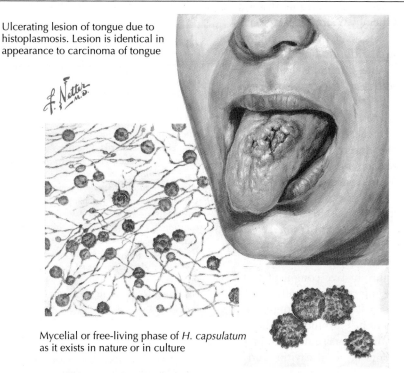

Ulcerating lesion of tongue due to histoplasmosis. Lesion is identical in appearance to carcinoma of tongue

Mycelial or free-living phase of *H. capsulatum* as it exists in nature or in culture

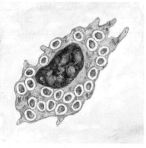

Spores of mycelial phase of *H. capsulatum*. Inhalation of these is source of infection

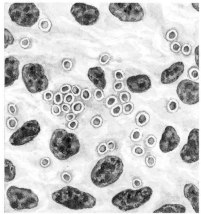

H. capsulatum in tissue

H. capsulatum in a macrophage. In this yeast or tissue phase, organism is not transmissible from person to person

such as pigeons and bats or is in an aerosolized form in caves. *H. capsulatum* is most commonly acquired by inhalation of the organism. The immune response is critical to control of the infection and requires interaction between CD4+ type 1 helper T cells that generate interferon-γ and macrophages that both activate T cells through interleukin-12 and control replication by the production of cytokines and reactive oxygen species. In humans, the organisms are contained in granulomas that are not sterile, leading to a high incidence of reactivation in T-cell-deficient individuals.

The clinical illness caused by *H. capsulatum* varies greatly depending on the immune status of the host and the expo-sure (Fig. 104-4). Most individuals exposed to *H. capsulatum* are either asymptomatic or develop a flu-like illness with fever, chills, headache, cough, and chest discomfort. An overwhelming exposure can lead to severe pneumonia with adult respiratory distress syndrome. A very small percentage of infected individuals develop chronic histoplasmosis, which has multiple varied manifestations. Chronic disseminated histoplasmosis is characterized by weight loss and fever and is often confused with mycobacterial infections such as tuberculosis. Subacute disseminated histoplasmosis is characterized by hepatosplenomegaly, peripheral blood count abnormalities, fever, and oral lesions. Acute disseminated histoplasmosis is seen in immunocompromised individuals and presents as a fulminant infection with a sepsis syndrome. Chronic disseminated histoplasmosis without therapy is almost always fatal. The diagnosis of histoplasmosis is made by identifying the yeast form in fluids or tissues. Antibody-based testing is helpful in the diagnosis of acute infections based on a fourfold rise in titers or based on the urinary histoplasmic antigen assay.

Infection with *Coccidioides immitis* is found predominantly in the United States in the Lower Sonoran Life Zone, which is found in the desert areas of Arizona, California, Nevada, New Mexico, and Texas. Outside of the United States, the organism is found in Mexico and in Central and South America. As in blastomycosis and histoplasmosis, infection is typically due to inhalation of the organism. Most patients infected with *C. immitis* are asymptomatic. Those who become sick after exposure most commonly develop a flu-like respiratory illness characterized by fever, chills, nonproductive cough, pleuritic chest pain, and fatigue. Acute infections typically resolve over 2 to 3 weeks; however, a small percentage of infected patients develop chronic infection. Chronic coccidioidomycosis can manifest as both a persistent pulmonary process characterized by the formation of cavities and as extrapulmonary manifestations including involvement of the meninges, skin and soft tissue, bone, and joints. Chronic coccidioidomycosis is typically fatal without prolonged specific therapy. Therapy is not typically required for immunocompetent patients who present with acute infection. However, any immunocompromised individual requires therapy for coccidioidomycosis (see Table 104-3).

Sporothrix schenckii is a fungus found in soil. Like the other fungi listed above, *S. schenckii* exists as a mycelium and yeast. Unlike the other organisms, *S. schenckii* causes infection throughout the world and is generally acquired by direct contact with soil or contaminated plants that cause puncture wounds. Clinically, patients with sporotrichosis present with local findings at the site of inoculation. The lesions are typically violaceous or red skin nodules that tend to ulcerate. Over time, direct extension of the organism to joints or bone occurs in some individuals. Disseminated sporotrichosis is typically found only in immunocompromised individuals. The diagnosis of sporotrichosis is made by culturing the organism from the site of infection. Antibody testing is available but not commonly used. The mainstay of treatment for skin or localized soft tissue sporotrichosis is azole therapy using either itraconazole (200 mg/day) or fluconazole (400 to 800 mg/day). Direct extension of sporotrichosis to bone or joint is typically treated with itraconazole.

Additional Resources

Doctor Fungus. Available at: http://www.doctorfungus.org/mycoses/index.htm. Accessed November 25, 2006.

This online reference focuses broadly on mycology.

Infectious Diseases Society of America. Standards, practice guidelines, and statements developed and/or endorsed by IDSA. Available at: http://www.idsociety.org/Content/NavigationMenu/Practice_Guidelines/Standards_Practice_Guidelines_Statements/Standards,_Practice_Guidelines,_and_Statements.htm. Accessed November 25, 2006.

This website provides consensus guidelines for the management of fungal infections from infectious disease experts.

Patterson T, Wingard J: Changing the treatment paradigm to improve fungal infection outcomes. Available at: http://www.projectsinknowledge.com/init/ID/1743/. Accessed November 25, 2006.

This excellent overview, part of the Projects in Knowledge website, addresses the treatment of invasive fungal infections with an emphasis on the treatment of Candida, Aspergillus, and Cryptococcus species from acknowledged experts in mycology.

Richardson MD: Changing patterns and trends in systemic fungal infections. J Antimicrob Chemother 56(Suppl 1):i5-i11, 2005.

This very good overview covers new trends in the prevalence and management of invasive fungal infections.

Stevens DA, Kan VL, Judson MA, et al: Practice guidelines for diseases caused by *Aspergillus*. Infectious Diseases Society of America. Clin Infect Dis 30(4):696-709, 2000.

This article includes the consensus guidelines from the Infectious Disease Society of America as part of their practice guidelines management tools for the diagnosis and management of aspergillus infections.

EVIDENCE

1. Anaissie E, McGinnis MR, Pfaller MA (eds): Clinical Mycology. London, Churchill Livingstone, 2003.

   This outstanding general reference deals in a comprehensive manner with fungal organisms and the infections that they cause.

2. Bennett JE: Introduction to mycoses. In Mandell GL, Bennett JE, Dolin R (eds): Principles and Practices of Infectious Diseases, 6th ed. London, Churchill Livingstone, 2005.

   Dr. Bennett is one of the leading experts in fungal infections. His chapter in this comprehensive textbook of infectious diseases summarizes basic mycology and provides an overview of significant fungal infections in humans.

3. Kauffman CA: The changing landscape of invasive fungal infections: Epidemiology, diagnosis, and pharmacologic options. Clin Infect Dis 43:S1-S39, 2006.

   This supplement provides the most recent and comprehensive update on invasive fungal infections encompassing epidemiology, diagnostics, and use of antifungal agents written by leading experts in the field.

4. Pappas PG, Rex JH, Sobel JD, et al: Guidelines for treatment of candidiasis. Clin Infect Dis 38(2):161-189, 2004.

   These consensus guidelines from the Infectious Diseases Society of America address the management of infections due to Candida species.

Mina C. Hosseinipour ▪ Douglas R. Morgan

105

Parasitic Infections

Introduction

Enteric parasitic infections remain an important cause of morbidity in developing countries. With the constant influx of immigrants, the growing number of travelers to developing countries, and immunosuppression related to HIV, transplantation, and chemotherapy, knowledge of parasitic diseases is of increasing importance. Parasitic diseases can be largely divided into two categories: those due to helminths (of which nematodes are a major category), and those due to protozoa.

Nematodes: Roundworms

Nematodes are categorized according to where the adult form of the worm resides. Intestinal nematodes are the most prevalent. Although intestinal nematode infections occur worldwide, most cases occur in tropical or subtropical countries and disproportionately afflict children. Poor sanitation plays a major role because maturation of eggs within the environment must occur to maintain the worm life cycle and human infections. Symptoms are highly dependent on the number of infectious organisms, the so-called worm burden. Infections involving a low worm burden (light infections) are generally asymptomatic, whereas those with a high worm burden (heavy infections) result in more severe symptoms and complications. Eosinophilia generally occurs with the tissue migration phase of the immature worm and may be absent when the adult worm resides in the intestine. Coinfections in individuals with intestinal worms are common.

Enterobiasis (Pinworm)

Etiology and Pathogenesis

Pinworm infection is caused by *Enterobius vermicularis* (Fig. 105-1). When infectious eggs are ingested, larvae mature within the intestine, and adult female worms lay eggs on the perianal skin. Immature eggs must mature in the environment to become infectious. Because the maturation of *Enterobius* eggs occurs within hours, reinfection of the child and infection of family members and close contacts is common.

Clinical Presentation

Nocturnal pruritus ani is the predominant symptom, particularly among children. Pruritus vulvae and genitourinary symptoms may occur in girls.

Differential Diagnosis

Other nematode infections or vaginal candidiasis can present similarly.

Diagnostic Approach

The cellophane tape test is the best diagnostic method. Cellophane tape pressed on the perianal skin in the morning will reveal eggs and possibly female worms. Fecal smears for ova and parasites are frequently negative and less useful in diagnosis.

Management and Therapy

Optimum treatment is a single dose of mebendazole, 100 mg; pyrantel pamoate, 11 mg/kg; or albendazole, 400 mg. Clothing and bedding should be washed to eradicate infectious eggs in the environment. The entire family should be treated simultaneously, and retreatment of all family members should occur within a 2-week period.

Trichuriasis (Whipworm)

Etiology and Pathogenesis

Whipworm infection is caused by *Trichuris trichiura*. This infection is also maintained through a direct life cycle.

Figure 105-1 Parasitic Diseases: Enterobiasis.

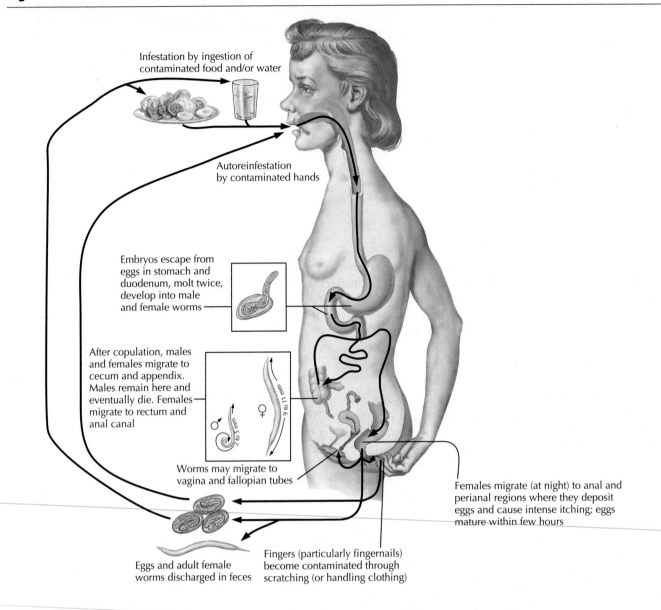

Infestation by ingestion of contaminated food and/or water

Autoreinfestation by contaminated hands

Embryos escape from eggs in stomach and duodenum, molt twice, develop into male and female worms

After copulation, males and females migrate to cecum and appendix. Males remain here and eventually die. Females migrate to rectum and anal canal

Worms may migrate to vagina and fallopian tubes

Females migrate (at night) to anal and perianal regions where they deposit eggs and cause intense itching; eggs mature within few hours

Eggs and adult female worms discharged in feces

Fingers (particularly fingernails) become contaminated through scratching (or handling clothing)

However, *Trichuris* eggs require weeks to months to mature; therefore, autoinfection (repeated infection of oneself) generally does not occur.

Clinical Presentation

Most infections are asymptomatic. Heavy infections in malnourished infants may result in diarrhea and rectal prolapse.

Differential Diagnosis

Other nematode infections should be considered.

Diagnostic Approach

A fecal smear for ova and parasites is the preferred diagnostic method.

Management and Therapy

Optimum treatment is either mebendazole, 100 mg twice daily for 3 days; mebendazole, 500 mg in a single dose; albendazole, 400 mg once daily for 3 days; or ivermectin, 200 µg/kg once daily for 3 days.

Figure 105-2 Parasitic Diseases: Ascariasis.

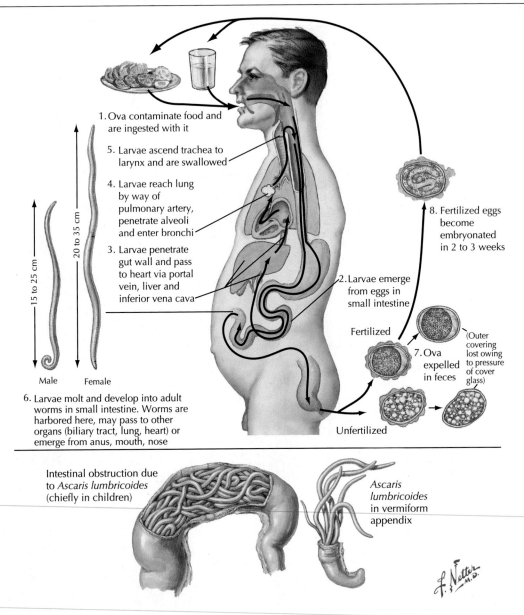

1. Ova contaminate food and are ingested with it

5. Larvae ascend trachea to larynx and are swallowed

4. Larvae reach lung by way of pulmonary artery, penetrate alveoli and enter bronchi

3. Larvae penetrate gut wall and pass to heart via portal vein, liver and inferior vena cava

2. Larvae emerge from eggs in small intestine

8. Fertilized eggs become embryonated in 2 to 3 weeks

Fertilized

7. Ova expelled in feces

(Outer covering lost owing to pressure of cover glass)

Unfertilized

20 to 35 cm

15 to 25 cm

Male   Female

6. Larvae molt and develop into adult worms in small intestine. Worms are harbored here, may pass to other organs (biliary tract, lung, heart) or emerge from anus, mouth, nose

Intestinal obstruction due to *Ascaris lumbricoides* (chiefly in children)

Ascaris lumbricoides in vermiform appendix

Ascariasis

Etiology and Pathogenesis

Ascaris lumbricoides infection occurs through a complex life cycle (Fig. 105-2). After ingestion of infectious eggs, the immature larvae migrate through the lungs before reaching the adult stage in the intestine.

Clinical Presentation

Pulmonary symptoms, such as cough, dyspnea, and wheezing with infiltrates and eosinophilia may occur during the lung migration phase. Low levels of infection are largely asymptomatic, whereas high worm burdens may cause gastrointestinal symptoms of abdominal pain, nausea, and small bowel obstruction. Rarely, ascarids may migrate into the biliary tract or pancreatic duct, causing symptoms consistent with biliary colic or pancreatitis. Occasionally, patients present with fecal passage of a large adult worm.

Differential Diagnosis

During the migration phase, pulmonary disorders such as asthma, eosinophilic pneumonia, and interstitial lung diseases may be considered. Peptic ulcer disease, biliary disease, or pancreatitis may be related to abdominal symptoms. Other nematode infections may also be considered.

Diagnostic Approach

A fecal smear for ova and parasites is generally positive because of the high egg output of this parasite.

Figure 105-3 Parasitic Diseases: Necatoriasis and Ancylostomiasis.

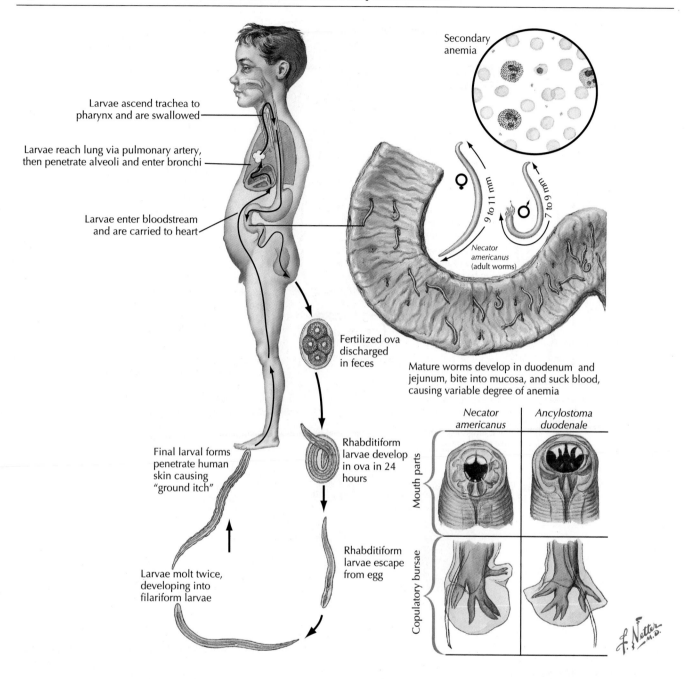

Secondary anemia

Larvae ascend trachea to pharynx and are swallowed

Larvae reach lung via pulmonary artery, then penetrate alveoli and enter bronchi

Larvae enter bloodstream and are carried to heart

♀ 9 to 11 mm

♂ 7 to 9 mm

Necator americanus (adult worms)

Fertilized ova discharged in feces

Mature worms develop in duodenum and jejunum, bite into mucosa, and suck blood, causing variable degree of anemia

Final larval forms penetrate human skin causing "ground itch"

Rhabditiform larvae develop in ova in 24 hours

	Necator americanus	*Ancylostoma duodenale*
Mouth parts		
Copulatory bursae		

Larvae molt twice, developing into filariform larvae

Rhabditiform larvae escape from egg

Management and Therapy

Optimum treatment is either mebendazole, 100 mg twice daily for 3 days; mebendazole, 500 mg in a single dose; albendazole, 400 mg in a single dose; pyrantel pamoate, 11 mg/kg in a single dose; or nitazoxanide, 500 mg twice daily for 3 days. After treatment, patients may experience the migration of adult worms from the nose or mouth, and reassurance may be required.

Hookworm Infections

Etiology and Pathogenesis

Hookworm infections are caused by either *Necator americanus* or *Ancylostoma duodenale* (Fig. 105-3). The hookworm life cycle begins with the percutaneous penetration of the infectious filariform larvae, usually through bare feet. The larvae migrate from the skin to the lung and eventually transit to the small intestine, where the adult worm resides

and releases eggs into the feces. The eggs must embryonate into rhabditiform larvae, then to filariform larvae before they are infectious again. The repetitive release and reattachment of the adult worm to intestinal mucosa may result in low-grade bleeding and anemia.

Clinical Presentation

A pruritic maculopapular rash may result after the penetration of the filariform larvae. Migration of the larvae through the lung is associated with cough, wheezing, pulmonary infiltrates, and eosinophilia. Abdominal symptoms include abdominal pain, diarrhea, and nausea and vomiting. Symptoms of iron-deficiency anemia such as fatigue, dyspnea, or pica may develop with chronic infection. Hypoproteinemia and growth retardation occur in children who have chronic infection.

Differential Diagnosis

During the migration phase, pulmonary disorders such as asthma, eosinophilic pneumonia, and interstitial lung diseases may be considered. Abdominal symptoms similar to those due to hookworm can result from peptic ulcer disease, biliary disease, or pancreatitis. Given the finding of iron-deficiency anemia in some cases, alternative causes of gastrointestinal blood loss (carcinoma, diverticular disease, peptic ulcer disease) should also be considered.

Diagnostic Approach

A fecal smear for ova and parasites is diagnostic.

Management and Therapy

Optimum treatment is either mebendazole, 100 mg twice daily for 3 days; mebendazole, 500 mg in a single dose; albendazole, 400 mg in a single dose; or pyrantel pamoate, 11 mg/kg once daily for 3 days. Iron supplementation may be necessary to correct the iron-deficiency anemia.

Currently, there is investigation into a hookworm vaccine. Until this is available, sanitation and ensuring the use of footwear are the key to prevention of this infection.

Strongyloidiasis

Etiology and Pathogenesis

Strongyloides stercoralis penetrates intact skin, transits the lung, and then resides in the small intestine as mature organisms. It is capable of maintaining an autoinfective cycle whereby rhabditiform larvae transform into the infectious filariform larvae within the host, allowing reinfection and persistence of the cycle for years. Autoinfection in an immunocompromised host can result in life-threatening disseminated illness known as *hyperinfection*. Those infected with human T-cell leukemia virus-1 are at increased risk for hyperinfection. In the southern United States, strongyloidiasis occurs at an estimated prevalence of 0.4% to 4%.

Clinical Presentation

Larva currens, a recurrent serpiginous urticarial rash usually around the buttocks, is suggestive of autoinfection. During the pulmonary transit phase, infected individuals may experience cough, wheezing, and pulmonary infiltrates. Abdominal symptoms include pain, diarrhea, nausea, and vomiting. Malabsorption and weight loss occur with heavier infections. Hyperinfection results in ileus, pneumonia, meningitis, polymicrobial gram-negative bacteremia, and multiorgan failure.

Eosinophilia, usually present, may be absent in hyperinfection.

Differential Diagnosis

During the migration phase, pulmonary disorders such as asthma, eosinophilic pneumonia, and interstitial lung diseases should be considered as alternative diagnoses. Peptic ulcer disease, biliary disease, or pancreatitis may be considered related to abdominal symptoms. Other nematode infections should also be considered.

Diagnostic Approach

A fecal smear is often negative, and multiple stool specimens using concentration techniques may be required for diagnosis. Alternatively, duodenal aspirate specimens from endoscopy or a string test can be used to make this diagnosis when necessary. In hyperinfection, sputum examination may reveal larvae. Patients from endemic areas planning immunosuppressive treatment such as chemotherapy or organ transplantation should have enzyme-linked immunosorbent assay (ELISA) serologic testing before initiating therapy, and individuals found to be infected should be treated appropriately.

Management and Therapy

Optimum therapy is ivermectin, 200 µg/kg/day for 1 to 2 days, which is highly efficacious and nontoxic for uncomplicated disease. Albendazole, 400 mg twice daily for 3 days, or thiabendazole, 25 mg/kg twice daily for 2 days, is also effective but has fallen from favor given the efficacy of ivermectin. For disseminated disease, treat with ivermectin, 200 µg/kg/day for 7 to 10 days.

Cestodes (Tapeworm)

Etiology and Pathogenesis

Tapeworm infection occurs in humans when uncooked or undercooked infected meat is ingested (Fig. 105-4). The infection transmitted depends on the meat consumed: beef, *Taenia saginata*; pork, *Taenia solium*; and fish, *Diphyllobothrium latum*.

Clinical Presentation

Infection is often asymptomatic, or individuals may sense the movement of the proglottids through the anus.

Figure 105-4 Parasitic Diseases: Taeniasis Solium (Cysticercosis Cellulosae).

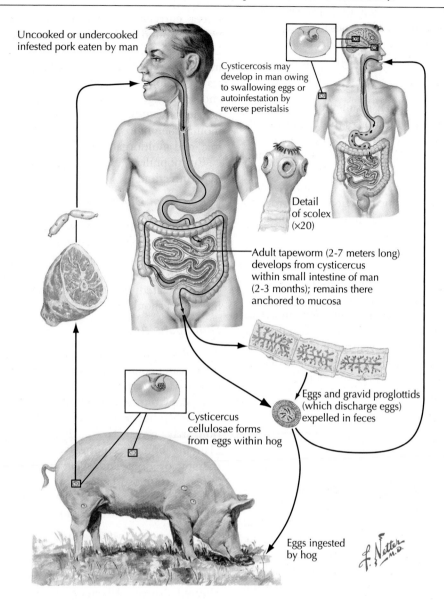

Uncooked or undercooked infested pork eaten by man

Cysticercosis may develop in man owing to swallowing eggs or autoinfestation by reverse peristalsis

Detail of scolex (×20)

Adult tapeworm (2-7 meters long) develops from cysticercus within small intestine of man (2-3 months); remains there anchored to mucosa

Eggs and gravid proglottids (which discharge eggs) expelled in feces

Cysticercus cellulosae forms from eggs within hog

Eggs ingested by hog

Infection with *D. latum* may result in megaloblastic anemia secondary to vitamin B_{12} deficiency.

Differential Diagnosis

Infection with other nematodes, particularly pinworm, should be considered.

Diagnostic Approach

Fecal demonstration of proglottids or eggs is diagnostic.

Management and Therapy

Optimum treatment is praziquantel, 10 mg/kg in a single dose, or niclosamide, 2 g in a single dose.

Cysticercosis

Etiology and Pathogenesis

The tapeworm *T. solium* has the potential to cause cysticercosis (see Fig. 105-4). When the egg of *T. solium* is ingested either directly through fecal contamination or through autoinfestation by reverse peristalsis, the larval form of the disease, cysticercus cellulosae, develops, and tissue cysts (cysticerci) may often develop in subcutaneous tissues, muscle, and brain.

Clinical Presentation

Subcutaneous nodules may be palpable. Neurologic symptoms vary widely according to the location and number of

cysts, stage of the infection, and the host response. Asymptomatic disease is common, particularly in the first years after infection. Seizure is the most common presenting symptom; headache, increased intracranial pressure, altered mental status, and focal neurologic findings occur less frequently.

Differential Diagnosis

Skin nodules may also occur with onchocerciasis. Primary epilepsy and infectious diseases of the central nervous system (toxoplasmosis, meningitis, tuberculosis, brain abscess) may be considered depending on the neurologic presentation.

Diagnostic Approach

Computed tomography (CT) scan and magnetic resonance imaging (MRI) are the primary methods to diagnose neurocysticercosis. MRI is more sensitive in the diagnosis of extraparenchymal cysts and inflammatory reactions to cysts. The enzyme-linked immunotransfer blot assay (serum titer) is highly specific for *T. solium* and highly sensitive in patients with multiple active cysts.

Management and Therapy

Treatment with antiparasitic agents should be individualized according to the location and activity of the cysts. Albendazole, 400 mg twice daily for 8 to 30 days with concomitant corticosteroids, may be effective if therapy is indicated. Praziquantel, 50 mg/kg daily for 15 days combined with corticosteroids, may also be effective. Consultation with an infectious disease physician is recommended.

Antiepileptic medication may be required even after successful treatment.

Intestinal Protozoa

Although several species of protozoa may be found in the human intestinal tract, many are regarded as nonpathogenic commensals. *Giardia lamblia* and *Entamoeba histolytica* cause most enteric protozoal diseases among immunocompetent individuals in the United States. *Cryptosporidium*, *Cyclospora*, *Microsporidia*, and *Isospora* species are important enteric protozoal diseases in patients with AIDS and are discussed elsewhere.

Giardiasis

Etiology and Pathogenesis

Giardia lamblia, the most common intestinal parasite worldwide, is a frequent cause of diarrhea and malabsorption. It is typically acquired through the ingestion of contaminated food and water or by person-to-person contact. Synonyms for *G. lamblia* include *G. intestinalis* and *G. duodenalis* (Fig. 105-5).

Giardiasis occurs in sporadic, epidemic, and endemic forms. Sporadic infections are seen with international travel, rural camping, or person-to-person contact. Outbreaks have been reported with community water systems and in institutions with close contact and the potential for fecal-oral contamination, such as day care centers. Giardiasis is endemic in the developing world. Studies based on stool specimens suggest that the prevalence is 2% to 5% in the developed world, compared with 20% to 30% in the developing world. Infection occurs year-round, with a small peak in the spring in the United States.

G. lamblia has two stages in its life cycle: cysts, the infectious form; and trophozoites, the replicating form. The cyst form is inert and environmentally resistant, viable for months outside the host. Water treatment, by filtration or boiling, prevents *G. lamblia* infections. Addition of iodine or chlorine to drinking water also inactivates cysts under appropriate concentrations and exposure duration. The trophozoite is the motile form, which is adherent to the small bowel mucosa. Replication occurs by binary fission within the intestine, with a doubling time of about 12 hours. Encystation occurs in the ileum, possibly triggered by exposure to bile, followed by cyst excretion in feces.

Clinical Presentation

Protracted diarrhea is a central feature of giardiasis. Typically, stools are loose and foul smelling and may contain mucus but not blood. Anorexia, nausea, abdominal cramping, bloating, and weight loss are common symptoms. Fever occurs in about 10% of patients. Patients chronically infected with *Giardia* often have malabsorption and weight loss.

Determinants of disease severity remain an enigma. Infected patients are either asymptomatic (60%), have acute infection (40%), or have a chronic infection (including 40% of those with acute infections). About 10% of asymptomatic patients have stool cysts and can transmit the disease. The infectious inoculum may be as low as 10 to 25 cysts. The incubation period is 1 to 2 weeks on average, with a range of 1 day to 6 weeks.

Differential Diagnosis

The primary focus in the evaluation of acute diarrhea is infectious agents. Important bacterial infections that should be included in the differential diagnosis are *Salmonella*, *Shigella*, *Campylobacter*, and *Yersinia* species, *Escherichia coli*, and *Clostridium difficile*. Other potential parasitic infections should also be included, particularly *Entamoeba histolytica* and *Cryptosporidium* species. Viral enteritides are also common and include rotavirus and the Norwalk agent. Dietary indiscretion, recent medication changes, and new-onset chronic diarrhea should also be considered.

Chronic diarrhea has a broad differential diagnosis with a variety of classification schemes. Other infectious diseases may be considered, particularly for the returning international traveler. The differential diagnosis includes

Figure 105-5 Giardiasis.

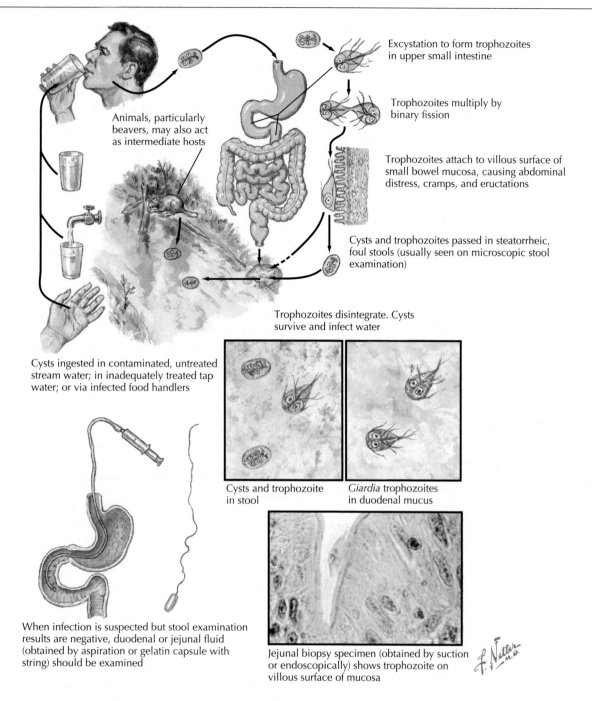

Excystation to form trophozoites in upper small intestine

Trophozoites multiply by binary fission

Trophozoites attach to villous surface of small bowel mucosa, causing abdominal distress, cramps, and eructations

Cysts and trophozoites passed in steatorrheic, foul stools (usually seen on microscopic stool examination)

Animals, particularly beavers, may also act as intermediate hosts

Trophozoites disintegrate. Cysts survive and infect water

Cysts ingested in contaminated, untreated stream water; in inadequately treated tap water; or via infected food handlers

Cysts and trophozoite in stool

Giardia trophozoites in duodenal mucus

When infection is suspected but stool examination results are negative, duodenal or jejunal fluid (obtained by aspiration or gelatin capsule with string) should be examined

Jejunal biopsy specimen (obtained by suction or endoscopically) shows trophozoite on villous surface of mucosa

the inflammatory diarrheas (e.g., Crohn's disease), maldigestion (e.g., pancreatic insufficiency), and malabsorption (e.g., bacterial overgrowth). Other considerations include systemic disease, lymphoma, medication side effects, and the rare tumor-related secretory diarrheas (e.g., gastrinoma, carcinoid tumor).

Diagnostic Approach

Examination of fecal specimens is the primary means for diagnosis. Cyst passage in stool is sporadic, and three samples are recommended as sensitivity increases from 60% to 90% with examination of one to three specimens. Many laboratories use *Giardia* antigen assays, using either immunofluorescent or ELISA technology, which typically have single specimen sensitivities greater than 90%.

Management and Therapy

Treatment is recommended for symptomatic patients and, in institutional settings, for asymptomatic patients to prevent the spread of disease. Metronidazole, 250 mg orally three times daily for 5 days; tinidazole, 2 g stat dose; and nitazoxanide, 500 mg twice daily for 3 days, are all

Figure 105-6 Amebiasis.

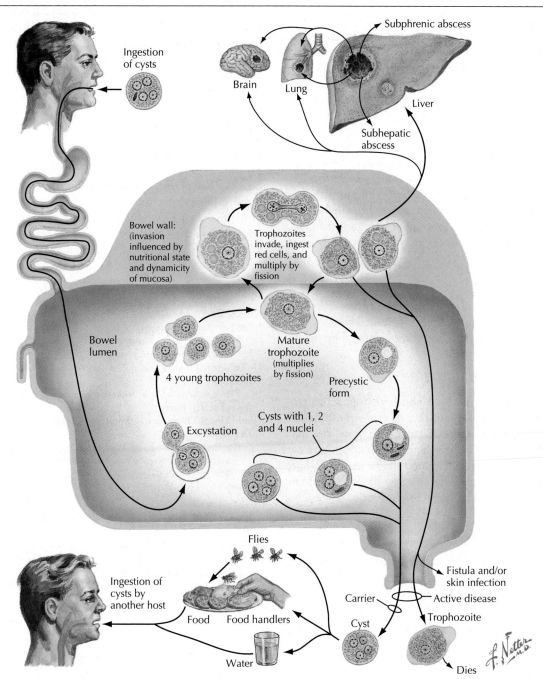

effective treatments. Treatment of giardiasis in pregnancy is difficult, and there are no consistent recommendations.

The prevention of *Giardia* outbreaks in community water systems depends on adequate sedimentation, filtration, and possibly a higher chlorine concentration within the treated water. For individuals who have been camping or for international travelers, boiling (at least 10 minutes), filtration (pore size less than or equal to 2 mm), or halogens (chlorine, iodine) are recommended. Within day care centers and other institutions, handwashing is important. Breast-feeding is recommended because maternal immu-

noglobulin A has been shown to be effective in preventing infection in infants.

Amebiasis

Etiology and Pathogenesis

Entamoeba histolytica infection is spread by fecal-oral contamination with infectious cysts (Fig. 105-6). Symptoms develop if the cysts become trophozoites capable of invading the colonic mucosa. *E. histolytica* cysts are morphologically indistinguishable from the nonpathogenic *Entamoeba dispar*.

Clinical Presentation

Most infected individuals with *Entamoeba* cysts in the stool are asymptomatic because most are actually infected with *E. dispar*. Symptomatic disease occurs in only 10% of *E. histolytica* cyst carriers. Among symptomatic patients, diarrhea with blood and mucus, and abdominal pain developing over 1 to 2 weeks are the predominant complaints. Rarely, patients present with a localized painful abdominal mass secondary to ameboma formation. Chronic amebic colitis presents with recurrent episodes of bloody diarrhea over years and may be confused with inflammatory bowel disease. Extraintestinal manifestations include abscess formation of the liver, lung, brain, or pericardium, with liver abscess the most common. Most patients with amebic liver abscess present with fever, right upper quadrant pain, and tenderness of the liver; others may present solely with fever.

Differential Diagnosis

Bacterial dysentery, giardiasis, inflammatory bowel disease, bacterial liver abscess, and biliary disease should all be considered in the differential diagnosis, depending on the presentation of the patient.

Diagnostic Approach

The finding of *Entamoeba* cysts and hematophagous trophozoites in a fresh stool wet mount is diagnostic of *E. histolytica*. In asymptomatic cyst passers, *E. histolytica* may be differentiated from *E. dispar* by the presence of positive amebic serology. Liver ultrasound, CT, and MRI are useful in the diagnosis of liver abscess. Biopsy of colonic tissue revealing trophozoites is diagnostic of amebic colitis.

Management and Therapy

Asymptomatic *E. dispar* cyst carriers do not require treatment. Asymptomatic *E. histolytica* cyst carriers should be treated with either iodoquinol, 650 mg thrice daily for 20 days, or paromomycin, 12 mg/kg orally thrice daily for 7 days. Amebic colitis is treated with metronidazole, 750 mg thrice daily for 10 days, or tinidazole, 2 g once daily for 3 days, followed with treatment with iodoquinol or paromomycin. Extraintestinal amebic disease is treated with metronidazole, 750 mg thrice daily for 10 days, or tinidazole, 2 g once daily for 5 days, followed with treatment with iodoquinol or paromomycin.

Future Directions

Efforts toward improving waste sanitation, food handling processes, animal husbandry processes, and ensuring quality control of water purification can virtually eliminate these enteric infections. Focused treatment of high-risk individuals, such as children in developing countries, in conjunction with improved sanitation remains a challenge and merits high priority as a global health initiative.

Additional Resources

Centers for Disease Control and Prevention. Available at: http://www.cdc.gov. Accessed December 20, 2006.

This website provides comprehensive information related to traveler's health related to geographic regions.

UpToDate Web site. Available at: http://www.uptodate.com. Accessed December 20, 2006.

This website provides a treatment summary for parasitic diseases not covered in this chapter.

World Health Organization. Available at: http://www.who.int. Accessed December 20, 2006.

Provides up-to-date information on general statistics and public health programs targeting control of parasite and soil transmitted helminths.

EVIDENCE

1. Guerrant RL, Walker DH, Weller PF (eds): Tropical Infectious Diseases: Principles, Pathogens, and Practice, 2nd ed. Philadelphia, Churchill Livingstone, 2006.

This textbook provides comprehensive chapters on tropical infectious diseases, including the parasitic infections highlighted in this chapter.

William C. Miller ▪ Jonathan J. Juliano

106

Malaria

Introduction

Malaria is a common and important infectious disease globally. An estimated 300 to 500 million cases of malaria occur worldwide each year, with more than 1 million deaths, primarily in Africa, Asia, and South and Central America (Fig. 106-1). Although once common in parts of the United States, most of the about 1300 cases reported in the United States each year are travelers to endemic regions. Cases have been reported from all 50 states, with most cases from New York City, California, and Maryland. More than half of the imported cases of malaria to the United States are *Plasmodium falciparum,* the most severe form of malaria.

Etiology and Pathogenesis

Malaria is caused by one of four species: *Plasmodium falciparum, Plasmodium vivax, Plasmodium ovale,* or *Plasmodium malariae.* The species are morphologically distinct, providing the basis for specific diagnosis.

The life cycles of the four species are similar (Fig. 106-2), but with important differences. Infection of humans begins with the inoculation of sporozoites from the salivary glands of an infected female *Anopheles* mosquito. The sporozoites rapidly invade hepatocytes and are largely cleared from the blood within 30 minutes of inoculation. In the liver, the parasite undergoes asexual multiplication to form hepatic or tissue schizonts. After a variable period of development, merozoites emerge from the liver cells into the bloodstream. The duration of the liver stage is typically 1 to 3 weeks, but is longer, 2 to 4 weeks, for *P. malariae.*

A critical difference between species is the existence of persistent liver forms, or hypnozoites, in *P. ovale* and *P. vivax* infections. In these species, hypnozoites form and can remain dormant for months or years before becoming active and causing relapse. Neither *P. falciparum* nor *P. malariae* have persistent liver forms. However, persistent, low-grade infections in the blood with *P. falciparum* or *P. malariae* may cause recrudescence of clinical disease.

The merozoites released from the liver attach to and invade erythrocytes. In the erythrocyte, ring forms with a small nucleus and a ring of pale cytoplasm develop. The parasite then develops into a trophozoite and finally into an erythrocytic schizont. Rupture of the schizont releases merozoites into the bloodstream, leading to another cycle of asexual development in fresh erythrocytes.

The parasite also undergoes a sexual cycle, which requires both humans and mosquitoes. In the erythrocyte, some merozoites develop into male and female gametocytes. These gametocytes are taken up during a blood meal by the female *Anopheles* mosquito. In the mosquito stomach, gametes form. Macrogametes are fertilized by microgametes forming zygotes, which then develop into ookinetes. The ookinetes invade the gut wall, form oocysts, and sporozoites develop within the oocysts. The sporozoites migrate to the salivary gland of the mosquito and await inoculation into the human host.

The cycle within the human host is affected by several host and parasite factors. *P. malariae* invades mature erythrocytes. *P. vivax* and *P. ovale* invade young erythrocytes. *P. falciparum* is capable of invading erythrocytes of any age. Thus, parasitemia is limited in *P. malariae, P. vivax,* and *P. ovale* infections but can reach extremely high levels in *P. falciparum* infections.

Persons with high levels of hemoglobin F and hemoglobin S have increased resistance to falciparum malaria due to reduced survival of the parasite in the erythrocytes. Persons with the heterozygous state of hemoglobin AS have a survival advantage and experience less severe falciparum malaria. Persons with glucose-6-phosphate dehydrogenase deficiency also appear to have increased resistance to falciparum malaria.

Persons lacking the Duffy group antigens on erythrocytes are resistant to infection with *P. vivax.* This trait,

Figure 106-1 Geographic Distribution of Malaria.

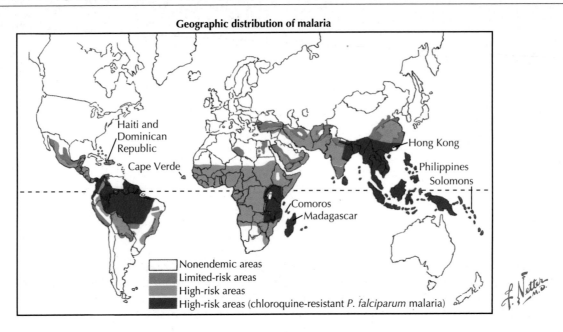

Geographic distribution of malaria

Figure 106-2 Life Cycle of Malaria Parasites (*Plasmodium vivax*).

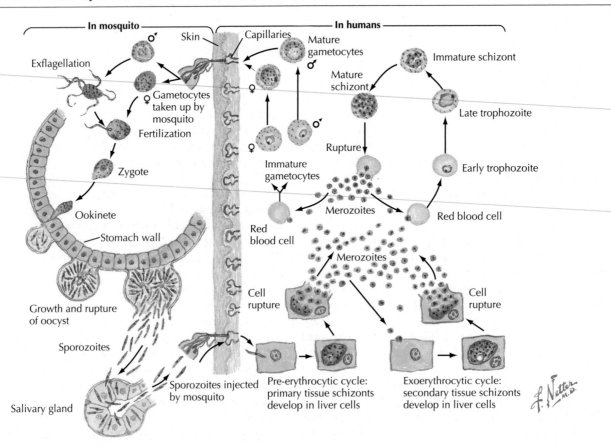

common throughout much of Africa, accounts for the low incidence of vivax malaria in Africa.

The symptoms, signs, and complications of malaria are due to the intraerythrocytic cycle. Fever occurs with schizont rupture. Anemia is common in all forms of malaria and is due primarily to destruction and phagocytosis of infected erythrocytes.

Falciparum malaria may be severe with life-threatening complications including cerebral malaria, acute renal failure, pulmonary edema and adult respiratory distress syndrome (ARDS), hyponatremia, and hypoglycemia. Cerebral malaria is caused, at least in part, by increased adherence of infected erythrocytes to capillary endothelial cells in the brain. Acute renal failure may result from volume depletion or acute tubular necrosis in the context of hyperparasitemia, intravascular hemolysis, and hemoglobinuria. Pulmonary edema may result from fluid administration. Pulmonary edema with an ARDS-like picture is more common, presumably because of increased capillary leakage secondary to cytokine production. Hyponatremia occurs secondary to inappropriate secretion of antidiuretic hormone. Hypoglycemia may be due to impaired hepatic gluconeogenesis. It is important to note that administration of quinine or quinidine may exacerbate hypoglycemia. Splenic rupture occurs with rapid rise in parasitemia. It is the primary cause of mortality in persons with *P. vivax* and *P. ovale* malaria.

Clinical Presentation

Many patients with malaria experience a prodrome with headache, decreased appetite, malaise, myalgias, and in some cases, low-grade fever. The prodrome may last 2 to 3 days but may be longer in persons with partial immunity or incomplete suppression due to prophylaxis.

Fever is the classic manifestation of malaria. The onset of a paroxysm of fever begins with abrupt onset of chills, often with teeth chattering and shivering. The subsequent fever, as high as 40° C to 41° C in falciparum malaria, typically lasts 2 to 4 hours and is followed by diaphoresis. The duration of the entire paroxysm is 8 to 12 hours. Between paroxysms, the patient may feel well.

The paroxysms of fever and chills are intermittent and may have periodicity (Fig. 106-3). Paroxysms associated with *P. vivax* and *P. ovale* infections occur every 48 hours, whereas with *P. malariae*, the interval interceding between episodes is 72 hours. The paroxysms of fever with these species are more common during the daylight hours. Fever is often irregular during the first few days of the illness. Periodicity is often absent in falciparum malaria but may occur with an interval of about 48 hours. Malaria cannot be excluded on the basis of the lack of periodicity.

Other symptoms, in addition to fever, include headache, backache, and myalgias. Nausea and vomiting commonly occur during the febrile paroxysm. Diarrhea may be present. Lightheadedness and postural hypotension may result from volume depletion. Confusion and delirium may also occur during the paroxysm of fever.

Physical findings in patients with malaria include fever, tachycardia, and orthostatic hypotension. Splenomegaly is typical, and tender hepatomegaly is often present. Jaundice and crackles in the lungs may be present.

Cerebral malaria is the most important and severe complication of falciparum malaria. Typically, it occurs after several days of illness, but it may also occur early in the course. Common initial manifestations include confusion and hallucinations, but coma is required for a true diagnosis of cerebral malaria. Physical examination may be nonfocal or have focal findings including disconjugate gaze, increased muscle tone, hemiparesis, and meningismus.

Splenic rupture may occur spontaneously or in association with minor trauma. Abdominal pain, possibly with radiation to the left shoulder, is typical. Hypotension and tachycardia result from the hemorrhage and rapid fall in blood volume. Rapid surgical intervention is essential.

A normocytic, normochromic anemia is typical, usually with evidence of hemolysis. Thrombocytopenia is also common. Hyponatremia, elevated blood urea nitrogen, bilirubinemia, and mildly elevated liver transaminase levels are also seen. Elevation of the serum creatinine level suggests acute renal failure due to hypovolemia or acute tubular necrosis.

The clinical presentation of malaria in adults from endemic regions is usually milder, manifested primarily by fever, headache, and gastrointestinal symptoms. This mild form of the illness is most often due to the acquisition of partial immunity. Immunity is not permanent and may wane after a prolonged period without exposure. In fact, natives to endemic regions represent one of the most common groups of travelers with imported malaria in the United States. Use of prophylaxis is uncommon among persons who have previously lived in malarious regions and are returning after a stay abroad.

Malaria during pregnancy is often more severe than in other adults. Mortality is increased, and the infection is associated with stillbirth, premature delivery, and low birth weight. Anemia is worse in malaria during pregnancy. Hypoglycemia is common in malaria during pregnancy, and as in other infected individuals, may be exacerbated by treatment with quinine or quinidine.

Differential Diagnosis

The clinical manifestations of malaria are nonspecific and may be present in a variety of other febrile illnesses. Common infections in the United States, such as influenza, bacteremia, viral gastroenteritis, viral hepatitis, viral encephalitis, and viral or bacterial meningitis, may present similarly. Febrile illnesses associated with travel that must be considered in the differential diagnosis include typhoid fever, relapsing fevers, yellow fever, leptospirosis, brucellosis, and traveler's diarrhea. Noninfectious causes of fever

Figure 106-3 Malaria: Clinical Course and Diagnosis.

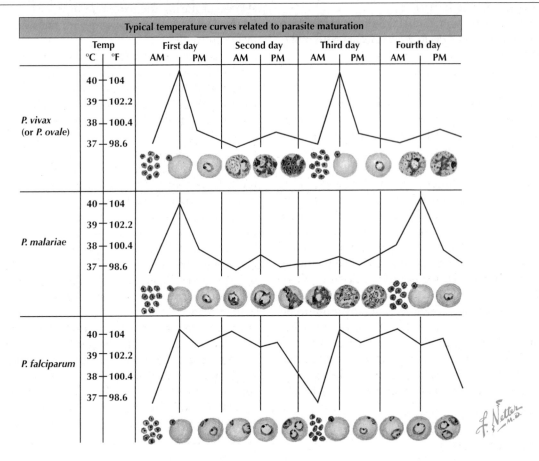

Typical temperature curves related to parasite maturation									

may also be considered, such as drug-induced fever with hemolysis.

Diagnostic Approach

Malaria must be considered in any person with fever and a history of travel to an endemic area. A carefully elicited travel history will assist in making the diagnosis and eliminating several of the other possible infectious causes of malaria. The travel history will provide insight into the likely species of *Plasmodium* and guide treatment choices. *P. falciparum* occurs throughout the malarious regions of the world but predominates in Africa, Haiti, and New Guinea. It is common in India, Southeast Asia, Oceania, and South America. *P. ovale* occurs primarily in Africa. *P. vivax* occurs in Central and South America, western Asia, and North Africa. *P. vivax* is rarely found in sub-Saharan Africa. *P. malariae* is widespread throughout the malarious regions of the world.

Throughout the world, including the United States, the primary diagnostic method is the use of blood films (Fig. 106-4). Thick films are prepared by placing a fresh drop of blood, preferably from a finger stick, on a microscope slide. After drying, the cells are lysed with distilled water, and the slide is stained with Giemsa or Wright-Giemsa stain. Thin films are prepared in the same manner as slides for examination of erythrocyte morphology. Preparation of thin films may be made from tubes of blood with anticoagulant, although the anticoagulant may distort parasite morphology. Thick films are more sensitive than thin films, but thin films are necessary for species identification. Speciation is critical for determining the appropriate therapy.

Thick and thin films may be falsely negative. Collection of specimens repeatedly is essential to ensure that the diagnosis is made. These specimens should be made at varying times of day to increase the likelihood of detecting the parasite. An experienced laboratory technologist should review the smears.

Maintenance of the microscopes and the quality of microscopy in resource-poor settings can lead to difficulty in accurately diagnosing malaria. Because of this, alternative methods of diagnosis have been developed. Several rapid diagnostic tests based on antigen capture techniques are now in use throughout the world. These methods are highly sensitive and specific for falciparum malaria and may eventually contribute immensely to improving malaria diagnosis.

Figure 106-4 Malaria: Clinical Course and Diagnosis.

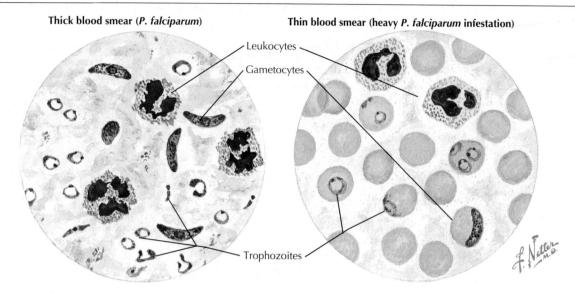

Thick blood smear (*P. falciparum*)   Thin blood smear (heavy *P. falciparum* infestation)

Leukocytes

Gametocytes

Trophozoites

Management and Therapy

The treatment decisions for malaria depend on the species and the severity of the illness (Fig. 106-5). Decisions concerning therapy have become much more complex over the past decade because of the increase in drug-resistant malaria. Guidelines for therapy of malaria are available from both the Centers for Disease Control and Prevention (CDC) and the World Health Organization (WHO). Malaria is a nationally reportable disease and should be reported to the state health department. The CDC also provides a 24-hour hotline for enquiries about malaria (770-488-7788 or 770-488-7100).

Optimum Treatment

Severe falciparum malaria requires parenteral therapy with quinine, quinidine, or an artemisinin derivative. Because intravenous quinine and artemisinin compounds are not routinely available in the United States, quinidine is the drug of choice. The CDC currently recommends that parenteral quinidine is paired with an oral agent: doxycycline, tetracycline, or clindamycin. In cases with high parasitemia (greater than 10% of erythrocytes infected), exchange transfusion can be considered as an adjunct to quinidine. However, there have been no comparative trials for the use of exchange transfusion, and the WHO does not make any recommendation for its use.

In uncomplicated falciparum malaria, treatment is guided by the location of acquisition of the infection. In most of the areas with endemic malaria, chloroquine resistance is common. However, *P. falciparum* in Central America, Haiti, the Dominican Republic, and the Middle East remains sensitive to chloroquine. In the past decade,

resistance to pyrimethamine-sulfadoxine has also become more widespread. For this reason, many countries around the world are attempting to introduce artemisinin combination therapy (ACT) for treatment of malaria. ACT is highly effective but will be limited for some time owing to the high costs and availability of the drugs. Artemisinin derivatives are not currently available in the United States.

Persons with travel history to areas where falciparum malaria is sensitive to chloroquine should be treated with chloroquine. If the species of malaria is unknown or travel occurred to regions with chloroquine-resistant *P. falciparum*, treatment should consist of oral quinine sulfate paired with one of the following drugs: doxycycline, tetracycline, or clindamycin. The CDC also recommends the use of atovaquone and proguanil in these patients. If neither of these options is available, the CDC recommends mefloquine as a third-line agent.

In infections due to *P. vivax, P. ovale,* and *P. malariae,* chloroquine is the drug of choice. Chloroquine does not treat the liver forms of *P. vivax* and *P. ovale.* Persons with infections by *P. vivax* and *P. ovale* must also receive primaquine to prevent relapse.

Cases of chloroquine-resistant *P. vivax* have been reported in Indonesia and Papua New Guinea. Treatment of persons with *P. vivax* acquired in these regions should consist of oral quinine sulfate with doxycycline or tetracycline and primaquine or mefloquine.

Avoiding Treatment Errors

A common treatment error is failure to use the correct antimalarial drug regimen. Before treatment, the species

Figure 106-5 Algorithm of Current Centers for Disease Control and Prevention Treatment Guidelines. AMS, altered mental status; ARDS, adult respiratory distress syndrome; DIC, disseminated intravascular coagulation; PNG, Papua New Guinea.

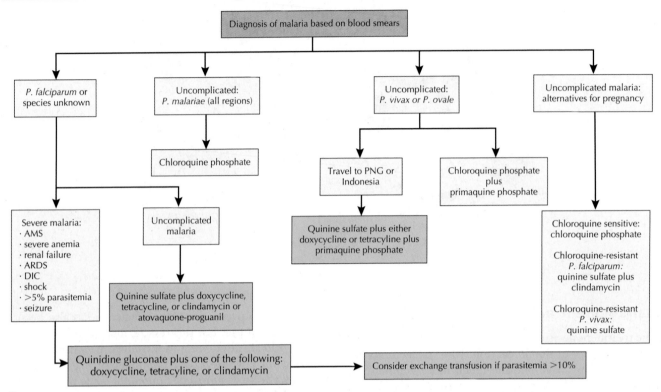

Dosages:
Quindine gluconate: 6.25 mg base/kg loading dose IV over 1-2 hr, then 0.0125 mg base/kg/min continuous infusion over at least 24 hr.
Chloroquine phosphate: 600 mg base PO loading dose, followed by 300 mg base PO at 6, 24, and 48 hr.
Quinine sulfate: 542 mg base PO tid for 3 to 7days (7days if infection from SE Asia or pregnant).
Doxycycline: 100 mg PO bid for 7days.
Tretracycline: 250 mg PO qid for 7days.
Clindamycin: 20 mg base/kg/day PO divided tid for 7 days.
Atovaquone-proguanil: 4 adult tabs PO qd for 3 days.
Primaquine phosphate: 30 mg base PO qd for 14 days.

and the region of acquisition must be identified for appropriate treatment. Furthermore, treatment of liver forms is essential for eradication of *P. vivax* and *P. ovale*.

The treatment of malaria is complicated primarily by medication side effects. Quinidine gluconate can cause hypotension, hypoglycemia, and widening of the QRS complex or lengthening of the QT interval. Cardiac complications may warrant temporary discontinuation of the drug or slowing of the intravenous infusion. Consultation with a cardiologist or a physician with experience treating malaria is recommended.

Prophylaxis

Chemoprophylaxis is a critical component of prevention of malaria for travelers to endemic regions. The choice of agent should be dictated by the location to which the patient travels. Recommendations are available by the CDC at their website. Chloroquine is effective for travel to areas with chloroquine-sensitive *P. falciparum* and the other species of *Plasmodium*. Mefloquine, atovaquone-proguanil or doxycycline are all acceptable for chemoprophylaxis for most other areas. However, the areas along the Thai-Cambodian and Thai-Burmese boarders have malaria resistant to mefloquine, and this drug should be avoided in those areas. In addition to chemoprophylaxis, personal protective measures such as insect repellant, treated bed nets, and long clothing are important in the prevention of malaria.

Future Directions

Malaria is likely to remain a problem worldwide for the foreseeable future. In the past decade, the malaria situation in sub-Saharan African has deteriorated owing to multiple factors including climate instability, global warming, civil disturbances, HIV, drug resistance, and insecticide resis-

tance. Consequently, several new initiatives for malaria control have been established, such as the Roll Back Malaria Partnership and the Gates Foundation. Other new resources include free online journals for dissemination of information on all areas of research, including vector control, drug resistance, and health policy.

Additional Resources

Gates Foundation. Available at: http://www.gatesfoundation.org. Accessed November 28, 2006.

The website for the Gates Foundation includes information about activities and research the foundation is currently funding.

Malaria Journal. Available at: http://www.malariajournal.com. Accessed November 28, 2006.

This free online journal has articles related to all areas of malaria research.

Roll Back Malaria Partnership. Available at: http://www.rbm.who.int/. Accessed November 28, 2006.

The website for the WHO Roll Back Malaria Partnership contains general information about their activities and research.

EVIDENCE

1. Centers for Disease Control and Prevention: Malaria topic home. Available at: http://www.cdc.gov/malaria. Accessed November 28, 2006.

   This CDC website has information specifically about malaria. The current treatment guidelines can be accessed through this site.
2. Centers for Disease Control and Prevention: Traveler's health. Available at: http://www.cdc.gov/travel. Accessed November 28, 2006.

   This CDC website has information for malaria prophylaxis and travel counseling.
3. Greenwood B, Bojang K, Whitty C, et al: Malaria. Lancet 365(9469):1487-1498, 2005.

   This article provides a recent review of current issues in malaria treatment and diagnosis.
4. White NJ: Malaria. In Cook G, Zumba A (eds): Manson's Tropical Diseases, 21st ed. London, WB Saunders, 2003, pp 1205-1295.

   This textbook chapter contains general information on malaria.
5. World Health Organization: Malaria. Available at: http://www.who.int/topics/malaria/en/. Accessed November 28, 2006.

   This WHO website has information on malaria as well as treatment recommendations for malaria in developing countries.

David J. Weber ▪ David A. Wohl ▪ William A. Rutala

Infectious Diseases in Travelers

Introduction

In 2004, there were about 700 million visits across international borders, an increase of about 75% over the course of 15 years. The health risks of international travelers are significant: 1% to 5% of travelers seek medical attention, 0.01% to 0.1% require medical evacuation, and 1 in 100,000 dies. This chapter reviews the medical hazards faced by travelers, methods for reducing the risks associated with travel, and evaluation of fever in the traveler returning from developing countries. The focus is on prevention and management of infectious diseases.

Prevention of Travel-Associated Illnesses

Health care providers should counsel travelers to less-developed countries on travel-related risks and methods to prevent illness. An accurate risk assessment requires information regarding the patient's medical condition (i.e., age, immunization history, underlying medical disorders, pregnancy status, allergies, and host defense abnormalities) and exact travel itinerary (i.e., locations to be visited, including exact length of stay, urban versus rural locales, and level of accommodations and activities such as freshwater exposure, contact with animals, and sexual relations). Special efforts should be made to identify and counsel travelers who are at high risk, such as those traveling to physically unsafe locations, persons planning a prolonged stay, those traveling off the usual tourist routes, persons providing medical care, and immunocompromised persons. Current information regarding prevention of travel-associated diseases is available on the website maintained by the Centers for Disease Control and Prevention.

General risk counseling includes advice on how to avoid the following:

- Accidents, trauma, and injuries
- Transportation-related injuries
- Altitude illness
- Heat-, humidity-, and sun-related illnesses
- Water-related illnesses

Special emphasis should be placed on the most common infectious diseases encountered by international travelers, including the following:

- Traveler's diarrhea (TD)
- Respiratory tract infections
- Arthropod-borne illnesses (especially malaria, dengue, yellow fever, and Japanese B encephalitis)
- Sexually transmitted diseases (especially HIV)
- Blood-borne illnesses (especially hepatitis B and HIV)
- Animal bites (especially rabies) and envenomations

All patients should have their immunization status reviewed, and if deficiencies are noted in universally recommended vaccines (e.g., measles, mumps, rubella, varicella, diphtheria, tetanus), the vaccinations should be provided. Travelers should be offered vaccines available to prevent travel-associated illnesses based on an individual risk assessment. Physicians prescribing vaccines must be familiar with indications, contraindications, and administration guidelines. Although immunoglobulin can be used to protect against hepatitis A, the hepatitis A vaccine is preferred provided there is time for immunity to develop before travel.

Etiology and Pathogenesis

Causes of Fever after Travel to Tropical Countries

Only limited data are available regarding the causes of fever in travelers returning from developing countries. A

recent series of patients evaluated in Australia from 1998 to 2004 reported the following frequency of diagnoses: malaria 27%, gastroenteritis 12%, upper respiratory tract infections 8%, dengue fever 7%, typhoid or paratyphoid fever 4%, pneumonia 4%, influenza A or B 4%, viral syndrome 4%, rickettsial disease 3%, urinary tract infection 3%, skin infection 2%, helminth infection 2%, and hepatitis A 1%. Only 7% of patients in this series had a febrile illness without a confirmed diagnosis. The same study evaluated infectious illnesses in immigrants and refugees. This group more typically has illnesses indigenous to their country of origin. The diagnoses reported were tuberculosis 50%, schistosomiasis 13%, helminth infections 10%, chronic hepatitis 9%, leprosy 6%, malaria 3%, gastroenteritis 2%, upper respiratory tract infections 2%, HIV 2%, eosinophilia 2%, amebiasis 1%, and other 9%. Thus, it is important to recognize the unique spectrum of diseases that most commonly present in short-term travelers who return to their country of origin with a fever, and that these are dramatically different from those of immigrants.

Researchers from 30 international sites that are specialized travel or tropical medicine clinics on six continents reported data on 17,353 ill returned travelers from 1996 through 2004. Reasons for travel included tourism 59%, business 14%, visit to friend or relative 15%, missionary or volunteer work 8%, and research or education 4%. Selected syndromes experienced by the travelers included systemic febrile illness 22.6%, acute diarrhea 22.2%, dermatologic disorder 17.0%, chronic diarrhea 11.3%, respiratory disorder 7.7%, genitourinary disorder 3.5%, adverse drug or vaccine reaction 1.2% and death 0.1%. Of the patients with a systemic febrile illness, the following specific disorders were diagnosed: malaria 35.2%, dengue fever 10.4%, mononucleosis 3.2%, rickettsial infection 3.1%, and typhoid or paratyphoid fever 2.9%. Among patients with acute diarrhea, the following disorders were diagnosed: giardiasis 17.3%, amebiasis 12.0%, campylobacteriosis 8.5%, shigellosis 4.1%, and paratyphoid fever 11.0%.

Diagnostic Approach

Fever in Returning Travelers

In evaluating fever in the returning traveler, checking the vital signs to assess whether the patient is medically stable is a crucial first step. If cardiorespiratory distress is present, initial therapy should be targeted toward stabilizing the patient. Next, one should assess whether the patient has a potentially communicable disease and determine the need for isolation and personal protective equipment. All patients should be evaluated using standard precautions, including the use of gloves when in contact with all body secretions or excretions (except sweat). Surgical masks should be worn if it is suspected that the patient has a droplet-transmitted (e.g., meningococcemia) or airborne-

transmitted (e.g., varicella) disease. An N-95 respirator should be worn if pulmonary tuberculosis, avian influenza, or a viral hemorrhagic fever is suspected.

Clinicians may find use of an algorithm helpful in establishing the differential diagnosis in returning travelers with fever. First, it is important to assess the patient for the presence of hemorrhagic manifestations given the potential severity of the likely pathogens. If hemorrhagic manifestations are present, viral hemorrhagic fevers (e.g., Ebola, Lassa, Marburg, Congo-Crimean, yellow fever), meningococcemia, gram-negative sepsis, and rickettsial infections should all be considered. If viral hemorrhagic fever is possible based on history, clinical presentation, and incubation period, one should proceed immediately with appropriate isolation precautions, expert consultation, and consideration of ribavirin therapy. Second, consider the diagnosis of malaria. If infection with *Plasmodium falciparum* is possible and the patient is acutely ill with signs of severe malaria, empiric therapy should be initiated. If the patient is not acutely ill, it is advisable that serial thick and thin blood smears be obtained and the decision how to treat be based on laboratory results (see Chapter 106). One should then perform a complete history and physical examination and obtain preliminary laboratory tests. If localized findings are present, pursue the appropriate differential diagnosis (Table 107-1). If no localizing findings are present enteric fever, dengue, rickettsial infections, leptospirosis, schistosomiasis, brucellosis, and noninfectious causes of disease should be considered.

Key historical questions include exact itinerary, immunization history, and prophylaxis. Physical examination should focus on a thorough dermatologic examination; inspection of the eyes for scleral icterus, conjunctival suffusion, or conjunctival petechiae; assessment for lymphadenopathy, splenomegaly, and hepatomegaly; auscultation of lungs for evidence of pneumonia; and neurologic evaluation for altered mental status. Altered mental status in a returned traveler represents a medical emergency. Initial laboratory examination includes a complete blood cell count; serum chemistries; liver function tests; urinalysis; cultures of blood, stool, and urine; and chest radiography. Additional tests are obtained as directed by the results of the history, physical examination, and preliminary laboratory results.

Caveats for the evaluation of fever in the returning traveler are as follows:

- The patient should be thoroughly evaluated for all causes of febrile illnesses, both travel- and non–travel-related (e.g., pneumonia, urinary tract infections) infections. Remember that fever after travel may be unrelated to exposures during travel.
- The most common tropical infections are malaria, respiratory tract infections, infectious gastroenteritis, dengue, typhoid and paratyphoid fever, viral hepatitis, and rickettsial infection.

Table 107-1 Possible Physical Findings in Selected Tropical Infections

Physical Finding	Infection or Disease
Rash	Acute HIV seroconversion disease, brucellosis, Ebola virus, cytomegalovirus, dengue fever, Epstein-Barr virus, gonorrhea, measles, syphilis, typhoid, typhus
Eschar	Anthrax, Borrelia species infection, Congo-Crimean fever, South African tick-bite fever, scrub typhus, tick typhus
Jaundice	Brucellosis, cytomegalovirus, leptospirosis, malaria, Q fever, relapsing fever, rickettsial diseases, viral hepatitis (A, B, C, D, E), yellow fever
Lymphadenopathy	Acute HIV seroconversion disease, brucellosis, cat-scratch disease, dengue fever, Lassa fever, leptospirosis, plague, secondary syphilis, tularemia, visceral leishmaniasis
Hepatomegaly	Amebiasis, leptospirosis, malaria, typhoid, viral hepatitis
Splenomegaly	Acute American trypanosomiasis, African trypanosomiasis, brucellosis, cytomegalovirus, dengue fever, Epstein-Barr virus, malaria, leptospirosis, Q fever, relapsing fever, trypanosomiasis, typhoid, tularemia, visceral leishmaniasis
Hemorrhagic fever	Congo-Crimean fever, dengue hemorrhagic fever, Ebola virus, epidemic louse-borne typhus, Hantaviruses, Lassa fever, Marburg virus, meningococcemia, Rift Valley fever, yellow fever
Neurologic findings	Arboviruses (including dengue, Japanese encephalitis), brucellosis, malaria, leptospirosis, meningococcemia, Q fever, rickettsial infections, typhoid fever

- Malaria is potentially fatal and may progress rapidly; it should be excluded as rapidly as possible in all travelers with a history of fever and epidemiologic exposure, even if the patient is afebrile when seen.
- Useful diagnostic points include travel history, travel itinerary, immunization and prophylaxis history, an assessment of incubation period (Box 107-1), and specific exposure history.

Clinical Presentation and Management of Traveler's Diarrhea and Typhoid Fever

Traveler's Diarrhea

Clinical Presentation

Traveler's diarrhea (TD) is characterized by a twofold or greater increase in the frequency of unformed bowel movements. Symptoms often include abdominal cramps, nausea, vomiting (about 15%), bloating, urgency, fever, and malaise. Episodes usually begin abruptly and are generally self-limited. The most important determinant of risk is the destination of the traveler; high-risk destinations include Latin America, Africa, the Middle East, and Asia. TD is almost always acquired through ingestion of fecally contaminated food or water. TD typically causes four to five loose or watery stools per day. The average duration of diarrhea is 3 to 4 days, but about 10% of cases persist longer than 1 week. Fever or bloody stools occur in 2% to 10% of cases. A causative pathogen is demonstrated in 50% to 75% of patients with diarrhea that lasts less than 2 weeks. The most common bacterial causes of TD are enterotoxigenic *Escherichia coli*, *Salmonella* species, *Shigella* species, *Campylobacter jejuni*, and *Vibrio parahaemolyticus*. Viral etiologies include rotavirus and norovirus. Although less common, parasitic enteric pathogens, including *Giardia*

Box 107-1 Differential Diagnosis of Fever in the Returning Traveler*

Short Incubation (<7 days)
- Arboviral infection (including dengue fever)
- Anthrax
- Enteric bacterial infections
- Influenza A and B
- Malaria
- Paratyphoid
- Plague
- Relapsing fever (*Borrelia* species)
- Typhus (louse-borne, flea-borne)
- Viral hemorrhagic fever (Ebola, Lassa, Marburg)

Medium Incubation (8-21 days)
- Anthrax
- Amebic liver abscess
- Brucellosis
- Hepatitis A, C, and E
- Leptospirosis
- Malaria
- Measles
- Q fever
- Scrub typhus
- Trypanosomiasis, American
- Trypanosomiasis, African
- Typhoid fever
- Typhus
- Viral hemorrhagic fever (Ebola, Lassa, Marburg)

Long Incubation (>21 days)
- Amebic liver abscess
- Brucellosis
- Filariasis
- Hepatitis A, B, and C
- HIV
- Malaria
- Melioidosis
- Schistosomiasis (Katayama fever)
- Tuberculosis
- Visceral leishmaniasis

*Lists are not exhaustive

Figure 107-1 Amebiasis.

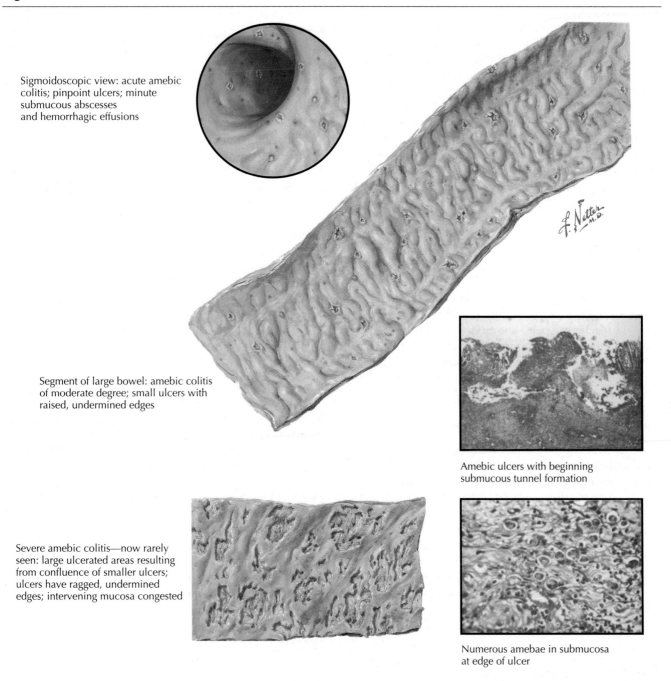

Sigmoidoscopic view: acute amebic colitis; pinpoint ulcers; minute submucous abscesses and hemorrhagic effusions

Segment of large bowel: amebic colitis of moderate degree; small ulcers with raised, undermined edges

Amebic ulcers with beginning submucous tunnel formation

Severe amebic colitis—now rarely seen: large ulcerated areas resulting from confluence of smaller ulcers; ulcers have ragged, undermined edges; intervening mucosa congested

Numerous amebae in submucosa at edge of ulcer

species, *Entamoeba histolytica* (Fig. 107-1), *Cryptosporidium parvum*, and *Cyclospora cayetanensis*, may cause TD.

Management and Therapy

Prevention of TD rests on three approaches: counseling regarding food and beverage consumption, use of non-antimicrobial medications, and use of prophylactic antibiotics. Bismuth subsalicylate decreases the incidence of diarrhea by about 60% but may result in temporary blackening of the tongue and stools, occasional nausea and constipation, and rarely, tinnitus. Bismuth subsalicylate should be avoided in infants and young children, persons with aspirin allergies, and persons taking anticoagulants, probenecid, or methotrexate. Several antibiotics (trimethoprim-sulfamethoxazole, doxycycline, trimethoprim alone, and fluoroquinolones) decrease the incidence of TD by 50% to 95%. However, their efficacy depends on local antibiotic resistance patterns. Antimicrobial prophylaxis is not recommended because of potential side effects. Prophylaxis is reasonable in travelers who are immunosuppressed, although no data directly support this practice.

Initial treatment of TD includes fluid replacement (oral or intravenous), bismuth subsalicylate, and antimotility agents (e.g., tincture of opium, diphenoxylate, loperamide). Antimotility agents should be avoided in persons with fever or bloody stools. In addition, antimotility agents should be discontinued if symptoms persist longer than 48 hours. Antibiotic therapy with a fluoroquinolone should be considered in patients with prolonged TD, severe TD, bloody stools, or fever. However, resistance to fluoroquinolones is a growing problem among *Campylobacter* species. When resistance is a problem, therapy with azithromycin should be considered. The diagnostic evaluation should include stool culture, stool for ova and parasites, and assessment for rotavirus and norovirus.

Typhoid Fever

Clinical Presentation

Typhoid fever is an acute, life-threatening febrile illness caused by *Salmonella typhi*. Clinical manifestations include fever, headache, malaise, anorexia, splenomegaly, and a relative bradycardia. Infection may result in mild symptoms. A clinical syndrome quite similar to typhoid fever can result from infection with other *Salmonella* species (paratyphoid disease) (Figs. 107-2 and 107-3).

Management and Therapy

Preventive measures include careful selection of food and drink and immunization. Immunization is recommended for travelers to high-risk destinations (e.g., Indian subcontinent and developing countries in Asia, Africa, and Central and South America).

Typhoid fever should be considered in any returned traveler with high fever and systemic disease. The diagnosis is confirmed by cultures of stool and blood. Treatment should be initiated with intravenous antibiotics, usually a third-generation cephalosporin or a quinolone. Because *S. typhi* may demonstrate antimicrobial resistance, susceptibility tests should be performed on all isolates.

Avoiding Treatment Errors

It is important to screen returning travelers for potential infectious disease exposures because postexposure prophylaxis or early treatment may be available. Screening questions should include contact with fresh water (schistosomiasis), sexual contacts (HIV, STDs), malaria prophylaxis and prevention, vaccinations, and animals bites or scratches (rabies). It is critical that returning febrile travelers be thoroughly evaluated for all causes of their illness, both travel-related and non–travel-related causes. Patients with a clinically febrile significant illness should be evaluated for malaria by thick and thin smears regardless of a history of malarial prophylaxis. Patients with

hemorrhagic manifestations should be evaluated for viral hemorrhagic fevers (e.g., Ebola, Lassa, Yellow fever), meningococcemia, rickettsial infections, and gramnegative sepsis. It is crucial to institute proper precautions (i.e., isolation and use of personal protective equipment) as soon as any person-to-person disease (e.g., meningococcemia, viral hemorrhagic fever) is possible. Clinically ill patients without localizing findings should also be evaluated for enteric fever, dengue, rickettsial infections, leptospirosis, and viral hepatitis.

A common mistake in evaluating returned travelers with fever who have been home for several days is failure to consider common infections acquired in the United States such as Rocky Mountain spotted fever, viral encephalitis, pneumonia, urinary tract infections, and intra-abdominal infections.

In severely ill patients, diagnostic tests should be rapidly performed. Critically ill patients may require empiric therapy directed against possible infectious agents.

Future Directions

The events of September 11, 2001 have raised the specter of bioterrorism. Although the ultimate impact remains to be seen, physicians must remain ever vigilant of this new threat. Because many of the potential agents of bioterrorism (with the exception of smallpox) represent potential infections in travelers, clinicians providing care to travelers should be familiar with these agents, including anthrax, plague, Q fever, tularemia, and botulism. In addition, physicians must be aware of potentially new and emerging diseases such as severe acute respiratory syndrome and avian influenza.

The most active research area that will affect travelers to developing countries is the worldwide effort to develop safe and effective vaccines for pandemic diseases, including HIV, malaria, and tuberculosis. It is hoped that such vaccines will become available within the next 10 years.

Additional Resources

Centers for Disease Control and Prevention: Health Information for International Travel 2005-2006. Atlanta, U.S. Department of Health and Human Services, 2005.

This excellent comprehensive text focuses on methods to prevent illness in travelers. It is an outstanding resource for health care providers on medical recommendations for travelers.

Freedman DO, Weld LH, Kozarsky PE, et al: Spectrum of disease and relation to place of exposure among ill returned travelers. N Engl J Med 354(2):119-130, 2006.

This is the largest study (30 sites, 17,353 ill travelers) published regarding the spectrum of illnesses reported in ill returned travelers.

MacLean JD, Libman M: Screening returning travelers. Infect Dis Clin North Am 12(2):431-444, 1998.

Figure 107-2 Typhoid Fever: Paratyphoid Fever, Enteric Fever.

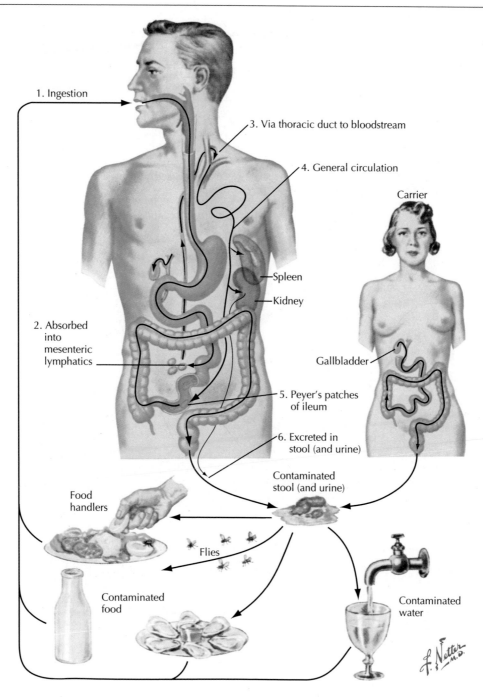

1. Ingestion

3. Via thoracic duct to bloodstream

4. General circulation

Carrier

Spleen

Kidney

2. Absorbed into mesenteric lymphatics

Gallbladder

5. Peyer's patches of ileum

6. Excreted in stool (and urine)

Contaminated stool (and urine)

Food handlers

Flies

Contaminated food

Contaminated water

The authors present an excellent overview of screening tests for infectious diseases in returned travelers.

O'Brien D, Leder K, Matchett E, et al: Illness in returned travelers and immigrants/refugees: The 6-year experience of two Australian infectious disease units. J Travel Med 13(3):145-152, 2006.

The authors report on more than 1000 patients evaluated for fever subdivided by returned travelers and immigrants.

Pigott DC: Emergency department evaluation of the febrile traveler. J Infect 54(1):1-5, 2007.

This concise review describes the appropriate emergency department evaluation of the febrile traveler.

EVIDENCE

1. Centers for Disease Control and Prevention. Available at: http://www.cdc.gov. Accessed February 4, 2007.

   This website contains current information regarding prevention of travel-associated diseases. The best source of up-to-date information for physicians and travelers planning trips abroad. Information is provided in a country-specific format.

2. Lo Re V 3rd, Gluckman SJ: Fever in the returned traveler. Am Fam Physician 68(7):1343-1350, 2003.

Figure 107-3 Typhoid Fever: Paratyphoid Fever, Enteric Fever.

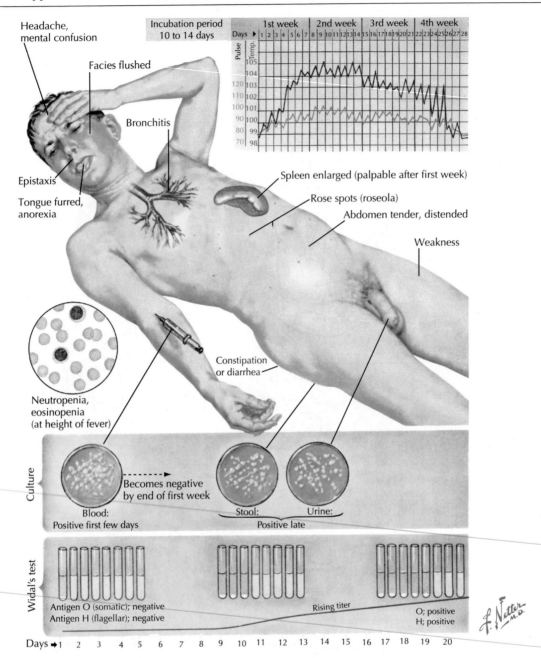

The authors present a short review of the appropriate evaluation of fever in the ill returned traveler.

3. Magill AJ: Fever in the returned traveler. Infect Dis Clin North Am 12(2):445-469, 1998.

   This review provides both an algorithm for evaluating ill returned travelers and review of the most common infections to consider.

4. Ryan ET, Wilson ME, Kain KC: Illness after international travel. N Engl J Med 347(7):505-516, 2002.

This review article addresses the most common or important infectious diseases that may cause fever in travelers.

5. Shlim DR: Update in traveler's diarrhea. Infect Dis Clin North Am 19(1):137-149, 2005.

   The author reviews the prophylaxis and treatment of traveler's diarrhea.

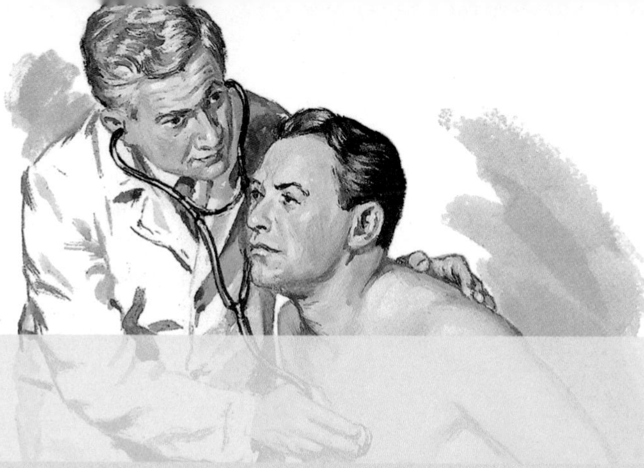

SECTION XI

Sexually Transmitted Diseases

David P. Fitzgerald ▪ Todd Correll ▪ Charles M. van der Horst

108

Acquired Immune Deficiency Syndrome (AIDS)

Introduction

Infection with HIV causes a continuum of diseases, from the acute (primary) HIV infection to prolonged periods of asymptomatic infection to AIDS. The diagnosis of AIDS implies that there has been significant damage to the immune system and is a surveillance case definition established by the Centers for Disease Control and Prevention (CDC) as part of the classification of the clinical status of HIV-infected patients.

To date, two types of HIV, HIV-1 and HIV-2, have been identified as the causative agents of AIDS. There are several subtypes (clades) of HIV-1 with varying distributions throughout the world, whereas HIV-2 is more prevalent in Western Africa. The pandemic of HIV continues to be a serious international problem. As of 2005, there were about 38.6 million people worldwide living with HIV/AIDS, with 2.8 million deaths in 2005 and 4 million people newly infected with HIV.

Etiology and Pathogenesis

HIV predominantly infects T cells bearing the CD4 surface protein and other cells associated with the immune system. HIV exhibits a cytopathic effect on most infected cells, but it can also establish a latent state in cells with a very long half-life, which makes eradication difficult if not impossible. Most patients with HIV experience a slow, progressive decline in the CD4+ T-cell count—the rate of which varies with plasma viral load—and become increasingly at risk for opportunistic infections and certain types of malignancies.

HIV is transmitted by blood and other blood-derived products, through sexual contact, and from infected mothers to infants during the intrapartum and perinatal periods or through breast-feeding. There is no evidence to suggest that HIV is transmitted by casual social contact.

Clinical Presentation

From 40% to 90% of patients with primary HIV infection present with symptomatic illness, including fever, fatigue, a rash (typically maculopapular), headaches, lymphadenopathy, pharyngitis, nausea, vomiting, and diarrhea. These symptoms usually last for less than 2 weeks (Fig. 108-1).

After these symptoms of acute illness abate, patients infected with HIV can remain asymptomatic for up to several years. Once the CD4+ cell count decreases to 200 to 500 cells/mL, certain infections may develop, including varicella zoster, oral hairy leukoplakia, molluscum contagiosum, oral thrush, reactivation of tuberculosis, increased frequency and severity of pneumococcal pneumonia, herpes simplex infections, and esophageal or vaginal candidiasis (Figs. 108-2, 108-3, and 108-4). These patients are also at higher risk for malignancies, including Kaposi's sarcoma and lymphoma, and may experience unexplained weight loss, sinusitis, diarrhea, and fatigue. Screening for HIV is always indicated in patients who present with these conditions. After the CD4+ T-cell count decreases to less than 200 cells/mL, patients are at greater risk for opportunistic infections (OIs) and certain malignancies. They can present with a number of symptoms, including fever, headache, weakness, cough, shortness of breath, nausea,

Figure 108-1 Sexually Transmitted Infections: Human Immunodeficiency Virus.
ELISA, enzyme-linked immunosorbent assay; CBC, complete blood count; G6PD, glucose-6-phosphate dehydrogenase; VDRL, venereal disease research laboratory; RPR, rapid plasma reagin test.

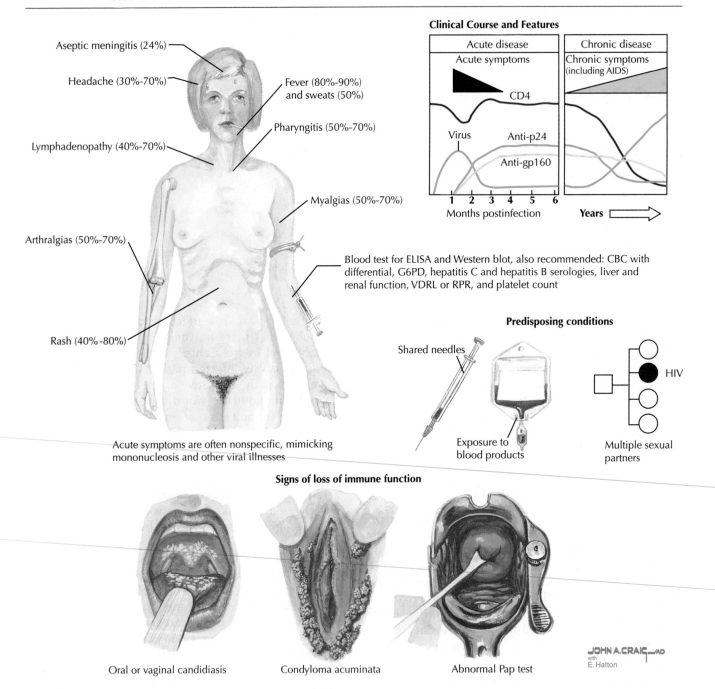

Clinical Course and Features

Aseptic meningitis (24%)

Headache (30%-70%)

Fever (80%-90%) and sweats (50%)

Pharyngitis (50%-70%)

Lymphadenopathy (40%-70%)

Myalgias (50%-70%)

Arthralgias (50%-70%)

Blood test for ELISA and Western blot, also recommended: CBC with differential, G6PD, hepatitis C and hepatitis B serologies, liver and renal function, VDRL or RPR, and platelet count

Rash (40%-80%)

Predisposing conditions

Shared needles

HIV

Exposure to blood products

Multiple sexual partners

Acute symptoms are often nonspecific, mimicking mononucleosis and other viral illnesses

Signs of loss of immune function

Oral or vaginal candidiasis   Condyloma acuminata   Abnormal Pap test

JOHN A. CRAIG—MD with E. Hatton

vomiting, and diarrhea. A careful history and physical examination are essential, and a high index of suspicion for HIV should be maintained because of the varied clinical presentation in HIV disease.

Differential Diagnosis

The presentation of primary HIV infection can mimic other viral diseases, including infectious mononucleosis due to Epstein-Barr virus or cytomegalovirus (CMV),

rubella, herpes simplex infection, and secondary syphilis. Patients with rare congenital immune deficiencies may present with opportunistic infections. However, the serologic tests for HIV generally allow a definitive diagnosis in those patients who are infected.

Diagnostic Approach

Early diagnosis of HIV is crucial. Currently, the CDC recommends that all persons between the ages of 13 and

Figure 108-2 Hairy Leukoplakia of the Tongue.
With permission from Mandel G (ed): Essential Atlas of Infectious Diseases, 2nd ed., Philadelphia, LWW, 2002, p 21.

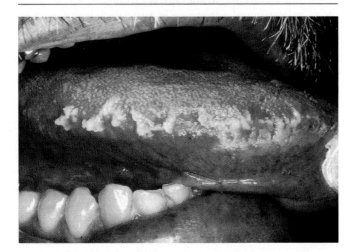

Figure 108-4 Pseudomembranous Candidiasis of the Palate.
With permission from Mandel G (ed): Essential Atlas of Infectious Diseases, 2nd ed., Philadelphia, LWW, 2002, p 27.

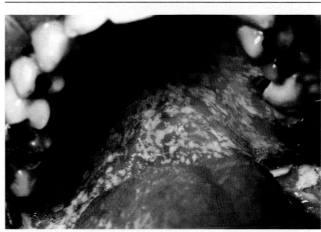

Figure 108-3 Disseminated Herpes Zoster.
With permission from Cohen PR, Beitrani VP, Grossman ME: Disseminated herpes zoster in patients with human immunodeficiency virus infection. Am J Med 84:1076-1080, 1988.

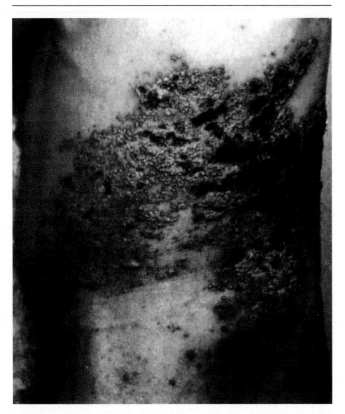

64 years be tested for HIV. In the absence of universal testing, the diagnosis of HIV infection requires a careful history to identify potential high-risk behavior and a physical examination to seek clinical evidence of opportunistic infections and malignancies.

Laboratory confirmation of chronic HIV infection requires detection of antibodies against HIV-derived proteins by enzyme-linked immunosorbent assay (ELISA) followed by a confirmatory Western blot. There are also U.S. Food and Drug Administration (FDA)-approved rapid ELISA tests that may be performed on whole blood, plasma, saliva, or urine.

At this time, the use of the HIV ribonucleic acid (RNA) polymerase chain reaction (PCR) test is not approved by the FDA for diagnosis of primary HIV infection, but it is routinely used by many clinicians. Patients with acute HIV usually have negative ELISA and Western blot test results.

The quantification of HIV RNA levels (viral load) and the CD4+ T-cell counts are used to assess prognosis and to monitor the effectiveness of antiretroviral therapy.

The diagnosis of AIDS is confirmed by diagnosis of opportunistic infections or a CD4 count less than 200 cells/mL in the presence of documented HIV infection. The 1993 revised CDC classification for AIDS in HIV-infected adults is shown in Box 108-1.

Management and Therapy

Therapy for HIV Infection

General Principles

There is no known cure for HIV infection. The current principle of therapy is the use of three or more antiretro-

Box 108-1   Conditions Included in the 1993 AIDS* Surveillance Case Definition

- Candidiasis of bronchi, trachea, lungs, or esophagus
- Cervical cancer, invasive
- Coccidioidomycosis, disseminated or extrapulmonary
- Cryptococcosis, extrapulmonary
- Cryptosporidiosis, chronic intestinal (>1 month duration)
- Cytomegalovirus disease (other than liver, spleen, or nodes; including cytomegalovirus retinitis with loss of vision)
- Encephalopathy, HIV related
- Herpes simplex: chronic ulcers (>1 month duration) or bronchitis, pneumonitis, or esophagitis
- Histoplasmosis, disseminated or extrapulmonary
- Isosporiasis, chronic intestinal (>1 month duration)
- Kaposi's sarcoma
- Leukoencephalopathy, progressive multifocal
- Lymphoma, Burkitt's (or equivalent form), immunoblastic (or equivalent form), or primary of brain
- *Mycobacterium avium* complex or *M. kansasii*, disseminated or extrapulmonary
- *Mycobacterium tuberculosis*, pulmonary or extrapulmonary
- Mycobacterium, other species or unidentified species, disseminated or extrapulmonary
- *Pneumocystis carinii*
- Pneumonia, recurrent
- *Salmonella* septicemia, recurrent
- Toxoplasmosis of brain
- Wasting syndrome due to HIV

*Patients infected with HIV and who have a CD4+ T-cell count <200 or CD4+ percent <14% are classified as having AIDS.

Adapted from 1993 Revised classification system for HIV infection and expanded surveillance case definition for AIDS among adolescents and adults. MMWR Recomm Rep 41(RR-17):1-19, 1992.

viral agents to maintain an undetectable viral load and thus allow some regeneration of the immune system. This approach prevents progression of HIV disease and significantly improves survival. Moreover, the concurrent use of multiple antiretroviral agents reduces the risk for early emergence of HIV that may be resistant to one or more agents.

Currently, there are four FDA-approved classes of antiretroviral agents: the nucleoside reverse transcriptase inhibitors (NRTIs), the non-nucleoside reverse transcriptase inhibitors (NNRTIs), the protease inhibitors (PIs), and the fusion inhibitors (Table 108-1). With the exception of the fusion inhibitors, almost all of these agents can cause nausea, vomiting, and diarrhea to varying degrees.

When to Start Treatment?

The most recent guidelines issued by the U.S. Department of Health and Human Services suggest that antiretroviral therapy be offered when the CD4+ T-cell count decreases below 350 cells/mL or with the occurrence of an AIDS-defining illness. In addition, all pregnant women, regardless of CD4+ count, should be offered antiretroviral treatment to reduce perinatal transmission and improve maternal health. The initiation of antiretroviral therapy is a major therapeutic decision that requires a mutual commitment between the patient and the physician to long-term, full adherence to therapy regardless of CD4 count. Poor antiretroviral adherence is associated with the rapid development of resistant virus and can limit future therapeutic options. Mental illness (especially depression) and addiction are potential barriers to full adherence that should be screened for and treated before initiation of HIV therapy.

Optimum Treatment

The choice of antiretroviral agents should consider multiple factors, including previous exposure to antiretroviral drugs (and thus a chance to harbor resistant strains of HIV), the status of the patient's immune system, the presence of coinfections, the patient's ability to adhere to drug treatment, the potential side effects, and drug-drug interactions. All newly diagnosed patients should have a genotype for resistance.

Currently, patients are usually started on at least two NRTIs, in combination with a PI or one of the NNRTIs (Table 108-2). Alternative regimens are available in the references. Combination tablets with two or more antiretroviral agents are available and should help simplify medication management and increase compliance. In many instances, low-dose ritonavir (100 to 200 mg orally once or twice daily) may be used to enhance the pharmacokinetic profile of other PIs.

Avoiding Treatment Errors

Antiretroviral treatment errors can range from drug-drug interactions to the inappropriate use of single drug regimens. In general, at least three antiretroviral agents should be administered at the appropriate dose and frequency. Antiretrovirals without overlapping side-effect profiles should be selected based on established guidelines or HIV resistance testing. Fusion inhibitors are not routinely used in treatment-naïve patients and should be reserved for treatment-experienced patients. Some drug combinations, such as zidovudine and stavudine, are to be avoided due to competitive antagonism. Drug interactions are common with PI- and NNRTI-containing regimens that may alter the efficacy and safety of concomitant medications as well as the antiretroviral regimen. Abacavir should never be restarted if a hypersensitivity reaction is suspected.

Particular attention must be paid to selecting appropriate regimens in pregnant patients and in patients with comorbidities such as tuberculosis, hepatitis B (HBV), and hepatitis C.

Patients coinfected with HIV and HBV should be evaluated for the need to treat the HBV. Three of the NRTIs are also active against HBV (emtricitabine, lamivudine, and tenofovir). In the coinfected patient, two different drugs active against HBV should be included as part of the three-drug regimen to prevent development of resistant

Table 108-1 Summary of Antiretroviral Agents

Drug	Usual Dosage	Major Side Effects (Besides Nausea, Vomiting, and Diarrhea)
Nucleoside and Nucleotide Reverse Transcriptase Inhibitors (NRTIs)		
Zidovudine (AZT)	300 mg by mouth twice a day	Anemia, granulocytopenia, headaches, myopathy
Lamivudine (3TC)	150 mg by mouth twice a day, or 300 mg every day	Pancreatitis (in pediatric trials), headaches, fat wasting, hepatitis B flares upon discontinuation
Abacavir (ABC)	300 mg by mouth twice a day, or 600 mg every day	Hypersensitivity reaction (including fever, respiratory symptoms, gastrointestinal upset, rash—*do not rechallenge*, headache
Didanosine (ddI)	▪ >60 kg: 400 mg enteric coated by mouth every day ▪ <60 kg: 250 mg enteric coated by mouth every day	Pancreatitis, peripheral neuropathy lactic acidosis
Stavudine (d4T)	▪ >60 kg: 40 mg by mouth twice a day ▪ <60 kg: 30 mg by mouth twice a day	Pancreatitis, peripheral neuropathy, lactic acidosis, fat wasting, dyslipidemia
Tenofovir (TDF)	300 mg by mouth every day	Asthenia, headaches, renal failure, osteopenia, hepatitis B flares upon discontinuation
Emtricitabine (FTC)	200 mg by mouth every day	Rash, photosensitivity, headache, hepatitis B flares upon discontinuation
Non-nucleoside Reverse Transcriptase Inhibitors (NNRTIs)		
Nevirapine (NVP)	200 mg by mouth every day ×2 weeks, then 200 mg by mouth twice a day	Hepatotoxicity, rash (including Steven-Johnson syndrome)
Delavirdine (DLV)	400 mg by mouth 3 times a day	Skin rash, headaches
Efavirenz (EFV)	600 mg by mouth every evening	Dizziness, insomnia, somnolence, abnormal dreams, rash (including Steven-Johnson syndrome) teratogenic, hepatotoxicity
Protease Inhibitors (PIs)		
Amprenavir (APV)	▪ >50 kg: 1200 mg by mouth twice a day ▪ <50 kg: 20 mg/kg twice a day	Rash
Indinavir (IDV)	800 mg by mouth every 8 hours, or 800 mg by mouth + ritonavir 100 mg every 12 hr	Nephrolithiasis, insomnia, rash
Nelfinavir (NFV)	1250 mg by mouth twice a day, or 750 mg by mouth 3 times a day ▪ Not to be used boosted with ritonavir	Rash, diarrhea
Ritonavir (RTV)	Mainly used for protease inhibitor boosting at low doses (100-200 mg every day to twice a day)	Bitter aftertaste, perioral paresthesias, dyslipidemias, hepatotoxicity
Saquinavir (SQV)	1000 mg by mouth + ritonavir 100 mg twice a day	Gastrointestinal disturbances
Lopinavir/Ritonavir (LPV/r)	400/100 mg (2 tablets) by mouth twice a day	Dyslipidemia, hepatotoxicity
Fosamprenavir (FPV)	1400 mg by mouth twice a day, or 1400 mg by mouth every day with ritonavir 200 mg by mouth every day, or 700 mg + ritonavir 100 mg by mouth twice a day	Rash, dyslipidemia, hepatotoxicity
Darunavir (DNV)	600 mg by mouth + ritonavir 100 mg by mouth twice a day ▪ Ritonavir boosting always required	Rash
Tipranavir (TPV)	500 mg + ritonavir 200 mg twice a day	Rash, hepatotoxicity, intracranial hemorrhage (use caution with anticoagulants, surgery, central nervous system lesions)
Atazanavir (ATV)	400 mg by mouth every day, or 300 mg by mouth + ritonavir 100 mg by mouth every day	Jaundice, asymptomatic hyperbilirubinemia, peripheral paresthesias, PR interval prolongation
Fusion Inhibitors (FIs)		
Enfuvirtide (T-20)	90 mg subcutaneous twice a day	Injection site/skin reaction

Table 108-2 Initial Antiretroviral Regimens Recommended by DHHS

	Non-nucleoside Reverse Transcriptase Inhibitor Based	Protease Inhibitor Based
Preferred	Efavirenz + (lamivudine or emtricitabine) + (zidovudine or tenofovir DF)*	Lopinavir/ritonavir + (lamivudine or emtricitabine) + zidovudine
Number of pills	2-3	6-7

* Except in pregnant women or women with high pregnancy potential.
DHHS, Department of Health and Human Services.

HBV strains. Discontinuation of HBV regimens can result in a severe hepatitis flare, and liver function tests should be monitored for several months after discontinuation.

Side Effects

Side effects associated with specific antiretroviral agents are listed in Table 108-1. More importantly, class-specific side effects have recently been noted. NRTIs have been implicated in mitochondrial dysfunction and rare but potentially life-threatening lactic acidosis and liver failure. Use of PIs and a subset of NRTIs has been associated with lipodystrophy with peripheral fat wasting and central fat accumulation and with hyperlipidemia in up to 50% of patients after 1 year of therapy. In a subset of these affected patients, type 2 diabetes mellitus has also been noted. Treatment of these metabolic side effects is similar to that of non–HIV-infected patients; however, special attention may be needed regarding drug interactions and concomitant side effects between these agents (i.e., statins) and antiretroviral agents.

An immune reconstitution syndrome is being increasingly recognized 1 to 8 weeks after initiation of highly active antiretroviral therapy (HAART). It presents as a paradoxical worsening of a patient's clinical, radiologic, or laboratory status (despite an improvement in viral load and CD4 count) and is due to restoration of immune responses to specific OIs or malignancies. Risk factors include a low baseline CD4+ count (<50 cells/mL) and a brisk virologic and immunologic response to HAART. Treatment is usually to continue HAART and OI treatment, with the occasional introduction of NSAIDs or steroids.

Follow-up

Ideally, HIV-viral load assays and CD4+ T-cell counts are obtained before therapy and 4 weeks and 8 to 12 weeks after initiation of treatment, and thereafter followed at 3- to 4-month intervals. If the treatment is effective, the viral load should decrease to less than 50 copies/mL within 4 to 6 months. Patients should be closely monitored for potential side effects of therapy. Consider performing the following laboratory studies at each clinic visit: serum chemistries, liver function tests, amylase, lipase, complete blood cell count with differential, viral load, and CD4+ T-cell count.

Prevention and Management of HIV-Associated Infections

The following baseline labs should be obtained before therapy: hepatitis A immunoglobulin G (IgG), hepatitis B surface antigen and antibody and hepatitis C IgG; CMV IgG; toxoplasma IgG; and rapid plasma reagin test (RPR). A tuberculin skin test should be done. A baseline Papanicolaou test should be performed, repeated at 6 months and annually thereafter with aggressive management of abnormal results.

The Pneumovax, HBV, and influenza vaccines are recommended for all HIV-infected patients. Hepatitis A vaccine is recommended in susceptible persons (those with negative anti-HAV antibody).

Based on the CD4 count, the following algorithm may be used in initiating prophylaxis for serious opportunistic infections in HIV-infected patients:

- CD4 count less than 200 cells/mL: obtain baseline ophthalmologic examination, start *Pneumocystis jiroveci* pneumonia (PCP) prophylaxis with trimethoprim-sulfamethoxazole (TMP-SMX), 1 double-strength tablet daily (preferred regimen); or dapsone, 100 mg orally once daily (check baseline glucose-6-phosphatase dehydrogenase); or atovaquone, 1500 mg daily.
- CD4 count less than 100 cells/mL: if toxoplasma IgG positive, start either TMP/SMX double-strength daily or dapsone, 50 mg daily, and pyrimethamine, 50 mg once weekly, with folinic acid, 25 mg once weekly.
- CD4 count less than 50 cells/mL: ophthalmologist examination every 3 months, prophylaxis against *Mycobacterium avium* complex (MAC) with azithromycin, 1200 mg weekly, or clarithromycin, 500 mg orally twice daily.

In evaluating HIV-positive patients, particularly those with a CD4 count of less than 200 cells/mL and the following clinical complaints, consider:

- Respiratory symptoms: bacterial pneumonia, PCP, tuberculosis, and histoplasmosis. Obtain chest x-ray, arterial blood gas, sputum culture, early referral for bronchoscopy if clinically warranted.

- Headache: computed tomography or magnetic resonance imaging, lumbar puncture. The differential diagnosis includes toxoplasmosis (if toxoplasma IgG positive and CD4 cell count <100 cells/mL), central nervous system lymphoma, meningitis (bacterial, cryptococcal, syphilis, tuberculosis).
- Diarrhea: *Salmonella*, *Giardia*, *Shigella*, *Campylobacter*, and *Yersinia* species. Obtain stool culture and ova/parasite screen; consider *Cryptosporidia*, *Isospora*, and *Microsporidia* species, *Mycobacterium-avium* complex, CMV, and *Clostridium difficile*.
- Rash: always consider drug-induced rash, most commonly from antiretroviral agents and TMP-SMX.

For specific treatments for these and other HIV-associated opportunistic infections, early referral to specialists is essential.

Prevention of Infection and Transmission

Physicians should emphasize preventive education to all patients, especially those who are sexually active or engage in high-risk behavior such as intravenous drug or crack cocaine use. Offer HIV testing (which requires patient consent) with pretest and post-test counseling to patients who request such tests and also to those at increased risk for HIV and other sexually transmitted diseases. Diagnosis of acute HIV infection requires an increased level of suspicion and testing must be done with HIV RNA PCR because HIV antibody testing has a window period following initial infection and will not be positive for several weeks to months. Patients with acute HIV infection generally have very high viral loads and the greatest risk for transmitting the virus is in this period.

HIV-infected patients should be carefully counseled to avoid transmission of HIV by practicing safer sexual behaviors and informing past and future partners of their HIV status, never sharing needles, and informing those involved in their care of their HIV status.

Future Directions

Management of HIV infection continues to change rapidly, as new potential therapeutic agents are being introduced and studied in clinical trials. Two new classes of antiretroviral medications, CCR5 receptor entry inhibitors (Maraviroc), and integrase inhibitors (Raltegravir), were approved for use in 2007. They are approved for use in treatment-experienced patients with resistant virus and are being studied in antiretroviral-naïve patients.

Analysis of viral genotype for mutations that confer resistance against specific antiretroviral agents is also available and should facilitate the selection of optimum therapeutic combinations in treatment-naïve and treatment-experienced patients. Numerous strategies to generate a vaccine against HIV are also being tested.

Additional Resources

AIDSinfo. Guidelines for the use of antiretroviral agents in HIV-1-infected adults and adolescents, October 10, 2006. Available at: http://www.aidsinfo.nih.gov. Accessed December 3, 2006.

This website is an excellent source for frequently updated guidelines on the evaluation and treatment of HIV-infected patients, in both general and specific populations.

Johns Hopkins POC-IT. HIV guide. Available at: http://www.hopkins-hivguide.org. Accessed December 3, 2006.

This is an excellent interactive website that is easy to browse and search and is up to date and accurate.

EVIDENCE

1. Kahn J, Walker B: Acute human immunodeficiency virus type 1 infection. N Engl J Med 339(1):33-39, 1998.

   This concise and accurate description of acute HIV infection should be read by all providers to aid in identification of acutely infected HIV patients.

2. National Institutes of Health: Recommendations for use of antiretroviral drugs in pregnant HIV-1-infected women for maternal health and interventions to reduce perinatal HIV-1 transmission in the United States. Available at: http://aidsinfo.nih.gov. Accessed December 3, 2006.

   These are important recommendations to review when initiating ARV therapy in pregnant women.

3. Revised recommendations for HIV testing of adults, adolescents, and pregnant women in health-care settings. MMWR Recomm Rep 55(RR-14);1-17, 2006.

   The new guidelines advocate universal opt-out HIV testing of all patients to aid in early detection of HIV infection.

Peter A. Leone

Nongonococcal Urethritis

Introduction

Urethritis, inflammation of the urethra, is a syndrome classically characterized by a urethral discharge and dysuria, but urethritis may also be asymptomatic. Urethritis is most accurately defined as the presence of an increased number of polymorphonuclear leukocytes (PMNs) from the anterior urethra. It is sexually acquired, primarily, and has many infectious etiologies. In general, the disease can be classified as either gonococcal or nongonococcal urethritis (NGU). The presence of gram-negative intracellular diplococci (GNID) on urethral smear correlates highly with gonorrhea infection. NGU is diagnosed when inflammation is present without GNID. Mucopurulent cervicitis (MPC) is the female equivalent. Noninfectious etiologies include chemical and physical irritants. As with most sexually transmitted infections, NGU is most prevalent in the 19- to 24-year age group, a time when changing sexual relationships are common. A minor disorder in most cases, MPC is clinically important for three reasons: (1) the potential for complications, particularly pelvic inflammatory disease (PID) associated with decreased fertility in female partners when *Chlamydia trachomatis* is the underlying pathogen; (2) its damaging influence on interpersonal relationships, especially when the condition is not adequately understood; and (3) prolonged anxiety when symptoms, although mild, are slow to resolve or when there are recurrences.

Etiology and Pathogenesis

C. trachomatis is the most common known causative organism and can be isolated from the urethra in 15% to 55% of men with NGU. Unlike most bacteria, this organism is dependent on the energy-producing metabolic activities of the host cells and thus is an obligate intracellular parasite. The prevalence of NGU caused by *C. trachomatis* infection varies by age, with lower prevalence in older age groups. Complications of NGU caused by *C. trachomatis* infection include prostatitis, epididymitis, and Reiter's syndrome.

Often, the causes of NGU are not elucidated, but recently defined pathogens include *Ureaplasma urealyticum*, *Mycoplasma genitalium*, *Trichomonas vaginalis*, *Candida* species, adenovirus, and *Neisseria meningitidis* (Fig. 109-1). Genital herpes simplex virus (HSV) can cause urethritis in about 30% of men with primary genital infection, but it is seen in a much lower percentage of men with recurrent genital HSV infection. Often, *Ureaplasma urealyticum* is isolated from the urethra of men with NGU, and differential antibiotic studies support the view that it sometimes has a pathogenic role. However, this organism is often isolated from the urethra in healthy men, and there is no simple way of identifying those cases in which it is patho-

genic. Between 20% and 30% of men with NGU have no detectable organisms. Recent observations have found an association of NGU with bacterial vaginosis and oral sex. Asymptomatic urethritis, without a visible discharge but with evidence of increased PMNs on smear, may have a different etiology from symptomatic disease. *C. trachomatis* is detected less frequently in this situation.

Noninfectious etiologies include chemical irritants (e.g., spermicides, bath products), physical irritants, urethral stricture, foreign bodies, bacterial urinary tract infections, repeated vigorous urethral stripping, and heavy crystalluria or calculous gravel in the urine.

Clinical Presentation

In the typical patient, symptoms include dysuria, urethral discharge (mucoid or purulent), and penile irritation. Urethral discharge, which may be present on examination or on a urethral smear in a significant number of asymptomatic individuals, is a sign of NGU (see Fig. 109-1).

The patient first notices symptoms from several days to several weeks after infection; 2 or 3 weeks is a common incubation period. Urethral inflammation will often give

Figure 109-1 Urethritis.
NGU, nongonococcal urethritis.

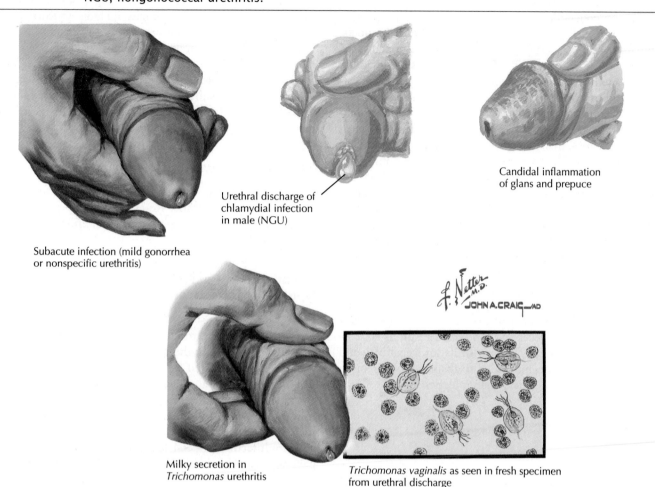

Subacute infection (mild gonorrhea or nonspecific urethritis)

Urethral discharge of chlamydial infection in male (NGU)

Candidal inflammation of glans and prepuce

Milky secretion in *Trichomonas* urethritis

Trichomonas vaginalis as seen in fresh specimen from urethral discharge

rise to a discharge and dysuria, and the patient may experience urinary frequency. When the posterior urethra is involved, symptoms are usually mild and may be intermittent or transient, lasting only 1 to 2 days. The absence of symptoms does not exclude the diagnosis of NGU. There is a high incidence of asymptomatic infection of the urethra with *C. trachomatis*.

Spotty balanitis caused by candidal overgrowth in uncircumcised men is the most common complication of NGU. Men presenting with balanitis should always be checked for NGU, even when there are no symptoms. Hyperglycemia should be excluded because diabetes mellitus sometimes presents with candidal balanitis. Other complications include epididymitis, orchitis, acquired reactive arthritis, and Reiter's syndrome.

Epididymitis occurs less commonly. Swelling and tenderness begins in the lower pole. The groove between the epididymis and the testis is accentuated at first but then becomes obscured as the condition progresses. Occasionally, patients complain of blood-stained semen due to seminal vesiculitis. Reiter's disease is a rare complication that presents 10 to 30 days after the sexual contact. Patients

may have an acute arthritis affecting one or more large peripheral joints. Conjunctivitis may also be present.

Diagnostic Approach

The diagnosis is confirmed by the demonstration of PMNs in the anterior urethra and by the absence of gram-negative diplococci on Gram stain with a negative culture or test result for *Neisseria gonorrhoeae*. Excessive PMNs can be confirmed by a Gram-stained urethral smear with more than 2 PMNs per high-power microscopic field (×1000), or a Gram-stained preparation from a first-pass urine specimen containing more than 9 PMNs per high-power microscopic field (×1000). Leukocyte esterase activity on first-pass urine correlates with the presence of urethritis but lacks sufficient sensitivity to be considered a reliable diagnostic test for NGU. The quality of the smear is dependent on how the specimen is collected.

Five or more PMNs per high-power field (×1000) is generally accepted as the criterion for urethritis. The absence of PMNs in a single urethral smear does not exclude the diagnosis, particularly if the patient urinated before the examination. There is no conclusive recommendation on the optimal time between micturition and specimen collection, but 2 to 4 hours is preferred, with a minimum of 30 minutes. Urethral specimens should be obtained using a 5-mm plastic loop or cotton-tipped swab. There is no information suggesting the superiority of either method, although the loop appears to be less physically and psychologically traumatic to the male patient.

Symptomatic patients without evidence of inflammation should be tested for an etiologic diagnosis. In most clinical settings, this includes testing for *N. gonorrhoeae* and *C. trachomatis*. Re-examination the following morning, having the patient not urinate overnight, may increase the diagnostic yield of the Gram stain. Empiric treatment is in order for those individuals with an observable purulent discharge, those at high risk for infection (e.g., patients in a sexually transmitted disease clinic, adolescent males in a juvenile detention center), or individuals unlikely to return for re-evaluation. The minimum time between exposure and the development of a detectable inflammatory response, by urethral smear or microscopic study of a urine sample, is not known, but it is reasonable to allow 1 week after a risk contact before accepting a negative result as conclusive. The two-glass test, because of its low sensitivity and specificity, is not recommended to diagnose NGU or to differentiate it from urinary tract infection.

Management and Therapy

Optimum Treatment

The diagnosis should be established by demonstrating that urethral inflammation is present and by excluding gonorrhea; all patients should have testing for *N. gonorrhoeae*. *C. trachomatis* testing, although preferable, may be deferred in men with inflammation on urethral smear when resources are limited. Urethral smears without evidence of significant PMNs should be tested for *C. trachomatis* in symptomatic men. The provider should take a detailed sexual history to identify all sexual partners requiring assessment and treatment and should treat sexual partners considered to be at risk even if there are no signs of infection. Chlamydial cervicitis or PID can develop suddenly and without warning in a female partner. It is better to treat unnecessarily if exposure to infection has occurred, rather than risk this complication. A full course of antibiotics should be completed even when the symptoms resolve within a few days. Alcohol in moderation will not affect the outcome. Sexual activity should be avoided until the inflammation has resolved.

Treatment should be administered at the time of diagnosis with medications that are highly effective against chlamydia (cure rate for *C. trachomatis* of more than 95%), are easy to use (preferably single-dose therapy, but not more then twice-daily therapy), have a low incidence of side effects, and minimally interfere with lifestyle. The preferred medication regimens are azithromycin, 1 g orally in a single dose, or doxycycline, 100 mg orally twice daily for 7 days. Alternative regimens include erythromycin, 500 mg orally 4 times daily for 7 days; erythromycin ethylsuccinate, 800 mg orally four times daily for 7 days; ofloxacin, 300 mg twice daily or 400 mg orally once daily for 7 days; or levofloxacin, 500 mg once daily for 7 days.

Trimethoprim-sulfamethoxazole (cotrimoxazole) is active against chlamydia but is not effective in the treatment of NGU and is, thus, *not* recommended.

Patient Follow-up

Patients should be instructed to abstain from sex for 7 days after initiation of therapy. Re-evaluation is not necessary unless signs or symptoms persist or recur after completion of therapy.

Recurrent or Persistent Nongonococcal Urethritis

In recurrent or persistent NGU, the urethral inflammation is usually mild and will resolve over several days with appropriate antibiotic therapy. Persistence occurs in 20% to 60% of men treated for acute NGU; however, resolution may take several weeks. Occasionally, relapse occurs, even in the absence of reinfection. Relapse is most common in the first 3 months after the initial episode. The pathologic basis of these relapses is not understood and is probably multifactorial. Persistence of signs and symptoms beyond 3 months should prompt the clinician to consider chronic prostatitis or chronic pelvic pain syndrome.

When relapse occurs in the context of a stable relationship, it is important to exclude the possibility of reinfection by confirming that the sexual partner has completed an appropriate course of antibiotics. Careful explanation is also necessary because relapse sometimes leads to the erroneous conclusion that there has been a sexual contact outside of the relationship.

Female partners of men with persistent or recurrent NGU do not appear to be at increased risk for the development of PID, provided they received appropriate therapy as a contact.

Minor sensations of urethral irritation may persist for some time after resolution of NGU, and the patient will often feel that the infection is still present. It is important to document definite urethral inflammation before prescribing another course of antibiotics.

After confirming persistent inflammation on urethral smear, alternative antibiotic therapy should be considered. If the patient has not adhered to initial therapy, consider switching to single-dose therapy. Azithromycin or doxycycline failure may be due to resistant *U. urealyticum* or to *T. vaginalis*. If the patient is symptomatic, was compliant with the initial regimen, and has not had sexual contact with an untreated partner, consider therapy with erythromycin, 500 mg orally 4 times daily for 7 days, plus a single oral dose of metronidazole, 2 g, or tinidazole, 2 g orally in a single dose. Some isolates of *U. urealyticum* are resistant to erythromycin but may respond to ofloxacin, 300 mg every 12 hours orally for 7 days. Persistent NGU following two courses of therapy requires other diagnostic considerations (i.e., cystitis and prostatitis) and urologic evaluation to rule out foreign bodies, strictures, and periurethral abscess. *M. genitalium* may cause persistent NGU and requires a 6-week course of erythromycin. If no cause for persistent NGU can be found, a 6-week course of empiric doxycycline or erythromycin is rational.

Sexual contacts and partners, including all partners and sexual contacts of symptomatic men 2 weeks before the onset of symptoms and those of asymptomatic men 6 months before diagnosis, should be evaluated and offered empiric therapy. The treatment regimen should be consistent with that used for the partner and, at a minimum, be effective for uncomplicated chlamydia infection. Female contacts of men with chlamydial urethritis should be treated regardless of the results of chlamydia testing. Concurrent treatment is preferred and may result in improved clinical response in men with chlamydia-negative NGU.

Referral to a specialist clinic is advisable if there is reluctance to give a detailed sexual history. Treatment of all partners who may be at risk, if symptoms persist after two courses of antibiotics or if complications develop, should be arranged.

Avoiding Treatment Errors

Whenever possible, single-dose, directly observed therapy for NGU is the best way to ensure adherence to treatment. The main cause of recurrent symptoms following treatment is reinfection from an untreated partner. NGU, like all bacterial sexually transmitted infections, requires referral for screening and treatment of partners. For patients in whom reinfection is not deemed the probable cause for persistent or recurrent infection, clinicians must consider antimicrobial resistance or the possibility of infection with pathogens not covered by the initial choice of therapy.

Future Directions

The use of urine-based nucleic acid amplification tests (NAATs) for the diagnosis of gonococcal and chlamydial urethral infections may warrant reclassification of urethritis into three categories: gonococcal, chlamydial, and nongonococcal-nonchlamydial urethritis. Diagnostic screening and testing for *C. trachomatis* will be strongly recommended for males as the cost of NAAT continues to decrease because chlamydia infection has significant public health implications. Other developments include clarification of the role of *M. genitalium* in NGU and the development of screening algorithms for men at increased risk for recurrent NGU.

Additional Resources

Carder C, Mercey D, Benn P: Chlamydia trachomatis. Sex Transm Infect 82(Suppl 4):iv10-12, 2006.

This excellent review of Chlamydia trachomatis is probably best suited to clinicians.

Centers for Disease Control and Prevention, National Center for HIV/AIDS, Viral Hepatitis, STD and TB Prevention: Male chlamydia screening consultation. Available at: http://www.cdc.gov/std/chlamydia/ChlamydiaScreening-males.pdf.

This website provides the latest recommendation for C. trachomatis screening in men. This sets the stage for the next level of community screenings in an attempt to lower prevalence of C. trachomatis infection.

Stamm WE, Koutsky LA, Benedetti JK, et al: Chlamydia trachomatis urethral infections in men. Prevalence, risk factors, and clinical manifestations. Ann Intern Med 100:47-51, 1984.

This important historical article addresses the role of C. trachomatis in NGU.

EVIDENCE

1. Arya OP, Mallinson H, Andrews BE, Sillis M: Diagnosis of urethritis: Role of polymorphonuclear leukocyte counts in gram-stained urethral smears. Sex Transm Dis 11:10-17, 1984.
   The article provides a historical reference for the diagnosis of NGU.
2. Janier M, Lassau F, Casin I, et al: Male urethritis with and without discharge: A clinical and microbiological study. Sex Transm Dis 22:244-252, 1995.
   This article provides an etiologic diagnosis in addition to the clinical diagnosis of NGU.
3. Podgore JK, Holmes KK, Alexander ER: Asymptomatic urethral infections due to Chlamydia trachomatis in male US military personnel. J Infect Dis 146:828, 1982.
   This historical reference underscores the rate of asymptomatic infection of chlamydia in males.
4. Root TE, Edwards LD, Spengler PJ: Nongonococcal urethritis: A survey of clinical and laboratory features. Sex Transm Dis 7:59-65, 1980.
   This historical reference set the criteria for NGU diagnosis.
5. Stamm WE, Hicks CB, Martin DH, et al: Azithromycin for empirical treatment of the nongonococcal urethritis syndrome in men. A randomized double-blind study. JAMA 274:545-549, 1995.
   This was the pivotal study on which the indication of azithromycin to treat NGU was based.
6. Taylor-Robinson D, Horner PJ: The role of Mycoplasma genitalium in non-gonococcal urethritis. Sex Transm Infect 77:229-231, 2001.
   This important article first described the growing role of Mycoplasma genitalium as a cause of NGU.
7. Workowski KA, Berman SM; Centers for Disease Control and Prevention: Sexually transmitted diseases treatment guidelines, 2006. MMWR Recomm Rep 55(RR-11):1-94, 2006.
   These guidelines provide the latest and best expert guidance for diagnosis and management of NGU.

Gonorrhea

Introduction

Gonorrhea is a sexually transmitted disease (STD) known since biblical times, for more than 2000 years, characterized by superficial or deep infection of mucosal surfaces, especially the genital mucosa, by the organism *Neisseria gonorrhoeae* (the gonococcus). Untreated infection often results in deeper complications, including salpingitis or epididymitis, and occasionally bacteremia and arthritis, meningitis, or endocarditis. Although antibiotic resistance is more common than in earlier decades, treatment is still highly efficacious. The primary problem is in case detection. Because some infections may have few symptoms, infected persons can be missed without attention to risk factors in a patient's history and knowledge of the epidemiology pertinent to gonorrhea. Excellent new noninvasive diagnostic tests are readily available in the United States.

Most cases of gonorrhea are sexually transmitted. Infection in neonates may be from the mother's birth canal. Infection of prepubescent children should be assumed to be the result of sexual abuse. Infection is most common in adolescents and young adults, with peak prevalence in women aged 15 to 19 and men aged 21 to 25 years. Prevalence is much higher in the United States among African Americans, which probably reflects a complex mixture of socioeconomic, behavioral, health care seeking, and health care access factors. Rates of infection are particularly high in many rural southeastern states and in certain large cities. In some inner cities, prevalence may approach 5%, but this is now uncommon. In general, risk is increased among the young and unmarried, and among those having a new sex partner or multiple sex partners or a sex partner with multiple partners. The prevalence of infection has declined in the past decade but is increasing in certain groups, including young men who have sex with men, among whom rectal gonococcus is increasing in some locales. Condoms probably are quite effective in prevention of transmission by genital sex. The risk for infection after unprotected genital sex with an infected partner is about 30% for men and 70% to 80% for women. Antibiotic-resistant strains are becoming more common, but distribution is uneven; multiple resistances including resistance to ciprofloxacin are found, particularly in isolates from persons from southeast Asia or parts of Africa.

Etiology and Pathogenesis

The gonococcus is a gram-negative diplococcus that grows only in humans and does not survive long outside of the body. It attaches to epithelial surfaces by several adherence ligands that interact with specific receptors. Attachment is followed by local invasion and sometimes by penetration of deeper tissues and bacteremia. Although much is known about molecular pathogenesis, there is no current vaccine candidate; earlier attempts to develop a vaccine based on the pilus adherence ligand failed. Strains may be typed on the basis of reactions with a panel of monoclonal antibodies against the porin (major outer membrane) protein (serotyping), or on the basis of DNA sequence differences in the *por* gene (genotyping), but these are only available in research laboratories.

Clinical Presentation

In men, purulent urethritis with dysuria and small amounts of yellow or greenish mucoid discharge develops, especially in the early morning before urination, within 2 to 7 days of exposure (Fig. 110-1). In 5% to 10% of men, a persistent low-grade or asymptomatic infection of the urethra may develop. These men do not present for health care and may transmit infection to their sexual partners. Epididymitis in men younger than 35 years is usually due to either gonococcal or genital chlamydia infection.

Figure 110-1 Urethritis in Men.

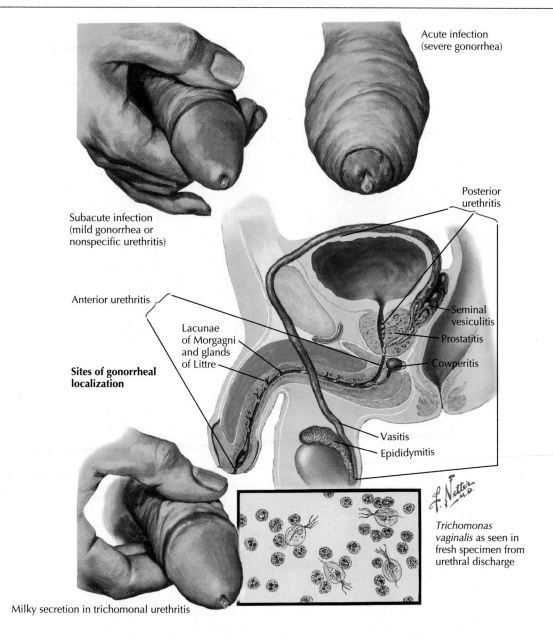

Acute infection
(severe gonorrhea)

Subacute infection
(mild gonorrhea or
nonspecific urethritis)

Posterior
urethritis

Anterior urethritis

Seminal
vesiculitis

Lacunae
of Morgagni
and glands
of Littre

Prostatitis

**Sites of gonorrheal
localization**

Cowperitis

Vasitis

Epididymitis

*Trichomonas
vaginalis* as seen in
fresh specimen from
urethral discharge

Milky secretion in trichomonal urethritis

Asymptomatic or oligosymptomatic cervical infection may develop in 50% of women; others have increased vaginal discharge or dysuria (Fig. 110-2). Physical examination often reveals mucopurulent cervical discharge. Low-grade infection of the endometrium is relatively common. About 10% to 15% of untreated genital infections in women are followed by salpingitis, with adnexal pain, and sometimes with fever and leukocytosis. Risk for salpingitis is increased in very young women (15 to 16 years) and in those who have had it previously. The severity of illness is variable, ranging from mild to acute; some patients may be treated as outpatients, whereas others require hospitalization. Physical examination may reveal cervical motion tenderness and adnexal tenderness or fullness. Salpingitis may be followed by tubal scarring and infertility, or increased risk for ectopic pregnancy (see Fig. 110-2).

Infection of the pharynx is found in up to 20% of patients with genital gonorrhea, but there usually are no symptoms. Rectal gonorrhea is found in up to 40% of women with cervical gonorrhea, also without symptoms and, presumably, reflecting spread of infection from the contiguous genital site. In contrast, rectal gonorrhea in men who have sex with men is often quite symptomatic with pain, discharge, and tenesmus.

Bacteremia develops in about 1% of patients, particularly in those infected by strains that are highly resistant to human serum complement. Persons with homozygous deficiency of late complement components are susceptible

Figure 110-2 Gonorrhea in Women.

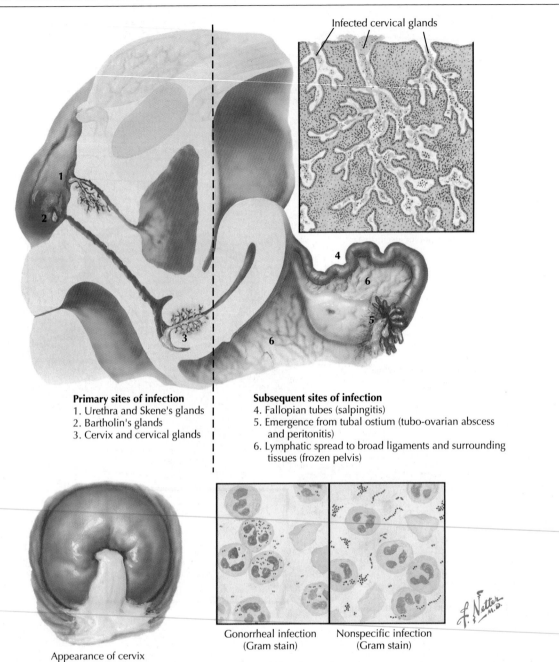

Infected cervical glands

Primary sites of infection
1. Urethra and Skene's glands
2. Bartholin's glands
3. Cervix and cervical glands

Subsequent sites of infection
4. Fallopian tubes (salpingitis)
5. Emergence from tubal ostium (tubo-ovarian abscess and peritonitis)
6. Lymphatic spread to broad ligaments and surrounding tissues (frozen pelvis)

Appearance of cervix
in acute infection

Gonorrheal infection
(Gram stain)

Nonspecific infection
(Gram stain)

to recurrent gonococcal or meningococcal bacteremias; about 5% of patients with the disseminated gonococcal infection (DGI) syndrome are lacking one of the late complement components C5 through C9. A CH50 test will detect such individuals, although it is best done after the acute infection has subsided. DGI presents in several forms, but patients usually are not acutely or severely ill, in contrast to meningococcal bacteremia. About half of patients with DGI do not have fever. Many have a typical rash distributed over the periphery, especially the hands, with a small number (fewer than 30) of pustular or hemorrhagic tender lesions. This may be accompanied by polyarticular arthralgias or monoarticular arthritis, typically involving major joints; rash may be absent in patients with arthritis. DGI frequently follows asymptomatic genital or pharyngeal infection.

Typically, infection in neonates presents as purulent conjunctivitis, which was a major cause of blindness but is now rare. Infection in young females most often presents as vulvovaginitis.

Differential Diagnosis

Gonococcal urethritis must be differentiated from *Chlamydia trachomatis* urethritis and from other causes of urethritis including *Mycoplasma genitalis* and, occasionally, herpes simplex virus or *Trichomonas vaginalis* (see Fig. 110-1). Gonococcal urethritis tends to have a more profuse and purulent discharge, but this is not helpful in individual patients. The differential diagnosis for epididymitis includes chlamydia epididymitis and testicular torsion. Gonococcal cervicitis with mucopurulent discharge must be differentiated from chlamydia cervicitis, which may produce an indistinguishable clinical picture. Many diseases, including ectopic pregnancy and appendicitis, may mimic salpingitis. The DGI syndrome may mimic Reiter's syndrome, bacterial endocarditis, and other types of acute arthritis.

Diagnostic Approach

The diagnosis of gonorrhea depends on awareness of patient risk factors, including a sexual history. Urethral discharge or mucopurulent cervicitis suggests gonococcal or chlamydial infection. In women, it is important to differentiate vaginal discharge and vaginitis from cervicitis; gonococci do not cause vaginitis except in prepubescent girls.

In men with purulent urethral discharge, a Gram stain showing intracellular gram-negative diplococci (see Fig. 110-2) is both highly sensitive and specific, and cultures or other tests are not usually necessary. In infected men without frank discharge, Gram stain is no more than 60% sensitive, and diagnosis is best achieved either by culture of a urethral swab or fresh urine sediment, or by use of a nucleic acid amplification test (NAAT) (polymerase chain reaction; transcription-mediated amplification; or DNA strand displacement assay). NAATs on urine or self-obtained vaginal swabs are more than 98% sensitive and 98% specific, and are as sensitive as cultures, but cost may be a limiting factor for some patients or practices. NAATS may be utilized for screening for both gonorrhea and chlamydia infection, and one combined test (Aptima Combo II) has a reported positive predictive value of greater than 95% in a population with prevalence of only 0.5% gonorrhea. Cultures are still required for pharyngeal or rectal infections because NAATs are not approved for such specimens. Despite their convenience, the NAATs do not preserve an isolate for testing susceptibility to antimicrobials, and they do not easily allow strain typing, which may be useful in medical-legal cases. Cultures should be plated on selective chocolate agar media containing antibiotics to inhibit the normal flora or placed in transport media for prompt transfer to the laboratory. There are no serologic tests for gonorrhea.

Women ordinarily require either cervical culture or a NAAT test of urine or vaginal introitus. Gram stains of cervical discharge are only 50% sensitive and not sufficiently specific for accurate diagnosis in most clinics. In patients with possible salpingitis, it may be helpful to seek consultation and to perform vaginal ultrasound to examine the anatomy of the fallopian tubes. Computed tomography of the pelvis and laparoscopy may be needed. Pregnancy tests should be obtained, and if culture materials are available from the fallopian tubes, they should be sent for testing for anaerobic and aerobic bacteria.

If DGI is suspected, culture specimens should be obtained from blood, genital, pharyngeal, and rectal sites, and NAAT performed on urine. Culture specimen results from infected joints are positive in only about one third of patients, and skin lesion culture results are rarely positive. Obtain a total serum hemolytic complement, especially in patients with recurrent DGI.

Sexual partners of patients with any type of gonorrhea should be seen or referred for proper diagnostic evaluation. Asymptomatic carriers are important vectors for transmission. Urine-based NAAT is the best test for detecting asymptomatic genital infection. Any patient with gonorrhea should be presumed to have other STDs, and appropriate tests should be undertaken, including a serologic test for syphilis and a screening test for HIV.

Management and Therapy

Optimum Treatment

For uncomplicated genital gonorrhea in adults, several regimens are highly effective, including a single intramuscular injection of 125 mg ceftriaxone, or a single oral dose of cefixime, 400 mg, or of cefpodoxime, 400 mg. These regimens provide adequate therapy for rectal or pharyngeal infection as well. Penicillins and tetracycline should not be used because resistance has increased substantially due to both plasmid-mediated genes and a variety of chromosomal mutations. Resistance to ciprofloxacin has become a clinical problem in Asia and Africa, and resistance has grown rapidly in the United States, spreading from Hawaii and California through the rest of the country in a west-to-east direction. In many regions, 20% or more of gonococcus isolates are resistant to fluorinated quinolones. Ciprofloxacin therapy therefore should be avoided. In most cases, therapy against chlamydia should be added because of the frequency of coinfection by genital chlamydia; this can be in the form of either a single oral dose of azithromycin of 1 g or doxycycline, 100 mg orally twice daily for 7 days. Directly observed therapy is preferred. For patients with complicated infections, including either salpingitis or DGI, consult standard texts for approaches to therapy.

Sex partners of patients should be screened and treated for probable gonorrhea. Many infections are transmitted by asymptomatically infected partners, who do not present voluntarily for diagnosis and treatment. Most health

departments do not have the resources to do contact tracing of partners for diseases other than syphilis and HIV, and the responsibility for partner diagnosis and treatment rests with the clinician and the index patient. If possible, diagnostic tests for gonorrhea as well as other STDs and HIV should be performed on contacts before treatment, but there may be circumstances in which it is most practical to provide medication for treatment of the partners. Many authorities advise expedited partner therapy in such circumstances, whereby the index patient is either given the drug for the partner or a prescription to give the partner. A randomized controlled trial showed that this was safe and effective for partners of patients with gonorrhea or chlamydial infection. Failure to treat infected sexual contacts results in repeated "ping-pong" infections. Infections should be reported to the public health authorities.

Every STD, including gonorrhea, is an opportunity to counsel patients about the risks of unprotected sex, particularly with multiple or high-risk partners. Proper counseling of such patients may prevent other more serious STDs, including HIV.

Avoiding Treatment Errors

There are no problems in regard to accurate choices of drugs as long as the treatment guidelines are followed.

Future Directions

Despite decades of research into the molecular basis of pathogenicity of gonorrhea, there is still no vaccine candidate in site. Previous attempts to create a vaccine against pilin protein failed, and more recent attempts to use porin protein as a vaccine have stalled in early stages of clinical development. A vaccine would be useful not only because gonorrhea is an important disease in its own right, especially regarding women's health, but also because it is a cofactor for transmission and acquisition of HIV.

Prevention depends on better sexual behaviors (abstinence, fewer partners, less risky partners, use of condoms in all but stable monogamous sexual relationships) and screening to detect infected persons who have yet to seek treatment. Implementation of screening in women was associated with better control of infection in the United States, but prevalence has stabilized and is increasing in certain communities and groups. Use of the urine-based NAAT test provides a noninvasive, patient-friendly means to screen groups at high risk, including adolescents, persons with a new sexual partner, and emergency room and jail populations.

Dramatic declines in the prevalence of gonorrhea in much of the industrialized world outside the United States show that vaccines are not necessary for disease control. The success of gonorrhea control in these other countries undoubtedly is multifactorial but includes better health care access and less inhibited use of media to promote healthy sexual behaviors, including use of condoms.

Additional Resources

Fleming DT, Wasserheit JN: From epidemiological synergy to public health policy and practice: The contribution of other sexually transmitted diseases to sexual transmission of HIV infection. Sex Transm Infect 75:3-17, 1999.
    This classic paper documents the roles of STDs in transmission of HIV.
Golden MR, Whittington WL, Handsfield HH, et al: Effects of expedited treatment of sex partners on recurrent or persistent gonorrhea or chlamydial infection. N Engl J Med 352(7):676-685, 2005.
    This randomized trial tests the efficacy of partner-delivered therapy as opposed to standard partner notification and treatment methods.
Handsfield HH, Sparling PF: Gonococcal infections. In Goldman L, Ausiello D (eds): Cecil Textbook of Medicine, 23rd ed. Philadelphia, WB Saunders, 2007.
    This is the most current general clinical chapter on gonorrhea with more coverage on treatment of DGI and salpingitis.
Sparling PF: Biology of Neisseria gonorrhoeae. In Holmes KK, Sparling PF, Stamm WE, et al (eds): Sexually Transmitted Diseases, 4th ed. New York, McGraw-Hill, 2007.
    This article is the most current review of gonococcal biology and pathogenesis.

EVIDENCE

1. Workowski KA, Berman SM; Centers for Disease Control and Prevention: Sexually transmitted diseases treatment guidelines, 2006. MMWR Recomm Rep 55(RR-11):1-94, 2006.
    The authors present the latest guidelines from the CDC, available also at http://www.cdc.gov/std/treatment/default.htm.

Pelvic Inflammatory Disease

Introduction

Pelvic inflammatory disease (PID) is a clinical syndrome defined as inflammation of the upper female genital tract, which may include endometritis, salpingitis, tubo-ovarian abscess, and pelvic peritonitis. The incidence of PID in the United States has been declining since the late 1980s. Still, an estimated 1 million women in the United States are diagnosed with PID annually at a cost of nearly $2 billion for treatment of PID and management of its sequelae. The reproductive complications of PID include infertility, ectopic pregnancy, and chronic pelvic pain. Clinical diagnosis is imprecise because there are no specific signs or symptoms for the diagnosis of PID. However, it is very important to make the diagnosis of PID because prompt recognition and initiation of effective therapy are critical for preserving fertility.

Etiology and Pathogenesis

PID is primarily due to sexually transmitted organisms, with *Neisseria gonorrhoeae* and *Chlamydia trachomatis* accounting for one third to one half of PID infections. However, organisms associated with the vaginal flora have also been associated with PID and include anaerobes, *Gardnerella vaginalis*, *Haemophilus influenzae*, enteric gram-negative rods, and *Streptococcus agalactiae*. Other organisms associated with PID are cytomegalovirus (CMV), *Mycoplasma hominis*, *Mycoplasma genitalium*, and *Ureaplasma urealyticum*. The polymicrobial nature of infection complicates both the choice of therapy and whether clinical or microbial end points should decide the duration of therapy.

PID primarily occurs with the accession of either one or more sexually transmitted pathogens or organisms present in vaginal flora, from the lower genital tract to the upper tract (Fig. 111-1). Risk factors for PID include those that are modifiable (use of condoms and number of sexual partners) and those related to demographics (i.e., age, race, ethnicity).

Adolescents are at particularly high risk for PID due to anatomic factors, the higher prevalence of *N. gonorrhoeae* and *C. trachomatis* among their male partners, the higher number of recent sexual partners, and the greater likelihood of partner concurrency (the overlap of sexual partners over a period of time). The adolescent cervix is believed to be at increased risk for sexually transmitted infection acquisition and hence the development of PID because of a larger proportion of columnar epithelium present on the ectocervix (ectopy) relative to that in older women. Columnar epithelial cells are the targeted cells for sexually transmitted infections. Additionally, changes in cervical mucus associated with persistent high-estrogen state seen in adolescence and lower endocervical immunity in those with recent sexual debut may increase the risk for PID.

The role of bacterial vaginosis (BV) as a cofactor for the development of PID is still unclear. The alteration in pH associated with the lack of H_2O_2-producing *Lactobacillus* species is associated with a higher vaginal concentration of anaerobes. The change in vaginal flora associated with BV increases the risk for infection by *N. gonorrhoeae* and *C. trachomatis*. Two studies found conflicting results regarding the risk for PID for women with BV. The PID evaluation and clinical health study (PEACH) found no association of BV with the development of PID. Ness and colleagues did find a twofold increased risk (relative risk = 2.0) associated with the presence of BV-associated microorganisms in the vaginal tract.

Figure 111-1 Pelvic Inflammatory Disease.

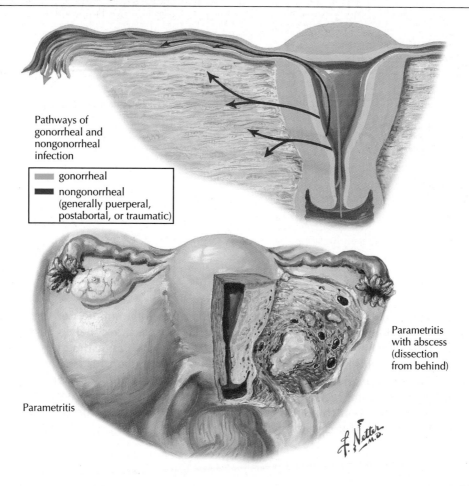

Pathways of gonorrheal and nongonorrheal infection

■ gonorrheal

■ nongonorrheal (generally puerperal, postabortal, or traumatic)

Parametritis

Parametritis with abscess (dissection from behind)

The most important risk factors associated with PID are recent infection with either *N. gonorrhoeae* or *C. trachomatis* or a past history of PID. In one study of women with acute PID, *N. gonorrhoeae* and *C. trachomatis* were isolated in 49% and 36% of women, respectively.

Clinical Presentation

The diagnosis of PID is imprecise, with a myriad of signs and symptoms and a wide spectrum in severity. Laparoscopy offers a high degree of sensitivity and allows for a precise microbiologic diagnosis but is limited by the invasiveness of the procedure and the inability to detect endometritis and mild to subclinical involvement of the fallopian tubes. No single clinical sign or symptom is pathognomonic for PID. Because delays in diagnosis can lead to further inflammation of the upper genital tract, there has been much interest in better diagnostic approaches to PID.

Unfortunately, any combination of findings that improves the specificity of a clinical diagnosis of PID tends to substantially lower sensitivity. As a result, clinicians must maintain a high index of suspicion for the diagnosis of PID and have a low threshold for the initiation of treatment. Therapy can be initiated while ruling out other potential causes of lower abdominal pain including ectopic pregnancy, acute appendicitis, endometriosis, ruptured ovarian cyst, irritable bowel syndrome, inflammatory bowel disease, and urinary tract infection. Considerations that will improve the performance of a clinical diagnosis include an adolescent population, sexually transmitted disease clinic patients, and populations with a high prevalence of chlamydia or gonorrhea.

Empiric antimicrobial therapy should be started in at-risk sexually active women with any of the following findings on pelvic examination: cervical motion tenderness, uterine tenderness, or adnexal tenderness.

The specificity of the minimum clinical findings increases when patients have evidence of lower genital tract inflammation such as abnormal cervical or vaginal mucopurulent discharge or elevated number of cells seen on vaginal wet mount.

Box 111-1 Differential Diagnosis of Pelvic Inflammatory Disease

Gynecologic
Endometriosis
Ruptured ovarian cyst
Ovarian torsion
Ovarian tumor
Ectopic pregnancy
Dysmenorrhea

Gastrointestinal
Appendicitis
Inflammatory bowel disease
Irritable bowel syndrome
Gastroenteritis

Urologic
Cystitis
Pyelonephritis

Differential Diagnosis

See Box 111-1 for the differential diagnosis of PID.

Diagnostic Approach

No laboratory tests are specific for the evaluation and diagnosis of PID. As mentioned, empiric treatment should be initiated when clinical findings are present. Evaluation for gonococcal or chlamydial infection of the endocervix should be obtained in all patients in whom PID is suspected. Evidence of white blood cells on vaginal saline microscopy and the presence of mucopurulent endocervical discharge increase the probability of PID in the presence of pain. Their absence should prompt investigation for an alternative diagnosis. Endometrial biopsy, transvaginal sonography, magnetic resonance imaging, or laparoscopy may be warranted in limited cases but are either costly or invasive and, in any case, must not delay initiation of therapy. As with all sexually transmitted infections, all patients with PID should be screened for HIV infection.

Other diagnostic tests to exclude alternative diagnoses and assess severity of illness include urinalysis and urine culture, serum or urine pregnancy test, total white blood cell count, and erythrocyte sedimentation rate or C-reactive protein.

Management and Therapy

Optimum Treatment

Treatment of PID must cover a broad spectrum of possible pathogens. All empiric regimens must contain antimicrobial agents effective against *N. gonorrhoeae* and *C. trachomatis* because these are the most common sexually transmitted infections associated with PID. Treatment directed against these organisms is not dependent on the detection of these organisms because negative cervical screening for these pathogens does not rule out an upper genital tract infection. A more controversial area is the need to take into account the possibility of anaerobic bacteria. Because a number of studies have found upper tract involvement with anaerobic bacteria in women with PID, many experts advocate the use of antimicrobial agents highly active against anaerobes. However, in a study of women with endometrial cultures, reproductive outcomes did not differ by the presence of anaerobes. Furthermore, the results of the PEACH trial, a study comparing intravenous cefoxitin and doxycycline for 48 hours followed by oral doxycycline for a total of 14 days of therapy with an outpatient regimen of a single dose of cefoxitin followed by 14 days of oral doxycycline, did not differ in superiority. This study calls into question the need to include anaerobic therapy in the treatment regimen for acute PID. These studies are limited by the short-term evaluation of cure rates and not the long-term reproductive outcomes, and at present, broader antibiotic regimens are still used preferentially by many experts.

The choice of inpatient or outpatient therapy depends on the severity of PID. Inpatient therapy is recommended when ectopic pregnancy and surgical emergencies have not been excluded, when outpatient management has failed or is not tolerated, in the presence of tubo-ovarian abscess, and for all pregnant women. In a study by Ness and colleagues, outpatient therapy for mild to moderate PID did not differ from inpatient therapy either in short-term clinical-microbiologic outcomes or long-term reproductive outcomes. Duration of therapy depends on clinical response but is recommended for a minimum of 14 days.

Recommended inpatient treatment regimens are shown in Box 111-2; recommended outpatient treatment regimens are shown in Box 111-3.

Management of Sexual Partners

The 2006 Centers for Disease Control and Prevention treatment guidelines recommend that men with sexual contact with women within 60 days of the onset of symptoms for PID should be evaluated for sexually transmitted infections including HIV. These partners should also be treated empirically for *C. trachomatis* and *N. gonorrhoeae*.

Avoiding Treatment Errors

The most important potential for treatment errors lies in failure to treat—that is, a lack of therapy for mild clinical presentations of PID or the delay of therapy. Clinicians must maintain a high index of clinical suspicion for PID and initiate immediate therapy on the basis of a clinical diagnosis. The hope in early initiation of therapy is to

---

Box 111-2   Recommended Parenteral Antibacterial Therapy for Acute Pelvic Inflammatory Disease*

Recommended Parenteral Regimen A

Cefotetan, 2 g IV every 12 hr,
or
Cefoxitin, 2 g IV every 6 hr,
plus
Doxycycline, 100 mg orally or IV every 12 hr

Recommended Parenteral Regimen B

Clindamycin, 900 mg IV every 8 hr,
plus
Gentamicin loading dose, IV or intramuscularly (2 mg/kg of body weight), followed by a maintenance dose (1.5 mg/kg) every 8 hr; single daily dosing may be substituted

Alternative Parenteral Regimens

1. Levofloxacin, 500 mg IV once daily,
or
Ofloxacin, 400 mg IV every 12 hr,
with or without
Metronidazole, 500 mg IV every 8 hr
2. Ampicillin-sulbactam, 3 g IV every 6 hr,
plus
Doxycycline, 100 mg orally or IV every 12 hr

*Based on the 2006 Centers for Disease Control and Prevention sexually transmitted diseases treatment guidelines.

Box 111-3   Recommended Oral Antibacterial Therapy for Acute Pelvic Inflammatory Disease*

Recommended Oral Regimen A

Levofloxacin, 500 mg orally once daily for 14 days,
or
Ofloxacin, 400 mg orally once daily for 14 days,
with or without
Metronidazole, 500 mg orally twice a day for 14 days

Recommended Oral Regimen B

Ceftriaxone, 250 mg intramuscularly in a single dose,
or
Cefoxitin, 2 g intramuscularly in a single dose; and probenecid, 1 g orally administered concurrently in a single dose,
or
Other parenteral third-generation cephalosporin (e.g., ceftizoxime or cefotaxime),
plus
Doxycycline, 100 mg orally twice a day for 14 days,
with or without
Metronidazole, 500 mg orally twice a day for 14 days

*Based on 2006 Centers for Disease Control and Prevention sexually transmitted diseases treatment guidelines.

---

avoid the long-term sequelae of PID, that is, tubal infertility and chronic pelvic pain.

Future Directions

Future studies are needed to evaluate the utility of monotherapies for PID, short (3 to 5 days) course of therapy, and the effectiveness of current antimicrobial regimens on subsequent reproductive morbidity. The emergence of resistant *N. gonorrhoeae* and anaerobes will require the continued evaluation of the efficacy of treatment regimens.

Additional Resource

U.S. Preventive Service Task Force. Chlamydial infection: Screening 2001. In Guide to Clinical Preventive Services. Alexandria, VA, International Medical Publishing, 2001, p 332.

These are the current recommendations for chlamydial screening. Chlamydia is the number one preventable cause of preventable tubal infertility. Screening for asymptomatic infection in young women is an effective strategy to reduce the incidence of PID.

EVIDENCE

1. Ness RB, Soper DE, Holley RL, et al: Effectiveness of inpatient and outpatient treatment strategies for women with pelvic inflammatory disease: Results from the Pelvic Inflammatory Disease Evaluation and Clinical Health (PEACH) randomized trial. Am J Obstet Gynecol 186:929-937, 2002.
    This important study serves as the basis for expansion in the use of outpatient therapy for PID.
2. Ness RB, Haggerty CL: Newest approaches to treatment of pelvic inflammatory disease: A review of recent randomized clinical trials. Clin Infect Dis 44:953-960, 2007.
    The authors present a well-written review of recent clinical trials for the treatment of PID.
3. Weisenfeld HC, Sweet RC, Ness RB, et al: Comparison of acute and subclinical pelvic inflammatory disease. Sex Transm Dis 32:400-405, 2005.
    This article is an important read in describing the significance of low-grade to subclinical PID.
4. Workowski KA, Berman SM; Centers for Disease Control and Prevention: Sexually transmitted diseases treatment guidelines, 2006. MMWR Recomm Rep 55(RR-11):1-94, 2006.
    This is the definitive reference for the diagnosis and management of PID.

Genital Warts

Introduction

Genital infection with human papillomavirus (HPV) is extremely common. Most infections are benign and result in no disease. The spectrum of genital HPV infection ranges from asymptomatic infection to warts and cervical cancer. More than 80 types of HPV have been identified, with more than 30 causing genital infection divided into low and high risk for the development of malignant cellular changes such as cervical and anal cancer. The clinical expression of low-risk types is genital warts, a problem that is increasing in incidence worldwide. The genital subgroups of HPV have a predilection for the anogenital squamous epithelium. Their primary mode of transmission is sexual, and genital warts are only one manifestation of a broad spectrum of clinical diseases associated with HPV, including a strong association with genital neoplasia.

Accurate incidence figures for genital warts in the United States are not available. It is estimated that 26.8% of U.S. females 14 to 59 years of age are infected with HPV. The highest prevalence was among those aged 20 to 24 years at 44.8%. More than 70% of the adult population have been or are currently infected with HPV. A 1996 report by the Centers for Disease Control and Prevention (CDC) estimated that 24 million Americans are infected with HPV and that 500,000 to 1 million new cases of condylomata acuminata occur annually. This means that about 1% of sexually active persons in the United States have visible genital warts at any one time. Most cases, about 80%, are caused by HPV-6. The prevalence rates for HPV-11 and HPV-5 in U.S. females 14 to 59 years of age were 0.1% and 1.3%, respectively. HPV-11 and HPV-6 account for more than 90% of genital warts. Epidemiologic studies indicate that independent risk factors for HPV infection include adolescents, young adults, marital status, and increasing number of lifetime and recent sex partners.

Etiology and Pathogenesis

HPV is a protein-encapsulated, nonenveloped icosahedral virus. It contains 8 to 10 genes that are circular, double-stranded DNA. The early region products control viral replication, transcription, and cellular transformation, and encode for the oncoproteins E6 and E7. The late region encodes for structural proteins, whereas the long-control region contains transcription enhancer genes and promoter elements.

HPV infects stratified squamous epithelial cells. HPV-containing cells do not undergo cell lysis and are shed from the surface of the skin. Upon infection with HPV, epithelial cells are transformed to proliferate into benign tumors known as *warts*. In nonkeratinized squamous epithelium, the exophytic growths are known as *condylomata acuminata*.

Clinical Presentation

In addition to the classic cauliflower-like proliferations, HPV infection may also manifest as smooth, flat lesions (pigmented or nonpigmented), papular warts (flesh-colored, dome-shaped papules), keratotic warts (thick, crust-like layer), or subclinical infections. The lesions most commonly are multiple but may be single, scattered, or confluent. They are seen most often in young adults. The incubation period is 2 to 3 months, although the latency period from exposure to disease development varies greatly.

Figure 112-1 Condyloma Acuminata of Penis.

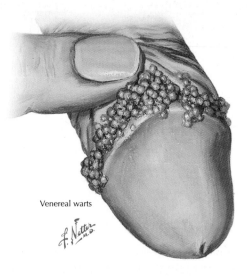

Venereal warts

Figure 112-2 Condylomata Acuminata in Females.

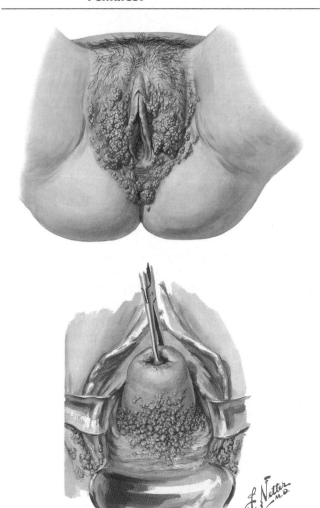

The entire genital tract, including the vulva, vagina, cervix, penis, perianal area, rectum, and urethra, is susceptible to HPV infection.

Clinical Features in Males

The classic condylomata acuminata (Fig. 112-1) predominate in moist areas, the inner surfaces of the prepuce, coronal sulcus, and frenum and may spread to the perianal area. More rounded papular warts are seen in drier areas of the penile shaft or perineal skin. Other clinically apparent lesions include sessile lesions and flat keratotic plaques with a roughened, variably pigmented surface. Condylomata may also involve the urethra and urethral meatus, resulting in hematuria and dysuria or discharge.

Clinical Features in Females

Condylomata usually first appear at the posterior part of the introitus and adjacent labia and may involve other parts of the vulva, perineum, and anus, but rarely the adjacent thighs. The vagina (upper and lower third) may be involved and, infrequently, the cervix (Fig. 112-2). More commonly, HPV infection of the cervix is subclinical, visible only after application of 5% acetic acid as flat acetowhite epithelium at colposcopy, or evident on Papanicolaou (Pap) tests (2% to 3% of which are currently positive for warty changes). Subclinical HPV infection can occur elsewhere in the genital tract. Vaginal warts are usually asymptomatic but occasionally present as vaginal discharge, pruritus, or post-coital bleeding.

In pregnancy and in immunosuppressed women, lesions may become exuberant. Occasionally, vaginal delivery may be threatened by obstruction or hemorrhage; however, lesions usually regress or disappear during the puerperium. The natural history of subclinical HPV infection of the

vulva and vagina is poorly understood; in the cervix, a proportion will regress, but a group will progress to dysplasia, intraepithelial neoplasia, or frank cancer.

Clinical Features in Children

Genital warts are rare in children. When present, there may be a history of maternal genital warts during pregnancy. In older children, molestation should be considered. Maternal genital warts during pregnancy may, in rare cases, cause laryngeal papillomatosis in infants. This may not become clinically apparent until the second decade of life.

Differential Diagnosis

Other papillomatous lesions that must be differentiated from anogenital warts include (1) anatomic variants (e.g., papillae coronae glandis or the pearly penile papules); (2)

infective conditions (e.g., condylomata lata of secondary syphilis [broader and flatter lesions; positive serologic test for syphilis and dark-field microscopy of lesions] and, in the tropics, donovanosis); and (3) benign and malignant neoplasias (e.g., intraepithelial carcinoma or invasive carcinoma).

Diagnostic Approach

HPV-associated lesions demonstrate specific changes recognized at colposcopy, cytology (Pap test of ectocervical and endocervical smears), and histology of biopsy materials. Although HPV cannot be cultivated in vitro, recent advances in molecular biologic techniques utilizing DNA probes can identify HPV DNA. Such techniques show that more than 100 different types of HPV exist, and a subgroup of these (HPV types 6, 11, 16, 18, and less often 31, 33, 35) specifically infects the genital area. HPV types 6 and 11 have a predilection for the external anogenital skin, usually producing the exophytic condyloma of the vulva and perianal area, although occasionally causing subclinical infections or condylomata on the cervix.

HPV types 16 and 18 are associated most often with subclinical lesions of mucosal surfaces, especially the cervix. They have been implicated in oncogenic progression of tissue changes (benign warty to dysplasia, to intraepithelial neoplasia, to invasive carcinoma) in the penis, vulva, vagina, and, especially, the cervix. Other cofactors apart from HPV are no doubt involved in oncogenicity.

Management and Therapy

- Other associated sexually transmitted infections should be excluded, especially condyloma lata of secondary syphilis.
- Warts should be treated as described later. All warts show unpredictable behavior and may regress spontaneously, enlarge and spread, or recur.
- Review weekly or biweekly for treatment and follow-up until lesions have resolved.
- It is important to evaluate for coexisting cervical dysplasia (Pap test). Repeat Pap test should be obtained every 6 to 12 months thereafter.
- Refer for colposcopy if there is evidence of cervical dysplasia or if there is persistent cervical HPV infection.
- Ensure examination of sexual partners and treat those with warts.
- Advise use of condoms until no lesions are apparent.
- Obtain a biopsy specimen of any atypical wart.

Pharmacologic Agents

There is no specific antiviral therapy available for HPV and no one method of treatment that is superior to all others. Therapy often involves methods that attempt to nonspecifically destroy infected tissue. Most of these cytodestructive therapies are painful and require multiple visits to a provider or require adherence to daily application of a medication. The efficacy of cytodestructive therapies has not been verified in placebo-controlled trials and has highly variable reported rates of success and high recurrence rates. Newer therapies involving pharmacologic approaches that stimulate immunologic or antiviral responses offer promise of higher response rates and lower rates of recurrence. Pharmacologic agents available for treatment include cytotoxic agents (podophyllin), destructive agents (trichloroacetic acid), and immunologic agents (interferon, imiquimod). Therapies can be divided into two categories: provider administered and patient applied.

Provider-Administered Therapies

Podophyllin resin is used for penile and vulvar warts. It should not be used in well-vascularized areas such as the vagina or anus. The major disadvantages of podophyllin are skin irritation, if not properly applied, and systemic toxicity and potential oncogenicity with use of large amounts or repeated application. Its use is contraindicated in pregnancy and if dysplasia or neoplasia is present. Given current treatment options and the toxicities associated with podophyllin therapy, there is little clinical indication for its use.

5-Fluorouracil (5-FU) is used topically as a 5% cream for treatment of vaginal lesions and urethral condylomata and for prophylaxis in immunocompromised patients. Its disadvantages are that an extensive erosive dermatitis may occur with incorrect application and that its use requires a reliable patient to follow instructions. Pregnancy is a contraindication to 5-FU treatment. The 2006 Sexually Transmitted Diseases Treatment Guidelines do not recommend the use of 5-FU for the treatment of genital warts.

Trichloroacetic acid (TCA) and dichloroacetic acid (DCA) are applied undiluted (25% to 85% solution) and washed off after 12 hours. They are weak destructive agents and are sometimes effective against small condylomata. They may be applied weekly for up to 6 weeks. Petroleum jelly or lanolin should be applied around the lesions to prevent spill onto surrounding normal tissue.

Interferon has antiviral, antiproliferative, and immunomodulating properties and has been used for persistent or resistant disease. It is administered by intralesional or intramuscular injection 3 times weekly. However, it is expensive, is nonspecific, and may cause multiple side effects (e.g., flu-like symptoms).

Patient-Applied Therapies

Imiquimod cream (5%) is an immune-response modifier capable of inducing a variety of cytokines, including interferon-α and tumor necrosis factor. It is applied 3 times weekly to affected areas and washed off after 8 hours.

Clinical response may take 2 to 8 weeks, and therapy may be continued for up to 16 weeks. Side effects include local inflammatory reactions with no systemic reactions.

Podofilox (0.5% solution or gel), an antimitotic agent purified from podophyllin resin, is less likely to cause systemic toxicity. It is approved for self-treatment in both men and women. It is applied twice daily for 3 days; this course can be repeated after 4 days and continued for up to 4 weeks if necessary. Safety for use in pregnant patients has not been established.

Other Treatment Methods

Other methods include electrocautery and curettage under local or general anesthesia, depending on the site and extent of the lesions. Cryotherapy is effective for both genital and anal warts, provided they are not too large. Treatment involves applying the cryocautery probe to each wart for 30 to 60 seconds (no anesthetic necessary). Alternatively, genital warts can be frozen with liquid nitrogen. Cautery and cryosurgery are the methods of choice for keratinized warts or for warts refractory to other forms of treatment. They can also be used as primary treatment of mucosal warts. Surgical excision or carbon dioxide laser destruction under general anesthesia may be used for extensive lesions.

Optimum Treatment

Exophytic Condylomata of External Genitals

If lesions are nonextensive, options should be discussed with the patient before therapy. The patient's ability to adhere to the treatment regimen as well as the location and number of warts should be considered. For provider-applied therapy, cryotherapy (weekly until lesions gone) or trichloroacetic or dichloroacetic acid (applied twice weekly) should be used. For patient-applied therapy, imiquimod 5% cream and podofilox 0.5% solution or gel are options as well. If lesions are extensive, laser therapy, cautery, or surgical excision are alternatives. In females, cervical HPV infection (cytology), and in men who have sex with men, rectal HPV infection (anoscopy and rectal cytology), should be excluded.

Cervical HPV Infection

Patients with cervical HPV infection should be referred for colposcopic evaluation with directed biopsy of abnormal areas.

Pregnant Patients

Trichloroacetic acid or cryotherapy should be used for isolated lesions, or laser therapy for extensive lesions. Careful cytologic and colposcopic follow-up is essential. Vaginal delivery, unless obstructed by lesions, is possible because cesarean birth does not prevent infant infection.

Specialist Referral

Referral is advisable for urethral or cervical warts; associated cervical HPV changes on cytology, dysplasia, or neoplasia; immunodeficient patients (who do not respond to conventional treatment); refractory warts; and condylomata in children.

Avoiding Treatment Errors

It is important to consider the potential for other sexually transmitted infections in patients with genital HPV. It is also important to test for pregnancy before considering systemic therapy.

Vaccines

Progress continues to be made on the development of prophylactic and therapeutic vaccines. Two vaccines against the most common HPV types associated with cervical cancer, HPV-16 and HPV-18, have been developed and tested in clinical trials. The first of the two vaccines to be approved is a quadrivalent vaccine (Gardasil) for HPV types 6, 11, 16, and 18. The second vaccine is a bivalent vaccine (Cervarix) for HPV types 16 and 18. Cervarix will be available the fourth quarter of 2007. The approach for both vaccines involved the use of a papillomavirus-like particle vaccine composed of a major structural viral protein, L1, to confer protection against infection. The efficacy of both vaccines for preventing HPV-16– or HPV-18–related cervical intraepithelial neoplasia (CIN) was 100%. Because only Gardasil is currently licensed by the U.S. Food and Drug Administration, recommendations for vaccination are limited to Gardasil. It is anticipated that similar recommendations will be made for Cervarix. Centers for Disease Control and Prevention and the Advisory Committee on Immunization Practices guidelines recommend that females 11 to 12 years of age be routinely vaccinated. Females aged 13 to 26 years of age are also recommended to be vaccinated. No guidelines currently recommend vaccination of young men, but approval for vaccination in men is likely. The duration of efficacy of the HPV vaccines is unknown, but the length of current follow-up and the rate of antibody decay suggest efficacy may be long lived. It is unknown whether vaccinating females alone will be sufficient to stop the HPV epidemic. Progress is also being made in the development of therapeutic vaccines that may prove effective against persistent HPV infection, warts, and premalignant lesions. There are no data to verify the safety of the vaccine in pregnancy; hence, pregnant women should not be vaccinated for HPV.

Future Directions

Future directions will primarily involve the expansion of the indications for HPV vaccination in older women and males. Future research will also explore the use of the current HPV vaccines for therapeutic benefits in HPV-related diseases.

Additional Resources

Beutner KR, Spruance SL, Hougham AJ, et al: Treatment of genital warts with an immune-response modifier (imiquimod). J Am Acad Dermatol 38:230-239, 1998.

Imiquimod is notable because it provides another option for patient-applied treatment of genital warts and is the first topically applied immune modulator for the treatment of genital warts.

Koutsky L: Epidemiology of genital human papillomavirus infection. Am J Med 102:3-8, 1997.

This outstanding overview of HPV epidemiology is also a good reference.

Langley PC, Richwald GA, Smith MH: Modeling the impact of treatment options in genital warts: Patient-applied versus physician-administered therapies. Clin Ther 21:2143-2155, 1999.

This paper provides a sound base for choosing treatment options for the treatment of genital warts.

EVIDENCE

1. Auborn KJ, Carter TH: Treatment of human papillomavirus gynecologic infections. Clin Lab Med 20:407-422, 2000.
    This is an excellent review for the treatment of HPV in women.

2. Beutner KR, Reitano MV, Richwald GA, Wiley DJ: External genital warts: Report of the American Medical Association Consensus Conference. AMA Expert Panel on External Genital Warts. Clin Infect Dis 27:796-806, 1998.
    This article presents a general review of the treatment of genital warts.

3. Dunne EF, Unger ER, Sternberg M, et al: Prevalence of HPV infection among females in the United States. JAMA 297(8):813-819, 2007.
    The authors report on the latest population-based survey of HPV infection among women.

4. Koutsky LA, Ault KA, Wheeler CM, et al: Proof of Principle Study Investigators. A controlled trial of a human papillomavirus type 16 vaccine. N Engl J Med 347(21)1645-1651, 2002.
    This is the landmark study for the HPV vaccine.

5. Markowitz LE, Dunne EF, Saraiya M, et al: Centers for Disease Control and Prevention Advisory Committee on Immunization Practices (ACIP): Quadrivalent Human Papillomavirus Vaccine: Recommendations of the Advisory Committee on Immunization Practices (ACIP). MMWR Recomm Rep 56(RR-2):1-24, 2007.
    These recommendations form the bases for current state and local HPV vaccine policies.

6. Workowski KA, Berman SM: Centers for Disease Control and Prevention. Sexually transmitted diseases treatment guidelines, 2006. MMWR Recomm Rep 55(RR-11):1-94, 2006.
    This article provides the latest and best expert guidance for diagnosis and management of HPV infection and HPV-related diseases.

Syphilis

Introduction

Syphilis, an infectious disease caused by *Treponema pallidum*, usually is sexually transmitted but may be transmitted transplacentally from an infected mother to her infant. Once very common, affecting as much as 10% or more of the general population, it became much less prevalent after the discovery of penicillin. Rates of infection declined steadily in the United States except for a rise among men having sex with men (MSM) at the onset of the HIV era and a brief period in the late 1980s and early 1990s due to an epidemic of trading heterosexual sex for crack cocaine. In the first years of the 21st century, however, there has been an increase in syphilis in the United States among MSM, including college students and others who use the Internet to find sexual partners. The infection continues to be a plague in much of the world, with prevalence of more than 10% in many sub-Saharan African countries. Early syphilis is a recognized cofactor for HIV transmission, warranting the serious attention of clinicians and investigators. In the United States, the infection is more common in some population groups, particularly African Americans who may have disease rates about 20 times those of whites. This probably reflects differences in several behaviors, including sexual and health-seeking behaviors, availability of appropriate health care access, and a complex mix of socioeconomic factors that help to determine behaviors. There has been recent progress in reducing the prevalence of syphilis in African Americans.

Etiology and Pathogenesis

T. pallidum is a spirochetal bacterium whose genome has now been sequenced. Although *T. pallidum* can be introduced in animals, it cannot be cultured in the laboratory and for this reason it is less well understood than many bacterial pathogens. It is a slender, spiral-shaped organism that cannot be seen by ordinary Gram stain but can be visualized by dark-field microscopy and has a characteristic motility that facilitates diagnosis from early infectious lesions. Relatively rare outer sheath proteins include proteins that are under intense current investigation because they appear to undergo rapid variation, possibly helping to account for the ability of the organism to persist in vivo despite an immune response. The organism does not survive drying, and its only natural host is humans, accounting for the usual necessity of contact with lesions in an infected sexual partner for disease transmission.

The median infective dose, the dose required to infect 50% of subjects, is about 10 organisms. Rate of growth in humans and animals is slow, with a doubling time of about 24 hours, which accounts for the slow progression of disease and helps explain the need for prolonged treatment to effect cure.

The intermittent, relapsing, slowly evolving nature of untreated syphilis suggests a delicate balance between the pathogen and the host immune system. There is partial immunity in late-acquired or congenital syphilis, as demonstrated in human prison volunteers 50 years ago. Immunity can be developed, albeit with difficulty, in experimental rabbit syphilis. Some of the lesions of late syphilis appear to be the result of a hypersensitivity response to infection, perhaps explaining the granulomatous reaction of some lesions (particularly gummas) of late syphilis. Typically, there is a vasculitis of the vasa vasorum, which may account for some late manifestations, including aortitis and some of the central nervous system (CNS) lesions.

Women may transmit infection transplacentally for up to 6 or 7 years after untreated infection, but during about the last 3 months of gestation only, owing to breakdown of placental barriers later in pregnancy. Routine testing and treatment of pregnant women during the first two trimesters should prevent congenital syphilis.

Clinical Presentation

Syphilis is generally divided into primary, secondary, latent, and late stages. The disease is the result of contact with infected lesions. *T. pallidum* enters the skin or mucosa and then disseminates early to many organs, including the skin, CNS, and others. The illness progresses from a lesion at the site of inoculation to a more generalized disease, punctuated by periods of clinical well-being. Primary and secondary syphilis are termed *early syphilis*. This is followed by a latent period with no abnormalities other than immunologic evidence of infection. Late or tertiary types of clinical disease develop in about one third of untreated persons. The interval between initial infection and recognized onset of late syphilis may be remarkably long, up to 20 years or more, depending on the type of syndrome.

Primary Syphilis

After an incubation period of about 10 to 21 days, there typically is a papule that evolves into a painless ulcer termed *chancre* (Fig. 113-1). About 10% of chancres are extragenital, especially around or in the mouth and anal areas (Fig. 113-2). A classic chancre has rolled margins and a clean nontender base, often with satellite adenopathy. Perirectal or oral chancres may have atypical presentations and may be missed without strong suspicion (see Fig. 113-2). Untreated infection heals spontaneously in about 3 weeks.

Secondary Syphilis

Lesions of secondary syphilis occasionally coincide with the primary lesion but more often occur weeks or months later, up to 6 months from onset of infection (Fig. 113-3). A primary lesion may not have been recognized. The secondary rash heals spontaneously in about 3 weeks but may relapse one or more times over the next 2 years if untreated. The cardinal sign of secondary syphilis is a rash on the mucosa or skin. Often, it starts on the trunk but spreads to involve much of the body, including the palms and soles. Early rash may be subtle and can be missed in persons with dark pigmentation. It varies from copper to brown macules to papulosquamous lesions to nodules but in adults almost never is vesicular or bullous or pruritic. Rash on moist mucosal surfaces may be hyperplastic (condyloma acuminata, or syphilitic warts) or may be flat plaques as in the gray mucous patches of the mouth or elsewhere. Mucosal lesions are quite infectious, but the cutaneous rash is minimally infectious. At this point, the disease is systemic, and there often is fever, sore throat, and generalized adenopa-thy. Meningitis with headache and a cerebrospinal fluid (CSF) mononuclear pleocytosis occurs in about 30% of patients. Occasional patients have clinical hepatitis or immune-deposit glomerulopathy.

Latent Syphilis

By definition, the latent stage is when the patient is infected and has positive serologic tests for syphilis but is clinically normal, including normal CSF findings. It is divided into early (first year) and late (more than 1 year) latency for epidemiologic reasons because the risk for transmission to sexual partners is essentially zero after 1 year of untreated infection. Untreated, about two thirds of patients do not progress beyond latency, but late syphilis develops in one third of patients.

Late Syphilis

Late syphilis may involve many organs but can be divided into three general types: gumma, neurosyphilis, and cardiovascular syphilis. Gumma usually presents as granulomatous or destructive ulcerative or mass lesions of the skin or viscera. Once common, it is now rare, probably because it responds readily to antibiotics. In the past decade, multiple cases have been documented in patients with HIV infection.

In cardiovascular syphilis, inflammation of the ascending aorta results in aortic wall weakness and aneurysm formation, which may lead to aortic valve insufficiency and, on occasion, occlusion of the coronary arteries. Clinical onset usually is a decade or more after infection, with presentation as aortic insufficiency.

Involvement of the nervous system takes many forms in neurosyphilis, with variable onset after initial infection. Meningitis (headache, stiff neck) may occur coincident with secondary syphilis or in the next 5 or 6 years. The CSF formula is indistinguishable from other causes of aseptic meningitis, but the CSF Venereal Disease Research Laboratory (VDRL) test is positive. Meningovascular syphilis occurs within the first 12 years of infection, with occlusion of small to medium vessels and stroke syndrome. It should be considered in young persons with no obvious cause for stroke. The form of stroke varies from isolated cranial nerve palsies, including the eighth cranial nerve, to hemispheric lesions. The CSF test results are abnormal, including a lymphocytic pleocytosis, and CSF serologic tests for syphilis usually are positive. General paresis occurs from 10 to 20 years after infection, with involvement of the cerebral hemispheres and various signs and symptoms including dementia, paranoia, and delusions of grandeur. Often, the CSF test results are abnormal, but there may not be a pleocytosis, and the serologic test results for syphilis are not always positive. Tabes dorsalis affects the posterior columns of the spinal cord, with loss of proprioception, often with associated severe sharp intermittent

Figure 113-1 Genital Lesions of Primary Syphilis.

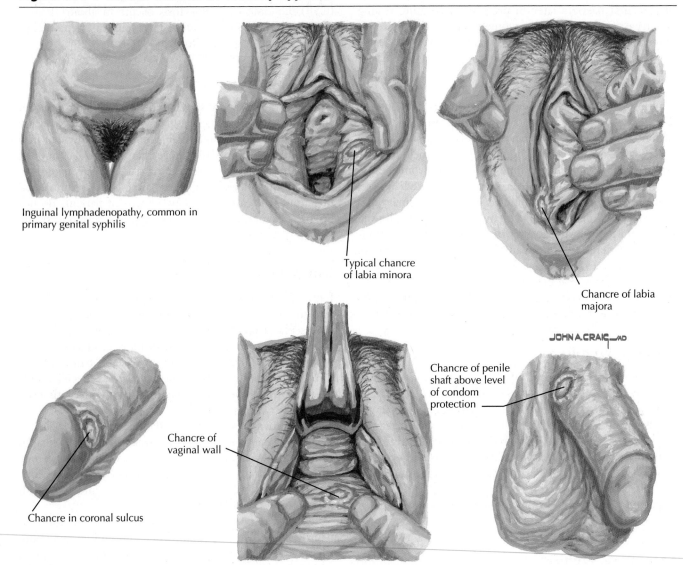

Inguinal lymphadenopathy, common in primary genital syphilis

Typical chancre of labia minora

Chancre of labia majora

JOHN A.CRAIG—AD

Chancre of penile shaft above level of condom protection

Chancre in coronal sulcus

Chancre of vaginal wall

radicular pains of the extremities or abdomen. There may be associated optic atrophy and Argyll-Robertson pupils (small pupils that accommodate but do not react to light). The CSF test results often are abnormal (high protein, increased mononuclear cells, positive VDRL), but one or more of these findings may be absent. Tabes typically has late onset. Some of the classic clinical forms may be indistinct or overlap.

Syphilis in Patients with HIV Infection

Anecdotal evidence suggests that syphilis presents differently in the presence of HIV, but there have been no confirmatory studies to substantiate this observation. Serologic tests and response to therapy approximate those in non–HIV-infected patients. Neurosyphilis may present a

particular dilemma, however, because patients with advanced HIV infection have myriad causes of abnormal CSF test results and neurologic illness.

Differential Diagnosis

In primary syphilis, the principal differential involves other causes of genital ulcer syndrome, particularly herpes simplex virus (HSV). HSV more often has multiple ulcers, and they are usually painful and tender, whereas the syphilitic chancre is painless unless secondarily infected (see Fig. 113-1). In other parts of the world, chancroid (*Haemophilus ducreyi*) is a common cause of single or multiple, usually tender, genital ulcers. Secondary syphilis has a very broad differential diagnosis, including mononucleosis, drug reactions, viral exanthems, hepatitis, and many more, depend-

Figure 113-2 Extragenital Lesions of Primary Syphilis.

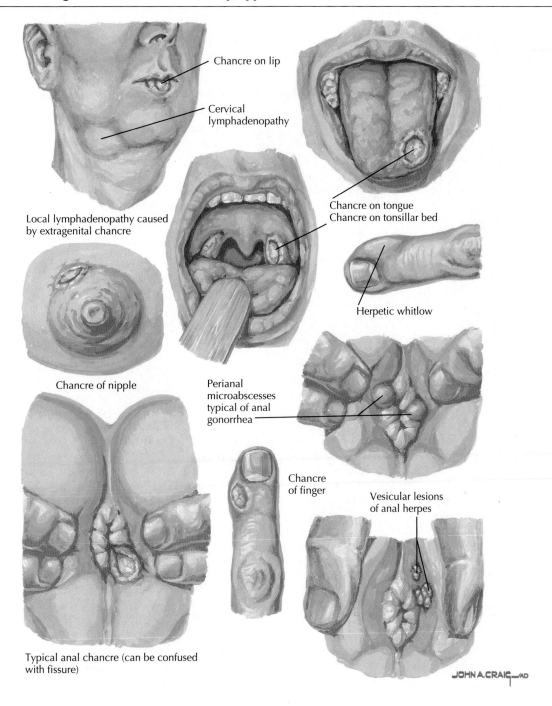

Chancre on lip

Cervical lymphadenopathy

Local lymphadenopathy caused by extragenital chancre

Chancre on tongue
Chancre on tonsillar bed

Herpetic whitlow

Chancre of nipple

Perianal microabscesses typical of anal gonorrhea

Chancre of finger

Vesicular lesions of anal herpes

Typical anal chancre (can be confused with fissure)

JOHN A. CRAIG—AD

ing on the particular presentation. Late syphilis also has a broad differential diagnosis, but in current practice, the usual problems are limited to neurologic diseases. CNS syphilis is a common question in elderly people with abnormal syphilis serology and abnormal CNS function, and the most extensive workup may not provide definitive answers because of the lack of sensitivity of many of the CSF tests for neurosyphilis.

Diagnostic Approach

There are two principal diagnostic tests: the dark-field examination, by which motile spirochetes may be seen in lesions from primary syphilis; and serology, by which various antibodies are detected. In many centers, it also is possible to obtain polymerase chain reaction molecular amplification tests for *T. pallidum*. Dark-field examination

Figure 113-3 Secondary Syphilis.

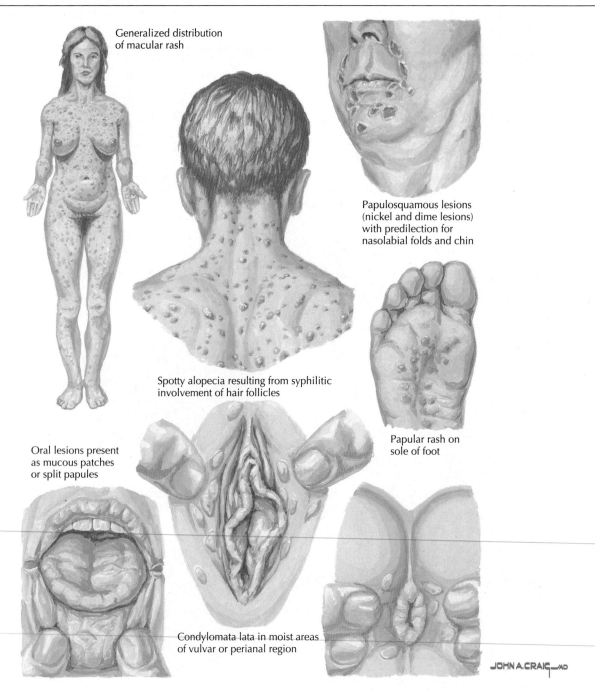

Generalized distribution of macular rash

Papulosquamous lesions (nickel and dime lesions) with predilection for nasolabial folds and chin

Spotty alopecia resulting from syphilitic involvement of hair follicles

Papular rash on sole of foot

Oral lesions present as mucous patches or split papules

Condylomata lata in moist areas of vulvar or perianal region

JOHN A.CRAIG—AD

requires a special microscope and is used less frequently than in earlier times. A mail-in variation that uses fluorescent antibodies to detect *T. pallidum* on slides has not been widely deployed.

Serologic tests are of two general types: those that detect nonspecific antibodies against diphosphatidyl glycerol, a normal tissue component, and those that detect specific antibodies against *T. pallidum*. Nonspecific tests include the VDRL and rapid plasma reagin (RPR) test. These tests are inexpensive and easy to use; the levels of antibodies detected rise in acute disease and fall after suc-

cessful treatment. Presumably, antibodies rise in syphilis because the spirochete binds host diphosphatidyl glycerol, increasing its immunogenicity. Reasons for false-positive test results include other infections and autoimmune diseases; in the latter, the test results are positive chronically (more than 6 months). Old age is another cause of a chronic false-positive VDRL test result, and a positive test result in a patient older than 80 years should ordinarily be ignored.

Specific tests include the fluorescent treponemal antibody absorbed (FTA-ABS) and the microhemagglutination against *T. pallidum* test. A variation on this test now widely used is the *T. pallidum* particle agglutination (TPPA) test. These tests are reported without titration, and the result is positive or negative. Once this antibody appears, it usually persists for life; thus, a positive test indicates present or prior infection with *T. pallidum*. There are few false-positive results, but because some studies showed that 1% of persons without any risks for sexually transmitted diseases had a positive FTA-ABS test result, these tests are not used as screening tests. These tests are not useful for following response to therapy.

In primary syphilis, the VDRL or RPR test results are positive in about 80% of patients, and the specific treponemal test results are positive in slightly more (about 85%). All test results are positive in blood in patients with secondary syphilis, and the treponemal test results remain positive in almost all patients with late syphilis. The nonspecific test results may be negative in some patients with late syphilis; therefore, a negative blood RPR or VDRL does not rule out late syphilis.

A diagnostic dilemma may occur in patients with possible neurosyphilis. A positive CSF VDRL test result in the absence of a traumatic tap is specific for neurosyphilis, but a negative test result does not rule out the diagnosis because as few as 30% to 40% of patients have a positive CSF VDRL test result. The CSF FTA-ABS appears to be more sensitive than the VDRL, but there are worries that this may reflect passive transfer from blood. Cells or protein may be normal in CSF of patients with neurosyphilis. Some experts use a negative CSF FTA-ABS test to help rule out syphilis of the CNS.

Management and Therapy

The first principle of management is to make a diagnosis, which requires consideration of syphilis in young or old persons with an ulcerative lesion, rash and adenopathy, unexplained stroke, or unexplained neurologic disease, among other syndromes. Assessment of risk is enhanced by a knowledgeable sexual history. In practice, a very common problem is how to diagnose and treat patients with nonspecific neurologic findings and a positive VDRL or TPPA test result and patients with positive serologic studies but no evidence of clinical syphilis. Careful examination and history, and examination of CSF, are helpful in management of problem cases.

Optimum Treatment

T. pallidum is sensitive to many antibiotics, and until recently there has been no evidence for antimicrobial resistance. In recent years, however, there have been reports of failure of therapy with azithromycin and DNA sequence evidence from *T. pallidum* recovered from patients of ribosomal resistance to azithromycin. Standard therapy of early syphilis is one intramuscular injection of 2.4 MU of benzathine penicillin; some experts give two injections a week apart. Alternatively, ceftriaxone, 1 g intramuscularly or intravenously daily for 8 to 10 days, may be given, although this is not completely safe in patients with penicillin allergy. Doxycycline, 100 mg orally twice daily for 14 days, is an acceptable substitute in patients who cannot tolerate penicillin or ceftriaxone. Use of azithromycin for treatment of early syphilis is discouraged based on the reports of failure, and of genetic evidence for resistance, even though there are reports of clinical trials showing that single-dose azithromycin may be very effective in treatment of early syphilis. Latent or late syphilis is treated with three intramuscular injections of 2.4 MU benzathine penicillin at weekly intervals.

If there is evidence of symptomatic neurosyphilis, most experts advocate intravenous aqueous crystalline penicillin G, 4 MU every 4 hours for at least 10 days, because benzathine penicillin provides low serum levels and undetectable CSF levels of penicillin. Similar considerations apply to patients with HIV who also have any type of neurosyphilis, including asymptomatic neurosyphilis, based on anecdotal evidence of poor response and persistent *T. pallidum* in CSF after benzathine penicillin therapy. There is good evidence that patients with early syphilis who are HIV negative are cured after benzathine therapy, even though one third have abnormal CSF. For this reason, HIV-negative patients with early syphilis ordinarily do not require a lumbar puncture (LP) to examine CSF. In patients with both syphilis and HIV infection, however, an LP may be wise, especially if the CD4 count is less than 350 or the RPR or VDRL titer is at least 1 : 32 because these are strong predictors of neurosyphilis. In patients allergic to penicillin, referral to experts for desensitization to penicillin is recommended because no other therapy has been proved efficacious.

Patients treated for syphilis should be observed at 3-month intervals for 6 months and then at 6-month intervals to complete a second year. In HIV infection, follow-up should be at 3-month intervals during the first year. VDRL or RPR titers decrease at least fourfold if therapy was successful and the patient did not reacquire infection. If titers persist unchanged or fall and then rise at least fourfold, retreatment should be given and CSF should be examined if not done previously. Some patients, especially those with latent or late disease, may continue to have persistently positive VDRL test results in low titer for years, unresponsive to repeated therapy. All infections should be reported to the public health authorities so that partners can be evaluated and treated.

Avoiding Treatment Errors

The only problems might come when prescribing Bicillin, which is a long-acting form of benzathine penicillin G. Other preparations containing shorter-acting penicillins have similar names; check to be sure Bicillin is used and that it contains only benzathine penicillin G.

Future Directions

Prevention requires adoption of better sexual behaviors by the at-risk public, including condom use, and better coordination between private and public medicine. Prevention campaigns focused on the highest risk groups, including MSM and African Americans from disadvantaged socioeconomic backgrounds, hope to essentially eliminate syphilis in this country, but eradication will require a vaccine to be effective. A vaccine may be possible in the distant future.

Additional Resources

Holmes KK: Azithromycin versus penicillin G benzathine for early syphilis. N Engl J Med 353(12):1291-1293, 2005.

The author presents a short discussion of the pros and cons of using azithromycin in therapy of early syphilis, concluding with a note of caution.

Sparling PF, Swartz, MN, Musher DM, Healy BP: Clinical manifestations of syphilis. In Holmes KK, Sparling PF, et al (eds): Sexually Transmitted Diseases, 4th ed. New York, McGraw-Hill, 2007 (in press).

This is the best current summary of syphilis in both HIV-negative and HIV-positive patients.

EVIDENCE

1. Workowski KA, Berman SM; Centers for Disease Control and Prevention: Sexually transmitted diseases treatment guidelines, 2006. MMWR Recomm Rep 55(RR-11):1-94, 2006.

    These are the latest guidelines from the CDC, available also at http://www.cdc.gov/std/treatment/default.htm.
2. Marra CM, Maxwell CL, Smith SL, et al: Cerebrospinal fluid abnormalities in patients with syphilis: Association with clinical and laboratory features. J Infect Dis 189(3):369-376, 2004.

    The authors present an analysis of the CSF findings that best predict who has neurosyphilis.

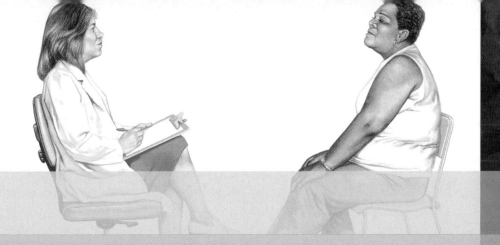

Disorders of the Reproductive System

M. Cristina Muñoz

Contraception

Introduction

Until recently, lack of access to effective methods of birth control meant that family planning was not feasible for most women. In the past 50 years, the development and dissemination of new methods of contraception—most notably the contraceptive pill—have led to a multiplicity of societal changes, including growing acceptance of premarital sexual relations, greater female participation in education and employment, and demographic changes like later age of marriage and smaller family size.

In family planning programs, contraceptives are effective tools. For example, contraception contributed to a decline in total fertility in Kenya from 8 births per woman in the late 1970s to less than 5 in 1998. Contraceptive use among reproductive-age women varies from 3.9% in Niger to 84% in China, with wide variations in rates of use of each method. China, with about one fifth of the world's population and one third of users, has an important impact on summary statistics, strongly affecting the prevalence of data on intrauterine devices (IUDs) and permanent sterilization, which are less commonly used in most countries (Table 114-1).

Benefits

Medical Benefits of Contraception

Beyond the social and economic benefits accrued by having a real choice of whether or when to parent, contraception offers direct medical benefits (attained by preventing pregnancy) and noncontraceptive benefits (beneficial side effects). Health benefits of pregnancy prevention are shown in Box 114-1.

Effectiveness and Failure Rates

Each contraceptive method has a risk for failure, resulting in pregnancy for some users. Contraceptives are most effective when directions for use are followed exactly, every time they are needed, for as long as pregnancy prevention is desired. In reality, most contraceptive failures are related to incorrect use or cessation of use of one contraceptive method before implementing a new method. Methods that do not require any work on the part of the user after the initial choice (IUDs, implants, sterilization) have use effectiveness that is similar to theoretical effectiveness. Providers can help guide patients to suitable methods, reassure patients about risks, instruct in proper use, and give anticipatory guidance about side effects. Nurse prac-

titioners, family planning clinic staff, and peer counselors may be able to spend more time with a patient than physicians and can be very effective, especially when counseling about behavioral issues. Table 114-2 demonstrates the effectiveness of most common methods.

Contraceptive Methods

Behavioral Methods

Abstinence is widely promoted as a method that is 100% effective. However, the use effectiveness of intended abstinence is poorly documented. Some experts have promoted alternate modes of sexual expression (masturbation or "outercourse") to reduce coital sexual behavior.

Periodic abstinence, or natural family planning (NFP), involves timing intercourse to avoid coitus during the "fertile window" when sex would likely result in conception. Studies have shown that intercourse up to 6 days before ovulation can result in pregnancy, with almost no conceptions from intercourse after the date of ovulation. Importantly, the timing of ovulation is more variable than previously thought. Modern NFP techniques include observation of physiologic changes associated with ovulation (temperature or cervical mucus changes). NFP is also used by couples desiring pregnancy to identify the most

Table 114-1 World Contraceptive Use, 2005

Method	Users (%)
Any method	60.5
Female sterilization	20.5
Male sterilization	3.4
Pill	7.5
Injectable or implant	4.8
Intrauterine device (IUD)	13.6
Male condom	4.8
Vaginal barrier methods	0.4
Rhythm	2.9
Withdrawal	3.1
Other methods	0.6

From United Nations, Department of Economic and Social Affairs, Population Division: World Contraceptive Use 2005.

Box 114-1 Health Benefits of Pregnancy Prevention

Help space births, resulting in:
- Lower rates of infant and child mortality
- Decreased risk for anemia in mothers
- More time to breast-feed, resulting in improved infant health and survival

Prevent high-risk pregnancies among:
- Very young adolescents
- Women in their late 30s and 40s
- Women who have had many births
- Women with preexisting medical conditions

Prevent unsafe abortion resulting from unwanted pregnancies, thereby reducing:
- Maternal deaths
- Ill health
- Infertility

Prevent maternal and infant deaths and ill health resulting from unwanted births

Facilitate screening for sexually transmitted infections and other health concerns

Noncontraceptive Benefits

Oral contraceptive pills:
- Protect against ovarian and endometrial cancers
- Decrease benign breast disease
- Decrease pelvic inflammatory disease requiring hospitalization
- Decrease ectopic pregnancy
- Treat menstruation-related iron-deficiency anemia
- Treat dysmenorrhea
- Treat menorrhagia
- Treat acne and hirsutism
- Decrease endometriosis pain

Nonhormonal intrauterine devices:
- Decrease endometrial cancer

Progestin-containing intrauterine devices:
- Decrease menorrhagia and anemia
- Prevent endometrial hyperplasia from tamoxifen or estrogen replacement
- Decrease hysterectomies for menstrual problems

Barrier methods:
- Prevent many sexually transmitted diseases

Data from Singh S, Darroch JE, Vlasoff M, Nadeau J: Adding it Up: The Benefits of Investing in Sexual and Reproductive Health Care. Washington DC and New York, The Alan Guttmacher Institute and UNFPA, 2004; Dayal M, Barnhart KT: Noncontraceptive benefits and therapeutic uses of the oral contraceptive pill. Semin Reprod Med 19(4):295-303, 2001; and Hubacher D, Grimes DA: Noncontraceptive health benefits of intrauterine devices: A systematic review. Obstet Gynecol Surv 57(2):120-128, 2002.

fertile days of the cycle. Withdrawal of the penis from the vagina before ejaculation has similar failure rates, with both typical and perfect use, as NFP.

Barrier Methods

Barrier methods, such as the male condom, female condom, diaphragm, and cervical cap, all work by preventing sperm from reaching the egg. With consistent, correct use they are quite effective, especially in mature, motivated individuals. Latex condoms are extremely important in fighting the spread of HIV infection as well as other sexually transmitted infections (STIs). Female condoms are expensive, but do not require the male partner to cooperate with putting on a condom. They also protect against infection. The diaphragm and cervical cap also reduce STIs, even though they do not prevent semen from coming in contact with the vagina.

Spermicides

Spermicides may be included in condoms, and contraceptive vaginal inserts, gels, film, and foams are also available. Spermicides are directly toxic to sperm. Current spermicides do not kill HIV and may increase the rate of HIV infection.

Hormonal Methods

Hormonal methods include progestin-only methods (implants, IUDs, injections, and minipills) and estrogen-progestin combinations (oral contraceptives, the patch, the vaginal ring, and injections) Progestin-only methods prevent pregnancy by thickening cervical mucus, thinning the uterine lining, and inhibiting ovulation, and include some of the most effective methods available. Emergency (postcoital) contraceptives may inhibit sperm transport or inhibit implantation of a fertilized egg.

Combination oral contraceptive pills (OCPs) have been available since the 1960s, but the dose and chemical composition have changed greatly since then. Combining estrogen and progestin increases efficacy when compared with the same dose of progestin alone, and allows a predictable withdrawal bleed (mimicking a menstrual period) every 28 days. Most current OCPs contain ethinyl estradiol, with doses ranging from 20 to 35 μg/day. There are several different progestins, with varying potencies and side effects. OCPs are used continuously (without a placebo

Table 114-2 Percentage of Women Experiencing an Unintended Pregnancy during the First Year of Typical Use and the First Year of Perfect Use of Contraception and the Percentage Continuing Use at the End of the First Year

Method	Women Experiencing an Unintended Pregnancy within the First Year of Use (%)		Women Continuing Use after 1 Year (%)
	Typical Use	Perfect Use	
No method	85	85	
Spermicides	29	18	
Withdrawal	27	4	42
Fertility awareness-based methods	25		43
Standard days method		5	51
Two-day method		4	
Ovulation method		3	
Sponge			
Parous women	32	20	46
Nulliparous women	16	9	57
Diaphragm	16	6	57
Condom			
Female (Reality)	21	5	49
Male	15	2	53
Combined pill and minipill	8	0.3	68
Evra patch	8	0.3	68
NuvaRing	8	0.3	68
Depo-Provera	3	0.3	56
Intrauterine device			
ParaGard (copper T)	0.8	0.6	78
Mirena (LNG-IUS)	0.2	0.2	80
Implanon	0.05	0.05	84
Female sterilization	0.5	0.5	100
Male sterilization	0.15	0.10	100

Note: Although not available in the United States, the Norplant and Norplant-2 have efficacy similar to Implanon, and the combined estrogen-progestin injection has similar efficacy to Depo-Provera.
LNG, levonorgestrel; IUS, intrauterine system (an IUD plus a drug delivery device).
From Trussell J: Contraceptive efficacy. In Hatcher RA, Trussell J, Nelson A, et al (eds): Contraceptive Technology, 19th revised ed. New York, Ardent Media, 2007, Table 27-1.

week) to prevent menstruation-associated illness such as anemia, menorrhagia, premenstrual symptoms, and menstrual exacerbations of migraine, seizures, or sickle cell crisis. Drug manufacturers are now producing extended cycle packs, allowing long-term suppression of menstrual bleeding.

The birth control patch is very similar to a combination OCP in its chemical composition and efficacy. It is applied to the skin once a week for 3 weeks. It is useful to women who have difficulty taking a daily pill. The total amount of drug delivered is higher than the comparable OCP, which may increase thromboembolic risk, but it may also improve efficacy.

The vaginal ring delivers less estrogen and a different progestin than the patch. It is designed to be used for 21 days out of 28 and is well tolerated by users. The amount of drug in the device is adequate to prevent conception for several days after the 21 days it is labeled for, so it can be used for up to 1 month at a time in a continuous cycle.

The combined estrogen-progestin injection is similar in efficacy to the progestin injection but is designed to give better control of bleeding. It is no longer available in the United States.

All contraceptives that contain estrogenic compounds induce hypercoagulability of the blood in a dose-dependent fashion, increasing the risk for deep venous thrombosis, myocardial infarction, and stroke. Thrombophilia including the increased clotting risk associated with diabetes, obesity, elevated serum lipids, and most importantly, smoking, can multiply the risk for cardiovascular events significantly, even with modern low-dose formulations. Hypertension may also be worsened by OCPs containing estrogen. Prolonged use of depo-medroxyprogesterone acetate, a progestin-only method, has been associated with osteopenia.

Intrauterine Devices

IUDs are devices implanted in the uterus to prevent pregnancy. The effectiveness of current devices is comparable to permanent sterilization but is easily reversible with removal of the device. Copper IUDs cause a local intrauterine inflammatory reaction that lyses sperm. IUDs containing progestins deliver a high dose of drug locally to the endometrium, thickening mucus, thinning the endometrial lining, and impairing sperm transport. IUDs have been associated with pelvic infections, such as pelvic inflammatory disease and septic abortion. Although current IUDs are much safer than previous designs, they are still not recommended for women at high risk for pelvic infection.

Permanent Sterilization

Couples who have completed their family size often choose permanent sterilization. Rates are influenced by insurance coverage and by availability of effective long-term methods. Vasectomy is easily performed in an outpatient setting with local anesthetic and is safer and more effective than tubal ligation. Bilateral tubal ligation can be done at cesarean delivery, immediately postpartum through a minilaparotomy incision, or laparoscopically. Risks include regret, especially in the very young and those who begin new relationships, surgical risks, and the risk for method failure (ectopic or intrauterine pregnancy).

Abortion

Abortion is not a primary method of controlling fertility because of its relatively high cost, poor availability, and social, emotional, and moral factors. However, medically supervised abortion, when used as a backup method, is important in reducing maternal morbidity and mortality, especially for women at high risk for pregnancy complications. The safety of the procedure is dependent on gestational age and on system factors such as skilled providers and adequate postabortion care.

Approach to the Patient

In clinical practice, it is common to learn a woman is having regular intercourse, does not want to have a child, and is not doing anything to prevent pregnancy. Reasons for this choice may include lack of access and ambivalence about sexual activity or parenting. Patients may be dissatisfied with available choices because of prior experiences with birth control, real or imagined risks, and side effects of available methods. Among those who do not currently want pregnancy, their goals might be to delay the birth of their first child, space births, or avoid future childbearing. These goals will affect their choice of birth control method. It is important to consider what methods are available regionally and for the patient individually. Some of the most effective and cost-effective methods of contraception, such as implants, IUDs, and permanent sterilization, may have high initial costs that put them out of reach.

Future Directions

Several current contraceptives are nearly 100% effective in preventing pregnancy, but unintended pregnancy is still a global problem because of limited access. Although novel methods of contraception (including male hormonal methods) may be developed in the future, in the next several years, progress will be made by increasing distribution of contraceptives to those who currently have poor access to them. Adherence is also poor for many methods, especially condoms, and research is needed to find the best ways to help women and men to use them consistently. For many women, the greatest risk of intercourse is not pregnancy, it is death from HIV/AIDS. Significant research is now being done on spermicides and microbicides that would be effective against both pregnancy and HIV.

Additional Resources

ACOG Committee on Practice Bulletins-Gynecology: ACOG practice bulletin. No. 73: Use of hormonal contraception in women with coexisting medical conditions. Obstet Gynecol 107(6):1453-1472, 2006.
   This paper describes medical conditions in which estrogen-progestin combination oral contraceptives or progestin-only pills can be safely used as well as their contraindications.
Dickey RP: Managing Contraceptive Pill Patients, 12th ed. Durant, OK, Essential Medical Information Systems, 2004.
   This book helps with rational explanations of the different pills available, different potencies and side effects of progestins, and detailed information on managing side effects. It also explains the use of extended-cycle pill regimens.
Hatcher RA, Zieman M, Cwiak C, et al: A Pocket Guide to Managing Contraception, 8th ed. Tiger, GA, The Bridging the Gap Foundation, 2005.
   The WHO Medical Eligibility Criteria for Starting Contraceptive Methods is included as an appendix, and it explains patient selection and medical contraindications for each method. The full text is available online as a free downloadable PDF at http://www.managingcontraception.com/cmanager/publish/.

EVIDENCE

1. Dayal M, Barnhart KT: Noncontraceptive benefits and therapeutic uses of the oral contraceptive pill. Semin Reprod Med 19(4):295-303, 2001.
   This article summarizes a number of medical benefits that accrue to pill users, and the use of the pill as therapy for different medical conditions.
2. Department of Economic and Social Affairs, Population Division: World Contraceptive Use 2005. Available at: http://www.un.org/esa/population/publications/contraceptive2005/WCU2005.htm. Accessed September 24, 2007.
   This comprehensive dataset on contraceptive use by reproductive-age women is downloadable as an Excel spreadsheet or as a wall chart. Differences in use by region and level of economic development are listed.
3. Edelman AB, Gallo MF, Jensen JT, et al: Continuous or extended cycle versus cyclic use of combined oral contraceptives for contraception. Cochrane Database Syst Rev 3:CD004695, 2005.
   This review of several studies comparing traditional oral contraceptive dosing to regimens using active pills for greater than 28 days showed

similar efficacy, safety, and patient satisfaction. Menstrual symptoms and bleeding patterns were better in the longer cycle regimens.

4. French R, Van Vliet H, Cowan F, et al: Hormonally impregnated intrauterine systems (IUSs) versus other forms of reversible contraceptives as effective methods of preventing pregnancy. Cochrane Database Syst Rev 3:CD001776, 2004.

   This meta-analysis showed that users of the levonorgestrel intrauterine system, IUDs containing more than 250 mm² of copper, and Norplant-2 had similar (very low) rates of pregnancy, but different effects on menstrual bleeding patterns.

5. Gallo MF, Grimes DA, Schulz KF: Skin patch and vaginal ring versus combined oral contraceptives for contraception. Cochrane Database Syst Rev 1:CD003552, 2003.

   This study found three randomized controlled trials comparing the combination contraceptive patch to a combination oral contraceptive, showing similar efficacy but more breast tenderness with the patch. Adequate trials comparing the ring to the pill were not found.

6. Gallo MF, Grimes DA, Schulz KF, et al: Combination injectable contraceptives for contraception. Cochrane Database Syst Rev 3: CD004568, 2005.

   In a meta-analysis, combination injectable contraceptives were associated with more regular bleeding patterns than progestin-only injectables were.

7. Hubacher D, Grimes DA: Noncontraceptive health benefits of intrauterine devices: A systematic review. Obstet Gynecol Surv 57(2):120-128, 2002.

   This review documents a large number of gynecologic conditions that are ameliorated by intrauterine devices.

8. Kulier R, Helmerhorst FM, O'Brien P, et al: Copper containing, framed intra-uterine devices for contraception. Cochrane Database Syst Rev 3:CD005347, 2006.

   This analysis of multiple studies showed that those containing a higher dose of copper are more effective in preventing pregnancy over a longer time period.

9. Nardin JM, Kulier R, Boulvain M: Techniques for the interruption of tubal patency for female sterilisation. Cochrane Database Syst Rev 4:CD003034, 2002.

   A review of nine trials found that all techniques studied (e.g., clips, rings, cautery, resection) effectively prevent pregnancy, although there were minor differences in morbidity with different techniques.

10. Singh S, Darroch JE, Vlasoff M, Nadeau J: Adding it Up: The Benefits of Investing in Sexual and Reproductive Health Care. Washington, DC and New York, The Alan Guttmacher Institute and UNFPA, 2004.

    This document describes in economic, medical, and social terms the recognized and potential benefits of family planning services worldwide, including contraception, maternal health services, and prevention and treatment of sexually transmitted infection.

11. Trussell J: Contraceptive efficacy. In Hatcher RA, Trussell J, Nelson A, et al (eds): Contraceptive Technology, 19th revised ed. New York, Ardent Media, 2007, Table 27-1.

    This chapter includes very detailed information about each method of contraception, including information for counseling patients. It also covers related health matters such as prevention of sexually transmitted infection, sexuality, and issues related to the study of family planning and population.

12. Wilcox AJ, Dunson D, Baird DD: The timing of the "fertile window" in the menstrual cycle: Day specific estimates from a prospective study. BMJ 321(7271):1259-1262, 2000; and Wilcox AJ, Weinberg CR, Baird DD: Timing of sexual intercourse in relation to ovulation: Effects on the probability of conception, survival of the pregnancy and sex of the baby. N Engl J Med 333(23):1517-1521, 1995.

    In a large cohort, a study showed that pregnancy could result from intercourse up to 6 days before ovulation, but not after ovulation, and the day of ovulation was more variable than previously believed.

M. Cristina Muñoz

Common Problems in Pregnancy

Introduction

Pregnancy is a time of extraordinary maternal adaptation. Some symptoms of pregnancy, such as nausea, breast tenderness, urinary frequency, low back pain, and fatigue, occur almost universally. These so-called minor discomforts of pregnancy cause significant morbidity. Benign conditions such as constipation, hemorrhoids, nasal congestion, peripheral swelling, and carpal tunnel syndrome are very common in pregnancy but are treated identically as in nonpregnant individuals. Common problems encountered in pregnancy are presented in Table 115-1, followed by a discussion of the use of medications in pregnancy.

Management and Therapy

Optimum Treatment

Rational Use of Medications in Pregnancy

Prescribing medications for pregnant women is difficult because the provider must tread a narrow path between excessively restrictive practices that deny women needed therapies and a casual approach that assumes most pregnancies will turn out fine. The following are general guidelines for treatment of women with routine pregnancies. Women with significant preexisting medical illness or complicated pregnancies should be referred to a perinatologist. It is never a mistake to call a specialist for management advice. Informal consultations give the consultant an opportunity to intervene early and to identify those cases where complex management and transfer of care are necessary.

Plan for Pregnancy

Ideally, the planning for use of medications in pregnancy begins before conception, especially in women with chronic illness. For conditions such as phenylketonuria, diabetes mellitus, hypertension, smoking, and obesity, the desire for a healthy baby may spur marked improvements in lifestyle and disease management. In these conditions, preconceptional improvements in maternal health status decrease problems such as miscarriage, fetal malformations, gesta-tional hypertension, or delivery complications. In diseases such as hypertension or diabetes mellitus, for which there are several effective therapies but some are believed to be safer in pregnancy, it is best to switch therapies before conception is attempted.

Expect the Unplanned Pregnancy

In all women of reproductive age, it is worthwhile to explore plans and desires for future pregnancy. In the United States, more than half of all pregnancies are unplanned. A realistic assessment of the risk for pregnancy, including sexual activity, contraceptive choice, and correct use of the method chosen, is helpful for those who do not desire pregnancy. Women who do not expect to become pregnant may have delayed entry into prenatal care and prolonged exposure to medications that may be harmful in pregnancy. Alternatively, women may discontinue medications in early pregnancy in hopes of protecting their child, although in some cases, this can be harmful to both the woman and the developing embryo. Generally, however, a multivitamin containing 400 µg of folic acid is recommended for reproductive-age women, to decrease neural tube defects that occur before recognition of pregnancy.

Current Prescriptions, Over-the-Counter Drugs, Herbs, and Drugs of Abuse

Pregnant women often assume that drugs they used before pregnancy, especially those sold over the counter, are safe

Table 115-1 Common Pregnancy Problems

Problem	Etiology, Pathogenesis	Clinical Presentation, Differential Diagnosis, Diagnostic Approach	Serious Conditions to Consider	Management and Therapy
First-trimester vaginal bleeding	Cervical bleeding: inflammation or polyp Uterine bleeding: implantation of zygote, threatened pregnancy loss	Ultrasound shows gestational sac, embryo, cardiac activity. Findings should correlate with quantitative β-hCG and gestational age In early gestation, β-hCG doubles every 48-72 hours; decreasing or plateauing level indicates abnormal pregnancy	Threatened, incomplete, or completed spontaneous abortion, ectopic pregnancy, ruptured hemorrhagic ovarian cyst. Pain and bleeding in early pregnancy equals ectopic till proven otherwise	Threatened abortion: observation; many continue with no sequelae Incomplete or inevitable abortion: vacuum aspiration Missed abortion or blighted ovum; expectant management, misoprostol, or aspiration. Ectopic: methotrexate or surgery
Third-trimester vaginal bleeding	Hemorrhage from placental separation Bloody show resulting from cervical changes in labor	Avoid digital examination of cervix if placental location is unknown. Doppler ultrasound may show vessels	Placenta previa, abruptio placentae, vasa previa, uterine rupture	For hemorrhage threatening mother or fetus, cesarean section, transfusion
Contractions	Uterine muscular activity	Braxton-Hicks contractions are painless and irregular; may increase with dehydration	Contractions leading to cervical change (often with bloody show or rupture of membranes) define labor.	For preterm labor, steroids given before birth improve neonatal outcome. Long-term tocolysis is ineffective, but short-term tocolytics may allow steroids to work
Rapid heartbeat	Increased cardiac output	Sustained tachycardia is usually of supraventricular origin	High-risk conditions include Marfan syndrome, aortic stenosis, pulmonary hypertension, and New York Heart Association class III or IV, regardless of etiology. Hyperthyroidism may cause tachycardia, palpitations, anxiety, and thyroid storm	Reassurance, caffeine restriction, and change in activities if transient or mild. Cardiology evaluation (electrocardiogram, Holter monitor) if severe/persistent. Abortion for cases with high risk for maternal mortality Treat hyperthyroidism with β blockers, propylthiouracil
Nausea and vomiting of pregnancy	Central effect of β-hCG, estrogen, vitamin side effect	Begins by 10 weeks, not accompanied by fever, headache, abdominal pain or jaundice	Hyperemesis gravidarum: weight loss >5% of prepregnancy weight, large ketonuria. May occur in multiple gestation or molar pregnancy	Frequent small, bland, or salty meals, high in carbohydrate, low in fat. Ginger or peppermint. Avoid rapid position changes, odors, iron pills. Acupuncture or acupressure wrist bands. Vitamin B₆, doxylamine, phenothiazines Severe vomiting: metoclopramide, ondansetron, droperidol, or corticosteroids. IV fluids, hyperalimentation as needed

Continued

Table 115-1 Common Pregnancy Problems—cont'd

Problem	Etiology, Pathogenesis	Clinical Presentation, Differential Diagnosis, Diagnostic Approach	Serious Conditions to Consider	Management and Therapy
Indigestion (heartburn, reflux)	Progesterone relaxes lower esophageal sphincter	Worse after meals, improved by keeping head elevated	HELLP (hypertension, elevated liver enzymes, low platelets) syndrome: right upper quadrant pain, nausea, vomiting from liver involvement, or fatty liver	Small meals, elevate head of bed. Antacids, H₂-receptor antagonists, metoclopramide, proton pump inhibitors
Dyspnea of pregnancy	Progesterone increases respiratory rate Large uterus restricts diaphragmatic excursion	Worse in late pregnancy, better with sitting	Cough or fever may indicate asthma or infection. Severe symptoms, blood-tinged sputum, or acute change may indicate pulmonary embolus	Reassurance. Asthma treatment is similar to nonpregnant; adequate treatment prevents intrauterine growth retardation, death
Fatigue, syncope	Decreased blood pressure. Hormonal effects	Worst in first and third trimesters. Screen for anemia if persistent	Hypovolemic shock (ectopic pregnancy, ruptured hemorrhagic cyst)	Arise slowly, remain well hydrated
Anemia	Volume expansion, iron use by fetus	Detected on routine screening	Screen for thalassemia or sickle cell disease in high-risk populations	Iron-containing foods, oral iron supplements
Gestational diabetes	Secretion of diabetogenic hormones by placenta	Detected on routine screening	Pregestational diabetes	Diet, glucose monitoring, moderate exercise, insulin when needed
Gestational hypertension	Preeclampsia is likely caused by placental growth factors	Measurement of blood pressure and urine protein at prenatal visits	Chronic hypertension, preeclampsia, eclampsia	Antihypertensives if severely elevated pressures; delivery is treatment for preeclampsia
Headache	Hormonal (vasodilation), postural	Headache frequency (including migraine) may increase or decrease in pregnancy	Preeclampsia: headache accompanied by hypertension, proteinuria	Rest, massage, postural change, acetaminophen, narcotics. (Avoid nonsteroidal anti-inflammatory drugs due to risk for bleeding and closure of fetal patent ductus arteriosus.)
Back pain	Mechanical strain	Worse in late pregnancy	Costovertebral angle tenderness may indicate pyelonephritis. Preterm contractions may be felt in low back	Erect posture, avoid high heels, use elastic support for uterus, acetaminophen
Abdominal or pelvic pain	Mechanical (stretching of round ligament and other structures)	Common with walking or arising	Ectopic pregnancy, preterm or term labor. Pain of appendicitis is noted in abnormal location (higher) in pregnancy	Reassurance, analgesics
Varicose veins, dependent edema	Expanded blood volume; uterus impedes venous return	Worse in late pregnancy	Deep venous thrombosis: unilateral pain, redness, swelling. Nerve compression may cause weakness or numbness in lower extremities	Elastic stockings, or pad to compress vulvar varices, rest in horizontal position

Table 115-1 Common Pregnancy Problems—cont'd

Problem	Etiology, Pathogenesis	Clinical Presentation, Differential Diagnosis, Diagnostic Approach	Serious Conditions to Consider	Management and Therapy
Leg cramps Respiratory infections	Cause unknown Viral or bacterial infection, may be more symptomatic in pregnancy	Worse in late pregnancy Incidence similar to nonpregnant state	Deep venous thrombosis Suspect pulmonary embolus if patient has been sedentary or symptoms are severe	Magnesium supplements May use acetaminophen, antihistamines, guaifenesin, saline nasal spray/neti pot. Pneumonia in pregnancy requires hospitalization
Urinary tract infections	Stasis caused by increased glomerular filtration rate, compression of ureters, relaxed smooth muscle tone, glycosuria	Frequent urination is normal in first and third trimester. Asymptomatic bacteriuria is common in pregnancy, diagnosed by routine urinalysis	Pyelonephritis with costovertebral angle tenderness and fever	Penicillins, cephalosporins are safe. Trimethoprim-sulfamethoxazole and nitrofurantoin are effective but may cause neonatal jaundice. Pyelonephritis in pregnancy requires hospitalization
Vaginal discharge	Estrogen increases physiologic discharge. Bacterial vaginosis is an alteration of vaginal flora	Vaginal pH, saline, and KOH prep and whiff test diagnose *Candida*, *Trichomonas*, and bacterial vaginosis	Amniotic fluid leakage may cause watery discharge	Topical azole antifungals for *Candida*. Metronidazole treats bacterial vaginosis or *Trichomonas*; some providers defer treatment until second trimester. Bacterial vaginosis increases risk for preterm rupture of membranes, preterm labor and delivery, and amnionitis
Dental problems	Edema and hyperemia of gums lead to gingivitis	Dental examination and radiography (with abdomen shielded) should be done as early as possible, so preventive care can begin	Periodontal infection may cause preterm labor	Dental cleaning, extractions, and other needed treatments may be done in pregnancy
Dermatologic problems	Hormonal changes cause hyperpigmentation, skin tags. Abdominal distention causes striae	Common dermatoses of pregnancy include pruritic urticarial papules and plaques of pregnancy, which cause an abdominal rash with intense itching and prurigo of pregnancy (itchy papules on extremities). Check liver function tests with itching to rule out cholestasis	Herpes gestationis (large blisters) may increase risk for premature delivery	Most changes improve after delivery. Antihistamines or topical fluorinated steroids are used for pruritus
Anxiety, depression	Multifactorial, including adjustment to new roles and body changes, hormonal influences, and social factors	Substance abuse is common in pregnancy; diagnosis often missed in nonminority patients. Domestic violence increases in pregnancy, in all social classes	Previous mood disorder or mental illness can recur in pregnancy or postpartum, with risk for suicide or infanticide	Reassurance and social support are needed in each pregnancy. Antidepressant, antipsychotic, or anxiolytic medications are used for mental illness that cannot be controlled without drugs. Victims of abuse may initially decline help, but later accept help from battered women's shelter, hospital, or police

β-hCG, β-Human chorionic gonadotropin.

in pregnancy. These often contain aspirin, nonsteroidal anti-inflammatory drugs, or other medications that are contraindicated in pregnancy. Combination medications, such as antihistamine-decongestant combinations, are also problematic because many prescribers are unaware of the exact components of these drugs. Popular cold remedies may contain six or more drugs, when a patient's symptoms could be treated with just one or two. Herbal preparations are also a concern because there is a dearth of research on their risks in pregnancy, and physicians may be unaware of the available data. Other drugs to consider include alcohol and illicit drugs, which have teratogenic or toxic effects. For many illnesses and discomforts of pregnancy, nonpharmacologic treatments are effective. These include foods, reassurance, social support, rest periods or alteration in working conditions, postural changes, local heat or ice, and use of braces or supports.

Use Minimum Effective Dose

Physiologic changes of pregnancy include increased plasma volume and cardiac output, increased glomerular filtration rate, decreased protein binding, delayed gastric transit, altered hepatic metabolism, and other changes that affect pharmacokinetics. These may require adjustment of drug doses. Use the minimum dose that works for the patient.

Stop Ineffective Drugs Rapidly

Prenatal visits in the first trimester are usually scheduled at 4- to 6-week intervals. When a drug is prescribed, the effectiveness of the therapy is often known in just a few days, but patients may obediently use an ineffective medication until the next scheduled visit. Rapid follow-up after starting a new medication is preferred, whether it is accomplished by a telephone call or an office visit.

Know a Few Drugs Well

Doctors who regularly care for pregnant women should have a personal formulary of treatments that they are comfortable prescribing. It is reasonable to start with a few drugs (e.g., acetaminophen, doxylamine, vitamin B_6, penicillins, cephalosporins, folic acid, and levothyroxine) and add only those drugs for which the literature shows effectiveness and not harm. The best approach favors drugs for which evidence has accumulated over years, rather than new drugs that have not previously been used in pregnancy.

Look Up What You Don't Know

There are excellent reference texts about drug risks in pregnancy and lactation as well as online resources such as REPROTOX. The Organization of Teratology Information Services and its member organizations in several states offer free information to providers and patients as well as informative fact sheets that can be printed directly from the Internet.

Well-known teratogens include alcohol; radioactive iodine; lithium; mercury; thalidomide; isotretinoin; angiotensin-converting enzyme inhibitors; coumarins; misoprostol; methimazole; penicillamine; tetracyclines; sex steroids, such as diethylstilbestrol and androgens; antiepileptic drugs, such as phenytoin, trimethadione, carbamazepine, and valproic acid; and many antineoplastic agents.

Although the developing fetus is at risk for teratogenesis, a policy of complete abstinence from drugs is dangerous. For certain diseases, the benefits of treatment may significantly outweigh the risks. The benefits may accrue to the fetus (e.g., treatment of severe maternal fever with antipyretics), to the mother (e.g., treatment of nausea and vomiting of pregnancy), or to both (e.g., treatment of asthma, varicella, thyroid disease, and HIV/AIDS). The risks of a drug should be compared to the risks of other possible disease treatments, the risks of untreated maternal disease, and the risks of preterm delivery to avoid fetal exposure to the drug. Even drugs that are known to cause fetal harm (antiepileptics, antineoplastic agents, anticoagulants) may be used in conditions in which risks of nonuse are extreme.

Avoiding Treatment Errors

Because hypertension is common, women with hypertensive disorders of pregnancy are occasionally misdiagnosed and treated with standard antihypertensive therapies. A pregnant or newly postpartum woman may present to an emergency room at night, away from her usual site of care, because of symptoms that indicate severe preeclampsia. These include severe headache, visual changes, and epigastric or right upper quadrant pain from liver damage. Other abnormalities in severe preeclampsia include blood pressure of 160/110 mm Hg or higher, oligohydramnios or intrauterine growth restriction, or HELLP (hemolysis, elevated liver enzymes, low platelets) syndrome. Although antihypertensives may be used in the management of preeclampsia, prompt delivery is the most important treatment for women near term and for women developing severe preeclampsia.

Peripartum cardiomyopathy is a rare disease that develops in the last month of pregnancy or within 6 months of delivery, in women with no previous cardiac disease. Initial symptoms include fatigue, chest pain, and shortness of breath. The patient may be tachycardic, with low blood pressure, which may prompt aggressive resuscitation with intravenous fluids. Although young, previously healthy women can usually tolerate rapid volume expansion, women with peripartum cardiomyopathy are in failure when they are diagnosed, and aggressive hydration may cause pulmonary edema and death. Echocardiogram, electrocardiogram, and chest x-ray help to diagnose the condition, which is treated with digoxin, diuretics, sodium restriction, β blockers, and afterload reduction.

Future Directions

Research on pregnant women had long been hampered by the perception that women's symptoms were minor discomforts and by hesitancy to include pregnant women and their fetuses in research trials. The generally good outcomes of pregnancies also contributed to acceptance of traditional methods of care without critical review. The current trend toward evidence-based medicine should help us determine what care is effective and what should be abandoned.

Additional Resources

Briggs GG, Freeman RK, Yaffe SJ: Drugs in Pregnancy and Lactation: A Reference Guide to Fetal and Neonatal Risk, 7th ed. New York, Lippincott Williams & Wilkins, 2005.

This book covers more than 1000 drugs commonly used by pregnant or nursing women, outlining the risks of each drug to the fetus and nursing infant. It is especially useful in determining which drug to choose when there are a number of treatments available.

European Network of Teratology Information Services. Available at: http://www.entis-org.com/. Accessed February 12, 2007.

This website rapidly provides information for providers on drugs that may affect the fetus or breast-feeding infant.

MotheRisk. Available at: http://www.motherisk.org/women/index.jsp. Accessed February 12, 2007.

This website provides online information on teratology and medical treatment during pregnancy for providers and patients.

EVIDENCE

1. Levichek Z, Atanackovic G, Oepkes D, et al: Nausea and vomiting of pregnancy. Evidence-based treatment algorithm. Can Fam Physician 48:267-268, 277, 2002.

   This article describes Motherisk's treatment algorithm, with supporting data on both safety and efficacy. Doxylamine with pyridoxine is a first-line therapy, with other drugs and tests used for refractory cases. The treatment algorithm is also described—"The Management of Nausea and Vomiting of Pregnancy"—and a tutorial is also presented at the Motherisk e-learning center: http://www.motherisk.org/prof/elearning. jsp#2. Accessed February 12, 2007.

2. Nanda K, Peloggia A, Grimes D, et al: Expectant care versus surgical treatment for miscarriage. Cochrane Database Syst Rev 2: CD003518, 2006.

   This meta-analysis found that women randomized to expectant management instead of surgical evacuation had a higher rate of incomplete abortion and a greater chance of unplanned surgery, but a lower risk for infection than women randomized to surgery, when the groups were followed for up to 2 weeks.

3. Roberts D, Dalziel S: Antenatal corticosteroids for accelerating fetal lung maturation for women at risk of preterm birth. Cochrane Database Syst Rev 3:CD004454, 2006.

   In 21 studies testing corticosteroids given to mothers at risk for preterm delivery, including studies of preterm rupture of membranes, treatment did not increase maternal infection. It did decrease neonatal respiratory distress, brain hemorrhage, necrotizing enterocolitis, and systemic infections in the first 48 hours of life.

Thomas S. Ivester

Diabetes in Pregnancy

Introduction

Diabetes mellitus (DM) is the most common medical complication of pregnancy. Diabetes may predate pregnancy (pregestational diabetes, PGDM) or may be diagnosed during gestation (gestational diabetes mellitus, GDM). DM complicates 2% to 5% of all pregnancies, with 90% of cases represented by GDM. However, a number of cases of GDM may represent an unmasking of previously undiagnosed diabetes. Despite improved understanding of the disease and its management, diabetes remains a significant cause of perinatal morbidity and mortality. Fetal effects may include major anomalies, as high as 22% if the HbA_1C exceeds 8.5%, involving the cardiovascular, central nervous, skeletal, and urinary systems; growth restriction; macrosomia; in utero demise; neonatal hypoglycemia; and respiratory distress. Most fetal anomalies are directly related to early antenatal glycemic control. Furthermore, 10% to 15% of mothers will have persistent glucose intolerance or overt DM after pregnancy, with more than 50% diagnosed with disease by 10 years. Unfortunately, only 23% to 45% of women undergo the recommended follow-up testing.

Etiology and Pathogenesis

The production of placental hormones including progesterone, estradiol, prolactin, and human somatomammotropin lead pregnancy to become a diabetogenic state (Fig. 116-1). Estrogen increases insulin binding at the cellular level; however, decreased binding secondary to progesterone and cortisol offsets this effect. A postbinding defect in insulin action is also caused by progesterone, cortisol, prolactin, and human somatomammotropin. In an effort to offset these changes, there is a marked increase in insulin secretion that peaks in the third trimester.

GDM shares many of the same features as type 2 DM. Hyperglycemia is related to two defects. First, there is a reduction in insulin secretion as compared with that in normal pregnancy. This is evidenced by a diminished first-phase insulin response and a delayed and reduced incremental response to a peak in serum glucose after oral loading. Second, insulin sensitivity is reduced to almost one third of the nonpregnant state.

Fetal effects are manifest through a number of pathways, with more implicated as research continues. Fetal glucose levels are typically 20 mg/dL lower than those in maternal serum. With significant hyperglycemia, decreased myoinositol and arachidonic acid, and aberrations in other eicosanoid biosynthetic pathways are present, leading to higher levels of free radicals and glucose within cells. Each of these may be implicated in the genesis of fetal anomalies, and interplay among them is most likely. Fetal hyperglycemia may also lead to acidosis, hypoxia, and hyperinsulinemia with consequent macrosomia. The effect of hyperglycemia on fetal cortisol levels has been implicated in decreased surfactant production by type II pneumocytes, leading to delayed pulmonary maturity.

Diagnostic Approach

Significant controversy remains regarding universal screening for GDM (Fig. 116-2). Low-risk women (<25 years old; not a member of an ethnic or racial group with a high prevalence of DM such as Hispanic, American Indian, South or East Asian, Pacific Islander, or African American; body mass index (BMI) <25; no history of abnormal glucose tolerance; no history of adverse obstetric outcomes related to GDM; and no first-degree relative with DM) probably do not need to be screened. Patients with high-risk factors, including morbid obesity, previous unexplained fetal death, a previous infant weighing more than 4 kg, and a history of GDM or glycosuria warrant screening at their first or

Figure 116-1 Diabetes in Pregnancy.

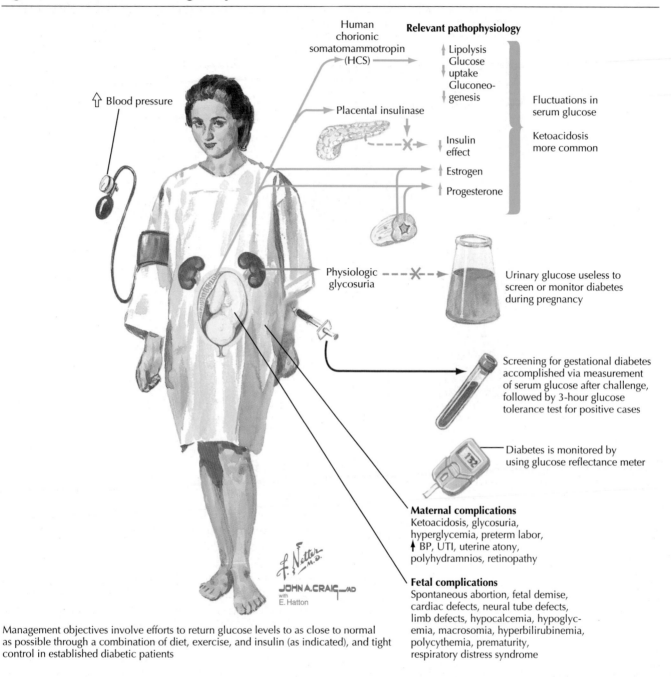

Human chorionic somatomammotropin (HCS)

Relevant pathophysiology

↑ Lipolysis
↓ Glucose uptake
↓ Gluconeo-genesis

Fluctuations in serum glucose

Ketoacidosis more common

↑ Blood pressure

Placental insulinase

↓ Insulin effect

↑ Estrogen

↑ Progesterone

Physiologic glycosuria

Urinary glucose useless to screen or monitor diabetes during pregnancy

Screening for gestational diabetes accomplished via measurement of serum glucose after challenge, followed by 3-hour glucose tolerance test for positive cases

Diabetes is monitored by using glucose reflectance meter

Maternal complications
Ketoacidosis, glycosuria, hyperglycemia, preterm labor, ↑ BP, UTI, uterine atony, polyhydramnios, retinopathy

Fetal complications
Spontaneous abortion, fetal demise, cardiac defects, neural tube defects, limb defects, hypocalcemia, hypoglycemia, macrosomia, hyperbilirubinemia, polycythemia, prematurity, respiratory distress syndrome

Management objectives involve efforts to return glucose levels to as close to normal as possible through a combination of diet, exercise, and insulin (as indicated), and tight control in established diabetic patients

second prenatal visit. If normal, such patients are screened again at 26 to 28 weeks. All other patients are usually screened once between 24 and 28 weeks' gestation.

Typically, a 50-g oral glucose load is given with a plasma glucose measurement performed 1 hour later. The patient need not be in the fasting state. A value of more than 140 mg/dL warrants evaluation with a 3-hour glucose tolerance test after a 100-g glucose load. Some centers choose to use a threshold of 130 mg/dL because the higher threshold is 10% less sensitive for the diagnosis of GDM. See Table 116-1.

Management and Therapy

Preconceptional Counseling

Patients with PGDM contemplating pregnancy should be under tight glucose control before conception. Because more than 50% of pregnancies are unplanned, the primary care physician caring for the woman of reproductive age must inquire about contraceptive practices and plans for conception at each visit. Hemoglobin A1C levels should be measured and be well within the normal range. A multivitamin containing a minimum of 0.4 mg of folate taken

Figure 116-2 Screening Algorithm for Gestational Diabetes.
BMI, body mass index; DM, diabetes mellitus; GDM, gestational diabetes mellitus; OB, obstetrics; OGTT, oral glucose tolerance test.

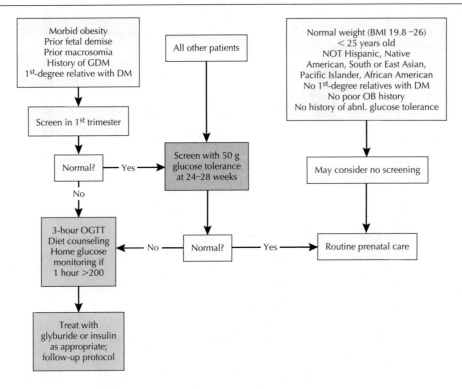

Table 116-1	Diagnostic Criteria for Gestational Diabetes	
Parameter	**National Diabetes Data Group***	**Carpenter and Coustan†**
Oral glucose dose (g)	100	100
Fasting	105	95
1 hr	190	180
2 hr	165	155
3 hr	145	140
Criteria for diagnosis	2 or more values exceeded	2 or more values exceeded

* Endorsed by the American College of Obstetricians and Gynecologists.
† Most commonly used in the United States.

daily for at least 3 months before conception has been shown to reduce the risk for neural tube defects, cleft lip, and certain congenital heart diseases. If the patient is taking an angiotensin-converting enzyme (ACE) inhibitor for coexisting hypertension, consider changing to a calcium channel blocker because ACE inhibitors are associated with fetal renal damage, especially if taken in the second trimester of pregnancy.

Glucose Control

Diet

The patient with PGDM or newly diagnosed GDM should undergo dietary counseling. Table 116-2 can be used to calculate the total caloric needs.

Although traditional recommendations call for 50% to 60% of calories to be in the form of carbohydrate, recent studies indicate that limiting carbohydrates to 40% of calories results in less fetal macrosomia. Protein should constitute about 20% of calories, with fats making up the remaining 40%. More frequent intake makes for smoother glycemic control, with one suggestion to distribute calories as follows: breakfast, 10% to 15%; morning snack, 0% to 10%; lunch, 20% to 30%; afternoon snack, 0% to 10%; supper, 30% to 40%; and bedtime snack, 0% to 10%.

Insulin

PREGESTATIONAL DIABETES MELLITUS. Patients taking oral hypoglycemics are usually switched to twice-daily insulin therapy using a combination of regular and neutral protamine Hagedorn (NPH) formulations, although recently patients are continuing oral hypoglycemics if they are taking glyburide, and occasionally if they are taking metformin. Typical needs include a total daily dose of 0.5 U/kg from conception until 12 weeks, 0.8 U/kg from

Table 116-2 Calculation of Caloric Needs for the Gestational Diabetic Patient

Weight Category	Body Mass Index*	Caloric Needs†
Underweight	<19.8	40 kcal/kg
Normal weight	19.8-26.0	30 kcal/kg
Obese	26.0-29.0	24 kcal/kg
Morbidly obese	>29.0	12 kcal/kg

* Actual weight at start of pregnancy divided by height in meters squared.
† Based on weight in pregnancy when diet is prescribed.

12 to 28 weeks, and 1 U/kg thereafter. Caution should be exercised in patients on insulin pump therapy. Decreased appetite in the first trimester and changing sleep patterns related to pregnancy place the patient at increased risk for hypoglycemia. Instructing patients on a protocol for oral glucose supplementation when they experience early signs of hypoglycemia is especially important. Family members should be educated on the proper use of a glucagon pen. Home glucose monitoring is undertaken daily with four to seven measurements. The motivated patient can use e-mail messages or fax to report her values weekly for insulin adjustment.

GESTATIONAL DIABETES MELLITUS. Many practitioners use once-weekly fasting and 1- or 2-hour postprandial plasma venous glucose determinations performed in the office, despite studies indicating a higher incidence of fetal macrosomia as compared with the use of home glucose monitoring. The decision to begin insulin therapy should be based on home capillary glucose monitoring using reflectance meters. The use of memory chips and computer software to calculate mean glucose values allows for ease and accuracy of reporting. A minimum of four daily values should be obtained fasting and 1 or 2 hours after each meal. The use of postprandial values to adjust the dose of insulin has proved more efficacious in preventing neonatal hypoglycemia and macrosomia than using preprandial values. A more intensive surveillance program includes preprandial values (seven determinations daily) with calculation of a daily mean glucose value. When measurements conducted on a daily basis confirm good control, the patient can decrease to determinations 3 times a week. Repetitive fasting values of more than 95 mg/dL or 1-hour postprandial values of more than 140 mg/dL warrant insulin therapy. A total insulin dose of 0.7 U/kg actual body weight is calculated and divided into 2 daily injections given before breakfast and before supper. The morning dose usually consists of a 2 : 1 ratio of regular and NPH insulin; the evening dose consists of a 1 : 1 mix of these preparations. On some occasions, a persistently elevated fasting value may require that the evening NPH dose be moved to bedtime and only regular insulin given before supper. Target capillary glucose values should include

fasting less than 95 mg/dL, preprandial less than 95 mg/dL, 1-hour postprandial less than 140 mg/dL, and mean glucose values of 90 to 100 mg/dL.

Oral Hypoglycemics

Until recently, oral hypoglycemics were not used in pregnancy because of concerns regarding fetal anomalies and neonatal hypoglycemia. The finding that GDM and type 2 diabetes have a similar pathophysiology has led to renewed interest in oral hypoglycemics for the treatment of GDM. Newer agents such as glyburide are tightly bound to protein and have a short elimination half-life, thereby minimizing fetal exposure. Recent studies in GDM have noted equivalent rates of macrosomia and neonatal hypoglycemia when compared with insulin therapy, with improved compliance and fewer hypoglycemic episodes. There is inadequate experience and data with other oral therapies to determine teratogenicity. Many studies to date have been unable to differentiate drug-related effects from those of poor glycemic control.

Other Prenatal Care

All PGDMs should undergo baseline ophthalmic examination to determine the presence of retinopathy. If proliferative changes are noted, photocoagulation can be undertaken during pregnancy. Benign retinopathy requires follow-up each trimester because institution of tight glycemic control has been associated with rapid deterioration. A baseline urine culture, as well as determination of 24-hour protein excretion and creatinine clearance, should be assessed early in gestation. Patients with DM of more than 10 years' duration should have an electrocardiogram, as should those with nephropathy or hypertension.

Fetal Surveillance

Because DM is associated with a higher incidence of congenital anomalies, a first-trimester hemoglobin A1C level should be obtained. All patients with DM should be offered serum and ultrasound-based screening for anomalies. First-trimester options include serum markers and ultrasound for nuchal translucency, associated with cardiac defects and aneuploidy. Second-trimester tests include alpha fetoprotein and comprehensive ultrasound at 18 to 20 weeks. If the hemoglobin A1C is elevated in the first trimester, a fetal echocardiogram at 22 weeks should be undertaken to assess for congenital heart disease. Cardiac lesions may include septal defects, transposition of the great vessels, tetralogy of Fallot, truncus arteriosus, and hypoplastic left heart. Antenatal testing may be warranted as early as 28 weeks' gestation in the patient with poorly controlled diabetes, vascular complications, or comorbidities. In most cases, testing is initiated by 32 weeks' gestation. Many centers use a modified biophysical profile consisting of a nonstress test (NST) performed in conjunc-

Figure 116-3 Brachial Plexus and Cervical Nerve Root Injuries at Birth (Erb's Palsy).

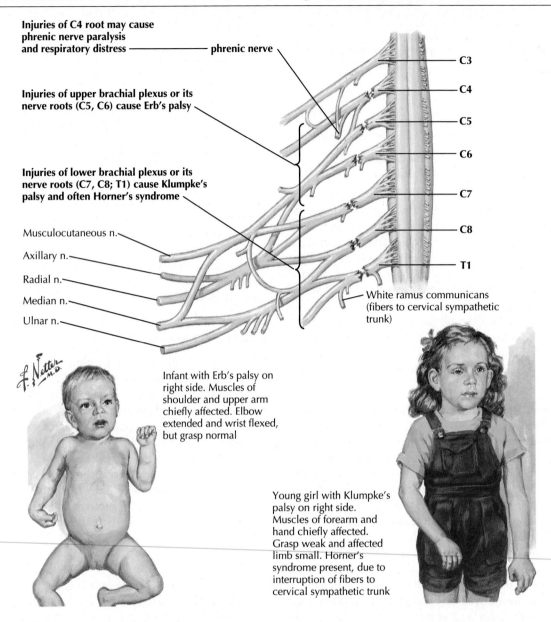

Injuries of C4 root may cause phrenic nerve paralysis and respiratory distress — phrenic nerve

Injuries of upper brachial plexus or its nerve roots (C5, C6) cause Erb's palsy

Injuries of lower brachial plexus or its nerve roots (C7, C8; T1) cause Klumpke's palsy and often Horner's syndrome

Musculocutaneous n.
Axillary n.
Radial n.
Median n.
Ulnar n.

C3
C4
C5
C6
C7
C8
T1

White ramus communicans (fibers to cervical sympathetic trunk)

Infant with Erb's palsy on right side. Muscles of shoulder and upper arm chiefly affected. Elbow extended and wrist flexed, but grasp normal

Young girl with Klumpke's palsy on right side. Muscles of forearm and hand chiefly affected. Grasp weak and affected limb small. Horner's syndrome present, due to interruption of fibers to cervical sympathetic trunk

tion with an ultrasound determination of amniotic fluid volume; others prefer to use the NST alone or full biophysical profile (BPP). Testing is undertaken at least weekly, although for the patient with type 1 DM or GDM requiring insulin, twice-weekly testing may be preferable.

Delivery

Optimal timing of delivery in the patient with diabetes is debated. In the case of poor metabolic control and documentation of fetal lung maturity by amniocentesis, induction of labor should be undertaken at 37 to 38 weeks' gestation. Some studies have confirmed a reduced incidence of fetal macrosomia with routine induction at 38

weeks' gestation. Most centers will not allow the diabetic patient (with PGDM or GDM) to proceed past 40 weeks' gestation even in light of good metabolic control and reassuring antenatal fetal testing.

Fetal macrosomia is among the most feared complications of diabetes secondary to its association with shoulder dystocia and possible brachial plexus injury in the neonate. Ten to 50% of fetuses who weigh more than 4500 g experience a shoulder dystocia at the time of vaginal delivery. Erb's palsy (Fig. 116-3) develops in 4% to 8% of macrosomic infants delivered vaginally, but only 10% to 20% of cases persist after age 1 year. Current clinical and ultrasonographic techniques are poor predictors of fetal macrosomia. However, because of medicolegal concerns, the

prevailing practice is to offer the diabetic patient delivery by cesarean birth if the estimated fetal weight is 4500 g or greater.

Neonatal hypoglycemia can be reduced when maternal glucose levels are tightly controlled in labor. A dextrose-containing intravenous fluid prevents ketosis. Continuous low-dose insulin infusion, in conjunction with hourly capillary glucose measurements, is then used to maintain the maternal glucose at 90-120 mg/dL.

Postpartum Care

Glucose Control

Because of the acute loss of placental hormones with delivery, the patient with type 1 DM is extremely sensitive to insulin in the first 24 hours postpartum. Permissive hyperglycemia is allowed with maintenance of glucose levels less than 200 mg/dL. Typically the patient will only require half of her prepregnancy dose in the first 24 hours; a sliding scale can be used for additional control. By the second postpartum day, she can be placed back on her full prepregnancy dose if oral intake is adequate. If the patient is nursing, caloric intake should be increased by 500 kcal over her pregestation caloric needs. Patients who were taking oral hypoglycemic agents before pregnancy are maintained on low-dose insulin while breastfeeding because these agents are readily excreted into the breast milk and can cause profound neonatal hypoglycemia.

The patient with GDM requiring insulin should continue glucose monitoring in the immediate postpartum period, which may be discontinued or reduced over time. For all others, a 75-g oral glucose tolerance test is recommended at the 6-week postpartum visit. A fasting value of more than 126 mg/dL or a 2-hour glucose measurement of more than 200 mg/dL is the provisional diagnostic criterion for diabetes. An impaired fasting glucose is defined as a value between 110 and 125 mg/dL, whereas impaired glucose tolerance is defined as a 2-hour postglucose value of 140 to 199 mg/dL. These patients require careful follow-up because they are at high risk for the development of overt diabetes.

Contraception

Today's oral contraceptives contain reduced amounts of estrogen and progestin and therefore have minimal effect on glucose control; their use in the diabetic patient is acceptable with monitoring of glucose and lipid levels. New intrauterine devices are not contraindicated in the diabetic patient. Injectable or implantable progestins can also be used. One study has indicated a higher rate of progression to type 2 DM in Hispanic patients with GDM who, because of concerns about milk production, were taking progestin-only birth control pills.

Optimum Treatment

Dietary therapy or modification is the primary foundation of the treatment regimen for the pregnant mother with diabetes. Intensive dietary counseling, education, and support are critical components of success. A general scheme of caloric needs is outlined in Table 116-2. However, even greater attention should be given to the proportions of specific macronutrients in the diet. Appropriate vigilance over blood glucose levels through home monitoring, to include fasting and postprandial values, is the basis on which key treatment decisions are made. Once threshold values are exceeded, treatment should be initiated early. Initial treatment with glyburide is recommended, however, for those with more severe hyperglycemia, insulin should be first line. Frequent assessment of glycemic control through visits every 1 to 2 weeks and review of logbook values should guide further adjustments. Surveillance of fetal growth with ultrasound is mandated in severe cases, and at least a one-time assessment is recommended in the latter third trimester for all diabetic mothers. Delivery should be effected before 40 weeks, and earlier with very poor control and fetal lung maturity, with cesarean birth reserved for those with estimated fetal weights beyond 4500 g. Fetal well-being should be assessed once or twice weekly with NST or BPPs. Postpartum, patients requiring insulin during pregnancy should continue to monitor blood glucose, and all patients should undergo a 2-hour oral glucose tolerance test between 2 and 4 months after delivery.

Avoiding Treatment Errors

Because of the increased risk for hypoglycemia in pregnancy, aggressive therapy with insulin early in the course of disease should be avoided. Some practitioners suggest starting with insulin doses of 0.5 to 0.7 U/kg, slightly lower than the typical doses listed earlier. Not only is hypoglycemia potentially harmful to mother and fetus, but also significant symptoms may impair future compliance. Also, not following through with dietary counseling and support, and not reinforcing home glucose monitoring are serious pitfalls to successful management. Initial therapy with glyburide will likely improve compliance and, thereby, treatment success. It is important to recognize key drug interactions with glyburide, such as aspirin, which displaces drug from protein, H_2 blockers that competitively inhibit metabolism, and β-blockers, which antagonize regulatory hormones.

Long-Term Outcome

Maternal

Women in whom GDM develops are at substantial risk for the subsequent development of type 2 DM. The rate of development is dependent on several factors, most notably

race and ethnic background. About 10% of white women with GDM have type 2 DM within the first decade postpartum; the rate increases to 30% to 40% by the third decade. In contrast, 50% of Latina women with GDM have type 2 DM within 5 years of delivery. Although parity does not appear to influence the risk, women with GDM in successive pregnancies are at further increased risk for the development of type 2 DM. Obesity also is a major risk factor. The risk for DM increases almost twofold with each 10-pound weight gain over postpartum weight. Thus, knowledge of a woman's health status during her pregnancies offers a unique window into her risk evaluation, enabling opportunities in preventing disease and in more optimally targeting screening activities.

Neonatal

Macrosomia, hypoglycemia, hyperbilirubinemia, and polycythemia are the short-term detrimental effects of poorly controlled maternal DM. More concerning are the results of long-term studies that indicate that in utero modeling occurs when there is poor maternal metabolic control. A higher incidence of obesity, persisting into adolescence; glucose intolerance; and even poorer intellectual and psychomotor development have been noted.

Future Directions

Randomized trials are desperately needed regarding therapeutic interventions in GDM and the relationship to short- and long-term neonatal outcome. In addition, newer treatment modalities such as intranasal insulin and new types of oral hypoglycemics should be studied in pregnancy.

Additional Resources

American College of Obstetricians and Gynecologists Committee on Practice Bulletins, Gabbe S: Pregestational diabetes mellitus. ACOG Practice Bulletin No. 60. Obstet Gynecol 105:675-685, 2005.

This article provides an excellent overview of pregestational diabetes in the setting of pregnancy and suggests practice guidelines. It encompasses an overview of the literature and provides consensus and expert opinion where evidence is lacking.

American College of Obstetricians and Gynecologists Committee on Practice Bulletins, Coustan D: Gestational diabetes. ACOG Practice Bulletin No. 30. Obstet Gynecol 98:525-538, 2001.

This article provides a brief overview of the current understanding of gestational diabetes and provides management guidelines based on evidence and supplemented by expert opinion where necessary.

Tran N, Hunter S, Yankowitz J: Oral hypoglycemic agents in pregnancy. Obstet Gynecol Surv 59:456-463, 2004.

The authors present a detailed review of the use, efficacy, and safety of various oral agents for the treatment of diabetes in pregnancy.

EVIDENCE

1. Ferrara A, Weiss N, Hedderson M, et al: Pregnancy plasma glucose levels exceeding the American Diabetes Association thresholds, but below the National Diabetes Data Group thresholds for gestational diabetes mellitus, are related to the risk of neonatal macrosomia, hypoglycemia, and hyperbilirubinemia. Diabetologia 50:298-306, 2007.

   This study demonstrates the elevated risk of pregnancy complications using the lower thresholds for 3-hour glucose tolerance testing endorsed by the ADA and originally proposed by Carpenter and Coustan.

2. Gabbe S, Graves C: Management of diabetes mellitus complicating pregnancy. Obstet Gynecol 102:857-868, 2003.

   This paper reviews key aspects and standards of care in management of pregnancies complicated by diabetes mellitus.

3. Langer O: Maternal glycemic criteria for insulin therapy in gestational diabetes mellitus. Diabetes Care 21(Suppl 2):B91-B98, 1998.

   This review of 58 clinical studies helps to establish criteria for initiating various therapies for diabetes in pregnancy. It demonstrates the increased risk for adverse pregnancy outcomes relative to the degree of glycemic control.

4. Langer O, Conway D, Berkus M, et al: A comparison of glyburide and insulin in women with gestational diabetes mellitus. N Engl J Med 343:1134-1138, 2000.

   This study demonstrates the efficacy of glyburide for glycemic control in pregnancies complicated by diabetes mellitus. It also shows a lower risk for hypoglycemic complications with glyburide compared with insulin therapy.

5. Miller E, Hare J, Cloherty J, et al: Elevated maternal hemoglobin A1c in early pregnancy and major congenital anomalies in infants of diabetic mothers. N Engl J Med 304:1331-1334, 1981.

   This study establishes the correlation between glycemic control in early pregnancy, as measured by glycosylated hemoglobin levels, and the risk for congenital anomalies. As hemoglobin A1C levels increase, the risk for major anomalies also increases.

6. Russell M, Phipps M, Olson C, et al: Rates of postpartum glucose testing after gestational diabetes mellitus. Obstet Gynecol 108(6):1456-1462, 2006.

   This retrospective study highlights that postpartum follow-up of pregnancies complicated by gestational diabetes is low, with less than 45% receiving appropriate testing. Among those who were tested, abnormal tests were discovered in more than one third.

7. Yang J, Cummings E, O'Connell C, Jangaard K: Fetal and neonatal outcomes of diabetic pregnancies. Obstet Gynecol 108:644-650, 2006.

   A population-based study that demonstrates an increased risk for poor pregnancy outcomes among pregestational diabetic patients compared with those without diabetes. Risks for adverse outcomes were 3 to 9 times more common, including perinatal mortality, congenital anomalies, and large-for-gestational-age infants.

8. Zhao Z, Reece A: Experimental mechanisms of diabetic embryopathy and strategies for developing therapeutic interventions. J Soc Gynecol Invest 12:549-557, 2005.

   The authors present a comprehensive review of the types and mechanisms of development for major congenital anomalies seen in diabetic pregnancies. Hyperglycemia, ketone bodies, and triglycerides and the secondary effects of increased oxidative stress have been shown to exert adverse effects on developing embryos.

Menstrual Disorders

Introduction

Menstruation, the periodic bleeding caused by shedding of the uterine lining at regular intervals, is a normal event. It signals sexual maturity, fertility, and good health for many women, but it may be accompanied by significant morbidity. Common menstrual complaints are excessive bleeding, bleeding that occurs too frequently or too infrequently, painful menstruation, and premenstrual syndrome (PMS).

The menstrual cycle (Fig. 117-1) is described both in terms of ovarian hormonal events and in terms of endometrial responses to hormonal changes. The first day of bleeding is defined as day 1 of the cycle. The ovarian cycle begins with the follicular phase. Several follicles (small cysts, each containing an oocyte surrounded by estrogen-producing granulosa cells) begin maturing in response to follicle-stimulating hormone (FSH) and luteinizing hormone (LH) secreted by the anterior pituitary gland. Through positive feedback, the follicle that secretes the most estradiol (the dominant follicle) becomes more sensitive to FSH stimulation and enlarges to about 2 cm in diameter, whereas the others atrophy. The hypothalamus and pituitary gland respond to ovarian hormones with a surge in LH and FSH secretion. Ovulation occurs within 24 to 48 hours of the LH surge. After ovulation, the granulosa and theca cells of the ovulatory follicle become the corpus luteum and produce estrogen and progesterone during the luteal phase. Rising ovarian hormone levels exert negative feedback on FSH and LH production. As FSH and LH fall (in the absence of pregnancy), the corpus luteum degenerates.

The uterus responds to ovarian or pharmacologic hormonal stimulation in a stereotypical fashion. During menstruation, there is shedding of the hormonally responsive upper zone of the endometrium, due to declining hormonal support. While the lining sheds down to its basal layer, new ovarian follicles are forming. Estrogen causes thickening of the lining and cessation of bleeding. This growth of glands and stroma that occurs before ovulation is the proliferative phase. After ovulation, progesterone and estrogen cause increased tortuosity of endometrial glands and secretion from the gland lumen, the secretory phase.

Normal menses occur every 24 to 35 days. The average is 28 days, with ovulation occurring on day 14. There is considerable variation in cycle length among women, and a significant chance that a woman will experience long or short cycles each year. Healthy women aged 20 to 40 years usually have regular cycles. The chance of irregular cycles is increased for 5 to 7 years after menarche and for several years before menopause.

In ovulatory cycles, bleeding averages 3 to 6 days, with the heaviest bleeding usually on day 2. Average blood loss is 30 to 40 mL per cycle.

DISORDERS OF TIMING AND AMOUNT OF BLEEDING

Menstruation may be excessive in amount, frequency, or duration, or a combination of these. Menorrhagia (hypermenorrhea) is prolonged (over 7 days) or heavy (greater than 80 mL/menses) bleeding, occurring at regular intervals. Polymenorrhea is regular menses occurring more often than every 21 days. Metrorrhagia is irregularly timed, frequent bleeding; menometrorrhagia is both frequent and heavy. Amenorrhea is the absence of bleeding. Oligomenorrhea refers to irregularly timed, infrequent periods. Dys-

Figure 117-1 Menstrual Cycle.

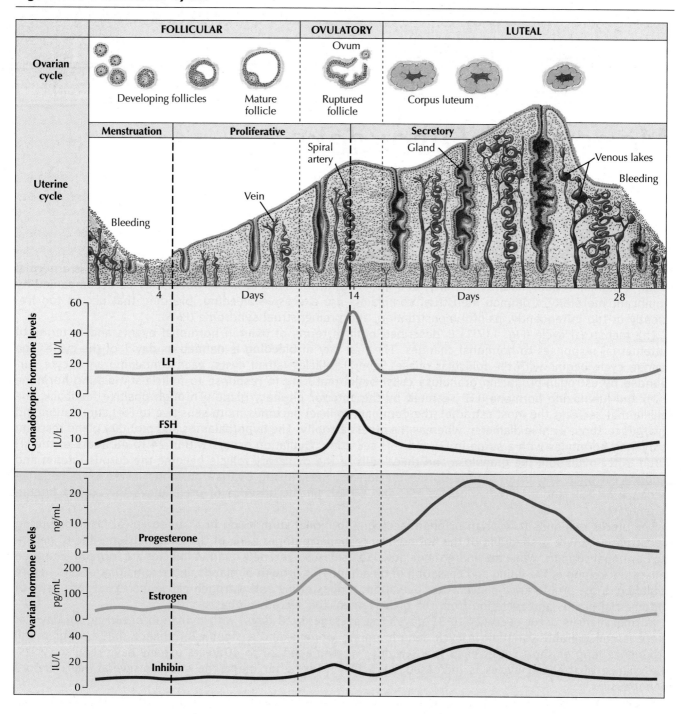

functional uterine bleeding refers to abnormal menstrual bleeding for which an organic cause cannot be found.

Etiology and Pathogenesis

Heavy regular bleeding is often due to an anatomic distortion of the uterus (Fig. 117-2). Uterine fibroids (submucous or large intramural leiomyomas), adenomyosis, and endometrial polyps cause heavy bleeding, possibly by increasing endometrial surface area. Nonhormonal intrauterine devices can also cause heavier, longer periods by creating a local foreign-body reaction. Inherited coagulation disorders (e.g., von Willebrand's disease) and alterations in clotting from use of anticoagulants or aspirin also increase menstrual blood loss.

Irregularly timed excessive bleeding may result from important pathologic circumstances. These include abnormal pregnancies—threatened or incomplete abortion,

Figure 117-2 Causes of Abnormal Uterine Bleeding.

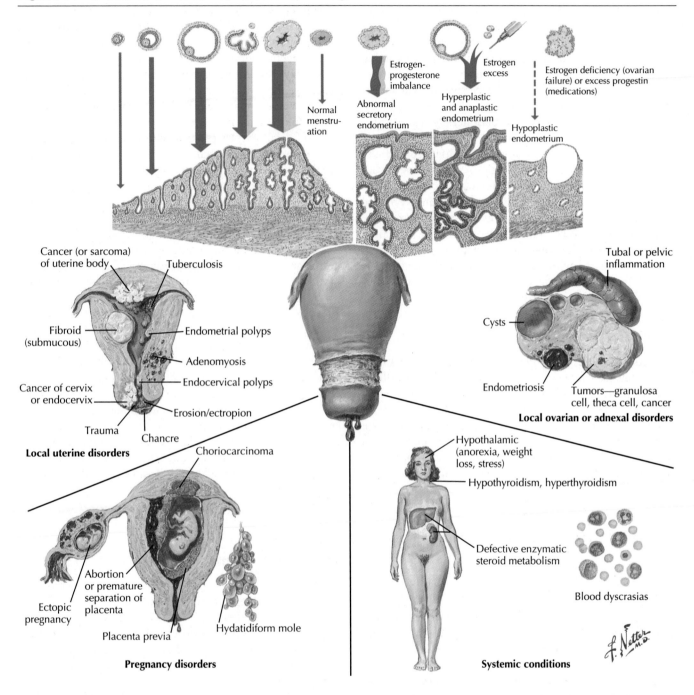

ectopic pregnancy, or molar pregnancy. Endometritis causes irregular uterine bleeding and uterine tenderness from inflammation. Anatomic distortions such as fibroids or polyps can cause irregular bleeding. Endometrial carcinoma is associated with irregular, sometimes heavy bleeding. Adenocarcinoma, the most common endometrial neoplasm, usually arises from cystic hyperplasia with atypia. This condition often causes bleeding, which may lead to evaluation and treatment before development of cancer. For this reason, prompt evaluation of irregular bleeding,

particularly in perimenopausal or postmenopausal women, is important.

Bleeding from the cervix or vagina (e.g., cervicitis, ectropion, invasive cancer, severe atrophic vaginitis, or trichomoniasis) may be confused with uterine bleeding. Rectal and anal bleeding and gross hematuria are occasionally misinterpreted as genital in origin.

Amenorrhea is most often caused by pregnancy. Other causes are hyperprolactinemia, hypothyroidism or adrenocorticotropic hormone deficiency, hypogonadotropic hypogonadism, menopause or premature ovarian failure, anorexia nervosa, sudden weight loss, severe stress, strenuous exercise, and numerous medications.

Prolonged anovulation may cause a period of amenorrhea, followed by heavy bleeding from uterine lining hyperplasia. In polycystic ovary syndrome (PCOS), elevated pituitary LH secretion and excessive ovarian androgens prevent follicle maturation in the ovary. Ovarian androstenedione is converted peripherally to estrone, which stimulates further LH release, and a vicious cycle ensues. Estrogens cause prolonged proliferation of the endometrium, but without ovulation—normal menstruation does not occur. Eventually the thick but fragile endometrium breaks down, causing heavy bleeding. Physical stigmata include obesity, acne, hirsutism, and multiple ovarian cysts in severe cases. Milder cases of hyperandrogenic oligo-ovulation may not have these signs. PCOS may be associated with elevated serum lipids, centripetal obesity, insulin resistance, and an increased risk for diabetes mellitus and heart disease.

Clinical Presentation

Patients complain when their menstrual pattern changes, when they pass large clots, or when bleeding overflows sanitary protection. Chronic menorrhagia also frequently causes iron deficiency anemia. Occasionally, women with severe anemia from menstrual bleeding do not recognize that their periods are abnormal. Absence of anemia does not exclude menorrhagia because women may compensate for significant losses by increasing iron consumption.

Differential Diagnosis

See Box 117-1 for the differential diagnosis of menstrual disorders.

Diagnostic Approach

A menstrual history should include an estimate of the timing, duration, and amount of bleeding (size of clots, the type of protection needed, and the time needed to soak a maxi pad or tampon.) Age at menarche and the presence of perimenopausal symptoms such as hot flashes and night sweats help to diagnose age-appropriate anovulatory cycles. The history should address diseases or medications that can affect the hypothalamic-pituitary-ovarian axis. Galactorrhea, hirsutism, acne, and weight gain and loss are important associated symptoms to consider. Rapidly progressive virilization (deepening voice, clitoral enlargement, temporal balding, and increased muscle mass or libido) raises concern about ovarian or adrenal neoplasms. A family history of menstrual disorders, hysterectomy, and bleeding disorders should be investigated for heritable causes of menstrual disorders. Physical examination should assess height, weight, blood pressure, hair distribution, and

acne. Speculum examination may demonstrate vaginal inflammation, cervical erosion, tumor, or cervical polyps. Bimanual examination reveals a firm lumpy texture with leiomyomas. Tenderness to uterine palpation may occur with infection or adenomyosis, and enlarged ovaries or cysts may develop in patients with anovulation. In obese patients, the ovaries are usually not palpable. In menopausal women, it is abnormal to palpate the ovaries; any palpable ovary must be evaluated by ultrasound.

Useful laboratory tests include a sensitive pregnancy test, complete blood cell count, ferritin and serum iron levels for women with menorrhagia, and prothrombin time and partial thromboplastin time in women suspected of bleeding disorders. In amenorrheic patients, measurement of β-human chorionic gonadotropin, prolactin, thyroid-stimulating hormone, FSH, and estradiol are helpful. When signs of excess androgen are present, check total testosterone and 17-hydroxyprogesterone (morning and fasting.) Because chronic anovulation may be associated with the metabolic syndrome, it is also important to measure serum lipids, and consider testing hyperinsulinemia and impaired glucose tolerance. Endometrial biopsy may show polyps, infection, endometrial hyperplasia, or carcinoma. Ultrasound shows the total uterine size and the thickness of the endometrial stripe, as well as leiomyomas and ovarian cysts or polycystic ovaries. Hydrosonography and hysterosalpingography are useful to outline lesions such as polyps in the endometrial cavity. Hysteroscopy allows visualization of the uterine cavity, and many lesions, such as submucous or pedunculated leiomyomas, or endometrial polyps, can be treated during the same procedure.

Management and Therapy

Optimum Treatment

Hormonal treatment is useful in treating excessive bleeding, even that due to nonhormonal causes. Estrogen stops bleeding by stimulating growth of new tissue to cover the denuded endometrium. Progestins mature the uterine lining, making it compact and ready to slough off after the drug is withdrawn, mimicking the normal changes that occur in the secretory phase of the menstrual cycle. Progestins are also used diagnostically in cases of amenorrhea because a withdrawal bleed induced by progestin (e.g., medroxyprogesterone acetate, 10 mg daily for 10 to 14 days) demonstrates adequate estrogen stimulation of the uterine lining and a patent outflow tract. In anovulation, cyclic use of progestins prevents the buildup of a thick endometrium by allowing regular withdrawal bleeding and prevents development of hyperplasia and carcinoma. High doses of combined (estrogen-progestin) oral contraceptive pills (e.g., 4 tablets a day for several days) will arrest heavy bleeding, and normal doses will establish predictable withdrawal bleeding every 28 days. The programmed "period"

Box 117-1   Differential Diagnosis of Menstrual Disorders

Menorrhagia

Leiomyomas
Endometrial or endocervical polyps
Endometrial hyperplasia or carcinoma
Anovulation (hypothalamic, pituitary, polycystic ovary
   syndrome, perimenopause)
Bleeding disorders (von Willebrand's disease, hemophilia,
   thrombocytopenia, anticoagulant use)
Hypothyroidism
Endometriosis
Endometritis
Systemic lupus erythematosus
Leukemia
Scurvy

Metrorrhagia

Pregnancy (intrauterine, ectopic, threatened abortion)
Anovulation
Breakthrough bleeding (progestin or estrogen-progestin
   contraceptives)
Endometrial or endocervical polyps
Leiomyomas
Adenomyosis
Endometritis
Endometrial hyperplasia or carcinoma
Bleeding disorders
Retained products of conception

Primary Amenorrhea

Müllerian anomalies (uterine or vaginal agenesis, vaginal
   septum, imperforate hymen)
Androgen insensitivity
Ovarian dysgenesis (Turner's syndrome, Swyer's syndrome,
   mosaicism)
Delayed puberty
Hypothyroidism, hyperthyroidism
Hypopituitarism
Pregnancy

Androgens
Androgen-producing tumors
Hysterectomy or oophorectomy
History of chemotherapy or radiation
Toxicities like lead, mercury, and alcohol
Malnutrition
Exercise
Chronic disease
Pituitary tumors like craniopharyngioma
Anorexia or depression

Secondary Amenorrhea

Pregnancy
Anovulation, polycystic ovary syndrome
Functional ovarian cyst
Menopause, premature ovarian failure
Hyperthyroidism, hypothyroidism
Elevated prolactin (normal lactation, prolactinoma)
Hypopituitarism (tumor, Sheehan's syndrome, genetic
   syndromes)
Hypothalamic (GnRH suppression from stress, anorexia
   nervosa, bulimia, acute weight loss, malnutrition,
   depression, strenuous exercise, chronic disease)
Drug effect (hormonal contraceptives, GnRH agonists,
   androgens, phenothiazines)
Heavy metal poisoning (lead, mercury)
Chemotherapy, radiation
Endometrial damage (Asherman's syndrome, tuberculosis,
   schistosomiasis)
Diabetes
Systemic lupus erythematosus
Vasculitis
HIV infection
Tuberculosis
Surgical causes of hypopituitarism
Hysterectomy or oophorectomy
Androgen-producing tumors

---

in pill users and breakthrough bleeding, are both effects of the drug, and they represent neither normal menstruation nor a menstrual abnormality. Oral contraceptives can be taken continuously (without placebos) to prevent withdrawal bleeding and blood loss. A levonorgestrel-containing intrauterine device and implanted or injected progestins also decrease menstrual blood loss, although irregular bleeding in the first months of use is expected. Nonsteroidal anti-inflammatory drugs (NSAIDs) decrease the total amount of uterine bleeding and pain associated with menses, and NSAIDs can be useful in conjunction with oral contraceptives or cyclic progestins. Tranexamic acid (not available in the United States) effectively reduces menstrual blood loss.

Surgical treatments include curettage, numerous procedures to ablate or resect the endometrial lining, myomectomy and destructive procedures for fibroids, and hysterectomy.

Avoiding Treatment Errors

The most serious error in treating abnormal bleeding is a missed diagnosis of endometrial cancer or precancer. Endometrial carcinoma has a long premalignant phase, and early-stage carcinoma is often curable with surgery. Endometrial biopsy will diagnose most endometrial cancer and precancer. False-negative results do occur, so in patients at high risk (those with family history of uterine cancer, obesity, diabetes mellitus, African American race, and those with prior concerning biopsy results), curettage should be considered if irregular bleeding does not resolve promptly with hormonal treatment.

Oral contraceptives and other hormones often cause breakthrough bleeding in the first several cycles of use. Patients should be advised of this, so that they do not stop therapy too soon. With prolonged use of progestins or estrogen-progestin combinations, the endometrial lining may become atrophic, so a woman who initially had too thick a lining can bleed when it becomes too thin. Ultrasound or hysteroscopy shows a very thin lining in such cases. Hormonal therapy works best in women with hormonal imbalance such as anovulation. When the anatomy is distorted by submucosal fibroids or polyps, hormonal treatment often improves symptoms, but surgery is more successful.

For severe endometriosis and adenomyosis, hysterectomy may provide welcome relief from symptoms, especially in women who have completed childbearing. When resources are limited, careful history taking will identify patients in greatest need of hysterectomy.

DYSMENORRHEA AND PREMENSTRUAL SYNDROME

Menstrual discomfort affects 30% to 60% of women. About 5% have symptoms severe enough to interfere with daily activities. PMS, a group of physical and emotional symptoms that occur in the luteal phase of the cycle, affects more than half of menstruating women intermittently, although severe symptoms occur in only 2% to 3% of women.

Etiology and Pathogenesis

Primary dysmenorrhea is caused by prostaglandin F2a, which causes uterine contractions. Secondary dysmenorrhea is caused by inflammation in acute or chronic pelvic infection, excessive prostaglandin production in endometriosis and adenomyosis, or cervical stenosis. The physical symptoms of PMS, such as bloating and breast tenderness, are hormonal in origin. Emotional symptoms, such as anger, irritability, and depression, are serotonin mediated.

Clinical Presentation

Presentation is straightforward because the patient notes a symptom pattern and requests treatment.

Differential Diagnosis

PMS and premenstrual dysphoric disorder (PMDD) must be distinguished from chronic mood disorders. Because mental illness is stigmatized, women with depression or anxiety often seek treatment for PMS. However, the emotional symptoms of PMS and PMDD occur only in the luteal phase, clearing during the menstrual and follicular phases. PMDD may be isolated, or a woman may have premenstrual exacerbations of an underlying mood disorder. In either case, the symptoms of depression, irritability, and inappropriate behaviors may cause severe impairment in a woman's work and family relationships and subsequent feelings of guilt and shame.

Diagnostic Approach

Menstrual history is important to elucidate the age at onset because symptom changes with age, contraceptive use, pregnancy and lactation, associated symptoms such as backache or dyspareunia, and response to previous treatments. For PMS, a menstrual calendar is used to document symptoms over several cycles. Family history of menstrual disorders may affect a woman's response to menstruation, whereas a history of endometriosis or adenomyosis increases suspicion of these conditions. Pelvic examination may demonstrate cervical motion tenderness or adnexal tenderness in infection, uterosacral nodularity in endometriosis, or a boggy, tender uterus in adenomyosis.

Management and Therapy

Optimum Treatment

Menstrual pain can be treated with NSAIDs, which decrease prostaglandin production, hypertonic uterine contractions, and menstrual blood loss. Oral contraceptives also decrease menstrual pain in 90% of users and can be used together with NSAIDs. Heat, transcutaneous electrical nerve stimulation, acupuncture, and acupressure are also effective. Severe pain refractory to treatment should be evaluated with laparoscopy, and endometriotic lesions can be fulgurated simultaneously. Presumed endometriosis can be empirically treated with gonadotropin-releasing hormone (GnRH) agonists. Improvement with this treatment does not confirm a diagnosis of endometriosis because ablation of menstruation treats several menstrual disorders. Pregnancy and vaginal delivery are associated with lower rates of dysmenorrhea, but the stress of parenting may increase PMS. Hysterectomy is effective in relieving pure dysmenorrhea. Chronic pelvic pain often recurs after hysterectomy even if the pain is localized to the uterus on examination.

The physical symptoms of PMS can be effectively treated with mild diuretics and analgesics. Emotional symptoms may improve with selective serotonin reuptake inhibitors (dosed continuously or in the luteal phase only), anxiolytics, tricyclic antidepressants, or suppression of menses with danazol, GnRH agonists, or oral contraceptives.

Avoiding Treatment Errors

Endometriosis, adenomyosis, and chronic pelvic inflammatory disease can all cause vague abdominal discomfort and bloating that are worse around the time of the menses. A careful pelvic exam and laparoscopy will help distinguish these conditions from the premenstrual syndrome.

A woman who is suspected of having premenstrual dysphoric disorder may have PMDD, depression, or both. Symptom charting will help distinguish among these possibilities. Misdiagnosis of depression as PMDD may lead to undertreatment because fewer drugs have been tested for PMDD than for depression. Ignoring the cyclic pattern of PMDD might lead to missed opportunities for therapy with hormonal or surgical ablation of the menstrual cycle.

Future Directions

For heavy and painful bleeding, hormonal contraceptives are often used. As the selection of delivery systems increases (intrauterine, implant, injection, patch, ring, or pill) and the dosing regimens are varied (from the traditional 21-day regimen to extended regimens), it will be important to know which methods have the most favorable effect on bleeding patterns and associated symptoms. Hysterectomy is 100% effective in stopping menstruation, but it is expensive and has significant operative morbidity. Many less invasive techniques to resect or ablate the endometrium have been developed. Research is needed to determine which among these is most safe, effective, and cost-effective.

As overweight and obesity become endemic around the world, the problem of anovulation and its relation to the metabolic syndrome will become more important. Primary prevention of these syndromes and the role of insulin-sensitizing agents, diet, exercise, and other treatments must be studied in detail.

Additional Resource

Speroff L, Fritz M: Clinical Gynecologic Endocrinology and Infertility, 7th ed. Philadelphia, Lippincott Williams & Wilkins, 2005, Chapters 6, 11, 12, and 14.

This text discusses all of the menstrual irregularities, with extremely thorough discussions of the biochemistry of normal and abnormal endocrine function, and with clinical applications.

EVIDENCE

1. Futterman LA, Rapkin AJ: Diagnosis of premenstrual disorders. J Reprod Med 51(4 Suppl):349-358, 2006.

    This review distinguishes premenstrual syndrome from premenstrual dysphoric disorder and documents the need for prospective symptom ratings.

2. Kroll R, Rapkin AJ: Treatment of premenstrual disorders. J Reprod Med 51(4 Suppl):359-370, 2006.

    This article discusses FDA-approved drugs for premenstrual syndrome and premenstrual dysphoric disorder, including selective serotonin reuptake inhibitors (SSRIs) and oral contraceptives containing drospirenone. Research on other treatments, such as exercise, cognitive behavioral therapy, dietary changes, and use of supplements, is described.

3. Lethaby A, Augood C, Duckitt K: Nonsteroidal anti-inflammatory drugs for heavy menstrual bleeding. Cochrane Database of Systematic Reviews 1998, Issue 3. Art. No.: CD000400. DOI: 10.1002/14651858.CD000400.

    This analysis of 16 randomized, controlled trials showed that NSAIDs reduced menstrual blood loss, although danazol and tranexamic acid were more effective.

4. Lethaby AE, Cooke I, Rees M: Progesterone or progestogen-releasing intrauterine systems for heavy menstrual bleeding. Cochrane Database of Systematic Reviews 2005, Issue 4. Art. No.: CD002126. DOI: 10.1002/14651858.CD002126.pub2.

    An analysis of 10 randomized controlled trials of the levonorgestrel-releasing intrauterine device (LNG IUS) showed that the LNG IUS was more effective than cyclic progestin treatment. It was less effective than surgical ablation and hysterectomy, but there was no difference in quality-of-life measures between these groups.

5. Lethaby A, Hickey M, Garry R: Endometrial destruction techniques for heavy menstrual bleeding. Cochrane Database of Systematic Reviews 2005, Issue 4. Art. No.: CD001501. DOI: 10.1002/14651858.CD001501.pub2.

    This meta-analysis lists a large number of techniques for destroying the endometrium. Women undergoing new techniques such as balloon, microwave, cryoablation, thermal laser, bipolar electrode ablation, and hydrothermal ablation had fewer complications than women undergoing traditional hysteroscopic ablation or resection.

6. Lord JM, Flight IHK, Norman RJ: Insulin-sensitising drugs (metformin, troglitazone, rosiglitazone, pioglitazone, D-chiro-inositol) for polycystic ovary syndrome. Cochrane Database of Systematic Reviews 2003, Issue 2. Art. No.: CD003053. DOI: 10.1002/14651858.CD003053.

    Multiple studies demonstrated that metformin increases ovulation in women with PCOS, and metformin with clomiphene increases ovulation more. Additionally, fasting insulin levels, blood pressure, and low-density lipoprotein cholesterol (LDL) all improved on metformin.

7. Marjoribanks J, Lethaby A, Farquhar C: Surgery versus medical therapy for heavy menstrual bleeding. Cochrane Database of Systematic Reviews 2006, Issue 2. Art. No.: CD003855. DOI: 10.1002/14651858.CD003855.pub2.

    In studies comparing oral therapy with hysterectomy, more than half the women randomized to medication eventually required hysterectomy. Studies of the levonorgestrel intrauterine system was less effective at controlling bleeding, but patient satisfaction was similar to that in women undergoing resection or hysterectomy.

Endometriosis

Introduction

A benign gynecologic condition with occasional invasive properties reminiscent of malignancies, endometriosis has long frustrated both physicians and patients. Defined as the presence and growth of both endometrial glands and stroma outside the endometrial cavity, endometriosis can lead to symptom manifestations of cyclical pelvic pain, dyspareunia, dysmenorrhea, and less frequently, abnormal uterine bleeding and gastrointestinal and urinary tract symptoms. There is speculation about the relationship between endometriosis and fertility.

The true incidence and prevalence of endometriosis are unknown because it is identified often incidentally at surgery for other indications. Estimates commonly cited include a 5% to 15% incidence in reproductive-aged women. Active endometriosis is found in about one third of women with chronic pelvic pain.

Etiology and Pathogenesis

No single theory has emerged as dominant for the pathogenesis of endometriosis. It is unclear why endometriosis develops in some, but not all, women. Proposed explanations include anatomic (retrograde menstruation, vascular and lymphatic dissemination), histologic (coelomic metaplasia), immunologic, genetic predisposition, and other theories.

Retrograde menstruation, found in up to 90% of women in any particular cycle, is clearly a common occurrence. Implantation of endometriotic cells shed during menstruation may lead to the development of endometriosis. Viable endometrial cells have been demonstrated in both menstrual effluent and in peritoneal fluid of reproductive-aged women. Supporting evidence for this theory includes work demonstrating endometriosis in women with genital tract outflow obstruction (up to 10% of teenagers with congenital outflow obstruction) and the fact that endometriotic implants most frequently appear in areas immediately adjacent to the tubal ostia and in the dependent regions of the pelvis (Figs. 118-1 and 118-2).

Endometriosis may arise from metaplasia of the multipotential coelomic epithelium. This epithelial metaplasia may occur in response to an inducing event such as expo-sure to menstrual effluent, estrogen, and progesterone. Supporting evidence includes ovarian surface epithelium differentiation into a variety of histologic cell types; peritoneal decidual reaction during pregnancy; and the rare occurrence of endometriosis in prepubertal girls and women with congenital absence of the uterus.

Research is continuing on the relationship between endometriosis and the immune response. The failure of the immune response may involve decreased cellular immunity with impaired natural killer cell cytotoxicity and decreased humoral response with impaired secretory product elaboration from B-cell lymphocytes. Combined, these defects in both cellular-mediated and humoral-mediated immunity likely contribute to faulty clearance of ectopic endometriotic implants and subsequent development of the disease. The exaggerated response may involve overactive peritoneal macrophages that secrete multiple growth factors and cytokines and exhibit impaired phagocytic properties in patients with endometriosis.

Lymphatic and vascular dissemination have been proposed to explain the development of endometriosis in sites distant from the pelvis including the lung, brain, and spinal column. Endometriotic involvement of pelvic lymph nodes has been reported in 30% of women with the disease. Iatrogenic spread has been implicated to explain the

Figure 118-1 Endometriosis: Laparoscopic Views.

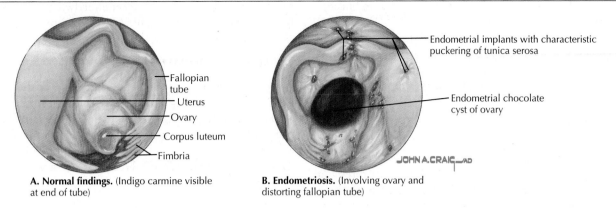

Fallopian tube
Uterus
Ovary
Corpus luteum
Fimbria

Endometrial implants with characteristic puckering of tunica serosa

Endometrial chocolate cyst of ovary

JOHN A.CRAIG_AD

A. Normal findings. (Indigo carmine visible at end of tube)

B. Endometriosis. (Involving ovary and distorting fallopian tube)

Figure 118-2 Endometriosis: Pelvis—Sites of Implantation.

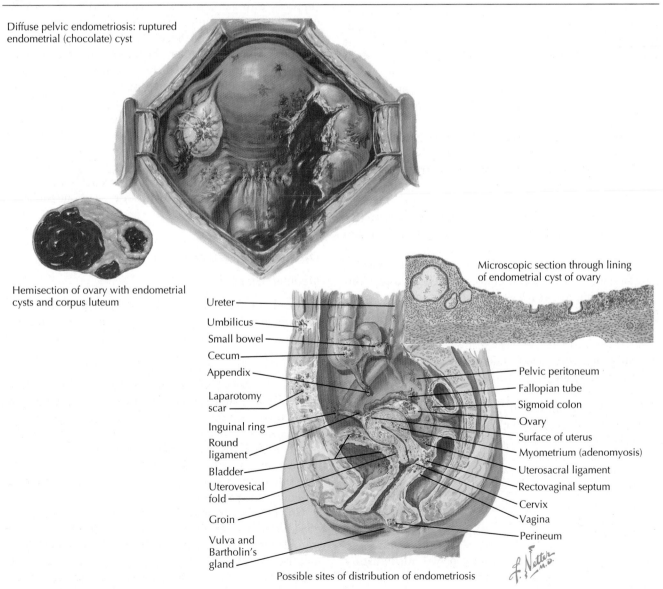

Diffuse pelvic endometriosis: ruptured endometrial (chocolate) cyst

Hemisection of ovary with endometrial cysts and corpus luteum

Microscopic section through lining of endometrial cyst of ovary

Ureter
Umbilicus
Small bowel
Cecum
Appendix
Laparotomy scar
Inguinal ring
Round ligament
Bladder
Uterovesical fold
Groin
Vulva and Bartholin's gland

Pelvic peritoneum
Fallopian tube
Sigmoid colon
Ovary
Surface of uterus
Myometrium (adenomyosis)
Uterosacral ligament
Rectovaginal septum
Cervix
Vagina
Perineum

Possible sites of distribution of endometriosis

F. Netter M.D.

appearance of endometriosis in the anterior abdominal wall after abdominal surgery and, more rarely, in episiotomy scar sites.

Genetic predisposition has also been described. A study has shown a sevenfold increase in the incidence of endometriosis in relatives of women with the disease and that 1 in 10 women with severe disease have a mother or sister with symptomatic disease.

Clinical Presentation

The heterogeneity of endometriosis symptom expression should not be overlooked, with as many as one third of patients lacking symptoms. The classic presentation is that of cyclical pelvic pain that develops 2 to 4 days before the onset of menses. A more traditional clinical picture of endometriosis includes secondary dysmenorrhea, dyspareunia, infertility, a fixed retroverted uterus, and tender nodularity of the cul-de-sac. However, in a Brisbane study, only 5% of 717 patients with endometriosis had this complete clinical picture. Moreover, clinicians have often observed an inverse relationship between the extent of observable endometriotic disease and the extent of pain.

Symptoms include cyclical pelvic pain, secondary dysmenorrhea, dyspareunia, abnormal uterine bleeding, constitutional symptoms, and infertility. Cyclical pelvic pain may result from cyclical swelling of endometriosis implants with blood extravasation into surrounding tissues. Secondary dysmenorrhea, described as a constant pain, may occur in 30% of patients and is a dominant symptom in adolescents. Dyspareunia, a deep pelvic pain during intercourse, occurs in about 30% of patients and may be secondary to immobility of pelvic organs or stretching of scarred tissues and uterine support tissues. Abnormal bleeding occurs in up to 15% of patients and may be secondary to ovulatory dysfunction, coincidental fibroids, or adenomyosis. Constitutional symptoms such as cyclical gastrointestinal complaints (cyclical diarrhea or constipation, abdominal pain) or urinary complaints (urinary frequency, hematuria, or dysuria) are experienced in as many as 15% of patients. Infertility may accompany endometriosis; however, in the work of O'Connor, it occurred in a minority of patients (13%).

Findings on examination include fixed uterine retroversion (up to 15% of patients); tenderness and nodularity in the cul-de-sac and rectovaginal septum (up to 30% of patients), best confirmed by rectovaginal examination; and uterine tenderness or enlargement with adnexal swelling (up to 20% to 30% of patients).

Differential Diagnosis

The differential diagnosis includes pelvic inflammatory disease, ovarian neoplasms, intermittent ovarian torsion, hemorrhagic ovarian cysts, uterine myomas with degeneration, adenomyosis, primary dysmenorrhea, and functional bowel disease such as irritable bowel syndrome.

Diagnostic Approach

Although symptoms are strongly suggestive of the disease process, definitive diagnosis requires biopsy samples taken at the time of laparoscopy or laparotomy to confirm the presence of extrauterine endometrial glands and stroma. Staging is based on the updated scoring system from the American Society for Reproductive Medicine.

Management and Therapy

The goal of therapy is relief of pain and preservation of fertility. Both medical and surgical options have been effective in relief of pain when compared with expectant management. Medical therapies available are designed to suppress estrogen synthesis, thereby inducing atrophy of endometriotic implants. Medical options include gonadotropin-releasing hormone (GnRH) agonists, oral contraceptives and other hormonal treatments, and danazol. Surgical options include ablation or excision of implants, excision of endometriomas, lysis of adhesions, and even appendectomy. The appendix is involved in up to 13% of cases. Presacral neurectomy and uterosacral nerve ablation provide additional options. The surgical approach can involve laparoscopy or laparotomy. Finally, definitive surgical management, when other alternatives have proved unsuccessful in symptom relief, requires total abdominal hysterectomy with or without bilateral salpingo-oophorectomy.

Optimum Treatment

Medical Therapy

Although the ultimate goal of endometriosis therapy is pain relief and protection of fertility, the goal of medical therapy is amenorrhea. Available medical therapies appear equally effective for treatment of symptoms and improvement in American fertility staging of disease scores and recurrence rates when compared with placebo. Recurrence rates after discontinuation of therapy have been reported as 5% to 15% in the first year and as high as 40% to 50% in 5 years. Recurrence appears directly related to the extent of the original disease, occurring in 35% in women with minimal disease and 75% in women with severe disease. The side-effect profile appears to be the primary factor in selection of the medical option used.

GnRH agonists bind to receptors leading to decreased gonadotropin secretion and subsequent decreased ovarian steroidogenesis. Therapy is usually recommended for 6 months. Agents available (leuprolide acetate, nafarelin acetate, and goserelin acetate) can be administered through intramuscular, intranasal, and subcutaneous routes. Medical oophorectomy leads to endometriosis pain relief in 75% to 90% of women with disease. Bothersome side effects include hot flashes, vaginal dryness, insomnia, headaches, diminished libido, mood swings, and breast changes. Bone density may decrease by 2% to 7% during the 6-month course of treatment but completely recovers by 12 to 24 months after completion of therapy. Add-back therapy with low doses of estrogen and progesterone has been used to ease side effects associated primarily with estrogen deficiency and appears to attenuate loss of bone mineral density while not interfering with the effectiveness of GnRH agonist therapy.

Oral contraceptives taken continuously to induce amenorrhea are effective therapy for endometriosis. Although 80% of women experience symptom improvement, side effects most common with this therapy include weight gain and breast tenderness. Other hormonal therapies include daily medroxyprogesterone (10-30 mg po qd) and depomedroxyprogesterone (150 to 200 mg intramuscularly every 3 months). The antiprogesterone mifepristone (RU486) has also demonstrated success in inducing amenorrhea, decreasing pain symptoms, and decreasing endometriotic lesion size. No large randomized controlled trial has been performed to date on the use of mifepristone in women with endometriosis.

Danazol, an attenuated androgen, is a derivative of 17α-ethinyltestosterone. Although its mechanism of action is not entirely clear, danazol binds to androgen and progesterone receptors as well as to sex hormone–binding globulin, inhibiting ovarian steroidogenesis as well as midcycle luteinizing hormone release. Amenorrhea is usually induced within 6 to 8 weeks of initiating therapy. Side effects include acne, hot flashes, depression, headaches, weight gain, and altered libido. Other androgen-related effects such as increased facial hair, clitoral hypertrophy, and voice changes are experienced by 80% of patients. As a result, 20% of women discontinue treatment.

Surgical Therapy

Surgical therapy is often used for diagnostic purposes and after the failure of medical therapy. Conservative therapy includes diagnostic laparoscopy accompanied by laser or electrocautery ablation of implants. Laser ablation has been effective in 95% of women at 18 months after surgery. Midline pelvic pain has been relieved by laparoscopic uterosacral nerve ablation and presacral neurectomy; however, there are no evidence-based studies comparing these procedures to placebo or sham procedures. More definitive surgical therapy includes hysterectomy with preservation of one or both ovaries for women in their 20s and 30s. In women for whom future fertility is not a consideration, definitive surgical therapy by total abdominal hysterectomy with bilateral salpingo-oophorectomy may be warranted.

Avoiding Treatment Errors

Contraindications to estrogen therapy include unexplained vaginal bleeding, the presence of breast or endometrial cancer, active liver disease, and active thrombophlebitis. Conservative therapy, particularly conservative surgical therapy, should be considered in all cases where future fertility is desired.

Future Directions

The remarkable heterogeneity of endometriosis provides both a diagnostic and management challenge. Although current therapy is focused on steroidogenesis suppression or surgical ablation or excision, future therapies may be directed toward some of the multiple immunologic mediators potentially involved in endometriosis development. Animal studies currently suggest that aromatase inhibitors, selective estrogen and selective progesterone receptor modulators, and immunomodulatory agents such as tumor necrosis factor-α may eventually have a role in therapy. Evidence-based medicine should guide therapy based on trials designed to study the effectiveness of current therapies, including the comparison of medical and surgical approaches. With this information, both the patient and her clinician can make better-informed treatment decisions in dealing with this common and at times disabling condition.

Additional Resource

Stenchever MA, Droegemueller W, Herbst AL, Mishell DR Jr: Comprehensive Gynecology, 4th ed. St Louis, Mosby, 2001.

EVIDENCE

All articles below provide a helpful overview perspective and data that remain timely to the overall understanding of endometriosis pathophysiology and the current science behind management options available to patients and providers at this time.

1. Farquhar C, Sutton C: The evidence for the management of endometriosis. Curr Opin Obstet Gynecol 10(4):321-332, 1998.
2. Fedele L, Parazzini F, Bianchi S, et al: Stage and localization of pelvic endometriosis and pain. Fertil Steril 53(1):155-158, 1990.
3. Ferrero S, Abbamonte LH, Anserini P, et al: Future perspectives in the medical treatment of endometriosis. Obstet Gynecol Surv 60(12):817-826, 2005.
4. Halme J, Hammond MG, Hulka JF, et al: Retrograde menstruation in healthy women and in patients with endometriosis. Obstet Gynecol 64(2):151-154, 1984.
5. Kruitwagen RF, Poels LG, Willemsen WN, et al: Endometrial epithelial cells in peritoneal fluid during early follicular phase. Fertil Steril 55(2):297-303, 1991.
6. O'Connor DT: Endometriosis (Current Reviews in Obstetrics and Gynaecology). Edinburgh, Churchill Livingstone, 1987.
7. Revised American Society for Reproductive Medicine classification of endometriosis. Fertil Steril 67(5):817-821, 1997.
8. Simpson JL, Elias S, Malinak LR, Buttram VC Jr: Heritable aspects of endometriosis. I. Genetic studies. Am J Obstet Gynecol 137(3):327-331, 1980.

Menopause

Introduction

Menopause is technically defined as the permanent cessation of menses, although the term is commonly used in association with the clinical manifestations and consequences of ovarian failure. Menopause is a physiologic event in the lives of all women. The clinical manifestations and consequences vary in type and intensity. The age of onset is genetically predetermined and independent of factors such as race, education, and socioeconomic status, as well as weight, height, and age at time of last pregnancy. Cigarette smoking has been shown consistently to hasten menopause by about 1 year. The average age of menopause in the United States is 51 years, and although this is normally distributed with 95% confidence limits between 45 and 55 years of age, about 1% of women experience menopause before age 40. The climacteric, the time during which women transition from reproductive years to postmenopausal years, usually lasts 4 years. The average life expectancy in the United States is 78 years; most women will live one third of their lives in the postmenopausal state. It is estimated that there are 60 million women in the United States older than 50 years.

Etiology and Pathogenesis

Ovarian failure leads to menopause (Fig. 119-1). Diminished ovarian function is present several years before the permanent cessation of menstruation. The number of ovarian follicles and follicular cell production of the glycoprotein inhibin, which functions to inhibit pituitary production of follicle-stimulating hormone (FSH), decrease with age, causing FSH levels to rise. Because FSH release is primarily controlled by inhibin, measurement of FSH levels is not a useful approach to determining therapeutic doses of postmenopausal estrogen replacement; FSH levels remain elevated even with the administration of large doses of exogenous estrogen. Granulosa and thecal cells degenerate, with ovarian estradiol secretion waning significantly up to 1 year before menopause, whereas stromal cells continue to produce the androgens androstenedione and testosterone.

Premature ovarian failure, or ovarian failure before the age of 40 years, occurs in up to 1% of women, with X chromosome abnormalities accounting for most cases. Women with a family history of early menopause may have as much as 6 times the likelihood of menopause before age 46 years, with the strongest association seen in women who had mothers or sisters undergoing menopause before age 40 years. Surgical removal of the ovaries and chemotherapy can induce menopause and associated postmenopausal symptoms.

Clinical Presentation

Although hot flushes and vaginal dryness are commonly associated with the postmenopausal state, change in menstrual cycle length is one of the first signs of menopause. A consequence of waning ovarian function, this change in cycle length reflects increasing anovulatory cycles and can occur up to 4 years before menopause.

Hot flushes, which occur in up to 50% of women, likely result from a central nervous system–mediated change in hypothalamic thermoregulation. The frequency and severity of this symptom corresponds to the magnitude of estrogen level fluctuation; the greater the estrogen level fluctuation, the more frequent and severe the hot flushes. The incidence of flushes declines with time, with only 20% of women reporting such symptoms 4 years after menopause. Obesity leads to fewer complaints of hot flushes given increased peripheral aromatization of androstenedione to estrone in adipose tissues.

Vaginal dryness and genitourinary atrophy are frequent complaints of women in the climacteric. Estrogen deficiency may lead to atrophy of vaginal epithelium, causing

Figure 119-1 Pituitary and Ovarian Hormone Changes in Menopause.

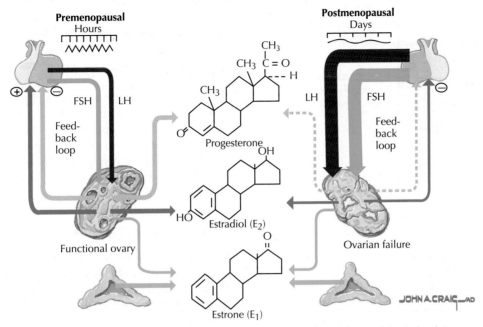

Hormone levels increase and decrease cyclically during menstrual cycle. Modulation occurs by pulsatile release of gonadotropins and positive and negative feedback loops.

In postmenopausal period, gonadotropin levels increase and ovarian hormone levels decrease secondary to ovarian failure. Endogenous estrogen is primarily of adrenal origin, and E_1/E_2 ratio is reversed.

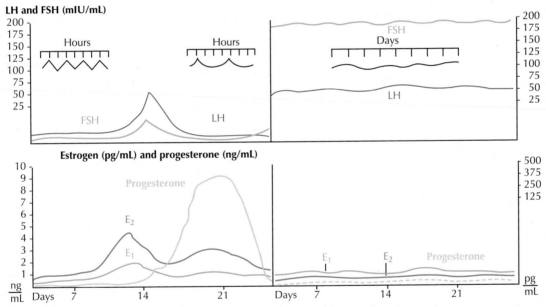

the symptoms of itching, light vaginal discharge, dyspareunia, and even vaginal bleeding (Fig. 119-2). Decreased libido has also been associated with menopause. Decreased collagen content associated with estrogen deficiency may lead to loss of support of the vaginal walls and uterus. Other estrogen-deficiency related symptoms include urinary urgency, frequency, nocturia, and dysuria as estrogen-dependent lower urinary tract epithelial tissues atrophy.

Menopause is also associated with change in body weight and total body fat. The randomized Postmeno-pausal Estrogen/Progestin Interventions study reported less weight gain in women on hormone replacement as compared with placebo. A reduced shift in body fat to the abdominal area was also noted, a factor associated with higher cardiovascular morbidity and mortality.

Other symptoms include increased insomnia, anxiety, mood lability, and depression. What is unclear is whether estrogen administration, which has been shown to improve such symptoms, works directly on the symptom of concern or alleviates hot flushes, allowing women to sleep better, thus leading to resolution of symptoms. Migraine head-

Figure 119-2 Target Organ Changes in Menopause.

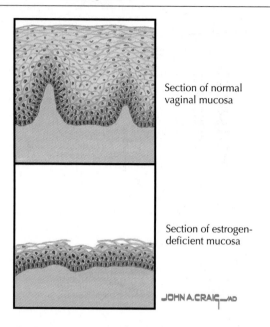

Section of normal vaginal mucosa

Section of estrogen-deficient mucosa

JOHN A.CRAIG_AD

aches may improve with menopause, whereas tension headaches typically remain unchanged. Cognitive function may also be affected. In one study, reported mental status examination scores of postmenopausal women taking estrogen were significantly higher than those of women not taking estrogen.

Differential Diagnosis

The differential diagnosis for menopausal symptoms is narrow. The most common additional diagnosis to consider is anxiety.

Diagnostic Approach

The diagnosis of menopause relies primarily on the history. Menstrual cycle irregularity secondary to oligo-ovulation or anovulation is commonly reported. Intermittent hot flushes secondary to fluctuating estrogen levels may lead to interrupted sleep, fatigue, irritability, anxiety, and depression. Personal and family history regarding cardiovascular and osteoporosis risk factors is important.

Physical examination should include weight, height, and blood pressure. Pelvic examination may reveal atrophic changes of the external genitalia, including thinning of the labial tissues and fusion of labial minora folds with the labia majora. Thinning of vaginal mucosa with loss of rugation commonly occurs, as does decreased vaginal pH. Serum FSH and luteinizing hormone concentrations are elevated.

Yearly mammograms should be obtained in all post-menopausal women older than 50 years presenting for annual care. It is difficult to set an upper age range for

cervical cancer screening. It is generally recommended that women older than 30 years who have had three consecutive negative Papanicolaou tests should be screened at 2- to 3-year intervals.

Management and Therapy

Why attempt to manage and treat a physiologic condition? This is a question posed to clinicians by many patients. The answer lies in the appreciation of the health problems of postmenopausal women and the preventative measures available. Two major health problems for which preventative measures are available include cardiovascular disease and osteoporosis.

Cardiovascular Disease

Cardiovascular disease is responsible for more postmenopausal deaths than all other causes of death combined. Cardiovascular disease is 3 times as common in men as in women before menopause. This ratio of myocardial infarction in women to men older than 50 years changes to 2 : 1. As such, it is important that postmenopausal women address cardiovascular risk factors aggressively, including control of hypertension, hypercholesterolemia, and diabetes mellitus, and cessation of cigarette smoking.

Controversy in the literature about the use of estrogens to reduce cardiac risk has existed for many years. On the basis of observational and epidemiologic studies and strong experimental data, estrogen therapy was long recommended for cardiac risk reduction in women. This recommendation came under question after the Women's Health Initiative Randomized Controlled Trial, in which a small increased cardiac risk of nominal statistical significance was seen in postmenopausal women taking combination (estrogen-progestin) hormone replacement therapy. However, estrogen-only therapy did not significantly affect the incidence of coronary heart disease (CHD). *Interestingly, younger women taking estrogen alone may have a reduced risk for CHD.* Thus, initiation of combination hormone replacement therapy solely for prophylaxis against myocardial infarction is not currently recommended. Estrogen-only therapy for CHD prophylaxis may have a role in younger postmenopausal women without preexisting heart disease.

Osteoporosis

Characterized by decreased bone mass, osteoporosis is usually asymptomatic and often not detected until fracture occurs. In the United States, about 800,000 fractures occur per year; 300,000 of these are hip fractures, with 15% of hip fractures in women older than 80 being fatal within 6 months. Fractures may occur many years after onset of the disease. The underlying pathophysiology in postmenopausal women is increased osteoclastic activity associated with a normal rate of bone formation. Dual-energy x-ray absorptiometry is currently the most accurate test for measurement of bone density, although 25% of bone needs to be lost before osteoporosis can be detected by routine examination. Markers of bone resorption, such as urinary excretion of collagen degradation products, are of limited use in the diagnosis of osteoporosis.

The most rapid phase of bone mass accrual occurs during puberty into the mid-20s. Bone mineral density may continue to improve until women reach their mid-30s, when peak bone mass is reached. After menopause, bone density decreases by 1% to 2% per year, more rapidly in trabecular than in cortical bone, with 25% of white and Asian women experiencing vertebral compression fractures by age 60 years if not taking hormone replacement. Risk factors include family history, race (white, Asian), body type, sedentary lifestyle, dietary calcium deficiencies, and tobacco use. Notably, these risk factors only identify 30% of women with osteoporosis.

Although weight-bearing exercise is important for overall health, exercise alone does not prevent postmenopausal bone loss. Recommendations from the National Institutes of Health (NIH) consensus panel of 1994 include that postmenopausal women take 1000 to 1500 mg of calcium per day along with vitamin D, 400 to 800 IU. Current data suggest that this level is too high and that calcium supplementation is necessary only for those women ingesting less than 500 mg per day if they are taking estrogen replacement therapy. NIH recommendations remain in place at this time.

Estrogen replacement appears to retard bone resorption. Estrogen and progesterone receptors have been identified in osteoblasts. Decreased postmenopausal bone loss and a decreased incidence of hip and spine fracture have been reported. The minimum estrogen dose observed to prevent bone loss was 0.625 mg of conjugated equine estrogens, 0.5 mg of esterified estrogens, or 0.3 mg of conjugated equine estrogen in the presence of 1500 mg of calcium each day, or 0.05 mg of transdermal estrogen. The addition of progestins to hormone replacement regimens does not appear to attenuate this bone-protective effect.

When hormone replacement is not an option, bisphosphonates such as alendronate and risedronate are available to decrease bone resorption and reduce fracture incidence. Calcitonin through nasal spray is also available for osteoporosis treatment and has been shown to increase vertebral bone mass. Finally, the selective estrogen receptor modulator (SERM) raloxifene has been shown to increase vertebral bone mass, although data available at this time do not demonstrate protective effects against hip fracture.

Optimum Treatment

Hormone Replacement Therapy

The importance of preventative measures has risen to new prominence since the publication of the Women's Health Initiative Randomized Controlled Trial. Such measures include balanced diet, multivitamin and calcium supplementation, and regular exercise. In some circumstances, selective serotonin reuptake inhibitors (SSRIs) may play a role in symptom relief, particularly relief from the estrogen deficiency symptom of hot flushes. Hormone replacement therapy (HRT) with either estrogen alone in those women who have undergone hysterectomy or with estrogen-progestin combination in women with an intact uterus continues to play a central role in postmenopausal medical management. HRT remains extremely effective for relief of estrogen deficiency symptoms such as hot flushes and for relief of symptoms of urogenital atrophy such as vaginal dryness, dyspareunia, and urinary frequency. HRT regimens are numerous. In the United States, continuous and cyclical regimens are most commonly used. The continuous regimen uses conjugated equine estrogen, 0.625 mg, and medroxyprogesterone acetate, 2.5 mg, given daily. The cyclical regimen uses 0.625 mg of conjugated equine estrogen given on days 1 to 25 and 5 mg of medroxyprogesterone acetate given on days 14 to 25. On the continuous regimen, women frequently have some degree of irregular spotting for up to 3 months after initiating therapy. On the cyclical regimen, most women demonstrate withdrawal bleeding.

Avoiding Treatment Errors

The area of most potential concern for patients and physicians is estrogen replacement therapy, and it is important to elicit a history of potential complications. Contraindications to estrogen replacement therapy include unexplained vaginal bleeding, the presence of breast or endometrial cancer, active liver disease, and active thrombophlebitis.

Future Directions

Postmenopausal health is affecting an ever-increasing number of women in the United States, and preventative health care is, at long last, becoming a focus for women and health care providers alike. The health benefits of hormone replacement have been outlined; however, concerns remain regarding breast cancer risks, particularly in long-term users. The Women's Health Initiative Randomized Controlled Trial has provided some insight into this problem. The development and longer-term use of agents such as the SERMs may also provide preventative health advantages without the potential adverse effects on endometrium and breast. Evidence-based medicine will continue to provide guidance in efforts to optimize the health care of postmenopausal women.

Additional Resource

Stenchever MA, Droegemueller W, Herbst AL, Mishell DR Jr: Comprehensive Gynecology, 4th ed. St Louis, Mosby, 2001.

EVIDENCE

All articles below provide helpful overview perspective and data that remain timely to the overall understanding of menopause physiology and the current science behind management options.

1. American College of Obstetricians and Gynecologists: Cervical cytology screening. ACOG Practice Bulletin No. 45. Obstet Gynecol 102:417-427, 2003.
2. Anderson GL, Limacher M, Assaf AR: Effects of conjugated equine estrogen in postmenopausal women with hysterectomy: The Women's Health Initiative randomized controlled trial. JAMA 291(14):1701-1712, 2004.
3. Cramer DW, Xu H, Harlow BL: Family history as a predictor of early menopause. Fertil Steril 64(4):740-745, 1995.
4. Effects of estrogen or estrogen/progestin regimens on heart disease risk factors in postmenopausal women. The Postmenopausal Estrogen/Progestin Interventions (PEPI) Trial. The Writing Group for the PEPI Trial. JAMA 273(3):199-208, 1995.
5. McKinlay SM, Brambilla DJ, Posner JG: The normal menopause transition. Maturitas 14(2):103-115, 1992.
6. Precis V: An Update in Obstetrics and Gynecology. Washington, DC, American College of Obstetricians and Gynecologists, 1994.
7. Rossouw JE, Anderson GL, Prentice RL, et al: Risks and benefits of estrogen plus progestin in healthy postmenopausal women: Principal results from the Women's Health Initiative Randomized Controlled Trial. JAMA 288(3):321-333, 2002.
8. Stanford JL, Hartge P, Brinton LA, et al: Factors influencing the age at natural menopause. J Chronic Dis 40(11):995-1002, 1987.
9. Steffens DC, Norton MC, Plassman BL, et al: Enhanced cognitive performance with estrogen in nondemented community-dwelling older women. J Am Geriatr Soc 47(10):1171-1175, 1999.

Erectile Dysfunction

Introduction

Erectile dysfunction (ED) is the inability to achieve or maintain an erection adequate for sexual intercourse. Based on extrapolated data from the Massachusetts Male Aging Study, ED affects some 20 to 30 million American men, most of whom are older than 50 years. This epidemiologic study of a homogeneous suburban Boston community surveyed 1709 men and reported that 52% of men aged 40 to 70 years had ED: 10% of the total sample had complete ED, 25% moderate, and 17% minimal. The prevalence of ED increases with age, with moderate and complete ED increasing most markedly. The percentages of ED were increased substantially in men with risk factors including cardiac disease, antihypertensive and vasoactive drug use, obesity, and tobacco use.

Physiology of Erections

Sexual stimulation causes release of the neurotransmitter nitric oxide (NO) from nerve endings in the corpus cavernosum, in turn increasing blood flow to the corpora cavernosa (Fig. 120-1). NO production results in relaxation of the corpus cavernosum smooth muscle tissue. The venous structures beneath the tunica albuginea are compressed, inhibiting venous outflow and producing a rigid erection. In the penis, NO is available from nitrergic nerve and endothelial cells. By stimulating the guanylate cyclase system and increasing cyclic guanosine monophosphate (cGMP), NO causes an efflux of calcium from the smooth muscle cell, producing relaxation. cGMP is broken down by the enzyme phosphodiesterase (PDE). The predominate PDE type in corpus cavernosum is type 5 (PDE5). The PDE5 inhibitors (PDE5i) such as sildenafil, tadalafil, and vardenafil, prolong the presence of cGMP and facilitate the relaxation of corpus cavernosum smooth muscle.

Etiology and Pathogenesis

ED has both organic and psychogenic etiologies, with 60% of patients having organic ED caused by vasculogenic, neurogenic, hormonal, or smooth muscle abnormalities (Fig. 120-2). Fewer than 40% of patients have pure psychogenic ED. The etiology of psychogenic ED remains controversial. Stress, anxiety disorders, and depression produce an overactivity of α agonists in the corpus cavernosum smooth muscle tissue, and this imbalance of α stimulation may inhibit smooth muscle relaxation.

Clinical Presentation

Risk Factors

Risk factors for ED include systemic diseases that produce vascular abnormalities, including hyperlipidemia, diabetes mellitus, the effects of hypertension and antihypertensive therapy, and atherosclerosis.

Neurogenic ED is seen with multiple sclerosis, diabetes mellitus, and paraplegia, and following radical pelvic surgery or radiation for pelvic malignancy such as prostate, colon, or bladder cancer.

Hormonal abnormalities and hypogonadism are also risk factors for ED, producing not only central nervous system abnormalities and low libido but also local changes in corpus cavernosum smooth muscle relaxation.

Psychologic causes are significant, and ED is frequently associated with depression, even of mild degree. Treatment of depression using selective serotonin reuptake inhibitors (SSRIs) further enhances ED by decreasing and delaying ejaculatory function.

Evaluation

A careful general and sexual history is the cornerstone in the evaluation and treatment of patients with ED. History

Figure 120-1 Cellular Mechanisms of Penile Smooth Muscle Relaxation.
cAMP, cyclic adenosine monophosphate; GTP, guanosine 5'-triphosphate.

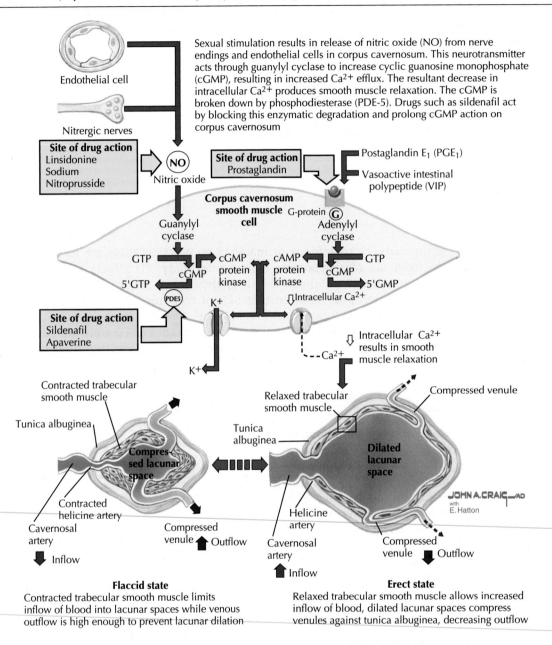

Sexual stimulation results in release of nitric oxide (NO) from nerve endings and endothelial cells in corpus cavernosum. This neurotransmitter acts through guanylyl cyclase to increase cyclic guanosine monophosphate (cGMP), resulting in increased Ca2+ efflux. The resultant decrease in intracellular Ca2+ produces smooth muscle relaxation. The cGMP is broken down by phosphodiesterase (PDE-5). Drugs such as sildenafil act by blocking this enzymatic degradation and prolong cGMP action on corpus cavernosum

Flaccid state
Contracted trabecular smooth muscle limits inflow of blood into lacunar spaces while venous outflow is high enough to prevent lacunar dilation

Erect state
Relaxed trabecular smooth muscle allows increased inflow of blood, dilated lacunar spaces compress venules against tunica albuginea, decreasing outflow

should include information regarding age of onset, associated lifestyle changes at onset, speed of onset, and the presence or absence of erections with other partners, during masturbation, and at night and in the early morning. Patients should be asked about ejaculatory function, postejaculatory pain, and ejaculatory volume. Careful questioning regarding decreased libido may suggest a hormonal cause but more often is associated with clinical depression. Because ED is highly associated with lower urinary tract symptoms, patients should be asked about voiding symptoms.

Patients who present with organic ED most often have a gradual onset beginning with intermittent loss of erec-

tions, decreased duration, and difficulty with maintaining erections until ejaculation. History is the most proficient method of identifying patients complaining of premature ejaculation who may also present for evaluation of ED.

Psychogenic ED most often begins with abrupt onset precipitated by psychological abnormalities such as depression, anxiety disorder, changes in lifestyle, or relationship problems. These men usually have preserved nocturnal and morning erections and may be functional with masturbation. Patients with organic ED also have secondary psychological ED. Patients with pure loss of libido or with other symptoms of androgen deficiency of the aging male can be identified by a hormone profile.

Figure 120-2 Etiology and Pathogenesis of Erectile Dysfunction.

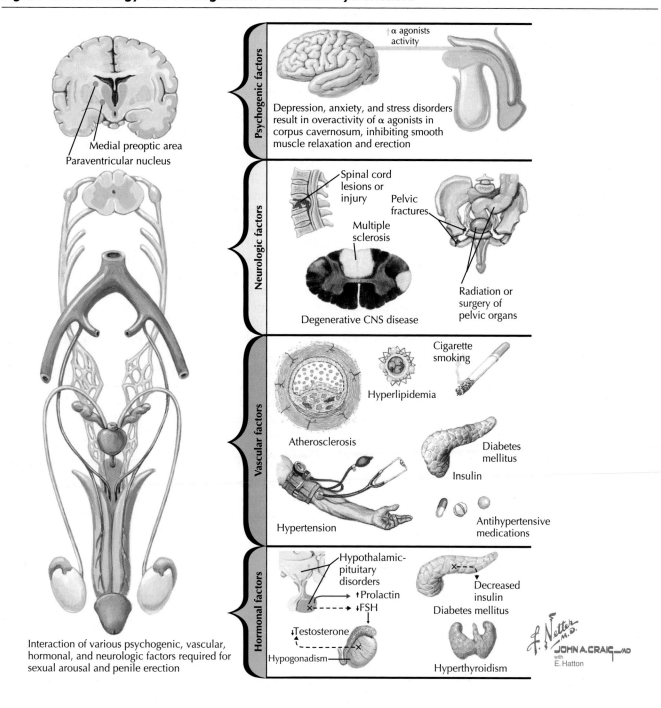

Medial preoptic area
Paraventricular nucleus

Interaction of various psychogenic, vascular, hormonal, and neurologic factors required for sexual arousal and penile erection

Psychogenic factors

↑α agonists activity

Depression, anxiety, and stress disorders result in overactivity of α agonists in corpus cavernosum, inhibiting smooth muscle relaxation and erection

Neurologic factors

Spinal cord lesions or injury

Pelvic fractures

Multiple sclerosis

Radiation or surgery of pelvic organs

Degenerative CNS disease

Vascular factors

Cigarette smoking

Hyperlipidemia

Atherosclerosis

Diabetes mellitus

Insulin

Hypertension

Antihypertensive medications

Hormonal factors

Hypothalamic-pituitary disorders

↑Prolactin

↓FSH

Decreased insulin

Diabetes mellitus

↓Testosterone

Hypogonadism

Hyperthyroidism

Physical Examination

The physical examination is focused on secondary sex characteristics, hair distribution, and genitalia. Evaluation of peripheral pulses, neurologic reflexes such as the bulbocavernosus reflex, and anal sphincter tone may help to identify some patients with peripheral neuropathy from nerve injury or diabetes. Changes in testicular size and consistency may be associated with primary hypogonadism. General physical examination of blood pressure, lower extremity reflexes and pulses, and visual fields (to evaluate pituitary tumors) may suggest underlying systemic causes for ED.

Differential Diagnosis

A careful history and laboratory studies are most important in the differential diagnosis. Differentiation of ejaculatory dysfunction and other nonerectile sexual dysfunction is imperative in recommending the best treatment. Many men complain of premature ejaculation (PE) as ED. Because the treatment for PE is an SSRI antidepressant, these must be differentiated. Androgen deficiency should also be excluded by history and a morning testosterone measurement. In couples with significant relationship issues, sexual counseling should be encouraged.

Diagnostic Approach

Because ED may be the first symptom of diabetes, hypercholesterolemia, hypertension, or other systemic disease, it is important to evaluate patients thoroughly for each of these disorders. A hormone profile should include a morning total testosterone. If the total testosterone is abnormal, a follow-up repeat total testosterone, free testosterone, luteinizing hormone, and prolactin may identify patients with androgen deficiency, pituitary tumors, or other causes of hypogonadism. Testosterone is typically low and prolactin high in patients who have pituitary tumors or chronic renal failure on hemodialysis. A lipid profile, hemoglobin A1C, and other general medical studies may be helpful.

For patients requiring additional investigation before surgical reconstruction or vascular bypass, specialized investigation such as Doppler penile blood flow studies following injection of vasoactive agents, nocturnal penile tumescence monitoring studies, and pelvic angiography may be helpful. Candidates for vascular bypass are usually young men with solitary pelvic artery lesions and a strong history of perineal or pelvic trauma. Vascular bypass surgery in older patients is rarely successful, especially if ED is associated with hypercholesterolemia, diabetes, hypertension, or smoking.

Nocturnal penile tumescence monitoring studies may be helpful in differentiating organic and psychogenic ED in some patients.

Management and Therapy

Initial treatment should focus on modifying medication and lifestyle abnormalities. Smoking cessation, managing diabetes, hypercholesterolemia, and hypertension may improve erectile function and facilitate medical treatment.

Modifying antihypertensive medications to include erection-hospitable agents such as α blockers, angiotensin-converting enzyme inhibitors, and calcium channel blockers may maintain antihypertensive therapy with restoration of erectile function. Patients with low testosterone levels should receive injectable or topical testosterone supplements.

If depression or relationship issues are a significant problem, sexual counseling may be helpful in addition to pharmacologic treatment. Office counseling with patient

and partner may facilitate understanding of the probable causes of erectile dysfunction, treatment alternatives, and expectations.

Optimum Treatment

First-Line Therapy

Oral agents such as sildenafil, tadalafil, and vardenafil are now established as first-line treatment of ED. These selective PDE5i agents facilitate cGMP concentration, duration, and subsequent corpus cavernosal smooth muscle relaxation. There is improvement in erectile function 30 to 60 minutes following ingestion of a PDE5i. The most popular starting dose is 50 mg sildenafil or 10 mg of vardenafil or tadalafil, although most patients respond best to 100 mg or 20 mg, respectively. As many as eight trials may be required for full success and effectiveness. Side effects include headache, dyspepsia, facial flushing, myalgias, and blue vision. PDE5i drugs have been reported to be significantly better in producing erections than placebo in patients with diabetes mellitus, spinal cord injury, hypercholesterolemia, depression, or cardiac disease, following radical prostatectomy, and in psychogenic erectile dysfunction. Although PDE5i drugs are effective in virtually all etiologies and severities of ED, they are least effective in patients with severe vascular disease. PDE5i agents are generally extremely safe; however, they do have additive affects with nitrate agents used for coronary artery disease, producing severe transient hypotension. For this reason, the use of PDE5i agents with nitrate drugs is contraindicated. In patients taking sildenafil after radical prostatectomy, results are best after a bilateral nerve-sparing radical prostatectomy. PDE5i treatment following non-nerve-sparing prostatectomy or pelvic radiation therapy is often unsuccessful.

Second-Line Therapy

Additional therapeutic alternatives are available if oral agents fail to improve erectile function. Intracavernosal pharmacotherapy is most effective in producing physiologic erections. This therapy can be carried out with prostaglandin E_1 (PGE$_1$) or a combination of papaverine and phentolamine. PGE$_1$ can be administered by intracavernosal injection or transurethral pellet.

Transurethral PGE$_1$ is available in 250-, 500-, or 1000-μg doses. Its effectiveness is about 30% in large clinical studies. A small applicator with a pellet of PGE$_1$ is placed in the urethra. After the pellet is deposited and the applicator removed, the patient stimulates the urethra to allow PGE$_1$ to enter the corpus cavernosum. Erection usually occurs in 10 to 15 minutes and is maintained for as long as 40 minutes. Rarely, side effects include prolonged erection or priapism, and significant penile pain, aching, and urethral burning can occur. Although this agent is an excellent addition to use of penile prostheses for further engorgement, its success in patients with ED of significant organic etiology has been disappointing.

Intracavernosal injection of PGE_1 has been widely used for more than two decades. It appears to be safe, although penile aching and occasional prolonged erections do occur. Initial dose of PGE_1 varies from 2.5 to 5 µg. Patients with significant vasculogenic ED require higher starting and maintenance doses. After an initial in-office titration to a dose that produces a firm erection satisfactory for sexual intercourse that lasts no longer than 60 minutes, many men may require at-home dose adjustment. If erections last more than 4 hours, patients should be advised to go to the emergency room for treatment using an α agonist such as intracavernosal phenylephrine or aspiration therapy. Although this complication is rare, early treatment will preserve future erectile function. If intracavernosal PGE_1 is ineffective or produces excessive pain, a combination of papaverine with or without phentolamine and PGE_1 may produce satisfactory erectile function with less penile discomfort. Side effects from this combination include prolonged erections and priapism, corpus cavernosum fibrosis, and occasional transient hypotension.

In addition to prolonged erections and priapism, side effects from PGE_1, as well as papaverine and phentolamine, include penile pain. This complication is most marked with PGE_1 and occurs in about 20% of injections. Patients may also observe hematoma, edema, and occasional corpus cavernosum fibrosis (<5%). Despite initial success rates in excess of 70%, few patients continue injection therapy for more than 3 to 4 years. The reasons for discontinuation include mental anxiety, inadequate erections, penile pain, and poor patient and partner satisfaction.

Avoiding Treatment Errors

Treatment errors include prescribing PDE5 inhibitors for PE because PE is best treated with SSRI agents. Also, many patients in whom PDE5 is unsuccessful require education about use of these drugs and may have improved response with normalization of decreased testosterone levels. PDE5 drugs are contraindicated in men using nitrate medications and in those with cardiovascular status that precludes moderate exercise tolerance.

Devices for Treatment of Erectile Dysfunction

For many years, vacuum erection devices have been used to stimulate, facilitate, and prolong duration of erections. These external devices create a vacuum around the penis to produce engorgement and tumescence, maintained by a constrictive ring placed at the base of the penis. Although the erections that ensue are less natural, they are satisfactory for vaginal penetration and sexual intercourse. The constriction devices may produce penile pain, bruising, scarring, and Peyronie's disease. They may also inhibit ejaculations. Although the cost is low, patient satisfaction is limited. Counseling and careful instruction before initiating use can increase patient satisfaction.

Implantation of penile prostheses is a successful, important method for restoring erectile function in severe ED and for reconstructing the penis of patients with significant Peyronie's disease or priapism. These surgically implanted devices are most often of the inflatable variety and consist of two hollow cylinders placed in the corpora cavernosa of the penis and connected to a small pump device placed in the scrotum. Fluid (normal saline) is supplied by a reservoir placed beneath the rectus muscles. Patients can feel and compress the pump device in the scrotum, fill the cylinders of the corpora cavernosa, and maintain an erection of normal sensation and rigidity throughout sexual intercourse. The device can then be deflated for concealment with excellent cosmetic results. The longevity of these devices is quite satisfactory, with 93% of devices functional at 3 years, 86% at 5 years, and 76% at 10 years after implantation. Mechanical malfunction is treated with device replacement. Patient and partner satisfaction has been reported in excess of 90%.

Androgen Replacement Therapy

In patients with androgen deficiency of the aging male or hypogonadism, testosterone replacement is necessary to enhance libido and facilitate other medical treatment. Testosterone replacement therapy is carried out using long-acting injectable agents, such as testosterone enanthate or cypionate, 200 mg every 2 to 3 weeks, and topical testosterone patches or gel. Topical treatment is more physiologic, with high testosterone levels in the morning and low in the evening, similar to the testosterone levels of young, sexually active males. Similarly, testosterone metabolites estradiol and dihydrotestosterone are maintained best with the topical preparations. The goal of testosterone replacement therapy is to restore testosterone levels to the normal physiologic range. The use of testosterone in eugonadal men with psychogenic erectile dysfunction, while raising testosterone beyond normal levels, is both ineffective and associated with significant potential complications. Testosterone supplementation can be associated with activation of carcinoma of the prostate, increased hematocrit and lipid levels, and increased benign prostatic hyperplasia. Patients treated with testosterone supplementation should be carefully evaluated twice yearly with digital rectal examination, prostate-specific antigen, lipid profile, and hematocrit. For patients with chronic renal failure or macroprolactinomas, normalization of prolactin before testosterone treatment is critical. Use of agents such as bromocriptine or cabergoline, in addition to testosterone replacement, will produce the best subsequent results.

Future Directions

The treatment of ED was revolutionized by the introduction of sildenafil in 1998. Newer agents are being investigated and will provide additional methods of treatment for patients with ED. Central nervous system–acting agents will be available for stimulating erections. The first of these agents, apomorphine SL (sublingual), is currently approved and in use in Europe, whereas the melanotropin agonist PT-141 is undergoing clinical trials. These agents, which stimulate dopamine receptors in the erectile center of the midbrain, have been demonstrated in clinical trials to be effective in producing erectile function. Side effects include nausea, vomiting, and syncope in small numbers of patients with predominate first-dose effect. Treatment of PE with the on-demand serotonin reuptake inhibitor dapoxetine has shown great promise in clinical trials.

Active research is underway to evaluate the feasibility and effectiveness of gene therapy for ED. Gene therapy to restore NO synthase concentrations, endothelial cell function, and potassium channel function in the corpus cavernosum smooth muscle appears, in animal models, to be an excellent method for restoring erectile function lost through diabetes, hypercholesterolemia, and other causes of vascular disease. This mode of therapy may provide a long-term solution for many patients with vasculogenic ED.

Despite the strides made in pharmacologic treatment, many patients will still require surgical reconstruction using penile prostheses. The currently available penile implant and prostheses have been modified and improved during the past 25 years to provide safe, reliable reconstruction for penile abnormalities and ED with low expected complications and morbidity and high patient satisfaction. Newer antibiotic-coated devices have reduced infection risks to less than 1%.

Additional Resource

Carson CC III, Kirby RS, Goldstein I (eds): Textbook of Erectile Dysfunction. Oxford, UK, Isis Medical Media, 1999.
   This textbook is a good general reference.

EVIDENCE

1. Carson CC, Lue TF: Phosphodiesterase type 5 inhibitors for erectile dysfunction. BJU Int 96(3):257-280, 2005.
   This comprehensive review addresses the pharmacology and clinical effects of the three currently available PDE5 inhibitors.
2. Feldman HA, Goldstein I, Hatzichristou DG, et al: Impotence and its medical and psychosocial correlates: Results of the Massachusetts Male Aging Study. J Urol 151:54-61, 1994.
   This most robust and extensive epidemiologic study of male sexual dysfunction has become the index paper from which many other epidemiologic data have been derived.
3. Kostis JB, Jackson G, Rosen R, et al: Sexual dysfunction and cardiac risk (the Second Princeton Consensus Conference). Am J Cardiol 15;96(2):313-321, 2005.
   This report from a consensus conference for the role of cardiovascular factors in erectile dysfunction includes caveats for treatment of men with erectile dysfunction with cardiac disease.
4. Mikhail N: Does testosterone have a role in erectile function? Am J Med 119(5):373-382, 2006.
   The author presents an excellent review of the place of testosterone in the sexual function of men, both physical and psychological.
5. Thompson IM, Tangen CM, Goodman PJ, et al: Erectile dysfunction and subsequent cardiovascular disease. JAMA 294(23):2996-3002, 2005.
   This report is on a study of the incidence of cardiac events and disease in men with erectile dysfunction followed for 5 years.
6. Wald M, Meacham RB, Ross LS, Niederberger CS: Testosterone replacement therapy for older men. J Androl 27(2):126-132, 2006.
   This article provides data on the safety and efficacy of testosterone replacement therapy in hypogonadal men.

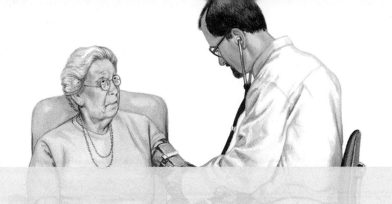
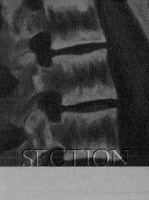

Neurologic Disorders

Disorders of Consciousness

Introduction

Consciousness is the state of being alert, aware, and responsive by thought and physical action to internal and external stimuli. Disorders of consciousness disrupt the level of consciousness, the content of consciousness, or both. More commonly, patients present with depressed levels of consciousness. This chapter focuses on the initial evaluation and treatment of patients presenting acutely with altered levels of consciousness. The etiologies of altered consciousness are varied, and great care must be taken to rapidly identify and treat acute causes, especially those that are potentially life-threatening.

Etiology and Pathogenesis

Anatomically, consciousness is the result of reciprocal interactions of ascending and descending systems. The reticular activating system (RAS) is a collection of nuclei and tracts originating in the medulla and projecting to the thalamus, and subsequent projections from the thalamus ascend to the cortex. Regions of the cortex send descending projections back to the thalamus in a feedback fashion. Arousal is generally attributed to the circuits of the RAS. Awareness is attributed to activity in the higher cortical centers. Impairments of either or both of the ascending and descending systems result in alterations of consciousness. Such impairments may be the result of focal or multifocal structural lesions that injure or compress vital areas of the brain or brainstem, or they may be the result of global neuronal dysfunction resulting from generalized medical disorders.

Clinical Presentation

Patients with disorders of consciousness present with variable degrees of disturbance of both the level and content of consciousness. Disturbances of the level of consciousness are characterized by impaired arousal and wakefulness. Such disturbances may be transient, resolving within seconds to minutes, or prolonged, lasting hours or much longer. Most disturbances of arousal make complete assessment of content of consciousness difficult. However, certain conditions disrupt content without altering the level of consciousness. The various dementias are conditions that may present in such a fashion. Lesions of the hippocampus may also present with isolated memory loss, and dominant hemisphere strokes may present with isolated aphasia.

Patients with altered levels of consciousness vary in the degree of response to stimuli. *Coma* is the most severe degree of depressed consciousness, and patients in coma are unresponsive and unarousable. Patients who are disoriented, sleepy, or inattentive are often described as *confused*, *clouded*, or *lethargic*. *Delirium* is used to describe patients with depressed consciousness and signs of elevated sympathetic tone, such as agitation, elevated heart rate and blood pressure, and hallucinations. *Obtunded* patients require repeated stimuli to maintain attention. *Stuporous* patients provide only minimal response to frequent or constant stimulation.

Other presenting features depend on the etiology of the alteration of consciousness. Patients may present with focal neurologic deficits, especially if the etiology is a structural lesion, and the nature and degree of these deficits depend on the location and size of the lesion or lesions

Figure 121-1 Differential Diagnosis of Altered Consciousness.

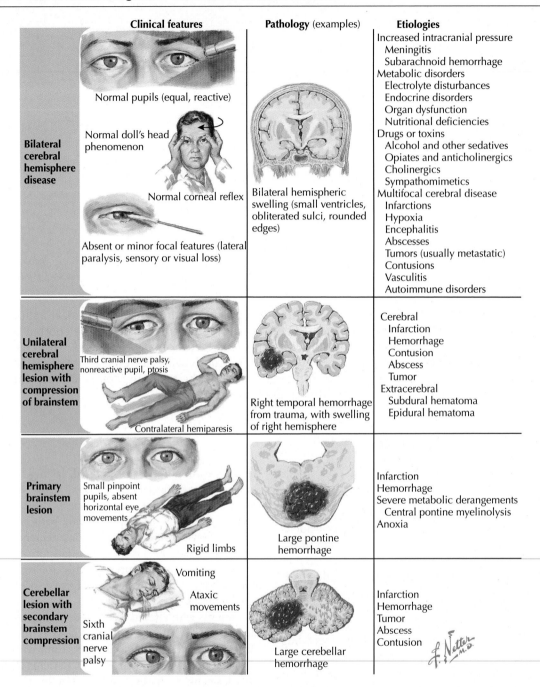

	Clinical features	Pathology (examples)	Etiologies
Bilateral cerebral hemisphere disease	Normal pupils (equal, reactive) — Normal doll's head phenomenon — Normal corneal reflex — Absent or minor focal features (lateral paralysis, sensory or visual loss)	Bilateral hemispheric swelling (small ventricles, obliterated sulci, rounded edges)	Increased intracranial pressure: Meningitis, Subarachnoid hemorrhage; Metabolic disorders: Electrolyte disturbances, Endocrine disorders, Organ dysfunction, Nutritional deficiencies; Drugs or toxins: Alcohol and other sedatives, Opiates and anticholinergics, Cholinergics, Sympathomimetics; Multifocal cerebral disease: Infarctions, Hypoxia, Encephalitis, Abscesses, Tumors (usually metastatic), Contusions, Vasculitis, Autoimmune disorders
Unilateral cerebral hemisphere lesion with compression of brainstem	Third cranial nerve palsy, nonreactive pupil, ptosis — Contralateral hemiparesis	Right temporal hemorrhage from trauma, with swelling of right hemisphere	Cerebral: Infarction, Hemorrhage, Contusion, Abscess, Tumor; Extracerebral: Subdural hematoma, Epidural hematoma
Primary brainstem lesion	Small pinpoint pupils, absent horizontal eye movements — Rigid limbs	Large pontine hemorrhage	Infarction; Hemorrhage; Severe metabolic derangements: Central pontine myelinolysis; Anoxia
Cerebellar lesion with secondary brainstem compression	Vomiting — Ataxic movements — Sixth cranial nerve palsy	Large cerebellar hemorrhage	Infarction; Hemorrhage; Tumor; Abscess; Contusion

(Fig. 121-1). Patients with generalized disorders may also present with focal signs. Isolated cranial nerve deficits can occur in patients with meningitis. Patients in postictal states may manifest transient weakness (Todd's paralysis).

Headache is a common symptom, especially when there is elevated intracranial pressure (ICP) or meningeal irritation. Patients with elevated ICP sometimes complain of visual disturbances and have papilledema or oculomotor abnormalities on examination. Elevated muscle tone is

another association. Cases of subarachnoid hemorrhage (SAH), meningitis, and meningoencephalitis may present with meningismus.

Signs of brainstem compression develop in patients with uncal herniation, brainstem lesions, and large cerebellar lesions. Depending on the severity of the compression, patients may have asymmetric pupils, a unilateral fixed and dilated ("blown") pupil, or bilateral fixed and dilated pupils. A third nerve palsy, hemiparesis, and flexor (decorticate) or extensor (decerebrate) responses to painful stimulation are other possible findings. The examiner should observe carefully for abnormal respiratory patterns (e.g., Cheyne-Stokes respirations, hyperventilation, and apneustic breathing). Patients presenting with evidence of brainstem compression require rapid confirmation of the diagnosis and treatment.

In cases of severe brain injury, patients may present with minimal clinical neurologic function on examination. In situations in which the proximate cause is known and demonstrably irreversible and when coma, absence of brainstem reflexes, and apnea are present, the condition is referred to as *brain death*. In the United States and many other countries, this condition is a legal form of death.

Differential Diagnosis

The causes of altered consciousness are numerous and varied (see Fig. 121-1). Conceptually, causes are often separated into structural lesions and generalized disorders. Structural lesions are divided into traumatic lesions and nontraumatic lesions and can be further divided by location: supratentorial (cerebral hemispheres), brainstem, and cerebellar. Epidural hematomas, subdural hematomas, contusions, and shear injuries occur secondary to trauma. Nontraumatic causes include ischemic strokes, intraparenchymal and intraventricular hemorrhages, SAH, tumors, and abscesses.

A large number of generalized disorders lead to altered consciousness: metabolic disorders, drug intoxication and withdrawal, hypoxia, central nervous system infections, sepsis, autoimmune diseases, hematologic disorders, diffuse vascular disorders (e.g., vasculitis), and seizure disorders (e.g., nonconvulsive status epilepticus and postictal states). Common metabolic causes to consider are electrolyte disturbances (hyponatremia, hypocalcemia, and hypercalcemia), endocrine disorders (hypoglycemia, hyperglycemia, diabetic ketoacidosis, hypothyroidism, hyperthyroidism, hypoadrenalism, and hyperadrenalism), organ dysfunction (uremia and hepatic encephalopathy), and nutritional deficiencies (Wernicke's encephalopathy). Drugs commonly associated with altered mental status include alcohol and other sedatives, opiates, cholinergics, anticholinergics, and sympathomimetics; however, many other drug associations have been reported. Meningitis is associated with many etiologies: bacteria, tuberculosis, syphilis, fungi, viruses, and metastases. Viruses, including herpes simplex virus (HSV), are also commonly associated with encephalitis.

Conditions Often Mistaken for Coma

In locked-in states, patients are fully alert and aware but have disrupted efferent pathways, leading to minimal motor output. Bilateral pontine infarcts resulting from basilar artery occlusion, pontine tumors, pontine hemorrhages, central pontine myelinolysis, brainstem encephalitis, severe myasthenia gravis, and severe acute inflammatory demyelinating polyneuropathy may present in this fashion.

Patients with akinetic mutism have preserved consciousness and retain the ability to move and speak but lack any initiative to respond to the environment. They often have brain lesions that disrupt reticular-cortical and limbic-cortical integration but spare corticospinal pathways. Abulia is a milder form of this condition.

Catatonia is often associated with psychiatric illnesses but may also be seen with metabolic derangements and drug intoxication. Patients may appear unresponsive to stimuli but will otherwise have a normal neurologic exam. Patients usually lie with their eyes open and may not blink to visual threat, but optokinetic responses are normal. Waxy flexibility of limbs is common, and features of catalepsy, such as rigid limbs and fixed postures, may be seen.

Psychogenic coma is a dissociative psychiatric disorder. Patients often have active resistance to passive opening of the eyelids, and eyelids may flutter when the eyelashes are stroked gently. Motor examination is often inconsistent and may reveal active resistance when examining tone or cogwheeling resistance with sudden "giving away." The patient may occasionally make voluntary movements or change body position in bed. Signs based on reflex self-protection may be seen, as when a hand held above the face drops to the side instead of hitting the face.

Diagnostic Approach

Acute alterations of consciousness should be approached as medical emergencies because the worst-case situations are generally life-threatening. An expedited medical history and physical should focus initially on excluding life-threatening conditions.

Because most patients with altered consciousness are unable to provide a detailed history, it is important to obtain information from available witnesses, family members, and emergency medical personnel. It is important to obtain information regarding details of the presenting event (e.g., Was there trauma? Did the patient have a seizure? Were there any precedent complaints or prodromes?); past medical history (i.e., diabetes, liver disease, renal failure, neurologic disorder, or psychiatric disorder); and medications (i.e., prescription medications and drugs of abuse).

On general physical examination, abnormal vital signs provide useful diagnostic clues and identify parameters (e.g., hypotension, high fever, and arrhythmias) that require immediate treatment. In cases of severely elevated ICP, an increase in systemic blood pressure, with simultaneous reduction in heart rate and respiration, may be seen (Cushing's phenomenon). General examination should also include evaluation for signs of head trauma, such as periorbital ecchymoses ("raccoon eyes"), postauricular ecchymoses (Battle's sign), hemotympanum, and cerebro-

Figure 121-2 Glasgow Coma Scale.

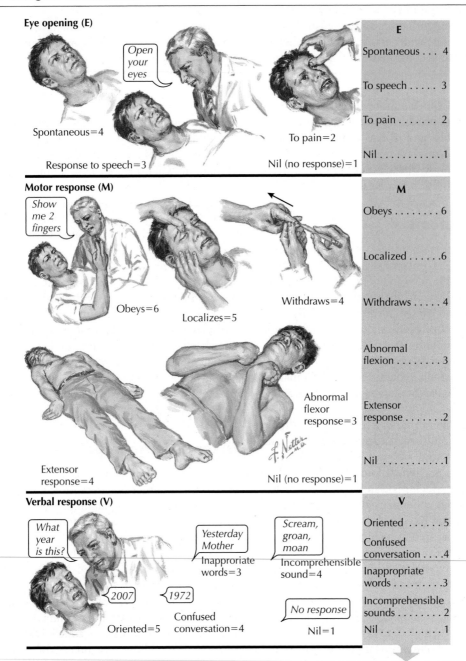

Coma score (E + M + V) = 3 to 15

spinal fluid (CSF) otorrhea or rhinorrhea. The neck should be evaluated for signs of injury and meningismus. Skin should be examined for rash, purpura, cyanosis, jaundice, and needle marks. Presence of organomegaly or lymphadenopathy may provide further insights into causation.

Neurologic evaluation of any patient with altered consciousness should begin with a quick assessment of the degree of the disturbance. The revised Glasgow Coma Scale (GCS) is a clinical score that quantifies the level of consciousness by assessing three parameters: eye opening, motor response to verbal commands or noxious stimuli,

and verbal response (Fig. 121-2). Although the 15-point scale was originally developed as a prognostic tool for traumatic brain injury, it has proved useful as a reproducible measure of level of consciousness in all patients. For patients with any scored abnormality (GCS score <15), brain imaging and observation are recommended in the acute setting. A GCS score of less than 9 is indicative of coma, and patients should be evaluated promptly for airway management. Additionally, a thorough neurologic examination should be performed, with greatest attention directed toward detecting signs of brainstem compression.

Presence of focal neurologic findings may provide clues to causation and assist in determining what additional studies are needed for diagnosis.

Blood samples should be drawn for glucose, serum electrolytes (including calcium and magnesium), complete blood counts, renal function tests, liver profile, coagulation studies, cardiac enzymes, and drug screens. When infection is suspected, blood cultures should be drawn, and a lumbar puncture should be performed to obtain CSF for cell count, glucose, protein, Gram stain, cultures, and HSV polymerase chain reaction. Secondary blood tests such as arterial blood gas, thyroid function tests, blood smear, ammonia, syphilis testing, and anticonvulsant drug levels may be indicated by the patient's history and examination findings. An electrocardiogram should be obtained, and the patient should have continuous cardiac monitoring.

Emergent imaging of the brain is generally indicated when the cause is uncertain, and computed tomography (CT) is the preferred modality in the acute setting because many structural etiologies may be identified quickly with this modality. If ischemic stroke or SAH is suspected, CT angiography is useful for identifying vessel occlusion or aneurysm, respectively. Magnetic resonance imaging is better for visualizing pathology of the brainstem and cerebellum, demonstrating acute infarcts, and detecting diffuse injuries such as encephalitis, laminar necrosis of hypoxia and ischemia, and the shear injuries seen with trauma; however, logistical issues, such as longer acquisition times and limited availability of scanners and specialists needed to interpret the images, often make use of this modality difficult in the acute setting.

An electroencephalogram (EEG) should be performed whenever seizures or status epilepticus is part of the differential diagnosis. EEG is also helpful in the diagnosis of toxic or metabolic encephalopathy, sedative overdose, and HSV encephalitis. EEG may be used to differentiate coma from locked-in states, psychogenic coma, and catatonia.

Management and Therapy

Optimum Treatment

Treatment of the patient should occur concomitantly with the diagnostic evaluation and should begin with evaluation of airway patency, breathing, and circulation. Effective ventilation and oxygenation may require the use of supplemental oxygen, mask ventilation, or intubation. The cervical spine should be immobilized until injury can be excluded. Hypotension, cardiac ischemia, and arrhythmias necessitate aggressive therapy. Hyperthermia must also be addressed definitively.

The empiric administration of thiamine, naloxone, and glucose will cover the immediately reversible causes of altered consciousness. Thiamine should be administered before glucose to avoid exacerbation or precipitation of

Wernicke's encephalopathy, and if possible, a blood sample should be sent for a glucose level to avoid glucose administration in cases of hyperosmolar coma.

Sepsis and meningitis are always suspect in febrile patients with altered consciousness. Blood cultures should be drawn immediately, and broad-spectrum antibiotics and acyclovir (for the possibility of HSV infection) should be administered intravenously. Evaluation for possible central nervous system (CNS) infection requires a lumbar puncture, but this procedure is often deferred until after brain imaging to exclude mass lesions.

If signs of significantly elevated ICP or herniation are seen on initial presentation, empiric treatment should not be delayed to obtain brain imaging. Treatment should begin with elevation of the head. Hyperventilation should be initiated because reduction of PCO_2 to 30 to 35 mm Hg rapidly lowers ICP by 25% to 30% in most patients. In cases in which cerebral edema is the suspected cause of elevated ICP, intravenous mannitol is an effective therapy. In most instances, acute administration of steroids is not recommended. Once medical treatment has been initiated, emergent brain CT imaging is useful for determining what additional interventions are warranted.

Other common interventions begun in the acute setting include placement of a urinary catheter and nasogastric tube. Arterial catheters and central venous access are useful in monitoring hemodynamic status. Invasive ICP monitors are helpful for patients who are at risk for elevated ICP but require sedatives that often make the neurologic exam difficult to follow.

Avoiding Treatment Errors

Delays in diagnosis and initiation of treatments are the most common and the most easily avoided errors. One should always keep in mind that even patients presenting with mild alterations in consciousness have the potential to deteriorate rapidly. Every patient should be evaluated emergently until life-threatening conditions have been excluded. The institution of critical care pathways for patients with depressed consciousness or coma facilitates rapid triage, evaluation, and treatment. Use of diagnostic algorithms may prevent omission of life-threatening conditions when generating the differential diagnosis.

Prognosis

In general, prognosis depends heavily on the degree of the disturbance and the underlying cause. Researchers have proposed various prognostic paradigms based on studies of patients with certain etiologies of coma. Paradigms and historical statistics exist for populations of patients with severe head trauma, nontraumatic coma, and hypoxic-ischemic coma. Although such studies provide a rough guide for clinicians, determining the prognosis for

Figure 121-3 Prognosis in Depressed Mental Status.

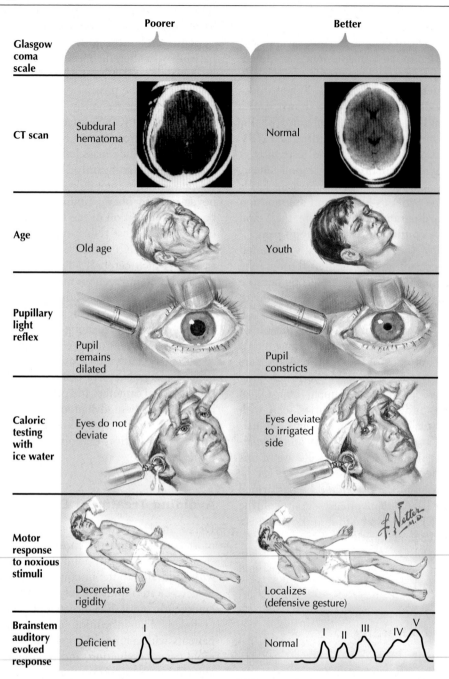

individual patients is much more difficult because other factors affect outcome and must be considered, including age and other comorbidities, severity of neurologic abnormalities on clinical exam, and findings on imaging or neurophysiologic testing (Fig. 121-3).

Patients presenting with low GCS score or with decreasing scores on subsequent examinations have a poorer prognosis. Most patients who are diagnosed with toxic or metabolic causes have a good likelihood of recovery, even if their neurologic illness is prolonged. Patients with normal brain imaging have better outcomes than patients with identified lesions. Patients with focal lesions on imaging (e.g., subdural hematomas) generally do better than patients with diffuse abnormalities (e.g., shear injuries from trauma or injuries due to hypoxia-ischemia). On neurologic testing, pupillary defects, other brainstem findings (e.g., abnormal cold water caloric testing), and abnormal posturing are associated with poorer prognosis. Abnormalities on EEG and evoked potentials are also associated with a lower likelihood of recovery.

Future Directions

Therapeutic hypothermia as a neuroprotective means to reduce injury has been studied in patients with stroke, traumatic brain injury, and hypoxia-ischemia. The most promising results have been seen in studies of patients who have been resuscitated after cardiac arrest. However, application of this technology has been limited to centers with neurointensive specialists, for the most part.

Neuroprotective agents have also been studied in ischemic stroke. Unfortunately, most attempts at limiting the extent of neuronal injury with these agents have been disappointing. Attempts to use neuroprotective agents for treatment of traumatic brain injury are in early stages of development and testing.

Additional Resources

Greer DM: Hypothermia for cardiac arrest. Curr Neurol Neurosci Rep 6(6):518-524, 2006.

This well-written article reviews the evidence for and use of hypothermia following cardiac arrest.

Levy DE, Caronna JJ, Singer BH, et al: Predicting outcome from hypoxic-ischemic coma. JAMA 253(10):1420-1426, 1985.

This study identifies predictors of outcome in cases of hypoxic-ischemic injury.

Practice parameters for determining brain death in adults (summary statement). The Quality Standards Subcommittee of the American Academy of Neurology. Neurology 45(5):1012-1014, 1995.

This paper presents guidelines for determining brain death.

EVIDENCE

1. Greenberg DA, Aminoff MJ, Simon RP: Disorders of consciousness. In Clinical Neurology, 5th ed. New York, Lange, 2002, pp 1-69.

   This is a well-written and well-organized survey of common disorders of consciousness.

2. Levy DE, Bates D, Caronna JJ, et al: Prognosis in non-traumatic coma. Ann Intern Med 94(3):293-301, 1981.

   This study identifies predictors of outcome in cases of nontraumatic coma.

3. Plum F, Posner JB: Diagnosis of Stupor and Coma, 3rd ed. Philadelphia, FA Davis, 1982.

   This classic volume focuses on diagnosis through understanding of the anatomic, biochemical, and physiologic disruptions that cause stupor and coma.

4. Stubgen JP, Caronna JJ: Altered mental status. In Samuels MA (ed): Hospitalist Neurology. Boston, Butterworth Heinemann, 1999, pp 27-43.

   The authors present a hospitalist approach to disorders of consciousness.

5. Teasdale GM, Jennett B: Assessment and prognosis of coma after head injury. Acta Neurochir (Wien) 34:45-55, 1976.

   This is the original description of the revised Glasgow Coma Scale.

Caroline M. Klein

Radiculopathies: Cervical, Lumbar, Spinal Stenosis

Introduction

Neck and low back pain are common symptoms leading patients to seek medical attention in the United States each year, with significant disability, loss of work, and medical expense. The estimated medical costs for patients with low back pain exceed $8 billion annually by some estimates. Up to 80% of the population will have at least one episode of low back pain during their lives. Radiculopathy, or disease of the spinal nerve roots, is a major cause for neck and low back pain, and may be due to a variety of etiologies, most commonly degenerative disease of the spine. Spinal stenosis, or anatomical narrowing of the central spinal canal or neuroforamina through which exiting spinal nerves traverse, is caused by congenital or acquired disease of the spine and may result in radiculopathy or spinal cord compression. Spinal stenosis may occur in either the cervical or lumbosacral spinal regions, with lumbar stenosis being the most common.

Etiology and Pathogenesis

Spinal Anatomy

Spinal nerves are formed by the joining of the dorsal and ventral nerve roots at the level of the intervertebral foramina of the spine, which are formed lateral to the central spinal canal, as the facet joints of adjacent vertebrae are joined together. There are 31 pairs of spinal nerves (8 cervical, 12 thoracic, 5 lumbar, 5 sacral, 1 coccygeal), each named according to the corresponding vertebral level at which it originates. However, the relationship between individual spinal nerves and the corresponding vertebrae changes depending on the level of the spinal cord being considered. In the cervical spine, spinal nerve roots exit at a level cephalad to the corresponding vertebra (C5 root exits between the C4 and C5 vertebrae); however, the C8 root exits between C7 vertebra and T1 vertebrae, with subsequent roots exiting caudad to the vertebra for which the root is named (i.e., T1 root exits between T1 and T2 vertebrae). The spinal nerve immediately divides into dorsal and ventral primary rami or branches, with the ventral primary rami joining in the brachial and lumbosacral plexus at the appropriate levels to form the peripheral nerves innervating the limbs and in the trunk forming segmental innervation to the trunk muscles and cutaneous structures. Cutaneous dermatomal innervation can be mapped according to this segmental innervation pattern based on the formation of the spinal nerve roots. The spinal cord itself ends typically at the L1-L2 vertebral level, and because of the differential growth of the spinal column relative to the spinal cord, the intrathecal lengths of spinal nerve roots progressively increase from cervical to lumbosacral levels. Above the C4 vertebral level, the spinal roots exit the spinal cord segment of their origin and enter the intervertebral foramen at a level basically perpendicular to the spinal cord level of origin; below C4, the distance from the spinal cord segment of origin and the intervertebral foramen of exit gradually increases, and below the L1 vertebral level, the nerve roots that exit at caudal intervertebral foramina extend for the greatest intrathecal distance and are together known as the cauda equina (Fig. 122-1).

Pathogenesis of Radiculopathy and Spinal Stenosis

Radiculopathy means injury or pathology affecting an individual spinal nerve or root and may involve any spinal nerve root, although certain nerve roots are more commonly involved clinically (Fig. 122-2). Pathophysiologic

Figure 122-1 Spinal Nerves and Sensory Dermatomes.

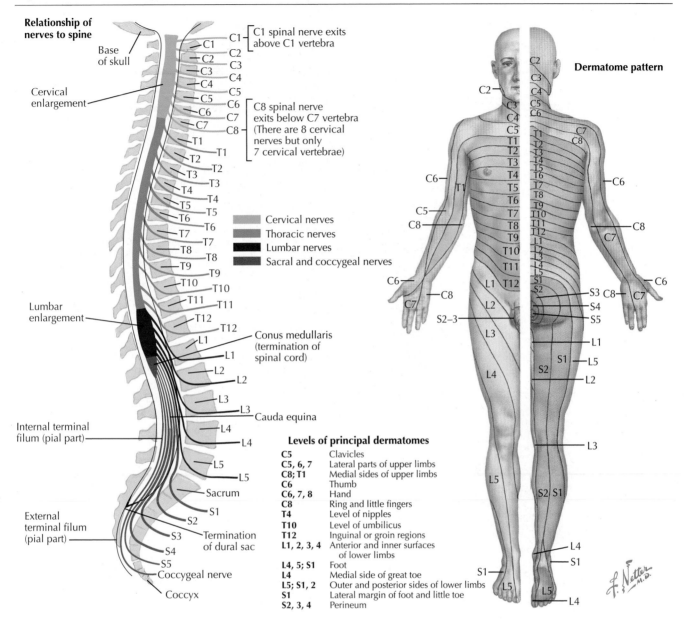

Relationship of nerves to spine

Base of skull

Cervical enlargement

C1 — C1 spinal nerve exits above C1 vertebra

C8 spinal nerve exits below C7 vertebra (There are 8 cervical nerves but only 7 cervical vertebrae)

Cervical nerves
Thoracic nerves
Lumbar nerves
Sacral and coccygeal nerves

Lumbar enlargement

Conus medullaris (termination of spinal cord)

Internal terminal filum (pial part)

Cauda equina

Sacrum

External terminal filum (pial part)

Termination of dural sac

Coccygeal nerve

Coccyx

Dermatome pattern

Levels of principal dermatomes

C5	Clavicles
C5, 6, 7	Lateral parts of upper limbs
C8; T1	Medial sides of upper limbs
C6	Thumb
C6, 7, 8	Hand
C8	Ring and little fingers
T4	Level of nipples
T10	Level of umbilicus
T12	Inguinal or groin regions
L1, 2, 3, 4	Anterior and inner surfaces of lower limbs
L4, 5; S1	Foot
L4	Medial side of great toe
L5; S1, 2	Outer and posterior sides of lower limbs
S1	Lateral margin of foot and little toe
S2, 3, 4	Perineum

mechanisms include inflammation or immune-mediated mechanisms, ischemia, tumor, or mechanical compression due to altered spinal anatomy (either congenital or acquired), the latter being most commonly seen. Congenital alterations in spinal column anatomy include congenital spinal stenosis. Acquired changes in the vertebral anatomy that may lead to spinal nerve root compression and a clinical radiculopathy include protrusion or herniation of intervertebral disks; spondylosis or degenerative changes in the facet joints between vertebrae; hypertrophy of ligaments such as the ligamentum flavum, which is present posteriorly within the spinal canal; and spondylolisthesis, or slippage of adjacent vertebrae relative to each other due to degeneration of the intervertebral disk between them and loss of spine mobility due to chronic mechanical stress.

The vertebral level of the herniated or protruded disk has implications in terms of which spinal root may be compressed and the neurologic symptoms and signs that result. For example, a herniated disk between C4 and C5 vertebrae most likely will affect the C5 root at that level; likewise, because of the normal anatomic changes described previously, a herniated disk in the lumbar spine, at L4-L5 will affect the L5 nerve root because the L4 root exits cephalad to that disk level. Also, depending on whether the protruding disk is central or lateral in location within the spinal canal, other nerve roots may become involved, particularly in the lower lumbar spine with the cauda equina, because the nerve roots at this level have an intrathecal course close together, such that a large disk protrusion can affect up to three or more roots. Ultimately, with progres-

Figure 122-2 Spinal Nerve Origin: Cross Sections.

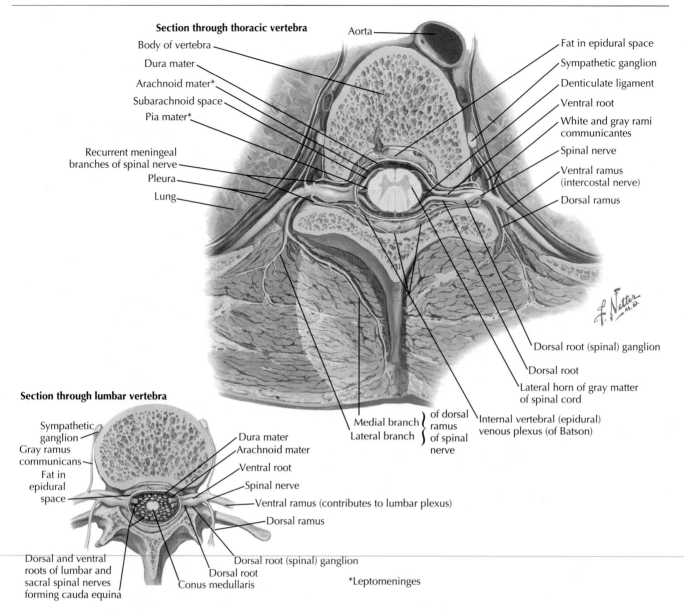

Section through thoracic vertebra

Aorta

Body of vertebra

Dura mater

Arachnoid mater*

Subarachnoid space

Pia mater*

Recurrent meningeal branches of spinal nerve

Pleura

Lung

Fat in epidural space

Sympathetic ganglion

Denticulate ligament

Ventral root

White and gray rami communicantes

Spinal nerve

Ventral ramus (intercostal nerve)

Dorsal ramus

Dorsal root (spinal) ganglion

Dorsal root

Lateral horn of gray matter of spinal cord

Medial branch } of dorsal ramus
Lateral branch } of spinal nerve

Internal vertebral (epidural) venous plexus (of Batson)

Section through lumbar vertebra

Sympathetic ganglion

Gray ramus communicans

Fat in epidural space

Dura mater

Arachnoid mater

Ventral root

Spinal nerve

Ventral ramus (contributes to lumbar plexus)

Dorsal ramus

Dorsal root (spinal) ganglion

Dorsal root

Conus medullaris

Dorsal and ventral roots of lumbar and sacral spinal nerves forming cauda equina

*Leptomeninges

sive encroachment by disease of the structural elements of the vertebral column into the central spinal canal or the lateral recesses leading into the intervertebral foramen, polyradiculopathy and spinal stenosis may develop and lead to neurologic compromise and symptoms. Spinal stenosis implies abnormal narrowing of the anatomical spaces where the neural elements are present.

Clinical Presentation

Radiculopathy

Cervical

Cervical radiculopathy most commonly involves the middle to lower cervical roots, from C5 to C8, usually due to intervertebral disk herniation. Clinical manifestations of cervical radiculopathy include neck pain with radiation into the posterior shoulder or arm in a dermatomal pattern, numbness and weakness, and associated loss of deep tendon reflexes in the affected upper limb. Radiating pain into the limb may be triggered or worsened by movement of the head, neck, or limb itself, or by Valsalva maneuvers during coughing, sneezing, or straining. The muscle weakness and sensory loss may follow a myotomal or dermatomal pattern, but it also may be difficult to discern on routine clinical examination because of the overlapping pattern of innervation of muscles by individual nerve roots. Weakness of the proximal shoulder girdle and the abductors of the shoulder, with radiating pain into the posterior scapular region and lateral shoulder with associated paresthesias,

Figure 122-3 Cervical Disk Herniation: Clinical Manifestations.

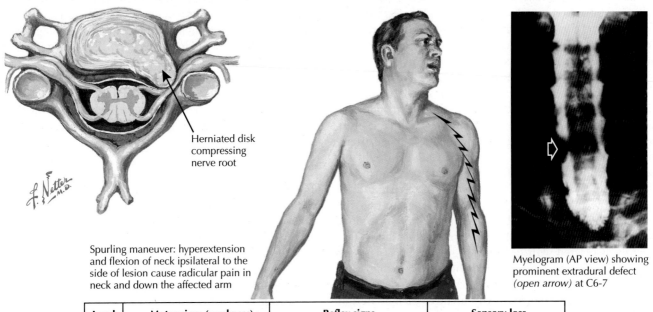

Spurling maneuver: hyperextension and flexion of neck ipsilateral to the side of lesion cause radicular pain in neck and down the affected arm

Myelogram (AP view) showing prominent extradural defect *(open arrow)* at C6-7

Level	Motor signs (weakness)	Reflex signs	Sensory loss
C5	Deltoid	0	
C6	Biceps brachii	Biceps brachii — Weak or absent reflex	
C7	Triceps brachii	Triceps brachii — Weak or absent reflex	
C8	Interossei	0	

suggests C5 radiculopathy. C6 radiculopathy presents as weakness of the biceps and other forearm flexors with radiating pain into the lateral forearm to the thumb. Weakness of the triceps and extensors of the fingers, with pain and tingling paresthesias radiating into the second and third digits, suggests C7 radiculopathy. Weakness of the intrinsic hand muscles and painful paresthesias in the medial forearm and fourth and fifth digits indicates C8, T1

radiculopathy. Asymmetrically diminished biceps and brachioradialis reflexes point to C6 root lesion, and a triceps reflex abnormality suggests C7 pathology (Fig. 122-3).

Lumbar

Lumbar radiculopathy predominantly involves lower lumbar segments, including L4 and L5, with upper roots being much less commonly affected clinically by such processes

as disk herniation leading to single-level radiculopathy. Clinically, patients may have acute low back pain with radiation into the buttocks and posterior hip and into the posterolateral thigh and leg into the foot. Lumbar radicular pain is typically worse with flexion of the lumbar spine and relieved with lying down (lumbar extension). L5 radiculopathy presents with painful sensory symptoms in the dorsomedial foot to the great toe and associated muscle weakness involving ankle dorsiflexion, inversion and eversion, and extension of the toes, particularly of the great toe. L4 radiculopathy may involve weakness of knee extension and pain and tingling in the anteromedial thigh and medial leg into the medial foot. Upper lumbar radiculopathies (L1, L2, L3) may present with low back pain radiating into the anterior thigh and inguinal or groin regions, with muscle weakness of hip flexion and hip adduction. Sacral radiculopathy, specifically S1 radiculopathy, is frequently associated with L5 root lesions, and also presents with low back pain radiating into the posterior thigh and leg and distally into the lateral and plantar foot regions. Weakness with S1 radiculopathy involves plantar flexion of the ankle and toes, as well as hip extension and knee flexion. Deep tendon reflexes affected include the knee jerk or patellar response with L4 radiculopathy and the ankle jerk or Achilles reflex with S1 radiculopathy. Straight-leg-raise maneuvers, with the patient in the supine position with passive flexion of the leg at the hip to between 30 and 70 degrees above the horizontal, may be helpful in confirming intraspinal pathology involving lower lumbar nerve roots if the maneuver leads to radiating pain into the lower extremity. Straight-leg-raise testing with the patient in a prone position, with reproduction of radicular pain into the anterior thigh, is more useful for diagnosis of upper lumbar radiculopathies.

Spinal Stenosis

Cervical

Cervical spinal stenosis is most commonly due to spondylosis, in which degenerative facet joint changes with osteophyte formation, degenerative disk disease with protrusion, and ligamentous hypertrophy combine to narrow the spinal canal and lateral recesses leading to the intervertebral foramina. Stenosis in the cervical spine may lead to multilevel cervical radiculopathies and, if severe, may also cause cervical myelopathy, or compression of the cervical spinal cord itself. The midsagittal cervical canal diameter is normally 18 to 21 mm, with the spinal cord itself measuring 7 to 11 mm in diameter. Significant narrowing or stenosis of the diameter of the spinal canal (12 mm in diameter or less) may lead to intermittent compression of the spinal cord with subsequent damage to the neural parenchyma. These changes are typically degenerative or acquired in nature but may be accelerated in patients with congenitally stenotic spinal canals. If myelopathy occurs, the clinical presentation may include upper motor neuron signs such as spasticity in addition to muscle weakness, hyperactive deep tendon reflexes with ankle clonus, and upgoing toes with plantar stimulation. These changes may involve both upper and lower extremities and may also lead to bowel and bladder dysfunction, including urinary retention and incontinence. Sensory changes may include not only those related to multiple cervical radiculopathies but also loss of vibratory and joint position sense in the distal lower extremities, as the myelopathy progresses (Fig. 122-4).

Lumbar

Lumbar spinal stenosis involves most commonly the lower lumbar spinal levels, and its incidence increases in patients older than 60 years. The most common cause is progressive degenerative spine disease with encroachment of the central spinal canal and resultant multiple lumbosacral radiculopathies. An important clinical feature of these patients is that they report worsening back and leg pain with extension of the spine, so that they experience pain with upright posture and ambulation, so-called neurogenic claudication or pseudoclaudication, to distinguish the syndrome from vascular claudication. If the patient's leg pain is due to a neurogenic lesion such as that observed in lumbar spinal stenosis, the leg pain is relieved with sitting and not with standing alone, as may occur with vascular claudication due to arterial insufficiency in the lower limbs. Patients may also note that the pain is worse when they lie down in a supine position at night, but improves if they lie in a lateral decubitus position with their knees flexed, which reduces the spinal stenosis and nerve root compression within the spinal canal. Patients with lumbar spinal stenosis may demonstrate a wide-based, antalgic gait with stooped posture and positive Romberg's sign.

A specific entity known as cauda equina syndrome occurs with compression of lumbosacral nerve roots within the spinal canal leading to bowel and bladder dysfunction. This is a rare condition (occurs in about 2% of cases of herniated lumbar disks) but requires immediate medical attention and treatment. Clinically, it may present with a gradual worsening over time of the chronic symptoms of lumbar spinal stenosis or, more typically, presents as an acute change in bowel or bladder function superimposed on a preceding history of symptoms of lumbar spinal stenosis. The latter clinical presentation is presumably due to an acute intervertebral disk herniation superimposed on lumbar spinal stenosis causing more severe narrowing of the spinal canal and compression of the sacral nerve roots. The earliest bladder symptom is usually urinary retention, which progresses to bladder incontinence. Patients with cauda equina syndrome also report altered sensation or anesthesia in the perineal or groin region (saddle anesthesia), corresponding to the lower sacral nerve roots being involved pathologically. Their leg pain and sensory symptoms, as well as motor weakness, may be asymmetric.

Figure 122-4 Cervical Spondylosis.

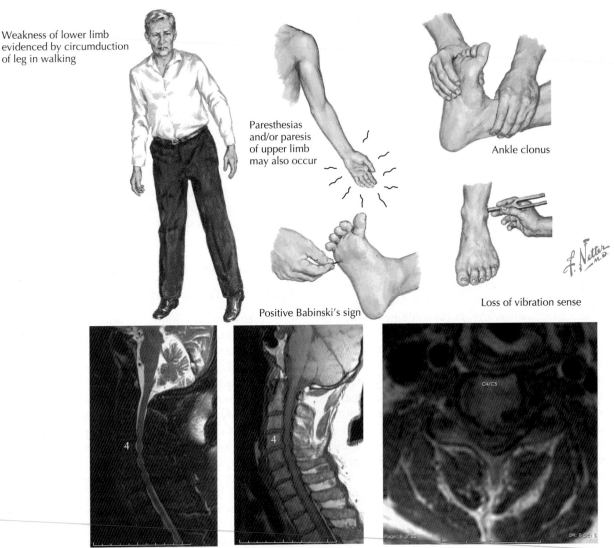

Weakness of lower limb evidenced by circumduction of leg in walking

Paresthesias and/or paresis of upper limb may also occur

Ankle clonus

Positive Babinski's sign

Loss of vibration sense

Degenerative disease with spinal cord compression. Idiopathic spinal stenosis with disk protrusion anteriorly and hypertrophy of ligamentum flavum posteriorly, most extreme at C4-5

Differential Diagnosis

The differential diagnosis of cervical or lumbosacral radiculopathies includes peripheral neuropathy or multiple mononeuropathies of the limbs, which may also present with pain, sensory and motor symptoms, and signs. Peripheral neuropathy includes distal polyneuropathy as well as polyradiculopathies that may result from a wide range of underlying acquired etiologies, such as inflammatory or immune-mediated, nutritional, diabetes, toxins, infectious causes, or tumor or cancer related. Radiculopathy related to malignancy may be due to tumor metastasis to the vertebral structures leading to nerve root compression or infiltration, or due to conditions in which the primary lesion is cancer infiltrating the nerve roots directly, such as may occur with lymphoma or carcinomatous meningitis.

Cancer should be strongly considered as the underlying cause of the patient's symptoms in patients who have unremitting back pain that is not relieved at night or with change in body position and in those who do not respond to conservative therapy after 6 to 8 weeks, particularly patients with a history of cancer that is known to metastasize to the spine (breast, prostate, lung, colon, melanoma, multiple myeloma). Likewise, in patients with back pain unresponsive to conservative therapy who have fever, elevated erythrocyte sedimentation rate, and white blood cell count, infectious causes for their symptoms, such as osteomyelitis of the spine or epidural spinal abscess, should be considered strongly. The differential diagnosis of cervical spondylotic myelopathy includes motor neuron disease, multiple sclerosis, syrinx, spinal cord tumor, or vascular malformation leading to cord compression.

Diagnostic Approach

Obtaining a detailed history regarding the onset and type of symptoms, triggering and relieving factors, and progression of symptoms since onset, is the most important initial first step in diagnosis. History of trauma, previous spinal injuries or surgeries, and other medical conditions such as diabetes or cancer may also be helpful. A careful neurologic examination, with particular focus on the neuromuscular examination, is the next step in localization of the underlying process that is causing the patient's symptoms. This will include testing muscle strength and tone, deep tendon reflexes, sensory examination with specific effort to demonstrate dermatomal loss of sensation to various modalities, gait testing including Romberg testing, and mechanical tests of range of motion of the trunk at the hip, palpation of the spine, and inspection of the spine for scoliosis or other osseous deformities.

After an isolated nerve root lesion or radiculopathy or multiple nerve root lesions (e.g., due to spinal stenosis) is suspected, additional laboratory testing and imaging studies should be ordered depending on the examiner's judgment regarding the underlying cause of the condition. Electrodiagnostic testing, specifically nerve conduction studies and electromyography, can be used to confirm the presence of a radiculopathy and exclude other potential diagnoses such as peripheral neuropathy or mononeuropathies, localize the segmental root levels involved, and provide information regarding the chronicity of the lesion and whether active denervation and reinnervation are present. In patients in whom multiple pathologies may be present, such as a diabetic patient with radiculopathy superimposed on an underlying peripheral neuropathy, or in patients with symptoms but limited objective findings on neurologic examination, electrodiagnostic testing can be particularly useful. Blood tests, including complete blood count and erythrocyte sedimentation rate, should be done immediately in patients with a suspected infectious process causing their radiculopathy, such as those with history of recent fever, other systemic infections, immunosuppression, or localized tenderness to palpation over spinous processes associated with acute or subacute onset of back or neck pain. In patients with a history of cancer, unexplained weight loss, or unremitting back pain unresponsive to conservative measures, neuroimaging with magnetic resonance imaging (MRI) of the involved spinal region is important, with contrast administration if possible. Additional testing may include cerebrospinal fluid examination in patients with a question of leptomeningeal metastasis (cerebrospinal fluid cytology) or infection (cell count and cultures). Patients with a history of recent trauma before the onset of the symptoms should undergo plain x-ray imaging, including anteroposterior and lateral views, as well as flexion and extension views of the spine. Plain x-rays are of limited value in the patient with spinal pain without a history of trauma; however, it should be remem-

bered that in elderly patients with a history of osteoporosis, minimal or unsuspected trauma may lead to vertebral fracture. For those patients in whom degenerative spine disease is present, who have progressive or severe symptoms and neurologic deficits despite a reasonable course of conservative therapy, MRI and possibly computed tomographic myelography should be considered. However, because many abnormalities found on imaging studies are nonspecific and can also be found in asymptomatic individuals, any results should be taken in the clinical context of the patient's history, physical examination, and electrodiagnostic test results. For those patients with possible cauda equina syndrome, neuroimaging with MRI should be done on an emergent basis because confirmation of this condition and institution of early treatment are important in terms of clinical outcome.

Management and Therapy

Optimum Treatment

The management options in patients with radiculopathy and spinal stenosis range from conservative therapy with physical therapy, analgesics, epidural steroid injections, and intermittent rest and limitation of physical activities that may aggravate the symptoms to spinal surgery for decompression. The natural history of radiculopathy is in part dependent on the cause of the nerve root lesion. In patients with infection or malignancy as a cause for the radiculopathy, aggressive treatment with antibiotics and possibly surgical drainage of a spinal abscess for the former, and surgery and possibly chemotherapy or radiation therapy for the latter, are indicated. For patients with degenerative spine disease as a cause for their radiculopathy or in patients with multilevel radiculopathies due to spinal stenosis, the optimal treatment is less clear, except for those patients with severe disease, in which case surgical intervention seems most reasonable because there appears to be a clinical benefit early after surgery (Fig. 122-5). Certainly, in patients with cauda equina syndrome, surgical intervention within 48 hours of onset of symptoms has been shown to result in better clinical outcomes compared with surgery after 48 hours. However, in patients with mild or moderate radiculopathy or spinal stenosis, the natural history appears to be that of stable or slowly progressive disease, in which case surgical treatment is controversial and has been shown to be of limited benefit in the short-term only in patients with moderate to severe spinal stenosis, for example. Most authors would agree that in most patients with mild or moderate disease, a period of conservative therapy of a minimum of 6 to 8 weeks to determine whether the patient's symptoms are persistent or progressive would be advisable. Additionally, the patient's preferences and confounding medical conditions in terms of being a surgical candidate should always be taken into consideration in decision making in regard to

Figure 122-5 Surgical Management of Spinal Stenosis.

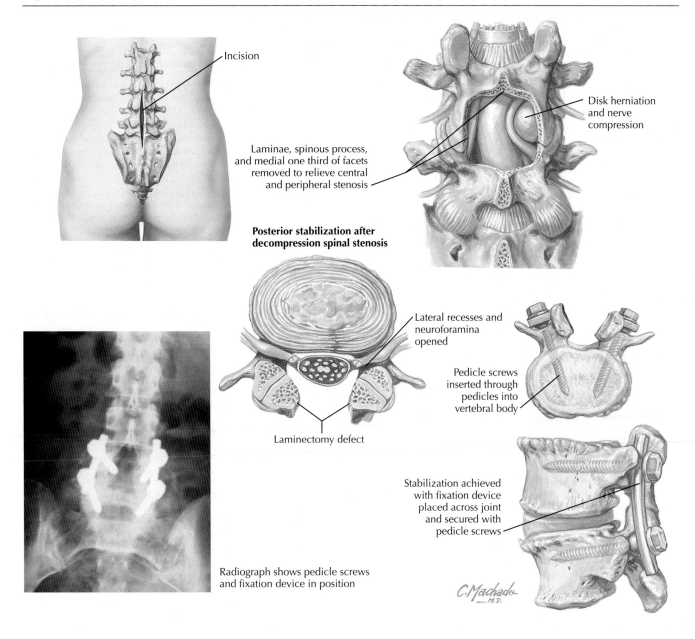

Incision

Laminae, spinous process, and medial one third of facets removed to relieve central and peripheral stenosis

Posterior stabilization after decompression spinal stenosis

Disk herniation and nerve compression

Lateral recesses and neuroforamina opened

Pedicle screws inserted through pedicles into vertebral body

Laminectomy defect

Stabilization achieved with fixation device placed across joint and secured with pedicle screws

Radiograph shows pedicle screws and fixation device in position

C. Machado M.D.

surgical intervention. Patients who develop signs of cervical myelopathy due to cervical spondylosis or canal stenosis should undergo surgical intervention to prevent further spinal cord damage.

Avoiding Treatment Errors

The most important management decisions regarding patients with possible radiculopathy or spinal stenosis are to evaluate the patient for potential "red flags" that would change dramatically the recommendations for the patient's treatment. These include symptoms and signs of possible infection or cancer, myelopathy, or cauda equina syn-

drome. These conditions, as causes of radiculopathy or as a consequence of spinal stenosis, require further evaluation and intervention as soon as possible. The risks of delay of evaluation and treatment are paraplegia and permanent incontinence. Currently available medical literature does not provide clear guidelines as to the relative benefit of surgical versus conservative therapy for radiculopathy or spinal stenosis that is mild or moderate because confounding factors exist such as nonspecific MRI abnormalities and the natural history of the disease, which may favor conservative therapy. According to the literature available currently, there does not seem to be a disadvantage to delaying surgical intervention in patients without red flags.

Future Directions

Improving the accuracy of the diagnosis of radiculopathy and spinal stenosis and determining optimal treatment protocols by means of prospective, blinded, randomized clinical trials are what is needed in the future to improve evaluation and treatment for patients with these conditions. Advances in imaging techniques, such as the ability to perform MRIs in patients in an upright position or posture that may be functionally significant for their disease process, will be helpful and are hopefully forthcoming. Likewise, expansion of currently available electrophysiologic testing, to include possibly magnetic nerve root stimulation, will also aid in diagnosis and localization of pathology. Increased understanding of the natural history of these diseases, relative risks and benefits of various surgical and conservative therapies, and predictors of outcome measures will help clinicians in the future make more informed recommendations to their patients about how to treat their condition.

Additional Resources

Chalk C: Diseases of spinal roots. In Dyck PJ, Thomas PK (eds): Peripheral Neuropathy, 4th ed. Philadelphia, Elsevier, 2005, pp 1323-1337.

This excellent overview of the anatomic and pathologic correlates of radicular spine disease also provides a comprehensive review of the differential diagnosis in terms of the various etiologies of nerve root disease.

Devereaux MW: Neck and low back pain. Med Clin North Am 87(3):643-662, 2003.

This is a basic overview of the clinical symptoms and signs in patients with cervical and lumbosacral radiculopathies and cervical myelopathy. It provides an excellent review of the anatomic features of the spine and their pathophysiologic correlates.

Katz JN, Sheon RP: Evaluation of low back pain in older subjects: Degenerative spinal disease and lumbar stenosis. Available at: http://www.uptodate.com. Accessed February 4, 2007.

This concise overview of the clinical features and therapeutic approaches for lumbar spinal stenosis specifically highlights important clinical "red flags" to be mindful of in an older patient population.

Kim SL, Lim RD: Spinal stenosis. Dis Mon 51(1):6-17, 2005.

This basic review of the anatomy and pathophysiology of lumbar spinal stenosis provides important guidelines regarding diagnostic evaluation and treatment.

Lehrich JR, Katz JN, Sheon RP: Approach to the diagnosis and evaluation of low back pain in adults. Available at: http://www.uptodate.com. Accessed February 4, 2007.

This comprehensive review of the clinical features, examination findings, and diagnostic and therapeutic approaches to consider in evaluation of patients with low back pain provides clear details of the clinical features and findings due to various radicular lesions.

Lehrich JR, Sheon RP: Laboratory evaluation of low back pain. Available at: http://www.uptodate.com. Accessed February 4, 2007.

This concise review of laboratory and radiographic tests available for evaluation of low back pain provides excellent guidelines regarding specific clinical features and their impact on the direction of the clinical evaluation.

Ronthal M: Cervical spondylosis, ankylosing spondylitis and lumbar disk disease. In Noseworthy JH (ed): Neurological Therapeutics: Principles and Practice. London, Martin Dunitz, 2005, pp 1597-1601.

The authors present a brief but concise review of the clinical features and therapeutic options for patients with cervical spondylosis or lumbar radiculopathy.

EVIDENCE

1. Ahn UM, Ahn NU, Buchowski JM, et al: Cauda equina syndrome secondary to lumbar disc herniation: A meta-analysis of surgical outcomes. Spine 25(12):1515-1522, 2000.

   This meta-analysis of 42 citations was used to determine the effect of the timing of surgical decompression after onset of clinical symptoms of cauda equina syndrome on clinical outcome. It also provides a review of the clinical presentation of cauda equina syndrome and which clinical features were associated with poor versus good surgical outcomes.

2. Atlas SJ, Keller RB, Wu YA, et al: Long-term outcomes of surgical and nonsurgical management of lumbar spinal stenosis: 8 to 10 year results from the Maine Lumbar Spine Study. Spine 30(8):936-943, 2005.

   A long-term observational study of patients with lumbar spinal stenosis treated either surgically or conservatively included data were from physician and patient questionnaires regarding symptoms and clinical course.

3. Fouyas IP, Statham PF, Sandercock PA: Cochrane review of the role of surgery in cervical spondylotic radiculomyelopathy. Spine 27(7):736-747, 2002.

   The authors report on a limited study (only two trials used for the analysis), but provide an important review of surgical intervention in cervical spondylotic myelopathy and its timing in relation to final clinical outcome.

4. Hall S, Bartleson JD, Onofrio BM, et al: Lumbar spinal stenosis. Clinical features, diagnostic procedures and results of surgical treatment in 68 patients. Ann Intern Med 103(2):271-275, 1985.

   The authors report on an important, early retrospective study from Mayo Clinic of the clinical features and surgical outcomes of 68 patients diagnosed with lumbar spinal stenosis, presenting an excellent review of the clinical presentation and laboratory results of patients with surgically confirmed lumbar spinal stenosis.

5. Kent DL, Haynor DR, Larson EB, Deyo RA: Diagnosis of lumbar spinal stenosis in adults: A meta-analysis of the accuracy of CT, MR and myelography. AJR Am J Roentgenol 158(5):1135-1144, 1992.

   In this review of various radiographic methods commonly available to diagnose lumbar spinal stenosis, the authors make specific reference to their sensitivity and correlation of various abnormalities with clinical presentation and features.

6. Niggemeyer O, Strauss JM, Schulitz KP: Comparison of surgical procedures for degenerative lumbar spinal stenosis: A meta-analysis of the literature from 1975-1995. Eur Spine J 6(6):423-429, 1997.

   The authors review data comparing clinical outcomes from various surgical treatments for lumbar spinal stenosis and the preoperative clinical variables that may influence clinical outcome after surgery.

7. Persson LC, Carlsson CA, Carlsson JY: Long-lasting cervical radicular pain managed with surgery, physiotherapy, or a cervical collar. A prospective, randomized study. Spine 22(7):751-758, 1997.

   This prospective, randomized clinical trial from Sweden compared clinical outcomes over a period of 1 year in patients with cervical radiculopathy treated with surgical or nonsurgical measures.

8. Weber H: Lumbar disc herniation: A controlled, prospective study with ten years of observation. Spine 8(2):131-140, 1983.

   The author reports on a comparative study at a single center of long-term clinical outcomes in patients with lumbar disk herniation who underwent either surgical or conservative therapy.

Peripheral Neuropathy

Introduction

Peripheral neuropathy is a condition that results from abnormalities in the structure and function of motor, sensory, or autonomic neurons or their peripheral processes. Neuropathies can be broadly classified into disorders that primarily affect myelin sheaths (demyelinating), those that affect the axonal process (axonopathies), and those that affect the neuronal cell body (neuronopathies or ganglionopathies). There are numerous hereditary and acquired causes of peripheral neuropathy within each subgroup. Neuropathies can also be classified based on their etiology and encompass those secondary to hereditary, toxic-metabolic, traumatic, entrapment, and systemic disease causes.

Etiology and Pathogenesis

The causes of neuropathy are diverse, and numerous pathogenic mechanisms exist. For both diagnostic and therapeutic purposes, neuropathies are usually categorized as either acquired or hereditary in origin.

There are many potential causes for acquired neuropathies. These include (1) metabolic disorders (e.g., critical illness polyneuropathy, diabetes mellitus, uremia, vitamin B_{12} deficiency, hypothyroidism) (Fig. 123-1); (2) toxic exposures (e.g., heavy metals, industrial toxins) (Fig. 123-2); (3) infectious causes (e.g., leprosy, herpes zoster, HIV disease, West Nile virus, hepatitis C); (4) pharmaceutical agents (e.g., vinca alkaloids, ddC, ddI, pyridoxine, amiodarone, cisplatin, allopurinol); (5) vasculitic and connective tissue disorders (e.g., lupus; rheumatoid arthritis; nonsystemic vasculitis affecting peripheral nerve; Sjögren's syndrome); (6) immune system aberrations (e.g., Landry-Guillain-Barré syndrome [GBS], chronic inflammatory demyelinating polyradiculoneuropathy [CIDP], brachial plexitis [Parsonage-Turner syndrome], neurosarcoidosis, amyloidosis); (7) underlying malignancy (e.g., paraproteinemias, lymphoma, a variety of solid cell tumors with paraneoplastic neuropathy); and (8) compressive-entrapment mononeuropathies (e.g., carpal tunnel and cubital tunnel syndromes, peroneal nerve compression at the fibular head).

Hereditary neuropathies are less common. Autosomal dominant, recessive, and X-linked inheritances have all been described. In some instances, the neuropathy is the major feature of the illness (e.g., Charcot-Marie-Tooth [CMT] disease or hereditary motor and sensory neuropathy). In other hereditary diseases, the neuropathy is only one manifestation of a more widespread disorder (e.g., metachromatic leukodystrophy, adrenoleukodystrophy, Fabry's disease, Refsum's disease).

Autonomic neuropathies are a special category in that they may also result from acquired (diabetes mellitus, Sjögren's syndrome, autoimmune autonomic neuropathy) or inherited (hereditary sensory and autonomic neuropathy [HSAN]) causes, which may or may not be associated with involvement of the somatic nervous system.

Clinical Presentation

The prototypical peripheral neuropathy is a distal, symmetrical process affecting motor and sensory nerves that produces a stocking more than glove distribution of sensory disturbance and muscle weakness. The clinical presentations of neuropathy are varied but often follow characteristic patterns of nerve involvement and fall under the broad categories of motor weakness, sensory disturbance, and autonomic dysfunction. The pattern of nerve involvement may be distal and symmetrical, proximal, or asymmetrical (Fig. 123-3).

The predominant motor symptom is muscle weakness and muscle atrophy, frequently with fasciculations. The pattern of distribution and severity depends on the cause of the neuropathy. Symptoms of weakness typically begin

Figure 123-1 Peripheral Neuropathies: Metabolic, Toxic, and Nutritional.

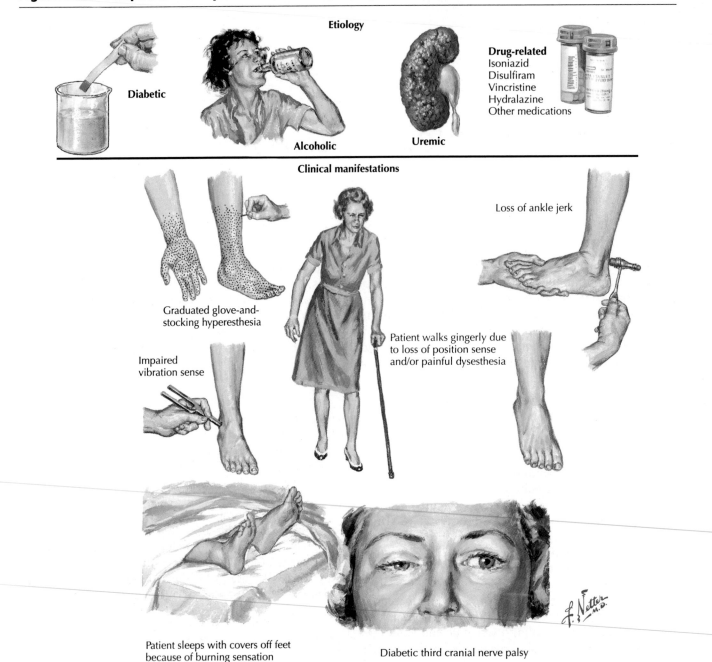

Etiology

Diabetic

Alcoholic

Uremic

Drug-related
Isoniazid
Disulfiram
Vincristine
Hydralazine
Other medications

Clinical manifestations

Graduated glove-and-stocking hyperesthesia

Impaired vibration sense

Patient walks gingerly due to loss of position sense and/or painful dysesthesia

Loss of ankle jerk

Patient sleeps with covers off feet because of burning sensation

Diabetic third cranial nerve palsy

distally with foot drop, which may cause the patient to trip, particularly when walking on uneven terrain, across door thresholds, or on rugs. There may be difficulties with fine motor movements of the fingers such as opening jars and manipulating small objects. More proximal motor nerve involvement often presents with trouble climbing up and down stairs or performance of motor tasks requiring the arms to be raised over the patient's head, such as combing the hair or reaching for objects from a high shelf.

Sensory symptoms can be quite varied. Positive symptoms include tingling, paresthesias (pins and needles),

neuropathic pain, and dysesthesias (unpleasant painful or uncomfortable symptoms). These symptoms may also include burning pains, especially in the feet or hands, or sharp, shooting, electrical shock–type pains in affected limbs. Negative symptoms include numbness or loss of sensation.

Autonomic dysfunction may present with subtle symptoms such as dry eyes or dry mouth, change in sweating, vasomotor skin changes, bowel and bladder dysfunction such as alternating diarrhea and constipation or incontinence, and erectile dysfunction, or more commonly with

Figure 123-2 Peripheral Neuropathy Caused by Heavy-Metal Poisoning.

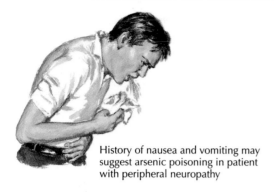

History of nausea and vomiting may suggest arsenic poisoning in patient with peripheral neuropathy

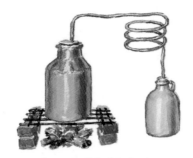

Antique copper utensils (e.g., still for bootleg liquor) and runoff waste from copper smelting plant may be sources of arsenic poisoning

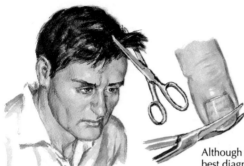

Although 24-hour urinalysis is the best diagnostic test for arsenic, hair and nail analysis may also be helpful

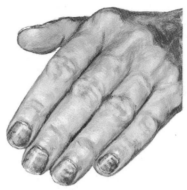

Mees' lines on fingernails are characteristic of arsenic poisoning

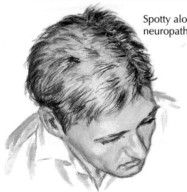

Spotty alopecia associated with peripheral neuropathy characterizes thallium poisoning

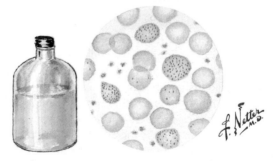

Lead poisoning, now relatively rare, causes basophilic stippling of red blood cells. 24-hour urinalysis is diagnostic test

symptoms of orthostatic intolerance or orthostatic hypotension leading to dizziness with standing and even syncope.

A distal symmetrical abnormality of motor and sensory function with associated diminution of muscle stretch reflexes is the most common pattern of involvement for a distal polyneuropathy. Weakness and muscle wasting predominate in the distal muscles of the hands and feet. Sensory loss follows the classic distal symmetrical (glove-stocking) distribution, and reflex loss follows a similar pattern. Other disorders have a proximal pattern of muscle weakness. GBS is the most well known, and it can be seen also in porphyric neuropathy or CIDP. Sensory loss is less

common in this pattern of abnormality, and the motor weakness is generally symmetric.

A predominant pattern of sensory involvement may occur with certain sensory neuropathies or ganglionopathies associated with occult malignancies, as in paraneoplastic syndrome, but may also be seen in diabetes, vitamin B_6 deficiency, leprosy, HIV, Sjögren's syndrome, and HSAN. Neuropathies that have motor involvement predominantly include GBS, multifocal motor neuropathy, diphtheria, and lead intoxication. Autonomic dysfunction is a feature of HSANs, diabetic polyneuropathy, amyloidosis, Sjögren's syndrome, and autoimmune autonomic neuropathy (Fig. 123-4). A multifocal pattern of

Figure 123-3 Signs and Symptoms Consistent with Neuropathy.

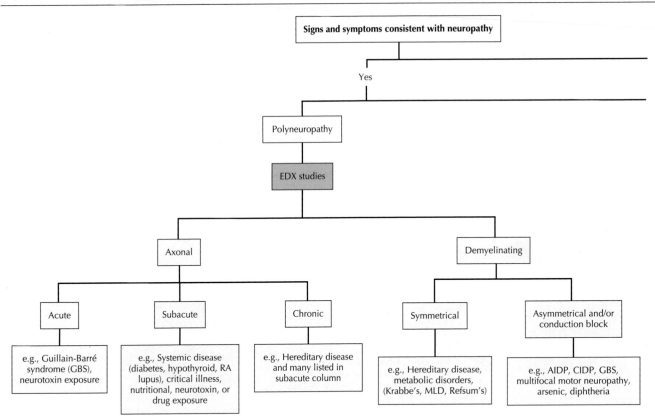

involvement may occur in mononeuritis multiplex that implies vasculitic or inflammatory and immune etiology, multiple entrapment mononeuropathies, hereditary neuropathy with liability to pressure palsy (HNPP), diabetic amyotrophy, or inherited brachial plexopathy (Fig. 123-5).

Some neuropathies progress very rapidly with a dramatic clinical course. These include GBS, vasculitic or ischemic neuropathies, and acute heavy metal intoxication (arsenic) typically. Rapidly evolving neuropathies may also follow acute compression resulting from hemorrhage (e.g., within the carpal tunnel or anterior compartment syndrome), direct trauma, or exposure to extreme cold. Subacute neuropathies, evolving over many days to a few weeks, are characteristic of chronic toxin or drug exposure, critical illness, Lyme disease, HIV, and nutritional disorders. A chronic time course is also typical of hereditary disorders, nutritional deficiencies, paraproteinemias, and some forms of inflammatory and HIV neuropathies.

Differential Diagnosis

The differential diagnosis is made easier once the neuropathy has been localized and characterized within the peripheral nervous system. This requires a carefully elicited history and a thorough neurologic examination to determine the pattern of nerve involvement, the population of nerve fibers affected, and the portion of the nerve that is involved in the neuropathic process. The presence of sensory loss and diminished or absent muscle stretch reflexes is the sine qua non of peripheral nerve disease. A neuropathy of childhood onset and insidious progression is likely to be of genetic origin. Similar progression in late adult life suggests a paraproteinemic disorder, although an inherited process should always be considered. Acute or subacute demyelinating neuropathies suggest an inflammatory process. Marked disturbances of sensation suggest diabetes, heavy metal intoxication, pyridoxine or vitamin B_{12} imbalance, paraneoplastic syndrome, or alcohol as the probable cause. Pure sensory neuropathies in an age-appropriate individual suggest a paraneoplastic disorder or connective tissue disease such as sicca or Sjögren's syndrome. A rapidly progressive painful sensory neuropathy with prominent autonomic features in an adult should raise the possibility of amyloidosis.

There are situations in which it may be difficult to distinguish primary sensory neuropathy from motor neuron diseases. For instance, spinal muscular atrophy, polio or postpolio syndrome, amyotrophic lateral sclerosis, and West Nile virus infection may be difficult to distinguish from axonal motor neuropathies. Likewise, diffuse motor polyradiculopathies due to cervical and lumbosacral spinal stenosis or degenerative disk disease with neuroforaminal

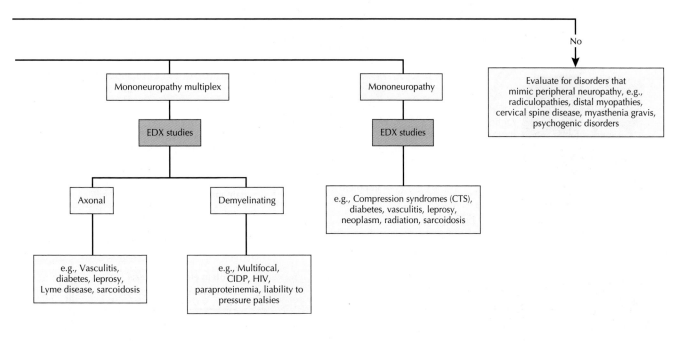

Mononeuropathy multiplex

EDX studies

Axonal

e.g., Vasculitis, diabetes, leprosy, Lyme disease, sarcoidosis

Demyelinating

e.g., Multifocal, CIDP, HIV, paraproteinemia, liability to pressure palsies

Mononeuropathy

EDX studies

e.g., Compression syndromes (CTS), diabetes, vasculitis, leprosy, neoplasm, radiation, sarcoidosis

No

Evaluate for disorders that mimic peripheral neuropathy, e.g., radiculopathies, distal myopathies, cervical spine disease, myasthenia gravis, psychogenic disorders

AIDP, acute inflammatory demyelinating polyneuropathy; CIDP, chronic inflammatory demyelinating polyneuropathy; CTS, carpal tunnel syndrome; EDX, electrodiagnostic; GBS, Guillain-Barré syndrome; HIV, human immunodeficiency virus; MLD, metachromatic leukodystrophy; RA, rheumatoid arthritis

stenosis may be difficult to distinguish from a motor neuropathy.

A careful history and electrodiagnostic and laboratory examination can help to differentiate these disorders. The initial presentation of a spinal cord syndrome may be confused for a sensory neuropathy because of the distal paresthesias. The presence of a definable truncal sensory limit and the presence of corticospinal tract involvement on careful examination can differentiate these entities. On rare occasions, isolated motor cranial neuropathies may be confused with myasthenia gravis. However, the tendency of the symptoms to worsen toward the end of the day in myasthenia gravis as well as electrodiagnostic and laboratory testing should aid in the proper diagnosis. Rarely, myopathies may present with a distal pattern of weakness. The preservation of muscle stretch reflexes, the absence of sensory abnormalities, and the typical laboratory (increased creatine kinase) and electrodiagnostic findings should clarify the problem. Autonomic neuropathies may be confused with primary cardiac disease as a cause for syncope or orthostatic intolerance. They may also be difficult to differentiate from central degenerative diseases of the autonomic nervous system, such as multisystem atrophy or Shy-Drager syndrome. However, careful history of autonomic symptoms and neurologic examina-

tion to detect central nervous system findings, as well as electrodiagnostic testing of autonomic nervous system reflex functioning, should allow for differentiation of these entities.

Diagnostic Approach

Nearly 75% of patients with neuropathic symptoms have a specific diagnosis if evaluated by physicians with experience in evaluation of patients with neuromuscular disease. Establishing a correct diagnosis is based on the optimal utilization of clinical, electrodiagnostic, and laboratory data. In some situations, pathologic examination of a peripheral nerve is necessary, or cerebrospinal fluid analysis is required.

The role of routine screening blood laboratory studies has not been established. The most useful studies include measurement of the vitamin B_{12} level, serum protein electrophoresis with immunofixation, complete blood count with differential, renal function tests, and glycosylated hemoglobin. Other routine studies may be of benefit in carefully screened patients to confirm a diagnosis, for example, thyroid function studies, vitamin B_6 levels, Lyme titer, 24-hour urine heavy metals, and collagen vascular studies such as erythrocyte sedimentation rate, antinuclear

Figure 123-4 Dysproteinemia: Amyloid Neuropathy.

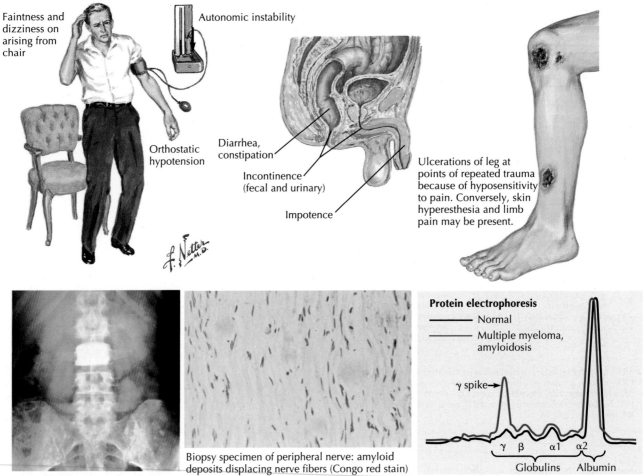

X-ray film showing osteosclerotic myeloma affecting isolated vertebra as seen in POEMS syndrome

Biopsy specimen of peripheral nerve: amyloid deposits displacing nerve fibers (Congo red stain)

POEMS, polyneuropathy-organomegaly-endocrinopathy-monoclonal gammopathy, skin changes.

antibody, extractable nuclear antigen, rheumatoid factor, and C-reactive protein. Other studies to consider include HIV and hepatitis C viral serologies. Finding of a serum monoclonal protein should lead to consideration of urine protein electrophoresis with immunofixation, myeloma bone survey, and possible bone marrow biopsy to rule out multiple myeloma.

Specific serum antibodies directed toward gangliosides and glycoproteins have been implicated in several motor and sensory neuropathies. These include antimyelin-associated glycoprotein (MAG), anti-GM1, anti-GM2, anti-GD1a and b, anti-GQ1b, antisulfatide, and paraneoplastic antibodies. Unfortunately, the diagnostic and prognostic value of these antibodies remains unclear. Although their presence enhances the likelihood of an immune-mediated or paraneoplastic neuropathy, many patients with identical clinical syndromes are seronegative, and some individuals with no clinical findings of neuropathy express low levels of these antibodies. Anti-GM1 antibody

is useful in situations of suspected treatable motor neuropathy that cannot be distinguished from amyotrophic lateral sclerosis, or in those patients in whom pure motor neuropathies are associated with a paucity of upper motor neuron findings and multifocal conduction block is demonstrated on electrodiagnostic studies of motor nerves. Anti-GQ1b antibodies may be helpful in confirming the suspected Miller-Fisher variant of GBS. Anti-Hu antibody is useful in patients with asymmetrical proximal sensory findings or in those patients with a predominantly sensory neuropathy and strong smoking history because this may be the earliest manifestation of an underlying malignancy. Anti-MAG antibodies may be associated with an immune-mediated sensory neuropathy.

Genetic testing should be considered in patients with a positive family history of peripheral neuropathy, as may be seen in patients with CMT disease or HNPP. Most currently known mutations for CMT involve the form of the disease that causes a demyelinating sensorimotor periph-

Figure 123-5 Mononeuritis Multiplex with Polyarteritis Nodosa.

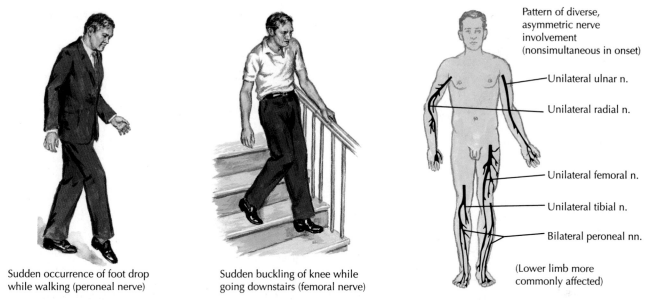

Sudden occurrence of foot drop while walking (peroneal nerve)

Sudden buckling of knee while going downstairs (femoral nerve)

Pattern of diverse, asymmetric nerve involvement (nonsimultaneous in onset)

Unilateral ulnar n.

Unilateral radial n.

Unilateral femoral n.

Unilateral tibial n.

Bilateral peroneal nn.

(Lower limb more commonly affected)

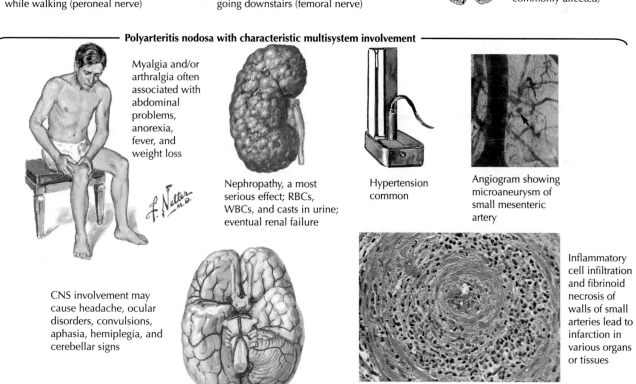

Polyarteritis nodosa with characteristic multisystem involvement

Myalgia and/or arthralgia often associated with abdominal problems, anorexia, fever, and weight loss

Nephropathy, a most serious effect; RBCs, WBCs, and casts in urine; eventual renal failure

Hypertension common

Angiogram showing microaneurysm of small mesenteric artery

CNS involvement may cause headache, ocular disorders, convulsions, aphasia, hemiplegia, and cerebellar signs

Inflammatory cell infiltration and fibrinoid necrosis of walls of small arteries lead to infarction in various organs or tissues

eral neuropathy (CMT type IA) (Fig. 123-6). A common genetic abnormality found in patients with CMT type IA involves duplication of the gene for PMP 22 protein, which is localized to chromosome 17. Interestingly, the genetic mutation seen most commonly in HNPP, which also has demyelinating features with superimposed compressive neuropathies at common entrapment sites, is a deletion in the same gene.

The electrophysiologic examination involves nerve conduction studies, needle electromyography (EMG), and in selected situations, autonomic reflex function testing. Electrodiagnostic studies provide information about the distribution of neuropathy and the elements involved (e.g., motor, sensory, autonomic, or combinations thereof). Electrodiagnostic testing can also help to determine whether the neuropathy primarily involves disease of

Figure 123-6 Hereditary Motor-Sensory Neuropathy Type I: Motor Nerve Conduction Velocity.

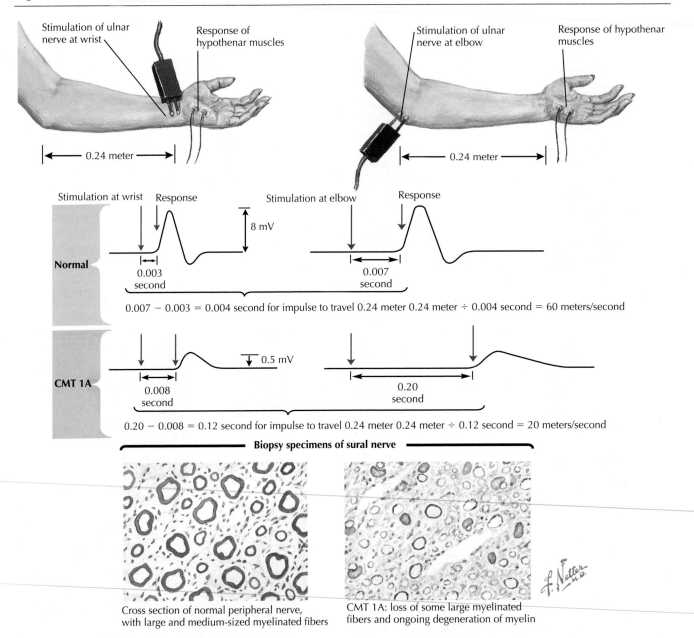

0.007 − 0.003 = 0.004 second for impulse to travel 0.24 meter   0.24 meter ÷ 0.004 second = 60 meters/second

0.20 − 0.008 = 0.12 second for impulse to travel 0.24 meter   0.24 meter ÷ 0.12 second = 20 meters/second

Biopsy specimens of sural nerve

Cross section of normal peripheral nerve, with large and medium-sized myelinated fibers

CMT 1A: loss of some large myelinated fibers and ongoing degeneration of myelin

myelination, nerve axons, or nerve cell bodies. Electrodiagnostic studies may also help distinguish between acquired and hereditary diseases. Disorders characterized by disease of myelin typically have modest to marked slowing of conduction velocities, whereas those of predominantly axonal origin preserve conduction velocity; or it is only minimally slowed but the amplitudes of the responses elicited by nerve stimulation are reduced. Needle EMG examination typically is relatively preserved in demyelinating disorders and demonstrates the findings of denervation and reinnervation in axonal processes. Autonomic reflex function testing examines reproducible autonomic pathways includ-

ing postganglionic sympathetic sudomotor axon reflexes to produce sweating, cardiovagal responses including heart rate response to deep breathing and Valsalva maneuver, and adrenergic nerve fiber function with beat-to-beat blood pressure responses during Valsalva maneuver and during head-up tilt-table testing. Some or all of these reflex pathways may be impaired in an autonomic neuropathy.

Nerve biopsy is useful in determining the underlying pathophysiology of neuropathy in selected circumstances. It is most helpful in acquired disorders such as vasculitis, sarcoidosis, and amyloidosis; in instances of tumor infiltration of the nerve sheath; and in small-fiber neuropathy in which electrodiagnostic studies are usually normal, as well as in the hereditary disorder of polyglucosan body neuropathy. The role of nerve biopsy in hereditary disorders will likely become less important as the molecular genetics of these disorders are elucidated. The sural nerve is the most common nerve biopsied, although in specialized centers, other nerves can undergo biopsy if needed. Because the sural nerve is a cutaneous sensory nerve, it may not be as useful in disorders that only affect motor or autonomic function.

Management and Therapy

Optimum Treatment

The treatment of neuropathy depends on its cause and can be directed either toward the underlying disease process or a specific symptom. Therapy directed toward the improvement of a particular symptom, usually pain or a skilled function that is impaired leading to disability, such as ankle-foot orthotic devices for patients with gait imbalance due to foot drop, can be very helpful for an affected patient. The symptomatic treatment of pain control is evolving and is also of importance. Many of the newer anticonvulsant agents have been shown to be beneficial in treating neuropathic pain in addition to the more common use of tricyclic antidepressants and certain topical anesthetic agents.

Entrapment neuropathies are best treated through discontinuation of those activities that worsen or precipitate symptoms. In some situations, surgical intervention is necessary. Many of the metabolic and toxic neuropathies require correction of the underlying problem (e.g., B_{12} replacement, control of diabetes mellitus or thyroid function status, treatment of collagen vascular disease, or removal or avoidance of the toxic agent or drug. Inflammatory (e.g., CIDP, GBS), vasculitic, or paraproteinemic neuropathies can be successfully treated with corticosteroids, intravenous immunoglobulin, immunosuppressive medications such as azathioprine or mycophenolate mofetil, or therapeutic apheresis. Physical and occupational therapies and the use of adaptive equipment are of benefit in more severe forms of neuropathies. Similarly, these modalities are all that are available in the management of hereditary neuropathies.

Patients with significant sensory loss as the result of their neuropathy are at risk for orthopedic and dermatologic injury of their limbs. The foot is most likely to be affected because patients are not able to perceive painful stimuli and their feet are subjected to repetitive trauma. The resulting painless, often overlooked, ulcers that develop may become secondarily infected resulting in cellulitis and osteomyelitis. Charcot's joints may develop in the most severe cases. These situations typically occur in patients with diabetic neuropathy or

HSAN, and patient and care provider vigilance is of critical importance.

Avoiding Treatment Errors

Careful diagnosis—confirmation of the presence of peripheral neuropathy as a cause for the patient's symptoms and findings, and its underlying cause—allows the clinician to provide the most appropriate treatment for each patient. Symptomatic treatment, such as medications for neuropathic pain and supportive care such as physical and occupational therapies, should be instituted in all patients with peripheral neuropathy as needed. However, a decision regarding appropriate treatment directed at the underlying cause of the peripheral neuropathy requires a careful and thorough investigation of each patient. Misdiagnosis of the underlying cause of the peripheral neuropathy can lead to administration of treatments that could be potentially dangerous to the patient, such as immunosuppressive therapies. Therefore, such treatments should only be considered in patients with a known immune-mediated neuropathy of a severity to justify such a therapeutic approach.

Future Directions

Advances in the treatment of neuropathy are evolving on three broad fronts: the identification of the gene mutations involved in hereditary neuropathies, which will hopefully lead to better diagnosis and ultimately gene therapy; the elucidation of the immunopathology in several immune-mediated acquired neuropathies; and the control of pain.

As understanding of the immune-mediated basis for several of the neuropathic disorders evolves, newer immunosuppressive regimens will be developed. The goal is to develop specific or targeted therapies that are nontoxic and that quickly and permanently remove the abnormal immune response in order to allow regeneration of the peripheral nerve and return of its normal function. The role of interferons and cytokines and the ability to interfere with antigen presentation or co-stimulatory processes are being studied. Because pain is a prominent feature of many neuropathies, extensive work is being carried out on the role of neural growth factors to modulate pain perception and to promote neuronal survival.

Additional Resources

Bromberg MB: Peripheral neurotoxic disorders. Neurol Clin 18(3):681-694, 2000.
   This excellent review of peripheral neuropathies caused by neurotoxic etiologies describes pharmacologic, environmental, and industrial causes for this subgroup of neuropathies.
Dyck PJ, Dyck PJ, Chalk CH: The 10 P's: A mnemonic helpful in characterization and differential diagnosis of peripheral neuropathy. Neurology 42(1):14-18, 1992.
   This landmark reference aims to provide clinicians from all backgrounds with an easily remembered working framework to the clinical approach needed

to diagnose and characterize peripheral neuropathy. It outlines a simple and basic approach to categorizing clinical features of peripheral neuropathy so that a focused investigation into its cause can be designed appropriately.

Dyck, PJ, Dyck PJ, Grant IA, Fealey RD: Ten steps in characterizing and diagnosing patients with peripheral neuropathy. Neurology 47(1):10-17, 1996.

This is an important reference for clinicians interested in designing an approach to diagnosis and characterization of peripheral neuropathy in their patients. It provides an outline of diagnostic approaches to peripheral neuropathy based on its clinical features and provides specific examples of common clinical cases.

England JD: Entrapment neuropathies. Curr Opin Neurol 12(5):597-602, 1999.

This review article highlights advances and interesting observations that cover a wide spectrum of such focal neuropathies. Selected disorders that can affect individual peripheral nerves and masquerade as entrapment neuropathies are also emphasized.

Keller MP, Chance PF: Inherited peripheral neuropathy. Semin Neurol 19(4):353-362, 1999.

This article is a comprehensive review of the spectrum of inherited neuropathies. It provides a logical approach to their diagnosis.

Leger JM, Salachas F: Diagnosis of motor neuropathy. Eur J Neurol 8(3):201-208, 2001.

This article is a comprehensive review of pure motor neuropathies and details distinguishing features between various causes of motor neuropathy and non-neuropathic etiologies.

EVIDENCE

1. England JD, Gronseth GS, Franklin G, et al: Distal symmetrical polyneuropathy: A definition for clinical research. Report of the American Academy of Neurology, the American Association of Electrodiagnostic Medicine, and the American Academy of Physical Medicine and Rehabilitation. Neurology 64(2):199-207, 2005.

This seminal article establishes the definition of a distal symmetrical polyneuropathy based on the available evidence and, where adequate evidence was not available, consensus of more than a dozen leading experts in the field of peripheral neuropathy. This definition will serve as the basis for defining patient populations for further clinical research studies.

2. Hughes RA, Bouche P, Cornblath DR, et al: European Federation of Neurological Societies/Peripheral Nerve Society guideline on management of chronic inflammatory demyelinating polyradiculoneuropathy. Report of a joint task force of the European Federation of Neurological Societies and the Peripheral Nerve Society. Eur J Neurol 13(4):326-332, 2006.

This article establishes guidelines for the definition, diagnosis, and treatment of chronic inflammatory demyelinating polyradiculoneuropathy (CIDP) based on the available evidence and, where adequate evidence was not available, consensus.

Kevin A. Kahn ▪ Alan G. Finkel

124

Migraine Headache

Introduction

Migraine is a prevalent disorder that has been documented throughout the record of human history. Neolithic humans (7000 BC) bore holes (trepanation) into the skulls of presumed headache sufferers, and the Egyptians (1200 BC) wrapped a clay crocodile around the heads of headache patients with cloth bearing the names of the gods. It was Arateus of Cappadocia (2nd century AD) who is given credit for first identifying many of the features of migraine described in later history. Galen (200 AD) named the illness using the Greek, *hemicrania*, from which the term *migraine* derives its name.

Today, we know migraine to be a disabling disorder with a lifetime prevalence of 18% among females and of 6% among all males in the United States. In 1988, the International Headache Society published guidelines for classification of all recognized headache types. Shortly thereafter, Stewart and Lipton published the American Migraine Study, recognized for its generalizability and reproducibility in other countries throughout the world.

Migraine disability has been estimated to cost the United States between $5 and $17 billion annually. Fifty percent of migraineurs miss work 2 days per month and have reduced work efficiency for 6 days per month. Two thirds of migraineurs recognize that the disease has adversely affected their family life. Classifiable migraine is physician diagnosed in only 52% of sufferers. These facts underscore the importance of the physician in recognizing, diagnosing, and treating migraine in the workplace and home.

Etiology and Pathogenesis

Migraine was considered a purely vascular disorder until the mid-1980s when Moskowitz proposed the *Trigeminovascular Theory* of migraine. Using animal models, he demonstrated that electrical stimulation of the trigeminal nucleus caudalis in the pons causes plasma protein extravasation from dural blood vessels. He concluded that the generation of migraine depended on serotonin-mediated increases in neuronal excitation, not on primary vascular reactivity. Thus the pain results in inflammation of blood vessels, although its source is a *neurogenic* cause localizable to trigeminal nuclear centers. In humans, trigeminal stimulation during neurosurgery has resulted in the expression of recognized inflammatory and pronociceptive substances (calcitonin gene–related peptide, neurokinin-A, substance P) within the extracranial circulation similar to that produced in the animal studies (Fig. 124-1).

Migraine aura occurs consistently in 15% to 25% of migraineurs (Figs. 124-2 and 124-3). Aura is a localizable and fully reversible neurologic deficit preceding head pain, which results from progressive, neuronal dysfunction spreading across the cerebral cortex. A similar spreading cortical depression occurs in experimental animals after chemical or electrical irritation of the brain surface. Studies including single-photon emission computed tomography, positron emission tomography, functional magnetic resonance imaging, phosphorous magnetic spectroscopy, and magnetoencephalography have bolstered this hypothesis. Decreased blood flow does not reach levels severe enough to qualify as ischemia. Other systems including serotonergic, noradrenergic, and dopaminergic pathways; hormones (e.g., estrogen); and hypothalamic and deep brainstem structures are involved in the ultimate expression of migraine. Thus, migraine can be described as neuronal sensitization and neurogenic inflammation in a milieu of multiple neurochemical influences. The goal of migraine treatment is to attenuate neuronal irritability and neurogenic inflammation while keeping in mind the importance of the contributions of these other central mechanisms.

Figure 124-1 Mechanisms in Migraine.

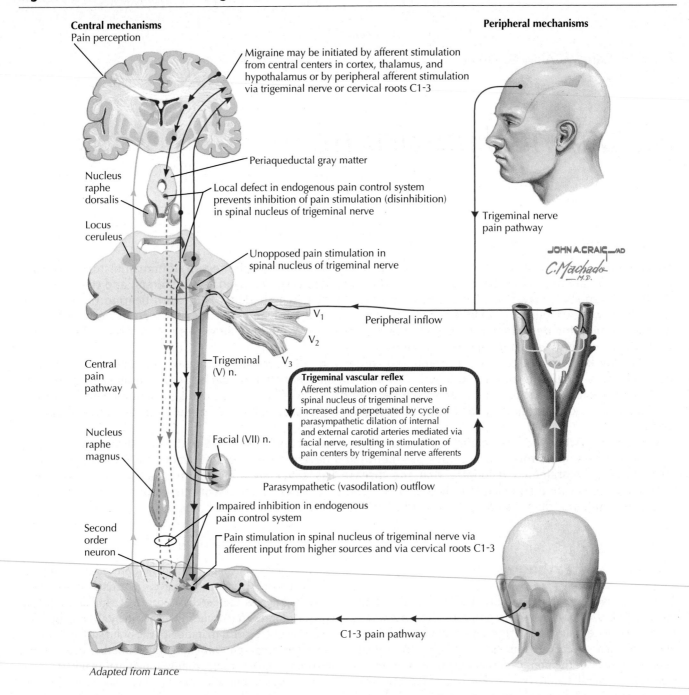

Central mechanisms
Pain perception

Migraine may be initiated by afferent stimulation from central centers in cortex, thalamus, and hypothalamus or by peripheral afferent stimulation via trigeminal nerve or cervical roots C1-3

Nucleus raphe dorsalis

Locus ceruleus

Periaqueductal gray matter

Local defect in endogenous pain control system prevents inhibition of pain stimulation (disinhibition) in spinal nucleus of trigeminal nerve

Unopposed pain stimulation in spinal nucleus of trigeminal nerve

Central pain pathway

V₁

V₂

Trigeminal (V) n.

V₃

Nucleus raphe magnus

Facial (VII) n.

Second order neuron

Impaired inhibition in endogenous pain control system

Pain stimulation in spinal nucleus of trigeminal nerve via afferent input from higher sources and via cervical roots C1-3

Peripheral mechanisms

Trigeminal nerve pain pathway

JOHN A. CRAIG—MD
C. Machado —M.D.

Peripheral inflow

Trigeminal vascular reflex
Afferent stimulation of pain centers in spinal nucleus of trigeminal nerve increased and perpetuated by cycle of parasympathetic dilation of internal and external carotid arteries mediated via facial nerve, resulting in stimulation of pain centers by trigeminal nerve afferents

Parasympathetic (vasodilation) outflow

C1-3 pain pathway

Adapted from Lance

Clinical Presentation

Migraine presents in a variable fashion, but it can be divided into two groups: with aura (classic migraine) and without aura (common migraine) (Fig. 124-4). A prodrome may occur up to 24 hours preceding headache. Prodromal features may include hunger, thirst, euphoria, mania, depression, drowsiness, psychomotor slowing, or irritability. Aura is present in only 15% to 25% of migraineurs. Aura symptoms may include visual scotomas (dark spots), photopsias (bright spots), fortification spectra (jagged bright lines), numbness, tingling, weakness, confusion, or aphasia. Triggers include environmental stimuli such as intense light, sound, and odors; certain foods (nitrates, sulfites, monosodium glutamate, alcohol); irregular sleep or nutrition; exercise; stress; and hormonal fluctuations (Fig. 124-5). The International Headache Society proposed guidelines in 1988 to diagnose migraine, shown in Boxes 124-1 and 124-2.

Figure 124-2 Migraine Prodromes and Attack.

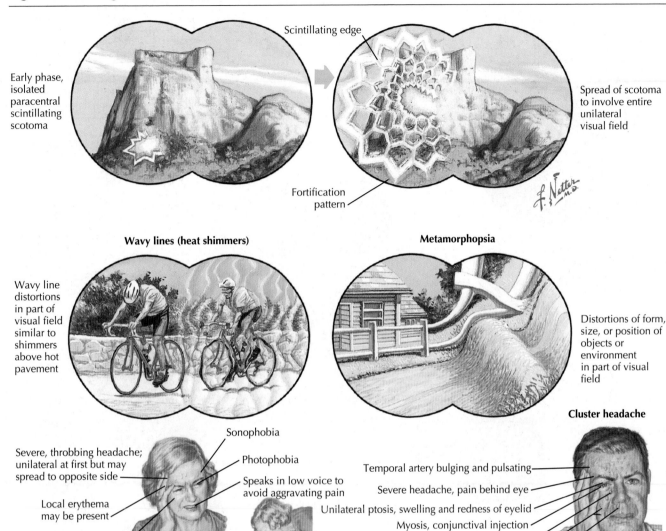

Early phase, isolated paracentral scintillating scotoma

Scintillating edge

Spread of scotoma to involve entire unilateral visual field

Fortification pattern

Wavy lines (heat shimmers)

Wavy line distortions in part of visual field similar to shimmers above hot pavement

Metamorphopsia

Distortions of form, size, or position of objects or environment in part of visual field

Severe, throbbing headache; unilateral at first but may spread to opposite side

Local erythema may be present

Pallor, perspiration

Sonophobia

Photophobia

Speaks in low voice to avoid aggravating pain

Vomiting may occur

Cluster headache

Temporal artery bulging and pulsating

Severe headache, pain behind eye

Unilateral ptosis, swelling and redness of eyelid

Myosis, conjunctival injection

Tearing

Flushing of side of face, sweating

Nasal congestion, rhinorrhea

Box 124-1   Diagnostic Criteria for Migraine without Aura (Common Migraine)

- No single feature required or sufficient for diagnosis
- At least five attacks lasting 4-72 hours
- Headache has at least two of the following characteristics:
  - Unilateral location
  - Pulsating quality
  - Moderate or severe intensity (inhibits or prohibits daily activities)
  - Aggravation by routine physical activity
- At least one of the following during headache:
  - Nausea or vomiting
  - Photophobia (light sensitivity)
  - Phonophobia (sound sensitivity)

History and exam do not support evidence of organic disease that could cause headaches, or if disease is present, then headaches should not have originated in close temporal relation to the disease.

Box 124-2   Diagnostic Criteria for Migraine with Aura (Classic Migraine)

- At least two attacks
- Aura must exhibit at least three of the following characteristics:
  - Fully reversible and indicative of focal cerebral cortical or brainstem dysfunction
  - Gradual onset
  - Lasts less than 60 minutes
  - Followed by headache with a free interval of less than 60 minutes
  - Headache may begin before or simultaneously with the aura

History and exam do not support evidence of organic disease that could cause headaches, or if disease is present, then headaches should not have originated in close temporal relation to the disease.

Figure 124-3 Basilar Artery Migraine.

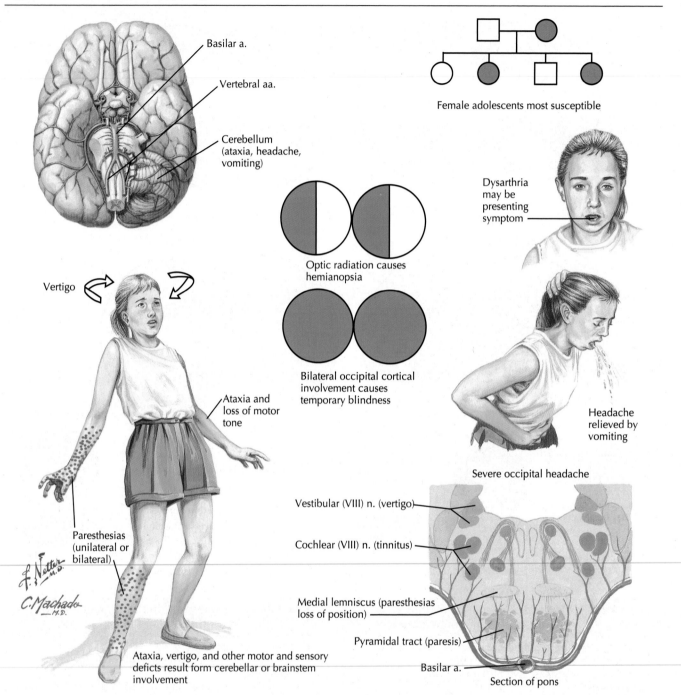

Basilar a.

Vertebral aa.

Cerebellum (ataxia, headache, vomiting)

Female adolescents most susceptible

Dysarthria may be presenting symptom

Optic radiation causes hemianopsia

Bilateral occipital cortical involvement causes temporary blindness

Vertigo

Ataxia and loss of motor tone

Paresthesias (unilateral or bilateral)

Ataxia, vertigo, and other motor and sensory deficts result form cerebellar or brainstem involvement

Headache relieved by vomiting

Severe occipital headache

Vestibular (VIII) n. (vertigo)

Cochlear (VIII) n. (tinnitus)

Medial lemniscus (paresthesias loss of position)

Pyramidal tract (paresis)

Basilar a.

Section of pons

Differential Diagnosis

Migraine must be differentiated from secondary causes of headache to rule out more lethal causes of severe head pain. Other primary headache disorders, tension-type headache, cluster headache, and cluster variants are often confused with migraine. Tension-type headache typically does not cause nausea and does not present with *both* photophobia and phonophobia. There is considerable debate about whether tension-type headache is an independent disorder or represents a part of a migraine continuum. Nevertheless, tension-type headache may coexist with migraine, and the presence of a tension headache does not preclude the possibility of migraine. Cluster headache derives its name from the pattern of recurrent groups of headaches within a finite period of days to months. It is characterized as an excruciating, typically retro-orbital or temporal pain with duration of 15 to 180 minutes and typically affects males more than females. The headache attack may recur at specific times of the day with remark-

Figure 124-4 Triggers of Migraine.

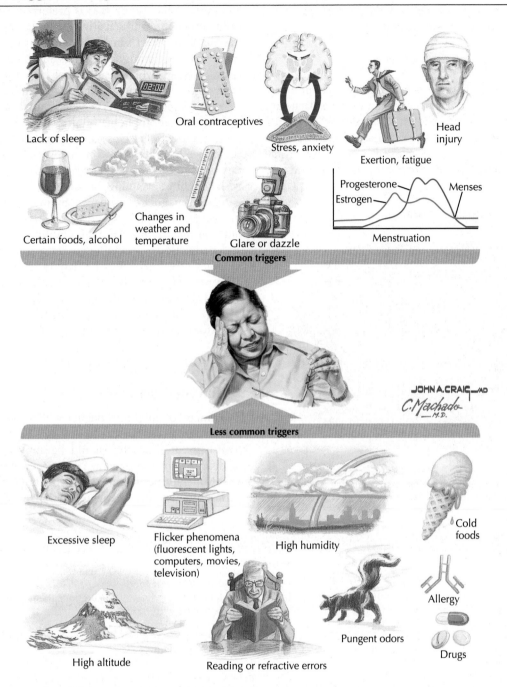

Lack of sleep

Oral contraceptives

Stress, anxiety

Exertion, fatigue

Head injury

Certain foods, alcohol

Changes in weather and temperature

Glare or dazzle

Progesterone

Estrogen

Menses

Menstruation

Common triggers

JOHN A. CRAIG—MD
C. Machado
—M.D.

Less common triggers

Excessive sleep

Flicker phenomena (fluorescent lights, computers, movies, television)

High humidity

Cold foods

Allergy

High altitude

Reading or refractive errors

Pungent odors

Drugs

able consistency. It is differentiated from migraine by its short duration and difference in behavior of the patient during the attack: the cluster patient cannot be still during the event, whereas the migraine patient prefers immobility and hibernation. In addition, it must present with at least one of the following features: lacrimation, rhinorrhea, ptosis, miosis, nasal congestion, conjunctival injection, eyelid edema, and forehead or facial sweating abnormalities. Cluster variants include those headaches with similar features to cluster but with shorter duration. Chronic par-

oxysmal hemicrania, a cluster variant, affects women more than men and has an absolute response to indomethacin.

Secondary causes of headache disorders include head trauma, vascular disorders (e.g., hemorrhage, stroke, vasculitis), intracranial disorders (e.g., neoplasm, increased or decreased intracranial pressure), substance withdrawal, infection, metabolic disorders (e.g., hypoxia, hypercapnia, hypoglycemia, dialysis), and disorders of other structures of the head and neck (e.g., cervical spine, eyes, ears, nose and sinuses, temporomandibular joints). Most of these can be elucidated by a careful history and exam; however, sometimes it is necessary to perform diagnostic procedures if suspicion for these disorders is raised.

Diagnostic Approach

There is no specific diagnostic test for migraine, but investigations are mandated if secondary causes of headache are of concern. Secondary headaches should be suspected when the patient reports a "worst headache," has an abnormal neurologic exam, has developed a new-onset headache, or when there has been a dramatic change in headache

Figure 124-5 Migraine Aura.

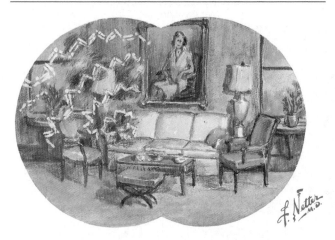

Visual disturbances, most common element of migraine aura: blurred cloudy vision, scotomas, scintillating zigzag lines (fortification spectrum), flashes of light, etc.

pattern. To rule out an acute hemorrhage, noncontrasted computed tomography scan is preferred because of speed of the procedure and sensitivity. Lumbar puncture may be necessary to detect xanthochromia in patients with negative computed tomography scans and high index of suspicion for bleed (worst headache of life). Lumbar puncture may also be helpful in assessing causes of headache related to pressure (position affects headache) or infection (nuchal rigidity plus photophobia or altered mental status). However, if intracranial masses are suspected, then magnetic resonance imaging with contrast is preferred. Abnormalities in the posterior fossae are associated with headaches with coughing, straining, bending, and so forth. Contrast-enhanced magnetic resonance angiogram may be helpful in assessing vasculitis or the presence of an aneurysm, but consider traditional angiography if suspicion is high and magnetic resonance angiogram is negative. Carotid Doppler assessment may be helpful in acute-onset headache with Horner's syndrome to rule out carotid dissection. Electroencephalography should be performed in those patients with paroxysmal headache with cognitive or behavioral changes to rule out epilepsy.

Management and Therapy

Optimum Treatment

Treatment of migraine begins with clear diagnosis and knowledge of its pathophysiology (Fig. 124-6). Acute treatment of headache should be stratified to the level of disability in the patient. Nonspecific therapies (Table 124-1) include nonsteroidal anti-inflammatory drugs, sympathomimetics (e.g., caffeine), or analgesics (acetamino-

Table 124-1 Nonspecific Acute Therapy for Migraine and Tension Headache*

Medication	Dose	Regimen	Comments
Aspirin	325 mg	1-2 PO every 6 hr PRN with food	
Acetaminophen	325 or 500 mg	1-2 PO every 6 hr PRN	Category B agent in pregnancy
Aspirin/caffeine	250 mg/65 mg	1-2 PO every 6 hr PRN with food	
Acetaminophen/caffeine	250 mg/65 mg	1-2 PO every 6 hr PRN	
Isometheptene/ dichloralphenazone/ acetaminophen	65 mg/100 mg/325 mg (1 capsule)	2 at headache onset; 1 every hour until headache remits	Maximum dose 5 capsules daily
Ergotamine/caffeine	1 mg/100 mg	2 at headache onset; 1 every 30 min until headache remits	Maximum dose 6 daily; category X agent in pregnancy
Ibuprofen	400, 600, or 800 mg	1 PO every 4-6 hr PRN with food	Category B agent in pregnancy
Indomethacin	25 or 50 mg	1 PO every 8 hr PRN with food	Category B agent in pregnancy
Ketoprofen	25 or 50 mg	1 PO every 8 hr PRN with food	Category B agent in pregnancy
Naproxen sodium	375 or 500 mg	1 PO every 8-12 h PRN with food	Category B agent in pregnancy
Lidocaine 4%	1 mL	0.5 mL per nostril every 4 hr PRN	Tilt head back during administration; supine position preferred; category B agent in pregnancy
Metoclopramide	10 mg	1 PO every 6 hr PRN	Use with other acute medications; category B agent in pregnancy
Prochlorperazine	5 or 10 mg	1 PO every 8 hr PRN	Use with other acute medications
Promethazine	25-50 mg	1 PO every 8 hr PRN	Use with other acute medications

* All nonsteroidal anti-inflammatory drugs are contraindicated during the third trimester of pregnancy.

phen, opiates). Frequent use of many of these has been associated with substance withdrawal headache and analgesic rebound. For moderate to severely disabling headache, specific medication should be used (Table 124-2). The most specific of these are triptans. They bind specifically to serotonin receptors on trigeminal nerve endings to halt neurogenic inflammation in addition to binding to dural blood vessels to reduce painful swelling. There is no class effect of triptans, and if one is not effective, another may be tried. They are contraindicated in patients with uncontrolled hypertension and a history of coronary artery disease but are generally safe and effective. Triptans are more costly than nonspecific therapy, but economic analyses point to cost savings and decreased disability when triptans are used in patients with moderate to severe headache.

Patients should be offered preventive treatment if untreatable headaches occur more than twice per month or if the patient is willing to use a daily medication to prevent headache. Preventive medication usually provides benefit after 2 to 3 months of administration. U.S. Food and Drug Administration–approved preventive treatment for migraine includes valproic acid, propranolol, and methysergide. There is evidence (Table 124-3) to support the use of other agents, including other anticonvulsants (decrease neuronal irritability), other β blockers (modulate noradrenergic system and vascular system), tricyclic antidepressants (modulate serotonin and norepinephrine), calcium channel blockers (vascular and central factors), and hormonal manipulation. Oral chelated magnesium, high-dose (400 mg/day) oral riboflavin, and coenzyme Q_{10} have been reported to be effective in double-blinded studies.

Nonpharmacologic approaches include the avoidance of migraine triggers (e.g., foods, missed meals), biofeed-back and self-hypnosis, psychological counseling to improve stress management skills, regular exercise, good sleep hygiene, and a balanced diet. All these measures serve to decrease neuronal irritability and thereby reduce the frequency of migraine.

Avoiding Treatment Errors

Acute Treatment Errors

Treatment errors are common among headache specialists and general practitioners alike. One common error is to treat migraine as a general pain disorder for which a step-based approach is often used. In this approach, a less-specific and often cheaper therapy is used followed by more sophisticated therapies if the initial therapy fails. It has been shown that a stratified approach to treatment is more effective for both reduction of disability and reduction of cost. In such an approach, patients with moderate to severe headache history are given migraine-specific therapy (triptans) first rather than waiting for them to fail nonspecific therapies (e.g., aspirin, caffeine, nonsteroidal anti-inflammatory drugs).

Another common error is to attempt to use acute treatment as a diagnostic tool. Although triptans are specific to the treatment of migraine, they do not have a class effect, so if one drug fails, another may still be effective. Thus, failure to respond to a given triptan does not exclude migraine as the underlying diagnosis.

Timing of therapy is a frequent pitfall in migraine acute treatment. Several studies have demonstrated that migraine is best treated within 1 to 2 hours of headache onset. Patients must be educated to treat their headaches when the first symptoms occur before the headache has a chance

Table 124-2 Migraine-Specific Acute Therapy			
Medication	**Dose**	**Regimen**	**Comments**
Ergot Derivatives			
Dihydroergotamine IV	1 mg	IV every 8 hr PRN	Administer antiemetic/antihistamine therapy before using this agent; category X agent in pregnancy
Dihydroergotamine intranasal spray	1 mg	1 spray in each nostril and repeat in 15 min every 2 hr PRN	FDA maximum dose 2 vials daily; must prime pump before administration; category X agent in pregnancy
Triptans			
Almotriptan	12.5 mg	1 PO every 2 hr PRN	FDA maximum dose 25 mg/d
Eletriptan	20 or 40 mg	1-2 PO every 2 hr PRN	FDA maximum dose 80 mg/d
Naratriptan	1 or 2.5 mg	1 PO every 4 hr PRN	FDA maximum dose 5 mg/d
Rizatriptan	5 or 10 mg	1 PO every 2 hr PRN	FDA maximum dose 30 mg/d
Sumatriptan PO	25, 50, or 100 mg	1 PO every 2 hr PRN	FDA maximum dose 200 mg/d
Sumatriptan intranasal spray	5 or 20 mg	1 spray to 1 nostril every 2 hr PRN	FDA maximum dose 40 mg/d
Sumatriptan injection	4 or 6 mg	1 injection SC every 2 hr PRN	FDA maximum dose 12 mg/d
Zolmitriptan PO	2.5 or 5 mg	2.5-5 mg PO every 2 hr	FDA maximum dose 10 mg/d
Zolmitriptan intranasal spray	5 mg	1 spray to 1 nostril every 2 hr	FDA maximum dose 10 mg/d

Table 124-3 Medications for Migraine Prevention (FDA Approved and Nonapproved)

Medication	Dose	Regimen	Comments
Tricyclic Antidepressants			
Amitriptyline; nortriptyline	10, 25, 50, 100, or 150 mg	10-150 mg PO qhs*	Titrate ≤25 mg per week; may cause dry mouth, blurred vision, drowsiness, and urinary retention
Ergot Derivatives			
Methysergide	2 or 4 mg	2-4 mg tid	*FDA-approved*; however, no longer available in the United States; titrate ≤2 mg every 2 days; taper after 4-6 months because of risk for retroperitoneal fibrosis; category D agent in pregnancy
Mitochondrial-Enhancing Agents			
Coenzyme Q$_{10}$	50, 100, 120, 200, or 300 mg	150-300 mg in 2 divided doses	Effective in about 50% of patients with migraine
Riboflavin	50 or 100 mg	400 mg PO qd with food	Effective in about 50% of patients with migraine
Miscellaneous			
Cyproheptadine	4 mg	1-6 tabs PO qhs*	Children with migraine should take low doses; adults with migraine with concurrent allergies should take higher doses
Magnesium oxide	200-250 or 400-500 mg	1 tab PO bid with food	Effective in menstrual migraine; 400 mg bid is preferred, but dose may be decreased to 200-250 mg bid if diarrhea occurs
β Blockers			
Atenolol	25-100 mg	qd or bid	Titrate slowly; contraindicated in patients with diabetes, asthma, and heart block; category D agent in pregnancy
Nadolol	40-120 mg	qd	*FDA-approved.* Titrate slowly; contraindicated in patients with diabetes, asthma, and heart block
Pindolol	5 mg	bid; titrate to 10-60 mg total daily	Titrate slowly; contraindicated in patients with diabetes, asthma, and heart block; category B agent in pregnancy
Propranolol LA	30-160 mg	qd or bid	*FDA-approved.* Titrate slowly; contraindicated in patients with diabetes, asthma, and heart block
Calcium Channel Blockers			
Verapamil	120-720 mg	qd or tid depending on total dose	High dose is often necessary; side effects may occur; titrate slowly; contraindicated in patients with congestive heart failure
Amlodipine	5-15 mg	qd or bid	Titrate slowly (every 2 wk) from 5 mg
Felodipine	5-15 mg	qd or bid	Titrate slowly from 5 mg
Nisoldipine	10-40 mg	qd or bid	Titrate slowly from 10 mg
Anticonvulsants			
Gabapentin	300, 400, 600, or 800 mg	1800-4800 mg/d in 3 divided doses	Titrate by 900-1200 mg every 2 wk; may cause fatigue or edema
Lamotrigine	25 or 100 mg	25-200 mg qhs* or divided bid	Titrate by 25 mg/wk; rapid titration may increase risk for rash
Levetiracetam	250, 500, or 750 mg	1000-4000 mg in 2 divided doses	Titrate by 250-500 mg/wk; may cause somnolence
Sodium valproate, sodium valproate ER	125, 250, or 500 mg (250 and 500 mg ER formulation)	500 mg bid; 1000 mg qhs* in ER formulation	*FDA-approved.* Begin at 250 mg total daily; titrate slowly over 2-4 weeks; women at risk for pregnancy should take folate supplements; category D agent in pregnancy; causes hair thinning in about 5% of patients; take selenium at a mealtime when sodium valproate is not administered; liver function testing is recommended after 1 and 3 months
Topiramate	15, 25, 50, or 100 mg	50-100 mg bid or 100-200 mg total qhs*	*FDA-approved.* May cause weight loss; reversible/transient side effects include tingling and drowsiness; contraindicated in patients with nephrolithiasis and glaucoma
Zonisamide	25, 50, or 100 mg	100-400 mg qhs*	Titrate extremely slowly by 25 mg/wk; may cause weight loss; reversible/transient side effects include tingling and drowsiness; contraindicated in patients with nephrolithiasis and glaucoma

* qhs, every night.
FDA, U.S. Food and Drug Administration.
Data from Krymchantowski AV, Bigal ME, Moreira PF: New and emerging prophylactic agents for migraine. CNS Drugs 16(9):611-634, 2002; and Silberstein SD: Practice parameter: Evidence-based guidelines for migraine headache (an evidence-based review). Report of the Quality Standards Subcommittee of the American Academy of Neurology. Neurology 55(6):754-762, 2002.

Figure 124-6 Approach to Migraine Treatment.

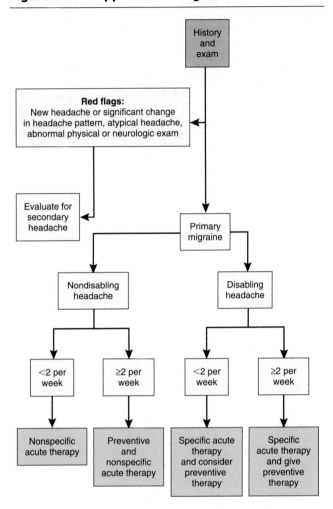

tive disk disease must be considered in refractory headache as well. If any one or any combination of these underlying problems is present, both acute and preventive medications will be less effective, and the patient will falsely conclude that potentially effective therapies have failed.

Future Directions

The future of migraine management lies in the development of pharmacologic and nonpharmacologic strategies that follow advances in migraine pathophysiology. Genetic studies have linked hemiplegic migraine (aura of reversible hemiplegia) to a defect on chromosome 19p13, which encodes voltage-gated P/Q type calcium channel. Genetic polymorphism studies have implicated alterations in the gene for serotonin receptors in migraine without aura and in dopamine receptors with migraine with aura. Such studies may provide clues to why migraineurs are predisposed to central sensitization and neurogenic inflammation. Neuroimaging studies may continue to provide links between the animal and human models. Nonpharmacologic therapies are just beginning to be subjected to evidence-based medicine trials. Pending such studies there will likely be a place in migraine therapy for neurohypnosis, acupuncture, music therapy, and other complementary medical approaches. Education of health care professionals is an important part of management of migraine because nearly half of all migraineurs remain undiagnosed. Proactive and educated health care providers will serve to improve the quality of life in migraineurs and will lessen the impact of this prevalent and disabling disease.

Additional Resources

Silberstein SD, Lipton RB, Goadsby PJ: Headache in Clinical Practice. Oxford, UK, Isis Medical Media, 1998.
  This text describes many of the principles of diagnosis and treatment outlined in this chapter as well as history of migraine.
Olesen J, Tfelt-Hansen P, Welch KMA: The Headaches. Philadelphia, Lippincott Williams & Wilkins, 2006.
  This book describes many of the principles of diagnosis and treatment outlined in this chapter.

to progress. This approach will increase the likelihood of drug efficacy and the chance for sustained headache relief. Early treatment decreases disability and decreases the cost of treating each headache.

Preventive Treatment Pitfalls

Patients who present with a long list of failed therapies often suffer the pitfall of attempting treatment without addressing causative or aggravating factors. In the setting of medication overuse headache (medication used on a near daily basis), the medication must be completely removed in order for prevention to be effective. The removal of caffeine is especially important if it is present in the offending medication or if it is a frequent component of the patient's diet. Other factors include the identification and treatment of sleep disorders such as sleep apnea or restless legs syndrome. Environmental sensitivities and dietary sensitivities are also issues that may perpetuate headache. The relationship of menstrual and ovulatory withdrawal of estrogen to headache must be considered. The presence of structural changes in the cervical spine secondary to degenerative arthritis or degenera-

EVIDENCE

1. Bigal ME, Lipton RB, Krymchantowski AV: The medical management of migraine. Am J Ther 11(2):130-140, 2004.
   The authors provide an evidence-based reference to the tables of medications used for treatment.
2. Burstein R, Collins B, Jakubowski M: Defeating migraine pain with triptans: A race against the development of cutaneous allodynia. Ann Neurol 55(1):19-26, 2004.
   This paper provides evidence-based support for early rather than late taking of medication in the acute treatment of migraine.
3. Calhoun AH: A novel specific prophylaxis for menstrual-associated migraine. South Med J 97(9):819-822, 2004.
   This reference speaks to the evidence-based relationship of estrogen to migraine.

4. Headache Classification Subcommittee of the International Headache Society: The International Classification of Headache Disorders, 2nd ed. Cephalalgia 24(Suppl 1):9-160, 2004.

This is the key literature reference for the diagnostic criteria for all the classifiable headaches mentioned in this chapter.

5. Krymchantowski AV, Bigal ME, Moreira PF: New and emerging prophylactic agents for migraine. CNS Drugs 16(9):611-634, 2002.

This article provides an evidence-based reference to the tables of medications used for treatment.

6. Lipton RB, Silberstein SD: The role of headache-related disability in migraine management: Implications for headache treatment guidelines. Neurology 56(6 Suppl 1):S35-S42, 2001.

This paper provides evidence-based support for stratified care in the acute treatment of migraine.

7. Lipton RB: American Migraine Study II. 42nd Annual Scientific Meeting of the American Headache Society, June 23, 2000.

This article is key to understanding the epidemiology of migraine.

8. Silberstein SD: Practice parameter: Evidence-based guidelines for migraine headache (an evidence-based review). Report of the Quality Standards Subcommittee of the American Academy of Neurology. Neurology 55(6):754-762, 2000.

This paper is very important for evidence-based use of medications presented in treatment table.

9. Warner JS: The outcome of treating patients with suspected rebound headache. Headache 41(7):685-692, 2001.

This evidence-based article discusses features of analgesic rebound headache and implications of its management.

David Y. Huang ▪ Albert R. Hinn

125

Stroke and Transient Ischemic Attacks

Introduction

Stroke is an illness of sudden onset causing brain injury as a result of occlusion or rupture of a cerebral blood vessel. Strokes can be further characterized as ischemic or hemorrhagic (Fig. 125-1). Transient ischemic attacks (TIAs) are brief episodes of neurologic dysfunction of vascular origin, with clinical symptoms typically lasting less than 1 hour, and without evidence of infarction. TIAs are strong predictors of future ischemic events, and the risk for having a stroke within 48 hours of a TIA is nearly 5%. This chapter will focus on ischemic strokes and TIAs, which account for nearly 85% of all strokes.

Etiology and Pathogenesis

Most ischemic strokes are thrombotic or embolic in origin, usually resulting from underlying atherosclerotic disease of extracranial or intracranial cerebral vessels or underlying cardiac disease. Lacunar strokes result from thrombosis of the small subcortical penetrating arteries of the brain and are most often associated with hypertension.

Well-documented, common stroke risk factors include hypertension, smoking, diabetes mellitus, atrial fibrillation, cardiac disease, carotid artery stenosis, dyslipidemia, physical inactivity, postmenopausal hormonal replacement therapy, and obesity. Other risk factors include alcohol and drug abuse, metabolic syndrome, hyperhomocysteinemia, hypercoagulability, and oral contraceptive use. A number of medical conditions (e.g., sickle cell disease, polycythemia vera, meningovascular syphilis, bacterial endocarditis) are much less commonly associated with stroke; however, such etiologies should be considered in patients when other risk factors are not present or when suggested by the medical history (Fig. 125-2).

Clinical Presentation

Symptoms and signs are a reflection of the cerebrovascular distribution of ischemia.

Carotid Artery Territory

Common symptoms and findings are monocular visual loss (amaurosis fugax), contralateral weakness or sensory disturbance, dysarthria, language impairment with dominant hemisphere involvement, neglect with nondominant hemisphere involvement, other higher cortical deficits, and contralateral homonymous visual loss (Fig. 125-3).

Vertebrobasilar Artery Territory

Common symptoms and findings are unilateral or bilateral weakness or sensory disturbance, crossed motor or sensory findings, dysarthria, pupil abnormalities, ophthalmoplegia, other cranial nerve deficits, Horner's syndrome, ataxia, various visual field deficits, and altered level of consciousness (Fig. 125-4). Several brainstem syndromes describe the findings seen with specific vascular distributions and are best understood in terms of the specific nuclei and anatomical pathways involved by the event.

Lacunar Strokes

A number of lacunar syndromes have been described, including pure motor hemiplegia, pure sensory stroke, clumsy hand–dysarthria syndrome, and ataxic hemiparesis.

Figure 125-1 Classification of Stroke Subtypes.

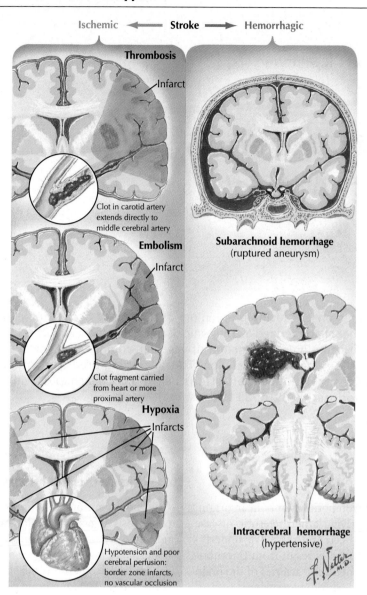

Differential Diagnosis

Many medical conditions may be confused for cerebrovascular events: partial seizures; migrainous auras; cardiac syncope and near-syncope; peripheral vestibulopathies; hypoglycemia; brain tumors, subdural hematomas, and other intracranial mass lesions; demyelinating diseases; spinal cord injuries or lesions; and somatoform disorders. One should also consider systemic infection, metabolic disorders, and medication intoxication or overdose in the patient with primarily generalized weakness or altered consciousness.

Diagnostic Approach

Rapid recognition and diagnosis are essential for treatment of acute strokes. Obtaining a time of symptom onset and a careful history are critical. Onset of symptoms is defined as the time since the patient was last known to be symptom free. For patients awakening with deficits, one must use the time they were last awake and without symptoms. Initial evaluation should include a careful history and neurologic examination. Many centers use the National Institutes of Health Stroke Scale to grade stroke severity.

Blood samples should be drawn for glucose, serum electrolytes, renal function tests, complete blood counts, coagulation studies, and sedimentation rate. Additional laboratory tests may be indicated to rule out systemic infection and medication intoxication or overdose. Emergent imaging of the brain is indicated because of the potential for therapeutic intervention. In general, computed tomography (CT) is the preferred modality for acute strokes, particularly if the patient is eligible for

Figure 125-2 Less Common Etiologic Mechanisms of Stroke.

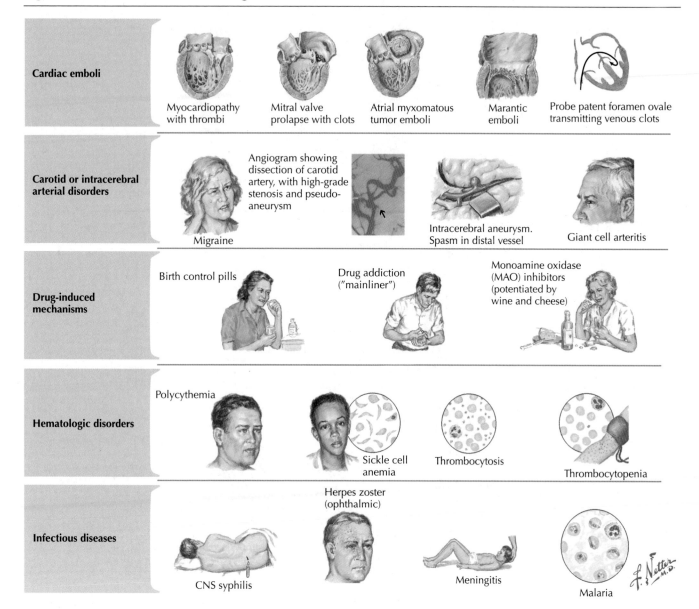

Cardiac emboli

Myocardiopathy with thrombi

Mitral valve prolapse with clots

Atrial myxomatous tumor emboli

Marantic emboli

Probe patent foramen ovale transmitting venous clots

Carotid or intracerebral arterial disorders

Migraine

Angiogram showing dissection of carotid artery, with high-grade stenosis and pseudo-aneurysm

Intracerebral aneurysm. Spasm in distal vessel

Giant cell arteritis

Drug-induced mechanisms

Birth control pills

Drug addiction ("mainliner")

Monoamine oxidase (MAO) inhibitors (potentiated by wine and cheese)

Hematologic disorders

Polycythemia

Sickle cell anemia

Thrombocytosis

Thrombocytopenia

Infectious diseases

Herpes zoster (ophthalmic)

CNS syphilis

Meningitis

Malaria

treatment with thrombolytic therapy. Magnetic resonance imaging with diffusion-weighted images is very useful in demonstrating acute infarcts, but logistical issues, such as longer acquisition times and limited availability of scanners and specialists needed to interpret the images, often make use of this modality difficult in the acute setting. At certain centers, CT or magnetic resonance angiography is performed acutely, if neurointerventionalists are available to provide endovascular therapies (see "Future Directions").

Following the initial acute assessment and treatment, or for patients presenting in the subacute period, the evaluation is focused on determining etiology and risk factors for secondary stroke prevention. Magnetic resonance imaging of the brain is most often performed in this period to confirm the diagnosis of stroke. Evaluation of cerebral vessels should be performed; carotid ultrasound, CT, or magnetic resonance angiography and conventional angiography are all acceptable studies. A cardiac evaluation should also be performed, including 12-lead electrocardiogram and echocardiography looking for sources of emboli or shunting. Electrocardiogram telemetry monitoring can be useful, particularly if concerns exist about undetected cardiac arrhythmias. Lipid and cholesterol panels, syphilis screening, homocysteine level, and high-sensitivity C-reactive protein level should be checked. In the young stroke patient, evaluation for hypercoagulable states may be indicated, including antithrombin III activity, protein C and S activity, sickle cell screen, lupus inhibitor, antinuclear antibody, and anticardiolipin antibody.

Figure 125-3 Ischemia in Internal Carotid Artery Territory: Clinical Manifestations.

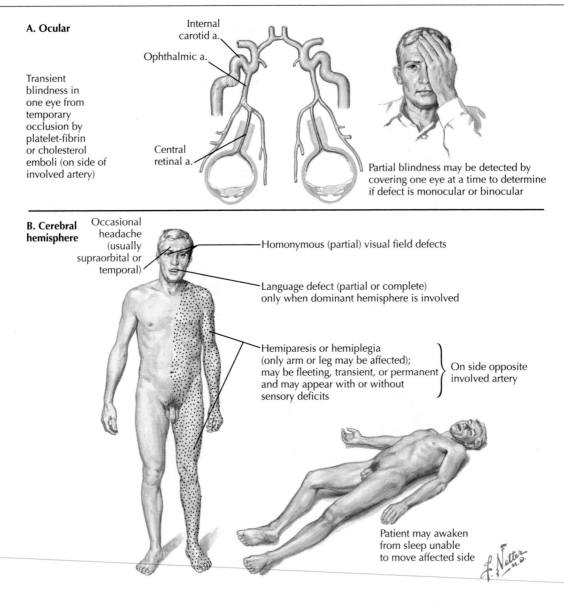

A. Ocular

Internal carotid a.

Ophthalmic a.

Central retinal a.

Transient blindness in one eye from temporary occlusion by platelet-fibrin or cholesterol emboli (on side of involved artery)

Partial blindness may be detected by covering one eye at a time to determine if defect is monocular or binocular

B. Cerebral hemisphere

Occasional headache (usually supraorbital or temporal)

Homonymous (partial) visual field defects

Language defect (partial or complete) only when dominant hemisphere is involved

Hemiparesis or hemiplegia (only arm or leg may be affected); may be fleeting, transient, or permanent and may appear with or without sensory deficits

On side opposite involved artery

Patient may awaken from sleep unable to move affected side

Management and Therapy

Optimum Treatment for Acute Strokes

In the acute setting, initial attention should be given to cardiopulmonary stabilization, and this stabilization should be achieved as rapidly as possible because all unnecessary delays to stroke treatment should be avoided. Currently, acute stroke therapy is centered on the use of intravenous thrombolytic therapy with recombinant tissue plasminogen activator (rt-PA), the only therapy approved by the U.S. Food and Drug Administration for the treatment of acute ischemic stroke. The National Institute of Neurological Disorders and Stroke study documented an approximately 30% relative and 12% absolute increase in patients having a good outcome with minimal to no disability at 3 months, when compared with the placebo group. This was despite an absolute increase of 6% in the occurrence of symptomatic intracerebral hemorrhage in the rt-PA treated patients. Treatment must be initiated within 3 hours after the onset of stroke symptoms and after careful consideration of the patient's eligibility (see Box 125-1 for guidelines). The recommended dose of rt-PA is 0.9 mg/kg (maximum of 90 mg) infused over 60 minutes with 10% of the total dose administered as an initial intravenous bolus over 1 minute.

Patients treated with rt-PA should be closely monitored for at least 24 hours. Neurologic examinations should focus on any signs of acute deterioration (e.g., progressing weakness and alterations in consciousness), which might suggest extension of the stroke or the development of an intracranial hemorrhage (ICH). If ICH is suspected, an emergency head CT scan should be obtained, and rt-PA

Figure 125-4 Ischemia in Vertebrobasilar Territory: Clinical Manifestations.

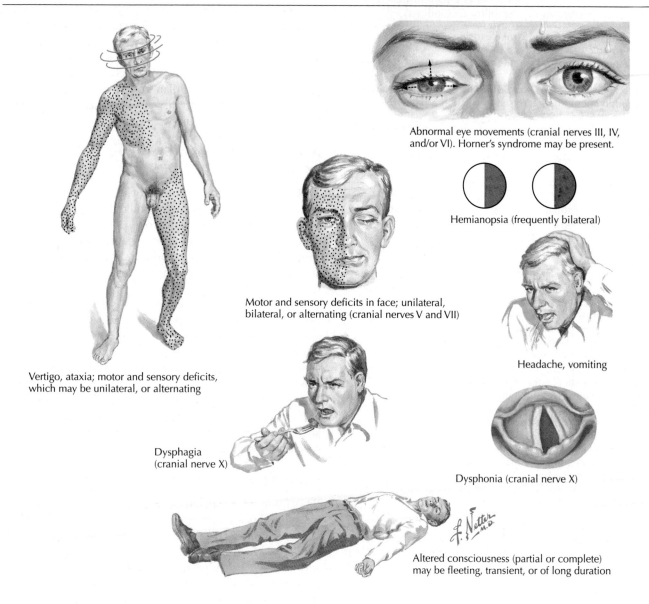

Abnormal eye movements (cranial nerves III, IV, and/or VI). Horner's syndrome may be present.

Hemianopsia (frequently bilateral)

Motor and sensory deficits in face; unilateral, bilateral, or alternating (cranial nerves V and VII)

Headache, vomiting

Vertigo, ataxia; motor and sensory deficits, which may be unilateral, or alternating

Dysphagia (cranial nerve X)

Dysphonia (cranial nerve X)

Altered consciousness (partial or complete) may be fleeting, transient, or of long duration

should be discontinued immediately. Blood should be drawn for complete blood counts, coagulation studies, fibrinogen level, and type and cross-match. If ICH is confirmed by CT, the administration of cryoprecipitate containing fibrinogen and factor VIII or fresh frozen plasma is suggested. Platelets and packed red blood cells should be transfused, if required. Neurosurgery should be consulted for possible hematoma evacuation.

After rt-PA administration, significant elevations in blood pressure should be actively controlled. The recommended upper limits for patients receiving thrombolytics are a diastolic blood pressure of 110 mm Hg and a systolic blood pressure of 185 mm Hg. Patients receiving rt-PA should not receive antiplatelet agents (e.g., aspirin, dipyridamole, clopidogrel, and abciximab) or anticoagulants (e.g., heparin and warfarin) during the first 24 hours.

In the event that rt-PA is not administered, most stroke and TIA patients should still be admitted to the hospital for further monitoring and evaluation and treatment of short- and long-term stroke risks. In general, aspirin should be given to patients within 24 to 48 hours of stroke onset. Aspirin should not be used as a substitute for other acute interventions, especially not in place of intravenous rt-PA. There are insufficient data with regard to the use of other antiplatelet agents, such dipyridamole, clopidogrel, or abciximab, in the acute setting.

Although anticoagulation with heparin has been used in the past for patients presenting with an acute ischemic stroke—especially for patients with progressing symptoms (so-called strokes in evolution)—there is no significant evidence for a clinical benefit and much evidence for an elevated bleeding risk from such an approach. It is possible

Box 125-1   Recombinant Tissue Plasminogen Activator Eligibility Guidelines

- Diagnosis of ischemic stroke causing measurable neurologic deficit
- The neurologic signs should not be clearing spontaneously
- The neurologic signs should not be minor and isolated
- Caution should be exercised in treating a patient with major deficits
- The symptoms of stroke should not be suggestive of subarachnoid hemorrhage
- Onset of symptoms <3 hours before beginning treatment
- No head trauma or prior stroke in previous 3 months
- No myocardial infarction in the previous 3 months
- No gastrointestinal or urinary tract hemorrhage in previous 21 days
- No major surgery in the previous 14 days
- No arterial puncture at a noncompressible site in the previous 7 days
- No history of previous intracranial hemorrhage
- Blood pressure not elevated (systolic <185 mm Hg and diastolic <110 mm Hg)
- No evidence of active bleeding or acute trauma (fracture) on examination
- Not taking an oral anticoagulant or if anticoagulant being taken, INR ≤1.7
- If receiving heparin in previous 48 hours, activated partial thromboplastin time must be in normal range
- Platelet count ≥100,000 mm^3
- Blood glucose concentration ≥50 mg/dL (2.7 mmol/L)
- No seizure with postictal residual neurologic impairments
- Computed tomography does not show a multilobar infarction (hypodensity greater than one third of cerebral hemisphere)
- The patient or family understand the potential risks and benefits of treatment

From Adams H, Adams R, Del Zoppo G, Goldstein LB: Guidelines for the early management of patients with ischemic stroke: 2005 Guidelines update. A Scientific Statement from the Stroke Council of the American Heart Association/American Stroke Association. Stroke 36:916-921, 2005.

that certain subsets of patients (e.g., patients with severe large vessel atherosclerosis or those perceived to be at high risk for recurrent embolism) might benefit from early anticoagulation, but additional research is needed.

An elevated blood pressure is commonly found in patients with acute and subacute strokes. If necessary, doses of outpatient antihypertensive drugs are reduced acutely to maintain perfusion to the ischemic penumbra. For patients not eligible for thrombolytic therapy, acute treatment of elevated blood pressures is generally only recommended for diastolic blood pressures greater than 120 mm Hg and systolic pressures greater than 220 mm Hg.

Deep venous thrombosis and pulmonary embolism can occur as a complication of immobility associated with strokes. For this reason, prophylaxis for deep venous thrombosis and pulmonary embolism is recommended in all stroke patients with immobility. Early mobilization of the patient is another important measure in preventing medical complications of acute stroke. The involvement of speech therapy, physical therapy, occupational therapy, and rehabilitative medicine are all important in preventing complications and maximizing recovery of the stroke patient. A rehabilitation plan is vital for reducing long-term morbidity and mortality after a patient is discharged from the acute care setting.

Avoiding Treatment Errors in Acute Stroke

Early recognition and treatment of stroke have been shown to improve functional outcome and reduce long-term morbidity and mortality after stroke. Delays in emergency transport should be minimized. Any suspected stroke should be given high triage priority at the treating facility, and initial evaluation and brain imaging should be performed as quickly as possible.

However, the pressures to treat quickly must also be balanced by a thorough review of the presenting history and a careful neurologic evaluation to exclude stroke mimics. Establishing a reliable time of onset is crucial to avoid treating a patient outside of the recommended time window. Familiarity with published guidelines for administering rt-PA in acute stroke will also reduce the likelihood of protocol deviations, and it is recommended that all treating facilities develop acute stroke care pathways based on these guidelines.

Secondary Stroke Prevention

Prevention of recurrent strokes should begin with risk factor modification. Hypertension and diabetes should be aggressively controlled. Statins are reasonable for all patients with stroke or TIA due to atherosclerotic disease and are recommended for all patients with dyslipidemia. All patients should be advised not to smoke, and smoking cessation should be recommended for current smokers.

Most patients with noncardioembolic strokes or TIAs should be placed on antiplatelet therapy. Aspirin, 50 to 325 mg once daily, the combination agent of aspirin, 25 mg and extended-release dipyridamole, 200 mg administered twice daily, and clopidogrel, 75 mg once daily are all acceptable initial options. The combination of clopidogrel and aspirin is frequently used for acute coronary syndrome; however, trials of this combination have not shown a significant benefit for stroke over the use of clopidogrel alone. One recent trial (the MATCH [Management of ATherothrombosis with Clopidogrel in High-risk patients with recent transient ischemic attacks or ischemic stroke] trial) reported a 1.3% absolute increase in life-threatening bleeding with clopidogrel plus aspirin compared with clopidogrel alone.

In treating stroke and TIA patients with cardiogenic embolic infarcts, anticoagulation with warfarin is effective, with a goal of an international normalized ratio in the range of 2.0 to 3.0. For patients with atrial fibrillation or paroxysmal atrial fibrillation, long-term anticoagulation with warfarin is generally recommended, and aspirin, 325 mg once daily, is recommended for patients unable to take warfarin. Other indications for anticoagulation include rheumatic mitral valve disease and prosthetic mechanical heart valves. For patients with acute myocardial infarction with left ventricular thrombus, anticoagulation for at least 3 months and up to a year is reasonable.

Surgical intervention may be indicated for patients found to have large-artery cerebrovascular disease. Carotid endarterectomy is recommended for stroke and TIA patients with severe (70% to 99%) ipsilateral carotid stenosis. A more moderate risk reduction is seen in patients with stenosis of 50% to 69%, and treatment decisions must take into consideration factors such as age, gender, comorbidities, and severity of the initial stroke or TIA. Carotid artery stenting may be considered for patients with severe stenosis who are considered high surgical risks.

Future Directions

Diagnostically, newer brain imaging modalities such as CT and magnetic resonance perfusion are being used to rapidly define the areas of cerebral perfusion abnormality and the degree of ischemic injury. These modalities will allow physicians to better define which patients might benefit from specific acute stroke therapies.

Acute interventional procedures for treating major vessel occlusions are being developed and evaluated. The Merci Retriever is an endovascular embolectomy system cleared by the U.S. Food and Drug Administration in 2005 for removal of blood clots from patients with ischemic stroke. The wire-based system was shown in a trial to be more successful in restoring the patency of occluded large intracranial vessels within 8 hours of stroke onset, at a rate of 46%, compared with a 18% spontaneous recanalization rate seen in a previous interventional study. However, use of this device is currently limited to centers with interventional facilities and trained operators. Interventional procedures involving intraarterial delivery rt-PA have been reported in case series and small trials, and larger trials are underway. Combination intravenous plus intra-arterial rt-PA strategies are also being tested.

Most attempts at limiting the extent of neuronal injury with neuroprotective agents have been disappointing. Some newer agents are in various stages of development and testing.

Additional Resources

Brott T, Adams HP Jr, Olinger CP, et al: Measurement of acute cerebral infarction: A clinical examination scale. Stroke 20:864-870, 1989.
  This is the original published description of the NIH Stroke Scale.
Diener HC, Bogousslavsky J, Brass LM, et al; MATCH investigators: Aspirin and clopidogrel compared with clopidogrel alone after recent ischaemic stroke or transient ischaemic attack in high-risk patients (MATCH): Randomised, double-blind, placebo-controlled trial. Lancet 364(9431):331-337, 2004.
  This article presents the MATCH trial results.
Goldstein LB, Adams R, Alberts MJ, et al: Primary prevention of ischemic stroke: A guideline from the American Heart Association/American Stroke Association Stroke Council. Stroke 37:1583-633, 2006.
  The authors present the general consensus guidelines from the American Heart Association/American Stroke Association for primary prevention of stroke.
Smith WS, Sung G, Starkman S, et al: Safety and efficacy of mechanical embolectomy in acute ischemic stroke: Results of the MERCI trial. Stroke 36(7):1432-1438, 2005.
  This article presents the MERCI trial results.

EVIDENCE

1. Adams HP Jr, Adams, RJ, Brott T, et al: Guidelines for the early management of patients with ischemic stroke. A scientific statement from the Stroke Council of the American Stroke Association. Stroke 34:1056-1083, 2003; and Adams H, Adams R, Del Zoppo G, Goldstein LB: Guidelines for the early management of patients with ischemic stroke: 2005 Guidelines update. A Scientific Statement from the Stroke Council of the American Heart Association/American Stroke Association. Stroke 36:916-921, 2005.
  These articles present the general consensus guidelines from the American Heart Association/American Stroke Association for acute and subacute (hospital admission) management of stroke.
2. Albers GW, Amarenco P, Easton JD, et al: Antithrombotic and thrombolytic therapy for ischemic stroke: The Seventh ACCP Conference on Antithrombotic and Thrombolytic Therapy. Chest 126(3 Suppl):483S-512S, 2004.
  This paper presents the American College of Chest Physicians guidelines for use of antiplatelets, anticoagulants, and thrombolytics for acute stroke and for secondary stroke prevention.
3. Sacco RL, Adams R, Albers G, et al: Guidelines for prevention of stroke in patients with ischemic stroke or transient ischemic attack: A statement for healthcare professionals from the American Heart Association/American Stroke Association Council on Stroke. Stroke 7:577-617, 2006.
  This paper presents the general consensus guidelines from the American Heart Association/American Stroke Association for secondary stroke and TIA prevention.

Bradley V. Vaughn ▪ Maha Alattar

Sleep Disorders

Introduction

Sleep is the reversible physiologic state of decreased responsiveness to the environment that is achieved by neuronal networks of the brain. Although the underlying purpose remains a mystery, sleep promotes higher levels of wakefulness and cognition, and sleep loss increases the likelihood of accidents, increases health costs, and lowers workplace productivity and quality of life.

One-in-three individuals will present with a sleep-related complaint to their physician. In the second edition of the International Classification of Sleep Disorders, sleep disorders are categorized into insomnias, hypersomnias, sleep-related breathing disorders, circadian rhythm disorders, parasomnias, sleep-related movement disorders, and other sleep disorders, including medical and psychiatric disorders. These disorders result in complaints of excessive daytime sleepiness and difficulty initiating or maintaining sleep or events associated with sleep (Boxes 127-1 and 127-2).

Etiology and Pathogenesis

The state of sleep is determined by symphony of neuronal processes. Sleep is typically divided into stages based on electroencephalogram (EEG) features, eye movements (electro-oculography), and muscle tone (electromyogram). Stages N1 to N3 are called collectively *non-rapid eye movement* (NREM) sleep. Stage N1 sleep is frequently associated with the perception of drowsiness and is characterized by EEG features of mild slowing and Vertex sharp waves. Stage N2 (light sleep) is characterized by the presence of K complexes or sleep spindles. In stage N3 (deep sleep), high-amplitude slow waves predominate the EEG activity. *Rapid eye movement* (REM) sleep or stage R is characterized by a low-amplitude, mixed-frequency pattern on EEG, absence of muscle tone in voluntary muscles, and intermittent REM. Dreams can occur in all stages of sleep but are more vividly recalled from REM sleep. All these stages have other physiologic correlates; NREM sleep has relatively constant respiration, cardiac rhythm, and autonomic function, whereas REM sleep demonstrates variation in respiration, cardiac function, and an absence of thermal regulation.

Healthy adults display a reproducible pattern of sleep organization. They enter sleep through stage N1, progress to stage N2, and after 20 to 30 minutes progress to stage N3, followed by reemergence of stage N2 sleep. The first REM sleep period occurs after 90 minutes. This pattern repeats about every 90 minutes throughout the sleep period with progressively less stage N3 sleep and longer periods of REM sleep in each cycle.

Both extrinsic and intrinsic factors may contribute to disordered sleep. Extrinsic factors disrupting sleep include environmental disturbances such as noise, uncomfortable setting, or bright light. Intrinsic disorders are prompted by an internal disruption associated with sleep. Obstructive sleep apnea (OSA) and periodic limb movements of sleep are excellent examples of disorders that become evident once the central nervous system (CNS) has entered the sleep state. OSA is associated with narrowing of the upper airway related to either a structural issue or relaxation of airway dilator muscles. Periodic limb movements of sleep appear to be related to unsuppressed excitation of spinal cord processes causing repetitive limb movement occurring every 10 to 120 seconds during sleep. Other sleep disorders such as narcolepsy are abnormalities in the mechanism of sleep-wake differentiation. Narcolepsy with cataplexy has a strong linkage to HLA DQB1*0602 and DR2 (DR15) major histocompatibility complex and is linked to a depletion of orexin-hypocretin-producing neurons in the hypothalamus.

Alteration of the circadian rhythm can also disrupt sleep-wake determination. This internal clock allows for the body to anticipate periods that are likely to be active

nerve that eventually encroach on other structures in the internal auditory canal and cerebellopontine angle. Typically, there is increased vestibular deficit and sensorineural hearing loss with increasing tumor size and local compression. Vestibular schwannomas most often present as progressive unilateral sensorineural hearing loss with symptoms of imbalance and tinnitus. The vestibular system often is able to compensate over time for the tumor growth, and thus, vertigo is often absent. The hearing loss may be sudden in up to 20% of patients. With large tumors, ipsilateral facial nerve function may be compromised. Vestibular schwannoma may be treated with surgical resection. Stereotactic radiotherapy is an alternative mode of treatment and may be considered if surgery is not desired or the patient would be at high risk for a general anesthetic.

Other brainstem neoplasms involving the cerebellopontine angle (meningiomas, epidermoids, lipomas, gliomas, astrocytomas) may cause vertigo. The etiology of the vertigo is usually compression of adjacent structures, either by direct extension of the neoplasm on the eighth nerve complex and brainstem or resulting hydrocephalus. Brainstem neoplasms presenting with vertigo tend to be large and have symptoms of cerebellar compression and hydrocephalus. Hearing loss is often associated, and patients may complain of otalgia, diplopia, and headaches. Brainstem neoplasms causing vertigo usually require resection and adjunctive therapy, the details of which depend on the histopathology of the neoplasm.

Avoiding Treatment Errors

The most important elements in the evaluation of the patient with dizziness are the clinical history and a thorough physical examination. Accurately distinguishing true vertigo from other types of dizziness such as unsteadiness, imbalance, or lightheadedness is the most critical aspect of the history and the most effective way to avoid an error in diagnosis and treatment. Once true vertigo is confirmed, it is important to have a detailed description of the episodes, most importantly the time course of the actual spinning sensation. When the neurotologic evaluation is negative, the patient should be evaluated for potential cardiovascular, metabolic, or neurologic pathologies.

Future Directions

A detailed understanding of the vestibular system and its pathophysiology is essential for the treatment of the vertiginous patient. The diagnosis still hinges heavily on the history of symptoms, but several areas show promise for future research. Reliable objective testing for perilymph fistula could streamline its diagnosis and treatment. Improved imaging modalities could pinpoint vascular lesions without the present risks of invasive angiography. Research into the underlying pathophysiology of Meniere's disease continues and may one day explain its constellation of findings. Even as more discoveries are made, patients with vertigo will continue to challenge the clinician's knowledge and skills.

Additional Resources

Eaton DA, Roland PS: Dizziness in the older adult, Part 1. Evaluation and general treatment strategies. Geriatrics 58(4):28-30, 33-36, 2003.
The authors present a good overview of the workup of the dizzy patient.

Eaton DA, Roland PS: Dizziness in the older adult, Part 2. Treatment for the four most common symptoms. Geriatrics 58(4):46, 49-52, 2003.
The authors describe the diagnosis and treatment of vertigo, presyncope, disequilibrium, and nonspecific dizziness.

EVIDENCE

1. Eaton DA, Roland PS: Dizziness in the older adult, Part 1. Evaluation and general treatment strategies. Geriatrics 58(4):28-30, 33-36, 2003.
The authors provide a good overview of the workup of the dizzy patient.
2. Eaton DA, Roland PS: Dizziness in the older adult, Part 2. Treatment for the four most common symptoms. Geriatrics 58(4):46, 49-52, 2003.
The authors describe the diagnosis and treatment of vertigo, presyncope, disequilibrium, and nonspecific dizziness.
3. Fetter M: Assessing vestibular function: Which tests, when? J Neurol 247(5):335-342, 2000.
The author presents a thorough review of diagnostic tests of vestibular function.
4. Luxon LM. The medical management of vertigo. J Laryngol Otol 111(12):1114-1121, 1997.
5. Shephard NT, Solomon D: Functional operation of the balance system in daily activities. Otolaryngol Clin North Am 33(3):455-469, 2000.
This article provides a good description of the physiology of the vestibular system.
6. Strupp M, Arbusow V: Acute vestibulopathy. Curr Opin Neurol 14(1):11-20, 2001.
This paper updates the etiology and treatment of peripheral and central vestibular disorders.
7. Strupp M, Zingler V, Arbusow V, et al: Methylprednisolone, valacyclovir or the combination for vestibular neuritis. N Engl J Med 351(4):354-362, 2004.
This prospective, randomized, double-blind trial examined the effectiveness of medical therapy in vestibular neuritis.
8. Weber PC, Adkins WY Jr: The differential diagnosis of Meniere's disease. Otolaryngol Clin North Am 30(6):977-986, 1997.
This article discusses how to correctly diagnose Meniére's disease by exclusion.

vative with bed rest, elevation of the head of the bed, and stool softeners. Many consider perilymph fistula a surgical entity which requires middle ear exploration and patching.

BPPV results from canalolithiasis, an accumulation of otoconial debris displaced into the semicircular canal system (typically the posterior canal), resulting in limited-duration gravity-dependent stimulation with changes in head position. BPPV typically presents as short-duration (seconds) vertiginous episodes associated with changes in head position. Careful questioning may reveal a latency in the onset of vertigo of up to 1 minute after head movement and that predictable changes in head position may routinely precipitate the symptom (e.g., rolling over in bed, looking up to the top shelf). Usually there is no hearing loss. Fatigable horizontal or torsional nystagmus with latency in onset may be reproduced by Dix-Hallpike positioning maneuvers. The Epley or Semont maneuvers can help relocate the debris from the semicircular canal. Patients are instructed to remain upright while sleeping for several days to avoid reaccumulation of displaced particles. In severe cases of BPPV unrelieved by repeated positioning maneuvers, posterior canal occlusion or singular neurectomy may be effective in controlling symptoms.

Chronic middle ear disease, either chronic infection or cholesteatoma, can cause vertigo by local destruction and erosion into the otic capsule, creating a fistula into the perilymph-filled system. The pathophysiology is similar to that of perilymph fistula described earlier. Additionally, serous labyrinthitis associated with the chronic suppurative process may exacerbate vertigo. Chronic middle ear disease classically presents as a persistently draining and painful ear, resistant to multiple courses of topical and systemic antibiotics. The otorrhea is often malodorous in the chronic state. The tympanic membrane is commonly heavily scarred with visible perforation. Pearly-white cholesteatoma matrix may be seen deep to the tympanic membrane remnant. As with perilymph fistula, pneumatic otoscopy may reproduce associated vertigo. Chronic middle ear disease treatment typically involves surgery to remove erosive cholesteatoma or infected tissue, repairing hearing loss and preventing further intratemporal or intracranial complications.

MS flares are often associated with vertigo. The etiology of MS-related vertigo may be plaque formation in the pontine region of the brainstem or proximal eighth nerve. Central vertigo may result from interruption of the medial longitudinal fasciculus, which causes disconjugate eye movements (internuclear ophthalmoplegia). MS is characterized by the episodic development of neurologic deficits. Vertigo and sensorineural hearing loss may fluctuate over time as plaques are formed. Nearly half of patients with MS present with vertigo at some point, and careful examination often reveals internuclear ophthalmoplegia, an ipsilateral adducting extraocular muscle deficit with

contralateral abducting nystagmus. An MS flare involving vertigo typically persists for days to weeks before adequate central compensation is achieved. MS often responds to high-dose pulse of corticosteroids with shortened duration of symptoms. Additionally, gabapentin may reduce resulting nystagmus and vertigo.

Migraine may produce vertigo through poorly understood mechanisms. Vertigo may precede the headache (aura equivalent) or replace it (migraine equivalent). Recent genetic discoveries in migraine research have implicated ion channel mutations as a potential link with the vestibular system; however, the definitive pathophysiologic explanation remains elusive. Vertigo associated with migraine is difficult to categorize. It may replace the aura of the migraine or the headache itself, or it may happen in the interval between headaches. The duration of migraine-associated vertigo is highly variable, lasting from hours to days and, in women, may show correlation to menstrual cycle. Severe cases may awaken the patient from sleep and are often associated with nausea and vomiting. There is usually a strong family history of migraines and no other neurologic deficits are typically noted during an episode. Migraine therapy involves behavioral as well as pharmacologic interventions. Serotonin receptor antagonists have proved effective as aborting agents and prophylaxis has been demonstrated for β-blockers, tricyclic antidepressants, valproic acid, and calcium channel blockers (see Chapter 124).

Vascular disease in the vertebrobasilar system may induce vertigo by compromising posterior circulation through occlusive or embolic processes. The most commonly affected arteries are the anterior-inferior cerebellar artery, posterior-inferior cerebellar artery, and superior cerebellar artery. Severe arthritic changes to the cervical spine are thought to be related to vascular insufficiency in the vertebrobasilar system. Additionally, there is evidence that aberrant vessel anatomy may compress the eighth nerve complex, resulting in vertigo and pulsatile tinnitus. Occlusive or embolic vascular disease affecting the posterior circulation often results in severe postural instability, direction-shifting nystagmus without suppression by visual fixation, and multiple neurologic findings, particularly if the brainstem is involved. Vascular insufficiency is typically associated with a lightheaded or presyncopal sensation exacerbated by neck extension with no related hearing loss. By contrast, vascular compression or impingement of the eighth nerve complex presents typically as pulsatile tinnitus with hypacusis, often exacerbated by head position. Vertigo in this case is a result of progressive functional loss and is usually less severe because of central compensation. Vertigo attributed to vascular disease requires addressing risk factors as well as instituting antiplatelet therapy. For significant stenosis, anticoagulation with warfarin may be considered.

Vestibular schwannomas (incorrectly called acoustic neuromas) are benign tumors arising from the vestibular

cholesteatoma or middle ear tumors. For soft tissue examination (e.g., cerebellopontine angle masses, vestibular schwannoma, MS plaques) magnetic resonance imaging is the study of choice. For suspected vascular disease, transcranial Doppler, magnetic resonance angiography, or selected arterial angiography may be diagnostic.

Management and Therapy

General Principles

The management of vertigo depends on the etiology and associated pathology. In general, however, acute control of symptoms is the same in all patients. The most commonly used class of medications includes the older antihistamines, such as meclizine, dimenhydrinate, and promethazine. These drugs help reduce the feeling of movement and instability as well as the associated gastrointestinal symptoms. Side effects are mostly limited to drowsiness. The newer generation antihistamines do not penetrate the central nervous system and are therefore not helpful in the management of vertigo. Other medications include anticholinergics such as scopolamine for motion sickness, antidopaminergics, and monoaminergics. Antidopaminergics help control the chemoreceptor trigger zone, whereas monoaminergics potentiate the effects of the antihistamines and can be used in severe cases.

Benzodiazepines, such as diazepam, are powerful vestibular suppressants that are very effective in the acute management of vertigo. Long-term use, however, can affect the natural compensatory processes that occur with the loss of one vestibular system and is therefore discouraged.

Vestibular rehabilitation therapy is usually performed on an outpatient basis. These exercises are designed to facilitate habituation and central compensation.

Optimum Treatment of the Most Common Entities

The following is a brief description of the most common etiologies of vertigo, both peripheral and central. These are also summarized in Table 126-1.

Acute vestibulopathy is the sudden failure of the balance system. A viral etiology has been postulated based on several lines of evidence. When associated with hearing loss, *labyrinthitis* is the commonly used term. When hearing is preserved, *vestibular neuritis* is the common terminology. Acute vestibulopathy typically presents as an attack of prolonged, incapacitating vertigo with nausea and vomiting that can persist for greater than 24 hours, gradually subsiding over the following days to weeks. Patients often describe a history of antecedent upper respiratory infection. In cases of vestibular neuritis, hearing is unaffected; however, in acute labyrinthitis, sensorineural hearing loss and tinnitus accompany the episode. About 20% of patients experience recurrent episodes that are often less severe than the initial presentation. Management is typically focused on control of the acute symptoms, in addition to bed rest and hydration. Corticosteroids have been shown to improve the recovery, whereas antivirals have shown no clear benefit. Vestibular suppressants should be withdrawn as soon as possible to allow effective central adaptation. Vestibular rehabilitation exercises and early mobilization improve final outcomes. One particular form of viral labyrinthitis, herpes zoster oticus or Ramsay Hunt syndrome, is due to a reactivation of the varicella-zoster virus. This has a unique clinical course that starts with a burning pain followed by a vesicular eruption; hearing loss, vertigo, and facial weakness can then follow. In addition to steroids, acyclovir can have a role in the treatment of this specific entity. Aggressive eye care in the presence of the facial paralysis is also warranted.

Endolymphatic hydrops (Meniere's disease) is believed to be caused by excessive accumulation of endolymph in the endolymphatic sac secondary to impaired resorption. The exact pathophysiologic mechanism in Meniere's disease remains unknown. Endolymphatic hydrops episodes are typically described as lasting for several hours and are characterized by fluctuating sensorineural hearing loss, vertigo, and tinnitus. Many patients report a sensation of aural fullness during or before an attack. Episodes occur at irregular intervals for many years and may become bilateral as the disease progresses. Late Meniere's disease is characterized by permanent severe sensorineural hearing loss and less severe vertiginous attacks. Treatment is again symptomatic during the acute attacks. Prevention starts with a low-salt (1 to 2 g/day) diet and a diuretic. Advanced cases can be treated with intratympanic gentamicin, shunting procedures, vestibular neurectomy, or labyrinthectomy depending on the progression, hearing, and status of the contralateral ear.

Episodic vertigo associated with perilymph fistula is believed to be caused by a leak of perilymph from the otic capsule, typically from a damaged oval or round window. The intermittent nature of the vertigo and associated sensorineural hearing loss reflects the intermittent leak from the defect and the subsequent exposure of the inner ear to ambient pressure changes. The recently described disorder of superior semicircular canal dehiscence is consistent with the findings of a perilymph fistula and may be considered together for the purposes of this text. The most common etiology for perilymph fistula is trauma to the ear—either direct, surgical, or barometric. Often the vertigo is least noticeable early in the morning or after lying down, then progresses with upright posture and activities through the day. Symptoms are exacerbated by Valsalva maneuvers (nose blowing, heavy lifting, straining, vomiting) and can often be reproduced with pneumatic otoscopy. An inciting traumatic event can often be elicited with a careful history (e.g., diving, head injury, direct ear trauma, childbirth, extreme straining or lifting). Initial management is conser-

Table 126-1   Clinical Features of the Most Common Causes of Vertigo

Clinical Features	Migraine	Vestibular Neuritis	Labyrinthitis	Meniére's Disease	Perilymph Fistula	BPPV	Vestibular Schwannoma	Chronic Otitis Media
Vertigo intensity and duration	Hours	Days	Days	Hours	Variable, worsens through day	Seconds	Imbalance	Variable
Nausea and vomiting	Yes	Yes	Yes	Yes	No	Yes	No	No
Hearing loss	No	No	SNHL	SNHL, fluctuates	Mild SNHL	No	SNHL, unilateral, progressive	CHL
Symptom-free interval	Yes	No	No	Yes	Lessens with rest, worsens with activity	Yes	No	No
Tinnitus present	No	No	No	Yes	Variable	No	Yes	Variable
Associated findings	Aura, vision changes	Hx of URI	Hx of URI	Aural fullness, diplacusis	(Baro) trauma	Positional	Facial numbness, ear numbness	Otorrhea, perforated tinnitus media
Study of choice	MRI	ENG	ENG	MRI	Pneumatic otoscopy	Dix-Hallpike	MRI	CT

BPPV, benign paroxysmal positional vertigo; CHL, conductive hearing loss; ENG, electronystagmography; Hx, history; MRI, magnetic resonance imaging; SNHL, sensorineural hearing loss; URI, upper respiratory infection.

Figure 126-4 Test for Positional Vertigo.

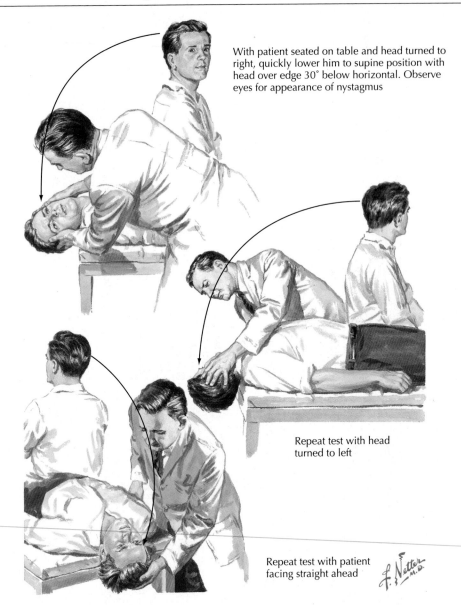

With patient seated on table and head turned to right, quickly lower him to supine position with head over edge 30° below horizontal. Observe eyes for appearance of nystagmus

Repeat test with head turned to left

Repeat test with patient facing straight ahead

Differential Diagnosis

A long differential diagnosis must be considered in patients with vertigo. However, it is possible to narrow the list of potential etiologies considerably based on the history and physical examination. Distinguishing factors are listed subsequently (Table 126-1; see Box 126-1).

Diagnostic Approach

Diagnostic testing is often required to distinguish between one of several possible clinical diagnoses. A pure tone audiogram should be performed to assess patients for related hearing loss. Electronystagmography can frequently identify unilateral vestibular weakness and help distinguish nystagmus of peripheral and central origin. Electrocochleography can be performed to aid in the diagnosis of Meniere's disease. Dynamic posturography may aid in localizing balance disorders when multiple systems are involved. Laboratory evaluation usually has a limited role in the diagnostic approach to vertigo and may include complete blood count, erythrocyte sedimentation rate, antinuclear antibody titers, rapid plasma reagin or VDRL screening, and evaluation of thyroid function. Cerebrospinal fluid analysis may aid in the diagnosis of multiple sclerosis (MS).

Radiographic imaging in patients with vertigo is sometimes useful. For middle ear disease and temporal bone pathology or trauma, computed tomography scan highlights bony anatomy and helps detect pathologies such as

Box 127-1   Sleep Disorders
Intrinsic Sleep Disorders
Obstructive sleep apnea
Primary central sleep apnea
Sleep-related hypoventilation
Narcolepsy with or without cataplexy
Recurrent hypersomnia
Idiopathic hypersomnia
Psychophysiologic insomnia
Paradoxical insomnia (sleep state misperception)
Idiopathic insomnia
Restless legs syndrome
Periodic limb movement disorder
Confusional arousals
Sleep walking
Sleep terrors
REM sleep behavior disorder
Recurrent isolated sleep paralysis
Nightmare disorders
Sleep-related leg cramps
Sleep-related bruxism
Extrinsic Sleep Disorders
High-altitude periodic breathing
Behavioral insomnia
Adjustment insomnia
Inadequate sleep hygiene
Hypersomnia due to drugs or substances
Behaviorally induced insufficient sleep syndrome
Insomnia due to drugs or substances
Circadian Rhythm Disorders
Delayed sleep phase type
Advanced sleep phase type
Free running type
Irregular sleep wake type
Jet lag syndrome
Shift work sleep disorder

REM, rapid eye movement.

Box 127-2   Common Medical and Psychiatric Disorders Associated with Sleep Disruption
Medical Disorders
Chronic pulmonary disease
Sleep-related asthma
Congestive heart failure
Gastroesophageal reflux
Diabetes mellitus
Infections
Fibromyalgia
Renal dysfunction
Iron deficiency
Neurologic Disorders
Cerebral degenerative disorders
Dementia
Parkinsonism
Headaches
Epilepsy
Stroke
Multiple sclerosis
Head trauma
Encephalitis
Psychiatric Disorders
Psychotic disorders
Mood disorders
Anxiety disorders
Panic disorder
Alcoholism and substance abuse

or inactive; thus, certain times of the day, such as 4:00 AM, are associated with a greater circadian pressure to sleep. A complex interaction of genes and proteins produce this chemical rhythm, which can be influenced by many external stimuli, including bright light, activity level, and social interactions.

Clinical Presentation

Typically, patients with sleep issues present with one of three major complaints: excessive daytime sleepiness; difficulty initiating or maintaining sleep; or unusual events occurring during the night. Patients may focus on one symptom yet have features that suggest several underlying processes. The following are commonly recognized sleep disorders.

Sleep Deprivation

Chronic reduction in total sleep time interferes with normal daytime function. Most commonly, sleep depriva-

tion is voluntary and a result of societal pressures for adults to perform more with less time for sleep. Sleep debt may accumulate over years. This unmet sleep need increases the likelihood for an individual to fall asleep at inappropriate times such as during work or driving, decreasing productivity and increasing risk for accidents. The physiologic effects of sleep deprivation also increase appetite, promote weight gain, and worsen mood.

Sleep Apnea

Sleep apnea is characterized by repetitive stoppage of breathing and sleep fragmentation. Typically, sleep apnea appears in two forms: obstructive and central. OSA is associated with narrowing of the upper airway, which causes turbulent air flow that results in snoring, loud snorts, or gasps during sleep. Typically, these patients are overweight, but many patients with OSA can have relatively normal body habitus. These patients may have large necks or crowded airways. The disorder is associated with increased risk for hypertension, diabetes, and recurrence of vascular events. Central sleep apnea, characterized by repetitive episodes of the absence of movement of the lower respiratory muscles, is associated with a pause in breathing. Both disorders may cause the patient to have

Figure 127-1 Sleep Disorders.

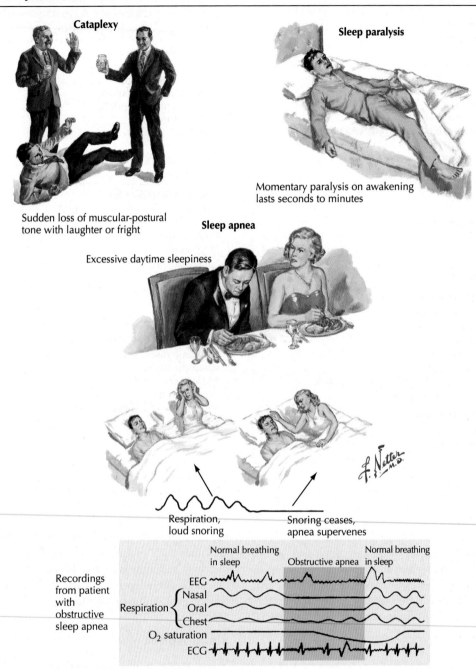

Cataplexy

Sudden loss of muscular-postural tone with laughter or fright

Sleep paralysis

Momentary paralysis on awakening lasts seconds to minutes

Sleep apnea

Excessive daytime sleepiness

Respiration, loud snoring

Snoring ceases, apnea supervenes

Recordings from patient with obstructive sleep apnea

Respiration { Nasal, Oral, Chest }

Normal breathing in sleep

Obstructive apnea

Normal breathing in sleep

EEG
O₂ saturation
ECG

hundreds of brief arousals per night, which lead to insomnia or excessive daytime sleepiness.

Narcolepsy

Narcolepsy is a disorder of the on/off control of NREM and REM sleep. This disorder is nonprogressive and typically appears in early adolescence. Patients have bouts of irresistible intrusions of sleep throughout the day. The traditional tetrad of symptoms is excessive daytime sleepi-

ness, cataplexy, sleep paralysis, and hypnagogic hallucinations (Fig. 127-1); however, insomnia and sleep disruption are common complaints. Excessive daytime sleepiness occurs despite a relatively normal total sleep time and may be described as uncontrollable bouts of sleep ("sleep attacks"). Cataplexy is an abrupt decrease in muscle tone without loss of consciousness and is provoked by strong emotional stimuli or exercise. Individuals may fall, or experience mild to severe degree of weakness. Sleep paralysis occurs in the transition from sleep to wakefulness with the retention of the atonia of REM sleep. These events can be accompanied with the feeling of impending doom and hallucinations. Hypnagogic hallucinations are visual imagery just before the onset of sleep that may be difficult to distinguish from reality. Most patients do not exhibit the complete tetrad.

Restless Legs Syndrome

Restless legs syndrome is a disorder associated with discomfort in the legs (less often, the arms) and includes sensations of crawling, wiggling, and electrical features. These symptoms must be worse with rest and improve with movement and are more prevalent during the evening. This disorder is sometimes associated with periodic limb movements. Periodic limb movements of sleep are repetitive stereotyped movements of the upper or lower extremities lasting 0.5 to 4.0 seconds, occurring at 20- to 120-second intervals, and sometimes associated with arousals. Patients may be unaware of the movements and have no sleep complaints, but bed partners may note the movements. Iron-deficiency anemia, uremia, peripheral vascular disease, arthritis, peripheral neuropathy, and spinal cord lesions have been associated with both disorders. The use of tricyclic antidepressants, selective serotonin reuptake inhibitors, dopamine antagonists, and caffeine may exacerbate sensory and motor phenomena.

Circadian Rhythm Disorders

The desynchronization of behavioral and neural sleep cycles may result in excessive daytime sleepiness or disrupted nocturnal sleep. Most individuals experience some of these symptoms with abruptly changing time zones or work schedule, but others have chronic desynchronization of the body clock with their surrounding environment. Delayed sleep phase type, characterized by an inability to fall asleep until past midnight and trouble waking in the morning, is seen commonly in adolescents. Advanced sleep phase type is more common among elderly individuals who fall asleep early in the evening and awake in the early morning hours. Individuals with a free running schedule have a lack of entrainment of the endogenous 24.3-hour circadian clock. This is most common in patients who are blind. Other patients with hypothalamic dysfunction may have an irregular sleep wake schedule owing to a loss of the rhythm generators.

Primary Disorders of Initiation or Maintenance of Sleep

Insomnia is the difficulty initiating or maintaining sleep, combined with daytime sleepiness, fatigue, or impairment of daytime performance. Most adults have occasional nights of poor sleep, which are often linked to daytime events or sudden changes in medical condition. For a smaller group of patients, insomnia persists for weeks, months, or years and leads to significant psychological and medical symptoms. Primary insomnias account for more than one third of insomnia cases. Psychophysiologic insomnia is characterized by somatized tension and learned sleep-preventing associations; individuals typically sleep well in a new environment away from associations that remind them of the difficulty of sleeping. Paradoxical insomnia is the inability to recognize the occurrence of sleep. Patients have normal sleep as measured by polysomnography, but report being unaware that they have slept. Idiopathic insomnia, an abnormality in the neuronal ability to attain adequate sleep, typically starts in childhood and persists as fragmented and unrefreshing sleep.

Nocturnal Events

Nocturnal events occur in about 3% of the adult population. Not all nocturnal events are parasomnias; some can be related to other non–sleep-related disorders. Parasomnias, however, present either as disorders of arousals from NREM sleep (sleep walking, sleep terrors, or confusional arousals) or REM-related events (REM sleep behavior disorder). The disorders of arousal typically occur as partial arousals from the deeper stages of NREM sleep. REM sleep behavior disorder is related to the loss of atonia during REM sleep. This disorder is associated with a higher risk for developing Parkinson's disease, Lewy body dementia, or multisystem atrophy. Other parasomnias can occur as events that are present during the transition from wake to sleep. Other disorders such as epilepsy or psychological events can occur at night as a result of changes in neurophysiology, which make those pathologic events more likely to appear.

Differential Diagnosis

The differential diagnosis is divided into intrinsic sleep disorders, extrinsic sleep disorders, and medical and psychiatric disorders (see Boxes 127-1 and 127-2). Patients with sleep apnea, periodic leg movements of sleep, and circadian rhythm disorders may or may not complain of sleepiness despite severe sleep disruption. Patients with medical disorders such as congestive heart failure, renal failure, arthritis, and pain syndromes may complain of poor sleep or fatigue. Psychiatric disorders are often preceded by insomnia; frequently, sleep disturbance outlasts the mood disturbance of affective disorders.

Nocturnal events may be difficult to distinguish. Key features such as time of the events, memory for the events, and stereotypic behavior help distinguish the events and allow for the clinician to guide the evaluation (Table 127-1). Clinicians should always be careful to screen these patients for other sleep disorders that may provoke nocturnal events.

Table 127-1 Distinguishing Features of Nocturnal Events

Feature	NREM Parasomnia	REM Behavior Disorder	Nocturnal Seizures	Psychogenic Events
Time of occurrence	First third of the night	During REM	Anytime	Anytime
Memory of event	Usually none	Dream recall	Usually none; may have memory	Usually none
Stereotypical movements	No	No	Yes	No
Polysomnographic findings	Arousals from deep NREM sleep	Excessive EMG tone during REM	Potentially epileptiform activity	Occur from awake state

EMG, electromyogram; NREM, non-rapid eye movement; REM, rapid eye movement.

Diagnostic Approach

The diagnostic evaluation should focus on several key points. Complaints should be separated into categories of excessive daytime sleepiness, insomnia, or unusual events at night. A detailed history is crucial, including information regarding the clinical course, the degree of impact, the sleep-wake pattern, perception of sleep quality, report from bed partner, dietary habits (especially caffeine and alcohol intake), activity changes, drug use (including over-the-counter agents, herbal and home remedies), and medical conditions. Clinicians should look for potential causes of sleep disturbance from four groups—intrinsic sleep disorder, extrinsic sleep disturbance, circadian rhythm disorder, and other medical, neurologic, or psychiatric disorders—and should consider the potential for multiple participating etiologies.

To sleep well, one needs a conducive environment, psychological preparedness for sleep, an adequate sleep period, and the neurophysiologic mechanisms for sleep. Most patients with chronic insomnia have a set of factors that predispose, initiate, and perpetuate insomnia. Gender, age, and coping mechanisms may predispose one to insomnia, whereas poor sleep hygiene, substance abuse, and performance anxiety may perpetuate it. Patients must be questioned for cardinal symptoms of sleep disorders, such as snoring, leg kicking, or sleep-related activities.

Many disorders can be elucidated with objective evaluation. Clinicians should consider referring patients with sleep complaints for polysomnography at a qualified sleep laboratory when they have symptoms suggestive of sleep-related breathing disorder (snoring, gasping), movement disorder, narcolepsy, paroxysmal arousals, or behaviors that are potentially injurious or atypical for parasomnia (Box 127-3). Patients being evaluated for excessive daytime sleepiness may require a multiple sleep latency test (MSLT) to measure the degree of daytime sleepiness and the potential to enter REM sleep inappropriately during the day such as in narcolepsy. Other tests such as the maintenance of wakefulness test (MWT) can measure the degree to which a subject can stay awake. This test is required for individuals with sleep disorders and certain occupations

Box 127-3 Primary Indications for Polysomnography

1. Snoring with complaint of excessive daytime sleepiness, insomnia, or nocturnal events
2. Snoring with history of vascular disease
3. Excessive daytime sleepiness despite adequate sleep time
4. Disruptive or potentially injurious nocturnal events
5. Intractable insomnia

(truck drivers, pilots). Although the MSLT and MWT are very similar tests, patients may have significant different abilities in falling asleep and remaining awake. Therefore, each test should be used to obtain specific information.

Management and Therapy

Optimum Treatment

The management of patients with sleep disorders requires close follow-up and clearly established therapeutic goals. Clinicians should identify and resolve issues of extrinsic sleep disruption before proceeding with expensive polysomnographic investigations. Through identification of underlying causes, directed therapeutic interventions are more likely to result in success. For example, OSA is traditionally treated with continuous positive airway pressure (CPAP) or, in more difficult cases, bilevel positive airway pressure. These therapies are dependent on the patient wearing the mask every night; thus, mask comfort is very important. Alternative therapies include oral devices and surgeries. These require identification of patients with characteristics favorable for each of these therapies but provide options for those patients unable to tolerate CPAP therapy. Patients with restless legs syndrome may be treated with an array of medications, including dopamine agonists, gabapentin, opiates, and benzodiazepines, but require close observation for worsening symptoms. CNS-active medications should be used to affect specific neurochemical processes. Stimulants, such as caffeine, methylphenidate, dextroamphetamine, and modafinil, have been used to treat the excessive sleepiness in narcolepsy or idiopathic hypersomnolence. Benzodiazepine receptor agonists (esopiclone, zolpidem, and zaleplon) and new melatonin agonists are approved for the treatment of insomnia with fewer psychomotor side effects and lower the chance of rebound insomnia compared with older hypnotics. For primary insomnia, behavioral modification and cognitive therapies show the greatest long-term success. Additionally, patients with circadian issues may augment or alter the sleep-wake clock by using bright light exposure and exercise at specific times to reinforce the timing of wakefulness. Most patients need clinical monitoring and education to reinforce therapies and behaviors conducive to good sleep.

Avoiding Treatment Errors

Our current societal view places low emphasis on adequate sleep. For some physicians, this view extends into their treatment of sleep disorders. Clinicians should view sleep complaints as opportunities to explore issues that may have long-term social and health consequences. These complaints should be approached with a logical delineation of the underlying etiologies, and treatment should be focused on those etiologies. Frequently, physicians may treat the symptoms of the disorder without adequately investigating the cause. Although the patients may initially derive benefit, long-term benefit is more likely to develop from a directed therapeutic approach.

Future Directions

Our understanding of the mechanisms involved in determining the sleep-wake state is rapidly expanding. Application of molecular biologic techniques to determine novel neuroactive substances and receptors has opened new understanding of state determination. Understanding these mechanisms provides opportunities for molecularly targeted therapies to manipulate sleep and wake states.

Additional Resource

Watson N, Vaughn BV (eds): Clinician's Guide to Sleep Disorders. New York, Taylor Francis, 2006.
This text provides an excellent clinical approach for primary care physicians caring for patients with sleep complaints.

EVIDENCE

1. Chesson AL, Ferber RA, Fry JM, et al: The indications for polysomnography and related procedures. Sleep 20(6);423-487, 1997.
This is an excellent review of when to order sleep studies and what type to order.
2. Chokroverty S (ed): Sleep Disorders Medicine: Basic Science, Technical Considerations, and Clinical Aspects. Boston, Butterworth-Heinemann Medical, 1999.
This excellent text reviews sleep disorders medicine.
3. Kryger MH, Roth T, Dement WC (eds): Principles and Practice of Sleep Medicine, 4th ed. Philadelphia, WB Saunders, 2005.
This text provides a comprehensive review of the basic and clinical knowledge in sleep medicine.

Bradley V. Vaughn ▪ Robert S. Greenwood

Epilepsy

Introduction

Epilepsy has been described for more than 2500 years. Hippocrates, in his manuscript "On the Sacred Disease," described detailed seizure types and localized seizures as a disorder of the brain. The term *epilepsy* is a derivative of the Greek word for "to take hold of": *epilepsia*. Throughout time, individuals with epilepsy have been regarded as having special powers or being possessed. Yet historical figures such as Julius Caesar, van Gogh, Napoleon, and Dostoyevsky, who lived with epilepsy, demonstrate that individuals with epilepsy can make tremendous contributions.

Etiology and Pathogenesis

The broad definition of seizure includes any sudden onset of morbid symptoms. This includes syncope, cataplexy, and even psychogenic events. However, epileptic seizures, a more narrowly defined paroxysmal form of seizures, are events resulting from excessive pathologic synchronous neuronal activity in a large population of neurons. Epileptic seizures are one of the most common symptoms of disturbed brain function. About 10% of the population will have a seizure by age 80 years. Some seizures are self-limited as part of an acute medical condition, illness, or exposure to epileptogenic substances, whereas other epileptic seizures are a sign of abnormal neuronal physiology and networks.

Epilepsy is a chronic disorder that is hallmarked by recurrent, unprovoked seizures. Thus, the diagnosis of epilepsy is based on historical features and can be made after the second unprovoked epileptic seizure. The patient with epilepsy may have multiple seizure types. A patient with juvenile myoclonic epilepsy, for example, may display absence, generalized tonic-clonic, and myoclonic seizures. Yet, all of these seizure types occur in one type of epilepsy.

Classification of Seizures

Seizures are classified by behavioral symptomatology (semiology) and electroencephalographic data (Box 128-1). Seizures are fundamentally of two types: focal onset (partial) and diffuse onset (primary generalized). About two thirds of epilepsy patients have partial seizures. Partial seizures are further divided into simple partial and complex partial. Simple partial seizures are defined by the retention of consciousness or memory. Complex partial seizures are defined by the impairment of consciousness or the loss of memory during the seizure. Focal-onset seizures may also evolve into generalized seizures, and these secondarily generalized seizures are the most common generalized seizures in adults.

Primary generalized seizures begin simultaneously across the whole brain and may comprise various types of behavior. Behavioral pauses associated with a three-per-second generalized spike-and-wave discharge characterize absence seizures. These seizures typically occur in children, last less than 20 seconds, and are associated with no postictal confusion. A sudden loss of muscle tone characterizes atonic seizures. An atonic seizure often causes patients to fall and sustain injuries. Tonic seizures are seizures that produce generalized stiffening. Patients with tonic seizures also frequently fall. The behaviors observed during clonic seizures are repetitive quick jerks with a slow relaxation phase. Tonic seizures may develop into clonic seizures, and clonic seizures may progress into tonic and then clonic seizures. Single quick jerks of the whole or a portion of the body characterize myoclonic seizures. The minority of myoclonus is of cortical origin, so that myoclonus often does not have an electroencephalogram (EEG) correlate. Only myoclonus with an EEG correlate is considered epileptic.

Box 128-1   Seizure Classification*

Generalized Seizures of Nonfocal Origin

Tonic-clonic
Tonic
Clonic
Absence
Atonic, akinetic
Myoclonic

Partial Seizures

Simple partial (without loss of consciousness)
- With motor symptoms
- With sensory symptoms
- With autonomic symptoms
- With psychic symptoms
- Compound forms

Complex partial (impaired consciousness)
- Simple partial onset followed by impairment of consciousness
- With impairment of consciousness at onset
- With or without automatisms

Partial seizures evolving to complex partial seizures or secondary generalization

Unclassified Seizures

*ILAE Commission on Classification (1985).

Adapted from Commission on the Classification and Terminology of the International League Against Epilepsy: Proposal for classification of epilepsies and epileptic syndromes. Epilepsia 26:268-278, 1985.

Box 128-2   Epilepsy Classification*

Localization Related (Focal)

Idiopathic, with age-related onset (presumed to be genetic and often associated with normal intelligence)
Symptomatic (epilepsies in which the seizures arise from a known lesion or site)
Cryptogenic (no identified symptomatic cause for the epilepsy)

Generalized

Idiopathic, with age-related onset
Cryptogenic or symptomatic
Symptomatic

Undetermined whether focal or generalized

Special syndromes

*Commission on Classification (1989).

Adapted from Commission on Classification and Terminology of the International League Against Epilepsy: Proposal for revised classification of epilepsies and epileptic syndromes. Epilepsia 30:389-399, 1989.

Classification of Epilepsy

The classification of the epilepsies is based on age, family history, the seizure types, associated clinical findings, and laboratory abnormalities, especially the EEG characteristics and neuroimaging abnormalities. Etiology, anatomic correlates, age at onset, associated neurologic signs, precipitating factors, prognosis, circadian cycles, and seizure type are important features used in the classification of epilepsy. The epilepsies are divided into two principle groups: localization-related and generalized events. Box 128-2 shows the current epilepsy classification. Plans are underway to revise this classification.

Causes of Seizures and Epilepsy

Focal seizures begin as an autonomous electrochemical discharge of a group of neurons that recruit surrounding neurons into a rhythmical firing pattern. Although many theories have been postulated about how focal seizures begin, most likely multiple factors are responsible. At the cellular level, the characteristic interictal abnormality of an epileptic focus is the paroxysmal depolarization shift (PDS). The PDS is an abnormal cellular event characterized intracellularly by a large membrane depolarization, which produces a burst of action potentials followed by hyperpolarization of the neuron. On the surface of the brain or scalp, the PDS is seen as a spike followed by a slow wave. With the occurrence of a seizure, the intracellular depolarization and bursting persist, and no hyperpolarization occurs. A clinical seizure occurs only when a large number of neurons synchronously display this activity. The spread of seizures from the focus is usually prevented by a surround inhibition manifested intracellularly by hyperpolarization of the neurons. This inhibition is mediated predominately by γ-aminobutyric acid. The mechanisms of the generalized epilepsies involve many neurons in a large portion of the brain.

Potential causes that lead to these epileptic changes can be potentially age dependent. The age of onset may give clues to the underlying cause of the seizures and epilepsy. Yet, any significant injury to cortical structures can produce seizures. These injuries may come in the form of tumor, stroke, hemorrhage, infection, or trauma (Fig. 128-1). More than two thirds of patients have no clear cause of their seizures. The most common identifiable causes are listed below by age (Box 128-3).

Most of the epilepsies with defined gene abnormalities have abnormalities of membrane channels. Only a few of the known genetic causes of epilepsy are abnormalities of neurotransmitters (Table 128-1).

Clinical Presentation

Individuals with epilepsy present with a wide variety of symptoms. The key clinical feature of a seizure is the paroxysmal nature of discrete stereotypic symptoms or signs. An accurate description of a seizure may require reports from many sources and at times even a videotape of the events because the patient may be unaware of the events and most seizures last less than 5 minutes.

Figure 128-1 Causes of Seizures.

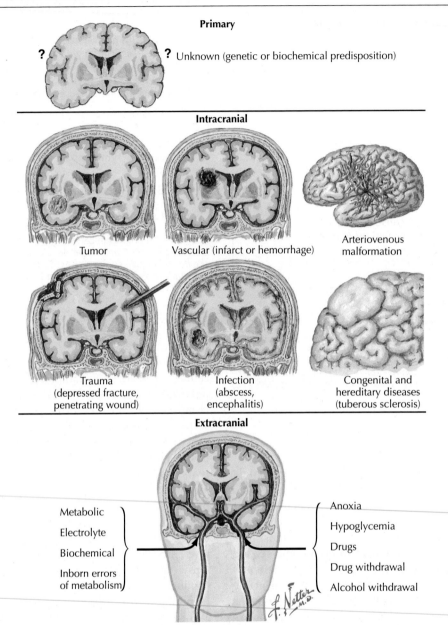

Primary

? ? Unknown (genetic or biochemical predisposition)

Intracranial

Tumor

Vascular (infarct or hemorrhage)

Arteriovenous malformation

Trauma (depressed fracture, penetrating wound)

Infection (abscess, encephalitis)

Congenital and hereditary diseases (tuberous sclerosis)

Extracranial

Metabolic
Electrolyte
Biochemical
Inborn errors of metabolism

Anoxia
Hypoglycemia
Drugs
Drug withdrawal
Alcohol withdrawal

Partial Seizures

The behavior exhibited during a seizure is determined by the pathophysiologic events in the region of affected brain (Fig. 128-2). Nearly any function performed by the brain may occur as part of a seizure. These symptoms range from motor and sensory involvement to complex automatisms or hallucinations. The symptoms or behaviors associated with the seizures are a manifestation of the area of brain being excited by the seizure. Thus, a patient with occipital lobe seizures may have visual symptoms, or a patient with temporal lobe seizures may smell something burning or have a rising sensation in their chest. Patients with frontal lobe seizures may have unusual motor manifestations such as turning or bicycling movements. Patients frequently may have automatisms. Automatisms are repetitive motor activities that are purposeless, undirected, and inappropriate and that can be done without awareness. Patients may exhibit lip smacking, sucking, swallowing, chewing, repetitive hand movement, picking at clothes, or fidgeting. Following the seizure, patients are frequently confused and disoriented; this is called the *postictal period*. These symptoms and behaviors are important in helping to define the seizure type and subsequent therapy.

Box 128-3 Causes of Seizures by Age

Newborn
- Perinatal hypoxia and ischemia
- Drug withdrawal
- Hypocalcemia
- Hypomagnesemia
- Hyperbilirubinemia
- Hypoglycemia
- Water intoxication
- Intracranial hemorrhage
- Intracranial birth injury
- Newborn errors in metabolism
- Pyridoxine deficiency
- Congenital malformations of the brain
- Central nervous system infection and inflammation (autoimmune diseases)
- Sepsis

Infancy
- Congenital defects
- Inborn errors in metabolism
- Brain tumor and other malignancy
- Central nervous system infection and inflammation (autoimmune diseases)
- Trauma
- Febrile convulsions
- Idiopathic

Childhood
- Trauma
- Brain tumor and other malignancy
- Congenital defects
- Intracranial hemorrhage, arterial venous malformation
- Central nervous system infection and inflammation (autoimmune diseases)
- Idiopathic

Adolescence and Young Adulthood
- Trauma
- Drug and alcohol withdrawal
- Intracranial hemorrhage, arterial venous malformation
- Brain tumor
- Idiopathic

Older Adulthood
- Alcoholism
- Brain tumor
- Cerebrovascular disease
- Trauma
- Metabolic disorders
- Uremia
- Hepatic failure
- Electrolyte abnormalities
- Hypoglycemia central nervous system infection, idiopathic

Primary Generalized Seizure

Generalized seizures involve both cerebral hemispheres from the onset. The expression of generalized seizures requires the interaction of cerebral hemispheres, thalamus, and possibly the brainstem.

Generalized seizures are subcategorized into several specific types. The most common form is generalized tonic-clonic convulsion (previously called grand mal) (Fig. 128-3). These seizures begin as tonic stiffening of the limbs in the extended position, followed by synchronous clonic jerking of the muscles. Occasionally, patients have pure tonic or pure clonic seizures. After the seizure, the patient is very lethargic, confused, and disoriented.

Absence seizures (previously called petit mal) are characterized by staring spells lasting less than 20 seconds and often associated with eye blinking (Fig. 128-4). Patients have no warning of oncoming seizures and also have no postictal period. Frequently, they have no memory of the event but may note a brief loss of time. Patients usually have hundreds of these per day. These seizures usually occur in children and many times are first noticed in school. Hyperventilation frequently can be used to provoke absence seizures. The characteristic generalized three-per-second spike-and-wave pattern on EEG is the hallmark for this seizure type.

Atonic seizures are composed of drop attacks or brief periods of loss of postural body tone. Patients may have clusters of atonic seizures causing injury from the falls. These patients frequently have to wear helmets to avoid serious head injury.

Myoclonic seizures are rapid, brief, usually bisynchronous contractions of the musculature. Patients may have frequent jerks occurring in bursts and have minimal impairment of consciousness.

Differential Diagnosis

The differential diagnosis for paroxysmal events can be divided into several categories: vasculature, endocrine, metabolic, neurologic, and psychiatric events (Table 128-2). The clinician should use a relatively wide differential before presuming the diagnosis. Frequently, nonepileptic paroxysmal events can be misinterpreted as epileptic seizures.

Diagnostic Approach

The goals of the evaluation of the patient with seizures are to identify the type of seizure that occurred, look for potential causes, elucidate possible risk factors that may promote recurrence, review the previous therapies, define the psychological and psychosocial impact of seizures on the patient, and recognize the patient's goals. The history is the most important feature of the evaluation. A clear description of the events as witnessed by an observer increases the likelihood of obtaining a correct diagnosis. The physician should pay particular attention to events leading up to the seizures, during the seizures, and following the seizures. The patients may have certain risk factors such as significant head trauma, stroke, family history of seizures, febrile seizures, or developmental delay. The physical examination should focus on the cardiac and

Table 128-1 Gene Defects in Genetic Epilepsy

Gene	Protein	Neuronal Function	Epilepsy
SCN1A	α1 Na Subunit	Membrane charge & action potential	Generalized epilepsy and febrile seizures (GEFs+)
SCN1B	β1 Na Subunit		
SCN2A	α2 Na Subunit	Membrane charge & action potential	Benign familial neonatal-infantile seizures
SCN1A	α1 Na Subunit	Membrane charge & action potential	Severe myoclonic epilepsy of infancy
GABRG2	GABA receptor	Inhibition	
GABRG2 γ2 subunit	GABA receptor	Inhibition	GEFs
GABRA1 α 1 subunit	GABA receptor	Inhibition	Juvenile myoclonic epilepsy
KCNQ2 KCNQ3	V-Sensitive K+ channel	Membrane charge & after hyperpolarization	Benign Familial Neonatal Seizures
KCNA1	Low V-Sensitive K+ channel	Membrane charge & after hyperpolarization	Familial Temporal Lobe
CNRN alpha 4 CHRNB2	Nicotinic α4 subunit Nicotinic β2 subunit	Excitation	Familial Frontal Lobe
KCNJ11 gene	Pore-forming subunit (Kir6.2) of the ATP-sensitive potassium (K_{ATP}) channel	Membrane charge & after hyperpolarization	Developmental delay, epilepsy, and neonatal diabetes—DEND
Cav2.1 subunit	voltage-gated Ca2+ channels	Excitation or inhibition	Absence

Table 128-2 Differential Diagnosis of Paroxysmal Disorders

Category	Cause
Vascular	Cardiac arrhythmia, transient ischemic attack, syncope, migraine, hyperventilation
Endocrine	Hypoglycemia, thyroid storm
Movement disorders	Paroxysmal vertigo, tics, alternating hemiplegia
Sleep disorders	Cataplexy, sleep paralysis, hypersomnia
Metabolic	Hypoxia, periodic paralysis
Toxic	Drugs
Psychiatric	Panic attacks, psychosis, conversion disorders, fugue states

vascular system, and a complete neurologic examination should be performed. Most patients with epilepsy have a normal neurologic examination, so the absence of neurologic deficits does not exclude the diagnosis.

All patients with epilepsy should have had an EEG. This study records the electrical fields generated over the scalp. Although about 40% of patients with epilepsy have a normal routine EEG, a second EEG performed with the subject asleep or sleep deprived increases the yield of abnormalities to 80%. The classic epileptiform abnormalities found on the EEG are spikes, sharp waves, or spike and slow wave complexes. These waveforms are the elec-

trical signature of epilepsy. Nevertheless, the incidence of these abnormalities in people without seizures may be as high as 2%.

Patients with possible focal-onset epilepsy should have an MRI study of the brain. This study can demonstrate the cortex in great detail and allow for the detection of small structural abnormalities.

Management and Therapy

Optimum Treatment

The goals for managing a patient with epilepsy are to have the patient completely seizure free, with no side effects of therapy, and to reverse any untoward effects of the epilepsy. These goals are not obtainable in all patients but should be strived for. Between 20% to 44% of patients with epilepsy do not achieve complete control of their seizures with medication. The general principles of medication therapy are to start a single medication at a low dose, slowly titrating the medication till one of two end points is reached: either the patient is seizure free, or the patient has untoward side effects that do not abate with drug manipulation. If the first medication does not succeed, a second medication is added and titrated to an efficacious dose before the tapering off of the first medication. Medications should be given ample trial time especially to allow side effects to improve with time. A list of medications is provided in Box 128-4.

If medications do not prove helpful, the physician should consider reevaluating the patient. Confirmation

Figure 128-2 Partial Motor and Somatosensory Seizures.

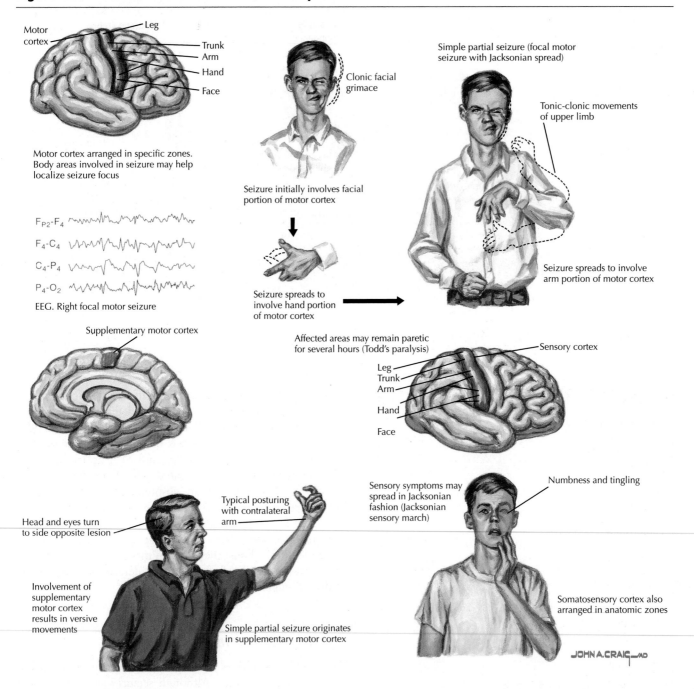

Motor cortex

Leg
Trunk
Arm
Hand
Face

Motor cortex arranged in specific zones. Body areas involved in seizure may help localize seizure focus

F_{P2}-F_4

F_4-C_4

C_4-P_4

P_4-O_2

EEG. Right focal motor seizure

Supplementary motor cortex

Head and eyes turn to side opposite lesion

Typical posturing with contralateral arm

Involvement of supplementary motor cortex results in versive movements

Simple partial seizure originates in supplementary motor cortex

Clonic facial grimace

Seizure initially involves facial portion of motor cortex

Seizure spreads to involve hand portion of motor cortex

Simple partial seizure (focal motor seizure with Jacksonian spread)

Tonic-clonic movements of upper limb

Seizure spreads to involve arm portion of motor cortex

Affected areas may remain paretic for several hours (Todd's paralysis)

Sensory cortex

Leg
Trunk
Arm
Hand
Face

Sensory symptoms may spread in Jacksonian fashion (Jacksonian sensory march)

Numbness and tingling

Somatosensory cortex also arranged in anatomic zones

JOHN A. CRAIG—AD

of the diagnosis with video EEG monitoring may prove helpful. Additionally, this monitoring may demonstrate whether the patient would be a candidate for potential evaluation for epilepsy surgery. Resection of the epileptic focus in some cases can cure the epilepsy. Success rates as high as 85% have been reported in resection of the seizure foci from the temporal lobes. Unfortunately, resections from other areas of the brain have not been as fruitful. Alternatively, neuronal stimulation therapy is available.

The vagus nerve stimulator is a proven therapy for patients with intractable epilepsy.

Avoiding Treatment Errors

The most common treatment error is that physicians fail to be aggressive enough to completely stop recurrent seizures. For patients to have a significant improvement in quality of life, they must be seizure free. Therefore, one

Figure 128-3 Generalized Tonic-Clonic Seizures.

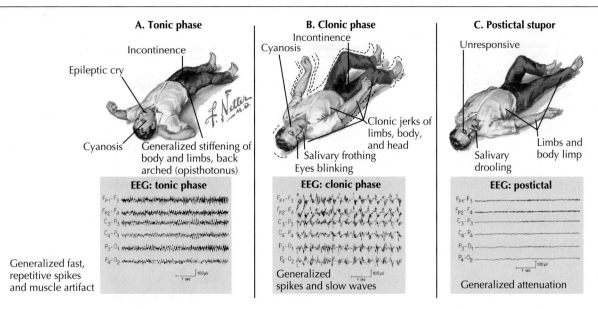

A. Tonic phase

Incontinence

Epileptic cry

Cyanosis   Generalized stiffening of body and limbs, back arched (opisthotonus)

EEG: tonic phase

F_{P1}-F_3
F_{P2}-F_4
C_3-P_3
C_4-P_4
P_3-O_1
P_4-O_2

Generalized fast, repetitive spikes and muscle artifact

B. Clonic phase

Incontinence
Cyanosis

Clonic jerks of limbs, body, and head

Salivary frothing
Eyes blinking

EEG: clonic phase

F_{P1}-F_3
F_{P2}-F_4
C_3-P_3
C_4-P_4
P_3-O_1
P_4-O_2

Generalized spikes and slow waves

C. Postictal stupor

Unresponsive

Limbs and body limp

Salivary drooling

EEG: postictal

F_{P1}-F_3
F_{P2}-F_4
C_3-P_3
C_4-P_4
P_3-O_1
P_4-O_2

Generalized attenuation

<table>
<tr><td colspan="2">Box 128-4   Medications for Treatment of Seizures</td></tr>
<tr><td colspan="2">Focal-Onset Seizures</td></tr>
<tr><td colspan="2">
Phenytoin
Carbamazepine
Phenobarbital
Primidone
Methsuximide
Valproate
Gabapentin
Lamotrigine
Felbamate
Topiramate
Tiagabine
Zonisamide
Oxcarbazepine
Levetiracetam
Pregabalin
Clorazepate
Clonazepam
Lorazepam
</td></tr>
<tr><td colspan="2">Primary Generalized Seizures</td></tr>
<tr><td colspan="2">
Valproate
Lamotrigine
Topiramate
Ethosuximide (for absence seizures)
Felbamate
Zonisamide
</td></tr>
</table>

seizure per year still impairs one's life. Antiepileptic medication should be gradually increased until the patient is seizure free or incurs a side effect. Physicians must also realize that serum drug levels only reflect the amount of drug in the blood, not the amount of drug in the brain, which is the organ being treated. The therapeutic range is only a guideline, not an absolute. Patients may have seizures while in the lower therapeutic range but remain seizure free with a higher level. Conversely, patients may experience side effects at a serum level below the therapeutic range. Thus, the clinician must follow the patient's symptoms and the clinical exam to determine whether the drug dosage needs to be changed.

Future Directions

Epilepsy research is striving toward curing epilepsy and the epileptic process. Although seizures are the defining component of the epilepsies, further research is needed to completely characterize the effect the epileptic process has on the brain and body. Development of new therapies that selectively treat the neurons participating in the seizure focus, while not altering normal brain function, will ultimately provide a key for us to unlock the mysteries of neuronal networking and plasticity. Additional approaches of gene manipulation and selective brain stimulation of epileptic networks using closed-loop computer integrated processors offer novel mechanisms to alter brain dysfunction and augment brain restoration.

Figure 128-4 Absence (Petit Mal) Seizures.

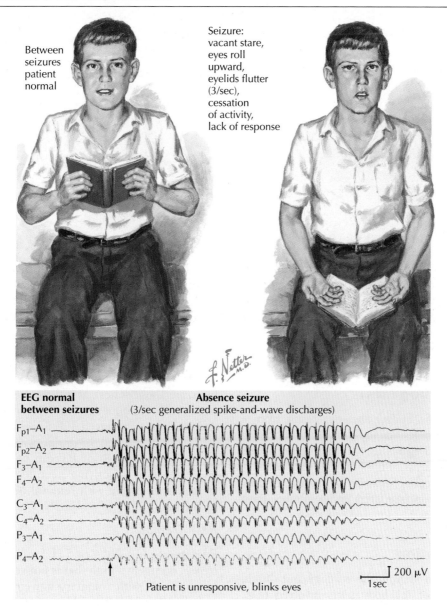

Between seizures patient normal

Seizure: vacant stare, eyes roll upward, eyelids flutter (3/sec), cessation of activity, lack of response

EEG normal between seizures

Absence seizure (3/sec generalized spike-and-wave discharges)

F_{p1}–A_1
F_{p2}–A_2
F_3–A_1
F_4–A_2
C_3–A_1
C_4–A_2
P_3–A_1
P_4–A_2

200 µV
1sec

Patient is unresponsive, blinks eyes

Additional Resource

Engel J Jr, Pedley TA (eds): Epilepsy: A Comprehensive Textbook. Philadelphia, Lippincott-Raven, 1998.
   This text provides an excellent overview of epilepsy.

EVIDENCE

1. Levy RH, Mattson RH, Meldrum BS, Perucca E (eds): Antiepileptic Drugs, 5th ed. Philadelphia, Lippincott Williams & Wilkins, 2002.
   This text provides an excellent review of the pharmacologic aspects of epilepsy.

2. Pellock JM, Dodson WE, Bourgeois BFD (eds): Pediatric Epilepsy: Diagnosis and Therapy, 2nd ed. New York, Demos, 2001.
   This text provides a comprehensive review of pediatric epilepsy.

3. Wyllie E (ed): Treatment of Epilepsy Principles and Practice, 4th ed. Baltimore, Williams & Wilkins, 2001.
   This book is an excellent resource for clinicians treating patients with epilepsy.

Tremor

Introduction

Tremor is defined as involuntary, rhythmical oscillations of a body part. The involved body part can be proximal (e.g., head tremor) or distal (e.g., hand tremors). The tremor may be fine or coarse, fast or slow; it may exist at rest, when maintaining a posture, or with movement. A unified clinical classification was lacking until the 1998 Movement Disorder Society consensus paper on clinical classification that serves as a guide for this chapter.

Etiology and Pathogenesis

Tremor is a nonspecific finding that can result from a variety of nervous system lesions and a number of underlying disease processes. Lesions in the basal ganglia, the cerebellum, or certain areas of the brainstem are particularly likely to result in tremor. Some fairly common tremors have no clear localization (see later) and a number have metabolic or toxic causes.

Clinical Presentation

Observation is a key to identify the etiology and should include a description of the body parts involved (e.g., upper or lower limbs, lips, tongue, neck, or voice), type of tremor (e.g., rest tremor, postural tremor, or action tremor), tremor frequency (e.g., low [<4 Hz], medium [4 to 7 Hz], or high [>7 Hz]), and the factors that exacerbate or suppress the tremor.

Phenomenology of Tremor

Physiologic Tremor

An 8- to 12-Hz tremor is inherent in the normal nervous system. It is the result of physiologic subtetanic recruitment of motor units and is not generally clinically obvious. When muscle contractions are maintained, as when the arms are held outstretched, especially with a paper on top, the physiologic tremor (PT) becomes visible to the naked eye. Enhanced PT involves more prominent responses in stressful situations (e.g., fatigue, anxiety, fever, and some hypermetabolic states), as well as after certain medications (e.g., sympathomimetic drugs, lithium, sodium valproate, and caffeine). Enhanced PT is easily visible when arms are held outstretched, or during writing or drinking from a cup. The diagnosis of PT can be made when there is no evidence of underlying neurologic disease, and if the tremor is reversible with removal of the offending factor or agent.

Rest Tremor

Rest tremor (usually 4 to 5 Hz), often called *parkinsonian tremor*, occurs in a limb that is not voluntarily activated. It is suppressed with voluntary movement, and may appear as "pill rolling" (thumb rubbing across the palm or fingers) (Fig. 129-1, upper panel). In early Parkinson's disease (PD), rest tremor can be intermittent and obvious only under emotional or physical stress. As with almost all movement disorders, it disappears with sleep.

Action Tremor

Accentuated by voluntary contraction of muscle, action tremors include postural, kinetic, and isometric tremors. Postural tremor is seen when maintaining a position, such as when the arms are held outstretched. Kinetic tremor occurs during voluntary movement and is subdivided into *simple kinetic tremor* (during non–target-directed movement), *intention tremor* (exacerbated as the hand or foot approaches the target of a voluntary movement, such as finger-to-nose), and *task-specific tremor*. Isometric tremor occurs with muscle contraction against a stationary object (squeezing the examiner's fingers).

Figure 129-1 Tremor.

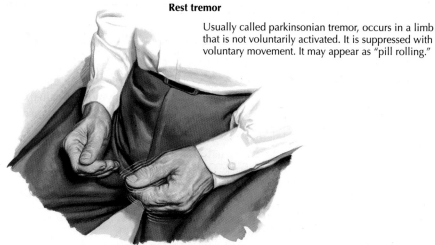

Rest tremor

Usually called parkinsonian tremor, occurs in a limb that is not voluntarily activated. It is suppressed with voluntary movement. It may appear as "pill rolling."

Action tremor (example: essential tremor)

Typically bilateral, this movement disorder is the most common. It may be accentuated with goal-directed movement of the limbs. Essential tremor affects the hands and facial musculature (in this order of prevalence). Most common presentation is the association of hand tremor and tremor in cranial musculature. Although considered benign, it can become incapacitating.

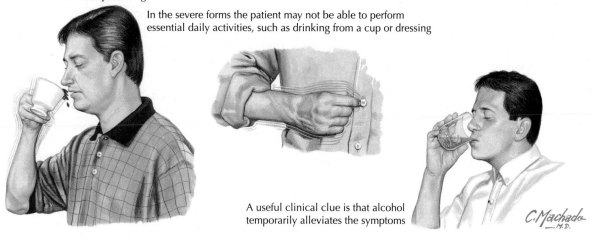

In the severe forms the patient may not be able to perform essential daily activities, such as drinking from a cup or dressing

A useful clinical clue is that alcohol temporarily alleviates the symptoms

Localization and Etiology of Different Clinical Tremor Syndromes

The tremor elements (discussed earlier) can be combined into the following clinical syndromes with specific etiologies that are useful for clinical diagnosis and treatment.

Rest Tremor (Parkinsonian Tremor)

This occurs most commonly with diseases of the basal ganglia, typically with idiopathic PD. The diagnosis of PD is usually established by concomitant findings, such as bradykinesia (e.g., slow movement, facial masking), rigidity (including cogwheel phenomenon from tremor superimposed on rigidity), and gait disorder (e.g., shuffling, lack of arm swing on walking). Other causes for rest tremor include both primary parkinsonism (e.g., progressive supranuclear palsy, multiple system atrophy) and secondary

parkinsonism (e.g., stroke lesions of the basal ganglia, carbon monoxide intoxication, mitochondrial diseases). Recently, benign monosymptomatic resting tremor has been recognized as an entity associated with neither the typical symptoms, nor the progressive course, of PD. It has been give a variety of names such as *benign tremulous PD* and *benign tremulous parkinsonism*, and the exact neuropathology of the condition is unknown.

Action Tremor (Cerebellar Tremor)

Postural and kinetic tremor is a common feature of disease involving the deep cerebellar nuclei and the cerebellar tracts in the brainstem. There may be a striking intention component that is particularly incapacitating. Other findings such as nystagmus, scanning dysarthria, dysrhythmia, and truncal ataxia help in cerebellar localization. Accompanying cranial nerve and pyramidal tract involvement also suggest brainstem disease. Many disease processes involving these structures may result in tremor, including neoplastic and paraneoplastic syndromes, hereditary and sporadic degenerative diseases, demyelinating diseases, trauma, infection, and cardiovascular disease. Alcohol is among the best-known toxicants causing this tremor.

Essential Tremor

Although of unknown etiology, essential tremor (ET) is the most common movement disorder (prevalence of 0.4% to 3.9%), presenting typically as bilateral, largely symmetric postural tremor that may be accentuated with goal-directed movement of the limbs. Severe ET also can manifest as rest tremor. ET most frequently affects the hands, and next most frequently, the cranial musculature. Although tongue, head, or voice may be affected in isolation, it is most common for the tremor in cranial musculature to occur in association with hand tremor. The legs and trunk are least affected, and usually only in the later stages of the illness. Our knowledge regarding the anatomic localization and pathologic mechanisms of ET is minimal. The cerebellum appears to be a prime candidate for the site of dysfunction based on animal model studies, and also the similarity in clinical signs and symptoms between advanced ET and patients with cerebellar disease. ET is currently thought to be a likely result of a central oscillator that can be enhanced or suppressed by reflex pathways.

ET may be sporadic or familial. It may appear at any age but is more frequent in early adulthood. The onset of ET may be earlier in the familial than the sporadic form. The course is unpredictable but may be static for many years or progress with a slow decline. Although usually considered benign, it can become incapacitating, particularly in occupations that require precise hand movements. In the severe form, patients may not be able to perform essential daily activities such as drinking from a cup or dressing. A family history will assist the diagnosis of ET, although the expression may be extremely varied in different members. A useful clinical clue in the diagnosis of ET is that alcohol may temporarily alleviate symptoms (Fig. 129-1, lower panel). As with most other tremors, ET remits during sleep.

Dystonic Tremor Syndrome

Dystonic tremor is described as postural, localized, and irregular, decreased during muscle relaxation, and accentuated by positioning the dystonic body part opposite to the direction of dystonia. The tremor caused by cervical dystonia is usually present as "no-no" kind of head shaking. The hand-and-head dystonic tremor can be difficult to differentiate from ET, but failure to respond to treatment for ET, or any dystonic feature in other body parts, may suggest the diagnosis. The etiology of dystonic tremor is unknown, however, but may be associated with basal ganglia dysfunction.

Primary Orthostatic Tremor

Primary orthostatic tremor (OT), also called *shaky leg syndrome*, is an uncommon condition that starts in late adulthood. The patient has a feeling of tremulousness in the legs when standing. This may lead to falls but generally disappears on movement and is not present when sitting or lying. The diagnosis is helped by specific surface electromyogram evaluation showing a 14- to 18-Hz oscillating tremor in the musculature of the legs when standing, disappearing with rest or movement. The etiology is unknown. Although suggested to be a variant of ET, it is probably a distinct entity because of the difference in age of onset, involvement of different parts (ET rarely affect legs), lack of family history, and lack of response to alcohol.

Holmes' Tremor

Holmes' tremor syndrome combines features of rest, intention, and postural tremor. The amplitude while resting may be small but may become uncontrollable while attempting to hold a posture, even worse when attempting a movement. In 1904, Holmes first described this as *rubral* tremor, but later it was called *midbrain* or *thalamic* tremor. Holmes' tremor is now preferred because the syndrome can occur with lesions affecting not only the red nucleus and rubral spinal tract in the brainstem but also the cerebellum and thalamus. The tremor may appear weeks to months after a known lesion (e.g., stroke), and some patients may have associated dystonia. Identifying this tremor always warrants evaluation for an underlying focal lesion.

Drug-Induced Tremor

A tremor is considered drug or toxicant induced if it occurs in a reasonable timeframe following ingestion or exposure. Drug-induced tremors can take any form, but the most common clinical manifestation is enhanced PT that can be caused by drugs such as sympathomimetic agents including bronchodilators, xanthines (e.g., caffeine), and epinephrine; centrally acting agents (e.g., valproate, lithium, tricyclic and other antidepressants, cocaine); antiarrhythmics (e.g., mexiletine, procainamide, and amiodarone); steroids (e.g., adrenocorticosteroids, tamoxifen, and progesterone); and cyclosporine and antimetabolites such as vincristine. Withdrawal from medications such as benzodiazepines or alcohol also may precipitate enhanced PT. Parkinsonian tremor can be caused by neuroleptic and dopamine-blocking drugs (e.g., haloperidol or metoclopramide), or dopamine-depleting agents (e.g., reserpine). Cerebellar tremor may occur after intoxication by lithium or alcohol. Environmental toxicants such as organophosphates and other insecticides, toxic metals, and some industrial chemicals also can cause or exacerbate tremor.

Tremor in Lower Motor Neuron Diseases and Peripheral Neuropathy

Tremor may accompany diseases of the anterior horn cell (e.g., amyotropic lateral sclerosis) and peripheral neuropathies. Demyelinating and particularly dysglobulinemic neuropathies are particularly likely to be associated with tremor, usually postural or kinetic. It is unclear whether tremor associated with peripheral neuropathy is due to enhanced PT secondary to weakness, to an abnormality in the central nervous system, or both.

Psychogenic Tremor

Psychogenic tremors can mimic nearly any type of tremor and, at times, can be difficult to diagnose. Psychogenic origin should be suspected when features of other recognized forms of tremor are not found. Clues to psychogenic etiology include sudden onset; bizarre fluctuations in the frequency and direction; increase when attention is drawn to the movement; history of secondary gain; and response to placebo. As always, it must be remembered that psychogenic disease may coexist in patients with organic disease.

Differential Diagnosis

Tremor must be differentiated from other movement disorders. Unlike tremor, clonus is increased by passive stretch of the muscle. Myoclonus, although difficult to distinguish, may have an electroencephalographic correlate, is generally more dysrhythmic, and has visible pauses between the jerks. Epilepsy partialis continua may continue through sleep and generally has electroencephalographic correlates. Asterixis (also called *negative myoclonus*) is characterized by a sudden loss of a maintained posture, followed by recovery, rather than an active movement.

Diagnostic Approach

The history should focus on the onset of tremor, family history, alcohol sensitivity, spreading sequence, associated disease, medication or chemical exposure, and possible drug abuse. The neurologic exam should assess akinesia and bradykinesia, muscle tone, postural abnormalities, dystonia, cerebellar signs, pyramidal signs, neuropathic signs, gait, and stance. Consideration should not be limited to the nervous system because tremor may result from other causes such as endocrine disease, hepatic failure, or neoplasm.

A history of relapsing and remitting neurologic symptoms, or the findings of other neurologic abnormalities associated with action tremor, may suggest evaluation for multiple sclerosis, mass lesions, or stroke. Effective treatments for some tremor-inducing conditions (thyroid dysfunction or Wilson's disease) make it reasonable to check thyroid function in all movement disorder patients and

ceruloplasmin levels in young patients. Holmes' tremor requires an extensive workup to identify local lesions in the brainstem, cerebellum, or thalamus pathway. If the tremor is bilateral and symmetric, but not associated with other clinical abnormalities, then imaging of the head is unlikely to be revealing.

Management and Therapy

Optimum Treatment

Effective treatment of the underlying disease is generally the most appropriate initial approach. Early in the course of PD, tremor may respond to anticholinergic medications (amantadine, trihexyphenidyl), or later to levodopa and dopamine agonists. ET may be responsive to propranolol (initially 80 mg/day in long-acting form, increased incrementally to 320 mg/day if required and tolerated), although primidone may also be effective (initially 50 mg/day, increasing to 250 mg twice a day or higher if required and tolerated). Topiramate has also been shown to be effective in treating ET (initially 25 mg/day, increasing to 100 mg twice a day or higher if required and tolerated). Isolated reports also suggest relief from gabapentin, clonidine, clozapine, acetazolamide, or methazolamide.

Primary OT is sometimes treated by clonazepam, phenobarbital, primidone, or valproate, although careful studies are not available. Neither alcohol nor propranolol is helpful. Treatment of dystonia with botulinum toxin often results in significant improvement of tremor (e.g., in cervical dystonia), but dystonic tremor may also respond to benzodiazepines (e.g., clonazepam, 0.25 to 2 mg/day). The overall treatment of cerebellar tremor remains unsatisfactory. Appending weights to the wrist may damp the amplitude of cerebellar, dystonic, and ET, but this rarely results in sustained functional improvement.

Stereotactic surgical ablation, or more commonly today, deep brain stimulation of the thalamus or basal ganglia is reserved for patients with severely disabling and medically intractable rest, essential, intention, dystonic, and rubral tremor. Trained and experienced multidisciplinary teams, appropriate patients, and clearly identified neuroanatomic targets are the critical factors for successful outcome.

Avoiding Treatment Errors

- Drugs are a common cause of tremor and can exacerbate existing milder tremor. It is important to address these drug issues before introducing new medication to treat the tremor.
- Different types of tremors can manifest in the same patients and require different approaches to treatment. For example, it is not uncommon that a patient with long-standing ET develops PD tremor at an older age. Introducing dopaminergic drugs is important to control the tremor and other associated PD symptoms.

- Tremor associated with dystonia is commonly misdiagnosed as ET. In some circumstances (e.g., head tremor with cervical dystonia), very satisfactory control can be obtained with periodic botulinum toxin injections. Looking for the dystonic component in evaluating tremor, especially in patients who fail to respond to ET treatment, is very important.

- Complete control of most tremors is not easily accomplished with current medications. The goal of treating tremor is not for the patient to be tremor free, but to maximize patient function within an acceptable range of drug side effects. Chasing the tremor-free goal may sometimes be medically futile, and even harmful to patients (especially elderly patients).

Future Directions

It is likely that deep brain stimulation will become increasingly useful as targets and methods are refined. Similarly, a wealth of new knowledge becoming available about the chemical neurocircuitry of the brain should also lead to better mechanistic understanding and to the discovery of new pharmacotherapeutic agents.

Additional Resources

Some very good websites about tremor and its treatment include the following:

http://www.ninds.nih.gov/disorders/tremor/detail_tremor.htm
http://www.wemove.org
http://www.medicinenet.com/tremor/article.htm
http://www.essentialtremor.org/
http://www.pdcaregiver.org/tremor.html

EVIDENCE

1. Britton TC, Thompson PD: Primary orthostatic tremor. BMJ 310:143-144, 1995.
   This short essay addresses the clinical presentation, diagnosis, and treatment of primary orthostatic tremor.
2. Deuschl G, Bain P, Brin M; Ad Hoc Scientific Committee: Consensus statement of the Movement Disorder Society on Tremor. Mov Disord 13(Suppl 3):2-23, 1998.
   This article includes a proposal of the Movement Disorder Society for a clinical classification of tremors. The classification is based on the distinction between rest, postural, simple kinetic, and intention tremor (tremor during target-directed movements).
3. Gross RE, Krack P, Rodriguez-Oroz MC, et al: Electrophysiological mapping for the implantation of deep brain stimulators for Parkinson's disease and tremor. Mov Disord 21(Suppl 14):S259-S283, 2006.
   This most recent review article discusses the techniques used in deep brain stimulation to treat Parkinson's disease and tremor.
4. Josephs KA, Matsumoto JY, Ahlskog JE: Benign tremulous parkinsonism. Arch Neurol 63:354-357, 2006.
   This article describes the features of a cohort of 16 patients with Parkinson's disease who developed moderate to severe rest tremor, but otherwise suffered less disability than is typical for Parkinson's disease. Authors proposed that "benign tremulous parkinsonism" may be a distinct clinical entity from classic Parkinson's disease.
5. Koller W, Hristova A, Brin M: Pharmacological treatment of essential tremor. Neurology 54(11 Suppl 4):S30-S38, 2000.
   This is an excellent overview of medical approaches to treating essential tremor.
6. Marsden CD: Origins of normal and pathological tremor. In Findley LJ, Capildeo R (eds): Movement Disorders: Tremor. London, Macmillan, 1984, pp 37-84.
   This is a classic, but still useful, overview of the physiology and pathology of various types of tremor.
7. Thanvi B, Lo N, Robinson T: Essential tremor—the most common movement disorder in older people. Age Ageing 35(4):344-349, 2006.
   The authors provide a review of the very common essential tremor.

Xuemei Huang ▪ Peter Lars Jacobson ▪ J. Douglas Mann

130

Parkinson's Disease

Introduction

Parkinson's disease (PD) is defined as a chronic, progressive neurodegenerative disorder of unknown etiology that can cause significant disability and early mortality if untreated. Parkinson's disease was first described in a classic monograph on "Shaking Palsy" in 1817 by James Parkinson. The disease affects about 1% of Americans older than 60 years, and its prevalence in the United States is expected to more than triple in the next 50 years as the U.S. population ages. The lifetime risk for PD is higher in men than in women—2.0% versus 1.3%. The estimated cost of PD in the United States is at least $6 billion annually in direct health-related costs, indirect disability-related costs, and lost productivity.

There have been significant advances in symptomatic treatment based primarily on dopamine replacement and, more recently, deep brain stimulation (DBS), that have dramatically improved the quality of life and life expectancy of patients with the disorder. Patients with this condition, however, continue to experience progressive motor and nonmotor deficits that impair their quality of life and are significant challenges for their caregivers.

Etiology and Pathogenesis

The most prominent pathologic change in PD is degeneration of melanin-pigmented dopamine neurons in the zona compacta of the substantia nigra (SNc) in the midbrain. Changes in the SNc are most pronounced in its ventrolateral region. Affected neurons also have intracellular inclusions known as Lewy bodies, which are now known to contain protein aggregates that, in some cases, are related to the cause of the disease. Neurodegenerative changes can also be found in the locus coeruleus, nucleus basalis of Meynert, pedunculopontine nucleus, cerebral cortex, and spinal cord.

Neurochemically, the hallmark of PD is a reduction in striatal dopamine. Less marked changes may also be seen in serotonergic, noradrenergic, and cholinergic systems. The most likely reason for the motor signs and symptoms is the dopamine deficiency or dysfunction in the basal ganglia, although there remains considerable uncertainty about the exact pathophysiologic basis of individual aspects of PD.

Genetic causes have been found only for familial PD, accounting for less than 5% of all patients. Mutations include several genes that produce proteins involved in synaptic function and protein processing. They have provided important research ideas, but not a specific cause for the much more common sporadic form of PD. Another landmark occurred when drug users injected MPTP (a byproduct of the production of an illicit opioid) intravenously and developed a rapidly progressive syndrome that was nearly identical to sporadic PD. Although the initial excitement around MPTP-like compounds in the environment playing a role in PD was not supported by later studies, this finding provided an impetus for the current hypothesis that sporadic PD results from the interactions between genetic and environmental factors.

Parkinson's disease is paradoxical in some interesting ways. For example, both smoking and coffee use have been consistently associated with a *lower* incidence of PD. Smoking certainly has proven health risks that make its association with a lower prevalence of PD surprising. Recently, there have been reports that the apolipoprotein ε2 allele, but not the ε4, is associated with an increased risk for PD. Generally, the apolipoprotein ε2 allele is linked to longevity and lower risk for Alzheimer's disease, whereas the ε4 allele is a major risk factor. If indeed sporadic PD is a result of complex genetic and environmental interactions, finding simple causes is unlikely.

Clinical Presentation

Cardinal Features

The cardinal clinical symptoms of PD are tremor, brady-kinesia, rigidity, and gait disorders (Fig. 130-1). At least two of the first three symptoms should be present to make a diagnosis.

Tremor typically occurs at rest and with a frequency of 4 to 7 Hz. Unlike essential tremor, in which postural and action components are predominant, PD tremor can be cosmetic, without affecting much function, because it disappears with use. Also, unlike essential tremor, the tremor of PD can affect the chin while not causing voice or head tremor.

Bradykinesia is a slowing of motor function. Rigidity is a finding of increased muscle tone with passive limb move-ment on examination. Varying degrees of bradykinesia and rigidity result in a spectrum of clinical presentations. Handwriting is affected, with difficulty initiating hand movement associated with a gradual reduction in the size of the words (micrographia). Ambulation is slowed, with decreased arm swing and reduced head turning. Poor turning ability, decreased reaction time, and a shuffling gait combine to increase the risk for falls. Facial expression is typically reduced (mask-like), and the frequency of spon-taneous eye blinks is decreased. Speech is slow, and vocal volume fades. Rigidity contributes to generalized immobi-lization and is a feature that leads to stooped posture when standing and walking (see Fig. 130-1, stage 3). Passive movement of the extremities often brings out cogwheel rigidity, a fine ratcheting feeling detected by the examiner in the muscles, which appears to be a product of intermixed rigidity and tremor. PD generally has an asymmetrical onset. Symmetrical disease early in the course is a red flag for other causes such as exposure to phenothiazines, hypo-thyroidism, or other causes of parkinsonism.

Mask-like facies, decreased eye blink, tremor at rest, cogwheel rigidity, micrographia, bradykinesia, decreased arm swing with walking, stooped posture, and shuffling gait can all be demonstrated by examination. There is also a significant absence of some findings such as abnormal tendon reflexes, lateralized weakness, sensory changes, and cerebellar signs. In recent years, it has been recognized that PD is often associated with (1) cognitive deficits such as impaired attention, executive function, and working memory, all related to frontal lobe function; and (2) dis-turbances in mood, sleep, olfaction, and autonomic nervous system function. These nonmotor deficits become espe-cially challenging when the disease progresses in these areas while motor symptoms are well managed with dopa-minergic replacement and deep brain stimulation (DBS).

Differential Diagnosis

Box 130-1 provides the differential diagnosis for Parkinson's disease.

> **Box 130-1　Differential Diagnosis of Parkinsonism**
>
> - Drug effects: medications, especially typical antipsychotics like the phenothiazines, can produce the findings of PD.
> - Depression: flat affect, psychomotor retardation, and pseudodementia may be present, but the primary findings of PD such as tremor and cogwheel rigidity are absent.
> - Head trauma: lateralized deep tendon reflexes, motor weakness, and sensory findings help to distinguish traumatic injury from PD (e.g., subdural hematomas).
> - Stroke: vascular injury to the brain can produce parkinsonian signs and symptoms that are generally sudden in onset and not progressive.
> - Wilson's disease: family history, Kayser-Fleischer rings on slit-lamp examination, liver dysfunction, abnormal serum ceruloplasmin, and elevated copper in serum and urine lead to the diagnosis.
> - Progressive supranuclear palsy (PSP): bradykinesia and rigidity may be present and the loss of voluntary eye movements, particularly upward gaze, is characteristic.
> - Intracranial tumors: the neurologic examination should help in identifying features that are not consistent with PD, leading to further diagnostic studies.
> - Viral and postviral factors: neurologic examination suggests more diffuse brain involvement with other physical symptoms and signs.
> - Normal-pressure hydrocephalus (NPH): gait is more suggestive of apraxia ("stuck foot"), and apathetic dementia and urinary incontinence are more evident.
> - Huntington's disease: a positive family history, choreiform movements, and dementia are predominant.
> - Multisystem atrophy (MSA), including Shy-Drager syndrome: parkinsonian features may be present, and autonomic insufficiency, including postural hypotension, is a major component.
> - Hypothyroidism: bradykinesia, skin thickening, constipation, cold intolerance, and low energy dominate the picture.

Diagnostic Approach

The diagnosis of PD is based on clinical criteria, including two of the classic triad (resting tremor, rigidity, and bradykinesia), asymmetry of symptoms and signs at initial presentation, and a significant positive response to levodopa. There are no reliable biologic markers of the disease. Although single-photon emission computed tomography and positron emission tomography are used in some research studies to determine the integrity of dopamine systems (i.e., dopamine transporters and fluoro-dopa uptake), they are not more accurate in diagnosing the disease than a trained clinician. Magnetic resonance imaging can help to eliminate other causes in the differen-tial diagnosis such as mass lesions, stroke, cerebellar pontine atrophy in multisystem atrophy, brain stem atrophy in progressive supranuclear palsy, and large ventricles in normal-pressure hydrocephalus. Laboratory tests should include thyroid and parathyroid function evaluation and,

Figure 130-1 Clinical Signs of Parkinson's Disease.

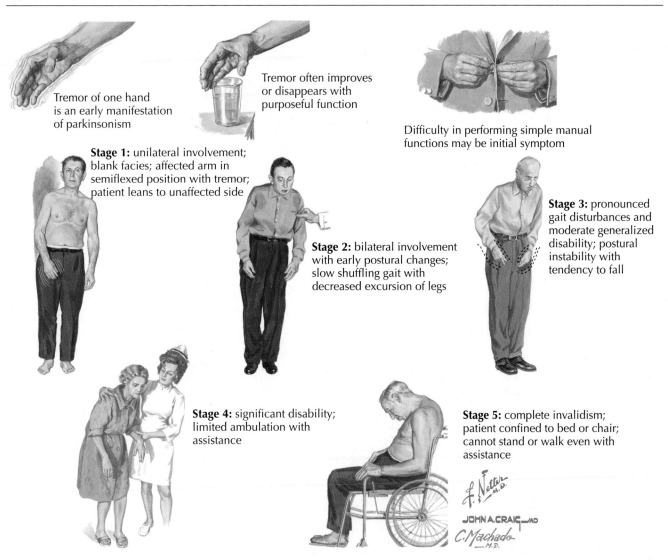

Tremor of one hand is an early manifestation of parkinsonism

Tremor often improves or disappears with purposeful function

Difficulty in performing simple manual functions may be initial symptom

Stage 1: unilateral involvement; blank facies; affected arm in semiflexed position with tremor; patient leans to unaffected side

Stage 2: bilateral involvement with early postural changes; slow shuffling gait with decreased excursion of legs

Stage 3: pronounced gait disturbances and moderate generalized disability; postural instability with tendency to fall

Stage 4: significant disability; limited ambulation with assistance

Stage 5: complete invalidism; patient confined to bed or chair; cannot stand or walk even with assistance

if onset is earlier than age 50 years, a serum ceruloplasmin for Wilson's disease.

Management and Therapy

Optimum Treatment

Medication

Levodopa, a precursor of dopamine, remains the most effective medication for symptom management, including all cardinal features of the disease. Levodopa is thought to allow the remaining dopamine neurons in the SNc to produce more dopamine, thereby resulting in near-normal dopamine receptor activation (Fig. 130-2). Almost all patients with PD will show a positive response to levodopa, and lack of such a response makes the diagnosis questionable. There is no evidence of benefit in delaying symptomatic treatment of PD. Early short-term and later long-term side effects are noted with levodopa. Early side effects include nausea, postural hypotension, confusion, hallucinations, and cardiac arrhythmias. Long-term use is associated with *wearing off* and dyskinesias. Wearing off results in the need for more frequent dosing of the drug. *On-off phenomena* are unpredictable, sudden, and usually brief losses of levodopa effectiveness in long-term users. Motor fluctuations occur in about half of patients after 5 years of levodopa therapy, increasing to 70% after 15 years. Carbidopa (aromatic amino acid decarboxylase inhibitor) is usually combined with levodopa to reduce the peripheral metabolic breakdown of levodopa. By decreasing the peripheral conversion of levodopa into dopamine, norepinephrine, and epinephrine, systemic side effects of levodopa, such as hypotension and cardiac dysrhythmias, are dramatically reduced. Blood tests are unnecessary with levodopa therapy.

Figure 130-2 Hypothesized Role of L-Dopa in Parkinson's Disease.

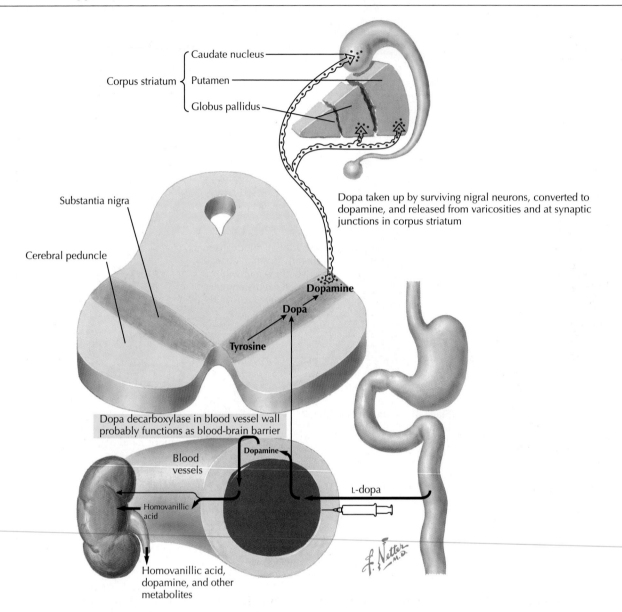

Corpus striatum
- Caudate nucleus
- Putamen
- Globus pallidus

Dopa taken up by surviving nigral neurons, converted to dopamine, and released from varicosities and at synaptic junctions in corpus striatum

Substantia nigra

Cerebral peduncle

Dopamine

Dopa

Tyrosine

Dopa decarboxylase in blood vessel wall probably functions as blood-brain barrier

Blood vessels

Dopamine

L-dopa

Homovanillic acid

Homovanillic acid, dopamine, and other metabolites

Dopamine agonists directly activate dopamine receptors in the brain without the need for bioconversion. When used with levodopa, benefits include reduction in fluctuating responses to levodopa and the pulsatile activation of dopamine receptors. There is clinical evidence that including a dopamine agonist in the treatment regimen may reduce dyskinesias associated with levodopa. The older dopamine agonists (bromocriptine and pergolide) are ergot derivatives with major side effects, including delusions, hallucinations, hypotension, and pulmonary and retroperitoneal fibrosis. Although the newer dopamine agonists, such as ropinirole and pramipexole, as nonergot derivatives, have significantly decreased risk for those problems, they can cause postural hypotension, peripheral edema, nausea, dyskinesias, confusion, and excessive somnolence.

Recently, compulsive behavior such as gambling has also been associated with use of dopamine agonists. Ropinirole and pramipexole may be helpful as an initial therapy in early PD, but their role is primarily adjunctive. Apomorphine, introduced in the U.S. market in 2005, can be given subcutaneously to treat severe PD freezing episodes.

Catechol-O-methyl transferase (COMT) inhibitors improve levodopa availability by reducing the peripheral conversion of levodopa to 3-O-methyldopa. COMT inhibitors reduce fluctuations in response to levodopa, resulting in more "on" time. The use of COMT inhibitors requires a 20% to 30% reduction in the daily dosage of levodopa to avoid side effects of excessive medication, such as dyskinesia. Tolcapone and entacapone are the available COMT inhibitors. Entacapone is more commonly used because it causes fewer hepatic side effects than tolcapone. The acute hepatic failure seen in a small number of patients taking tolcapone requires monitoring of liver function tests before and up to 6 months after the start of therapy. Other tolcapone side effects include diarrhea, abdominal pain, sleep disturbance, and postural hypotension. Despite these limitations, tolcapone appears to have superior effectiveness, probably because it penetrates the blood-brain barrier to a greater extent, thereby increasing the duration of action of dopamine.

Amantadine is effective in PD, but improvement may be transient. It is the only drug proven to be effective in the treatment of dyskinesias. The mode of action is likely to be through its effects on N-methyl-D-aspartate glutamate receptors. Although the drug is generally well tolerated, side effects may include peripheral edema, urinary retention, livedo reticularis, restlessness, confusion, dizziness, vivid dreams, and insomnia.

The *monoamine oxidase B inhibitors* selegiline and rasagiline have been suggested to be neuroprotective, slowing disease progression. Because both drugs have small beneficial effects on the primary symptoms, it has been difficult to get unequivocal data confirming neuroprotection. Selegiline and rasagiline may reduce both fluctuations in levodopa responsiveness and the daily dose of levodopa. Although they do not require the dietary restrictions of monoamine oxidase A inhibitors, they do adversely interact with some drugs, including meperidine, tricyclic antidepressants, and selective serotonin reuptake inhibitors. Selegiline is associated with more side effects, such as hallucinations and sleep disturbance, possibly because it is metabolized to L-amphetamine. The newer agent rasagiline has fewer side effects in this older population.

The *anticholinergic agents* benztropine and trihexyphenidyl, may relieve tremor and may also reduce drooling. The dosing range is limited because of the significant side effects, commonly including blurred vision, urinary retention, memory disturbance, hallucinations, and confusion.

Diet

Restricting dietary protein improves the gastrointestinal uptake of levodopa and also improves transport of levodopa across the blood-brain barrier. High protein diets increase amino acids that compete with levodopa for transport and may produce fluctuations in nervous system levodopa levels. Although vitamin E (tocopherol) acts to limit the effects of free radicals and is theoretically neuroprotective, a single large study did not confirm benefits in PD.

Physical Therapy and Exercise

There is evidence that regular exercise decreases the risk for PD and improves long-term quality of life in those with the condition. Regular exercise and physical therapy help maintain flexibility and strength. Speech therapy may help with volume and clarity.

Neurosurgical Approaches

A variety of ablative neurosurgical procedures used previously for control of tremor and rigidity have largely been replaced by DBS with implanted electrodes, resulting in better efficacy coupled with lower morbidity and mortality. DBS has become established during the past 5 years as an important part of the therapeutic armamentarium for use in selected patients who can no longer be managed medically. DBS may improve both motor fluctuations and dyskinesias, while decreasing the required doses of medication that cause many nonmotor side effects. The benefits of DBS have been reported to persist for up to 10 years in some cases. The potential side effects, in addition to perioperative stroke and infection, include disorganization of thought processes, speech impairment, visual and sensory disturbances, gait disturbance, incoordination, headaches, seizures, and depression. Medical centers performing DBS for PD are growing in number as the requisite interdisciplinary skills and experience are acquired.

Avoiding Treatment Errors

- Avoid using antipsychotic medications that can worsen PD. These drugs include typical antipsychotic drugs (e.g., haloperidol) as well as some atypical ones (e.g., olanzapine and risperidone). It is preferable to use those atypical antipsychotic drugs that are less likely to worsen PD (clozapine and quetiapine) if needed.
- Avoid antiemetic drugs that can worsen PD. These drugs include prochlorperazine, metoclopramide, and promethazine. Instead, use trimethobenzamide or ondansetron if needed.
- PD is a slowly progressive disorder. Many stressors, both medical (e.g., infection) and social (e.g., divorce, loss of spouse), can exacerbate PD symptoms acutely. These factors should be considered and managed during acute exacerbations of PD.
- Treating PD often involves polypharmacy because many patients are elderly. Carefully explaining the regimen to patients, family, and caregivers and writing down the treatment plan legibly can play a crucial role in the successful implementation of treatment.
- Starting medications at low doses and tapering upward slowly is the rule to minimize side effects for all PD medications.
- Treating nonmotor symptoms (e.g., depression, sleep disorder, cognitive and behavioral impairment) that are commonly associated with PD is critical to provide the best quality of life for the patients and their families.

Future Directions

Based on a variety of research approaches, a host of neuroreceptor targets have been suggested as playing a role in the development of PD. Several new dopamine agonists are being tested that either are delivered in novel ways (e.g., sublingually and transdermally) or target different populations of dopamine receptors. In addition, adenosine and glutamate receptor antagonists, as well as several other classes of drugs, are in development. Currently, a moratorium has been placed on experiments using transplantation of embryonic neurons for severe PD. However, there is a major research effort to determine whether genetically engineered stem cells may have treatment utility. There is also major interest in neuroprotective strategies, including both small molecules and gene therapeutics. Although the goals of either neuroprotection or curative procedures remain unmet, the current level of research activity in these arenas offers significant promise of success.

Additional Resources

Some very good websites on Parkinson's disease and its treatment include the following:

http://www.ninds.nih.gov/funding/research/parkinsonsweb/index.htm
http://www.parkinson.org
http://www.apdaparkinson.org
http://www.pdf.org
http://www.parkinsonsinfo.com
http://www.parkinsonsdisease.com/
http://www.mdvu.org
http://www.wemove.org/par/
http://www.michaeljfox.org

EVIDENCE

1. Davis GC, Williams AC, Markey SP, et al: Chronic parkinsonism secondary to intravenous injection of meperidine analogues. Psychiatry Res 1:249-254, 1979.

   This article provides the first description of acute, permanent, and dramatic parkinsonism caused by injection of MPTP, a compound made accidentally by addicts seeking to synthesize a meperidine congener. The subject responded to antiparkinson medication and, at necropsy, had pathologic changes remarkably similar to PD. This led to the most useful animal model of PD.

2. Dubois B, Pillon B: Cognitive deficits in Parkinson's disease. J Neurol 244:2-8, 1997.

   Cognitive deficits are seen in some patients with PD, including impaired executive function, defective memory storage, and impaired visuospatial processing. Evidence is reviewed for possible causes and underlying neural mechanisms.

3. Edwards LL, Pfeiffer RF, Quigley EM, et al: Gastrointestinal symptoms in Parkinson's disease. Mov Disord 6:151-156, 1991.

   This controlled clinical study in 98 subjects with PD supports direct involvement of gastrointestinal function by the primary disease process that is not explained by medication side effects or other factors. Symptoms that were greater in PD subjects included abnormal salivation, dysphagia, nausea, constipation, and defecatory control.

4. Elbaz A, Bower JH, Maraganore DM, et al: Risk tables for parkinsonism and Parkinson's disease. J Clin Epidemiol 55:25-31, 2002.

   This epidemiologic study found that lifetime risk for developing parkinsonism from birth was 4% for men and 3.7% for women in Olmsted County, Minnesota. For PD, the figures were 2% for men and 1.3% for women. These figures provide useful information in discussions with patients and their families.

5. Garcia-Borreguero D, Larrosa O, Bravo M: Parkinson's disease and sleep. Sleep Med Rev 7:115-129, 2003.

   Sleep disturbance is found in almost two thirds of those with PD and includes excessive daytime sleepiness, parasomnias, and problems with initiation or maintenance of sleep. This is an important area of clinical inquiry and management because quality of life can be severely affected by poor sleep in this population.

6. Hornykiewicz O, Kish SJ: Biochemical pathophysiology of Parkinson's disease. Adv Neurol 45:19-34, 1987.

   Our basic understanding of the pathophysiology of PD is reviewed. Complex interrelationships of neuroanatomy and neurochemistry are explained and explored.

7. Huang X, Chen PC, Poole C: APOE-ε2 allele associated with higher prevalence of sporadic Parkinson disease. Neurology 62:2198-2202, 2004.

   A meta-analysis revealed that APOE-ε2 allele, but not the ε4 allele, is positively associated with sporadic PD. This contrasts to Alzheimer's disease, for which the APOE-ε4 allele increases the prevalence of the disease and the APOE-ε2 allele is protective, underscoring that neurodegenerative diseases differ.

8. Katzenschlager R, Lees AJ: Olfaction and Parkinson's syndromes: Its role in differential diagnosis. Curr Opin Neurol 17:417-423, 2004.

   Loss of olfactory function is common in PD, dementia with Lewy bodies, and some of the spinocerebellar syndromes, but not in PSP, corticobasal degeneration, or vascular parkinsonism. Testing olfaction has become more standardized and can lead to early diagnosis in some movement disorders, including PD.

9. Kish SJ, Shannak K, Hornykiewicz O: Uneven pattern of dopamine loss in the striatum of patients with idiopathic Parkinson's disease: Pathophysiologic and clinical implications. N Engl J Med 318:876-880, 1988.

   Eight patients with PD undergoing necropsy were found to have severe losses in dopamine in major portions of the putamen, but highly focal and individualized, restricted losses in the caudate nucleus.

10. Langston JW, Ballard PA Jr. Parkinson's disease in a chemist working with 1-methyl-4-phenyl-1,2,5,6-tetrahydropyridine. N Engl J Med 309:310, 1983.

    This is another early case report of MPTP exposure leading to parkinsonism.

11. Nussbaum RL, Ellis CE: Alzheimer's disease and Parkinson's disease. N Engl J Med 348:1356-1364, 2003.

    This article compares and contrasts these two neurodegenerative disorders from the perspectives of phenotypic expression, genetics, neuropathology, neurochemistry, and functional neuropharmacology.

12. Parkinson J: An Essay on the Shaking Palsy. London, Sherwood, Neely, and Jones, 1817.

    This was the first description of PD.

13. Sherer TB, Betarbet R, Greenamyre JT: Pathogenesis of Parkinson's disease. Curr Opin Investig Drugs 2:657-662, 2001.

    This review of the role of mitochondrial dysfunction in the development of PD considers genetic and environmental factors as well as oxidative stress and excitotoxicity.

14. Tanner CM, Goldman SM: Epidemiology of Parkinson's disease. Neurol Clin 14:317-335, 1996.

    The authors presents PD as a multifactorial disorder with both environment and genetics playing a role in the development of the disease. They stress early detection as important in successful disease management and prolongation of function.

15. Tanner CM, Goldman SM, Ross GW: Etiology of Parkinson's disease. In Jankovic J, Tolosa E (eds): Parkinson's Disease and Movement Disorders. Philadelphia, Lippincott Williams & Wilkins, 2002, pp 90-103.

    This chapter is an updated review of the etiology of PD from the 1996 article.

Karen Kölln ▪ Jeffrey LaCour ▪ Harold C. Pillsbury III

Bell's Palsy

Introduction

The muscles of facial expression are intimately involved in our ability to communicate emotions with those around us. Acute unilateral facial palsy, also known as Bell's palsy after Sir Charles Bell who described the disorder in 1821, is the most common cause of facial weakness and the most common cranial neuropathy. Bell's palsy has traditionally been a diagnosis of exclusion and attributed to idiopathic origins; however, recent investigations have implicated herpetic viral infection with associated inflammation as the source of the paresis or paralysis. Bell's palsy is the most common cause of unilateral lower motor neuron facial palsy, accounting for 60% to 75% of all peripheral facial nerve palsies. Bell's palsy shows no gender or seasonal predilection and occurs with an incidence of about 20 to 30 per 100,000 population. As many as 71% of untreated patients recover completely, whereas 84% achieve near-normal facial function. Poor prognostic indicators for return of function include older age, hypertension, impairment of taste, pain other than in the ear, and complete facial nerve palsy.

Etiology and Pathogenesis

An understanding of the anatomy of the facial nerve is critical to the understanding of Bell's palsy. The facial nerve primarily carries fibers for motor control to the muscles of facial expression, the stapedius muscle, and the posterior belly of the digastric muscle. In addition to these motor fibers, sensory branches and parasympathetic fibers course within the facial nerve. Taste sensation from the anterior two thirds of the tongue joins the facial nerve through the chorda tympani branch. Parasympathetic fibers reach the lacrimal and submandibular glands through the greater superficial petrosal nerve and the chorda tympani, respectively. Loss of nerve conduction in the facial nerve can potentially disrupt all these fibers (Fig. 131-1).

The facial nerve travels through the temporal bone housed in a bony canal (fallopian canal), entering the temporal bone at the internal auditory canal and exiting from the stylomastoid foramen. The narrowest segment of the bony canal is located at the lateral end of the internal auditory canal. Acute unilateral facial palsy has been postulated to arise from an inflammatory process causing the facial nerve to swell within the bony canal surrounding it.

Although still a controversial topic, a large body of evidence implicates herpes simplex virus (HSV) infection as the primary cause of acute unilateral facial palsy. Nucleic acids from HSV have been found to be present in the geniculate ganglion of the facial nerve, and HSV DNA has been detected in the endoneural fluid of the facial nerve in patients with acute paralysis undergoing surgical decompression. An animal model of facial paralysis has been developed by inoculating mouse tongues or auricles with HSV. It is hypothesized that primary HSV may result in the entrapment of the virus within the geniculate ganglion, and its reactivation causes the inflammatory process causing the seventh nerve neuropathy. Another herpes virus, varicella-zoster virus, is known to be associated with acute facial nerve palsy in the setting of Ramsey Hunt's syndrome.

Clinical Presentation

The onset of Bell's palsy is typically acute, with the progression of weakness in several hours to overnight (Fig. 131-2). Bell's palsy may present as a complete hemifacial paralysis or, more commonly, as an incomplete palsy that may or may not progress to complete paralysis over several days. Many patients describe pain behind the affected ear as a prodrome and a sensation of numbness on the affected side of the face, although this sensation appears to be

Figure 131-1 Facial (VII) Nerve.

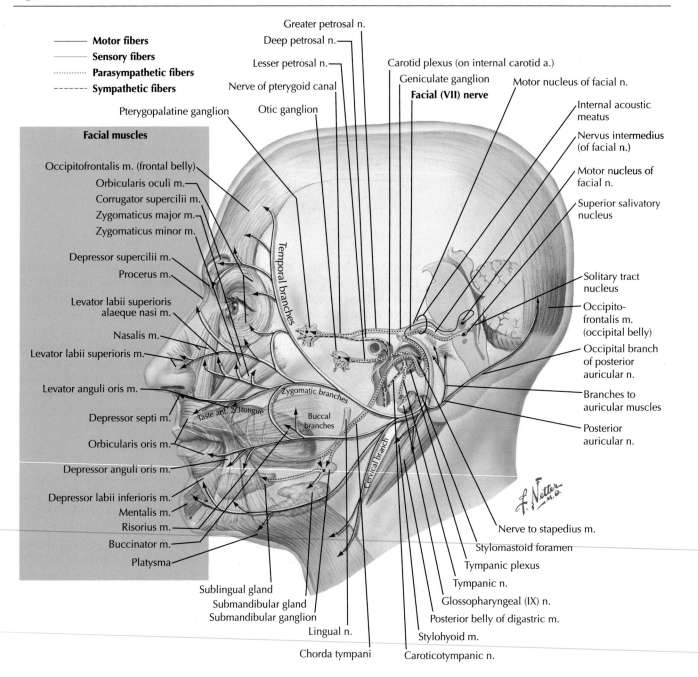

Motor fibers
Sensory fibers
Parasympathetic fibers
Sympathetic fibers

Facial muscles

Greater petrosal n.
Deep petrosal n.
Lesser petrosal n.
Nerve of pterygoid canal
Pterygopalatine ganglion
Otic ganglion

Carotid plexus (on internal carotid a.)
Geniculate ganglion
Facial (VII) nerve
Motor nucleus of facial n.
Internal acoustic meatus
Nervus intermedius (of facial n.)
Motor nucleus of facial n.
Superior salivatory nucleus
Solitary tract nucleus
Occipito-frontalis m. (occipital belly)
Occipital branch of posterior auricular n.
Branches to auricular muscles
Posterior auricular n.

Occipitofrontalis m. (frontal belly)
Orbicularis oculi m.
Corrugator supercilii m.
Zygomaticus major m.
Zygomaticus minor m.
Depressor supercilii m.
Procerus m.
Levator labii superioris alaeque nasi m.
Nasalis m.
Levator labii superioris m.
Levator anguli oris m.
Depressor septi m.
Orbicularis oris m.
Depressor anguli oris m.
Depressor labii inferioris m.
Mentalis m.
Risorius m.
Buccinator m.
Platysma

Temporal branches
Zygomatic branches
Taste ant. 2/3 tongue
Buccal branches
Cervical branch

Nerve to stapedius m.
Stylomastoid foramen
Tympanic plexus
Tympanic n.
Glossopharyngeal (IX) n.
Posterior belly of digastric m.
Stylohyoid m.
Caroticotympanic n.

Sublingual gland
Submandibular gland
Submandibular ganglion
Lingual n.
Chorda tympani

secondary to the lack of motion. Dysgeusia (disturbed taste), hyperacusis (sounds are too loud in the affected ear), and difficulty drinking are also common complaints.

Physical examination reveals unilateral paresis or paralysis of the muscles of facial expression. An important distinction is that the unilateral paresis or paralysis involves both the upper and lower face on the affected side (lower motor neuron lesion pattern). When severe, the affected hemiface shows no voluntary movements and obvious asymmetry at rest. The degree of facial paralysis is often quantified using the House-Brackmann scale, which incor-

porates gross facial appearance, symmetry at rest, and symmetry of the forehead, eye, and mouth in motion (Table 131-1). The skin surrounding the affected side of the mouth is displaced to the opposite side with smiling, and often the affected eye cannot be completely closed with maximal effort. When attempts are made to close the affected eye, the globe is seen to roll upward into the orbit, revealing sclera (Bell's phenomenon).

Thorough history taking and a complete physical examination with cranial nerve testing is critical to establishing the diagnosis. The parotid glands must be palpated for

Figure 131-2 Bell's Palsy.

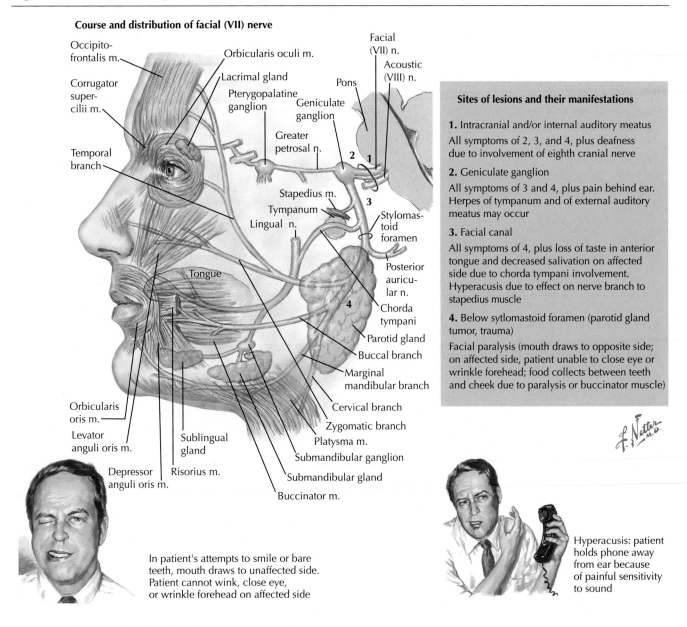

Course and distribution of facial (VII) nerve

Occipito-frontalis m.

Orbicularis oculi m.

Corrugator super-cilii m.

Lacrimal gland

Pterygopalatine ganglion

Temporal branch

Geniculate ganglion

Greater petrosal n.

Facial (VII) n.

Acoustic (VIII) n.

Pons

Stapedius m.

Tympanum

Lingual n.

Tongue

Stylomas-toid foramen

Posterior auricu-lar n.

Chorda tympani

Parotid gland

Buccal branch

Marginal mandibular branch

Cervical branch

Zygomatic branch

Platysma m.

Submandibular ganglion

Submandibular gland

Buccinator m.

Orbicularis oris m.

Levator anguli oris m.

Sublingual gland

Depressor anguli oris m.

Risorius m.

Sites of lesions and their manifestations

1. Intracranial and/or internal auditory meatus

All symptoms of 2, 3, and 4, plus deafness due to involvement of eighth cranial nerve

2. Geniculate ganglion

All symptoms of 3 and 4, plus pain behind ear. Herpes of tympanum and of external auditory meatus may occur

3. Facial canal

All symptoms of 4, plus loss of taste in anterior tongue and decreased salivation on affected side due to chorda tympani involvement. Hyperacusis due to effect on nerve branch to stapedius muscle

4. Below sytlomastoid foramen (parotid gland tumor, trauma)

Facial paralysis (mouth draws to opposite side; on affected side, patient unable to close eye or wrinkle forehead; food collects between teeth and cheek due to paralysis or buccinator muscle)

In patient's attempts to smile or bare teeth, mouth draws to unaffected side. Patient cannot wink, close eye, or wrinkle forehead on affected side

Hyperacusis: patient holds phone away from ear because of painful sensitivity to sound

masses, and the otoscopic examination must establish clear tympanic membranes with no evidence of infection or lesions. Examination of the tongue will often reveal inflammation of the fungiform papillae on the affected side. Lacrimation may be decreased in the affected eye. Audiometric assessment will often reveal stapedial muscle dysfunction and hyperacusis on the affected side.

Other etiologies of facial nerve palsy should be explored in the following scenarios: a history of recurrent facial palsy, other cranial nerve involvement, facial twitching, no recovery after 3 to 6 weeks or only partial recovery after 3 to 6 months, and a slowly progressive palsy lasting longer than 3 weeks.

Differential Diagnosis

Bell's palsy is a diagnosis of exclusion. The reported incidence of misdiagnosing facial palsy as Bell's palsy is between 13% and 20%. The differential diagnosis for unilateral facial palsy must include infectious causes, neoplasms, trauma, inflammatory processes, and metabolic disorders; symptoms also may result from a central insult, such as cerebrovascular accident or multiple sclerosis (Table 131-2).

Infectious etiologies include Lyme disease, Ramsey Hunt's syndrome (varicella-zoster), HIV, and otitis media or mastoiditis. Varicella-zoster virus facial paralysis

Table 131-1 House-Brackmann Facial Nerve Grading System

Grade	Description	Findings
I	Normal	Normal facial function in all areas
II	Mild dysfunction	Gross: slight weakness on close inspection, very slight synkinesis At rest: normal symmetry and tone In motion: forehead—moderate to good function; eye—complete closure with minimal effort; mouth—slight asymmetry
III	Moderate dysfunction	Gross: obvious but not disfiguring difference between sides, noticeable but not severe synkinesis At rest: normal symmetry and tone In motion: forehead—slight to moderate movement; eye—complete closure with effort; mouth—slightly weak with maximal effort
IV	Moderately severe dysfunction	Gross: obvious weakness or disfiguring asymmetry At rest: normal symmetry and tone In motion: forehead—no movement; eye—incomplete closure; mouth—asymmetrical with maximal effort
V	Severe dysfunction	Gross: barely perceptible motion At rest: asymmetry In motion: forehead—no movement; eye—incomplete closure; mouth—slight movement
VI	Total paralysis	No movement

Table 131-2 Differential Diagnosis of Peripheral Facial Palsy

Category	Signs and Symptoms
Infectious	
Lyme disease	History of tick bite, other neurologic symptoms, and constitutional symptoms (asthenia, anorexia, headache)
Ramsey Hunt's syndrome (varicella zoster)	Painful vesicular lesions on external ear or within ear canal; occasional lesions on soft palate
Human immunodeficiency virus (HIV)	History of HIV
Otitis media, mastoiditis	Evidence of middle ear purulence on otoscopy; postauricular erythema, edema
Neoplastic	
Middle ear tumor	Lesion seen on otoscopy
Parotid tumor	Mass palpated on physical examination
Cerebellopontine angle tumor (acoustic neuroma)	Sensorineural hearing loss, vertigo, facial hypesthesia (impingement of cranial nerve V)
Cholesteatoma	History of chronic draining ear, otoscopic examination with squamous debris
Traumatic	
Temporal bone fracture	History of trauma, possible sensorineural hearing loss, computed tomography scan demonstrating fracture along course of facial nerve
Middle ear trauma	History of penetrating trauma to middle ear, tympanic membrane perforation
Inflammatory	
Sjögren's syndrome	Sicca complex—dryness of mucous membranes of eyes and mouth
Amyloidosis	Possible proteinuria, hepatomegaly, heart failure, arrhythmia
Sarcoidosis	History with pulmonary symptoms
Guillain-Barré syndrome	Caudal to cranial progression of weakness, tingling starting in lower extremities
Metabolic	
Diabetes mellitus	History of diabetes; visual or renal problems
Preeclampsia	Pregnant patient with hypertension and proteinuria
Central Insult	
Multiple sclerosis	Visual changes, vertigo, weakness or numbness
Cerebral vascular accident	Hemiparesis, hemisensory loss, hemineglect with sparing of the forehead on the affected side

(Ramsey Hunt's syndrome) is the second most common cause of hemifacial palsy. Typical varicella-zoster infection is associated with skin blistering or blebs involving the tympanic membrane, external auditory canal, or post-auricular skin. Often these patients complain of severe pain around the affected auricle and may experience sensorineural hearing loss. The severity and prognosis for recovery of facial function is much graver in varicella-zoster infection.

Other infectious sources of unilateral facial palsy merit consideration. Acute otitis media may present as unilateral facial palsy. This is believed to be secondary to inflammation at natural dehiscences of the fallopian canal through the middle ear cavity. Suppurative or coalescent mastoiditis may alter neural conduction through the facial nerve in its vertical segment in the temporal bone. Interestingly, the most common head and neck manifestation of Lyme disease is facial nerve paralysis. HIV-associated facial nerve paralysis has also been reported.

Parotid gland neoplasms may present with hemifacial paresis or paralysis, as can paragangliomas involving the middle ear cavity. Temporal bone malignancy, primary or metastatic, may also present in a similar fashion. Cholesteatoma may also erode the fallopian canal, causing paresis of the facial nerve. A cerebellopontine angle tumor such as an acoustic neuroma may present with facial weakness as well as with hearing loss, vertigo, and facial hypesthesia.

Traumatic injury to the facial nerve, either in its intratemporal course or after exiting the stylomastoid foramen, must be excluded. This would include recent surgeries involving the parotid gland, middle ear, or internal auditory canal as well as trauma violating the tympanic membrane or resulting in a temporal bone fracture.

Inflammatory causes of facial palsy include Sjögren's syndrome, amyloidosis, sarcoidosis, and Guillain-Barré syndrome. Presentation of a patient with bilateral palsies should raise suspicion of these diagnoses.

Patients with metabolic disorders such as diabetes mellitus and preeclampsia have been noted to have a higher incidence of facial palsy of various etiologies.

Central nervous system insults such as cerebrovascular accident and multiple sclerosis may present with facial paralysis. These lesions typically present as an upper motor neuron lesion pattern without involvement of the upper face musculature on the affected side.

Diagnostic Approach

An imaging study is indicated if there is no improvement in facial paresis after one month, hearing loss, multiple cranial neuropathies, or if there signs of limb paresis or sensory loss. A CT of the temporal bones is indicated if trauma is suspected or if an intratemporal facial nerve tumor is suspected. Magnetic resonance imaging with gadolinium is the test of choice to rule out a cerebellopontine angle tumor, multiple sclerosis, or other structural lesions. An audiogram with stapedial reflexes should be obtained if hearing loss is reported to help rule out an acoustic neuroma.

If a patient has evidence of systemic symptoms such as fever, weight loss, rash, or a progressive facial weakness without improvement, a complete blood count with differential helps rule out lymphoreticular malignancy. Blood glucose (or hemoglobin A1C) should be ordered if diabetes is suspected. Serum antibodies against varicella zoster and *Borrelia burgdorferi* should be obtained if these entities are high on the differential list. Serum calcium and angiotensin-converting enzyme levels should be ordered if sarcoidosis is suspected.

Management and Therapy

The management of acute unilateral facial palsy is directed toward decreasing presumed inflammation influencing the facial nerve, preventing potential complications, and establishing prognosis for recovery.

Optimum Treatment

Optimum treatment for Bell's palsy includes a regimen of corticosteroids equivalent to 1 mg/kg prednisone daily for 1 week, tapering to off over a second week of therapy. This has been demonstrated to improve return of facial function. Antiviral therapy has also been shown to improve outcome when given in conjunction with corticosteroids, and a typical dose equivalent to 1000 mg of acyclovir daily is often used for 7 to 10 days. Early treatment (within 3 days of onset) is necessary for acyclovir-prednisone therapy to have the greatest effects.

Meticulous eye protection and care is critical in patients unable to fully close the affected eye (House-Brackmann grade IV or higher). This should consist of the liberal use of artificial tears and lubricating ointment multiple times daily until the protective function of eye closing returns. In addition, the affected eye should be taped or patched in the closed position before sleeping to avoid inadvertent damage or desiccation to the exposed cornea during sleep. Rarely, a tarsorrhaphy may be required to prevent eye damage.

Electrical testing can be used as an aid to predict prognosis in acute facial paralysis. Unlike many other nerves, the facial nerve cannot easily be stimulated proximal to the presumed site of inflammation or edema. Instead, stimulation of the trunk of the facial nerve as it exits the stylomastoid foramen with measurement of compound muscle action potential amplitude at the muscles of facial expression has been shown to be helpful in establishing prognosis. This test, called electroneurography (ENOG), is only beneficial between days 3 and 21 after complete loss of voluntary movements. In patients with more than 90% degeneration on ENOG compared with the contralateral side and no evidence of motor unit potentials on electromyography by day 14 of paralysis, a poorer prognosis for return of facial function can be given and surgical decompression considered.

The role of surgical decompression of the facial nerve in acute paralysis has generated much debate. Surgical decompression undertaken in carefully selected patients with clearly defined electrical findings has been shown to improve final outcome of facial nerve function. The approach for this surgery involves a middle cranial fossa craniotomy with selected decompression of the perigeniculate region of the facial nerve by an experienced otolaryngologist or neurosurgeon. This directed decompression is focused on the regions of the facial nerve with the most restrictive bony canal anatomy and has been shown to improve final House-Brackmann grade of facial nerve function.

Avoiding Treatment Errors

The best way to avoid treatment errors is to be thorough in the evaluation of patients with facial palsy, considering all possible etiologies before placing the patient on an acyclovir-prednisone regimen. A serious medical condition or tumor may otherwise be missed.

Recovery

Generally, recovery from paresis or paralysis of the facial nerve is satisfactory. For patients with poor recovery 3 to 6 months after onset of weakness and no other discoverable cause, several surgical procedures may help restore function. For patients with poor recovery of eye-closing function, upper eyelid gold weight implantation may be considered to enhance corneal protection. For patients with poor recovery of the muscles of facial expression, a variety of reanimation and reinnervation operations have been developed in recent years.

Future Directions

Although the current evidence linking HSV infection to Bell's palsy is strong, our understanding of when and why the latent infection causes symptoms is poorly understood. In order to demonstrate that the reactivation of HSV virus from its latent to lytic state, a study performing reverse transcriptase polymerase chain reaction aimed at detecting lytic state-specific messenger ribonucleic acids should be performed. A recent article has also reported facial palsy following the administration of the inactivated intranasal influenza vaccine, indicating that other viruses can be pathogenic.

Additional Resources

American Academy of Otolaryngology—Head and Neck Surgery. Available at: http://www.entnet.org. Click on Bell's Palsy. Accessed October 9, 2006.

This site provides a basic overview of the facial nerve anatomy and function. It offers a one-page summary of diagnosis, treatment, and prognosis.

Bell's Palsy Information Site. Available at: http://www.bellspalsy.ws/. Accessed October 9, 2006.

This website provides the most frequent questions from physicians and patients, with corresponding answers.

eMedicine: Bell's Palsy. Available at: http://www.emedicine.com/EMERG/topic56.htm. Accessed October 9, 2006.

This site provides the physician with a more comprehensive approach to the diagnosis and treatment of patients with Bell's palsy.

EVIDENCE

1. Adour KK, Ruboyianes JM, Von Doersten PG, et al: Bell's palsy treatment with acyclovir and prednisone compared with prednisone alone: A double-blind, randomized, controlled trial. Ann Otol Rhinol Laryngol 105(5):371-378, 1996.

    This trial demonstrated that treatment with acyclovir-prednisone is statistically more effective in returning volitional muscle motion and in preventing partial nerve degeneration than placebo-prednisone treatment.

2. Ahmed A: When is facial paralysis Bell palsy? Current diagnosis and treatment. Cleve Clin J Med 72(5):398-401, 405, 2005.

    This article provides a broad differential diagnosis for facial palsy and discusses appropriate tests to order as well as treatment options.

3. Alaani A, Hogg R, Saravanappa N, Irving RM: An analysis of diagnostic delay in unilateral facial paralysis. J Laryngol Otol 119(3):184-188, 2005.

    This analysis demonstrates how Bell's palsy has commonly been misdiagnosed when there is an underlying cause for the facial palsy.

4. Gilden DH: Clinical practice: Bell's palsy. N Engl J Med 351(13):1323-1331, 2004.

    This article emphasizes the likely viral etiology of Bell's palsy: herpes simplex virus type I. It also provides a detailed diagram of the facial nerve and physical findings associated with central and peripheral facial weakness.

5. Linder T, Bossart W, Bodmer D: Bell's palsy and herpes simplex virus: Fact or mystery? Otol Neurotol 26(1):109-113, 2005.

    This article questions herpes simplex virus as the etiology of all Bell's palsy; the authors recommend a study in the future to demonstrate the identification of an active replicating virus in Bell's palsy patients to confirm the causality.

6. Ramsey MJ, DerSimonian R, Holtel MR, Burgess LP: Corticosteroid treatment for idiopathic facial nerve paralysis: A meta-analysis. Laryngoscope 110(3 Pt 1):335-341, 2000.

    This meta-analysis indicates that corticosteroid treatment improves complete facial motor recovery for individuals with complete idiopathic facial nerve paralysis.

Alim M. Ladha ▪ Wesley Caswell Fowler ▪ Elizabeth Bullitt

Trigeminal Neuralgia

Introduction

Trigeminal neuralgia (TGN), also known as *tic douloureux*, is a clinical entity defined by episodes of brief, lancinating facial pain in the sensory distribution of the trigeminal nerve. Painful episodes are usually triggered by specific sensory stimuli such as chewing, light touch, or shaving. No other symptoms accompany the pain episodes, and their presence should alert the examiner to question the diagnosis. The finding of a neurologic deficit on clinical exam should trigger a more exhaustive workup for other etiologies. Most cases occur in patients in their fifth decade or beyond, with an incidence ranging from 1 to 4 per 100,000 persons per year, and with females predominating over males in some reports in a 2 : 1 ratio.

Etiology and Pathogenesis

The exact cause of TGN is unclear. In 1934, Walter Dandy published a series of 215 cases of TGN. Although Dandy did not discuss presenting symptoms, he found that in most cases there was vascular compression of the sensory component of the trigeminal nerve, most commonly by the superior cerebellar artery, or no obvious abnormality. Currently, the leading etiologic theory is that the sensory root entry zone of the trigeminal nerve is particularly susceptible to mechanical compression, most commonly by the superior cerebellar artery. Microscopically, the root entry zone adjacent to the brainstem provides an area of transition from central to peripheral myelin. Pathophysiologically, mechanical disturbance as a result of vascular compression may result in ephaptic transmission and the conduction of painful stimuli.

Clinical Presentation

Patients presenting with idiopathic TGN complain of brief, recurrent episodes of lancinating pain confined to one or more divisions of the trigeminal nerve (Fig. 132-1). Most commonly, the V2 (maxillary) and V3 (mandibular) divisions are involved unilaterally. Fewer than 6% of cases involve V1 (ophthalmic). The pain is often induced by touch of the affected dermatome. Long periods of spontaneous remission are common. Episodes tend to become more frequent and more severe with time, which may lead to malnutrition and poor hygiene of the affected region. Bilateral symptoms occur in about 5% of patients and should alert the examiner to the possibility of multiple sclerosis. The presentation of patients with TGN is often quite stereotypical and includes paroxysmal lancinating pain, triggers based on chewing or touch to a trigger area, and presence during the day and absence during sleep. Many authors also include response to a trial of carbamazepine as diagnostic, with failure of response indicative of a need to search for other etiologies.

Differential Diagnosis

The presence of any neurologic deficit should alert the physician to consider diagnoses other than idiopathic TGN. Facial pain, accompanied by neurologic deficits, may be caused by a variety of mass lesions, including tumors, infection, aneurysms, other vascular malformations or even multiple sclerosis. A small minority of patients with underlying mass lesions may present without neurologic deficit, complaining only of lancinating, paroxysmal pain episodes inseparable from those of TGN. The differential diagnosis is broad (Box 132-1). The diagnosis is made by careful history and physical examination. Any deviation from the stereotypical presentation outlined earlier or the presence of other accompanying symptoms and findings should prompt an evaluation for other diagnoses.

Diagnostic Approach

Strict attention to the clinical history and physical examination is the key to successful diagnosis of both primary

Figure 132-1 Typical Distribution Patterns of Trigeminal Neuralgia and Relevant Anatomy.

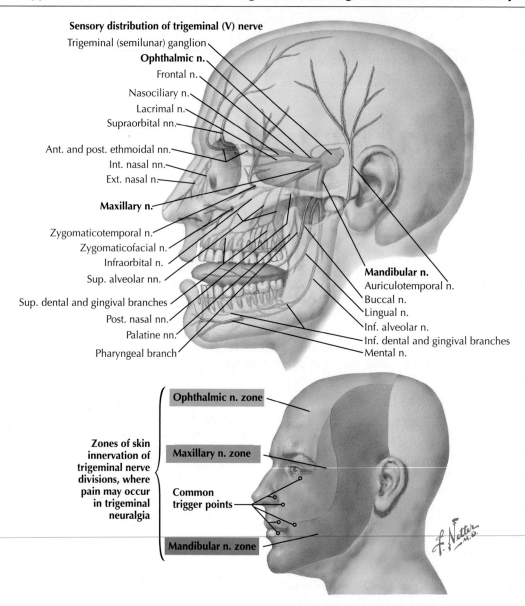

Sensory distribution of trigeminal (V) nerve
Trigeminal (semilunar) ganglion
Ophthalmic n.
Frontal n.
Nasociliary n.
Lacrimal n.
Supraorbital nn.
Ant. and post. ethmoidal nn.
Int. nasal nn.
Ext. nasal n.
Maxillary n.
Zygomaticotemporal n.
Zygomaticofacial n.
Infraorbital n.
Sup. alveolar nn.
Sup. dental and gingival branches
Post. nasal nn.
Palatine nn.
Pharyngeal branch

Mandibular n.
Auriculotemporal n.
Buccal n.
Lingual n.
Inf. alveolar n.
Inf. dental and gingival branches
Mental n.

Ophthalmic n. zone
Maxillary n. zone
Zones of skin innervation of trigeminal nerve divisions, where pain may occur in trigeminal neuralgia
Common trigger points
Mandibular n. zone

and secondary TGN. Specifically, attention to the defining characteristics of the pain is critical. The exact location, the precise quality, the duration and timing, and the triggering and alleviating factors of pain should all be noted. Pain that is atypical for TGN (constant, dull, or throbbing; a pain that awakens the patient from sleep or is in an unusual distribution) should prompt consideration of other etiologies because any of these characteristics make the diagnosis of TGN suspect. Furthermore, any neurologic deficit found on physical examination should point to diagnoses other than that of idiopathic TGN. Finally, most TGN patients respond to carbamazepine at least briefly. Given the broad range of diseases that present similarly to TGN, magnetic resonance imaging (MRI) of the brain should be performed ■ to help eliminate other causes of facial pain. An otherwise negative MRI helps confirm the diagnosis of TGN and may demonstrate vascular compression of the trigeminal nerve. There are no laboratory tests that help make the diagnosis, although such tests can be helpful in narrowing the differential diagnosis as suggested by the history and physical examination.

Management and Therapy

Optimum Treatment

The goal of optimum treatment is to alleviate the patient's pain with a minimum of side effects. Initial treatment is almost always pharmacologic. First-line therapy is carbamazepine, which provides initial relief in more than 80%

Neuralgias
Trigeminal neuralgia
Geniculate neuralgia
Glossopharyngeal neuralgia
Occipital neuralgia
Sphenopalatine neuralgia

Infectious
Herpes zoster

Demyelinating
Multiple sclerosis

Tumor
Intracranial tumors
Cerebellopontine angle masses
Head and neck cancers

Tooth and Jaw
Dental disease
Temporomandibular disease

Eyes, Orbits, and Sinuses
Glaucoma
Iritis
Optic neuritis
Sinusitis

Vascular
Temporal arteritis
Aneurysms
Vascular malformations

Headache syndromes
Cluster headache
Migraines

Psychiatric
Atypical facial pain

of patients. Over time, the effectiveness of carbamazepine declines in many patients, and up to 40% of patients have some type of side effect. Furthermore, carbamazepine is an inducer of hepatic metabolism and can interact with many other pharmacologic agents. The usual initial dose is 200 mg/day and is titrated upward to the usual therapeutic range, 800 to 1200 mg/day. Side effects can include dizziness, sedation, nystagmus, hepatic and bone marrow toxicity, syndrome of inappropriate antidiuretic hormone secretion, congestive heart failure, and rashes. Periodic monitoring of complete blood count, platelet count, and liver function tests is mandatory. Gabapentin is often the second agent added to or substituted for carbamazepine. It should begin at 300 mg, then, on the second day, 300 mg twice a day, followed by 300 mg 3 times a day. The dosage may then be titrated up to 2.4 g/day. Phenytoin is also used, although it has not been demonstrated to be as effective as carbamazepine and should be considered only after other therapies fail. If there is no response to anticonvul-

sants or if breakthrough pain occurs, baclofen may be added or substituted. However, the long-term response rate of baclofen is less than 50%. Dosing should begin at 5 mg 3 times a day, increasing 5 mg per dose every 3 days to a maximum of 80 mg per day. Clonazepam has been shown to be effective but is often too sedating to use in clinical practice.

Surgical Approaches

Failure to respond to medical therapy or the presence of intolerable side effects mandates surgery. Surgical approaches fall into three categories: percutaneous ablative procedures, microvascular decompressive procedures, and stereotactic radiosurgical procedures.

Various ablative procedures have been used for the treatment of TGN. All result in some degree of facial numbness. The most common procedures include percutaneous retrogasserian glycerol injection, percutaneous balloon compression of the trigeminal ganglion, and percutaneous radiofrequency trigeminal rhizotomy (PTR). In each procedure, the foramen ovale is cannulated percutaneously through a needle introduced through the cheek ipsilateral to the patient's symptoms. Patient selection includes those who have failed medical management, are older than 70 years, are in poor health, are willing to tolerate facial numbness, and have symptoms excluding the V1 distribution. Of patients treated by ablation of the trigeminal nerve, 99% experience initial pain relief after one procedure. Forty-six percent of patients experience postoperative facial analgesia, 42% dense hypalgesia, and 17% mild hypalgesia, however. Dysesthesia develops in 36% of patients with postoperative analgesia, in 15% of patients with dense hypalgesia, and in 7% of patients with mild hypalgesia. Pain recurrence occurs in 18% of patients with postoperative analgesia, 21% of patients with dense hypalgesia, and 47% of patients with mild hypalgesia. Mortality is rare.

Microvascular decompression (MVD) of the trigeminal nerve is more invasive than the percutaneous procedures but offers the advantage of preserving facial sensation. This treatment modality should be entertained in younger patients, in patients with symptoms in the V1 distribution, and in patients expressing unwillingness to tolerate facial numbness. Based on several reports, in 75% of cases, the superior cerebellar artery compresses the trigeminal root, whereas a vein accounts for compression in an additional 12% of cases. Immediate pain relief occurs in 82% of patients. Ten years after surgery, 70% continue to have excellent pain relief. The rate of facial numbness is 1% and that of dysesthesia requiring treatment, 0.3%. Major complications in a study involving 1185 subjects included two deaths (0.2%), one brainstem infarction (0.1%), and 16 cases of ipsilateral hearing losses (1%). Factors predictive of long-term operative success include male gender, duration of preoperative symptoms less than 8 years, absence of venous compression, and immediate postoperative relief.

Reported success rates for the treatment of TGN demonstrate that immediate relief of pain for all procedures is excellent, ranging from 91% for glycerol rhizotomy to 98% for MVD and PTR. The recurrence rate is highest for glycerol injection (54%) and lowest for MVD (15%), with PTR having a 20% to 23% recurrence rate. Major dysesthesia occurs in 2% to 10% of PTR procedures, 55% of glycerol injections, and 0.3% of MVD procedures. Perioperative mortality is 0.6% for MVD and close to 0% for percutaneous procedures.

Recently, stereotactic radiosurgery (SRS) has been used in the treatment of TGN. SRS, the least invasive of the surgical approaches, consists of focused-beam radiation therapy. Emerging evidence suggests that this is an effective technique, although recurrence rates are unknown. The most common side effect is facial numbness. Effectiveness is decreased if the patient has undergone previous surgical treatment. The major advantage of SRS is its lack of invasiveness. The major disadvantage of SRS is that, unlike the other surgical treatment options, pain relief is not immediate but may take weeks or months to appear. SRS is therefore not suitable for the patient with severe TGN who is unable to eat, but may be the treatment of choice for patients with less severe disease.

In summary, the diagnosis of TGN should be made based on careful history and physical examination and with the aid of MRI. Pharmacologic therapy should then be initiated, usually with carbamazepine if there is no contraindication. Failure to respond to carbamazepine requires additional therapy with other anticonvulsants or baclofen. When all medical therapies have been exhausted, surgical therapy can be entertained; the choice of surgical therapy depends on the distribution of the pain, patient characteristics, and patient preference.

Avoiding Treatment Errors

Treatment errors fall into two broad categories. The first is related to making the correct diagnosis and initiating treatment. Any instance in which the history and physical findings are not characteristic should trigger a search for other etiologies. Subsequent to that, patients should be followed for improvements and medication tolerance. The second broad category is failure to consider surgical treatment in selected patients. Newer procedures are promising and should be considered in symptomatic patients who have failed all potential medical therapies or who are unable to function because of debilitating symptoms, such as anorexia.

Future Directions

TGN remains a debilitating disease. Medical treatment is currently the clear mainstay of therapy. However, surgical treatment can provide effective results in patients who have failed a reasonable trial of drug therapy. MVD is relatively safe, is well tolerated, provides immediate relief, and may be definitive. Surgical therapy can provide immediate relief of symptoms, and should be considered early, particularly in patients who are unable to function because of severe symptoms such as anorexia. One other avenue of investigation is the efficacy and safety of SRS. Recent data in small studies have shown that repeat SRS is effective but also seem to indicate that some sensory loss is necessary for SRS to be effective. The primary advantage of SRS is that it can be performed noninvasively and apparently repeatedly. Furthermore, debilitated patients unable to tolerate surgical procedures may remain good candidates for radiosurgery.

Additional Resources

UpToDate Website: Trigeminal Neuralgia. Available at: http://www.uptodate.com. Accessed October 11, 2006.
This website provides an excellent overview of disease diagnosis and medical treatment.

eMedicine: Trigeminal Neuralgia. Available at: http://www.emedicine.com/EMERG/topic617.htm. Accessed December 8, 2006.
This website provides a very brief overview.

EVIDENCE

1. Dworkin RH, Backonja M, Rowbotham MC, et al: Advances in neuropathic pain: Diagnosis, mechanisms, and treatment recommendations. Arch Neurol 60(11):1520, 2003.
   This article contains recent treatment recommendations for pharmacologic management of TGN.
2. IRSA: Stereotactic radiosurgery for patients with intractable typical trigeminal neuralgia who have failed medical management. In Radiosurgery Practice Guideline Report, No. 1-3. Harrisburg, PA, IRSA, 2003.
   This paper outlines an algorithm for treatment and patient selection for radiosurgical treatment of TGN.
3. Lopez BC, Hamlyn PJ, Zakrzewska JM: Systematic review of ablative neurosurgical techniques for the treatment of trigeminal neuralgia. Neurosurgery 54(4):973-983, 2004.
   This review of the literature discusses ablative surgical techniques. These techniques are often underutilized and are deemed appropriate in debilitated patients and those desiring to avoid an open procedure.
4. Wiffen PJ, McQuay HJ, Moore RA: Carbamazepine for acute and chronic pain. Cochrane Database Syst Rev 3:CD005451, 2005.
   This article reviews carbamazepine and its current usage.

Silva Markovic-Plese ▪ Susan A. Gaylord ▪ J. Douglas Mann

Multiple Sclerosis

Introduction

Multiple sclerosis (MS) is a disease of central nervous system (CNS) white matter that afflicts young adults, with a peak incidence between ages 20 and 30 years. Prevalence of the disease in the United States is close to 300,000. The impact of MS is considerable given the age at onset, lost work and family time, and the overall reduction in quality of life.

The diagnosis of MS is based on a careful history and neurologic examination combined with a diagnostic magnetic resonance imaging (MRI) scan and, in some cases, a confirmatory lumbar puncture (LP). Recent advances in the treatment of MS have come through a better understanding of immune-mediated damage to the nervous system leading to effective immunomodulatory therapies designed to block specific steps in disease development. During the past 10 years, six immunomodulatory therapies have been approved for MS and are now routinely used in most patients with relapsing-remitting (R-R) disease. They effectively decrease new lesion formation, relapse rate, and disability accumulation.

Etiology and Pathogenesis

MS is a chronic inflammatory CNS disease. Most of the studies suggest an autoimmune etiology of the disease that results in perivascular demyelination of CNS white matter through an autoimmune inflammatory process. Mechanisms of remyelination are incompletely effective, accounting for partial recovery and accumulation of deficits with repeated attacks over time. The specific mechanisms responsible for initiation, maintenance, and cessation of attacks are under intensive investigation.

Genetic and environmental factors play a role in the disease development. Although individuals with the major histocompatibility subtypes HLA-DR2, B7, and A3 at greater risk for developing MS, it is likely that many genes are involved in the disease. Genetic factors influencing disease onset are reflected in twin studies, in which the monozygotic concordance rate is 35%. The rate of concordance in dizygotic twins is only 5%. First-degree relatives carry at least a 10% increased risk for the disease compared with an age-matched unrelated population.

Older epidemiologic studies reported that risk for developing MS is based in part on geographic location during the first 15 years of life. The condition is progressively more common with distance from the equator in both hemispheres. Those of northern European ancestry are at relatively high risk, whereas African Americans exhibit half the risk of whites. Asians and Hispanics in the United States carry a low overall risk. Whether the geographic risk of developing MS is more related to environment or genetics remains unknown.

Although seasonal variations in disease activity have been reported, the pace of the illness is largely independent of environmental factors. Physical trauma, emotional stress, and upper respiratory infections have been implicated and may precipitate attacks. Elevated body temperature temporarily brings out latent and reversible neurologic deficits secondary to impaired neural transmission through partially demyelinated axons.

Clinical Presentation

Typically, multiple attacks occur over a period of years, involving multiple areas of CNS white matter in a process of plaque formation (Fig. 133-1). Several patterns of attack are encountered. R-R MS occurs in about 85% of cases, is more common in younger females, and often starts with prominent sensory-visual symptoms (Fig. 133-2). The average attack frequency is less than one per year in that group. R-R MS is not only the most prevalent subtype of MS. It is also the only subtype of MS that responds

Figure 133-1 Multiple Sclerosis: Central Nervous System Plaques.

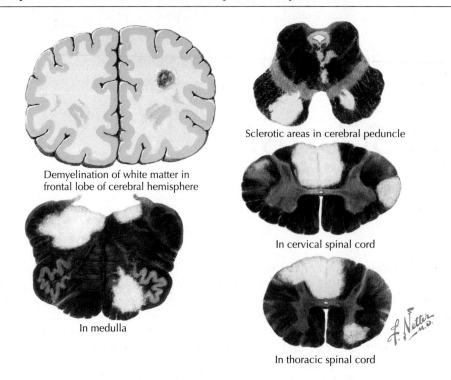

Demyelination of white matter in frontal lobe of cerebral hemisphere

In medulla

Sclerotic areas in cerebral peduncle

In cervical spinal cord

In thoracic spinal cord

favorably to the immunomodulatory therapies. Chronic progressive MS without remitting features is seen in up to 10% of patients, typically later in onset and more frequently in males. A progressive component of the illness develops in half of those with R-R MS after 10 years, termed *secondary progressive MS*. A fulminant course without remission is encountered rarely. Cases of single attacks without further progression have been reported. Patients with clinically isolated syndrome, or first clinical attack suggestive of MS, who have, in addition, an MRI scan consistent with MS, have an 80% risk for developing clinically definite MS within 2 years. Recently, efforts have focused on starting immunomodulatory therapy as early as possible to reduce long-term disability. This approach requires early diagnosis of the disease, and this has been possible with advances in MRI.

Symptoms in the R-R form develop over hours to days and are followed by variable recovery over days to weeks. Sensory symptoms, muscle weakness, monocular blindness, double vision, vertigo (see Fig. 133-2), incoordination, and bladder dysfunction are among the most common presentations of MS. Multiple symptoms, reflecting involvement of multiple areas of white matter, can appear during a single attack. First attacks, especially if not associated with visual or motor deficits, tend to be unnoticed except in retrospect, being attributed to viral causes, stress, or minor trauma. Some patients will experience recurrent episodes involving the same brain region. Diffuse symptoms, including fatigue, cognitive deficits, diffuse pain, and depression, usually follow the initial attacks. The timing

of attacks and degree of recovery are highly variable and are best predicted by the clinical course during the first 2 years, by the accumulation of lesions noted on MRI and by the presence of contrast-enhancing lesions on MRI, suggestive of acute inflammatory changes.

Pain at presentation is uncommon, although two thirds of patients with MS will have significant pain at some time during their illness. Pain syndromes include central neuropathic pain with burning dysesthesias and radicular pain similar to trigeminal neuralgia. Lhermitte's sign is a painful shock-like sensation, usually experienced in the neck, upper back, or limbs, occurring spontaneously or with neck movement. Spasticity can lead to painful muscle contractions. Autonomic nervous system impairment can lead to painful distention of the bladder. Headache is more common (27%) in individuals with MS than in an age-matched population (12%). Optic neuritis can be painful before and during the episode. There is an increase in seizures in individuals with MS—with a frequency twice that of a matched population—but overall seizures are uncommon. Constipation and bladder dysfunction often require careful management. Emotional lability and cognitive deficits are associated with accelerated cortical atrophy noted in some patients with MS.

Prognosis

The average duration of R-R MS is 5 to 10 years from diagnosis. Limited resolution in the wake of repeated exacerbations leads to the accumulation of disability that char-

Figure 133-2 Multiple Sclerosis.

Ocular manifestations of multiple sclerosis

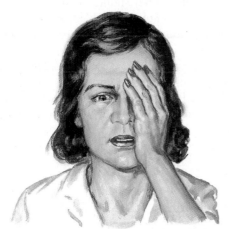

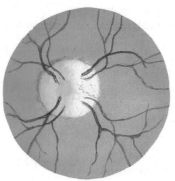

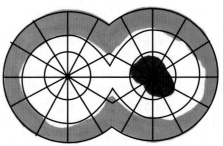

Sudden unilateral blindness, self-limited (usually 2 to 3 weeks). Patient covering one eye, suddenly realizes other eye is partially or totally blind.

Temporal pallor in optic disc, caused by delayed recovery of temporal side of optic (II) nerve

Visual fields reveal central scotoma due to acute retrobulbar neuritis

Internuclear ophthalmoplegia

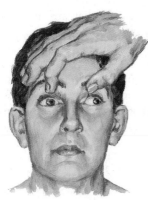

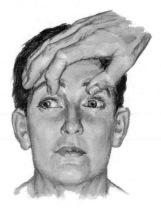

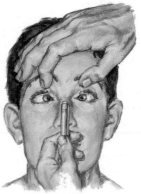

Eyes turned to left, right eye lags

Eyes turned to right, left eye lags (to lesser degree)

Convergence unimpaired

acterizes the secondary progressive phase. Overall life expectancy is reduced only by 5 to 7 years. Death from complications of MS is more common in males with progressive forms of the illness. Pneumonia and loss of respiratory drive are associated causes in those patients. Depression is common. The suicide rate is increased sevenfold, especially when the diagnosis is first established, and later when there is advanced disability.

MS is benign 40% of the time, with few limiting deficits after 15 years. Favorable prognostic factors include younger age at onset, dominance of sensory and visual symptoms, female gender, an R-R pattern of attacks, and sparing of spine and bladder. Poor prognosis is associated with age at onset older than 35 years, early motor impairment, male gender, a chronic progressive pattern, and cerebellar and spinal involvement.

MRI is the best predictor of risk for clinical exacerbations in the ensuing 6 to 12 months. It reveals disease about 10 times more often than the clinical exam. Predictors of clinical flares include significant accumulation of visualized lesions over time and the presence of gadolinium-enhancing lesions on MRI.

Differential Diagnosis

Recurrent exacerbations of CNS vasculitis can mimic MS. Atypical features for MS, such as psychosis, seizures, and gray matter lesions on MRI, assist in making the correct diagnosis. CNS systemic lupus erythematosus (SLE) is characterized by disseminated lesions in subcortical perivascular areas. However, SLE with CNS involvement generally does not have a relapsing-remitting clinical course, and there is often an elevated serum antinuclear antibody titer along with evidence of systemic involvement not seen in MS. Behçet's disease and Sjögren's syndrome can manifest as multifocal CNS disease. Behçet's disease is suspected when there are multiple cranial nerve deficits in combination with oral or genital ulcers, uveitis, and meningoencephalitis. A diagnosis of Sjögren's syndrome can be made with a lip or parotid gland biopsy. Vitamin B_{12} deficiency can present with progressive spinal cord symptoms that correlate with white matter lesions in the posterior columns seen with MRI. Adrenoleukodystrophy and tropical spastic paraparesis can also resemble MS, but these entities are rare. Vascular disease with multiple transient ischemic attacks or infarctions generally occurs in an older population, or in those with significant risk factors for vascular disease, and is not often mistaken for MS. Sarcoid, lues, and tumors must also be considered in the differential diagnosis. They can be distinguished by a combination of MRI and cerebrospinal fluid (CSF) studies when suspected. The diagnosis of MS can be quite difficult in the case of a first attack that has atypical features.

Diagnostic Approach

The diagnosis of MS rests on a history of multiple episodes of CNS dysfunction, occurring over a period of months to years with variable recovery, combined with a neurologic examination revealing abnormal signs referable to multiple CNS locations. MRI is invariably used to confirm diagnosis of MS and demonstrates multiple disseminated hyperintense T2 and fluid-attenuated inversion recovery (FLAIR) intensity changes in periventricular distributions. Lesions are typically larger than 0.5 cm, round or oval in shape, and oriented perpendicularly to the corpus callosum and lateral ventricles. LP and evoked potential studies are useful in confirming the clinical impression and ruling out other conditions (Figs. 133-3 and 133-4).

Definitive MS is characterized by the history of two distinct attacks with two or more lesions confirmed by clinical examination or supportive laboratory studies. MRI of brain and spinal cord, with and without gadolinium, is used to define active lesions (contrast positive) and to assess total lesion load visualized on T2-weighted and FLAIR MRI images. An absence of MRI-visualized lesions is incompatible with diagnosis of MS. The CSF is usually positive for oligoclonal bands or elevated immunoglobulin G/albumin CSF/serum ratios in 95% of confirmed cases when the disease has been present for more than 1 year. The CSF may be normal with the first attack, and repeated LPs may be needed to identify the presence of antibodies synthesized within the CNS (see Fig. 133-3).

Evoked potential electroencephalograms are useful in uncovering clinically silent white matter lesions that may confirm the diagnosis by establishing multiple sites of CNS involvement (see Figs. 133-3 and 133-4).

Management and Therapy

It is helpful for patients to know the variable and progressive nature of the disease. They should be informed about the high degree of variability of attack and recovery patterns in MS that make outcome predictions regarding disability for a given individual very difficult.

Immunomodulatory therapy is recommended for all patients with a clinically isolated syndrome suggestive of MS and for definitive R-R MS. Although immunomodulatory agents have not been shown to have efficacy in primary and secondary progressive MS, many symptomatic therapies that contribute to improved quality of life can be offered.

Optimum Treatment

Optimum treatment includes involvement of caregivers familiar with the all the different manifestations of the disease, the primary medications for acute exacerbations as well as those that directly influence the long term prognosis, dietary and stress management recommendations, and the various treatment strategies for the many symptoms that can develop. There are many choices in therapy (see later), and those therapies that are most highly recommended are listed first.

Acute Exacerbations

High-dose, pulsed corticosteroids have immediate antiinflammatory effects and can significantly shorten clinical attacks. Side effects of short-term intravenous steroids are limited. Chronic oral steroids have no beneficial effects on the long-term progression of the disease and must be avoided.

Optimum therapy for acute attacks is methylprednisolone, given daily, 1 g intravenously for 5 consecutive days. Steroids are most effective if administered within 2 weeks of the onset of new symptoms. Although positive effects of steroids may be immediate, in some individuals the beneficial responses are delayed by a month or more.

Long-Term Therapy

Several medications have been shown to have efficacy in suppression of disease activity over years. The choice of agent is often determined by the fewest side effects and the preference of the patient in terms of route and time of administration.

Interferon (IFN)-β1a and IFN-β1b reduce the number of attacks in R-R forms of MS by an average of 35%. They also reduce the number of MRI-documented new lesions by up to 85%. The mechanism of action of interferons is complex. In MS, IFN-β1a and 1b likely inhibit inflammatory cell activity and T-cell migration across the blood-brain barrier. Dosing is either by weekly intramuscular injection (IFN-β1a) or every-other-day subcutaneous injection (IFN-β1a and 1b). Side effects include flu-like

Figure 133-3 Multiple Sclerosis: Diagnostic Tests I.

Somatosensory evoked response (SER)

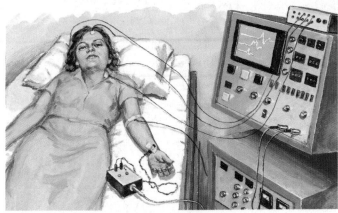

Patient with stimulating electrode over median nerve at wrist; ground at cubital fossa. Responses recorded from electrodes placed at (1) Erb's point for supraclavicular brachial plexus, (2) spinous process of C2 and C7 for cervical spinal cord and cervicomedullary junction, and (3) contralateral side of head for cortical response

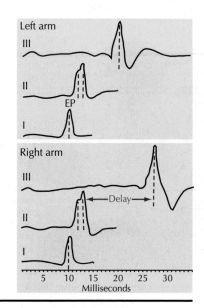

Cerebrospinal fluid electrophoresis

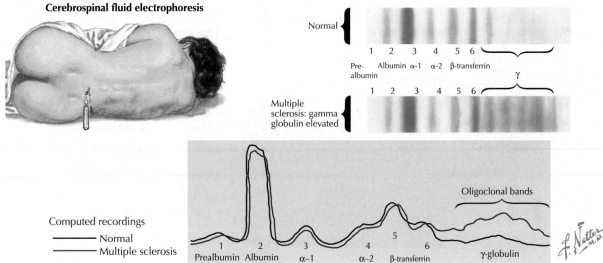

Computed recordings
— Normal
— Multiple sclerosis

symptoms, headache, injection-site reactions, and possibly worsening of depression. Neutralizing antibodies occur in 5% to 45% of patients and are associated with reduction in treatment efficacy. Liver enzyme abnormalities and blood count changes occur in 5% to 20% of treated patients and require close follow-up for the duration of therapy.

Glatiramer acetate (copolymer 1, COP-1) is a mixture of four amino acids that are over-represented in the immunodominant epitope of the presumed autoantigen, myelin basic protein. It has been proposed that glatiramer acetate induces tolerance against myelin antigens that trigger autoimmune responses. Given daily by subcutaneous injection, it reduces exacerbations by one third in R-R MS. It is well tolerated with minimal side effects.

Mitoxantrone (Novantrone) is an immunosuppressive agent approved for patients with aggressive MS with

clinical disease progression despite the first-line therapy with IFN or glatiramer acetate. Intravenous infusions are administered every 3 months. Mitoxantrone is cardiotoxic and requires monitoring of cardiac ejection fraction. It also induces neutropenia with increased risk for infection. Patients receiving mitoxantrone need to be carefully monitored and also treated before each treatment with antiemetic medications.

Natalizumab (Tysabri) is a recently approved immunomodulatory therapy. It is a humanized monoclonal antibody against adhesion molecules expressed on activated mononuclear cells. Natalizumab blocks the migration of activated mononuclear cells from the peripheral circulation into the CNS. The efficacy of natalizumab is somewhat higher than IFN treatment. However, upon initial approval of the drug, three fatal cases of progressive

Figure 133-4 Multiple Sclerosis: Diagnostic Tests II.

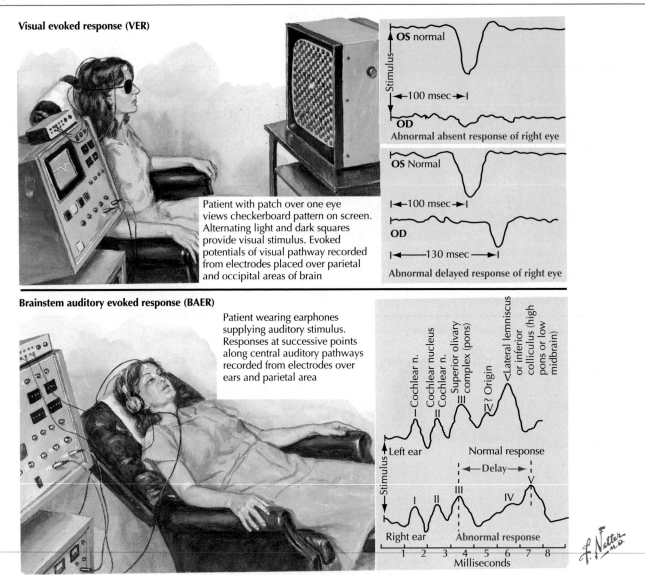

Visual evoked response (VER)

Patient with patch over one eye views checkerboard pattern on screen. Alternating light and dark squares provide visual stimulus. Evoked potentials of visual pathway recorded from electrodes placed over parietal and occipital areas of brain

OS normal

◄—100 msec—►

OD
Abnormal absent response of right eye

OS Normal

◄—100 msec—►

OD

◄—130 msec—►
Abnormal delayed response of right eye

Brainstem auditory evoked response (BAER)

Patient wearing earphones supplying auditory stimulus. Responses at successive points along central auditory pathways recorded from electrodes over ears and parietal area

Cochlear n.
Cochlear nucleus
Cochlear n.
Superior olivary complex (pons)
? Origin
Lateral lemniscus or inferior colliculus (high pons or low midbrain)

Stimulus
Left ear   Normal response
◄—Delay—►

Stimulus
I II III IV V
Right ear   Abnormal response
1 2 3 4 5 6 7 8
Milliseconds

multifocal leukoencephalopathy were associated with its use. Therefore, it is restricted to a subset of patients with very aggressive disease who are willing to accept the risk.

Intravenous immunoglobulin and plasmapheresis are used in patients with neuromyelitis optica, a subset of MS mediated by antibodies.

Azathioprine, methotrexate, cladribine, cyclophosphamide, and cyclosporine have limited benefit in patients with rapidly progressive MS, and these agents are only rarely considered because of the significant side-effect profile that limits their use.

Dietary Therapies

Dietary recommendations currently include the supplemental use of vitamin D and adopting a diet low in saturated fats. Epidemiologic studies suggest that regular intake of vitamin D from supplements, but not from food, may protect against developing MS. Older studies show that lowering saturated fats in the diet can reduce the number of exacerbations.

Additional studies around fats in the diet have yielded mixed results. One randomized, controlled clinical trial that compared supplements of a vegetable oil mixture containing either linoleate or oleate for 2 years found a greater severity of clinical relapses in patients taking oleate than those receiving the linoleate. Another randomized clinical trial compared four groups using lower and higher dosages of linoleic and oleic acid and reported marginally shorter, and less severe, exacerbations in those taking a higher dose of linoleic acid.

Stress Management

Stress management is an important element in successful management of MS. One study showed that MS relapse

James F. Howard, Jr.

Myasthenia Gravis

Introduction

Myasthenia gravis (MG) is the most common primary disorder of neuromuscular transmission. The usual cause is an acquired immunologic abnormality, but some cases result from genetic abnormalities related to proteins, receptors, and hormones critical for normal function of neuromuscular junctions. The estimated incidence of MG is 9 per million per year with a prevalence of 200 per million population; however, MG is probably under-diagnosed. Previous studies showed that women are more often affected than men. The most common age at onset is the second and third decades in women and the seventh and eighth decades in men. With aging of the population, the average age of onset of MG has also increased. Today males are more often affected than females, and the onset of symptoms is usually after age 50 years.

Etiology and Pathogenesis

The normal neuromuscular junction releases acetylcholine (ACh) from the motor nerve terminal in discrete packages (quanta). These ACh quanta diffuse across the synaptic cleft and bind to specific receptors on the folded muscle end-plate membrane. Stimulation of the motor nerve releases many ACh quanta that depolarize the muscle end-plate region and the muscle membrane, causing muscle contraction. In acquired MG, the postsynaptic muscle membrane is distorted and simplified, having lost its normal folded shape. ACh receptor (AChR)-specific antibodies attach to the membrane, and as a result, the concentration of AChRs is reduced on the muscle end-plate membrane. ACh is released normally, but its effect on the postsynaptic membrane is reduced as a result of these abnormalities, lessening the probability that any nerve impulse will cause a muscle action potential.

Thymic abnormalities are associated with MG, but the nature of the association is uncertain. Ten to 15% of patients with MG have a thymic tumor, and 70% have hyperplastic changes (germinal centers) that indicate an active immune response. These hyperplastic changes occur in areas within lymphoid tissue where B cells interact with helper T cells to produce antibodies. Because the thymus is the central organ for immunologic self-tolerance, it is reasonable to suspect that thymic abnormalities cause the breakdown in tolerance that produces an immune-mediated attack on AChR in MG. The thymus contains all the necessary elements for the pathogenesis of MG: myoid cells that express the AChR antigen, antigen-presenting cells, and immunocompetent T cells. Thymus tissue from patients with MG produces AChR antibodies when implanted into immunodeficient mice. It remains to be elucidated whether the role of the thymus in the pathogenesis of MG is primary or secondary.

Most thymic tumors in patients with MG are benign, well differentiated, and encapsulated and can be removed completely at surgery. It is unlikely that thymomas result from chronic thymic hyperactivity because MG can develop years after thymoma removal, and the human leukocyte antigen haplotypes that predominate in patients with thymic hyperplasia are different from those in patients with thymomas. Patients with thymoma usually have more severe disease, higher levels of AChR antibodies, and more severe electromyographic (EMG) abnormalities than patients without thymoma. Almost 20% of patients with MG whose symptoms began between the ages of 30 and 60 years have thymoma; the frequency is much lower when symptom onset is after age 60 years.

Clinical Presentation

Patients with MG complain of specific muscle weakness rather than generalized fatigue. Ocular motor disturbances, ptosis or diplopia, are the initial symptom of MG in two thirds of patients; almost all have both symptoms within

Figure 134-1 Myasthenia Gravis.

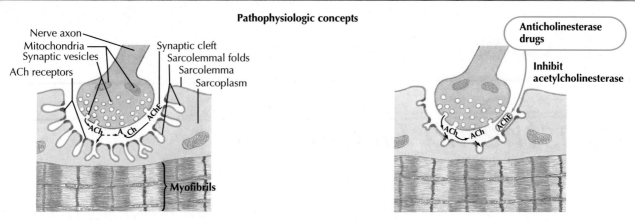

Pathophysiologic concepts

Normal neuromuscular junction: Synaptic vesicles containing acetylcholine (ACh) form in nerve terminal. In response to nerve impulse, vesicles discharge ACh into synaptic cleft. ACh binds to receptor sites on muscle sarcolemma to initiate muscle contraction. Acetylcholinesterase (AChE) hydrolyzes ACh, thus limiting effect and duration of its action

Myasthenia gravis: Marked reduction in number and length of subneural sarcolemmal folds indicates that underlying defect lies in neuromuscular junction. Anticholinesterase drugs increase effectiveness and duration of ACh action by slowing its destruction by AChE

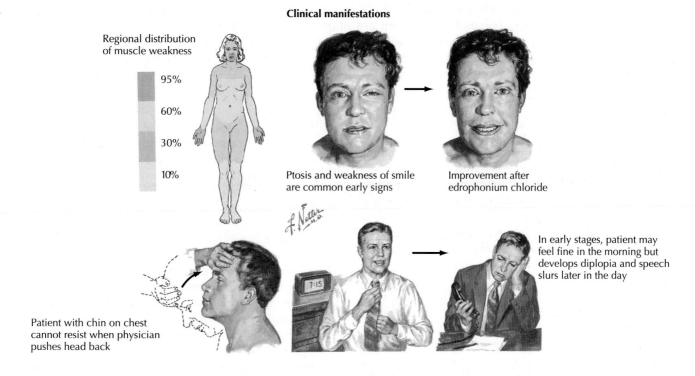

Clinical manifestations

Regional distribution of muscle weakness

95%
60%
30%
10%

Ptosis and weakness of smile are common early signs

Improvement after edrophonium chloride

Patient with chin on chest cannot resist when physician pushes head back

In early stages, patient may feel fine in the morning but develops diplopia and speech slurs later in the day

---

2 years (Fig. 134-1). Oropharyngeal muscle weakness (difficulty chewing, swallowing, or talking) is the initial symptom in one sixth of patients. Limb weakness occurs in only 10%. Initial weakness is rarely limited to single muscle groups such as neck or finger extensors or hip flexors. The severity of weakness fluctuates during the day, usually being least severe in the morning and worse as the day progresses, especially after prolonged use of affected muscles.

The course of disease is variable but usually progressive. Weakness is restricted to the ocular muscles in about 10%

of cases. The rest have progressive weakness during the first 2 years involving oropharyngeal and limb muscles. Maximum weakness occurs during the first year in two thirds of patients. Before corticosteroids were used for treatment, about one third of patients improved spontaneously, one third became worse, and one third died of the disease. Without treatment, spontaneous improvement can occur early in the course of the disease, but typically symptoms fluctuate over a relatively short time and then became progressively severe for several years. Treatment (see later) has improved the course and prognosis of MG.

Myasthenic symptoms are made worse by emotional upset, systemic illness (especially viral respiratory infections), hypothyroidism or hyperthyroidism, pregnancy, the menstrual cycle, drugs affecting neuromuscular transmission, and increases in body temperature.

Differential Diagnosis

The differential diagnosis of muscle weakness is broad; however, in typical cases, the diagnosis is apparent to the clinician. Variable eyelid ptosis and fluctuating ophthalmoparesis are unique to MG. In less typical cases, one must consider diseases of the motor neuron and the muscle membrane (mitochondrial myopathies). Rarely, neurotoxins, central nervous system disorders involving the brainstem, and cavernous sinus thrombosis must be considered. Careful neurologic examination and appropriate diagnostic testing should clarify each diagnosis.

Diagnostic Approach

Weakness caused by abnormal neuromuscular transmission characteristically improves after intravenous administration of edrophonium chloride. Often, it is diagnostic in patients with ptosis or ophthalmoparesis, but it is less useful when other muscles are weak. Some patients, particularly infants and children, who do not respond to intravenous edrophonium chloride, may respond to intramuscular neostigmine because of the longer duration of action. In some patients, a therapeutic trial of daily oral pyridostigmine produces improvement that cannot be appreciated after a single dose of edrophonium chloride or neostigmine.

Serum antibodies that bind human AChR are found in 70% to 90% of patients with acquired generalized myasthenia and 50% to 75% with ocular myasthenia. The serum concentration of these anti-AChR antibodies varies widely among patients with similar degrees of weakness and cannot predict the severity of disease. About 10% of patients, who do not have binding antibodies, have other antibodies that modulate the turnover of AChR in tissue culture. The concentration of anti-AChR antibodies may be low or absent at symptom onset and become elevated later. Anti-AChR antibodies are rarely increased in patients with systemic lupus erythematosus, inflammatory neuropathy, amyotrophic lateral sclerosis, rheumatoid arthritis and taking D-penicillamine, and thymoma without MG, and in normal relatives of patients with MG. False-positive test results are reported when blood is drawn within 48 hours of a surgical procedure using general anesthesia and muscle relaxants. An elevated concentration of AChR-binding antibodies in a patient with compatible clinical features confirms the diagnosis of MG, but normal antibody concentrations do not exclude the diagnosis. Antibodies to muscle-specific receptor tyrosine kinase (MuSK), a surface membrane component essential in the development of the neuromuscular junction, are found in up to 50% of MG patients who are seronegative for AChR antibodies.

The amplitude of the compound muscle action potential elicited by repetitive nerve stimulation (RNS) is normal or only slightly reduced in patients without MG. The amplitude of the fourth or fifth response to a train of low-frequency nerve stimuli falls at least 10% from the initial value in myasthenic patients (Fig. 134-2). This decremental response to RNS is seen more often in proximal muscles, such as the facial muscles, biceps, deltoid, and trapezius, than in hand muscles, and becomes more marked as the disease progresses. A significant decrement to RNS is found in about 60% of patients with MG.

Single-fiber EMG (see Fig. 134-2), the most sensitive clinical test of neuromuscular transmission, shows increased jitter in some muscles in almost all patients with MG. Jitter is greatest in weak muscles but may be abnormal even in muscles with normal strength. In mild or purely ocular muscle weakness, increased jitter may be in facial muscles only. Increased jitter is a nonspecific sign of abnormal neuromuscular transmission and is seen in other motor unit diseases. Normal jitter in a weak muscle excludes abnormal neuromuscular transmission as the cause of weakness.

Management and Therapy

There are numerous treatment options for MG. All recommended regimens are empirical, and there is no consensus opinion among experts on a specific treatment of choice. Treatment decisions should be based on knowledge of the natural history of disease in each patient and the predicted response to a specific form of therapy. Treatment goals must be individualized according to the severity of disease, the patient's age and gender, and the degree of functional impairment. The response to any treatment is difficult to assess because the severity of symptoms fluctuates. Spontaneous improvements, even remissions, occur without specific therapy, especially during the early stages of the disease.

Cholinesterase (ChE) inhibitors retard the enzymatic hydrolysis of ACh at cholinergic synapses so that ACh accumulates at the neuromuscular junction and its effect is prolonged. ChE inhibitors cause considerable improvement in some patients and little to none in others. Strength rarely returns to normal. Pyridostigmine bromide and neostigmine bromide are the most commonly used ChE inhibitors. No fixed dosage schedule suits all patients. The need for ACh inhibitors varies from day to day and during the same day in response to infection, menstruation, emotional stress, and hot weather. Different muscles respond differently; with any dose, certain muscles get stronger, others do not change, and still others become weaker.

Gastrointestinal complaints (queasiness, loose stools, nausea, vomiting, abdominal cramps, and diarrhea) are common. Increased bronchial and oral secretions are a

Figure 134-2 Complementary Exams.

Thymus gland abnormality in myasthenia gravis

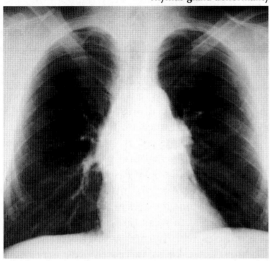

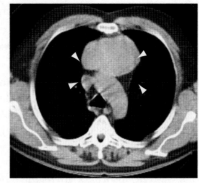

CT scan clearly demonstrates same large tumor anterior to aortic arch *(arrowheads)*

X-ray film shows large mediastinal tumor, which localized to anterior compartment (view not shown)

Repetitive nerve stimulation

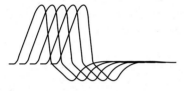

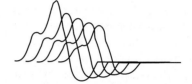

No decremental response is seen to slow rates of stimulation in normal individuals

Decremental responses are seen to slow rates of stimulation in patients with abnormal synaptic transmission

Single fiber electromyography

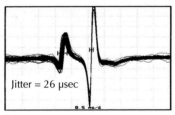

Jitter = 26 μsec

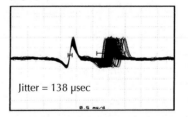

Jitter = 138 μsec

Normal neuromuscular jitter (variation in single action potential intervals) in normal individuals

Increased neuromuscular jitter in patients with abnormal synaptic transmission

serious problem in patients with impaired swallowing or respiratory insufficiency. These adverse effects of ChE inhibitors likely result from ACh accumulation at muscarinic receptors on smooth muscle and autonomic glands and at nicotinic receptors of skeletal muscle. Central nervous system side effects are rarely seen at the ChE inhibitor doses typically used to treat MG. Symptoms of muscarinic overdosage may indicate that nicotinic overdosage (weakness) is also occurring. Excessive nicotinic receptor overdosage results in myasthenic crisis characterized by severe generalized weakness and respiratory failure.

Thymectomy is recommended for most patients with MG. Unfortunately, there are few studies that have directly correlated the severity of weakness before surgery with the timing or degree of improvement after thymectomy. In general, however, the maximal favorable response to thymectomy occurs 2 to 5 years after surgery. However, this time frame is relatively unpredictable, and significant impairment may continue for months or years after surgery. The best responses to thymectomy are in young people early in the course of their disease, but improvement can occur even after 30 years (or more) of symptoms. Patients with disease onset after the age of 60 rarely show substantial improvement from thymectomy. Patients with thymomas do not respond as well to thymectomy as do patients without thymoma.

Marked improvement or complete relief of symptoms occurs in more than 75% of patients treated with prednisone, and even the remaining 25% of treated individuals

experience some improvement. Much of the improvement in symptoms occurs in the first 6 to 8 weeks, but strength may increase to total remission in the months that follow. The best responses occur in patients with recent onset of symptoms, but patients with chronic disease may also respond. The severity of disease does not predict the ultimate improvement. Patients with thymoma have an excellent response to prednisone before or after removal of the tumor. The most predictable response to prednisone occurs when treatment begins with a daily dose of 1.5 to 2 mg/kg/day. About one third of patients become weaker temporarily after starting prednisone, usually within the first 7 to 10 days, and lasting for up to 6 days. Treatment can be started at low dose to minimize exacerbations; the dose is then slowly increased until improvement occurs. Exacerbations may also occur with this approach, and the response is less predictable. The major disadvantages of chronic corticosteroids are their side effects.

Several other immunosuppressive medications are used in treatment of MG. Mycophenolate mofetil and azathioprine reverse symptoms in most patients. The effect is delayed by 4 to 8 months with azathioprine. Once improvement begins, it is maintained for as long as the drug is given, but symptoms recur 2 to 3 months after the drug is discontinued or the dose is reduced below therapeutic levels. Patients who do not respond favorably to corticosteroids may respond to other immunosuppressive drugs, and the reverse is also true. Some patients respond better to combination treatment with corticosteroids and another immunosuppressive drug than to either alone. Because the response to azathioprine is delayed, both drugs may be started simultaneously with the intent of rapidly tapering prednisone when azathioprine becomes effective. About one third of patients have mild dose-dependent side effects that may require dose reductions but do not require stopping treatment.

Cyclosporine inhibits predominantly T-lymphocyte-dependent immune responses and is sometimes beneficial in treating MG. Most patients improve 1 to 2 months after starting cyclosporine, and improvement is maintained as long as therapeutic doses are given. Maximum improvement is typically achieved 6 months or longer after starting treatment. After achieving the maximal response, the dose should be gradually reduced to a minimum dose that maintains improvement. Renal toxicity and hypertension are the most concerning adverse reactions. Many drugs interfere with cyclosporine metabolism and should be avoided or used with caution.

Cyclophosphamide can also be used intravenously and orally for the treatment of MG. More than half of patients become asymptomatic after 1 year. Side effects are common. Life-threatening infections are an important risk in immunosuppressed patients and patients with invasive thymoma. The long-term risk for malignancy is not established.

Therapeutic apheresis (plasma exchange) is used as a short-term intervention for patients with sudden worsening of myasthenic symptoms for any reason, to rapidly improve strength before surgery, and as a chronic intermittent treatment for patients who are refractory to all other treatments. The need for plasma exchange and its frequency of use is determined by the clinical response. Almost all patients with acquired MG improve temporarily following plasma exchange. Maximum improvement may be reached as early as after the first exchange or as late as after 14 exchanges. Improvement lasts for weeks or months, and then the effect is lost unless the exchange is followed by thymectomy or immunosuppressive therapy. Most patients who respond to the first plasma exchange will respond again to subsequent courses. Repeated exchanges do not have a cumulative benefit.

Favorable response to high-dose (2 g/kg infused over 2 to 5 days) infusions of intravenous immunoglobulin (IVIG) has been reported. Improvement occurs in 50% to 100% of patients, usually within 1 week, and clinical improvement often lasts for several weeks or months. The common adverse effects of IVIG are related to the rate of infusion. The precise mechanism of action is not known but most likely involves a nonspecific down-regulation of antibody production.

Avoiding Treatment Errors

Treatment errors can be avoided when the treating clinician has a thorough understanding of the predicted course of disease in each patient, the predicted response to a specific treatment, and the potential side effects of treatment decisions. Treatment goals must be individualized according to the severity of disease, the patient's age and gender, and the degree of functional impairment. Successful treatment of MG requires close medical supervision and long-term follow-up. Return of weakness after a period of improvement should be considered a herald of further progression that requires reassessment of current treatment and evaluation for underlying systemic disease or thymoma.

Future Directions

The future of MG treatment lies in the elucidation of the molecular immunology of the anti-AChR response with the goal of developing a rational treatment for the illness that will cure the abnormality in the immune system that results in the AChR immune response. To this end, six broad categories of theoretical treatment strategies need to be explored: first, treatments that target the antigen-specific B cells; second, treatments that target the antigen specific CD4+ T cells; third, treatments that interfere with co-stimulatory response for antigen presentation; fourth, treatments aimed at inducing tolerance or anergy of the CD4+ T cell to the autoantigen or the CD4+ epitopes;

fifth, treatments designed to stimulate those immunologic circuits that activate CD8+ cells specific for the activation antigens expressed by CD4+ cells; and sixth, treatments that intervene with cytokine function and discourage auto-immune-mediated inflammatory responses.

Additional Resources

Conti-Fine BM, Protti MO, Bellone M, Howard JF: Myasthenia Gravis: The Immunology of an Autoimmune Disease. Austin, TX, RG Landes, 1997.

This comprehensive reference provides a thorough understanding of current knowledge on the immunologic mechanisms of myasthenia gravis. This monograph serves as a source reference for additional readings on the topic.

Howard JF: Structure and function of the neuromuscular junction. In Stalberg E (ed): Clinical Neurophysiology of Disorders of Muscle and Neuromuscular Junction, Including Fatigue. St. Louis, Elsevier, 2003, pp 27–46.

This article provides an overview of the anatomy and physiology of the neuromuscular junction and will complement readings on the clinical aspects of myasthenia gravis.

Howard JF Jr: Adverse drug effects on neuromuscular transmission. Semin Neurol 10:89–102, 1990.

This article provides a comprehensive review of the adverse effects of pharmaceuticals on neuromuscular transmission and disorders of the neuromuscular junction. Many drugs have the potential to acutely and severely worsen the strength of myasthenic patients, and in some instances this may be life threatening. The reader is also referred to http://www.myasthenia.org/docs/MGFA_MedicationsandMG.pdf.

Howard JF Jr, Sanders DB, Massey JM: The electrodiagnosis of myasthenia gravis and the Lambert-Eaton myasthenic syndrome. Neurol Clin 12(2):305–330, 1994.

In this comprehensive review of the tools available for the diagnosis of disorders of neuromuscular transmission, attention is focused on the electrodiagnostic principles, methodology, anticipated findings, and pitfalls.

Sanders DB, Howard JF Jr: Disorders of neuromuscular transmission. In Bradley WG, Daroff RB, Fenichel GM, Jankovic J (eds): Neurology in Clinical Practice: Principles of Diagnosis and Management, 4th ed. Boston, Butterworth-Heinemann, 2004, pp 2441–2461.

This is the most current review of the clinical features of myasthenia gravis, its pathophysiology, diagnosis, and treatment, based on the 30 years of experience with nearly 2600 patients.

Vincent A: Immunology of disorders of neuromuscular transmission. Acta Neurol Scand Suppl 183:1–7, 2006.

This is a recent review of the immunology of disorders of synaptic transmission by one of the leading experts in the field.

EVIDENCE

1. Benatar M, Kaminski H: Medical and surgical treatment for ocular myasthenia. Cochrane Database of Systematic Reviews 2006, Issue 2. Art. No.: CD005081. DOI: 10.1002/14651858.CD005081. pub2.

   This is a comprehensive review of evidence-based literature regarding the treatment of ocular myasthenia gravis.

2. Gajdos P, Chevret S, Toyka K: Plasma exchange for myasthenia gravis. Cochrane Database of Systematic Reviews 2002, Issue 4. Art. No.: CD002275. DOI: 10.1002/14651858.CD002275.

   This is a comprehensive review of evidence-based literature regarding the use of plasma exchange in the treatment of myasthenia gravis.

3. Gajdos P, Chevret S, Toyka K: Intravenous immunoglobulin for myasthenia gravis. Cochrane Database of Systematic Reviews 2006, Issue 2. Art. No.: CD002277. DOI: 10.1002/14651858. CD002277.pub2.

   This is a comprehensive review of evidence-based literature regarding the use of intravenous human immunoglobulin in the treatment of myasthenia gravis.

4. Hart I, Sathasivam S, Sharshar T: Immunosuppressive agents for myasthenia gravis. (Protocol) Cochrane Database of Systematic Reviews 2005, Issue 2. Art. No.: CD005224. DOI: 10.1002/14651858.CD005224.

   This is a comprehensive review of evidence-based literature regarding the use of immunomodulatory agents in the treatment of myasthenia gravis.

5. Schneider-Gold C, Gajdos P, Toyka KV, Hohlfeld RR: Corticosteroids for myasthenia gravis. Cochrane Database of Systematic Reviews 2005, Issue 2. Art. No.: CD002828. DOI: 10.1002/14651858.CD002828.pub2.

   This is a comprehensive review of evidence-based literature regarding the use of corticosteroids in the treatment of myasthenia gravis.

6. Zinman L, Ng E, Beil V: IV immunoglobulin in patients with myasthenia gravis: a randomized controlled trial. Neurology 13;68(11):837–841, Mar 2007.

   A randomized controlled trial evaluating the effectiveness of IV immunoglobulin in patients with MG.

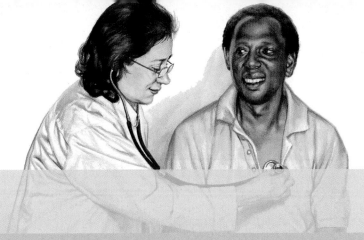

Disorders of the Kidney and Urinary Tract

Philip J. Klemmer ▪ William D. Mattern

135

Urinary Tract Infection

Introduction

Urinary tract infection (UTI) is a broad term describing microbial colonization of the urine and infection of any of the components of the urinary tract, including the urethra, bladder, ureters, renal pelvis, and kidneys. UTI is among the most common reasons for office visits in general medical practice; it is also among the most common predisposing causes of bacteremia and sepsis in hospitalized patients. UTI is divided into four categories: asymptomatic bacteriuria (AB), uncomplicated UTI, complicated UTI, and acute pyelonephritis. Uncomplicated UTIs are those that occur in otherwise healthy adult women who are not pregnant and who do not have underlying abnormalities of the urinary tract. Complicated infections are all others.

Etiology, Pathogenesis, Clinical Presentation, Differential Diagnosis, and Diagnostic Approach

Asymptomatic Bacteriuria

In adult, nonpregnant, healthy women of childbearing age, the prevalence of AB is about 6%, using a urine culture cutoff of more than 10^5 colony forming units/mL. The most common infecting organism is *Escherichia coli*. Epidemiologic studies have shown that AB may resolve spontaneously, but it is sometimes associated with an increased incidence of symptomatic UTI with the onset of sexual activity. Treatment is not indicated unless there is a history of recurrent UTI.

Screening and treatment for AB are an essential part of prenatal care because, untreated, it is associated with a 40% risk for UTI and a 20% to 60% risk for acute pyelonephritis in late pregnancy. AB is also associated with prematurity and low birth weight.

In diabetic women, the incidence of AB may be as high as 18%. Treatment is still not generally recommended because recurrence is extremely high, and no long-term benefit can be documented. Treatment is also not recommended in elderly people who live independently because no adverse effects have been documented. In those with long-term indwelling catheters who are colonized, treatment tends to select out resistant strains and will not eradicate bacteriuria while the catheter remains in place.

Uncomplicated Urinary Tract Infection

Acute cystitis is extremely common. About one half of adult women report having had at least one UTI. Young, sexually active women have about 0.5 episodes per person year. *E. coli* is responsible for infection in about 80% of episodes in healthy adult women, whereas *Staphylococcus saprophyticus* accounts for most of the rest. Cystitis develops when fecal flora from the rectum colonize the vaginal introitus and periurethral zone, colonize the urethra, ascend into and invade the bladder mucosa, proliferate in the urine, and incite an inflammatory response (Fig. 135-1). The shorter urethra in women may help explain why women are more susceptible than men, but not why some women are more susceptible than others. Studies have indicated that uropathogens, such as *E. coli*, have special characteristics that facilitate this process of colonization and invasion, whereas other studies indicate that host factors also play a role. Of particular interest are the studies examining the role of behavioral or mechanical factors. In women otherwise predisposed to UTI, the frequency of sexual intercourse and the use of spermicide-containing contraceptives, particularly the diaphragm-spermicide combination, are clearly associated, as is a history of UTI. Perineal hygiene and the direction of wiping have not been shown to be associated.

The usual symptoms of cystitis are dysuria, along with frequency, urgency, suprapubic discomfort (and tenderness), and hematuria. The diagnosis is made by the history,

Figure 135-1 Factors in Etiology of Cystitis.

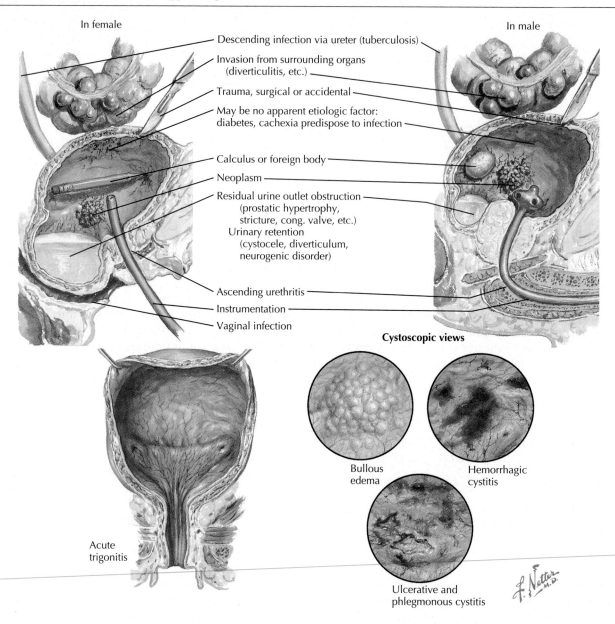

In female

In male

Descending infection via ureter (tuberculosis)

Invasion from surrounding organs (diverticulitis, etc.)

Trauma, surgical or accidental

May be no apparent etiologic factor: diabetes, cachexia predispose to infection

Calculus or foreign body

Neoplasm

Residual urine outlet obstruction (prostatic hypertrophy, stricture, cong. valve, etc.)
Urinary retention (cystocele, diverticulum, neurogenic disorder)

Ascending urethritis

Instrumentation

Vaginal infection

Cystoscopic views

Bullous edema

Hemorrhagic cystitis

Acute trigonitis

Ulcerative and phlegmonous cystitis

physical examination (temperature, abdominal exam, and evaluation for costovertebral angle tenderness), and examination of the urine. Although the gold standard for pyuria is the finding of 10 to 20 leukocytes/mm³ in an unspun, midstream urine using a counting chamber, examination of the urine sediment for white blood cells and bacteria is more routinely done. In practice, urine dipsticks that detect leukocyte esterase, indicating significant pyuria, provide a reliable method for excluding and a rapid method for confirming the likelihood of infection. Dipsticks also allow testing for nitrite, which, when positive, indicates the presence of Enterobacteriaceae, which convert nitrate to nitrite. Urine cultures are not routinely done with uncomplicated UTI, unless it fails to resolve with treatment,

relapses quickly after treatment, or frequently recurs. Imaging studies of the urinary tract are also unnecessary.

Patients presenting with dysuria as their predominant symptom have the broadest differential diagnosis. Hematuria makes cystitis more likely. Urethritis due to *Neisseria gonorrhea* or *Chlamydia trachomatis* is suggested by a history of sexually transmitted disease (STD), a new partner or one with urethral symptoms, a more gradual or uneven onset of symptoms, and the presence of pyuria with negative urine culture results. Pelvic examination is indicated to look for discharge from the urethral or cervical os. Although Gram stain and culture of discharge are still valuable in the diagnosis of gonococcal infection, DNA amplification tests on urine have emerged as highly sensitive and specific for detection of both *Chlamydia* and *N. gonorrhea*. In patients with dysuria, particularly when it is perceived as an external burning and is accompanied by symptoms of vaginitis (vaginal discharge or odor, pruritus, and dyspareunia), infection with *Candida albicans*, *Trichomonas vaginalis*, and *Gardnerella vaginalis*, especially in young, sexually active women, is more likely. Patients with vaginitis usually have a negative urine culture, and pyuria is less common. Pelvic examination to detect and characterize the vaginal discharge is indicated, as well as microscopic examination of the discharge to distinguish among the three common infecting organisms and to guide treatment.

Recurrent Urinary Tract Infection

Most recurrent UTIs in otherwise healthy women represent reinfection, not relapse or recurrence with the same strain. The epidemiology, organisms, clinical presentation, and treatment regimens are the same as those for initial episodes. Most recurrences occur within 3 months, and single recurrences are quite common. In those predisposed, the frequency of sexual intercourse and the use of the diaphragm-spermicide combination are strongly associated, as is recent antibiotic use and a history of UTI.

Complicated Urinary Tract Infection

Complicated UTIs are those that occur during pregnancy, in the presence of structural or functional abnormalities of the urinary tract (obstruction, stones, or indwelling urinary catheters), in patients with underlying diseases such as diabetes who are immunosuppressed, in institutionalized elderly patients, in men, and in children (see Fig. 135-1).

In pregnancy, the focus is on detecting asymptomatic bacteriuria by urine culture and preventing the significant morbidity of UTI and acute pyelonephritis later in pregnancy. The same uropathogens are involved as in uncomplicated UTI. Predisposing factors include dilation of the ureters and forward displacement of the bladder as the uterus enlarges, along with incomplete emptying.

In men, UTI may be asymptomatic or present with symptoms of cystitis, prostatitis, epididymitis, or pyelonephritis. Bacteriuria and symptomatic infections are uncommon in males younger than 50 years in the absence of urinary tract instrumentation or prostatitis. Organisms that persist in the prostate gland and intermittently colonize the bladder urine usually cause recurrent UTI in younger men. Prostatic infections are difficult to eradicate, especially when prostatic stones are present. In older men, the organisms are those associated with complicated infection, usually in association with obstructive symptoms or the use of indwelling catheters.

Patients with diabetes usually have uncomplicated UTI. However, some diabetic patients, mostly women with a history of recurrent UTI due to multidrug-resistant organisms, have an increased risk for severe acute cystitis and acute pyelonephritis, complicated by papillary necrosis, perinephric abscess, and bacteremia. Predisposing factors in these patients include impaired bladder emptying, impaired leukocyte function, and focal damage to the kidney as a consequence of diabetic microangiopathy.

Patients with spinal cord injuries and demyelinating diseases such as multiple sclerosis suffer high morbidity and mortality because of urosepsis associated with neurogenic bladders. Chronic indwelling catheters should be avoided in these patients in favor of intermittent (4 times/day) in-and-out catheterization.

UTI in the more debilitated elderly patient is usually complicated, often by concomitant disease, by bladder malfunction, incontinence, or indwelling catheters. UTI accounts for more than 50% of episodes of bacteremia in institutionalized elderly patients, often in those with long-term indwelling catheters.

Acute Pyelonephritis

Acute pyelonephritis presents with fever, flank pain, costovertebral angle tenderness, leukocytosis, pyuria with white cell casts in the urine sediment, positive urine culture results, and frequently, bacteremia (Figs. 135-2 and 135-3). The risk factors for pyelonephritis are similar to those for acute and recurrent cystitis, which supports the concept that pyelonephritis is caused by the ascent of organisms from the bladder. Specific variables associated with pyelonephritis include frequency of intercourse, new sexual partners, spermicidal use, diabetes, history of previous UTI, and stress incontinence. With regard to specific sexual practices, anal sex was marginally associated with acute pyelonephritis, but oral sex was not. The most common (85%) organism causing acute pyelonephritis is *E. coli*. Most uncomplicated episodes occur in young women and respond to treatment with no residual damage. In all others, renal and bladder ultrasound studies are standard. These studies are rapid, noninvasive, and less expensive than other radiologic screening procedures, show the extent of renal involvement, eliminate obstruction and stones, and indicate the ability to empty the bladder. The differential diagnosis includes renal or ureteral stones, acute cholecystitis, appendicitis, diverticulitis, tubo-ovarian abscess, and acute pancreatitis (Box 135-1).

Box 135-1 Differential Diagnosis of Acute Pyelonephritis

- Acute appendicitis
- Acute salpingitis
- Nephrolithiasis
- Acute cholecystitis
- Psoas or paravertebral abscess
- Cyst hemorrhage in polycystic kidney disease
- Acute pancreatitis

Figure 135-2 Pyelonephritis.

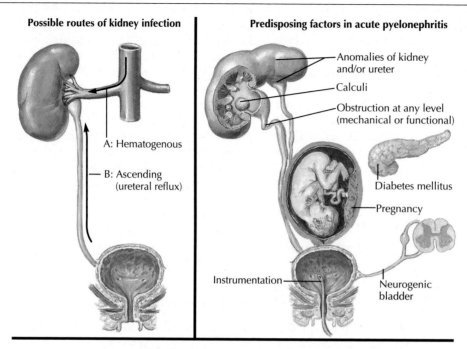

Possible routes of kidney infection

A: Hematogenous

B: Ascending
(ureteral reflux)

Predisposing factors in acute pyelonephritis

Anomalies of kidney and/or ureter

Calculi

Obstruction at any level (mechanical or functional)

Diabetes mellitus

Pregnancy

Instrumentation

Neurogenic bladder

Common clinical and laboratory features of acute pyelonephritis

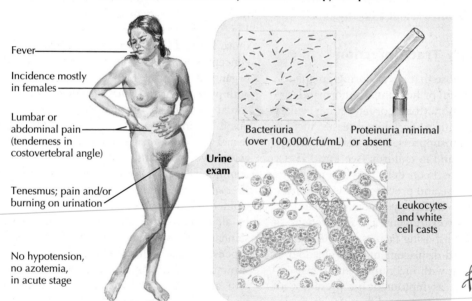

Fever

Incidence mostly in females

Lumbar or abdominal pain (tenderness in costovertebral angle)

Tenesmus; pain and/or burning on urination

No hypotension, no azotemia, in acute stage

Urine exam

Bacteriuria (over 100,000/cfu/mL)

Proteinuria minimal or absent

Leukocytes and white cell casts

Management and Therapy

Optimum Treatment

Uncomplicated Urinary Tract Infection

For cystitis, 3-day, short course antibiotic regimens for uncomplicated UTI using trimethoprim-sulfamethoxazole, trimethoprim, or the fluoroquinolones (ofloxacin, ciprofloxacin, norfloxacin) are more effective than 1-day regimens, and equally as effective as 7-day regimens with lower cost and better compliance. Nitrofurantoin, for 7 days, remains an established alternative. Many do not recommend the fluoroquinolones as initial drugs because of concerns about cost and the emergence of resistance. The increasing resistance of *E. coli* to trimethoprim-sulfamethoxazole needs to be kept in mind. No adverse effects on renal function or long-term morbidity have been documented as a consequence of uncomplicated UTI.

Figure 135-3 Acute Pyelonephritis: Pathology.

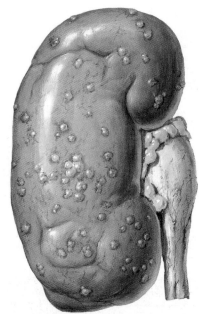

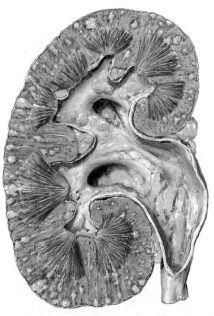

Surface aspect of kidney: Multiple minute abscesses (surface may appear relatively normal in some cases)

Cut section: Radiating yellowish gray streaks in pyramids and abscesses in cortex; moderate hydronephrosis with infection; blunting of calyces (ascending infection)

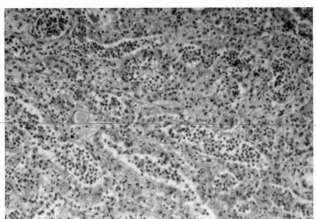

Acute pyelonephritis with exudate chiefly of polymorphonuclear leukocytes in interstitium and collecting tubules

Recurrent Urinary Tract Infection

Highly recurrent infections, more than two within a year, indicate the need to consider preventive and prophylactic measures. Successful approaches, using trimethoprim-sulfamethoxazole, trimethoprim, or the fluoroquinolones (ofloxacin, ciprofloxacin, norfloxacin) have been reported using three regimens: continuous daily treatment for at least 6 months, and sometimes for an additional 2 years in the event of relapse; postcoital single-dose treatment if the episodes are temporally related to intercourse; and intermittent self-treatment at the first onset of symptoms in reliable, highly motivated patients. Decisions on which to use are based on physician and patient preference. Imaging studies are almost always unrevealing, and no long-term adverse consequences have been noted.

Complicated Urinary Tract Infection

The presence of underlying structural abnormalities determines the nature of invading organisms and choice of therapy. Treatment of complicated infections remains difficult; it is more important to relieve obstruction, remove foreign bodies, such as stones and catheters, and restore complete emptying than to eradicate organisms. The usual pathogens include the more resistant strains of *E. coli*, enteric gram-negative organisms, *Pseudomonas*, *Staphylococcus aureus*, enterococci, yeast, and fungi.

Figure 135-4 Algorithm for Treatment of Uncomplicated UTI.

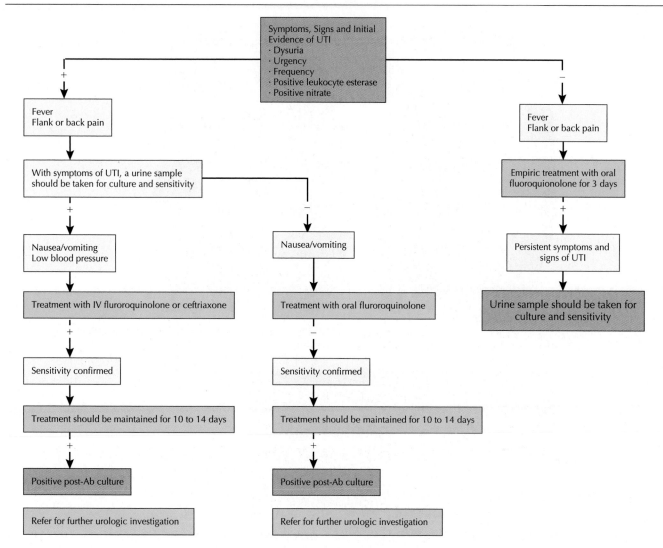

Treatment during pregnancy is complicated by the fact that trimethoprim and the quinolones are not approved for use, and tetracycline is contraindicated because it concentrates in bone and teeth. The β-lactam antibiotics and nitrofurantoin are highly effective. A single course of therapy is not always effective, and follow-up cultures are mandatory, including in the postpartum period when risk remains high. Abdominal and renal ultrasound studies are indicated in those in whom treatment repeatedly fails.

Antibiotic selection in men should be guided by urine culture. Nitrofurantoin and β lactams may not achieve predictable tissue concentrations. The fluoroquinolones provide the best initial coverage and adequate tissue levels. The site of infection, severity of symptoms, and frequency of recurrence determine the duration of therapy. Imaging studies are indicated, except in younger males with uncomplicated presentations.

Diabetes mellitus is an indication for initial therapy with a fluoroquinolone. Subsequent therapy is guided by cultures and imaging studies of the urinary tract and kidneys. Recurrences are difficult to prevent while impaired emptying persists.

In elderly patients who live independently and void normally, UTI is usually uncomplicated and responds to treatment without increased morbidity or mortality. However, it is complicated in the more debilitated elderly patients by septic shock in one third of cases, and the fatality rate in patients with bacteremia approaches 20%. These infections may be resistant to multiple antibiotics and are difficult to treat if the underlying abnormalities are not corrected. Incontinence occurs in 5% to 10% of elderly people living independently and in 50% of those in long-term facilities. It should be managed without a catheter whenever possible, using prompted voiding in the more

responsive or diapers in women and condom catheters in men. The indwelling catheter is an independent risk factor for premature death.

Acute Pyelonephritis

Hospitalization and intravenous drugs (guided by urine culture along with ultrasound studies) are indicated for hypotensive septic patients as well as those with nausea who cannot be treated at home; oral treatment is indicated otherwise. The usual duration of treatment is 10 to 14 days, and the fluoroquinolones are recommended for empiric therapy until cultures are available to guide treatment. If enterococcus is not documented on culture, ceftriaxone (1 g intravenously daily) is an effective and inexpensive agent.

Avoiding Treatment Errors

It is important to differentiate between lower (cystitis) and upper (pyelonephritis) UTI because pyelonephritis frequently requires more aggressive antibiotic therapy. The presence of costovertebral angle tenderness, fever, tachycardia, and hypotension is consistent with a diagnosis of pyelonephritis, which requires treatment with parenteral antibiotics (Fig. 135-4). Failure to recognize and treat urodynamic abnormalities (e.g., neurogenic bladder, vesicoureteral reflux, prostatic obstruction) will frequently result in failure to eradicate UTI on a long-term basis. The removal of infected struvite stones is indicated before antibiotic therapy and is effective in preventing recurrent infection. Finally, in patients with chronic indwelling Foley catheters, long-term suppression therapy is ill advised because it frequently selects out antibiotic-resistant organisms.

Future Directions

The need for a better understanding of the factors that predispose to urethral colonization and bladder infection, particularly in otherwise healthy women, is obvious. There is also a clear need, particularly in institutionalized elderly patients, to develop methods to restore function of the urinary tract that do not predispose to complicated infection. As resistance emerges to today's standard antibiotic regimens, the importance of developing new antibiotics will continue. Lactobacillus probiotics represent a new innovation in the treatment of institutionalized females. These lower the pH of the periurethral area and thereby decrease the risk for colonization by coliforms.

Additional Resources

Graham JC, Galloway A: ACP Best Practice No. 167: The laboratory diagnosis of urinary tract infection. J Clin Pathol 54:911-919, 2001.

This article reviews laboratory and specimen handling procedures that will quickly exclude patients who do not have UTI.

Hooton TM: Recurrent urinary tract infection in women. Int J Antimicrob Agents 17:259-268, 2001.

The author discusses risk factors for recurrent UTI in young women as well as preventive strategies.

Regal RE, Pham CQ, Bostwick TR: Urinary tract infections in extended care facilities: Preventive management strategies. Consult Pharm 21:400-409, 2006.

This paper provides useful information about the approach to management in this special group of patients.

Stamm WE, Hooton TM: Management of urinary tract infections in adults. N Engl J Med 329:1328-1334, 1993.

This article presents a useful general review.

EVIDENCE

1. Ebell MH: Point-of-care guides: Treating women with suspected UTI. Am Fam Physician 73:293-296, 2006.

   Validated clinical decision rules have been combined with patient historical, physical, and laboratory findings to assist in correctly diagnosing UTI.

2. Hooton TM, Stamm WE: Diagnosis and treatment of uncomplicated urinary tract infection. Infect Dis Clin North Am 11:551-581, 1997.

   This is an excellent review of the epidemiology of uncomplicated UTI in young and middle-aged adults.

3. Kunin CM: Urinary Tract Infections: Detection, Prevention, and Management, 5th ed. Baltimore, Lippincott Williams & Wilkins, 1997.

   This text provides a good general review.

4. Saint S, Kaufman SR, Rogers MA, et al: Condom versus indwelling urinary catheters: A randomized trial. J Am Geriatr Soc 54:1055-1061, 2006.

   Condom catheter use was found to be superior to indwelling catheters.

5. Scholes D, Hooton TM, Roberts PL, et al: Risk factors for recurrent urinary tract infection in young women. J Infect Dis 182:1177-1182, 2000.

   The authors review risk factors associated with lower UTI.

6. Scholes D, Hooton TM, Roberts PL, et al: Risk factors associated with acute pyelonephritis in healthy women. Ann Intern Med 142:20-27, 2005.

   Multivariate models of risk factors associated with the development of acute upper UTI are developed in this group of young and middle-aged women.

7. Schooff M, Hill K: Cochrane for physicians: Antibiotics for recurrent urinary tract infections. Am Fam Physician 71:1301-1302, 2005.

   This article presents an evidence-based examination of prevention and treatment of UTI in women.

8. Warren JW, Abrutyn E, Hebel JR, et al: Guidelines for antimicrobial treatment of uncomplicated acute bacterial cystitis and acute pyelonephritis in women. Infectious Diseases Society of America (IDSA). Clin Infect Dis 29:745-758, 1999.

   This article provides useful guidelines for treatment in women with UTI.

Bladder Function Disorders

Introduction

Bladder symptoms are a common presenting complaint in the primary care setting. Many of these symptoms are the result of infectious or inflammatory processes of the lower urinary tract. Others represent abnormalities in bladder storage and emptying. Urinary incontinence is a common and distressing symptom within this group, affecting between 25% and 38% of the female population. Many women do not seek treatment because of embarrassment and lack of knowledge of treatment options.

Adequate bladder storage and emptying depend on the anatomic relationships of the lower genitourinary system and the neurologic control of micturition. These bladder functions are also influenced by other systemic medical conditions and medications.

Etiology and Pathogenesis

Continence requires that the urethral closure pressure exceeds the intravesical pressure (Fig. 136-1). Urethral closure pressure is maintained by smooth and striated muscle, urethral vasculature, and the elasticity of the urethral tissue. It is also influenced by abdominal pressure due to the intra-abdominal location of the proximal urethra. Intravesical pressure increases with increases in intra-abdominal pressure and with detrusor contractions. With normal pelvic anatomy, intra-abdominal pressure is transmitted equally to the bladder and proximal urethra.

Neurologic control of urethral closure depends on stimulation of α receptors within the smooth muscle of the urethral sphincter by the sympathetic nervous system. In addition, the sympathetic system aids in storage of urine by relaxing the detrusor through stimulation of β receptors by norepinephrine. The parasympathetic system aids in voiding by contracting the detrusor muscle through stimulation of receptors by acetylcholine.

Control of micturition depends on a system of complex neurologic loops that interconnect the cerebral cortex, brainstem, sacral micturition center, detrusor muscle, and urethral sphincter. The integrity of these loops is necessary for proper storage and emptying of the bladder. Consequently, varied neurologic disorders, systemic diseases, and medications can affect the neurologic pathways involved.

Clinical Presentation

When evaluating a patient who complains of urinary incontinence, a thorough guided history and physical examination are essential. Important information includes duration, frequency, estimated volume, nocturia, enuresis, sensation of incomplete emptying, postvoid dribbling, impact on quality of life, history of urinary tract infections or urolithiasis, dysuria, hematuria, and associations with the loss of urine (e.g., coughing, laughing, running water). Pertinent parts of the history include medications; general medical history; previous surgeries, particularly gynecologic or urologic procedures; and an obstetric history including methods of delivery, birth weights, and delivery complications. A functional status evaluation is important to determine whether a patient is able to get to the toilet and to comply with treatment options. Smoking, caffeine, and alcohol intake are important variables to consider. A review of systems should include the gastrointestinal system, with particular emphasis on history of constipation. A review of systems should also probe for underlying neurologic or medical diseases that can affect proper bladder function. The patient should document a 3- to 7-day diary that tracks the amount and kind of fluid intake as well as the timing and volume of urinary voids and leaking episodes.

A complete pelvic examination should include testing pelvic floor muscle strength, reflexes, and sensation. The

Figure 136-1 Bladder Function.

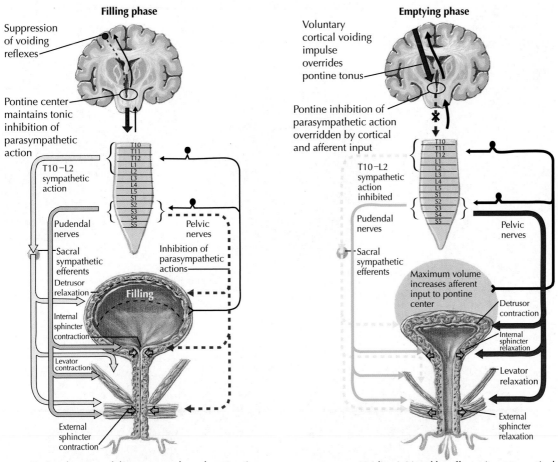

Filling phase

Suppression of voiding reflexes

Pontine center maintains tonic inhibition of parasympathetic action

T10−L2 sympathetic action

Pudendal nerves

Sacral sympathetic efferents

Detrusor relaxation

Internal sphincter contraction

Levator contraction

External sphincter contraction

Inhibition of parasympathetic actions

Filling

Tonic relaxation of detrusor muscle and contraction of sphincters and levator muscles allow bladder filling. Accomplished via parasympathetic inhibition and stimulation of sympathetic and pudendal nerves

Emptying phase

Voluntary cortical voiding impulse overrides pontine tonus

Pontine inhibition of parasympathetic action overridden by cortical and afferent input

T10−L2 sympathetic action inhibited

Pudendal nerves

Sacral sympathetic efferents

Pelvic nerves

Maximum volume increases afferent input to pontine center

Detrusor contraction

Internal sphincter relaxation

Levator relaxation

External sphincter relaxation

Voiding initiated by afferent input to cortical centers from stretch receptors in bladder wall. Parasympathetic inhibition released by pontine center. Sphincter and levator relaxation with detrusor contraction culminate in voiding

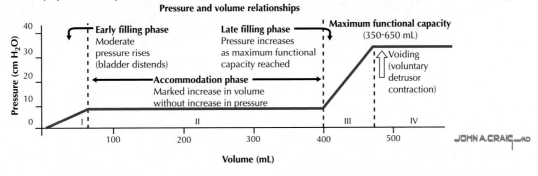

Pressure and volume relationships

Early filling phase Moderate pressure rises (bladder distends)

Late filling phase Pressure increases as maximum functional capacity reached

Maximum functional capacity (350-650 mL)

Voiding (voluntary detrusor contraction)

Accommodation phase Marked increase in volume without increase in pressure

Pressure (cm H_2O)

Volume (mL)

JOHN A.CRAIG—AD

presence and degree of pelvic organ prolapse are important to assess. The bimanual examination should evaluate for gynecologic disorders and should include palpating the urethra for masses or tenderness. A Q-tip test is performed by placing the cotton end of a cotton swab through the urethra to the level of the vesical neck. The angle between the cotton swab and the horizontal when the patient is lying flat is measured at rest and with Valsalva maneuvers; 30 degrees or greater with strain indicates hypermobility of the urethrovesical angle. A rectal examination should

exclude a fecal impaction. A lower extremity neurologic examination is also essential.

Differential Diagnosis of Storage and Emptying Disorders

Urodynamic stress incontinence (USI) is defined by the observation of involuntary urine loss through the urethra with an increase in abdominal pressure in the absence of a detrusor contraction. Patients complain of loss of urine

Figure 136-2 Urinary Incontinence: Stress Incontinence.

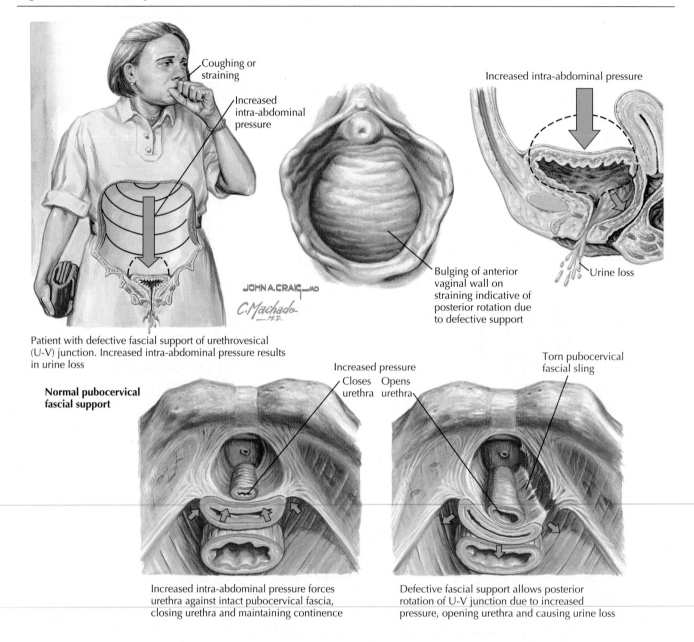

Coughing or straining

Increased intra-abdominal pressure

Increased intra-abdominal pressure

JOHN A. CRAIG—AD
C. Machado—M.D.

Bulging of anterior vaginal wall on straining indicative of posterior rotation due to defective support

Urine loss

Patient with defective fascial support of urethrovesical (U-V) junction. Increased intra-abdominal pressure results in urine loss

Normal pubocervical fascial support

Increased pressure
Closes urethra   Opens urethra

Torn pubocervical fascial sling

Increased intra-abdominal pressure forces urethra against intact pubocervical fascia, closing urethra and maintaining continence

Defective fascial support allows posterior rotation of U-V junction due to increased pressure, opening urethra and causing urine loss

with maneuvers such as coughing, sneezing, or running. Inadequate support of the proximal urethra, usually as a result of childbirth, repeated Valsalva maneuvers, or atrophy due to advancing age, is the usual underlying cause. The proximal urethra is displaced inferiorly out of its normal intra-abdominal location. Consequently, an increase in intra-abdominal pressure causes a greater increase in the intravesical pressure than the intraurethral pressure, thus favoring incontinence. Physical examination often reveals a cystourethrocele (Fig. 136-2). The Q-tip test reveals hypermobility of the urethrovesical angle.

Intrinsic sphincter deficiency (ISD) is urinary incontinence associated with a urethra that does not coapt properly to prevent leakage of urine. Urethral closure pressure

is diminished. Patients complain of frequent loss of urine even with small increases in intra-abdominal pressure. ISD can be caused by denervation injury, radiation, neurologic disorders, or scarring. The Q-tip test can show a normal or hypermobile urethrovesical junction with strain. Diagnosis requires more sophisticated testing than office cystometrics.

Detrusor overactivity (DO) is due to uninhibited detrusor contractions during the filling phase. Patients often complain of large volumes of urine loss, nocturia, urinary frequency (more than 7 times a day with normal fluid intake), enuresis, and a sense of urgency with fear of urinary leakage. DO can be idiopathic or neurogenic. Possible etiologies include decreased central nervous system inhibi-

Figure 136-3 Other Causes of Incontinence.

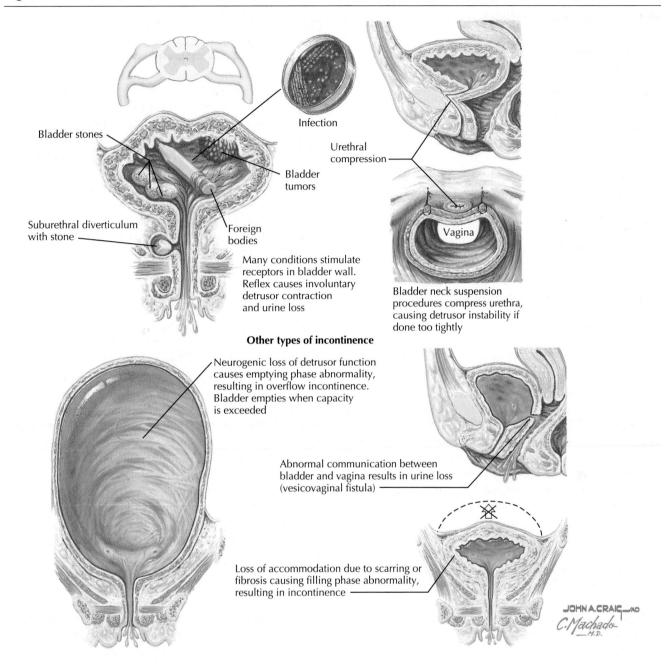

Infection

Bladder stones

Urethral compression

Bladder tumors

Suburethral diverticulum with stone

Foreign bodies

Vagina

Many conditions stimulate receptors in bladder wall. Reflex causes involuntary detrusor contraction and urine loss

Bladder neck suspension procedures compress urethra, causing detrusor instability if done too tightly

Other types of incontinence

Neurogenic loss of detrusor function causes emptying phase abnormality, resulting in overflow incontinence. Bladder empties when capacity is exceeded

Abnormal communication between bladder and vagina results in urine loss (vesicovaginal fistula)

Loss of accommodation due to scarring or fibrosis causing filling phase abnormality, resulting in incontinence

JOHN A. CRAIG —MD
C. Machado —M.D.

tion due to disease or tumor, spinal lesions, or dietary irritative substances. Secondary causes include infection, foreign body, stone or tumor in the bladder, or surgical compression of the urethra after bladder neck suspension procedures (Fig. 136-3). Detrusor overactivity with impaired contractility is a condition found in elderly patients in which detrusor overactivity coexists with incomplete bladder emptying on volitional voids due to detrusor weakness.

Overflow incontinence (OI) occurs when incomplete emptying and decreased sensation of fullness are present and result in the bladder being filled to maximum capacity from which the patient constantly leaks. A high postvoid residual (usually greater than 300 mL) supports this diagnosis. Patients may complain of a sense of incomplete emptying, a slow urine stream, or the need to use abdominal strain to void. OI can be due to obstruction such as with an enlarged prostate gland or due to an inadequate detrusor contraction. The latter can be due to neurologic diseases, diabetes mellitus, medications, or aging.

Functional incontinence occurs in individuals who have normal emptying capabilities but are incontinent because of decreased mobility or decreased cognitive function. Congenital ectopic ureters may present in children who

---

Box 136-1   Systemic Illnesses That Can Affect Bladder Function

Diabetes mellitus
Myasthenia gravis
Parkinson's disease
Multiple sclerosis
Cerebrovascular disease
Central nervous system mass
Spinal cord injury or mass
Dementia

Box 136-2   Medications That Can Affect Bladder Function

Alcohol
α or β Blockers
Anticholinergic agents
Antidepressants
Antipsychotics
Caffeine
Calcium channel blockers or agonists
Diuretics
Narcotic analgesics
Sedative-hypnotics

---

are not able to toilet train. Urinary tract fistulas can result from pelvic surgery and inflammatory conditions such as inflammatory bowel disease and can present as incontinence. Patients complain of constant loss of urine from the vagina. Orange coloring on a tampon in the vagina after a patient has taken oral Pyridium can document the vaginal fluid as urine. Urethral diverticula are outpocketings of the urethral mucosa that can fill with urine during micturition and then drain when the patient stands up, thus presenting with postvoid dribbling. On physical examination, urethral diverticula can occasionally be palpated, or purulence can be milked from the urethra. Often a double-balloon radiologic study is necessary to confirm the diagnosis.

Systemic illnesses or medications can disrupt the neurologic loops that control micturition and storage (Boxes 136-1 and 136-2).

Diagnostic Approach

Initial evaluation should include a urinalysis and urine culture. A pad test to quantify the amount of leaking involves placing a pad on the patient's perineum for 1 hour while maneuvers are performed. An increase in the weight of the pad by 2 g indicates incontinence. Pyridium can be used to confirm that the fluid is urine. Office cystometrics are performed as follows: The patient voids, and a postvoid residual (PVR) is obtained by transurethral catheterization. A PVR of less than 50 mL is normal, whereas a PVR of greater than 200 mL represents inadequate bladder emptying. The bladder is filled with water by gravity through this catheter using a 50-mL syringe without the

plunger. During filling, sensation and capacity are documented. In the absence of an increase in abdominal pressure, a rise in the column of water in the open syringe during filling, usually associated with urgency, indicates a detrusor contraction. The catheter is then removed, the patient coughs while standing, and any leaking is noted.

Multichannel urodynamic studies are commonly performed at academic institutions and provide more detailed information. Patients who warrant referral for these studies include those who describe mixed symptoms or have a history of failed anti-incontinence surgery. Other indications include the desire to rule out detrusor overactivity when the history is suggestive of its presence but simple cystometry is negative, to identify risk factors for surgical failure (e.g., ISD), and to determine the voiding mechanism to attempt to predict those who will have postoperative urinary retention. Cystourethroscopy may identify bladder lesions, foreign bodies, urethral diverticula, fistulas, strictures, and ISD.

Management and Therapy

Optimum Treatment

Conservative measures for genuine stress urinary incontinence (GSI) include pelvic floor muscle exercises (Kegel exercises), biofeedback with or without electrical stimulation, weighted vaginal cones, and placement of a vaginal pessary. Surgical procedures to correct GSI stabilize the urethrovesical angle. Urethropexy and pubovaginal slings are the preferred surgical procedures for GSI.

Intrinsic sphincter deficiency with hypermobility of the urethrovesical junction requires surgical management with creation of a pubovaginal sling to help support and coapt the urethra. ISD without urethrovesical hypermobility is an indication for injection of periurethral bulking agents such as collagen.

The management of detrusor overactivity and urge incontinence includes pelvic floor muscle exercises, bladder retraining programs, and behavioral techniques based on patterns identified from the voiding diary. Bladder infections are treated with antibiotics. The avoidance of bladder irritants such as alcohol, caffeine, carbonated drinks, and acidic foods or drinks is often helpful. Anticholinergic medications can decrease frequency and incontinence episodes and are available in extended-release oral and transdermal forms. Common side effects include dry mouth and constipation. Nocturia, often associated with DO, can also be due to mobilization of lower extremity edema in the supine position. Elevation of the legs during the day or compression stockings can decrease this problem.

Overflow incontinence due to obstruction requires correction of the obstruction. OI due to an acontractile bladder usually is an indication for self-catheterization, Credé's maneuver, or an abdominal strain technique (see Fig. 136-3). The approach to functional incontinence

Box 136-3 Treatments for Incontinence

Urodynamic Stress Incontinence
- Pelvic floor muscle exercises
- Incontinence ring (pessary)
- Urethropexy or sling

Intrinsic Sphincter Deficiency
- Without urethral hypermobility—periurethral bulking agents
- With urethral hypermobility—sling

Detrusor Overactivity
- Behavioral therapy
- Pelvic floor muscle exercises
- Dietary restrictions
- Anticholinergic medications

Overflow Incontinence
- Remove obstruction
- Void/catheter regimen

Functional Incontinence
- Bedside commode
- Assistance with ambulation
- Verbal prompts

Nocturia
- Decrease evening fluids
- Support stockings
- Improve sleep pattern
- Evening dosing of anticholinergics or tricyclic antidepressants

includes providing assistance in the form of a bedside commode, assistance with mobility, or verbal prompts to void. Fistulas and bladder diverticula are indications for surgical excision and repair. Underlying neurologic and medical diseases require an optimal treatment regimen, including the dosage or timing of medications. For all forms of urinary incontinence, the initial approach is to try conservative methods, followed by surgical procedures (Box 136-3) if medical therapy fails.

Avoiding Treatment Errors

The anterior colporrhaphy and needle suspension procedures, once commonly performed for USI, are no longer preferred because of a high rate of failure. Conservative treatments such as pelvic floor muscle exercises for ISD are often not as successful as when used for USI and DO. DO is best managed with a combination of behavioral and dietary changes along with medication as needed. Failures are commonly due to lack of compliance to these measures, inadequate dosing or duration of medication use, or discontinuation of medications because of side effects. Treatment of DO with anticholinergics requires assessment of the PVR before and during treatment to prevent retention and OI.

Future Directions

Surgical outcomes research is ongoing, including comparisons of Burch urethropexy with sling for treatment of USI and the effectiveness of different mesh slings and laparoscopic and robotic suspension procedures. Sacral nerve stimulators to modulate reflexes may improve emptying or storage of urine in patients who have incomplete emptying or detrusor overactivity. Other periurethral bulking agents are available that may last longer than the originally used collagen for ISD. Botulinum toxin (Botox) injections have shown promise in controlling detrusor overactivity in initial studies.

Additional Resources

The American Urogynecological Society Website. Available at: http://www.augs.org.
This website contains educational materials and resources for physicians and patients. It also identifies urogynecologists by practice location.

The National Association for Continence Website. Available at: http://www.nafc.org.
The National Association for Continence promotes newsletters, an online forum, advocacy, educational materials, and products to serve the needs of men and women with continence problems.

The National Institute of Diabetes and Digestive and Kidney Diseases Website. Available at: http://www.niddk.nih.gov.
This site provides excellent patient educational materials on incontinence.

The Simon Foundation for Continence Website. Available at: http://www.simonfoundation.org.
This site similarly provides resources for individuals, families, and health care providers in areas of incontinence education and treatment.

EVIDENCE

1. Bo K, Talseth T, Holme I: Single blind, randomized controlled trial of pelvic floor exercises, electrical stimulation, vaginal cones, and no treatment in management of genuine stress incontinence in women. BMJ 318:487-493, 1999.
   This article provides a comparison of commonly used behavioral therapies for genuine stress incontinence.
2. Burgio KL, Goode PS, Locher JL, et al: Behavioral training with and without biofeedback in the treatment of urge incontinence in older women: A randomized controlled trial. JAMA 288:2293-2299, 2003.
   This article demonstrates the techniques and efficacy of behavioral therapy and the additional benefit of biofeedback in the treatment of urge incontinence.
3. Goode PS, Burgio KL, Locher JL, et al: Effects of behavioral training with or without pelvic floor electrical stimulation on stress incontinence in women: A randomized controlled trial. JAMA 290:345-352, 2003.
   This paper documents the additional benefits of electrical stimulation in the treatment of women with stress incontinence.
4. Urinary incontinence in women. ACOG Practice Bulletin No. 63. American College of Obstetricians and Gynecologists. Obstet Gynecol 105:1533-1545, 2005.
   This article summarizes the current concepts in the diagnosis and management options for women with incontinence and reviews behavioral, medical, and surgical therapy.

Scott L. Sanoff ▪ Patrick H. Nachman

Hematuria

Introduction

Hematuria is a clinical sign requiring careful evaluation because it may be the earliest manifestation of serious underlying processes such as renal or bladder carcinoma or glomerulonephritis. Classified as gross versus microscopic, depending on appearance of the urine, and upper tract versus lower tract, based on the site of bleeding, hematuria can also reflect benign processes such as menstrual bleeding or recent strenuous exercise. Prevalence estimates of microscopic hematuria vary widely from less than 1% to more than 16%, depending on the population studied and screening methodology. With a diversity of causes, each patient requires an individualized evaluation plan that considers the anatomic source of bleeding as well as the individual's risk factors for disease.

Etiology and Pathogenesis

Blood may enter the urine at any point along the urinary tract from the kidneys to the urethra. Considering the urinary tract in two parts, the upper tract (kidneys, renal collecting system) and the lower tract (ureters, bladder, prostate, urethra), helps the clinician organize a differential diagnosis and focus the evaluation. Gross bleeding is often from the lower tract, whereas microscopic hematuria can be more difficult to localize (Fig. 137-1).

Upper Tract

Urine is produced by filtering blood through the layers of the glomerulus: the capillary endothelium, basement membrane, and epithelium (Fig. 137-2). An intact glomerulus allows passage of plasma ultrafiltrate, such as urea, while preventing essential proteins and cells from passing through, such as albumin and red blood cells (RBCs). Damage to the glomerular endothelium from inflammation, as in vasculitis and crescentic glomerulonephritides, can permit passage of RBCs into the urine. Similarly, a change in the structure of the basement membrane may allow RBC passage into the urine. Such is the case in the hereditary conditions of Alport's disease and thin basement membrane disease, in which the basement membrane is altered by mutations in its collagen components. Isolated damage to glomerular epithelium rarely produces hematuria. Minimal change disease, a condition characterized by changes limited to the epithelium, is notable for profound proteinuria in the absence of hematuria.

Urine is further modified as it courses through the tubular system of the kidney into the more proximal collecting ducts. Injury to the tubules from ischemia (e.g., arterial thrombosis or hypotension in sepsis) or toxin injury (e.g., aminoglycoside toxicity) may cause acute tubular necrosis (ATN) with subsequent RBC passage into the urine. Additionally, damage to the collecting ducts, calices, or renal pelvis from nephrolithiasis, renal cell carcinoma, or pyelonephritis can cause hematuria.

Lower Tract

Urine flows out of the kidney into the ureters, where it is transported to the bladder. Nephrolithiasis, urothelial tumors, and ascending infection can damage the lining of this transport system with resultant bleeding. Damage to the bladder wall by tumors, infection, or foreign bodies can also cause hematuria. In men, hematuria may result from inflammation of a highly vascular prostate gland secondary to prostate cancer or infection. Finally, blood may enter the urine more distally, as in the case of urethritis or contamination from menses.

Clinical Presentation

Gross hematuria describes a visible change in the color of the urine to red, pink, or brown. It is often brought to the

Figure 137-1 Sources of Microscopic and Macroscopic Hematuria.

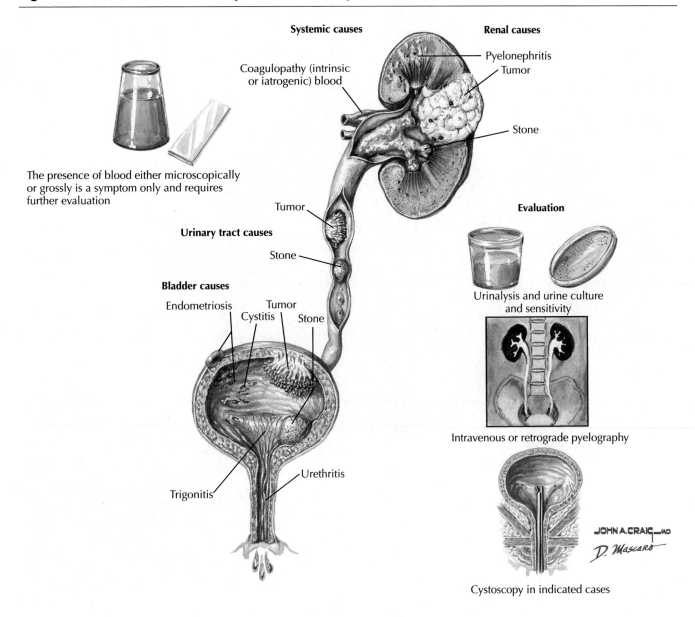

Systemic causes

Coagulopathy (intrinsic or iatrogenic) blood

The presence of blood either microscopically or grossly is a symptom only and requires further evaluation

Urinary tract causes

Tumor

Stone

Bladder causes

Endometriosis

Tumor

Cystitis

Stone

Trigonitis

Urethritis

Renal causes

Pyelonephritis

Tumor

Stone

Evaluation

Urinalysis and urine culture and sensitivity

Intravenous or retrograde pyelography

JOHN A. CRAIG_AD
D. Mascaro

Cystoscopy in indicated cases

attention of a physician by a concerned patient. Red or pink urine that is opaque is consistent with a urinary tract source, whereas brown (tea-colored) translucent urine is suggestive of glomerular bleeding. Microscopic hematuria, undetectable by the unaided eye, is commonly discovered by urine dipstick or automated urinalysis. Hematuria may present amid a complex of localizing symptoms, such as unilateral colicky flank pain associated with nephrolithiasis. It may be discovered unexpectedly (asymptomatic hematuria) such as during screening of a diabetic patient for proteinuria, an early sign of diabetic nephropathy. Because dipstick assays lack specificity, it is important to confirm the diagnosis of microscopic hematuria by repeat testing and microscopic examination of the urine (see "Diagnostic Approach"). As always, a focused history and physical exam are mandatory to guide the workup and limit the differential diagnosis.

History

A focused history should begin with a complete description of the chief complaint, paying particular attention to associated symptoms and risk factors for underlying disease. It is helpful to structure the interview around an age-appropriate, anatomically organized differential diagnosis that considers the epidemiology of hematuria.

When gross hematuria is first identified by the patient, it is important for the clinician to understand the timing of the first episode as well as the frequency of subsequent episodes. Cyclical hematuria coinciding with menstruation

Figure 137-2 Structure of the Glomerulus.

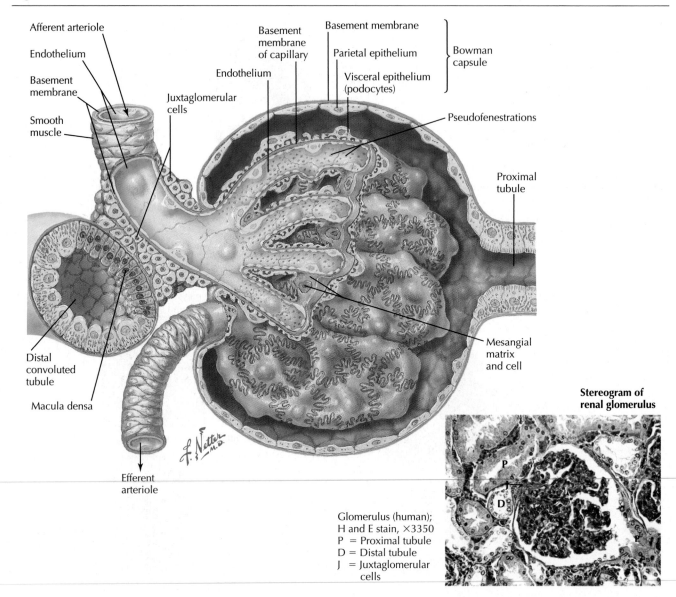

Afferent arteriole

Endothelium

Basement membrane

Smooth muscle

Juxtaglomerular cells

Basement membrane of capillary

Endothelium

Basement membrane

Parietal epithelium

Visceral epithelium (podocytes)

Bowman capsule

Pseudofenestrations

Proximal tubule

Mesangial matrix and cell

Distal convoluted tubule

Macula densa

Efferent arteriole

f. Netter M.D.

Stereogram of renal glomerulus

Glomerulus (human); H and E stain, ×3350
P = Proximal tubule
D = Distal tubule
J = Juxtaglomerular cells

may reflect endometriosis in the urinary tract or contamination of the sample. Although clinically significant blood loss is rare (unless clots obstruct the urinary tract), one should attempt to quantify hematuria by assessing the quality of the urine (e.g., was the urine bright red with clots, light pink, brown?).

For both gross and microscopic hematuria, it is important to identify preceding events or illnesses that may suggest a source (e.g., recent trauma, exercise, sexual activity, menstruation, or upper respiratory tract infection—a common predecessor to glomerulonephropathy). One should pay particular attention to the location and quality of associated pain (e.g., dysuria associated with a urinary tract infection [UTI]; lower abdominal pressure associated with UTI or tumor; or colicky flank pain associated with nephrolithiasis or pyelonephritis), evidence of infection

(e.g., fever, chills, sweats), symptoms of obstruction (e.g., urinary hesitancy, urgency, incontinence), symptoms of renal insufficiency (e.g., oliguria, nausea, loss of appetite), and symptoms that may point to systemic illness (e.g., fatigue; respiratory tract, gastrointestinal, or musculoskeletal symptoms; or rashes). The presence of flank pain along with fever or dysuria should prompt an emergent evaluation to rule out obstruction-related infection, which can lead to life-threatening sepsis syndrome.

A detailed medication history is important, with special attention given to nonsteroidal anti-inflammatory drugs (e.g., analgesic nephropathy, papillary necrosis), antibiotics (e.g., interstitial nephritis), drugs known to change urine color (e.g., rifampin), and anticoagulants. Importantly, hematuria in the setting of anticoagulation still requires a complete evaluation. A comprehensive past medical history should identify previously diagnosed renal disease (e.g., glomerulonephritis, medullary sponge kidney), past UTI or pyelonephritis, nephrolithiasis, cancer (with particular attention to chemotherapy exposure and radiation), sickle cell disease (e.g., papillary necrosis), and bleeding disorders. Family history should identify others with hematuria or known renal disease (e.g., thin basement membrane disease, Alport's syndrome, or polycystic kidney disease). Additionally, one should elicit a complete travel history, assessing risk factors for regional infections (e.g., schistosomiasis, tuberculosis), and consider exposure to mutagens such as tobacco, phenacetin, cyclophosphamide, and industrial chemicals as risk factors for genitourinary cancers.

Physical Examination

The purpose of the physical exam is to search for clues that localize the source of hematuria or suggest a causative process. Hypertension and edema are common in glomerular diseases of many kinds. Nephrotic range proteinuria (>3 g/day), common in many glomerular diseases, is associated with edema and is an independent risk factor for renal vein thrombosis. Oral sores, scleral injection, swollen joints, and rash can be found in various vasculitic and autoimmune processes. Cachexia, swollen lymph nodes, and flank or abdominal tenderness may reflect a cancer or chronic infection. Atrial fibrillation and valvular vegetations (often first identified by cardiac murmur) increase risk for renal artery embolism. A tender or asymmetric prostate or testicle may also reflect an underlying cancer or infection.

Differential Diagnosis

A comprehensive anatomically based differential grounded in basic epidemiology and prioritized by the most threatening conditions should guide the diagnostic evaluation (Box 137-1). Examples illustrating the importance of this balance are glomerulonephritides and urinary tract cancers.

Glomerular diseases are a common cause of hematuria in children but account for only 5% of hematuria in adults. However, one must immediately consider a glomerular process in any patient with hematuria and renal insufficiency because an untreated, rapidly progressive glomerulonephropathy often advances quickly to end-stage renal disease and the need for dialysis. Meanwhile, isolated glomerular hematuria (hematuria in the absence of proteinuria or renal insufficiency) in an adult is most commonly caused by immunoglobulin A nephropathy, Alport's syndrome (i.e., hereditary nephritis), or thin basement membrane disease (i.e., benign familial hematuria). It is critical to check the renal function of anyone with a new diagnosis of hematuria early in their evaluation.

A second example is that of urinary tract malignancies. These are an important cause of hematuria in adults, accounting for up to 15% of cases, two thirds of which are due to bladder cancer. However, they are rare in patients younger than 35 years of age (about 1 in 100,000).

Diagnostic Approach

Because microscopic hematuria is often transient and may be secondary to a benign process (e.g., vigorous exercise, recent sexual activity, or menstruation), it is often helpful to evaluate a second urine sample collected several days after the first, avoiding confounding activities around the time of collection. It is important to note, however, that transient hematuria in those with an appreciable risk for malignancy may warrant a complete evaluation in the absence of positive follow-up testing. Ideally, urine samples are collected midstream in the absence of external bleeding, such as menses, and examined within 1 hour. Those with gross hematuria require a thorough evaluation of the upper and lower urinary tract.

One should start by considering all information provided by the urinalysis. Concurrent positive tests for leukocyte esterase or nitrites in the right clinical setting should prompt a urine culture. Evidence of proteinuria should be followed with a urine protein-to-creatinine ratio for estimation of the 24-hour protein excretion (a ratio >0.2 reflects abnormal proteinuria and likely glomerular disease). Alternatively, a 24-hour urine collection may be sent for protein quantification. It is also important to assess the renal function of all patients with newly diagnosed hematuria with a measure of the serum urea nitrogen and creatinine. Any elevation of these tests should prompt an urgent evaluation for obstruction and intrinsic renal disease.

Substances such as myoglobin (e.g., from rhabdomyolysis) and hemoglobin (e.g., from hemolysis) can produce gross color change of the urine and false-positive results on dipstick assays. Therefore, it can be helpful to centrifuge urine for gross examination and repeat dipstick testing of the supernatant. It is important to perform microscopic evaluation of the sediment.

Samples should be prepared by centrifugation of 10 mL of urine at 2000 rpm for 5 minutes. Hematuria from intact RBCs in the absence of lysis will produce a clear supernatant and sediment with a reddish hue, depending on the volume of cells. Most dipstick assays can detect as few as 1 or 2 RBCs per high-power field, although hematuria is often defined as more than 2 RBCs per high-power field. If the supernatant remains red, it should be retested with a dipstick. A positive test may reflect myoglobinuria or hemoglobinuria. A red supernatant negative for blood on dipstick testing may reflect phenazopyridine or porphyria.

The supernatant is then discarded, and the sediment is resuspended for examination under low- and high-power light microscopy. Identification of intact RBCs in the absence of contamination (often indicated by the presence of multiple squamous cells) confirms the diagnosis of hematuria.

Box 137-1   Causes of Hematuria Organized Anatomically*

Renal

Glomerular

Immunoglobulin A nephropathy (the most common primary glomerulonephritis, often occurs within 1-3 days of an upper respiratory infection)
Poststreptococcal glomerulonephritis (most commonly occurs >10 days after streptococcal pharyngitis)
Genetic diseases of glomerular basement membrane (e.g., thin basement membrane disease, or Alport's syndrome)
Lupus nephritis
Goodpasture's syndrome
Wegener's granulomatosis
Microscopic polyangiitis
Henoch-Schönlein purpura

Tubulointerstitial

Interstitial nephritis (commonly associated with drugs such as penicillins, cephalosporins, trimethoprim-sulfamethoxazole, and nonsteroidal anti-inflammatory drugs)
Sarcoidosis
Medullary sponge kidney
Polycystic disease
Acute tubular necrosis
Renal cell carcinoma (most commonly occurring in the renal cortex)

Collecting System

Nephrolithiasis (may precipitate and obstruct anywhere along the urinary tract)
Pyelonephritis
Hydronephrosis (often due to obstruction occurring lower in the urinary tract)
Urothelial cell neoplasm (most commonly transitional cell carcinoma)

Vascular

Renal artery thrombosis with infarction
Renal vein thrombosis
Arteriovenous malformations
Sickle cell disease
Papillary necrosis
Nutcracker syndrome

Extrarenal

Ureters

Urothelial cell neoplasm (most commonly transitional cell carcinoma)
Nephrolithiasis (may precipitate and obstruct anywhere along the urinary tract)

Bladder

Transitional cell carcinoma
Infectious cystitis
Radiation-induced cystitis
Bladder diverticulum
Bladder stone
Bladder neck contracture

Urethra

Urethritis
Urethral stricture

Male Specific

Prostate cancer
Prostatitis
Benign prostatic hyperplasia
Epididymitis

Female Specific

Endometriosis
Menstrual contamination

Nonspecific

Strenuous exercise
Genitourinary tuberculosis
Genitourinary trauma
Factitious
Foreign bodies
Perineal irritation
Sexual intercourse
Schistosomiasis (consider if travel to endemic area, e.g., Africa)
Loin pain hematuria syndrome

*In some cases (e.g., nephrolithiasis), the anatomic distinction is somewhat artificial because the process may occur in multiple sites along the urinary tract.

Dysmorphic erythrocytes (acanthocytes) and RBC casts on light microscopy are virtually diagnostic of glomerular disease, an important finding that can often make a lower tract evaluation unnecessary. Evidence of proteinuria would support this diagnosis. Demonstration of other formed elements, such as white blood cell casts, granular casts, and pigmented casts, suggests a tubular or interstitial process such as pyelonephritis, interstitial nephritis, or ATN. An elevated serum creatinine would support a renal source of blood as well.

When glomerular bleeding is thought to be unlikely, it is important to image the upper tract for evidence of neoplasm, stones, obstruction, or polycystic kidney disease. Selecting the appropriate imaging modalities requires an understanding of their various performance characteris-

tics. Ultrasound, a noninvasive procedure, is often less expensive then others tests, but is limited in the detection of small tumors. Computed tomography (CT) scans without contrast are ideal for the evaluation of stones. Excretory urography, which introduces the risks associated with intravenous contrast administration (e.g., nephrotoxicity and allergic reaction), can be helpful to diagnose medullary sponge kidney or to assess for stones when CT is unavailable. CT and magnetic resonance imaging with contrast provide the most detailed images of the renal parenchyma but should be used cautiously in those with renal insufficiency.

Urine cytology is indicated on a first morning void for those at risk for a urinary tract neoplasm. Test performance is determined by the quality of the sample, experience of the pathologist, and differentiation of the tumor cells. Cytology is more sensitive for cancers of the bladder than those of the upper urinary tract, such as transitional cell carcinoma. In general, cytology is relatively insensitive, although specific.

Cystoscopy, visualization of the lower urinary tract through a fiberoptic camera inserted into the bladder, warrants consideration for those at risk for bladder cancer. This includes men older than 40 years (although there is disagreement about the appropriate age cutoff) and patients with a history of phenacetin use or analgesic abuse, significant smoking history, exposure to mutagenic dyes, exposure to cyclophosphamide, or persistent or recurrent episodes of gross hematuria. Specific cases may require specialty consultation or review of available guidelines.

In many cases, a complete workup will yield no definitive source of bleeding. The most common cause in these instances is an indolent glomerular disease. However, because malignancy may eventually become evident, particularly for those at higher risk, it is important to have an appropriate follow-up plan.

Management and Therapy

Optimum Treatment

Appropriate management of hematuria and the need for subsequent therapy is dictated by the underlying cause and need for subspecialty evaluation. For those with evidence of glomerular disease or polycystic kidney disease, referral to a nephrologist is appropriate. Evidence of progressive renal insufficiency in the setting of glomerular disease warrants urgent referral for consideration of a renal biopsy. Referral to a urologist should be made for those with gross hematuria, an identified mass, or persistent hematuria, and those at high risk for malignancy.

Avoiding Treatment Errors

It is important to consider the etiology of hematuria carefully in all patients in whom it is detected. Early assessment of renal function in each case will help ensure timely diagnosis of progressive glomerulonephropathy, a condition that requires immediate evaluation by a nephrologist. A thorough evaluation of the urinary tract for those at greatest risk for malignancy, and a timely referral to the appropriate subspecialist when indicated, will ensure the best possible outcome. Contacting a subspecialist with questions about the necessity or timing of a referral will help avoid unnecessary errors.

Future Directions

With continued development and improvement of noninvasive imaging technologies and urinary markers for disease, the elimination of invasive evaluations and the use of contrast with its associated comorbidities may ultimately be possible. The availability of more sensitive and specific low-risk testing will undoubtedly change the clinical approach to the evaluation of hematuria.

Additional Resource

Agency for Health Care Research and Quality (AHRQ) National Guideline Clearinghouse Website. Available at: http://www.guideline.gov. Accessed October 2, 2007.

  This website provides the recommendations of various professional groups for the evaluation and management of hematuria and many associated conditions.

EVIDENCE

1. Brenner BM, ed. Brenner & Rector's The Kidney, 7th ed. Philadelphia, WB Saunders, 2004, pp 1128-1131.

  This comprehensive textbook offers a concise evaluation strategy for the patient with hematuria as well as multiple well-referenced chapters reviewing related conditions.

2. Cohen RA, Brown RS: Microscopic hematuria. N Engl J Med 348(23):2330-2338, 2003.

  This commonly sited, clinically based review of the epidemiology, evaluation, and management of patients with microscopic hematuria includes a flow diagram as a quick summary of the suggested evaluation process.

3. Khadra MH, Pickard RS, Charlton M, et al: A prospective analysis of 1,930 patients with hematuria to evaluate current diagnostic practice. J Urol 163(2):524-527, 2000.

  This analysis of a large prospective cohort describes the epidemiology of microscopic and macroscopic hematuria in patients seen in a hematuria clinic. Presented tables clearly illustrate the prevalence of associated tumors by age and gender.

4. Yun EJ, Meng MV, Carroll PR: Evaluation of the patient with hematuria. Med Clin North Am 88(2):329-343, 2004.

  This thorough, evidenced-based discussion of the evaluation and management of patients found to have hematuria provides an especially helpful review of relevant testing and a concise algorithm for patient evaluation.

Cynthia J. Denu-Ciocca ▪ Romulo E. Colindres

Urinary Stone Disease (Nephrolithiasis)

Introduction

Nephrolithiasis is a common disorder with an annual incidence of 0.1% to 0.5%. The peak age at onset is 20 to 30 years, and males are affected more than females through most of adult life until about the sixth decade, when the incidence increases in women and tends to decrease in men. Rates of stone formation may be affected by genetic, nutritional, and environmental factors. The relative risk for nephrolithiasis for patients with a positive family history may be as great as 2.5. In the United States, the prevalence of stones has risen over the past 20 years from 3.2% to 5.2%. Wide geographic variations exist, and in the United States, prevalence is greatest among those who live in the southern latitudes. This may be due to differences in diet and water composition, as well as ambient and sunlight exposure. An estimated 28% to 50% of patients experience a recurrence at 5 years.

Etiology and Pathogenesis

Calcium Stones

About 75% to 80% of all kidney stones contain calcium. Most are composed of calcium oxalate alone or in combination with calcium phosphate. Calcium oxalate stones are brown or gray, small, and well circumscribed on radiographs. Calcium oxalate crystals may appear as dumbbells or pyramids (Fig. 138-1). Calcium phosphate stones are beige or white and form apatite and brushite crystals. Calcium oxalate stones are thought to arise and grow from Randall's plaques. These are plaque-like aggregates that originate in the basement membrane of the thin loop of Henle and spread; they can protrude into the uroepithelium in the renal papillae and serve as a nidus for crystal aggregation and growth. Calcium crystals may form in urine that is supersaturated from excess excretion of calcium, oxalate, or uric acid. Diminished citrate in the urine may also lead to calcium stone formation. Hypercalciuria, the most common metabolic disorder in people in whom stones form, affects 50% of patients. Hypercalciuria may be broadly classified as absorptive, renal leak, or hormonal.

Absorptive Hypercalciuria

Absorptive hypercalciuria is the most common cause of abnormal calcium excretion. These patients have a tendency to absorb and excrete a higher proportion of dietary calcium than normal people. The disorder is familial and affects both sexes equally.

Renal Leak

Renal leak or renal hypercalciuria is a syndrome of inappropriate renal wasting of calcium. This wasting leads to the stimulation of parathyroid hormone and subsequently 1,25-OH vitamin D in efforts to normalize the serum calcium.

Hormonal Hypercalciuria

Hormonal hypercalciuria develops in the setting of hyperparathyroidism of both primary and paraneoplastic origin. Granulomatous disorders such as sarcoidosis may also lead to hypercalciuria due to increased levels of 1,25-OH vitamin D.

Figure 138-1 Unorganized Elements That May Be Found in Urinary Sediment.

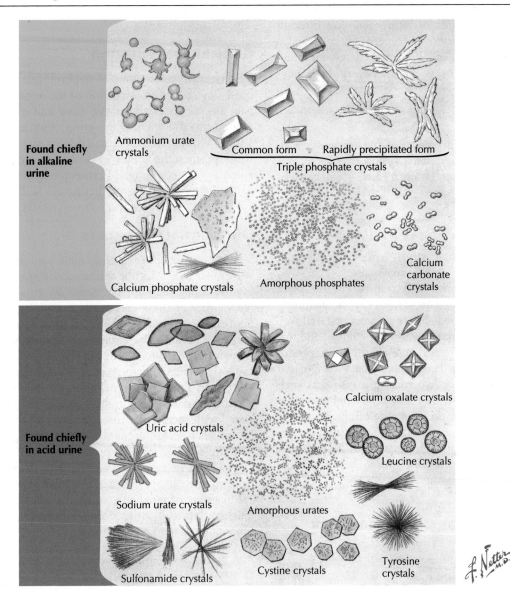

Found chiefly in alkaline urine

Ammonium urate crystals

Common form   Rapidly precipitated form
Triple phosphate crystals

Calcium phosphate crystals

Amorphous phosphates

Calcium carbonate crystals

Found chiefly in acid urine

Uric acid crystals

Calcium oxalate crystals

Leucine crystals

Sodium urate crystals

Amorphous urates

Sulfonamide crystals

Cystine crystals

Tyrosine crystals

Hypocitraturia

Citrate is an inhibitor of calcium stone formation that complexes with calcium, reducing its free urinary concentration, and subsequently decreases the saturation of calcium oxalate and calcium phosphate. Hypocitraturia may be idiopathic or secondary to metabolic acidosis, a metabolic state that reduces urinary citrate excretion by increasing its proximal reabsorption. Type I renal tubular acidosis is a defect in hydrogen ion secretion that leads to metabolic acidosis and inability to acidify the urine. More than half of these patients have nephrolithiasis, nephrocalcinosis, or both. Increased bone turnover due to the metabolic acidosis leads to increased filtration of calcium and phosphorus. The metabolic acidosis decreases calcium reabsorption and increases citrate reabsorption. Finally, the alkaline urine pH leads to supersaturation of calcium phosphate.

Hyperoxaluria

Primary hyperoxaluria types I and II are rare genetic disorders caused by enzyme deficiencies that lead to massive oxaluria. Patients may excrete up to 300 mg per day and deposit calcium oxalate in multiple tissues, including kidneys, heart, and blood vessels. Enteric hyperoxaluria occurs when small bowel absorption is altered from any mechanism. This results in increased intraluminal bile salts and fatty acids, which increase the permeability of the colonic mucosa to oxalate and bind to calcium. The end result is an increase in the free oxalate available for absorption. This is accompanied by a markedly reduced urinary citrate due to additional bicarbonate loss through the bowel and systemic acidosis. Hyperoxaluria may also occur from ingestion of a diet high in oxalate-containing foods such as spinach, beets, chocolate, rhubarb, and nuts.

Hyperuricosuria

There is an increased incidence of hyperuricosuria in calcium stone formers. Uric acid crystals may serve as a nidus for heterogeneous nucleation; 5% to 10% of calcium stones contain a uric acid core.

Uric Acid Stones

Uric acid stones account for 5% to 10% of stones, although in Mediterranean countries, they may cause up to 30%. They are yellow or orange and transparent on plain radiography. Urate crystals take various shapes, including rhomboids, rosettes, needles, or amorphous material (see Fig. 138-1). Hyperuricosuria, low urinary volume, and low urine pH predispose to uric acid nephrolithiasis. Excessive urinary excretion of uric acid may be secondary to increased dietary intake of purines or hyperuricemic disorders such as tumor lysis syndrome, or they may be related to certain medications. Urine pH is the major determinant of uric acid supersaturation; an increase to 6.5 can increase the solubility markedly and possibly dissolve existing stones. Decreased urinary volume also increases uric acid supersaturation.

Struvite Stones (Magnesium Ammonium Phosphate)

Infection stones (10% to 15% of all stones), the most common cause of staghorn calculi, are more prevalent in women (Fig. 138-2). They are light brown and appear laminated on radiograph. Struvite crystals have the classic coffin-lid appearance (see Fig. 138-1). They are associated with infections of the urinary tract by urease-producing bacteria. Hydrolysis of urea sets up a cascade of events that leads to supersaturation of magnesium ammonium phosphate.

Cystine Stones

Less than 2% of all stones are composed of cystine. They are yellow-green and homogeneous on radiograph. Cystine crystals take a hexagonal form, and the stones are often bilateral and may cause staghorn calculi (see Fig. 138-2). Cystinuria is an autosomal recessive disease in which there is a tubular defect in dibasic amino acid transport. Affected patients excrete excessive amounts of cystine, ornithine, arginine, and lysine. Cystine has a low solubility

(300 mg/L), and affected patients may excrete 480 to 3600 mg/day.

Clinical Presentation

The typical presentation of nephrolithiasis is renal colic caused by an acute obstruction of the urinary tract. Severe pain begins suddenly in the flank and radiates laterally around the abdomen to the groin, testicles, or labia (Fig. 138-3). Urinary frequency and dysuria may occur when the stone reaches the ureterovesicular junction. Nausea and vomiting are common. Microscopic hematuria occurs in 75% of patients, and gross hematuria in 20% or less.

Differential Diagnosis

Various diseases causing abdominal pain may be confused with renal colic. An abdominal aortic aneurysm or acute intestinal obstruction may cause severe abdominal pain, but neither of these conditions is usually associated with hematuria. In females of childbearing age, ectopic pregnancy is in the differential, and testing with serum β-human chorionic gonadotropin is indicated. Disorders that cause significant hematuria may produce clots that obstruct the ureter, mimicking renal colic. Occasionally, renal cell carcinoma may present in this manner, but hematuria associated with glomerular diseases does not produce enough hematuria to cause ureteral obstruction.

Drug-seeking patients presenting for medial attention may self-inflict injury to cause hematuria. Unfortunately, patients with history of nephrolithiasis may also present complaining of renal colic in an attempt to obtain narcotics. Imaging to identify stones within the ureter and not the kidney can aid management.

Diagnostic Approach

The usual diagnostic approach is to obtain an imaging study. Radiography of the kidneys, ureters, and bladder reveals most stones, with the exception of uric acid stones. Ultrasound of the urinary tract is noninvasive, identifies all stone types including uric acid stones, and can assess the presence of obstruction. Unfortunately, ureteral stones are not well visualized. Intravenous pyelography provides information on the structure and function of the urinary tract and determines the cause, site, and severity of obstruction. Unenhanced helical computed tomography (CT) has become the standard radiologic test for evaluating patients with acute renal colic. CT requires less time to perform, has an excellent sensitivity and specificity (96% and 99%, respectively), obviates the risks of intravenous contrast material, and detects extraurinary diseases that may present with symptoms similar to renal colic. Given the higher exposure to radiation with CT, however, ultrasonography may still be the preferred imaging choice in children. Once

Figure 138-2 Renal Calculi.

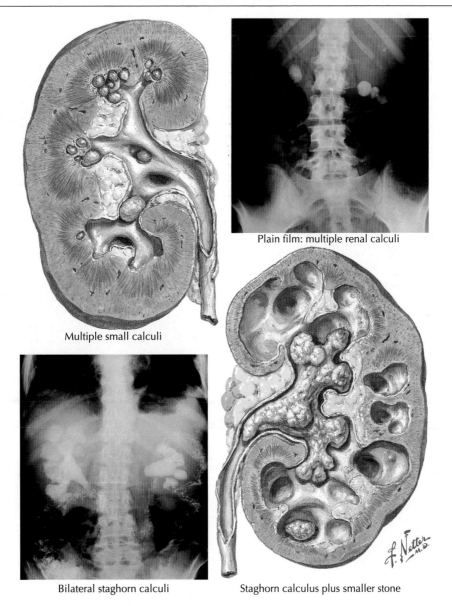

Multiple small calculi

Plain film: multiple renal calculi

Bilateral staghorn calculi

Staghorn calculus plus smaller stone

a diagnosis of nephrolithiasis has been made, an evaluation should be performed as outlined in Box 138-1.

Although some recommend further metabolic screening for all patients with nephrolithiasis, it is generally accepted that patients with recurrent stone disease, those with nephrocalcinosis, first stone formers with a moderate to high risk for recurrent disease, and all children should undergo a 24-hour urine collection to establish risk factors for nephrolithiasis. Obtaining at least two 24-hour urine samples on a normal diet is optimal. The normal values of all the constituents that should be tested are listed in Table 138-1.

Management and Therapy

Optimum Treatment

In the acute phase of renal colic, the goal of management is to relieve pain, treat infection, establish the size and location of the stone and the presence of obstruction, and facilitate stone passage. Most ureteral stones 4 mm in diameter or smaller pass spontaneously. There is a gradual decrease in the spontaneous passage rate for stones larger than 4 mm. For patients with urosepsis, acute renal failure, intractable pain, and nausea or vomiting, immediate urologic consultation is indicated. Outpatient urology referral

Figure 138-3 Calculous Urinary Obstruction.

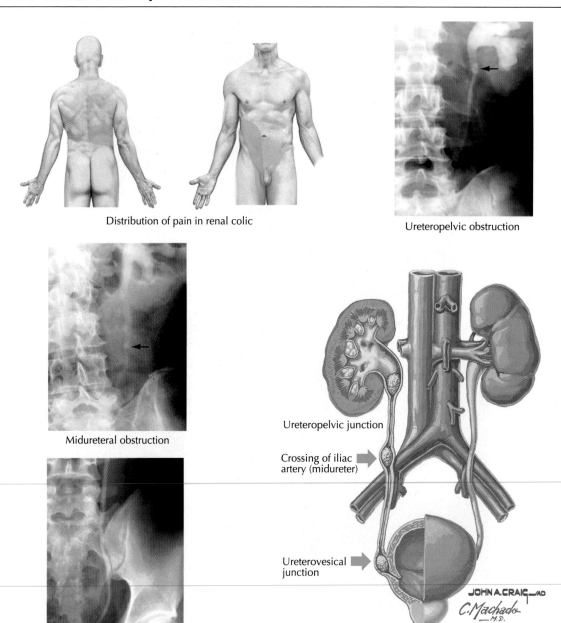

Distribution of pain in renal colic

Ureteropelvic obstruction

Midureteral obstruction

Distal ureteral obstruction

Ureteropelvic junction

Crossing of iliac artery (midureter)

Ureterovesical junction

Common sites of obstruction

should be made for patients who fail to pass the stone with conservative therapy and for those in whom the stone is larger than 10 mm. Further urologic management may include extracorporeal shock wave lithotripsy, ureteroscopic removal, or percutaneous nephrolithotomy.

To decrease the incidence of stone recurrence, all patients should be treated with nonspecific therapy. Urinary volume should exceed 2 L/day. Increased urinary volume alone has been shown to reduce the incidence of recurrent nephrolithiasis. Certain dietary restrictions have been shown to change urine constituents favorably. A

low-protein diet (0.8 g/kg/day) is recommended for stone formers because a high-protein diet (2.0 g/kg/day) increases uric acid and calcium excretion and reduces citrate excretion. Multiple studies have shown that high dietary sodium intake increases sodium and calcium excretion, and low-sodium diets have the opposite effect; therefore, a modest sodium dietary restriction (2 to 3 g/day) is recommended. Generalized dietary restriction of calcium is no longer recommended to prevent calcium stones. Studies have shown a decreased risk for nephrolithiasis in patients with normal calcium intake. This is related to the decreased

Box 138-1	Evaluation of Patients with Nephrolithiasis

History

Stone history
Medical diseases associated with stone disease: sarcoidosis, inflammatory bowel disease, malignancy
Family history: age at onset, type of nephrolithiasis
Medications: loop diuretics, indinavir
Social history: occupation
Diet: fluids, protein, purine, sodium, calcium, oxalate

Laboratory Studies

Stone analysis
Urinalysis and culture
Serum electrolytes, blood urea nitrogen, creatinine, calcium, phosphorous, uric acid, parathyroid hormone if the calcium is elevated

Adapted from Bushinsky DA: Nephrolithiasis. J Am Soc Nephrol 9(5):918-924, 1998; and Monk RD: Clinical approach to adults. Semin Nephrol 16(5):375-388, 1996.

Table 138-1 Normal 24-Hour Urinary Values

Volume	>2-2.5 L
Calcium	<300 mg in men, <250 mg in women
Uric acid	<800 mg in men, <750 mg in women
Oxalate	<40 mg
Citrate	>320 mg
Phosphorus	<1000 mg
Sodium	<200 mEq
pH	5.0-7.0

Adapted from Monk RD: Clinical approach to adults. Semin Nephrol 16(5):375-388, 1996.

availability of oxalate to be absorbed in the gut due to binding with calcium. Dietary oxalate should be restricted. In addition to conservative measures, specific therapy should be tailored to patients with recurrent stone disease.

Calcium Stones

In hypercalciuria, thiazide diuretics decrease urinary calcium excretion by reducing intestinal calcium absorption and increasing renal tubular reabsorption. Thiazides are the first line of treatment for patients with renal leak syndrome and have been shown to be effective in reducing stone recurrence in patients with idiopathic hypercalciuria. Adding potassium citrate may be helpful to avoid associated hypokalemia, as well as offering the benefit of increasing citraturia. Parathyroid surgery is the treatment of choice for patients with primary hyperparathyroidism and nephrolithiasis. In hypocitraturia, potassium alkali salts significantly reduce the rates of stone recurrence. Potassium citrate at doses from 15 to 30 mEq 2 to 3 times daily up to 100 mEq daily may be required. The goal of treatment of calcium phosphate stones due to type I renal

tubular acidosis is to reduce systemic metabolic acidosis, which in turn decreases bone resorption and urinary calcium excretion and increases citraturia. Potassium citrate or potassium bicarbonate may be used, but large doses are often required. A thiazide diuretic may be added if hypercalciuria persists. Primary oxaluria is treated with dietary oxalate restriction and increased urinary volume. Some patients may benefit from pyridoxine therapy. For enteric hyperoxaluria, calcium supplementation with meals will bind dietary oxalate. A low-fat diet and cholestyramine to bind bile acids may decrease oxalate absorption. For patients with metabolic acidosis due to diarrhea, potassium citrate may be a helpful adjuvant therapy. Dietary purine restriction and increasing urinary volume are first-line treatments for hyperuricosuria. If it persists, allopurinol should be added.

Uric Acid Stones

Conservative therapy, including increased urinary volume and dietary restriction of protein and purine products, may decrease uric acid supersaturation. Urinary alkalinization with potassium citrate or potassium bicarbonate to a pH of 6.0 to 7.0 may help dissolve existing stones and prevent recurrence. Add allopurinol if urinary pH remains low or if hyperuricosuria persists despite dietary modification.

Struvite Stones

Therapy is aimed at removing existing calculi, which harbor the urease-producing bacteria, and eradicating infection. Acetohydroxamic acid, an inhibitor of urease production, has been shown to reduce the rate of stone growth but is poorly tolerated because of its multiple side effects.

Cystine Stones

The goal of therapy is to increase the solubility of cystine in the urine with hydration and alkalinization (pH 6.5 to 7.0). For patients with severe disease, more specific therapy with chelating agents may be necessary to reduce cystine excretion.

Avoiding Treatment Errors

Caution must be used when treating calcium stone–forming patients with potassium citrate. Although this therapy has been shown to reduce the incidence of stone recurrence and is standard therapy for patients with hypocitraturia, follow-up 24-hour urine collections to assess efficacy are recommended. Calcium stone–forming patients may suffer from more than one urinary risk factor. Citrate therapy may result in a significant elevation of the urine pH. Although urinary citrate may improve, this may predispose to calcium phosphate stone formation, especially in patients who also have hypercalciuria.

Generalized treatment recommendations were made in the text, but it is important to reiterate several points.

Although drug therapies are effective at reducing the incidence of stone recurrence, excessive reliance on these agents should be avoided, and emphasis should be placed on dietary alteration, which also reduces recurrent nephrolithiasis, such as increased fluid intake and avoiding calcium restriction in the diet. High doses of thiazide diuretics are often necessary to reduce hypercalcemia; therefore, it is prudent that patients undergo serial monitoring to assess for potential side effects, including hyponatremia, hypokalemia, and hyperuricemia. Finally, sodium bicarbonate should be avoided in patients with renal tubular acidosis given the increased hypercalciuria associated with sodium-containing therapy. Potassium citrate or potassium bicarbonate should be used to treat associated metabolic acidosis and hypocitraturia.

Future Directions

There have been many advances in the surgical management of nephrolithiasis, including improved ability to access the different areas of the kidney by creation of smaller-caliber endoscopes and improved ureteral access sheaths, leading to less trauma of the ureter. Although surgical therapy continues to play a major role in management of nephrolithiasis, further research in the pathologic mechanisms determining stone formation may provide insights into additional treatment options. Measurement of crystal surface adhesion forces in stone formers may aid the design of agents that can block crystal aggregation. Other areas that require further research include the role of crystal-binding molecules such as hyaluronan in crystal retention and growth.

Additional Resources

Bushinsky DA: Nephrolithiasis. J Am Soc Nephrol 9(5):917-924, 1998.
This comprehensive review of nephrolithiasis includes pathophysiology, etiology, and treatment guidelines.
Coll DM, Varanelli MJ, Smith RC: Relationship of spontaneous passage of ureteral calculi to stone size and location as revealed by unenhanced helical CT. AJR Am J Roentgenol 178:101-103, 2002.
The prospective study analyzed the rate of stone passage depending on stone size and location.
Curhan GC, Willett WC, Rimm EB, Stampfer MJ: Family history and risk of kidney stones. J Am Soc Nephrol 8:1568-1573, 1997.
The authors report on a study of the significance of family history on kidney stone formation in a cohort.
Parks JH, Coe FL: Pathogenesis and treatment of calcium stones. Semin Nephrol 16(5):398-411, 1996.
The authors review nephrolithiasis with a focus on specific treatments aimed toward the specific stone type and underlying etiology.

EVIDENCE

1. Borghi L, Schianchi T, Meschi T, et al: Comparison of two diets for the prevention of recurrent stones in idiopathic hypercalciuria. N Engl J Med 346(2):77-84, 2002.
This randomized trial compared the effects of a low-calcium diet with those of a normal-calcium, low-protein, low-sodium diet in patients with recurrent calcium stones. The trial demonstrated the benefit of a normal-calcium, low-protein, and low-sodium diet in decreasing the incidence of recurrent nephrolithiasis.
2. Chen MY, Zagoria RJ, Saunders HS, Dyer RB: Trends in the use of unenhanced helical CT for acute urinary colic. AJR Am J Roentgenol 173(6):1447-1450, 1999.
This prospective study evaluated the potential uses of unenhanced helical CT in evaluating patients with typical renal colic and unspecified flank pain and verified the accuracy of uncontrasted CT for detection of nephrolithiasis.
3. Moe OW: Kidney stones: Pathophysiology and medical management. Lancet 367(9507):333-344, 2006.
This in-depth review of nephrolithiasis concentrates on the pathophysiology and management of the disease. The authors focus on advances in genetics, medical and surgical interventions, and potential directions for further therapeutic options.
4. Monk RD: Clinical approach to adults. Semin Nephrol 16(5):375-388, 1996.
The author presents a systematic review of the evaluation and medical treatment of nephrolithiasis.
5. Pearle M, Roehrborn C, Pak CYC: Meta-analysis of randomized trials for medical prevention of calcium oxalate nephrolithiasis. J Endourol 13(9):679-685, 1999.
An analysis of 14 randomized, controlled trials investigated drug therapy for the prevention of renal stone recurrence. Drug therapy significantly reduced recurrent stone disease.
6. Verkoelen CF: Crystal retention in renal stone disease: A crucial role for glycosaminoglycan hyaluronan? J Am Soc Nephrol 17(6):1673-1687, 2006.
The author discusses various proposed mechanisms involved in the development of nephrolithiasis.

Chronic Kidney Disease

Introduction

Chronic kidney disease (CKD) is a common diagnosis, affecting about 12% of the U.S. population. CKD is broadly defined as the presence of renal dysfunction for longer than 3 months and is classified according to the degree of functional impairment in the glomerular filtration rate (GFR) (Table 139-1). Patients with a normal GFR who have persistent urinary sediment abnormalities, abnormal kidney structure as documented radiographically, or abnormal renal biopsies are categorized as having stage 1 CKD. The serum creatinine concentration alone is frequently a misleading indicator of GFR, a fact that has led to the routine use of equations such as the Modification of Diet in Renal Disease (MDRD) and the Cockcroft-Gault equations. These should be routinely used when estimating renal function from the serum creatinine concentration (Table 139-2).

The number of patients with stage 5 CKD (end-stage renal disease [ESRD]) continues to grow in the United States, with a total prevalent population of 452,957 patients as of 2003. About 45% of incident ESRD patients have diabetes mellitus. About 70% of the ESRD patients are maintained on dialysis, whereas only about 30% have a functioning transplant. The annual incidence rates of stage 5 CKD appear to be stabilizing following 15 years of a steady increase, possibly as a result of efforts to delay progression of CKD with measures such as the treatment of hypertension. Spending for the ESRD program continues to grow, accounting for about 7% of all Medicare expenditures. The aging of the population and the growing burden of diabetes mellitus have had a significant impact on the increasing prevalence of ESRD, which has a projected prevalence of 2.24 million in the United States by 2030. Cardiovascular disease is the most important cause of mortality and morbidity in patients with CKD. Life expectancy for ESRD patients is only 16% to 37% of that of age-, gender- and race-matched controls. It is hoped that this can be improved with earlier detection of CKD, permitting aggressive risk factor modification and timely treatment of complications.

Etiology and Pathogenesis

Prevalent causes of ESRD in 2003 according to the U.S. Renal Data System were as follows:

Diabetes mellitus (36.2%)
Hypertension (24.5%)
Glomerulonephritis (19.9%)
Cystic, hereditary, or congenital (6.7%)
Interstitial nephritis (4.7%)
Neoplasms or tumors (0.9%)
Miscellaneous or uncertain causes (7.1%)

Renal function inexorably declines once the GFR has fallen below about 50 mL/min/1.73 m² of body surface area. In the Modification of Diet in Renal Disease (MDRD) study, 85% of patients with nondiabetic renal disease demonstrated a persistent decline in GFR averaging 4 mL/minute/year. The decline in GFR in patients with untreated diabetic nephropathy approaches 12 mL/minute/year. Several common pathologic and physiologic factors have been identified in all patients with CKD regardless of the cause of the initial insult. Intraglomerular hypertension, afferent arteriolar vasodilation, and decreased extracellular matrix turnover driven in part by increased angiotensin II interact to promote glomerular and vascular sclerosis, tubulointerstitial fibrosis, and progressive nephron loss. Studies have demonstrated that angiotensin-converting enzyme (ACE) inhibitors and angiotensin receptor blockers (ARBs) not only reduce blood pressure but also decrease intraglomerular hypertension and tubulointerstitial fibrosis. These drugs have been shown to attenuate and in some cases halt progression of renal failure and to reduce mortality.

Table 139-1 Stages of Chronic Kidney Disease

Stage	Description	GFR, mL/min per 1.73 m^2	Action
1	Kidney damage with normal or increased GFR	≥90	Treatment of comorbid conditions; slowing progression; cardiovascular disease risk reduction
2	Kidney damage with mild decreased GFR	60-89	Estimating progression
3	Kidney damage with moderate decreased GFR	30-59	Evaluating and treating complications
4	Severely decreased GFR	15-29	Preparation for renal replacement therapy
5	Kidney failure	<15	Renal replacement therapy

GFR, glomerular filtration rate.
Modified from National Kidney Foundation: K/DOQI clinical practice guidelines for chronic kidney disease: Evaluation, classification, and stratification. Kidney Disease Outcome Quality Initiative. Am J Kidney Dis 39:S1-S266, 2002.

Table 139-2 Methods for Calculating Creatinine Clearance and Estimated Glomerular Filtration Rate

Method	Equation
Cockcroft-Gault (conventional units)	$C_{cr} \text{ (mL/min)} = \dfrac{(140 - \text{age}\{yr\}) \times \text{weight}\{kg\} \times (0.85 \text{ if female})}{72 \times S_{cr}\{mg/dL\}}$
Cockcroft-Gault (SI units)	$C_{cr} \text{ (mL/min)} = \dfrac{(140 - \text{age}\{yr\}) \times \text{weight}\{kg\} \times (0.85 \text{ if female})}{S_{cr}\{\mu mol/L\}}$
Four-variable MDRD equation (conventional units)	$\text{eGFR (mL/min/1.73 m}^2) = 175 \times (S_{cr}\{mg/dL\})^{-1.154} \times (\text{age } \{yr\})^{-0.203} \times (0.742 \text{ if female}) \times (1.21 \text{ if black})$
Four-variable MDRD equation (SI units)	$\text{eGFR (mL/min/1.73 m}^2) = 175 \times (S_{cr}\{\mu mol/L\}/88.4)^{-1.154} \times (\text{age } \{yr\})^{-0.203} \times (0.742 \text{ if female}) \times (1.21 \text{ if black})$

C$_{cr}$, creatinine clearance; eGFR, estimated glomerular filtration rate; MDRD, Modification of Diet in Renal Disease; S$_{cr}$, serum creatinine concentration; SI, standardized international.

Cardiovascular Disease in Chronic Kidney Disease

Excess cardiovascular risk has been well documented in patients with ESRD and is believed to be mediated in part by a proinflammatory state. The prevalence of elevated C-reactive protein levels in hemodialysis patients is about 50%. Factors that may contribute to this proinflammatory state include decreased renal clearance of inflammatory cytokines, metabolic acidosis, increased oxidant stress, and volume overload. Other factors, including effects of the hemodialysis membrane and dialysate contamination with bacterial products such as lipopolysaccharide, may also account for accelerated atherosclerosis in ESRD patients on hemodialysis. Recently, the role of altered calcium-phosphorus metabolism has gained considerable attention as a significant risk factor in cardiovascular disease and mortality. Elevated serum concentrations of both calcium and phosphorus contribute to increased vascular calcification and have been associated with higher mortality rates in the ESRD population.

Excess cardiovascular disease burden has been demonstrated in patients with CKD before the onset of ESRD. Traditional risk factors such as hypertension and dyslipidemia, as well as nontraditional risk factors such as vascular calcification and chronic inflammation, have been implicated to explain the observed excess mortality. ACE inhibitors, ARBs, and statins have been found to partially ameliorate the microinflammatory state of CKD. The effects of aspirin and antioxidants such as vitamin E have been less convincing.

Clinical Presentation

Clinical features of CKD vary depending on the underlying cause and stage of the kidney disease. Patients with incipient diabetic nephropathy may present with asymptomatic microalbuminuria, whereas those with advanced nephropathy associated with nephrotic-range proteinuria are often edematous with evidence of retinopathy and neuropathy. Patients with ischemic renal disease frequently have bruits over the renal arteries, as well as in other vascular beds. CKD is often diagnosed in the clinical evaluation of hypertension, and it is worth noting that renal parenchymal disease remains the leading cause of secondary hypertension. Patients with adult polycystic kidney disease can present with abdominal masses and hypertension. The family history will indicate an autosomal dominant pattern of inheritance. Many patients present with nonspecific symptoms of fatigue due to progressive anemia and azotemia. Unfortunately, the symptoms and clinical findings of CKD are often subtle and go unnoticed until the GFR decreases to 5 to 10 mL/minute, at which point the uremic syndrome (Box 139-1) becomes apparent, and renal replacement therapy (RRT) is necessary to maintain life.

Differential Diagnosis and Diagnostic Approach

The etiology of CKD is often apparent after obtaining a careful history and performing a detailed physical examination (Box 139-2; Fig. 139-1). Patients with longstanding diabetes mellitus and hypertension with clinical evidence of end-organ damage in other vascular beds such as retinopathy have a high likelihood of diabetic nephropathy. The evaluation of patients with CKD should begin with a detailed examination of the urinary sediment as well as renal ultrasonography (Fig. 139-2). Serologic studies such as antinuclear antibodies, serum complement levels, and protein electrophoresis are particularly helpful in patients presenting with systemic vasculitis, proteinuria, or hematuria. Nephrologic consultation and renal biopsy are often required in these cases to arrive at a specific diagnosis.

Management and Therapy

Optimal Treatment

Treatment of CKD patients starts disease-specific therapy. Immunosuppressive therapy should be started when indicated in patients with lupus nephritis. Attention should be paid to glycemic control in patients with diabetes mellitus. Intensified glycemic control delays or prevents progression from normal urinary albumin excretion to microalbuminuria, clinical proteinuria, and overt nephropathy. The hemoglobin A1C should ideally be maintained close to 6%.

Aggressive control of cardiovascular risk factors such as dyslipidemia should be initiated from the outset in all CKD patients. The low-density lipoprotein cholesterol should be maintained at less than 100 mg/dL (2.6 mmol/L), or less than 80 mg/dL (2 mmol/L) if atherosclerosis is present or suspected. Other recommendations include discontinuation of tobacco products, avoidance of nephrotoxic agents such as nonsteroidal anti-inflammatory

---

Box 139-1   Uremic Syndrome: Clinical Alterations

Nervous System
Stupor, coma
Polyneuritis
Fatigue
Seizures
Dementia
Motor weakness
Malaise
Asterixis
Sleep disturbances
Headache
Cramps
Restless legs

Gastrointestinal System
Stomatitis
Nausea, vomiting
Gastritis
Ulcers
Anorexia

Hematologic System
Anemia
Bleeding

Cardiovascular System
Pericarditis
Hypertension
Atherosclerosis
Cardiomyopathy
Edema
Diastolic dysfunction

Pulmonary System
Pleuritis
Pulmonary edema
Uremic lung

Skin
Pruritus
Melanosis
Retarded wound healing
Nail atrophy

Bone Disease
Osteodystrophy
Amyloidosis
Hyperparathyroidism
Adynamic bone disease

Miscellaneous
Thirst
Uremic fetor
Weight loss
Hypothermia
Erectile dysfunction

Adapted from Greenberg A, Coffman TM, Cheung AK, et al: Uremic syndrome: Clinical alterations. In Primer on Kidney Disease, 3rd ed. Philadelphia, Elsevier, 2001, p 392.

Box 139-2	Differential Diagnosis of Chronic Kidney Disease

A. Diabetic Kidney Disease

B. Nondiabetic Kidney Disease
Glomerular Disease
- Autoimmune
- Systemic infection
- Myeloma-related glomerular disease

Vascular Disease
- Hypertensive nephrosclerosis
- Ischemic renal disease

Tubulointerstitial Disease
- Nephrosclerosis
- Chronic urinary tract obstruction
- Chronic interstitial nephritis
- Severe ischemic or nephrotoxic tubular injury
- Myeloma cast nephropathy

Cystic Disease
- Autosomal dominant polycystic kidney disease
- Medullary cystic disease

Structural Abnormality
- Renal dysplasia
- Obstructive nephropathy

drugs, cyclooxygenase-2 inhibitors, and iodinated radiocontrast.

Treatment of Hypertension

Control of blood pressure is the single most important therapeutic intervention currently available to retard the progression of CKD. The blood pressure should ideally be maintained at less than 130/80 mm Hg, with a goal of less than 120/80 mm Hg for patients with greater than 1 g of daily urinary protein excretion. ACE inhibitors or ARBs are preferred, especially in patients with proteinuria. Diabetic patients with microalbuminuria should be treated with ACE inhibitors or ARBs even when the blood pressure is in the normal range. Up to a 30% increase in the serum creatinine is acceptable after initiation of ACE inhibitors or ARBs. One study demonstrated sustained renoprotective benefit of continued ACE inhibitor therapy in patients with stage 3 and 4 CKD, and thus ACE inhibitors should be continued in patients with CKD whenever possible. Once-daily dosing of a low-dose ACE inhibitor or ARB should initially be employed to limit the risk for hyperkalemia. The serum potassium and serum creatinine concentration should be measured every 7 to 10 days during the initial dose titration and then every 2 to 3 months.

Most patients with advanced CKD generally require at least two to three agents to achieve blood pressure goals. Preferred agents (Fig. 139-3) should be added initially in a stepwise fashion. Therapy may also need to be tailored to individual patient needs, such as β blockade in the patient with angina. Patients with persistent proteinuria greater than 500 mg/day despite control of hypertension may benefit from combination ACE inhibitor and ARB therapy.

Correction of Anemia

Most patients with stage 3 to 4 CKD develop normocytic and normochromic anemia due to reduced erythropoietin production. Anemia is a risk factor for the development of left ventricular hypertrophy, hospitalization, and worsened cardiovascular outcomes in patients with CKD. Correction of anemia in patients with CKD has been demonstrated to improve quality of life. Recombinant erythropoietin or darbepoetin should be considered for patients with hemoglobin levels less than 11 g/dL (110 g/L), with a goal of maintaining the hemoglobin in the 11 to 12 g/dL (110 to 120 g/L) range. Care should be taken to avoid hemoglobin levels above 13 g/dL (130 g/L) owing to an associated increased risk of cardiovascular events. Patients should also receive concurrent iron supplementation.

Calcium, Phosphorus, and Bone Metabolism

As the GFR decreases to less than 60 to 80 mL/min, the excretion of phosphorus decreases, leading to hyperphosphatemia. This results in a transient decrease in the serum calcium that is exacerbated by decreased calcium absorption as a result of low levels of 1,25-dihydroxyvitamin D. Hypocalcemia, hyperphosphatemia, and decreased 1,25-dihydroxyvitamin D all lead to secondary hyperparathyroidism. Although increased parathyroid hormone (PTH) restores the serum calcium concentration to the normal range, it does so at the expense of increased bone turnover. Persistent untreated hyperparathyroidism leads to a distinct form of bone disease characterized by increased bone turnover and fibrosis termed *osteitis fibrosa cystica* (Fig. 139-4). Once established, this bone disorder is essentially irreversible. Prevention, therefore, remains the best therapeutic strategy.

Treatment of secondary hyperparathyroidism previously relied on the use of calcium-based phosphate binders and vitamin D analogues. There has been a growing concern about the risk for arterial calcification in patients with CKD treated with calcium-based phosphate binders and vitamin D analogues. Vitamin D analogues also have the untoward effect of increasing phosphate absorption and worsening hyperphosphatemia. Studies have demonstrated an association, albeit not a causal one, between serum phosphorus levels greater than 3.5 mg/dL (1.13 mmol/L) and increased cardiovascular mortality.

Dietary phosphorus restriction is generally not effective in preventing hyperphosphatemia, and therefore oral phosphate binders such as calcium carbonate or acetate,

Figure 139-1 Etiology of Chronic Renal Failure.

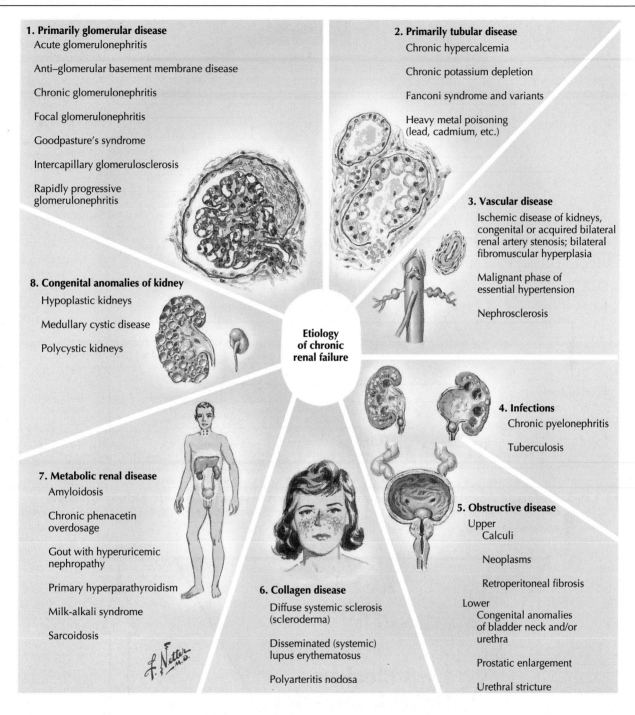

1. Primarily glomerular disease
  Acute glomerulonephritis

  Anti–glomerular basement membrane disease

  Chronic glomerulonephritis

  Focal glomerulonephritis

  Goodpasture's syndrome

  Intercapillary glomerulosclerosis

  Rapidly progressive
  glomerulonephritis

8. Congenital anomalies of kidney
  Hypoplastic kidneys

  Medullary cystic disease

  Polycystic kidneys

7. Metabolic renal disease
  Amyloidosis

  Chronic phenacetin
  overdosage

  Gout with hyperuricemic
  nephropathy

  Primary hyperparathyroidism

  Milk-alkali syndrome

  Sarcoidosis

6. Collagen disease
  Diffuse systemic sclerosis
  (scleroderma)

  Disseminated (systemic)
  lupus erythematosus

  Polyarteritis nodosa

**Etiology
of chronic
renal failure**

2. Primarily tubular disease
  Chronic hypercalcemia

  Chronic potassium depletion

  Fanconi syndrome and variants

  Heavy metal poisoning
  (lead, cadmium, etc.)

3. Vascular disease
  Ischemic disease of kidneys,
  congenital or acquired bilateral
  renal artery stenosis; bilateral
  fibromuscular hyperplasia

  Malignant phase of
  essential hypertension

  Nephrosclerosis

4. Infections
  Chronic pyelonephritis

  Tuberculosis

5. Obstructive disease
  Upper
    Calculi

    Neoplasms

    Retroperitoneal fibrosis

  Lower
    Congenital anomalies
    of bladder neck and/or
    urethra

    Prostatic enlargement

    Urethral stricture

sevelamer, and lanthanum carbonate are usually necessary. When calcium-based binders are used, the total dose of elemental calcium should not exceed 2000 mg/day in order to avoid positive calcium balance. Oral vitamin D analogues such as calcitriol, doxercalciferol, and paracalcitol can be administered to suppress PTH secretion and retard the development of renal bone disease. The goal of therapy is to maintain intact parathyroid hormone levels at 35 to 70 ng/L for patients with stage 3 disease, 70 to 110 ng/L in stage 4 disease, and 150 to 300 ng/L in stage 5 disease.

Careful monitoring, initially every 4 to 8 weeks, then quarterly, is important to prevent development of hypercalcemia or oversuppression of PTH. The serum calcium and phosphorus should be maintained at less than 9.5 mg/dL (2.37 mmol/L) and 4.7 mg/dL (1.52 mmol/L), respectively. Cinacalcet suppresses PTH secretion by acting primarily on the calcium-sensing receptor in the parathyroid glands and is effective in lowering the serum PTH and decreasing serum phosphorus concentrations in ESRD patients with secondary hyperparathyroidism. The role of

Figure 139-2 Diagnostic Evaluation of Chronic Kidney Disease.

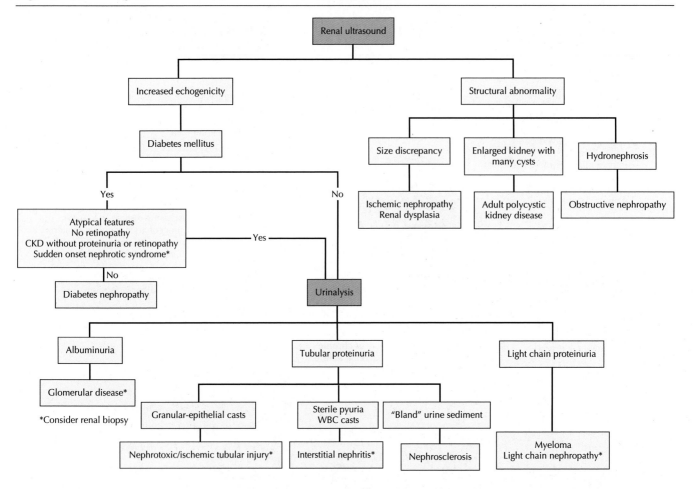

Figure 139-3 Preferred Agents for the Treatment of Hypertension in Chronic Kidney Disease. ARB, angiotensin receptor blocker; CCB, calcium channel blocker; ACE-I, angiotensin-converting enzyme inhibitor.

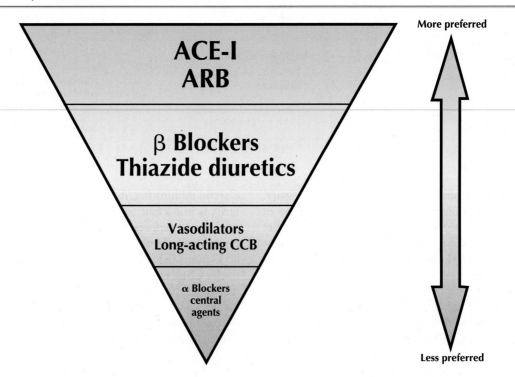

Figure 139-4 Vascular and Soft Tissue Calcification in Secondary Hyperparathyroidism of Chronic Renal Disease.

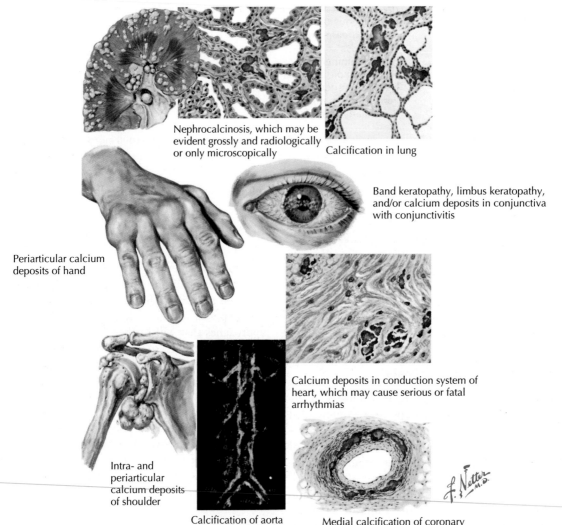

Nephrocalcinosis, which may be evident grossly and radiologically or only microscopically

Calcification in lung

Band keratopathy, limbus keratopathy, and/or calcium deposits in conjunctiva with conjunctivitis

Periarticular calcium deposits of hand

Intra- and periarticular calcium deposits of shoulder

Calcium deposits in conduction system of heart, which may cause serious or fatal arrhythmias

Calcification of aorta and/or other large vessels

Medial calcification of coronary and/or other small arteries

this agent in pre–ESRD CKD patients in optimizing bone and mineral metabolism remains to be determined pending further clinical trials.

Preparation for Renal Replacement Therapy

Discussions regarding the need for RRT and choice of modality should begin at least 1 year before the anticipated start of dialysis. The appropriate mode of dialysis should be determined as well as suitability for transplantation. Patients electing peritoneal dialysis (PD) should have a PD catheter inserted 3 to 4 weeks before the anticipated need for dialysis. Patients who choose hemodialysis should have a functioning, permanent vascular access at the time RRT is initiated. Native arteriovenous fistulas have excellent long-term patency rates and, compared with other forms of vascular access, are consistently associated with the lowest mortality risk. Fistula maturation occurs over several months, and patients should therefore be referred for fistula creation once the serum creatinine concentration is 4 mg/dL (305 μmol/L) or greater, or once GFR falls to less than 30 mL/min/1.73 m². Use of cephalic veins for phlebotomy or intravenous cannulation can prevent successful fistula placement. Thus, physicians caring for patients with chronic kidney failure must educate patients and medical personnel to strictly avoid venipuncture and intravenous cannulation above the level of the hands, particularly in the nondominant extremity. Peripherally inserted central catheters and subclavian catheters can also impair the creation or function of arteriovenous fistulas and are contraindicated in patients with CKD. When central venous access is required, the internal jugular site is preferred.

Table 139-3   Factors Influencing Decision of Timing of Initiation of Dialysis

Renal clearance	Creatinine clearance <15 mL/min/1.73 m²
	Urea clearance <8 mL/min/1.73 m²
Nutritional status	Spontaneous dietary protein intake <0.8 gm/kg/day (can be estimated based on 24-hr urine urea nitrogen excretion)*
	Weight loss
	Hypoalbuminemia
Congestive heart failure	Not amenable to usual medical interventions
Uremic symptoms	Nausea, dysgeusia, cognitive impairment, pruritus
Uremic complications	Pericarditis, peripheral neuropathy, acidosis, hyperkalemia
Quality of life considerations	Particularly in the elderly

*Estimated dietary protein intake = 6.25 (daily urinary urea nitrogen [g] + {30 mg/kg × weight [kg]/1000 mg/g}).

Kidney transplantation remains the treatment of choice for most patients with ESRD. Outcomes with transplantation are more favorable in all groups when compared with dialysis, with diabetic patients gaining the greatest survival advantage through transplantation. Patient and allograft survival advantages have been demonstrated for preemptive transplantation and for transplantations performed after shorter periods of dialysis. This highlights the importance of early referral of patients with progressive CKD to facilitate timely identification of potential living donors.

Timing of Initiation of Dialysis

The National Kidney Foundation Kidney Disease Outcomes Quality Initiative work group has recommended that RRT be considered when the renal clearance of creatinine falls to less than 15 mL/min/1.73 m². This level of renal function generally precedes the onset of uremic complications. RRT can be delayed, however, in patients with stable edema-free body weight and nutritional status, and complete absence of clinical signs or symptoms attributable to uremia. The early-start approach was initially advocated to improve mortality, but subsequent studies have shown no evidence to support this hypothesis. Other factors such as nutritional status and quality of life clearly need to be weighed in decisions regarding the timing of dialysis initiation (Table 139-3). Generally, younger patients and those with diabetes mellitus have the greatest benefit from earlier initiation of dialysis.

Avoiding Treatment Errors

Every effort should be made to initiate and continue ACE inhibitor or ARB therapy throughout the course of progressive CKD. Hyperkalemia can often be minimized by using these agents once daily in conjunction with dietary potassium restriction and loop diuretics. Hemoglobin levels should be monitored at least monthly in patients receiving erythropoietin or darbepoetin to permit appropriate titration of these agents to the target range. Every time a serum creatinine concentration is measured, GFR should be estimated to facilitate appropriate and timely initiation of interventions such as placement of vascular access.

Future Directions

Although considerable advances have been made in understanding mechanisms leading to CKD, future research is required to further elucidate the pathogenesis of progressive nephron loss. It is hoped that this will lead to new approaches that will further retard loss of renal function. The pathogenesis of accelerated cardiovascular disease needs to be further characterized in CKD populations to help identify new therapeutic strategies. The management of mineral and bone metabolism is in evolution, and the optimal therapeutic approach remains to be determined. Competing concerns of abnormal bone metabolism must be balanced with adverse cardiovascular outcomes. Finally, the impact of cardiovascular screening and interventions needs to be studied in CKD populations with the hope of ultimately decreasing excess cardiovascular mortality.

Additional Resources

Levey AS, Coresh J, Balk E, et al: National Kidney Foundation practice guidelines for chronic kidney disease: Evaluation, classification, and stratification. Ann Intern Med 139:137-147, 2003.
   This is an excellent summary of the National Kidney Foundation clinical practice guidelines.
National Kidney Disease Education Program. Available at: http://www.nkdep.nih.gov/professionals/gfr_calculators/idms_con.htm.
   This website provides a tool for calculating estimated GFR using the MDRD equation.
National Kidney Foundation—Kidney Disease Outcomes Quality Initiative Clinical Practice Guidelines. Available at: http://www.kidney.org/professionals/kdoqi/guidelines.cfm.
   This website provides the most comprehensive and updated compilation of practice guidelines for CKD patients.

EVIDENCE

1. Brenner BM, Cooper ME, de Zeeuw D, et al; the RENAAL Study Investigators. Effects of losartan on renal and cardiovascular outcomes in patients with type 2 diabetes and nephropathy. N Engl J Med 345:861-869, 2001.

This well-designed randomized placebo-controlled trial demonstrated the renoprotective effect of losartan beyond the effect of hypertension control.

2. Go AS, Chertow GM, Fan D, et al: Chronic kidney disease and the risks of death, cardiovascular events, and hospitalization. N Engl J Med 351:1296-1305, 2004.

   This article underscores the importance of progressive CKD as an independent risk factor for increased mortality and cardiovascular events.

3. Kestenbaum B, Sampson JN, Rudser KD, et al: Serum phosphate levels and mortality risk among people with chronic kidney disease. J Am Soc Nephrol 16:520-528, 2005.

   The authors present evidence for an association between increased serum phosphorus levels and mortality in the pre–end-stage kidney disease population.

4. Klahr S, Levey AS, Beck GJ, et al: The effects of dietary protein restriction and blood-pressure control on the progression of chronic renal disease. Modification of Diet in Renal Disease Study Group. N Engl J Med 330:877-884, 1994.

   This large, well-designed trial did not document benefit of protein restriction on decreasing the rate of progressive renal failure; it is best known for validation of the MDRD equation for estimation of GFR in the CKD population.

5. Lewis EJ, Hunsicker LG, Bain RP, Rhode RD: The effect of angiotensin-converting enzyme inhibition on diabetic nephropathy. The Collaborative Study Group. N Engl J Med 329:1456-1462, 1993.

   This classic study demonstrated the salutary effects of ACE inhibitors in treating type 1 diabetes with overt nephropathy.

6. Nakao N, Yoshimura A, Morita H, et al: Combination treatment of angiotensin-II receptor blocker and angiotensin-converting-enzyme inhibitor in non-diabetic renal disease (COOPERATE): A randomised controlled trial. Lancet 361:117-124, 2003.

   This was the first well-designed clinical trial documenting that combination therapy with an ACE inhibitor and an ARB may be superior to either agent alone in slowing progressive renal failure in nondiabetic kidney disease.

7. National Kidney Foundation K/DOQI clinical practice guidelines for chronic kidney disease: Evaluation, classification, and stratification. Kidney Disease Outcome Quality Initiative. Am J Kidney Dis 39:S1-S266, 2002.

   This paper includes comprehensive evidence-based clinical practice guidelines for CKD patients.

8. Ruggenenti P, Fassi A, Ilieva AP, et al; the Bergamo Nephrologic Diabetes Complications Trial (BENEDICT) Investigators: Preventing microalbuminuria in type 2 diabetes. N Engl J Med 351:1941-1951, 2004.

   ACE inhibitors were shown to prevent onset of microalbuminuria in diabetic patients with hypertension and normoalbuminuria. It was not clear, however, whether this was due to an effect of the ACE inhibitor or to better blood pressure control in the ACE inhibitor group.

9. United States Renal Data System (USRDS) 2006 Annual Report. Atlas of End-Stage Renal Disease in the United States. Bethesda, National Institutes of Health, National Institute of Diabetes and Digestive and Kidney Diseases, Division of Kidney, Urologic and Hematologic Diseases, 2006. Available at: http://www.usrds.org/2006/ref/H_morte_06.pdf. Accessed September 23, 2006.

   This is the most complete and authoritative database for characteristics and outcomes of CKD and end-stage kidney disease patients in the United States.

William F. Finn

Acute Kidney Injury

Introduction

The term *acute renal failure* has been applied to a variety of situations in which the function of the kidneys declines over a period of hours to days. In the most severe cases, this leads to a prolonged increase in plasma concentrations of urea and creatinine, disruption of fluid and electrolyte balance, abnormalities in acid-base metabolism, and impairment of renal endocrine function.

There are many instances, however, in which there is a less severe impairment of renal function without overt failure. It is now known that even a minor elevation in the serum creatinine concentration (S_{Cr}) has a negative impact on both short-term and long-term mortality. Consequently, the term *acute kidney injury* (AKI) is now considered more appropriate, with further separation into stages depending on its severity (Table 140-1).

The actual incidence of AKI is difficult to determine because of the ambiguity in the definition of AKI itself. One definition considers renal function to be compromised with a more than 25% increase in S_{Cr} or an increase of 0.5 mg/dL. An increase in S_{Cr} of 50% or more above baseline or 1.0 mg/dL indicates serious renal impairment.

AKI that is hospital acquired may affect 5% of all inpatients; ischemic injury and exposure to nephrotoxic agents are the leading causes. AKI occurs in a much higher percentage of patients in intensive care units. When dialysis is necessary in these patients, the mortality rate exceeds 50%. AKI also may be community acquired, with alterations in systemic hemodynamics and urinary tract obstruction leading the list of causes. In all cases, the most susceptible patients are those with chronic kidney disease (CKD), with the risk increasing as the CKD worsens.

Etiology and Pathogenesis

AKI is often classified as prerenal, postrenal, or intrinsic, which is in turn further categorized on the basis of the proximate cause of the renal injury. Each of these conditions has different mechanisms of injury.

Prerenal Acute Kidney Injury

Prerenal AKI is marked by a reduction in the glomerular filtration rate (GFR) due to a disturbance in systemic or renal hemodynamics. Absolute volume depletion in severe dehydration, blood loss, or septic shock is a frequent cause of prerenal AKI. In other circumstances, there is a functional rather than an absolute decrease in the effective blood volume that leads to acute changes in renal function. In situations such as decompensated liver disease or congestive heart failure, the picture is complicated by an increase in renal vascular resistance (RVR) that results in a decrease in renal blood flow (RBF) and GFR.

In advanced liver disease, the fall in GFR may decline to such an extent that renal replacement therapy (RRT) with dialysis is necessary. This often is an indication of the development of the hepatorenal syndrome (Fig. 140-1). Overall prognosis is poor unless the liver failure resolves or liver transplantation occurs. Prerenal AKI may develop in individuals with congestive heart failure as the combined result of a decrease in cardiac output and an increase in RVR. Prerenal AKI may also complicate therapy with certain medications, especially diuretics, angiotensin-converting enzyme inhibitors, and nonsteroidal anti-inflammatory drugs. In these situations, the kidney is responding to an altered internal environment. However, if the decrease in RBF is severe or prolonged, ischemic injury may occur.

Table 140-1 Classification and Staging System for Acute Kidney Injury

Stage	Creatinine Criteria	Urine Output Criteria
1	Increase serum creatinine ≥0.3 mg/dL (≥26.4 μmol) or increase to ≥150% to 200% from baseline	<0.5 mL/kg/hr for >6 hr
2	Increase serum creatinine to >200% to 300% (>2- to 3-fold) from baseline	<0.5 mL/kg/hr for >12 hr
3	Increase serum creatinine to >300% (>3-fold) from baseline or serum creatinine ≥4.0 mg/dL (≥354 μmol/L) with an acute rise of at least 0.5 mg/dL	<0.3 mL/kg/hr × 24 hr or anuria × 2 hr

Figure 140-1 Kidney Injury in Liver Disease.

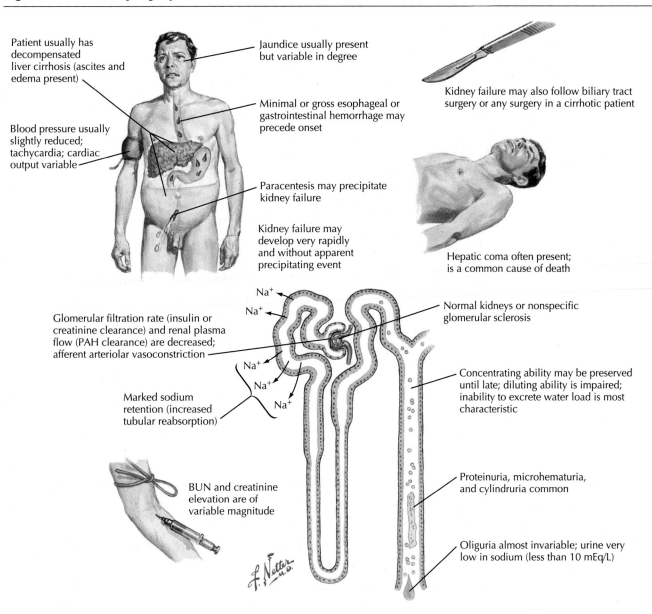

Patient usually has decompensated liver cirrhosis (ascites and edema present)

Blood pressure usually slightly reduced; tachycardia; cardiac output variable

Jaundice usually present but variable in degree

Minimal or gross esophageal or gastrointestinal hemorrhage may precede onset

Paracentesis may precipitate kidney failure

Kidney failure may develop very rapidly and without apparent precipitating event

Kidney failure may also follow biliary tract surgery or any surgery in a cirrhotic patient

Hepatic coma often present; is a common cause of death

Glomerular filtration rate (insulin or creatinine clearance) and renal plasma flow (PAH clearance) are decreased; afferent arteriolar vasoconstriction

Marked sodium retention (increased tubular reabsorption)

BUN and creatinine elevation are of variable magnitude

Normal kidneys or nonspecific glomerular sclerosis

Concentrating ability may be preserved until late; diluting ability is impaired; inability to excrete water load is most characteristic

Proteinuria, microhematuria, and cylindruria common

Oliguria almost invariable; urine very low in sodium (less than 10 mEq/L)

Figure 140-2 Obstructive Uropathy: Etiology.

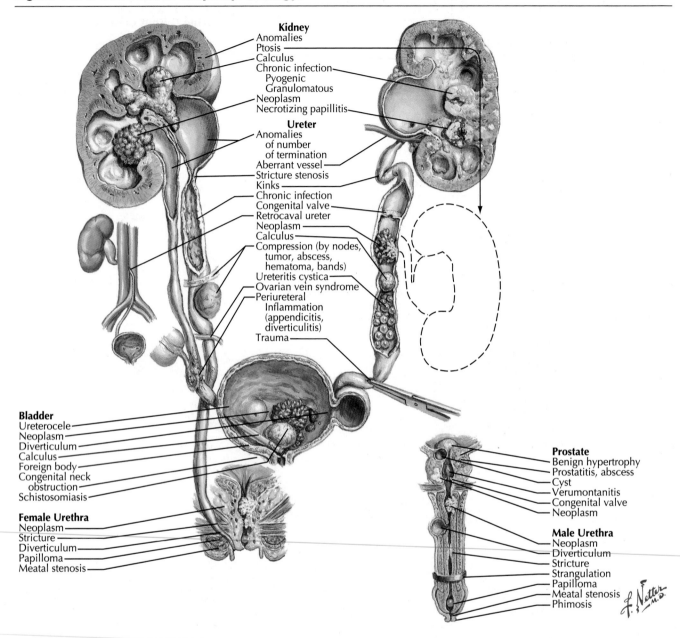

Kidney
Anomalies
Ptosis
Calculus
Chronic infection
  Pyogenic
  Granulomatous
Neoplasm
Necrotizing papillitis

Ureter
Anomalies
  of number
  of termination
Aberrant vessel
Stricture stenosis
Kinks
Chronic infection
Congenital valve
Retrocaval ureter
Neoplasm
Calculus
Compression (by nodes,
  tumor, abscess,
  hematoma, bands)
Ureteritis cystica
Ovarian vein syndrome
Periureteral
  Inflammation
  (appendicitis,
  diverticulitis)
Trauma

Bladder
Ureterocele
Neoplasm
Diverticulum
Calculus
Foreign body
Congenital neck
  obstruction
Schistosomiasis

Female Urethra
Neoplasm
Stricture
Diverticulum
Papilloma
Meatal stenosis

Prostate
Benign hypertrophy
Prostatitis, abscess
Cyst
Verumontanitis
Congenital valve
Neoplasm

Male Urethra
Neoplasm
Diverticulum
Stricture
Strangulation
Papilloma
Meatal stenosis
Phimosis

Postrenal Acute Kidney Injury

Postrenal AKI may result from obstruction at any point along the urinary tract system (Fig. 140-2) and is not an infrequent cause of AKI. Excluding individuals with solitary kidneys and those with significantly impaired renal function due to underlying renal parenchymal disease, ureteral obstruction must be bilateral to produce clinically apparent abnormalities. If the obstruction is partial, urine flow may remain normal as a result of elevated pressures proximal to the site of the obstruction. A calculus, mass lesion, or sloughed papilla in papillary necrosis may cause ureteral obstruction. Papillary necrosis may complicate sickle cell disease, diabetes mellitus, and excessive analgesic use. Urethral obstruction occurs more commonly in men with prostatic hypertrophy.

Intrinsic Acute Kidney Injury

The pathogenesis of AKI-associated ischemic and nephrotoxic injury is complex. In both ischemic and nephrotoxic AKI, renal tubular epithelial (RTE) cells are injured, and some may undergo necrosis or apoptosis. With severe tubular injury, debris accumulates within tubules and may obstruct fluid flow and compress adjacent peritubular capillaries. Necrosis of the tubular epithelium permits passage of filtrate into the renal interstitium. In most circum-

Figure 140-3 Hemolytic-Uremic Syndrome.

Intravascular coagulation, hemolytic-uremic syndrome, and thrombotic microangiopathy

Common electron microscopic findings: Deposits (D) and mesangial cell cytoplasmic processes (M) in the subendothelial space; endothelium (E) swollen; both mesangial (MC) and endothelial cells (EN) contain many vacuoles and dilated rough endoplasmic reticulum; lumen (L) narrowed (may be slit-like); red blood cells (RC) may or may not be present; basement membrane (B) often wrinkled; epithelial foot processes (F) partly fused

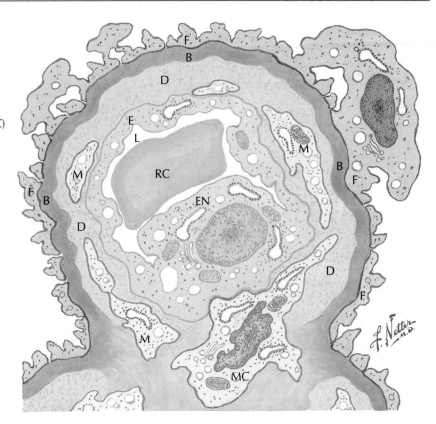

Clinical Presentation

The clinical course of AKI is highly variable, ranging from a transient, self-limited disturbance of kidney function to prolonged and often life-threatening renal failure. The classic pattern involves three phases: initial, maintenance, and recovery. The initial phase begins with a specific renal insult and continues until functional abnormalities of the kidney develop. The time from injury to renal impairment during the initial stage depends on the severity of the injury. Oliguria (urine volume <500 mL/day) or anuria (urine volume <100 mL/day) may accompany the maintenance phase. In some instances, however, the urine volume remains normal, although the quality of the urine is poor, the GFR is severely reduced, and the blood urea nitrogen (BUN) and S_{Cr} rise. Characteristically, the maintenance phase lasts for 10 to 14 days, depending on the nature of the renal injury, although longer courses have been described. The final phase of AKI is the recovery phase.

stances, there is an increase in RVR and decrease in RBF. Finally, the permeability of the glomerular capillary membranes may change, contributing to the AKI. The injured kidney has the capacity to recover. Recent studies indicate that it may be possible to influence the extent to which this occurs.

If the patient had been oliguric, there may be a dramatic increase in urine volume at a relatively constant rate, ranging anywhere from hours to days. The degree of the diuresis is dependent on the volume status of the individual and inversely related to the duration of the maintenance phase. In nonoliguric individuals, improvement in the quality rather than the quantity of the urine heralds recovery. Late in recovery, glomerular and tubular function is restored, and the renal function returns to or toward the preexisting level. The likelihood of complete renal recovery is influenced by many factors. Poor prognostic indicators include the presence of preexisting renal disease, advanced age at the onset of renal injury, and persistent oliguria. As many as 10% to 15% of individuals do not recover adequate renal function, and chronic kidney disease develops in up to one third of patients.

Differential Diagnosis

Ischemic injury and exposure to nephrotoxic agents account for a significant proportion of cases of AKI among the conditions that may precipitously disrupt renal function. Injury resulting in AKI may involve any or all of the histologic components of the kidney, including glomeruli, tubules, interstitium, and vasculature (Box 140-1).

Box 140-1 Causes of Acute Kidney Injury

Diseases of the Renal Vasculature

Renal artery occlusion
  Thromboemboli
  Atheroemboli
  Thrombosis
  Dissecting aortic aneurysm
  Renal artery stenosis
  Vasculitis
Renal vein thrombosis
  Dehydration (infants)
  Hypercoagulable state
  Neoplasms

Diseases of the Renal Cortex

Bilateral cortical necrosis
  Obstetrical accidents
  Abruptio placentae
  Placenta previa
Gram-negative septicemia
Ischemia
Hyperacute renal allograft rejection
Gastroenteritis (children)

Acute Tubulointerstitial Diseases

Acute pyelonephritis
Acute allergic interstitial nephritis
Hypokalemic nephropathy
Hypercalcemia
Acute uric acid nephropathy
Multiple myeloma

Acute Glomerular Diseases

Acute glomerulonephritis
  Postinfectious glomerulonephritis
  Bacterial endocarditis
  Henoch-Schönlein purpura
  Hypersensitivity angiitis
Rapidly progressive glomerulonephritis
  Systemic lupus erythematosus
  Wegener's granulomatosis
  Goodpasture's syndrome

Thrombotic Microangiopathy

Thrombotic thrombocytopenic purpura
Hemolytic-uremic syndrome
Scleroderma
Malignant hypertension

Diseases of the Renal Medulla

Bilateral papillary necrosis
Analgesic abuse
Sickle cell disease
Diabetes mellitus

Urinary Obstruction

Intrarenal abnormalities
Ureteral obstruction
Diseases of bladder or urethra

Postischemic Acute Kidney Injury

Nephrotoxic Acute Kidney Injury

Sustained episodes of prerenal AKI due to protracted decreases in arterial blood pressure and RBF may evolve into postischemic AKI, in which tubular injury predominates. With profound ischemia, glomerular damage and cortical necrosis may further complicate the clinical picture. Cortical necrosis can also result from intraglomerular microthrombi, as occurs with the hemolytic-uremic syndrome or other types of thrombotic microangiopathies (see Fig. 140-3). Other instances of postischemic AKI complicate severe crushing injuries from trauma, resulting in rhabdomyolysis and myoglobinuria. Nontraumatic rhabdomyolysis with AKI may occur as a side effect of prescription and nonprescription drugs, including cholesterol-lowering agents and cocaine. Heat stress can also precipitate rhabdomyolysis.

AKI is associated with hemolysis and hemoglobinuria. A number of substances (xenobiotics) have been identified as capable of producing significant renal injury. The most common agents causing nephrotoxic AKI are medications, including antibiotics, especially the aminoglycosides, antifungal and chemotherapeutic agents; diagnostic agents such as iodinated radiocontrast media; and environmental substances including organic solvents and heavy metals. Analgesics, certain antibiotics, and several diuretics may be associated with a diffuse acute interstitial nephritis that differs from postischemic and nephrotoxic AKI because of evidence of an allergic reaction. Less frequently intrinsic AKI develops in the setting of multiple myeloma where light chains and uric acid deposit in the renal tubules, resulting in cast nephropathy.

Diagnostic Approach

The diagnosis of AKI requires a careful and systematic approach to identifying and managing potentially reversible conditions. After a careful history and physical examination, urine and plasma measurements are useful for further investigation of the etiology. The urine examination includes a microscopic exam of the urinary sediment and electrolyte measurements. The urine sediment is typically normal in prerenal and postrenal AKI except for the presence of hyaline casts. In intrinsic AKI, the urine sediment is often quite active, with muddy brown granular casts, free RTE cells and casts, white blood cells, and red blood cells.

The urinary sodium concentration and osmolality help to differentiate prerenal failure from AKI due to intrinsic renal disease. In prerenal AKI, the fractional excretions of sodium (FE_{Na}) and urea are low, and the urinary osmolality and specific gravity are high. The urine-to-plasma creatinine ratio (U/P_{creat}) is generally above 20 : 1. In postischemic and nephrotoxic AKI, the urinary sodium is high, the urinary osmolality and specific gravity are closer to that of plasma and, the U/P_{creat} may be less than 20 : 1. Intrinsic AKI is associated with a high FE_{Na}, usually greater than

1% and often more than 3%, which helps to distinguish it from the prerenal causes of AKI. Plasma measurements of electrolytes, BUN, and S_{Cr} indicate the severity of the AKI. These may be accompanied by the appearance of tubular aquaporins and the sodium transporter NHE-3 in the urine.

Renal ultrasonography is highly recommended early in the evaluation of AKI because of the importance of diagnosing postrenal AKI quickly. Less commonly, plain radiographs of the abdomen are performed to look for urinary calculi. Renal biopsy is indicated if the diagnosis of the AKI is in question, if a systemic illness is suspected, and to help guide therapy.

Management and Therapy

Optimum Treatment

The management and therapy of AKI, once largely supportive, now requires more specific attention. To begin, for patients with underlying CKD, the risk for developing AKI requires assessment followed by appropriate actions to minimize the risk. The first step is to estimate the baseline GFR using the formula from the modification in diet renal disease study. The use of the S_{Cr} alone is not acceptable. The risk for AKI increases in stepwise fashion with CKD 3 (GFR 30 to 60 mL/min), CKD 4 (GFR 15 to 30 mL/min), and CKD 5 (GFR <15 mL/min). On this basis, the dose and dosing interval of nephrotoxic agents such as aminoglycoside antibiotics must be adjusted and deficiencies in intravascular volume or systemic hemodynamics corrected. The need for prophylaxis is most obvious in preventing contrast-induced nephropathy (CIN), the third most common cause of hospital-acquired renal failure. CIN develops in about 3% of the general population. The risk for CIN may be as high as 50% in at-risk patient subsets, including those with CKD, diabetes mellitus, or both. Although the decline in renal function is usually reversible, it is associated with an increase in mortality rates.

When AKI occurs, all potentially reversible causes require urgent identification and correction. In prerenal AKI, volume repletion to correct circulatory abnormalities will restore renal function. In all patients, the cessation of nephrotoxic agents is essential. For mild cases of AKI that fail to resolve quickly, conservative medical management is often all that is required. This includes careful monitoring of fluid and electrolyte intake, in addition to prescribing potassium-binding resins and sodium bicarbonate for non–life-threatening hyperkalemia and metabolic acidosis, respectively. For persistent oliguria following volume repletion, loop diuretics are commonly employed, although their use is not associated with improved mortality or renal recovery but may be associated with shorter duration of RRT. There is overwhelming evidence that there is no role for "renal-dose" or "low-dose" dopamine in the prevention

of AKI from any cause, nor does it affect the need for dialysis or mortality.

The use of RRT with either intermittent hemodialysis (IHD) or continuous renal replacement therapy (CRRT) is often essential. The use of CRRT may be associated with better renal recovery than IHD; however, mortality rates are similar. Based on published reports, daily IHD, as compared with alternate-day therapy, is associated with improved survival; nevertheless, the current recommendation is to perform dialysis at least three times per week and to monitor the adequacy of dialysis to ensure that clearance and ultrafiltration goals are achieved. Few parameters are helpful in predicting the severity or prognosis of AKI; however, a prompt diagnosis and an aggressive treatment strategy are mandatory to preserve renal function and to avoid serious complications.

Avoiding Treatment Errors

During the course of AKI, monitoring sequential changes in urine quality rather than urine volume is often more valuable. In this way, the recovery of tubular function may be observed by an increase in the U/P_{urea} ratio and a decrease in the FE_{Na}. At times, a delay in recovery is a result of the superimposition of a state of volume depletion due to overaggressive ultrafiltration and intravascular volume depletion. A fall in blood pressure in a patient with AKI is likely to result in a proportional fall in RBF because of an inability of the injured kidney to compensate by a reduction in RVR. To avoid additional injury, it is important to choose a dialysis modality that minimizes the risk for intradialytic hypotension. This should be part of an overall dialysis prescription, which should include a program of nutritional support. It is important to record the amount delivered versus that prescribed to avoid otherwise unrecognized underdialysis and malnutrition.

Future Directions

The continued high mortality rate in individuals with AKI and the failure of many who survive to recover normal renal function have placed considerable importance on understanding the mechanisms by which the kidney responds to injury. There is considerable interest in the development of one or more biomarkers to judge the events occurring within the kidney. These include kidney injury molecule-1 (KIM-1), neutrophil gelatinase-associated lipocalin (NGAL), and urine interleukin-18 (IL-18). The quest for a pharmacologic therapy that could improve survival has been largely unsuccessful. Additional insight into the details of the cell cycle and the application of the tools of molecular biology may eventually lead to the development of pharmacologic agents that protect the kidney from injury or promote its full recovery. Increasing evidence suggests that at least three mechanisms contribute to the regenerative capacity of the kidney. These include the ability of RTE cells to differentiate, proliferate, and repopulate the tubule; the possibility that specific renal progenitor stem cells within the kidney serve the same purpose; and the more recent data that bone marrow–derived stem cells may contribute to the regeneration of the renal parenchyma.

Additional Resources

Bell M, Granath F, Schön S, et al: Continuous renal replacement therapy is associated with less chronic renal failure than intermittent haemodialysis after acute renal failure. Intensive Care Med 33(5):773-780, 2007.

The authors suggest that recovery from AKI is improved with continuous versus intermittent hemodialysis.

Friedrich JO, Adhikari N, Herridge MS, Beyene J: Meta-analysis: Low-dose dopamine increases urine output but does not prevent renal dysfunction or death. Ann Intern Med 142(7):510-524, 2005.

The authors present definitive data concerning the controversial use of low-dose dopamine for AKI.

Kale S, Karihaloo A, Clark PR, et al: Bone marrow stem cells contribute to repair of the ischemically injured renal tubule. J Clin Invest 112(1):42-49, 2003.

This article introduces the concept that stem cells—in addition to tubular epithelial cells—contribute to the recovery from renal ischemic injury.

Kellum JA, Mehta RL, Angus DC, et al: ADQI Workgroup. The first international consensus conference on continuous renal replacement therapy. Kidney Int 62(5):1855-1863, 2002.

The authors discuss the indications for and advantages of continuous versus intermittent renal replacement therapy for AKI.

Nguyen MT, Devarajan P: Biomarkers for the early detection of acute kidney injury. Pediatr Nephrol, March 30, 2007 [ePub ahead of print].

This is an excellent discussion of the ideal properties of renal biomarkers with emphasis on NGAL, Cystatin C, KIM-1, and IL-18.

Schiffl H, Lang SM, Fischer R: Daily hemodialysis and the outcome of acute renal failure. N Engl J Med 346(5):305-310, 2002.

This article represents an early proponent of daily hemodialysis for AKI.

Trof RJ, Di Maggio F, Leenreis J, Groeneveld ABJ: Biomarkers of acute renal injury and renal failure. Shock 26:245-253, 2006.

This article presents an extensive review and categorization of a broad range of renal biomarkers with a discussion of the corresponding pathophysiology.

EVIDENCE

1. Bellomo R, Ronco C, Kellum JA, et al: Acute renal failure—definition, outcome measures, animal models, fluid therapy and information technology needs: The Second International Consensus Conference of the Acute Dialysis Quality Initiative (ADQI) Group. Crit Care 8(4):R204-R212, 2004.

   The authors provide consensus statements for the physiologic and clinical principles for defining acute renal failure, selection of animal models, methods of monitoring fluid therapy, and choice of physiologic and clinical end points for trials.

2. Chertow GM, Burdick E, Honour M, et al: Acute kidney injury, mortality, length of stay, and costs in hospitalized patients. J Am Soc Nephrol 16(11):3365-3370, 2005.

   The authors describe the effects of AKI on in-hospital mortality, length of stay, and costs associated with AKI.

3. Mehta RL, Kellum JA, Shah SV, et al: Acute Kidney Injury Network (AKIN): Report of an initiative to improve outcomes in acute kidney injury. Crit Care 11(2):R31, 2007 [ePub ahead of print].

   The authors propose uniform standards for the diagnosis and classification of AKI.

Patrick H. Nachman ▪ Ronald J. Falk

Glomerulonephritis

Introduction

Glomerulonephritis refers to a typically inflammatory injury of glomeruli that results in hematuria, proteinuria, edema, hypertension, and azotemia. Of the numerous glomerular diseases, each characterized by its own pathologic features, natural history, and response to treatment, many can present with the same clinical syndrome. For instance, asymptomatic microscopic hematuria is a consequence of several disparate pathologic entities, most commonly thin basement membrane nephropathy and immunoglobulin A (IgA) nephropathy. Thus, when evaluating patients with glomerulonephritis, it is helpful to first determine to which general clinical category they belong, and then to dissect the different diseases within each group as described in Box 141-1.

Etiology and Pathogenesis

There are several pathogenic mechanisms of glomerulonephritis. The most common is an inflammatory glomerular injury that results from immune complex formation or deposition within the glomerular basement membrane or the mesangium. These immune complexes initiate many phlogistic pathways, in particular, complement activation, cytokine, and chemokine generation and release. In response, circulating inflammatory cells, including neutrophils, monocytes, and lymphocytes infiltrate the glomeruli and the surrounding tubulointerstitial compartments. Immune deposits may develop in the glomeruli in three basic ways: the deposition of circulating immune complexes (e.g., lupus nephritis), the deposition of antigens with subsequent in situ immune complex formation (e.g., peri-infectious disorders), or the presence of circulating antibodies that react to intrinsic components of the glomerulus (e.g., anti-glomerular basement membrane [anti-GBM] diseases) (Fig. 141-1). The mesangial cell response to injury is marked by proliferation, production, and deposition of extracellular matrix, and, eventually, glomerular scarring. Glomerular endothelial cells are the target of injury in some diseases, such as hemolytic-uremic syndrome and the vasculitides.

Hereditary nephritides, including Alport's syndrome and thin basement membrane disease, are the result of mutations in type IV collagen. Genetically, Alport's syndrome may result from mutations in the α5 chain of type IV collagen (X-linked transmission), or mutations of the α3 or α4 chains associated with autosomal recessive or dominant patterns of transmission. Thin basement membrane disease, a relatively common autosomal dominant disorder, is also related to mutations of the α3 or α4 chains. Although both syndromes present with asymptomatic glomerular hematuria, they diverge in their natural history. Thin basement membrane disease (also referred to as *benign familial hematuria*) is associated with an excellent long-term outcome, whereas Alport's syndrome causes a progressive loss of renal function. Some kindred with Alport's syndrome may also present with sensorineural deafness, ocular anomalies, mental retardation, or leiomyomatosis.

Clinical Presentation

The clinical expression of disease correlates with the pathologic features; the more aggressive the pathologic injury, the more severe the illness. Some patients present with asymptomatic hematuria and recurrent gross hematuria. Hematuria, defined as more than three red blood cells per high-power field observed in centrifuged urine sediment, can be of either glomerular or nonglomerular origin (Fig. 141-2). Chemical stress on red blood cells as they pass along the nephron result in morphologic changes and dysmorphic red cells. The most diagnostic of these, acanthocytes (Mickey Mouse cells), are virtually pathognomonic of glomerular bleeding. In combination with red blood cell casts, other cylindruria, and proteinuria, these

Box 141-1 Clinical Presentation of Various Glomerulonephritides

Asymptomatic Microscopic Hematuria

Thin basement membrane nephropathy
Immunoglobulin A (IgA) nephropathy
Mesangioproliferative glomerulonephritis (GN)
Alport's syndrome

Recurrent Gross Hematuria

Thin basement membrane nephropathy
IgA nephropathy
Alport's syndrome

Acute Nephritis

Acute diffuse proliferative GN
Poststreptococcal GN
Poststaphylococcal GN
Focal or diffuse proliferative GN
IgA nephropathy
Lupus nephritis
Membranoproliferative GN

Rapidly Progressive Nephritis

Crescentic GN
Anti-glomerular basement membrane (anti-GBM) GN
Immune complex GN
Anti-neutrophil cytoplasmic autoantibodies (ANCA) GN

Pulmonary-Renal Vasculitic Syndrome

Goodpasture's (anti-GBM) syndrome
Immune complex vasculitis
Lupus nephritis
ANCA vasculitis
  Microscopic polyangiitis
  Wegener's granulomatosis
  Churg-Strauss syndrome

Renal-Dermal Vasculitic Syndromes

Immune complex vasculitis
ANCA vasculitis
Cryoglobulinemia
Henoch-Schönlein purpura

Chronic Renal Failure

Chronic sclerosing GN

abnormalities suggest a glomerular as opposed to a urinary tract source of hematuria.

The most common causes of asymptomatic hematuria are listed in Box 141-1. Patients with IgA nephropathy present with one of three syndromes. About half have a history of episodes of macroscopic hematuria associated with an upper respiratory tract infection that may recur, with subsequent episodes of pharyngitis, febrile illness, or heavy exertion. Patients are typically asymptomatic; hypertension and peripheral edema are uncommon. Asymptomatic microscopic hematuria with proteinuria, the second most common presentation, is associated with the worst long-term prognosis. A third presentation is part of the vasculitic syndrome, Henoch-Schönlein purpura, which develops most commonly in children. The postinfectious

nephritic syndrome of IgA nephropathy is differentiated from poststreptococcal glomerulonephritis in that it occurs only 1 to 2 days after the onset of the infection, as opposed to after the 10- to 14-day delay in poststreptococcal glomerulonephritis.

Acute glomerulonephritis usually presents with the sudden onset of proteinuria, hematuria, and urine sediment containing dysmorphic red blood cells, red blood cell casts, and cellular debris. Patients typically have edema, hypertension, oliguria, and renal insufficiency. In the most severe form, rapidly progressive glomerulonephritis (RPGN), the serum creatinine concentration rises in a matter of days to weeks, resulting in profound renal insufficiency. Structurally, RPGNs are usually associated with the formation of glomerular crescents that result from the proliferation of both glomerular epithelial cells and mononuclear phagocytes in Bowman's space. Crescents are not indicative of a specific cause of glomerular injury but may result from many different pathogenetic mechanisms.

All forms of acute nephritis, including RPGN, may be a consequence of streptococcal or staphylococcal infections or immunologic diseases. The illness is characterized by the sudden onset of edema and by oliguria with heavy proteinuria and hematuria (Fig. 141-3). Hypertension, cardiac enlargement, and pulmonary edema may complicate the clinical course. In the Western world, the types of infections resulting in postinfectious glomerulonephritis have changed so that patients with underlying immunocompromised states, including cirrhosis, malignancy, and transplantation, develop glomerulopathies associated with a variety of gram-negative organisms.

Recently, the role of hepatitis C virus was recognized in the pathogenesis of membranoproliferative glomerulonephritis type I and cryoglobulinemia. A clinical syndrome of mixed cryoglobulins is characterized by purpura, weakness, arthralgias, and in some cases, glomerular disease.

Systemic lupus erythematosus (SLE) is the prototypic cause of acute nephritis associated with immunologic injury. The characteristic renal lesion of lupus is a consequence of the accumulation of immune complexes in the mesangium and along the glomerular capillary wall. Lupus nephritis ranges from almost no pathologic abnormality to a severe diffusely proliferative and crescentic lesion; the clinical spectrum of disease ranges from normal renal function with minimal proteinuria (<1 g/24 hours) to RPGN and severe proteinuria. Almost all patients have hematuria. Other causes of diffuse proliferative glomerulonephritis include IgA nephropathy and membranoproliferative glomerulonephritides.

The most common causes of RPGN associated with crescent formation include the immune complex–mediated diseases, diseases associated with antineutrophil cytoplasmic autoantibodies (ANCA) or with anti-GBM. The presence of pulmonary hemorrhage in addition to anti-GBM–mediated nephritis defines Goodpasture's syndrome. There is a bimodal age distribution of patients with

Figure 141-1 Hypothesis of Pathogenesis of Acute Glomerular Injury by Circulating Immune Complexes (Schematic).

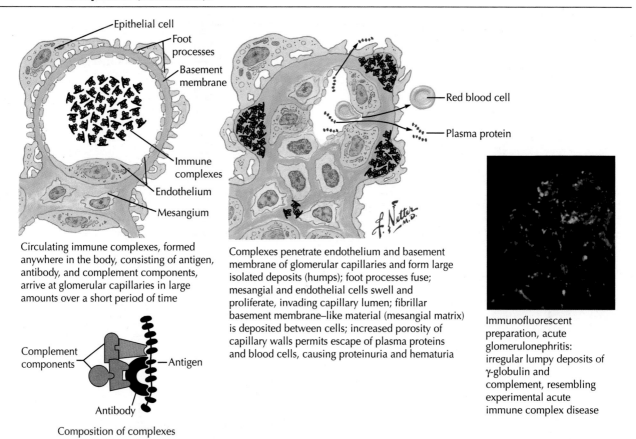

Epithelial cell

Foot processes

Basement membrane

Immune complexes

Endothelium

Mesangium

Red blood cell

Plasma protein

Circulating immune complexes, formed anywhere in the body, consisting of antigen, antibody, and complement components, arrive at glomerular capillaries in large amounts over a short period of time

Complexes penetrate endothelium and basement membrane of glomerular capillaries and form large isolated deposits (humps); foot processes fuse; mesangial and endothelial cells swell and proliferate, invading capillary lumen; fibrillar basement membrane–like material (mesangial matrix) is deposited between cells; increased porosity of capillary walls permits escape of plasma proteins and blood cells, causing proteinuria and hematuria

Immunofluorescent preparation, acute glomerulonephritis: irregular lumpy deposits of γ-globulin and complement, resembling experimental acute immune complex disease

Complement components

Antigen

Antibody

Composition of complexes

Goodpasture's syndrome with peaks in the third and sixth decades. One third of patients have isolated glomerular disease. Malaise, fatigue, and weight loss are common.

In a patient with a glomerulonephritis, it is most important to determine whether the renal disease is part of a systemic disorder resulting from an infection or is caused by an immunologic disorder. One approach is to determine whether a patient has a pulmonary-renal or dermal-renal syndrome. Pulmonary-renal vasculitic syndromes include Goodpasture's syndrome, the ANCA vasculitides (including microscopic polyangiitis, Wegener's granulomatosis, and Churg-Strauss syndrome), or immune complex vasculitis, especially SLE and cryoglobulinemia. In renal-dermal vasculitic syndromes, the glomerulonephritis is associated with a number of skin manifestations, including petechiae, purpura, hives, livedo reticularis, and ecchymoses. These diseases are usually attributable to SLE, ANCA vasculitis, Henoch-Schönlein purpura, or cryoglobulinemia.

Differential Diagnosis

The differential diagnosis of glomerulonephritis is broad and includes other causes of hematuria and azotemia. Glomerulonephritides account for only about 5% of hematu-

ria in the adult population where urinary tract stones, infections, and malignancies predominate. Azotemia may be caused by tubulointerstitial disease (e.g., acute tubular necrosis or acute interstitial nephritis), thrombotic microangiopathies or urinary tract obstruction. The presence of dysmorphic erythrocyturia, red blood cell casts, and proteinuria more than 500 mg/day are strong clues for a glomerular cause of hematuria. Extrarenal manifestations of disease identified on a thorough review of systems and physical examination provide clues to the presence of systemic infections or autoimmune diseases associated with glomerulonephritis.

Diagnostic Approach

The initial diagnostic approach in anyone with kidney disease is to examine the urine for the presence of glomerular hematuria, proteinuria, or other formed elements. This simple study allows the inclusion or exclusion of many renal processes. Multisystem disease is usually associated with constitutional signs and symptoms of inflammation, including arthralgias, myalgias, fever, and weight loss. The pattern and character of organ involvement provide clues for a differential diagnosis. The eyes, ears,

Figure 141-2 Urinary Sediment: Organized Elements.

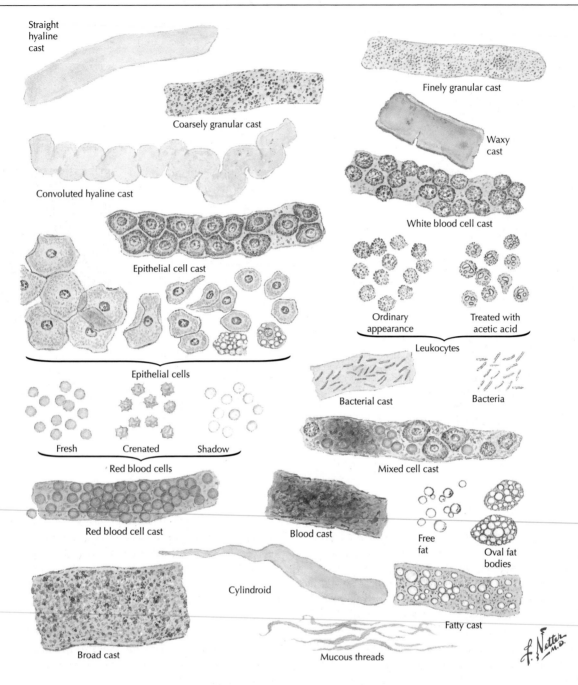

sinuses, upper respiratory tract, lungs, gastrointestinal tract, central and peripheral nervous system, and skin may be involved in the various vasculitides associated with glomerulonephritis. Serologic tests help in the diagnosis of glomerular diseases. It is possible to separate glomerular diseases on the basis of whether the patient has circulating immune complexes such as cryoglobulins; antibodies to nuclear antigens including anti-double-stranded DNA, ANCA, anti-GBM antibodies, and hypocomplementemia; or evidence for infectious diseases including assays for hepatitis C, hepatitis B, and streptococcal disease, includ-

ing deoxyribonuclease-B and anti-streptolysin O testing (Fig. 141-4).

The evaluation of pathologic features on a renal biopsy specimen is usually required for diagnosis. Light, immunofluorescence, and electron microscopy are used to establish the precise pattern of injury. The definitive diagnosis frequently depends on an integrated synthesis of the clinical features of disease, serologic tests, and pathologic findings. For example, glomerulonephritides associated with proliferative lesions are attributable to infections, lupus nephritis, or IgA nephropathy and require serologic tests

Figure 141-3 Clinical Course of Acute Glomerulonephritis.

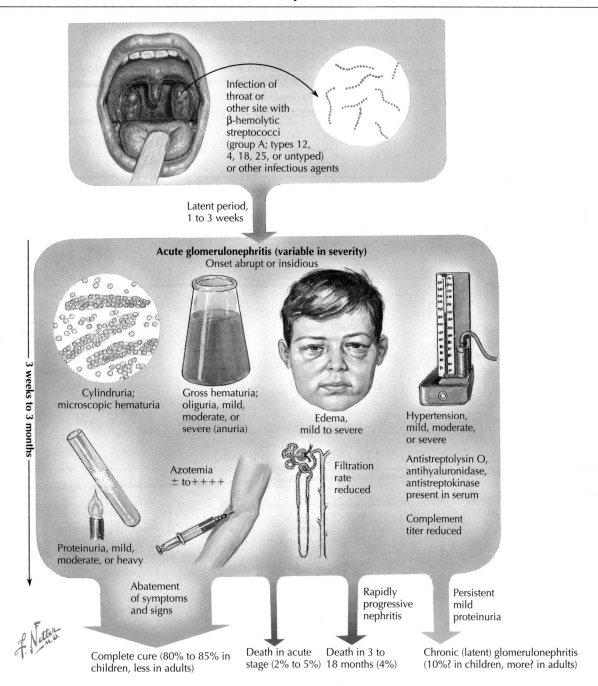

Infection of throat or other site with β-hemolytic streptococci (group A; types 12, 4, 18, 25, or untyped) or other infectious agents

Latent period, 1 to 3 weeks

Acute glomerulonephritis (variable in severity)
Onset abrupt or insidious

3 weeks to 3 months

Cylindruria; microscopic hematuria

Gross hematuria; oliguria, mild, moderate, or severe (anuria)

Edema, mild to severe

Hypertension, mild, moderate, or severe

Azotemia ± to++++

Filtration rate reduced

Antistreptolysin O, antihyaluronidase, antistreptokinase present in serum

Complement titer reduced

Proteinuria, mild, moderate, or heavy

Abatement of symptoms and signs

Rapidly progressive nephritis

Persistent mild proteinuria

Complete cure (80% to 85% in children, less in adults)

Death in acute stage (2% to 5%)

Death in 3 to 18 months (4%)

Chronic (latent) glomerulonephritis (10%? in children, more? in adults)

to differentiate among them. In addition to its diagnostic value, the renal biopsy also allows estimation of prognosis and treatment options. Generally, a renal biopsy is indicated in any patient with renal disease when the cause cannot be adequately determined by the clinical pattern of disease or laboratory findings, the differential diagnosis results in differing prognoses and treatment, or signs and symptoms suggest intrinsic renal disease that can be diagnosed by the biopsy (Fig. 141-5).

Contraindications to renal biopsy include the presence of a solitary kidney, an uncooperative patient, bleeding disorders of any kind, severe hypertension, multiple cysts within the kidney, obstructive uropathy, renal neoplasm, and a very thin cortex (usually indicative of end-stage renal disease) in which case a biopsy is no longer useful.

Management and Therapy

Optimum Treatment

All forms of glomerular disease require supportive care. The treatment of hypertension is a cornerstone of therapy.

Figure 141-4 A serologic approach to glomerulonephritis.

The *purple boxes* denote diseases limited to the kidney; *yellow boxes* denote systemic diseases. ANCA, anti-neutrophil cytoplasmic autoantibody; anti-GBM, anti-glomerular basement membrane; IF, immunofluorescence microscopy; Ig, immunoglobulin; GN, glomerulonephritis; anti-HCV, anti-hepatitis C virus antibodies; anti-HBV, anti-hepatitis B virus antibodies. HBV serologies should include HBV surface antigen, and antibodies to the HBV core antigen; H-S purpura, Henoch-Schönlein purpura, MPGN, membranoproliferative glomerulonephritis; SLE, systemic lupus erythematosus. *From Falk RJ, Jennette JC, Nachman PH: Primary glomerular disease. In: Brenner BM (ed): Brenner & Rector's The Kidney, 6th ed. Philadelphia, WB Saunders, 2004, pp 1293-1380.*

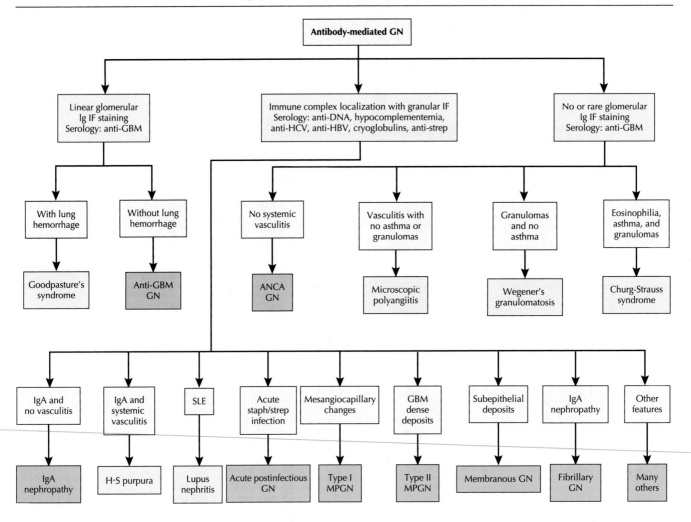

Angiotensin-converting enzyme inhibitors or angiotensin receptor blockers are the agents of choice because they control blood pressure, reduce proteinuria, and slow the rate of decline of creatinine clearance. Other supportive measures include management of edema with diuretics, diminution of hyperlipidemia, prevention of osteoporosis from glucocorticoids, and a moderate restriction of protein intake (avoiding protein malnutrition in patients with severe proteinuria).

Some diseases require observation alone, including thin basement membrane disease, Alport's syndrome, and mild glomerular injury. Poststreptococcal glomerulonephritis typically resolves spontaneously, but other peri-infectious diseases may require specific treatment of the underlying infection, including antiviral therapy in hepatitis C–associated conditions. Glucocorticoid therapy, usually given orally, is useful in patients with many types of acute nephritis, especially those in which renal impairment may ensue. Glucocorticoids are usually started at 1 mg/kg/day of prednisone (<80 mg/day) for 4 weeks, and then rapidly titrated to an alternate-day regime, and discontinued by the end of 3 to 4 months. This approach is used in treating lupus nephritis, ANCA glomerulonephritis, and milder forms of other types of glomerulonephritis. The use of cyclophosphamide is indicated for patients with severe lupus nephritis, anti-GBM disease,

Figure 141-5 Clinical Course of Chronic Glomerulonephritis.

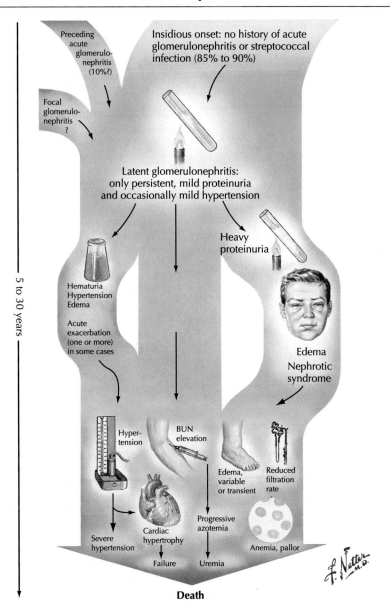

Goodpasture's syndrome, and ANCA glomerulonephritis or vasculitis. The method in which cyclophosphamide is administered has varied, although monthly intravenous doses for at least 6 months have been recommended for the treatment of lupus nephritis. A consolidation treatment is extended for an additional 18 months to preserve a renal remission in severe lupus nephritis. Similarly, both intravenous cyclophosphamide and oral cyclophosphamide have been used in the treatment of ANCA glomerulonephritis. The duration and intensity of therapy must match the intensity and severity of the underlying glomerular-systemic inflammation. Data do not allow for specific recommendations, but generally 6 to 12 months is sufficient for almost all forms of glomerulonephritis.

Some conditions are life threatening as a consequence of pulmonary hemorrhage or RPGN. In these most aggressive forms of disease, induction therapy with intravenous methylprednisolone at a dose of 7 mg/kg (<1000 mg/day) on 3 consecutive days is useful adjunctive therapy. Patients presenting with pulmonary hemorrhage or severe renal failure are treated with plasmapheresis in addition to glucocorticoids and cyclophosphamide. Daily plasma exchange is indicated for patients with anti-GBM disease and Goodpasture's syndrome.

Avoiding Treatment Errors

The outcome of patients with aggressive forms of glomerulonephritis depends on prompt diagnosis and the early institution of therapy. The lower the serum creatinine at the time of initiation of therapy, the smaller is the risk for progression to end-stage renal disease. Delay in diagnosis and therapy adversely affects long-term outcome in all forms of glomerular inflammation.

Whenever immunosuppressive therapy is instituted, it is important to pay close attention to the prevention and early detection of potential infectious and metabolic complications. The use of high-dose glucocorticoids should be accompanied by measures to prevent bone loss with calcium, vitamin D, and when appropriate, the use of bisphosphonates. Close monitoring is necessary for the early detection and management of steroid-induced diabetes mellitus. The prophylactic use of trimethoprim-sulfamethoxazole should be considered in all patients undergoing therapy with cyclophosphamide. Monitoring of the peripheral white cell count during treatment with cyclophosphamide (especially 2 weeks after an intravenous dose) is necessary to adjust its dosage and avoid severe leukopenia.

Future Directions

Very little is known about the precise pathogenesis of any form of glomerulonephritis, so it is difficult to target therapy on the basis of the pathogenic mechanisms of these disorders. New pharmaceutical agents that target specific portions of the immune system's effector arm, such as cytokines, complement activation, lymphocyte co-stimulatory molecules, and effector immune cells, are under various stages of development. Agents that inhibit T and B cells are available and have been experimentally used in glomerular diseases, including cyclosporine, tacrolimus, and mycophenolate mofetil. The precise role of these agents in the treatment of glomerular disease remains under investigation.

Precisely targeted therapy awaits the understanding of proximate causes of glomerular inflammation, whereas the ultimate goal will be their prevention. Assessment of populations at risk will require a careful understanding of the genes and environmental conditions that spawn glomerular injury.

Additional Resources

Falk RJ, Jennette, JC, Nachman PH: Primary glomerular disease. In Brenner BM (ed): Brenner & Rector's The Kidney, 7th ed. Philadelphia, WB Saunders, 2004, pp 1293-1380.
  This extensive review of primary glomerulonephritides, covers clinical, pathogenetic, pathologic, and therapeutic aspects.
Jennette JC, Falk RJ: Glomerular clinicopathologic syndromes. In Greenberg A (ed): Primer on Kidney Diseases, 4th ed. Philadelphia, WB Saunders, 2005, pp 150-164.
  The authors present a succinct review of the general aspects of glomerulonephritis.
Mandal AK, Jennette JC: The syndrome of glomerulonephritis. In Mandal AK, Jennette JC (eds): Diagnosis and Management of Renal Disease and Hypertension, 2nd ed. Durham, NC, Carolina Academic Press, 1994.
  This chapter provides a comprehensive review of glomerulonephritides.

EVIDENCE

1. Levy JB, Turner AN, Rees AJ, Pusey CD: Long-term outcome of anti-glomerular basement membrane antibody disease treated with plasma exchange and immunosuppression. Ann Intern Med 134(11):1033-1042, 2001.
  This important article describes the optimal therapy of anti-GBM disease.
2. Jayne D, Rasmussen N, Andrassy K, et al: A randomized trial of maintenance therapy for vasculitis associated with antineutrophil cytoplasmic autoantibodies. N Engl J Med 3;349(1):36-44, 2003.
  The authors describe their landmark study on the management of ANCA vasculitis.
3. Weening JJ, D'Agati VD, Schwartz MM, et al: The classification of glomerulonephritis in systemic lupus erythematosus revisited. Kidney Int 65(2):521-530, 2004.
  This important study defines the new approach to the classification of lupus nephritis.

Nephrotic Syndrome

Introduction

The nephrotic syndrome represents a diverse group of diseases that share the clinical hallmark of proteinuria of 3.5 g/day per 1.73 m² body surface area or more, accompanied by hypoalbuminemia, edema, hyperlipidemia, and lipiduria. Although the nephrotic syndrome can occur at all ages, certain forms primarily affect children and young adults (minimal change glomerulopathy [MCG] and membranoproliferative glomerulonephritis), and others are more common among older adults (membranous glomerulopathy [MGN]).

Etiology and Pathogenesis

The diseases that present with the nephrotic syndrome have various etiologies and pathogeneses (Fig. 142-1). In general, they can all present as a primary (idiopathic) renal disease or be secondary to an underlying systemic disease. Diabetes mellitus is the most common cause of secondary nephrotic syndrome. Other causes are infections, malignancies, connective tissue diseases, exposure to drugs or environmental agents, and hemodynamic or genetic abnormalities (Table 142-1).

The exact mechanisms leading to the severe proteinuria are poorly understood in most cases of primary and secondary nephrotic syndrome (Fig. 142-2).

Clinical Presentation

Edema is the most common presenting symptom. Reduced plasma oncotic pressure has long been considered the proximate cause of intravascular depletion resulting in salt and water retention by the kidney (Fig. 142-3). This concept is challenged by the fact that some patients have an increased plasma volume and hypertension. Furthermore, in children with a relapse of MCG, sodium retention may precede the reduction in serum protein concentrations, and natriuresis can start before the hypoalbuminemia has resolved with treatment. Enhanced tubular sodium reabsorption is instead more likely a function of multiple mediator systems, including the activation of the renin-angiotensin aldosterone, sympathetic nervous, and vasopressor systems.

The hypercholesterolemia and hypertriglyceridemia are thought to be the consequence of both increased synthesis and decreased catabolism and may persist well after clinical remission has occurred. Hypercholesterolemia is largely a result of hepatic overproduction of lipoproteins and appears to be stimulated by the fall in oncotic pressure. An acquired defect in the low-density lipoprotein (LDL) receptor results in a diminished clearance of LDL. Lipiduria is reflected by the presence of free lipid droplets, hyalofatty casts, and oval fat bodies in the urine. The latter are sloughed tubular epithelial cells engorged with the excess lipids and lipoproteins in the urine. Hypoalbuminemia is a consequence of urinary losses and of an increased albumin catabolism, whereas hepatic albumin synthesis is increased. Although proteinuria and lipiduria are the hallmark urinary findings of the nephrotic syndrome, microscopic hematuria may be present in patients with focal segmental glomerulosclerosis (FSGS), MGN, and membranoproliferative glomerulonephritis (MPGN).

As a consequence of the urinary losses of immunoglobulins and defects in the complement cascade, nephrotic patients have an increased susceptibility to infection, particularly peritonitis.

Several abnormalities of the coagulation system may result in venous and, less frequently, arterial thrombi. Thrombi may occur in virtually any venous bed but have a predilection for the renal veins. The hypercoagulability is attributed to urinary losses of anticoagulant factors such as proteins C and S and antithrombin III, as well as to intravascular consumption.

Figure 142-1 Multiple Etiologies of Nephrotic Syndrome.

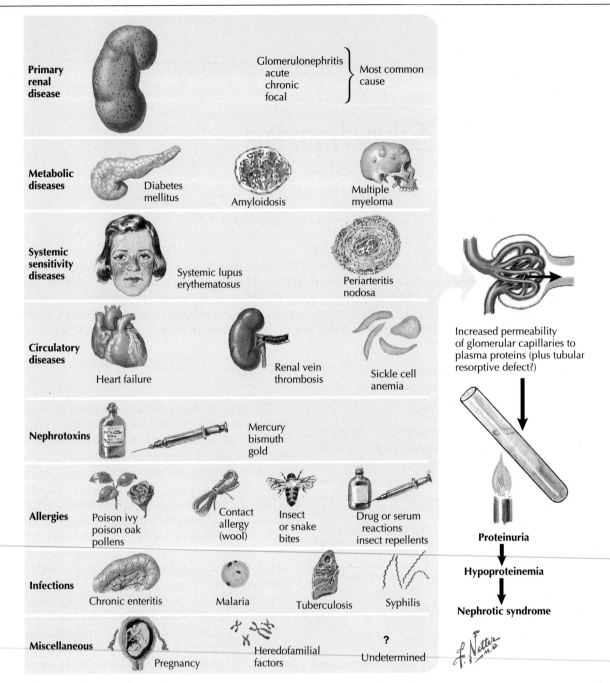

Major Forms of Primary Nephrotic Syndrome

Minimal Change Glomerulopathy (MCG)

MCG is most common in children, accounting for 70% to 90% of nephrotic syndrome cases in children younger than 10 years, and 10% to 15% of primary nephrotic syndrome in adults. MCG has no glomerular lesions by light microscopy and no staining with antisera specific for immuno-globulins or complement by immunofluorescence microscopy (Fig. 142-4). Electron microscopy reveals effacement of visceral epithelial cell foot processes. Primary MCG is thought to be mediated by an as yet unidentified T-cell lymphokine that increases glomerular permeability to protein. The cardinal clinical feature of MCG is the abrupt onset of the nephrotic syndrome. Hypertension and renal insufficiency, although rare in children, may be seen in older adults.

Table 142-1 Underlying Causes of the Nephrotic Syndrome and Associated Pathologic Findings

Underlying Cause	Disease
Infections	
HIV	Collapsing FSGS
Hepatitis C virus	MPGN > MGN
Hepatitis B virus	MGN > MPGN
Subacute bacterial infections (endocarditis, osteomyelitis)	MPGN, MGN
Malaria	Proliferative glomerulonephritis > MGN
Syphilis	MGN > MPGN
Autoimmune	
Autoimmune thyroiditis	MGN
Systemic lupus erythematosus	MGN, MPGN
Allergic	
Food allergies	MCG
Malignancies	
Hodgkin's lymphoma	MCG
Non-Hodgkin's lymphoma, leukemia	MGN
Solid tumors	MGN
Metabolic and Hemodynamic	
Diabetes mellitus	Diabetic nephropathy
Obesity	FSGS
Sickle cell disease	FSGS
Cyanotic congenital heart disease	FSGS
Congenital pulmonary disease	FSGS
Nephron loss	FSGS
Exposures	
NSAIDs	MCG
Penicillamine, gold	MGN
Heroin, intravenous drug abuse	Collapsing FSGS
Genetic	Familial FSGS

FSGS, focal segmental glomerulosclerosis; MCG, minimal change glomerulopathy; MGN, membranous glomerulopathy; MPGN, membranoproliferative glomerulonephritis; NSAID, nonsteroidal anti-inflammatory drugs.

Focal Segmental Glomerulosclerosis

FSGS is a clinical-pathologic syndrome that likely encompasses diseases of multiple etiologies and pathogenic mechanisms. The incidence of FSGS has increased over the past two decades, and it is the most common cause of nephrotic syndrome among African Americans. FSGS may be a primary renal disease, or it may be associated with a variety of other conditions (see Table 142-1). On histology, it is characterized by focal and segmental glomerular sclerosis. Although many specimens have nonspecific patterns of sclerosis, at least three major structural variants are recognized (Fig. 142-5).

The perihilar variant is characterized by sclerotic lesions that have a predilection for the glomerular perihilar segments and are accompanied usually by hyalinosis and adhesions to Bowman's capsule. There is no staining for immunoglobulins or complement by immunofluorescence microscopy. Electron microscopy reveals focal foot process effacement.

The collapsing glomerulopathy occurs in HIV nephropathy, with intravenous drug abuse, or as an idiopathic process. The characteristic feature is focal segmental or global collapse of glomerular capillaries with obliteration of capillary lumens. Visceral epithelial cells that overlie collapsed segments usually are enlarged and contain conspicuous resorption droplets.

The glomerular tip lesion variant is characterized by consolidation of the glomerular segment that is adjacent to the origin of, and may project into the lumen of, the proximal tubule. Visceral epithelial cells adjacent to the consolidated segment are enlarged and contain clear vacuoles and hyaline droplets.

The pathogenesis of FSGS is poorly understood. Many theories suggest that podocyte injury is a component of the pathogenic process. FSGS may result from the loss of nephrons, which causes compensatory intraglomerular hypertension and hypertrophy in the remaining glomeruli, although data from long-term studies of uninephrectomized individuals have demonstrated either none or only a small increase in mild proteinuria and systolic hypertension. An as yet poorly characterized permeability factor has been described in some patients with primary FSGS, especially in those with recurrent FSGS after transplantation.

Figure 142-2 Pathophysiologic Factors in the Etiology of Nephrotic Edema.
ADH, antidiuretic hormone.

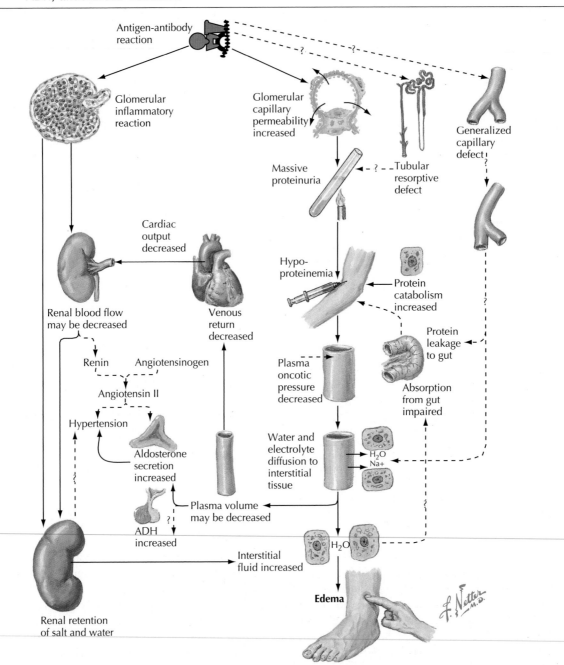

Microscopic hematuria occurs in more than half of FSGS patients, and about one third of patients present with some degree of renal insufficiency or hypertension. The collapsing variant often presents with more severe proteinuria and renal insufficiency and carries a poorer prognosis than the perihilar variant. The glomerular tip lesion variant often presents with rapid onset of edema similar to MCG.

Membranous Glomerulopathy (MGN)

MGN, the most common cause for nephrotic syndrome in white adults, is uncommon in children. The peak incidence is in the fourth or fifth decade. It occurs as an idiopathic (primary) or secondary disease (see Table 142-1). Infectious and autoimmune causes are more frequent in children, whereas underlying malignancies are found in 20% to 30% of patients older than 60 years. The characteristic histologic abnormality is diffuse global capillary wall thickening associated with subepithelial immune complex deposits, in the absence of significant glomerular hypercellularity (Figure 142-4). By immunofluorescence microscopy, there is diffuse global granular capillary wall staining for immunoglobulin and complement. In idiopathic MGN, the nature of the antigens involved in the subepithelial

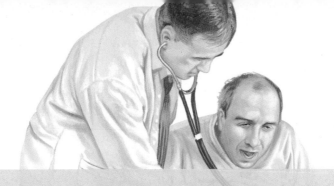
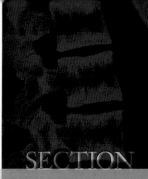

Disorders of the Immune System, Connective Tissue, and Joints

Focal Segmental Glomerulosclerosis

The treatment of patients with FSGS remains controversial. Although some older studies suggested that only 15% of patients responded to corticosteroids, more recent reports suggest that 40% to 55% of adult patients may attain some form of remission with the prolonged use of high-dose corticosteroids. The data currently available do not take into account a careful assessment of the risk-benefit ratio of such treatments. Cyclosporine therapy has been used with varying degrees of success and is complicated by an elevated rate of relapse.

Membranous Glomerulopathy

Because of the variable course of MGN, the choice of therapy must be individualized based on an assessment of each patient's risks for progressive disease. A pooled analysis of randomized and prospective studies demonstrated a lack of benefit of corticosteroids alone in inducing a remission of the nephrotic syndrome or on renal survival of patients. The current approaches shown to lead to complete or partial resolution of proteinuria include the use of chlorambucil or cyclophosphamide in combination with corticosteroids or cyclosporine. The rate of relapse after discontinuation of cyclosporin is high.

Membranoproliferative Glomerulonephritis

The treatment of patients with type I MPGN is based on the underlying cause of the disease process. In children, corticosteroid therapy improves renal survival. The addition of anticoagulant therapy with dipyridamole, aspirin, and warfarin is of questionable benefit. Unfortunately, evidence for an effective therapy for type II MPGN is currently very limited.

Avoiding Treatment Errors

Whenever glucocorticoids are prescribed in the management of nephrotic syndrome, it is important to implement measures to reduce the risk for osteoporosis with calcium, vitamin D, and when appropriate, bisphosphonate therapy. The optimal dose of cyclosporine in the management of nephrotic syndrome is not well established. To avoid the adverse effects of cyclosporine therapy, it is advisable to initiate treatment at a modest dose (about 2 mg/kg/day in two divided doses) and titrate the dose up while monitoring drug levels and the development of hypertension, hyperlipidemia, and a decrease in glomerular filtration rate (GFR). Several formulations of cyclosporine are currently available. Because of their different pharmacokinetic profiles, switches from one formulation to another may be accompanied by significant changes in drug levels and adverse effects, and are best avoided.

Future Directions

Recent advances in genetics have vastly increased our definition of the molecular anatomy of the glomerular podocytes and the role of these cells in pathogenesis of nephrotic syndrome. Advances in diagnosis and treatment will depend on a better understanding of the precipitating agents (e.g., infections or toxins for secondary forms) and the pathogenetic mechanisms involved. Current research holds the promise of more specifically targeted therapies that will avoid the need for aggressive immunosuppression.

Additional Resource

Falk RJ, Jennette, JC, Nachman PH: Primary glomerular disease. In Brenner BM (ed): Brenner & Rector's The Kidney, 7th ed. Philadelphia, WB Saunders, 2004, pp 1293-1380.
  This extensive review of primary glomerulonephritides covers clinical, pathogenetic, pathologic, and therapeutic aspects.

EVIDENCE

1. Cattran D: Management of membranous nephropathy: When and what for treatment. J Am Soc Nephrol 16(5):1188-1194, 2005.
   This is an excellent review of the management of membranous nephropathy.
2. D'Agati VD, Fogo AB, Bruijn JA, Jennette JC: Pathologic classification of focal segmental glomerulosclerosis: A working proposal. Am J Kidney Dis 43(2):368-382, 2004.
   This landmark article describes the new approach to the classification of focal segmental glomerulosclerosis.
3. D'Amico G, Ferrario F: Mesangiocapillary glomerulonephritis. J Am Soc Nephrol 2(10 Suppl):S159-S166, 1992.
   This article reviews mesangioproliferative glomerulonephritis.
4. Donckerwolcke RA, Vande Walle JG: Pathogenesis of edema formation in the nephrotic syndrome. Kidney Int Suppl 58:S72-S74, 1997.
   The authors review the mechanisms of edema formation in nephrotic syndrome.
5. Glassock RJ: Secondary membranous glomerulonephritis. Nephrol Dial Transplant 7(Suppl 1):64-71, 1992.
   The author reviews the underlying causes of membranous glomerulopathy.
6. Kerjaschki D: Pathogenetic concepts of membranous glomerulopathy (MGN). J Nephrol 13(Suppl 3):S96-S100, 2000.
   The author reviews the pathogenic mechanisms of membranous glomerulopathy.
7. Passerini P, Ponticelli C: Treatment of focal segmental glomerulosclerosis. Curr Opin Nephrol Hypertens 10(2):189-193, 2001.
   The authors present an expert review of the treatment of focal segmental glomerulosclerosis.
8. Shankland SJ: The podocyte's response to injury: Role in proteinuria and glomerulosclerosis. Kidney Int 69(12):2131-2147, 2006.
   This is an excellent review of new information on the role of podocytes in glomerular disease.
9. Thomas DB, Franceschini N, Hogan SL, et al: Clinical and pathologic characteristics of focal segmental glomerulosclerosis pathologic variants. Kidney Int 69(5):920-926, 2006.
   This article presents a description of clinical characteristics of the pathologic variants of focal segmental glomerulosclerosis as classified according to the new proposed system described in Am J Kidney Dis 43(2):368-382, 2004.

Figure 142-5 Histologic Variants of Focal Segmental Glomerulosclerosis.
Courtesy of Charles Jennette, MD.

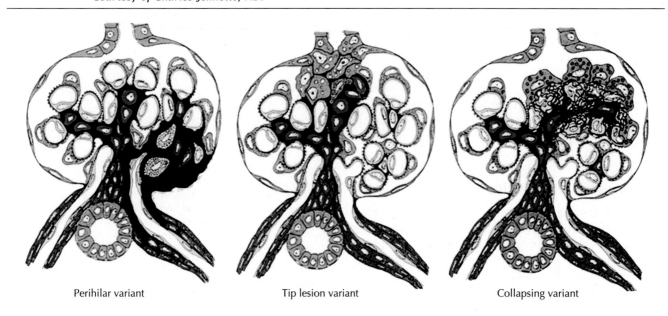

Perihilar variant   Tip lesion variant   Collapsing variant

Diagnostic Approach

The diagnosis of the nephrotic syndrome begins with quantifying the proteinuria using a 24-hour urine collection measurement of protein and creatinine excretion. The excreted creatinine verifies the adequacy of the collection; the normal 24-hour creatinine excretion is 20 to 25 mg/kg/day for males and 15 to 20 mg/kg/day for females.

Unless an underlying systemic disease is evident, a renal biopsy is required in adults to establish the specific diagnosis of the nephrotic syndrome and assess the severity and acuity of the renal disease. A detailed history and serologic workup that includes testing for hepatitis B and C, HIV, syphilis, antinuclear antibody, cryoglobulins, and hypocomplementemia are essential in evaluating secondary forms of nephrotic syndome. Based on the clinical presentation, testing for chronic infections such as subacute bacterial endocarditis is necessary. The search for occult malignancies is warranted, especially for older adults.

Management and Therapy

Optimum Treatment

Treatments aimed at the reduction or elimination of proteinuria is essential to the management of nephrotic syndrome. In most forms of the disease, even a partial reduction in proteinuria is associated with a beneficial effect on outcome. For this reason, angiotensin-converting enzyme inhibitors, angiotensin receptor blockers, or both deserve consideration in all adult patients, with upward dosage titration as tolerated (avoiding hypotension and hyperkalemia).

The management of edema requires dietary restriction of sodium intake and the judicious use of diuretics. An overzealous diuresis is contraindicated because intravascular depletion, hypotension, and acute renal failure may result.

The hyperlipidemia of the nephrotic syndrome predisposes to atherosclerotic cardiovascular disease and may contribute to the progression of renal disease. The treatment of hyperlipidemia is difficult; the most useful agents are the HMG-CoA reductase inhibitors and bile acid sequestrants.

The treatment of secondary forms of nephrotic syndrome depends on the underlying disease process. When associated with the use of medications such as nonsteroidal anti-inflammatory drugs, the proteinuria may resolve with cessation of the offending agent. Similarly, peri-infectious nephrotic syndrome typically responds to treatment of the underlying infection.

For the primary diseases that cause the nephrotic syndrome, various therapies apply depending on the pathologic diagnosis.

Minimal Change Glomerulopathy

MCG is treated primarily with corticosteroids. Proteinuria abates in more than 90% of children within 4 to 6 weeks but may take up to 15 weeks in adults. After the clinical response to initial treatment, as few as 25% of patients have a long-term remission, 25% to 30% have infrequent relapses (one per year or less), and the remainder have frequent relapses, steroid dependence, or steroid resistance. Frequently, relapsing or steroid-dependent nephrotic patients may require the use of cyclophosphamide. Cyclosporine may lead to a partial or complete remission in up to 90% of patients with steroid-resistant MCG, but relapses are frequent once the drug is discontinued.

Figure 142-4 Pathology of the Nephrotic Syndrome.

Pathology of the nephrotic syndrome

Minimal disease

Epithelial cell
Basement membrane
Foot processes fused
Subendothelial "fluff"

Glomerular capillary lumen

Endothelial cell
Mesangial cell

Electron microscopic findings: Only fusion of epithelial foot processes and some subendothelial fluff

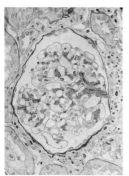

Light microscopic findings: Glomerulus appears normal; protein may be present in tubule lumina and lipoid droplets in tubule cells (PAS, ×250)

Membranous disease

Subepithelial deposits
Basement membrane thickened
Foot processes fused

Electron microscopic findings: Electron-dense deposits beneath epithelial cells, thickening of basement membrane, and fusion of foot processes

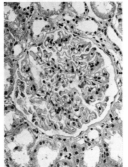

Light microscopic findings: Basement membrane thickened and eosinophilic; prominence but no numerical increase of epithelial, endothelial, and mesangial cells (H&E, ×250)

Proliferative disease

Epithelial cell proliferation
Endothelial cell proliferation
Foot processes fused

Fibrinoid
Basement membrane–like material
Mesangial cell proliferation

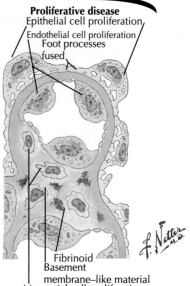

Electron microscopic findings: Epithelial, endothelial, and mesangial cell proliferation; little or no thickening of basement membrane, but variable amount of basement membrane–like material (mesangial matrix) deposited in mesangium; foot processes fused

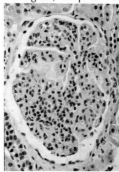

Light microscopic appearance: Cellular proliferation – epithelial, endothelial, and mesangial; very little, if any, basement membrane thickening (H&E, × 250)

deposited immune complexes or complement results in the proliferation of mesangial and endothelial cells and the recruitment of inflammatory cells, including neutrophils and monocytes.

Hypocomplementemia is a frequent feature of all types of MPGN. Complement activation occurs through the classic pathway initiated by immune complex formation in type I MPGN and by the alternate pathway in type II MPGN. C3 nephritic factor, an autoantibody that binds to C3 convertase and prevents its inactivation, is found in more than 60% of patients with MPGN type II.

The clinical features of all forms of MPGN are usually that of the nephrotic syndrome, but about 30% of patients (especially patients with type II) present with an acute nephritic syndrome with hematuria, hypertension, and renal insufficiency. In general, one third of patients with type I MPGN have a spontaneous remission, one third have progressive disease, and one third have a disease process that will wax and wane but never completely disappear. The prognosis for type II disease is worse than that for type I, and clinical remissions are rare. MPGN is associated with hepatitis C virus infection (and the presence of cryoglobulins), other infections, and autoimmune diseases.

Differential Diagnosis

In the evaluation of patients with proteinuria, nonglomerular causes such as functional or transient proteinuria and orthostatic proteinuria should be excluded. These types of proteinuria rarely exceed 500 mg/day.

Figure 142-3 Clinical and Laboratory Findings that May Be Present in Nephrotic Syndrome.

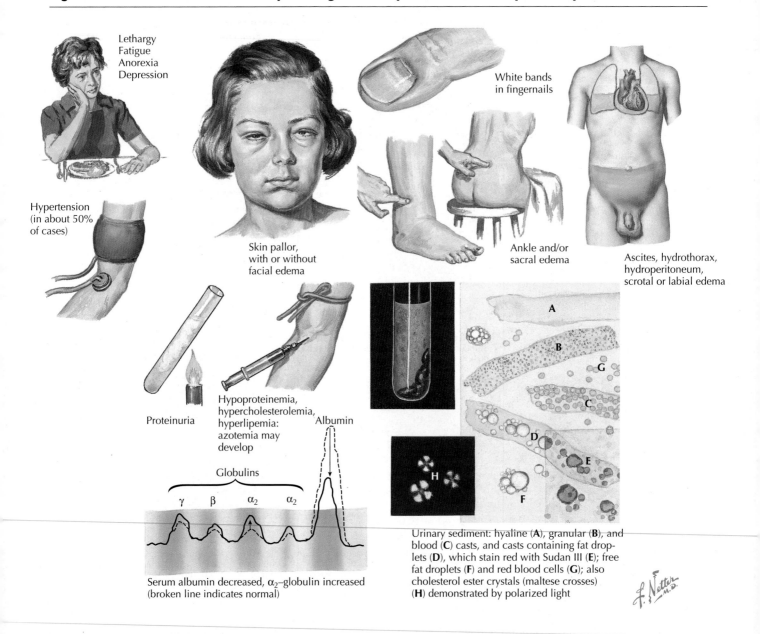

Lethargy
Fatigue
Anorexia
Depression

White bands
in fingernails

Hypertension
(in about 50%
of cases)

Skin pallor,
with or without
facial edema

Ankle and/or
sacral edema

Ascites, hydrothorax,
hydroperitoneum,
scrotal or labial edema

Proteinuria

Hypoproteinemia,
hypercholesterolemia,
hyperlipemia:
azotemia may
develop

Albumin

Globulins

γ   β   α₂   α₂

Serum albumin decreased, α₂–globulin increased
(broken line indicates normal)

Urinary sediment: hyaline (**A**), granular (**B**), and
blood (**C**) casts, and casts containing fat droplets (**D**), which stain red with Sudan III (**E**); free
fat droplets (**F**) and red blood cells (**G**); also
cholesterol ester crystals (maltese crosses)
(**H**) demonstrated by polarized light

immune complexes is unknown. The immune complexes
activate the complement pathway, leading to the formation
of the C5b-C9 membrane attack complex and injury to the
epithelial cells. Patients usually present with normal or
slightly decreased renal function. If progressive renal insufficiency develops, it is usually relatively indolent, resulting
in end-stage renal disease in 25% of patients. Twenty-five
percent of patients may have a complete spontaneous
remission of proteinuria within 5 years.

Membranoproliferative
Glomerulonephritis

Type I MPGN is characterized by diffuse global capillary
wall thickening and endocapillary hypercellularity with

infiltrating mononuclear leukocytes and neutrophils.
Immunofluorescence microscopy reveals a characteristic
pattern of peripheral granular to band-like staining for
complement, especially C3, and usually immunoglobulins.
Electron microscopy demonstrates prominent subendothelial immune complexes with associated subendothelial
mesangial interposition. The identity of the antigens
involved in the immune complexes is unknown in most
cases.

Type II MPGN, also named *dense deposit disease*, is characterized by discontinuous electron-dense bands within
glomerular basement membranes. Immunofluorescence
microscopy demonstrates intense capillary wall band-like
staining for C3, with little or no staining for immunoglobulin. These pathologic findings suggest that the

Osteoarthritis

Introduction

Osteoarthritis (OA) is the most common form of arthritis, affecting about 21 million adults in the United States. Symptomatic knee and hip OA is the leading cause of joint replacement surgery, disability, and diminished quality of life among older individuals. The onset of OA before the fifth decade is unusual, and prevalence increases with age. Before the age of 50 years, men with OA outnumber women, but after this age, women are more likely to have OA than men, particularly at the hand and knee.

OA may be the final common pathway of many different disease processes. Although commonly defined radiographically, radiographic change can exist without corresponding symptoms. The causes of pain and disability from OA are complex and include comorbid conditions, muscle weakness, and psychosocial factors, as well as radiographic severity.

Etiology and Pathogenesis

Formerly regarded as primarily a disorder of articular cartilage, OA affects the entire joint, including cartilage, subchondral bone, ligaments, synovium, and surrounding muscle. The earliest pathologic changes are increased hydration and loss of proteoglycan content of cartilage, with subchondral bony thickening or sclerosis. With progression, cartilage frays or fibrillates with the development of focal ulcerations, sometimes leading to exposure of subchondral bone. Growth of bony osteophytes, a hallmark of the condition, occurs at joint margins, and mild synovitis may also ensue. Laxity of ligaments and weakness of surrounding muscle, formerly believed to be the result of disuse, may actually precede some of these disease processes (Figs. 143-1 and 143-2).

The cause of these events is unknown, but risk factors for the occurrence and progression of OA have been identified, although their relative importance may vary for different populations and for different joints. For example, increased body mass index is associated with knee and hand OA, but less strongly with hip OA. Further, these associations may be stronger in women, in whom weight loss has been shown to decrease the risk for developing symptomatic knee OA. The role of hormonal status and bone mineral density in OA is complex, with the incidence of OA in women increasing greatly with the onset of menopause. Genetics may account for as much as 65% of OA. Other risk factors include joint injury, occupational and sports physical demands, and possibly quadriceps weakness.

Clinical Presentation

OA has a characteristic joint distribution with symptoms dependent on the joint involved (Fig. 143-3). The most commonly involved joints are the knees, hands, feet, hips, and spine. The usual presenting complaint in OA is pain, initially activity related, with pain at rest occurring with advanced disease. Stiffness after inactivity (gel phenomenon) is prominent, but morning stiffness is of shorter duration and intensity than in systemic inflammatory arthropathies.

On clinical examination, the affected joint demonstrates hard, bony enlargement with or without soft tissue swelling, crepitus, tenderness, and limited range of motion. Synovial fluid, when present, is typically noninflammatory or only mildly inflammatory, and may have associated calcium pyrophosphate crystals.

Clinical Involvement: Knee

Knee OA is characterized by insidious onset of pain, gelling, limited motion, and difficulty with walking, transferring, and stair climbing (Fig. 143-4). Physical examination reveals crepitus and bony enlargement with pain along the medial or lateral joint line with or without effusion. Varus deformity is not uncommon, and flexion deformity

Figure 143-1 Normal Joint and Articular Surface; Early Degenerative Changes.

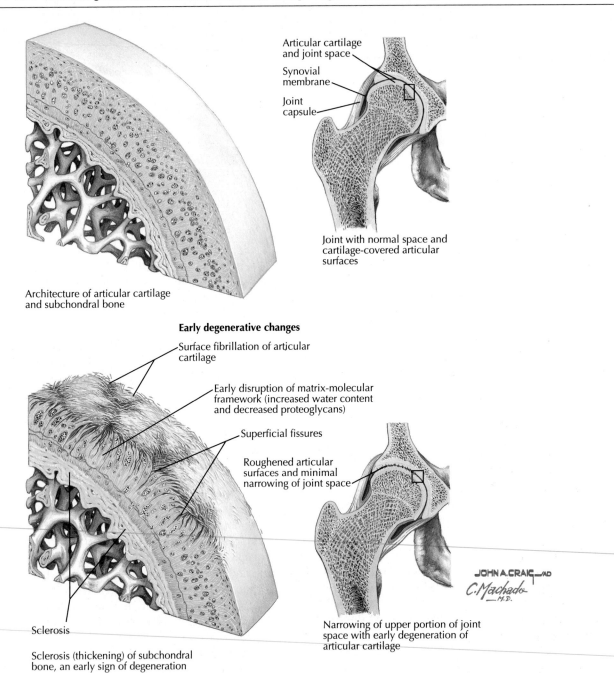

Architecture of articular cartilage and subchondral bone

Articular cartilage and joint space
Synovial membrane
Joint capsule

Joint with normal space and cartilage-covered articular surfaces

Early degenerative changes

Surface fibrillation of articular cartilage

Early disruption of matrix-molecular framework (increased water content and decreased proteoglycans)

Superficial fissures

Roughened articular surfaces and minimal narrowing of joint space

Sclerosis

Sclerosis (thickening) of subchondral bone, an early sign of degeneration

Narrowing of upper portion of joint space with early degeneration of articular cartilage

JOHN A. CRAIG—MD
C. Machado
—M.D.

and joint instability are signs of severity. Quadriceps weakness may occur early and may contribute to progression.

Clinical Involvement: Hip

Hip OA usually presents with groin pain, but pain can be felt in the thigh, buttock, or knee. Pain and limitation of motion in walking, bending, and transfer can be severe. On examination, painful limitation of internal rotation can be an early sign. Deformity and limitation of hip flexion indicate advanced disease (Fig. 143-5).

Clinical Involvement: Hand

Bony enlargement of the distal interphalangeal joints (Heberden's nodes) and proximal interphalangeal joints (Bouchard's nodes) can begin with an acute inflammatory phase, but the joints may become less symptomatic after

Figure 143-2 Advanced and End-Stage Degenerative Changes.

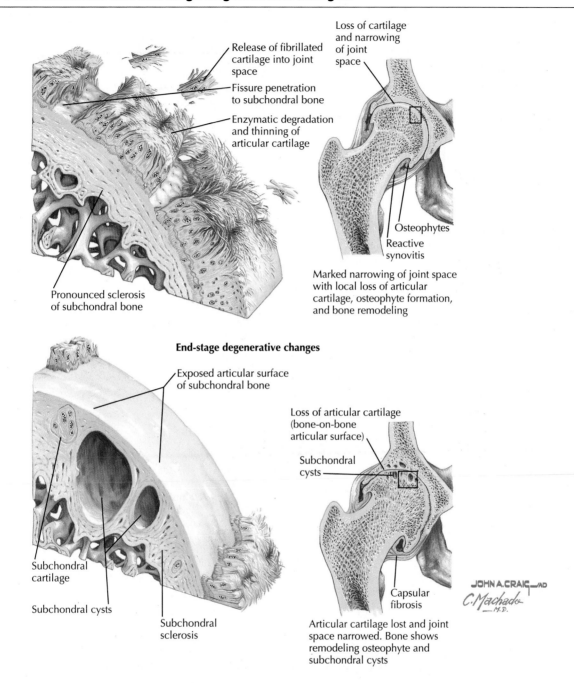

Release of fibrillated cartilage into joint space

Fissure penetration to subchondral bone

Enzymatic degradation and thinning of articular cartilage

Pronounced sclerosis of subchondral bone

Loss of cartilage and narrowing of joint space

Osteophytes

Reactive synovitis

Marked narrowing of joint space with local loss of articular cartilage, osteophyte formation, and bone remodeling

End-stage degenerative changes

Exposed articular surface of subchondral bone

Loss of articular cartilage (bone-on-bone articular surface)

Subchondral cysts

Subchondral cartilage

Subchondral cysts

Subchondral sclerosis

Capsular fibrosis

Articular cartilage lost and joint space narrowed. Bone shows remodeling osteophyte and subchondral cysts

JOHN A. CRAIG—AD
C. Machado
—M.D.

the initial inflammation has subsided. A subset of patients may have erosive osteoarthritis of hand joints, which presents as episodes of inflammation, pain, and swelling. Involvement of the first carpometacarpal joint can be associated with significant pain and limited function (Fig. 143-6). Bilateral involvement of multiple joints within and across joint groups is frequent. Metacarpophalangeal joints are affected more commonly than previously recognized; nonetheless, prominent involvement of these joints in the OA process should prompt consideration of secondary causes (see "Differential Diagnosis").

Clinical Involvement: Spine

Radiographic OA in the cervical and lumbar spine, frequently with degenerative disk disease, is very common in those older than 45 years, but may not be associated with symptoms. Clinical symptoms in the cervical spine can include pain in the neck and occiput, with radiation down the arm, weakness, or paresthesia occurring from compression of cervical nerves from osteophytic encroachment on intervertebral foramina. An analogous process can occur in the lower thoracic and lumbosacral spine.

Figure 143-3 Distribution of Joint Involvement in Osteoarthritis.

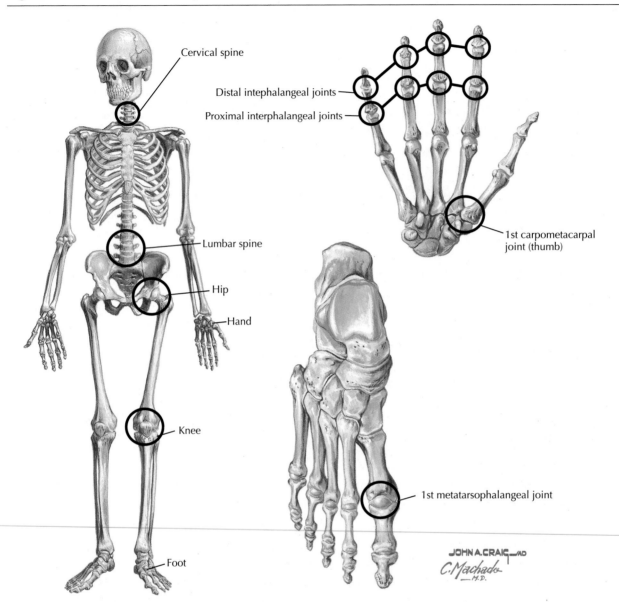

Cervical spine

Distal intephalangeal joints

Proximal interphalangeal joints

Lumbar spine

Hip

Hand

Knee

Foot

1st carpometacarpal joint (thumb)

1st metatarsophalangeal joint

JOHN A. CRAIG—MD
C. Machado
—M.D.

Radiographic changes (by joint) in oseoarthritis
(%/100 population)

Age (yr)	Hand	Foot	Knee	Hip
18-24	1.6	2.8		
25-34	3.4	7.0		
35-44	14.3	14.1	1.6	
45-54	36.4	23.9	3.0	
55-64	63.0	36.9	5.7	2.7
65-74	74.5	44.2	13.8	3.5

Figure 143-4 Clinical Findings.

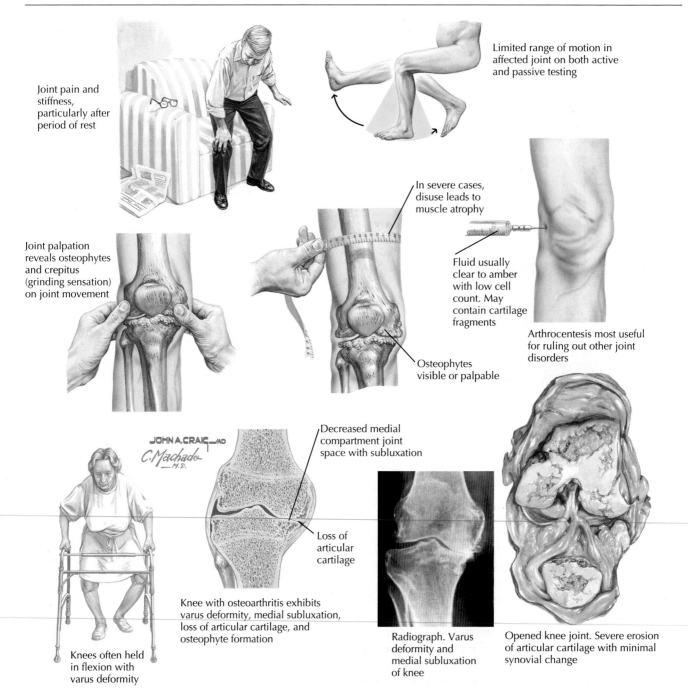

Joint pain and stiffness, particularly after period of rest

Limited range of motion in affected joint on both active and passive testing

Joint palpation reveals osteophytes and crepitus (grinding sensation) on joint movement

In severe cases, disuse leads to muscle atrophy

Fluid usually clear to amber with low cell count. May contain cartilage fragments

Osteophytes visible or palpable

Arthrocentesis most useful for ruling out other joint disorders

Decreased medial compartment joint space with subluxation

Loss of articular cartilage

Knees often held in flexion with varus deformity

Knee with osteoarthritis exhibits varus deformity, medial subluxation, loss of articular cartilage, and osteophyte formation

Radiograph. Varus deformity and medial subluxation of knee

Opened knee joint. Severe erosion of articular cartilage with minimal synovial change

Differential Diagnosis

General

Diagnosis of OA is usually made clinically, but other disorders need to be considered, depending on the joints involved. OA in individuals younger than 45 years frequently has an antecedent cause, such as hereditary conditions, prior trauma, or congenital or developmental conditions such as Legg-Perthes disease. OA typically has an insidious onset; an acute onset should prompt investigation for crystal arthropathies, infection, or trauma. OA does not have systemic inflammatory features nor prolonged morning stiffness. If these are present, systemic inflammatory arthropathies such as rheumatoid arthritis, systemic lupus erythematosus, malignancy, or infection should be considered.

Hip Osteoarthritis

Patients may mistakenly refer to the lumbar spine, pelvis, or greater trochanter as the "hip." The differential diagnosis of hip OA thus includes fracture, avascular necrosis,

Figure 143-5 Hip Joint Involvement in Osteoarthritis.

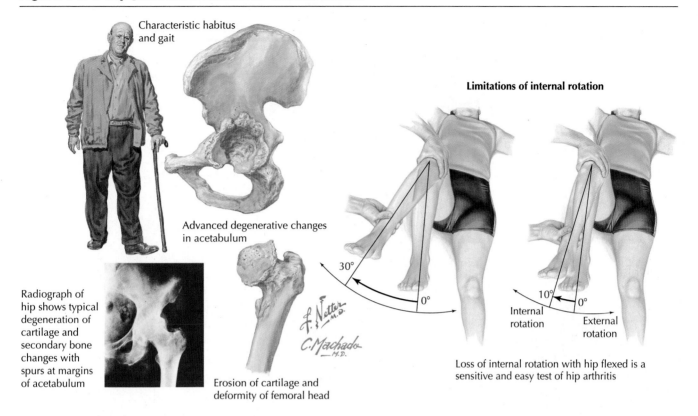

Characteristic habitus and gait

Advanced degenerative changes in acetabulum

Radiograph of hip shows typical degeneration of cartilage and secondary bone changes with spurs at margins of acetabulum

Erosion of cartilage and deformity of femoral head

Limitations of internal rotation

30°

0°

10°

0°

Internal rotation

External rotation

Loss of internal rotation with hip flexed is a sensitive and easy test of hip arthritis

inflammatory arthropathies, and pathologies involving the lumbar spine and pelvis or surrounding structures. Trochanteric bursitis is characterized by discomfort in the hip region, particularly with stair climbing and lying on the offending side. Palpation over the greater trochanter reproduces the patient's pain, and groin pain and painful limitation of hip rotation are absent. Low back pain with radiation, weakness, numbness, and paresthesia help differentiate hip OA from lumbar spine disorders.

Hip fracture usually presents acutely after trauma, but in the frail and osteoporotic patient, it can occur without such history. Clinical suspicion should be high in such patients, particularly if severe pain on hip motion or a posture of hip flexion and external rotation are present. Avascular necrosis of the hip should be considered in the patient with sickle cell disease, diabetes mellitus, a history of corticosteroid use, or alcohol.

Hand Osteoarthritis

Because hand OA is common, especially in women, hand complaints should be evaluated with the purpose of eliminating an accompanying, superimposed inflammatory condition. Involvement of the metacarpophalangeal joints with significant soft tissue swelling should suggest an inflammatory arthropathy, such as rheumatoid arthritis or calcium pyrophosphate dihydrate deposition. Involvement of the metacarpophalangeal joints with bony enlargement can occur in hand OA, but such findings may also indicate other disorders, such as hypothyroidism, hemochromatosis, hyperparathyroidism, or calcium pyrophosphate dihydrate deposition.

Foot Osteoarthritis

Involvement of the first metatarsophalangeal joint in the foot may mimic gout if sufficient erythema and swelling exist. Involvement of multiple metatarsophalangeal joints may indicate inflammatory arthropathy, such as rheumatoid arthritis, particularly if accompanied by prolonged morning stiffness and involvement of the small joints of the hands.

Diagnostic Approach

There are no definitive tests for OA, and the diagnosis remains a clinical one. A thorough history and physical to elicit the presence of other conditions should be performed. Unless clinical suspicion exists for a systemic inflammatory arthropathy or systemic autoimmune condi-

Figure 143-6 Hand Involvement in Osteoarthritis.

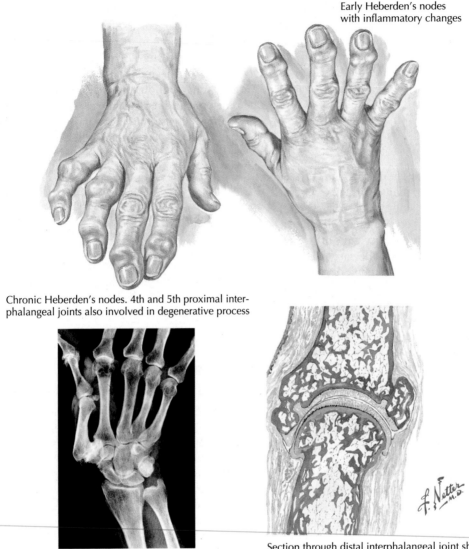

Early Heberden's nodes with inflammatory changes

Chronic Heberden's nodes. 4th and 5th proximal interphalangeal joints also involved in degenerative process

End-stage degenerative changes in carpometacarpal articulation of thumb

Section through distal interphalangeal joint shows irregular, hyperplastic bony nodules (Heberden's nodes) at articular margins of distal phalanx

tions, there is little purpose in measuring rheumatoid factor, antinuclear antibodies, or other serologic tests. Assessment of complete blood count, electrolytes with glucose and creatinine, and liver function tests should be checked before beginning pharmacologic therapy, especially in the older individual with comorbid medical conditions. In cases of atypical appearance of the hands, particularly with involvement of the metacarpophalangeal joints, evaluation for hypothyroidism and hemochromatosis may be warranted.

Radiographs typically show osteophytes, joint space narrowing, sclerosis of subchondral bone, cysts, and joint deformity. They can confirm a diagnosis and exclude others, particularly in those cases with an unclear clinical picture or when alternate diagnoses, such as inflammatory

arthropathy, hip fracture, avascular necrosis, infection, or malignancy, may exist. In the erosive variant of OA, radiographs may show central erosion and "gull deformity" of the interphalangeal joints. Radionuclide scans, magnetic resonance imaging, and other modalities may be useful in certain situations, but are not routinely needed in clinical practice.

Management and Therapy

Optimum Therapy

There is no cure for OA, nor are there pharmacologic agents available at this time that definitively affect the underlying pathologic process. Optimal medical management

consists of nonpharmacologic modalities and pharmacologic agents to relieve pain and improve function and health-related quality of life, with the goal of avoiding complications of therapy. In more severe cases, surgical intervention, particularly joint replacement, can be effective. Recently, similar guidelines for the treatment of hip and knee osteoarthritis were published by the American College of Rheumatology and the European League against Rheumatism.

Nonpharmacologic Therapy

Physical and occupational therapy should be mainstays of the treatment approach of most patients with OA. Assessment of gait disturbances, leg length discrepancy, and functional and other difficulties is critical in developing an individualized treatment plan. Ambulatory aids, orthotics, splints, and other assistive devices can alleviate pain and improve function by correcting malalignment, distributing weight more evenly to decrease stress on a particular joint, and altering abnormal joint biomechanics. Instruction in joint protection and energy saving techniques, aerobic exercise, muscle strengthening, and range-of-motion exercises can help the patient regain, maintain, or improve function. Weight loss should be prescribed for overweight OA patients and can be more effective in combination with exercise in reducing pain.

Pharmacologic Therapy

If the above measures prove insufficient, pharmacologic therapy (oral, topical and intra-articular) can be considered.

Acetaminophen and nonopioid analgesics, such as tramadol, can be helpful in the patient with mild to moderate or intermittent pain. Nonsteroidal anti-inflammatory drugs (NSAIDs) can be used in those in whom acetaminophen is ineffective. However, the potential for serious side effects, including gastrointestinal ulceration and bleeding, exacerbation of hypertension, and fluid retention, particularly in older individuals with comorbidities, limit their use. Although selective cyclooxygenase-2 inhibitors provided analgesia similar to traditional NSAIDs and were less likely to be associated with gastrointestinal ulceration and bleeding, concerns about their renal and cardiovascular safety have restricted their availability and utilization. Opioids should be reserved for those with severe pain that cannot be controlled otherwise.

The use of glucosamine and chondroitin, nutraceuticals that have demonstrated possible symptom- and disease-modifying properties in OA, remains popular but controversial. A recent clinical trial showed that the combination of glucosamine and chondroitin may be effective in relieving moderate to severe pain from knee osteoarthritis.

Other studies have had mixed results. Topical methylsalicylate, capsaicin, and NSAIDs can be useful as adjunctive or sole therapy in some patients.

Intra-articular corticosteroid therapy can relieve pain and inflammation in patients with OA. The need for repeated corticosteroid injections should prompt re-evaluation of the medical regimen and consideration of surgical intervention. Intra-articular hyaluronan can be administered in a series of injections for knee OA; although no definite disease modification has been shown for such agents, there may be a pain-relieving effect that can last several months.

With improved imaging methodology to measure cartilage loss, several agents have been studied recently to evaluate their effect on OA disease progression. Two trials have suggested that glucosamine sulfate may be associated with less joint space narrowing than placebo in knee OA. Other agents aimed at inhibition of catabolic processes in the joint and bone turnover, including diacerein, doxycycline, and bisphosphonates, have been or are currently under evaluation for their potential to modify the disease process. Future studies will reveal their significance and usefulness in clinical practice.

Avoiding Treatment Errors

Treatment errors in OA include (1) failure to recognize superimposed inflammatory arthritis, such as rheumatoid arthritis or gout, which would prompt different therapy; (2) inadequate attention to effective nonpharmacologic interventions such as weight loss, exercise, lifestyle modification, and biomechanical and assistive devices; (3) use of medications with a poor safety profile in susceptible individuals; and (4) failure to recognize potential drug interactions between OA therapy and concomitant medications. For example, the use of NSAIDs in older individuals and in those with cardiac, hepatic, or renal disease can be particularly problematic. Because of the risk for gastrointestinal ulceration with the use of NSAIDs, prophylactic therapy for ulcers should be considered as concomitant therapy in many patients. Use of any pharmaceutical should prompt careful periodic evaluation for side effects such as renal, electrolyte, hepatic, and gastrointestinal toxicity.

Future Directions

Therapy in OA at this time modifies symptoms without altering the underlying disease process, which may have progressed considerably by the time symptoms occur. The goals of future research are to develop better means to identify individuals at increased risk for OA for early intervention and to develop interventions to influence the disease process. Avenues for exploration in this regard include genetics, advanced imaging such as magnetic

resonance imaging, and biomarkers in serum, urine, and synovial fluid. For those in whom OA has already progressed, future research also endeavors to improve techniques and materials for joint replacement and to develop new ways to grow, modify, and implant cartilage into diseased joints.

Additional Resources

American College of Rheumatology. Available at: http://www.rheumatology.org.
  This website has information for health care professionals, patients, and the public about osteoarthritis, services available, and links to further information.
Arthritis Foundation. Available at: http://www.arthritis.org.
  This website has information for health care professionals, patients, and the public about osteoarthritis, medications, services, upcoming educational and advocacy events, and links to further information.

EVIDENCE

1. American College of Rheumatology Subcommittee on Osteoarthritis Guidelines: Recommendations for the medical management of osteoarthritis of the hip and knee. 2000 update. Arthritis Rheum 43(9):1905-1915, 2000.
    This article provides evidence-based recommendations for the treatment of hip and knee OA.

2. Clegg DO, Reda DJ, Harris CL, et al: Glucosamine, chondroitin sulfate, and the two in combination for painful knee osteoarthritis. N Engl J Med 354(8):795-808, 2006.
    The authors report on a randomized, double-blind, placebo and active comparator-controlled multicenter trial to evaluate glucosamine hydrochloride and chondroitin sulfate, alone and in combination, in the treatment of symptomatic knee OA. The combination of glucosamine and chondroitin was associated with significant pain reduction in those with moderate to severe pain.

3. Hochberg MC: Nutritional supplements for knee osteoarthritis-still no resolution. N Engl J Med 354(8):858-860, 2006.
    This editorial on the strengths and weaknesses of the above study addresses multiple relevant points in the current debate about the use of glucosamine and chondroitin in OA.

4. Jordan KM, Arden N, Doherty M, et al: EULAR recommendations 2003: An evidence based approach to the management of knee osteoarthritis. Report of a Task Force of the Standing Committee for International Clinical Studies Including Therapeutic Trials (ESCISIT). Ann Rheum Dis 62(12):1145-1155, 2003.
    This evidence-based article evaluates various treatment options for knee OA, classifying them into four broad categories: nonpharmacologic, pharmacologic, intra-articular, and surgical. The authors emphasize that recommendations should be tailored to the individual patient.

5. Zhang W, Doherty M, Arden N, et al: EULAR evidence based recommendations for the management of hip osteoarthritis. Report of a task force of the EULAR Standing Committee for International Clinical Studies Including Therapeutics (ESCISIT). Ann Rheum Dis 64(5):669-681, 2005.
    The authors provide 10 key recommendations for the treatment of hip OA, based on evidence from literature and expert opinion.

Low Back Pain in Adults

Introduction

Low back pain is a common and remitting ailment for most adults. About 80% of adults have an episode sufficiently severe that they cannot do their usual daily activities for at least 1 day at some time in their lives. About 8% of individuals have an episode in a given year, and about 3% to 4% have the very disabling syndrome of chronic low back pain. Most patients with low back pain can be treated at the primary care level.

Etiology and Pathogenesis

Adult vertebrae are complex anatomic and biomechanical structures (Fig. 144-1). Usually, these structures function extraordinarily well under various loads, postures, and torque, and after mild to moderate trauma. Most back pain occurs in the lumbar area, and 95% of intervertebral disk problems occur at the L-2 through L-5 areas.

The pain generator for most cases of back pain is unclear. The annulus fibrosus of the intervertebral disk is richly innervated, and many cases of back pain are undoubtedly diskogenic. Facet joints, ligaments, and muscles can all cause chronic back pain. Leg pain is more likely to be related to pressure on the intervertebral disk, but can occur as a result of bone spurs or pressure on the nerve roots related to spinal stenosis. Sciatica is generally defined as radiation of pain to the level of the knee or below. Classic diskogenic pain is more prominent in the leg than in the back. In spinal stenosis, a variation of nerve root impingement, the patient's thigh pain becomes worse on walking or prolonged standing (pseudoclaudication). The pathogenesis of pseudoclaudication appears to relate to a congenitally narrow spinal canal combined with bony overgrowth around the facet joints.

More than 85% of cases of acute back pain are not related to sciatica, spinal stenosis, or serious causes such as malignancy or abdominal aortic aneurysm. Cases of nonspecific chronic back pain are usually the most difficult to manage and require a great deal of skill in both communicating with patients and coordinating care.

Clinical Presentation

Because most patients have a relatively nonspecific diagnosis, it is important to identify the minority of patients who do have a specific cause of their back pain. Patients with acute back pain generally present after 2 weeks of symptoms. The onset of the pain is usually not substantial trauma; most often, it occurs with activities of daily living such as lifting, bending, or twisting. Often, patients are fearful that the cause of their back pain is serious and will result in chronic pain or permanent disability. Eliciting these fears by asking, "What do you think is causing your back pain?" can lead to productive reassurance.

Differential Diagnosis

The history should include a search for red-flag factors, described below, relating to the patient's back pain in order to make the correct diagnosis and rule out important, potentially correctable, causes of back pain.

Cauda Equina Syndrome

In the cauda equina syndrome, the acute onset of urinary retention or fecal incontinence, loss of anal sphincter tone, and perianal anesthesia are typical and may occur with bilateral leg weakness. Immediate magnetic resonance imaging (MRI) and referral to an orthopedic surgeon or neurosurgeon is indicated. The etiology is most commonly related to a metastatic malignancy and rarely to a large central disk herniation.

Infectious Diskitis and Osteomyelitis

Back pain associated with fever, sweats, and weight loss may occur with infectious diskitis or osteomyelitis. These patients generally have an elevated erythrocyte sedimenta-

Figure 144-1 Lumbosacral Spine and Ligaments.

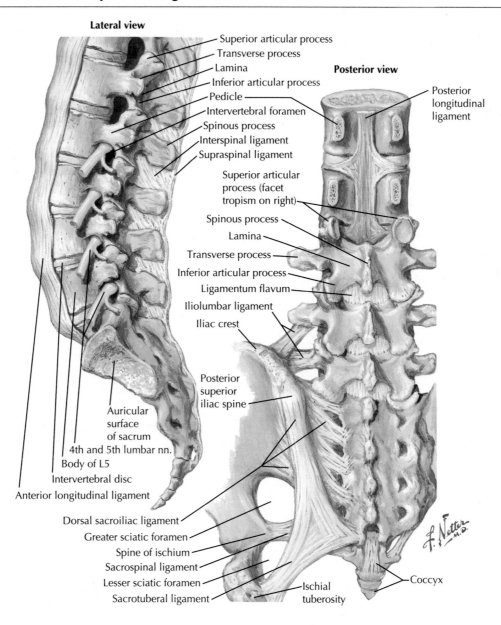

Lateral view

Superior articular process
Transverse process
Lamina
Inferior articular process
Pedicle
Intervertebral foramen
Spinous process
Interspinal ligament
Supraspinal ligament

Posterior view

Posterior longitudinal ligament

Superior articular process (facet tropism on right)
Spinous process
Lamina
Transverse process
Inferior articular process
Ligamentum flavum
Iliolumbar ligament
Iliac crest
Posterior superior iliac spine

Auricular surface of sacrum
4th and 5th lumbar nn.
Body of L5
Intervertebral disc
Anterior longitudinal ligament
Dorsal sacroiliac ligament
Greater sciatic foramen
Spine of ischium
Sacrospinal ligament
Lesser sciatic foramen
Sacrotuberal ligament
Ischial tuberosity
Coccyx

tion rate and may be immunocompromised or have a nidus of infection, such as a chronic urinary tract infection. Plain film radiographs have only about a 70% sensitivity in the early phases of diskitis.

Metastatic Cancer

Progressive and unrelenting back pain can be a sign of prostate, breast, or lung cancer. Multiple myeloma may also initially present as back pain. A history of cancer other than skin cancer in the previous 5 to 10 years requires plain film radiographs, measurement of erythrocyte sedimentation rate, or advanced imaging such as bone scan, MRI, or computed tomography (CT) scan.

Trauma

Trauma, especially in a patient with or at risk for osteoporosis, should raise concern regarding fracture.

Ankylosing Spondylitis and Other Syndromes

Pain made worse with morning stiffness in younger men and relieved by exercise may be indicative of ankylosing spondylitis, an uncommon but important cause of back pain.

Back pain may occasionally present as referred pain from an abdominal or retroperitoneal source. This may include the burning pain of early shingles (herpes zoster), back pain secondary to an abdominal aortic aneurysm, or pyelonephritis.

The red-flag syndromes described previously are very important to recognize because some causes of back pain may lead to an irreversible neurologic deficit. The chance of a patient presenting with back pain having one of these serious red-flag problems is low in an ambulatory practice but is higher in emergency room settings or tertiary care centers.

A brief evaluation for yellow flags is also indicated. These social factors include litigation through personal injury or worker compensation, intense preoccupation with the pain, or anger toward the employer, all of which may indicate a worse prognosis from back pain. The presence of one of these factors does not indicate that the patient is malingering. The physician's perspective should be attuned to encouraging improved functioning and psychosocial support.

Diagnostic Approach

The physical examination can be brief in most cases. Examination of the abdomen may pick up bruits or pulsating masses in cases of abdominal aneurysm; this is especially important in males older than 50 years with a smoking history and other signs of atherosclerosis. Palpation of the back can sometimes find tender areas or trigger points. Usually, these findings are quite nonspecific; however, it is important to touch the part of the patient that hurts in order to assure the patient that he or she is receiving a thorough evaluation. Examination of the knee and ankle jerk reflexes can pick up nerve root impingement (Figs. 144-2, 144-3, and 144-4). Testing of dorsiflexion foot

Figure 144-2 Sensory and Motor Innervation of Lower Limb.

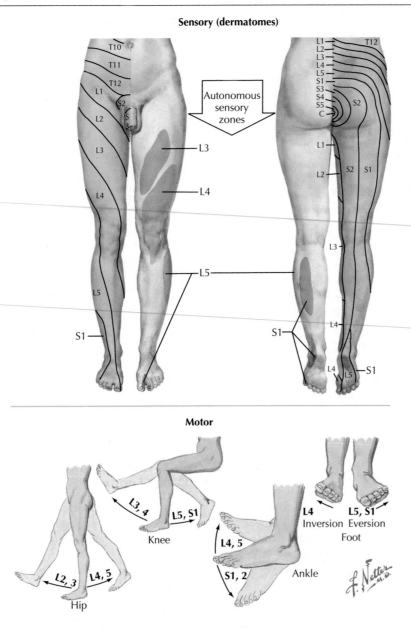

Figure 144-3 Clinical Features of Herniated Lumbar Nucleus Pulposus.

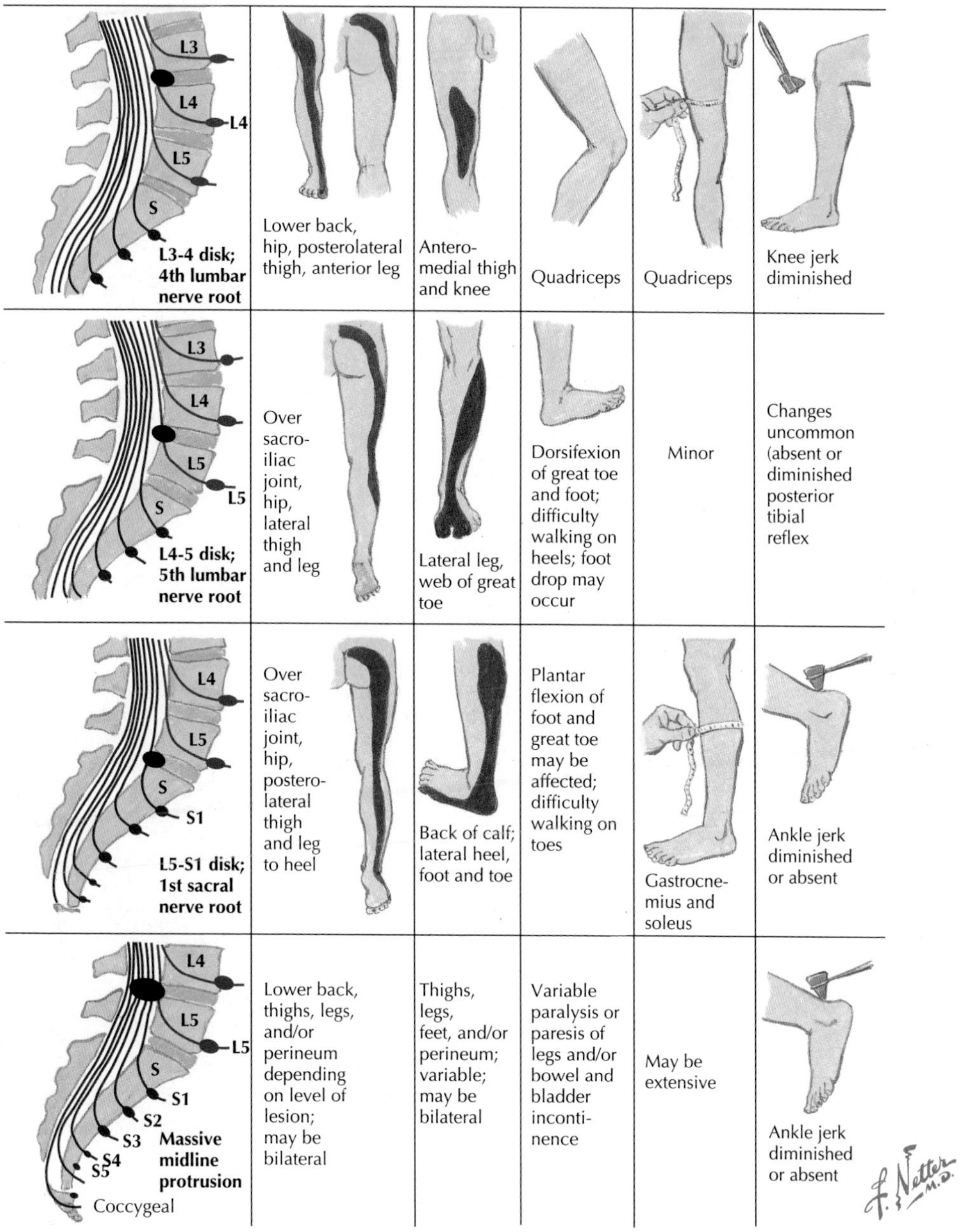

Level of herniation	Pain	Numbness	Weakness	Atrophy	Reflexes
L3-4 disk; 4th lumbar nerve root	Lower back, hip, posterolateral thigh, anterior leg	Antero-medial thigh and knee	Quadriceps	Quadriceps	Knee jerk diminished
L4-5 disk; 5th lumbar nerve root	Over sacro-iliac joint, hip, lateral thigh and leg	Lateral leg, web of great toe	Dorsifexion of great toe and foot; difficulty walking on heels; foot drop may occur	Minor	Changes uncommon (absent or diminished posterior tibial reflex
L5-S1 disk; 1st sacral nerve root	Over sacro-iliac joint, hip, postero-lateral thigh and leg to heel	Back of calf; lateral heel, foot and toe	Plantar flexion of foot and great toe may be affected; difficulty walking on toes	Gastrocnemius and soleus	Ankle jerk diminished or absent
Massive midline protrusion	Lower back, thighs, legs, and/or perineum depending on level of lesion; may be bilateral	Thighs, legs, feet, and/or perineum; variable; may be bilateral	Variable paralysis or paresis of legs and/or bowel and bladder incontinence	May be extensive	Ankle jerk diminished or absent

strength can assess the L-4 to L-5 nerve root. The ankle-jerk reflex assesses L-5 to S-1. More than 90% of nerve root impingements occur at one of these two levels. The dorsum of the foot may have hypoesthesia in impingement of the L-4 to L-5 disk space.

The straight-leg-raising sign is relatively specific but not very sensitive for nerve root impingement. For this maneuver, the leg is elevated passively, and when positive, the patient has pain on the affected side that radiates to the level of the knee or below.

Rectal examination is indicated when there is concern about carcinoma of the prostate gland (prolonged pain, older men) or potential cauda equina syndrome (bilateral leg weakness, incontinence, or retention of urine or stool).

Exaggerated pain behavior and reproduction of pain by pressing on the top of the head (axial loading, which transmits essentially zero force to the lumbar spine) are associated with a strong psychological component to pain. These patients tend to do poorly with surgery and require greater attention to psychosocial issues.

Most patients do not require immediate imaging studies. Lumbar spine radiographs are indicated when there is concern regarding trauma, in the presence of red flags, or

Figure 144-4 Pain Patterns in Lumbar Disease.

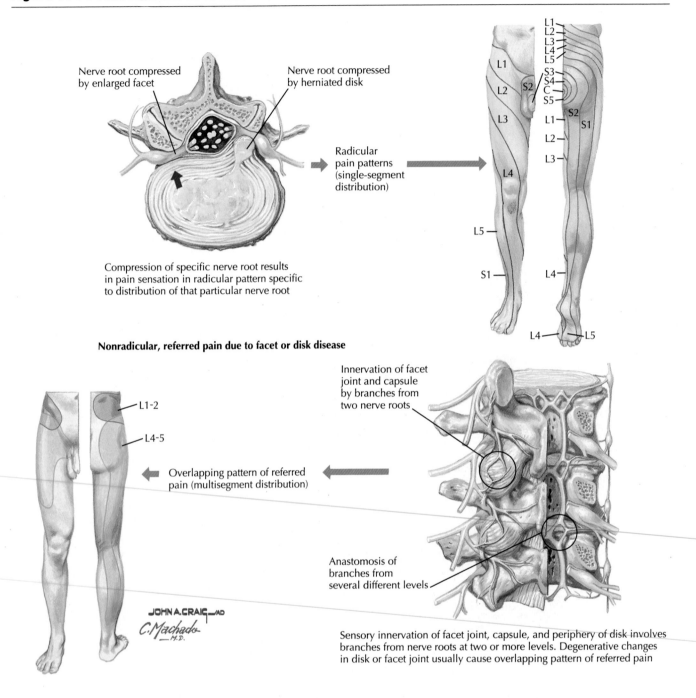

Nerve root compressed by enlarged facet

Nerve root compressed by herniated disk

Radicular pain patterns (single-segment distribution)

Compression of specific nerve root results in pain sensation in radicular pattern specific to distribution of that particular nerve root

Nonradicular, referred pain due to facet or disk disease

Innervation of facet joint and capsule by branches from two nerve roots

L1-2

L4-5

Overlapping pattern of referred pain (multisegment distribution)

Anastomosis of branches from several different levels

JOHN A. CRAIG, AD
C. Machado, M.D.

Sensory innervation of facet joint, capsule, and periphery of disk involves branches from nerve roots at two or more levels. Degenerative changes in disk or facet joint usually cause overlapping pattern of referred pain

if the patient has not attained functional recovery within 4 to 6 weeks. There is no consensus regarding indications for advanced techniques such as CT or MRI. Such tests should be urgently performed when there is concern regarding metastasis or infection. In general, such advanced imaging techniques are indicated only when a red flag is present or an operation is under active consideration. Although these tests are highly sensitive, nonspecific findings are common, herniated disks may be found in 20% to 30% of asymptomatic individuals. MRI evidence of spinal stenosis has been demonstrated in more than 20% of individuals older than 60 years without symptoms.

Management and Therapy

When a serious cause of low back pain is found (metastatic malignancy, diskitis), specific treatment is urgently indicated. However, this is unusual, and most cases of non-emergent back pain can be divided into three broad categories: nonspecific back pain, nerve root impingement related to herniated disk, and spinal stenosis.

Nonspecific Low Back Pain

More than 80% of patients present with nonspecific or mechanical low back pain. This lack of specificity is often frustrating for both doctors and patients. It is important to provide patients with an explanatory model of what is going on with their back so that they can live with their symptoms and know that, given the natural history of back pain, they will likely improve. Patients often relate well to phrases such as "it's like a flu in your back" or "strained ligaments" because these common syndromes have a relatively benign prognosis.

Ninety-five percent of patients with nonspecific acute back pain (less than 2 months of symptoms) return to their usual daily functioning within 3 months of conservative treatment.

Optimum Treatment

Reassurance, appropriate analgesia, and advice to resume usual daily activities as quickly as possible are the most effective treatments. Bed rest for more than 48 hours appears to be counterproductive. Acetaminophen, nonsteroidal anti-inflammatory drugs, and, possibly, a muscle relaxant provide adequate symptom relief for most patients. Those with very severe initial symptoms may benefit from a short course of a narcotic analgesic. It is important to encourage patients to return to work as quickly as possible because prolonged time off work appears to worsen rather than improve back-related disability. A note or conversation with a patient's supervisor regarding avoiding heavy lifting or awkward postures for a designated period can be helpful and is often indicated. Patients often benefit from a telephone call or return office visit within 2 weeks. If the patient is off work after 2 weeks, more specific treatment such as a physical therapy referral may be in order. Spinal manipulative therapy may be performed by doctors of chiropractic medicine, osteopathic physicians, and some physical therapists. Randomized trials of spinal manipulation have yielded somewhat conflicting results; more recent studies have demonstrated marginal, if any, benefit when compared with conventional conservative medical therapy.

Herniated Lumbar Disk

Diagnostic clues of a herniated disk include true sciatica and presence of suggestive neurologic findings (Fig. 144-5). In the absence of red flags, a supportive approach is indicated. Ninety percent of patients with sciatica improve with conservative therapy over a 3-month period.

Optimum Treatment

Some patients benefit from a brief (1 to 2 days) period of bed rest. Patients often are quite fearful of resuming usual activities, and a physical therapy referral may be helpful to coach the patient to maintain activities such as walking, even when uncomfortable. If a patient has persistent predominant leg pain as the primary back symptom, especially if combined with asymmetrical reflexes or mild weakness in dorsiflexion of the foot, limited evidence suggests that the patient may benefit from an advanced imaging technique and consideration of operative microdiskectomy.

Spinal Stenosis

Cohort studies have demonstrated that, over several years, one third of patients stay the same, and one third worsen. Some patients become severely impaired with nearly constant pain and limited ambulation.

Optimum Treatment

Analgesics and physical therapy may offer only modest benefit. Because walking is often limited by the nature of the disease, swimming or stationary bicycling may be helpful. Surgical decompression appears to offer substantial relief of leg symptoms and improved walking distance, although most patients continue to have back pain and some limitation in walking distance. Older age leads to greater risk for cardiac complications at the time of surgery.

Chronic Back Pain

Many patients with chronic low back pain have no radiculopathy or anatomic abnormalities that clearly explain their symptoms. Patients with 2 months of continuous symptoms have more than a 50% chance of having significant back symptoms 1 to 2 years later. No single therapy appears to be beneficial for their symptoms. Lumbar spinal fusion may provide some relief, but it is a significantly morbid procedure with high failure rates, which provides relief of symptoms in less than half of patients. After an acute episode of worsened back pain is resolved, chronic back pain patients who can adhere to an exercise regimen (as recommended by a physical therapist) have less back pain and fewer exacerbations.

Optimum Treatment

Intensive exercise regimens reduce pain and improve functioning. As noted earlier, reinforcement of exercise needs to take place on an ongoing basis. Tricyclic antidepressant medications or antiseizure medications such as gabapentin are useful adjuncts. Long-term opioid therapy is favored by some authorities. One small, randomized trial showed that opioids reduced pain; however, activity levels were not improved, and side effects such as sedation and constipation may be substantial. Patients with disabling chronic

Figure 144-5 Intervertebral Disk.

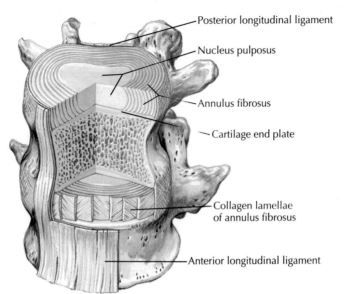

Posterior longitudinal ligament

Nucleus pulposus

Annulus fibrosus

Cartilage end plate

Collagen lamellae of annulus fibrosus

Anterior longitudinal ligament

Intervertebral disk composed of central nuclear zone of collagen and hydrated proteoglycans surrounded by concentric lamellae of collagen fibers

Pump mechanism of disk nutrition

Nonload bearing   Load bearing

Movement-driven pump mechanism alternately compresses and relaxes pressure on disk, pumping water and waste products out and water and nutrients in. Baseline turgor maintained by hydrophilic proteins. Failure of pump mechanism may result in biochemical changes, causing back pain

JOHN A. CRAIG _AD
C. Machado
_M.D.

Disk rupture and nuclear herniation

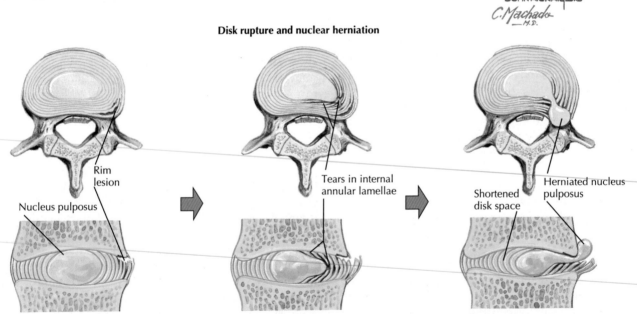

Rim lesion

Nucleus pulposus

Tears in internal annular lamellae

Shortened disk space

Herniated nucleus pulposus

Peripheral tear of annulus fibrosus and cartilage end plate (rim lesion) initiates sequence of events that weaken and tear internal annular lamellae, allowing extrusion and herniation of nucleus pulposus

pain may benefit from referral to a multidisciplinary pain center.

Avoiding Treatment Errors

Problems with back pain care can occur in nonrecognition of serious pathology, such as not imaging a patient with a history of severe low back pain and a history of breast cancer. Errors are also common through provision of *too many* diagnostic tests or recommendation of inappropriate treatments. When patients with nonspecific back pain receive an MRI, they may be told they have degenerated or bulging disks, when in fact they have a typical imaging test for age, resulting in markedly increased anxiety and fear of activity. Recommendation of therapies for which there is limited evidence of benefit, such as intradiskal electrothermal therapy or prolonged courses of traction, may also result in wasted time, additional cost, and exposure to complications. One must also be cautious in recommending surgical intervention for chronic back pain because the patient rarely obtains long-term benefit and often requires subsequent procedures.

Future Directions

The use of an initial clinical diagnostic evaluation and a stepped care approach to back pain can reduce provider and patient frustration and result in improved outcomes, including improved functional status and earlier return to work. Basic research in identifying the pain generator in a larger portion of cases will improve diagnosis and better guide treatment. Randomized trials, currently underway, should give clinicians better information regarding which patients may benefit from diskectomy, spinal fusion, and spinal decompressive surgery.

Additional Resource

Deyo RA, Weinstein JN: Low back pain. N Engl J Med 344:363-370, 2001.

This is an excellent overall review of diagnostic and treatment options.

EVIDENCE

1. Assendelft WJ, Morton SC, Yu EI, et al: Spinal manipulative therapy for low back pain. A meta-analysis of effectiveness relative to other therapies. Ann Intern Med 138:871-881, 2003.

This very complete review and meta-analysis indicates that spinal manipulation is not superior to conventional medical treatments, but may be helpful in some circumstances.

2. Atlas SJ, Keller RB, Wu YA, et al: Long-term outcomes of surgical and nonsurgical management of sciatica secondary to lumbar disc herniation: 10 year results from the Main Lumbar Spine Study. Spine 30:927-935, 2005.

In this long-term cohort study, patients receiving surgical treatment for sciatica had greater improvement in symptoms than patients who chose nonoperative treatments. However, at 10 years, the work and disability outcomes were similar regardless of treatment chosen. This is the best evidence at present until new randomized trials are reported.

3. Hayden JA, van Tudler MW, Tomlinson G: Systematic review: Strategies for using exercise therapy to improve outcomes in chronic low back pain. Ann Intern Med 142:776-785, 2005.

Exercise of longer duration and programs that were individually tailored to the patient had the greatest benefit. The magnitude of benefit for the best-performing exercise regimens was both clinically and statistically significant.

4. Jamison RN, Raymond SA, Slawsby EA, et al: Opioid therapy for chronic noncancer back pain. A randomized prospective study. Spine 23:2591-2600, 1998.

This article describes one of the very few true randomized controlled trials of opioid use for nonmalignant pain. Pain scores were improved by opiates, but patient functional status was not.

John B. Winfield

Fibromyalgia

Introduction

Fibromyalgia is a chronic disorder occurring predominately in females; the female-to-male ratio is 10 : 1. It is characterized by pain amplification (manifest as widespread pain) and psychological distress (manifest as fatigue, poor sleep, and in some patients, anxiety, depression, and numerous somatic complaints) (Fig. 145-1). Fibromyalgia overlaps with other illnesses that remain unexplained after usual clinical and laboratory assessment, such as chronic fatigue syndrome, irritable bowel syndrome (IBS), temporomandibular joint pain, and other regional pain syndromes. Advances in our understanding of the genetic, neurophysiologic, neuro-endocrinologic, and environmental events that underlie the development of such illnesses are impelling a unifying reclassification as central sensitivity syndromes (CSS) (Box 145-1).

Otherwise unexplained chronic pain and fatigue are extremely prevalent in the general population in the United States and Europe, especially among women and persons of lower socioeconomic status: regional pain, 20%; widespread pain, 11%; fibromyalgia by American College of Rheumatology (ACR) criteria, 3% to 5% in females and 0.5% to 1.6% in males; and chronic fatigue, about 20%. Fibromyalgia may develop in both children and older persons.

Etiology and Pathogenesis

Although many of the biologic and psychological variables that contribute to chronic pain and fatigue in fibromyalgia and other CSS have been identified, clinical expression of illness in fibromyalgia is best viewed from the perspective of the biopsychosocial model, in which health status and outcomes are influenced by the interaction of a series of biologic, psychological, and sociologic variables.

Biologic Elements

Biologic elements in fibromyalgia that were so lacking for most of this century, such as structural pathology in muscles, have recently been identified and partially characterized. These include gender, genes, central and peripheral mechanisms of pain amplification, abnormal sleep, and dysregulation of the stress response system. Female gender is a likely modifier of the interaction between genetic and environmental factors that influence vulnerability to pain amplification and psychological distress. For example, compared with males, females exhibit higher pain sensitivity; lack certain pain inhibitory mechanisms; exhibit greater sympathetic nervous system, neuroendocrine, and psychological responses to stressful or aversive stimuli; and are at greater risk for chronic pain conditions. The number of specific genetic variants that influence vulnerability to pain amplification and psychological distress is expanding exponentially as a result of high-throughput genetic analyses. The neurophysiologic and neuroendocrinologic bases for pain amplification involve multiple abnormalities in pronociceptive and antinociceptive pathways in the central nervous system. These include glial activation; increased levels of inflammatory cytokines and excitatory amino acids; decreased availability of serotonin, norepinephrine, and enkephalins; and deficiency of biogenic amines that normally regulate the release of substance P, to list a few. Nonrestorative sleep is related to intrusion of α waves into the brain's electrical field during restorative stage 3 and 4 non-rapid eye movement sleep and to several other well-characterized sleep abnormalities. Dysregulation of the stress response system is manifest by hypofunctional sympathetic reflex response to stressors and by abnormalities of the hypothalamic-pituitary-adrenal axis as well as other neuroendocrine axes, including growth hormone secretion in response to exercise.

Figure 145-1 Faces of Fibromyalgia.

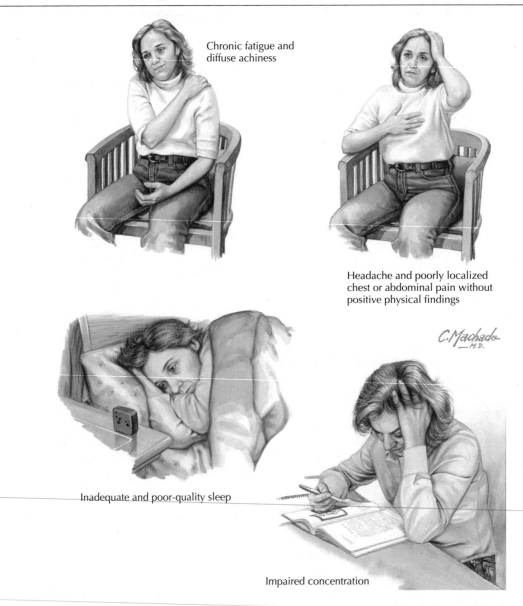

Chronic fatigue and diffuse achiness

Headache and poorly localized chest or abdominal pain without positive physical findings

Inadequate and poor-quality sleep

Impaired concentration

Psychological (Cognitive-Behavioral) Variables

Psychological distress, especially in association with depression, anxiety, post-traumatic stress disorder, and personality disorders, is prevalent in fibromyalgia and other CSS. When vulnerable individuals who express various combinations of genetic susceptibility haplotypes encounter environmental situations of unrelieved stress and distress, functional alterations of the stress response system may result. Other psychological variables that play a role in the overall symptomatology and clinical impact of fibromyalgia include pain beliefs and attributions regarding environmental causation of the illness, pain behaviors,

hypervigilance, coping strategies, and the degree of perceived self-efficacy for pain control.

Sociologic (Environmental and Sociocultural) Variables

Sociologic variables consist of experiences influenced by life and culture that interact with gender and genetic vulnerabilities in the clinical expression of fibromyalgia, such as psychosocial experiences during childhood, family support, work environment, job satisfaction, and ethnologic factors. Particularly important with respect to the development of chronic pain in adulthood are adverse

---

Box 145-1   Currently Proposed Members of the Central Sensitivity Syndromes

Fibromyalgia (overlaps strongly with chronic fatigue syndrome)
Irritable bowel syndrome (includes functional dyspepsia)
Temporomandibular disorders
Myofascial pain syndrome, regional soft tissue pain syndrome
Periodic limb movements in sleep
Multiple chemical sensitivity
Female urethral syndrome, interstitial cystitis (possibly may also include vulvodynia)
Post-traumatic stress syndrome
Depression

Table 145-1   Differential Diagnosis of Fibromyalgia

Major Disorder Group	Selected Specific Disorders
Rheumatologic	Systemic lupus erythematosus*
	Rheumatoid arthritis, Sjögren's syndrome*
	Polyarticular osteoarthritis, degenerative spondylosis
	Polymyalgia rheumatica*
	Polymyositis, statin myopathy
	Regional pain syndromes*
	Osteomalacia
	Hypermobility syndromes
Neurologic	Carpal tunnel syndrome*
	Cervical radiculopathy*
	Metabolic myopathies
	Multiple sclerosis*
	Cervical cord compression
Chronic infection	Subacute bacterial endocarditis
	Brucellosis
	Hepatitis
	HIV
Endocrine	Hypothyroidism*
	Diabetes mellitus type 2
	Hyperparathyroidism
Neoplastic	Metastatic (e.g., breast, lung, prostate)
	Myeloma
Psychiatric	Pain disorder associated with psychological factors* (formerly, somatoform pain disorder)
	Somatization disorder (hysteria, Briquet's syndrome)

*Common alternative diagnoses.
From Winfield JB: Fibromyalgia. In Dale DC (ed): ACP Medicine. New York, WebMD Professional Publishing, 2006, pp 1412-1418.

---

experiences during childhood, such as poor family environment or childhood sexual abuse, as has been particularly well studied in IBS.

Clinical Presentation

Fibromyalgia presents with widespread pain, fatigue, subjective weakness, insomnia, and in many patients, depression and anxiety, "like I have flu all the time." Pain radiates diffusely from the axial skeleton and is localized to muscles and muscle-tendon junctions of the neck, shoulders, hips, and extremities. The pain may be described as "exhausting," "miserable," or "unbearable," and there often is the complaint that even gentle touch is unpleasant (allodynia). Fatigue may dominate the clinical picture. Cognitive complaints, such as difficulties with concentration and memory, may be prominent. Many patients express numerous somatic complaints that remain unexplained after careful clinical assessment. Significant functional impairment in activities of daily living is usually present, as is deconditioning due to lack of exercise. Indeed, there often is fear and avoidance of exercise because of exacerbation of symptomatology following excessive activity on "good days." Fibromyalgia frequently coexists with inflammatory disorders of defined structural pathology, such as systemic lupus erythematosus (SLE), rheumatoid arthritis, ankylosing spondylitis, Crohn's disease, and ulcerative colitis. Optimum therapeutic outcomes require recognition and treatment of both fibromyalgia and associated disease.

As in IBS, patients with more severe fibromyalgia may exhibit a history of childhood abuse, major psychosocial stressors, post-traumatic stress disorder, personality disorder, or major depressive disorder. Such patients require counseling and psychiatric consultation. Prognosis varies among three fairly distinct subsets of patients. Adaptive copers, many of whom do not seek care for fibromyalgia, do well with respect to self-reported pain, disturbed sleep, and fatigue. Interpersonally distressed patients also respond to a comprehensive interdisciplinary therapeutic approach.

Dysfunctional patients, who exhibit high levels of pain, anxiety, functional impairment, and a history of opioid dependence, respond poorly to therapeutic intervention, as do patients with pending litigation.

Differential Diagnosis

Although the differential diagnosis of fibromyalgia is broad (Table 145-1), extensive diagnostic testing should not be done unless the patient exhibits objective signs of structural disease on physical or neurologic examinations. It is not helpful clinically to distinguish fibromyalgia from chronic fatigue syndrome (refer to Chapter 6) or the many regional pain syndromes. However, giving patients a name for their illness has therapeutic value in that it enables them to concentrate on getting better, rather than on continuously searching for a cause and a cure.

Figure 145-2 Fibromyalgia Tender Points.

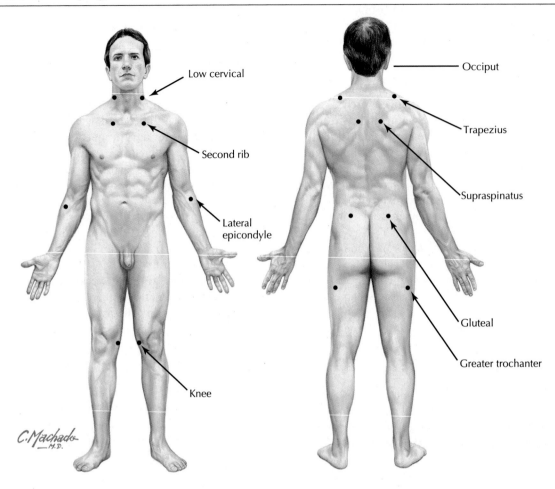

Diagnostic Approach

There are no generally accepted diagnostic criteria for fibromyalgia, although the ACR classification criteria designed and validated for selection of research subjects provides a reminder for two key features: widespread pain and painful tender points (Fig. 145-2) on physical examination. In practice, consider fibromyalgia when a patient presents with widespread pain for longer than 3 months, fatigue associated with usual daily activities, poor sleep, and multiple symptoms that cannot be easily explained. Except for painful tender points (perhaps five is sufficient), the physical and neurologic examinations will be unremarkable unless coexisting disease is present. Routine diagnostic testing should be limited to a few screening tests to exclude or confirm the presence of diseases that can be confused with fibromyalgia or that frequently coexist with fibromyalgia (Box 145-2).

Key Elements in the History

- Assess the onset, location, and nature of pain, together with ameliorating and exacerbating factors.

Box 145-2 Routine Diagnostic Testing
Complete blood count and differential
Creatine kinase
Thyroid-stimulating hormone (TSH)
Erythrocyte sedimentation rate (ESR)
Antinuclear antibodies (ANAs)
Rheumatoid factor
Other tests that may be considered:
Laboratory sleep assessment if sleep does not improve with usual conservative measures
Consider screening with a serum transferrin saturation and a serum ferritin concentration in patients aged 40-60 years because diffuse arthralgias and myalgias have been described in patients with hemochromatosis
Pressure algometry (dolorimetry) to assess pressure pain detection thresholds at four tender points associated with fibromyalgia (i.e., both lateral epicondyles, midpoints of the trapezii) is useful both as an aid in diagnosis and as a semiquantitative guide to therapy. Normal values are ≥4 kg/cm²

- Inquire about sleep quality, impairment in activities of daily living, ongoing and past stressors, feelings of anxiety or depression, marital adjustment, and perceived levels of social support. Recognition of difficulties in these areas is essential in the overall management of fibromyalgia.
- Ask "how was your childhood?" This inquiry often reveals adverse childhood experiences, such as abuse, that have increased the patient's vulnerability to chronic pain (consequences of abuse are not limited to children; adult domestic violence is an important antecedent of fibromyalgia).
- Determine the presence of regional pain syndromes that overlap with fibromyalgia and frequently coexist in the same patient, such as temporomandibular joint pain, IBS, and chronic pelvic pain.
- Inquire about previous treatment for pain and insomnia, which can guide the physician in developing a therapeutic plan. Dependency on opioids and unsuccessful prior referrals to multidisciplinary pain centers suggest a poor prognosis.
- Ask about use of complementary and alternative medicine (CAM). Some CAM agents are not safe, and many have the potential to interact with conventional medicines.

A simple self-report form that incorporates validated scales for physical and psychological health status; visual analog scales for pain and fatigue, cognitive performance, and self-efficacy; and a checklist of current symptoms can be completed in just a few minutes in the waiting room. Easily adaptable to a busy practice, such information is invaluable in the comprehensive assessment of fibromyalgia.

Physical Findings

With the exception of painful tender points, the physical and neurologic examinations are normal in the absence of comorbid disease. Pressure algometry at several fibromyalgia tender point sites to assess pain detection threshold (normal is about 4 kg/cm^2) at the initial visit and in follow-up visits provides a guide to therapeutic response. Moreover, algometry can serve as an effective starting point for patient education regarding the nature of their illness.

Diagnostic Testing

Although there are no specific laboratory test abnormalities in fibromyalgia, limited screening for commonly associated disorders and for other diseases that can cause pain and fatigue is useful. These include antinuclear antibody, complete blood count, erythrocyte sedimentation rate or C-reactive protein, thyroid-stimulating hormone, creatine kinase, aspartate aminotransferase, and alanine aminotransferase. Tests for viral infection, autonomic dysfunction (tilt-table test), nerve conduction velocity and electromyography, and imaging studies are usually unnecessary.

Diagnostic Pitfalls

Missed diagnosis of coexisting disease: Do not automatically attribute all symptoms to fibromyalgia, and remember that patients with fibromyalgia can develop intercurrent diseases. Fibromyalgia frequently coexists with other disorders of defined structural pathology, such as SLE or rheumatoid arthritis, and optimum therapy requires recognition of both fibromyalgia and comorbid disease.

Excessive diagnostic testing: Conversely, avoid large-scale diagnostic testing based on symptoms alone, which is both nonproductive and a potential barrier to optimum therapeutic outcome.

Failure to recognize coexisting nociceptive or neuropathic pain: Identify pain generators (e.g., coexisting osteoarthritis or degenerative disk disease with sciatica) that exacerbate fibromyalgia and must be treated separately.

Failure to recognize symptom exaggeration and malingering: In situations of potential secondary gain, such as personal injury litigation, the physician may encounter symptom exaggeration and overt malingering. For example, certain otherwise healthy claimants are well informed regarding the location of tender points. Firm pressure over the trapezii or posterior thorax with a stethoscope, rather than a finger, can provide insight in such cases.

Management and Therapy
General Considerations

Four principles govern the treatment of fibromyalgia: (1) validation of distress, (2) diagnostic and therapeutic conservatism, (3) an individualized combination of pharmacologic and nonpharmacologic measures, and (4) *care* rather than *cure*. Validation of the patient's symptoms and distress begins with the initial history and physical examination. Comments like "it's all in your mind" or "there is nothing really wrong with you" serve only to perpetuate illness and may constitute an insurmountable barrier to treatment. An overarching goal of therapy is the promotion of self-efficacy—the patient's firmly held belief that he or she can control symptoms of pain and fatigue.

Although much current treatment is empirical, abundant data from randomized controlled trials suggest that pain, fatigue, nonrestorative sleep, depression, and anxiety respond to a multifaceted therapeutic approach combining drug therapy with physical, psychological, and behavioral interventions. Consultative referral to a rheumatologist familiar with fibromyalgia is indicated when the diagnosis is unclear, when fibromyalgia is complicated by comorbid

autoimmune or musculoskeletal disease, and when response to therapy is poor. Psychiatric referral is essential for comorbid psychosis and for severe depression with suicidal ideation.

Optimum Treatment

Drug Therapy

For the diffuse pain of fibromyalgia, initial therapy with low-doses of a tricyclic agent (TCA), for example, 10 to 50 mg amitriptyline at bedtime, improves pain, sleep, and overall sense of well-being in about one third of patients, but patient acceptance may be limited by anticholinergic and sedative effects. Selective serotonin reuptake inhibitors, such as fluoxetine or citalopram, and dual-action serotonin-noradrenaline reuptake inhibitors, such as venlafaxine and duloxetine, are of proven efficacy for pain control irrespective of comorbid depression and may be used in combination with a TCA (at initiation of therapy, carefully monitor patients for worsening depression and suicidal thoughts). Addition of an antiepileptic drug, such as gabapentin, topiramate, tiagabine, or pregabalin, is indicated in patients with severe allodynia and hyperalgesia. Centrally acting skeletal muscle relaxants (e.g., cyclobenzaprine, baclofen, tizanidine) generally are less effective. Topical capsaicin is useful when gently massaged into painful areas twice a day. Opioids generally should be avoided, but a subset of patients can achieve a reasonable quality of life and maintain daily functioning in no other way. Pain from comorbid disease is treated in a stepwise fashion with nonsteroidal anti-inflammatory drugs with or without opioid or nonopioid analgesics.

Fatigue generally improves with effective treatment of pain, depression, and sleep disturbances in combination with a graded aerobic exercise program. Modafinil may benefit patients in whom overwhelming fatigue is a persistent complaint. Sleep disturbances should be managed aggressively, beginning with instruction in the elements of good sleep hygiene. Most patients require medication, such as alprazolam, cyclobenzaprine, temazepam, trazodone, or doxepin, either singly or in combination with a nonbenzodiazepine hypnotic, such as zolpidem, zaleplon, or esopiclone. Clonazepam or ropinirole at bedtime is effective for frequently comorbid restless legs syndrome. A formal sleep study is indicated when the simple measures described previously are ineffective. Comorbid depression also requires aggressive pharmacologic management, perhaps in conjunction with formal or informal psychotherapy.

Nonpharmacologic Management

Many nonpharmacologic treatments are of proven benefit with respect to physical capacity, pain reduction, and global well-being and should be combined with drug therapy. Effective modalities include graded aerobic exercise, medi-

tation, yoga, biofeedback training alone or in combination with relaxation training and aerobic exercise, psychotherapeutic counseling, and participation in support groups. Efficacy may be limited by poor motivation, however. High-intensity fitness programs, trigger-point injections, ultrasound, laser therapy, sphenopalatine blocks, vegetarian diets, magnet therapies, manipulative therapy, and referral to anesthesia pain clinics either have no place in the treatment of fibromyalgia or are of questionable benefit.

Treatment in Older Persons and Children

Treatment of diffuse pain in older persons and in children requires special approaches. Accurate pain assessment and effective management are difficult in older persons, who fear diagnostic testing, may be reluctant to report pain, have lower self-efficacy, and use fewer cognitive coping methods. In the pediatric population, unexplained diffuse or localized pain is most common in preadolescent to adolescent girls, often in association with incongruent affect; disproportionate impairment of performance in school; and psychological distress in the patient, the family, or both. Medications should be discontinued, and a program of aerobic exercise should be instituted. A psychological evaluation and psychotherapy may be necessary in some cases. Fortunately, most children do well.

Avoiding Treatment Errors

Failure to recognize pseudoaddiction: Be aware that drug-seeking behavior may be a sign of inadequate symptom control (pseudoaddiction) rather than drug dependency.

Iatrogenic exacerbation: An unsympathetic, uninformed physician who is dismissive of fibromyalgia as a diagnostic entity or who fails to validate suffering can be a major perpetuating factor in this illness.

Converting an acute injury into a chronic pain condition: In the management of an acute injury, for example, a neck strain incurred in a minor traffic accident avoid diagnostic waffling, open-ended referral for physical therapy, prolonged release from work, prescription of a neck brace, and use of the term *post-traumatic fibromyalgia*.

Future Directions

Future directions are rapidly being defined by enormous progress in four areas. First, it is now recognized that fibromyalgia and multiple other regional pain disorders, such as IBS and chronic headaches, frequently coexist, share common pathophysiologic features, and can all be classified as CSS. Second, pain amplification and psychological distress have been identified as the two primary pathways of vulnerability in such disorders. Third, we have a much deeper understanding of the neurophysiologic mechanisms and pathways that underlie pain amplification. Finally, high-throughput genotyping methods are giving us profound insights into both the genetic contributions to chronic pain and psychological disorders and the bases for individual differences in clinical disease expression. Progress in these areas will impel clinician acceptance of fibromyalgia and related syndromes as "real" diseases and will provide a rational guide for improved therapy and drug development.

Additional Resources

American College of Rheumatology. Available at: http://www.rheumatology.org/patients/factsheets/fibromya.html. Accessed December 2, 2006.

This is an excellent source of information from a rheumatologist's perspective.

Arthritis Foundation. Available at: http://www.arthritis.org/conditions/DiseaseCenter/Fibromyalgia/fibromyalgia.asp. Accessed December 2, 2006.

This is an excellent source of practical information for patients and their families.

Medlineplus Health Information. Available at: http://www.nlm.nih.gov/medlineplus/fibromyalgia.html. Accessed December 2, 2006.

This website provides insight into how the federal government is approaching the fibromyalgia problem.

National Fibromyalgia Association. Available at: http://www.fmaware.org/. Accessed December 2, 2006.

This website provides very practical information from the leading fibromyalgia advocacy organization.

EVIDENCE

1. Burckhardt CS, Goldenberg D, Crofford L, et al: Guideline for the Management of Fibromyalgia Pain in Adults and Children. APS Clinical Practice Guidelines Series. No. 4. Glenview, IL, American Pain Society, 2005.

   This comprehensive guide represents the consensus of the American Pain Society regarding current management of fibromyalgia.

2. Diatchenko L, Nackley AG, Slade GD, et al: Idiopathic pain disorders—pathways of vulnerability. Pain 123(3):226-230, 2006.

   This brief and insightful review summarizes recent advances in the genetics of chronic pain disorders and conceptualizes how genes and environmental influences interact in fibromyalgia and other central sensitivity syndromes.

3. Winfield JB. Fibromyalgia. In Dale DC (ed): ACP Medicine. New York, WebMD Professional Publishing, 2006, pp 1412-1418.

   The author provides a detailed and practical approach to fibromyalgia, its diagnosis, and its management.

4. Yunus MB: Fibromyalgia and overlapping disorders: The unifying concept of central sensitivity syndromes. Semin Arthritis Rheum 36(6):339-356, 2007.

   Dr. Yunus exhaustively reviews the clinical features and neurobiology of fibromyalgia and allied chronic pain disorders. The literature in this area is critically reviewed and combined with the author's own vast experience.

Gout

Introduction

Crystal arthropathies are diseases caused by precipitation of the phlogistic crystals within the synovial or tenosynovial spaces. *Phlogism* is the capability of a biologic compound to produce inflammation when present in its crystalline form within the body. In the musculoskeletal system, the most common phlogistic crystal is sodium urate, which produces the disease gout. This chapter discusses the pathophysiology of the formation of uric acid crystals within synovial spaces, the different clinical presentations of gout, and the respective therapies for these entities.

Etiology and Pathogenesis

The cumulative incidence of gout over a 20-year follow-up period is about 8%, with a male predominance. The risk for an acute attack of gout relates to the serum level of uric acid, the risk increasing as the serum urate level rises. At a serum urate level of 9 mg/dL, the risk for developing gout is about 5 times that in a person with a normal serum uric acid level. Although most patients have an elevated serum uric acid level, this value may be falsely low, particularly during an acute exacerbation of the disease, when uric acid is being consumed within the synovial spaces by the crystallization process.

Uric acid forms as a consequence of the purine breakdown biochemical pathway and is eliminated primarily by renal excretion and secretion. Elevation of the serum uric acid concentration and resultant gout occurs by one of the following three etiologies: uric acid underexcretion by the kidney, genetic defects causing overproduction of uric acid, or high cell turnover.

Underexcretion by the kidney causes 85% to 90% of cases of clinical gout. In some cases, underexcretion is due to a presumed genetic defect in renal handling of uric acid. Underexcretion of uric acid may also occur as a result of tubular renal disease (with normal creatinine clearance) or any disease that results in a decrease in overall renal function. Drugs and ingestions decreasing renal excretion of uric acid, such as thiazide and loop diuretics, cyclosporine, ethambutol, alcohol, lead, and low-dose aspirin, all may lead to underexcretion and hyperuricemia.

Genetic defects in the biochemical purine elimination pathway resulting in overproduction of uric acid cause 5% of cases of clinical gout (Fig. 146-1). Increased activity of PRPP synthetase (alcohol use also results in increased activity of this enzyme) and partial or complete deficiency of the purine scavenger pathway enzyme HGPRT are the most common enzyme abnormalities causing this mechanism of hyperuricemia. Complete deficiency of the HGPRT enzyme results in Lesch-Nyhan syndrome with its neurologic sequelae. Lesch-Nyhan syndrome is seen almost exclusively in children.

High cell turnover states resulting in the overproduction of uric acid in patients with normal purine pathway biochemistry (secondary gout) can occur in a variety of settings. Most notable are in the presence of hematologic malignancies, particularly multiple myeloma in elderly patients; during chemotherapeutic treatment of malignancies (either hematologic or metastatic carcinoma) or during the onset of treatment of pernicious anemia; and with exfoliative skin disorders such as psoriasis (see Fig. 146-1).

Clinical Presentation

Acute Gout

Classic acute gout usually involves the metatarsophalangeal joint of the great toe. This acute monarthritis, known as podagra, occurs with an abrupt onset usually in the early morning hours. Erythema, warmth, and acute pain occur over the dorsal aspect of the joint and may involve the extensor tendons and surrounding tissue. The pain is usually quite severe and out of proportion to the clinical exam, and patients frequently describe podagra as the

Figure 146-1 Purine Elimination Biochemical Pathway.

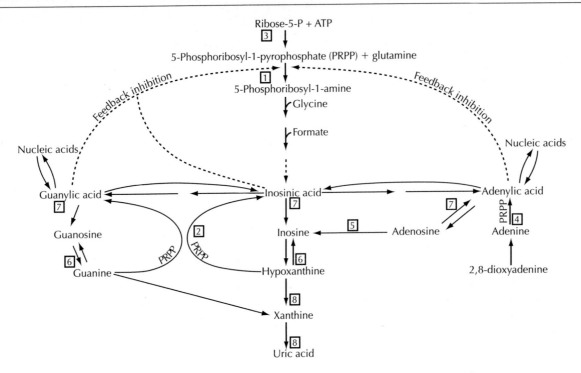

worst pain they have ever experienced. Patients describe not being able tolerate a thin bed sheet or cool air moving over the top of the involved joint. Without treatment, the attack may last from 5 to 7 days, and resolve with scaling of the superficial dermis over the involved joint. Recurrent attacks are common and may occur as frequently as monthly or sporadically, with attacks every few years.

Acute gout may affect any joint in the body. Most commonly involved are the knees, wrists, shoulders, and metacarpophalangeal and proximal or distal interphalangeal finger or toe joints. The axial skeleton, including the hips, is less commonly involved, but acute gout has been reported in the sacroiliac joints and the sternoclavicular joints. Attacks may be limited to tenosynovial sheaths alone and may be confused with other causes of tendonitis, particularly overuse musculoskeletal syndromes. Polyarticular attacks involving two or more joints or tendons are not uncommon and may mimic other systemic rheumatic diseases. Fever and malaise are common in polyarticular acute gout, but less so in monoarticular attacks.

On physical exam, the patient usually cannot move the affected joint or tendon without severe pain. Tendon involvement can be elicited by stretching the suspected muscle-tendon unit without moving the underlying joint. Large tense joint effusions are common in knees, shoulders, or ankles during an acute gout attack. Occasionally, a posterior popliteal cyst (Baker cyst) may form as a result of acute gout in the knee and then, in some cases, rupture down the posterior calf and mimic the physical findings of deep venous thrombosis.

Laboratory findings during the acute attack may include an elevated white blood cell count with a left shift, elevated sedimentation rate (sometimes greater than 100 mm/hr, Westergren method) and increased levels of other acute-phase reactants such as ferritin and C-reactive protein. Synovial fluid contains large numbers of polymorphonuclear leukocytes and may appear grossly purulent. Serum uric acid may be normal and is of no value in the diagnosis of gout. Radiographs are almost always normal other than illustrating soft tissue swelling and effusion in the larger joints, unless the involved joint has had damage from recurrent attacks or the patient has chronic gout.

Chronic Gout

Patients present with a chronic, sometimes deforming, arthritis affecting hands, wrists, feet, knees, and shoulders (Fig. 146-2). It can produce ulnar deviation, swan neck deformities, and other hand and foot deformities, and as a result, can commonly be misdiagnosed as rheumatoid arthritis. Patients may describe episodic acute attacks of swelling, redness, and pain in the involved joints or a more indolent history of chronic swelling and pain. On physical examination, common findings are of chronic synovitis, most often involving the hands and feet and usually asymmetrical (unlike rheumatoid arthritis). Joint deformities and decreased range of motion may be present.

Laboratory evaluation can compound the confusion with rheumatoid arthritis because 20% to 25% of patients with chronic gout have a positive serum rheumatoid factor.

Figure 146-2 Gouty Arthritis: Natural History.

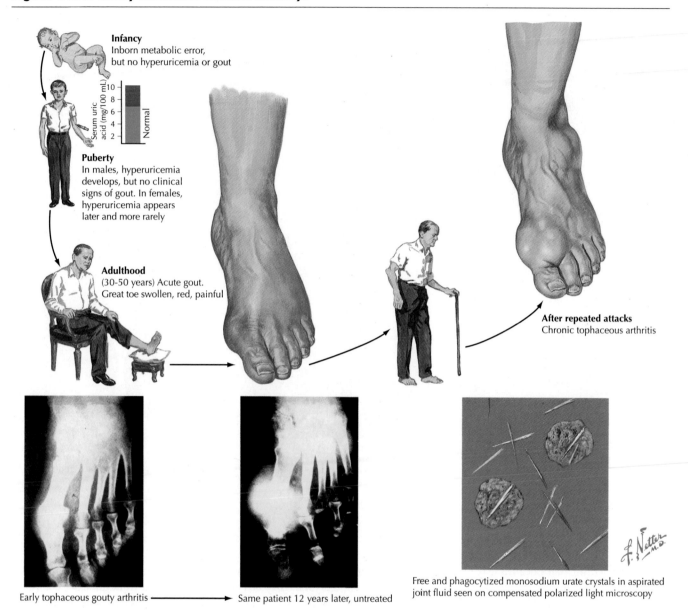

Infancy
Inborn metabolic error, but no hyperuricemia or gout

Puberty
In males, hyperuricemia develops, but no clinical signs of gout. In females, hyperuricemia appears later and more rarely

Adulthood
(30-50 years) Acute gout. Great toe swollen, red, painful

After repeated attacks
Chronic tophaceous arthritis

Early tophaceous gouty arthritis ⟶ Same patient 12 years later, untreated

Free and phagocytized monosodium urate crystals in aspirated joint fluid seen on compensated polarized light microscopy

Serum uric acid is usually elevated but may be normal. The sedimentation rate is usually modestly elevated. Radiographs show erosive destructive disease similar to rheumatoid arthritis, but an experienced bone radiologist may discern more cystic periarticular erosions with new bone formation that help distinguish the findings of chronic gout from rheumatoid arthritis.

Tophaceous Gout

Some patients, almost always with the chronic form of gout, develop subcutaneous deposits of uric acid known as *tophi*. These deposits form nodules, usually over the extensor surfaces of the elbows, in the Achilles tendons, over the extensor surfaces of the hands and feet, and within the pinnae of the ears (Fig. 146-3). Their appearance on physical examination is identical to that of rheumatoid nodules, and they can only be distinguished by the presence of uric acid crystals when examined with cross-polarized compensated microscopy. Crystals can be found in joint aspirates or biopsy samples of nodules. Patients who abuse homemade alcohol (moonshine) made by using older-model automobile batteries containing lead may develop a severe form of tophaceous gout know as *saturnine gout*.

Differential Diagnosis

The most common mistake in acute gout is to miss a septic joint. This can be avoided by prompt arthrocentesis of any acutely inflamed joint. If uric acid crystals are seen, the

Figure 146-3 Tophaceous Gout.

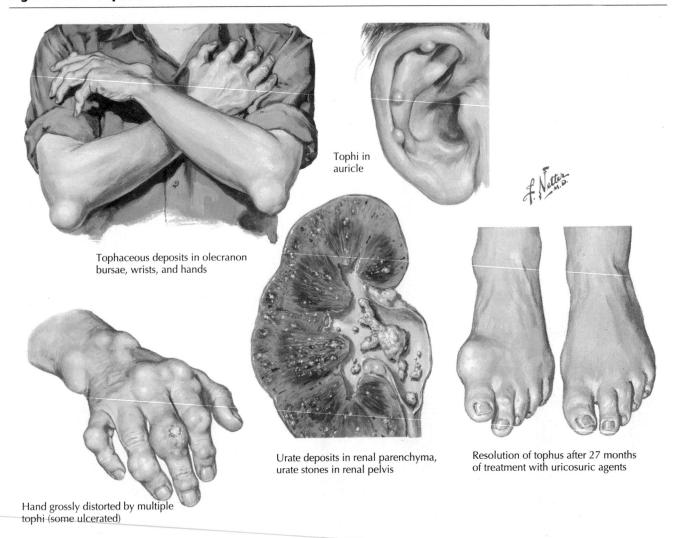

Tophaceous deposits in olecranon bursae, wrists, and hands

Tophi in auricle

Hand grossly distorted by multiple tophi (some ulcerated)

Urate deposits in renal parenchyma, urate stones in renal pelvis

Resolution of tophus after 27 months of treatment with uricosuric agents

diagnosis is confirmed because it is extremely uncommon for bacteria and uric acid crystals to be present in the same joint. Occasionally, the HLA-B27 diseases, particularly Reiter's syndrome, may present in the same manner as acute gout. Tophaceous gout has very commonly been diagnosed as rheumatoid arthritis because, as mentioned earlier, the nodules appear clinically identical to rheumatoid nodules and 20% of patients with chronic gout are rheumatoid factor positive. This mistake can be avoided by aspirating a nodule, which in gout will contain pure uric acid.

Diagnostic Approach

Diagnosis of any of the forms of gout can only be made by demonstration of negatively birefringent, needle-shaped uric acid crystals in synovial, tenosynovial, or nodule fluid obtained by aspiration of the involved joints, tendons, or subcutaneous nodules. In acute gout, these crystals are both extracellular and intracellular within polymorphonuclear leukocytes. In chronic and tophaceous gout, free uric acid crystals may be present without any inflammatory cell reaction. Most commercial laboratories are able to examine synovial fluid under crossed-polarized compensated microscopy, and uric acid crystals remain observable in synovial fluid samples for up to 7 days. Planar bone radiography may be helpful in establishing a diagnosis of gout.

Management and Therapy

Acute Gout

Nonsteroidal anti-inflammatory drugs (NSAIDs) remain the mainstay of treatment of the acute attack. Indomethacin was the first of this group to be used for acute gout. The typical initial dose is between 100 mg and 200 mg/day orally in divided doses, depending on the severity of the attack and the weight of the patient. Some relief of symptoms should occur within 2 hours. The dosage should be decreased gradually over 3 to 4 days as the acute gout

resolves. Other NSAIDs, such as naproxen (500 mg, 2 to 3 times daily) or ibuprofen (800 mg 4 times a day), are also effective. Aspirin is contraindicated because it produces increased serum uric acid at onset of usage. Long-acting NSAIDs with delayed time to steady-state concentrations (e.g., piroxicam and nabumetone) should be avoided. NSAIDs should be avoided in patients with preexisting renal disease with altered renal hemodynamics, in whom hyperkalemia and deterioration of renal function may be precipitated. The newer cyclooxygenase-2 selective NSAIDs are equivalent in efficacy to the nonspecific NSAIDS in acute gout.

If NSAIDs are contraindicated, patients can receive oral colchicine. There is no current role for intravenous administration of colchicine for acute gout. Colchicine is effective in acute gout, and a clear response to this drug may be valuable in supporting the diagnosis. However, doses close to toxic levels are needed. For this reason, the following regimen is usually recommended: 1.2 mg initially, followed by 0.6 mg every 2 hours until there is either diarrhea or vomiting or the patient obtains relief of pain. The total dose required usually ranges between 4 and 8 mg. Relief may not occur for some hours after the toxic features have developed and may not be complete.

Intra-articular injection of steroids can be used if both colchicine and NSAIDs are contraindicated. Oral steroids may also be considered for those patients who have too many joints involved for intra-articular injections.

Chronic Gout and Recurrent Acute Gout

Patients with chronic gout or episodic recurrent acute gout should receive prophylactic treatment with agents that lower serum uric acid. The decision to use these drugs in episodic acute gout should be based on an individual patient's desires because some patients will tolerate four to five attacks yearly and use only NSAIDs during each attack, whereas others prefer long-term prophylaxis. Low purine diets are unpalatable and rarely tolerated as a method to lower serum uric acid. Uric acid–lowering agents should never be started during an acute attack because they will worsen and prolong the course of the attack. Patients with episodic acute gout should be asymptomatic for at least 4 to 6 weeks before uric acid–lowering agents are begun. Patients with chronic gout should take an NSAID or daily colchicine (0.6 mg twice daily) when prophylactic treatment is started.

The choice of prophylactic agent is based on whether the patient is an underexcreter or overproducer of uric acid. Ninety percent of patients with gout are underexcreters of uric acid and should receive the less toxic uricosuric agents. Allopurinol is reserved for overproducers of uric acid. A 24-hour urine collection for uric acid will establish which group the patient is in. Therapy should be based on the urine uric acid excretion level determined. A serum uric acid level should be determined at onset of

prophylaxis and used as a guide to adjust dosing of the drug chosen, with a goal of lowering the serum uric acid to the range of 5 to 7 mg/dL. Historically, colchicine (0.6 mg twice daily) has been added to any prophylactic regimen to prevent breakthrough attacks.

Probenecid, the original uricosuric agent, is used as initial therapy in patients who underexcrete uric acid. It acts by inhibiting reabsorption of urate from the renal tubule and thus increasing urinary urate excretion. It is contraindicated in patients with nephrolithiasis and is not effective in patients with decreased renal function. Its effect is decreased by the concurrent administration of aspirin. The initial dose is 500 mg twice daily, and the drug is available in a combination form with 0.6 mg of colchicine. Sulfinpyrazone (200 mg twice daily), also an effective uricosuric drug, may be used in lieu of probenecid. Angiotensin receptor–blocking antihypertensive drugs such as losartan also act as uricosuric agents and are a convenient way to treat hypertension and gout with a single agent.

Allopurinol, which is rapidly metabolized to oxypurinol, acts by inhibiting the enzyme xanthine oxidase, thereby reducing the production of uric acid. It should be used only in overproducers of uric acid or when uricosuric agents are contraindicated or ineffective. The initial dose should be 100 mg/day, and depending on the risk of precipitating acute gout, the dose can then be increased each week by 100 mg/day until a dose of 300 mg/day is reached. Occasionally, dosages approaching 600 mg/day are required in patients who have genetic causes of overproduction of uric acid. The main complications of using allopurinol are allergic reactions, which may range from a minor skin rash to a severe, life-threatening toxic epidermolysis with interstitial nephritis. About 30% of patients beginning allopurinol develop a rash. If a rash is observed, allopurinol should be immediately discontinued. The dose should be reduced in the presence of renal insufficiency (by about 100 mg/day for a 30-mL/minute decrease in creatinine clearance).

Tophaceous Gout

The goal of therapy for tophaceous gout is to reduce serum uric acid and mobilize and dissolve the nodular deposits of uric acid. This is accomplished by using uricosuric agents with allopurinol in patients who can tolerate this regimen. These patients do not require 24-hour urine collection for uric acid because both classes of drugs are employed in combination. Allopurinol is instituted first with a 6-week interval before beginning the uricosuric agent. After the tophaceous deposits have disappeared (this may take years), the uricosuric agent may be stopped.

Future Directions

Newer, nonpurine xanthine oxidase inhibitors without the cutaneous side effects of allopurinol are in trials, as are

uricases that convert uric acid to water, carbon dioxide, and hydrogen peroxide. Because of the peroxide radicals, these agents are still too toxic for clinical use. It is hoped that, in the future, therapies will be developed that result in increased metabolism of uric acid and improved outcomes in patients with a propensity to develop gout.

Additional Resources

National Institute of Arthritis and Musculoskeletal and Skin Disease: Questions and Answers about Gout. Available at: http://www.niams.nih.gov/hi/topics/gout/gout.htm. Accessed October 11, 2006.

This excellent review geared toward patients addresses the pathogenesis and treatment of gout.

National Library of Medicine: Gout and Pseudogout. Available at: http://www.nlm.nih.gov/medlineplus/goutandpseudogout.html. Accessed October 11, 2006.

This overview of both crystal diseases includes a summary of causation, symptoms, and treatment. The discussion is geared more toward physicians, but patients will understand most of the information as well.

EVIDENCE

1. Lee SJ, Terkeltaub RA: New developments in clinically relevant mechanisms and treatment of hyperuricemia. Curr Rheumatol Rep 8(3):224-230, 2006.

The authors discuss the newest treatments of hyperuricemia with non–purine-based xanthine oxidase inhibitors and uricases.

2. Nuki G: Treatment of crystal arthropathy—history and advances. Rheum Dis Clin North Am 32(2):333-357, 2006.

The authors provide an excellent overview of history and past and current treatments of an ancient disease.

Calcium Crystal Diseases

Introduction

Crystal arthropathy disease, in addition to gout, can be caused by precipitation of the phlogistic crystals of calcium pyrophosphate and the basic calcium phosphate (BCP) group of crystals within the synovial or teno-synovial spaces. Although each of these crystals produces a distinct clinical syndrome, they share the common phlogistic potential to induce local inflammation within affected joints. The focus of this chapter is on calcium pyrophosphate and the BCP diseases, but it is important to note that many other types of crystals have been seen within synovial spaces by crystallography and cross-polarized compensated microscopy. These range from calcium oxalate in patients with primary oxalosis or on hemodialysis, cholesterol and lipid liquid crystals, to cryoglobulins, hemoglobin, cystine, and Charcot Leyden crystals. In some cases, these rare crystals almost certainly cause a primary inflammatory response, but in other cases, they may just be epiphenomena to other primary disease processes.

CALCIUM PYROPHOSPHATE DEPOSITION DISEASE

Etiology and Pathogenesis

Calcium pyrophosphate deposition disease is a disease caused by precipitation of crystals of calcium phosphate dihydrate (CPPD) within the synovial, tenosynovial, or cartilaginous spaces. Unlike uric acid crystals, which almost always produce clinical inflammation, CPPD crystals may deposit in cartilaginous tissue, particularly in elderly patients, and produce no apparent clinical symptoms. These deposits appear within the joint spaces on routine radiographs of knees or wrists in about 30% of patients older than 80 years and in 10% of patients between the ages of 60 and 75 years. Only a small percentage of these patients have any of the clinical manifestations of CPPD that are described later. The biochemical mechanism or defects producing the articular deposits of calcium pyrophosphate have yet to be established. Despite the lack of understanding of the pathophysiology of CPPD, certain diseases have an absolute association with the entity and should be pursued as coexisting whenever a patient first presents with clinical manifestations of CPPD. These can be remembered as the five Hs: hyperparathyroidism, hemochromatosis, hypothyroidism, hypomagnesemia, and hypophosphatasia. Early appearance of CPPD (before age 40 years) may be associated with any of these conditions, or in some cases may be the result of a rare inherited familial form of CPPD.

Clinical Presentation

Acute Pseudogout

Classic acute CPPD is known as *pseudogout* because of the abrupt clinical presentation of an acute monoarthritis or oligoarthritis. This form of CPPD affects older women preferentially and usually occurs in the knees, shoulders, or wrists (Fig. 147-1). Its presentation mimics that of gout (although it rarely affects the toes and fingers) or septic arthritis.

On physical exam, as in gout, the patient usually cannot move the affected joint without severe pain. Large tense joint effusions are common in knees or shoulders during the acute attack. Patients will have redness and heat over the joint and may have a low-grade fever. Laboratory findings during the acute attack may include an elevated white blood cell (WBC) count with a left shift, elevated sedimentation rate, and increased levels of other acute-phase reactants such as ferritin and C-reactive protein. The synovial fluid is usually mildly to moderately inflammatory, containing mostly polymorphonuclear leukocytes. Synovial fluid may appear grossly purulent. Radiographs may or may not show chondrocalcinosis within the involved joint (Fig. 147-2).

Figure 147-1 Pseudogout.

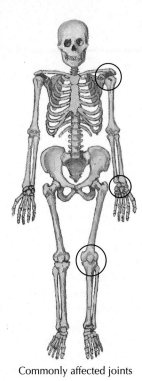

Acute pseudogout
Abrupt clinical onset, usually in older women. Typically a mono- or oligoarthritis affecting knees, shoulders, or wrists

Osteoarthritic form
Chronic, deforming arthritis primarily affecting knees, shoulders, and wrists. M-P joints may also be involved

Hand may be involved in osteoarthritic and pseudorheumatoid forms

Pseudorheumatoid form
Rare—mimics rheumatoid arthritis as symmetrical acute or chronic polyarthritis particularly of hands and wrists

Many patients exhibit radiographic evidence of CPPD deposition but are clinically asymptomatic

Commonly affected joints

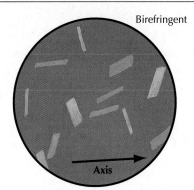

Birefringent

Axis

Diagnosis made on basis of demonstration of weakly positive birefringent, rhomboid-shaped calcium pyrophosphate dihydrate crystals in synovial fluid aspirate of involved joints

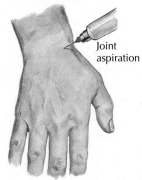

Joint aspiration

Wrist involvement is common in pseudogout, but rare in osteoarthritis, and helps to differentiate the two conditions

**Associated conditions
(The 5 "H"s)**

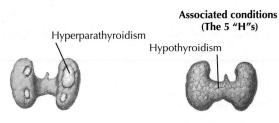

Hyperparathyroidism

Hypothyroidism

Hemochromatosis

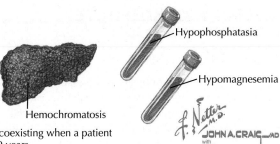

Hypophosphatasia

Hypomagnesemia

Certain conditions show an absolute association and should be pursued as coexisting when a patient first presents with clinical manifestations—especially when younger than 40 years

Osteoarthritic Calcium Phosphate Dihydrate

Patients with the osteoarthritic form of CPPD present with a chronic, sometimes deforming, arthritis primarily affecting the knees, wrists and shoulders, and metacarpophalangeal joints. Patients may describe episodic acute attacks of swelling, redness, and pain in the involved joints or a more indolent history of chronic noninflammatory pain. The physical examination reveals changes consistent with osteoarthritis, with joint crepitance, deformities, and decreased range of motion of the involved areas. The knee may have valgus deformities ("windswept knees") instead of the more common varus deformities seen in pure osteoarthritis. Because the wrist is almost never involved in pure osteoarthritis, when wrist deformities are present in a patient with other areas of osteoarthritis, the diagnosis of

CPPD should be considered. Laboratory evaluation is generally not helpful. The sedimentation rate is usually normal. Radiographs of involved joints usually show osteoarthritis, although the presence of chondrocalcinosis, particularly in the wrist ulnar triangular fibrocartilage, may be helpful to discriminate this form of CPPD from routine osteoarthritis.

Pseudorheumatoid Calcium Phosphate Dihydrate

This rare form of CPPD can mimic rheumatoid arthritis. The presentation is a symmetrical acute or chronic polyarthritis, particularly of the hands and wrists. Serum rheumatoid factor may sometimes be positive. Occasionally, patients with this form of CPPD may be quite ill, with fever, polyarticular inflammation, and sedimentation rates

Figure 147-2 Articular Chondrocalcinosis (Pseudogout).

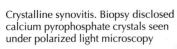

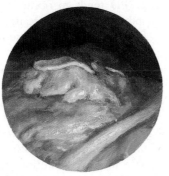

Crystalline synovitis. Biopsy disclosed calcium pyrophosphate crystals seen under polarized light microscopy

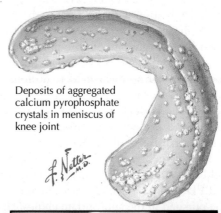

Deposits of aggregated calcium pyrophosphate crystals in meniscus of knee joint

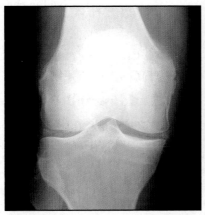

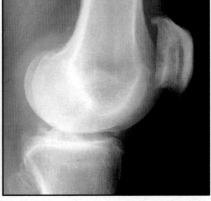

Anteroposterior radiograph of knee reveals densities due to calcific deposits in menisci

In lateral radiograph, calcific deposits in articular cartilage of femur and patella appear as fluffy white opacities

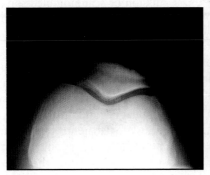

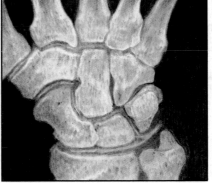

Axial ("skyline") view of knee joint in flexion demonstrates calcinosis of articular cartilages of patella and femur

Drawing of radiograph shows calcific deposits in articular cartilages of carpus as fine lines between carpal bones and in radiocarpal joint

above 100 mm/hr (Westergren method). Radiographs (particularly of the hands) may discriminate this entity from classic rheumatoid arthritis.

Differential Diagnosis and Diagnostic Approach

Diagnosis of any of the forms of pseudogout can only be made by demonstration of weakly positively birefringent, rhomboidal calcium pyrophosphate dihydrate crystals in synovial fluid obtained by aspiration of the involved joints. Most commercial laboratories can examine synovial fluid under cross-polarized compensated microscopy. However, unlike uric acid crystals, calcium pyrophosphate crystals may remain observable in synovial fluid samples for only 48 to 72 hours before redissolving, making prompt examination of synovial fluid mandatory. These crystals are much smaller than uric acid crystals (about one fourth the diameter of a neutrophil) and may be shed into the synovial fluid as a result of another process that is primarily responsible for the joint inflammation. For this reason, the presence of calcium pyrophosphate crystals (even intracellular) in synovial fluid cannot entirely rule out the possibility of coexistent infectious arthritis. And, if the time from joint aspiration to examination of synovial fluid is prolonged, the lack of calcium pyrophosphate crystals does not rule out a role for CPPD. If a high clinical index of suspicion for infectious arthritis is present, the patient should be managed for bacterial arthritis until culture results return. Serum calcium, phosphate, and thyroid-stimulating hormone levels should be obtained in all patients with the first presentation of CPPD, and genetic markers for hemochromatosis should be pursued in the appropriate clinical situation (if other findings suggestive of hemochromatosis are present).

Management and Therapy

Acute Pseudogout

The most effective, least toxic therapy for acute pseudogout involving one or two joints is local intra-articular corticosteroid injection. A long-acting steroid preparation such as triamcinolone hexacetonide should be used. These crystalline branched-chain esters of cortisol will be present and have anti-inflammatory effects within the synovial space for 2 to 3 months. Patients with acute polyarticular pseudogout should be treated with rapidly acting nonsteroidal anti-inflammatory drugs (NSAIDs). Long-acting NSAIDs with delayed time to steady-state concentrations (piroxicam and namebutone) should be avoided. The newer cyclooxygenase-2 selective NSAIDs have not been studied for use in acute pseudogout. Low-dose oral prednisone with subsequent rapid taper may be employed in patients in whom NSAIDs are contraindicated. Oral colchine does have some beneficial effect in acute pseudogout but should be reserved for the rare patient who cannot receive any of the other therapies discussed previously.

Osteoarthritic Calcium Phosphate Dihydrate

Patients with the osteoarthritic form of chronic disease should be managed similarly to any patient with osteoarthritis. Because of the inflammatory basis of the arthropathy, NSAIDs (not acetaminophen) should be used as first-line agents. Oral corticosteroids are usually not effective, and surgical joint replacement may be required if severe joint destruction is present.

Pseudorheumatoid Calcium Phosphate Dihydrate

Patients with pseudorheumatoid disease may be tried on an NSAID as initial therapy but frequently require moderate doses of oral corticosteroids for control of their joint disease. Unlike true rheumatoid arthritis, this form of CPPD tends to occur in the form of acute attacks that spontaneously resolve after weeks to months, thus allowing for episodic use of corticosteroids.

Future Directions

The therapies for control of CPPD disease are less than optimal. Because the biochemical defects that result in the formation of calcium pyrophosphate dihydrate crystals are unknown, no preventative pharmacologic agents are available for this condition. Ongoing research into the biochemistry and physical chemistry of CPPD should result in effective control of this disease, similar to what has already been achieved in the management of gout.

BASIC CALCIUM PHOSPHATE CRYSTALS

Etiology and Pathogenesis

BCP crystals (previously thought to be only calcium hydroxyapatite) have been isolated from patients with calcific periarthritis, tendonitis, bursitis, and occasionally acute monoarthritis. On rare occasions, they have been associated with a chronic arthritis or periarthritis, but in these cases, it is not completely clear whether their presence is causative or an epiphenomena. BCP crystals are not birefringent and can only be reliably identified by transmission or scanning electron microscopy. They are much smaller than sodium urate or CPPD. Their crystalline shape and chemical formula depend on the calcium-to-phosphate-to-water ratio (Table 147-1).

The pathogenic mechanism of how and whether these crystals cause an inflammatory response is inconclusive. In some cases (discussed later), such as hydroxyapatite pseudopodagra and Milwaukee shoulder syndrome, high intrasynovial neutrophil counts may be seen along with intracellular ingestion of crystals (by electron microscopy), strongly suggesting that these BCP crystals can cause primary acute inflammation. On the other hand, 30% to 60% of osteoarthritic knee synovial fluids have been found to contain BCP crystals with low neutrophil counts,

Table 147-1 Basic Calcium Phosphate Crystals

Crystal	Chemical Formula	Ca/P Ratio
Hydroxyapatite	$Ca_5(PO_4)_3OH2H_2O$	1.67
Octacalcium phosphate	$Ca_8H_2(PO_4)_65H_2O$	1.33
Tricalcium phosphate (whitlockite)	$Ca_3(PO_4)_2$	1.50

suggesting that these crystals are "fellow travelers" with the chronic loss of cartilage of this disease.

Clinical Presentation

The three most common presentations of BCP arthropathy are calcific periarthritis, pseudopodagra and other acute monoarthropathies, and Milwaukee shoulder syndrome. Calcifications around the shoulder rotator cuff are very common radiographically and are almost always made up of coalesced BCP crystals. Attacks of acute pain, redness, swelling, and heat around these areas are the hallmark of symptomatic calcific periarthritis. Most patients have marked limited range of motion of the shoulder, particularly in abduction, and point tenderness just below the lateral curve of the acromion. Pseudopodagra presents as a gout-like attack of acute inflammation of the great toe metatarsophalangeal joint. Unlike gout, pseudopodagra is more common in women than in men. Acute inflammatory effusions of other joints where BCP crystals have been found are less common but do occur, involving the knee, hip, ankle, wrist, or elbow. Milwaukee shoulder is a chronic destructive cuff arthropathy in older women in which BCP crystals have been implicated as pathogenic. This entity presents with either chronic or acute rupture (sometimes with hemarthrosis) of the rotator cuff and classic physical exam signs of cuff rupture, with the patient unable to keep the arm in active abduction at 70 degrees.

Differential Diagnosis

The differential diagnosis of the BCP crystal diseases is the same as in acute gout in regard to the acute arthropathies caused by these crystals. As in gout, it is important to rule out sepsis as a cause of the arthropathy. In fact, because BCP crystals are not birefringent, patients should be treated with antibiotics until cultures return. Whether this treatment is administered intravenously with an inpatient admission or orally is dependent on clinical judgment. If the patient is febrile, has an elevated peripheral WBC count, or has any other signs of toxicity, an inpatient admission is justified.

Diagnostic Approach

Because the BCP crystals are not visible under polarized light and synovial cell counts may be normal, examination of synovial fluid may be normal. Because the involvement may be periarticular and not intra-articular, the mainstay of diagnosis is planar radiography or, in the case of Milwaukee shoulder, magnetic resonance imaging (MRI) of the rotator cuff. If calcification is seen in the area of patient complaint and correlates with the physical examination, then the diagnosis can be strongly supported. MRI evidence of complete rotator cuff tear along with cuff cal-

cification is strong evidence for the diagnosis of Milwaukee shoulder in an elderly woman.

Management and Therapy

Unfortunately, other than calcific periarthritis, which responds to aspiration and corticosteroid injection, to NSAIDs, or in medically unresponsive cases, to surgical removal (Fig. 147-3), there is no effective therapy for the other entities of BCP crystal disease. Intra-articular steroids or NSAIDs should be attempted for these other forms of disease, but physician and patient expectations for pain relief should be low to moderate. Milwaukee shoulder

Figure 147-3 Calcium Crystal Diseases.

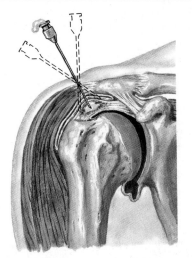

Aspiration of calcific shoulder bursitis

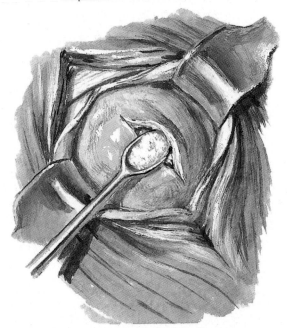

Surgical removal of calcium deposit in shoulder bursae

in many cases can only be treated with surgical reconstruction of the rotator cuff.

Future Directions

Similar to CPPD, the biochemical defects that result in the formation of BCP crystals are unknown, and no preventative pharmacologic agents are available for this condition. Like CPPD, the answer will lie in better understanding the physical chemistry and biologic effects of these crystals and how to prevent formation or dissolve BCP crystals.

Additional Resource

National Library of Medicine: Gout and Pseudogout. Available at: http://www.nlm.nih.gov/medlineplus/goutandpseudogout.html. Accessed October 12, 2006.

This overview of both crystal diseases includes a summary of causation, symptoms, and treatment. The discussion is geared more towards physicians, but patients will understand most of the information as well.

EVIDENCE

1. Ea HK, Liote F: Calcium pyrophosphate dihydrate and basic calcium phosphate crystal-induced arthropathies: Update on pathogenesis, clinical features, and therapy. Curr Rheumatol Rep 6(3):221-227, 2004.

    This is the latest review on primarily pseudogout but with some discussion of the basic calcium crystal arthropathies,

2. Molloy ES, McCarthy GM: Basic calcium phosphate crystals: Pathways to joint degeneration. Curr Opin Rheumatol 18(2):187-192, 2006.

    This review concentrates solely on the basic calcium crystals and theories and whether or not calcium crystals are a major cause of osteoarthritis. The article stimulates thought on mechanisms of primary osteoarthritis.

3. Molloy ES, McCarthy GM: Calcium crystal deposition diseases: Update on pathogenesis and manifestations. Rheum Dis Clin North Am 32(2):383-400, 2006.

    The authors discuss the latest thinking on the etiopathogenesis of all the calcium crystal diseases, with excellent sections on clinical manifestations and symptoms.

Autoinflammatory Syndromes

Introduction

The inherited autoinflammatory syndromes are a group of rare genetic disorders characterized by recurrent bouts of systemic inflammation in the absence of autoantibodies, antigen-specific T cells, or identifiable infection. Most of these diseases fall into the category of hereditary periodic fever disorders, which include familial Mediterranean fever (FMF), tumor necrosis factor receptor–associated periodic syndrome (TRAPS), hyper–immunoglobulin D syndrome (HIDS) with periodic fever, and the cryopyrinopathies. Recently, the genetic basis of these disorders has been elucidated, resulting in improved understanding of pathophysiology, more accurate diagnosis, and newer targeted therapies.

Additional rare monogenic inflammatory disorders are often included in the category of autoinflammatory syndromes. These include a disease characterized by pyogenic arthritis with pyoderma gangrenosum and acne and a disease characterized by granulomas known as Blau syndrome. These disorders, which are not discussed in this chapter, are characterized by recurrent inflammation and are pathogenetically associated with, but not clinically related to, the periodic fevers. Other more common inflammatory diseases, including Crohn's disease and gout, have also been classified as autoinflammatory diseases, and are discussed elsewhere in this book.

Etiology and Pathogenesis

Identification of the responsible genes for the inherited autoinflammatory syndromes has begun to elucidate the etiology of these disorders. A common theme underlying the pathogenesis of these diseases is dysregulation of innate immunity. Each of the mutations results in increased cytokine-mediated inflammation at various steps of innate immune pathways (Fig. 148-1).

The innate immune system is an evolutionarily ancient part of the immune system that allows for a rapid and relatively nonspecific response to infection or danger signals, but does not require prior exposure to the inciting agent. Like the adaptive immune system, there are cellular and humoral factors that make up the innate immune response. Instead of lymphocytes, the primary cells involved are those of the myeloid lineage, including monocyte-macrophages and granulocytes. These cells migrate to the site of infection under the direction of chemokine-chemoattractants and are able to phagocytose pathogens. Monocytes and macrophages possess extracellular and intracellular pathogen-sensing receptors called toll-like receptors and nucleotide-binding domain leucine-rich repeat (NLR) proteins that detect danger signals or pathogen-associated molecules such as lipopolysaccharide, bacterial-derived ribonucleic acid (RNA), double-stranded RNA, and peptidoglycan-derived products. Activation of these innate mediators leads to the production and release of cytokines such as interleukin-1β (IL-1β) and tumor necrosis factor-α (TNF-α). These humoral factors have direct and indirect effects on pathogen survival and attract additional inflammatory cells to the site of inflammation.

Although mutations in genes involved in the adaptive immune system often result in immunodeficiency, mutations in several genes that regulate the innate immune response result in increased or uncontrolled cytokine-mediated inflammation with associated fever and tissue specific symptoms. One common result of chronic

Figure 148-1 Innate Immune System Pathways Involved in the Autoinflammatory Syndromes.

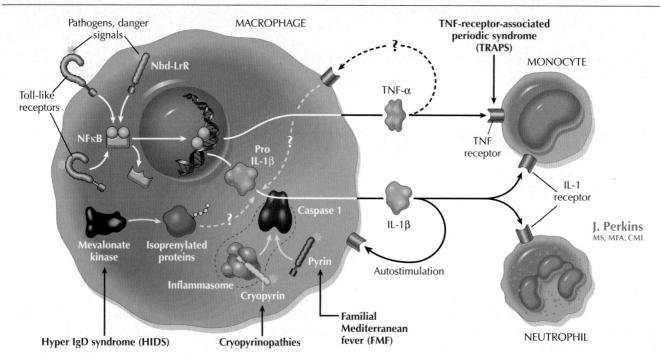

unregulated inflammation is the development of amyloidosis, a comorbidity observed at different frequencies in each of the autoinflammatory syndromes. The mechanisms underlying the specific clinical features of each syndrome have not yet been elucidated.

Genetic and Molecular Basis

Familial Mediterranean Fever

MEFV, the gene mutated in FMF, encodes the protein pyrin. Pyrin is mainly expressed as a cytoplasmic protein in neutrophils and monocytes. Its exact role in the clinical manifestations of FMF has not been fully elucidated, but pyrin has been associated with caspase-1 regulation and therefore with IL-1β processing. Mutations in *MEFV* have also been associated with other inflammatory diseases, such as Behçet's disease, and may also have a modifying effect on the severity of rheumatoid arthritis.

Tumor Necrosis Factor Receptor–Associated Periodic Syndrome

TRAPS results from mutations in the *TNFRSF1A* gene, which encodes TNFRSF1A, the 55-kD receptor for tumor necrosis factor (TNF). In some cases, mutations cause impaired receptor shedding, leading to increased or prolonged signaling through the TNF receptor and to a reduced generation of soluble TNF-receptor (sTNFRSF1A), the natural antagonist of TNF-α. However, not all patients show defective receptor shedding, suggesting additional mechanisms behind the fever attacks in TRAPS.

Mutations with a low penetrance may lead to more general inflammatory disorders.

Hyper–Immunoglobulin D syndrome (HIDS)

Mutations in the gene that codes for mevalonate kinase (MVK) were found to be the cause of HIDS. Previously, mutations in the same gene were associated with a more severe phenotype of MVK deficiency known as mevalonic aciduria. MVK is an enzyme in the cholesterol biosynthesis pathway. It is unclear how the metabolic defect leads to the clinical manifestations of HIDS, but evidence suggests that the shortage of specific isoprenylated proteins can induce IL-1β-mediated inflammation.

Cryopyrinopathies

Cryopyrin is coded for by the gene *NLRP3 (CIAS1)*. Cryopyrin, an intracellular NLR protein expressed in monocytes and neutrophils, shares some structural features with pyrin and has also been implicated in the regulation of cytokine production, particularly IL-1β, by activating caspase-1. Cryopyrin and other intercellular adaptor proteins form a protein complex known as the inflammasome, which has been implicated in responses to molecules associated with pathogens and danger signals such as gout crystals. Mutations appear to gain function, resulting in increased cytokine-mediated inflammation.

Clinical Presentation

Patients with autoinflammatory syndromes present with episodes of fever alternating with disease-free periods. Systemic inflammatory symptoms involving the joints, skin,

Figure 148-2 Patient Evaluation and Clinical Presentation.

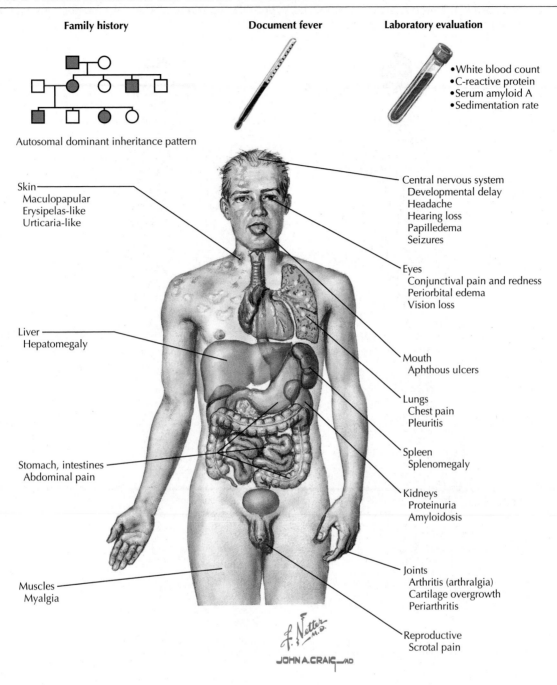

Family history

Autosomal dominant inheritance pattern

Document fever

Laboratory evaluation
- White blood count
- C-reactive protein
- Serum amyloid A
- Sedimentation rate

Skin
Maculopapular
Erysipelas-like
Urticaria-like

Liver
Hepatomegaly

Stomach, intestines
Abdominal pain

Muscles
Myalgia

Central nervous system
Developmental delay
Headache
Hearing loss
Papilledema
Seizures

Eyes
Conjunctival pain and redness
Periorbital edema
Vision loss

Mouth
Aphthous ulcers

Lungs
Chest pain
Pleuritis

Spleen
Splenomegaly

Kidneys
Proteinuria
Amyloidosis

Joints
Arthritis (arthralgia)
Cartilage overgrowth
Periarthritis

Reproductive
Scrotal pain

eyes, or abdomen are also characteristic of episodes. Each of these disorders has unique clinical features, which when combined with appropriate genetic testing, may aid in making the correct diagnosis and guide the choice of specific therapies (Figs. 148-2, 148-3, and 148-4).

Clinical Features of Individual Syndromes

Familial Mediterranean Fever (FMF)

FMF is the most prevalent and well known of the hereditary autoinflammatory diseases. It affects more than 10,000 patients worldwide, mostly from the Mediterranean area, including Armenians, Arabs, Turks, and Sephardic Jews. It is almost always inherited in an autosomal recessive fashion. Patients with FMF suffer from recurrent fever attacks with acute monoarthritis, abdominal pain, and serositis such as peritonitis, pleuritis, or pericarditis. Some patients have an erysipelas-like rash, and a few develop chronic erosive arthritis. Symptoms usually present in childhood, with about 80% of patients having their first attack before the age of 20 years. While the attacks usually last 1 to 3 days, patients are well between attacks, with symptom-free

Figure 148-3 Cutaneous Findings.
FMF, familial Mediterranean fever; HIDS, hyper-IgD syndrome; TRAPS, tumor necrosis factor receptor–associated periodic syndrome.

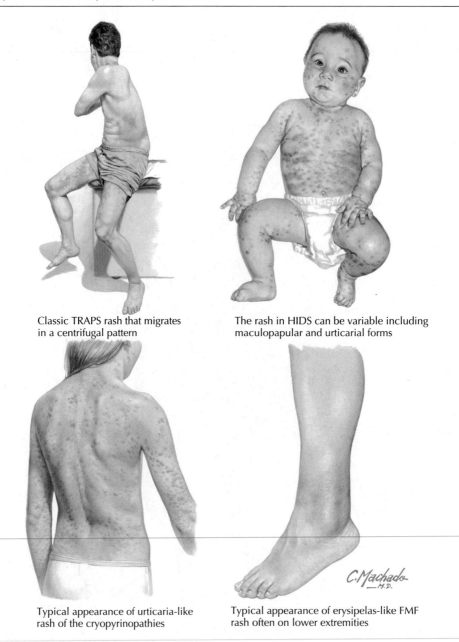

Classic TRAPS rash that migrates in a centrifugal pattern

The rash in HIDS can be variable including maculopapular and urticarial forms

Typical appearance of urticaria-like rash of the cryopyrinopathies

Typical appearance of erysipelas-like FMF rash often on lower extremities

intervals sometimes lasting many months or even years. Long-term prognosis depends on the development of amyloidosis, which can result in renal failure.

Tumor Necrosis Factor Receptor–Associated Periodic Syndrome (TRAPS)

TRAPS (MIM#142680) was originally called familial Hibernian fever when it was first reported in 1982 in a large family of Irish and Scottish descent. Since then it has been described in more than 20 families from many ethnic groups. TRAPS is transmitted in an autosomal dominant manner, and most patients have their first symptoms in childhood, but the age of onset is between a few weeks and 50 years of age. TRAPS episodes include fever, conjunctivitis, periorbital swelling, migratory rash, abdominal pain, myalgias, and monoarthritis lasting several days to weeks and recurring a few times a year. Attacks can be set off by emotional stress, minor infections, or vigorous exercise, but often are unprovoked. The main determinant for poor prognosis is the development of amyloidosis.

Figure 148-4 Joint and Central Nervous System Findings.

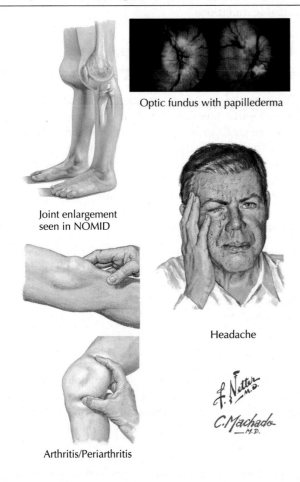

Optic fundus with papilledema

Joint enlargement seen in NOMID

Headache

Arthritis/Periarthritis

Hyper–Immunoglobulin D Syndrome (HIDS)

HIDS is an autosomal recessive disease affecting about 200 patients worldwide. HIDS is relatively common in the Netherlands owing to a founder effect. The recurrent fever attacks of HIDS last 3 to 5 days and usually return with some periodicity every 3 to 6 weeks. Episodes are almost always characterized by painful cervical lymphadenopathy as well as abdominal pain, vomiting, and diarrhea. Other symptoms, including skin rashes, mucosal ulcers, myalgias, arthralgias, and headaches, may also occur. Ninety percent of HIDS patients will experience their first attack within the first year of life, but the fever episodes tend to become less frequent and less severe with age. Usually, there is no obvious trigger, but episodes are occasionally provoked by infection, vaccinations, or minor trauma. Although fever may disappear after a few days, malaise and arthritis may take longer to resolve. Between attacks, patients are well.

Cryopyrinopathies

The cryopyrinopathies include familial cold autoinflammatory syndrome (FCAS), Muckle-Wells syndrome (MWS), and neonatal-onset multisystem inflammatory disease (NOMID). These diseases were previously thought of as distinct disorders, but now they are considered a spectrum of one systemic inflammatory disease with varying severity. The exact prevalence of these rare autosomal dominant inherited diseases is unknown; however, more than 300 patients with FCAS, MWS, and NOMID have been reported worldwide.

FCAS patients present with recurrent episodes of urticaria-like rash, fever, chills, and joint pain precipitated by generalized cold exposure. Attacks are also characterized by conjunctivitis, sweating, drowsiness, headache, extreme thirst, and nausea. Symptoms usually develop 1 to 2 hours after exposure, peak about 6 to 8 hours later, and resolve in less than 24 hours. Although significant cold exposure can trigger attacks, air conditioning is a common precipitant of episodes. Many patients have daily rash and fatigue that begin in the afternoon, peak at night, and resolve by morning, regardless of cold exposure during the day. Ninety-five percent of patients experience symptoms by 6 months of age, and most present with neonatal rash.

Attacks associated with MWS are very similar to those with FCAS, except episodes often have no clear trigger. Occasionally, attacks may be precipitated by cold, heat, exercise, and stress. Acute episodes last less than 24 to 48 hours, but there are often daily symptoms of rash, fatigue, and joint pain. Disease symptoms present in early childhood, but sensorineural deafness, one characteristic feature of MWS, develops in up to two thirds of patients in later childhood and progresses through adulthood. Systemic amyloidosis develops in up to 25% of MWS patients and often leads to renal failure in adulthood.

NOMID, also known as chronic infantile neurologic cutaneous articular syndrome, is the most severe of the cryopyrin-associated phenotypes. Patients present in the neonatal period with urticaria-like rash but also develop chronic multisystem inflammatory symptoms, including persistent fever, chronic meningitis leading to neurologic impairment and complications, and progressive joint and cartilage abnormalities. One characteristic finding is cartilage overgrowth around the knee. Patients have evidence of chronic inflammation but also have intermittent acute flares. Most cases are sporadic, but autosomal dominant inheritance has been reported. Amyloidosis has been reported in older patients.

Differential Diagnosis

There are a few apparently nonhereditary conditions that also present with recurrent fever and inflammation, such as Behçet's disease and periodic fever with aphthous stomatitis, pharyngitis, and adenitis (PFAPA). Behçet's disease is characterized by recurrent mucosal ulcers (oral and genital), uveitis and other inflammatory eye diseases, and erythema nodosum, as well as other rashes. It is prevalent in the same ethnic populations as FMF. Onset occurs usually in childhood or young adulthood, and although there is some association with human leukocyte antigen types, there is no clear genetic association. The pathophysiology of Behçet's disease is not well understood.

PFAPA is the most common cause of periodic fever in children. It is a nonhereditary autoinflammatory disease characterized by recurrent episodes of fever with one or more inflammatory symptoms including pharyngitis, cervical adenitis or adenopathy, and aphthous stomatitis. Additional symptoms are similar to those seen in many of the hereditary disorders, including headache, malaise, abdominal pain, arthralgia, and myalgia. Onset is usually between 2 and 5 years of age, and attacks last between 3 and 6 days. Episodes are often extremely predictable, occurring every 3 to 8 weeks, and are separated by completely asymptomatic periods with normal growth and development. Unlike the hereditary disorders, this condition is self-limited, and most children with PFAPA have a complete remission after 2 to 6 years of symptoms with no long-term morbidity. PFAPA symptoms are usually sensitive to systemic corticosteroid therapy.

Diagnostic Approach

Periodic fever syndromes are all characterized by recurrent inflammation. The first diagnostic step, therefore, is to examine the patient during an attack and to document fever, systemic symptoms, and acute-phase response including leukocytosis, erythrocyte sedimentation rate, C-reactive protein, or serum amyloid A protein. (This assay is unfortunately not commercially available in the United States.) A careful evaluation should be performed for occult infection. Another characteristic of the periodic fever syndromes (except NOMID) is recovery between attacks. If the patient does not fully recover, chronic or recurrent infections, autoimmune diseases, and occult malignancies must be ruled out.

In some cases, the clinical findings, such as age of onset, length of attacks, precipitating factors, associated symptoms, and family history, are adequate to distinguish a known periodic fever syndrome. In patients with clinical findings consistent with HIDS, serum immunoglobulin D and urine mevalonate may provide additional support for this diagnosis. However, in many patients, there is no straightforward diagnosis, so the combination of epidemiology, signs, symptoms, and disease course can lead to a tentative diagnosis, which may then be supported by genetic testing. Appropriate genetic testing is available at several commercial laboratories internationally, but in some cases, comprehensive testing of certain genes can only be performed in specialized research labs. Unfortu-

nately, there are some patients with classic presentation of each of the autoinflammatory syndromes who do not have identifiable mutations.

Management and Therapy
Avoiding Treatment Errors

The diagnosis of an autoinflammatory syndrome should be confirmed when possible with genetic testing. Discussion with or referral to a specialist is advisable. Adequate response to therapy includes decreased frequency or severity of episodes and decreased laboratory markers of chronic inflammation, such as C-reactive protein and serum amyloid A that may lead to amyloidosis.

Optimum Treatment

Because of the relative rarity of the disorders discussed in this chapter, there are no regulatory agency–approved therapies for most of these diseases, and knowledge of therapy comes from anecdotal case reports and case series of a few patients.

Familial Mediterranean Fever

The standard approved treatment of FMF is colchicine, which prevents inflammatory attacks in about 60% of the patients and significantly reduces the number of attacks in another 20% to 30%. Colchicine treatment has been shown to reduce the incidence of amyloidosis from more than 60% to less than 5%. Its mode of action in FMF is poorly understood but may be because of its effects on neutrophil motility. Nonsteroidal anti-inflammatory drugs (NSAIDs) are often used for pain.

Tumor Necrosis Factor Receptor–Associated Periodic Syndrome

TRAPS can be treated with NSAIDs and glucocorticoids to alleviate the symptoms associated with the flare of disease, but these drugs do not affect the frequency of attacks or the development of amyloidosis. Anecdotal experience with etanercept and recombinant interleukin-1 (IL-1) receptor antagonist has been more successful, resulting in a reduction in frequency, duration, and severity of attacks in many patients and reversal of amyloidosis in some.

Hyper–Immunoglobulin D Syndrome

HIDS is resistant to therapy. Colchicine, thalidomide, and immunosuppressive agents seem largely ineffective. Treatment with simvastatin may induce a modest improvement, and there have been case reports of successful treatment with etanercept. Recently, studies have begun with the recombinant IL-1 receptor antagonist.

Cryopyrinopathies

Treatment, until recently, has been limited to avoidance of cold exposure and NSAIDs for FCAS patients, and high-dose steroids for more severe cryopyrinopathy patients. Recently, numerous case reports and a few controlled studies have demonstrated the effectiveness of the IL-1 targeted therapies in all three diseases, pointing to an essential role for IL-1 in these disorders.

Future Directions

In the past decade, there have been significant advances in diagnosis and treatment of the periodic fever disorders. The identification of the genes responsible for these disorders has allowed for better characterization of the clinical features, improved diagnosis, and novel treatment. Cytokine-targeted therapies hold great promise for these patients. Further study of this field will likely yield additional diseases, genes, and inflammatory pathways that may be involved in more common inflammatory diseases such as gout.

Additional Resources

Brydges S, Kastner DL: The systemic autoinflammatory diseases: Inborn errors of the innate immune system. Curr Top Microbiol Immunol 305:127-160, 2006.

The authors provide an excellent review of autoinflammatory diseases and pathogenesis.

Church LD, Churchman SM, Hawkins PN, McDermott MF: Hereditary auto-inflammatory disorders and biologics. Springer Seminars in Immunopathology 27:494-508, 2006.

The article reviews inherited autoinflammatory syndromes with a focus on new therapies.

Infevers Mutation Database for Autoinflammatory Syndromes. Available at: http://fmf.igh.cnrs.fr/infevers. Accessed March 5, 2007.

This comprehensive online database catalogs mutations reported in autoinflammatory diseases.

Janeway CA, Medzhitov R: Innate immune recognition. Annu Rev Immunol 20:197-216, 2002.

This is an excellent review of innate immunity.

Martinon F, Tschopp J: NLRs join TLRs as innate sensors of pathogens. Trends Immunol 26:447-454, 2005.

This comprehensive review covers new proteins involved in pathogen sensing.

EVIDENCE

1. Dinarello CA, Wolff SM, Goldfinger SE, et al: Colchicine therapy for familial Mediterranean fever. A double-blind trial. N Engl J Med 31;291(18):934-937, 1974.

   The authors report on the first double-blind clinical trial of colchicines in FMF.

2. Drewe E, McDermott EM, Powell PT, et al: Prospective study of anti-tumour necrosis factor receptor superfamily 1B fusion protein, and case study of anti-tumour necrosis factor receptor superfamily 1A fusion protein, in tumour necrosis factor receptor associated periodic syndrome (TRAPS): Clinical and laboratory findings in a series of seven patients. Rheumatology (Oxford) 42(2):235-239, 2003.

   The authors report on a clinical trial of etanercept in TRAPS.

3. Federici L, Rittore-Domingo C, Kone-Paut I, et al: A decision tree for genetic diagnosis of hereditary periodic fever in unselected patients. Ann Rheum Dis 65(11):1427-1432, 2006.

   The authors provide a rational approach to genetic diagnosis of periodic fever disorders.

4. Goldbach-Mansky R, Dailey NJ, Canna SW, et al: Neonatal-onset multisystem inflammatory disease responsive to interleukin-1beta inhibition. N Engl J Med 10;355(6):581-592, 2006.

   The authors report on a large clinical trial of IL-1 receptor antagonist in NOMID.

5. Kallinich T, Haffner D, Niehues T, et al: Colchicine use in children and adolescents with familial Mediterranean fever: Literature review and consensus statement. Pediatrics 119(2):e474-483, 2007.

   This article presents a comprehensive analysis of colchicine therapy in FMF.

6. Leslie KS, Lachmann HJ, Bruning E, et al: Phenotype, genotype, and sustained response to anakinra in 22 patients with autoinflammatory disease associated with CIAS-1/NALP3 mutations. Arch Dermatol 142(12):1591-1597, 2006.

   The authors report on the largest therapeutic trial of IL-1 receptor antagonist in cryopyrinopathy patients.

7. Simon A, van der Meer JW, Vesely R, et al: International HIDS Study Group. Approach to genetic analysis in the diagnosis of hereditary autoinflammatory syndromes. Rheumatology (Oxford) 45(3):269-273, 2006.

   This article presents a logical approach to the diagnosis of autoinflammatory syndromes.

8. Stojanov S, Kastner DL: Familial autoinflammatory diseases: Genetics, pathogenesis and treatment. Curr Opin Rheumatol 17:586-599, 2005.

   This article presents a complete review of inherited autoinflammatory syndromes.

Carla M. Nester ▪ Ronald J. Falk

Vasculitis

Introduction

The vasculitides are a heterogeneous group of disorders characterized by leukocyte infiltration, inflammation, and destruction of blood vessel walls. The inciting events causing inflammation vary among disease groups and are largely unknown (Box 149-1). In general, infectious and immunologic abnormalities are the predominant cause postulated. A genetic predisposition to disease is likely in some forms of vasculitis. Blood vessels of all sizes are involved, from the large vessels (aorta) to the tiniest of veins (postcapillary venules). Consequently, a myriad of clinical and pathologic presentations occurs. Although specific diseases may have a predilection for certain organs (e.g., coronary vessel involvement in Kawasaki's disease), most vasculitides, especially the small vessel vasculitides, affect virtually any vascular bed. The clinical diagnosis involves careful clinical assessment, specific laboratory and radiographic tests, and tissue samples of targeted organs. The internationally accepted Chapel Hill Consensus Conference definitions of the systemic vasculitides allow for the standardized characterization of the various systemic vasculitides (Table 149-1).

The most significant recent advances in vasculitis are in the use of the immunobiologicals for treatment (i.e., rituximab and infliximab) and in the continued struggle toward minimizing toxicities of standard therapies. Basic and clinical research advances have increased our understanding of the pathogenetic mechanisms of the systemic vasculitides and subsequently given some insight into improving remission rates, alternative therapies for resistant disease, reducing the toxicities of therapy, predicting relapse, and identifying prognostic markers of long-term outcome.

Etiology and Pathogenesis

The unifying feature of all vasculitides is the activation of inflammatory mediators within vessel walls. Virtually all components of the effector arm of the immune system may be affected. For instance, T-cell-mediated inflammation has been implicated as a causative feature in giant cell arteritis and Takayasu's arteritis. In immune complex–mediated vasculitides, circulating antibody-antigen complexes deposit within the vessel wall or form within the vessel wall itself (in situ immune complex formation). Direct antibody binding to antigens integral to vessel walls occur in Goodpasture's syndrome secondary to anti–glomerular basement antibodies, and in Kawasaki's disease because of antiendothelial antibodies. Regardless of how they are deposited within the vasculature, immune complexes, complement, coagulation, and kinin systems act as inflammatory (phlogistic) stimulants for neutrophils and monocytes. These cells then release toxic oxygen metabolites and enzymes that damage the vasculature.

Pauci-immune vasculitides are characterized by lacking either immune complexes or direct antibody binding to the vessel wall. They are closely associated with antineutrophil cytoplasmic antibodies (ANCA). Although the role of ANCA is not certain, a large body of evidence suggests that these antibodies are pathogenic agents (Fig. 149-1). In the presence of stimulatory cytokines, ANCA antigens (myeloperoxidase and proteinase 3) are translocated to the surface of neutrophils and monocytes, allowing binding of ANCA to their target antigens. Alternatively, release of these antigens from leukocytes and endothelial cells may result in damage from immune complex formation with ANCA or by the direct effect of leukocyte serine protein, causing endothelial cell death.

Table 149-1 Names and Definitions of Vasculitis Adopted by the Chapel Hill Consensus Conference on the Nomenclature of Systemic Vasculitis

Name	Large Vessel Vasculitis*
Giant cell (temporal arteritis)	Granulomatous arteritis of the aorta and its major branches, with a predilection for the extracranial branches of the carotid artery. Often involves the temporal artery. Usually occurs in patients older than 50 years and often is associated with polymyalgia rheumatica
Takayasu's arteritis	Granulomatous inflammation of the aorta and its major branches. Usually occurs in patients younger than 50 years
	Medium-Sized Vessel Vasculitis*
Polyarteritis nodosa (classic polyarteritis nodosa)	Necrotizing inflammation of medium-sized or small arteries without glomerulonephritis or vasculitis in arterioles, capillaries, or venules. Kawasaki's disease arteritis involving large, medium-sized, and small arteries and associated with mucocutaneous lymph node syndrome. Coronary arteries are often involved. Aorta and veins may be involved. Usually occurs in children
	Small Vessel Vasculitis*
Wegener's granulomatosis[†,‡]	Granulomatous inflammation involving the respiratory tract and necrotizing vasculitis affecting small to medium-sized vessels, e.g., capillaries, venules, arterioles, and arteries. Necrotizing glomerulonephritis is common
Churg-Strauss syndrome[†,‡]	Eosinophil-rich and granulomatous inflammation involving the respiratory tract and necrotizing vasculitis affecting small to medium-sized vessels and associated with asthma and blood eosinophilia
Microscopic polyangiitis (microscopic polyarteritis)[†,‡]	Necrotizing vasculitis with few or no immune deposits affecting small vessels, i.e., capillaries, venules, or arterioles. Necrotizing arteritis involving small and medium-sized arteries may be present. Necrotizing glomerulonephritis is very common. Pulmonary capillaritis often occurs
Henoch-Schönlein purpura[‡]	Vasculitis with immunoglobulin A–dominant immune deposits affecting small vessels, i.e., capillaries, venules, or arterioles. Typically involves the skin, gut, and glomeruli and is associated with arthralgias or arthritis
Essential cryoglobulinemic vasculitis[‡]	Vasculitis with cryoglobulin immune deposits affecting small vessels, i.e., capillaries, venules, or arterioles, and associated with cryoglobulins in serum. Skin and glomeruli are often involved
Cutaneous leukocytoclastic angiitis	Isolated cutaneous leukocytoclastic angiitis without systemic vasculitis or glomerulonephritis

* *Large artery* refers to the aorta and the largest branches directed toward major body regions (e.g., to the extremities and the head and neck); *medium-sized artery* refers to the main visceral arteries (e.g., renal, hepatic, coronary, and mesenteric arteries); and *small artery* refers to the distal arterial radicals that connect with arterioles (e.g., renal arcuate and interlobular arteries). Note that some small and large vessel vasculitides may involve medium-sized arteries; but large and medium-sized vessel vasculitides do not involve vessels smaller than arteries.
† Strongly associated with antineutrophil cytoplasmic autoantibodies (ANCA).
‡ May be accompanied by glomerulonephritis and can manifest as nephritis or pulmonary-renal vasculitic syndrome.
Adapted from Jennette JC, Falk RJ, Andrassy K, et al: Nomenclature of systemic vasculitides. Proposal of an international consensus conference. Arthritis Rheum 37(2):187-192, 1994.

Box 149-1 Causes of Vasculitis

Direct infection of vessels
Immunologic injury
 ■ Immune complex mediated
 ■ Direct antibody attack mediated
 ■ Antineutrophil cytoplasmic autoantibody associated and possibly antineutrophil cytoplasmic antibody mediated
 ■ Cell mediated
Unknown

Clinical Presentation

Most patients present with constitutional symptoms, including fever, anorexia, fatigue, weight loss, and arthralgias. Organ-specific manifestations may be strongly suggestive of vasculitis, but these signs may lag for weeks behind the systemic complaints. The clinical features are markedly variable and depend on the type of vasculitis, the size of involved vessels, and the organs affected.

The large vessel vasculitides typically present with ischemia of the involved tissues. The most common symptom seen with Takayasu's arteritis is claudication, particularly in the upper extremities, with absent or asymmetrical pulses and bruits. Renovascular hypertension develops in 40% of patients. Important epidemiologic features include the predominance of Takayasu's arteritis in women and in those younger than 50 years. Giant cell arteritis, on the other hand, is usually seen in patients older than 50 years, who have headache, jaw claudication, swollen and tender temporal arteries, and vision loss. About half of patients with giant cell arteritis have polymyalgia rheumatica.

Medium vessel vasculitides often manifest with infarctions of affected organs. Polyarteritis nodosa causes

Figure 149-1 Vasculitis.

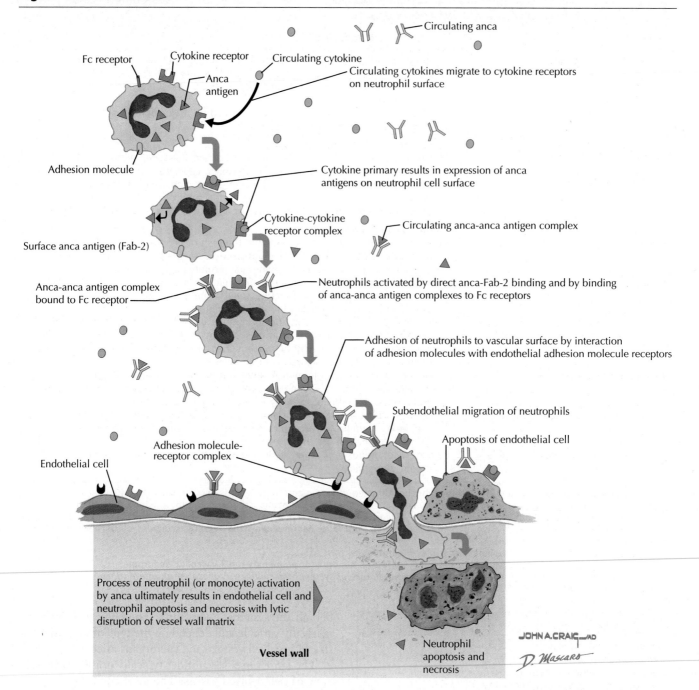

ischemia involving the vasa nervosum resulting in mono-neuropathies and polyneuropathies. Aneurysms and infarctions of the renal circulation result in renal insufficiency and hypertension, whereas disease in other vascular beds, such as the mesentery, results in symptoms of bowel ischemia (Fig. 149-2). Many cases of polyarteritis nodosa are associated with hepatitis B, and it is considered a disease of middle-aged or older adults, with a peak in the sixth decade of life. There appears to be a 1.5 : 1 male predominance for polyarteritis nodosa. Alternatively, Kawasaki's

disease occurs almost exclusively in children and is characterized by involvement of the axillary, iliac, and coronary vessels. Previously referred to as the mucocutaneous lymph node syndrome, the cardinal features include fever, conjunctivitis, adenopathy, mucosal lesions, and a desquamating rash.

Small vessel vasculitis is the most common of the vasculitides and can be classified as immune complex mediated (e.g., systemic lupus erythematosus, Henoch-Schönlein purpura [HSP]) or as pauci-immune. The pauci-immune

Figure 149-2 Renal Involvement in Classic Form of Polyarteritis Nodosa.

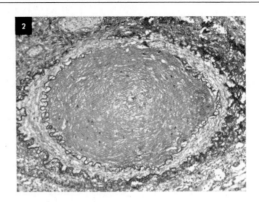

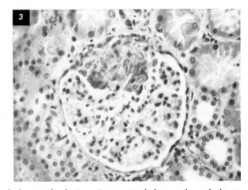

Almost complete obliteration of lumen of arcuate renal artery by intimal fibrosis; fragmentation of internal elastic membrane and medial fibrosis (elastic van Gieson stain, ×100)

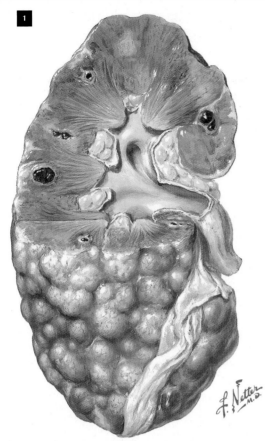

Coarsely nodular, irregularly scarred kidney: Cut section reveals organizing infarcts and thrombosed aneurysms in corticomedullary region

Focal glomerular lesion: Segment of glomerular tuft destroyed by necrotic process with much fibrin and some cellular reaction; patient died from intestinal perforation (H&E stain, ×200)

Box 149-2 Signs and Symptoms of Necrotizing Small Vessel Vasculitis

- Cutaneous purpura, nodules, and ulcerations
- Peripheral neuropathy (mononeuritis multiplex)
- Abdominal pain and blood in stool
- Hematuria, proteinuria, and renal insufficiency
- Hemoptysis and pulmonary infiltrates or nodules
- Necrotizing (hemorrhagic) sinusitis
- Myalgias and arthralgias
- Muscle and pancreatic enzymes in blood
- Iritis and uveitis

---

nomenclature results from the paucity or lack of immune complex deposition viewed by indirect immunofluorescence microscopy of affected tissues.

These diseases are typically associated with ANCA and include Wegener's granulomatosis, Churg-Strauss syndrome, and microscopic polyangiitis. Patients can present with inflammation of single or multiple organs. Many patients present with skin disease caused by leukocytoclastic vasculitis. The cutaneous manifestations of dermal vasculitis include purpura, livido reticularis, nodules, ulcers,

and hives. Similarly, many patients present with kidney disease because of the small blood vessels that make up the glomerulus, resulting in glomerulonephritis. Glomerular inflammation results in hematuria, proteinuria, hypertension, and in some cases, rapidly progressive renal insufficiency (Box 149-2).

The most common cause of a renal-dermal vasculitic syndrome in adults is the small vessel vasculitis associated with ANCA (ANCA-SVV), especially microscopic polyangiitis. In children, the most common systemic vasculitis that causes a renal-dermal vasculitic syndrome is HSP, frequently occurring after a respiratory tract infection. HSP is characterized by cramping abdominal pain, purpura, and arthralgias (Fig. 149-3). Cryoglobulinemia, another cause of renal dermal vasculitic syndrome, has a significant association with hepatitis C.

Glomerulonephritis and pulmonary disease are found in Goodpasture's syndrome (Fig. 149-4), Wegener's granulomatosis, Churg-Strauss syndrome, and microscopic polyangiitis. Respiratory symptoms range from fleeting pulmonary infiltrates to gross hemoptysis. Many patients with small vessel vasculitis have upper respiratory

Figure 149-3 Nephropathy in Anaphylactoid Purpura (Henoch-Schönlein's Disease).

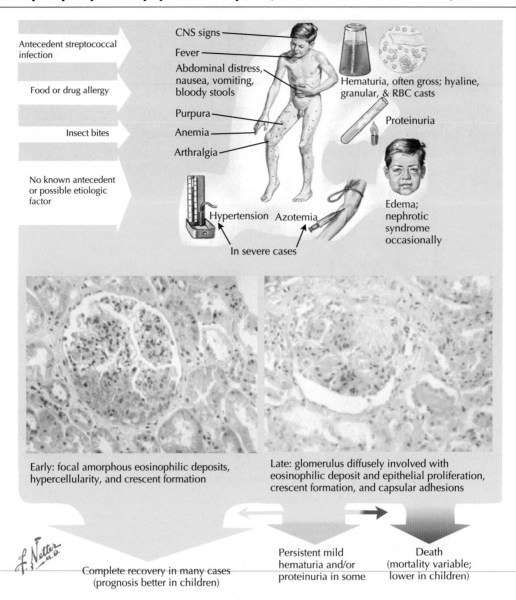

Early: focal amorphous eosinophilic deposits, hypercellularity, and crescent formation

Late: glomerulus diffusely involved with eosinophilic deposit and epithelial proliferation, crescent formation, and capsular adhesions

Complete recovery in many cases (prognosis better in children)

Persistent mild hematuria and/or proteinuria in some

Death (mortality variable; lower in children)

symptoms, including sinus pain, epistaxis, and occasional stridor from tracheal involvement. Pulmonary involvement in Wegener's granulomatosis results in nodules and cavities. Churg-Strauss syndrome less frequently has renal involvement. Asthma is one of the disease-defining findings; allergic rhinitis is also a common finding.

Differential Diagnosis

The systemic inflammatory nature of the vasculitic process and the shared elements of the vasculitides in general often represent a diagnostic dilemma. Diseases in the differential diagnosis include systemic infections such as endocarditis, bacteremia with sepsis, and other connective tissue forms of vascular illness.

This is compounded by the fact that many of the features of the vasculitides are nonspecific. Purpura, consid-

ered a classic sign, may be seen in meningococcemia, viral illnesses, and thrombocytopenic disorders. Pulmonary abnormalities can be difficult to differentiate from respiratory infections. Glomerulonephritis can be seen with other primary renal diseases such as membranoproliferative glomerulonephritis and immunoglobulin A (IgA) nephropathy. Mononeuritis multiplex is one of the more specific findings in vasculitis, and only rarely can be mimicked by asymmetric presentations of other neuropathies such as diabetic neuropathy.

Diagnostic Approach

A clinical history and examination remain helpful diagnostic tools, but serologic tests, imaging, and often biopsy are needed for definitive diagnosis. ANCA serologies (both by immunofluorescence and enzyme-linked immunosorbent

Figure 149-4 Lung Purpura with Nephritis (Goodpasture's Syndrome).

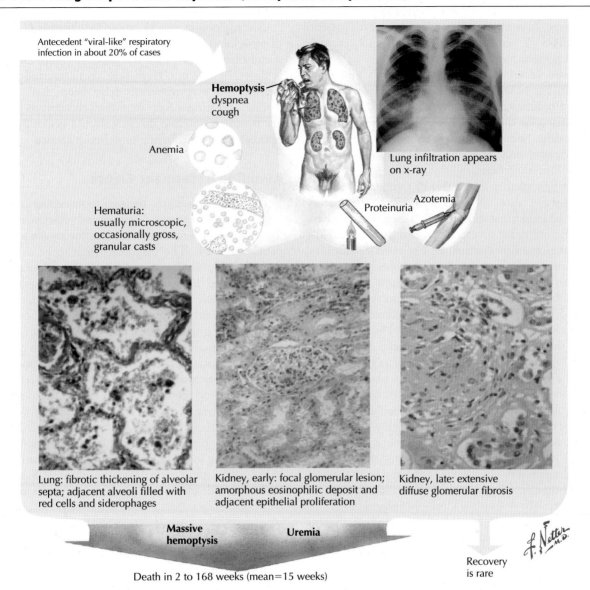

Antecedent "viral-like" respiratory infection in about 20% of cases

Hemoptysis dyspnea cough

Anemia

Lung infiltration appears on x-ray

Hematuria: usually microscopic, occasionally gross, granular casts

Proteinuria

Azotemia

Lung: fibrotic thickening of alveolar septa; adjacent alveoli filled with red cells and siderophages

Kidney, early: focal glomerular lesion; amorphous eosinophilic deposit and adjacent epithelial proliferation

Kidney, late: extensive diffuse glomerular fibrosis

Massive hemoptysis   **Uremia**

Recovery is rare

Death in 2 to 168 weeks (mean=15 weeks)

assay) are essential for ruling in or out the pauci-immune small vessel vasculitides. Other serologic tests that may be useful include those for hepatitis B and C, antinuclear antibodies, anti–glomerular basement membrane antibodies, cryoglobulins, and evaluation of complement components C3 and C4. A urinalysis looking for hematuria is crucial.

Radiographic studies also have a valuable role in the diagnosis of vasculitides. Chest radiographs may demonstrate infiltrates or hemorrhage. Computed tomography scans are often needed for better evaluation of nodules and cavities. For large and medium vessel vasculitides, angiography may be useful; magnetic resonance angiography may allow a noninvasive diagnosis. Demonstration of aneurysms is critical in confirming the diagnosis of polyarteritis nodosa when no specific evidence of small vessel vasculitis can be found.

Biopsy of the affected organs is one of the most important tests. Biopsy specimens of purpuric skin lesions typically demonstrate leukocytoclastic vasculitis. Although this confirms the presence of vasculitis, it does not differentiate between diseases. Biopsy of the lungs or kidneys can be very helpful, especially if immunohistology is performed. Immune-mediated vasculitides will demonstrate granular deposits of immunoglobulin, such as in IgA or HSP, or linear staining, such as in Goodpasture's syndrome. ANCA-associated diseases generally demonstrate vascular necrosis without the presence of immune complexes.

Management and Therapy

Optimum Treatment

Treatment must be designed for each patient based on the severity of disease and the specific diagnosis. The natural history of each vasculitis varies considerably. Some vasculitides are mild in nature and never cause any major end-organ damage. In contrast, the standard of care for patients with ANCA-SVV requires glucocorticoid and cytotoxic therapy to prevent morbidity or mortality.

The large vessel vasculitides, Takayasu's and giant cell arteritis, generally respond to high-dose corticosteroids. Prednisone, at 1 mg/kg daily (maximum, 60 mg), is used for the acute phase and then tapered over several months. Some patients may require maintenance low-dose prednisone. Steroid-resistant disease may be treated with methotrexate.

Henoch-Schönlein purpura (HSP) frequently requires only supportive care. Nonsteroidal anti-inflammatory drugs may be used for associated arthralgias. Steroids have shown some utility for severe abdominal pain and rapidly progressive glomerulonephritis. Unlike most vasculitides, Kawasaki's disease is not treated with steroids because they may worsen coronary artery disease. Instead, intravenous immunoglobulin and aspirin are the mainstays of therapy.

ANCA-SVV is treated with high-dose steroids and typically with a cytotoxic agent such as cyclophosphamide. Induction therapy involves pulse intravenous methylprednisolone, 7 mg/kg (maximum, 500 mg) IV every day for 3 days. In the case of pulmonary bleeding, plasmapheresis should be included as part of the induction therapy (grade A). Plasmapheresis should also be considered as part of the treatment regimen when patients present with dialysis-dependant acute renal failure. Prednisone is then given orally at 1 mg/kg daily (maximum, 60 mg) for the first month and tapered to alternate-day therapy by the end of the second month. Glucocorticoids are gradually tapered over the next 3 to 4 months. Cyclophosphamide may be given as an intravenous infusion monthly (grade A), beginning at 0.5 g/m^2 body surface area (BSA). The dose is increased to 1 g/m^2 BSA based on nadir white blood cell counts. These are drawn 2 weeks after each dose, with a goal of maintaining the white blood cell count above 3000/mm^3. An alternative is oral cyclophosphamide used at 2 mg/kg per day. This regimen exposes the patient to a higher cumulative dose of cyclophosphamide, and increased side effects may result. The required duration of treatment with cyclophosphamide is somewhat variable from patient to patient, but recent evidence (grade A) suggests that azathioprine may be substituted for cyclophosphamide 3 months after induction, if the patient is in remission. Indicators of relapse that may warrant more aggressive therapy or extended length of therapy include proteinase-3 positivity, persistent high-titer ANCA at the time of placement on maintenance therapy, and the presence of upper or lower airway disease.

The use of trimethoprim-sulfamethoxazole, 1 single strength tablet each day, has been shown to reduce upper airway disease recurrence and may play a role in protecting the vasculitis patient from opportunistic infections. Goodpasture's syndrome is treated similarly to the ANCA-associated vasculitides with plasmapheresis as part of the induction regimen.

If cryoglobulinemia is caused by hepatitis C, treatment of cryoglobulinemic vasculitis should consist of interferon-α and ribavirin, provided the patient's creatinine clearance is above 50 mL/min. High-dose corticosteroids, cytotoxic agents, and plasmapheresis have been used for severe disease. Treatment for vasculitides thought to be secondary to other systemic diseases should generally focus on optimal treatment for the underlying disease.

Avoiding Treatment Errors

In the case of vasculitis, the two most common treatment errors involve incorrect diagnosis and reluctance to use the toxic therapies sometimes required for an adequate therapeutic response. The diagnosis needs to be as precise as possible using laboratory and radiologic evidence and biopsies reviewed by experienced histopathologists familiar with the disease process before treatment is initiated. The diffuse nature of the vasculitides makes practitioner experience in recognizing signs and symptoms an important factor. Because the potential for relapse is often present, the physician must be constantly alert to this problem and ready to reinstitute aggressive therapy as needed at the earliest sign of recrudescence. Despite the potential for toxicity with many of the current therapies, it would be an error to be inappropriately cautious in selecting a gentler pharmacologic plan than would be ideal, or to delay treatment too long in the hope that things may improve on their own. Careful attention to dosing and close observation of the patient for side effects and beneficial effects is mandatory.

Future Directions

Studies are ongoing to determine whether alternative agents such as mycophenolate mofetil (Cellcept) may be used effectively for induction therapy. This regimen may offer less toxicity compared with cyclophosphamide. Preliminary studies using infliximab [a monoclonal antibody with tumor neurosis factor (TNF) inhibitory activity] for induction are ongoing. The recent results obtained with Rituximab (an anti-CD20 monoclonal antibody) for the treatment of resistant vasculitis patients have been encouraging. For both of these agents (infliximab and rituximab), randomized controlled trials will be necessary to document unequivocal success or equivalence of these modes of therapy.

Ideally, research should be aimed at prevention of vascular inflammation in order to avoid end-organ damage. Toward this end, basic science must continue to identify causative agents. Detecting populations at risk using genetic markers may allow for close scrutiny and earlier detection in specific individuals. Until such detection tools are available, however, early diagnosis of disease before end-organ damage occurs should be the overriding goal. Education of patients and physicians to consider the

Figure 149-5 Distribution of Specific Vasculitis Syndromes.

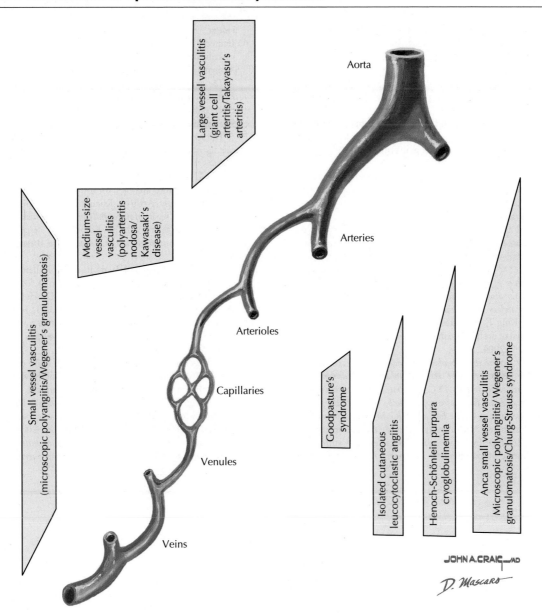

spectrum of vasculitis and to order the appropriate laboratory tests is vital (Fig. 149-5). Once the diagnosis is made, early treatment with drugs that specifically target pathogenetic factors without suppressing the entire immune system should be the goal. Clinical science must continue to focus on refining existing treatments such that baseline toxicities are reduced, while testing new therapies that have better toxicity profiles.

Additional Resources

European Vasculitis Study Group. Available at: http://www.vasculitis.org/. Accessed November 26, 2006.

The European Vasculitis Study group is a group whose intention is to perform multicenter studies of therapy in systemic vasculitis. Their focus is on European Union–supported clinical trials.

National Library of Medicine and the National Institutes of Health: Vasculitis. Available at: http://www.nlm.nih.gov/medlineplus/vasculitis.html. Accessed November 26, 2006.

This vasculitis resource is for both health professionals and consumers.

National Organization for Rare Disorders. Vasculitis: Available at: http://www.rarediseases.org/search/rdbdetail_abstract.html?disname=Vasculitis. Accessed November 26, 2006.

This site provides both disease reports and associated organizations and support groups for each disease.

UNC Kidney Center. Available at: http://www.unckidneycenter.org/patients.htm. Accessed November 26, 2006.

This site is a patient and caregiver resource.

EVIDENCE

1. Booth A, Harper L, Hammad T, et al: Prospective study of TNFalpha blockade with infliximab in anti-neutrophil cytoplasmic antibody-associated systemic vasculitis. J Am Soc Nephrol 15(3):717-721, 2004.

   The authors report that TNF-α blockade with infliximab was effective at inducing remission in antibody-associated systemic vasculitis.

2. de Groot K, Adu D, Savage CO; EUVAS (European Vasculitis Study Group). The value of pulse cyclophosphamide in ANCA-associated vasculitis: Meta-analysis and critical review. Nephrol Dial Transplant 16(10):2018-2027, 2001.

   This meta-analysis on the three prospective, randomized controlled trials indicated that pulse cyclophosphamide is less toxic than continuous cyclophosphamide and is an equally potent inductor of remission in ANCA-associated vasculitides.

3. Hogan SL, Falk RJ, Chin H, et al: Predictors of relapse and treatment resistance in antineutrophil cytoplasmic antibody-associated small-vessel vasculitis. Ann Intern Med 143(9):621-631, 2005.

   An evaluation of a cohort of 350 ANCA patients shows that the increased risk for disease relapse appears to be related to the presence of lung or upper airway disease and anti-PR3 antibody seropositivity.

4. Huber AM, King J, McLaine P, et al: A randomized, placebo-controlled trial of prednisone in early Henoch Schonlein purpura. BMC Med 2:7, 2004.

   This article reports that females and blacks, as well as those with severe kidney disease, may be resistant to initial treatment more often than other patients with ANCA-associated small vessel vasculitis and that increased risk for relapse appears to be related to the presence of lung or upper airway disease and anti-PR3 antibody seropositivity.

5. Jayne D, Rasmussen N, Andrassy K, et al: A randomized trial of maintenance therapy for vasculitis associated with antineutrophil cytoplasmic autoantibodies. N Engl J Med 349(1):36-44, 2003.

   This article reports that the withdrawal of cyclophosphamide and the substitution of azathioprine after remission did not increase the rate of relapse.

6. Jennette JC, Falk RJ, Andrassy K, et al: Nomenclature of systemic vasculitides. Proposal of an international consensus conference. Arthritis Rheum 37(2):187-192, 1994.

   The authors propose definitions of the systemic vasculitides.

7. Leib ES, Restivo C, Paulus HE: Immunosuppressive and corticosteroid therapy of polyarteritis nodosa. Am J Med 67(6):941-947, 1979.

   This series report shows improved outcome when an immunosuppressive agent is added to corticosteroid therapy in treating polyarteritis nodosa.

8. Specks U, Fervenza FC, McDonald TJ, Hogan MC: Response of Wegener's granulomatosis to anti-CD20 chimeric monoclonal antibody therapy. Arthritis Rheum 44(12):2836-2840, 2001.

   This is a case report of successfully inducing remission with the use of rituximab in a patient with chronic, relapsing cytoplasmic antineutrophil cytoplasmic antibody (cANCA)–associated Wegener's granulomatosis (WG).

9. Stegeman CA, Tervaert JW, de Jong PE, Kallenberg CG: Trimethoprim-sulfamethoxazole (co-trimoxazole) for the prevention of relapses of Wegener's granulomatosis. Dutch Co-Trimoxazole Wegener Study Group. N Engl J Med 335(1):16-20, 1996.

   This article presents uncontrolled data indicating the efficacy of co-trimoxazole in reducing the incidence of relapses in patients with Wegener's granulomatosis in remission.

10. Newburger JW, Takahashi M, Gerber MA, et al: Diagnosis, treatment and long-term management of Kawasaki disease: A statement for health professionals from the Committee on Rheumatic Fever, Endocarditis and Kawasaki Disease, Council on Cardiovascular Disease in the Young, American Heart Association. Circulation 110(17):2747-2771, 2004.

    This paper reports on a multidisciplinary committee of experts' recommendations for diagnosis, treatment, and long-term management of Kawasaki's disease.

Toby Bates ▪ Mary Anne Dooley

Polymyalgia Rheumatica and Giant Cell Arteritis

Introduction

Polymyalgia rheumatica (PMR) and giant cell arteritis (GCA) are linked conditions. PMR develops in up to one half of patients with GCA. On the other hand, GCA develops in only 15% of patients with PMR. Both conditions can present simultaneously or develop sequentially, with delayed onset of symptoms reported 10 years after the initial illness. PMR and GCA affect individuals older than 50 years and more often women than men. Prevalence increases with age. The incidence varies with ethnicity. High-risk populations, such as individuals of Northern European descent older than 50 years, have an incidence of PMR and GCA of 20 to 53 per 100,000 and 15 to 25 per 100,000, respectively. In contrast, African-American and Hispanic populations have an incidence of PMR of 1 to 2 per 100,000. In both conditions, markers of inflammation, such as erythrocyte sedimentation rate (ESR), are typically elevated. Elevations in interleukin-6 and association with human leukocyte antigen DR4 have also been found.

Etiology and Pathogenesis

The etiology of PMR and GCA is unknown. Several potential mechanisms, including infections, local degenerative processes, genetic susceptibility, and endocrinopathies, have been proposed as instigators of a cellular autoimmune process. Specific autoantibodies, hypergammaglobulinemia, and the presence of B cells in vascular lesions have yet to be identified. GCA is a vasculitis of medium and large vessels that often involves the cranial arterial branches originating from the aortic arch. The vasculitis is transmural with mononuclear cell infiltrate, destruction of the internal and external elastic lamina, and intimal proliferation. Multinucleated giant cells and granuloma formation may be absent.

Mortality rates of GCA are similar to those of the general population; however, there appears to be an increase in ischemic events (myocardial infarction, cerebrovascular accident) early in the disease course. There does not appear to be an increase of malignancy in patients with GCA.

Clinical Presentation

Polymyalgia Rheumatica

Symptoms consist of severe myalgia and stiffness of the neck, shoulders, and hip girdles. The pain is symmetric, often beginning in the shoulders, and may be abrupt in onset. Oligoarticular synovitis may be present. Constitutional symptoms, including weight loss, malaise, and depression, can occur; however, spiking fevers are rare. Muscle strength is normal but can appear diminished because of pain. Active rather than passive motion is limited by pain. There is often a disparity between the severity of pain and the clinical findings.

Giant Cell Arteritis

Signs and symptoms of vascular insufficiency or systemic inflammation may be the predominate complaints in subsets of GCA patients. Cranial arteritis presents with headaches of variable intensity that are localized to the

Figure 150-1 Giant Cell (Temporal) Arteritis, Polymyalgia Rheumatica.

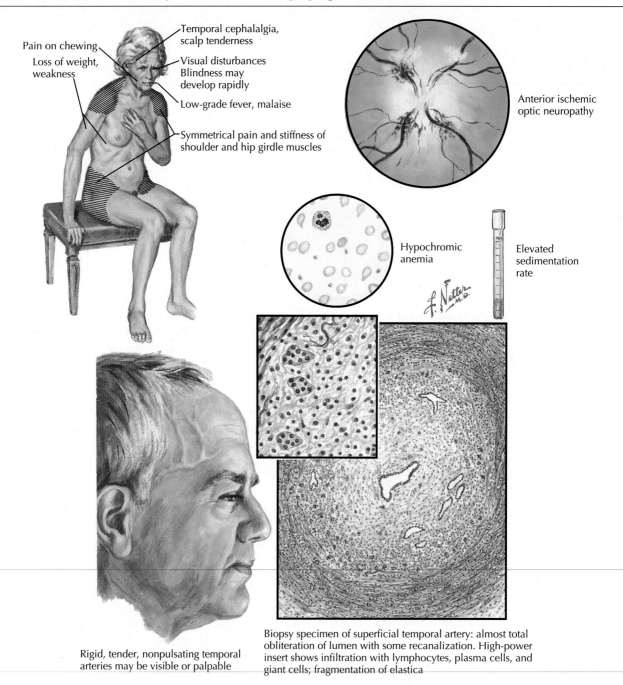

Pain on chewing

Loss of weight, weakness

Temporal cephalalgia, scalp tenderness

Visual disturbances Blindness may develop rapidly

Low-grade fever, malaise

Symmetrical pain and stiffness of shoulder and hip girdle muscles

Anterior ischemic optic neuropathy

Hypochromic anemia

Elevated sedimentation rate

Rigid, tender, nonpulsating temporal arteries may be visible or palpable

Biopsy specimen of superficial temporal artery: almost total obliteration of lumen with some recanalization. High-power insert shows infiltration with lymphocytes, plasma cells, and giant cells; fragmentation of elastica

temporal or occipital area in two thirds of patients. Temporal artery tenderness or decreased pulsation with scalp tenderness is often but not always present (Fig. 150-1). An abnormal temporal artery on exam is a clinical predictor of ischemic complications. On the other hand, anemia is a negative predictor of severe ischemic events. Jaw claudication is specific for GCA but is found in only half of patients. Patients can present with trismus rather than fatigue of the muscles of mastication. Tongue claudication and odynophagia have also been reported.

Constitutional symptoms are observed more frequently in GCA than in PMR and are present in up to 50% of patients at the onset of disease. Fever of unknown origin, with high-grade spiking temperatures, is seen in 15% of patients with GCA. Anorexia, weight loss, night sweats, chills, and depression may be presenting complaints.

Visual symptoms are diverse and include blurry vision, diplopia, eye pain, visual hallucinations, partial visual loss, and amaurosis fugax. Bilateral or unilateral blindness, often without any previous visual symptoms, occurs in 15% to

20% of patients. Unilateral eye disease, if left untreated, can progress to involve the contralateral eye. Arteritis of the posterior ciliary ophthalmic arteries results in ischemic optic neuropathy that can be visualized on funduscopic examination. An elevated ESR is associated with a reduced incidence of visual ischemic events.

Neurologic manifestations occur in up to 30% of patients and consist of transient ischemic attacks, stroke, and neuropathies. Large vessel vasculitis can present with arm claudication, pulselessness, or Raynaud's phenomenon. Thoracic aortic aneurysms are complications of long-standing disease and may be up to 17 times more common in patients with GCA. Fatalities from myocardial infarction (coronary arteritis) or ruptured aortic aneurysm, although rare, may occur.

Differential Diagnosis

Underlying infection and malignancy need to be excluded in all patients for whom the diagnosis of PMR or GCA is contemplated. Infections, such as hepatitis C, subacute bacterial endocarditis, Lyme disease, tuberculosis, and brucellosis, may cause diagnostic confusion. Multiple myeloma may present similarly; however, patients with PMR do not have a paraprotein on serum and urine electrophoresis. Amyloidosis can mimic GCA with jaw or arm claudication.

Hypothyroidism, spondyloarthropathy, polymyositis, rheumatoid arthritis (RA), and rarely amyotrophic lateral sclerosis can present in a similar pattern to PMR. Unlike PMR, polymyositis classically presents with muscle weakness and less commonly muscle pain. Early RA may initially be diagnosed as PMR and with time will clearly declare itself. Synovitis in RA is usually more pronounced and symmetrical. Complete and rapid resolution of synovitis on low-dose steroids is indicative of PMR. Erosive arthritic changes are common in RA but not PMR.

Diagnostic Approach

PMR is a clinical diagnosis supported by nonspecific laboratory findings. The diagnosis should be considered in patients older than 50 years complaining of greater than 1 month of morning stiffness (>30 minutes) and bilateral shoulder and hip girdle pain in the presence of elevated markers of inflammation. For some physicians, a rapid response to low-dose corticosteroids confirms the diagnosis of PMR.

The diagnosis of GCA should be considered in patients older than 50 years who present with symptoms of new or changing headaches, vision loss, PMR, or arterial occlusion in the extracranial vascular territory. Diagnostic confirmation of arteritis should take place with minimal delay. Temporal artery biopsy is the gold standard for the diagnosis. The temporal artery biopsy specimen is abnormal in up to 80% to 90% of GCA cases. The lesions of GCA are patchy, and thus a larger biopsy of 3 to 5 cm is ideal. A recent study found that a 1-cm postformalin fixed arterial segment was associated with increased diagnostic yield for GCA. If the biopsy is negative, the contralateral temporal artery may be resected. The temporal artery biopsy of GCA reveals fragmentation of the elastica lamina, luminal narrowing, intimal edema, granulomas with multinucleated giant cells, and a monocellular infiltrate.

There is no single diagnostic test for PMR or GCA. ESR is usually, but not always, elevated over 40 mm/hr. Some authors suggest that up to 25% of patients with positive results on temporal artery biopsy may have a normal ESR. Other acute-phase reactants may also be elevated, such as C-reactive protein. Other findings include normochromic normocytic anemia, thrombocytosis, and abnormal liver function tests, particularly alkaline phosphatase and an elevated von Willebrand factor. Rheumatoid factor, antinuclear antibodies, and other autoantibodies such as antineutrophil cytoplasmic antibodies are negative. Complement levels are typically normal.

Magnetic resonance imaging with magnetic resonance angiography are used to assess vessel involvement, particularly large vessel involvement in GCA. Reports suggest that these changes may be present for weeks after initiation of corticosteroid therapy. Color Doppler ultrasonography (CDS) of the temporal arteries appears promising in identifying GCA. The findings of a bilateral halo have been noted to be highly specific for GCA. CDS may be a less invasive method to confirm GCA; however, results are extremely operator dependent and thus patients at this time still warrant a biopsy. 18-Fluorodeoxyglucose positron emission tomography (PET) can be helpful in the diagnosis of GCA of large arteries with an atypical presentation. PET is less accurate for smaller vessels such as the temporal artery. PET scan findings improve with corticosteroid treatment and thus may indicate a role for PET in monitoring for disease reactivation. Such scans have shown activity in the aorta in patients with PMR without clinical features of GCA. The implications of these findings are presently under study. Besides needing further validation, PET scans are limited by their availability and cost.

Management and Therapy
Optimum Therapy

Corticosteroids are the drugs of choice for the treatment of GCA and PMR. Both PMR and GCA respond dramatically and rapidly to corticosteroids. Unfortunately, steroid-sparing therapy such as methotrexate has not been uniformly effective. Pulse methylprednisolone has been evaluated to reduce overall steroid exposure.

In GCA, the initial prednisone is 1 mg/kg, usually 60 mg or less per day. There is no clear marker identifying the appropriate time to initiate tapering of steroid therapy. Often this decision is based on a combination of clinical symptoms and normalizations of markers of inflammation. Prednisone may be decreased by 5 mg every 2 to 4 weeks until a dose of 10 mg/day and subsequently decreased by 1 mg every 2 to 4 weeks. Patients are often maintained on low-dose therapy for at least 1 to 2 years. Disease relapse or the appearance of PMR is common during the tapering of steroids. ESR and C-reactive protein do not always reflect disease activity, and recurrence of symptoms should be treated seriously.

In PMR, response to lower doses of prednisone is common. At onset of treatment, only one third of patients receive doses above 20 mg daily. Typically, patients can taper the dosage by 5-mg increments every 2 to 4 weeks. Once 10 mg/day is obtained, the dose is decreased by 1 mg every month. Although PMR is generally a self-limited process, prednisone is usually not discontinued for 1 year and may be continued in some patients for 2 years or longer. Some patients may require 1- to 2-mg doses long-term to avoid relapse. Patient symptoms, not just laboratory results, guide the steroid taper. Nonsteroidal anti-inflammatory drugs can be used in conjunction with steroids in mild PMR. This may be associated with gastrointestinal intolerance and bleeding. If a patient develops a symmetric polyarthritis, consider the diagnosis of seronegative RA. An anticitrillunated peptide antibody and hand-foot films may be helpful. Synovitis in PMR is nonerosive.

Patients with PMR should understand the importance of reporting any symptoms of GCA immediately. Along with symptoms, markers of inflammation can help determine whether a patient is having a flare. Change in treatment is not based solely on markers of inflammation. Patients should receive prophylaxis for steroid-induced osteoporosis. This should include calcium and vitamin D supplementation. A baseline bone densitometry is helpful in future decision making. Patient monitoring for steroid-associated complications of diabetes or hypertension is also important. Because patients will be on corticosteroids for over 3 months, bisphosphonate therapy warrants consideration.

Additional Therapies

The efficacy of methotrexate and azathioprine as steroid-sparing agents has not been clearly demonstrated in either PMR or GCA. Several recent trials of methotrexate in GCA reached opposite conclusions. Cyclophosphamide, an alkylating agent, has been used in large vessel vasculitis, and there are case reports of use of these drugs in severe GCA. There are encouraging case reports of therapy with antitumor necrosis factor (TNF)-α inhibitors; however, controlled trials are needed. Anti-CD20 therapy has been described as an adjunct therapy in a case report of GCA.

The use of aspirin or warfarin may have beneficial effects in GCA. A retrospective trial found a decrease in cranial ischemic events; however, this effect was not seen in another trial.

Avoiding Treatment Errors

GCA is considered a medical emergency because of the potential risk for blindness. Corticosteroid treatment should not be delayed until after temporal artery biopsy. A biopsy performed within several days of starting steroids should not substantially lower the likelihood of obtaining a positive biopsy. Recovery of vision loss with high-dose methylprednisolone has been described; however, this approach is usually unsuccessful in preventing visual loss.

Future Directions

PMR and GCA often require at least 1 year of therapy with corticosteroids. Long-term corticosteroid use has numerous complications, and thus the search for possible steroid-sparing agents remains essential for patients unable to discontinue steroids and for those who have severe complications or who are refractory to steroid therapy. Anti-TNF agents appear promising yet need further structured randomized trials. The risk for malignancy needs further investigation with larger patient groups. Some researchers have indicated that treatment targeting interferon-γ may be useful because it is produced locally, correlating with ischemic complications. Finally, further study of the utility of aspirin therapy is needed.

Additional Resources

American College of Rheumatology. Available at: http://www.rheumatology.org. Accessed December 2, 2006.
  This is the home site for the American College of Rheumatology. It has up-to-date information for patient and providers on rheumatic diseases and resources. There is a directory of rheumatologist members that provides contact information by name and by location.
Arthritis Foundation. Available at: http://www.arthritis.org. Accessed December 2, 2006.
  This website offers continually updated information on a wide variety of rheumatic diseases.
Hunder GG: Giant cell arteritis and polymyalgia rheumatica. Med Clin North Am 81:195-219, 1997.
  This is an excellent clinical reference on the features of GCA.
Koopman WJ (ed): Arthritis and Allied Conditions: A Textbook of Rheumatology, 14th ed. Philadelphia, Lippincott Williams & Wilkins, 2001.
  This text is a good general reference.
National Institute of Arthritis and Musculoskeletal and Skin Diseases. Available at: http://www.niams.nih.gov. Accessed December 2, 2006.
  This site is the branch of the NIH that includes rheumatic disease. Information on current clinical trials, research studies, and access to search PubMed for further information is available.
Ruddy S, Harris ED Jr, Sledge CB, et al: Kelley's Textbook of Rheumatology, 6th ed. Philadelphia, WB Saunders, 2001.
  This text is a good general reference.
Weyand CM, Goronzy JJ: Arterial wall injury in giant cell arteritis. Arthritis Rheum 42(5):844-853, 1999.
  The authors provide a good review of the immunologic and clinical features of GCA for the generalist.

EVIDENCE

1. Blockmans D, de Ceuninck L, Vanderschueren S, et al: 18F-fluorodeoxyglucose positron emission tomography in giant cell arteritis: A prospective study of 35 patients. Arthritis Rheum 55:131-137, 2006.

FDG uptake in the large vessels is a sensitive marker for GCA. Shoulder uptake at diagnosis correlated significantly with the presence of polymyalgia rheumatica. Results of prior PET scintigraphies do not predict relapses of GCA.

2. Jover JA, Hernandez-Garcia C, Morado IC, et al: Combined treatment of giant-cell arteritis with methotrexate and prednisone: A randomized, double-blind, placebo-controlled trial. Ann Intern Med 134:106-114, 2001.

The study shows the combination of methotrexate with corticosteroid therapy for giant cell arteritis therapy does not decrease a patient's steroid exposure.

3. Karahaliou M, Vaiopoulos G, Papaspyrou S, et al: Colour duplex sonography of temporal arteries before decision for biopsy: A prospective study in 55 patients with suspected giant cell arteritis. Arthritis Res Ther 8(4):R116, 2006.

Color duplex sonography (CDS) is an inexpensive and noninvasive method that allows a directional biopsy with an increased probability to confirm the clinical diagnosis of GCA. The authors report that biopsy is not necessary in a substantial proportion of patients in whom bilateral halo signs can be found by CDS, although the technique is highly operator dependent.

4. Mazlumzadeh M, Hunder GG, Easley KA, et al: Treatment of giant cell arteritis using induction therapy with high-dose glucocorticoids: A double-blind, placebo-controlled, randomized prospective clinical trial. Arthritis Rheum 54:3310-3318, 2006.

Initial treatment of GCA with pulse intravenous methylprednisolone allows for more rapid tapering of oral prednisone and was associated with an increased proportion of patients with sustained remission of their disease.

5. Spiera RF, Mitnick HJ, Kupersmith M, et al: A prospective, double-blind, randomized, placebo controlled trial of methotrexate in the treatment of giant cell arteritis (GCA). Clin Exp Rheumatol 19(5):495-501, 2001.

No corticosteroid-sparing benefit could be attributed to the combination of methotrexate and corticosteroid therapy for the treatment of patients with giant cell arteritis.

6. Torrente SV, Güerri RC, Pérez-García C, et al: Amaurosis in patients with giant cell arteritis: Treatment with anti-tumour necrosis factor-α; Intern Med J 37:280-281, 2007.

The authors report on a patient with blindness due to ischemic optic neuritis during a GCA flare that does not respond to high-dose corticosteroid therapy, but improves significantly with antitumor necrosis factor-α therapy.

Mary Katherine Farmer-Boatwright ▪ Mary Anne Dooley

Systemic Lupus Erythematosus

Introduction

Systemic lupus erythematosus (SLE) is a chronic inflammatory autoimmune disease that can affect multiple organ systems and is characterized by non–organ-specific autoantibodies, including antinuclear antibody (ANA), anti–double-stranded DNA (anti-dsDNA), antiphospholipid antibodies, and the marker autoantibody, anti-Smith (anti-Sm). Significant health consequences include renal failure, vasculitis, arthritis, and neuropsychiatric complications. The clinical symptoms and immunologic manifestations of SLE are diverse, and the clinical course involves periods of flares and remissions, requiring therapy that includes the extensive use of corticosteroids and other immunosuppressants. There is a striking female predominance (8 to 9 : 1), with a peak incidence during the reproductive years, but SLE can strike at any age. Concordance in monozygotic twins is 25% to 50%, reflecting a strong genetic component. African Americans have a threefold increase in incidence, tend to have onset at an earlier age, and have increased mortality when compared with whites. Those of Hispanic and Asian descent have an increased prevalence of SLE and associated nephritis. Despite investigative attention, racial differences in lupus expression remain poorly understood.

There are several forms of lupus in addition to SLE. Chronic cutaneous lupus and subacute cutaneous lupus are limited to the skin. Drug-induced lupus is self-limited and resolves when the offending drug is discontinued. Procainamide and hydralazine are commonly recognized offenders; antihistone antibodies are seen in most cases. Neonatal lupus is characterized by a transient rash or congenital heart block in the newborn and is due to maternal anti-Ro (anti-SSA [anti-Sjögren's syndrome A]) that crosses the placenta.

Etiology and Pathogenesis

The cause of SLE is unknown and is likely the result of interactions between susceptibility genes and environmental triggers. Such triggers may include endogenous factors, such as sex hormones, stress, and diet, as well as exogenous triggers, such as silica or sunlight exposure. Other triggers include infections or environmental toxins that have yet to be identified. B-cell hyperactivity, abnormal recognition of self antigens, autoantibody formation, and failure of normal tolerance are some of the reported abnormalities in immune system function. T-cell defects also occur, including excessive T-cell helper function and defects in cell-mediated immunity.

Clinical Presentation

Manifestations of SLE are protean and can affect any organ system (Fig. 151-1).

Musculoskeletal Disease

Musculoskeletal involvement is one of the earliest and most common manifestations of SLE. Arthralgias and tendonitis are more frequent than synovitis. Jaccoud's arthritis, a nonerosive but deforming arthropathy due to ligamentous laxity, can develop. Myositis is infrequent (<15%) and mild to moderate in severity. Myopathy may also develop as a result of therapy with corticosteroids or

Figure 151-1 Lupus Erythematosus of the Heart.

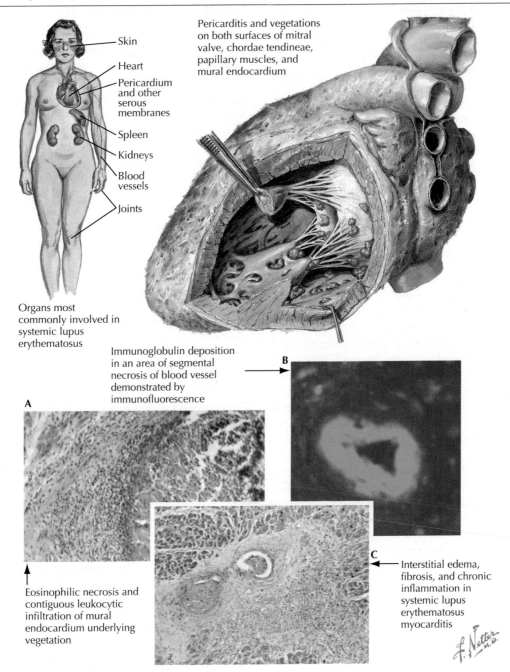

Skin

Heart

Pericardium and other serous membranes

Spleen

Kidneys

Blood vessels

Joints

Organs most commonly involved in systemic lupus erythematosus

Pericarditis and vegetations on both surfaces of mitral valve, chordae tendineae, papillary muscles, and mural endocardium

Immunoglobulin deposition in an area of segmental necrosis of blood vessel demonstrated by immunofluorescence

A

B

C

Eosinophilic necrosis and contiguous leukocytic infiltration of mural endocardium underlying vegetation

Interstitial edema, fibrosis, and chronic inflammation in systemic lupus erythematosus myocarditis

rarely antimalarials. Osteonecrosis or avascular necrosis develops in up to 5% to 10% of SLE patients and frequently affects the femoral heads bilaterally. This complication is often related to the duration and peak of corticosteroid exposure.

Cutaneous Disease

The mucocutaneous system is affected in 80% to 90% of patients with SLE and includes oral and nasal ulcers as well as skin manifestations. Discoid lupus is the skin finding most commonly seen, affecting 15% to 30% of patients.

The specific lupus erythematosus (LE) skin findings in SLE include acute cutaneous LE (with malar erythema or a generalized bullous or photosensitive rash). The nonspecific features are protean and range from a florid cutaneous small vessel vasculitis to panniculitis or even livedo reticularis.

Cardiopulmonary Disease

Pleuritis (serositis) is the most frequently encountered cardiopulmonary complication caused by lupus. A syndrome of progressive loss of lung volume or "shrinking lung" due to diaphragmatic dysfunction is being increasingly recognized. The symptoms of chest pain and shortness of breath have a broad differential in patients with SLE, including pulmonary embolus, myocardial ischemia, pericardial effusion, and pleural effusion. Immunosuppressive therapy increases the risk for bacterial pneumonia. Accelerated atherosclerosis accounts for the second peak of the recognized bimodal curve of lupus mortality. Interestingly, the ongoing inflammatory process appears to be an independent cardiovascular risk factor distinct from hypertension, hypercholesterolemia, corticosteroid therapy, and diabetes mellitus. Elevated serum homocysteine is another risk factor in lupus patients.

Renal Disease

Clinically, lupus nephritis can range from mild asymptomatic proteinuria to rapidly progressive glomerulonephritis associated with end-stage renal disease. Renal involvement in SLE is highly variable in histologic presentation (Fig. 151-2). Early onset of renal disease is a poor prognostic indicator. Youth, male gender, persistent azotemia, and high activity and chronicity scores on renal biopsy are other prognostic features that correlate with a poorer outcome. SLE is not a contraindication to renal transplantation because lupus patients do not differ from others in frequency of rejection or graft maintenance. The risk for recurrence of lupus nephritis in the transplanted kidney is less than 10%.

African Americans have a threefold increased incidence of SLE, more frequently develop nephritis, and have increased morbidity and mortality compared with other races. Although mortality rates from SLE have been relatively stable among whites since the 1970s, they have increased among African Americans during this time span. The progression of diffuse proliferative nephritis to end-stage renal disease is much faster in African Americans than in whites as well, even with comparable cytotoxic therapy. Progression is independent of age, duration of lupus, history of hypertension or control of hypertension, and activity or chronicity indexes on renal biopsy.

Neuropsychiatric Disease

Neuropsychiatric manifestations of lupus are protean and include both acute and chronic forms, vasculitis, and cerebritis. All levels of the central and peripheral nervous system may be involved. Headaches, seizures (focal and diffuse), and various aberrations of the psyche (affective disorders, psychoses, and organic brain disease) are the most common manifestations of central nervous system involvement. Secondary pathophysiologic mechanisms related to infection, uremia, and drugs (particularly corticosteroids) must be excluded.

Pregnancy and Systemic Lupus Erythematosus

Surprisingly, fertility in uncomplicated SLE is normal. The frequency of lupus flares during pregnancy remains controversial because lupus exacerbations have not been found to be uniformly more frequent or severe during pregnancy. There is, however, an increased frequency of midtrimester spontaneous abortions (15%), prematurity (20%) and stillbirth (5%). Lupus activity at the time of conception is a predictor of pregnancy outcome. The neonatal lupus syndrome may present with rash, transient thrombocytopenia, and complete heart block, often irreversible. Estrogen-containing contraceptives and synthetic estrogen receptor antagonists should not be used in those with antiphospholipid antibodies due to an increased risk for thrombosis. The Safety of Estrogens in Lupus Erythematosus National Assessment (SELENA) trial, reported in 2005, noted that oral contraceptives did not increase the risk for flares in patients with stable SLE, although postmenopausal hormone replacement therapy was associated with an increased risk for mild to moderate, but not severe, flares.

Differential Diagnosis and Diagnostic Approach

The criteria for classification of SLE shown in Table 151-1 were most recently revised in 1997 by the American College of Rheumatology (ACR). It is important to remember that these criteria allow comparison of patients in clinical studies and are not meant to be used as diagnostic criteria. Patients may present with less than four features and clearly have SLE without developing other clinical or serologic features; patients with primary antiphospholipid antibody syndrome may meet four or more criteria and not have SLE. Interestingly, the ACR criteria do not include hypocomplementemia or pathology on renal biopsy, which are useful to evaluate disease activity and guide treatment. These criteria are currently under review by several groups proposing diagnostic criteria.

Antinuclear antibodies (ANA) are the most sensitive screening test; more than 95% of patients will be ANA positive when the test is performed with a substrate containing human nuclei such as HEP-2 cells. A positive test for ANA is not specific for SLE, and positive ANAs may occur in normal individuals. In fact, about 15% of those older than 65 years have a positive ANA, often low titer (i.e., 1 : 80). Positive ANAs are also associated with other autoimmune diseases that can be confused with SLE, including rheumatoid arthritis, Sjögren's syndrome, scleroderma, and isolated Raynaud's syndrome. Organ-specific autoimmune diseases such as idiopathic thrombocytopenic purpura, autoimmune thyroid disease, and hemolytic anemia can also be associated with ANA. Family members of SLE patients frequently manifest an ANA without developing clinical features of SLE. Many autoimmune

Figure 151-2 Renal Lesions in Systemic Lupus Erythematosus (SLE).

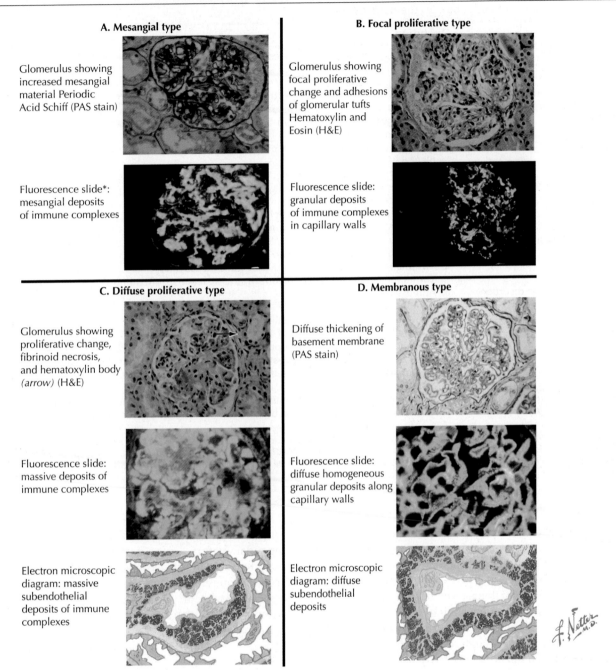

A. Mesangial type

Glomerulus showing increased mesangial material Periodic Acid Schiff (PAS stain)

Fluorescence slide*: mesangial deposits of immune complexes

B. Focal proliferative type

Glomerulus showing focal proliferative change and adhesions of glomerular tufts Hematoxylin and Eosin (H&E)

Fluorescence slide: granular deposits of immune complexes in capillary walls

C. Diffuse proliferative type

Glomerulus showing proliferative change, fibrinoid necrosis, and hematoxylin body *(arrow)* (H&E)

Fluorescence slide: massive deposits of immune complexes

Electron microscopic diagram: massive subendothelial deposits of immune complexes

D. Membranous type

Diffuse thickening of basement membrane (PAS stain)

Fluorescence slide: diffuse homogeneous granular deposits along capillary walls

Electron microscopic diagram: diffuse subendothelial deposits

* All fluorescence slides stained with fluorescein-labeled rabbit antihuman γ-globulin

diseases may have overlapping features, which makes strict classification difficult. The presence of antibodies to the Sm (Smith) antigen is pathognomonic for a diagnosis of SLE, although found in only 30% of patients.

Drug-induced lupus is associated with a number of medications, including procainamide and hydralazine. More recently, minocycline, interferon-α, and tumor necrosis factor inhibitors have been associated with ANA and anti-dsDNA antibody formation, and with development of SLE.

Management and Therapy

Optimum Treatment

Lupus is a clinically heterogeneous disorder; some patients experience troubling skin or joint complaints, whereas others are affected by life-threatening renal or neurologic compromise. Treatment is based on each patient's individual clinical manifestations. Determination of disease activity (active versus quiescent) and severity is essential to choose appropriate therapy and to establish the potential

Table 151-1 The 1997 Revised American College of Rheumatology Criteria for Systemic Lupus Erythematosus

Criterion	Definition
1. Malar rash	Fixed malar erythema, flat or raised
2. Discoid rash	Erythematous raised patches with keratotic scaling and follicular plugging; atrophic scarring may occur in older lesions
3. Photosensitivity	Skin rash as an unusual reaction to sunlight, by patient history or physician observation
4. Oral ulcers	Oral or nasopharyngeal ulcers, usually painless, observed by physician
5. Arthritis	Nonerosive arthritis involving two or more peripheral joints, characterized by tenderness, swelling, or effusion
6. Serositis	a. Pleuritis (convincing history of pleuritic pain or rub heard by physician or evidence of pleural effusion), *or* b. Pericarditis (documented by electrocardiogram or rub or evidence of pericardial effusion)
7. Renal disorder	a. Persistent proteinuria: >0.5 g/day or >3+, *or* b. Cellular casts of any type
8. Neurologic disorder	a. Seizures (in the absence of other causes) b. Psychosis (in the absence of other causes)
9. Hematologic disorder	a. Hemolytic anemia b. Leukopenia (<4000/mm^3 on two or more occasions) c. Lymphopenia (<1500/mm^3 on two or more occasions) d. Thrombocytopenia (<100,000/mm^3 in the absence of offending drugs)

10. Immunologic disorder	a. Anti-dsDNA, *or*
	 b. Anti-Sm, *or*
	 c. Positive finding of antiphospholipid antibodies based on:
	   (1) An abnormal serum level of IgG or IgM anticardiolipin antibodies, *or*
	   (2) A positive test result for lupus anticoagulant using a standard method, *or*
	   (3) A false-positive serologic test for syphilis known to be positive for 6 months and confirmed by *Treponema pallidum* immobilization or fluorescent treponemal antibody absorption test

11. Antinuclear antibody	An abnormal titer of ANA by immunofluorescence or an equivalent assay at any time and in the absence of drugs known to be associated with "drug-induced lupus syndrome"

From Tan EM, Cohen AS, Fries JF, et al: The 1982 revised criteria for the classification of systemic lupus erythematosus (SLE). Arthritis Rheum 25:1271-1277, 1982; and Updating the American College of Rheumatology revised criteria for the classification of systemic lupus erythematosus (letter). Arthritis Rheum 40:1725, 1997. Reprinted with permission of Wiley-Liss, Inc., a subsidiary of John Wiley & Sons, Inc.

for involvement of vital organs. Evidence for an inflammatory process may prompt immunosuppressive therapy versus anticoagulation for thrombotic or embolic events. Patient education is a vital part of the treatment of SLE, especially in terms of long-term outcomes, recognizing clinical changes, and understanding risks.

Patients should understand the importance of avoiding excessive ultraviolet (UV) light exposure by wearing a sunscreen with a high sun protective factor (SPF; 30 or higher). Mexoril, a UVA and UVB protectant, recently received U.S. Food and Drug Administration. Fluorescent light sources should be screened for patients who experience photosensitivity. Lupus patients are at increased risk of infection even in the absence of corticosteroids; fevers should be fully assessed rather than attributed initially to SLE. Fatigue is common in SLE and can be severe. Consideration of other causes, including thyroid disease, coexisting fibromyalgia, depression, and adrenal insufficiency following steroid taper, is important. Regularly scheduled long-term follow-up is absolutely essential and should include regular urinalyses because renal involvement can be asymptomatic until well established. The increased risk

for premature cardiovascular disease secondary to underlying inflammatory disease warrants aggressive treatment of hypertension and hyperlipidemia. Patients should also receive counseling about tobacco abstinence. Lupus is associated with an increased risk for osteoporosis even without steroid therapy, and prevention or treatment of bone loss is important.

Key points in the management of SLE include the following:

1. SLE is a disease of remissions and exacerbations. Patients who are in clinical remission should not be treated.

2. Cyclophosphamide should not be employed in non–life-threatening situations because of the severity of its side effects, including gonadal ablation, alopecia, bladder hemorrhage, and malignancy.

3. Plasma exchange or plasmapheresis has not shown benefit in severe lupus nephritis, but there have been anecdotal reports of response in acute life-threatening situations such as systemic vasculitis and thrombotic thrombocytopenia (TTP) associated with SLE.

4. Sunscreen with an SPF of 30+ should be encouraged.
5. Risk factors for atherosclerosis, including hypertension, hyperlipidemia, and smoking cessation, should be addressed, as previously emphasized.

Pharmacologic Agents Available for Treatment

Nonsteroidal Anti-inflammatory Drugs

Nonsteroidal anti-inflammatory drugs are useful for controlling joint symptoms, serositis (pleuritis and pericarditis), and headaches. The selective cyclooxygenase (COX)-2 inhibitors have not been studied specifically in SLE but are likely to show the same decreased gastrointestinal toxicity demonstrated in other patient populations. The side effects of COX-2 and nonselective COX inhibitors include adverse effects on kidney, liver, and central nervous system function that may mimic increased SLE activity.

Corticosteroids

Many of the clinical features of SLE respond to corticosteroids. Dosing is based on organ involvement, with higher doses in acute renal disease and myositis, and lower doses for arthralgias and fatigue. Numerous routes and formulations are available. Skin lesions can be injected, and intra-articular injections are often helpful in arthritis. Oral and intravenous routes are also used for delivery. The risks with long-term use include increased susceptibility to infection, cataracts, hypertension, diabetes, osteoporosis, and avascular necrosis of bone.

Antimalarial Drugs

These agents are most useful when cutaneous, joint, pleural, or pericardial features are predominant, and when patients experience severe fatigue associated with SLE. Hydroxychloroquine (Plaquenil) is the most commonly prescribed medication in this group, but chloroquine and quinacrine are sometimes used as well. Regular ophthalmology exams for monitoring possible toxicity are essential. The risk for ocular toxicity with hydroxychloroquine is low if the recommended doses are employed. Benefits include lipid-lowering and possible antithrombotic effects.

Immunosuppressive Drugs

Additional immunosuppressants are frequently used for more severe disease and for their steroid-sparing effects. Drugs in this group include azathioprine, cyclophosphamide, mycophenolate mofetil, and cyclosporine. Methotrexate has been increasingly used for severe arthritis or skin disease. Potential toxicities make close monitoring mandatory and are specific to each drug. Contraception is required during therapy because of the risk for teratogenicity associated with most of these medications.

Avoiding Treatment Errors

Given the wide range of clinical presentations in patients with SLE, there is a critical need to consider new symptoms as possible manifestations of SLE. The consideration of other medical etiologies should follow. Appropriate laboratory testing and biopsies to confirm organ involvement must always occur before the initiation of immunosuppressive therapy. SLE patients are most likely to develop new disease features within the first few years of onset; thus, close follow-up is important. Recent studies confirm the benefits of hydroxychloroquine for prevention of disease flares and for decreasing cardiovascular and thrombotic risks. The patient should continue hydroxychloroquine long term, even during periods of immunosuppressive therapy. The dose should remain no greater than 6.5 mg/kg, reduced by half in patients with renal insufficiency. Gastrointestinal intolerance may occur with generics, which are not enteric coated.

Future Directions

Previous investigators demonstrated an association between lower socioeconomic status measures and higher morbidity and mortality in SLE. This relationship is complex and a focus of long-term assessment in the Lumina cohort. Environmental risks for developing lupus have been addressed in the Carolina Lupus Study, a case-controlled population-based study of lupus patients in the southeastern United States. Exposure to silica was a strong risk in this population.

Several new agents are under investigation for SLE therapy. Mycophenolate mofetil and intermittent intravenous cyclophosphamide are being compared as initial therapy for proliferative glomerulonephritis. Shorter courses of cyclophosphamide are being evaluated in the EuroLupus Trial as well. Monoclonal antibodies to inhibit costimulatory pathways for T-cell and B-cell activation are currently in clinical trials. Several drugs approved for use in rheumatoid arthritis are also being evaluated in clinical trials for use in lupus. An oral tolerogen, JPJ 394, has shown promise in delaying initial renal flare in patients with high-titer anti-dsDNA antibodies through downregulation of their production. Autologous hematopoietic stem cell transplantation has been performed in patients with SLE; seven patients were disease free at a median follow-up of 25 months, but the durability of response remains unknown. Immunoablative high-dose cyclophosphamide without stem cell transplantation (thus decreasing the risk for graft-versus-host disease) is being evaluated for therapy of severe refractory SLE.

Additional Resources

American College of Rheumatology. Available at: http://www.rheumatology.org.

This website includes a geographic directory of rheumatologists, patient information, and additional links.

Arthritis Foundation. Available a: http://www.arthritis.org.

This website offers continually updated information on a wide variety of rheumatic diseases and includes patient educational materials.

Lupus Foundation of America. Available at: http://www.lfa.org.

This website contains valuable patient information and references to patient support groups and national lupus centers.

National Institutes of Health. Available at: http://www.nih.gov/institutes/niams.

The website for the branch of the NIH that focuses on rheumatic diseases provides helpful links to multiple sites, including other organizations, literature, current research, and clinical trials.

EVIDENCE

1. Buyon JP, Petri MA, Kim MY, et al: The effect of combined estrogen and progesterone hormone replacement therapy on disease activity in systemic lupus erythematosus: A randomized trial. Ann Intern Med 142:953-962, 2005.

This randomized, placebo-controlled trial evaluates the effect of hormonal replacement therapy on SLE disease activity. The authors conclude that a short course of hormonal replacement therapy is associated with a 10% increase in risk for mild to moderate disease activity among postmenopausal women with lupus. Most flares that did occur were mild.

2. Koopman WJ (ed): Arthritis and Allied Conditions, 15th ed. Philadelphia, Lippincott Williams & Wilkins, 2005.

This text provides a thorough review of recent therapies and pathogenesis of SLE.

3. Petri M, Kim MY, Kalunian KC, et al: Combined oral contraceptives in women with systemic lupus erythematosus. N Engl J Med 353(24):2550-2558, 2005.

This pivotal clinical trial concludes that oral contraceptives do not increase the flare rate of SLE in young, antiphospholipid antibody-negative women with SLE.

4. Wallace D, Hahn B (eds): Dubois' Lupus Erythematosus, 7th ed. Philadelphia, Lippincott Williams & Wilkins, 2006.

This excellent comprehensive review of past and current information on causes and treatments of lupus manifestations includes a useful annotated reference list.

Box 152-1 Causes of Thrombophilia

Inherited

Factor V Leiden mutation
Prothrombin gene mutation
Protein C deficiency
Protein S deficiency
Antithrombin deficiency
Hyperhomocysteinemia

Acquired

Malignancy, myeloproliferative disorders
Trauma, surgery, vascular catheters
Pregnancy
Immobilization
Oral contraceptives, hormone replacement therapy,
  tamoxifen
Congestive heart failure
Inflammatory bowel disease
Behçet's disease
Nephrotic syndrome
Hyperviscosity syndromes

---

history of SLE, APS, or both; in the other half, the catastrophic syndrome is the first manifestation of APS. Catastrophic APS is fatal in nearly 50% of reported cases. Major causes of death are cardiac (myocardial infarction, myocardial microthrombi, heart block) and pulmonary (acute respiratory distress syndrome, pulmonary embolism) manifestations. Apparent precipitating events (e.g., infection, surgery, trauma, or withdrawal of anticoagulant medication) are identifiable in many cases.

Differential Diagnosis

When considering the diagnosis of APS in a patient with thrombosis, it is important to consider other causes of thrombophilia (summarized in Box 152-1).

Recurrent pregnancy loss should be evaluated by a high-risk obstetrician or a reproductive endocrinology and infertility expert to exclude anatomic, hormonal, metabolic, and chromosomal causes. Inherited thrombophilic disorders (see Box 152-1) are also associated with recurrent pregnancy loss.

Catastrophic APS may mimic several conditions, including thrombotic thrombocytopenic purpura and lupus vasculitis.

Diagnostic Approach

The diagnosis of APS rests on the demonstration of persistently positive tests for one or more aPL in a patient with a history of thrombosis or recurrent pregnancy loss. The diagnosis of APS based on other clinical manifestations (in the absence of thrombosis or pregnancy loss) is more controversial. International consensus criteria for the classification of definite APS are useful for clinical trials but have little practical use in the care of individual patients.

Laboratory Tests for aPL

Anticardiolipin Antibodies

Standard anticardiolipin antibody testing remains a key first-line test for aPL. Persistently positive tests for immunoglobulin G (IgG) or IgM anticardiolipin antibodies, at medium or high titer, are strongly associated with the clinical manifestations of APS. Transiently positive tests and low-titer antibodies are more difficult to assess. Isolated IgA anticardiolipin antibodies may also be associated with APS but are relatively rare.

Lupus Anticoagulant

Lupus anticoagulants are antibodies detected based on their ability to inhibit phospholipid-dependent coagulation reactions. Testing involves one or more screening tests. Common screening tests include an activated partial thromboplastin time optimized for the detection of lupus anticoagulants (lupus aPTT) and the dilute Russell viper venom time (dRVVT). If one of these tests is prolonged, two types of screening tests are performed. A mixing study helps to exclude a coagulation factor deficiency. Mixing patient plasma with normal plasma will correct a factor deficiency but not a lupus anticoagulant. The second type of confirmatory test is demonstration of phospholipid dependency; that is, excess phospholipid corrects prolongation of the coagulation assay.

Protein-Based Immunoassays

As discussed, most aPL are directed against β_2-GPI and prothrombin, not negatively charged phospholipids. In patients with APS, most antibodies detected in anticardiolipin assays are specific for β_2-GPI. Lupus anticoagulant assays detect certain anti–β_2-GPI antibodies and antibodies to prothrombin. Anti–β_2-GPI immunoassays are available and appear to be more specific for clinical manifestations of APS than conventional anticardiolipin tests. At present, anti–β_2-GPI assays are considered to be second-line tests, to be utilized if initial anticardiolipin and lupus anticoagulant tests are negative or inconclusive. Antiprothrombin assays (some using a combination of prothrombin and phosphatidylserine) are being developed.

Antibodies to Other Phospholipids

Testing for antibodies to a panel of phospholipids (e.g., phosphatidylinositol, phosphatidic acid, phosphatidylcholine) is controversial. In general, these tests are poorly standardized, and their clinical significance in patients with negative anticardiolipin, lupus anticoagulant, and anti–β_2-GPI tests has not been established.

Recommendations for aPL testing are summarized in Box 152-2.

Figure 152-3 Libman-Sacks Endocarditis.

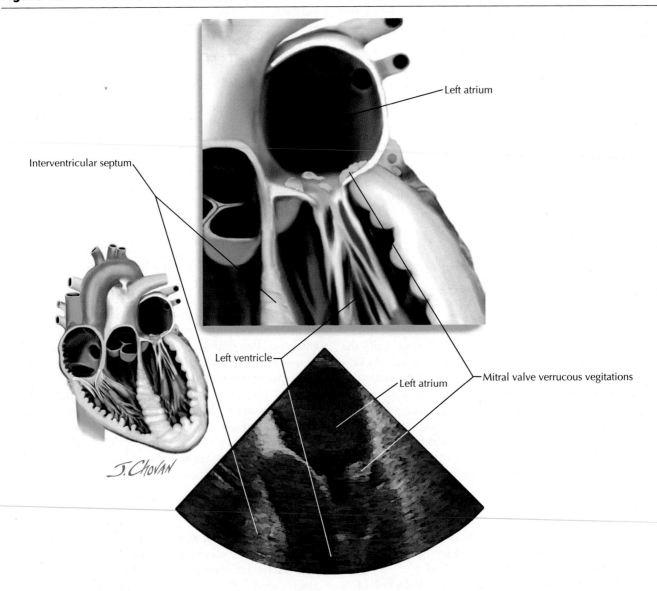

Left atrium

Interventricular septum

Left ventricle

Left atrium

Mitral valve verrucous vegitations

J. CHOVAN

is usually moderate and not associated with hemorrhage. Interestingly, low platelet counts do not appear to protect APS patients from thrombosis.

Valvular Heart Disease

Libman-Sacks endocarditis, noninfective verrucous vegetations, are associated with aPL in patients with and without SLE (Fig. 152-3). These vegetations may embolize, causing ischemic events such as stroke.

Neurologic Manifestations

As noted, stroke is the major neurologic manifestation of APS. Recurrent strokes may lead to multi-infarct dementia. Transient ischemic attacks may also occur. A number of neurologic events that are not clearly stroke related may also be associated with aPL, although the evidence-based data are weaker than for stroke. These include transverse myelitis, multiple sclerosis–like syndromes, chorea, and cognitive dysfunction.

Catastrophic Disease

Catastrophic APS is a syndrome of multiple thromboses occurring over a relatively short period of time (days to weeks). The thromboses typically involve small vessels supplying several major organs (heart, lung, kidney, brain, liver), leading to severe organ system dysfunction or failure. Large vessel thromboses, such as deep venous thrombosis, are less common. Several hundred cases of catastrophic APS have been reported. About half the patients have a

Figure 152-1 Livedo Reticularis.

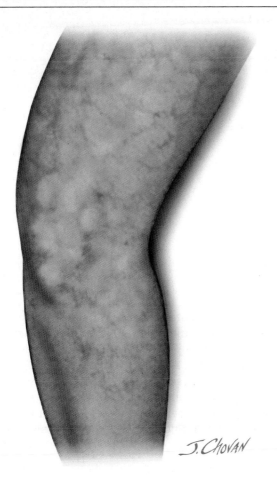

Figure 152-2 Livedo Racemosa.

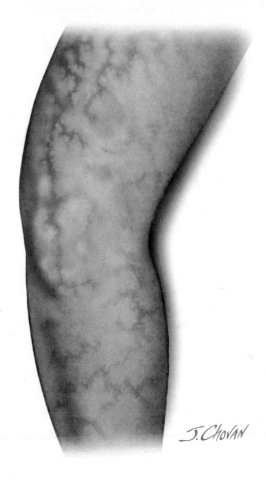

Thrombosis

Thrombosis is a major clinical manifestation of APS and has been reported in nearly every location in the vasculature. The most common sites of venous thrombosis are the deep and superficial veins of the lower extremities. Pulmonary embolism occurs in up to half the cases of deep venous thrombosis. Stroke is the most common form of arterial thrombosis in APS. Thrombosis is probably the underlying pathophysiologic process in a number of other clinical manifestations of APS (e.g., placental thrombosis and infarction leading to pregnancy loss, and thrombosis of dermal blood vessels leading to cutaneous ulcers).

Pregnancy Loss and Morbidity

The type of pregnancy loss that is most strongly associated with aPL is fetal death occurring from the late first trimester onward. Earlier losses (less than 10 weeks' gestation) also occur; however, the statistical association is weaker because of the high incidence of such early losses in the general population. Various types of pregnancy morbidity are also associated with aPL. These include fetal growth impairment, oligohydramnios, preeclampsia and eclamp-

sia, fetal distress, premature delivery, and maternal thrombotic events in the postpartum period.

Cutaneous Manifestations

Livedo reticularis, a latticework of blue to red subcutaneous mottling, is often present in patients with aPL. Some authors make a distinction between two major patterns of livedo: livedo reticularis (Fig. 152-1) and livedo racemosa (Fig. 152-2). The latter is a more open, streak-like pattern and may have greater pathologic significance. Sneddon's syndrome, the association of livedo and stroke, is associated with aPL in many instances.

Cutaneous ulcers and skin necrosis have also been reported in association with aPL.

Thrombocytopenia

In SLE patients, thrombocytopenia is associated with aPL, occurring in about 40% of patients with aPL, as compared with only 10% of patients without aPL. aPL are also present in about one third of patients with chronic autoimmune thrombocytopenia. Thrombocytopenia in APS

The Antiphospholipid Syndrome

Introduction

The antiphospholipid syndrome (APS) is the association of a group of autoantibodies having an apparent specificity for anionic phospholipids with thrombosis and pregnancy morbidity or pregnancy loss. Other clinical manifestations include thrombocytopenia, livedo reticularis, a form of valvular heart disease (Libman-Sachs endocarditis), cutaneous ulcers, and certain nonstroke neurologic problems. Antiphospholipid antibodies (aPL) are present in about one third of patients with systemic lupus erythematosus (SLE), and about one third of these patients (10% to 15% of SLE patients) have one or more clinical manifestations of APS. APS may also occur as a primary syndrome in the absence of SLE or other autoimmune diseases. Primary APS is a relatively common form of acquired thrombophilia in the general population, accounting for 15% to 20% of all cases of venous thromboembolism, up to one third of stroke in younger individuals (younger than 50 years of age), and 10% to 15% of women with recurrent pregnancy losses.

Etiology and Pathogenesis

The underlying events leading to the development of aPL are not known. It is likely that genetic factors play a role. A number of familial cases of APS have been reported; however, specific genes contributing to the development of aPL and APS have not yet been identified.

Although aPL were originally thought to be directed against anionic phospholipids, such as cardiolipin and phosphatidylserine, the major targets of these autoantibodies are now thought to be certain phospholipid-binding plasma proteins. The two most important antigens appear to be β_2-glycoprotein I (β_2-GPI) and prothrombin. β_2-GPI is a normal plasma glycoprotein with an unknown physiologic function. Inherited deficiency of β_2-GPI is not associated with a disease phenotype. β_2-GPI may interact with certain other molecules (e.g., coagulation factor XI, oxidized low-density lipoproteins), and cells (e.g., vascular endothelial cells, monocytes, apoptotic cells). Prothrombin, of course, plays a key role in blood coagulation.

Research suggests that aPL are not merely markers of this condition but play an important role in the pathophysiology of hypercoagulability and pregnancy loss. For example, a number of monoclonal and polyclonal antibodies to β_2-GPI have been shown to be procoagulant or to induce pregnancy loss in animal models. Numerous mechanisms have been proposed. Certain aPL inhibit normal anticoagulant pathways, particularly the protein C pathway. Additionally, aPL may bind to and activate vascular endothelial cells or blood monocytes, leading to a procoagulant phenotype, including the expression of tissue factor and of intercellular adhesion molecules. Animal models also suggest that the pathologic effects of aPL require activation of the complement system.

It is likely that aPL are risk factors for thrombosis, that is, that they cause or contribute to a hypercoagulable state, but are not themselves the proximate trigger of a thrombotic event. In individuals with aPL, the antibodies are constantly present in the circulation, but a thrombotic event occurs only rarely, if ever, and at a particular site in the vasculature.

Clinical Presentation

The clinical presentations of APS are varied and depend on the particular clinical manifestation.

This website includes a geographic directory of rheumatologists, patient information, and additional links.

Arthritis Foundation. Available a: http://www.arthritis.org.

This website offers continually updated information on a wide variety of rheumatic diseases and includes patient educational materials.

Lupus Foundation of America. Available at: http://www.lfa.org.

This website contains valuable patient information and references to patient support groups and national lupus centers.

National Institutes of Health. Available at: http://www.nih.gov/institutes/niams.

The website for the branch of the NIH that focuses on rheumatic diseases provides helpful links to multiple sites, including other organizations, literature, current research, and clinical trials.

EVIDENCE

1. Buyon JP, Petri MA, Kim MY, et al: The effect of combined estrogen and progesterone hormone replacement therapy on disease activity in systemic lupus erythematosus: A randomized trial. Ann Intern Med 142:953-962, 2005.

This randomized, placebo-controlled trial evaluates the effect of hormonal replacement therapy on SLE disease activity. The authors conclude that a short course of hormonal replacement therapy is associated with a 10% increase in risk for mild to moderate disease activity among postmenopausal women with lupus. Most flares that did occur were mild.

2. Koopman WJ (ed): Arthritis and Allied Conditions, 15th ed. Philadelphia, Lippincott Williams & Wilkins, 2005.

This text provides a thorough review of recent therapies and pathogenesis of SLE.

3. Petri M, Kim MY, Kalunian KC, et al: Combined oral contraceptives in women with systemic lupus erythematosus. N Engl J Med 353(24):2550-2558, 2005.

This pivotal clinical trial concludes that oral contraceptives do not increase the flare rate of SLE in young, antiphospholipid antibody-negative women with SLE.

4. Wallace D, Hahn B (eds): Dubois' Lupus Erythematosus, 7th ed. Philadelphia, Lippincott Williams & Wilkins, 2006.

This excellent comprehensive review of past and current information on causes and treatments of lupus manifestations includes a useful annotated reference list.

4. Sunscreen with an SPF of 30+ should be encouraged.
5. Risk factors for atherosclerosis, including hypertension, hyperlipidemia, and smoking cessation, should be addressed, as previously emphasized.

Pharmacologic Agents Available for Treatment

Nonsteroidal Anti-inflammatory Drugs

Nonsteroidal anti-inflammatory drugs are useful for controlling joint symptoms, serositis (pleuritis and pericarditis), and headaches. The selective cyclooxygenase (COX)-2 inhibitors have not been studied specifically in SLE but are likely to show the same decreased gastrointestinal toxicity demonstrated in other patient populations. The side effects of COX-2 and nonselective COX inhibitors include adverse effects on kidney, liver, and central nervous system function that may mimic increased SLE activity.

Corticosteroids

Many of the clinical features of SLE respond to corticosteroids. Dosing is based on organ involvement, with higher doses in acute renal disease and myositis, and lower doses for arthralgias and fatigue. Numerous routes and formulations are available. Skin lesions can be injected, and intra-articular injections are often helpful in arthritis. Oral and intravenous routes are also used for delivery. The risks with long-term use include increased susceptibility to infection, cataracts, hypertension, diabetes, osteoporosis, and avascular necrosis of bone.

Antimalarial Drugs

These agents are most useful when cutaneous, joint, pleural, or pericardial features are predominant, and when patients experience severe fatigue associated with SLE. Hydroxychloroquine (Plaquenil) is the most commonly prescribed medication in this group, but chloroquine and quinacrine are sometimes used as well. Regular ophthalmology exams for monitoring possible toxicity are essential. The risk for ocular toxicity with hydroxychloroquine is low if the recommended doses are employed. Benefits include lipid-lowering and possible antithrombotic effects.

Immunosuppressive Drugs

Additional immunosuppressants are frequently used for more severe disease and for their steroid-sparing effects. Drugs in this group include azathioprine, cyclophosphamide, mycophenolate mofetil, and cyclosporine. Methotrexate has been increasingly used for severe arthritis or skin disease. Potential toxicities make close monitoring mandatory and are specific to each drug. Contraception is required during therapy because of the risk for teratogenicity associated with most of these medications.

Avoiding Treatment Errors

Given the wide range of clinical presentations in patients with SLE, there is a critical need to consider new symptoms as possible manifestations of SLE. The consideration of other medical etiologies should follow. Appropriate laboratory testing and biopsies to confirm organ involvement must always occur before the initiation of immunosuppressive therapy. SLE patients are most likely to develop new disease features within the first few years of onset; thus, close follow-up is important. Recent studies confirm the benefits of hydroxychloroquine for prevention of disease flares and for decreasing cardiovascular and thrombotic risks. The patient should continue hydroxychloroquine long term, even during periods of immunosuppressive therapy. The dose should remain no greater than 6.5 mg/kg, reduced by half in patients with renal insufficiency. Gastrointestinal intolerance may occur with generics, which are not enteric coated.

Future Directions

Previous investigators demonstrated an association between lower socioeconomic status measures and higher morbidity and mortality in SLE. This relationship is complex and a focus of long-term assessment in the Lumina cohort. Environmental risks for developing lupus have been addressed in the Carolina Lupus Study, a case-controlled population-based study of lupus patients in the southeastern United States. Exposure to silica was a strong risk in this population.

Several new agents are under investigation for SLE therapy. Mycophenolate mofetil and intermittent intravenous cyclophosphamide are being compared as initial therapy for proliferative glomerulonephritis. Shorter courses of cyclophosphamide are being evaluated in the EuroLupus Trial as well. Monoclonal antibodies to inhibit costimulatory pathways for T-cell and B-cell activation are currently in clinical trials. Several drugs approved for use in rheumatoid arthritis are also being evaluated in clinical trials for use in lupus. An oral tolerogen, JPJ 394, has shown promise in delaying initial renal flare in patients with high-titer anti-dsDNA antibodies through downregulation of their production. Autologous hematopoietic stem cell transplantation has been performed in patients with SLE; seven patients were disease free at a median follow-up of 25 months, but the durability of response remains unknown. Immunoablative high-dose cyclophosphamide without stem cell transplantation (thus decreasing the risk for graft-versus-host disease) is being evaluated for therapy of severe refractory SLE.

Additional Resources

American College of Rheumatology. Available at: http://www.rheumatology.org.

Management and Therapy

Optimum Treatment

Prevention of Recurrent Thrombosis

Long-term anticoagulation, rather than immunosuppression, is the mainstay of therapy. Warfarin anticoagulation at a high target international normalized ratio (INR) (3.0 to 4.0) was previously recommended. More recently, a randomized trial suggested that a target INR of 2.0 to 3.0 is adequate, and many experts in the field have adopted this recommendation. Anticoagulation with unfractionated or low-molecular-weight heparin may be used in some cases. In general, anticoagulation is for an indefinite period of time. Of course, long-term full anticoagulation carries a significant risk for bleeding complications, and the decision to institute such therapy must be individualized and take into account the patient's age, compliance, and comorbid conditions. In some patients, aPL tests may become negative after months or years. It is not known whether it is safe to discontinue anticoagulation in this situation.

Prevention of Pregnancy Loss

In women with a prior pregnancy loss related to aPL, the chance of an untreated subsequent pregnancy resulting in a live birth is only about 20%. Treatment with low-dose aspirin alone increases the live birth rate significantly, to about 40%. Treatment with heparin and low-dose aspirin is even more effective, increasing the chance of a live birth to about 80%.

Candidates for treatment are women with persistent medium or high positive tests for aPL and one or more fetal losses (>10 weeks' gestation) or a history of thrombosis. Women with early pregnancy losses (<10 weeks' gestation) or low levels of aPL are at lower risk for subsequent pregnancy loss, and the treatment decision is more difficult.

For women with obstetric APS without a prior history of thrombosis, typical treatment regimens are minidose or low-dose unfractionated heparin (5,000 to 10,000 units every 12 hours) or prophylactic doses of low-molecular-weight heparin. Anticoagulation is held around the time of delivery but is recommended during the postpartum period (6 weeks) to prevent maternal thrombosis.

Asymptomatic aPL

Unless contraindicated, low-dose aspirin is recommended for asymptomatic individuals with aPL, including women with a history of obstetric APS who are not pregnant. This recommendation is not strongly evidence based; however, low-dose aspirin is likely to lower the risk for thrombosis, has a low incidence of adverse side effects, and is inexpensive.

Other Therapeutic Agents

In patients with SLE and aPL, hydroxychloroquine appears to lower the risk for thrombosis. The role of antiplatelet agents, such as clopidogrel, in APS is unknown. Rituximab therapy in a small number of cases of APS has produced mixed results. Intravenous immune globulin (IVIG) has been used in several cases of pregnancy loss, previously refractory to heparin and aspirin. In a small randomized trial, however, IVIG did not add benefit. HMG-CoA reductase inhibitors (statins) have a number of beneficial vascular effects in addition to lowering cholesterol. In animal models of APS, statins have shown some benefit.

Avoiding Treatment Errors

Given the considerable risks of long-term anticoagulation, it is especially important to carefully determine which patients clearly have aPL and require such treatment. Ideally, the presence of aPL, either the lupus anticoagulant or medium to high levels of anticardiolipin or anti–β_2-GPI antibodies, should be confirmed on two or more occasions, at least 2 to 3 months apart. Care should also be taken to ensure that lupus anticoagulant testing is complete and includes the necessary confirmatory tests. A prolonged routine aPTT alone is not sufficient evidence to establish the presence of a lupus anticoagulant. Finally, panels of tests for antibodies to multiple phospholipids are not recommended and, if performed, should be interpreted with caution. As noted, most of these tests are not well standardized, and their significance, if standard antiphospholipid tests are negative, is questionable.

Future Directions

Research is rapidly shedding light on the immunology of aPL and the pathophysiology of the associated hypercoagulability. The elucidation of these mechanisms may suggest therapeutic approaches that are effective but much safer than full anticoagulation. For example, a β_2-GPI-specific B-cell toleragen has been developed and may be able to specifically decrease levels of anti–β_2-GPI autoantibodies.

Additional Resources

APS Foundation of America. Available at: http://apsfa.org. Accessed March 17, 2007.

This new nonprofit organization provides information and support to patients.

Antiphospholipid Syndrome Collaborative Registry (APSCORE). Available at: http://www.apscore.org. Accessed March 17, 2007.

APSCORE is a national disease registry begun by the National Institutes of Health. The website contains information for physicians and patients.

Hughes Syndrome Website. Available at: http://www.hughes-syndrome.org/overview.htm. Accessed March 17, 2007.

This website is a good general source for information on the antiphospholipid syndrome.

Rare Thrombotic Disease Consortium. Available at: http://rarediseasesnetwork.epi.usf.edu/rtdc/index.htm. Accessed May 21, 2007.

The "Information for Physicians" section contains good reviews on the antiphospholipid syndrome in general and on catastrophic antiphospholipid syndrome.

EVIDENCE

1. Crowther MA, Ginsberg JS, Julian J, et al: A comparison of two intensities of warfarin for the prevention of recurrent thrombosis in patients with the antiphospholipid antibody syndrome. N Engl J Med 349:1133-1138, 2003.

   The authors describe a key randomized trial of warfarin for the prevention of recurrent thrombosis in APS.
2. Derksen RHWM, Khamashta MA, Branch DW: Management of the obstetric antiphospholipid syndrome. Arthritis Rheum 50:1028-1039, 2004.

   This is an excellent evidence-based review.
3. Miyakis S, Lockshin MD, Atsumi T, et al: International consensus statement on an update of the classification criteria for definite antiphospholipid syndrome (APS). J Thromb Haemost 4:295-306, 2006.

   Although the criteria themselves are of limited clinical use, this consensus statement summarizes a large body of evidence-based data on the clinical manifestations of APS.

Beth L. Jonas ▪ Robert A.S. Roubey

153

Rheumatoid Arthritis

Introduction

Rheumatoid arthritis (RA) is a multisystem inflammatory disorder with a worldwide prevalence rate in the population of about 1%. The peak age of onset is between 40 and 50 years, with females being affected significantly more often than males; however, with increasing age, the male-to-female ratio equilibrates.

Etiology and Pathogenesis

The etiology of RA is not completely established and is likely to be multifactorial. It is clear that genetic makeup, the immune responses of the individual, and an inciting agent, possibly of bacterial or viral origin, all play a role. RA is associated with a conserved sequence in the hypervariable region of the human leukocyte antigen (HLA)-DR gene; the so-called shared epitope. The presence of the shared epitope is associated with both susceptibility to and severity of RA in some populations. A putative arthrogenic antigen has not been elucidated, although it is likely that numerous exogenous or endogenous antigens may trigger the disease.

Pathologically, synovitis is the hallmark of the disease. New blood vessel formation is prominent in early disease, and the normally thin synovial membrane becomes hypertrophic. Synovial inflammation is characterized by the influx of CD4+ cells. Release of cytokines locally helps mediate tissue destruction with cartilage degradation and, ultimately, erosion of bone.

Clinical Presentation

The diagnosis of RA is important particularly now that early treatment with disease-modifying antirheumatic drugs (DMARDs) and the newer biologic agents has been shown to improve outcomes. The diagnostic criteria of the American College of Rheumatology are shown in Box 153-1. Eventually, a symmetrical inflammatory polyarthritis with small joint involvement develops in all patients. Most patients present with an insidious onset over weeks to months, but some patients (about 10%) have an acute onset over a few days. The small joints of the hand and wrist are most commonly involved early, but some patients may present with a monoarthritis. The diagnosis can be difficult in the early stages, and patients with chronic joint pain need to be reassessed on a regular basis.

Signs and symptoms include joint pain; joint swelling with synovitis (synovial thickening and fluid); joint stiffness, worse in the mornings; joints that are usually warm, and occasionally erythematous; limited range of motion; nodule formation on the extensor aspect of the forearm; low-grade fever in some cases; and malaise and fatigue (Fig. 153-1). Extra-articular manifestations occur in patients with more severe disease and may include Sjögren's syndrome, episcleritis or scleritis, pleurisy, pulmonary nodules, pulmonary fibrosis, pericarditis, rheumatoid vasculitis, and Felty's syndrome (Fig. 153-2).

Initial laboratory test results may be normal but can show a thrombocytosis, leukocytosis, mild anemia (normochromic, normocytic, or microcytic), elevated erythrocyte sedimentation rate, and high C-reactive protein. Immunoglobulin M rheumatoid factor is present in about 50% of cases at presentation, and in 70% to 75% of cases over time. Antibodies to cyclic citrullinated peptide (CCP) are a more sensitive marker and may be seen in early disease. Aspiration of inflammatory fluid from the joint often reveals a high white blood cell count with polymorphonuclear leukocytes predominating. Synovial fluid analysis is particularly important in early disease to rule out crystalline arthropathies, or in the case of a monoarthritis to rule out infection.

Differential Diagnosis

Box 153-2 provides the differential diagnosis of rheumatoid arthritis.

Diagnostic Approach

Patients with recent onset of inflammatory polyarthralgia or polyarthritis should have a complete history and physical examination. Although RA is common, elements of the history or physical examination that might suggest another cause require special attention. Swollen or tender joints should be surveyed to document true synovitis and to form a baseline examination to assess progress in future visits. Radiographs are often normal in early disease. The presence of periarticular osteopenia is sometimes helpful in differentiating inflammatory from noninflammatory causes of joint pain. Radiographs of the hands (and feet if clinically indicated) can be useful to establish a baseline. The presence of erosions on the baseline radiograph is a poor

prognostic factor and indicates the need for an aggressive approach. Synovial fluid analysis is performed to document the inflammatory nature of the joint disease and rule out other causes of synovitis, including gout, calcium pyrophosphate deposition disease, and septic arthritis. Other laboratory tests include rheumatoid factor, anti-CCP, complete blood cell count, chemistry profile, and some acute-phase reactants such as the erythrocyte sedimentation rate or C-reactive protein. Serologic testing for parvovirus or other viral illnesses deserves consideration in the case of an acute presentation.

Management and Therapy

Disease-Modifying Antirheumatic Drugs

The most commonly used DMARDs include hydroxychloroquine, sulfasalazine, methotrexate, and leflunomide. The mechanism of action of these drugs is complex, but they all inhibit inflammatory responses and suppress synovitis. Hydroxychloroquine is useful in very early and mild disease. Because it is laid down in pigment tissue, ophthalmologic assessment is recommended at baseline and annually. There is little or no risk for long-term ocular sequelae if standard dose regimens are adhered to (200 to 400 mg daily) and routine monitoring is performed. Sulfasalazine is given orally; the dosage should be increased slowly from 500 mg to 2 g daily. Some patients might require a trial of up to 4 g daily for 4 to 6 weeks if there is no response. Side effects include indigestion, abnormal liver function tests, leukopenia, anemia, and skin rashes. Required monitoring includes complete blood cell count and liver function tests on a regular basis, at least for the first 3 months of therapy, and periodically thereafter.

Methotrexate, the most commonly used member of this group, is given orally in a dose of 10 to 25 mg once a week. Side effects include indigestion, oral ulcers, hair loss, occasional blood dyscrasias, and abnormal liver function tests. The risk for hepatic fibrosis with long-term administration now appears sufficiently small to preclude routine liver biopsy, except in patients with preexisting liver disease. Treatment of patients who have a regular moderate alcohol intake, history of liver disease, diabetes, or obesity requires great care and vigilance. Patients should be screened for chronic infection with hepatitis B and C before instituting therapy with methotrexate. The drug is contraindicated in pregnancy. The addition of folic acid, 1 mg daily, is recommended to reduce toxicity. Monitoring of blood cell counts and liver function tests is recommended every 8 weeks, although less frequent monitoring can be done in patients who have been taking a long-term stable dose without a history of toxicity.

Leflunomide is given orally in a dose of 20 mg daily after a 3-day loading dose of 100 mg daily. It has been shown to slow the radiographic progression of disease. Common side effects include diarrhea, elevated transami-

Figure 153-1 Early and Moderate Hand Involvement in Rheumatoid Arthritis.

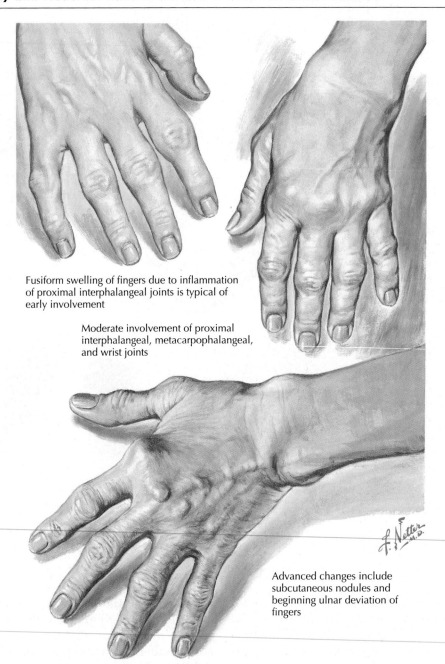

Fusiform swelling of fingers due to inflammation of proximal interphalangeal joints is typical of early involvement

Moderate involvement of proximal interphalangeal, metacarpophalangeal, and wrist joints

Advanced changes include subcutaneous nodules and beginning ulnar deviation of fingers

nase levels, reversible alopecia, and rash. Leflunomide is teratogenic in animals. Women who wish to become pregnant and men who want to father a child must first discontinue the drug and take cholestyramine (8 g 3 times daily for 11 days) to eliminate the drug. Use of leflunomide in reduced dose (10 mg daily) in combination with methotrexate is an alternative, but long-term safety has not been established. Monitoring of blood cell counts and liver function tests is recommended every 8 weeks.

Biologic Agents

Etanercept is a recombinant dimeric fusion protein of the soluble human tumor necrosis factor (TNF) receptor. Etanercept, 50 mg subcutaneously weekly, has been shown to be effective in RA when there has been an inadequate response to other DMARDs. Injection-site reactions are common but rarely limit therapy. Infliximab is a monoclonal antibody that binds TNF and neutralizes its activity.

Figure 153-2 Extra-articular Manifestations of Rheumatoid Arthritis.

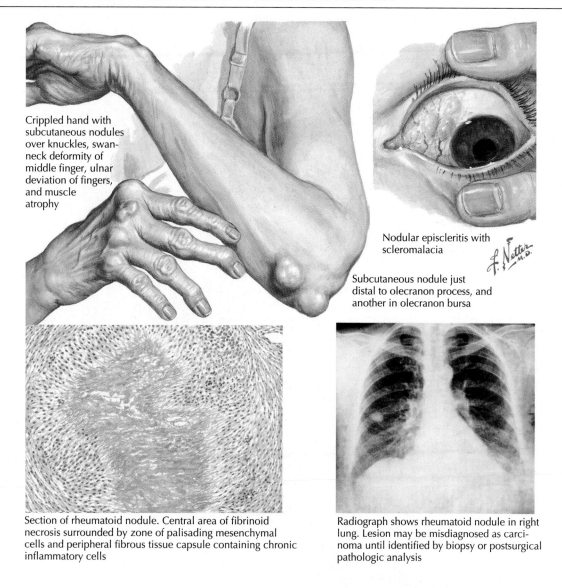

Crippled hand with subcutaneous nodules over knuckles, swan-neck deformity of middle finger, ulnar deviation of fingers, and muscle atrophy

Nodular episcleritis with scleromalacia

Subcutaneous nodule just distal to olecranon process, and another in olecranon bursa

Section of rheumatoid nodule. Central area of fibrinoid necrosis surrounded by zone of palisading mesenchymal cells and peripheral fibrous tissue capsule containing chronic inflammatory cells

Radiograph shows rheumatoid nodule in right lung. Lesion may be misdiagnosed as carcinoma until identified by biopsy or postsurgical pathologic analysis

Like etanercept, it is indicated in RA unresponsive to traditional DMARDs. Administration is by intravenous infusion at weeks 0, 2, and 6 and then every 8 weeks. Infusion reactions may occur but are usually mild. The newest anti-TNF agent, adalimumab, is a fully humanized monoclonal antibody given subcutaneously, 40 mg every other week. Infections, some life-threatening, have been reported and warrant caution in debilitated patients. Severe infections have been reported, particularly tuberculosis. Therefore, a pretreatment purified protein derivative (PPD) tuberculin is recommended for patients starting anti-TNF therapy. The U.S. Food and Drug Administration has approved anakinra, an interleukin-1 receptor antagonist, for RA. It is given subcutaneously, 100 mg daily. Efficacy appears to be modest, but it may be an option for patients who have not responded to other, more effective therapies. Injection-site reactions can be severe but usually wane after 4 to 6 weeks of therapy.

In patients who have had an inadequate response to DMARDs or TNF-α inhibitors, two new agents with unique mechanisms may provide good clinical efficacy. Rituximab is an anti-CD20 monoclonal antibody that results in B-cell depletion. It is given by intravenous infusion, two doses separated by 2 weeks. Because of the drug's ability to effectively deplete B cells for a long period, dosing occurs no more frequently than every 6 months. Abatacept is a selective costimulation modulator with inhibitory activity on T cells. The drug is given monthly by the intravenous route.

Corticosteroids

Systemic corticosteroids are effective in the treatment of RA, but significant short- and long-term toxicity limits their use. Doses of prednisone should be kept below 10 mg

daily if possible, with the majority of the dose given in the morning. Corticosteroids should be aggressively tapered once effective DMARDs have been instituted if at all possible. At times, intra-articular injections are extremely useful in controlling inflammation in individual joints. However, they should not be given at intervals of less than 3 months and are contraindicated in the presence of local infection.

Nonsteroidal Anti-inflammatory Drugs

Nonsteroidal anti-inflammatory drugs (NSAIDs) interfere with the production of prostaglandins and therefore reduce pain and inflammation. NSAIDs produce a plethora of adverse reactions, the most common being peptic ulceration. The newer selective cyclooxygenase-2 inhibitors may have some advantage over traditional NSAIDs because the relative risk for gastrointestinal ulceration is lower. However, recent concerns regarding potential cardiovascular toxicity require careful consideration when choosing an agent. All NSAIDs have significant renal adverse effects, particularly in elderly patients, including acute renal failure and fluid retention. As a rule, NSAIDs should be used as an adjunct to DMARD therapy and never as monotherapy in patients with established RA because they do not have any disease-modifying properties.

Drug Therapy

NSAIDs are suitable first-line agents for the management of active disease. Consider low-dose prednisone (10 mg daily) in patients who are not adequately controlled on NSAIDs, at least until effective DMARD therapy can be achieved. Most patients with RA will require DMARDs, and therapy with these drugs should begin as soon as the diagnosis of RA is established. Delay will lead to irreversible joint destruction in most patients with moderate or severe disease activity. Patients may not respond to DMARD therapy for up to 3 months after a therapeutic dose is achieved. The evaluation of efficacy requires frequent monitoring of disease activity. If there is no evidence of disease suppression, then the drug should be changed. Periodic radiographic assessment is recommended even in those patients with an adequate clinical response because progression of erosive disease warrants intensification of therapy. When response to methotrexate is incomplete, the patient may benefit from combinations of methotrexate with other agents such as sulfasalazine, leflunomide, or a TNF inhibitor. If general control is achieved but individual joints continue to show active inflammation, intra-articular corticosteroid injections can be considered. These might need to be repeated on occasion, but preferably no more than 3 times per year in a single joint. A joint requiring more frequent injections may indicate the need for more aggressive systemic therapy or, in the case of a persistent monoarthritis, a surgical approach.

Surgical Treatment

The major reason for surgery is pain relief or restoration of function. Surgical options include synovectomy (of joint or tendons), arthroplasty, and arthrodesis. Synovectomy can be performed on the knees, wrists, metacarpophalangeal joints, or other joints unresponsive to medical therapies. The synovium might well grow back into the joint if disease activity continues, but patients can experience some pain relief for a number of years. Arthroplasty with joint replacement is commonly used in the hips, knees, and metacarpophalangeal and interphalangeal joints. Shoulder and elbow joint replacements are now gaining acceptance; wrist and ankle replacements are still in their infancy. Use of new prosthetic materials and cementless prostheses is likely to improve long-term morbidity. Although joint replacement should be put off as long as possible, great relief can be afforded appropriate patients. Arthrodesis remains an option for intractable wrist or ankle disease.

Avoiding Treatment Errors

The diagnosis of inflammatory joint disease should be confirmed. Whether the pain is due to active synovitis or to secondary degenerative changes should be determined. This is particularly important in those patients with chronic disease when the question of DMARD therapy is raised. It is critically important to maintain awareness of potential drug interactions and to continually reassess patients and change drugs or other treatments if there is no response to treatment. Referring patients to a rheumatologist on diagnosis is advisable, particularly for educational purposes. Also consider referral if there is deteriorating function, when the patient appears generally ill and systemic corticosteroids are contemplated, if there is persistent inflammation in a joint (this could lead to deformity), or if a surgical procedure is contemplated.

Optimum Treatment

Psychological factors are important in patients who have chronic pain and inflammatory joint disease. These need to be addressed and demand a combined approach with allied health professionals including the physiotherapist, occupational therapist, social worker, nurse, and the patient's family. Patient education and self-management skills are extremely important.

Future Directions

Research in RA has made significant strides with the understanding of the role of genetic factors in disease onset and progression, the cytokine profile in active disease, and the introduction of targeted therapies based on these discoveries. The TNF inhibitors, B-cell-targeted therapies, and co-stimulation modulation have made a large contribution to our armamentarium of antirheumatic therapies.

There is an explosion of new biologic compounds on the horizon. These include new TNF inhibitors, anti-interleukin-6 therapy, newer agents directed against interleukin-1, and many more. New targets for therapy are being sought and found. The next decade will bring further work on mechanisms of inflammation that may contribute to disease activity and the development of novel therapeutic targets.

Additional Resources

The Arthritis Foundation. Available at: http://www.arthritis.org.

This website contains extensive information about RA and has excellent resources for patients.

Furst DE, Breedveld FC, Kalden JR, et al: Updated consensus statement on biological agents for the treatment of rheumatic diseases, 2006. Ann Rheum Dis 65:2-15, 2006.

This consensus document is based on a meeting of 143 rheumatologists and scientists who have reviewed the indications, efficacy, and safety of the biologic agents for all the rheumatic diseases. There is an informative section on recommendations for future research.

Harris ED: Clinical features of rheumatoid arthritis. In Kelly's Textbook of Rheumatology, 7th ed. Philadelphia, Elsevier Saunders, 2005.

The text chapter is a good resource on the clinical presentation of rheumatoid arthritis.

EVIDENCE

1. Choy EHS, Panayi GS: Mechanisms of disease: Cytokine pathways and joint inflammation in rheumatoid arthritis. N Engl J Med 344:907-916, 2001.

The authors provide a comprehensive review of the current understanding of the etiology and pathogenesis of rheumatoid arthritis.

2. Machold KP, Nel V, Stamm T, et al: Early rheumatoid arthritis. Curr Opin Rheum 18(3):282-288, 2006.

This paper reviews some of the most up-to-date information on the importance of timely and aggressive intervention in early RA.

3. O'Dell JR: Drug therapy: Therapeutic strategies for rheumatoid arthritis. N Engl J Med 350:2591-2602, 2004.

This is an excellent review of the therapeutic principles for the treatment of RA. The article includes clear and concise algorithms and guidelines for monitoring drug therapy.

Scleroderma

Introduction

Scleroderma encompasses a heterogenous group of chronic autoimmune disorders characterized by inflammation and fibrosis in the skin (Fig. 154-1). Systemic involvement and treatment response may correlate with the extent of skin involvement. Systemic sclerosis is classified into three major clinical subtypes: limited cutaneous scleroderma (lcSSc), diffuse cutaneous scleroderma (dcSSc), and overlap. These subtypes are distinguished from each other primarily on the basis of the extent and degree of skin involvement. Localized or limited scleroderma consists of morphea and linear scleroderma, sclerotic lesions of the skin without visceral involvement. Systemic sclerosis sans scleroderma is characterized by visceral involvement only. Diffuse scleroderma includes two syndromes: CREST (calcinosis cutis, Raynaud phenomenon [RP], esophageal dysmotility, sclerodactyly, and telangiectasias) and diffuse systemic sclerosis. In addition to the skin, systemic sclerosis involves the blood vessels, joints, skeletal muscle, and frequently internal organs such as the gastrointestinal tract, heart, kidney, and lungs. In the United States, the incidence is about 20 to 30 new cases per million people annually, with a prevalence of 105 to 138 per 1 million. The female-to-male incidence ratio is 3 : 1, and the peak age of onset is 40 to 60 years. No significant racial differences in disease onset or expression have been found.

Etiology and Pathogenesis

The etiology of scleroderma remains unknown. Monozygotic twin concordance rates are lower than those of other rheumatic diseases such as rheumatoid arthritis and lupus, suggesting an important role for environmental exposure in pathogenesis. Prior investigation suggests that scleroderma is a multigenic, complex disorder. An individual with a susceptible genetic background may encounter an inciting factor such as infection, organic solvents, drugs, or environmental agents. Implicated environmental agents include silica dust exposure, certain solvents, drugs, and chemotherapeutic agents. Several retrospective studies do not show an increased risk in women with silicone breast implants.

Clinical expression includes vascular, fibrotic, and immunologic features. Pathogenic events include endothelial cell injury and vascular obliteration, increased matrix deposition by dermal and visceral fibroblasts, and activation of cellular and humoral immune responses. Genetic factors play a role in disease susceptibility, but no single major histocompatibility complex allele is associated with an increased risk for scleroderma in all ethnic groups.

Microchimerism (the persistence of fetal cells in the maternal circulation) may contribute to immune activation in this autoimmune disorder. Complete remission in diffuse scleroderma is rare.

Clinical Presentation

Limited Cutaneous Scleroderma

There is restricted skin fibrosis affecting the distal extremities and face and occasional late development of pulmonary arterial hypertension, pulmonary fibrosis, or small bowel malabsorption. The CREST syndrome that presents with findings of calcinosis, RP, esophageal dysfunction, sclerodactyly, and telangiectasia is closely analogous to lcSSc. The 10-year survival is more than 70%.

Diffuse Cutaneous Scleroderma

Widespread skin fibrosis affects distal and proximal extremities (proximal to elbow), trunk, and face. There is a tendency to rapid progression of skin thickening and early occurrence of visceral disease affecting the gastro-

Figure 154-1 Progressive Systemic Sclerosis (Scleroderma).

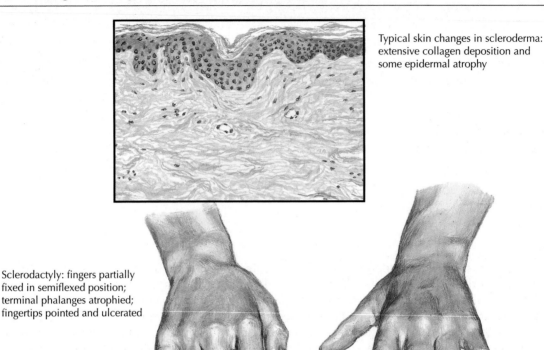

Typical skin changes in scleroderma: extensive collagen deposition and some epidermal atrophy

Sclerodactyly: fingers partially fixed in semiflexed position; terminal phalanges atrophied; fingertips pointed and ulcerated

intestinal tract, lung, heart, and kidneys. Palpable tendon friction rubs and flexion contractures are frequently associated. The 10-year survival rate is usually less than 70%.

Scleroderma Sans Sclerodactyly

Some patients with scleroderma may have no detectable skin thickening and present with pulmonary fibrosis or renal, cardiac, or gastrointestinal disease. RP may be present.

Overlap

Scleroderma overlap includes either diffuse or limited skin fibrosis and typical features of one or more of the connective tissue diseases such as rheumatoid arthritis, systemic lupus erythematosus, polymyositis, dermatomyositis, or Sjögren's syndrome.

Raynaud's Phenomenon

RP, an episodic and reversible vasospasm precipitated by cold exposure or emotional stress, occurs in about 95% of scleroderma patients at some time during the disease. It is accompanied by color changes of pallor (white), acrocyanosis (blue), and reperfusion hyperemia (red). Typically, it affects the fingers, toes, nose, and ears but can also affect the heart, lungs, and kidneys. Ischemic necrosis may occur, leading to ulceration of the fingertips in up to 15% to 25% of patients. Gangrene or superinfection may occur in these areas of tissue necrosis.

Skin

In lcSSc, skin thickening is minimal over several years and does not correlate with development of visceral disease. Calcinosis from intracutaneous or subcutaneous calcific deposition of hydroxyapatite is commonly present on the digital pads and extensor surface of the forearms, elbows, and knees. Occasionally, it is more widespread. Telangiectasias, most typical of lcSSc, are usually present on the fingers, face, lips, and anterior chest. On nail-fold capillary microscopic examination, dilated loops of capillaries are seen in both diffuse and limited subsets of scleroderma. In dcSSc, a paucity of nail-fold vessels or "drop out" may be seen.

In dcSSc, patients may complain early in the disease of puffy, edematous hands (edematous phase). This is followed by thickening and tightening over subsequent weeks to months (indurative phase). Hypopigmentation and hyperpigmentation of the skin may occur. Over several years, the skin may revert to normal thickness or become thin (atrophic phase). Perioral involvement leads to thinning of the lips, puckering, and reduced oral aperture. In early dcSSc, skin sclerosis progresses rapidly, peaking in the first 2 years. It is closely associated with progression of visceral disease and development of joint contractures. Skin scores are employed in clinical trials to assess these changes. Notably, the natural history of the skin involvement is to decrease over time even without treatment.

Musculoskeletal

Arthralgias and joint stiffness may affect the small and large joints. Tendon friction rubs commonly palpated over the flexor or extensor tendons due to fibrinous tenosynovitis and tendinitis are specific for dcSSc. They are associated with increased skin thickness, renal involvement, and reduced survival. The patient may lose a significant degree of range of motion in the joints due to the progression of skin fibrosis or to bridging calcinosis. Erosive joint disease is also seen. Patients may also develop proximal muscle weakness that is associated with electromyographic and pathologic evidence of myositis.

Gastrointestinal Tract

Esophageal dysfunction eventually develops in about 80% of patients. The most frequent symptoms are heartburn and substernal dysphagia. Conventional barium swallow shows hypomotility of the distal portions of the esophagus. Classic manometric findings consist of an incompetent lower esophageal sphincter and low-amplitude contractions in the distal smooth muscle portion of the esophagus. Small bowel dysfunction has been reported in 20% to 60% of patients. Reduced peristalsis leads to stasis and intestinal dilation, which favors bacterial overgrowth, causing fat malabsorption and eventually malnutrition. Pseudo-obstruction is a rare complication that presents with severe postprandial bloating and cramps. Hypomotility of the small intestine results in a functional ileus with symptoms simulating a mechanical obstruction. Constipation often complicates impaired peristalsis of the colon, either alone or alternating with diarrhea. Patchy atrophy of the muscular wall leads to development of wide-mouthed diverticula on the antimesenteric border of the transverse and descending colon. The liver, biliary tract, and pancreas are rarely involved. Primary biliary cirrhosis, the liver disorder seen most frequently with limited cutaneous scleroderma, is strongly associated with the presence of the antimitochondrial antibody (AMA).

Lung

Pulmonary involvement occurs in more than 70% of patients with systemic sclerosis (diffuse cutaneous scleroderma) and is the most common cause of disease-related mortality (Fig. 154-2). Interstitial lung disease (ILD) and pulmonary vascular disease complicated by pulmonary hypertension are the main clinical manifestations. The most common symptoms of interstitial lung disease are dyspnea on exertion and dry cough. Dry, bibasilar end-inspiratory rales are usually present, and chest radiographs show reticular interstitial changes or fibrosis, most prominent in the lower lung fields. A restrictive ventilatory defect is commonly noted. High-resolution computed tomography (CT) identifies a ground-glass appearance representing active alveolitis. Bronchoalveolar lavage (BAL) is helpful to determine whether there is active inflammation (alveolitis) characterized by an overall increase in alveolar macrophages and granulocytes recovered by BAL, as well as an increased percentage of granulocytes (neutrophils >3% or eosinophils >2.2% of total cells). Interstitial alveolitis may progress to fibrosis with irreversible scarring, secondary pulmonary hypertension, and hypoxia. The factors associated with the highest risk for severe restrictive disease are black race, male gender, younger age in patients with diffuse cutaneous disease, and the presence of anti-topoisomerase I antibody.

Pulmonary hypertension characterized by rapidly progressive dyspnea and accentuation of the pulmonic component of the second heart sound occurs in about 5% of patients with lcSSc, typically 10 to 30 years after onset of RP. Occasionally, it is seen in patients who have anti-U3 ribonucleoprotein (anti-U3RNP) antibody. The diffusing capacity is severely reduced, and the electrocardiogram (ECG) shows evidence of right heart dysfunction. The prognosis is poor; a median survival of less than 2 years may be affected by intravenous or subcutaneous prostacyclin, sildenafil given three times daily, inhaled iloprostacyclin, or the endothelin receptor antagonists. Many patients receive a combination of these therapies.

Heart

Clinically symptomatic pericardial disease is infrequent (5% to 16%). The echocardiogram detects small effusions in about 41% of asymptomatic patients with scleroderma. A large pericardial effusion (>200 mL) can lead to cardiac tamponade and is a marker for poor outcome with an increased risk for subsequent renal crisis. Myocarditis is rare but occurs in patients with systemic scleroderma and concomitant skeletal myositis. Systolic or diastolic dysfunction may develop in this setting as a result of myocardial fibrosis. About 37% of patients (both diffuse and limited cutaneous) have abnormalities on resting ECG. Supraventricular and ventricular arrhythmias are found more frequently in patients with diffuse cutaneous scleroderma. Cardiac arrhythmias are strongly associated with

Figure 154-2 Progressive Systemic Sclerosis (PSS; Scleroderma); Lung Involvement.

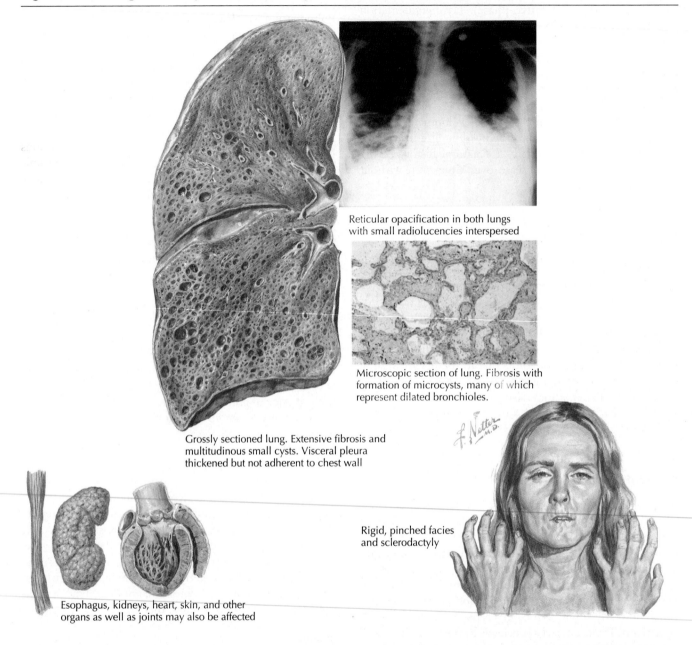

Reticular opacification in both lungs with small radiolucencies interspersed

Microscopic section of lung. Fibrosis with formation of microcysts, many of which represent dilated bronchioles.

Grossly sectioned lung. Extensive fibrosis and multitudinous small cysts. Visceral pleura thickened but not adherent to chest wall

Rigid, pinched facies and sclerodactyly

Esophagus, kidneys, heart, skin, and other organs as well as joints may also be affected

mortality and are related to the severity of cardiopulmonary and renal involvement.

Kidney

Twenty-five percent of patients with dcSSc may develop renal crisis, in contrast to only 1% of patients with lcSSc. Scleroderma renal crisis (SRC) is defined as the new onset of accelerated hypertension and rapidly progressive oliguric renal failure. These patients have elevated plasma renin activity and may have an active urinary sediment (microscopic hematuria, proteinuria) or features consistent with ischemic renal injury (acute tubular necrosis) with muddy-brown casts or inactive urinary sediment. Microangiopathic hemolytic anemia and thrombocytopenia are

prominent hematologic features. Some patients present with congestive heart failure, ventricular arrhythmias, or large pericardial effusions. Factors helpful in identifying patients with dcSSc at risk for developing SRC are rapid progression of skin thickening, disease duration less than 4 years, anti-RNA polymerase III antibody, antecedent high-dose steroid use (>20 mg daily), and serum creatinine level higher than 3 mg/dL. All these factors are indicators of a poor prognosis.

Clinical Outcomes

Recent 5- and 10-year survival rates are 80% to 85% and 60% to 65%, respectively. Prognosis is worse for diffuse scleroderma (10-year survival rate of 40% to 60%) than for limited scleroderma (>70%), primarily because of greater risk for early visceral involvement. Other poor prognostic indicators include later age at onset, African American or Native American race, absence of RP, and presence of tendon friction rubs. Limited scleroderma may be relatively benign at onset, but visceral involvement usually develops over time, most notably pulmonary hypertension.

Differential Diagnosis

The differential diagnosis requires consideration of several scleroderma-like disorders. These include localized scleroderma with fibrosis involving distinct areas, different levels of the skin, and sometimes the underlying soft tissue, muscle, or bone. Women and children are more commonly affected. Subtypes include isolated or generalized morphea, linear scleroderma, nodular (keloid) scleroderma, and, rarely, localized bullous lesions. Diffuse scleroderma with eosinophilia (eosinophilic fasciitis) is associated with swelling, stiffness, and restricted range of motion, but usually spares the hands and face. There is sometimes an association with preceding trauma.

Other disorders may mimic systemic scleroderma (SSc). Sclerodactyly and fibrosis of the palmar fascia occur in insulin-dependent diabetes mellitus, particularly juvenile-onset type—a condition called *diabetic chiropathy*. A newly described disorder, nephrogenic fibrosing dermopathy, may develop in patients with renal insufficiency following exposure to gadolinium contrast administered for magnetic resonance imaging procedures. This disorder is not autoimmune but may occur in dialysis patients or in patients with renal insufficiency from any cause. The disorder may improve or resolve in some, but not all, patients if renal function improves, following medical therapy or renal transplantation. The disorder is associated with prominent and often quite rapid systemic involvement and is generally fatal because of infectious complications of skin involvement or organ dysfunction. The disease process is often very painful and rapidly produces disability due to joint contractures that may progress over days. Chronic graft-versus-host disease, particularly after bone marrow grafts, may produce many common clinical, biochemical, and histologic features of SSc. Environmental exposures (inhalation of epoxy resins, vinyl chloride, silica dusts, organic solvents and pesticides; ingestion of toxic rape seed cooking oil; or injection of paraffin or bleomycin) may produce features of SSc. Miscellaneous and rare conditions that may lead to diagnostic confusion include Sézary's syndrome, scleredema, carcinoid syndrome, Werner's syndrome, porphyria cutanea tarda, progeria, phenylketonuria, local lipodystrophies, and POEMS syndrome (plasma cell dyscrasia, polyneuropathy, organomegaly, monoclonal spikes, and scleroderma-like skin changes).

Diagnostic Approach

The diagnosis of systemic scleroderma is approached systematically by evaluating the patient for evidence of auto-antibody formation and for involvement of major target organs. Features of other connective tissue disorders such as lupus or dermatomyositis require careful review.

Autoantibodies associated with diffuse cutaneous scleroderma are antitopoisomerase I (Scl 70) or anti-RNA polymerase I and III antibodies. Anticentromere antibody is found in up to 90% of patients with limited cutaneous systemic scleroderma and 5% of those with diffuse cutaneous scleroderma. Additional helpful testing includes radiographs of the hands (acral osteolysis and calcification), chest (bibasilar pulmonary fibrosis), and esophagus (barium swallow showing hypomotility). Pulmonary function testing demonstrating decreased diffusion capacity with a restrictive pattern and high-resolution chest CT showing ground-glass opacities are more sensitive indicators of early lung disease. A skin biopsy in an affected area that demonstrates a progressive increase in dermal collagen with loss of appendages can establish the diagnosis.

Management and Therapy

There is no proven therapy for scleroderma. The primary focus is preservation of end-organ function to prolong survival and to enhance quality of life. Aggressive antihypertensive therapy with ACE inhibitors has improved survival rates following onset of renal crisis to more than 2 years. Skin changes in diffuse scleroderma commonly peak in 3 to 5 years and then stabilize; musculoskeletal symptoms and well-being usually improve after this initial period. Skin changes in limited scleroderma are usually very gradual and irreversible, but may start as generalized skin patches, which then retreat to the face and hands. Localized scleroderma generally fades away in 3 to 5 years, but dark skin patches and muscle weakness may persist. After many years, the skin in diffuse scleroderma usually softens and returns to normal thickness, or thins and atrophies; hair and sweat glands always remain absent.

Skin

In the early stages, pruritus may be treated with antihistamines, topical doxepin, 1% hydrocortisone cream, or psoralen plus ultraviolet A (PUVA) therapy. Later, topical emollients help to lubricate sclerotic skin. A recent placebo-controlled study of therapeutic D-penicillamine versus low-dose D-penicillamine failed to show a difference in skin score or mortality rate. Considering the toxic side-effect profile, late onset of action, and lack of proven efficacy, enthusiasm for D-penicillamine treatment in scleroderma has greatly diminished.

Raynaud's Phenomenon

The most effective method of preventing RP is avoidance of cold exposure. Patients should wear warm protective clothing and avoid tobacco use. Long-acting calcium channel blockers (nifedipine, amlodipine, felodipine) are safe and effective vasodilators. Other vasodilators such as nitrates and prazosin are used alone or in combination with calcium channel blockers. One coated aspirin (81 mg daily) is recommended to inhibit platelet activation and occlusion. Intravenous prostaglandins (epoprostenol, iloprost), which reduce the severity of RP and may prevent digital ulceration, are effective when given acutely for critical digital ischemia. The endothelin receptor antagonist, bosentan, has also been shown to be effective as a rescue therapy. Newer more selective inhibitors are under development. Selective digital sympathectomy has been successful in cases that are not responsive to medical management. Oral antibiotics with good staphylococcal coverage are indicated if lesions become infected. Deeper soft tissue infections or osteomyelitis require treatment with intravenous antibiotics, debridement of devitalized tissue, and, if necessary, amputation.

Calcinosis

No therapies have been uniformly successful in treating this rare and often severe involvement of the affected skin. Colchicine (7- to 10-day course) may be useful in suppressing the local inflammation surrounding the areas of calcinosis. Anticoagulation with warfarin, bisphosphonates, and local drainage have been reported effective in series or pilot studies.

Gastrointestinal Disease

Esophageal dysfunction symptoms can be minimized with small, frequent meals, elevation of the head of the bed, and use of proton pump inhibitors. Patients with persistent symptoms require upper gastrointestinal endoscopy to exclude stricture and Barrett's metaplasia. Small bowel dysmotility symptoms can be managed by increasing dietary fiber, avoiding drugs that affect motility (narcotics), and administering empiric antibiotic therapy for bacterial overgrowth. Octreotide has been used as a small bowel prokinetic agent with variable results. In refractory disease, parenteral hyperalimentation may be needed to improve nutrition.

Pulmonary Hypertension

Conventional therapies such as vasodilators, diuretics, and anticoagulation are recommended. Epoprostenol (prostacyclin), administered by continuous intravenous or subcutaneous infusion, has been demonstrated to improve the clinical and hemodynamic measurements in patients with scleroderma. The endothelan-1 receptor inhibitor (bosentan) and sildenafil have been approved for treatment of pulmonary hypertension.

Interstitial Lung Disease

Patients with active alveolitis had improvement or stabilization in lung function when treated with oral or monthly intravenous cyclophosphamide for 12 to 18 months. The role for bronchoalveolar lavage to diagnose alveolitis is less clear. Resting or exertional hypoxia is an indication for supplemental oxygen. Patients with scleroderma who are recipients of lung transplantation experience similar rates of survival 2 years after the procedure as patients with idiopathic pulmonary fibrosis or idiopathic pulmonary hypertension. Lung transplantation may represent a therapeutic option for patients with end-stage lung disease due to scleroderma.

Renal Disease

SRC is a medical emergency. A rapid-acting angiotensin-converting enzyme (ACE) inhibitor should be titrated to normalize blood pressure promptly. Some patients may not respond and progress to renal failure requiring dialysis. Patients requiring dialysis for 12 to 18 months for SRC may recover renal function with continued ACE inhibitor therapy.

Cardiac Disease

The dual endothelin receptor antagonist, bosentan, diminishes the vasoconstrictive and profibrotic effects of endothelin. Reports have documented that bosentan decreases vascular resistance and reduces progression of sclerosis in patients treated for pulmonary hypertension. Increased myocardial perfusion and function have been demonstrated by magnetic resonance imaging and tissue Doppler echography during bosentan therapy.

Musculoskeletal Disease

Nonsteroidal anti-inflammatory drugs may help associated arthralgias. A regular exercise program can improve joint range of motion. Active myositis is treated with methotrexate, azathioprine, or other immunosuppressive agents. Corticosteroid therapy should be avoided, or used in low dose if required, because of the increased the risk for SRC.

Avoiding Treatment Errors

The increased risk for SRC in patients given high-dose steroids cannot be overemphasized. Patient evaluation must exclude scleroderma or scleroderma overlap before committing to prednisone dosing. When it is essential to treat with steroids, particularly during the edematous phase, the lowest dose that effectively controls symptoms, preferably less than 20 mg of prednisone daily, is prescribed. To reduce the risk for SRC, treatment with ACE inhibitors is essential provided the patient can tolerate these agents.

Future Directions

There are no proven effective therapies for systemic scleroderma. There have been few randomized controlled trials (RCTs) in pulmonary fibrosis in SSc. A recently published RCT investigated the effects of intravenous cyclophosphamide followed by azathioprine treatment in pulmonary fibrosis in SSc. Primary outcome measures were change in percentage of predicted forced vital capacity and change in single-breath diffusing capacity for carbon monoxide. Secondary outcome measures included changes in appearance on high-resolution computed tomography and dyspnea scores. The trial did not demonstrate significant improvement in the primary or secondary end points. Recent trials of methotrexate and cyclosporine have not shown convincing efficacy. A large multicenter trial of relaxin (an insulin-like protein secreted by the corpus luteum during pregnancy that decreases collagen synthesis by fibroblasts) did not demonstrate improvement in skin score. New therapies under investigation include an oral endothelin-1 inhibitor (bosentan), subcutaneous infusion of prostacyclin, and intravenous interferon-γ infusion. Distinctive fibrotic features and data from translational research consistently place transforming growth factor-β (TGF-β) as a central mediator in SSc. A pilot study of a systemic anti–TGF-β1 drug, CAT-192, showed no evidence of efficacy. Interleukin-4 and interleukin-13 are other fibrotic mediators produced during immune activation that might be targeted for SSc therapy, and therapeutics targeting these interleukins are also being developed. Immune dysregulation, leading to overproduction of these or other fibrotic mediators, might respond to currently available immunosuppressive agents, including mycophenolate mofetil, cyclosporine, tacrolimus, or sirolimus, alone or in combination.

Additional Resources

Poormoghim H, Lucas M, Fertig N, Medsger TA Jr: Systemic sclerosis sine scleroderma: Demographic, clinical, and serologic features and survival in forty-eight patients. Arthritis Rheum 43:444-451, 2000.

This helpful article addresses the subset of patients with visceral involvement and no skin disease.

Yu BD, Eisen AZ: Scleroderma. In Freedberg IM, Eisen AZ, Wolff K, et al (eds): Fitzpatrick's Dermatology in General Medicine, 6th ed. New York, McGraw-Hill Medical, 2003.

This chapter includes a useful general review of the skin findings of scleroderma.

EVIDENCE

1. American College of Rheumatology. Available at: http://www.rheumatology.org. Accessed March 2, 2007.

   This website includes a geographic directory of rheumatologists, patient information, and additional links.

2. Arthritis Foundation. Available at: http://www.arthritis.org. Accessed March 21, 2007.

   This website is an excellent source for patient educational materials and information on local resources.

3. Clements PJ, Roth MD, Elashoff R, Tashkin DP, et al: Scleroderma Lung Study (SLS): Differences in the presentation and course of patients with limited versus diffuse systemic sclerosis. Ann Rheum Dis May 7, 2007 [Epub ahead of print].

   This article provides a current update of the subgroups of scleroderma.

4. Ioannidis JP, Vlachoyiannopoulus PG, Haidich AB, et al: Mortality in systemic sclerosis: An international metaanalysis of individual patient data. Am J Med 118:2-10, 2005.

   The authors provide an excellent review of recent mortality risks.

5. National Institute of Arthritis and Musculoskeletal and Skin Diseases. Available at: http://www.niams.nih.gov. Accessed March 20, 2007.

   This site provides timely and up-to-date information on available clinical trials and current research efforts in scleroderma.

6. Sanchez-Guerrero J, Colditz GA, Karlson EW, et al: Silicone breast implants and the risk of connective-tissue diseases and symptoms. N Engl J Med 332:1666-1670, 1995.

   This is a timely review of the topic given the recent approval for new devices by the FDA.

Beth L. Jonas ▪ Robert A.S. Roubey

Spondyloarthropathies

Introduction

The spondyloarthropathies are a group of systemic inflammatory disorders with similar musculoskeletal findings, extra-articular manifestations, and immunogenetic associations. The major conditions and syndromes are ankylosing spondylitis (AS), reactive arthritis (formerly Reiter's syndrome), enteropathic arthritis, psoriatic arthritis, and juvenile spondyloarthropathy. Although these diagnostic entities are useful and important, it may be more useful to regard the spondyloarthropathies not so much as a group of four or five distinct entities, but as arthropathies characterized by combinations of findings, including sacroiliitis, with or without spondylitis; peripheral inflammatory arthritis, which is often asymmetrical and affects the lower limbs predominantly; enthesopathy, especially at the heels and around the pelvis; certain extra-articular features, including iritis, and some mucocutaneous lesions; absence of rheumatoid factor; and familial aggregation and increased prevalence of human leukocyte antigen (HLA)-B27.

Etiology and Pathogenesis

Most of the spondyloarthropathies are associated with inheritance of the HLA-B27 histocompatibility antigen (Table 155-1). HLA-B27 is particularly associated with spondylitis, sacroiliitis, and eye involvement. Epidemiologic data and transgenic animal models support the role of HLA-B27 in disease pathogenesis. HLA-B27 diseases are closely associated with intestinal bacteria or inflammation. Reactive arthritis is associated with *Yersinia*, *Salmonella*, *Shigella*, and *Campylobacter* species gastrointestinal infections, as well as with *Chlamydia* species genitourinary infection. Although intact organisms are not present in inflamed joints, bacterial antigens have been identified in affected synovium. In inflammatory bowel disease, increased intestinal permeability and exposure to normal intestinal flora may play a role in the development of enteropathic arthritis. Microscopic, and usually asymptomatic, gastrointestinal inflammation is present in patients with AS and infection-associated reactive arthritis.

Clinical Presentation

The musculoskeletal features that characterize the spondyloarthropathies as a group include inflammatory back pain, axial arthritis, and enthesopathy.

Inflammatory back pain and axial arthritis are characterized by an insidious onset, radiation of pain to the buttocks and thighs that sometimes alternates from side to side, prominent stiffness, and relief with activity rather than rest. Initially, pain is worse in the low back, but later it may involve the thoracic and cervical areas, sometimes with pain around the thoracic cage. In established disease, there may be loss of normal lumbar lordosis, restriction of lumbar movements in all directions, restriction of chest expansion, and sacroiliac joint and sternal tenderness.

Enthesopathy is inflammation at the site of ligamentous attachments to bone (the enthesis). In spondyloarthropathy, enthesopathy commonly causes plantar fasciitis, Achilles tendonitis, and pain at other sites, including the attachment of the thigh adductors at the pelvis, intercostal muscle insertions, ischial tuberosities, and pelvic brim.

Ankylosing Spondylitis

AS usually presents with inflammatory back pain and stiffness in a young adult, although 20% of patients present with peripheral joint involvement, and more than 50% have joints other than the spine affected at some stage. The disease is 3 times more common in males than females (Figs. 155-1 and 155-2). Enthesopathy is a common association, as previously described.

Table 155-1 HLA-B27 Frequency in Spondyloarthropathies

Disorder	HLA-B27 frequency
Ankylosing spondylitis	90%
With uveitis or aortitis	Nearly 100%
Reactive arthritis	50%-80%
With sacroiliitis or uveitis	90%
Juvenile spondyloarthropathy	80%
Inflammatory bowel disease	Not increased
With peripheral arthritis	Not increased
With spondylitis	50%
Psoriasis	Not increased
With peripheral arthritis	Not increased
With spondylitis	50%
Unaffected whites	6%-8%

Iritis (uveitis) occurs in 25% to 30% and may present with severe throbbing pain, usually unilateral, associated with lacrimation, photophobia, and blurring of vision (see Fig. 155-2). Cardiac involvement occurs in 1% to 4% and includes aortic insufficiency, conduction defects, and pericarditis (see Fig. 155-2). HLA-B27 is present in 90% of patients (nearly 100% of patients with uveitis or aortitis).

Reactive Arthritis

Nonseptic arthritis and often sacroiliitis develop after an acute infection with certain venereal or dysenteric organisms (Fig. 155-3). HLA-B27 is positive in 60% to 80% of cases. Onset is usually abrupt, with urethritis or diarrhea, and conjunctivitis, followed 1 to 3 weeks later by arthritis. The knees and ankles are usually affected, but radiologic sacroiliitis occurs in about 20% to 40% of cases, and a small subset of patients develop a condition indistinguishable from AS.

Mucocutaneous lesions, including keratoderma blennorrhagicum and circinate balanitis, may occur. Cardiac disease develops in 5% to 10% of cases.

Psoriatic Arthritis

Some form of psoriatic arthropathy develops in about 5% of patients with psoriasis. There are several patterns of arthritis.

Monoarticular or oligoarticular disease is the most common (70% to 80%). The distribution is asymmetrical, affecting a large joint, such as the knees, and a few scattered distal interphalangeal joints, proximal interphalangeal joints, and metacarpophalangeal joints. There may be diffuse swelling of one or more involved fingers and toes (sausage digits).

Some patients present with a symmetrical polyarthritis that may resemble rheumatoid arthritis. Arthritis mutilans, a particularly aggressive form of the disease with osteolysis of affected joints, occurs in about 5% of patients with psoriatic arthritis.

Spondyloarthropathy occurs in about 10% of patients. Sacroiliitis may be less symmetrical than AS, and unilateral spinal changes may be seen. HLA-B27 is present in about 60% of patients with spondylitis. It is not associated with psoriasis or with peripheral psoriatic arthritis (Fig. 155-4).

Enteropathic Arthritis

Both peripheral and axial involvement can occur in patients with inflammatory bowel disease (ulcerative colitis and Crohn's disease). Peripheral arthritis occurs in 10% to 20% of patients. Joint disease may precede the onset of bowel symptoms and the diagnosis of inflammatory bowel disease, particularly in Crohn's disease. Arthritis may be acute and migratory. Knees, ankles, and feet are most frequently affected.

Spondylitis and sacroiliitis occur in about 10% of patients with inflammatory bowel disease. They may resemble AS and are occasionally asymptomatic.

HLA-B27 is present in 50% of inflammatory bowel disease patients with axial joint disease, but not frequently in patients with peripheral joint disease.

Juvenile Spondyloarthropathy

A subgroup of patients with juvenile-onset arthritis present with pauciarticular onset, often later than other forms. The age of onset is in the early teens, affecting boys more than girls. Hips, knees, and ankles are affected. Acute iritis is common, and HLA-B27 is usually positive. An arthropathy indistinguishable from AS develops in about half of these patients in young adult life.

Differential Diagnosis
Spondylitis and Sacroiliitis

Mechanical low back pain may be difficult to differentiate. Features suggestive of inflammatory back pain and the spondyloarthropathies include an insidious onset, younger age, pain lasting longer than 3 months, and improvement with exercise. Lumbosacral disk disease may have similar clinical characteristics; however, neurologic signs of nerve root compression are uncommon in the spondyloarthropathies. Osteoarthritis occurs in older patients and can usually be differentiated radiographically.

Diffuse idiopathic skeletal hyperostosis occurs in older patients and may involve all levels of the spine. This disease is characterized by large spurs and ossification along the anterolateral aspect of multiple contiguous vertebrae.

Peripheral Arthritis

Acute monoarthritis should be differentiated from septic arthritis, gout, or pseudogout by synovial fluid examina-

Figure 155-1 Ankylosing Spondylitis.

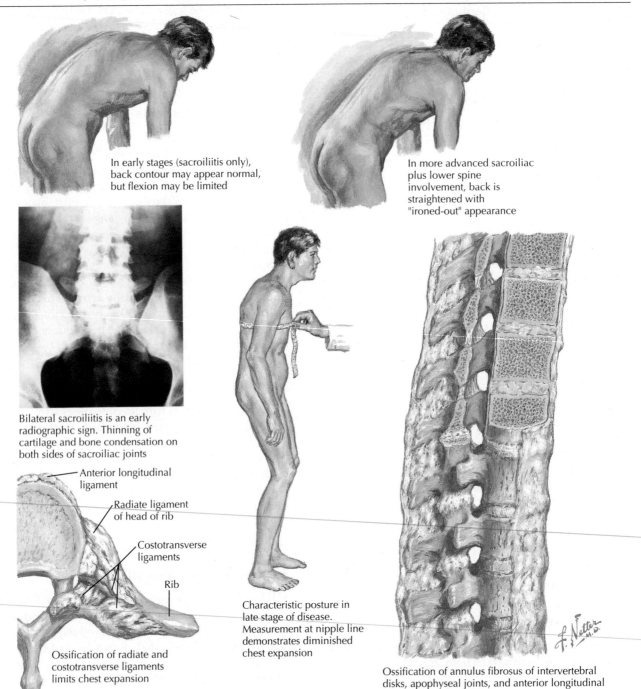

In early stages (sacroiliitis only), back contour may appear normal, but flexion may be limited

In more advanced sacroiliac plus lower spine involvement, back is straightened with "ironed-out" appearance

Bilateral sacroiliitis is an early radiographic sign. Thinning of cartilage and bone condensation on both sides of sacroiliac joints

Anterior longitudinal ligament

Radiate ligament of head of rib

Costotransverse ligaments

Rib

Ossification of radiate and costotransverse ligaments limits chest expansion

Characteristic posture in late stage of disease. Measurement at nipple line demonstrates diminished chest expansion

Ossification of annulus fibrosus of intervertebral disks, apophyseal joints, and anterior longitudinal and interspinal ligaments

tion. Psoriatic arthritis resembling rheumatoid arthritis may be differentiated by distal and asymmetrical interphalangeal joint involvement, the absence of rheumatoid factor, and the presence of psoriatic skin and nail lesions.

Distinguishing between different types of spondyloarthropathy may be difficult, especially early in the course of the disease. For example, spondylitis preceding the development of inflammatory bowel disease may be indistinguishable from AS. Cutaneous lesions of reactive arthritis may be indistinguishable from pustular psoriasis. The presence of other extra-articular manifestations of reactive arthritis is helpful.

Diagnostic Approach

The diagnosis of the spondyloarthropathies is largely based on the history, physical examination, and radiography. Laboratory tests rarely confirm or refute the diagnosis.

Figure 155-2 Ankylosing Spondylitis.

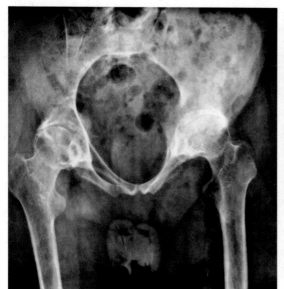

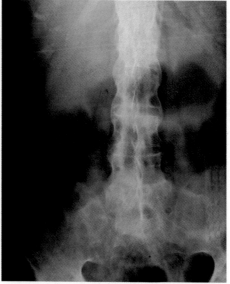

Radiograph shows complete bony ankylosis of both sacroiliac joints in late stage of disease

"Bamboo spine." Bony ankylosis of joints of lumbar spine. Ossification exaggerates bulges of intervertebral disks

Complications

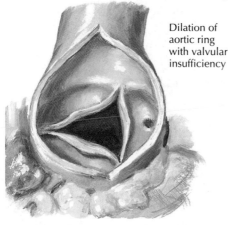

Dilation of aortic ring with valvular insufficiency

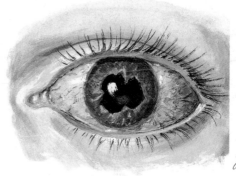

Iridocyclitis with irregular pupil due to synechiae

The patient's history is critical. Characteristic features include inflammatory back pain in younger patients, asymmetrical peripheral arthritis, pain at one or more entheses, extra-articular features or precipitation of the arthritis by enteric or sexually acquired infection, and a positive family history.

The physical examination may not demonstrate obvious physical signs of spondylitis in early or mild disease. Forward flexion can be measured by the Schober test, in which the examiner marks 2 points on the patient's back, one at the lumbosacral junction (sacral dimples) and one 10 cm above. Forward flexion in normal individuals increases the distance between the 2 points by at least 5 cm. Any loss of lumbar lordosis should be noted. Costovertebral involvement is manifested by decreased chest expansion (<5 cm chest expansion on inspiration, measured at the nipple line). However, these signs frequently do not become positive until there has been significant damage. Tenderness over the sacroiliac joints and other signs of sacroiliitis such as pelvic compression and the Gaenslen sign (pain on involved side hip hyperextension with the opposite hip in flexion) may be helpful, but are not uniformly reliable. Enthesitis at one or more sites (e.g., plantar fasciitis, Achilles tendonitis, epicondylitis) may be present. A thorough search for extra-articular manifestations is especially important, including examination of the skin, nails, genitalia, heart, and eyes.

Radiographic studies may demonstrate syndesmophytes as evidence of sacroiliitis or spondylitis. Periostitis and new bone formation may occur at sites of enthesitis or around affected joints. Radiographic features of psoriatic arthritis include asymmetrical erosions of interphalangeal joints,

Figure 155-3 Reactive Arthritis.

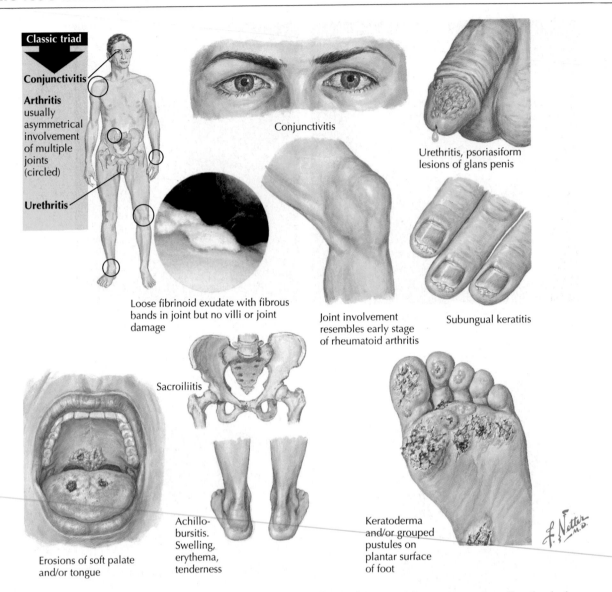

Classic triad

Conjunctivitis

Arthritis usually asymmetrical involvement of multiple joints (circled)

Urethritis

Conjunctivitis

Urethritis, psoriasiform lesions of glans penis

Loose fibrinoid exudate with fibrous bands in joint but no villi or joint damage

Joint involvement resembles early stage of rheumatoid arthritis

Subungual keratitis

Sacroiliitis

Erosions of soft palate and/or tongue

Achillobursitis. Swelling, erythema, tenderness

Keratoderma and/or grouped pustules on plantar surface of foot

including the distal interphalangeal joints, and pencil-in-cup appearance of the distal interphalangeal joints (see Fig. 155-4). Synovial fluid analysis is nonspecific but useful in excluding infection and crystal-induced arthritis. Tests for rheumatoid factor and antinuclear antibodies are characteristically negative. HLA-B27 testing is generally not necessary, but in selected cases, it may be useful in decreasing the uncertainty of the diagnosis. The test does not help distinguish between AS and other spondyloarthropathies. In reactive arthritis, identification of persistent pathogens by urethral and stool culture or polymerase chain reaction (e.g., *Chlamydia*) is recommended.

Management and Therapy

Optimum Treatment

It is important to identify the active elements in the disease (spondylitis, peripheral arthritis, enthesopathy) because their relative activity and severity affect both the treatment and prognosis. The management of the spondyloarthropathies has advanced considerably over the past decade. The primary goals of therapy are to limit joint damage and to maintain functional status. Management has two main components: drugs to control pain and stiffness and to limit joint damage and physical therapy to prevent range-of-motion limitation and to maintain muscle power.

The diagnosis and prognosis should be discussed with the patient, stressing the importance of early and appropriately aggressive therapy. For most patients, there is effective, but noncurative, treatment, but the long-term prognosis is generally fairly good.

Nonsteroidal anti-inflammatory drugs (NSAIDs) are important in controlling symptoms of spondylitis and peripheral arthritis. Indomethacin (25 to 50 mg 3 to 4 times daily) is usually effective. The extended-release

Figure 155-4 Psoriatic Arthritis.

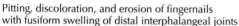

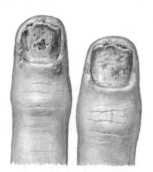

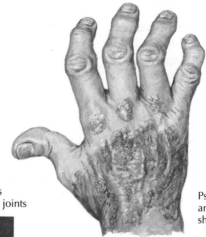

Pitting, discoloration, and erosion of fingernails with fusiform swelling of distal interphalangeal joints

Psoriatic patches on dorsum of hand with swelling and distortion of many interphalangeal joints and shortening of fingers due to loss of bone mass

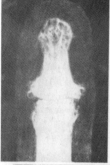
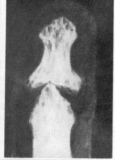

Radiographic changes in distal interphalangeal joint. Left: in early stages, bone erosions seen at joint margins. Right: in late stages, further loss of bone mass produces "pencil point in cup" appearance

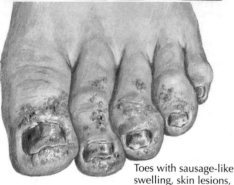

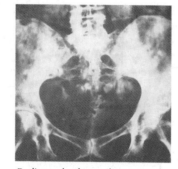

Toes with sausage-like swelling, skin lesions, and nail changes

Radiograph of sacroiliac joints shows thin cartilage with irregular surface and condensation of adjacent bone in sacrum and ilia

capsule or a nighttime suppository may be given to counter early morning stiffness. Several agents may be tried to find the best tolerated drug.

Sulfasalazine is effective in treatment of the peripheral arthritis of spondyloarthropathy. Side effects include nausea, rash, reversible reduction in sperm count, and rarely, agranulocytosis. Regular hematologic monitoring is required, at least in the early stages. Despite side effects, if NSAIDs have failed, sulfasalazine is a useful drug (2 to 3 g daily in divided doses). Intra-articular corticosteroid injections are useful for selected peripheral joints. Systemic corticosteroids are not indicated.

Methotrexate is an effective treatment for the skin and joint manifestations of psoriasis. Typically, therapy is initiated with a single weekly oral dosage of 10 mg. The weekly dosage may be gradually increased in 2.5- or 5.0-mg incre-

ments to 25 mg per week. Methotrexate may also be useful in other forms of spondyloarthropathy when peripheral joint disease predominates. The axial joint disease is usually not responsive to methotrexate.

Antibiotics should be given to patients with proven *Chlamydia* urethritis. A number of studies also suggest that antibiotics may decrease the duration of disease in patients with *Chlamydia*-induced reactive arthritis. The use of antibiotics in postdysenteric reactive arthritis is controversial.

Inhibition of tumor necrosis factor-α (TNF-α) is useful in patients not responsive to other agents. All three TNF-α inhibitors (etanercept, infliximab, and adalimumab) have demonstrated effectiveness in controlling symptoms of disease activity in AS and psoriatic arthritis. In addition, the TNF inhibitors slow the progression of joint damage in psoriatic disease.

In axial disease, the major aims of early therapy are to relieve pain and stiffness and to maintain normal posture and mobility. The inflamed painful spine may feel more comfortable in the flexed position, but fusion in this position can be functionally disastrous. Physical therapy aims to reduce rigidity and ensure that, if ankylosis does occur, the spine is in a nonflexed position. Regular supervision is usually required, and participation in classes may be helpful. Various modalities, including ultrasound, may be helpful in relieving pain due to enthesopathy.

Appropriate orthotic devices may be helpful (e.g., insoles for plantar fasciitis). Uveitis, cardiac, pulmonary, and severe cutaneous involvement should be assessed by appropriate specialists.

Avoiding Treatment Errors

The diagnosis of an active seronegative spondyloarthropathy should be confirmed. If the diagnosis is in question, or if biologic therapy is considered, a consultation with a rheumatologist should be sought. Careful workup to assess the activity of the disease before instituting disease-modifying antirheumatic drug (DMARD) therapy is essential. Periodic evaluation of the patient to determine efficacy and to assess for drug toxicity is also important. Early involvement of other health care providers such as physical therapists, occupational therapists, and psychologists can help the patient manage chronic illness and decrease long-term morbidity.

Future Directions

Ongoing investigations in the seronegative spondyloarthropathies include studies of the pathophysiology of the diseases, specifically with respect to the role of pathogenic bacteria; the immunogenetics of the diseases; and the role of the new biologic response modifiers in the treatment of severe disease.

Additional Resources

The Arthritis Foundation. Available at: http://www.arthritis.org.
  This website contains extensive information about all kinds of arthritis and has excellent resources for patients.
Furst DE, Breedveld FC, Kalden JR, et al: Updated consensus statement on biological agents for the treatment of rheumatic diseases, 2006. Ann Rheum Dis 65:2-15, 2006.
  This consensus document is based on a meeting of 143 rheumatologists and scientists and reviews the indications, efficacy, and safety of the biologic agents for all the rheumatic diseases. It includes a section on recommendations for future research.

EVIDENCE

1. Khan A (ed): Ankylosing spondylitis: Burden of the illness, diagnosis and effective treatment. J Rheum Suppl 78:1-31, 2006.
   This very practical journal supplement includes three papers: one on epidemiology of the disease, one on diagnosis, and one on treatment.
2. Mease P: Current treatment for psoriatic arthritis and other spondyloarthritides. Rheum Dis Clin North Am 32(Suppl 1):11-20, 2006.
   This comprehensive review of psoriatic arthritis includes disease features, immunopathology, classification, outcome measures, and treatment.
3. Smith JA, Marker-Herman E, Colbert RA: Pathogenesis of ankylosing spondylitis: Current concepts. Best Pract Res Clin Rheumatol 20(3):571-591, 2006.
   This excellent review of the current knowledge of the pathogenesis of ankylosing spondylitis includes the importance of HLA-B27, the innate immune system, and the role of inflammation of the gut.

Toby Bates ▪ Teresa K. Tarrant

Polymyositis and Dermatomyositis

Introduction

Polymyositis (PM) and dermatomyositis (DM) are idiopathic inflammatory myopathies. Both diseases may present with an insidious onset of proximal symmetric muscle weakness. Extramuscular disease may manifest as cardiac, gastrointestinal, pulmonary, cutaneous, or arthritic symptoms. PM and DM can occur in association with other autoimmune diseases and malignancies.

The true incidence of these diseases is difficult to ascertain because of their rarity. The estimated annual incidence is 2.18 to 7.7 cases per million per year with a bimodal age distribution. The onset in children occurs between 10 and 15 years of age and in adults between 45 and 60 years of age. DM is more common than PM, particularly in children. As with most autoimmune diseases, women are affected disproportionately (2 : 1 female-to-male ratio), and there appears to be an increased incidence in African Americans compared with whites. An overall increase in incidence has been suggested; however, improved diagnostic criteria and elevated awareness may account for this trend.

Etiology and Pathogenesis

The etiology and pathogenesis of PM and DM remain unclear. Reports of idiopathic inflammatory muscle disease in multiple members of a single family and in monozygotic twins implicate a possible genetic predisposition. Correlations have been observed with human leukocyte antigen (HLA)-DRB1*0301 in whites with PM and with HLA-DQA1*0501 in juvenile DM. Myositis-specific antibodies unique to these diseases have been identified; however, whether these antibodies play a pathogenic role remains unclear. Three groups of myositis-specific antibodies have been well studied, and clinical profiles have been described for each group (Table 156-1).

Although PM and DM have similar presentations, the immunologic process of the underlying disease pathogenesis appears quite different. DM results in microangiopathy, destruction of endomysial capillaries, and muscle ischemia from humoral-mediated injury. B cells predominate in the inflammatory perivascular infiltrate, and immunoglobulins and complement split products are deposited in the blood vessels. In contrast, the inflammation of PM occurs through a cell-mediated mechanism. Muscles expressing major histocompatibility complex (MHC) class I are infiltrated with CD8+ cytotoxic cells.

Inflammatory myopathies can occur as a part of a heterogeneous connective tissue diseases complex with overlapping features of scleroderma, systemic lupus erythematosus (SLE), mixed connective tissue disease, or Sjögren's syndrome. Less commonly, PM and DM are seen in association with rheumatoid arthritis, adult-onset Still's disease, or Wegener's granulomatosis. Muscle weakness is often a prominent symptom in these overlap syndromes.

The risk for malignancy is increased in both PM and DM, but DM has a greater relative risk. Prototypic malignancies associated with these inflammatory myopathies are ovarian, breast, stomach, colon, and non-Hodgkin's lymphoma, although any neoplasm is possible. The risk for malignancy is highest within the first year of the diagnosis and then decreases but never reaches that of the normal population.

Clinical Presentation

PM and DM are defined by the insidious onset of symmetrical proximal muscle weakness over weeks to months,

Table 156-1 Myositis Specific Antibodies

Autoantibody	Clinical Manifestations	Treatment Outcomes
Anti–aminoacyl tRNA synthetase (Anti–Jo-1 most common)	Increased risk for interstitial lung disease. *Antisynthetase syndrome:* fever, arthritis, interstitial lung diseases, Raynaud's phenomenon, and mechanic hands	Variable
Anti–Mi-2 Anti–signal recognition particle (SRP)	Acute onset of dermatomyositis often with shawl sign Polymyositis Acute severe illness Possible association with necrotizing myositis	Good Poor

Table 156-2 Cutaneous Manifestations of Dermatomyositis

Cutaneous Manifestation	Description
Gottron's papules	Pathognomonic for DM. Flat or raised, violaceous to dusky red papules on dorsal aspect of MCP, PIP joints. Can occur over wrist, elbows, knees, and malleoli. SLE differs in that the rash occurs between MCP and PIP joints (see Fig. 156-2)
Heliotrope rash	Highly characteristic of DM. Lilac/purple colored rash often periorbital with edema. Can involve chin, forehead and malar region. Unlike SLE does not spare nasolabial folds (see Fig. 156-2)
V sign	Less specific. Violaceous, erythematous, and confluent macular lesions of the neck and anterior chest
Shawl sign	Less specific. Violaceous, erythematous macular lesions involving the nape of the neck, upper back, and posterior shoulders
Holster sign	Less specific. Violaceous, erythematous macular lesions over the lateral aspects of the thighs
Mechanic hands	Hyperkeratosis, scaling and fissuring of the lateral portion of the fingers and palms. This can be associated with antisynthetase syndrome
Calcifications	Subcutaneous, fascial, and intramuscular. Predominately seen in juvenile DM. Can be extensive, debilitating, and independent of inflammatory muscle involvement
Nail-fold telangiectasias, periungual erythema, and cuticular overgrowth	Nonspecific findings seen in both DM and PM, as well as other connective tissue disorders

DIP, distal interphalangeal; DM, dermatomyositis; MCP, metacarpophalangeal; PIP, proximal interphalangeal; PM, polymyositis; SLE, systemic lupus erythematosus.

which often delays patients from seeking medical attention and thus a definitive diagnosis. Classically, painless muscle weakness is the hallmark of disease; however, myalgia accompanies weakness in up to 30% of cases.

Patients may complain of difficulty getting up from a chair or toilet on their own or without the use of their hands (Fig. 156-1). Proximal lower extremity weakness results in an unsteady, waddling gait. Stairs and steps become a challenge, especially if there is no handrail available. Involvement of the shoulder girdle causes weakness that manifests as complaints of trouble shampooing and combing hair (see Fig. 156-1). The central muscles of the trunk and neck can be involved, making it difficult to rise from a supine position or raise the head from the pillow. Over time, patients may develop distal muscle weakness, but facial and ocular involvement is extremely rare.

As the name implies, the differentiating clinical feature of DM from PM is cutaneous involvement (Table 156-2; Fig. 156-2), which can precede, develop simultaneously, or occur after muscle manifestations. The rashes are often photosensitive. A minority of patients develop classic skin findings without muscle involvement, referred to as *amyopathic dermatomyositis* or *dermatomyositis sine myositis*.

PM and DM are systemic diseases and can involve multiple organ systems. The prevalence rate of interstitial lung disease varies widely from 5% to 65% and can occur at any time in the course of the disease. Symptoms range from asymptomatic (27%) or dry cough to frank dyspnea. Having anti–histidyl-tRNA synthetase antibodies (anti–Jo-1) is associated with an increased risk for interstitial lung disease. However, dyspnea in inflammatory muscle disease may not always be interstitial lung disease and can result from weakness of the thoracic muscles or chronic aspiration from esophageal dysfunction.

Cardiac involvement typically manifests as asymptomatic electrocardiogram changes in up to 50% of cases. Significant arrhythmias, myocarditis, and congestive heart failure are rare.

Dysphagia occurs in up to one third of cases. This is either from weakness of the oropharyngeal muscles or from involvement of the striated muscles of the upper one third of the esophagus. Aspiration pneumonia, nasal regur-

Figure 156-1 Signs of Inflammatory Myopathies.

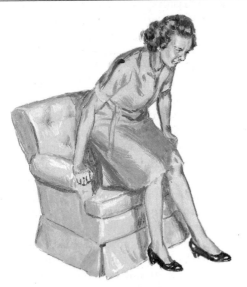

Difficulty in arising from chair, often early complaint

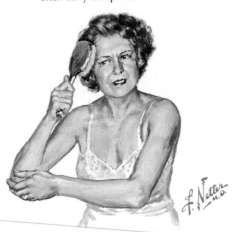

Difficulty in raising arm to brush hair

Figure 156-2 Classic Cutaneous Findings of Dermatomyositis.

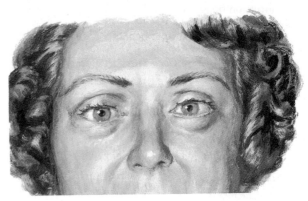

Edema and heliotrope discoloration around eyes are a classic sign. More widespread erythematous rash may also be present

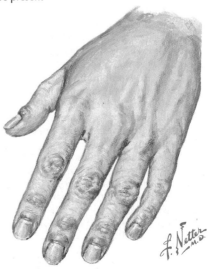

Erythema and/or scaly, papular eruption around fingernails and on dorsum of interphalangeal joints

gitation, and dysphonia can result from oropharyngeal or esophageal muscle weakness. Although rare in adults, gastrointestinal bleeding can occur in juvenile dermatomyositis secondary to vasculitic lesions.

A non-deforming, rheumatoid-like arthritis may occur, which is typically mild. In contrast, anti–Jo-1–positive patients and those with antisynthetase syndrome may have a destructive arthritis involving the hands. The term *floppy thumb* describes the destruction of the first interphalangeal joint in these patients.

Differential Diagnosis

Patients presenting with muscle weakness require a complete history and physical examination. PM and DM are rare diseases, and thus one must look for findings indica-

tive of other etiologies (Box 156-1). Differentiating PM from inclusion body myositis clinically may be difficult (Table 156-3), which is why muscle biopsy is usually recommended for a definitive diagnosis.

Diagnostic Approach

PM and DM can overlap with other connective tissue diseases, especially scleroderma and SLE, so an extensive review of systems is essential. All medications need to be examined as potential causes of weakness (see Box 156-1). Documentation of activities that cannot be performed is useful. For instance, testing proximal lower extremity strength by having a patient rise from a seated position without the use of the arms or having the patient squat and

Box 156-1 Differential Diagnosis of Muscle Weakness

1. Inclusion body myositis
2. Infection
   a. Viral—influenza A, B; hepatitis B, HIV, Coxsackie virus, mononucleosis
   b. Bacterial—*Staphylococcus, Streptococcus*
   c. Parasite—*Trichinella, Toxoplasma*
3. Endocrine
   a. Hypothyroid, hyperthyroid
   b. Hyperthyroid, hypoparathyroid
   c. Hypokalemia, hypocalcemia
4. Medications: partial list
   a. Hydroxymethyl glutaryl–coenzyme A reductase inhibitors (statins)
   b. Corticosteroids
   c. Colchicine
   d. Hydroxychloroquine
   e. Cimetidine
   f. Ethanol, cocaine, heroin
   g. Zidovudine
   h. Fibric acid derivatives
5. Genetic muscular dystrophies:
   a. Limb-girdle muscular dystrophy
   b. Duchenne's, Becker's
   c. Facioscapulohumeral
6. Glycogen storage myopathies: adult-onset acid maltase deficiency, McArdle's disease
7. Lipid storage myopathies: carnitine deficiency, palmityltransferase deficiency
8. Neurology
   a. Myasthenia gravis
   b. Amyotrophic lateral sclerosis
   c. Chronic inflammatory demyelinating polyneuropathy (CIPD)
9. Amyloidosis
10. Acute myopathy of intensive care

stand will clearly define the patient's strength and provides an easy way of measuring response to treatment.

Initial laboratory work should consist of a complete blood count with differential, chemistries and electrolytes, liver function tests, creatine kinase (CK), aldolase, erythrocyte sedimentation rate (ESR), thyroid-stimulating hormone, antinuclear antibody (ANA), and serum protein electrophoresis. The most sensitive muscle enzyme is CK, which is elevated before detectable weakness and should normalize before a discernable response to therapy. Elevations of aldolase, aspartate, and alanine aminotransferases can also be observed, and these typically are markers of muscle breakdown. Commonly, but not always, there are increases in markers of inflammation (ESR, C-reactive protein). ANA can be found in up to 80% of patients.

Electromyography (EMG) is a sensitive, yet nonspecific, test for inflammatory muscle disease. Infections and metabolic disorders can have similar EMG findings as DM and PM. Because not all muscles are necessarily involved, several sites should be evaluated, particularly because EMG is useful for guiding the location for biopsy. Typical findings on EMG are spontaneous fibrillations, needle insertion irritability, low-amplitude polyphasic motor units of short duration, and early recruitment. EMG is also useful during the interval management of these patients because it can differentiate between steroid myopathy (chronic steroids are used in the treatment of DM and PM) and persistently active inflammatory disease.

Because muscle enzymes and EMG findings can be abnormal in a variety of muscular disorders (see Table 156-3), a muscle biopsy is the gold standard for the diagnosis of both PM and DM. Traditionally, this has been

Table 156-3 Differentiating Characteristics of Polymyositis, Dermatomyositis, and Inclusion Body Myositis

	Polymyositis	Dermatomyositis	Inclusion Body Myositis
Age	>2nd decade	Any age (bimodal)	>50 years of age
Sex	Female-to-male ratio of 2 : 1	Female > male	Male > female
Muscle weakness	Symmetrical and proximal	Symmetrical and proximal	Asymmetrical, proximal, and distal. Muscle atrophy of quadriceps and finger flexors
ANA	Common	Common	Uncommon
Cutaneous	No	Yes	No
CK	≤50 times normal	≤50 times normal	Often ≤5 times normal
Anti-Jo-1 antibody	Up to 20%	Yes	No
Muscle biopsy	Cell mediated, CD8+, endomysial infiltrate	Humoral-mediated, CD4+ infiltrate, perivascular, and interfascicular Perifascicular atrophy	CD8+ infiltrate, vacuolated muscle fibers, intracellular amyloid deposits
Multiple organ system involvement?	Yes	Yes	No
Treatment	Responsive	Responsive	Often refractory

ANA, antinuclear antibody; CK, creatine kinase.

Figure 156-3 Treatment Paradigm for Polymyositis and Dermatomyositis.
IVIG, intravenous immunoglobulin; TNF, tumor necrosis factor.

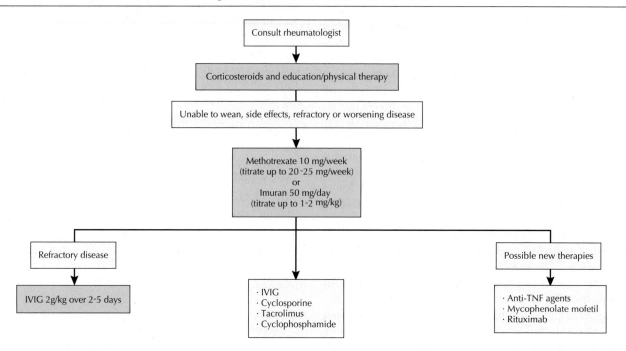

done as an open biopsy; however, percutaneous needle biopsies are now being performed because they are less invasive and multiple samples can be obtained to increase the sensitivity of the diagnosis. To rule out muscular dystrophies, glycogen and lipid storage diseases, the muscle biopsy requires immunohistochemical, biochemical, and genetic evaluation.

The muscle biopsy of PM will demonstrate scattered necrotic, regenerating fibers. Inflammation will be localized around individual muscle fibers, with a predominance of CD8+ cells. Class I major histocompatibility complex is not normally expressed on muscles. Further immunocytochemical staining and genetic testing are important because the pathology described in PM can be seen in muscular dystrophies and inclusion body myositis. DM, which is a humorally mediated process, will have perivascular and interfascicular inflammation with associated microinfarctions and perifascicular atrophy.

After a diagnosis of either DM or PM is made, it is important to evaluate for extramuscular involvement. A baseline chest radiographic examination and spirometry with diffusion capacity is a part of the initial workup for pulmonary involvement. High-resolution chest computed tomography or bronchoalveolar lavage may be indicated if symptoms or screening abnormalities suggest interstitial lung disease. Screening for anti–Jo-1 antibodies can predict the risk for developing interstitial lung disease because up to 70% of anti–Jo-1–positive patients develop this complication. Esophageal dysmotility is common, and thus one should have a low threshold for obtaining a barium swallow in the workup of dysphagia and dyspnea. Age-appropriate cancer screening should be performed given the association with malignancy.

Management and Therapy

Optimum Treatment

Corticosteroids are first-line therapy (Fig. 156-3). For severe disease, pulse intravenous steroids are given for 3 days at 1 g/day and then switched to oral steroids at 1 mg/kg/day. More commonly, oral steroids are initiated at 1 mg/kg/day. Titration of corticosteroids begins once the muscle exam and enzymes normalize, which may take several months. Currently, there are no clinical trials to guide the titration of corticosteroids, but consensus opinion recommends a taper of 20% every 3 to 4 weeks. Once the patient is weaned to 10 mg/day, this dose is continued for about 1 year. The American College of Rheumatology recommends the initiation of bisphosphonates for patients who will require corticosteroids for more than 3 months. When a patient has esophageal dysmotility, intravenous pamidronate is the bisphosphonate of choice. Early incorporation of physical therapy into the treatment regimen of patients with inflammatory myositis is essential.

A steroid-sparing agent can be added to the treatment regimen when corticosteroids are unable to be decreased or are incompletely effective. These agents are typically added early in disease to minimize the exposure and complications from high-dose corticosteroids. Azathioprine or methotrexate is most commonly used during active treatment or maintenance of remission. A prospective placebo-

controlled trial of the combination of azathioprine and corticosteroids found improved functional outcomes and ability to wean corticosteroids compared to placebo. A retrospective series found that 71% to 88% of patients with DM and PM improved with the addition of methotrexate to prednisone therapy. However, because of the idiosyncratic side effect of pulmonary involvement with methotrexate, azathioprine is preferred in patients with interstitial lung disease and in anti–Jo-1–positive patients.

Intravenous immunoglobulin (IVIG) is used in the setting of critically ill patients with pulmonary or cardiac disease. IVIG is also used as a second-line agent for patients refractory to prednisone, azathioprine, or methotrexate. In DM, a double-blind, placebo-controlled trial found improved muscle strength and functional status using IVIG compared with placebo.

Other immunosuppressive agents used in inflammatory muscle disease include cyclosporine, tacrolimus, and cyclophosphamide. The use of these medications is driven by failure to respond to the aforementioned medications, by the severity of disease, or by extramuscular involvement. Cyclosporine and tacrolimus have been shown to improve muscle strength and functional status. Both medications, in case series, appear beneficial for inflammatory myositis, associated interstitial lung disease, and antisynthetase syndrome. More recently, there are case series showing benefits of mycophenolate mofetil, tumor necrosis factor-α antagonists, rituximab, and leflunomide, but further controlled studies are needed to assess the efficacy of these medications.

Avoiding Treatment Errors

As with any disease, the diagnosis should be confirmed before initiating a treatment regimen. After treatment is started, monitoring for toxicity is essential. Most medications used in DM and PM result in significant immunosuppression and increase the risk for infection. Consequently, worsening symptoms such as weakness and dyspnea do not necessarily reflect disease activity. Specifically, prolonged steroid therapy can result in weakness secondary to a steroid myopathy. If this is not recognized, it may lead to an unnecessary exposure to further immunosuppression and toxicity. In another example, increased dyspnea could result from the known pulmonary manifestations of DM and PM but could also reflect secondary pulmonary infections or hypersensitivity pneumonitis from therapy (i.e., methotrexate).

Creatine kinase and aldolase, markers of muscle breakdown, are often used to monitor for disease activity in a stable patient. Often, there is a delay between the initial rise in these markers and the detectable onset of weakness. Although treatment should not be changed based on laboratory values alone, an increased vigilance by the patient and physician is indicated if this is observed.

Future Directions

In 2000, the International Myositis Outcome Assessment Collaboration Study (IMACS) group was created to help standardize trial design and outcome assessment. The group has defined measurements of disease activity for outcomes assessment, proposed a definition for clinical improvement, and proposed consensus guidelines for clinical trials in myositis. Several initiatives to determine the utility of newer medications are either enrolling or awaiting approval. These studies evaluate B-cell therapy in idiopathic myopathy, etanercept in adult DM, infliximab in DM and PM, methotrexate in PM and DM, and interleukin-1 receptor antagonists in chronic inflammatory myopathy. The results of these trials may broaden the treatment options significantly.

Additional Resources

American College of Rheumatology. Available at: http://www. rheumatology.org.
  This website offers information directed at patient education.
Klippel JH: Primer on the Rheumatic Diseases, 12th ed. Atlanta, Arthritis Foundation, 2001, pp 369-376.
  The author provides a basic overview of epidemiology, pathology, and clinical findings.

EVIDENCE

1. Briani C, Doria A, Sarzi-Puttini P, Dalakas MC: Update on idiopathic inflammatory myopathies. Autoimmunity 39(3):161-170, 2006.
    This in-depth review of inflammatory myopathies expands beyond discussion of DM and PM.
2. Choy EHS, Hoogendijk JE, Lecky B, Winer JB: Immunosuppressant and immunomodulatory treatment for dermatomyositis and polymyositis. The Cochrane Database of Systemic Reviews 2005, Issue 3. Art. No.: CD003643.pub2. DOI:10.1002/14651858. CD003643.pub2.
    This article provides a concise review of the available studies on the treatment of DM and PM.
3. Choy EHS, Isenberg DA: Treatment of dermatomyositis and polymyositis. Rheumatology 41:7-13, 2002.
    The authors provide a concise review and discussion of treatment options.
4. Christopher-Stine L, Plotz PH: Adult inflammatory myopathies. Best Pract Res Clin Rheumatol 18(3):331-344, 2004.
    This review of inflammatory myopathies includes a section on inclusion body myositis.
5. Dalakas MC, Illa I, Dambrosia JM, et al: A controlled trial of high-dose intravenous immunoglobulin infusions as treatment for dermatomyositis. N Engl J Med 329:1993-2000, 1993.
    This double-blind, placebo-controlled, crossover trial of 15 patients whose dermatomyositis was refractory to treatment investigates whether IVIG may be an important therapy for patients with severe disability.
6. Okada S, Weatherhead E, Targoff IN, et al: Global surface ultraviolet radiation intensity may modulate the clinical and immunologic expression of autoimmune muscle disease. Arthritis Rheum 48:2285-2293, 2003.
    The authors investigate whether geoclimatic factors may influence the nature and frequency of DM, PM, and associated autoantibodies around the world.

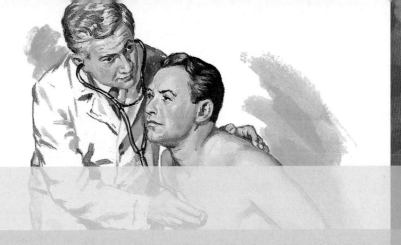

Ocular Diseases

Myopia and Common Refractive Disorders

Introduction

Ocular refractive disorders, or ametropias, are defined as aberrant focusing of entering light rays away from the optimal plane of the retinal macula. Ametropias include myopia, hyperopia, astigmatism, and presbyopia. These conditions represent a significant public health issue in the United States. A 1980 survey of vision correction in the United States estimates that more than half of the population older than 3 years have refractive errors corrected with spectacles or contact lenses. Myopia alone afflicts about 70 million Americans, with associated costs of up to $4.6 billion per year.

Etiology and Pathogenesis

In basic optical terms, the human visual system is made up of the cornea, crystalline lens, and ocular axial length. Each of these anatomic components must develop in precise balance to produce sharp optical focus on the retina.

Emmetropia (Fig. 157-1) is vision devoid of optical defects, and emmetropization is the developmental process of growth and integration of ocular components, which optimally leads to normal vision. Until age 3 years, cornea and lens curvatures (refractive powers) are adjusted through a poorly understood mechanism to correlate with changes in axial length. The result is that greater than 95% of eyes end up with a refraction close to emmetropia (between +4 and −4 diopters of refractive error).

Myopia (nearsightedness) (see Fig. 157-1) is the most common refractive error, with a prevalence of 80% of ametropias. In simple terms, myopia occurs when light from distant objects is focused anterior to the retina. The refractive power of the eye is too strong for its axial length. Myopia can be classified as simple juvenile onset, adult onset, and degenerative.

Simple myopia accounts for more than 85% of all myopia. It is estimated that 15% to 25% of the U.S. population has or will have juvenile-onset myopia. Typically, it begins after age 5 years with gradual increases in severity until around age 16 years, when 75% stabilize in prescription. Others may experience an increase in severity into their 20s and 30s. Increases of −.25 to −.75 per year are common, but higher rates are not unusual.

Generally, earlier onset of myopia leads to higher refractive error at maturity. There is evidence of gender difference; females tend to begin progression of myopia and stabilize 1 or 2 years before males. Controversy exists regarding the exact etiology of myopia (heredity versus use-abuse), but recent research has reinforced the theory that positive family history is the primary risk factor for developing myopia. Studies indicate that children of parents who both have myopia have a 30% to 40% prevalence of myopia, and when only one is afflicted, a 20% to 25% prevalence. If neither parent has myopia, there is a less than 10% chance of developing myopia. Research involving prediction of myopia indicates that at third-grade age, 60% of individuals with a cycloplegic refraction of +.5 (hyperopia) or less will become myopic by eighth grade.

Adult-onset myopia affects individuals in high near-point stress environments, such as graduate students, and usually begins around 20 years of age. The disorder has an unpredictable end point in terms of time and severity but usually ends in low to moderate myopia. It is possible for previously stable myopic individuals to experience an increase in myopia years later in times of increased near-point activity. It has been hypothesized that a new process

Figure 157-1 Myopia and Other Refractive Errors.
IOL, intraocular lens.

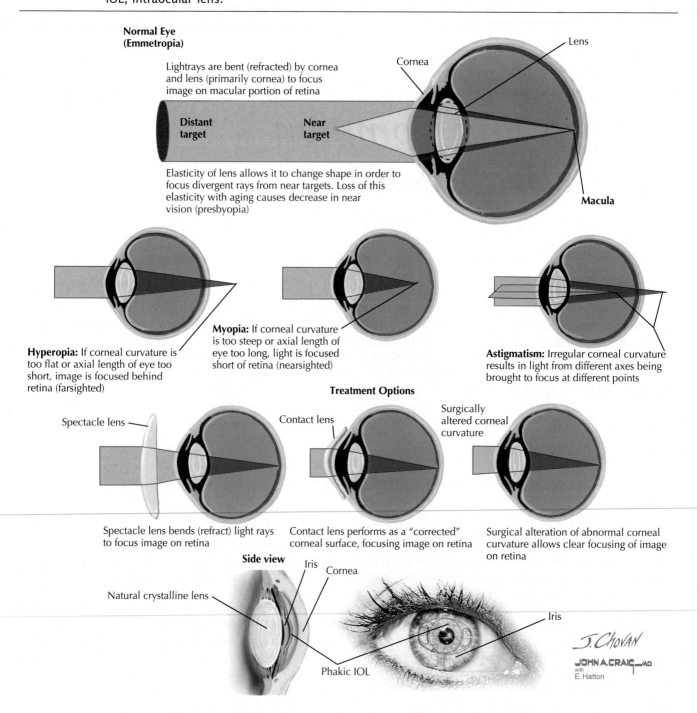

Normal Eye (Emmetropia)

Lightrays are bent (refracted) by cornea and lens (primarily cornea) to focus image on macular portion of retina

Distant target

Near target

Cornea

Lens

Macula

Elasticity of lens allows it to change shape in order to focus divergent rays from near targets. Loss of this elasticity with aging causes decrease in near vision (presbyopia)

Hyperopia: If corneal curvature is too flat or axial length of eye too short, image is focused behind retina (farsighted)

Myopia: If corneal curvature is too steep or axial length of eye too long, light is focused short of retina (nearsighted)

Astigmatism: Irregular corneal curvature results in light from different axes being brought to focus at different points

Treatment Options

Spectacle lens

Contact lens

Surgically altered corneal curvature

Spectacle lens bends (refract) light rays to focus image on retina

Contact lens performs as a "corrected" corneal surface, focusing image on retina

Surgical alteration of abnormal corneal curvature allows clear focusing of image on retina

Side view

Natural crystalline lens

Iris

Cornea

Phakic IOL

Iris

J. Chovan

JOHN A. CRAIG—AD
with
E. Hatton

of emmetropization occurs, developing an optical focus for near, which induces myopic progression.

Degenerative myopia is rare (1% to 2% of all myopia) and is a far more serious form in which the eye elongates at a rapid, pathologic rate. As the eye elongates, the retina thins, increasing the incidence of retinal degeneration and detachment. Tears in the retina can occur at the level of Bruch's membrane, with secondary hemorrhages and scarring at the macula leading to permanent visual distortion and blindness. Degenerative myopia is developmental in origin and progresses most rapidly at puberty.

Other causes of temporary myopic shifts are variations in blood sugar levels, nuclear sclerotic cataract progression, or introduction of various pharmaceutic agents (pilocarpine, tetracycline, adrenergic agents, phenothiazines, corticosteroids, oral contraceptives). These myopic tendencies are usually reversible.

Hyperopia (farsightedness) (see Fig. 157-1) is characterized by a weaker than normal refractive power or a shorter axial length, both of which cause light to focus posterior to the retina in the unaccommodated eye. Its incidence is directly related to age. Most full-term infants begin life with low hyperopia, but the condition diminishes rapidly with the emmetropization process of flattening of lens and cornea in conjunction with growth-related elongation of the eye. The amount of hyperopia in individuals younger than 30 years is often difficult to measure because of the ability of the accommodative system to produce positive refractive power, in essence correcting hyperopia. This aberrant use of the accommodative system can cause symptoms of headache and eyestrain as well as other binocular integration and general eye disorders. There is a strong association between moderate to high hyperopia in childhood and development of esotropia and amblyopia.

Astigmatism (see Fig. 157-1) is a refractive disorder in which the cornea has a nonspherical shape, with different powers at individual meridians or axes. This causes entering light rays to focus at multiple locations instead of a single point. Lenticular astigmatism is an unusual variant caused by abnormal tilting of the crystalline lens. Astigmatism follows a course similar to myopia, manifesting at about 8 years of age and stabilizing in the middle teen years. There is no gender difference, and both distance and near vision are affected. Astigmatism affects about 25% to 40% of the population and is commonly found in conjunction with myopia or hyperopia.

Presbyopia involves the progressive loss of accommodative ability in middle age leading to difficulty focusing on near objects. Accommodation, the ability to change shape and power of the crystalline lens by contraction of the ciliary body, develops maximum amplitude early in childhood. With advancing age, hardening of the crystalline lens reduces flexibility and decreases accommodative amplitude. Although hyperopia is often confused with presbyopia, hyperopia is relatively uncommon, whereas presbyopia will cause noticeable effects in everyone by age 45 years. Other eye disorders such as accommodative insufficiency may cause identical symptoms at an earlier age.

Clinical Presentation

The clinical presentation of all ametropias involves blurred vision at one or more viewing distances. In myopia, distance vision is affected, whereas near vision remains intact. Frequently, an individual will seek eye care when having difficulty driving at night or watching television. Unfortunately, children often tolerate very poor vision without complaint, so attention should be given to apparent difficulty seeing the classroom blackboard or while playing sports. Frequently, individuals with myopia report that squinting (creating a pinhole effect) improves vision.

Hyperopia is less straightforward in presentation. Theoretically, it is the opposite of myopia, leading to the assumption of blurred near and intact distance vision, but that is rarely the case. The accommodative system is able to provide optical correction for low amounts of hyperopia without much difficulty until ages 30 to 40 years. Individuals under this age are rarely aware of their refractive error and are resistant to the notion of refractive correction. Eventually, the accommodative system wanes, and the farsighted person has difficulty seeing all distances and must resort to wearing spectacles or contact lenses.

Astigmatism is usually less visually disturbing unless it develops concurrently with another refractive error. Those afflicted can function well for years without correction, and as with myopia, squinting improves vision. Common complaints include visual halo distortions while driving at night, or monocular diplopia.

Presbyopia is easily recognized in individuals 40 years and older. It manifests as gradual and progressive loss of near focusing ability, usually worse at the end of the day. As the accommodative demand for near work exceeds the accommodative reserve, blurred vision, headaches, fatigue, and eyestrain occur. Hyperopes typically have an earlier onset than myopes, and astigmatism can exacerbate symptoms.

Diagnostic Approach

Diagnosing refractive error is relatively straightforward and can be accomplished using Snellen or other visual acuity charts for near and far. The Snellen equivalent optotype system is based on a standard normal acuity measurement of 20/20, which equates to a letter height of 8.7 mm measured at 20 feet. All other sizes of letters for different acuity levels are extrapolated from this standard. The numerator in the acuity fraction corresponds to the distance a standard letter can be seen by a tested individual (usually 20 feet), and the denominator corresponds to the distance the same letter can be seen by a normal observer. An acuity level of less than 20/20 at distance with normal acuity at near indicates some level of myopia. Normal acuity at distance with difficulty focusing at near indicates hyperopia. Astigmatism causes a generalized reduction of acuity at near and far, and presbyopia is similar to hyperopia in middle-aged or older individuals.

The most accurate method of measuring refractive error is to perform cycloplegic refraction to best-corrected acuity. This procedure requires instillation of pharmaceutical agents (e.g., cyclopentolate) for paralysis of the ciliary body and the accommodative system. Cycloplegia is especially important when assessing refractive error in children because of their high accommodative amplitude and its effortless use. In-office use of specialty ophthalmic equipment such as phoropter and automated refractor enable quick and efficient measurement of refractive error and simulates spectacle-corrected vision.

Management and Therapy

There are many treatments (see Fig. 157-1) available for the correction of ametropias, running the gamut from very basic to extremely high-tech. Corrective options are generally classified as nonsurgical or surgical.

Optimum Treatment

Nonsurgical Methods

Nonsurgical corrective options, including spectacles and contact lenses, are most widely used and are reversible. Spectacles, the most common option, provide economical, safe, and exacting correction of all ametropias. Limitations include facial discomfort, lack of peripheral vision, and cosmesis issues. Nonetheless, with the advent of high-index materials, improved progressive bifocal designs, and newer frame designs, spectacle use has increased in popularity. Plastic polymers are the most widely used materials in the fabrication of ophthalmic lenses because they are lighter weight and safer than glass. Recent estimates of contact lens use in the United States are as high as 10% to 15%. Soft hydrogel contact lens wearers make up 85% of the population wearing contact lenses with the remainder using rigid gas permeable or polymethyl methacrylate (PMMA). With current technology, contact lenses can be used to correct virtually any refractive condition. Advantages include improved cosmesis, intact peripheral vision, and correction of irregular corneal disorders not correctable with spectacles (e.g., keratoconus). Disadvantages include expense, risk for infection or other pathology, and required diligence in care.

Surgical Methods

Current surgical corrective options include laser procedures and intraocular lens (IOL) implantation. Of these, laser procedures are most widely used. They offer an ever-expanding level of precision sculpting of corneal tissues to provide refractive correction.

Photorefractive keratectomy (PRK) uses a computer-guided excimer laser (193 nm wavelength) to reshape the corneal stroma to a desired curvature for refractive correction. PRK requires removal of stromal tissue, so unusually thin corneas can limit the amount of correction. Because epithelial tissue must be disrupted for laser access to the stroma, a bandage contact lens is applied directly after surgery to decrease pain and protect healing epithelium. Mild to moderate discomfort may be reported for 2 to 3 days as re-epithelialization occurs. PRK usually takes only 1 to 2 minutes to perform and can currently be used to correct 1 to 12 diopters of myopia, 1 to 6 diopters of hyperopia, and up to 4 diopters of astigmatism. Approved by the U.S. Food and Drug Administration in 1995, PRK has proved most accurate in correction of low to moderate myopia (up to –6 diopters) with a postoperative acuity of 20/40 or better in 90% to 95% of procedures. Major complications, aside

from undercorrection or overcorrection, include a transient visual disturbance described as foggy or hazy vision that is most noticeable at night and dry-eye symptoms.

Laser-assisted in situ keratomileusis (LASIK) is a refractive procedure that combines PRK with the surgical creation of a corneal flap by an instrument called a microkeratome. This precise instrument cuts a thin, circular flap in the stromal and epithelial layers of the cornea, leaving a hinge on one side. Once the flap is folded away, PRK is performed on the exposed stroma. The flap is then carefully placed back in its original position, completing the procedure. Like PRK, LASIK can be used to treat myopia, hyperopia, and astigmatism. The accuracy of postoperative correction has been greatly enhanced by employing wavefront-guided laser paradigms that can compensate for higher-order optical aberrations, yielding extremely acute vision.

The advantages of LASIK over PRK are faster vision rehabilitation and less discomfort. Complications of LASIK include surgical flap creation errors, loss of best-corrected acuity, and reduced corneal sensitivity, which can lead to a chronic irritation similar to dry-eye syndrome. Both PRK and LASIK can be performed several times on the same eye (enhancements) for refinement of surgical correction or naturally occurring refractive changes.

Phakic IOLs are surgically implanted anterior to the natural crystalline lens and are available for medium to extremely high amounts of myopic correction (–5 to –20 D). Postoperative acuity has been excellent, especially in higher myopic corrections. Potential complications include glaucoma, cataracts, and infection.

Avoiding Treatment Errors

The process of identifying appropriate candidates for refractive surgery has evolved and improved significantly as the surgical techniques have become more precise. Mandatory use and careful examination of corneal topography and corneal pachometry have greatly reduced the possibility of postsurgical complications such as ectasia or keratoconus. Treatment of dry-eye with punctal occlusion, anti-inflammatory agents, and tear supplements along with improved lid hygiene before surgery have also reduced complications of discomfort and visual distortions after the procedure.

Future Directions

The future of laser-refractive correction lies in increased accuracy of correction and improved safety profiles of surgical techniques. The focus of current research is safer flap creation in LASIK and nonlamellar (no stromal flap) advanced surface ablations, including laser epithelial keratomileusis (LASEK) and Epi-LASIK. The epithelium is retained in the advanced ablation techniques and removed in PRK. These newer refractive procedures have the potential to greatly reduce complication rates from those of lamellar procedures (LASIK).

Other nonlaser surgical options on the horizon are scleral expansion and accommodative IOLs for the correction of presbyopia. Of all the refractive disorders, the permanent correction of presbyopia appears to be the most difficult to achieve.

Additional Resources

Michaels DD: Visual Optics and Refraction, 3rd ed. St. Louis, CV Mosby, 1985.

This authoritative resource addresses topics regarding refraction or refractive errors.

Ophthalmic Hyperguide. Available at: www.ophthalmic.hyperguides. com. Accessed December 9, 2006.

This is an excellent searchable source for current research and the latest articles regarding eye disease and treatment.

EVIDENCE

1. Goss DA, Jackson TW: Clinical findings before the onset of myopia in youth: 4. Parental history of myopia. Optom Vis Sci 73(4):279-282, 1996.

   The authors present research for predicting myopia in children using parental myopia as a variable.

2. Zadnik K: The Glenn A. Fry Award Lecture (1995). Myopia development in childhood. Optom Vis Sci 74(8):603-608, 1997.

   The author presents an excellent review and compilation of current myopia genesis theory.

3. Zadnik K, Mutti DO, Friedman NE, et al: Ocular predictors of the onset of juvenile myopia. Invest Ophthalmol Vis Sci 40(9):1936-1943, 1999.

   This article reviews current research regarding predicting myopia.

Common Anterior Segment and Red Eye Problems for the Primary Care Specialist: Diagnosis and Management

Introduction

Primary care specialists and other non-ophthalmologists frequently encounter patients who complain of a red eye. The primary purpose of this chapter is to provide an approach to the differential diagnosis and management of conditions that cause red eye. An additional goal is to give the primary care physician guidance in dealing with the following: Which conditions require immediate treatment? In which is a delay in therapy acceptable pending a second opinion from an ophthalmologist? Which conditions require treatment by an ophthalmologist, which can the primary care physician treat without referral, and which require no treatment?

Etiology

Potential causes of ocular and periocular erythema include trauma, chemicals, infection, allergy, systemic conditions, and surgery. Red eye disorders are generally subcategorized as vision threatening or non–vision threatening. Those that threaten vision include corneal infections, perforating trauma, hyphema, endophthalmitis, orbital cellulitis, scleritis, iritis, and acute glaucoma. These require immediate referral to an ophthalmologist. Non–vision-threatening disorders include subconjunctival hemorrhage, hordeolum, chalazion, blepharitis, dry eye, conjunctivitis, and most corneal abrasions. These are commonly and appropriately managed by primary care professionals.

Clinical Presentation

Subjective ocular complaints may be categorized by the mnemonic RSVP: redness, sensitivity to light, vision decrease, or pain. Specific symptoms may help reveal the underlying cause of the red eye (Table 158-1).

Diagnostic Approach

To evaluate the red eye optimally, the primary care physician needs a Snellen visual acuity chart or near card, topical anesthetic drops, a fluorescein filter paper dye strip, and a penlight with a blue filter cap. The exam should begin with a recording of visual acuity at 20 feet using a Snellen chart, which is usually available in most offices. A near card is an acceptable alternative. Patients who normally wear spectacles or contact lenses should wear these for testing, if possible. Patients older than 40 years are likely presbyopic, and although they may have good distance vision, they probably still need magnifying spectacles for good near vision. When no vision loss is detected, most red eye disorders are treatable without ophthalmology referral. If

Table 158-1 Causes of Subjective Ocular Complaints

Symptom	Cause
Itching	Allergy
Photophobia	Corneal abrasions or surface breakdown, contact lens–related infiltrates or overwear, keratitis, iritis, acute glaucoma, corneal ulceration
Burning, scratchiness	Commonly dry eye but also blepharitis, foreign body material, and trichiasis
Deep intense pain	Corneal abrasions, corneal ulceration, scleritis, iritis, endophthalmitis, severe keratitis, severe surface epitheliopathy, acute angle-closure glaucoma
Localized lid tenderness	Hordeolum, chalazion, meibomitis, cellulitis
Foreign body sensation	Corneal surface breakdown, retained foreign body or debris, trichiasis, surface filaments from dry eye
Halo vision	Corneal edema of any cause (especially contact lens overwear syndrome and acute glaucoma)

Box 158-1 History: Important Questions and Considerations

Are one or both eyes affected? Vision at the time of exam? Is there a decrease in vision?

Vision before trauma?

Onset sudden or progressive?

What is the timeline of symptoms? Hours or days? Intermittent?

Any family members with red eye recently? Recent upper respiratory infection?

Recent eye surgery? (If yes, *refer immediately*.)

History of contact lens use? Do they sleep in them? (If yes, then patients have a 10 times greater risk for cornea ulcer.)

Pain? Foreign body sensation? Itchiness? Sensitivity to light?

Discharge? Scant or profuse? Watery or purulent? Chronic or acute?

Use of any eye medications, past or present, including over the counter?

Any history of trauma? Environmental associations? Systemic conditions?

reduced visual acuity is noted, serious ocular disease is likely, and referral to an eye care specialist is essential. Notably, conjunctivitis is extremely unlikely to reduce visual acuity (Box 158-1).

After the history and visual acuity are recorded, a systematic anatomic exam of the eye and adnexa should be performed. First, the face, lids, preauricular lymph nodes, and orbital area are inspected. Next, the extraocular movements, confrontational visual fields, and pupils are evaluated, followed by examination of the globe, paying particular attention to the conjunctiva, cornea, and sclera. A slit lamp biomicroscope is especially valuable for evaluating the anterior chamber for iritis, hyphema, or angle-closure glaucoma. If a slit lamp is not available, a penlight is a useful alternative. The smoothness and clarity of the corneal surface and the light reflex are especially important components of the exam. A drop of sterile fluorescein dye, when applied to the lower tarsal conjunctiva using a wetted

fluorescein strip, is especially helpful in detecting denuded areas of the corneal epithelium. During blinking, the dye spreads over the corneal surface and adheres only to epithelial defects, which light up with a bright green color under the cobalt blue–capped penlight. Following the fluorescein exam, an intraocular pressure (IOP) measurement is easily performed using either a Tono-Pen or Goldmann applanation tonometry. Gentle digital palpation provides a gross assessment as to whether the globe is very hard due to high pressure from acute glaucoma or painfully tender due to scleritis, acute glaucoma, iritis, or other anterior-segment inflammatory process. Palpation of the globe is contraindicated if there is a history of trauma and if globe rupture is suspected (Fig. 158-1).

Differential Diagnosis

A guide to differentiating common red eye features is shown in Table 158-2.

Management and Therapy

Ocular Adnexal Disorders of the Lids, Lashes, and Lacrimal Apparatus

Hordeolum and Chalazion

Inflamed or impacted lid margin sebaceous glands may present with local nodular swelling, tenderness, lid injection, and localized or diffuse cellulitis of the lid. A hordeolum is an inflamed lesion on the lid margin, whereas a chalazion presents as a nodule in a more central lid location. Treatment includes hot compresses to the eyelids four times daily for 3 to 5 minutes when the lesion is acute or subacute. Following hot compress application, the patient should massage the lid and lash line in hopes of achieving drainage. This treatment may take several weeks to be effective. If discharge is noted or infection is suspected, a topical antibiotic ointment (e.g., bacitracin, gentamicin, bacitracin-neomycin-polymyxin B) should be applied to the lash line and over the affected area 3 to 4 times daily. Occasionally, oral antibiotics are necessary if

Figure 158-1 Diagnostic Approach.

Foreign bodies

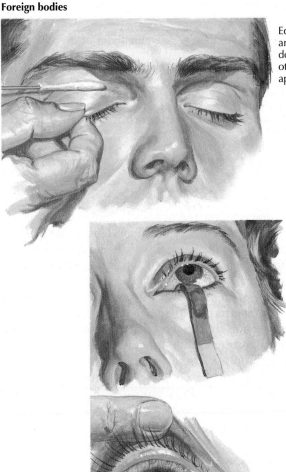

Edge of upper lid grasped
and drawn outward and
downward; applicator or
other rod-like device
applied at tarsal fold

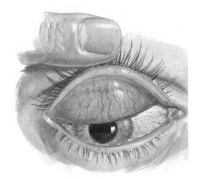

Lid everted,
exposing foreign
body which may
then be wiped off

Keratitis (inflammation of the cornea)

Technique of applying
fluorescein strip in
previously anesthetized eye

Dendritic keratitis
(herpes simplex)
demonstrated by
fluorescein

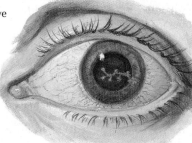

Treatment of corneal scars

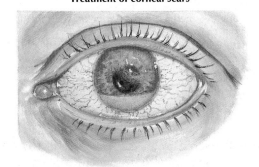

Acute keratitis
(ciliary injection,
irregular corneal surface)

Corneal ulcer stained with fluorescein
hypopyon (pus in anterior chamber)

the accompanying meibomian gland dysfunction reveals marked inspissation or impaction. In these instances, the treatment of choice is doxycycline, 100 mg administered twice daily for 1 month, then tapered to once daily for at least 2 months or longer. Meibomian gland dysfunction is particularly common in white middle-aged men and often accompanies rosacea.

If a chalazion fails to resolve and becomes chronic (i.e., nontender and localized, or persists more than 3 to 4 weeks), then referral to an ophthalmologist is indicated. A persistent or recurring lid mass is an indication for biopsy because it may represent a rare sebaceous gland carcinoma or squamous cell carcinoma of the lid (Fig. 158-2).

Blepharitis

Blepharitis is chronic lid margin inflammation that is associated with staphylococcal infection, seborrhea, or dry eyes. Its symptoms and signs may include burning; foreign body or gritty sensation; red, thickened lid margins; lash matting and crusting; and sticky lids on awakening in the morning. Blepharitis may also be asymptomatic.

Table 158-2 Differentiating Common Red Eye Features

	Conjunctivitis	Keratitis (Corneal Inflammation or Foreign Body)	Iritis	Acute Angle-Closure Glaucoma
Vision	Normal or intermittent blurring that clears with blinking	Slightly blurred	Slightly blurred	Marked blurring
Discharge	Prominent, often crusting of lashes; purulent indicates bacterial infection; clear, watery indicates viral infection*; stringy, scant mucus indicates allergy	None to mild	None	None
Pain	None or minor and superficial	Sharp, severe foreign body sensation	Moderately severe; aching and photophobia	Very severe, frequently nausea and vomiting
Injection pattern	Diffuse	Circumcorneal	Circumcorneal, ciliary flush	Diffuse, with prominent circumcorneal injection
Corneal appearance	Clear	Dull or altered light reflex; positive fluorescein staining; opacification present	Clear or slightly hazy	Hazy, steamy, clouded; altered light reflex
Intraocular pressure	Normal	Normal	Normal to low	Very high
Pupil size	Normal	Normal or slightly constricted	Constricted	Fixed, mid-dilated
Pupillary response to light	Normal	Normal	Minimal further constriction	Usually no reaction
Anterior chamber depth	Normal	Normal	Normal	Shallow
Referral advisable	No (unless hyperpurulent)	Yes	Yes	Yes

*Preauricular lymph nodes are characteristic of viral conjunctivitis.

Figure 158-2 Disorders of the Lid.

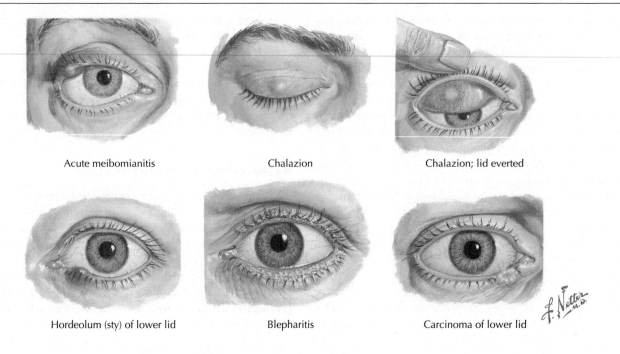

Acute meibomianitis

Chalazion

Chalazion; lid everted

Hordeolum (sty) of lower lid

Blepharitis

Carcinoma of lower lid

Treatment includes warm compresses to loosen crusts and proper eyelid hygiene, including eyelid scrubs applied to the base of the eyelashes to remove scurf and collarettes. The patient may use dilute baby shampoo on a small wash-cloth. Commercially available eyelid scrub kits work particularly well and are recommended. Topical ophthalmic antibiotic ointment applied nightly after the lid hygiene measures for 2 to 6 weeks is necessary if there is associated infection or significant bacterial colonization. Rarely, cultures and susceptibility testing are warranted. Additional dry eye treatment may also be essential to effect control because eye dryness is a contributing factor.

Cellulitis of Extraocular Structures

Preseptal (Anterior) Cellulitis

The symptoms and signs of anterior cellulitis include eyelid erythema, tense edema, warmth, tenderness, and fluctuant lymphedema or swelling that may extend over the nasal bridge to the opposite eyelids. The patient is often unable to open the eyelids because of severe edema, but the eye itself is relatively uninvolved, with minimal to no conjunctival injection. Often there is a history of sinusitis, insect bite, dacryocystitis, local skin abrasion, laceration, or puncture wound. Preseptal cellulitis is usually accompanied by low-grade fever and an elevated white blood cell count. Vision, pupils, and ocular motility are normal, and there is no proptosis and no pain with eye movement.

Treatment includes checking a complete blood count with differential in addition to taking a culture of any open wound, purulent nasal drainage, conjunctival discharge, or weeping vesicles. In mild cases without localized abscess, administration of a broad-spectrum oral antibiotic for 10 days is indicated (e.g., amoxicillin-clavulanate, cefaclor, or trimethoprim-sulfamethoxazole). If secondary conjunctivitis is present, the application of a topical antibiotic ointment (gentamicin, bacitracin, ciprofloxacin, erythromycin, or neomycin-bacitracin-polymyxin B), $1/2$-inch ribbon 3 to 4 times daily, is indicated. A computed tomography (CT) scan of the orbits and sinuses is essential in moderate to severe cases in children younger than 5 years and in those who have no noticeable improvement after a few days of oral antibiotics. These patients may require hospital admission and intravenous antibiotics (ceftriaxone, cefuroxime, ampicillin-sulbactam, or vancomycin). If indicated because of a traumatic facial lesion, tetanus toxoid should be administered per Centers for Disease Control and Prevention (CDC) guidelines. If a fluctuant mass or abscess is present, wound exploration, débridement, or drainage may be necessary.

Orbital (Posterior) Cellulitis

The symptoms and signs of posterior orbital cellulitis include eye pain, blurred vision, headache, double vision, eyelid edema, eyelid erythema, eyelid warmth, eyelid tenderness, and proptosis. Conjunctival chemosis and injection, restricted ocular movement, and pain on attempted eye movement are the critical signs that help differentiate orbital from preseptal cellulitis. Fever, purulent discharge, decreased periorbital sensation, decreased vision, and retinal venous congestion are worrisome signs. A computed tomography (CT) scan often demonstrates sinusitis (commonly ethmoid sinusitis). The periorbital area may be relatively uninflamed. Optic nerve involvement presents with optic disc edema, decreased vision, and an afferent papillary defect.

Treatment includes hospitalization, immediate eye consultation, blood culture, imaging studies (orbit and sinus CT with contrast or magnetic resonance imaging with contrast), ear-nose-throat consultation if sinus disease is present, and broad spectrum intravenous antibiotics. The antibiotics are required for at least 72 hours, followed by oral medication for 1 week. *Staphylococcus* species, *Streptococcus* species, *Haemophilus influenzae*, bacteroides, and gram-negative rods (especially after trauma) are the most commonly associated microorganisms. Infectious disease and pediatric specialist consultation may help to confirm the most current antibiotics and dosages. Ceftriaxone, 1 to 2 g every 12 hours, plus vancomycin, 1 g intravenously every 12 hours, for adults is reasonable initial therapy; however, doses require adjustment based on renal function. The addition of metronidazole, 15 mg/kg intravenously every 6 hours, is necessary for chronic orbital cellulitis or when an anaerobic infection is suspected (not to exceed 4 g/day). Fungal infection must be excluded in immunosuppressed patients because, if confirmed, surgical débridement by an ear-nose-throat specialist is indicated. *Phycomycosis (mucormycosis) is a life-threatening disease that must be considered in all diabetic and immunocompromised patients. Immediate débridement is usually indicated.*

If there is not a rapid response to intravenous antibiotics, or if a subperiosteal abscess is present, surgical intervention is the next step. All patients require careful monitoring for complications, including cavernous sinus thrombosis and meningitis. Severe proptosis is an indication for the use of topical antibiotic ointment 4 times daily to reduce corneal exposure and prevent corneal ulceration.

Nasolacrimal Duct Obstruction

The symptoms and signs of nasolacrimal duct obstruction include: a wet-appearing eye with tears flowing over the eyelid, moist or dried mucoid matter with crusting principally on the medial eyelashes, punctal reflux material expressible with digital pressure on the lacrimal sac (the region between the medial canthus and nose), medial lower eyelid erythema, and swelling of the medial canthus region. If mucopurulent discharge is expressible with palpation of the lacrimal sac, the patient may have an associated dac-

ryocystitis (infected tear sac). The etiology of nasolacrimal duct obstruction is congenital or acquired.

Congenital obstruction is usually due to an imperforate membrane (valve of Hasner) at the distal end of the nasolacrimal duct. It occurs clinically in 2% to 4% of full-term infants and is diagnosed at 1 to 2 weeks of age. Treatment consists of having the parent apply digital index-finger pressure with downward strokes to the common canaliculus and lacrimal sac region 2 to 4 times daily. Ninety percent open spontaneously with this treatment by 1 year of age. If there is no resolution in 6 to 8 months, referral to an ophthalmologist for probing and irrigation is indicated. *If no reflux from the sac occurs with pressure or if the patient keeps the eye closed when exposed to light, timely referral to a pediatric ophthalmologist is necessary.* Rarely, preseptal cellulitis or dacryocystitis may develop.

Acquired nasolacrimal duct obstruction results from chronic nasal or sinus disease, dacryocystitis, previous surgery, tumor, or naso-orbital trauma. Involutional stenosis is the most common cause in older individuals. Treatment includes systemic antibiotics if dacryocystitis is present. In afebrile children who have mild cases and a reliable parent, treatment with cefaclor, 20 to 40 mg/kg/day orally in three divided doses, is usually effective. Fever in children with moderate to severe obstruction and an unreliable parent are indications for hospitalization and administration of intravenous cefuroxime, 50 to 100 mg/kg/day in three divided doses. In afebrile adults with mild disease, cephalexin, 500 mg orally every 8 hours, is appropriate. Febrile adults who appear acutely ill require hospitalization and therapy with intravenous cefazolin, 1 g every 8 hours. Supplemental topical antibiotic drops (moxifloxacin, gatifloxacin, neomycin, or gentamicin) 4 times daily plus warm compresses and gentle massage to the inner canthal region 4 times daily may aid treatment in all patients. *Use of steroids requires evaluation and supervision by an ophthalmologist.* A pointing abscess is an indication to consider incision and drainage of the lacrimal sac by an ophthalmologist. If the obstruction is chronic or recurrent, referral to an ophthalmologist is also appropriate. Surgical correction by dacryocystorhinostomy with silicone intubation is usually needed once the acute episode has resolved.

Anterior Segment Disorders of the Conjunctiva, Sclera, and Cornea, Including Dry Eye and Trauma

Conjunctivitis

Conjunctivitis can be an isolated problem or can occur in association with any type of ocular inflammation. Symptoms and signs of conjunctivitis include a diffuse pattern of injection (redness) over the bulbar conjunctiva or the palpebral, or tarsal, conjunctiva. In conjunctivitis, the pattern of erythema is not sectoral. Pain is usually not associated (as opposed to episcleritis or scleritis) but may

occur with irritation or a foreign body sensation. In adult patients, both infectious and noninfectious inflammation of the conjunctiva is usually associated with ocular discharge. The characteristics of the discharge imply specific etiologies:

- Bacterial: purulent discharge
- Viral: serous, watery discharge
- Allergic: watery discharge with grayish, scant, stringy mucus

BACTERIAL (NONGONOCOCCAL) CONJUNCTIVITIS. Bacterial (nongonococcal) conjunctivitis presents with a purulent discharge of mild to moderate degree and tarsal conjunctival papillary inflammation. Involvement may be unilateral or bilateral. Common organisms include *Staphylococcus* species, *Streptococcus* species, and *Haemophilus* species (in children). No preauricular lymph node is palpable unless hyperpurulent discharge is present due to *Neisseria gonorrhoeae.*

Treatment includes topical antibiotic drops: moxifloxacin, gatifloxacin, levofloxacin, gentamicin, tobramycin, neomycin–polymyxin B–gramicidin, or sulfacetamide 4 times daily for 5 to 7 days. Alternatively, ointments including bacitracin, gentamicin, ciprofloxacin, neomycin–bacitracin–polymyxin B, or polymyxin B–bacitracin, $^{1}/_{2}$-inch ribbon 4 times daily for 5 to 7 days, may be used.

The patient requires follow-up every 2 days initially, then every 3 to 5 days until resolution. If there is no improvement in 3 days, or if vision worsens, referral to an ophthalmologist is indicated. Copious purulent discharge is an indication to perform a Gram stain and culture to exclude gonococcal infection. Referral to an ophthalmologist is wise in this situation. In children, the accepted treatment for *H. influenzae* conjunctivitis is oral amoxicillin-clavulanate, 20 to 40 mg/kg/day in three divided doses, given the risk for development of otitis media, pneumonia, or meningitis.

VIRAL CONJUNCTIVITIS. Viral conjunctivitis is highly contagious because it is usually caused by an adenovirus. Often there is a history of recent upper respiratory infection, contact with someone who had an upper respiratory infection or red eye contact exposure in the prior 5 to 14 days before developing symptoms. Both eyes are affected simultaneously or in sequence (up to 3 days apart). Symptoms and signs include eye irritation or itchiness, a palpable preauricular lymph node, and an inferior palpebral conjunctival follicular or folliculopapillary reaction. Follicles are the macroappearance of aggregated lymphocytes surrounded by mast and plasma cells in the conjunctival stroma. Pseudomembranes (inflammatory debris and fibrin) or true conjunctival membranes herald severe involvement. Small subconjunctival hemorrhages are noted in 43% of adenoviral conjunctivitis cases. Typically, viral conjunctivitis gets worse for the first 4 to 7 days after onset and may not resolve for 2 to 3 weeks. Punctate keratitis may be detected in 2 days to 1 week. Subepithelial opacities may develop in 7 to 14 days and result in decreased vision, reduced contrast sensitivity, photosensitivity, and glare or haloes around bright lights.

Treatment includes taking steps to prevent transmission and complications as well as to provide symptomatic relief. Patients with suspected viral conjunctivitis should be examined in a separate area to avoid spread of infection to other patients and minimize surface contact within the physician's office. Cleaning and disinfection of all equipment handled during the exam is mandatory. Doorknobs or objects the patient touches in the office should be disinfected as well. Chlorine-releasing solutions (such as 2% sodium hypochlorite solution) and povidone-iodine are effective in eliminating viral pathogens. Recently prepared chlorine solutions should be used because activity is rapidly lost after dilution. Isopropyl alcohol is not effective in disinfecting adenoviral contaminated surfaces. Patients are instructed to avoid personal contacts and the sharing of towels, pillows, or any personal item that could be contaminated by ocular secretions. Patients should wash their hands after touching their eyes. Health care professionals with viral conjunctivitis should not have direct hand-to-patient contact for a minimum of 14 days after onset of symptoms. Chilled artificial tears or cool compresses may help alleviate symptoms. Similarly, antiallergy drops or topical nonsteroidal drops may offer some relief if the itchiness is severe. Topical antibiotics should be prescribed in patients with large epithelial defects or after the removal of membranes or pseudomembranes.

Topical corticosteroids should only be used by eye care professionals in patients with membranous or pseudo-membranous conjunctivitis, severe keratitis, or persistent subepithelial infiltrates with visual loss. *Corticosteroids enhance viral replication and promote superinfection. Their use delays viral clearance and can result in a much greater number of infected patients in community epidemics.*

ALLERGIC CONJUNCTIVITIS. Symptoms and signs of allergic conjunctivitis include itching, burning, bilateral presentation, mild conjunctival injection, possible eyelid or conjunctival edema (chemosis), papillary conjunctival reaction, and possible whitish stringy mucus. A seasonal presentation is commonly seen with an associated history of airborne allergies (e.g., animal dander, pollens, ragweed, dust, or mold spores).

Treatment is symptomatic. Elimination of the inciting agent and the use of cool compresses or chilled artificial tears are helpful measures. For cases of moderate severity, useful topical agents include dual antihistamine–mast cell stabilizer agents (olopatadine, epinastine, ketotifen, azelastine); pure topical antihistamines (levocabastine, emedastine); pure mast cell stabilizers (cromolyn, lodoxamide, nedocromil, pemirolast); and decongestant combinations (naphazoline plus pheniramine). The addition of a topical nonsteroidal medication (nepafenac, ketorolac, bromfenac) can be helpful. Severe cases and those refractory to treatment require referral to an ophthalmologist. *Topical steroids are reserved for severe cases and should only be used after evaluation by an ophthalmologist* (Fig. 158-3).

Subconjunctival Hemorrhage

Usually occurring spontaneously without known cause, subconjunctival hemorrhages (SCHs) may appear after Valsalva episodes (e.g., coughing, sneezing, straining during a bowel movement or with heavy lifting). SCHs are often noted upon awakening. One theory is that tiny blood vessels bridging cystic, thin conjunctiva easily shear or rupture with eye rubbing or pressure from the pillow during sleep. There is a possible association with anticoagulants, aspirin, high-dose vitamin E, accelerated hypertension, or bleeding diathesis—particularly if the hemorrhages occur bilaterally or are recurrent. Patients typically present with an acute, painless, flat, unilateral, dense, blood-red discoloration of the subconjunctival space. There is no loss of vision.

Treatment includes careful examination to rule out traumatic causes (perforating injury or globe rupture). Suspicion of penetration is an indication to shield the eye (using a hard shield, not a soft patch) and to obtain an immediate ophthalmologic evaluation. If there is no perforating injury or globe rupture, no treatment is needed except time (often 2 to 3 weeks before clearing) and reassurance of the excellent prognosis. Re-evaluation is indicated if the hemorrhage does not clear in 3 weeks or if it recurs.

Dry Eye Syndrome

Dry eye syndrome (DES), a tear film deficiency (keratoconjunctivitis sicca), is extremely common in the aging population, especially in women older than 40 years. Symptoms often exceed what can be found on physical exam. Symptoms and signs may include burning, irritation, grittiness, foreign body sensation, mild conjunctival redness, intermittent visual blurring, and reflex tearing. Patients often protest that they cannot have dry eye syndrome because their eyes are constantly tearing. However, the tear film is mostly oil (about 85% mucin and lipid), with the central aqueous portion making up only 15%. Therefore, educating the patient on the difference between poor tear film lubrication (lack of surface oil) and the body's compensatory response of watery reflex tearing to make up for the oil deficiency is often helpful. Typically patient's symptoms worsen as the day progresses.

DES symptoms are often exacerbated by prolonged reading, staring at the television, or working at the computer because of the decreased blink rate and increased evaporative loss associated with these activities. Symptoms are aggravated by smoke, high-airflow environments (e.g., car air conditioner or vent fan), low-humidity conditions (especially during the winter months when heaters are on), and fatigue due to lack of sleep.

Figure 158-3 Conjunctivitis, Subconjunctival Hemorrhage, Episcleritis.

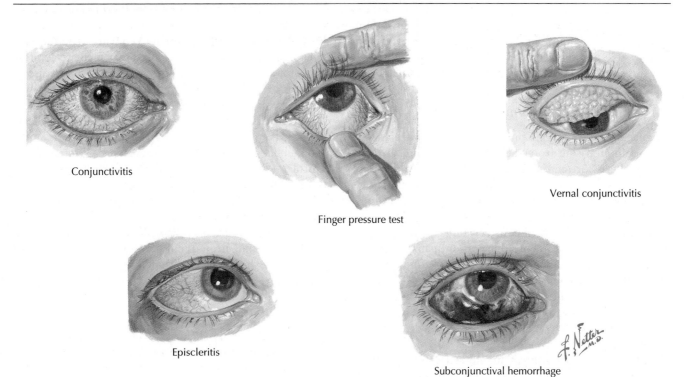

Conjunctivitis

Finger pressure test

Vernal conjunctivitis

Episcleritis

Subconjunctival hemorrhage

Bilateral low tear meniscus (height of the tear lake measured as less than 0.3 mm at the inferior eyelid margin), rapid tear break-up time (discontinuity in the precorneal tear film recorded as less than 10 seconds), and punctate epithelial erosions (PEE) of the conjunctiva or cornea (best visualized with fluorescein dye or lissamine green staining using slit lamp biomicroscopy) are hallmarks of the disorder. Excess mucus, tear film debris, corneal filaments, and lid margin froth (denoting staphylococcal colonization) may also be noted. Visual blurring or glare occurs when PEE are in the optical pathway (i.e., in the pupil area), and these symptoms tend to be intermittent and variable.

Associated conditions abound. Dry eye after laser-assisted in situ keratomileusis (LASIK) is very common. This is due to relative corneal denervation disrupting the normal corneal sensation and feedback loop to the lacrimal gland with subsequent reduced tear production. Confocal microscopy has demonstrated that the number of stromal nerve fiber bundles decreases by 90% immediately after LASIK. By 1 year, their numbers improve, but remain less than half of their original value.

Connective tissue diseases such as Sjögren's syndrome, rheumatoid arthritis, Wegener's granulomatosis, and systemic lupus erythematosus may manifest significant dry eye keratopathy. Conjunctival scarring disorders that often have associated DES include ocular cicatricial pemphigoid (typically severe), Stevens-Johnson syndrome, trachoma, and chemical burns. DES may be a side effect of drugs, including diuretics, antihistamines, antidepressants, dermatologic drying agents, and anticholinergics.

Incomplete lid closure resulting in increased corneal exposure and DES may occur as a result of Bell's palsy, thyroid-related (Graves') exophthalmopathy, or scarred or malpositioned eyelids. Miscellaneous causes of DES include vitamin A deficiency, infiltration of the lacrimal glands (sarcoidosis, tumor), and postirradiation fibrosis of the lacrimal glands.

Initial treatment measures may include artificial tears instilled every 2 to 4 hours, cyclosporine 0.2% drops twice daily, and lubricating gels or ointment at bedtime. If corneal exposure is present when the patient is asleep, taping the eyelids closed during sleep or wearing a pair of moisture-chamber eye goggles (e.g., tranquileyes and goggles by eyeeco) is often helpful. Patients should not patch their eyes closed because the eyelids may creep open under the patch, thereby potentiating an abrasion. Lubricating gels are typically preferred over ointments because they cause less visual blurring. Humidifiers at the bedside may also prove helpful. Oral omega-3 fatty acids (wild-caught fish oil brands recommended), about 2000 mg/day, are also useful for improving the quality (oily mucin layer) of the precorneal tear film.

If the DES is severe or unresponsive to the above measures, ophthalmology referral for punctal plugs to help the patient retain more natural tears is the next step. *(Intracanalicular style plugs should never be used because bacterial biofilm may develop and induce canaliculitis.)* If the patient does not develop epiphora with plugs in place, plug removal with punctal cautery may prove especially beneficial. Long-term retention or utilization of punctal plugs is discouraged owing to loosening and bacterial biofilm formation. In profound DES, upper and lower punctal cautery closure may become necessary. Adjunctive preservative-free hydroxypropyl cellulose lubricant lacrisert inserts (3.5 mm long by 1.27 mm diameter, placed in the lower lateral fornices) stabilize and thicken the precorneal tear film and are useful in moderate to severe dry eye syndromes.

Pinguecula and Pterygium

Pingueculae and pterygia are benign masses of elastotic degeneration arising from the interpalpebral bulbar conjunctiva (nasal or temporal) caused by actinic (ultraviolet light) exposure, wind, dust, dry eye, or chronic irritation. Pingueculae are yellow-white nodules, typically asymptomatic, and confined to conjunctiva. Pterygia are triangular fibrovascular growths that extend onto the cornea.

Treatment includes ocular lubrication management as in dry eye, starting with artificial tears 4 to 6 times per day plus protection from ultraviolet light or irritants (e.g., sunglasses or safety goggles if appropriate). Topical nonsteroidal anti-inflammatory drugs (NSAIDs) are useful to alleviate inflammation (e.g., nepafenac 3 times daily, ketorolac 4 times daily, or bromfenac 2 times daily) for 2 weeks. An actively enlarging pterygium and refractory or severe inflammation are indications for referral to an ophthalmologist.

Corneal Abrasion

Symptoms and signs characteristic of corneal abrasion include sharp pain, photophobia, foreign body sensation, tearing, redness, a history of scratching the eye, and an epithelial defect that stains bright green with fluorescein. If there is no recent history of trauma and if symptoms occurred upon awakening, then recurrent erosion syndrome is likely.

Treatment should begin by using fluorescein dye to map the size and location of the epithelial defect. Except for the defect, the cornea should be clear. Evaluation for infiltrate, corneal laceration, penetrating trauma, and anterior chamber reaction is essential. If corneal haze is present, a superinfection is possible, and an ophthalmology consultation is needed. The eyelid should be everted to ensure that no retained foreign body is present. Pain may be relieved with cycloplegic drops (1% cyclopentolate, 5% homatropine). Oral analgesics with codeine or other appropriate narcotic agent can be prescribed if the patient's pain is marked. *Topical anesthetics are contraindicated!* They are used only to aid the exam and to confirm the diagnosis because immediate relief occurs within seconds of their instillation.

Topical antibiotics are recommended for infection prophylaxis. Contact lens wearers must have *Pseudomonas* species coverage (e.g., ciprofloxacin, tobramycin, gentamicin, moxifloxacin, gatifloxacin) and should have daily follow-up until the epithelial defect resolves. Drops are used 4 times daily; ointments should be used every 2 to 4 hours.

Ointments offer better barrier function between eyelid and abraded surface, but they blur vision. If drops are used concurrently with ointments, then drop instillation should always occur before the ointment to enhance penetration.

Taping the patient's eyelid closed may increase comfort but is not advised in contact lens wearers. Also, the use of patching or taping is contraindicated if the abrasion was due to trauma by plant matter (e.g., tree branch), vegetable matter, or false fingernails. To promote healing and alleviate pain, the patient should keep the eye closed as much as possible. Topical NSAIDs (nepafenac 3 times daily, ketorolac 4 times daily, or bromfenac 2 times daily) enhance comfort but can retard epithelial healing.

If the abrasion is not healed within 24 to 48 hours, referral to an ophthalmologist is indicated. Central or large abrasions must be followed daily. If infiltrates are noted at any time, prompt cultures and an ophthalmology consultation should be instituted because these patients require more aggressive therapy.

Chemical Injury

ACID INJURY. Acids such as car battery acid (H_2SO_4), bleach, refrigerant (H_2SO_3), fruit preservatives, and glass-etching chemicals precipitate tissue proteins and do not penetrate the cornea as deeply as alkali substances. However, acids do cause immediate corneal damage.

Treatment of acid injuries begins with immediate copious irrigation, preferably with saline or Ringer's lactate, for at least 30 minutes. It is helpful to place topical anesthetic and an eyelid speculum or a Morgan irrigating lens in the eye to facilitate irrigation. Five to 10 minutes after irrigation, the pH of the inferior conjunctival cul-de-sac is measured to ensure that a neutral pH (7.0) has been achieved. If not, irrigation must continue. The volume needed to neutralize the pH may range from 2 to 8 liters. If there is a persistently abnormal pH, sweeping the fornices with a moistened cotton-tipped swab is effective in removing retained particulates that may be lodged in the deep forniceal space.

Acid injuries are treated the same as corneal abrasions, and referral to an ophthalmologist is necessary.

ALKALINE INJURY. Alkali injuries from lye (NaOH), caustic potash (KOH), and ammonia (NH_4) tend to have worse outcomes than those from fresh lime $Ca(OH)_2$ or magnesium hydroxide $Mg(OH)_2$. Household cleaners, fertilizers, and refrigerants contain ammonia. Cement, mortar, plaster, and whitewash contain fresh lime. Flares and sparklers contain magnesium hydroxide. Alkali injuries cause both immediate and delayed damage to the eye because of deeper substrate penetration as compared with acid burns. Alkali burns also have a greater potential for serious ocular damage.

Treatment of alkaline injuries begins with immediate copious irrigation as for acid injury. Immediacy is imperative, even if nonsterile water is the only irrigation solution available! The timeliness of irrigation is the most important therapeutic and sight-saving measure. Acidic solutions should never be used to neutralize alkaline burns (or vice versa). Alkaline injuries require immediate referral to an ophthalmologist after appropriate irrigation has been commenced.

Contact Lens Overwear Syndrome

Hypoxic stress to the corneal epithelium leads to the same symptoms and complications as corneal abrasions, which include pain, tearing, and photophobia. This syndrome is often associated with sleeping in contact lenses or a tight contact lens fit and presents with corneal edema, blurred vision, conjunctival hyperemia, and occasional corneal infiltrates. The inciting factor is often poor tear exchange and clearance of metabolic byproducts from beneath the lens.

Treatment is the same as for corneal abrasion. Contact lens wear must be discontinued, and monitoring for potential corneal ulcer or infiltrates is essential. Re-evaluation should occur daily with referral to an ophthalmologist if there is no improvement within 1 to 2 days.

Infectious Keratitis

Infectious keratitis results from destruction of corneal epithelium and stroma due to inflammation from an infectious organism. It is typically unilateral. Risk factors include contact lens wear, trauma, dry eyes, chronic ocular surface disease, topical corticosteroids, lid abnormalities, exposure, and corneal hypesthesia.

Symptoms of *bacterial* infectious keratitis include redness with mild to severe pain, photophobia, decreased vision, and purulent discharge. A discrete gray or white corneal opacity (infiltrate) is visible with penlight or slit lamp examination. Urgent referral to an ophthalmologist is indicated for diagnosis and treatment.

Viral infectious keratitis is most commonly caused by recurrent herpes simplex virus type 1. Associations include sun exposure, stress, illness, trauma, menses, and immunosuppression. Symptoms and signs include red eye with watery discharge and foreign body sensation. A dendrite, or branching figure, is the characteristic epithelial lesion of the cornea and is best seen with fluorescein staining (see Fig. 158-1). Urgent referral to an ophthalmologist is indicated. Topical steroids should never be used in the setting of possible herpes keratitis.

Other etiologies of keratitis are multiple, but infectious etiologies more commonly include: fungal (particularly common after trauma with plant or vegetable matter) and parasitic (e.g., acanthamoeba, which is particularly painful and commonly seen with poor soft contact lens hygiene or hot tub use).

Hyphema

Hyphema is blood in the anterior chamber, usually following blunt trauma. The patient may present with pain, redness, blurred vision, and red blood cells, either suspended (microhyphema: cells only detectable by slit lamp) or layered along the dependent portion of the anterior chamber (usually at 6-o'clock position and detectable by penlight). The pupil may be irregular, peaked, or sluggish on the affected side (Fig. 158-4).

Evaluation includes confirmation of visual acuity, if possible, and performance of an initial screening exam with minimal globe manipulation because concurrent injury may be present. If the hyphema is reported as occurring spontaneously in a child, child abuse is always suspected. Treatment includes shielding the eye and keeping the patient at rest with the head elevated at least 30 degrees. NSAIDs or aspirin products are contraindicated. The patient should not read because the associated eye movement may promote rebleeding. Television watching is okay. Immediate ophthalmology referral is indicated.

Episcleritis and Scleritis

Symptoms and signs of *episcleritis* include acute onset of redness (70% sectoral, 30% diffuse) in one or both eyes, typically in young adults, which blanches on application of topical phenylephrine 2.5% (unlike scleritis, which does not); mild pain described as a dull ache localized to the eye; normal vision; and no ocular discharge. A history of recurrent episodes is common.

Most cases of episcleritis are self-limited and resolve in about 3 weeks. However, referral to ophthalmology is necessary for confirmation. Some cases require topical NSAIDs (nepafenac 3 times daily), oral NSAIDs, or both. Resistance to treatment may signify systemic disease and the need for a systemic workup by the primary care specialist.

Scleritis usually has a gradual onset. The hallmark symptom is severe and boring eye pain that may radiate to the brow, forehead, temple, or jaw. Pain may awaken the patient at night. Redness does not blanch with phenylephrine 2.5%, and the eye has a bluish hue in natural light by gross inspection. Vision is normal or mildly decreased. Photophobia is prominent because 30% have associated iritis. Tearing may be present, but there is no ocular discharge. Of patients with scleritis, 25% to 50% have underlying systemic disease, commonly connective tissue disorders such as rheumatoid arthritis, Wegener's granulomatosis, or relapsing polychondritis. Less commonly, the underlying disease is ankylosing spondylitis, systemic lupus erythematosus, polyarteritis nodosa, inflammatory bowel disease, gout, post–herpes zoster ophthalmicus, sarcoidosis, Lyme disease, tuberculosis, Reiter's syndrome, or microbial (bacterial or parasitic) infection. Hence, a thorough workup by rheumatology or an internal medicine specialist is needed.

Patients with scleritis require an ophthalmology evaluation because vision-threatening complications can occur. A team approach between the internist or rheumatologist

Figure 158-4 Hyphema.

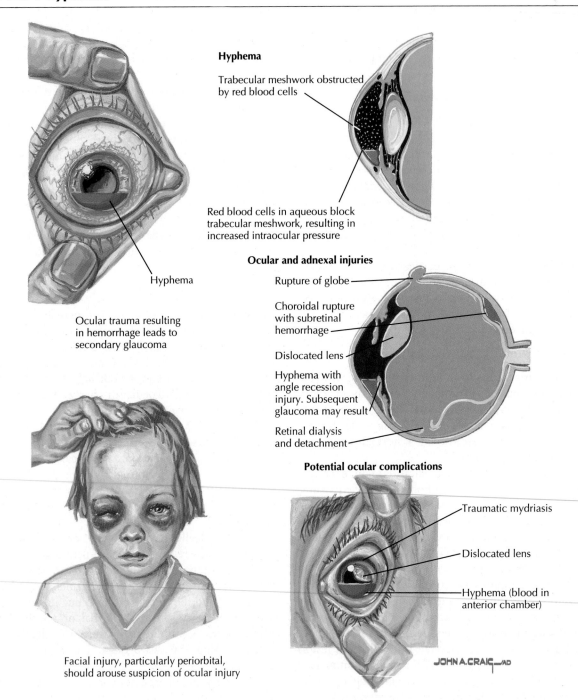

Hyphema

Trabecular meshwork obstructed by red blood cells

Red blood cells in aqueous block trabecular meshwork, resulting in increased intraocular pressure

Hyphema

Ocular trauma resulting in hemorrhage leads to secondary glaucoma

Ocular and adnexal injuries

Rupture of globe

Choroidal rupture with subretinal hemorrhage

Dislocated lens

Hyphema with angle recession injury. Subsequent glaucoma may result

Retinal dialysis and detachment

Potential ocular complications

Traumatic mydriasis

Dislocated lens

Hyphema (blood in anterior chamber)

Facial injury, particularly periorbital, should arouse suspicion of ocular injury

JOHN A. CRAIG—AD

and the ophthalmologist is essential to guide the systemic therapy. The ophthalmologist reports on the persistence of ocular inflammation and the internist or rheumatologist prescribes and monitors the systemic immunosuppressive agents.

Iritis

Iritis is inflammation of the anterior chamber. Its symptoms and signs include circumlimbal redness, eye pain, headache (described as a boring pain), photophobia, decreased vision, miosis (small pupil, may be fixed or poorly reactive due to posterior adhesions), hypopyon (layering of white blood cells in anterior chamber), and keratic precipitates. Possible associated conditions are arthritis, infections, sarcoidosis, urethritis, and inflammatory bowel disorders. If there is a history of blunt ocular trauma, onset of iritis may be delayed 1 to 3 days. Complications of iritis include elevated eye pressures, chronic angle-closure glaucoma, and cataract. Prompt referral to an ophthalmologist is indicated (Fig. 158-5).

Figure 158-5 Iritis.

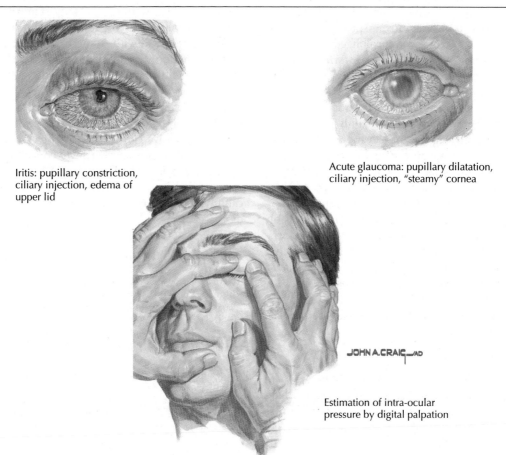

Iritis: pupillary constriction, ciliary injection, edema of upper lid

Acute glaucoma: pupillary dilatation, ciliary injection, "steamy" cornea

JOHN A.CRAIG—AD

Estimation of intra-ocular pressure by digital palpation

Acute Angle-Closure Glaucoma

Acute angle-closure glaucoma is due to an acute blockage of aqueous outflow from the eye. It is characteristically seen in persons with narrow angles who experience an acute rise in IOP when the pupil dilates. Predisposing factors include dim light, topical mydriatics, some systemic medications, and emotional stress. Typically unilateral, acute angle-closure glaucoma presents with severe ocular pain, eye redness, a mid-dilated nonreactive pupil, corneal cloudiness, blurred vision, frontal headache, haloes around lights, nausea, or vomiting. The affected eye may be firm or hard to palpation.

Optimal treatment requires referral to an ophthalmologist immediately. If treatment by the ophthalmologist is to be delayed by 1 hour or more, initial treatment should include the following:

- Pilocarpine 2%, 1 drop, then repeat in 15 minutes
- Timolol maleate 0.5%, 1 drop (if no asthma or heart failure)
- Apraclonidine 0.5%, 1 drop
- Acetazolamide, 500 mg by mouth or intravenously (if no contraindications)
- Consider intravenous mannitol 20% solution if no contraindications.

Avoiding Treatment Errors: Therapeutic Warnings

Topical Anesthetics

Topical anesthetics should never be prescribed or dispensed for analgesia. First, they inhibit the growth and healing of the corneal epithelium. Second, they eliminate the protective blink reflex and lead to exposure, dehydration, and epithelial breakdown, predisposing the patient to infection and corneal melting (ulcerative breakdown). Third, they create a punctate epitheliopathy that degrades vision. Finally, they have the tendency to be abused by health care workers and patients alike.

Topical Corticosteroids

Topical corticosteroid drops or ointments (alone or in combination with an antibiotic) should never be administered or prescribed by primary care physicians unless under the direct supervision and close monitoring of an ophthalmologist. This recommendation is based on several observations. First, topical corticosteroids inhibit wound healing, delay re-epithelialization, and can lead to perforation in neurotrophic conditions such as herpes zoster keratitis. They can mask inflammation, leading the patient to have a false sense of security, when in fact an ulcerative breakdown may be developing. Further, topical steroids potentiate fungal and herpes simplex keratitis and promote posterior subcapsular cataract formation with prolonged use.

Corticosteroid-induced glaucoma is a form of open-angle glaucoma caused by prolonged use of topical, periocular (including skin creams), inhaled, or systemic corticosteroids. About one third of all patients demonstrate some steroid responsiveness, but only a small percentage have a clinically significant elevation in IOP. The type and potency of the agent, the agent's route and frequency, and the intrinsic susceptibility of the patient all affect the duration of time before the IOP rises and the extent of the rise. If the pressure rise is severe, then asymptomatic optic nerve damage and permanent loss of vision can occur. Hence, when the primary care specialist prescribes systemic steroids, it is recommended that patients have their eye pressure monitored by an eye care specialist about every 3 months. When topical steroids are stopped, the IOP elevation may persist for many months. When systemic steroids are stopped, the IOP usually normalizes to pretreatment levels within a few days.

Future Referral Considerations

Any pupillary inequality in a patient with red eye is a warning sign of serious ocular disease and merits ophthalmology referral. Further, if vision is acutely and significantly decreased, then a diagnosis of conjunctivitis is extremely unlikely and ophthalmology referral is indicated. Finally, if a patient with red eye wears soft contact lenses, referral to ophthalmology is strongly advised because an experienced interpretation of slit lamp findings is crucial to differentiate complications. Close communication and cooperation between the primary care specialist and the ophthalmologist is essential for early diagnosis and successful management of the red eye.

Future Directions

Viral conjunctivitis (especially secondary to adenovirus) remains a common red eye problem and a substantial source of ocular morbidity. Viral isolation by culture is currently the gold standard for the direct detection of adenovirus, but results are typically not available for several days or weeks. As a consequence, cultures are of no use for clinical therapeutic decision making. Current polymerase chain reaction testing provides the accuracy needed for the diagnosis of adenoviral conjunctivitis but lacks the speed and simplicity needed for a useful and widely deployable office-based test. The medical community needs a rapid and highly accurate method to identify adenoviral conjunctivitis in a relatively short time span (with results available in less than 30 minutes) in order to be clinically useful and potentially curtail widespread community outbreaks. Furthermore, efficient topical antiviral agents need to be developed that can shorten the course of the viral disease,

reduce viral replication, and decrease viral antigen load. At the time of this writing, the only standard commercially available topical antiviral drop is trifluridine (Viroptic), which is preserved with thimerosal, a mercurial derivative that is commonly irritative. In a prospective masked trial involving trifluridine, there was no difference between the treatment group and the group receiving artificial tear therapy. Other tests under development lack sensitivity. Until these future advances are realized, health care professionals involved in direct patient contact who acquire epidemic keratoconjunctivitis will continue to be restricted in their activities for a minimum of 14 days. Adults should also avoid close contact during periods of high communicability, or at least during periods of significant ocular discharge.

Additional Resources

American Academy of Ophthalmology (Preferred Practice Patterns): Primary Angle Closure Glaucoma; Primary Open Angle Glaucoma; and Comprehensive Adult Medical Evaluation. San Francisco, American Academy of Ophthalmology, 2005.

These preferred practice guidelines available from the American Academy of Ophthalmology are designed to identify the characteristics and components of quality eye care based on the best available scientific knowledge. They are a good review of the titled subject and are often updated on a 5-year cycle.

Pavan-Langston D (ed): Manual of Ocular Diagnosis and Therapy, 5th ed. Philadelphia, Lippincott Williams & Wilkins, 2002.

This is a good resource for the primary care professional.

Tasman WJ, Jaeger EA (eds): Duane's Clinical Ophthalmology, revised ed. Philadelphia, Lippincott Williams & Wilkins, 2004.

This is a time honored, comprehensive, multivolume, detailed review of ophthalmology.

EVIDENCE

1. American Academy of Ophthalmology: External Disease and Cornea. Basic and Clinical Science Course, vol 8; Intraocular Inflammation and Uveitis, vol 9; and Glaucoma, vol 10. San Francisco, American Academy of Ophthalmology, 2006-2007, updated annually.
   The BCSC (Basic and Clinical Science Course) is a 14-volume series of foundational texts available from the American Academy of Ophthalmology that provide ophthalmologists with the core information needed to pass their board certification exam. Each volume is an excellent overview of the titled subject and includes many photos, diagrams, and instructive illustrations. They are not intended to be an exhaustive review, but rather an excellent source of core information.
2. American Academy of Ophthalmology (Preferred Practice Patterns): Bacterial Keratitis; Blepharitis; Conjunctivitis; Dry Eye Syndrome. San Francisco, American Academy of Ophthalmology, 2003 (Bacterial Keratitis: 2005).
   Preferred practice guidelines available from the American Academy of Ophthalmology are designed to identify the characteristics and components of quality eye care based on the best available scientific knowledge. They are a good review of the titled subject and are often updated on a 5-year cycle.
3. Albert DM, Jakobiec F (eds): Principles and Practice of Ophthalmology, 2nd ed. Philadelphia, WB Saunders, 2000.
   This is a good multivolume comprehensive ophthalmic reference.
4. Ang RT, Dartt DA, Tsubota K: Dry eye after refractive surgery. Curr Opin Ophthalmol 12(4):318-322, 2001.

This article reviews the dry eye syndrome that can complicate refractive surgery.

5. Avellon A, Perez, P, Aguilar JC, et al: Rapid and sensitive diagnosis of human adenovirus infections by a generic polymerase chain reaction. J Virol Methods 92(2):113-120, 2001.
   This article reviews PCR as a diagnostic test of adenovirus infections.

6. Bradford CA (ed): Basic Ophthalmology for Medical Students and Primary Care Residents, 8th ed. San Francisco, American Academy of Ophthalmology, 2004.
   This text is an excellent clinical reference for primary care providers.

7. Darougar S, Grey RG, Thaker U, McSwiggan DA: Clinical and epidemiological features of adenovirus keratoconjunctivitis in London. Br J Ophthalmol 67:1-7, 1983.
   This is a useful review of adenoviral ophthalmic infections.

8. Garg A, Pandey SK (eds): Textbook of Ocular Therapeutics, 2nd ed. New Delhi, Jaypee Brothers, 2003.
   Chapters are organized to serve as a quick reference to ophthalmologists, with attempts to include advances in ocular therapeutics.

9. Green SM: Tarascon Pocket Pharmacopoeia. Lompoc, CA, Tarascon Publishing, 2007.
   This handy quick reference guide was designed to assist the practitioner in prescribing pharmaceuticals outside of his or her specialty. It is subdivided by extremely useful specialty headings (such as ophthalmology and dermatology) and by pertinent categories (such as analgesics and antimicrobials). Both trade and generic listings are indexed alphabetically.

10. Johns KJ (ed): Eye Care Skills. CD-ROM. San Francisco, American Academy of Ophthalmology, 2005.
    This CD-ROM includes eight topical PowerPoint educational training presentations for non-ophthalmic physicians and allied health care providers. It is available from the American Academy of Ophthalmology, PO Box 7424, San Francisco, CA 94120-7424.

11. Kaiser PK, Friedman NJ, Pineda R (eds): The Massachusetts Eye and Ear Infirmary Illustrated Manual of Ophthalmology, 2nd ed. Philadelphia, WB Saunders, 2004.
    This handy full-color guide provides on-the-go clinical information. It includes hundreds of clinical photographs and is a concise general ophthalmology manual that is particularly useful for primary care providers and practitioners in training.

12. Kawana R, Kitamura T, Nakagomi O, et al: Inactivation of human viruses by povidone-iodine in comparison with other antiseptics. Dermatology 195:29-35, 1997.
    This article addresses the effectiveness of povidone-iodine as an antiseptic.

13. Krachmer JH, Mannis MJ, Holland EJ (eds): Cornea, 2nd ed, vol. 2. Philadelphia, Elsevier Mosby, 2005.
    This is the best comprehensive text available for cornea and external disease. It is well illustrated and referenced.

14. Kunimoto DY, Kanitkar KD, Makar MS (eds): The Wills Eye Manual: Office and Emergency Room Diagnosis and Treatment of Eye Disease, 4th ed. Philadelphia, Lippincott Williams & Wilkins, 2004.
    This excellent quick reference information manual covers nearly every ocular disorder commonly encountered in the office, hospital, or emergency room. Key differentiating features are emphasized to aid the practitioner in accurate diagnosis.

15. Lee BH, McLaren JW, Erie JC, et al: Reinnervation in the cornea after LASIK. Invest Ophthalmol Vis Sci 43(12):3660-3664, 2002.
    This article provides information on corneal denervation following LASIK.

16. Palay DA, Krachmer JH (eds): Ophthalmology for the Primary Care Physician, 1st ed. St. Louis, Mosby, 1997.
    This is a good single-volume ophthalmic reference for the primary care provider.

17. Romanowski EG, Yates KA, Gordon YJ: Topical corticosteroids of limited potency promote adenovirus replication in the Ad5/NZW rabbit ocular model. Cornea 21(3):289-291, 2002.
    This article addresses adenoviral infection as a complication of topical corticosteroids.

18. Tabery H: Corneal epithelial changes due to adenovirus type 8 infection. Acta Ophthalmol Scand 78:45-48, 2000.
    This article documents the pathology of adenovirus type 8 infection.

19. Toda I, Asano-Kato N, Komai-Hori Y, Tsubota K: Dry eye after laser in situ keratomileusis. Am J Ophthalmol 132(1):1-7, 2001.
    This article reviews dry eye complicating LASIK.

20. Ward JB, Siojo LG, Waller SG: A prospective, masked clinical trial of trifluridine, dexamethasone, and artificial tears in the treatment of epidemic keratoconjunctivitis. Cornea 12:216-221, 1993.
    This article reviews the effectiveness of trifluridine in epidemic keratoconjunctivitis.

21. Wilson SE, Ambrosio R: Laser in situ keratomileusis-induced neurotrophic epitheliopathy. Am J Ophthalmol 132(3):405-406, 2001.
    This article reviews neurotrophic epitheliopathy complicating LASIK.

Cataract Evaluation and Management

Introduction

Cataracts are the leading cause of blindness worldwide and may develop as a result of aging, various diseases, certain medical therapies, genetic anomalies, or can be congenital in origin. Because a normal lens is transparent, any opacification or discoloration in the lens capsule or substance, irrespective of its size or the amount of induced visual impairment, is technically defined as a cataract. However, clinically the term *cataract* is used to describe lens opacities that reduce or affect vision.

Most patients over the age of 70 are expected to have some degree of cataract formation or lenticular aging changes. Age-related cataract occurs in 50% of patients between the ages of 65 and 74 and in approximately 70% of patients over age 75. The prevalence roughly doubles each 10 years of age after age 30. In the United States, cataracts are the leading cause of decreased vision not correctable by spectacles and are the most common reason for Medicare beneficiary visits to ophthalmologists. Approximately 1.6 million cataract surgeries with the implantation of an intraocular lens are performed annually in the US. Cataract surgery is arguably one of the most successful surgical procedures in medicine (in terms of reducing morbidity and improving quality of life). A prospective study demonstrated that cataract removal was associated with a 50% drop in motor vehicle accidents. Furthermore, uncorrected chronic vision loss in elderly residential care patients has been associated with an increased risk of falls and tumbling-related injuries. The Framingham study noted an increase in the relative risk of hip fracture over 10 years with moderate vision impairment (1.54 if overall vision is reduced to 20/30 to 20/80) and severe vision loss (2.17 if vision is worse than 20/100). Moderate vision loss in only one eye demonstrated a relative risk of 1.94, which underscores the significance of maintaining good stereoscopic vision in potentially preventing falls and related fractures. When decreased vision affects a patient's activities of daily living by limiting the ability to drive safely, read, participate in hobbies such as knitting or other recreational activities, then the practitioner needs to consider referral for cataract evaluation after ensuring that other more serious causes of visual loss have not been overlooked.

Etiology and Pathogenesis

Etiologies of acquired cataract are shown in Box 159-1.

Clinical Presentation

Patients' symptoms include image blur initially followed by slowly progressive visual loss over months to years affecting one or both eyes (Fig. 159-1). Additionally, patients may experience glare in bright sunlight or at night (especially with oncoming car headlights), image ghosting or distortion, brownish or yellowish discoloration of objects, star-bursting around images, multiple images, mildly decreased color discrimination, and, sometimes, the surprising ability to read at near without glasses that were previously required. This unexpected visual improvement is referred to as *second sight* and is due to increased nuclear sclerosis of the lens, which leads to increased refractive power and a myopic shift. Reduced color perception, dyschromatopsia, does not occur to the same degree as in optic neuropathies, and a cataract alone does not cause a relative afferent pupillary defect as is observed in optic neuropathy. A patient's particular symptoms are based on the location and density of the lens opacification (Fig. 159-2).

Cataracts are most commonly classified by morphology but also can be classified according to maturity. The morphologic classification includes nuclear, subcapsular, cortical, and the uncommon "Christmas tree" cataract. The maturity classification scheme includes immature, mature, hypermature, and morgagnian cataracts.

Nuclear cataracts demonstrate yellow or brown discoloration of the central portion of the lens on slit lamp biomicroscopy. These typically blur distance vision more than near vision. They are typical of aging and generally take many years to advance and become visually significant. Cortical cataracts may involve the anterior, posterior, or equatorial cortex and are often asymptomatic until the changes extend into the optical axis. The opacities start as tiny clefts and small vacuoles between the outer lens fibers due to hydration of the cortex. With time, these progressively enlarge to become radial, gray, spoke-like opacities densest in the lens periphery. They remain visually asymptomatic until they encroach on the central pupillary region. Subcapsular cataract opacities may appear near the anterior lens capsule but more commonly appear near the posterior aspect of the lens, often forming a plaque-like opacification. They may develop rapidly over a few months or a few years and are best visualized by retroillumination against a red fundus reflex with slit lamp biomicroscopy or direct ophthalmoscopy. Posterior subcapsular cataracts may be associated with prolonged steroid use, diabetes, trauma, ocular inflammation, or radiation and commonly occur in patients younger than 50 years.

The maturity classification is not commonly used except to describe the most severe forms of lens opacification such as the mature, hypermature, or morgagnian cataracts. An immature cataract is one in which the lens is partially opaque and a posterior segment view is possible. In a mature cataract, the lens is completely opaque, and no posterior segment view is possible. A hypermature cataract is a mature cataract with a shrunken and wrinkled capsule due to leakage of water out of the lens. Total liquefaction of the outer cortex allows the hardened central nucleus to sink inferiorly and form a hypermature morgagnian cataract.

Diagnostic Approach

A patient with decreasing vision requires a complete examination to determine the etiology. Evaluation of the visual significance of a cataract must also include an evaluation of the optic nerve and retina to detect coexisting diseases that might also be the cause of decreased vision. For example, if patients complain of either difficulty with near work or metamorphopsia (waviness or distortion of central vision), special analysis is directed toward the central macula or fovea. If the lens is densely cataractous, the direct ophthalmoscope may not afford an adequate view of fundus detail to permit a reliable assessment of optic nerve or retinal pathology. If a patient has diabetic retinopathy in one eye and decreased vision in the contralateral eye, but the presence of a cataract precludes adequate examination of the fundus, a high level of suspicion for diabetes-related visual loss in the cataractous eye should be maintained. Removal of the cataract is often warranted to permit evaluation and possible treatment of retinal pathology, even if cataract surgery may not improve the patient's visual acuity.

The following are the appropriate steps for the patient's workup (Fig. 159-3):

1. *Obtain an accurate history of visual decline.* Ask about timing, onset, ocular disease, or poor vision in youth or young adulthood (before the cataract), side affected (unilateral or bilateral), ocular trauma, medications, and systemic diseases.

2. *Record a distance visual acuity using a Snellen chart.* Usually, vision is tested at a distance of 20 feet, or 6 meters, because 20 feet is equated with optical infinity for the eye. If a patient uses glasses for distance vision, these should be worn. The right eye is tested and recorded first, with the left eye occluded. The patient is asked to read the smallest line in which more than one half of the letters can be distinguished. Record the acuity measurement as a notation (e.g., 20/20) in which the numerator represents the distance at which the test is performed and the denominator represents the numeric designation for the line read. This is repeated for the left eye. If the vision is 20/40 or less in one or both eyes, have the patient view the chart through a pinhole occluder and record the results. The pinhole occluder may be used over the patient's glasses. If an illiterate E chart is used, have the patient point in the same direction in

Figure 159-1 Cataract Symptoms.

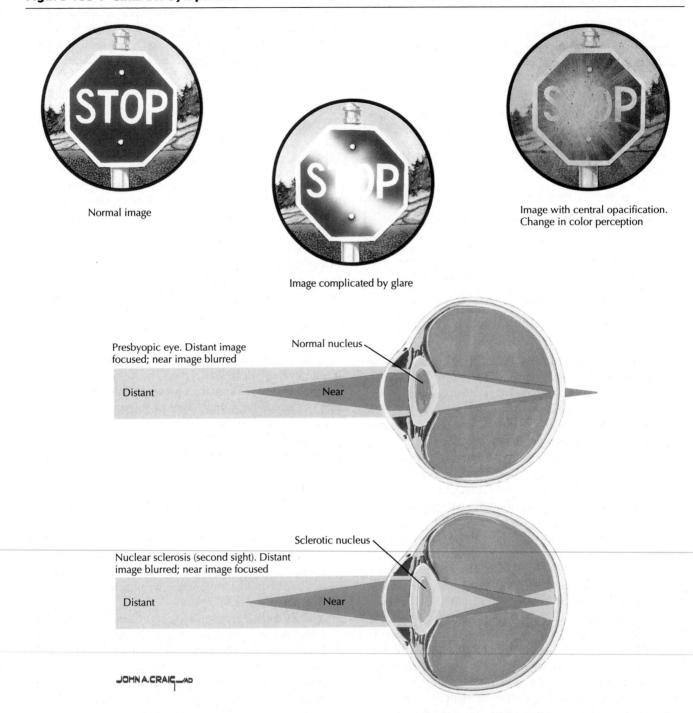

Normal image

Image complicated by glare

Image with central opacification.
Change in color perception

Presbyopic eye. Distant image
focused; near image blurred

Normal nucleus

Distant

Near

Sclerotic nucleus

Nuclear sclerosis (second sight). Distant
image blurred; near image focused

Distant

Near

JOHN A.CRAIG—AD

which the strokes of the E point. If the patient cannot see the largest Snellen letters, reduce the distance between the patient and the chart. Record the new distance as the numerator of the acuity designation (e.g., 10/400 or 5/400). If the patient is unable to see the big E (20/400) at 3 feet, hold up 1or 2 fingers and record the distance at which counting fingers is done accurately (e.g., CF at 1 ft). If the patient cannot count fingers, record whether vertical and horizontal hand motion can be accurately detected (e.g., HM at 3 ft). If hand motion cannot be detected, use a penlight to determine whether the patient can detect the direction or perception of light. Record as LP (light perception), either with projection (patient able to determine direction of the light source) or without projection, or NLP (no light perception).

Figure 159-2 Age-Related Cataracts.

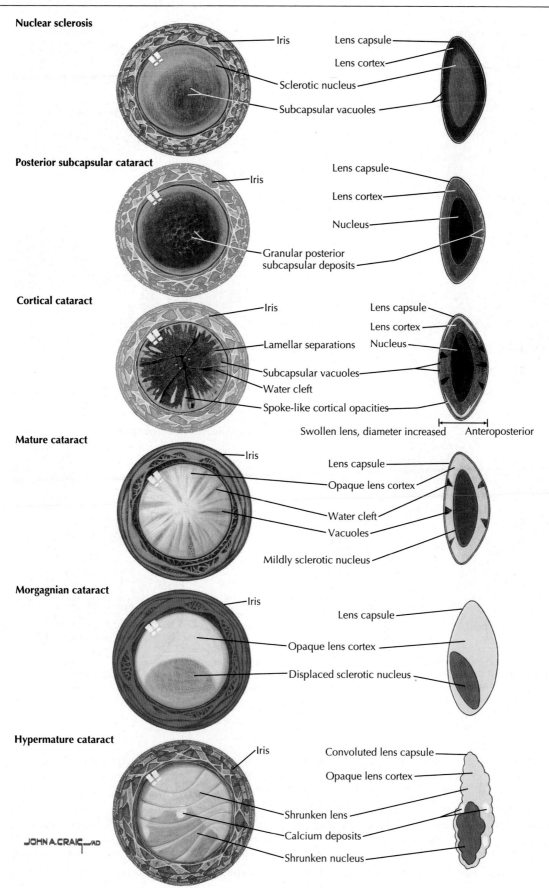

Nuclear sclerosis

Iris

Lens capsule
Lens cortex
Sclerotic nucleus
Subcapsular vacuoles

Posterior subcapsular cataract

Iris

Lens capsule
Lens cortex
Nucleus
Granular posterior subcapsular deposits

Cortical cataract

Iris
Lamellar separations
Subcapsular vacuoles
Water cleft
Spoke-like cortical opacities

Lens capsule
Lens cortex
Nucleus

Swollen lens, diameter increased   Anteroposterior

Mature cataract

Iris

Lens capsule
Opaque lens cortex
Water cleft
Vacuoles
Mildly sclerotic nucleus

Morgagnian cataract

Iris

Lens capsule
Opaque lens cortex
Displaced sclerotic nucleus

Hypermature cataract

Iris

Convoluted lens capsule
Opaque lens cortex
Shrunken lens
Calcium deposits
Shrunken nucleus

JOHN A.CRAIG—MD

Figure 159-3 Diagnostic Evaluation.

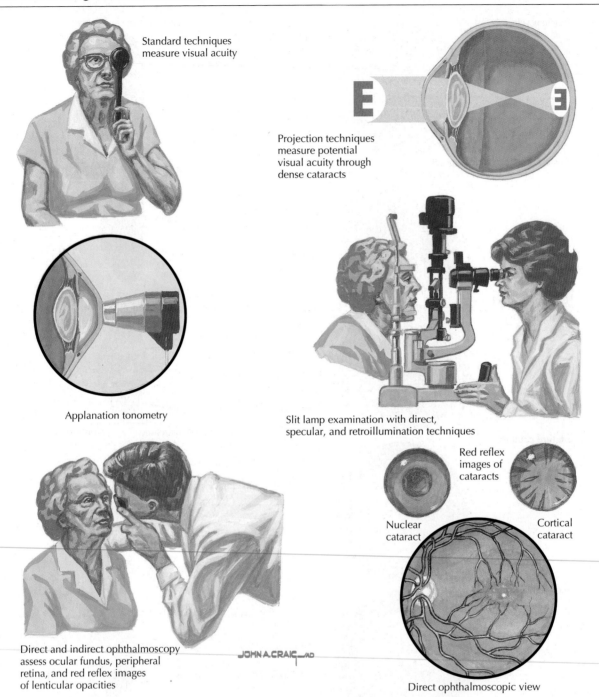

Standard techniques measure visual acuity

Projection techniques measure potential visual acuity through dense cataracts

Applanation tonometry

Slit lamp examination with direct, specular, and retroillumination techniques

Red reflex images of cataracts

Nuclear cataract

Cortical cataract

Direct and indirect ophthalmoscopy assess ocular fundus, peripheral retina, and red reflex images of lenticular opacities

JOHN A. CRAIG—MD

Direct ophthalmoscopic view

Near vision testing is performed only if distance testing is difficult or impossible (exam confined to bedside). It is only valid if the test is done at the recommended distance with a standard near-vision card. If the patient is older than 40 years, reading glasses may be necessary to accurately see the near card.

3. *Evaluate pupillary responses, being careful to use a bright-enough light source to rule out a relative afferent pupillary defect (RAPD).* Advanced cataracts do not produce a RAPD.

4. *Ophthalmoscopy of the lens, retina, and optic nerve.* Pharmacologic dilation of the pupils greatly facilitates this examination. Recommended agents include phenylephrine hydrochloride 2.5% and tropicamide 1%. Dilation should not be done if assessment of anterior chamber depth suggests a narrow angle or shallow chamber

because an attack of angle-closure glaucoma could result. The examiner's view into the eye should be about the same as the cataract patient's visual acuity (i.e., the physician's view into the patient's eye through the direct ophthalmoscope will be degraded to about the same extent as the patient's view out). Special attention is concentrated on the macula and fovea.

5. An eye physician will also routinely do a refraction to assess a patient's best corrected visual acuity and perform a slit lamp examination, which provides a magnified stereoscopic view of the cornea, lens, macula, and optic nerve. If the fundus is obscured by a dense cataract, B-scan ultrasonography is performed to rule out posterior-segment pathology such as a tumor or retinal detachment. Typically, cataract surgery is indicated if a patient has functional visual symptoms and visual acuity that has decreased to a level of 20/50 or worse by means of standard Snellen acuity testing or by Brightness Acuity Testing (BAT). BAT indicates the level of vision degradation in glare or sunlight conditions that may be experienced by a patient while driving a car. In addition, the potential acuity meter or laser interferometry can be used to estimate the patient's vision potential before cataract surgery when there is concurrent posterior segment disease. When cataract surgery is planned, additional measurements, including axial length of the eye (done with A-scan ultrasonography) and keratometry (corneal curvature readings), are required to determine the power of the desired intraocular lens to be implanted at the time of surgery. Specular microscopy and pachymetry are occasionally needed to evaluate the status and health of the corneal endothelium and its ability to withstand intraocular surgery (Fig. 159-4).

Management and Therapy

Optimum Treatment

Cataract surgery is typically performed to improve visual function or to facilitate examination and management of posterior segment disease (e.g., diabetic retinopathy, glaucoma) (Fig. 159-5). In some instances, cataract surgery is performed because the cataract itself is causing another ocular disease (e.g., uveitis, phacolytic glaucoma). Phacoemulsification or extracapsular cataract extraction techniques with the implantation of an intraocular lens are constantly evolving and improving and enjoy a success rate greater than 95% for *routine* cataract surgery.

If the patient declines cataract surgery, refractive errors are corrected by spectacles to the extent possible given the limitations involved. In some patients with small central opacities, a trial of mydriatic therapy (tropicamide 1% with or without phenylephrine 2.5% 3 times daily) may be temporarily helpful to allow the patient to view around the central visual axis opacities until the opacities enlarge

further in the rare instances when a patient cannot undergo surgery. Patients who decline surgery are generally reexamined yearly but may be reevaluated sooner if there is a symptomatic decrease in vision or if they have other associated ocular diseases.

After cataract extraction, about 50% of patients develop posterior capsule opacification (PCO) causing decreased vision, glare, or symptoms described as a film or smudging of vision. Some patients may complain of diminished contrast or even monocular diplopia. Treatment involves a painless opening of the posterior capsule with the neodymium : yttrium-aluminum-garnet (Nd : YAG) laser. Anterior capsule opacification or fibrosis can result in constriction of the capsular opening (phimosis) and may similarly require YAG capsulotomy enlargement. PCO treatment has led to the popular misconception among patients that a cataract can be removed with a laser (Fig. 159-6).

Perspective

The operating surgeon needs to do a preoperative examination on all patients contemplating cataract surgery and discuss the risks, benefits, alternatives, and potential complications. Using an eye model greatly facilitates a patient's understanding of the eye and how vision works. In an established university eye practice, greater than 50% of the time patients incorrectly guessed where the lens, cornea, retina, or optic nerve was located. Most patients do not know what a cataract is and are too embarrassed to admit this to their physician. Hence, it is very important never to assume that patients know the most basic ocular anatomy or understand the physiology of vision. Physicians need to remember that patients cannot begin to comprehend explanations or the need for surgical referral if they have not had a review of the most basic ocular anatomy and vision principles.

Avoiding Treatment Errors

Obtaining an accurate visual acuity measurement in each eye is essential because visual loss is a common symptom of cataracts as well as many other ophthalmic conditions. The patient's subjective description of the loss often correlates poorly with objective findings. Some patients with profound loss of vision present long after the onset of their symptoms and may have relatively minor complaints. Others may have minimal visual disturbance and overstate their complaints. Others inaccurately report the onset and timing of their symptoms. For example, a patient may have chronic ocular disease and vision loss in one eye, yet not recognize the problem until some vision decrease occurs in the other eye. The patient then mistakenly interprets the problem as acute bilateral visual loss because each eye is now being assessed individually. Hence, all reports of vision loss need to be evaluated.

Figure 159-4 Intraocular Lens (IOL) Studies.

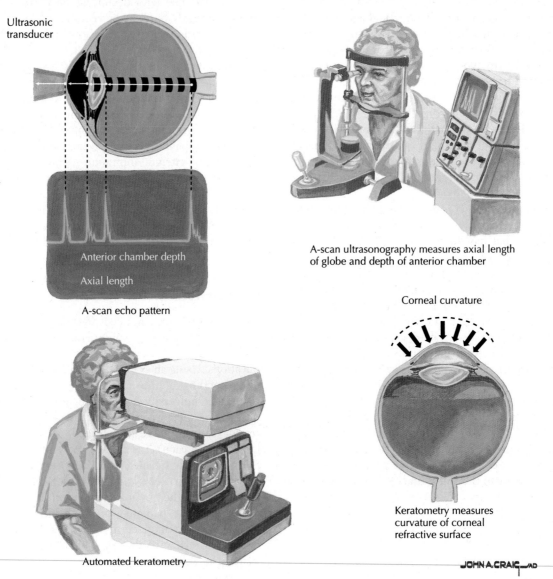

Ultrasonic transducer

Anterior chamber depth

Axial length

A-scan echo pattern

A-scan ultrasonography measures axial length of globe and depth of anterior chamber

Corneal curvature

Keratometry measures curvature of corneal refractive surface

Automated keratometry

JOHN A.CRAIG—AD

Accurate measurement of corneal curvature, anterior chamber depth, and axial length of globe needed to calculate correct power for IOL

If an RAPD is noted, visual loss is likely due to either optic nerve disease (e.g., optic neuritis or ischemic optic neuropathy) or widespread retinal damage. Only rarely is a mild RAPD seen with a cataract or dense ocular media opacity (e.g., vitreous hemorrhage in a diabetic patient). The primary care physician should also remember to perform confrontational visual field testing because hemianopic defects (blindness involving half of the visual field) may have normal visual acuity. Furthermore, color vision should be assessed because, if it is aberrant, optic nerve or central retinal disease is likely.

If transient vision loss is reported and tends to fluctuate with blinking, dry eye is likely the cause, and the ocular surface tear film needs to be improved. Other causes of visual fluctuation may be due to new-onset diabetes from elevations in blood glucose levels causing swelling of the lens and progressive nearsightedness. Uncorrected presbyopia should be suspected when patients older than 40 years report blurring when they change focus from distance to near, or vice versa. If a patient reports a 2- to 5-minute dimming of vision with either a curtain or cloud over the visual field, amaurosis fugax is likely, and a cardiovascular and neurologic assessment is indicated. Transient visual changes associated with carotid artery or vertebrobasilar insufficiency may be precipitated by movements of the neck, especially extension. Increased intracranial pressure may cause papilledema, resulting in transitory, bilateral visual blurring or loss lasting a few seconds. Finally, many systemic medications, particularly those associated with hypotension as a side effect, may cause transitory visual symptoms.

Figure 159-5 Phacoemulsification and Insertion of Flexible Intraocular Lens (IOL).

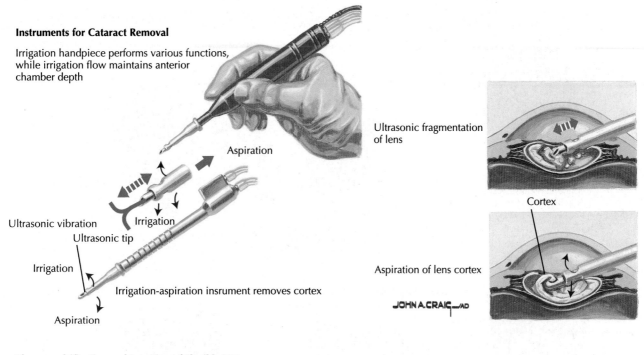

Instruments for Cataract Removal

Irrigation handpiece performs various functions, while irrigation flow maintains anterior chamber depth

Aspiration

Ultrasonic vibration

Irrigation

Ultrasonic tip

Irrigation

Aspiration

Irrigation-aspiration insrument removes cortex

Ultrasonic fragmentation of lens

Cortex

Aspiration of lens cortex

JOHN A. CRAIG—AD

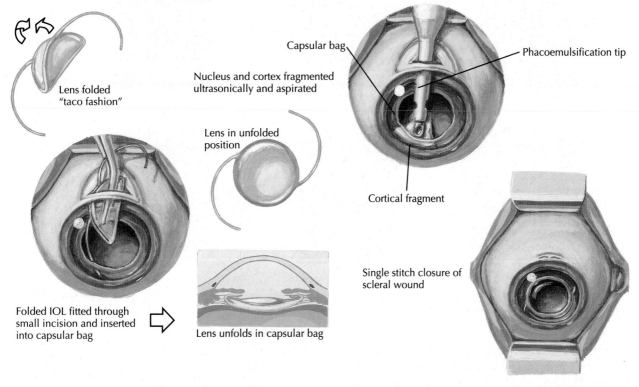

Phacoemulsification and Insertion of Flexible IOL

Lens folded "taco fashion"

Nucleus and cortex fragmented ultrasonically and aspirated

Lens in unfolded position

Capsular bag

Phacoemulsification tip

Cortical fragment

Folded IOL fitted through small incision and inserted into capsular bag

Lens unfolds in capsular bag

Single stitch closure of scleral wound

If the visual loss is painful and acute, immediate referral is necessary. Discussion and management of these common anterior segment and red eye problems are reviewed in Chapter 158. If the visual loss is chronic and progressive, cataracts or a refractive error is likely. However, the primary care specialist should remember that glaucoma, atrophic macular degeneration, and brain tumor are also possible causes. Brain tumor patients may report headache,

nausea upon awakening, or variable neurologic symptoms. It is important to remember that only rarely are ocular problems a source of headache.

Future Directions

Cataract surgery is arguably one of the most effective surgeries in medicine. Smaller incision sizes made possible by

Figure 159-6 Posterior Capsule Opacification.

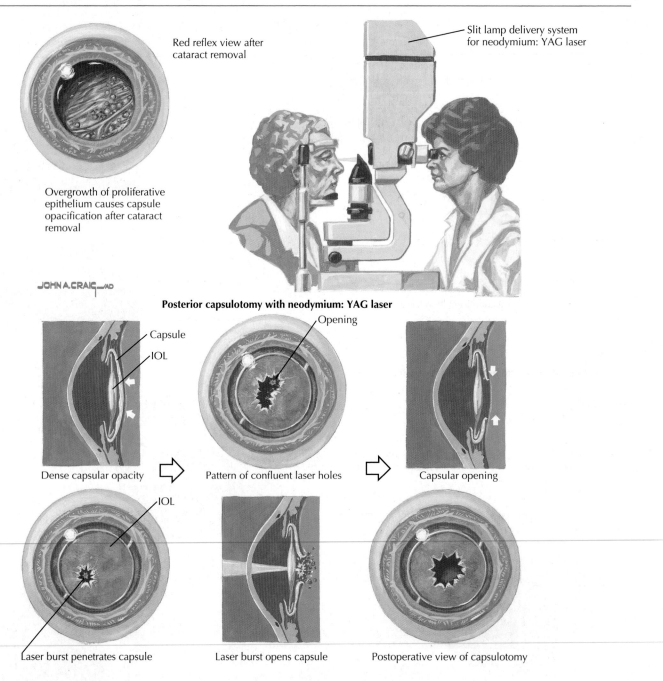

Red reflex view after cataract removal

Overgrowth of proliferative epithelium causes capsule opacification after cataract removal

Slit lamp delivery system for neodymium: YAG laser

JOHN A.CRAIG—AD

Posterior capsulotomy with neodymium: YAG laser

Capsule
IOL
Opening

Dense capsular opacity

Pattern of confluent laser holes

Capsular opening

IOL

Laser burst penetrates capsule

Laser burst opens capsule

Postoperative view of capsulotomy

improved lens fragmentation technologies along with advancements in intraocular lens technology continue to evolve and facilitate rapid visual recovery. Laser-adjusted intraocular lenses, multifocal lenses, and refractive lens implants are being refined and offer promise for the future to help correct myopia, hyperopia, astigmatism, and presbyopia. In fact, lens implantation technologic advances may one day compete favorably with laser vision correction surgery as an excellent alternative to spectacles or contact lenses for correction of refractive error.

Additional Resources

Johns KJ (ed): Eye Care Skills. CD-ROM. San Francisco, American Academy of Ophthalmology, 2005.

This CD-ROM includes eight topical PowerPoint educational training presentations for nonophthalmic physicians and allied health care providers. Available from the American Academy of Ophthalmology, PO Box 7424, San Francisco, CA 94120-7424.

Tasman WJ, Jaeger EA (eds): Duane's Clinical Ophthalmology, revised ed. Philadelphia, Lippincott Williams & Wilkins, 2004.

This text is a time-honored, comprehensive, multivolume and detailed review of ophthalmology.

EVIDENCE

1. Albert DM, Jakobiec F (eds): Principles and Practice of Ophthalmology, 2nd ed. Philadelphia, WB Saunders, 2000.

   This text is a good multivolume comprehensive ophthalmic reference.

2. American Academy of Ophthalmology: Section 2: Fundamentals and Principles of Ophthalmology. Basic and Clinical Science Course, Vol. 2; Section 3: Optics, Refraction and Contact Lens. Basic and Clinical Science Course, Vol. 2; and Section 11: Lens and Cataract. Basic and Clinical Science Course, Vol. 11. San Francisco, American Academy of Ophthalmology, 2006-2007; updated annually.

   The BCSC (Basic and Clinical Science Course) is a 14-volume series of foundational texts available from the American Academy of Ophthalmology that provide ophthalmologists with the core information needed to pass their board certification exam. Each volume is an excellent overview of the titled subject and includes many photos, diagrams, and instructive illustrations. They are not intended to be an exhaustive review, but rather an excellent source of core information.

3. Bradford CA (ed): Basic Ophthalmology for Medical Students and Primary Care Residents, 8th ed. San Francisco, American Academy of Ophthalmology, 2004.

   This is an excellent clinical reference for primary care providers.

4. Felson DT, Anderson JJ, Hannan MT, et al: Impaired vision and hip fracture. The Framingham Study. J Am Geriatr Soc 37(6):495-500, 1989.

   This article reviews the role decreased visual acuity plays in hip fracture risk.

5. Kaiser PK, Friedman NJ, Pineda R (eds): The Massachusetts Eye and Ear Infirmary Illustrated Manual of Ophthalmology, 2nd ed. Philadelphia, WB Saunders, 2004.

   This handy full-color guide provides on-the-go clinical information. It includes hundreds of clinical photographs and is a concise general ophthalmology manual that is particularly useful for primary care providers and practitioners in training.

6. Ledford JK (ed): Handbook of Clinical Ophthalmology for Eyecare Professionals, 1st ed. Thorofare, NJ, Slack, 2001.

   This text is a basic reference for eye care professionals in training.

7. Newell FW: Ophthalmology: Principles and Concepts, 8th ed. St. Louis, Mosby, 1996.

   This classic general ophthalmic text is very readable and a good overview of basic ophthalmology. It does not include the most current advances, however.

8. Palay DA, Krachmer JH (eds): Ophthalmology for the Primary Care Physician, 1st ed. St. Louis, Mosby, 1997.

   This is a good single-volume ophthalmic reference for the primary care provider.

9. Trobe JD: The Physicians' Guide to Eye Care, 2nd ed. San Francisco, American Academy of Ophthalmology, 2001.

   This text is a good guide to eye care.

10. Wilmer Eye Institute: Eye Diseases Alert: Primer on Cataracts. Johns Hopkins Health Alerts: Vision and Eye Care. Medletter Associates, LLC, 2006.

    This is a good primer on cataracts.

11. Wilmer Eye Institute: Eye Care Alert: Diagnosing Cataract Diseases. Johns Hopkins Health Alerts: Vision and Eye Care. Medletter Associates, LLC, 2006.

    This text provides helpful information about cataracts.

12. Yoder DM, Fowler WC, Lloyd AH: Anatomic eye models as a patient education modality. Ophthalmic Pract 17(1):12-18, 1999.

    This important article underscores the usefulness of eye models in explaining concepts of vision to patients.

Sandra M. Johnson

Glaucoma

Introduction

Glaucoma, a leading cause of blindness in the United States and the world, is defined as an optic neuropathy with characteristic visual field defects, often associated with elevated intraocular pressure (IOP). About 80,000 Americans are blind due to glaucoma, and it is the leading cause of blindness in African Americans. Primary open angle glaucoma (POAG) is the most common form in the United States, Europe, and Africa. Referral of at-risk patients for early detection and treatment is essential because only advanced and irreversible vision loss is recognized by an afflicted patient. Traditional risk factors include African American ancestry, family history of the disease, elevated intraocular pressure, and age. Ocular parameters such as baseline cup-to-disc ratio and corneal thickness are important in the assessment of the risk for damage from elevated eye pressure. Glaucoma is also associated with the vascular risk factors of diabetes mellitus and hypertension, as well as myopia, or nearsightedness. In the United States, the number of cases is increasing because of the aging population.

Etiology and Pathogenesis

As we age, IOP characteristically elevates within the normal range of 10 to 21 mm Hg. IOP level is primarily determined by the rate of aqueous production and the resistance to outflow across the trabecular meshwork (Fig. 160-1). Elevated IOP is usually caused by increased resistance to outflow, but glaucoma without elevated IOP does exist. Because patients can have both pressure-dependent and pressure-independent glaucoma, other poorly understood factors are thought to predispose optic nerve axons to damage. Factors under consideration include structure of the lamina cribrosa and optic nerve blood flow.

In primary open angle glaucoma, the anterior segment angle structures all appear normal. The angle, which is the junction between the cornea and iris, contains the trabecular meshwork. The use of special lenses in a technique referred to as *gonioscopy* provides a view of the angle. In secondary open angle glaucoma, the angle is open, but a cause of malfunction or obstruction is detected on examination or in the history. For example, corticosteroid use may increase resistance to outflow in about one third of patients, with a minority demonstrating a clinically significant rise in IOP. A higher percentage of glaucoma patients will demonstrate elevation of IOP. Elevated episcleral venous pressure, which may be idiopathic or secondary, causes secondary open angle glaucoma. Conditions leading to elevated episcleral venous pressure include carotid-dural fistulas, Sturge-Weber syndrome, thyroid ophthalmopathy, retrobulbar tumors, and superior vena cava syndrome. Trauma may also lead to malfunction of an open angle.

Closed or narrow angle glaucoma, as defined by gonioscopy, is the other major category of glaucoma and is more prevalent in Asian populations and increases with aging. This may result from baseline anatomic factors such as anterior chamber depth, which lead to pupillary block. Angle closure may also be secondary to a disease process that pulls the iris over the trabecular meshwork, such as neovascular glaucoma or to a process, such as an intraocular tumor, that pushes the iris forward causing obstruction of the angle.

Clinical Presentation

There is some variation in the presentation of glaucoma. In significant open angle glaucoma, the presentation is one of painless vision loss. A patient with acute angle closure glaucoma will present dramatically with a red painful eye, blurred vision, nausea, and vomiting (Fig. 160-2). Neovascular glaucoma secondary to retinal vascular disease such as proliferative diabetic retinopathy may present in much

Figure 160-1 Intraocular Pressure.

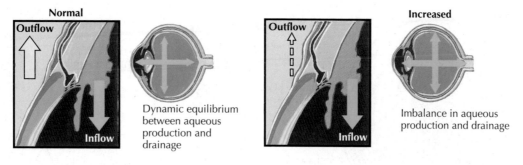

Normal

Outflow

Inflow

Dynamic equilibrium between aqueous production and drainage

Increased

Outflow

Inflow

Imbalance in aqueous production and drainage

Schiötz (indentation) tonometry

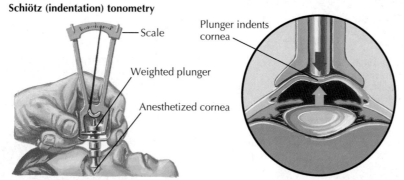

Scale

Weighted plunger

Anesthetized cornea

Plunger indents cornea

Intraocular pressure measured by amount of corneal indentation produced by known weight

Goldmann (applanation) tonometry

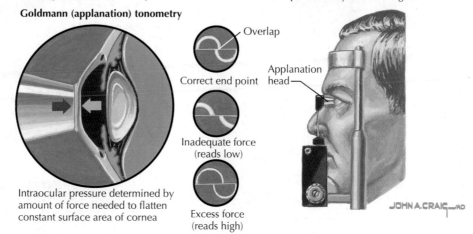

Overlap

Correct end point

Inadequate force (reads low)

Excess force (reads high)

Applanation head

Intraocular pressure determined by amount of force needed to flatten constant surface area of cornea

JOHN A. CRAIG─AD

the same as acute angle closure. Both of these types of glaucoma involve angle closure and acute elevation of IOP, which results in their shared symptoms. An infant may be born with a developmental defect in the outflow system leading to congenital glaucoma with characteristic photophobia, tearing, and a cloudy cornea.

Differential Diagnosis

The differential diagnosis of glaucoma based on a patient's symptoms is broad. A patient with painless loss of vision could have a retinal detachment, macular degeneration, cataract, or artery occlusion. The differential of acute angle closure is that of a red eye and includes conditions such as infectious keratitis, conjunctivitis, orbital cellulitis, and uveitis.

The differential diagnosis of glaucoma based on ocular examination includes other optic neuropathies, including acute ischemic optic neuropathy, toxic optic neuropathies such as vitamin B_{12} deficiency, and previous optic neuritis. Pituitary adenomas can cause optic nerve and visual field defects that resemble glaucoma. In general, other optic neuropathies display more pallor than cupping when compared with glaucoma, in which loss of ganglion cells leads to cupping or thinning of the neuroretinal rim much more than pallor.

Figure 160-2 Primary Closed Angle Glaucoma.

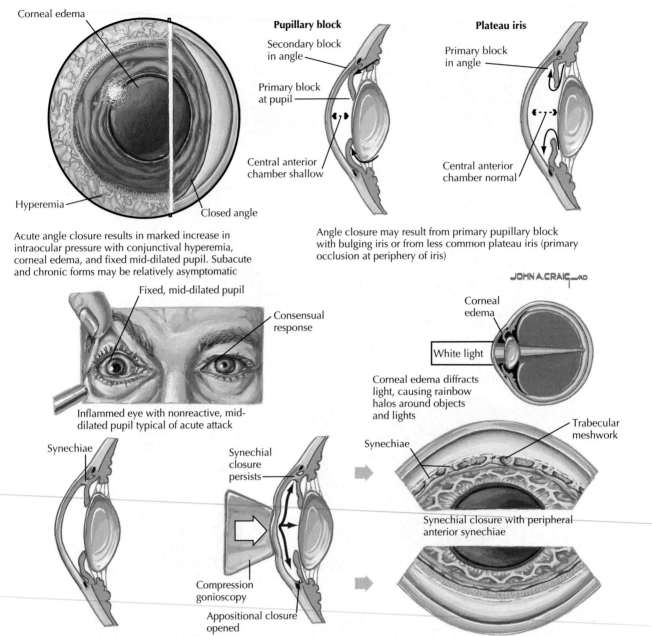

Corneal edema

Hyperemia

Closed angle

Acute angle closure results in marked increase in intraocular pressure with conjunctival hyperemia, corneal edema, and fixed mid-dilated pupil. Subacute and chronic forms may be relatively asymptomatic

Pupillary block

Secondary block in angle

Primary block at pupil

Central anterior chamber shallow

Plateau iris

Primary block in angle

Central anterior chamber normal

Angle closure may result from primary pupillary block with bulging iris or from less common plateau iris (primary occlusion at periphery of iris)

Fixed, mid-dilated pupil

Consensual response

Inflammed eye with nonreactive, mid-dilated pupil typical of acute attack

JOHN A. CRAIG—AD

Corneal edema

White light

Corneal edema diffracts light, causing rainbow halos around objects and lights

Synechiae

Synechial closure persists

Compression gonioscopy

Appositional closure opened

Long-term angle closure may result in synechiae that can permanently close angle. Compression gonioscopy differentiates appositional closure from synechial closure

Synechiae

Trabecular meshwork

Synechial closure with peripheral anterior synechiae

Appositional closure opened by compression gonioscopy

Diagnostic Approach

The diagnosis requires a complete eye examination, including gonioscopy and automated visual field testing. Gonioscopy determines whether the glaucoma is an open or a closed angle type or is likely to progress to a closed angle. Examination of the intraocular structures establishes whether a patient has a secondary cause of glaucoma. IOP is measured, and the optic nerve is closely inspected. Automated visual field testing is done to assess the function of the optic nerve and to measure relative scotomas not detected on confrontational visual field testing. Central corneal thickness is measured to help assess the risk for glaucomatous damage from elevated IOP. The type of correlation seen between the disc features and visual field findings are depicted in Figure 160-3.

Management and Therapy

Most glaucoma cases in the United States are treated medically with topical drug therapy (Table 160-1), followed by laser, then incisional surgery.

Figure 160-3 Optic Disc and Visual Field Changes in Glaucoma.

Early

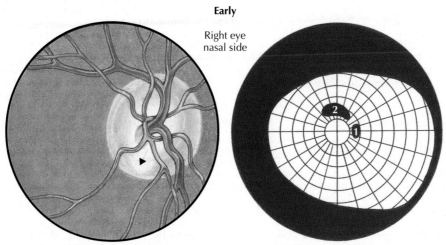

Right eye
nasal side

Funduscopy: notching of contour of physiologic cup in optic disc with slight focal pallor in area of notching; occurs almost invariably in superotemporal or inferotemporal (as shown) quadrants

Perimetry: slight enlargement of physiologic blind spot (1) development of secondary, superonasal field defect (2) which corresponds to nerve fiber damage in area of inferotemporal notching

Minimally advanced

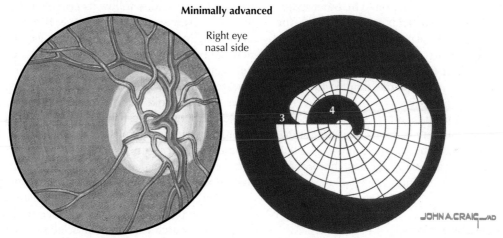

Right eye
nasal side

JOHN A.CRAIG—AD

Funduscopy: increased notching of rim of cup; thinning of rim of cup (enlargement of cup); deepening of cup; lamina cribrosa visible in deepest areas

Perimetry: localized constriction of superonasal visual field (3) because of progessive damage to inferotemporal fibers; superior arc-shaped scotoma (Bjerrum's scotoma) develops (4)

Optimum Treatment

The principle that guides the aggressiveness of treatment is the concept of target IOP. After the clinical assessment is complete, the ophthalmologist chooses a treatment goal that is the level of IOP that he or she believes will not cause further glaucomatous damage. This level of IOP is guided by many major National Eye Institute–sponsored glaucoma clinical trials. The overall choice of treatment involves noting the patient's medical history and taking quality-of-life issues into account. If a patient progresses, then the IOP target is reassessed. Progression versus stability is determined by visual field and optic disc evaluations.

For open angle glaucoma, laser trabeculoplasty is used when medical therapy fails. Its effect can last from months to years. Some patients receive multiple treatments per eye.

After the IOP has been decreased as much as possible by medications, the management of angle closure glaucoma is laser peripheral iridotomy (LPI). This procedure uses a laser to create an opening in the superior peripheral iris to permit an alternate route of aqueous flow from the posterior to anterior chamber. LPI, like trabeculoplasty, is an office procedure with minimal pain and a high success rate.

Patients who have failed both the maximum tolerated medical therapy and laser therapy often progress to incisional surgery. In the most common filtering surgery, trabeculectomy, a small hole is created through which aqueous fluid can flow from the anterior chamber to the subconjunctival space. The fluid collection, under the upper lid,

Table 160-1 Commonly Used Topical Medicines for Management of Glaucoma

Drug Class	Members	Major Systemic Interactions	Common Ocular Side Effects*
β Blockers	Timolol, metipranolol, carteolol, betaxolol, levobunolol	Bradycardia, exacerbate lung disease, depression, malaise	Nonspecific
Prostaglandin analogues	Latanoprost, travoprost, bimatoprost, unoprostone	Rare	Lash thickening or darkening, caution in inflammation, iris darkening
Topical carbonic anhydrase inhibitors	Dorzolamide, brinzolamide	Avoid in true sulfa allergy	Nonspecific
Adrenergic agents	Brimonidine, apraclonidine	Hypotension, sleepiness, dry mouth	Allergy, including lids

*All eye drops can cause ocular irritation manifested by foreign body sensation, hyperemia, or stinging or burning.

is termed a *bleb*. The bleb wall is thinned conjunctiva. In many circumstances, it is a thin barrier against penetration of bacterial organisms that can gain access to the intraocular space and cause a significant infection. Any patient who has had filtration surgery and in whom a red eye develops should have prompt evaluation. The other major filtering procedure, used for patients with or at risk for conjunctival scarring, involves placing a plate in a superior quadrant with a small tube from the plate placed into the anterior chamber. These devices, referred to as glaucoma shunts or tube implants, shunt aqueous fluid to the plate and then into the subtenon's space.

Developmental glaucoma in infants is a surgical disease like acute angle closure. Surgery is done after some stabilization of pressure by medications. Angle surgery, called *goniotomy* or *trabeculotomy*, is usually the first-line procedure and is curative in many infants.

Avoiding Treatment Errors

The most common source of treatment error in choosing topical therapy is disregard for the patient's medical history. One of the most frequent underlying misconceptions is that eye drops are not true medications that can be absorbed and produce systemic effects. The most common systemic interactions result from topical β-blocker use. Table 160-1 provides an overview of the major systemic interactions for the common classes of glaucoma medications.

Future Directions

Research in glaucoma includes identifying the genetics of the disorder and more elegantly understanding the process by which the trabecular meshwork develops sclerosis. Exploring whether there are optic nerve structural or vascular characteristics that are inherited and predispose individuals to glaucomatous optic neuropathy is especially important. One gene, present in about 16% of POAG patients, has been identified, and a screening test can now

be used clinically in select cases. Another large area of study is optic nerve head blood flow, which, given its anatomic location and number of vascular supplies, has been difficult to image to date. Technology to image the retinal ganglion cell layer and the optic nerve, to reliably screen for the disease, and to follow its progression more precisely and objectively continues to evolve. Progress continues in understanding the cascade leading to ganglion cell death, new knowledge that may lead to the development of new approaches to pharmacologic neuroprotection. This research overlaps with other neurobiology studies of diseases such as stroke and Alzheimer's disease.

Research on medical therapy will continue to focus on improving patient compliance through the development of simpler medical regimens and newer pharmacologic agents, such as the prostaglandin analogues, which only require daily dosing. Most other topical agents can now be used twice daily. The development of combination drugs is also likely to improve patient compliance and convenience. Surgical research includes procedures that shunt the aqueous past the obstruction of the trabecular meshwork into the Schlemm canal, a more physiologic route.

Additional Resources

American Academy of Ophthalmology Preferred Practice Pattern, 2005. Available at: http://www.aao.org/education/library/ppp/poag_new.cfm.
   This website outlines the current practice patterns in glaucoma care and serves as a reference for practitioners.
Cantor LB (ed): Section 10: Glaucoma. In Basic and Clinical Science Course 2002. San Francisco, American Academy of Ophthalmology, 2002.
   This paper was written by a panel of experts who review the literature and provide a summary of the current understanding of ophthalmic subspecialties such as glaucoma.

EVIDENCE

1. Colomb E, Nguyen TD, Bechetoille A, et al: Association of a single nucleotide polymorphism in the TIGR/MYOCILIN gene

promoter with the severity of primary open-angle glaucoma. Clin Genet 60(3):220-225, 2001.

This work on the myocilin gene has been the major breakthrough in the genetic study of glaucoma.

2. Jampel HD, Quigley HA, Kerrigan-Baumrind LA, et al: Risk factors for late-onset infection following glaucoma filtration surgery. Arch Ophthalmol 119:1001-1008, 2001.

These authors reviewed 131 cases of bleb-associated endophthalmitis to identify risk factors for infection. The risks included use of mitomycin during surgery and continued use of topical antibiotics after surgery.

3. Kass MA, Heuer DK, Higgenbotham EJ, et al: The Ocular Hypertension Treatment Study: A randomized trial determines that topical ocular hypotensive medication delays or prevents the onset of primary open-angle glaucoma. Arch Ophthalmol 120(6):701-713, 2002.

This study identifies risk factors for the development of glaucoma in patients with elevated intraocular pressures. It provided evidence on the utility of central corneal thickness and cup-to-disc ratio assessments in assessing risk for glaucoma in these patients.

4. Sommer A, Tielsch JM, Katz J, et al: Relationship between intraocular pressure and primary open angle glaucoma among white and black Americans. The Baltimore Eye Survey. Arch Ophthalmol 109(8):1090-1095, 1991.

This study illustrates the increased risk for glaucoma with black race and age. It also shows that intraocular pressure measurements alone are not definitive in the diagnosis of glaucoma.

Diabetic Retinopathy

Introduction

Diabetic retinopathy is the most significant cause of visual loss in working-age adults in the United States. Nearly all persons who have had diabetes for 20 years or more develop diabetic retinopathy, a startling statistic because as many as 16 million patients in the United States are affected with diabetes mellitus. Diabetic retinopathy becomes more common with increased duration of the disease. The Early Treatment Diabetic Retinopathy Study (ETDRS) developed and popularized a classification scheme that recognizes that diabetic retinopathy goes through a number of discrete stages until it reaches a severity leading to visual loss. The earliest stages are termed *nonproliferative retinopathy*. These stages can be subdivided into mild, moderate, moderately severe, and severe. *Proliferative retinopathy*, a later stage, occurs when abnormal blood vessels grow on the surface of the retina or the optic nerve and can be differentiated into early and high-risk phases.

Etiology and Pathogenesis

The precise sequence of events in diabetic retinopathy is complex and, despite multiple studies, is not entirely understood. Hyperglycemia is the major driving force in the development of the many abnormalities that ultimately result in visual loss in untreated patients. With increased blood glucose, hemoglobin A1C is increased, as is growth hormone. Intracellular sorbitol increases. Basement membrane thickening is an early pathologic change and can be seen in the ciliary body epithelium. Capillary basement membranes develop thickening, and there is a selective loss of the mural cells (pericytes). Endothelial cells proliferate in some capillaries, whereas others become acellular. With the progression of disease, some areas deteriorate to a nonperfused capillary bed consisting of acellular strands of thickened basement membrane. Microaneurysms consisting of outpouchings of the capillary wall develop in other areas of the retina. Eventually microaneurysms become hypercellular, obliterated, and sometimes thrombosed.

Blood flow within the retina changes as the disease progresses. Retinal blood vessels are not directly regulated by the autonomic nervous system and instead are governed by an autoregulation process that is lost as the disease progresses. Systemic hypertension often further damages the retinal vascular system and is associated with an increased risk for diabetic retinopathy incidence, progression, and visual loss.

As focal hypoxia occurs, two significant concomitant processes begin to involve the retina. Vascular endothelial growth factor (VEGF) contributes to a breakdown of the blood retinal barrier in early diabetic retinopathy. Of special note from the therapeutic standpoint (see later), VEGF kinase inhibitors have been shown to decrease this VEGF-induced blood retinal barrier breakdown. Increased permeability of the vascular capillaries leads to *macular edema*. When this edema involves the central macular area, mild to moderate visual loss begins to occur.

The second major process is the development of abnormal new blood vessels called *proliferative diabetic retinopathy* or neovascularization. These new vessels are most often seen on the optic nerve and on the retinal surface but in extreme cases may grow on the iris and over the trabecular meshwork, producing neovascular glaucoma in eyes with marked retinal ischemia. VEGF has been shown to be sufficient for the development of retinal neovascularization, and induced expression of VEGF in the retina results in neovascularization. However, when VEGF kinase inhibitors are administered in an experimental setting, retinal neovascularization is blocked.

Figure 161-1 Diabetic Retinopathy.
IRMA, intraretinal microvascular abnormalities.

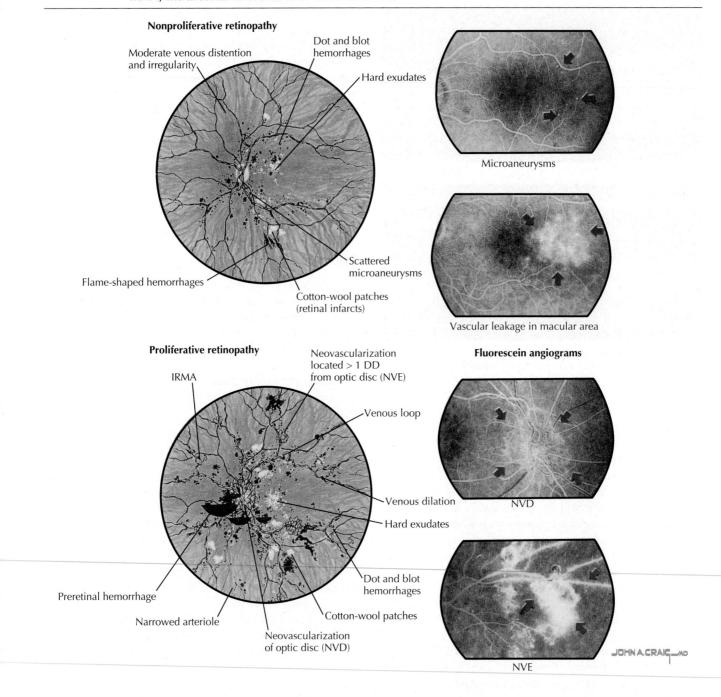

Nonproliferative retinopathy

Moderate venous distention and irregularity
Dot and blot hemorrhages
Hard exudates
Scattered microaneurysms
Flame-shaped hemorrhages
Cotton-wool patches (retinal infarcts)

Microaneurysms

Vascular leakage in macular area

Proliferative retinopathy

IRMA
Neovascularization located > 1 DD from optic disc (NVE)
Venous loop
Venous dilation
Hard exudates
Dot and blot hemorrhages
Cotton-wool patches
Neovascularization of optic disc (NVD)
Narrowed arteriole
Preretinal hemorrhage

Fluorescein angiograms

NVD

NVE

JOHN A. CRAIG—AD

Clinical Presentation and Diagnostic Approach

The earliest manifestations of diabetic retinopathy are microaneurysms or small round red dots in the retina created by outpouchings of the capillary walls (Fig. 161-1). Injection of a fluorescent dye into the antecubital veins allows photographs of the inner eye to light up these areas of microaneurysms and demonstrate that more are present than can be seen through simple fundus ophthalmoscopic examination. Small intraretinal hemorrhages called *dot-and-blot hemorrhages* are the next manifestation. These circular hemorrhages tend to occur in the outer plexiform layer where bipolar and Mueller cells are oriented vertically. Closer to the optic nerve where the nerve fiber layers are tightly packed, the hemorrhages may be more superficial and, by following the nerve fiber layer, assume a flame-shaped appearance.

As capillary permeability breaks down further, fluid accumulates within the retina, typically in the middle

Figure 161-2 Ocular Coherence Tomograms.

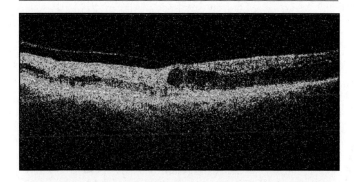

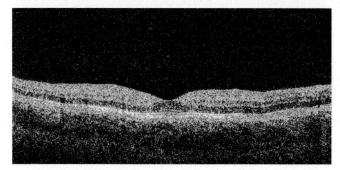

An ocular coherence tomography image of a macula with diabetic macular edema (*top*) and a normal macula (*bottom*) for comparison.

retinal layers, and is seen ophthalmoscopically as a thickening of the retina. When the thickening involves the macula, the central area takes on a cystic appearance (*cystoid macular edema*) and is associated with mild to moderate visual loss. Greater degrees of altered permeability cause deposition of lipoprotein in the middle retinal layers leading to the formation of *hard exudates*, patchy yellow accumulations within the retina often associated with areas of thickening and edema. These macular changes are seen dramatically using a new retinal imaging device, called *ocular coherence tomography* (Fig. 161-2).

At the later stages (often associated with severe systemic hypertension), focal nerve fiber layer infarcts called *cotton-wool patches* (soft, white, superficial changes in the retina with fluffy indistinct borders) develop. When a fluorescein angiogram is performed, these areas correspond to areas of capillary obstruction and capillary dropout. As ischemia develops, the veins take on multiple focal areas of irregularity called *beading*. Arteries become narrowed, and on a gross level, loops may occur in the major veins. Smaller intraretinal changes at the small vessel and capillary level consist of dilation of microvasculature, referred to as *intraretinal microvascular abnormalities* (IRMA).

The development of hypoxia then leads to elaboration of vasogenic factors including VEGF, which stimulates the formation of neovascular tufts on the retinal surface and optic nerve surface (Fig. 161-3). These small new abnormal vessels break through the internal limiting membrane of the retina and begin to grow on the posterior hyaloid face using the hyaloid as a scaffold. These vessels are fragile and are prone to rupture and hemorrhage, particularly in association with vitreous traction. As vessels grow more exuberantly, they begin to be accompanied by fibrous tissue in their development. The hyaloid then contracts, elevating the fibrovascular tissue and sometimes exerting sufficient force on the retina to produce *traction retinal detachment*. Vision may be lost either from vitreous hemorrhage, blocking access of visual images to the retina, or by the detachment of the macula by the fibrovascular proliferation. Typically, many of these findings are in the fundus at one time. The precise findings, their severity, and their extent throughout the fundus are combined into the grading scale that is used in clinical studies.

Management and Therapy

Optimum Treatment

Management of diabetic retinopathy encompasses three strategies: (1) systemic control of diabetes and its complications to prevent the occurrence and progression of diabetic retinopathy; (2) regular ocular examinations to detect lesions that become vision threatening; and (3) direct ocular management, including laser photocoagulation, pars plana vitrectomy surgery, and local administration of therapeutic agents through the vitreous cavity or sub-Tenon's space.

The Diabetes Control and Complications Trial (DCCT) and the United Kingdom Prospective Diabetes Study (UKPDS) demonstrated conclusively that intensive glycemic control in patients with type 1 and type 2 diabetes has beneficial effects for preventing vision loss associated with diabetic retinopathy. Patients placed on intensive insulin therapy in the DCCT had a slight initial worsening of retinopathy that reversed after 18 months. Subsequently, patients with intensive glycemic control fared considerably better on every measurement, with a 76% risk reduction on onset of retinopathy, a 63% reduction of progression of retinopathy, and a 56% reduction in need for laser treatment. These benefits persisted 4 years after the period when intensive control was instituted. In a study of type 2 patients, the UKPDS demonstrated a reduction in aggregate microvascular end points with improved glycemic control.

An association between hypertension and diabetic retinopathy has been demonstrated in multiple studies. In the UKPDS, intensive blood pressure control significantly reduced the need for photocoagulation, reduced the risk for diabetic retinopathy progression, and reduced moderate visual loss. Elevated total cholesterol, high-density lipids, and triglycerides have been associated with the faster development of hard exudates in the retina; more extensive hard exudates are correlated with a higher risk for moderate visual loss. Definite improvement of retinopathy by administration of lipid-lowering agents has not

Figure 161-3 Complications of Proliferative Diabetic Retinopathy.

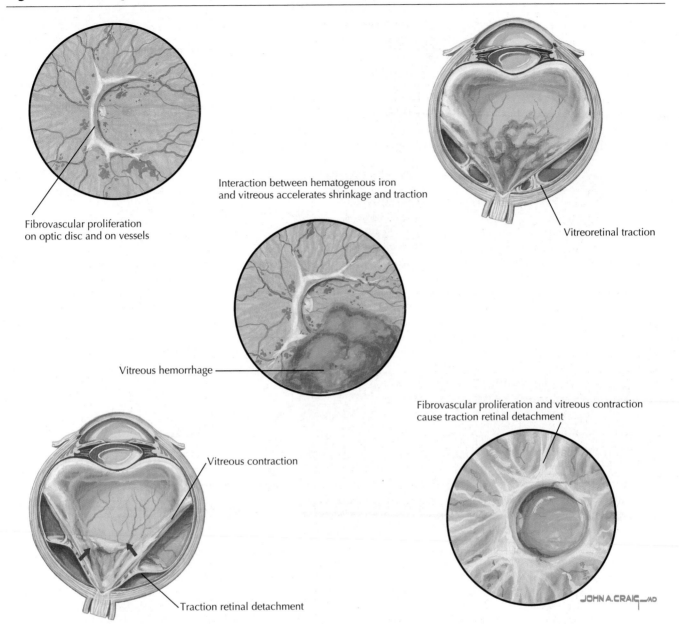

Fibrovascular proliferation on optic disc and on vessels

Interaction between hematogenous iron and vitreous accelerates shrinkage and traction

Vitreoretinal traction

Vitreous hemorrhage

Fibrovascular proliferation and vitreous contraction cause traction retinal detachment

Vitreous contraction

Traction retinal detachment

JOHN A.CRAIG

been demonstrated but appears reasonable in view of the positive effects on cardiovascular morbidity.

Regular ocular examinations are important to detect diabetic retinopathy in its early stages and allow early intervention when high-risk characteristics occur. Earlier intervention has a strong correlation with a better prognosis for avoiding moderate visual loss. Numerous studies indicate that only 60% of the American population is being appropriately screened at regular intervals.

Laser photocoagulation performed as an office procedure is the mainstay of treatment of proliferative diabetic retinopathy and diabetic macular edema (Fig. 161-4). Using either a fundus contact lens or indirect ophthalmoscopy, brief laser pulses are emitted and focused onto the retina. The laser acts by inducing thermal damage (a "burn") after absorption of the energy by tissue pigments. In the case of argon wavelengths, the light energy is absorbed by hemoglobin pigment and hence acts at the level of small vascular structures. When treating microaneurysms, this burn seals the microaneurysm and decreases the leakage. Most energy from krypton, argon, and diode wavelengths is absorbed by melanin in the retinal pigment epithelium and by choroidal melanocytes.

When abnormal blood vessels proliferate on the optic nerve surface or the retinal surface, a panretinal or full scatter photocoagulation is carried out. In this treatment, about 1200 to 1600 laser burns are diffusely placed throughout the peripheral retina avoiding the nerve, the macula,

Figure 161-4 Photocoagulation.

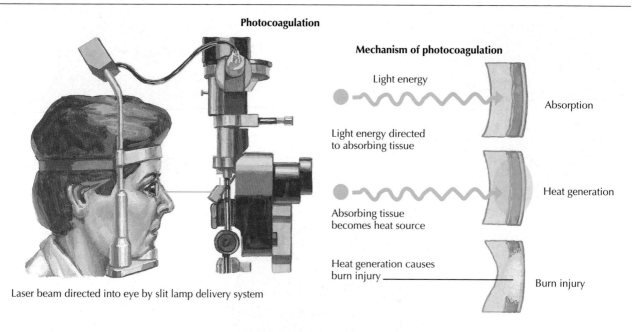

Photocoagulation

Laser beam directed into eye by slit lamp delivery system

Mechanism of photocoagulation

Light energy → Absorption

Light energy directed to absorbing tissue

Absorbing tissue becomes heat source → Heat generation

Heat generation causes burn injury → Burn injury

Wavelength (nm)	Light energy emission by source (nm)				Light energy absorption		
	Xenon	Argon	Ruby	Krypton	Hemoglobin	Xanthophyll	Melanin
Ultraviolet <400							
Violet 400–450							
Blue 450–480				478			
B-green 480–510		488					
Green 510–550		514		530			
Y-green 550–565							
Yellow 565–590				568			
Orange 590–630							
Red 630–700			694	647			
Infrared >700							

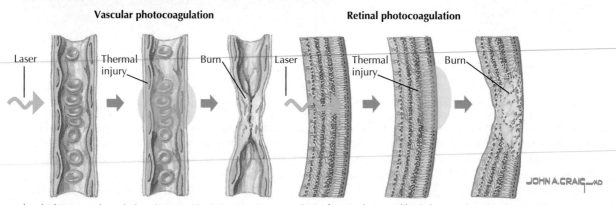

Vascular photocoagulation

Laser → Thermal injury → Burn

Abnormal or leaking vessels sealed or destroyed by light wavelengths absorbed by hemoglobin (argon, 514 nm, or krypton, 568 nm)

Retinal photocoagulation

Laser → Thermal injury → Burn

Retinal areas destroyed by light wavelengths absorbed by melanin and retinal xanthophyll (argon, 488 nm and 514 nm)

JOHN A. CRAIG—AD

and large vessels (Fig. 161-5). Burn sizes range from 200 to 500 μm in diameter. It is possible that by ablating a large area of ischemic retinal tissue in this manner, less VEGF is secreted, thereby decreasing the stimulus for neovascularization. The risk for visual loss correlates with the number of risk factors present. When one or two risk factors are present, the 2-year risk for severe visual loss is reduced from 7% to 3%. When three or four risk factors are present, the risk for severe visual loss is reduced from 26% to 11%.

Figure 161-5 Panretinal Photocoagulation.
NVD, neovascularization of disc.

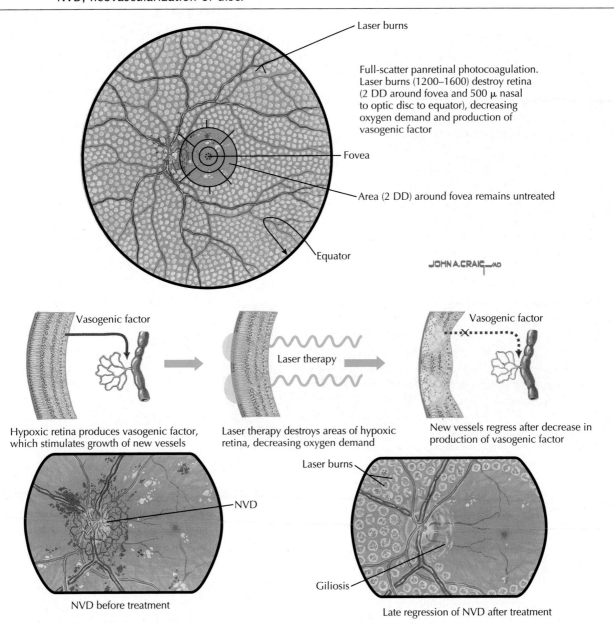

Laser burns

Full-scatter panretinal photocoagulation. Laser burns (1200–1600) destroy retina (2 DD around fovea and 500 μ nasal to optic disc to equator), decreasing oxygen demand and production of vasogenic factor

Fovea

Area (2 DD) around fovea remains untreated

Equator

JOHN A.CRAIG—AD

Vasogenic factor

Laser therapy

Vasogenic factor

Hypoxic retina produces vasogenic factor, which stimulates growth of new vessels

Laser therapy destroys areas of hypoxic retina, decreasing oxygen demand

New vessels regress after decrease in production of vasogenic factor

NVD

NVD before treatment

Laser burns

Gliosis

Late regression of NVD after treatment

Clinically significant diabetic macular edema has been defined as (1) retinal thickening within 500 μm of the fovea, (2) hard exudates associated with thickening within 500 μm of the fovea, or (3) a disc area of edema within one disc diameter of the fovea. The decision for treatment is made on the basis of the thickening noted on ophthalmoscopic examination (see Fig. 161-6). Treatment is then directed at leaking microaneurysms within 500 μm of the center of the fovea. Laser burn size is generally 50 to 100 μm. Most physicians now will treat even 20/20 eyes if the position of the aneurysm seems favorable and the risk for treatment can be minimized. Appropriate and timely laser photocoagulation for macular edema can reduce the risk for severe visual loss by more than 95% and reduce the risk for moderate visual loss from 25% to 12%.

Although laser photocoagulation has dramatically improved visual outcome and decreased the need for vitrectomy in diabetic patients, there remains a subset of patients in whom diabetic retinopathy persists or progresses. The need for further improvement has led to widespread local administration of steroid and anti-VEGF compounds. Ranibizumab and bevacizumab are anti-VEGF agents initially approved for macular degeneration and colorectal cancer, respectively. Reports of rapid resolution of neovascularization have generated increased off-label use of these agents. A small volume (50 μL) of the

Figure 161-6 Focal Photocoagulation for Macular Edema.

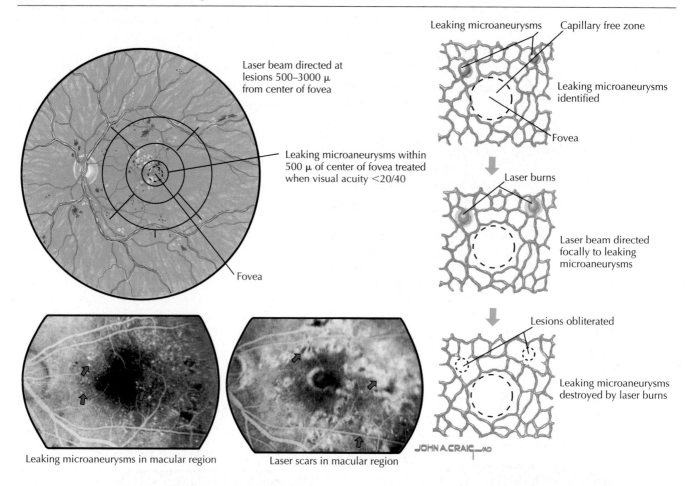

Laser beam directed at lesions 500–3000 μ from center of fovea

Leaking microaneurysms within 500 μ of center of fovea treated when visual acuity <20/40

Fovea

Leaking microaneurysms   Capillary free zone

Leaking microaneurysms identified

Fovea

Laser burns

Laser beam directed focally to leaking microaneurysms

Lesions obliterated

Leaking microaneurysms destroyed by laser burns

JOHN A. CRAIG—AD

Leaking microaneurysms in macular region

Laser scars in macular region

agent is injected directly into the vitreous cavity using a small-gauge needle.

Triamcinolone acetonide has grown in popularity for treatment of diabetic macular edema refractory to laser photocoagulation. This steroid has been injected directly into the vitreous cavity as well as into the sub-Tenon's space, adjacent to the posterior scleral wall. Intravitreal placement of long-acting steroid depots are also currently under investigation. Several multicenter, randomized control clinical trials are underway to assess these agents.

When early treatment of proliferative disease is not carried out or is ineffective, vitreous hemorrhage or traction retinal detachment may develop. Surgical intervention is then indicated with the goals of removing the blood, reattaching the retina, and arresting the proliferative process. Specific instrumentation has been developed that can cut and suck out the blood and vitreous from the internal eye under microscopic control. A variety of scissors, knives, and other instruments have been devised to cut proliferative tissue away from the retina, allowing retinal reattachment. When necessary, intraocular photocoagulation can be performed once the retina is visualized and reattached. Because of the success in controlling the proliferative process, surgical intervention is sometimes

indicated before vision is lost when fibrovascular proliferation is growing in a particularly aggressive fashion.

Avoiding Treatment Errors

The most common treatment error in diabetic retinopathy is delay in diagnosis and treatment. It is therefore imperative that patients at risk for complications from diabetic retinopathy be evaluated at regular intervals by an experienced ophthalmologist. Worsening of macular edema and a decrease in vision can follow either panretinal photocoagulation or focal laser treatment. It is customary to perform macular laser first and then to wait about 1 month before performing panretinal ablation to reduce the likelihood of this risk. Wrong-sided procedures may be avoided by having efficient systems in place to ensure correct-sided laser or vitrectomy surgery. A thorough informed consent process should be undertaken before any procedure.

Future Directions

Future directions in the management of diabetic retinopathy will center on improved early detection, medical management of the systemic condition, development of medications that may control vascular proliferation and vascular permeability, and improved laser and surgical strategies particularly for macular edema. Efforts are underway to ensure that a higher percentage of diabetic patients are screened so that early disease may be detected and managed properly. These include mandated screening programs by health maintenance organizations and special screening initiatives put forward through a collaboration of Medicare and eye care provider organizations. Tele-medicine screening initiatives are being studied in which photographs may be taken through nondilated pupils and referred to expert reading centers where detection of retinopathy can be achieved without an actual dilated examination by a trained ophthalmic examiner.

Improved cooperation between internists and ophthalmologists will undoubtedly lead to better management of diabetic retinopathy. The end-organ effects of hypertension and elevated lipids may be viewed directly in the fundus examination by the ophthalmologist, who can then emphasize to the patient and the treating physician the importance of better control of these parameters. Patients will often value the advice of a second physician who reinforces the diabetic care provider's recommendations regarding the importance of good blood glucose control.

Compounds that block the protein kinase C pathways may reduce the progression of retinopathy to the proliferative stage. Anti-VEGF compounds reduce vascular permeability and continue to be studied in clinical trials. Macular edema remains the main cause of visual loss from diabetic retinopathy, and new strategies are being devised for its management. At this time, direct injection of intraocular steroids, implantation of intraocular steroid devices, sustained-release intraocular steroid devices, and surgery removing the internal hyaloid membrane are investigational approaches to achieve better control and reduction of macular edema.

Additional Resources

American Diabetes Association: Diabetic retinopathy: Position statement. Diabetes Care 21:157-159, 1997.
This is the position statement from the American Diabetes Association.
Diabetic Retinopathy Clinical Research Network. Available at: http://public.drcr.net. Accessed August 22, 2006.
A multicenter, collaborative research group participate in multiple trials concerning diabetic retinopathy.

EVIDENCE

1. Aiello LP, Cahill MT, Wong JS: Systemic considerations in the management of diabetic retinopathy. Am J Ophthalmol 132:760-776, 2001.
   The authors provide an authoritative literature review of seminal articles on the topic.
2. Diabetes Control and Complications Trial Research Group: The effect of intensive treatment of diabetes on the development and progression of long-term complications in insulin dependent diabetes mellitus. N Engl J Med 329:977-986, 1993.
   This landmark multicenter, prospective, single-masked trial provides conclusive evidence that the complications of diabetes mellitus are related to elevation of the plasma glucose concentration.
3. Diabetic Retinopathy Study Research Group: Photocoagulation treatment of proliferative diabetic retinopathy. Clinical application of Diabetic Retinopathy Study (DRS) findings, DRS Report #8. Ophthalmology 88:583-600, 1998.
   This report is on the clinical relevance of one of the first National Eye Institute-sponsored multicenter, prospective, interventional studies investigating the effect of laser treatment on proliferative diabetic retinopathy.
4. Early Treatment Diabetic Retinopathy Study Research Group: Photocoagulation of diabetic macular edema. Early Treatment Diabetic Retinopathy Report #1. Arch Ophthalmol 103:1796-1806, 1985.
   This report on a National Eye Institute–sponsored multicenter, randomized, prospective trial investigating the effect of laser treatment on macular edema defined the term clinically significant macular edema.

rage or by rapid, unpredictable changes in mood. Judgments on whether an emotion is appropriate depend on understanding the patient's perspective, but tendencies such as hostility toward all members of the opposite sex or rage reactions to any criticism would clearly be a mismatch to the situation.

Problems in *social interaction* can range from inhibitions to imbroglios. Tendencies to get into power struggles, to expect and provoke abandonment, or to take advantage of others are all examples of such problems. Excessive neediness, repetitive attractions to unavailable people, or ingratiating submission also suggests a personality disorder. Peculiar tendencies in communication such as vagueness or verbosity might represent another form of impaired social interaction.

Impulse control is frequently weak or inconsistent in a person with a personality disorder. Acting on thoughts of self-hatred by cutting or burning one's self frequently brings personality disordered patients to acute medical attention. Patterns of overcontrol alternating with bursts of ill-advised behaviors such as alcohol or drug binges, sexual promiscuity, or angry outbursts demonstrate poor impulse control.

These four categories encompass most of the traits and behavioral patterns typically disturbed with a personality disorder. As mentioned previously, some tendencies appear to cluster together often enough that we can usefully speak of specific personality disorders. The specific personality disorders are defined by *DSM-IV* or ICD 10 using various criteria. For simplicity, the following descriptions are based on the *DSM-IV*. The *DSM-IV* personality disorders are commonly grouped into three clusters: cluster A (the *odd* cluster), cluster B (the *erratic* cluster), and cluster C (the *anxious* cluster). To repeat, all descriptions are based on prototypes of purity when in reality admixtures are the rule.

Cluster A includes paranoid, schizoid, and schizotypal personality disorders. Those with *paranoid* personality dwell on doubts about others and on suspicions of loyalty or exploitation. Feeling victimized, they bear grudges, counterattack when they perceive insults, and avoid confiding for fear others will take advantage. The person with a *schizoid* personality prefers solitude, lacks close or sexual relationships, and appears cold and indifferent. Lacking social graces, the person seems indifferent to the feelings of others. Those with *schizotypal* personality also have few close relationships and vague suspicions of others, but in addition they strike others as peculiar in manner or appearance. They may hold unusual beliefs that do not reach delusional proportions. Schizotypal personality may represent subsyndromal or prodromal schizophrenia.

Cluster B includes antisocial, narcissistic, histrionic, and borderline personality disorders. The person with *antisocial* personality demonstrates disregard for others through deceit, exploitation, manipulation, and reckless pursuit of immediate pleasures. This person does not honor commitments and threatens harm as a way to influence others. Frequently living on the wrong side of the law, such individuals often manifest little empathy and express no remorse. Furthermore, they tend to blame others for their misdeeds. Those with *narcissistic* personality manifest grandiosity by considering others as an audience to their specialness and by seeking preferential treatment. Lacking empathy, they require excessive attention and recognition while disregarding the emotional desires of others and expressing arrogance. Those with *histrionic* personality also seek to be the center of attention commonly by employing exaggerated emotions, seduction, or other provocative behaviors. Seen as shallow and suggestible by others, they rapidly develop unrealistic expectations in relationships.

Borderline personality subsumes a broad range of patients commonly seen in clinical practice. They may be emotionally labile, frequently threatening or attempting self-harm when inconsolable, thereby engaging others in the regulation of their emotions. They also may engage others through power struggles, expressing hostility and contrarian ways while feeling powerless and mistreated. Fears of abandonment fuel such maladaptive engagements with others and lead to intense entanglements that can also include idealizations of the other party. Such expressions as "the help-rejecting complainer" and "I hate you; don't leave me" capture the type of engagements frequently seen with borderline personality disorder. Often impulsive and reckless, they may lack a stable sense of self or identity, leading to searches for ways to feel belonging and fight empty feelings. Borderline personality is also associated with dissociation and brief psychosis under stress.

Cluster C includes avoidant, dependent, obsessive-compulsive personality disorders. The person with *avoidant* personality expresses a sense of inferiority and shame through inhibited social interactions, avoidance of risk, and preoccupation with humiliation or rejection. Reserved and awkward, this person feels inept and inadequate. Those with *dependent* personality submit themselves to relationships in which another person may make their decisions and even abuse them. Requiring frequent reassurances from others, they avoid disagreements and consent to unpleasant activities for fear of losing the other and subsequently being left to care for themselves. Those with *obsessive-compulsive* personality prefer orderliness, rules, productivity, and standards. Conscientious, stubborn, and perfectionistic, they get bogged down in details and hesitate to delegate. Seen as miserly, they hoard money and objects.

Differential Diagnosis

Personality disorders are not diagnosed when it is judged that the personality features of concern are caused by other psychiatric or medical problems. For example, personality changes can frequently follow psychotic illnesses, head

Personality Disorders

Introduction

Personality refers to each individual's enduring patterns of behavior, mental state, and interaction with others. Although each personality is unique, attempts have been made throughout history to categorize types of personality. Presently the nomenclatures of the *Diagnostic and Statistical Manual of Mental Disorders,* 4th edition (*DSM-IV*) and the International Statistical Classification of Diseases and Related Health Problems, 10th revision (ICD 10) use similar categories for personality pathologies that create functional impairment. When evaluating personality, the borders of normality and pathology may blur, so diagnosis relies on clinical judgments about the degree of impairment and associated distress, including distress to others. A recent representative survey of the U.S. civilian, noninstitutionalized population aged 18 years and older found that 15% met criteria for at least one personality disorder. Personality disorders have an untold impact on society given the underdiagnosis and undertreatment of these complex conditions and given that the impact of personality disorders spreads out through families and other social networks.

Etiology and Pathogenesis

All aspects of the human experience can influence the development of personality. Biologic temperaments and vulnerabilities, the intentions of caregivers, and the vagaries of fate—all levels of accumulating personal experience shape the individual personality. In every facet of development, harmful factors (or a lack of beneficial factors) can impede personality development and potentially lead to a personality disorder. Clearly, damaging events such as abuse, neglect, poverty, and war can scar a developing mind, but no personality development can be reduced to a sum of positive and negative experiences. During development, each person is increasingly an agent in his or her own personal growth. Each of the innumerable theories of personality development adds a perspective to this complex ontogeny.

In clinical psychiatry, the diagnosis of a personality disorder is one of the most common comorbidities with almost every other adult diagnosis. A personality disorder, given its usually early roots, could be seen as a risk factor for the development of any subsequent psychiatric disorder during the life of the individual.

Clinical Presentation

The common features of all personality disorders include deviation from cultural norms in the areas of social cogni-

tion, emotional expression, social interaction, and impulsivity. Such deviations must be strong tendencies of the individual, not just occasional events or the products of personality regression at times of great stress. These deviations must also interfere with function. Specific personality disorders are defined by specific criteria relating to these four areas.

Social cognition refers to the person's patterns of perceiving and interpreting the social world, including one's own place in that world. Common abnormal findings related to social cognition include idealizing or devaluing one's self or other people. A person might tend to see all problems as catastrophes, to feel like an outsider in every situation, or to believe all his or her problems are caused by external circumstances. Strong tendencies to misunderstand one's place in the world through such distortions in thinking are characteristic of personality disorders.

Emotional expression varies widely across cultures and families. When a person's emotional expression is maladaptive in its range, intensity, volatility, and mismatch to the situation, a personality disorder is likely. Limitations of range might be exemplified by incapacity to feel anger or empathy or by the tendency to express all emotions through somatic symptoms. Intensity of emotional expression is a problem when one expresses emotion in an exaggerated or theatrical fashion. Emotional volatility or mood lability is manifested by spiraling extremes of anxiety or

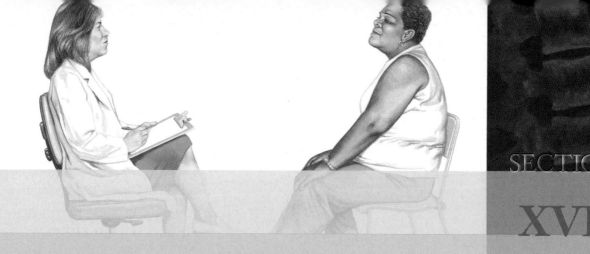

Psychiatric Disorders

injuries, or heavy metal poisoning. Likewise, substances of abuse can induce personality changes during intoxication and sometimes during prolonged withdrawal. Mental retardation can globally affect personality function. All such personality pathology attributable to another specific cause is viewed as secondary to that primary problem.

Many patients with a personality disorder prefer to think of their problems as primarily a biologic illness over which they can exert no control. For example, commonly patients with borderline personality will identify with bipolar disorder. Bipolar disorder is a psychiatric illness characterized by *episodes* of mood disturbance and impulsivity followed by interepisode periods of stable euthymia and good impulse control. Rapid-cycling bipolar disorder is defined in *DSM-IV* by four episodes of depression, mania, or hypomania in a 12-month period. Chronic mood swings in the course of the day are far more likely to be symptoms of a personality disorder than rapid-cycling bipolar disorder. Yet commonly such patients pursue aggressive treatment regimens for bipolar disorder despite deriving minimal benefit rather than pursuing treatment plans designed for personality disorders.

Diagnostic Approach

A detailed psychiatric evaluation is required to make the diagnosis of a personality disorder with confidence. The symptoms of personality disorder may be initially too subtle to be detected by a limited contact. Many experienced clinicians can make a presumptive diagnosis based on observations of personality functioning in a clinical situation, but the differential diagnosis should retain all other possibilities until they are reasonably excluded.

Psychological testing can provide additional evidence for a diagnosis based on self-reported tendencies, rated behaviors, or inferences from responses to projective tests. Like any other testing, psychological testing must be interpreted in the clinical context, but it can be invaluable in some cases in which pathology is not obvious.

Management and Therapy

Most personality disorders are untreated or undertreated. Typically others around the patient feel more burden and distress than the patient does, and effective treatment can be reasonably conducted only with patients motivated to make changes for their own reasons. Those patients who engage in treatment should expect to engage in difficult work for extended periods in order to reap realistic change.

Some personality disorders more frequently than others reach the point of intervention and treatment. This is due to unequal prevalences of the disorders, to their relative likelihoods of coming to clinical attention, and to differing prognoses with treatment. Undoubtedly, borderline personality disorder is the most commonly diagnosed and treated personality disorder. Narcissistic, histrionic, and the cluster C personality disorders also frequently present for treatment usually with other psychiatric comorbidity such as a mood or anxiety disorder. However, cluster A and antisocial personality disorders are more rarely targeted. Antisocial personality disorder in particular does not respond well to any known treatment.

Optimum Treatment

The appropriate treatment of personality disorders relies primarily on psychosocial interventions, although medications can play an adjunctive role in some cases. A range and variety of psychotherapeutic interventions can offer substantial benefit, and matching the patient to the proper therapy involves not only careful assessment of the targeted pathology but also an awareness of the strengths and resources that the patient can bring to bear as a collaborative partner in the process. One generalization about treatment relates to the level of impulse control the patient possesses. More impulsive patients should be in treatment situations that can contain them through predictable and more focused agendas. Those with stronger impulse control can withstand and benefit from more anxiety-provoking treatments such as exploratory psychotherapies.

Although treatment of the personality disorder itself may not always be pursued, such patients are commonly encountered in all clinical arenas, and the treatments required for their more acute conditions can be compromised or disrupted by the patient's personality disorder. Noncompliance, refusal of treatment, inordinate consumption of resources, and clashes with providers can make these patients a challenge in any clinical setting. Management of the personality disorder becomes an essential part of a comprehensive treatment plan for whatever other problems are being addressed more directly. The basis of such management relies on avoiding common errors.

Avoiding Treatment Errors

Patients with personality disorders typically evoke strong feelings from others, ranging from annoyance, dread, and hatred to unusual attraction. When faced with strong emotions, care providers understandably make missteps in the management of these patients (Fig. 162-1). These patients draw others into interactions that can be detrimental to both parties.

The general principles of managing patients with personality disorders include recognition of heightened emotion and tension in the relationship along with impartial assessment of what is best recommended for the acute condition being treated. In other words, the maintenance of objectivity in the face of an emotional challenge is the goal (Fig. 162-2). That means withstanding temptations to avoid, to rescue, to control, to punish, or to react to provocation with retaliation. Robotic detachment is not in order,

Figure 162-1 Patients with Personality Disorders Provoke Strong Feelings That Physicians Must Manage Internally.

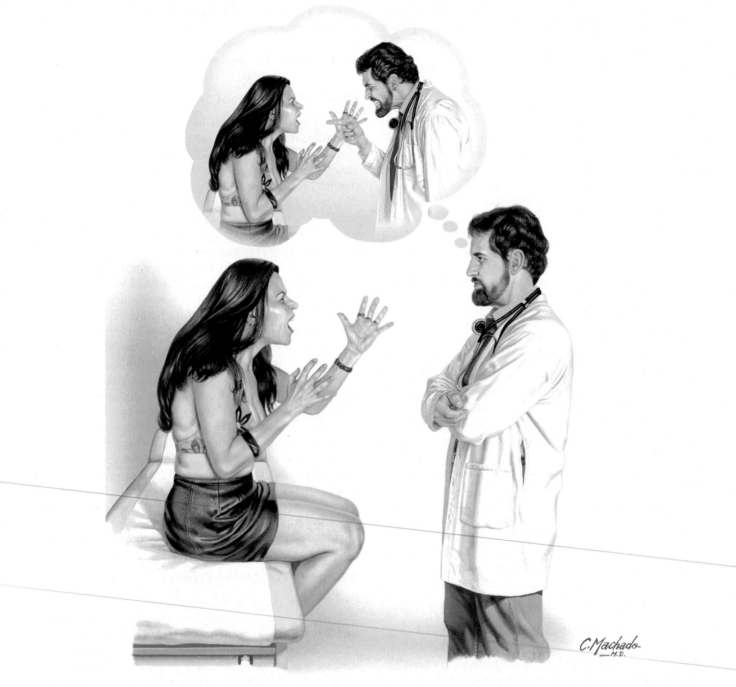

but management of patients with personality disorders often requires bearing strong emotions internally while keeping the focus on the needs (not the desires or demands) of the patient.

Clinicians (and others) frequently conceptualize such patients as willfully oppositional, morally weak, or less worthy of care. It is vital to understand that personality develops to adapt to the environment. Patients with a personality disorder have adapted to early situations (or at least perceived situations) that called for their currently maladaptive tendencies. Recognizing that the behaviors have meaning related to other contexts can allow the clinician to avoid taking those behaviors personally. Patients are usually doing their best based on what they have learned in life.

In the rapidly moving clinical world where doctors often terminate clinical interactions with prescriptions, it is tempting to hope that psychopharmacology will provide a buffer from the patient who is too demanding, irrational, or emotionally charged. Some medications show limited

Figure 162-2 Physicians Must not Disregard the Medical Needs of Patients with Personality Disorders.

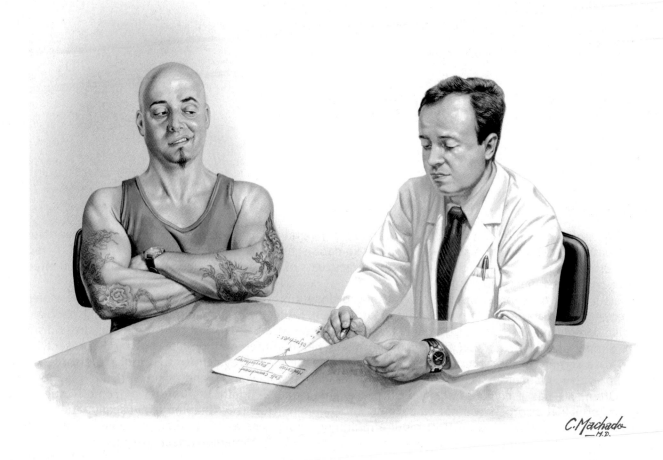

efficacy (such as selective serotonin reuptake inhibitors in borderline personality), but expectations should be tempered. Benzodiazepines in particular are generally contraindicated in patients with impulsivity or hostility.

Given the sensitivities of these patients or the hopelessness sometimes felt by the clinician, personality problems are not easily brought into discussion in most clinical settings. Most clinicians offer treatment or referral when the patient requests help, but patients with a personality disorder infrequently ask directly for help. When they do, they often expect a medication or some other "magical" relief. Referrals for psychotherapeutic interventions can be delicate, but most patients can handle the recommendation of "talking to someone." Thus, the referral to mental health providers should not be avoided.

Future Directions

Research into personality disorders and effective treatments has lagged behind in the era of biologic research in psychiatry. There is growing interest in outcomes research

for therapies that can address the challenges in treating personality disorders.

Additional Resources

Gunderson JG: Borderline personality disorder: A clinical guide. Washington, DC, American Psychiatric Publishing, 2001.
This single-authored book written by a leader in the field focuses on all aspects of diagnosis and the full range of accepted treatments for the most clinically prevalent personality disorder.

Haas LJ, Leiser JP, Magill MK, Sanyer ON: Management of the difficult patient. Am Fam Physician 72(10):2063-2068, 2005.
This pithy article offers many practical tips on managing difficult patients, including those with personality disorders, in primary care settings.

EVIDENCE

1. Oldham JM, Skodol AE, Bender DS: The American Psychiatric Publishing Textbook of Personality Disorders. Washington, DC, American Psychiatric Publishing, 2005.
With contributions from dozens of authors, this comprehensive text covers each personality disorder in detail, including etiology, clinical evaluation, treatment, and research.

Matthew N. Goldenberg · Lea C. Watson · B. Anthony Lindsey

Anxiety and Panic

Introduction

Most patients with psychiatric symptoms are seen in the general medical setting exclusively. This is particularly true for patients with anxiety disorders, in whom somatic symptoms often predominate. Although detection of these disorders remains poor, the direct and indirect costs of untreated anxiety are enormous, and effective evidence-based treatments are available.

Anxiety is tension or apprehension that is disproportional to the actual stimulus (Fig. 163-1). There are five principal anxiety disorders in adults: panic disorder (PD) with or without agoraphobia, social phobia (SP), obsessive-compulsive disorder (OCD), generalized anxiety disorder (GAD), and post-traumatic stress disorder (PTSD). Simple phobias (e.g., specific fear of storms or heights) are common also but rarely present in the primary care setting. In the general medical setting, PD is the most prevalent of the principal disorders. The lifetime prevalence is nearly 5%, with a twofold increased risk for women, and onset in the 20s is most frequent. Often, PD has a complicated medical presentation and a significant burden of comorbidities. The remaining principal disorders will not be covered in detail here. OCD (see Chapter 167) usually requires early psychiatric referral. GAD, SP, and PTSD require multimodal therapies and are often too time intensive to be exclusively managed in the general medical setting. Table 163-1 summarizes these disorders.

Etiology and Pathogenesis

As with most psychiatric disorders, it is likely that psychological and environmental triggers unmask a biologic predisposition to PD.

Neurobiologic

There is an explosion of research in this area, including the study of the fear and anxiety centers in the brain, such as the amygdala, locus ceruleus, and hippocampus. Preliminary neuroimaging studies highlight deficits in these neuroanatomic areas. Provocative agents, including sodium lactate, carbon dioxide, caffeine, yohimbine, m-chlorophenylpiperazine, fenfluramine, and cholecystokinin, can induce panic states in patients with PD. Supporting neurochemical hypotheses is the fact that similar states cannot be induced in normal control subjects. No specific etiologic determinants have emerged in this likely heterogeneous disorder. Family studies also suggest that PD is familial, with increased risk for first-degree relatives of those with the disorder.

Cognitive-Behavioral

Progressive fear of recurrent attacks is a large part of PD and is even more important when agoraphobia (avoidance of activities secondary to fear of having an attack) occurs. Many believe that this conditioning leads to catastrophic misinterpretation of bodily sensations starting a cycle of escalating anxiety.

Clinical Presentation

Given the primacy of their somatic symptoms, most patients with PD (85%) make their initial contact in the medical setting, most often in the emergency department, followed by visits to their primary care physician. Onset of PD usually occurs in the third or fourth decade. The criteria for a panic attack (Box 163-1) should be differentiated from PD (Box 163-2) because panic attacks can occur in the context of multiple illnesses and do not necessarily represent PD.

The hallmark difficulty in recognizing PD is that patients usually do not complain of anxiety, but instead present with as many as 10 to 15 somatic symptoms, several

Figure 163-1 Panic Disorder.

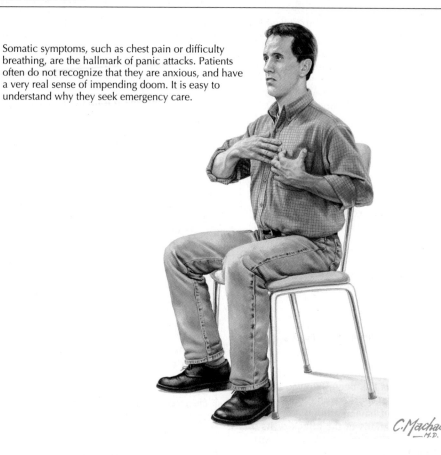

Somatic symptoms, such as chest pain or difficulty breathing, are the hallmark of panic attacks. Patients often do not recognize that they are anxious, and have a very real sense of impending doom. It is easy to understand why they seek emergency care.

Table 163-1	Other Common Anxiety Disorders		
	Social Phobia	**Generalized Anxiety Disorder**	**Post-traumatic Stress Disorder**
Defining features	Excessive fear of public scrutiny in single or multiple situations; may have panic attacks	Unrealistic or excessive worry about common life circumstances; chronic autonomic hyperarousal	Occurs after threat to life or body, followed by intrusive memories, avoidance, and hyperarousal
Lifetime prevalence	5%-13%	5% (2 : 1 female)	1%-14% (varies with specific trauma)
Common comorbidities	Depression, substance abuse	Depression, substance abuse, panic disorder	Substance abuse, depression, somatoform disorders
Treatment	*SSRI, benzodiazepines, venlafaxine, CBT	*SSRI, benzodiazepines, venlafaxine	*SSRI, antiadrenergic agents (clonidine, propranolol)
Referral threshold	Low: therapy enhances medications	Depends on symptom severity and number of comorbidities	Low: patients are usually time intensive

*See Table 163-2 for SSRI and benzodiazepine dosing.
CBT, cognitive behavioral therapy; SSRI, selective serotonin reuptake inhibitor.

of them quite dramatic. The most common cluster of symptoms is cardiac, including chest pain and tachycardia. Gastrointestinal and pulmonary symptoms are also common, and nearly half of PD patients report neurologic symptoms (headache and dizziness are the most frequent). PD may also be complicated by agoraphobia (Box 163-3).

Differential Diagnosis

Psychiatric

Major depression and bipolar disorder often present with predominant anxiety symptoms and should always be considered as a primary diagnosis in the differential diagnosis of the anxious patient. Depression also develops later in

---

Box 163-1 Panic Attack Diagnostic Criteria

A discrete period of intense fear or discomfort, in which four (or more) of the following symptoms develop abruptly and reach a peak within 10 minutes:

1. Palpitations, pounding heart, or accelerated heart rate
2. Sweating
3. Trembling or shaking
4. Sensations of shortness of breath or smothering
5. Feeling of choking
6. Chest pain or discomfort
7. Nausea or abdominal pain
8. Feeling dizzy, unsteady, lightheaded, or faint
9. Paresthesias (numbness or tingling sensations)
10. Chills or hot flushes
11. Derealization (feelings of unreality) or depersonalization (being detached from oneself)
12. Fear of losing control or going crazy
13. Fear of dying

Adapted from American Psychiatric Association: Diagnostic and Statistical Manual of Mental Disorders, 4th ed, text rev. Washington, DC, American Psychiatric Association, 2000.

Box 163-2 Panic Disorder Diagnostic Criteria

1. Both (A) and (B):
   A. Recurrent unexpected panic attacks
   B. At least one of the attacks has been followed by 1 month (or more) of one (or more) of the following:
      ▪ Persistent concern about having additional attacks
      ▪ Worry about the implications of the attack or its consequences (e.g., losing control, having a heart attack, going crazy)
      ▪ A significant change in behavior related to the attacks
2. The panic attacks are not due to the direct physiologic effects of a substance (e.g., a drug of abuse, a medication) or a general medical condition (e.g., hyperthyroidism).
3. The panic attacks are not better accounted for by another mental disorder, such as social phobia, specific phobia, obsessive-compulsive disorder, or post-traumatic stress disorder.

Box 163-3 Agoraphobia Diagnostic Criteria

1. Anxiety about being in places or situations from which escape might be difficult (or embarrassing) or in which help may not be available in the event of having an unexpected or situationally predisposed panic attack or panic-like symptoms. Agoraphobic fears typically involve characteristic clusters of situations that include being outside the home alone, being in a crowd or standing in a line, being on a bridge, or traveling in a bus, train, or automobile.
2. The situations are avoided (e.g., travel is restricted) or else are endured with marked distress or with anxiety about having a panic attack or panic-like symptoms, or require the presence of a companion.

Adapted from American Psychiatric Association: Diagnostic and Statistical Manual of Mental Disorders, 4th ed, text rev. Washington, DC, American Psychiatric Association, 2000.

Box 163-4 Common Medical Conditions Associated with Anxiety or Panic Symptoms

Anemia
Angina
Arrhythmias
Asthma
Congestive heart failure
Electrolyte disturbance
Hyperthyroidism
Hypoxia
Hypoglycemia
Myocardial infarction
Parathyroid disorder
Pulmonary embolism
Seizures
Transient ischemic attacks
Vertigo

---

life in one third to one half of patients with PD. Many drugs of abuse, including cocaine, marijuana, amphetamines, and caffeine, may also induce panic states independent of PD.

Medical

PD and anxiety symptoms coexist with one third or more of several common conditions, including atypical chest pain, Parkinson's disease, irritable bowel syndrome, and chronic obstructive pulmonary disease (Box 163-4). The diagnosis of PD should not be conceptualized as mutually exclusive from "medical" illness. Current medications, including sympathomimetic medications such as cold and allergy preparations, should also be investigated as causes of anxiety symptoms. Alcohol and other sedative withdrawal can also cause anxiety symptoms.

Diagnostic Approach

A high index of suspicion for PD and related disorders should be maintained for patients who are young, have multiple somatic complaints, and visit the doctor frequently. A search for PD, as well as comorbid depression and substance abuse, should be a priority. (PD sufferers are more than 4 times as likely to abuse alcohol.) If a primary anxiety disorder seems likely, defer extensive system-specific workups (e.g., endoscopy, cardiac catheterization). A thorough medical, psychiatric, family, and social history will usually lead to the correct diagnosis.

The medical workup includes physical examination, with a thorough neurologic examination; medication history (include over-the-counter medications); electrocardiogram (if older than 40 years, having current chest

Table 163-2 Medications for Panic Disorder

Class	Agent	Starting Dose	Maintenance
SSRI			
	Citalopram[†]	10 mg/day	20-40 mg/day
	Escitalopram[†]	5-10 mg/day	10-20 mg/day
	Fluoxetine*	5-10 mg/day	20-80 mg/day
	Fluvoxamine	25 mg/day	50-300 mg/day
	Paroxetine	10 mg/day	20-60 mg/day
	Sertraline[†]	25 mg/day	50-200 mg/day
SNRI			
	Venlafaxine XR	37.5mg/day	75-300mg/day
Benzodiazepines			
	Alprazolam	0.25-0.5 mg tid	2-6 mg/day total
	Clonazepam	0.5 mg bid to tid	1-4 mg/day total
	Lorazepam[†]	0.5-1.0 mg bid to tid	2-10 mg/day total

*Fluoxetine has a long half-life and may not be the best choice for a patient with known sensitivity to drug side effects.
[†]These medications are used to treat panic disorder, but do not have that specific U.S. Food and Drug Administration indication.
SNRI, serotonin norepinephrine reuptake inhibitor; SSRI, selective serotonin reuptake inhibitor.

pain, or with a significant family history of heart disease); and selected laboratory tests, including complete blood count, chemistry panel, and thyroid-stimulating hormone. If the patient is older than 40 years, nonpsychiatric medical diagnoses should be suspected and excluded.

Management and Treatment

Significant evidence has emerged to guide the treatment of anxiety disorders, specifically PD. The greatest challenge remains in detecting these disorders and in prescribing adequate treatment (Table 163-2). Most importantly, clinicians must routinely consider the possibility of a PD diagnosis. Once detected, the goals of treatment include reduction of the frequency and intensity of symptoms and management of the anticipatory anxiety associated with panic attacks.

Optimum Treatment

Both medications and behavioral therapy have proved equally efficacious in psychiatric populations. Pharmacotherapy in PD has been well studied, with similar monotherapeutic efficacy among the tricyclic antidepressants, monoamine oxidase inhibitors, high-potency benzodiazepines, a serotonin norepinephrine reuptake inhibitor (venlafaxine XR), and selective serotonin reuptake inhibitors (SSRIs). However, side effects, potential drug interactions, dietary restrictions, and risk for dependence have limited the utility of the first three classes. SSRIs have supplanted these older agents for first-line therapy due to a more favorable side-effect profile, whereas venlafaxine is routinely considered a second-line agent. The 3- to 4-week latency in response to pharmacologic treatment of depression may be shorter for PD (2 to 3 weeks), but PD patients generally have greater sensitivity to side effects.

Benzodiazepines, which have a rapid onset of action (several days), are best used adjunctively in the acutely ill patient to bridge delayed response to SSRIs or venlafaxine. Alprazolam, clonazepam, and lorazepam have the most data supporting their use. Adequate standing doses of benzodiazepines should be prescribed, as opposed to as-needed doses.

Use of medication in the treatment of anxiety disorders should begin at the lowest possible dose and should be titrated slowly but assertively to the maximum dose necessary for symptom improvement, which is often higher than that required for depression (start low, go slow, but go . . . and go). Adequate duration of this dose is 6 weeks before determining medication failure.

Cognitive behavioral therapy (CBT; e.g., psychoeducation, symptom monitoring, breathing training, cognitive restructuring focusing on correction of catastrophic misinterpretations of bodily sensations, and exposure) designed to address panic symptoms has proven efficacy but requires trained therapists and committed patients. This may be an important referral point for patients desiring a nonpharmacologic intervention. Patients should be informed that studies show that the best success is seen with the combination of medications and CBT.

Response rates vary, but controlled trials suggest that 50% to 60% patients become panic free during most proven treatments, with improved outcomes as treatment is extended. Venlafaxine has been shown to reduce severity of panic and agoraphobic symptoms, but was no better than placebo in achieving a panic-free state. PD is a chronic illness usually requiring maintenance therapy and often characterized by residual symptoms. Optimal length of treatment has not been fully elucidated, and relapse is common, particularly without maintenance therapy. Agoraphobia and other psychiatric comorbidities are thought to be predictors of poorer outcomes. PD, particularly in association with depression and substance abuse, also places the patient at increased risk for suicide.

Optimal management of PD includes assessing for suicide risk, evaluating and acknowledging the degree of functional impairment, establishing and maintaining a therapeutic alliance, providing patient and family education, communicating with other physicians (which plays a large role in preventing unnecessary diagnostic tests), and helping the patient learn how to address early signs of relapse. Patients should be encouraged to limit consumption of caffeine and sympathomimetic drugs and to abstain from use of illicit substances.

Recent studies suggest that a model of collaborative care based in the primary care setting is a more effective and cost-efficient way to treat PD. The model includes algorithm-based medication management by the primary care physician (with guidance available from a psychiatrist) supplemented by six sessions of CBT and telephone follow-up provided by a midlevel behavioral health specialist.

Consider referral to a psychiatrist for diagnostic clarification (consultation); for suicidal patients; after two trials of first-line treatment have failed; for treatment of agoraphobia; when psychotherapy is indicated (e.g., significant life stressors, limited support systems); when patients have psychiatric comorbidity that is unstable (e.g., unremitting depressive symptoms, active substance abuse); or when optimal management exceeds the time constraints of the primary care setting.

Avoiding Treatment Errors

The primary treatment errors encountered with panic disorder are under-recognition and undertreatment. Pharmacologic treatment should be both long enough (6 weeks) and at a high enough dose (up to maximum) before a therapeutic trial is considered a failure. Educating the patient that they may experience a weeks-long delay in symptom response to treatment is important. Furthermore, evidence suggests that a combination of pharmacologic and psychotherapeutic interventions is more successful than either treatment modality alone, so making a referral to a therapist can be an important adjunct to drug therapy. Physicians should also be cautious in the long-term use of benzodiazepines, especially given the risk for dependency.

Future Directions

The complexity and challenge presented by anxious patients must be embraced and integrated into primary care. Researchers should continue their search for new therapeutic agents, especially given that 40% to 50% of patients may not respond to current therapies. More research on collaborative care and self-help models of care (including Internet-based resources) is being pursued. Neuroimaging technologies are quickly evolving to help answer some of these questions, and psychotherapeutic principles are being equally explored. Efficient and feasible methods to detect these common disorders must also be further investigated. Interdisciplinary communication and multimodal interventions will continue to be crucial in the successful management of the anxious patient.

Additional Resources

American Psychiatric Association: Diagnostic and Statistical Manual of Mental Disorders, 4th ed., text rev. Washington, DC, American Psychiatric Association, 2000.

Anxiety Disorders Association of America. Available at: http://www.adaa.org. Accessed December 13, 2006.

National Alliance on Mental Illness. Available at: http://www.nami.org. Accessed December 13, 2006.

National Institute of Mental Health (NIMH). Available at: http://www.nimh.nih.gov. Accessed December 13, 2006.

Work Group on Panic Disorder: Practice guideline for the treatment of patients with panic disorder. American Psychiatric Association. Am J Psychiatry 155(5 Suppl):1-34, 1998.

EVIDENCE

1. Ballenger JC: Current treatments of the anxiety disorders in adults. Biol Psychiatry 46(11):1579-1594, 1999.
   The author presents a comprehensive overview of the evidence for treatments of several anxiety disorders.
2. Ballenger JC: Panic disorder in the medical setting. J Clin Psychiatry 58(Suppl 2):13-19, 1997.
   This editorial review argues for and advises on improved detection of panic disorder in the general medical setting.
3. Goddard AW, Charney DS: Toward an integrated neurobiology of panic disorder. J Clin Psychiatry 58(Suppl 2):4-12, 1997.
   The authors propose a functional neuroanatomic model of fear and anxiety and provide a review of brain imaging studies of panic disorder.
4. Katon W: Clinical practice. Panic disorder. N Engl J Med 354(22):2360-2367, 2006.
   This article presents a current, clinically based review of the diagnosis and evidence-based treatment of panic disorder.
5. Roy-Byrne PP, Craske MG, Stein MB: Panic disorder. Lancet 368(9540):1023-1032, 2006.
   This current review of the literature on the epidemiology, etiology, diagnosis, and treatment of panic disorder includes a discussion of the evidence for various treatment delivery systems such as a collaborative care model.

John J. Haggerty, Jr. ▪ Micah J. Sickel

Depression

Introduction

The word *depression* signifies a common and nonpathologic emotional experience. It also signifies a specific biopsychological disorder. The two are not the same. Depression, the illness, is a coherent syndrome with a constellation of specific signs, symptoms, and features. A lifelong recurrent disorder, it occurs in 10% to 20% of the population worldwide. It interferes with work and family life and has a mortality rate of 15%.

Etiology and Pathogenesis

Depression results from disturbances in monoamine neurotransmission. It may be maintained by secondary neurohormonal changes involving the hypothalamic-pituitary-thyroid and hypothalamic-thyroid axes. These combined changes ultimately result in altered nucleic acid transcription. The strongest etiologic factor is inheritance. Risk for depression can also be acquired through early life trauma, which may "wire-in" exaggerated neurohormonal stress responses. Other medical illnesses or interventions may cause a secondary depressive syndrome, most notably hypothyroidism, and medications such as antihypertensive agents that affect central monoamine neurotransmission. A variety of substances may also induce secondary depression during intoxication or withdrawal, most notably alcohol, cocaine, and stimulants.

Clinical Presentation

Although clinically evident depression presents in the third or fourth decade typically, the initial onset of depression can occur at any point in the life cycle, including early childhood. The presentation varies from individual to individual and across the life cycle, but the core features are always present during an episode (Figs. 164-1 and 164-2). As codified in the *Diagnostic and Statistical Manual of Mental Disorders*, 4th edition (*DSM-IV*), these include depressed mood, or anhedonia (required); increased or decreased appetite; increased or decreased sleeping; slowed activity; fatigue; exaggerated self-criticalness, worthlessness, or guilt; decreased libido; mental slowing, decreased memory, or inattention; and recurrent thoughts of death or suicide.

DSM-IV requires five signs or symptoms concurrently for at least 2 weeks for an unequivocal diagnosis, but most clinicians recognize that patients can qualify for the diagnosis with as few as three or four symptoms. Depressed mood is not always the most prominent symptom and may even be absent. Often the presenting symptom is insomnia, nervousness, somatic pain, or memory change. Depression is often accompanied by anxiety and may be complicated by striking symptoms of psychosis such as auditory hallucinations and delusions of impoverishment or guilt. Depressive episodes may occur with or without evident stressors, and reported stressors often are actually the result of incipient depression rather than the cause.

Differential Diagnosis

Adjustment Disorder

In adjustment disorder, depressed mood follows clear-cut stressors, but the full depressive syndrome is not present or is transient (<2 weeks). Adjustment disorder does not respond to antidepressant medication.

Bipolar Disorder, Depressed Phase

About 20% of individuals who present with depression actually have unrecognized bipolar mood disorder. The recognized forms of bipolar disorder, bipolar I and bipolar II, differ primarily in the severity of the manic phase. Bipolar I requires the occurrence of full-blown mania at some point in the life cycle. Bipolar II requires only the occurrence of hypomania. Because hypomania is often transient and nondysfunctional, it can be easily overlooked.

Figure 164-1 The Face of Depression.

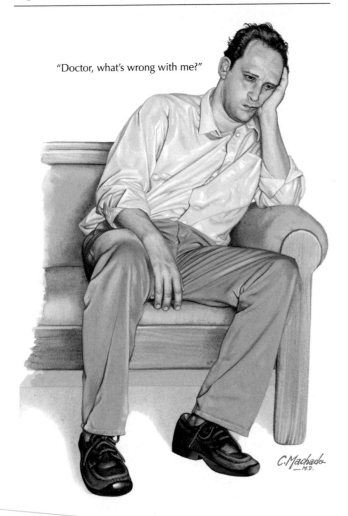

"Doctor, what's wrong with me?"

C. Machado —M.D.

Because the depressed phase of bipolar disorder is usually indistinguishable from simple depressive disorder (unipolar), bipolar II disorder can easily masquerade as unipolar depression. This distinction is important because bipolar disorder requires a different treatment approach, emphasizing mood stabilizers over antidepressants.

Substance-Induced Depression

Depression can be a direct result of substance use, but it can also exist as an independent comorbid condition complicating substance abuse. Depression that is purely secondary to a substance clears within several days to a week of substance discontinuation. If depression does not resolve within this time frame, it requires treatment in its own right. Comorbid substance use disorder affects the occurrence, course, and treatment of depression. Depression is frequently comorbid with alcohol, cocaine, and opiate addiction. With alcoholism comes an increased risk for suicide, and all individuals who present with depression and alcoholism should have a suicide assessment. Alcohol dependence increases the odds that one would have a major

depression, and conversely, major depression increases the lifetime odds of having alcohol dependence. Treatment of depression that is comorbid with cocaine dependence requires both an antidepressant as well as a therapy that focuses on the addiction. Treatment of opiate dependence typically results in improvement in the comorbid depression. However, similar to antidepressant treatment of a depression that is comorbid with other drug addictions, treatment of depression in the setting of untreated opiate dependence yields mixed results.

Depression Secondary to Medical Illness

Depression secondary to a medical condition should be considered whenever depressive mood changes accompany a medical condition known to be associated with depression. A partial list includes hypothyroidism, Addison's or Cushing's disease, pancreatic cancer, AIDS, tuberculosis, multiple sclerosis, stroke, Alzheimer's disease, Parkinson's disease, and diabetes mellitus. Sometimes depression may be the first manifestation of undetected systemic illness, and for this reason, medical history and reasonable medical assessment should be part of the standard evaluation of all new cases of depression. Depression may also be induced by a variety of commonly used medications, including glucocorticoids and interferon. Evidence fails to support the belief that β-blockers commonly induce depression.

Diagnostic Approach

Consider depression not just in patients who present with depressed mood, but also in those who primarily complain of insomnia, anxiety, decreased energy, chronic pain, or cognitive changes. The diagnosis is established purely on the basis of history and observation of symptoms and signs consistent with the diagnostic criteria. Excellent self-administered screening tools such as the Zung, Beck, or PHQ-9 depression inventories are available. Information from family members or close associates is invaluable in substantiating the diagnosis when the onset of symptoms has been insidious. Diagnostic evaluation must include enumeration of the frequency and timing of prior episodes, and an exploration for past episodes of elevated mood. This information is necessary for later treatment planning, including decisions about the duration of treatment. Every evaluation must include queries about suicide risk. The simplest way to begin this inquiry is to ask, "Have you had thoughts of death or of harming yourself in any way?" Thoughts of dying or committing suicide are extremely common in depression. Most frequently, they remain at the thought level and can be managed on an outpatient basis. However, in a significant minority of patients, thoughts are accompanied by intent or specific suicidal plans, which require rapid psychiatric consultation or hospitalization. History of a suicide attempt and the presence of psychosis, substance use, or significant isolation raise the risk for suicide.

Figure 164-2 Depression (Unipolar).

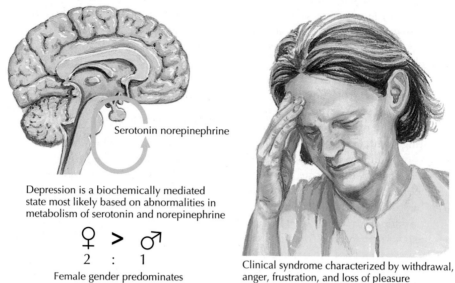

Serotonin norepinephrine

Depression is a biochemically mediated
state most likely based on abnormalities in
metabolism of serotonin and norepinephrine

♀ > ♂
2 : 1
Female gender predominates

Clinical syndrome characterized by withdrawal,
anger, frustration, and loss of pleasure

Associated symptoms and comorbidities

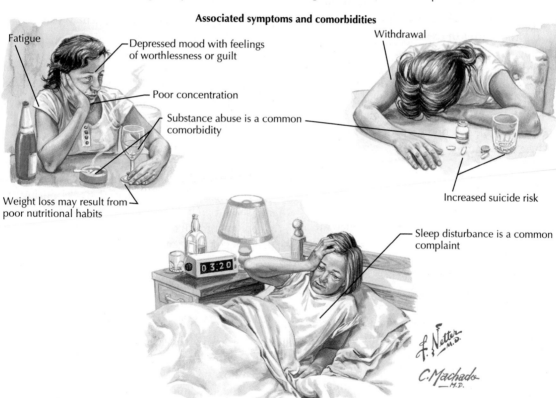

Fatigue

Depressed mood with feelings
of worthlessness or guilt

Poor concentration

Substance abuse is a common
comorbidity

Weight loss may result from
poor nutritional habits

Withdrawal

Increased suicide risk

Sleep disturbance is a common
complaint

Management and Therapy

The most important principle for the management of
depression is to view it as a lifelong disorder that recurs
at a rate of at least 50% following a single episode. The
recurrence rate climbs with each subsequent episode, as
does the rate of chronic residual symptoms between major
episodes. Treatment planning must take into account
patient education and duration of treatment. The second
most important principle is that, although all antidepressant agents have similar efficacy rates, there is significant
variability in terms of response and tolerance among
patients. Many patients try more than one antidepressant
before finding one that works for them.

Initial medication treatment usually starts with a member
of the serotonin-specific reuptake inhibitor (SSRI) class of
antidepressants, which includes fluoxetine, sertraline, paroxetine, citalopram, and escitalopram. If there is a personal

or family history of preferential response to a particular antidepressant of any class, then this should be the first choice. A generic member of the older tricyclic class of antidepressants is an equally good choice if cost is an issue. Sixty to 70% of patients have at least partial response to the initial choice. Evidence-based algorithms exist to guide treatment when it is necessary to move beyond this step (see Texas Medication Algorithm Project website). The usual sequence is to (1) increase the dose every 1 to 2 weeks as tolerated; (2) add either lithium or tri-iodothyronine (25 to 50 mcg) as an augmenting agent; (3) switch to a different member of the same class or switch to a member of a different class (bupropion, venlafaxine, duloxetine, mirtazapine, tricyclic, monoamine oxidase inhibitor); (4) combine antidepressants (SSRI + bupropion or tricyclic; venlafaxine + mirtazapine); and (5) consider electroconvulsive therapy, which has the highest response rate of all somatic treatments for depression. Recently approved vagal nerve stimulation, which uses an implantable device to deliver deep brain stimulation through the vagus nerve, may induce remission in up to 30% of individuals who are completely refractory to all other forms of treatment.

Psychotherapy is equally as effective as medication in mild to moderate depression, but not in severe depression. Psychotherapies specifically designed for depression, cognitive behavioral therapy, and interpersonal psychotherapy in particular have been shown to have the highest effectiveness. A combination of psychotherapy plus medication provides the best coverage.

Optimum Treatment

Optimum treatment of depression requires a systematic approach using routine screening, algorithm-guided medication management targeting full symptom remission, and adequate duration of treatment.

Routine and universal screening for depression, followed by prompt psychoeducation and medication management, has been shown to be feasible and effective in decreasing morbidity in general medical settings and is a necessary starting point for successful management. Any of the brief self-administered tools mentioned earlier will work.

The goal of antidepressant therapy needs to be full remission rather than partial symptom reduction. With time and effort, this is feasible in at least 70% of depressed individuals. However, only 25% achieve full remission after the initial medication trial and 50% after the first two interventions. Therefore, reaching this end point requires routine monitoring of all symptoms at each evaluation (ideally using one of the symptom rating scales mentioned previously) and a systematic approach to advancing treatment if benchmarked improvement does not occur within a specified interval. The Texas Medication Algorithm Project provides an excellent detailed example of this process.

Optimally, antidepressant treatment should continue at least 6 to 12 months after a single episode to prevent relapse. Evidence shows that indefinite maintenance treatment with antidepressants, psychotherapy, or both is safe and significantly decreases the future relapse rate. It should be strongly considered in individuals with more than one episode of depression or in those who experience chronic interepisode depressive symptoms.

Avoiding Treatment Errors

Reluctance to Treat

The U.S. Food and Drug Administration (FDA) black-box warnings about possible treatment-associated emergent suicide can be misinterpreted as a caution against starting an antidepressant. Evidence continues to emerge that the risk for not treating outweighs treatment-associated risks. The more important message in the FDA warnings is to monitor adequately once treatment is initiated (see below).

Failure to Recognize Depression as Part of Bipolar Disorder

Patients with bipolar depression may respond initially to antidepressants, but are unlikely to sustain their response, and frequently worsen over time owing to antidepressant-driven mood cycling. These individuals require mood stabilizers and are often best served by psychiatric consultation.

Inadequate Monitoring

Issues affecting safety and treatment adherence typically occur during the first 4 to 6 weeks on medication. Monitoring, which can be either in person or by phone, should occur no less than every 1 to 2 weeks during this period and should include assessment of medication tolerance and response (or worsening) and education about importance of daily compliance.

Future Directions

Further Delineation of Pathogenesis and Inheritance

One or more genes affecting catecholaminergic neurotransmission show promise for predicting risk for depression following stressful life events. With time, these findings may lead to clinically useful biologic markers for mood disorders. Research using functional brain imaging and molecular biology will significantly improve our understanding of the neural circuitry of depression and of what happens between the synapse and the cell nucleus during initiation, maintenance, and recovery from depression.

Development of Antidepressant Treatments with Novel Mechanisms of Action

There are many individuals who do not respond to available treatments, all of which tend to focus on synaptic activity. Examples of treatments under investigation include agents that block the exaggerated hypothalamic-pituitary-adrenal axis response in depression, transcranial magnetic stimulation, and other forms of deep brain stimulation.

Public Education and Stigma Reduction

Failure to seek treatment is the single most important impediment to reducing morbidity and mortality in depression. Public education about depression lags far behind health information efforts for other common illnesses. Investment of public resources in the development of organized, ongoing screening and health education programs for depression will have an impact on the burden of depression that is equal to if not greater than biologic advances.

Additional Resources

American Psychiatric Association: Practice guidelines. Available at: http://www.psych.org/psych_pract/treatg/pg/prac_guide.cfm. Accessed March 12, 2007.

The APA treatment guidelines represent the most comprehensive expert guidelines for depression and other psychiatric disorders.

National Institute of Mental Health: Depression. Available at: http://www.nimh.nih.gov/healthinformation/depressionmenu.cfm. Accessed March 12, 2007.

This frequently updated site is an excellent source of information for patients and families. It summarizes and links to significant research advances, including Sequenced Treatment Alternatives to Relieve Depression (STAR*D).

Texas Department of State Health Services: Texas implementation of medication algorithms. Available at: http://www.dshs.state.tx.us/mhprograms/TIMA.shtm. Accessed March 12, 2007.

These are the most frequently used and best tested medication algorithms for mood disorders and other psychiatric conditions.

EVIDENCE

1. Duval F, Mokrani MC, Monreal-Ortiz JA, et al: Cortisol hypersecretion in unipolar major depression with melancholic and psychotic features: Dopaminergic, noradrenergic and thyroid correlates. Psychoneuroendocrinology 31(7):876-888, 2006.

   Comparison of responses in depressed patients versus healthy controls to a number of chemical stressors gives some validation to the theory that HPA dysregulation affects dysregulation of the catecholamine and HP-thyroid systems.

2. Fava M, Rush AJ, Wisniewski SR, et al: A comparison of mirtazapine and nortriptyline following two consecutive failed medication treatments for depressed outpatients: A STAR*D report. Am J Psychiatry 163(7):1161-1172, 2006.

   Remission rates in sequenced antidepressant trials drop at each stage and are only 12% to 20% following two failed trials.

3. Kendler KS, Kuhn JW, Vittum J, et al: The interaction of stressful life events and a serotonin transporter polymorphism in the prediction of episodes of major depression: A replication. Arch Gen Psychiatry 62(5):529-535, 2005.

   Susceptibility to depression can now be linked to specific relevant genotypes. Individuals with two short alleles of the serotonin transporter gene (5-HTTLPR) have a greater likelihood than those with other variants to develop depression following stressful life events.

4. Kessler RC, Berglund P, Demler O, et al: The epidemiology of major depressive disorder: Results from the national com-morbidity survey replications (NCS-R). JAMA 289:3095-3105, 2003.

   The most current national epidemiologic data show an annual prevalence of 6.6% and a lifetime prevalence of 16% for depression. Only 50% of annual cases receive treatment, and only 42% of these receive adequate treatment.

5. Ko DT, Hebert PR, Coffey CS, et al: Beta-blocker therapy and symptoms of depression, fatigue, and sexual dysfunction. JAMA 288(3):351-357, 2002.

   The authors cull randomized trials using β-blockers and look for adverse effects including depressed mood. There are 15 randomized trials that include more than 35,000 patients. A significant increase in depressed mood was not found.

6. Lima MS, Reisser AA, Soares BG, Farrell M: Antidepressants for cocaine dependence. Cochrane Database Syst Rev 2:CD002950, 2003.

   The Cochrane Collaboration focuses on randomized controlled trials that examine the use of antidepressants in the treatment of cocaine dependence. They find no evidence to support the use of antidepressants in cocaine dependence.

7. Nunes EV, Sullivan MA, Levin FR: Treatment of depression in patients with opiate dependence. Biol Psychiatry 56(10):793-802, 2004.

   This review article looks at the comorbidity of depression and opiate dependence and how to effectively treat both disorders using psychosocial interventions in addition to pharmacotherapy.

8. Reynolds CF 3rd, Dew MA, Pollock BG, et al: Maintenance treatment of major depression in old age. N Engl J Med 354(11):1130-1138, 2006.

   Maintenance antidepressant treatment safely and effectively reduces recurrence rate. More than half of previously depressed individuals followed without antidepressant treatment over 2 years experienced recurrence. Maintenance paroxetine treatment cut recurrence rate nearly in half.

9. Rush AJ, Trivedi MH, Wisniewski SR, et al: Bupropion-SR, sertraline, or venlafaxine-XR after failure of SSRIs for depression. N Engl J Med 354(12):1231-1242, 2006.

   Of patients who failed to respond to first-line treatment with an SSRI in the STAR*D study, 25% reached remission when switched to another antidepressant. Switch to a different class of antidepressant was no more effective than switch to another SSRI.

10. Sher L: Alcoholism and suicidal behavior: A clinical overview. Acta Psychiatr Scand 113(1):13-22, 2006.

    This author reviews the literature on alcoholism and increased suicide risk with the final recommendation that all those with alcohol abuse and dependence be assessed for suicide risk.

11. Simon GE, Savarino J, Operskalski B, Wang PS: Suicide risk during antidepressant treatment. Am J Psychiatry 163(1):41-47, 2006.

    In a large cohort study including more than 65,000 individuals receiving antidepressants, serotonin reuptake inhibitor use did not increase risk over time for suicide attempt or suicide.

12. Slattery DA, Hudson AL, Nutt DJ: Invited review: The evolution of antidepressant mechanisms. Fundam Clin Pharmacol 18(1):1-21, 2004.

    This review article examines the 50-year history of the monoamine theory of depression, citing numerous supporting research studies

13. Trivedi MH, Rush AJ, Wisniewski SR, et al: Evaluation of outcomes with citalopram for depression using measurement-based care in STAR*D: Implications for clinical practice. Am J Psychiatry 163(1):28-40, 2006.

    Structured treatment in real-world settings, including primary care, can achieve results approaching that of highly selective efficacy studies. In the STAR*D study, which accepted psychiatric and medical comorbidity, 47% of patients responded to first-line treatment, and 28% reached remission.

Burton R. Hutto

Grief

Introduction

The loss of a love object triggers a complex set of biologic, psychological, and social reactions. Definitions vary, but generally, grief refers to the psychological response, bereavement to the loss itself, and mourning to the social expression of grief. Social expressions differ widely among cultures and families, and grief can vary depending on the bereaved person's psychological makeup and the nature of the lost relationship. Grief can also be a psychological reaction to any loss. A person may grieve misspent youth and missed opportunities or the loss of any cherished object such as a pet or even an inanimate object. Grieving the loss of a loved person typically evokes more pronounced and clinically relevant responses, but other losses should not be dismissed. This chapter focuses on grief and pathologic variants of grief following a death.

Etiology and Pathogenesis

The risk for pathologic outcome in grief is increased by factors related to the loss and by factors related to the psychology of the grieving person. Sudden, unanticipated, and untimely deaths are more likely to be associated with adverse outcomes. If such losses are horrific (e.g., violent deaths, deaths in disaster or accidents), the bereaved person may suffer post-traumatic stress symptoms that interfere with grief. Other types of losses are more difficult to bear. The loss of a spouse or child, or the loss of a parent during childhood or adolescence, is a major life event that is often traumatic. Multiple losses, suicide, or murder-related deaths add to the complications of grief. Concurrent life crises and stresses, such as accidents, illness, separation from family, relationship difficulties, unemployment, or the consequences of trauma, may be so severe that the bereaved person is completely occupied with psychological survival and may not have the energy to withstand the process of grief.

Some individuals may be more vulnerable to pathologic grief. A perceived lack of social support worsens outcomes. A history of psychiatric disorder and a history of suicidal behavior specifically should alert the clinician to monitor closely for difficulty in the process of grief. The nature of the relationship that is lost can also contribute to pathology in grief. The loss of ambivalent or dependent relationships can be problematic. With ambivalence, acknowledgment of satisfaction with the death of the person who is also beloved can provoke extreme guilt. The loss of either partner of a dependent relationship may require such an unusual degree of sudden development toward independence and autonomy that such persons may instead quickly establish new similar relationships before completing a process of grief.

Clinical Presentation

Normal grief can manifest in a myriad of ways. Initial responses to a death often include a sense of shocked disbelief and numbness. The bereaved person engages in searching behaviors that include seeing the lost loved one, hearing his or her voice, or feeling his or her touch (Fig. 165-1). Such hallucinatory experiences may last weeks or sometimes months and are not considered pathologic. Following the initial shock, a period of intense anguish and emotionality ensues. All conceivable emotions can be experienced with rapid fluctuation. Many of the neurovegetative symptoms of depression such as low energy, loss of appetite with weight loss, and insomnia can last for months. The final stage of grief includes a reorganization of the psychological life that may take years. Although most bereaved people await closure and a return to normal, some losses lead to psychological changes that last a lifetime.

Generally, experts agree that these stages of grief do occur, yet the individual variance is so wide that boundaries of normal grief can be hard to define. The time frame cannot be specified or predicted for any individual, and

Figure 165-1 Grief.

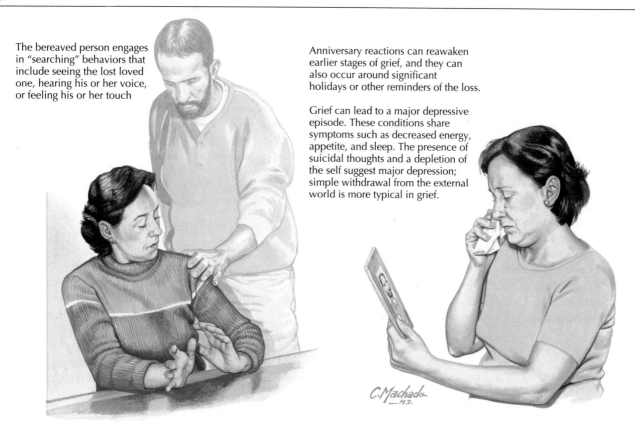

The bereaved person engages in "searching" behaviors that include seeing the lost loved one, hearing his or her voice, or feeling his or her touch

Anniversary reactions can reawaken earlier stages of grief, and they can also occur around significant holidays or other reminders of the loss.

Grief can lead to a major depressive episode. These conditions share symptoms such as decreased energy, appetite, and sleep. The presence of suicidal thoughts and a depletion of the self suggest major depression; simple withdrawal from the external world is more typical in grief.

attenuated experiences of any of the stages or nonlinear progression through them does not always signify pathology. Stage models provide a broad outline that does not account for the variables of psychological differences, personal history, or cultural expectations. Most people avoid pain and will attempt to suppress expressions of grief. What emerges is a compromise between this suppression and the underlying pain. Such partial expressions of the depth of the pain can be perceived not only as unwanted but also as "out of the blue."

Anniversary reactions can reawaken earlier stages of grief, and they can occur not only at the anniversary of the loss but also around significant holidays or other reminders of the loss. When a bereaved person reaches the age at which a parent died, often there is some pause of grief. Such anniversary reactions can be unconscious to the person, who experiences only the symptoms without understanding their context.

Biologic changes can accompany grief. There is evidence to suggest that numerous physiologic changes occur, including impairment of immunity, increased adrenocortical activity, increased prolactin, and increased growth hormone. The clinical significance of such changes is not clear. Studies of relative risk for diagnosable morbidity following grief have been inconclusive. Several studies have demonstrated an increased relative risk for mortality in bereaved spouses, but the absolute risk remains low.

Differential Diagnosis

Grief has pathologic forms marked by abnormalities of time course or intensity. Absent grief or rigid denial occurs when expression of grief is much less than expected. Delayed grief is another abnormality of time course in which the expression of grief is somehow postponed or suspended. The grief may follow a typical course after the delay. Chronic grief can continue for years, remain extremely intense, and block personal growth and the establishment of new attachments. Pathologic grief characterized by such abnormalities of time course or intensity can border on normal grief. Pathologic grief is, thus, distinguished by the degree of functional impairment.

Grief can also lead to a major depressive episode, and grief and depression share some symptoms, including decreased energy, appetite, and sleep. Because of these shared symptoms, differentiating the two can be difficult. Symptoms characterized by a depletion of the self, such as the presence of undue guilt, suicidal thoughts, or feelings of worthlessness, suggest a major depression. Simple withdrawal from the external world is more typical of normal grief. Severe psychomotor retardation and hallucinations, other than brief contacts with the lost one, suggest a possible depressive episode complicating the grief. The number of depressive symptoms present at 1 month after the loss is a strong predictor of an unremitting depression.

In addition, sleep studies may distinguish depression from grief. Medications, alcohol, and illicit substances can be abused in the effort to avoid painful effects of grief. Substance abuse requires aggressive treatment to prevent its progression and the development of further consequences.

Grieving patients commonly seek medical advice for vague symptoms of somatic distress such as dull aching pains. Such somatic expressions of grief can be psychologically mediated or related to the biologic response to loss.

Management and Therapy

Most commonly, grief will run its own course with little need for intervention by a clinician. Inquiry about perceived supports and education to help the patient anticipate the process of grief are almost always justified. Sensitivity to the circumstances and psychological meaning of the particular loss will guide further management. Availability and sensitivity will facilitate uncomplicated grief. When a complication occurs or is anticipated, more specific measures can be taken. One intervention that may be indicated is a more involved level of bereavement counseling.

Optimum Treatment

The goal of bereavement counseling is to facilitate the grieving process or to convert pathologic grief to normal grief. Bereavement counseling has been established as being effective in a number of studies. Key elements include having the patient review (1) the period leading up to the death and the immediate afterward, including perceptions, rituals, and reactions; (2) the history of the lost relationship, including its good and bad aspects; (3) what has happened since the loss, including social responses and support, and other stressors; (4) the impact on and needs of other family members and their relationship to the bereaved person; and (5) relevant experience and coping, including earlier losses and personal styles. Such explorations are designed to assist the bereaved person in expressing grief and reassessing the lost relationship, two important aspects of the resolution process. If a grieving person is unwilling or unable to move forward from the loss, an exploration of the block he or she is experiencing, such as trauma, depression, or dependent needs, may be necessary. Some bereaved people need permission from a perceived authority to stop mourning after sufficient expression of grief.

Information, education, books, and videos about grief may help the bereaved anticipate their reactions. The opportunity to explore concrete memories, places, and objects associated with the deceased (e.g., by looking at and discussing photographs or visiting the gravesite) may help overcome resistance to grieving. Self-help associations for general bereavement or the specific form of loss (Sudden

Infant Death Association, Compassionate Friends [for loss of a child], Stillbirth and Neonatal Death Support Groups, and spousal support groups) can provide support, education, role models, and practical assistance. Writing about the loss (e.g., keeping a diary or journal) or giving testimony builds mastery and may be of value for some bereaved people. Referral to a psychiatrist with skills in this area is sometimes appropriate. Indications include severe, unremitting grief; a traumatic loss (especially if the bereaved develops symptoms of post-traumatic stress disorder); major depression or suicidal ideation; and children who have lost a parent or sibling, especially if a surviving parent is depressed.

Avoiding Treatment Errors

The role of any caregiver is to facilitate normal grief and not to intervene in any way that might interfere with grief such as giving ill-conceived advice or suggesting any religious or other prescriptive formulas for grieving. Nor should a clinician prevent the bereaved from undertaking adaptive tasks such as viewing the deceased or attending the funeral or memorial service.

Medication is not part of the management of normal or pathologic grief unless specific indications exist. If sedation is initiated, it should be prescribed for a few nights while support and counseling are also provided. Sedation can impair the memory of important events such as viewing the body, family gatherings, or funeral services that may provide the patient comfort in the future. If major depression develops, antidepressant medication is indicated.

Additional Resources

Prigerson HG, Jacobs SC: Caring for bereaved patients: "All the doctors just suddenly go." JAMA 286:1369-1376, 2001.
  This article illustrates how complicated grief is to diagnose and recommends how physicians can interact with bereaved patients and families.
Raphael B: The Anatomy of Bereavement. New York, Basic Books, 1983.
  This handbook for professionals reviews the topic of bereavement and covers a variety of situations such as losses of spouses and children as well as the experience of grief for children and adolescents.

EVIDENCE

1. Parkes CM: Bereavement in adult life. BMJ 316:856-859, 1998.
     This brief, excellent review includes further details and suggestions for dealing with death in medical practice.
2. Shear K, Frank E, Houck PR, Reynolds CF: Treatment of complicated grief: A randomized controlled trial. JAMA 293:2601-2608, 2005.
     This study compares two forms of psychotherapy for grief patients. It describes details of the treatment techniques.
3. Woof WR, Carter YH: The grieving adult and the general practitioner: A literature review in two parts (part 1). Br J Gen Pract 47:443-448, 1997.
     This literature review summarizes the psychology of grief and research on morbidity and mortality related to grieving.

Post-traumatic Stress Disorder

Introduction

Post-traumatic stress disorder (PTSD) occurs after an event in which an individual either has personally been subjected to risk for death or serious injury or has witnessed or been confronted with the same circumstances involving another person. In addition, PTSD usually occurs only if the individual's response to the event involves a sense of intense fear, helplessness, or horror. A wide range of events can produce the symptoms of PTSD, and several populations have been identified as having an increased incidence and prevalence of PTSD. Among these are war veterans, motor vehicle crash survivors, rape and incest survivors, and survivors of natural and human-made disasters.

There are three major symptom clusters of PTSD: (1) re-experiencing the traumatic event, (2) avoidance and emotional numbing, and (3) increased arousal. Re-experiencing phenomena such as flashbacks and nightmares are the hallmarks of PTSD. Almost anything can trigger flashbacks, even when its connection to the traumatic event goes unrecognized by the individual. For example, a rape survivor might not understand why she cannot stand the odor of lilacs until she recalls that there was a vase of the fresh cut flowers in the room where she was attacked.

Avoidance symptoms, including emotional numbing, are frequently viewed as attempts to control or protect against the negative affect and arousal associated with re-experiencing the event. For survivors, it can become extreme, as in cases in which the individual becomes agoraphobic and refuses to leave his or her home for years. Emotional numbing can include suppression of positive affective responses and an increased sensitivity to negative events and emotions. Increased arousal symptoms can include such things such as hypervigilance and an exaggerated startle reaction. Sleep disturbance, difficulty concentrating, and memory impairment are also commonly reported by individuals suffering from PTSD.

Symptoms of PTSD usually develop within 3 months of the event but occasionally emerge years afterward, and not every person who experiences a traumatic event will develop PTSD. The symptoms must last more than a month to be considered PTSD. There is a high degree of variability as to the course of PTSD. Some people recover within 3 months (acute PTSD), whereas others have symptoms that last much longer (chronic PTSD).

PTSD affects about 7.7 million American adults, but it can occur at any age, including childhood. Women are more likely to develop PTSD than men, and there is some evidence that susceptibility to the disorder may run in families. PTSD is often accompanied by depression, substance abuse, or one or more of the other anxiety disorders. Among men, the traumas most commonly associated with PTSD are combat exposure and witnessing someone being badly injured or killed. Among women, rape and sexual molestation are the traumas most commonly associated with PTSD.

Etiology and Pathogenesis

As with many psychiatric disorders, there is not one specific factor or set of factors involved in the etiology of PTSD. It is likely that a combination of psychological, biologic, and environmental factors contribute to its development. Learning theorists speculate that the major symptoms of PTSD are caused by classical conditioning to fear. For example, a patient with PTSD may experience increased anxiety or fear when traveling in a car, after having been involved in a traumatic car accident. Avoidance of motor vehicles only serves to reinforce the fear of cars, which is to say that when a car is not present, neither is the anxiety or fear.

From a biologic viewpoint, lasting changes in brain chemistry are often evident in patients diagnosed with PTSD. People with PTSD have heightened physiologic responses (e.g., an exaggerated startle reflex) to any physical stress, not just to reminders of the trauma. When the sympathetic nervous system is activated to prepare for an emergency, the locus coeruleus releases the catecholamine neurotransmitters norepinephrine and epinephrine. Many studies have shown that patients with PTSD may have characteristic catecholamine abnormalities. Some studies have found that a high norepinephrine-to-cortisol ratio is present in individuals with PTSD.

Clinical Presentation

PTSD develops after a traumatic event. A person who develops PTSD may have been the one who was harmed, the harm may have happened to a loved one, or the person may have witnessed a harmful event that happened to someone else.

PTSD was first brought to public attention in relation to war veterans, but it can result from a variety of traumatic events. Patients with PTSD can startle easily, become emotionally numb, lose interest in most things they used to enjoy, have trouble feeling affectionate, be irritable, become more aggressive, or even become violent toward others. They avoid situations that remind them of the trauma, and anniversaries of the incident are often very difficult. Most people with PTSD repeatedly relive the trauma in their thoughts during the day and in nightmares when they sleep (Fig. 166-1). Some patients experience flashbacks—intense, highly realistic memories of a trauma. Flashbacks may consist of images, sounds, smells, or feelings and are often triggered by ordinary occurrences, such as a door slamming or a car backfiring on the street. In some cases, the person with PTSD having a flashback may lose touch with reality and believe that the traumatic incident is happening all over again.

Differential Diagnosis

A diagnosis of PTSD cannot be made without a clear history of a traumatic event. Other conditions cause many of the symptoms experienced in PTSD, and these conditions must be ruled out. Conditions such as substance abuse and depression develop as complications of PTSD. Ultimately, the distinguishing factor is the fact that the patient has experienced a severe trauma. Some of the conditions that must be ruled out include adjustment disorder, depression, panic disorder, and substance abuse or dependence disorder. Furthermore, malingerers—in this case, people who falsely claim to be traumatized—sometimes feign PTSD symptoms to win money in a court case as compensation for emotional suffering.

Acute stress disorder (ASD) is similar to PTSD in that it occurs after exposure to a traumatic event. Symptoms of ASD appear within 4 weeks of the trauma and last from 2 days to 4 weeks. As with PTSD, they include re-experiencing, avoidance, and increased arousal. However, fewer symptoms are required in each category to make a diagnosis. ASD is distinguished from PTSD by having more dissociative symptoms; that is, patients describe feeling "as if they're in a daze," or have temporary amnesia about the trauma. ASD may progress to PTSD but is more responsive to treatment, emphasizing the need for early recognition and intervention.

Diagnostic Approach

Diagnosing PTSD in an office visit can be challenging. The diagnosis is frequently missed because patients do not typically volunteer information about traumatic events they may have experienced or readily disclose symptoms associated with PTSD. Although direct questioning is necessary, making the diagnosis requires more than checking off a list of symptoms.

To ensure that the diagnosis is not missed, a brief trauma history should be included in all evaluations for anxiety or depression. Traumatic events of adulthood can be asked about directly, for example, "Have you ever been physically attacked or assaulted? Have you ever been in a severe accident? Have you ever been in combat or a disaster?" A positive response should alert the clinician to inquire further about the relationship between the event and any current symptoms. Traumatic childhood experiences require reassuring statements of normality to put the patient at ease: "Many people continue to think about frightening aspects of their childhood. Do you?"

The mnemonic DREAMS can help elicit pertinent details after the trauma history has been obtained (Box 166-1). With each event, the examiner should determine if the person appears emotionally *d*etached (called alexithymia), either from the event or in relationships with others. It may also manifest as a general numbing of emotional responsiveness. The individual *r*e-experiences the event in the form of nightmares, recollections, or flashbacks. The event involved substantial *e*motional distress, with threatened death or loss of physical integrity, and feelings of helplessness or disabling fear. The person avoids

Figure 166-1 Post-traumatic Stress Disorder.

Individuals with PTSD may relive traumatic events in their thoughts during the day and in nightmares when they sleep.

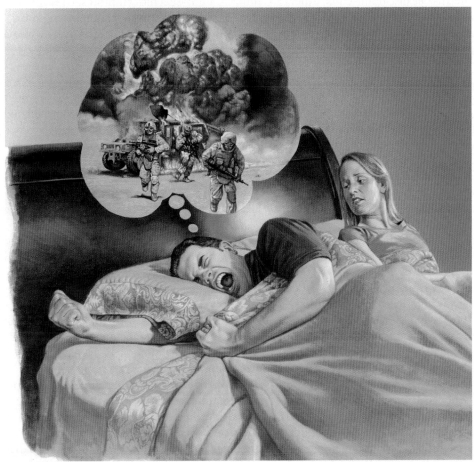

C. Machado
—M.D.

Box 166-1   DREAMS: A Mnemonic for Screening
Patients with Post-traumatic
Stress Disorder

Detachment
Re-experiencing
Emotional distress
Avoidance
Month's duration of symptoms
Sympathetic hyper-reactivity or hypervigilance

---

places, activities, or people that remind him or her of the event. The symptoms need to have been present longer than one *m*onth, and the individual should experience *s*ympathetic hyperactivity or hypervigilance, which may include insomnia, irritability, and difficulty concentrating. As with all psychiatric interviews, assessing imminent danger of the patient to self or others is essential.

More formal means of assessing traumatic events and PTSD with tests and diagnostic interviews are also available. Selection of tests and diagnostic instruments should include an examination by the clinician of the relevant data on their psychometric properties, such as rates of false-positive and false-negative results, sensitivity, and specificity.

It is standard practice in clinical research settings to use structured diagnostic interviews to ensure that PTSD symptoms are reviewed in detail. The use of structured diagnostic interviews in the clinical setting is less common, with perhaps the exception of clinical forensic practice.

Several self-report measures have been developed as a time- and cost-efficient method for assessing PTSD symptoms. These measures are widely used because of their ease of administration, but are also useful as adjuncts to the structured diagnostic interviews. They are often used as screening measures for PTSD, but specific cutoff scores on some instruments can be used to derive a diagnosis of PTSD.

Research on biologically based measures of PTSD has grown tremendously during the past 15 years. Studies have shown that PTSD alters a variety of physiologic functions and may also affect structural regions of the brain. Findings in this area point to the capacity of psychophysiologic indices to identify and classify cases of PTSD on the basis of reactivity to audio-, audiovisual-, and imagery-based cues. Measures have included heart rate, blood pressure, skin conductance, and electromyography. Psychophysiologic assessment is costly in terms of time, patient burden, and cost. It is unlikely that this form of assessment will be widely adopted by clinicians because of the costs, expertise required, and success of other, more economical measures such as the diagnostic interviews and self-report measures that are currently available.

Management and Therapy

Optimum Treatment

Treatment of PTSD typically begins with a detailed evaluation and the development of a treatment plan that meets the unique needs of the patient. Generally, PTSD-specific treatment is started when the patient is not in crisis. Crises that need to be addressed before the initiation of PTSD-specific treatment include: problems such as the patient is currently being exposed to trauma, for example, ongoing domestic violence, abuse, or homelessness; severe depression or suicidal ideation, extreme panic or disorganized thinking; or the need of alcohol or drug detoxification. The important components of treatment for PTSD include (1) educating trauma survivors and their families about the likely causes of PTSD, how PTSD affects survivors and their loved ones, and other problems that commonly occur with PTSD symptoms; (2) exposure to the traumatic event through imagery, which allows the survivor to re-experience the event in a safe, controlled environment, while also carefully examining his or her reactions and beliefs in relation to that event; (3) having the patient examine and resolve strong feelings such as anger, shame, or guilt, which are common among survivors of trauma; and (4) teaching the patient to cope with post-traumatic memories, reminders, reactions, and feelings without becoming overwhelmed or emotionally numb. Trauma-related memories usually do not go away entirely as a result of therapy but become manageable with the mastery of new coping skills. The steps outlined here represent only a portion of the several therapeutic approaches commonly used to treat PTSD.

Cognitive-behavioral therapy (CBT) involves working on thoughts (cognitions) and how those cognitions influence emotions and behaviors. Exposure therapy is one form of CBT that is unique to trauma treatment. It uses careful, repeated, detailed imagining of the trauma (exposure) in a safe, controlled context to help the survivor face and gain control of the fear and distress that were overwhelming during the trauma. In some cases, trauma memories or reminders can be confronted all at once, an approach referred to as *flooding*. For other individuals or traumas, it is preferable to work up to the most severe trauma gradually by using relaxation techniques and by starting with less upsetting life stresses, or by taking the trauma one piece at a time. This approach is called *systematic desensitization*.

Along with exposure, CBT for trauma includes learning skills for coping with anxiety (such as breathing retraining or relaxation training), and negative thoughts (cognitive restructuring), anger management training, preparing for stress reactions (stress inoculation training), coping with future trauma-specific symptoms, coping with urges to use alcohol or drugs when trauma symptoms occur, and communicating and relating effectively with people (social skills training or couples therapy).

Pharmacotherapy can reduce the anxiety, depression, and insomnia often experienced with PTSD, and in some cases, pharmacotherapy may help relieve the distress and emotional numbness caused by trauma-related memories. Several kinds of antidepressant drugs have been shown to contribute to patient improvement in most (but not all) clinical trials, and it is possible that other classes of drugs will be useful based on preliminary studies. At this time, however, the only drug approved by the U.S. Food and Drug Administration for the specific treatment of PTSD is sertraline (Zoloft).

Eye movement desensitization and reprocessing (EMDR) involves elements of exposure therapy and CBT combined with techniques (eye movements, hand taps, or sounds) that create an alternation of attention back and forth across the person's midline. Although the theory and research are still evolving for this form of treatment, there is some evidence that the therapeutic element unique to EMDR, attentional alternation, may facilitate the accessing and processing of traumatic material.

Group treatment is often an ideal therapeutic setting because trauma survivors are able to share traumatic material within the safety, cohesion, and empathy provided by other survivors. As group members achieve greater understanding and resolution of their trauma, they often feel more confident and able to trust. As they discuss and share how they cope with trauma-related shame, guilt, rage, fear, doubt, and self-condemnation, they prepare themselves to focus on the present rather than the past. Telling one's story (the "trauma narrative") and directly facing the grief, anxiety, and guilt related to trauma enable many survivors to cope with their symptoms and memories and other aspects of their lives.

Brief psychodynamic psychotherapy focuses on the emotional conflicts caused by the traumatic event, particularly as they relate to early life experiences. Through the retelling of the traumatic event to a calm, empathic, compassionate, and nonjudgmental therapist, the survivor achieves a greater sense of self-esteem, develops effective ways of thinking and coping, and learns to deal more successfully with intense emotions. The therapist can help the survivor identify current life situations that set off traumatic memories and worsen PTSD symptoms as well as help identify coping mechanisms.

Avoiding Treatment Errors

The first step in effectively treating PTSD is an accurate diagnosis. Not all patients will spontaneously disclose that they have experienced a traumatic event, especially one that they may perceive as particularly stigmatizing such as childhood trauma, sexual assault, or domestic violence. Additionally, many patients with a history of trauma and PTSD present with somatic complaints, depression, anxiety, or substance abuse that is comorbid with their trauma symptoms. It is important that clinicians routinely screen patients for a history of trauma and assess the individual for symptoms of PTSD if a traumatic event is present in the individual's history. Once a diagnosis of PTSD has been established, the second step in effectively treating PTSD is to assess the patient's symptoms and level of functional impairment to see if pharmacotherapy is indicated or to refer the patient for trauma-focused therapy.

Future Directions

The primary prevention of PTSD is vital and should include support and advocacy of community and national efforts to prevent violence and curb its sequelae. Gun control and educational efforts to prevent rape, child abuse, and domestic violence are primary preventive strategies that may reduce the incidence of PTSD.

Biologic and treatment outcome research has been largely restricted to combat veterans. Similar types of studies need to be conducted on survivors of other types of trauma such as natural disasters, sexual assault, and industrial accidents. Future trauma studies are needed to clarify whether the subjective, behavioral, and biologic responses to different types of trauma are the same as the responses to combat-related trauma. Other issues that merit further study include investigation of whether there are gender-specific factors that may promote a different trauma response in women than men, how PTSD is expressed differently in people from different cultures and nationalities, and whether there are other psychiatric syndromes resulting from traumatic exposure that may have a unique cluster of symptoms distinguishable from PTSD.

Additional Resources

International Society for Traumatic Stress Studies (ISTSS). Available at: http://www.istss.org/. Accessed August 22, 2006.

This website is maintained by an international multidisciplinary, professional membership organization that promotes advancement and exchange of knowledge about severe stress and trauma. It provides information on professional and public education, treatment guidelines, worldwide networking and support, fact sheets, and information for the media.

National Center for PTSD. Available at: http://www.ncptsd.va.gov/. Accessed August 22, 2006.

This website is oriented primarily to military veterans, although there are many readings of value to families and trauma survivors. There are also assessment tools, fact sheets, and a very large index to trauma-related literature.

National Crime Victims Treatment and Research Center (NCVC). Available at: http://www.musc.edu/cvc/. Accessed August 22, 2006.

The NCVC is devoted to achieving a better understanding of the impact of criminal victimization on adults, children, and their families. The program activities of the NCVC are focused in four major areas: scientific research, evidence-based treatment, professional education, and consultation.

EVIDENCE

1. Davidson JR: Pharmacological treatment of acute and chronic stress following trauma. J Clin Psychiatry 67(Suppl 2):34-39, 2006.

   This article reviews pharmacologic treatment options for post-traumatic stress disorder (PTSD), focusing on goals of pharmacotherapy and the clinical trial evidence for drug treatments available for PTSD.

2. Foa EB, Keane TM, Friedman MJ: Guidelines for treatment of PTSD. J Trauma Stress 13(4):539-588, 2000.

   This article describes treatment guidelines developed by the PTSD Treatment Guidelines Task Force of the ISTSS based on an extensive review of the clinical and research literature. These guidelines are intended to inform the clinician about what are considered to be the best practices in the treatment of individuals with a diagnosis of PTSD.

Linda M. Nicholas

Obsessive-Compulsive Disorder

Introduction

Obsessive-compulsive disorder (OCD) is a well-defined, often debilitating illness characterized by obsessions, compulsions, or both. First described 150 years ago, the conceptualization of OCD has undergone profound changes over the past 2 decades. Once considered a rare psychogenic syndrome with treatment based on the exploration of early childhood conflict, OCD is now understood as a prominent, neuropsychiatric disease with abnormal brain circuitry and neurotransmitter dysfunction. Unfortunately, OCD continues to be a hidden, often unrecognized illness with an average 5- to 10-year lag from onset of symptoms to appropriate diagnosis and treatment. Because effective treatment is highly specific and nonspecific treatments are ineffective, many are left to suffer needlessly.

OCD affects 2% to 3% of the U.S. population, and cross-national studies have found a remarkably similar prevalence across diverse geographic and cultural sites. Men and women are equally likely to be affected. Age of onset is typically during late adolescence or early adulthood, although childhood onset is not uncommon, with as many as one third of patients recalling the emergence of symptoms before age 15 years. Males tend to have an earlier age of onset than females.

Etiology and Pathogenesis

Remarkable advances have been made in our understanding of the genetic and neurologic underpinnings of OCD. The observation that the tricyclic antidepressant, clomipramine, a serotonin reuptake inhibitor (SRI), is effective in treating patients with OCD, whereas antidepressants with primarily noradrenergic reuptake activity (e.g., desipramine) are not, led to the hypothesis that serotonin plays a major role in the mediation of OCD. Results of neuroendocrine, metabolite, and platelet-binding studies also suggest dysregulation of serotonin function in OCD.

Studies using modern neuroimaging techniques strongly implicate basal ganglia circuitry in the mediation of OCD symptoms. Corticostriatal pathways involve both serotonergic and dopaminergic neurons. Several structural studies have found decreased basal ganglia volumes in OCD patients compared with those in healthy controls. Functional studies using positron emission tomography have shown increased resting activity in the frontal lobes, basal ganglia, and cingulum of patients with OCD, with normalization of these findings following successful pharmacologic or behavioral intervention. Neuropsychological and neurosurgical studies are also consistent with the importance of the basal ganglia in OCD.

Family and twin studies indicate a genetic contribution to the etiology of OCD. There is increased risk for OCD in first-degree relatives of affected patients, as well as increased concordance in monozygotic compared with dizygotic twins.

Clinical Presentation

The clinical description of OCD has changed little over the past 150 years. The core clinical symptoms are obsessions or compulsions that either are time consuming or cause functional impairment or distress, and are not due to another psychiatric or medical illness (Box 167-1).

Obsessions are persistent thoughts, images, or impulses that are experienced as intrusive, distressing, and inappropriate. Most studies have found that the most common

Figure 167-1 Obsessive-Compulsive Disorder.

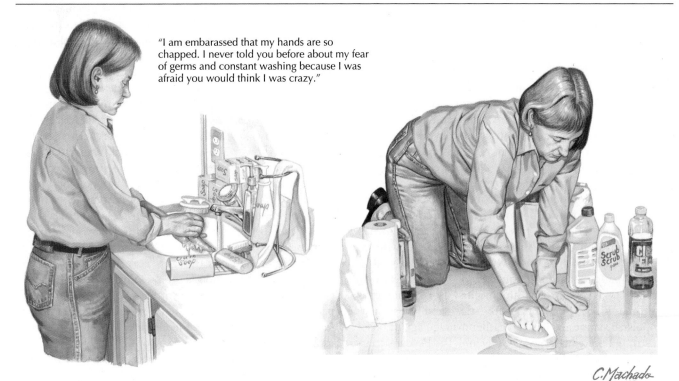

"I am embarassed that my hands are so chapped. I never told you before about my fear of germs and constant washing because I was afraid you would think I was crazy."

Box 167-1 *DSM-IV* Criteria for Obsessive Compulsive Disorder
Either obsessions or compulsions
Symptoms cause marked distress
Not simply excessive worries about real life problems
Attempts to ignore, suppress, neutralize
Recognition that thoughts, impulses, and images are product of one's own mind
Behaviors or mental acts are aimed at preventing or reducing distress or preventing some dreaded event; however, they either are not connected in a realistic way with what they are meant to neutralize or prevent, or are clearly excessive
Symptoms recognized as excessive at some point (*does not apply to children*)
Obsessions or compulsions result in one of the following:
■ Cause marked distress
■ Are time consuming (take more than an hour a day)
■ Significantly interfere with the person's normal routine, occupational or academic functioning, or usual social activities or relationships
Content not restricted to another Axis I disorder
Not due to the direct effects of a substance (e.g., a drug of abuse, a medication) or a general medical condition

obsessional theme in both adults and children is that of contamination, typified by fear of dirt, germs, toxins, environmental hazards, or bodily secretions (Fig. 167-1). Patients may fear spreading disease or contracting an illness, and such worries are often associated with elaborate and time-consuming washing or bathing compulsions. Other obsessions include pathologic doubt, whereby one worries that his or her actions may cause harm or disastrous consequences; somatic obsessions; sexual or aggressive thoughts and images; and need for symmetry, order, or exactness.

Compulsions are repetitive behaviors or mental acts that an individual feels driven to perform to reduce anxiety or to prevent some dreaded event or outcome, even though the event may be totally unrelated to the behavior. Common compulsions are checking, washing (often associated with contamination obsessions), counting, needing to ask or confess, repeating, hoarding, and ordering or arranging. In clinical samples, the presence of pure obsessions or compulsions is rare. Often patients who appear to have only obsessions also have covert reassurance rituals or mental compulsions, such as repeating or praying rituals.

Traditionally, the obsessions and compulsions in OCD have been characterized as *ego dystonic* (i.e., patients typically view their thoughts and behaviors as senseless and excessive). However, more recent studies and field trials have reported a subset of patients who at times lack insight and display conviction about the reasonableness of their obsessions and necessity of their rituals. It is more likely that insight in OCD may span a spectrum from good to delusional thinking.

Several studies have found that about two thirds of OCD patients have a lifetime diagnosis of a comorbid psychiatric disorder. Major depression is common (50% to 67%), as are other anxiety disorders, including social anxiety disorder, specific phobia, panic disorder, and generalized anxiety disorder (GAD). OCD rarely occurs with mania. Some patients with schizophrenia have coexisting obsessions and compulsions, and concurrent OCD may be associated with a poorer outcome of schizophrenia.

There is a high degree of bidirectional overlap between tic disorders and OCD. Almost 25% of patients with tic disorders meet full criteria for OCD, and conversely, 20% of OCD patients have a lifetime history of multiple tics, with 5% to 10% having a lifetime history of Tourette's syndrome (TS). Patients with tics and obsessive-compulsive symptoms have an earlier average age of onset and strong family histories of OCD and TS. Psychostimulants (e.g., methylphenidate or dextroamphetamine) may exacerbate both tics and obsessive-compulsive symptoms in susceptible individuals.

Recent research has focused on the concept of an obsessive-compulsive spectrum, based on the observation that a series of possibly related disorders are similar in phenomenology, associated features (age of onset, clinical course, neurobiology), familial transmission, and clinical response to specific pharmacologic and behavioral interventions. These include eating disorders, certain somatoform disorders (hypochondriasis, body dysmorphic disorder), and disorders of impulse control (trichotillomania, pathologic gambling).

Differential Diagnosis

There are a number of medical disorders that can produce syndromes resembling OCD, including diseases of the basal ganglia such as Huntington's disease, certain tumors, postencephalitic conditions, and traumatic brain injury. Because OCD characteristically presents in the teens and 20s, new onset of symptoms in an older individual should raise questions considering the possibility of neurologic conditions.

Swedo and colleagues observed a high prevalence of obsessions and compulsions in children in whom Sydenham's chorea developed. Sydenham's chorea is a neurologic variant of rheumatic fever following a group A β-hemolytic streptococci infection. Because there is evidence that Sydenham's chorea may be an autoimmune response involving antibodies to the basal ganglia, this association has led to intriguing work on this phenomenon that has come to be called *pediatric autoimmune neuropsy-*

chiatric disorder associated with *Streptococcus* and treatment with immunologic interventions, such as plasmapheresis or intravenous immunoglobulin therapy. This syndrome tends to present more acutely, in contrast to the more insidious onset in other cases of childhood OCD.

The clinician must also rule out other psychiatric conditions in which obsessive-compulsive behavior might be found. Major depressive disorder is frequently comorbid with OCD and may be characterized by obsessive ruminations. The two conditions may be differentiated by the course of illness. Obsessive symptoms associated with depression are only present during the depressive episode, whereas true OCD symptoms persist independently of a depressive episode. Additionally, depressed patients do not see their thoughts as absurd or senseless. It can also be difficult to distinguish OCD from the worry and anxious apprehension seen in GAD. In patients with GAD, the content of the anxious thoughts is realistic, although the worry is excessive. OCD is often confused with obsessive-compulsive personality disorder (OCPD). Although patients with OCD may display perfectionism and indecisiveness, they are no more likely than healthy controls to exhibit the features characteristic of OCPD, such as rigidity, restricted ability to express warmth, or excessive devotion to work.

Psychotic symptoms may sometimes result in obsessions and compulsions that are difficult to distinguish from OCD with poor insight. In most instances, however, patients with OCD will be able to acknowledge the unreasonable nature of their symptoms. Additionally, psychotic disorders, such as schizophrenia, are characterized by other symptoms that are not present in OCD, such as hallucinations, disorganized speech, or flattened affect.

Diagnostic Approach

The failure to properly diagnose OCD is most likely due, in part, to the shame and humiliation that many patients feel about the symptoms and the fear that they will be seen as crazy. Adults and children can be very secretive about their symptoms, and often OCD is not apparent until secondary symptoms (e.g., dermatologic problems from excessive washing and cleaning) reveal themselves or until families complain. However, lack of suspicion on the part of clinicians, as well as failure to ask appropriate screening questions, also play a role in the failure to recognize this disorder. The primary method of establishing a diagnosis is a clinical interview with specific questions designed to elicit a history of intrusive thoughts or behavioral rituals.

Because OCD typically presents in adolescence or early adulthood, screening questions should be asked of any patient in this age group who presents with anxiety, depression, or secondary symptoms, or whose family complains of odd rituals and preoccupations. Sample questions might include, "Do you experience thoughts or images that you find disturbing but cannot seem to keep out of your head?"

Table 167-1 Comparison of Antidepressant Treatment of Depression versus Obsessive-Compulsive Disorder

	Depression	**Obsessive-Compulsive Disorder**
Drug	Drugs with different profiles of monoamine uptake effective	Only serotonergic drugs effective
Time to response	Adequate trial usually 4-6 weeks for treatment response	Trial of 8-12 weeks for response
Treatment goal	Remission	Symptom reduction
Relapse rate	Variable upon discontinuation of medication (30%-50% within 2 months)	Higher relapse rate upon medication discontinuation (90% within 2 months)

and "Are there actions you feel you must do over and over even though you don't want to?" A patient-administered diagnostic instrument, as well as relevant information about OCD is available on the Obsessive Compulsive Foundation website.

Management and Therapy

Pharmacotherapeutic advances have revolutionized the treatment of OCD. Serotonin reuptake inhibitors (SRIs), including the tricyclic antidepressant clomipramine and the selective serotonin reuptake inhibitors (SSRIs), are the first-line treatment for OCD. Treatment of OCD is specific; antidepressants other than SRIs are ineffective. Additionally, the therapeutic lag time is longer (8 to 12 weeks), and higher doses are often needed for patients with OCD compared with those with other conditions. Failure to recognize these differences in appropriate treatment of OCD versus depression can result in major treatment errors and therapeutic response failures (Table 167-1).

A case report in 1967 provided the first hint that clomipramine might be effective for OCD. Its efficacy was later confirmed by multicenter placebo-controlled trials. Clomipramine also has norepinephrine and dopamine reuptake properties and is associated with the adverse effects typical of tricyclic antidepressant agents, including anticholinergic, antihistaminergic, α-adrenergic side effects; quinidine-like cardiac properties; sexual dysfunction; increased risk for seizures; and lethality in overdose. SSRIs are better tolerated than clomipramine and are also effective in treating obsessive-compulsive spectrum disorders. Fluvoxamine, sertraline, fluoxetine, and paroxetine have been shown to be effective in large, multicenter, placebo-controlled trials. There is also evidence that citalopram and escitalopram are effective. SRIs may effectively treat comorbid mood and anxiety disorders (Table 167-2).

A review of studies suggests that 65% to 70% of OCD patients have a clinically significant response to initial SRI treatment and that as many as 90% of patients respond with sequential trials. Thus, patients who do not respond to one SRI may respond to a different one. Generally, treatment provides a 30% to 60% relief of symptoms but does not induce a full remission. Symptoms tend to re-

Table 167-2 First-Line Pharmacologic Treatment for Obsessive-Compulsive Disorder

Drug (Serotonin Reuptake Inhibitor)	Usual Dose Range (mg)	Average Daily Dose (mg)
Clomipramine	100-300	200
Fluoxetine	20-80	50
Sertraline	75-225	150
Paroxetine	20-60	50
Fluvoxamine	100-300 (divided)	200
Citalopram	20-60	—
Escitalopram	10-40	—

emerge upon discontinuation of therapy, thus requiring long-term treatment for most patients. Long-term data suggest that efficacy is maintained and may even increase over time.

Because as many as 40% to 60% of patients do not have an adequate response to SRI treatment, augmentation strategies are important in managing OCD. A number of pharmacologic agents, including a second SRI, lithium, buspirone, clonazepam, and trazodone, have been used to augment SRIs, but data confirming their usefulness are limited. Dopamine antagonists, such as haloperidol, have been found to be helpful, particularly in patients with comorbid tic disorders or poor insight. More recently, the combination of an SRI and the atypical antipsychotic risperidone seems to hold some promise. Electroconvulsive therapy has not been shown to be effective. Neurosurgery, particularly cingulotomy, has been effective in treating severe, refractory OCD, and deep brain stimulation is being studied.

Cognitive Behavioral Therapy

Behavioral therapy has consistently been shown to be helpful in reducing the symptoms of OCD, and studies have shown techniques are based on exposure and response prevention. Patients are increasingly exposed to the feared situation or avoided stimuli and prevented from performing the associated rituals. Compulsions are more amenable to behavioral treatment than obsessions. Cognitive therapy may be particularly useful for pathologic doubt, aggressive obsessions, and scrupulosity. Because traditional psychodynamic psychotherapy is not effective for OCD, patients should be referred to a mental health professional trained in these techniques.

Optimum Treatment

Treatment of OCD should always include cognitive behavioral therapy, and mild to moderate cases may respond to this modality alone. A combination of pharmacotherapy and behavioral therapy is considered the standard of care for more severe or disabling cases and is associated with earlier response and reduced risk for relapse.

Avoiding Treatment Errors

Misdiagnosis accounts for many of the treatment errors made in the management of OCD. A mistaken diagnosis of psychosis may result in unnecessary and potentially harmful treatment with antipsychotic drugs. Treatment of major depression without recognition of comorbid OCD may result in ineffective drug choice, as well as inadequate dosing and duration of treatment. Failure to include a behavioral therapy component to treatment may deprive the patient of an optimal chance of recovery.

Future Directions

As our understanding of the brain continues to advance, the exact nature of the pathogenesis and etiology of OCD should become more apparent, enabling more precise detection and treatment. More work should be done identifying subtypes of OCD as well as exploring alternative and adjunctive treatment for patients with treatment resistance. Exciting developments clarifying this important disorder will certainly continue over the coming years.

Additional Resources

March JS, Frances A, Carpenter D, Kahn DA (eds): Expert consensus guideline series. Treatment of obsessive compulsive disorder. Available at: http://www.psychguides.com/ocgl.html. Accessed December 24, 2006.

This consensus paper provides excellent guidelines for evidence-based and stepwise treatment of OCD for the clinician.

Obsessive Compulsive Foundation. Available at: http://www.ocfoundation.org. Accessed December 24, 2006.

The Obsessive Compulsive Foundation provides an informative website for physicians, therapists, and patients with OCD and their families. There are many resources provided, including literature and educational materials, a guide to finding a therapist, and research opportunities.

EVIDENCE

1. Fineberg NA, Gale TM: Evidence-based pharmacotherapy of obsessive-compulsive disorder. Int J Neuropsychopharmacol 8(1):107-129, 2005.

   This excellent synthesis of randomized trials, meta-analyses, and consensus guidelines addresses pharmacologic treatment of OCD.

2. Hollander E, Kaplan A, Allen A, Cartwright C: Pharmacotherapy for obsessive-compulsive disorder. Psychiatr Clin North Am 23(3):643-656, 2000.

   The authors provide an excellent review of the nuances associated with OCD management as well as the evidence for alternative strategies in the face of nonresponse or inadequate response to SRIs.

3. Swedo SE, Leonard HL, Garvey M, et al: Pediatric autoimmune neuropsychiatric disorders associated with streptococcal infections: Clinical description of the first 50 cases. Am J Psychiatry 155:264-271, 1998.

   Swedo's characterization of the OCD-like symptoms associated with Sydenham's chorea is fascinating and sheds light on the neurobiology of OCD.

Schizophrenia

Introduction

Schizophrenia describes a heterogeneous group of chronic relapsing psychotic disorders with a lifetime incidence of about 1% worldwide. Schizophrenia is a disease that often significantly affects the ability of an individual to function in a number of different ways. The overt clinical symptoms typically present in late adolescence or early adulthood, at a time when one is establishing independence from family, beginning higher education or employment, and establishing adult relationships. Males have an earlier onset, more severe symptoms, poorer treatment response, and a more chronic course. Childhood-onset schizophrenia is a rare, more severe form of the adult-onset illness. About 10% of new-onset psychosis occurs after the age of 40 to 45 years, designated as late-life schizophrenia.

Schizophrenia is, at its core, a disorder of altered reality perception, characterized by hallucinations and delusions (Fig. 168-1). However, its onset, presentation, clinical course, and presumably its causes are remarkably heterogeneous. The course is characterized by acute episodes of psychotic symptoms with intervening periods of relative stability that have a varying degree of residual symptoms and functional impairment. The chronic course is variable. In some individuals, symptoms are minimal between acute psychotic episodes, and there is little functional impairment. At the opposite extreme, hallucinations and delusions persist, and there is profound functional impairment.

Etiology and Pathogenesis

There is clearly a genetic component to schizophrenia. The incidence in the first-degree relatives of an affected individual is about 10%. The concordance rate in monozygotic twins is about 45%. The search for genes that confer risk for schizophrenia has been somewhat disappointing because a contribution of any single gene to risk for schizophrenia is small. Regions on several chromosomes have been identified, and it is most likely that schizophrenia is a polygenic disorder with multiple susceptibility genes.

Environmental factors contribute to the risk for schizophrenia in an individual. Prenatal exposure to maternal infection, perinatal hypoxia, and other obstetric complications increase risk. Birth in an urban area and late winter or early spring birth are more frequent in people in whom schizophrenia develops, perhaps a result of toxic, nutritional, or infectious exposures.

Structural neuroimaging studies find subtle abnormalities of the brain, including mild enlargement of the lateral and third ventricles and gray matter reductions in the frontal and temporal lobes, as well as reductions in the volume of the hippocampus. There is evidence that white matter is also abnormal. Functional imaging studies such as positron emission tomography (PET), magnetic resonance imaging (MRI), and magnetic resonance spectroscopy reveal abnormalities in frontal cortex and temporal structures, including the hippocampus. Abnormalities in the cerebellum, thalamus, and striatum have also been described.

Postmortem studies reveal subtle abnormalities as well, including changes in neuron number, alteration of various synaptic protein densities, and reduced density of dendritic spines. Abnormalities in several neurotransmitter systems have been implicated by postmortem, PET, and preclinical studies as well as by the mechanism of action of antipsychotic medications. The dopamine, glutamate, and serotonin systems are all of importance in schizophrenia.

Currently, schizophrenia is conceptualized with a two-hit model, in which genetic risk factors interact with perinatal environmental risk factors to cause subtle abnormalities

Figure 168-1 Schizophrenia.

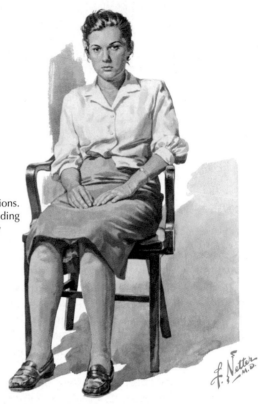

Schizophrenia is a heterogeneous disorder with a wide range of symptomatology. This patient demonstrates the flat affect that is common in schizophrenia. She appears to be responding to internal stimulation—perhaps attending to auditory hallucinations. Alternatively, she may have significant negative symptoms, including anhedonia, amotivation, and poverty of speech. Finally, she may have parkinsonism secondary to antipsychotic medication.

in brain structure and connectivity between neurons. Age-dependent neurodevelopmental events during adolescence such as synaptic pruning and myelination unmask abnormal functional circuits in the brain and give rise to clinical symptoms.

Clinical Presentation

There are three main domains of symptoms associated with schizophrenia: (1) positive symptoms, (2) negative symptoms, and (3) cognitive dysfunction. Positive symptoms are the classic symptoms of psychosis and include delusions and hallucinations. Delusions, false beliefs that are held with conviction despite evidence to the contrary, are present in more than 90% of patients. Delusions can take many forms; paranoid, persecutory, and religious are common. Hallucinations, perceptual disturbances that can occur in any sensory modality, are present in about 50% of patients. Of these, auditory and visual hallucinations are the most common.

Negative symptoms are abnormalities of volition and include restricted or flat affect, anhedonia, poverty of speech, apathy, amotivation, and asociality. About 25% of patients with schizophrenia have the deficit syndrome, or primary negative symptoms, which may be a true subtype of schizophrenia. In other patients, negative symptoms, although common, are secondary to the positive symptoms

(i.e., a paranoid person would be asocial and amotivated), depression, anxiety, demoralization, an understimulating environment, or side effects of the medication used to treat psychosis.

Patients typically have cognitive dysfunction, which is increasingly recognized as a major reason for functional impairment. A variety of neurocognitive functions including attention, memory, and executive function are impaired. Patients often present with disorganized thinking and speech, as a result of cognitive dysfunction, as well as positive and negative symptoms.

Differential Diagnosis

The differential diagnosis of psychosis (Box 168-1) is long and begins with substance abuse (amphetamines, cocaine, phencyclidine, marijuana, hallucinogens) or withdrawal (alcohol, sedative-hypnotic). Psychosis is often seen in a hospital setting in the form of delirium resulting from a variety of causes. Medical conditions include acute intermittent porphyria, Cushing's syndrome, hypocalcemia and hypercalcemia, hypoglycemia, hypothyroidism and hyperthyroidism, hepatic encephalopathy, and paraneoplastic syndromes. Neurologic conditions include partial complex seizures, brain tumors, multiple sclerosis, degenerative disorders (Alzheimer's, Pick's, Huntington's disease), infections (HIV, neurosyphilis, herpes simplex), lupus cerebritis,

---

Box 168-1 Differential Diagnosis of Psychosis

Drugs and Toxic Exposure

Substance abuse (amphetamines, cocaine, phencyclidine, marijuana, hallucinogens)
Withdrawal (alcohol; sedative-hypnotics)
Side effects of prescribed medication (steroids, L-dopa, isoniazid, many others)
Heavy metals (lead, mercury)

Medical Conditions

Delirium
Acute intermittent porphyria
Cushing's syndrome
Hypothyroidism, hyperthyroidism
Hypocalcemia, hypercalcemia
Hypoglycemia
Hepatic encephalopathy
Paraneoplastic syndrome

Neurologic Conditions

Partial complex seizures
Brain tumors
Multiple sclerosis
Degenerative disorders (Alzheimer's, Pick's, Huntington's disease)
Infections (HIV, neurosyphilis, herpes simplex)
Ischemia, infarcts
Lupus cerebritis

Nutritional Deficiencies

Folate
Niacin
Thiamine
Vitamin B_{12}

Psychiatric Conditions

Bipolar disorder
Major depression

Box 168-2 Diagnostic and Statistical manuals of Mental Disorders, Fourth Edition (*DSM-IV*) Criteria for Schizophrenia

A. Characteristic symptoms
   Two or more present for a month or more:
   1. Delusions
   2. Hallucinations
   3. Disorganized speech
   4. Grossly disorganized or catatonic behavior
   5. Negative symptoms
B. Social and occupational dysfunction
   For a significant portion of the time since onset, one or more major areas of functioning such as work, interpersonal relations, or self-care are marked below the level achieved before onset.
C. Duration: continuous signs of the disturbance persist for at least 6 months.
D. Schizoaffective disorder and mood disorders have been ruled out.
E. Substance and general medical condition have been ruled out.
F. Relationship to a pervasive developmental disorder
   If there is a history of autism or another pervasive developmental disorder, the additional diagnosis of schizophrenia is made only if prominent delusions or hallucinations are also present for at least 1 month.

---

stroke, and Wilson's disease. Nutritional deficiencies of folate, niacin, thiamine, and vitamin B_{12} can present with psychosis. Many prescribed medications, heavy metals, and other toxic agents can cause psychotic symptoms. Psychotic symptoms are present in other psychiatric disorders, including mania, severe depression, brief psychotic disorder, delusional disorder, and schizoaffective disorder.

Diagnostic Approach

The diagnosis is a clinical one based on symptoms present during an interview and by history (Box 168-2). Diagnostic criteria for schizophrenia include the presence of two of the following for 1 month: delusions, hallucinations, disorganized speech, grossly disorganized or catatonic behavior, and negative symptoms. In addition, significant social and occupational impairment and duration of symptoms of at least 6 months are needed to make a diagnosis of schizophrenia. Symptoms that meet criteria for schizophrenia but have not lasted as long as 6 months are designated as *schizophreniform disorder*. Patients often believe that their psychotic experiences are real and do not recognize that they are ill. Acutely psychotic patients are frequently disorganized, responding to internal stimuli, and unable to attend to questions. Therefore, it is necessary to get collaborative history from a friend or family member.

New-onset psychosis requires a careful workup, including a physical and neurologic examination to rule out medical and neurologic causes and substance abuse. Basic laboratory tests include a drug screen; complete blood count; and blood chemistries, including calcium, thyroid function tests, HIV, VDRL, and measurement of vitamin B_{12} and folate levels. Additional laboratory work including ceruloplasmin, heavy metals, and autoantibody titers, should be pursued based on relevant history, physical examination, and clinical suspicion. Neuroimaging (computed tomography, MRI) is typically done in the workup to rule out a brain tumor and other central nervous system abnormalities.

Management and Therapy

Hospitalization is indicated when the patient is disorganized and is unable to care for himself or herself or unable to participate in treatment as an outpatient. Suicidal ideation is common. As many as 50% attempt suicide, and 10% are successful. Less frequently, patients with schizophrenia harbor homicidal thoughts based on their delusions. The presence of suicidal and homicidal ideation should be carefully assessed. Hospitalization is indicated when the patient is a danger to himself or herself or to others.

The mainstay of treatment is antipsychotic medications. There are a number of antipsychotic medications, now designated as the older *typical* antipsychotics or the newer *atypical* antipsychotics. Although antipsychotics have different receptor-binding profiles, all have dopamine D_2 receptor antagonist properties that are thought to underlie their antipsychotic action. All antipsychotics are equally efficacious in the treatment of psychosis; choice is based on side-effect profile, prior treatment response, and physician or patient preference. Clozapine has been shown to be more effective than other antipsychotics in patients with treatment-resistant schizophrenia (those who have failed two other antipsychotic trials of adequate dose and duration). Cognitive dysfunction and disorganization may make it difficult for a patient to consistently take medication. In these situations, long-acting injectable antipsychotics can be given every 2 to 4 weeks.

Antipsychotic side effects represent a significant challenge in the management of schizophrenia. Acute extrapyramidal syndromes such as parkinsonism, dystonias, akathisia, and acute dyskinesia are most common. Tardive dyskinesia is a long-term effect consisting of involuntary choreoathetoid movements of the mouth, hands, or trunk. Neuroleptic malignant syndrome, a rare but potentially fatal syndrome, is characterized by fever, muscular rigidity, and mental status changes and can also include autonomic instability, leukocytosis, and elevated creatinine kinase. Other side effects include sedation, orthostatic hypotension, electrocardiogram changes (especially prolongation of the Q-T interval), agranulocytosis, hyperprolactinemia, and sexual dysfunction. Many of the newer atypical antipsychotics are associated with development of the metabolic syndrome, including significant weight gain; elevation of glucose, cholesterol, and triglycerides; and development of type 2 diabetes mellitus.

Optimum Treatment

Schizophrenia is a chronic, complex disorder that is best treated by a team of professionals who work together to address all aspects of the illness. Patients with schizophrenia frequently have comorbid psychiatric disorders that need to be recognized and treated to improve the course of schizophrenia and the patient's overall functioning. The most common are substance abuse, depression, and obsessive-compulsive disorder.

Although medication is the foundation of treatment, other psychosocial treatment modalities play an important role in helping the patient deal with the impact of schizophrenia on his or her life. Supportive, psychoeducational, and cognitive-behavioral therapies, as well as family psychoeducation and intensive community-based outreach programs, all improve outcome and level of functioning in patients. Rehabilitative strategies are used to help patients compensate for deficits in cognitive and social functioning.

Avoiding Treatment Errors

The diagnosis of schizophrenia can be made only after other organic causes of psychosis are ruled out. Psychosis also occurs in severe depression and bipolar illness; these and other psychiatric conditions should be considered when making the diagnosis. It often takes several weeks for antipsychotic treatment to achieve its full benefit, so the temptation to escalate the dose of an antipsychotic prematurely should be avoided. All antipsychotics can have severe and life-threatening side effects; the treating physician should be aware of and carefully monitor for the presence of side effects of the prescribed antipsychotic. Many of the newer atypical antipsychotics are associated with the metabolic syndrome, which can cause significant long-term morbidity and mortality; weight, serum glucose, cholesterol, and triglycerides should be routinely monitored.

Management of Medical Illness

Medical illness is common in patients with schizophrenia, and the recognition and treatment of medical illness presents a challenge to clinicians. Individuals with schizophrenia have high rates of morbidity and mortality related to a variety of medical conditions, including cardiovascular disease, infections, endocrine disorders, and cancer. This high rate of morbidity and mortality is probably related to the side effects of antipsychotic medications (especially the newer atypical antipsychotics), high rates of smoking, low physical activity, poor nutrition, and high levels of chronic stress.

Psychiatrists and other physicians fail to diagnose medical conditions in one third to one half of patients with schizophrenia and a comorbid medical disorder. Psychotic symptoms and cognitive dysfunction, as well as elevated pain thresholds associated with schizophrenia, interfere with symptom recognition, symptom reporting, and seeking help on the part of the patient. From the physician's perspective, a frightening, unhygienic patient with imaginary voices and delusions may be assumed to have imaginary medical problems. Physicians must be alert to high rates of unreported and unrecognized medical illness in patients with schizophrenia. Once a medical illness is diagnosed, it is important to anticipate how the positive and negative symptoms and cognitive dysfunction of schizophrenia might affect a patient's ability to participate in treatment.

Future Directions

There is a clear need for improved pharmacologic treatment of schizophrenia. Only 35% to 45% of patients with schizophrenia have their positive symptoms well controlled by antipsychotic medication, and an estimated 33% are considered to be treatment resistant. In addition, available antipsychotics have potentially serious side effects. Medications that treat negative symptoms and cognitive dysfunction have the potential to improve functional outcome. There is new interest in recognizing and treating schizophrenia before the onset of gross psychotic symptoms with the hope of preventing the progression of the illness and improving long-term outcome. Continuing advances in understanding brain development and functioning from basic neuroscience studies will ultimately improve our ability to define the causes and pathogenesis of schizophrenia and should lead to improved preventive and therapeutic efforts.

Additional Resources

Hwang MY, Bermanzohn PC (eds): Schizophrenia and Comorbid Conditions. Washington, DC, American Psychiatric Press, 2001.

This broad overview covers comorbid medical and psychiatric conditions associated with schizophrenia.

Lehman AF, Lieberman JA, Dixon LB, et al: Practice guideline for the treatment of patients with schizophrenia, 2nd ed. Am J Psychiatry 161(2 Suppl):1-56, 2004.

The authors provide an excellent summary of treatment approaches for the person with schizophrenia.

Lieberman JA, Stroup TS, Perkins DO (eds): Textbook of Schizophrenia. Washington, DC, American Psychiatric Publishing, 2006.

This in-depth consideration of all aspects of schizophrenia includes neurobiology, pathophysiology, and treatment.

Marder SR, Essock SM, Miller AL, et al: Physical health monitoring of patients with schizophrenia. Am J Psychiatry 161(8):1334-1349, 2004.

Consensus recommendations address identifying and monitoring the medical complications that may result from chronic antipsychotic use.

EVIDENCE

1. Lieberman JA, Stroup TS, McEvoy JP, et al: Effectiveness of antipsychotic drugs in patients with chronic schizophrenia. N Engl J Med 353(12):1209-1223, 2005.

This is the initial report from the Clinical Antipsychotic Trials of Intervention Effectiveness (CATIE) study, a landmark study of antipsychotic effectiveness in a large sample of patients with a real-world design, with broad inclusion and minimal exclusion criteria.

2. McEvoy JP, Lieberman JA, Stroup TS, et al: Effectiveness of clozapine versus olanzapine, quetiapine, and risperidone in patients with chronic schizophrenia who did not respond to prior atypical antipsychotic treatment. Am J Psychiatry 163(4):600-610, 2006.

Phase 2 of the CATIE study evaluates treatment for patients with a poor response to the initial trail of antipsychotics.

Emotional and Behavioral Problems among Adolescents and Young Adults

Introduction

Emotional and behavioral problems among adolescents and young adults are associated with substantial morbidity, mortality, and health care costs. Young people experiencing these problems are more likely to participate in behaviors leading to negative outcomes such as injuries, sexually transmitted infections, and unwanted pregnancy. Frequently such problems herald the onset of psychiatric disorders including major depression, bipolar affective disorder (BPAD), and schizophrenia that will require lifelong treatment. Emotional and behavior problems may complicate management of chronic illness in youth by influencing choices about adherence to treatment plans. In all these situations, individuals' life trajectories may be affected by the establishment of maladaptive patterns of behavior and negative influences on major life decisions about education, work, and family. Finally, adolescents and young adults with emotional and behavioral problems are at increased risk for suicide and homicide, the second and third leading causes of death in this age group.

Etiology and Pathogenesis

A broad spectrum of emotional and behavioral problems are seen among adolescents and young adults. The etiology of most problems appears to be multifactorial, with genetic, biologic, social, and developmental factors contributing to varying degrees.

Clinical Presentation

Many adolescents and young adults with emotional and behavioral problems first present in medical rather than mental health care settings. Common presentations include the following:

- Physical symptoms directly related to underlying mental health problems
- Mental status changes that raise questions about underlying medical versus mental illness
- Negative health outcomes of behaviors precipitated by underlying mental health problems
- Worrisome symptoms elicited during routine health care evaluation, which should include a psychosocial history asking about family and peer relationships, school and vocation, alcohol and other drug use, sexual behaviors, emotional health, and body image

Youth experiencing emotional or behavioral problems that are seriously affecting their life and functioning are usually not "just going through a phase" of normal development, and evaluation must include a physical examination and assessment for psychiatric disorders.

Depressive Disorders

The prevalence of major depressive disorder (MDD) in adolescence is estimated at 4% to 8% with a male-to-female ratio of 1 : 2. Symptoms include the following:

- At least 2 weeks of marked change in mood or loss of interest and pleasure
- Significant changes in patterns of appetite, weight, sleep, activity, concentration, energy level, or motivation

Symptoms must impair relationships or performance of activities. Comorbid psychiatric conditions are common, including anxiety disorders, learning problems, attention-deficit/hyperactivity disorder (ADHD) and substance abuse. Adolescents tend to display more irritability and behavioral problems and fewer neurovegetative symptoms than adults with MDD. Hallucinations are also more frequent. Clinical variants include atypical depression with increased sleep and weight gain, seasonal affective disorder, and dysthymia with chronic changes in mood and motivation but few neurovegetative symptoms. About 25% of youth with major depression will attempt suicide within 5 years.

Anxiety Disorders

There are several different anxiety disorders seen in youth, with estimated prevalence ranging from 0.3% to 4.6%. These include panic disorder (0.6% prevalence), post-traumatic stress disorder (PTSD) (about 1%), generalized anxiety disorder (4.6%), obsessive-compulsive disorder (1.9%), and various phobias. Distribution by gender varies by disorder and age of onset.

In each of these disorders, there are unwanted, disturbing thoughts or worries that negatively affect the youth's functioning. Panic disorder is characterized by the presence of panic attacks with at least four somatic symptoms, including palpitations, dyspnea, nausea, dizziness, sweating, paresthesias, and gastrointestinal discomfort. Early onset of panic disorder is associated with greater morbidity. Youth with PTSD often have experienced recurrent traumas and may have difficulty identifying a clear precipitant.

Bipolar Affective Disorder

The overall prevalence of BPAD is 2%, with one third of adults reporting onset during adolescence. There are no significant gender differences. The diagnosis requires the presence of at least one episode with manic symptoms including the following:

- Significantly elevated, expansive, or irritable mood associated with functional impairment
- Significant distractibility, pressured speech, racing thoughts, grandiosity, agitation, and decreased need for sleep

Mixed manic and depressed episodes are common. Youth tend to have more frequent, but shorter, episodes with more severe psychotic symptoms than adults. Youth with bipolar disorder are at even greater risk for suicide than those with major depression. They are also likely to be involved in dangerous sexual and physical activities with numerous health risks.

Substance Use Disorders

Substance use is very common among adolescents and young adults, especially the use of alcohol. To be considered a problem, substance use must produce dysfunction in one or more domains of a patient's life and cause clinically significant levels of distress or impairment. The most common features among adolescents are impairment in psychosocial and academic functioning. Substance use disorders are often associated with other psychiatric disorders and significantly increase the risk for suicide in those disorders.

Eating Disorders

Estimates of the lifetime prevalence of anorexia nervosa range from 0.5% to 3.7% and of bulimia nervosa range from 1.1% to 4.2%. Eating disorders are more common in females (male-to-female ratio of 1:6 to 1:10), and onset usually occurs during adolescence and young adulthood.

Symptoms of anorexia nervosa include the following:

- Refusal to maintain weight at or above a minimally normal weight or failure to gain weight during a period of expected growth
- Intense fears of gaining weight
- Disturbance in body image
- Absence of at least three spontaneous menstrual cycles in postmenarchal females

Symptoms of bulimia nervosa include the following:

- Recurrent episodes of binge eating characterized by eating large amounts of food in a short period and inability to control eating
- Recurrent inappropriate compensatory behavior to prevent weight gain (e.g., self-induced vomiting, misuse of medications, fasting, or excessive exercise)
- Binge eating and inappropriate compensatory behaviors have both occurred at least twice a week for 3 months
- Self-evaluation is unduly influenced by body shape and weight

Patients with anorexia nervosa often present to medical settings with weight loss or amenorrhea. Patients with either disorder may present with complications of severe electrolyte disturbances. Occasionally patients present with constipation or esophageal tears. Rates of comorbid psychiatric diagnosis among patients with eating disorders are high (50% to 75%). Mortality rates vary according to age of onset, length of disease, and presence of purging behaviors. Death is typically from cardiac arrhythmia or suicide. In general, younger adolescents have the best and adults have the worst outcomes.

Schizophrenia Spectrum Disorders

Schizophrenia affects 1% of the adult population. Sixty percent of those affected have symptoms during adolescence. Although equal numbers of males and females are affected, males typically have earlier onset with more severe symptoms. At least two of the following symptoms are required for diagnosis:

- Delusions
- Hallucinations
- Disorganized or illogical speech
- Catatonia or grossly disorganized behavior
- Negative symptoms (social withdrawal, apathy, and poverty of speech)

Frank symptoms are often preceded by transient hallucinations or delusions, social isolation, or deterioration in social and academic functioning. Substance use may trigger symptoms in biologically vulnerable individuals or may reflect efforts to self-medicate. Youth tend to have less systematized delusions and more complex hallucinations than adults. The main variant is schizoaffective disorder with intermittent affective symptoms but persistent psychotic symptoms. One in ten individuals with schizophrenia commits suicide.

Attention-Deficit/Hyperactivity Disorder

The estimated prevalence of ADHD is 5% in the school-age population with male-to-female ratios ranging from 4 : 1 to 9 : 1. As many as 80% have symptoms persisting into adolescence and 65% into adulthood. Infrequently ADHD is diagnosed in adolescents and young adults, although there should be a history of attentional difficulties in childhood.

Symptoms may be predominately inattention, predominately hyperactivity with impulsiveness, or a combination of both. Symptoms typically are present in situations that are unstructured, boring, or require sustained mental effort. Adolescents often complain of restlessness rather than hyperactivity. Other psychiatric illnesses such as major depression and schizophrenia may also reduce attention.

Differential Diagnosis

When evaluating emotional and behavioral disorders in adolescents and young adults, it is important to recognize that the same symptoms may occur in different disorders. For instance, striking changes in appetite and weight may be seen in anorexia nervosa, major depression, schizophrenia, and substance abuse. Generally the diagnosis is dependent on the constellation of symptoms observed and their developmental course. It is also essential to consider nonpsychiatric etiologies of the symptoms such as medical illness or reactions to medications.

Diagnostic Approach

The evaluation and management of adolescents and young adults should be conducted in a developmentally

appropriate manner. Issues to consider include chronologic age, cognitive development, psychosocial development, and parental relationships. Youth often provide more accurate reports about their affective state, anxieties, and cognitive processes than their parents, but may have difficulty recognizing behavioral, functional, and social problems. Legal, ethical, and professional guidelines have been developed for managing confidentiality when providing health care to minor adolescents.

The general approach to diagnosis of emotional and behavioral problems in youth includes the following:

- Complete history and physical examination, including a detailed neurologic examination
- Gathering additional information from family and other sources (e.g., school personnel)
- Judicious use of laboratory tests to exclude primary medical conditions
- Consultation with or referral to a mental health professional as needed

All adolescents and young adults with emotional and behavioral problems should be assessed for risk for suicide. Factors that place youth at highest risk for suicide include male gender, previous suicide attempt, substance abuse, MDD, agitation, psychosis, and family history of suicide.

Management and Therapy

Optimum Treatment

The American Academy of Child and Adolescent Psychiatry publishes Practice Parameters guiding the treatment of adolescents with emotional and behavioral disorders.

General management strategies encourage the adolescent or young adult to take an active role in treatment. Health care providers and families should provide support and guidance. Treatment often includes the following:

- Individual cognitive, behavioral, and supportive therapy
- Family therapy and education
- Psychopharmacology

Cognitive therapy has been demonstrated to be particularly effective in the treatment of anxiety disorders and milder cases of depression. Behavior therapy is often essential for the treatment of eating disorders, substance abuse disorders, ADHD, and BPAD. Education about the illnesses and their treatments are essential in all disorders.

Medication treatments are effective in adolescents. Serotonin reuptake inhibitors are typically the first line of treatment for major depression and anxiety disorders and may also be useful in the treatment of some eating disorders. Some of the newer antidepressants may be alternatives. Tricyclic medications have been established to be ineffective antidepressants in youth. Antidepressants are associated with increased suicidal thoughts and behavior in about 4% of treated youth (particularly during the early phases of treatment) regardless of diagnosis.

Concerns about the safety of antidepressants in adolescents need to be weighed against clear risks for inadequately treated depression.

Mood stabilizers, including lithium, valproic acid, carbamazepine, and many newer antiepileptic agents, are the cornerstone of treatment for BPAD. Each of these agents can have significant systemic side effects, including renal, liver, and hematologic changes. Increasingly, newer antipsychotics are being used for first-line treatment of BPAD without psychotic features. Antipsychotic medication is essential for youth with psychotic symptoms, whether associated with depression, BPAD, or schizophrenia. The newer antipsychotics have relatively few extrapyramidal side effects but often result in considerable weight gain and increased risk for diabetes and lipid abnormalities. Some antipsychotics, particularly risperidone, cause prolactin elevations that may lead to amenorrhea and increased risk for osteopenia in females.

Management of patients who are at high risk for suicide includes measures to ensure their acute safety and treatment for associated emotional disorders. Those at highest risk may need to be hospitalized. Those who do not require hospitalization need to have adequate supervision and support from a responsible adult and a safe home environment. It is essential that firearms be removed from the home and that access is limited to medications.

All adolescents and young adults with emotional and behavioral problems should continue receiving routine health care to monitor for possible health consequences of psychotropic medications and to assess emerging health needs.

Avoiding Treatment Errors

It is particularly important to monitor adolescents' clinical response to medication because the emergence of symptoms of lifelong psychopathology often occurs during this stage of development and definitive diagnoses may not yet be clear. For example, an adolescent who will eventually be diagnosed as having BPAD may first present as an adolescent with clinical signs and symptoms of MDD; treatment with antidepressants may precipitate the first manic episode.

Future Directions

Adolescents and young adults with psychiatric disorders are much less likely to be identified and treated than older adults. Better identification depends on improving community education about major mental illnesses in youth, recognition in schools, and diagnosis by primary care physicians. Future research needs to focus on prevention, early intervention, and treatment of emotional and behavioral disorders specifically in adolescent and young adult populations. Focus on mental health issues in this age group has the potential to substantially reduce morbidity, mortality, health care costs, and the individual and societal burden of psychiatric illness among youth and across the life cycle.

Additional Resources

National Institute of Mental Health. Antidepressant medications for children and adolescents: information for parents and caregivers. Available at: http://www.nimh.nih.gov/healthinformation/antidepressant_child.cfm. Accessed February 25, 2007.

This site contains information about the potential risks and benefits of antidepressant medication in adolescents.

National Institute on Drug Abuse. NIDA Infofacts: High school and youth trends. Available at: http://www.nida.nih.gov/Infofax/HSYouthtrends.html. Accessed February 25, 2007.

This site provides a recent summary of substance use among adolescents in the United States.

Ozer EM, Park MJ, Paul T, et al: America's adolescents: Are they healthy? National Adolescent Health Information Center. Available at: http://nahic.ucsf.edu. Accessed February 25, 2007.

This website provides an overview of adolescent health in the United States.

EVIDENCE

1. American Academy of Child and Adolescent Psychiatry: Practice parameters. Available at: http://www.aacap.org/page.ww?section=Practice+Parameters&name=Practice+Parameters. Accessed February 25, 2007.

   This reference site provides management and treatment guidelines specific to adolescent mental health problems that are based on evidence and professional consensus.

2. Ford C, English A, Sigman G: Confidential health care for adolescents: A position paper of the society for adolescent medicine. J Adolesc Health 35(2):160-167, 2004.

   The authors review legal, policy, and practical issues influencing the provision of confidential adolescent health care services.

3. March J, Silva S, Petrycki S, et al: Fluoxetine, cognitive-behavioral therapy, and their combination for adolescents with depression. Treatment for Adolescents with Depression Study (TADS) randomized controlled trial. JAMA 292(7):807-820, 2004.

   This article presents evidence supporting the effectiveness of antidepressant medication in treatment of MDD in adolescents.

4. Wolraich ML: The classification of child and adolescent mental diagnosis in primary care. In Diagnostic and Statistical Manual for Primary Care (DSM-PC) Child and Adolescent Version. Elk Grove Village, IL, American Academy of Pediatrics, 1996.

   This classification provides specific criteria for diagnosis of mental health problems in adolescents.

James C. Garbutt ▪ Robert E. Gwyther ▪ John M. Thorpe, Jr.

Alcohol and Substance Dependence and Abuse

Introduction

Humans have used psychoactive substances for thousands of years. Nature has provided most of our psycho-active drugs, including ethanol, morphine, cocaine, and marijuana. However, human ingenuity has enabled us to also develop synthetic molecules with potent psychoactive properties, such as fentanyl, oxycodone, and methamphetamine. Although most cultures accept the use of some psychoactive drugs, which drugs are used and the patterns of use differ across cultures. For example, alcohol consumption is common in the United States, with 60% to 70% of the U.S. population reporting use.

Psychoactive substances can produce medical harm in many ways, but the two principal causes of harm are direct effects of the substance (e.g., cocaine-induced arrhythmia) and behavioral consequences of seeking and using the substance (e.g., missing work recovering from alcohol or activities related to procuring psycho-active substances). Most psychoactive substances share a unique ability to produce addiction in vulnerable individuals. Addiction, or substance use dependence, represents the most severe form of dysfunctional use of psychoactive substances. Addiction is characterized by a compulsive need to use the drug, loss of control over the use of the drug, continued use despite negative consequences, and—particularly for alcohol, opiates, and the sedative-hypnotics—development of physical dependence.

Unhealthy substance use, including addiction, is common. At least 15% of outpatients, 25% to 40% of in-patients, and more than 50% of some specialty unit patients (e.g., psychiatry, burn unit) have a substance abuse problem. Alcohol and tobacco use causes most of these encounters; however, the use and abuse of other drugs is substantial. Concurrent use of two or more psychoactive drugs is common. In some cases, this can lead to unique problems. For example, the metabolic production of cocaethylene after alcohol and cocaine consumption can produce serious arrhythmias and necrotizing vasculitis. Physicians need to understand the consequences of the use of alcohol and drugs of abuse and develop an open-minded approach that considers these agents as potential contributors in every patient encounter.

Etiology and Pathogenesis

Alcoholism, as a disease syndrome, was described independently in 1785 by the American physician Dr. Benjamin Rush and the British physician Dr. Thomas Trotter. Although considerable societal stigma remains, many studies have demonstrated the therapeutic importance of regarding alcohol and drug abuse through a disease concept with both genetic and environmental components. Adoption and twin studies have revealed that genetic factors contribute about 50% to the etiology of substance use disorders. No single gene is dominant, and multiple genes are being identified, many affecting neurobiologic function.

Significant advances have occurred in understanding the neurobiologic actions of addictive drugs and how these contribute to the disease process. Two components have emerged from the many studies on addiction and the development of the compulsive use pattern that character-izes addiction. First, positive reinforcement occurs from all addictive drugs—these drugs activate the classic dopamine reward pathways from midbrain to nucleus accumbens and prefrontal cortex. Thus, drugs take on behavioral significance for an individual, and the sensitivity to this effect is likely genetically influenced. Second, over time, alcohol and other drugs produce neuroadaptation such that when the drug is stopped, acute and protracted withdrawal can occur. Acute withdrawal is well understood (see later). Protracted withdrawal, a relatively new concept, lasts for months. Although the symptom profile of protracted withdrawal is still being defined, it likely includes insomnia, stress sensitivity, anxiety, decreased ability to experience pleasure, and other symptoms. These are negatively reinforcing and are significant factors in relapse to use.

Alcoholism and drug addiction are progressive and, not uncommonly, fatal illnesses. Individuals may have cycles of treatment and relapse, never receive treatment, or achieve significant improvement with, or even without, treatment.

Clinical Presentation

The clinical presentation of alcoholism is extremely varied. In a general medical practice or hospital setting, the medical or traumatic consequences of alcoholism are the most common reasons an individual with an alcohol problem comes to a physician's attention. Alcohol has toxic effects on most organ systems, and individuals may present with any of a number of end-stage medical problems (e.g., cirrhosis, pancreatitis), behavioral problems, including depression and insomnia, and a number of less severe medical problems that are exacerbated by alcohol or drug use (Fig. 170-1). Patients in surgical and medical units frequently go into alcohol withdrawal after admission with symptoms of autonomic activation, tremor, confusion, fever, seizures, agitation, and hallucinations. Withdrawal delirium is one of the most common reasons for psychiatry consultations. At the less severe end of the spectrum, alcohol use is known to increase the risk for common medical problems such as essential hypertension, hypertriglyceridemia, and gout. A connection between alcohol use and presenting physical symptoms is commonly not offered. Therefore, physicians should always consider the possible role of alcohol and other drugs of abuse in their clinical evaluation of patients who are acutely ill and hospitalized or who are outpatients with less severe problems.

The clinical presentation of drugs of abuse is also quite varied and can include the following:

- Stimulants: tachycardia, increased blood pressure, ischemia of brain or heart, delusions, grandiose behavior
- Opioids: bradycardia, decreased respiratory rate, miotic pupils, decreased consciousness
- Sedative-hypnotic drugs: bradycardia, hypotension, decreased respiratory rate, decreased consciousness, ataxia
- Hallucinogens: hallucinations, disorientation, anxiety, psychosis

These general findings on presentation are as useful as a more comprehensive list of presenting signs and symptoms, given the very large number of agents and their association with numerous diseases. There are a number of additional red flags for substance abuse that reflect the physical and social effects of addiction, infection related to intravenous drug abuse, clinical syndromes resulting from accelerated atherothrombosis (from cocaine and other stimulants), and laboratory or physical findings resulting from alcohol or drug-induced end-organ damage. These include the following:

Historical factors: violence, trauma, hematemesis, acute mental status changes, acute psychosis, previous drug abuse, homelessness, criminal behavior, financial deterioration, job loss, seeking a specific controlled substance

Physical findings: increased or decreased pulse, respirations or blood pressure; poor hygiene; odor of alcohol; jaundice, splinter hemorrhages, needle tracks or spider hemangiomas; miosis or mydriasis; perforated nasal septum; new heart murmur; ataxia, hyperreflexia; combativeness, decreased consciousness; findings inconsistent with the stated level of pain

Diagnostic test results: positive drug screen; ethanol level >0.10 g/dL; elevated liver enzymes; elevated mean corpuscular volume; positive cardiac enzymes in a young person; electrocardiograms showing rapid rhythms; evidence of myocardial infarction (MI) in a young person; computed tomography or magnetic resonance imaging evidence of stroke in a young person

Differential Diagnosis

The differential diagnosis of alcohol use and other drug disorders can be conceptualized as separating the consequences of unhealthy alcohol or drug use from true alcohol or drug addiction, wherein loss of control and compulsive use commonly lead to severe consequences. The diagnosis of alcohol dependence (alcoholism), or drug dependence, as defined by the *Diagnostic and Statistical Manual of Mental Disorders*, 4th edition, includes a maladaptive pattern of substance use, leading to clinically significant impairment or distress, as manifested by three or more of the following, occurring in the same 12-month period (Fig. 170-2):

- Tolerance as evidenced by requiring more alcohol (or drug) to achieve intoxication or less of an effect with continued use of the same quantity of alcohol (or drug)
- Withdrawal symptoms when alcohol (or drug) is stopped
- Alcohol (or drug) taken in greater quantities or for a longer time than intended
- Persistent desire or unsuccessful efforts to reduce use
- A great deal of time spent in using and recovering from alcohol (or drug)
- Important activities given up or reduced because of alcohol (or drug) use
- Alcohol (or drug) use continued despite adverse consequences

Figure 170-1 Effects of Alcohol on End Organs.

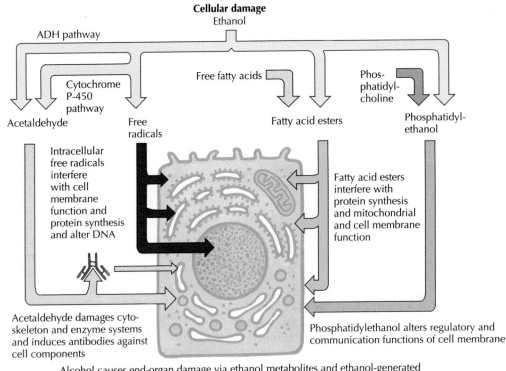

Cellular damage
Ethanol

ADH pathway

Cytochrome P-450 pathway

Free fatty acids

Phos-phatidyl-choline

Acetaldehyde

Free radicals

Fatty acid esters

Phosphatidyl-ethanol

Intracellular free radicals interfere with cell membrane function and protein synthesis and alter DNA

Fatty acid esters interfere with protein synthesis and mitochondrial and cell membrane function

Acetaldehyde damages cyto-skeleton and enzyme systems and induces antibodies against cell components

Phosphatidylethanol alters regulatory and communication functions of cell membrane

Alcohol causes end-organ damage via ethanol metabolites and ethanol-generated compounds, which alter structure and function of cell components

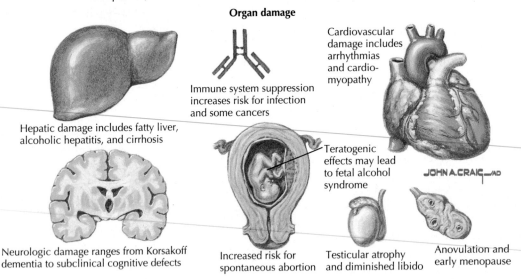

Organ damage

Immune system suppression increases risk for infection and some cancers

Cardiovascular damage includes arrhythmias and cardio-myopathy

Hepatic damage includes fatty liver, alcoholic hepatitis, and cirrhosis

Teratogenic effects may lead to fetal alcohol syndrome

JOHN A. CRAIG—AD

Neurologic damage ranges from Korsakoff dementia to subclinical cognitive defects

Increased risk for spontaneous abortion

Testicular atrophy and diminished libido

Anovulation and early menopause

Alcohol and drugs of abuse may be the underlying cause of disease in patients not previously known to be abusers. Because known drug abusers are often malnourished, have underlying organ damage, and experience events such as falls or tracheal aspiration while intoxicated, it is common for them to develop other mental and physical illnesses. For these reasons, drug abuse should be a part of the differential diagnoses for most common medical and psychiatric diagnoses.

Some general considerations for drug-related problems are (1) when the working diagnoses are ruled out, think about drugs; (2) when young patients suffer ischemia (e.g., transient ischemic attacks or MI), consider cocaine or the combination of cocaine and alcohol; (3) when treating a substance abuser (e.g., delirium in a withdrawal syndrome) without getting the expected response, look for a complication (e.g., subdural hematoma); (4) toxic manifestations of one drug (e.g., agitation, tachycardia in cocaine intoxication) mimic the withdrawal symptoms of another (e.g., agitation, tachycardia in barbiturate withdrawal); and (5) drug use is associated with perinatal problems (e.g., premature labor, placental abruption with cocaine abuse) and

Figure 170-2 Alcohol Dependence.

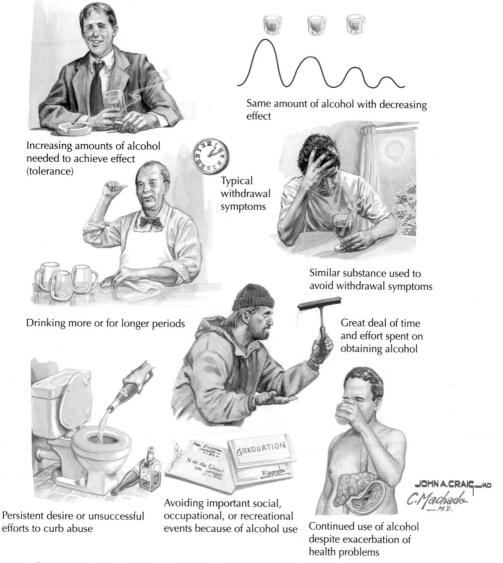

Increasing amounts of alcohol needed to achieve effect (tolerance)

Same amount of alcohol with decreasing effect

Typical withdrawal symptoms

Similar substance used to avoid withdrawal symptoms

Drinking more or for longer periods

Great deal of time and effort spent on obtaining alcohol

Persistent desire or unsuccessful efforts to curb abuse

Avoiding important social, occupational, or recreational events because of alcohol use

Continued use of alcohol despite exacerbation of health problems

JOHN A. CRAIG—MD
C. Machado—M.D.

Three or more incidences during 1 year indicate pattern of physical dependence

newborn complications (e.g., HIV, opiate withdrawal in infants of heroin-addicted mothers).

Diagnostic Approach

The diagnosis of alcohol and drug use disorders depends on the documentation of signs and symptoms (see previous criteria and Fig. 170-3). Because the diagnosis is based primarily on the history, it is important to gather data on alcohol and drug use patterns and related problems from the patient, as well as from collateral sources of information such as a spouse. In a nonjudgmental fashion, ask the patient about the type, amount, and frequency of substances used. After determining use, its consequences should be explored, including physical symptoms, relationship and employment problems, and emotional and psychological issues.

Screening tests have been developed, including the CAGE (4 questions) and the Alcohol Use Disorders Identification Test (AUDIT, 10 questions), which are easy to administer and provide good sensitivity for detection of alcohol problems (Box 170-1). The AUDIT-C, the first three questions of the AUDIT, focuses just on consumption—how often do you have a drink, how many drinks on a typical day, how often have you had six or more drinks on one occasion—and has shown very good sensitivity and specificity as a simple screening tool. The higher the score on the AUDIT-C, the greater the likelihood that the individual has alcohol-related problems.

Laboratory tests for alcoholism have suffered from a lack of specificity. For example, γ-glutamyl transpeptidase is a reasonably sensitive test of recent heavy alcohol use but is not specific for alcohol use. Recently, carbohydrate-

Figure 170-3 Signs Suggestive of Alcohol Abuse.

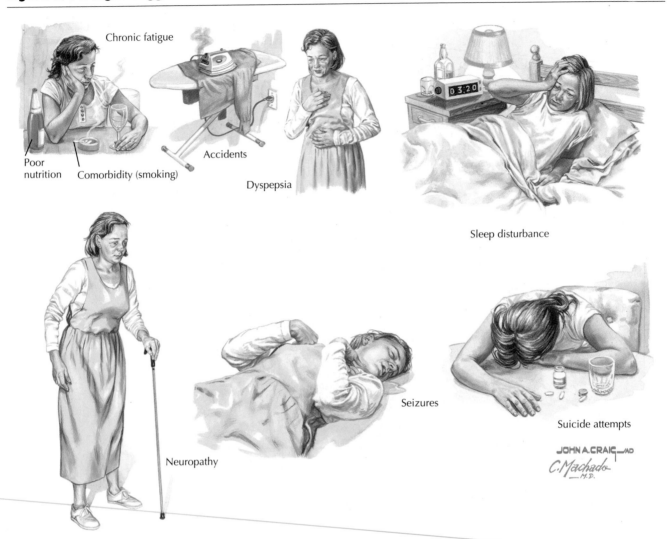

deficient transferrin has emerged as a test with improved specificity for heavy alcohol use, and it may be useful when heavy drinking is suspected.

Blood testing for drugs is quantitatively accurate and necessary for managing critical problems but has the diagnostic disadvantage of a relatively narrow window of positivity. Urine drug screens are qualitatively accurate and offer a longer window of positivity (e.g., 48 to 72 hours for cocaine users, 2 to 4 weeks for regular marijuana users). Hair testing is helpful in documenting remote use and use over time. However, hair testing is not quantitatively accurate or readily available, and is expensive.

Laboratory testing may be necessary to make diagnoses; properly manage patients' medical conditions; monitor patients in addiction treatment; screen job applicants; and monitor federal personnel involved in the Departments of Transportation (e.g., pilots, truck drivers) and Defense (e.g., the Army). The federal screening panel includes amphetamines, cannabinoids, cocaine, opioids, and phencyclidine. Laboratories are regulated by strict criteria;

certified medical review officers interpret positive results, taking patient histories into account.

Legal and ethical dilemmas of laboratory drug testing include the following:

- *Informed consent.* Ideally, patients should understand the ramifications of getting tested for drug use. Yet, some patients are unconscious on presentation and cannot give consent. Others are minors living in states where parents can demand tests even though the child refuses. Some refusals may be ignored, especially when a patient is intoxicated and not competent to refuse. Inevitably, drug tests sometimes are performed without patient consent.

- *Criminal and civil justice.* For a drug test to be admissible in a criminal court, the following must happen: (1) a chain of custody must be established from the time the sample is collected until the results are introduced into evidence; and (2) the methodology required by the state's courts must be used.

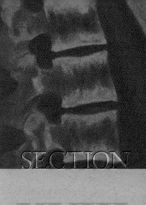

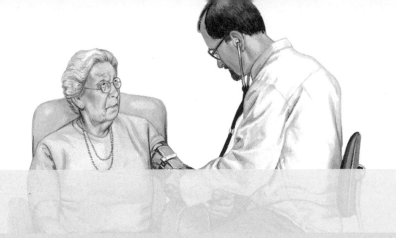

Disorders of the Skin

Grant BF, Dawson DA, Stinson FS, et al: The 12-month prevalence and trends in DSM-IV alcohol abuse and dependence: United States, 1991-1992 and 2001-2002. Drug Alcohol Depend 74(3):223-234, 2004.

The authors present one of the more recent epidemiologic studies of the prevalence of alcohol use disorders.

Koob GF, Roberts AJ: Brain reward circuits in alcoholism. CNS Spectr 4:23-37, 1999.

The authors review the neurochemical circuits that may mediate the reinforcing effects of alcohol.

Mayo-Smith MF: Pharmacological management of alcohol withdrawal. A meta-analysis and evidence-based practice guideline. American Society of Addiction Medicine Working Group on Pharmacological Management of Alcohol Withdrawal. JAMA 278(2):144-151, 1997.

The author summarizes clinical trials of medication treatment for alcohol withdrawal.

O'Brien CP, McLellan AT: Myths about the treatment of addiction. Lancet 347(8996):237-240, 1996.

This article provides a perspective on addictive disorders as chronic illnesses that can respond to treatment.

Prescott CA, Kendler KS: Genetic and environmental contributions to alcohol abuse and dependence in a population-based sample of male twins. Am J Psychiatry 156(1):34-40, 1999.

This is one of the key papers showing the role of genetics in contributing to alcohol use disorders.

Saitz R: Clinical practice. Unhealthy alcohol use. N Engl J Med 352(6):596-607, 2005.

The author provides a recent summary of the range of alcohol use problems.

Saunders JB, Aasland OG, Babor TF, et al: Development of the Alcohol Use Disorders Identification Test (AUDIT): WHO Collaborative Project on Early Detection of Persons with Harmful Alcohol Consumption—II. Addiction 88(6):791-804, 1993.

The AUDIT is another useful screening instrument for alcohol use disorders.

Sullivan JT, Sykora K, Schneiderman J, et al: Assessment of alcohol withdrawal: The revised Clinical Institute Withdrawal Assessment for Alcohol scale (CIWA-Ar). Br J Addict 84(11):1353-1357, 1989.

This article describes probably the most widely used scale to assess alcohol withdrawal.

EVIDENCE

1. Bouza C, Angeles M, Munoz A, Amate JM: Efficacy and safety of naltrexone and acamprosate in the treatment of alcohol dependence: A systematic review. Addiction 99(7):811-828, 2004.

   This recent article updates the efficacy of naltrexone and acamprosate for alcohol dependence.

2. Garbutt JC, West SL, Carey TS, et al: Pharmacological treatment of alcohol dependence: A review of the evidence. JAMA 281(14):1318-1325, 1999.

   The authors review the efficacy of pharmacotherapies, including lithium, SSRIs, disulfiram, naltrexone, and acamprosate for alcohol dependence.

3. Mattick RP, Kimber J, Breen C, Davoli M: Buprenorphine maintenance versus placebo or methadone maintenance for opioid dependence. Cochrane Database Syst Rev 3:CD002207, 2004.

   This article reviews the efficacy of buprenorphine for opiate dependence.

4. Miller WR, Wilbourne PL: Mesa Grande: A methodological analysis of clinical trials of treatments for alcohol use disorders. Addiction 97(3):265-277, 2002.

   The authors thoroughly review the efficacy of multiple psychosocial and medical therapies for alcoholism.

as methadone, a partial opioid agonist such as buprenorphine, or an α_2-noradrenergic agonist such as clonidine. Once opiate withdrawal is complete, patients need to be engaged in psychosocial treatment. Some patients may need longer-term agonist treatment with either methadone or buprenorphine in order to achieve stabilization. Buprenorphine may be prescribed by specially licensed physicians in their office, whereas methadone must be provided by a certified clinic. The advantage to agonist therapy is that it has been shown to significantly reduce HIV conversion, legal problems, and use of illegal opiates.

Benzodiazepines and Barbiturates

Benzodiazepine and barbiturate withdrawal can be severe and life threatening. Withdrawal symptoms can include agitation, anxiety, insomnia, tremor, tinnitus, nausea, delirium, hallucinations, tachycardia, hypertension, fever, and in severe cases, seizures and death. The onset of withdrawal is rapid for short-acting drugs such as alprazolam but can be delayed until up to 7 to 10 days for long-acting drugs such as clonazepam or diazepam. Management of withdrawal is usually done with a long-acting benzodiazepine or phenobarbital. No medications are approved for long-term management of benzodiazepine or barbiturate addiction.

Cocaine and Stimulants

Cocaine or stimulant withdrawal is not life threatening and, by itself, is not an indication for hospitalization. Withdrawal symptoms include depression, oversleeping, tiredness, increased appetite, increased dreaming, and drug craving. After withdrawal, patients should be engaged in counseling and encouraged to attend 12-step meetings. No medications are approved for treatment of cocaine or stimulant addiction.

Cannabinoids

Cannabinoid withdrawal in a heavy user does occur and can include irritability, strange dreams, anxiety, and decreased appetite. There are no treatments for cannabinoid withdrawal. The discovery of antagonists for brain cannabinoid receptors (e.g., rimonabant) is of theoretical interest for treatment of cannabinoid dependence, but no large-scale clinical trial data are available.

General Issues

Most clinicians have recovering patients in their practices. Physicians should follow certain principles in the treatment of these patients: use appropriate, nonpharmacologic therapies when possible; be wary of treating anxiety, insomnia, pain, and allergies with sedative-hypnotic drugs or opioids, which may provoke relapse; treat depression and anxiety with drugs that are not addictive (e.g., selective serotonin reuptake inhibitors, buspirone). When an analgesic is needed, the physician and the patient should contract specifically for pain relief. Finally, it is very important for physicians to offer ongoing support for the patient's recovery.

Avoiding Treatment Errors

The first error to avoid is failure to identify substance misuse as an important factor in a patient's health problems. It is important to be aware that more than one substance is often used by patients. For this reason, it is important to gather additional history and use toxicology screens to enhance the accuracy of the diagnosis. Identification of multiple drug use is important for detoxification and long-term management.

The clinician should remain flexible with regard to the level of care that a patient may need. If a patient is failing less intense outpatient treatment, consider more intense outpatient treatment or residential care.

Compliance with medication use is a common problem. Monitor for compliance by using collateral information and talking to the patient. For patients who have problems with compliance, consider a long-acting formulation where available, such as intramuscular naltrexone.

Future Directions

The development of the disease concept of addictive disorders has been a significant advance for understanding and treating alcohol and drug use disorders. The past 30 years have seen a much more sophisticated description of the biologic and psychosocial forces that lead to addiction. However, far too many individuals remain undiagnosed and untreated. Science will continue to provide new and unexpected insights into the genetic and pathophysiologic basis of addiction, and undoubtedly more effective medications will emerge. Yet, for the benefits of science to be translated to the care of patients, health care providers, policy makers, and the general public will need to realize that the treatment of addiction is not only effective but the most efficient manner in which to use society's scarce resources. Clinicians will be key players in the effort to reduce the stigma of substance use disorders through education and to advocate for adequate resources for treatment.

Additional Resources

Edenberg HJ, Foroud T: The genetics of alcoholism: Identifying specific genes through family studies. Addict Biol 11(3-4):386-396, 2006.
The authors review recent developments in the identification of genes that contribute to the risk for alcohol dependence.
Ewing JA: Detecting alcoholism. The CAGE questionnaire. JAMA 252(14):1905-1907, 1984.
This is the original simple screening tool to identify patients who may have alcohol use disorders.
Fleming MF, Barry KL, Manwell LB, et al: Brief physician advice for problem alcohol drinkers. A randomized controlled trial in community-based primary care practices. JAMA 277(13):1039-1045, 1997.
This well-conducted trial demonstrates that brief interventions can be effective in alcohol use disorders.

nature of addiction, nor are they fully aware of the health-related consequences of heavy alcohol use. In these circumstances, patient education is valuable.

The decision whether to medically detoxify a patient depends on the risk for serious withdrawal (i.e., seizures, delirium tremens [DTs]). Factors that increase the likelihood of serious withdrawal include history of seizures or DTs, concomitant medical illness, old age, and to some extent, quantity and frequency of alcohol consumption. Patients who do not have risk factors can be monitored for signs of significant withdrawal. The Clinical Institute Withdrawal Assessment of Alcohol Scale Revised is a useful instrument to quantify withdrawal severity. Patients with risk factors or significant withdrawal symptoms require medical detoxification, and this should be completed in a residential medical setting unless an established outpatient detoxification program is available. Benzodiazepines have been recommended as the treatment of choice for alcohol withdrawal and are highly effective in reducing withdrawal symptoms and in reducing the risk for seizures or DTs. However, DTs develop in some patients despite benzodiazepine treatment. Thiamine should be given parenterally to prevent the development of Wernicke's encephalopathy (confusion, ataxia, ophthalmoplegia) or permanent memory impairment (Korsakoff's syndrome).

Detoxification has been referred to as the first step in alcoholism treatment. Many approaches have been tried to help the alcoholic or alcohol abuser to change his or her drinking behavior, ranging from long-term residential care to brief outpatient visits. To date, no clear algorithms are available to guide the clinician on what specific form of treatment should be recommended for a given patient. However, patients with milder forms of alcohol problems may show improvement in a primary care setting with very brief interventions that provide education, feedback, and encouragement to alter drinking patterns. Patients with more severe alcohol problems usually require more specialized treatment that may include a period of residential care, intensive outpatient treatment, encouragement to attend Alcoholics Anonymous (AA), and medication. The strategies employed in these settings include motivational therapy, cognitive-behavioral relapse prevention therapy, and engagement in the 12 steps of AA. An important element in working with the alcoholic patient is to provide care over time and to avoid therapeutic nihilism. In fact, outcome studies suggest that 50% or so of alcoholics will have at least a 50% reduction in alcohol use 6 months after treatment.

The question of abstinence versus reduced use commonly comes up in early discussions of treatment. For some drugs, such as cocaine and heroin, there is no question that abstinence is the necessary path. For alcohol, the picture can be less clear. For patients with alcoholism and severe consequences, abstinence is the appropriate objective. For patients with unhealthy alcohol use and resistance to abstinence, it is appropriate for the clinician to work with the patient to reduce use and evaluate the role alcohol plays in the patient's life. Maintaining a therapeutic relationship is more important than demanding a patient endorse lifelong abstinence. Over time, many patients will move toward abstinence.

Medication management of alcoholism is in the midst of significant change that should enhance treatment. For years, the only medication to treat alcoholism was disulfiram, an inhibitor of aldehyde dehydrogenase. Disulfiram produces an aversive reaction (ranging from flushing and headache to profuse vomiting, tachycardia, chest pain, confusion, and other symptoms) when alcohol is consumed and provides a psychological deterrent to alcohol consumption. Its efficacy is related to compliance, and it is particularly valuable in highly motivated patients or with supervised administration. In the United States, disulfiram is usually given as 250 mg/day once a patient is detoxified from alcohol.

Naltrexone represents a newer class of medications for the treatment of alcoholism that do not act by aversive deterrence. Naltrexone is an opioid antagonist that has been shown to reduce the risk for relapse to heavy drinking and, possibly, enhance the likelihood of abstinence. Naltrexone is thought to work by counteracting the "high" experienced after drinking alcohol so that patients are less likely to lose control. Naltrexone is usually started after several days of sobriety and continued for at least several months in combination with psychosocial treatment. In 2006, the U.S. Food and Drug Administration approved a long-acting injectable formulation of naltrexone that is administered once per month. This formulation has been shown to reduce heavy drinking frequency and, in patients with a period of abstinence before injection, to enhance abstinence.

Acamprosate, another relatively new agent, is thought to attenuate overactive N-methyl-D-aspartate activity in the brain that may occur after alcohol withdrawal. Acamprosate has been shown to significantly reduce the frequency of drinking and enhance the likelihood of abstinence.

Because of the added value provided by medications and the overall positive risk-to-benefit ratio, clinicians should strongly consider the use of medications along with psychosocial therapy in the treatment of alcoholism.

These broad treatment concepts are also applicable to the management of other drugs of abuse. However, there are specific issues with different classes of drugs about which physicians should be aware.

Opiates

Opiates produce a classic physical withdrawal syndrome that can include diarrhea, nausea, restlessness, piloerection, mydriasis, rhinorrhea, tachycardia, hypertension, fever, insomnia, and drug craving. Serious medical consequences to opiate withdrawal are rare; however, relapse to opiate use is high. Pharmacologic management of opiate withdrawal involves the use of either an opiate agonist such

Box 170-1   CAGE and AUDIT Questions

CAGE: One positive answer on the CAGE should raise suspicion; two positive answers on the CAGE is highly predictive of alcohol dependence.

Cut
1. Ever felt you ought to cut down on your drinking?
   Annoyed
2. Have people annoyed you by criticizing your drinking?
   Guilt
3. Ever felt bad or guilty about your drinking?
   Eye Opener
4. Ever had an eye opener to steady nerves in the morning?

AUDIT: A score of 8 or greater on the AUDIT indicates that additional screening should be conducted for alcohol problems. (points in parentheses)

1. How often do you have a drink containing alcohol?
   Never (0)
   Monthly or less (1)
   2-4 times a month (2)
   2-3 times a week (3)
   4 or more times a week (4)
2. How many drinks containing alcohol do you have a typical day when you are drinking?
   1-2 (0)
   3-4 (1)
   5-6 (2)
   7-9 (3)
   10 or more (4)
3. How often do you have 6 or more drinks on one occasion?
   Never (0)
   Less than monthly (1)
   Monthly (2)
   Weekly (3)
   Daily or almost daily (4)
4. How often during the last year have you found you were not able to stop drinking once you had started?
   Never (0)
   Less than monthly (1)
   Monthly (2)
   Weekly (3)
   Daily or almost daily (4)

5. How often during the last year have you failed to do what was normally expected from you because of drinking?
   Never (0)
   Less than monthly (1)
   Monthly (2)
   Weekly (3)
   Daily or almost daily (4)
6. How often during last year have you needed a first drink in the morning to get yourself going after a heavy drinking session?
   Never (0)
   Less than monthly (1)
   Monthly (2)
   Weekly (3)
   Daily or almost daily (4)
7. How often during the last year have you had a feeling of guilt or remorse after drinking?
   Never (0)
   Less than monthly (1)
   Monthly (2)
   Weekly (3)
   Daily or almost daily (4)
8. How often during the last year have you been unable to remember what happened the night before because you had been drinking?
   Never (0)
   Less than monthly (1)
   Monthly (2)
   Weekly (3)
   Daily or almost daily (4)
9. Have you or someone else been injured as a result of your drinking?
   No (0)
   Yes, but not in the last year (2)
   Yes, during the last year (4)
10. Has a relative, friend, doctor, or other health worker been concerned about your drinking or suggested that you should cut down?
   No (0)
   Yes, but not in the last year (2)
   Yes, during the last year (4)

Cage test from Ewing JA: Detecting alcoholism. The CAGE questionnaire. JAMA 252(14):1905-1907, 1984.
Audit test from Babor TF, de la Fuente JR, Saunders J, Grant M: AUDIT: The Alcohol Use Disorders Identification Test. Guidelines for use in primary health care. Geneva, World Health Organization, 1992.

- *Medicolegal liability.* There is legal risk for physicians treating drug abusers without definitive diagnoses. If a patient suffers a bad outcome from a medical condition caused by use of illicit drugs (defined in most states as the fault of the user), but drug use testing was never considered or performed, the treating physician may be held responsible.

Management and Therapy

The treatment of alcoholism and drug use disorders should involve a long-term management approach similar to the treatment of diabetes or hypertension. O'Brien and McLellan have articulated this perspective of a harm-reduction model viewing substance use disorders as a chronic disease. In this model, the clinician is aware that there will be ups and downs in the course of treatment but that over time many patients will have significant reductions in their use of the substance and fewer substance-related problems.

Optimum Treatment

Alcohol

The initial step in alcoholism treatment is for the clinician to identify alcohol as a problem for the patient and attempt to work collaboratively with the patient on ways to modify drinking behavior. Most patients do not understand the

Box 171-1   Disorders Associated with Urticaria or Angioedema

Acquired angioedema
Adrenergic urticaria
Atopy
Autoimmune anti-IgE or anti-FceRI
Bacterial infections
  Dental abscess
  Genitourinary infection
  Helicobacter pylori
  Mycoplasmal infection
  Sinus infection
  Streptococcal infections
Endocrine disorders
  Hyperthyroidism
  Progesterone
Fungal infections
  Candida
  Dermatophytosis
Hematologic disorders
  Iron deficiency anemia
  Paraproteinemia
Infestation and parasites
  Amebiasis
  Ascaris
  Filariasis
  Giardiasis
  Hookworm
  Malaria
  Scabies
  Schistosomiasis
  Strongyloides
  Trichomonas

Hereditary disorders and syndromes
  Arthritis, hives, angioedema
  C3b inactivator deficiency
  Cold-induced autoinflammatory syndrome
  Erythropoietic protoporphyria
  Familial cold urticaria
  Hereditary angioedema
  Muckle-Wells syndrome (urticaria, deafness, amyloidosis)
  Schnitzler's syndrome
Malignancy
  Carcinoma
  Leukemia
  Lymphoma
  Myeloma
  Polycythemia vera
Rheumatologic disorders
  Necrotizing vasculitis
  Polymyositis
  Rheumatoid arthritis
  Rheumatic fever
  Sjögren's syndrome
  Still's disease
  Systemic lupus erythematosus
Viral infections
  Coxsackie virus
  ECHO virus
  Cytomegalovirus
  Epstein-Barr virus
  Hepatitis B and C viruses
  HIV
  Mononucleosis

Box 171-2   Substances Associated with Urticaria or Angioedema

Blood products
Contactants
  Animal dander and saliva
  Arthropods
  Foods
  Latex
  Marine forms
  Medications (topical)
  Plants
  Textiles
  Toiletry items
Drugs*
  Anesthetics
  Angiotensin-converting enzyme inhibitors
  Antiepileptic agents
  Aspirin
  Bromides
  Cephalosporins
  Chloroquine
  Dextran
  Diuretics
  Isoniazid
  Nonsteroidal anti-inflammatory drugs
  Opioids
  Penicillins
  Polymyxin B
  Quinidine
  Sulfa drugs
  Radiographic contrast media
  Vancomycin

Foods
  Berries
  Cheese
  Chocolate
  Eggs
  Fish
  Gluten
  Milk
  Nuts
  Shellfish
  Tomatoes
Food additives
  Sulfites
  Tartrazine
Implants
  Amalgam fillings
  Intrauterine devices
  Orthodontic bands
  Platinum
  Tantalum staples
Insect and arthropod stings and bites
Inhalants
  Animal dander
  Cigarette smoke
  Dusts
  Flour
  Mold
  Pollen

* Almost any prescription or over-the-counter medication can cause urticaria.

Urticaria

Introduction

Urticaria is often a source of great frustration to patients and physicians alike. Although the list of reported associations is extensive, many patients have idiopathic urticaria with no obvious cause defined after an extensive evaluation. Also, urticaria is not infrequently recalcitrant to treatment, leading to therapeutic trials of many agents.

Etiology and Pathogenesis

Urticaria results from fluid transudation from tiny cutaneous blood vessels, often with mast cells and histamine acting as mediators. It is subclassified into immunologic and nonimmunologic categories. Physical urticaria is nonimmunologic; urticaria associated with food, drugs, or insect stings is often immunologic. The most common allergic mechanism is the type I hypersensitivity state mediated by immunoglobulin E (IgE). Type III (immune complex) reactions can also induce urticaria with activation of classic or alternative complement cascades, as in serum sickness. In nonimmunologic urticaria, physical factors or substances cause nonspecific histamine release from mast cells. Genetic factors may predispose individuals to urticaria as evidenced by the hereditary syndromes in Box 171-1. Angioedema is similar to urticaria but involves deeper dermal and subcutaneous tissues. The plasma kinin–generating system may play an important role in types of angioedema. Recent reports have identified autoimmune chronic urticaria as the etiology in about 30% of patients with chronic idiopathic urticaria. In this condition, an anti-IgE antibody of the IgG (immunoglobulin G) class or anti-FceRIa (Fc-epsilon-RI receptor antibody) cross-links adjacent mast cell receptors or IgE molecules. Many disorders and substances are reported, but not necessarily proven, to be associated with urticaria or angioedema (Boxes 171-1 and 171-2). In chronic urticaria, an etiologic diagnosis is established in less than 20% of patients.

Clinical Presentation

Intensely itching wheals with smooth, elevated, usually white centers and surrounding erythema characterize urticaria (Fig. 171-1). The lesions range in size from pinpoint to several centimeters and are circular, annular, or serpiginous in shape (Fig. 171-2). Typically, lesions appear in widely distributed crops over the body surface. Variations in presentation of the physical urticarias are given in Table 171-1. Chronic urticaria and physical urticaria can coexist. Contact urticaria is most prominent where the inciting substance has contacted the skin. Adrenergic urticaria presents with a halo of white skin around a small papule and is associated with stress. A single wheal tends to last less than 24 hours. Usually no constitutional symptoms are present; however, nausea, vomiting, abdominal cramping, headache, salivation, wheezing, and syncope may accompany urticaria.

Angioedema presents as an area of painful swelling, often initially around the eyelids, lips, or on a limb, that can persist for several days. In hereditary angioedema, an autosomal dominant condition, episodes of nonpruritic swelling occur either spontaneously or after minor trauma. Erythema may develop before the swelling occurs, but typically urticaria is absent. Laryngeal edema, which is often life threatening, and gastrointestinal involvement can complicate the clinical presentation.

Differential Diagnosis

If individual lesions last more than 24 hours, have a violaceous hue, show hyperpigmentation, are painful and nonblanching, or are associated with signs and symptoms of a rheumatologic disease, a biopsy is indicated to rule out urticarial vasculitis. In urticaria pigmentosum or mastocytosis, patients can develop pruritic urticarial-type wheals

Table 171-1 Physical Urticaria

Type of Urticaria	Clinical Appearance	Method to Test for Presence
Aquagenic	Small punctate pruritic wheals in a follicular pattern on an erythematous background	Wet compresses at 35° to 36° C for 30 minutes
Cholinergic	Small (2-3 mm), very pruritic papules on a large erythematous background (Fig. 171-3)	Use methacholine skin test or immerse in hot bath of 42° C, raising body temperature 0.7° C
Cold	Wheal assumes the shape of the stimulus with surrounding erythema	Wheal and flare within 10 to 15 minutes at the site of application of an ice cube, maintained for 5 minutes
Dermatographism	Linear cutaneous wheal greater than 3 mm long, surrounded by a flare	Stroke skin on back firmly with tongue blade or dermatographometer
Delayed pressure	Raised, painful, erythematous, deep-seated swellings that develop in areas 4 to 8 hours after pressure exposure	Use 15 pounds of weight slung over the shoulder for 15 minutes with the patient walking during the test
Local heat	Erythema, pruritus, urticaria	Apply warm compress to forearm
Solar	Urticaria in exposed areas (Fig. 171-4)	Expose skin to defined wavelengths of light
Vibration-induced angioedema	Pruritus, erythema, and local swelling in the area confined to application of a vibratory stimulus	Gently apply lab vortex to forearm for 4 minutes

Figure 171-1 Urticaria.

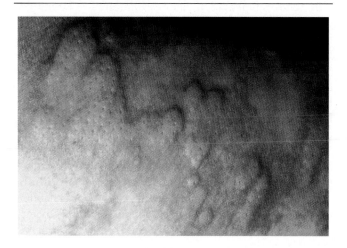

Figure 171-2 Annular and Serpiginous Urticaria.

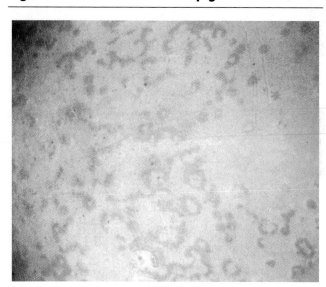

Figure 171-3 Cholinergic Urticaria.

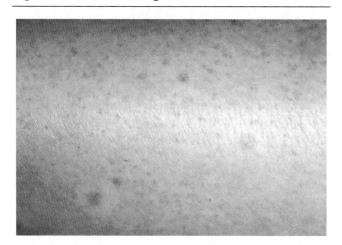

Figure 171-4 Solar Urticaria.

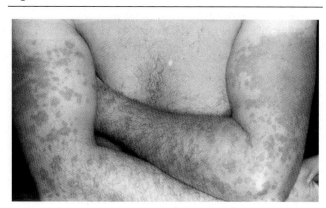

at the sites of the mast cell infiltrates in the skin. The skin lesions, however, are often persistent red-brown papules or macules that can urticate with stroking (the Darier sign). Pruritic urticarial papules and plaques of pregnancy, typically seen in the third trimester, are characterized by pruritic erythematous papules and urticarial plaques with onset typically in the striae distensae of the abdomen. In papular urticaria, a hypersensitivity syndrome, lesions are more persistent, typically on the lower extremities, and thought to be caused by insect bites. Erythema multiforme and the urticarial phase of bullous pemphigoid are often also considered in the differential diagnosis. Serum sickness occurs 8 to 10 days after administration of a foreign protein; fever, lymphadenopathy, arthralgias or arthritis, splenomegaly, and nephritis may develop in addition to urticaria. Laboratory findings include leukopenia, hypocomplementemia, and albuminuria.

Diagnostic Approach

A thorough history and review of systems are key, with emphasis on timing of attacks, provoking factors, and associated signs and symptoms (Box 171-3). The timing of urticaria in comparison with a list of exposures is helpful in determining an underlying cause. Often a diary of food intake and exposures will help determine any associations. Almost any medication may cause urticaria, so trials off medication are often necessary. To exclude urticarial vasculitis, characterized by urticarial lesions lasting longer than 24 hours, a wheal should be circled and observed. A skin biopsy, done at the edge of a wheal, will clarify the diagnosis. If a particular allergen is suspected, scratch, intradermal, or radioallergosorbent testing is helpful. Aeroallergens, dermatophytes, foods, and candida can be tested. Allergy to aeroallergens warrants consideration if there is a history of rhinitis or asthma.

Urticaria is defined as chronic if it persists for 6 weeks or longer. The laboratory workup for chronic urticaria includes a white blood cell count, differential count, and sedimentation rate. Other tests to consider include a thyroid-stimulating hormone level and thyroid microsomal (peroxidase) and thyroglobulin antibodies. In the case of chronic urticaria, testing for *Helicobacter pylori* infection could also be considered. Additional tests, based on history and physical examination, may include urinalysis and urine culture, liver function tests, hepatitis B and C serologies, antinuclear antibody, complement levels, serum IgE, streptococcal throat culture, monospot, stool for parasites, vaginal smears for *Candida* and *Trichomonas* species, and chest radiograph. If serum sickness is suspected, urinalysis, CBC and sedimentation rate are indicated. The autologous serum skin test is the only in vivo method to test for functional autoantibodies to FceRIa or IgE. In vitro testing for functional autoantibodies is not widely available.

In hereditary angioedema, C4 levels, which remain depressed between attacks, are a reliable screening test, but hereditary angioedema must be confirmed by C1 inhibitor level and function. An IgE-mediated allergic or drug reaction or a parasitic infection is high on the differential list if eosinophilia or elevated IgE is present. An elevated erythrocyte sedimentation rate suggests a systemic disease or urticarial vasculitis. Testing for physical urticaria is done as described in Table 171-1. In cold urticaria, laboratory testing may include cryoglobulins, cryofibrinogens, VDRL, cold hemolysis, and α_1-antitrypsin. Adrenergic urticaria is diagnosed by intracutaneous injection of noradrenaline.

Management and Therapy

General Management

General recommendations for allergen avoidance and assistance by the patient in determining possible causes are important (Box 171-4). Ideally, the cause of the urticaria is determined and eliminated. In physical urticaria, the associated physical factor should be avoided. Because aspirin and nonsteroidal anti-inflammatory medications can function as histamine releasers and cause exacerbation of urticaria, they should be discontinued. Patients with physical urticaria, such as cold urticaria, should be warned that intense exposure to the inciting agent (such as diving into a cold pool) can result in massive angioedema and anaphylaxis.

Box 171-3   Diagnosis

- Obtain a thorough history and physical exam and tailor evaluation based on individual clues.
- Perform a physical exam to look for urticaria and angioedema. Check for dermatographism.
- Consider examination for the physical urticaria in atypical cases.
- If individual lesions last more than 24 hours, have a violaceous hue, show hyperpigmentation, are painful or nonblanching, or are associated with signs and symptoms of a rheumatologic disease, a biopsy is indicated to rule out urticarial vasculitis.
- If urticaria is chronic:
  - Consider obtaining a white blood cell count, differential count, and sedimentation rate.
  - Consider also obtaining thyroid-stimulating hormone level and thyroid microsomal (peroxidase) and thyroglobulin antibodies.
  - Consider testing for *Helicobacter pylori* infection.
  - Overall, tailor diagnostic testing to the individual history and examination.
- Obtain complement studies if isolated angioedema is present or if hypocomplementemic vasculitis is being considered.
- A C4 level can be used as a screen for C1 esterase inhibitor deficiency, which may be associated with a family history of angioedema.

- Urticaria accompanied by asthma, laryngeal edema, or circulatory collapse is treated as a medical emergency.
- Adrenaline emergency packs should be prescribed for patients with a history of severe urticaria or angioedema.
- Advise patients to avoid aspirin and nonsteroidal anti-inflammatory medications.
- Advise patients to avoid foods known for being allergens such as nuts, peanuts, and shellfish.
- Ask patients to keep a food and hive diary.
- For chronic urticaria, consider an elimination diet.

Box 171-5 Antihistamines Used for Urticaria

- Cetirizine, 10 mg once daily
- Chlorpheniramine, 4 mg every 4-6 hours
- Cyproheptadine, 2-4 mg every 6-8 hours
- Desloratadine, 5 mg once daily
- Diphenhydramine, 25-50 mg every 6 hours
- Doxepin, 10-25 mg every 12-24 hours
- Fexofenadine, 120-180 mg daily
- Hydroxyzine, 25-50 mg every 6 hours
- Loratadine, 10 mg once daily

Drug Therapy

Acute urticaria is usually treated with antihistamines and, if severe, with corticosteroids. An acute episode of urticaria, accompanied by asthma, laryngeal edema, or circulatory collapse, is treated as a medical emergency with epinephrine, systemic corticosteroids, oxygen, intravenous fluids, or even airway intubation. The prescription of adrenaline emergency packs is critical for patients with a history of severe urticaria or angioedema.

H_1 blockers are often the first-line treatment (Box 171-5). Treatment with the tricyclic antidepressant doxepin takes advantage of its combination of H_1 and H_2 blockade. Alternatively, the addition of an H_2 blocker like ranitidine (150 mg orally every 12 hours) or cimetidine (300 mg orally every 8 hours) to an H_1 blocker offers some advantages.

For chronic urticaria, it is best to avoid prescribing corticosteroids whenever possible. Other treatments that may have value include mycophenolate mofetil, antileukotrienes, cyclosporine-attenuated anabolic steroids, nifedipine, dapsone, sulfasalazine, colchicine, methotrexate, hydroxychloroquine, cyclosporine, ultraviolet B, and psoralen plus ultraviolet light of A wavelength. Some clinicians use estrogen therapy for autoimmune progesterone urticaria. In patients with autoimmune thyroiditis, urticaria has been reported to respond to thyroxine, even when the patient is euthyroid.

Cyproheptadine is effective for cold urticaria in some patients. In physical urticaria, induction of tolerance is sometimes possible. Adrenergic urticaria responds to β-blocker therapy.

Acute treatment and short- and long-term prophylaxis of hereditary angioedema are important, and the treatment must be tailored to the severity. Agents, available in the United States, that have shown some efficacy are fresh-frozen plasma, attenuated androgens, and epsilon amino-caproic acid.

Avoiding Treatment Errors

The diagnostic workup for chronic urticaria is important in an attempt to identify and eliminate any underlying causes; however, the testing must be carefully tailored to the patient's history and physical exam findings. In chronic urticaria, the use of long-term corticosteroids should be avoided whenever possible.

Optimum Treatment

Nonsedating H_1 blockers are often preferred in chronic urticaria. It is not unusual for H_1 blockers to be used at increased dosages, for two H_1 blockers to be given in combination, or both. H_2 blockers added to the regimen may improve control. A variety of corticosteroid-sparing immunosuppressive agents have been studied for their use in urticaria and may be helpful for certain patients.

Future Directions

Further study of autoimmune chronic urticaria and development of a reliable commercial test of functional autoantibodies implicated in this process seem important for better classification of these patients. Also, whether proposed disease associations such as chronic urticaria and *H. pylori* are real or merely coincidental remains to be determined. Latex allergy is important as a cause of urticaria and anaphylaxis. The future should bring better control of the use of latex in our environment and better preventive measures to avoid sensitization of individuals.

New antihistamines are undergoing testing and may result in improved treatments. Recently, two distinct mast cell populations have been identified, and their homeostasis between inhibition and activation is under study. Research is likely to lead to drugs directed against these specific subtypes. Better classification of patients with autoimmune urticaria may allow improved diagnosis and appropriate treatment of this entity with immunosuppressive agents. Several promising drugs to treat hereditary angioedema, including drugs to replace the C1 inhibitor protein and others to decrease bradykinin-mediated vascular permeability, are undergoing testing in the United States.

Additional Resources

Crawford MB: Urticaria. Available at: http://www.emedicine.com/emerg/topic628.htm. Accessed March 13, 2007.
   This website provides information on workup and treatment, including dosing of antihistamines.

Gompels MM, Lock RJ, Abinun M, et al: C1 inhibitor deficiency: Consensus document. Clin Exp Immunol 139:379-394, 2005.

This consensus document addresses the diagnosis and management of C1 inhibitor deficiency.

Grattan CEH, Sabroe RA, Sabroe RA, Greaves MW: Chronic urticaria. J Am Acad Dermatol 46:654-657, 2002.

This CME article on chronic urticaria discusses classification, assessment, and management.

Leung DY, Diaz LA, DeLeo V, Soter NA: Allergic and immunologic skin disorders. JAMA 278:1914-1923, 1997.

This review chapter includes information on the immunology of urticaria and angioedema.

Litt JZ: Drug Eruption Reference Manual, 13th ed. New York, Informa Healthcare, 2007.

This is a reference for drugs that have been reported to cause urticaria.

Metzger WJ: Urticaria, angioedema, and hereditary angioedema. In Grammer LC, Greenberger PA (eds): Patterson's Allergic Diseases, 6th ed. Philadelphia, Lippincott Williams & Wilkins, 2002.

This is a helpful review chapter.

Nettis E, Dambra P, Loria MP, et al: Mast-cell phenotype in urticaria. Allergy 56:915, 2001.

This article discusses the science of mast-cell phenotypes.

Sabroe RA, Greaves MW: Chronic idiopathic urticaria with functional autoantibodies. Br J Dermatol 154:813-819, 2006.

This review article discusses the literature regarding functional autoantibodies.

Schocket AL: Chronic urticaria: Pathophysiology and etiology, or the what and why. Allergy Asthma Proc 27:90-95, 2006.

This review article on chronic urticaria discusses potential etiologies and possible screening tests, including a discussion of autoimmune thyroiditis.

EVIDENCE

1. Buss YA, Garrelfs UC, Sticherling M: Chronic urticaria: Which clinical parameters are pathogenetically relevant? A retrospective investigation of 339 patients. J Dtsch Dermatol Ges 5(1):22-27, 2007.

   This retrospective chart review examines laboratory and clinical data of 339 patients with chronic urticaria.

2. Di Lorenzo G, Pacor ML, Mansueto P, et al: Is there a role for antileukotrienes in urticaria? Clin Exp Dermatol 31:327-334, 2006.

   This article reviews the literature for use of antileukotrienes in urticaria and finds it to be mainly anecdotal.

3. Hook-Nikanne J, Varjonen E, Harvima RJ, Kosunen TU: Is Helicobacter pylori infection associated with chronic urticaria? Acta Derm Venereol 80:425-426, 2000.

   In this study of 231 Finnish patients, no difference was found in the prevalence rate of H. pylori infection in chronic urticaria patients compared with controls, and eradication of H. pylori did not have marked influence on the course of chronic urticaria. The article also provides references on other studies, including those that agree and conflict with this study.

4. Kozel MM, Bossuyt PM, Mekkes JR, Bos JD: Laboratory tests and identified diagnoses in patients with physical and chronic urticaria and angioedema: A systematic review. J Am Acad Dermatol 48:409-416, 2003.

   Based on the review of 29 studies involving 6462 patients, a clinical flow sheet is presented.

5. Shahar E, Bergman R, Guttman-Yassky E, Pollack S: Treatment of severe chronic idiopathic urticaria with oral mycophenolate mofetil in patients not responding to antihistamines and/or corticosteroids. Int J Dermatol 45:1224-1227, 2006.

   The authors report on an open-label, uncontrolled trial of nine patients with chronic urticaria with poor response to antihistamines and/or corticosteroids who improved with mycophenolate mofetil.

6. Vena GA, Cassano N, Colombo D, et al; Neo-I-30 Study Group. Cyclosporine in chronic idiopathic urticaria: A double-blind, randomized, placebo-controlled trial. J Am Acad Dermatol 55(4):705-709, 2006.

   The authors report on a double-blind, randomized, three-armed study of cyclosporine for chronic urticaria.

Kelly C. Nelson • Dean S. Morrell • David S. Rubenstein

172

Eczema and Other Common Dermatoses

Introduction

Eczema is a term broadly applied to many inflammatory skin conditions or dermatoses, characterized by the presence of pruritus, erythema, scaling, macules, papules, plaques, or vesicles. Evaluation of the patient with eczema or dermatitis should include a thorough history focusing on onset (acute versus chronic), inciting and exacerbating factors, associated medical conditions, and family history of similar or related diseases. On physical examination, attention is paid to individual lesion morphology, pattern, and distribution. A potassium hydroxide preparation of skin scrapings is often helpful in differentiating superficial fungal infection from other causes of scaling dermatitides. Punch biopsy can also be helpful in identifying specific dermatoses. A complete description of each of the clinical entities that can cause eczematous dermatitis is beyond the scope of this chapter, but many excellent resources are available for in-depth study of this reaction pattern.

ATOPIC DERMATITIS

Etiology and Pathogenesis

Atopic dermatitis is an immune-mediated disease. Most patients have a personal or family history of atopic disease (allergic rhinitis, asthma, and atopic dermatitis). In affected areas, a predominance of T-helper type 2 cells produce interleukins that cause elevated immunoglobulin E and eosinophil levels. Controversy exists on the role of potential food and other environmental allergens in the pathogenesis of atopic dermatitis.

Clinical Presentation

The major feature of atopic dermatitis is pruritus. In adults, chronic flexural involvement with lichenified erythematous plaques is common (Fig. 172-1). The plaques are distributed symmetrically on the face, neck, and antecubital and popliteal fossae. However, significant involvement of the dorsal hands and feet can occur. Exacerbations typically occur during dry weather and episodes of stress. Even during periods of relative remission, individuals usually have dry and sensitive skin. Secondary bacterial or viral infections involving the affected areas should always be considered during acute exacerbations that are unresponsive to previously effective therapy.

Differential Diagnosis

The intense pruritus and symmetric distribution distinguish atopic dermatitis from other scaling eruptions. Seborrheic dermatitis, irritant dermatitis, and contact dermatitis should be considered.

Diagnostic Approach

Bacterial and viral cultures can dictate therapy in secondarily infected plaques. Skin biopsies are rarely necessary.

Management and Therapy

Optimum Treatment

Affected skin has an impaired barrier to transcutaneous water loss. Therefore, efforts to improve and maintain skin hydration are helpful. Daily bathing can be useful in rehydration if a gentle soap (Cetaphil, Dove) is used sparingly and moisturizers are applied after bathing. Immediate (within 3 minutes) application of thicker moisturizers like petrolatum, Eucerin, and Aquaphor is effective during winter months, whereas lighter products (Cetaphil cream) are better tolerated in warmer weather. Recent U.S. Food and Drug Administration–approved topical emollients are claimed to repair barrier function by including ceramides. Regardless of the vehicle, emollients should be applied twice daily, following application of topical steroids, if indicated.

Figure 172-1 Atopic Dermatitis.
Lichenified plaques of the antecubital fossa are typical.

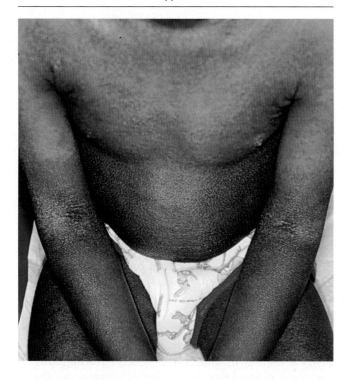

Oral antihistamines can be quite effective in controlling episodes of pruritus. Awareness of possible sedation with the use of these products is important.

Topical corticosteroids are the mainstay of treatment. The location and thickness of the plaque should guide the choice of an agent. Corticosteroids are best used in pulsed applications such that a particular agent significantly improves the area in 1 week. Topical pulsing avoids the chronic use of topical steroids and reduces the risk for steroid atrophy and striae. Low-potency steroids can be used intermittently on the face and neck. Potent and ultra-potent steroids are occasionally necessary for thickened, lichenified plaques on the extremities. With all topical corticosteroids, ointments are more potent than creams, which are more potent than lotions.

Crusted and weeping lesions frequently demonstrate secondary bacterial infection. Topical soaks or compresses with aluminum acetate (Domeboro) are indicated for these lesions, followed by steroid application. Oral antibiotics (antistaphylococcal, antistreptococcal) may be necessary for multiple areas of infection. Given the increasing rates of community-acquired oxacillin-resistant *Staphylococcus aureus* infections, a low threshold for surface culture to provide directed antibiotic therapy is recommended.

Other Therapies

Conclusive safety data remain elusive for topical calcineurin inhibitors, such as tacrolimus (Protopic) and pimecrolimus (Elidel). Reported malignancies after use of topical immunomodulators are not typical of calcineurin inhibitors used systemically, and these malignancies likely existed before use of the topical medication. The current recommendation is to use these preparations as second-line therapy in patients 2 years of age or older. Long-term studies and clinical experience will better address potential side effects of this class of medication. When topical agents fail, the next step is systemic therapy, such as phototherapy, azathioprine, or cyclosporine.

CONTACT DERMATITIS

(Refer to Chapter 173 for a more complete review.)

Etiology and Pathogenesis

Contact dermatitis may develop secondary to an allergic or an irritant response. Allergic contact dermatitis represents a cell-mediated immune response to haptens, small molecules that modify endogenous macromolecules in the skin. Re-exposure to antigen results in repeated bouts of cutaneous inflammation as a result of the generation of antigen-specific memory T cells. In contrast, irritant contact dermatitis represents a response to a non-immune-mediated injury to the skin from prolonged or repeated exposures to noxious substances. Soaps, detergents, and organic solvents are typical agents that cause irritant contact dermatitis.

Clinical Presentation

Acute contact dermatitis is a very pruritic eruption characterized by erythema, papules, vesicles, and bullae corresponding to the pattern and exposure of the contactant (Fig. 172-2). An acute vesicular eruption in a geometric pattern is essentially pathognomonic for acute contact dermatitis. Chronic contact dermatitis presents as lichenified, scaling, erythematous, hyperpigmented or hypopigmented papules, plaques, or both.

Differential Diagnosis

Contact dermatitis should be distinguished from other eczematous processes, including atopic dermatitis, nummular eczema, seborrheic dermatitis, and lichen simplex chronicus.

Diagnostic Approach

The onset, distribution, and pattern of the reaction are helpful in identifying responsible contactants. Biopsy is rarely indicated.

Management and Therapy

Optimum Treatment

Identification and removal of the offending agent is necessary. Frequently this requires eliciting an extensive history to determine the relationship of the patient's exposures to

Figure 172-2 Contact Dermatitis.
Linear distribution of erythematous papules and vesicles characterizes contact dermatitis to poison ivy.

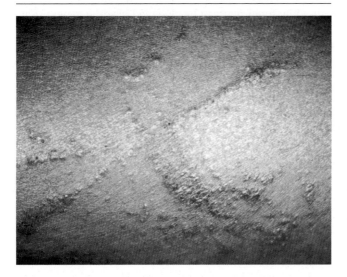

the onset, exacerbations, and ameliorations of the dermatitis. For example, eyelid dermatitis is often an allergic contact dermatitis to nail polish (transferred when the patient rubs the eyelids), and ear lobe involvement is often caused by nickel in earrings. Patch testing may be helpful in identifying potential allergic contactants. High-potency topical corticosteroids, emollients, and antihistamines will generally be sufficient to resolve the condition once the exposure has been identified and eliminated. For vigorous, generalized, acute contact dermatitis, such as can be seen in response to poison ivy, systemic corticosteroids may be indicated. Prednisone (40 to 60 mg by mouth daily) tapered over 2 to 3 weeks prevents flares experienced with shorter-duration oral corticosteroid dose packs.

SEBORRHEIC DERMATITIS

Etiology and Pathogenesis

The etiology of seborrheic dermatitis is uncertain. Individuals appear to have an exuberant response to increased numbers of *Malassezia furfur* in lesional skin; however, the exact role of this organism in the pathogenesis is unclear.

Clinical Presentation

Seborrheic dermatitis is a chronic inflammatory disease with periods of remissions and exacerbations. It is characterized by greasy scale overlying erythematous patches involving the eyebrows, nasal bridge, and nasolabial folds. Extension to the forehead and postauricular areas is often seen (Fig. 172-3). On the scalp, diffuse dry scale (dandruff) is common. Intertriginous areas (axillae and groin) can have sharply demarcated erythematous patches with yel-

Figure 172-3 Seborrheic Dermatitis.
Erythema and greasy yellow scale of the forehead, eyebrows, nasal bridge, and nasolabial folds.

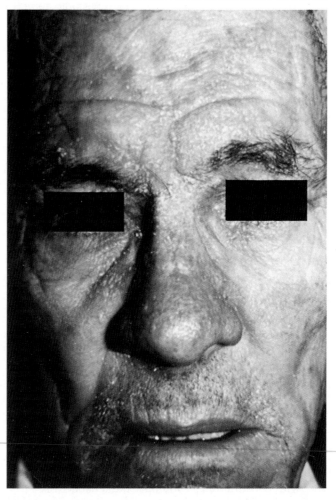

lowish, greasy, or waxy scale. Progression to exfoliative erythroderma is a rare event.

Differential Diagnosis

In some patients, seborrheic dermatitis can be difficult to distinguish from psoriasis. Intertrigo, candidal infection, and atopic dermatitis should also be considered.

Diagnostic Approach

Cultures of intertriginous lesions will differentiate candidal intertrigo.

Management and Therapy

Optimum Treatment

Generally, seborrheic dermatitis is more responsive to treatment than psoriasis. Treatment for 3 to 5 days is

usually adequate to control flares. Shampooing with zinc pyrithione (Head and Shoulders, DHS Zinc), selenium sulfide 1% or 2.5% (Selsun Blue), salicylic acid (T/Sal), or ketoconazole 1% or 2% can decrease scalp scale. Facial and intertriginous areas typically respond to periodic application of 1% or 2.5% hydrocortisone, 1% or 2% ketoconazole cream, or sulfur-based products (sulfacetamide lotion, 5% or 10%). Resistant cases may need brief application (twice daily for 5 to 7 days) of medium-potency corticosteroids (fluocinolone .01% or .025%) and should be evaluated for possible secondary bacterial or fungal infections.

STASIS DERMATITIS

Etiology and Pathogenesis

Poor venous return leads to edema, which affects the diffusion barrier of oxygen and nutrients to the epidermis. These chronic changes result in inflammation.

Clinical Presentation

Typically, stasis dermatitis occurs on the lower extremities of elderly patients as a bilateral, pruritic, erythematous, scaling macular and sometimes papular eruption. Chronic stasis dermatitis can result in pigment deposition from hemosiderin and from postinflammatory hyperpigmentation. Pitting edema is present. Chronic stasis dermatitis can progress to ulceration.

Differential Diagnosis

Potassium hydroxide preparation of skin scrapings aids in differentiating stasis dermatitis from dermatophytosis. Cellulitis is usually unilateral, acute in onset, and associated with constitutional symptoms and leukocytosis.

Diagnostic Approach

Usually, the clinical presentation is quite characteristic. When ulceration is present, other causes of ulcer formation should be considered, including arteriolar disease, vasculitis, infection, malignancy, and pyoderma gangrenosum. If warranted by clinical suspicion, biopsy may be helpful in excluding nonstasis entities.

Management and Therapy

Optimum Treatment

Decreasing lower extremity edema by leg elevation, daily compression stockings, and medical management of underlying cardiovascular disease is essential. Low- to mid-potency topical corticosteroids reduce cutaneous inflammation and pruritus. Frequent emollients aid in preventing exacerbations after the inflammation has resolved. Stasis ulcers respond well to Unna boots, a medicated compression dressing.

DERMATOPHYTOSIS

Etiology and Pathogenesis

The superficial mycoses of the skin, hair, and nails are caused by fungi that can be classified in three genera: *Epidermophyton*, *Microsporum*, and *Trichophyton*. The fungi are transmitted from multiple sources, including soil (geophilic), animals (zoophilic), and humans (anthropophilic). Genetic susceptibility and immunosuppression promote dermatophytosis. Once infected, the incubation period can be as little as 2 to 4 days before skin lesions are evident.

Clinical Presentation

Tinea faciei and corporis present similarly with annular, erythematous, scaling patches and plaques (Fig. 172-4). The borders are described as active, with more erythema and elevation, whereas the centers tend to be clear and flat. Tinea pedis can be quite inflammatory with weeping and vesiculation or noninflammatory with dry, scaling, minimally erythematous patches. Onychomycosis presents as a thickened nail plate with subungual debris. The plate will often separate from the underlying nail bed.

Tinea capitis is unusual in individuals after adolescence. Inflammatory lesions can develop into boggy, indurated, erythematous plaques called *kerions*. Noninflammatory lesions present with scaling papules and patches with broken-off hairs. Pruritus and occipital lymphadenopathy are common findings with tinea capitis.

Differential Diagnosis

Tinea faciei can be confused with lupus erythematosus, seborrheic dermatitis, contact dermatitis, and atopic dermatitis. Onychomycosis must be distinguished from psoriasis, atopic or contact dermatitis, lichen planus, chronic paronychia, and trachyonychia. Tinea capitis should be

Figure 172-4 Tinea Faciei.
Serpiginous bordered, erythematous plaque with central clearing.

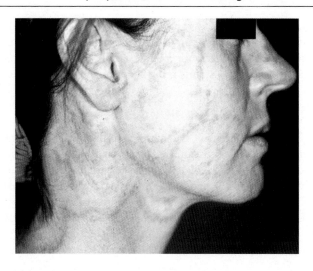

differentiated from pediculosis, atopic dermatitis, seborrheic dermatitis, psoriasis, and bacterial infection.

Diagnostic Approach

The performance of a potassium hydroxide preparation of the scale, hair, or nail from affected lesions is essential in the diagnosis of dermatophytosis. Cultures can also be obtained from affected areas and placed on Mycosel or dermatophyte test medium culture. Alternatively, skin scrapings or brushings may be submitted for a dermatophyte screen, which will also provide speciation. In cases in which nail clippings fail to identify a fungal etiology, nail plates can be clipped and fixed in formalin for histologic evaluation with periodic acid–Schiff staining. Rarely, skin biopsies are needed to diagnose dermatophytosis. Wood lamp illumination of the scalp is no longer helpful in the diagnosis of tinea capitis because the more common fungi do not fluoresce.

Management and Therapy

Optimum Treatment

Multiple antifungal preparations are available for topical and oral dosing. Consideration of the extent and location of the infection dictates the route. Localized tinea faciei, corporis, pedis, and cruris can be treated effectively with topical agents (clotrimazole, miconazole, econazole, oxiconazole, ketoconazole, terbinafine, naftifine, ciclopirox, and butenafine) twice daily for 1 week after the eruption resolves. Extensive skin disease is more effectively treated with oral therapy (terbinafine, itraconazole, or fluconazole). Regular use of antifungal powders can be useful in preventing recurrences of tinea cruris and pedis. Erosive tinea pedis may be secondarily infected with gram-negative organisms; therefore, topical or oral antibacterial therapy should be considered as an adjunct to antifungal therapy.

Involvement of hair or nails requires systemic therapy. Griseofulvin is still the drug of choice for childhood tinea capitis at 20 to 25 mg/kg/day (micronized) or 15 to 20 mg/kg/day (ultramicronized) for 8 to 12 weeks. As more literature and experience are available, the newer allylamines (terbinafine) and triazoles (itraconazole, fluconazole) may replace griseofulvin with easier dosing and shorter treatment duration. Onychomycosis requires 3 to 4 months of therapy (terbinafine or itraconazole). Most insurance companies will not approve the course of therapy for onychomycosis until diagnosis is confirmed through culture or potassium hydroxide examination. Rare cases of hepatic failure have been reported with several of the oral antifungal agents. Patients should be screened for underlying hepatic disease before the use of these systemic medications. Recurrences are not unusual; preventative measures (antifungal cream or powder) may be helpful after a course of oral therapy. Combining systemic antifungal medications with topical antifungal medications may result in slightly higher mycologic and clinical cure rates.

Avoiding Treatment Errors

It is essential to distinguish noninfectious inflammatory dermatoses such as atopic dermatitis and contact dermatitis from tinea. Physicians treating these disorders should have a low threshold for performing a potassium hydroxide preparation and be comfortable interpreting the results.

Future Directions

Corticosteroids have been the therapeutic mainstay for treatment of eczema and dermatitis; however, chronic use results in dermal atrophy and tachyphylaxis. Extensive investigations by numerous researchers have led to a more precise understanding of the molecular and cellular events that are required to generate cutaneous inflammation. Using this information, nonsteroidal drugs are being developed that target specific components of the immune response. For example, bioengineered macromolecules that modify immune cell responses by disrupting antigen presentation and cytokine secretion profile will likely broaden the therapeutic armamentarium available to treat particularly recalcitrant eczema and dermatitis.

Additional Resources

American Academy of Dermatology. Available at http://www.aad.org. Accessed December 6, 2006.
> *This website can be helpful in identifying physicians with clinical expertise in eczematous dermatitis.*

Rietscel RL, Fowler JR Jr (eds): Fischer's Contact Dermatitis, 4th ed. Baltimore, Williams & Wilkins, 1995.
> *This comprehensive textbook catalogues the many agents responsible for contact dermatitis.*

Society for Investigative Dermatology. Available at http://www.sidnet.org. Accessed December 6, 2006.
> *This website can be helpful in identifying scientists with research expertise in skin disease.*

EVIDENCE

1. Alaiti S, Kang S, Fiedler VC, et al: Tacrolimus (FK506) ointment for atopic dermatitis: A phase I study in adults and children. J Am Acad Dermatol 38(1):69-76, 1998.
   > *This is one of the initial reports describing the use of tacrolimus 0.3% ointment for atopic dermatitis.*
2. Griffiths CE: Ascomycin: An advance in the management of atopic dermatitis. Br J Dermatol 144(4):679-681, 2001.
   > *The author provides a commentary on the value of noncorticosteroid topical anti-inflammatory agents and the potential of ascomycins as topical immunomodulators.*
3. Reitamo S, Wollenberg A, Schopf E, et al: Safety and efficacy of 1 year of tacrolimus ointment monotherapy in adults with atopic dermatitis. The European Tacrolimus Ointment Study Group. Arch Dermatol 136(8):999-1006, 2000.
   > *This study reported the 1-year safety and efficacy data for 0.1% tacrolimus in the treatment of atopic dermatitis.*
4. Van Leent EJ, Graber M, Thurston M, et al: Effectiveness of the ascomycin macrolactam SDZ ASM 981 in the topical treatment of atopic dermatitis. Arch Dermatol 134(7):805-809, 1998.
   > *This placebo-controlled trial shows the efficacy of topical ascomycins in the treatment of atopic dermatitis.*

173

Emily J. Schwarz ▪ Susan Riggs Runge

Allergic Contact Dermatitis

Introduction

Allergic contact dermatitis (ACD) is a common skin disorder characterized by pruritic erythematous papules and vesicles that develop after repeated contact with an allergen. ACD accounts for 20% of occupational contact dermatitis and is the second most frequent dermatologic diagnosis. Worldwide, the most common contact allergen is nickel.

Etiology and Pathogenesis

ACD occurs from exposure to environmental allergens, usually small-molecule substances. These allergens bind to class II molecules on the antigen-presenting cells of the skin, primarily Langerhans cells, and are subsequently presented to effector T lymphocytes in the lymph nodes. Initial sensitization may take 7 to 14 days for a specific antigen. Once sensitization has occurred, the antigen may elicit a clinical response within hours to days through a delayed-type hypersensitivity reaction. However, individuals can also become sensitized by low levels of chronic exposure to certain antigens over years, such as cement workers chronically exposed to low levels of chromium.

ACD is more common in women, presumably because of allergens in jewelry, especially nickel. ACD can affect all ages, and allergen exposure also varies with age. The top four allergens in the United States are nickel sulfate, neomycin sulfate, balsam of Peru, and fragrance mix.

Clinical Presentation

Acute ACD may manifest as very pruritic erythematous papules and vesicles days after exposure to the sensitizing agent. Chronic ACD presents as lichenified plaques with scale over a longer period of time. In areas of thin skin such as the eyelids, penis, and scrotum, edematous lesions may appear.

The location of the lesions provides important diagnostic clues (Fig. 173-1). Classic ACD caused by the plant allergen urushiol in poison ivy and poison oak is characterized by linear streaks of vesicles that are usually seen on the extremities. Patients who present with well-demarcated hand dermatitis on the dorsal aspect may be reacting to chemicals in rubber gloves. Sensitization to nail products, ophthalmologic preparations, and airborne allergens may manifest as eyelid dermatitis. Topical preparations such as benzocaine lead to perianal ACD in susceptible patients. ACD to hair dyes containing paraphenyldiamine often presents with lesions on the adjacent face and ears. ACD over the dorsal feet is often a reaction to rubber accelerators or potassium dichromate in tanned leather. Table 173-1 shows important contact allergens, sources of contact, and usual ACD sites.

A widespread autosensitization eruption may develop from local sites of contact to the offending agent and lead to erythroderma.

Differential Diagnosis

The differential diagnosis of ACD includes irritant contact dermatitis, atopic dermatitis, nummular eczema, dyshidrotic eczema, and even tinea corporis. When scale is present, a potassium hydroxide (KOH) prep should be performed to rule out dermatophytosis. In contrast to ACD, tinea pedis usually involves the interdigital spaces and is associated with onychomycosis. Psoriasis of the palms and soles can be confused with ACD but usually has accompanying nail changes and psoriatic plaques elsewhere. In the setting of ACD-induced autosensitization

Figure 173-1 Allergic Contact Dermatitis.

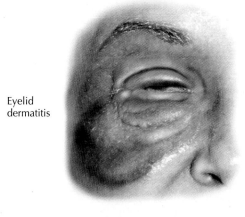

Eyelid
dermatitis

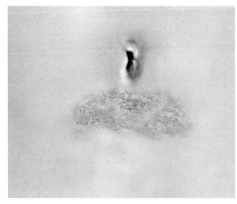

Nickel
dermatitis
(around the
umbilicus)

Poison Ivy

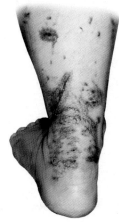

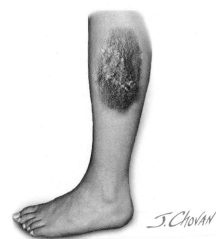

J. Chovan

Table 173-1   Contact Allergens, Sources, and Locations

Allergen	Source	Location
Nickel sulfate	Jewelry, clothing snaps	Earlobes, neck, umbilicus
Neomycin sulfate	Topical antibiotic	Wounds
Balsam of Peru	Fragrance, adhesives	Neck
Chromates	Leather and cement	Dorsal feet from leather boots
Paraphenylenediamine	Hair dye	Adjacent face and ears
Toluene sulfonamide	Nail lacquer	Eyelids

with erythroderma, other causes to consider include cutaneous T-cell lymphoma. A skin biopsy provides very useful information: in ACD, microscopy demonstrates epidermal spongiosis and a superficial, perivascular, lymphohistiocytic dermal infiltrate.

Diagnostic Approach

When ACD is suspected, a thorough exploration of the patient's work exposures and hobbies is essential. When occupational exposure is likely, asking whether the condition improves away from the workplace is key. A review of personal care products is also very important. The critical role of a detailed history cannot be overemphasized.

Patch testing remains the gold standard in the diagnosis of ACD. U.S. Food and Drug Administration–approved ready-to-use-skin patch tests are used for the diagnosis of contact dermatitis by most dermatologists. The TRUE (Allerderm) and TROLAB (Hermal) patch test kits are two commonly used commercial products that allow testing for many allergens simultaneously. Some dermatologists and allergy clinics prefer customized skin patch tests (Fig. 173-2). There are also specific allergen panels when occupational exposure is suspected, including a hairdressing tray or a florist tray. Chemicals that patients bring in should not be used because the substances may cause severe skin damage and all ingredients may not be known.

Figure 173-2. Patch Test.

Patch test placement

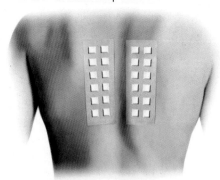

Positive patch test

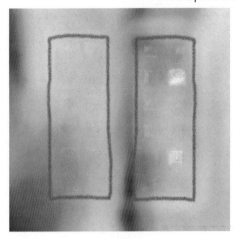
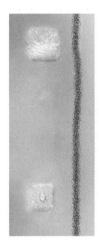

J. Chovan

When a specific allergen is suspected, the patient should be considered for confirmatory patch testing. The most common site for application is the upper back. The patient should not have a sunburn or other significant rash in the test area and should not have used topical corticosteroids on the patch test site for at least 1 week and oral corticosteroids at a dose greater than 15 mg for 1 month before patch testing. Both topical and systemic steroids decrease the patient's ability to produce a positive response.

Once patch testing is planned, the TRUE test strips are applied to the upper back and then reinforced with paper tape. The patient should keep the area dry for at least 48 hours and refrain from activities that cause excessive sweating. Whether oral antihistamines will affect the test results remains controversial. After 48 to 72 hours, the patient should return, the outline of the tests marked, and the patches removed for the first reading. After the initial reading, the patient should ideally return for a second reading 5 to 7 days after the initial patch test placement. The second reading is necessary because some allergens, including gold and disperse blue dye, take a longer time to induce a response.

The patch test is graded by the International Grading System (Box 173-1) and should be interpreted in the context of the patient's current exposures. For example, the clinical significance of a positive reaction to thimerosal

Box 173-1	International Grading System

±, Doubtful reaction, faint macular erythema
+, Weak, nonvesicular reaction with erythema, infiltration, and papules
++, Strong, vesicular reaction with erythema, infiltration, and papules
+++, Spreading bullous reaction
−, Negative reaction
IR, Irritant reaction

may be minimal because many people are sensitized in their childhood through routine vaccinations. When interpreting the patch test, clinical correlation is recommended. False-positive reactions may occur secondary to *excited skin syndrome*. True allergic reactions tend to itch more than irritant ones. The second reading is particularly important in elderly patients, who may take longer to react. False-negative reactions occur because of a low concentration of the suspected substance, failure to perform a later reading, wet patches, or the influence of corticosteroids.

Management and Therapy

Once the diagnosis of ACD is made, the mainstay of therapy is allergen avoidance. With the TRUE patch test, information sheets on substances that test positive are provided to the patient. Unfortunately, some allergens are not listed on the label of the offending product. Patients and physicians should also be aware of cross-reacting substances, such as poison ivy and mangos.

For a few allergens, a test kit is available to determine product content. For example, in patients allergic to nickel, the dimethylglyoxime test is commercially available so that patients can test products before purchasing them to determine whether they contain nickel. The feasibility and usefulness of a nickel-free diet are debatable. The elimination of nickel from the diet is very difficult, and little information is available on dietary recommendations for individuals with a true nickel allergy. Canned foods and acidic foods prepared in stainless steel cookware can contain nickel, as can a variety of uncooked foods, such as leafy green vegetables.

Optimum Treatment

In addition to antigen avoidance, therapy should focus on symptomatic care. Patients with ACD to poison ivy manifested by an acute vesicular eruption benefit from using a drying agent such as Burow solution 2 to 3 times per day and from lukewarm oatmeal baths. Patients with lesions that are more chronic in nature should use an emollient such as petrolatum. When significant pruritus is present, oral antihistamines are helpful, such as hydroxyzine, 10 to 25 mg every 6 to 8 hours, plus a longer-acting agent such as cetirizine, 10 mg every 24 hours. Do not use topical antihistamines because they can produce an additional ACD. The presence of superinfected lesions with crusting is an indication for oral antibiotics. Patients should also be advised to cleanse with gentle agents like Cetaphil.

Topical glucocorticoids are indicated in most cases of ACD. For thicker skin areas, including the hands and feet, and for severe cases, a class 1 steroid such as clobetasol ointment can be used twice a day for 3 weeks. A class VI to VII steroid such as hydrocortisone valerate should be used twice a day on thinner skin such as the face and intertriginous regions. For lesions on other body areas, a medium-potency steroid such as triamcinolone 0.1% ointment twice a day will often suffice. In general, ointments are better vehicles to use than creams or gel formulations because they contain fewer ingredients and therefore fewer possible allergens. For ACD inside the oral cavity, a mid-potency steroid gel is better suited. For suspected cases occurring on the scalp, mid- to high-potency steroids are available in solution formulations.

Involvement of greater than 25% of the body surface area by allergic contact dermatitis warrants a course of oral glucocorticoids. Prednisone, 40 to 60 mg daily tapered over a 2-week period, is usually sufficient. If steroid therapy is contraindicated, patients should be referred to a dermatologist for possible narrow-band ultraviolet B treatment

or immunosuppressive medications. The complete clearing of ACD lesions may take as long as 6 weeks.

Avoiding Treatment Errors

One pitfall in the treatment of ACD is the failure to use the appropriate strength of topical glucocorticoid for a given body region. For instance, a 2.5% hydrocortisone ointment will likely not be strong enough to treat an ACD of the hands caused by mercaptobenzothiazole found in rubber gloves. Patients also need to use the topical steroid often and for a long enough period of time. They need to be reminded that results are not apparent overnight. Another common pitfall is the failure to identify the responsible allergen. The result is repeated patient exposure to the antigen during the treatment period with little apparent benefit. A thorough history and significant investigative work are important in avoiding treatment errors.

Future Directions

ACD is a subspecialty of dermatology in which the marriage of history and physical exam is extremely important. Although patch testing remains the gold standard for diagnosis, there are many allergens not contained in currently available commercial patch test kits. There are more than 3700 potential environmental allergens. Future editions of patch tests will most likely contain more allergens to help guide therapy and allow avoidance of the offending agent. Tolerance induction is also an exciting area of research in this area.

Additional Resource

American Academy of Dermatology. Available at: http://www.AAD.org.
This website is largely devoted to patient education and contains a significant number of patient resources, including patient support groups.

EVIDENCE

1. Belsito D: Allergic contact dermatitis. In Freedburg IM, Eisen AZ, Wolff K, et al (eds): Fitzpatrick's Dermatology in General Medicine, 6th ed. New York, McGraw-Hill, 2003, pp 1164-1176.
   This chapter is a short introduction to the pathogenesis of ACD, including a few interesting tables concerning contact allergens.
2. Hogan D: Contact dermatitis: Allergic. Available at: http://www.emedicine.com. Accessed January 12, 2005.
   This article provides a general overview of ACD and includes information about specific allergens.
3. Mowad C, Marks J Jr: Allergic contact dermatitis. In Bolognia JL, Jorizzo JL, Rapini RP (eds): Dermatology. St. Louis, Mosby, 2003, pp 227-239.
   This textbook chapter contains details about patch testing.
4. Rietchel RL, Fowler JF (eds): The pathogenesis of allergic contact hypersensitivity; and practical aspects of patch testing. In Fisher's Contact Dermatitis, 5th ed. Philadelphia, Lippincott Williams & Wilkins, 2001, pp 1-26.
   This reference is the authoritative textbook on all aspects of allergic contact dermatitis and devotes chapters to specific types of contact allergens.

Heidi T. Jacobe ▪ Daniel J. Parsons ▪ David S. Rubenstein

Psoriasis

Introduction

Psoriasis is a chronic, relapsing disorder of the skin characterized by sharply demarcated, red plaques with silvery scale in a characteristic distribution. It occurs in 1% to 3% of the population. The lesions are usually distinctive, allowing diagnosis based on physical findings alone. A seronegative destructive arthritis can be seen in association with the skin disease and is more common in patients whose psoriasis begins in childhood.

Etiology and Pathogenesis

Increasing research into the molecular mechanisms of psoriasis has led to an increased understanding of disease pathogenesis. Evidence of a genetic predisposition includes an increased incidence in relatives and children of affected patients and a high rate of concordance in monozygotic twins. To date, six psoriasis susceptibility loci (Psor1-6) have been described. The genes mapped to these regions encode proteins involved in inflammation and epithelial differentiation. For example, Psor1 encodes the major histocompatibility complex, which is involved in antigen presentation. Psor2 has been mapped to the RunX1 transcription factor binding site that regulates transcription of two genes whose protein products regulate association of cytoskeletal proteins and transmembrane proteins. The genes for S100A8 and S100A9, two chemotactic proteins, have been mapped to Psor4. Psor6 has recently been mapped to JunB, a component of the activator protein-1 (AP-1) transcription factor. The polygenic nature of psoriasis may explain its variable presentation.

Psoriasis is currently believed to represent an aberrant immune response in which cytokines and chemokines secreted by inflammatory cells stimulate the keratinocytes to proliferate and differentiate in a pattern suggestive of wound repair. The increased proliferation and altered differentiation manifest histologically as thickened epidermis and parakeratosis, corresponding to the thickened skin plaques with adherent silvery scale observed clinically. Therapies targeting components of this inflam-matory cascade, including such drugs as cyclosporine or the newer biologics, are very effective in treating psoriasis.

Clinical Presentation

Psoriasis affects men and women equally. It usually begins in the third decade but can develop at any age. It is clinically distinctive. Psoriasis begins as red, scaly papules that coalesce to form sharply demarcated plaques with adherent silvery white scale (Fig. 174-1). The extent of scaling varies with the body part involved and treatment. Scaling can be quite thick in the scalp and minimal in intertriginous areas and treated sites (Fig. 174-2). The plaques are deep red underneath the scale.

Psoriasis has a predilection for certain cutaneous sites, including elbows, knees, gluteal cleft, scalp, fingernails, and toenails (Fig. 174-3). Nail involvement most commonly appears as pits in the surface of the nail plate; less commonly, oil stains (brown discoloration), onychodystro-phy, and onycholysis occur (Fig. 174-4). It has a tendency to spread to sites of skin trauma (Koebner's phenomenon). Lesions may be asymptomatic or extremely pruritic. Most disease is limited to the sites listed previously, but there are many other clinical presentations of psoriasis (Box 174-1).

Psoriatic arthritis follows the onset of the cutaneous manifestations most commonly but may occur at any time. It usually presents as asymmetric arthritis involving one or more joints of the fingers and toes. The affected digit is

Figure 174-1 Psoriasis.

Plaque psoriasis

Section of skin lesion
Histopathologic features

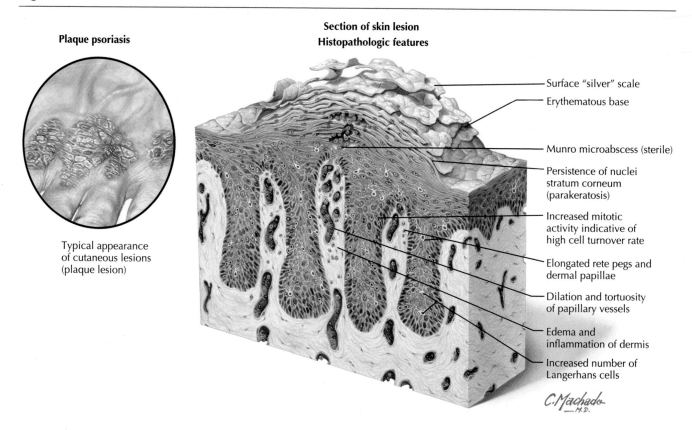

Typical appearance
of cutaneous lesions
(plaque lesion)

Surface "silver" scale

Erythematous base

Munro microabscess (sterile)

Persistence of nuclei
stratum corneum
(parakeratosis)

Increased mitotic
activity indicative of
high cell turnover rate

Elongated rete pegs and
dermal papillae

Dilation and tortuosity
of papillary vessels

Edema and
inflammation of dermis

Increased number of
Langerhans cells

C. Machado
—M.D.

Figure 174-2 Psoriasis in the Genital Area.

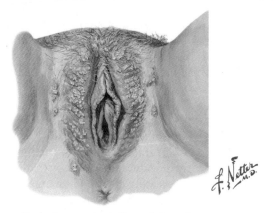

Typical appearance of intertriginous lesion.
Note minimal scale

acutely hot and swollen and eventually develops soft tissue
swelling producing the so-called sausage digit. There is a
5% incidence of psoriatic arthritis in the psoriatic population; men and women are affected equally. The usual age
of presentation is between 20 and 40 years. About 80% of
patients have nail involvement. Psoriatic arthritis can be
progressive and deforming. Rheumatoid factor and antinuclear antibody test results are usually negative.

Box 174-1   Clinical Presentations of Psoriasis
Chronic plaque psoriasis
Guttate psoriasis—acute eruptive psoriasis following streptococcal pharyngitis
Pustular psoriasis
Erythrodermic psoriasis
Psoriasis of the palms and soles
Inverse psoriasis (flexural areas)

Differential Diagnosis

The differential diagnosis often depends on the morphology of the psoriatic lesions. Classic plaque psoriasis is quite
distinctive but may occasionally be difficult to distinguish
from nummular eczema, mycosis fungoides, atopic dermatitis, or tinea corporis. Guttate psoriasis should be differentiated from secondary syphilis, pityriasis lichenoides et
varioliformis, and pityriasis rosea. Scalp psoriasis can be
confused with seborrheic dermatitis or eczema. One distinguishing characteristic of scalp psoriasis is its tendency
to move onto the forehead. Inverse psoriasis resembles
seborrheic dermatitis, tinea, or candidal infection.

Figure 174-3 Psoriasis: Typical Distribution.

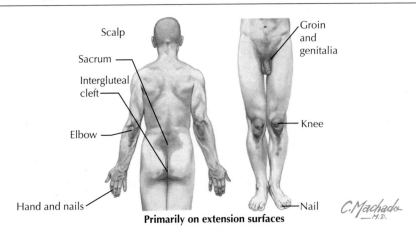

Primarily on extension surfaces

Figure 174-4 Psoriatic Nail Involvement.

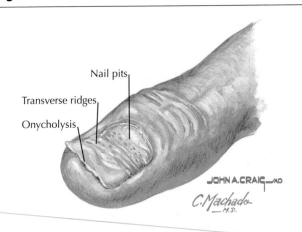

Diagnostic Approach

Classic plaque psoriasis is usually diagnosed clinically. Guttate psoriasis is differentiated from secondary syphilis through serologic testing. Pityriasis rosea is excluded by history and histologic examination. When tinea or candida is suspected, potassium hydroxide preparation of scale is helpful. In difficult cases, a punch biopsy can be done for histologic examination. HIV type 1 should be considered in patients with a particularly explosive onset of widespread psoriasis, including assessment of risk factors for HIV infection. HIV testing should be offered to all these patients.

Management and Therapy

Optimum Treatment

Management of psoriasis is determined by several factors:

Amount of body surface area involved: Generally, patients with less than 10% body surface area involvement can be treated topically; greater than 10% body surface area involvement requires treatment with ultraviolet (UV) light or systemic therapy.

Area of involvement: Select topical medications based on where they will be applied. Potency is guided by the characteristics of the skin being treated. Some topical preparations (calcipotriene and tazarotene) can irritate the face or intertriginous areas. Systemic therapy is also guided by the distribution of lesions. For example, UV light therapy is not a good choice for intertriginous or scalp psoriasis.

Degree of plaque inflammation: Inflammatory, red plaques are irritated and worsened by certain topical therapies, including tar, anthralin, and calcipotriene.

Patient health and mental status: Some patients are unable or unwilling to follow a complicated regimen that includes multiple topical medications. Other patients may not be candidates for systemic therapy. It is important to tailor treatment to the individual needs of the patient.

Topical Therapy Options

Topical steroids offer the advantage of quick response with rapid improvement in inflammation and itching. Tolerance develops fairly quickly, and patients who did very well initially will note decreasing efficacy over time. This often leads to overuse of the preparation in an attempt to recapture the initial dramatic improvement. Patients should be educated regarding this aspect of steroid use. The specific steroid preparation needs to be tailored to the area where it will be applied and the thickness of the psoriatic plaque. Treat the face and intertriginous areas with a class V to VII steroid cream or ointment (Table 174-1). The extremities and trunk can be treated with class IV to I steroid creams or ointments depending on the thickness of the plaques. Hands and feet have thick skin and usually require a class I or II steroid ointment. Ointments have better absorption, making them more effective, but are less well

Table 174-1 Steroid Potency in Psoriasis

Group	Potency	Medication
I	Super high	Clobetasol propionate 0.05% (cream, ointment, scalp solution)
II	High	Fluocinonide 0.05% (cream, ointment, scalp solution)
III	Intermediate	Betamethasone diproprionate 0.05% (cream)
III	Intermediate	Betamethasone-17-valerate 0.1% (ointment)
IV	Intermediate	Fluocinolone acetonide 0.025% (ointment, scalp solution)
V	Low-intermediate	Hydrocortisone butyrate 0.1% (cream)
VI	Low	Desonide 0.05% (cream, lotion)
VII	Very low	Hydrocortisone 1, 2.5% (cream, ointment)

tolerated. Scalp psoriasis can be treated with a class IV to I steroid solution. Most topical steroids are designed for twice-a-day use. Class I steroids can induce atrophy and striae very quickly and cause adrenal axis suppression if applied to a large body surface area. Most practitioners use a class I steroid for 2 weeks, alternating with a 1-week rest period. As patients improve, they can taper the frequency of steroid use. Long-term steroid use should be discouraged. Application twice a week for maintenance is acceptable. Systemic steroids should not be used for psoriasis. Although they rapidly control the disease, withdrawal produces a rebound effect and potential conversion to pustular psoriasis, which requires hospitalization.

Vitamin D analogues including calcipotriene ointment, cream, and solution inhibit the proliferation of keratinocytes and normalize their maturation. These drugs can be effective as single agents, but better results are achieved when they are used along with a potent topical steroid. A typical regimen begins with once-a-day application of calcipotriene and of a class I steroid, which is continued until the plaques begin to thin, usually 2 to 3 weeks. Subsequently, calcipotriene is applied twice a day Monday through Friday, and the class I steroid is applied twice a day on the weekend. This phase can be continued for several weeks or even months. The goal is to use calcipotriene once or twice a day for maintenance as a single agent. Calcipotriene benefits include reduced time to clearance, decreased steroid use, less tolerance to steroids, and prolonged improvement. The most common side effect is irritation at the site of application. It should not be used on the face and intertriginous areas. There have been no reported effects on bone or calcium metabolism if less than 100 g/week is used. Acidic substances such as salicylic acid should be avoided because they inactivate calcipotriene.

Tazarotene (0.05% or 0.1% gel) is a retinoid developed specifically for use in psoriasis. It can be irritating and should only be used in noninflamed stable plaque psoriasis. Topical steroids can be used to help decrease inflammation. Tazarotene is rated pregnancy category X and should not be used in pregnant women. Use in intertriginous sites should be avoided. The advantages of tazarotene are that it is a once-daily dosage that can be used on the scalp, it decreases steroid use, and it often provides a prolonged response.

Psoriatic plaques frequently develop thick, adherent scale that limits the absorption and efficacy of topical medications, particularly on the scalp. Keratolytics including salicylic acid, urea, and lactic acid are available to remove the scale. A lotion or cream containing one of these agents can be applied to psoriatic plaques either concomitantly with other topical medications or separately. The scalp responds well to a lotion or solution containing a keratolytic applied under a shower cap overnight followed by a shampoo in the morning and the application of corticosteroid solution. Improvement within 1 to 2 weeks is typical, allowing for the discontinuation of the keratolytic. Patients should then be instructed to restart keratolytics whenever scale starts to build up.

Systemic Therapies

Systemic therapies should be considered in patients who fail topical medications, those with more than 10% total body surface involvement or palmar plantar involvement, or those with associated arthritis. Narrow-band UV-B phototherapy can rapidly clear patients with extensive skin disease; however, joint disease is not responsive to phototherapy. Care must be taken during administration of these treatments to avoid burning the patient. Additionally, UV-B phototherapy is associated with an increased risk for photodamage and photoaging and skin cancers. This risk appears to be cumulative, and patients who have received phototherapy should be monitored for the development of skin cancer.

Oral medications, including antimetabolites, systemic retinoids, and immunosuppressive agents are very effective at treating psoriasis. These agents should be used with caution and by those experienced with their toxicities and side effects. Methotrexate is an antimetabolite that inhibits dihydrofolate reductase. It is effective in treating both the skin and joint manifestations of psoriasis. Methotrexate can suppress the bone marrow, and patients should be regularly monitored. Additionally, methotrexate can cause hepatotoxicity. Serologic liver function tests and periodic liver biopsies are used to monitor for the hepatotoxic effects of methotrexate. Rare adverse effects, including pulmonary fibrosis, have been reported. Typical doses of methotrexate used for psoriasis are 7.5 to 25 mg weekly.

Supplementation with folate can be helpful in reducing methotrexate-associated gastrointestinal distress and may also lower the risk for cardiovascular disease that has recently been reported to be increased in psoriasis patients. Methotrexate is renally excreted and should be used with caution in patients with renal insufficiency. Nonsteroidal anti-inflammatory agents can decrease renal excretion of methotrexate, and patients should be cautioned on the concomitant use of these medications.

Acitretin is a systemic retinoid used for psoriasis. Because of the potent teratogenic effects, this medication should not be used in women of child-bearing potential. Systemic retinoids are particularly effective for pustular psoriasis but have efficacy in large-plaque psoriasis as well. Side effects, such as dryness, alopecia, and arthralgias, can often be limiting. Regular serologic monitoring includes fasting triglycerides, liver enzymes, and complete blood counts because of the potential for systemic retinoids to cause hypertriglyceridemia, hepatic inflammation, and rarely leukopenia.

Cyclosporine is very effective at treating psoriasis; however, systemic toxicities such as bone marrow suppression and nephrotoxicity limit its chronic use. In our practice, we typically limit the use of this potent immunosuppressive medication to the short-term treatment of acute exacerbations and psoriatic flares. To minimize nephrotoxicity, dosing should not exceed 5 mg/kg/day. Monitoring should include measurement of blood pressure, a complete blood count, liver function panels, renal function (blood urea nitrogen and creatinine), serum electrolytes, uric acid and magnesium.

Biologic agents represent a relatively new class of drugs that have added significantly to the therapeutic armamentarium. These agents are recombinant proteins produced in biologic expression systems and subsequently purified to homogeneity. The limiting factor tends to be the cost, typically being between $12,000 and 25,000 per year depending on the agent and the dosing regimen. Several drugs are currently approved for the treatment of psoriasis and psoriatic arthritis, including the tumor necrosis factor-α blocking agents etanercept, adalimumab, and infliximab. Efalizumab, a monoclonal antibody directed against the CD11a subunit of LFA-1 (lymphocyte function-associated antigen), disrupts antigen presentation and the ability of lymphocytes to bind to vascular endothelium and keratinocytes. It is self-administered as weekly subcutaneous injections.

Special Considerations

Patients with scalp psoriasis should use medicated shampoos in addition to the agents discussed previously. Formulations with additives such as salicylic acid, zinc pyrithione, selenium sulfide, or coal tar can be helpful. Psoriasis in intertriginous sites is frequently superinfected with candida. The addition of a topical antifungal with yeast coverage is helpful in these patients.

There is a correlation between the severity of psoriasis and the degree of stress the patient is experiencing. Minimizing stress can also improve psoriasis.

Certain drugs, including lithium, β-blocking drugs, antimalarials, and systemic steroids can exacerbate psoriasis and should be avoided.

If the patient has greater than 10% body surface area involvement or remains unresponsive to topical therapy, consider referral to a dermatologist. Dermatologists use UV light, methotrexate, acitretin, cyclosporine, and a variety of other systemic medications to control severe, widespread psoriasis.

Avoiding Treatment Errors

Physicians may underestimate the time and inconvenience associated with use of topical therapies for patients with significant body surface area involvement. Patients may not necessarily admit to not using their topical medications; in this case, the physician assumes that the patient requires more potent medications. Treatment needs to be individualized to the patient with consideration of the patient's lifestyle in order to be optimally effective.

Future Directions

Decades of investigation into the detailed mechanisms of psoriatic inflammation have been translated into new mechanism-based therapies. Additional molecules are currently being investigated and developed to treat patients with psoriasis and psoriatic arthritis. These medicines will continue to improve our ability to care for patients suffering from this very common skin disease.

Additional Resources

American Academy of Dermatology. Available at: http://www.aad.org. Accessed December 22, 2006.
   Patient-specific information and physicians with expertise in psoriasis can be found here.
National Psoriasis Foundation. Available at: http://www.psoriasis.org. Accessed December 22, 2006.
   This website describes patient experiences, treatment options, and listings of physicians with expertise in treating psoriasis.

EVIDENCE

1. Camisa C: Handbook of Psoriasis. Malden, MA, Blackwell Science, 1998.
   This excellent and detailed monograph reviews the diagnosis and treatment of psoriasis.
2. Fitzpatrick TB: Psoriasis. In Freedberg IM, Eisen AZ, Wolff K, et al (eds): Fitzpatrick's Dermatology in General Medicine, 5th ed. New York, McGraw-Hill, 1999.
   This text chapter reviews the pathophysiology, clinical presentation, and natural history of psoriasis as well as current treatment considerations.

Bullous Skin Disease

Introduction

Blisters are classified by etiology or location; intraepidermal, dermal-epidermal junction, or subepidermal. Primary causes of blistering include inherited defects in cell adhesion proteins or diseases in which cell adhesion proteins are the target antigens for autoimmune responses. Autoimmune bullous skin disease typically presents in adults and tends to persist in the absence of clinical intervention. Secondary causes include infectious, traumatic, and inflammatory processes. Blistering as a secondary event is often acute in onset, is transient, and resolves with treatment of the underlying disease.

The clinical manifestations of bullous genodermatoses are apparent at birth or shortly thereafter, and similarly affected family members may be identified. Laboratory examination is critical to making a correct diagnosis and should include biopsy for (1) routine histology to determine the plane of cleavage within the skin and the presence or absence and nature of the inflammatory infiltrate, and (2) direct immunofluorescence to identify the nature and location of immunoreactants in the skin. Additional diagnostic studies include indirect immunofluorescent studies, Western blot analysis, immunoprecipitation, enzyme-linked immunosorbent assay, and immunoelectron microscopy (Box 175-1).

BULLOUS PEMPHIGOID

Etiology and Pathogenesis

Bullous pemphigoid (BP) is an autoimmune disease in which immunoglobulin G (IgG) autoantibodies target the basal keratinocyte hemidesmosome proteins BP180 (BP antigen 2) and BP230 (BP antigen 1). Passive transfer of BP180 IgG to neonatal mice causes subepidermal blister formation, demonstrating that the antibodies are pathogenic (Fig. 175-1).

Clinical Presentation

BP typically affects adults in the fifth to sixth decades of life with tense bullae on either a noninflammatory or an erythematous base (Fig. 175-2). BP may be localized or widespread. An urticarial phase may precede the development of frank blisters by 2 to 4 weeks. BP may resolve spontaneously within 2 to 6 years.

Differential Diagnosis

BP can be distinguished from other bullous dermatoses, particularly epidermolysis bullosa acquisita (EBA), by immunofluorescent studies on salt split skin (see Fig. 175-1).

Diagnostic Approach

Punch biopsy should be performed for routine histologic studies and direct immunofluorescence. Histologic analysis of BP demonstrates a subepidermal blister with an eosinophilic infiltrate. Direct immunofluorescence demonstrates linear staining of the basement membrane with IgG and C3. In BP, immunoreactants localize to the blister roof on salt split skin. About 80% of patients with active disease demonstrate immunoreactants by indirect immunofluorescence.

Management and Therapy

Optimum Treatment

Localized BP may respond to ultrapotent topical or intralesional corticosteroids. Initial management should utilize systemic corticosteroids with the subsequent addition of a steroid-sparing agent such as azathioprine. Higher doses of prednisone or additional immunosuppressive agents

Figure 175-1 Autoantibody-Mediated Blisters: Location of Cleavage Plane.
BP, bullous pemphigoid; Col VII, type VII collagen; CP, cicatricial pemphigoid; Dsg 1, desmoglein 1; Dsg 3, desmoglein 3; EBA, epidermolysis bullosa acquisita; HG, herpes gestationis; PF, pemphigus foliaceous; PV, pemphigus vulgaris; LABD, linear immunoglobulin A bullous dermatosis.

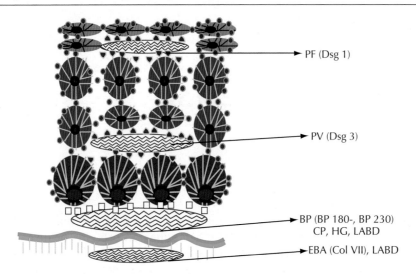

PF (Dsg 1)

PV (Dsg 3)

BP (BP 180-, BP 230)
CP, HG, LABD

EBA (Col VII), LABD

Box 175-1   Differential Diagnosis of Bullous Skin Disease

Infection
- Herpes simplex
- Herpes zoster
- Bullous impetigo
- Staphylococcal scalded skin syndrome
- Bullous tinea pedis

Injury or Trauma
- Burn (thermal, solar)
- Cryoinjury
- Friction
- Ischemia
- Pressure

Inflammatory
- Acute allergic contact dermatitis
- Dyshidrotic eczema
- Lichen planus
- Toxic epidermal necrolysis

Bullous Genodermatoses
- Epidermolysis bullosa simplex
- Junctional epidermolysis bullosa
- Dystrophic epidermolysis bullosa
- Hailey-Hailey (benign familial pemphigus)

Autoimmune
- Erythema multiforme
- Bullous pemphigoid
- Cicatricial pemphigoid
- Herpes gestationis
- Linear immunoglobulin A bullous dermatoses
- Epidermolysis bullosa acquisita
- Pemphigus vulgaris
- Pemphigus foliaceus
- Paraneoplastic pemphigus
- Dermatitis herpetiformis

---

such as cyclosporine may be necessary to control severe disease. Some patients respond to tetracycline and niacinamide. These agents are particularly useful in the elderly patient with focal stable disease and medical problems exacerbated by prednisone.

BULLOUS PEMPHIGOID–LIKE DISEASES

Related autoimmune diseases in which autoantibodies target the hemidesmosome complex include cicatricial pemphigoid (CP), herpes gestationis (HG), and linear IgA bullous dermatoses (LABD). CP is a group of chronic, progressive diseases in which autoantibodies target the β_4-integrin subunit, BP180, or laminin 5. HG is an autoimmune blistering disease of pregnant women. In LABD, a disease of adults and children, IgA antibodies to BP180 and to type VII collagen have been described. These processes present as subepidermal blistering diseases. The workup should include biopsies for routine histologic analysis and for direct immunofluorescence. Immunosuppressive agents, including prednisone, azathioprine, and cyclophosphamide, are used for treatment. For CP, the

Figure 175-2 Bullous Pemphigoid.

Tense bulla and urticarial plaques in bullous pemphigoid. *Courtesy of Dr. Walter Barkey.*

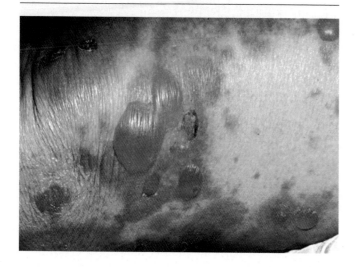

risk for blindness with ocular disease and stenosis with esophageal and laryngeal disease warrants aggressive therapy with high-dose systemic corticosteroids and adjunctive agents (azathioprine or cyclophosphamide). Less aggressive disease with minimal mucosal involvement should be treated with dapsone or ultrapotent topical corticosteroids. HG resolves postpartum; therefore, the goals of therapy are symptom relief and decreased blister formation. Mild disease can often be controlled with antihistamines and topical corticosteroids, whereas aggressive disease may require systemic corticosteroids. LABD is often self-limited in children, spontaneously resolving within several years. In adults, the disease may persist for many years. Dapsone or systemic corticosteroids can be used to control disease. Mucosal disease, particularly involving the eyes, is an indication for aggressive therapy.

EPIDERMOLYSIS BULLOSA ACQUISITA

Etiology and Pathogenesis

In this autoimmune process, patients make antibodies against type VII collagen, which is the major protein component of anchoring fibrils.

Clinical Presentation

EBA is a disease of middle-aged adults characterized by noninflammatory vesicles, bullae, and erosions on trauma-prone areas (knees, elbows, extensor hands and fingers, sacrum). It heals with scar and milia formation. Permanent nail dystrophy or loss and scarring alopecia may result. A BP-like variant of EBA presents with blisters and vesicles on an inflammatory base.

Differential Diagnosis

Porphyria cutanea tarda can be distinguished by the presence of photoexacerbation, hirsutism, and positive urine porphyrins. Bullous lupus can present with vesicles and bullae identical to those seen in EBA. However, in addition to collagen VII autoantibodies, patients have a positive antinuclear antigen and other more typical lupus erythematosus lesions. The BP-like variant of EBA is distinguished from BP by immunofluorescence on salt split skin.

Diagnostic Approach

Biopsy specimens reveal a subepidermal blister in which the presence of an inflammatory infiltrate is variable. Direct immunofluorescence demonstrates linear staining of IgG with or without C3, IgA, and IgM along the basement membrane zone. Incubating perilesional skin biopsies in 1M NaCl (salt split skin) results in separation of the epidermis from the dermis by cleavage formation within the lamina lucida. In EBA, immunoreactants localize to the dermal side of salt split skin. In BP, the immunoreactants localize to the epidermal side. Indirect immunofluorescence is positive in greater than 50% of patients with EBA. Immunoelectron microscopy demonstrates the localization of immunoreactants below the lamina densa.

Management and Therapy

Immunosuppressive therapy does not alter the course. Avoidance of trauma, hot environments, and wound care are beneficial.

PEMPHIGUS VULGARIS

Etiology and Pathogenesis

Pemphigus vulgaris (PV) is an autoimmune disease in which autoantibodies target the desmosomal cadherin desmoglein-3 (dsg-3). Passive transfer of anti-dsg-3 PV IgG to neonatal mice reproduces the clinical and histologic findings of PV, demonstrating that the IgG is pathogenic. Studies in both human skin cultures and the PV mouse model suggest that PV IgG triggers intracellular signaling mediated by p38 mitogen-activated protein kinase (MAPK) and heat-shock protein 27. Pharmacologic inhibition of p38MAPK prevents PV IgG-induced blistering in the mouse model.

Clinical Presentation

Patients in their 50s and 60s present with flaccid vesicles, bullae, and erosions of the skin with prominent mucosal lesions (Fig. 175-3). Examination for ocular lesions is imperative; scarring can result in loss of vision. Most patients have oral lesions, often as the initial presentation.

Figure 175-3 Pemphigus Vulgaris.
Flaccid vesicles and erosions of pemphigus.

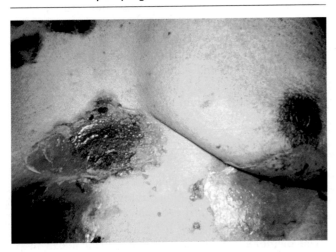

Figure 175-4 Pemphigus Foliaceus.
Crusted erosions of the trunk in pemphigus foliaceus.

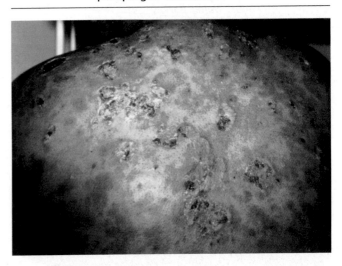

Lesions are painful, but not usually pruritic. Severe oral pain can lead to decreased oral intake and dehydration. Loss of skin barrier function places these patients at risk for secondary infection and fluid and electrolyte disturbances. Skin fragility is demonstrated by Nikolsky's sign, in which minimal mechanical traction causes lateral movement of the epidermis relative to the underlying structures.

Differential Diagnosis

Histologic studies and immunofluorescence distinguish PV from erythema multiforme major and toxic epidermal necrolysis.

Diagnostic Approach

Biopsy specimens reveal suprabasal acantholysis, which is a loss of cell-cell adhesion just above the basal layer (see Fig. 175-1). Direct immunofluorescence demonstrates IgG outlining keratinocyte cell membranes.

Management and Therapy

Optimum Treatment

PV is life threatening. Untreated, the mortality rate approaches 60%. Rapid therapeutic response necessitates high-dose systemic corticosteroids. Consider adjunctive steroid-sparing agents (azathioprine or cyclophosphamide). Mycophenolate mofetil, as a single agent or as a steroid-sparing agent, is successful in treating PV, pemphigus foliaceus (PF), and paraneoplastic pemphigus (PNP). Ocular involvement should be managed with an ophthalmologist.

PEMPHIGUS FOLIACEUS

Etiology and Pathogenesis

In this autoimmune disease, autoantibodies target desmoglein-1 (dsg-1), a major component of suprabasal keratinocyte desmosomes. Anti-dsg-1 PF IgG is pathogenic; passive transfer to neonatal mice reproduces the clinical and histologic findings of PF. Endemic PF, fogo selvagem, occurs in native populations of Brazil. Both hereditary susceptibility and environmental factors likely combine to incite the production of autoantibodies in susceptible individuals.

Clinical Presentation

Acantholysis in the upper epidermis results in fragile vesicles that are often not identified clinically. Examination reveals painful or burning, scaling, and crusted erosions of the scalp, face, and trunk (Fig. 175-4).

Differential Diagnosis

PF is distinguished from exfoliative dermatitis by histologic studies and direct immunofluorescence.

Diagnostic Approach

Biopsy specimens reveal acantholysis in the subcorneal and granular layers of the epidermis (see Fig. 175-1). Direct immunofluorescence shows IgG outlining keratinocyte cell membranes. Indirect immunofluorescence on skin substrates demonstrates antikeratinocyte IgG in 80% to 90% of patients. A highly sensitive and specific enzyme-linked immunosorbent assay is available to detect anti-dsg-1 IgG in PF sera.

Management and Therapy

Optimum Treatment

Local disease is managed with potent topical corticosteroids. Widespread disease is managed with systemic prednisone. Steroid-sparing agents (azathioprine or cyclophosphamide) are added to lower the prednisone dose or if patients fail to respond adequately to prednisone alone.

PARANEOPLASTIC PEMPHIGUS

Etiology and Pathogenesis

Paraneoplastic pemphigus (PNP) is a blistering disease associated with an underlying lymphoproliferative disorder. The autoantibody response may represent an immune response to tumor antigens and includes antibodies to desmoplakin I (250 kD), desmoplakin II, BP antigen 1 (230 kD), envoplakin (210 kD), periplakin (190 kD), dsg-3, and dsg-1. Passive transfer experiments show that the anti-dsg-3 IgGs cause acantholysis.

Clinical Presentation

PNP aggressively involves the oral and ocular mucosa. Pulmonary and esophageal epithelia may be similarly affected. Patients present with painful oral erosions and ulcerations and a variety of cutaneous lesions that may mimic the flaccid bullae and erosions of PV, the crusted plaques of PF, the dusky targetoid lesions of erythema multiforme, or even the widespread erythema and skin necrosis of toxic epidermal necrolysis.

Differential Diagnosis

PNP is distinguished from PV, PF, ulcerative oral lichen planus, erythema multiforme major, and toxic epidermal necrolysis by indirect immunofluorescence on bladder epithelia and by immunoprecipitation studies.

Diagnostic Approach

Biopsy specimens demonstrate variable features, including suprabasilar acantholysis; keratinocyte necrosis, a dense lichenoid infiltrate at the dermoepidermal junction; and subepidermal blistering. Direct immunofluorescence shows IgG and C3 staining of keratinocyte cell membranes. Features consistent with BP include IgG or C3 staining of the basement membrane zone. Differentiation of PNP from other variants of pemphigus is made by (1) indirect immunofluorescence of patient sera on rat bladder epithelium substrates (positive in 75% to 85% of PNP patients, but unusual in PV and PF); and (2) the presence of periplakin and envoplakin autoantibodies in PNP, but not PV nor PF. PNP can affect the palms and soles, which is unusual in PV.

Management and Therapy

Optimum Treatment

Patients with PNP should be evaluated for the presence of an underlying neoplasm. Surgical excision for benign tumors often results in clearing of the disease within 6 to 18 months. When associated with malignancy, PNP is difficult to treat. Numerous therapies have been tried, including treatment of the underlying malignancy, prednisone, azathioprine, cyclophosphamide, cyclosporine, dapsone, and plasmapheresis. However, none is uniformly successful. Most patients with PNP and malignant neoplasms die within 2 years of the onset of PNP. Involvement of the pulmonary epithelium can result in respiratory failure.

DERMATITIS HERPETIFORMIS

Etiology and Pathogenesis

Dermatitis herpetiformis (DH) is an autoimmune blistering disease associated with gluten-sensitive enteropathy; IgA autoantibodies can be identified in the papillary dermis.

Clinical Presentation

DH is a chronic disease that typically affects people in the second to fourth decades and presents as extremely pruritic, grouped vesicles symmetrically distributed on extensor surfaces, typically the scalp, back, elbows, knees, and buttocks. Scratching often makes it difficult to find intact vesicles on physical examination. Examination may reveal only secondary grouped, crusted lesions.

Differential Diagnosis

DH is differentiated from linear IgA disease, BP, HG, scabies, and erythema multiforme by histologic and immunofluorescent studies.

Diagnostic Approach

Biopsy specimens reveal a subepidermal vesicle with papillary dermal neutrophils and variable numbers of eosinophils. Direct immunofluorescence shows granular deposits of IgA at the tips of the dermal papilla.

Management and Therapy

Optimum Treatment

Dapsone is the treatment of choice. Patients respond within 1 to 2 days with decreased pruritus and no new lesion formation. Once control is achieved, the dose should be titrated down to the lowest level that controls disease. The risk for agranulocytosis necessitates monitoring the complete blood cell count when initiating therapy. Dapsone can cause hemolysis and methemoglobinemia, which can be severe in patients with glucose-6-phosphate dehydrogenase (G6PD) deficiency. For this reason, G6PD status should be determined before beginning dapsone. Patients on dapsone should be monitored for the development of peripheral neuropathy. Sulfapyridine is an alternative to dapsone. Clearing of DH lesions can occur with gluten-free diets; however, most patients do not tolerate restrictive diets and may take up to 1 year for the skin to clear.

Avoiding Treatment Errors

Many of the blistering disorders described in this chapter are treated with potent systemic or immunosuppressive agents. Use of these agents requires familiarity with their potential side effects. Constant vigilance and thorough monitoring is essential for reducing the risk for adverse events.

Future Directions

Current research on autoimmune blistering disease is aimed at (1) determining the mechanism by which autoantibodies cause loss of keratinocyte adhesion, (2) developing treatments that prevent the loss of cell adhesion without the need for global immunosuppression, and (3) identifying the triggers that incite the autoantibody response. For example, PV IgG trigger activation of p38MAPK within the target keratinocytes and pharmacologic inhibitors of p38MAPK block the ability of PV IgG to induce blistering in the PV mouse model. Several companies are developing inhibitors of p38MAPK. Should these drugs prove safe, p38 inhibitors may prove effective in the treatment of PV. Additionally, ongoing studies of fogo selvagem, the endemic form of PF, have revealed close associations between certain environmental triggers that lead to host cross-reactive immune responses. Studies of fogo selvagem are likely to yield insights into the biology of autoimmunity that extend far beyond cutaneous pathology.

Additional Resources

Current patient-specific information and physicians with expertise in the disorders discussed in the chapter can be found on the following websites:

American Academy of Dermatology. Available at: http://www.aad.org. Accessed December 6, 2006.

Dystrophic Epidermolysis Bullosa Research Association of America (DebRA). Available at: http://www.debra.org. Accessed December 6, 2006.

International Pemphigus and Pemphigoid Foundation. Available at: http://www.pemphigus.org. Accessed December 6, 2006.

Society for Investigative Dermatology. Available at: http://www.sidnet.org. Accessed December 6, 2006.

EVIDENCE

1. Anhalt GJ, Diaz LA: Prospects for autoimmune disease: Research advances in pemphigus. JAMA 285(5):652-654, 2001.

   This article reviews the structural features of the major histocompatibility complex class II gene–peptide–T-cell receptor complex involved and of the environmental and genetic factors that induce autoimmunity against desmoglein 1.

2. Anhalt GJ, Kim SC, Stanley JR, et al: Paraneoplastic pemphigus: An autoimmune mucocutaneous disease associated with neoplasia. N Engl J Med 323(25):1729-1735, 1990.

   This is the initial clinical, histologic, and immunobiologic description of this variant of pemphigus that is associated with underlying neoplasms.

3. Berkowitz P, Hu P, Liu Z, et al: Desmosome signaling: Inhibition of p38MAPK prevents pemphigus vulgaris IgG-induced cytoskeleton reorganization. J Biol Chem 280(25):23778-23784, 2005.

   This article reports the identification of signaling induced within target skin cells by anti-desmoglein-3 antibodies from PV patients. Blocking PV IgG-induced phosphorylation of p38MAPK and HSP27 prevents early cytoskeletal changes that precede loss of adhesion, suggesting a mechanistic role for p38MAPK and HSP27 in pemphigus acantholysis.

4. Berkowitz P, Hu P, Warren S, et al: p38MAPK inhibition prevents disease in pemphigus vulgaris mice. Proc Natl Acad Sci U S A 103(34):12855-12860, 2006.

   This article reports that PV IgG activates keratinocyte signaling through p38MAPK and HSP25 in the in vivo passive transfer mouse model and that pharmacologic blockade of these events prevents PV IgG-induced blistering in vivo. Combined with the previous reference, these two papers establish a role for p38MAPK as a drug-treated target in pemphigus.

5. Diaz LA, Giudice GJ: End of the century overview of skin blisters. Arch Dermatol 136(1):106-112, 2000.

   This well-written and compact review of the pathophysiology of adhesive defects in autoimmune and inherited blistering disorders of the skin presents the target structural proteins for each blistering disorder and their location within the epidermis in both diagrammatic and table formats.

6. Rubenstein DS, Diaz LA: Pemphigus antibody induced phosphorylation of keratinocyte proteins. Autoimmunity 39(7):1-10, 2006.

   A recent review of the data suggests that pemphigus autoantibodies cause loss of cell-cell adhesion by activating biochemical signaling events within the target keratinocytes.

7. Stanley JR: Pemphigus and pemphigoid as paradigms of organ-specific, autoantibody-mediated diseases. J Clin Invest 83(5):1443-1448, 1989.

   The author reviews the work leading to the identification of the pathophysiologic target antigens desmoglein-3 and desmoglein-1 in pemphigus and BP180 in bullous pemphigoid.

8. Woodley DT, Briggaman RA, Gammon WR: Acquired epidermolysis bullosa. A bullous disease associated with autoimmunity to type VII (anchoring fibril) collagen. Dermatol Clin 8(4):717-726, 1990.

   This article reviews the data supporting epidermolysis bullosa acquisita (EBA) as a chronic subepidermal autoimmune blistering disease of the skin caused by antibodies to type VII collagen.

Diem N. Wu ▪ David S. Rubenstein

176

Alopecia

Introduction

Hair loss results from a number of pathologic and physiologic processes (Fig. 176-1). Identification of the causative agents of hair loss enables the clinician to design a rational approach to treatment. This chapter will briefly familiarize the reader with the basic diagnostic tools and treatment options for common causes of hair loss (Box 176-1).

NONSCARRING ALOPECIA

Nonscarring alopecia is hair loss in the setting of a normal-appearing scalp. The hair-pull test will differentiate breaking from shedding.

The hair-pull test is performed by taking 50 to 100 hairs and gently pulling from the scalp. Repeat this several times all over the scalp. If more than a few hairs come out from the roots, the test result is positive. The hair bulbs should be examined under the microscope to determine whether the hairs are anagen or telogen hairs (Fig. 176-2). This will help differentiate between different causes of nonscarring alopecia.

In the patient with brittle hair, the hair pull test will reveal broken off hair with no visible bulb. Patients with brittle hair should be questioned regarding hair care. Improper hair care is the most common cause of brittle hair in adults. Treatment is gentle hair care. Brittle hair in children, in the absence of tinea capitis, can be the result of a heritable structural defect of the hair shaft. These patients should be referred to a dermatologist.

ALOPECIA AREATA

Etiology and Pathogenesis

The precise etiology of alopecia areata is unknown. However, a genetic predisposition and autoimmunity appear important. Alopecia areata is associated with a number of autoimmune disorders, including atopy, autoimmune thyroid disease, vitiligo, diabetes mellitus, Addison's disease, pernicious anemia, systemic lupus erythematosus, and rheumatoid arthritis.

Clinical Presentation

Alopecia areata is most common in children and young adults. It affects men and women equally. Patients note a sudden loss of hair in oval patches (Fig. 176-3). Nonscalp hair-bearing areas are rarely affected. Regrowth occurs after 1 to 3 months. Hair loss may occur in new areas while regrowth occurs.

Examination reveals 1- to 4-cm oval patches of alopecia with a smooth scalp or short stubs of hair (exclamation point hairs). Nail pitting occurs in 3% to 30% of patients.

Differential Diagnosis

Secondary syphilis is in the differential diagnosis.

Diagnostic Approach

The diagnosis is usually clinical. The hair-pull test shows dystrophic anagen and telogen hairs. Serologic testing should be performed to check for thyroid disorders. Biopsy is rarely necessary.

Management and Therapy

Optimum Treatment

Limited alopecia areata frequently resolves spontaneously, and treatment is not always necessary. The therapy of choice is intradermal injection of triamcinolone acetonide repeated every 4 weeks until regrowth is achieved. Atrophy is the major side effect. Potent topical steroids (clobetasol propionate) in cycles of 2 weeks on and 1 week off are an

Figure 176-1 Hair Loss.

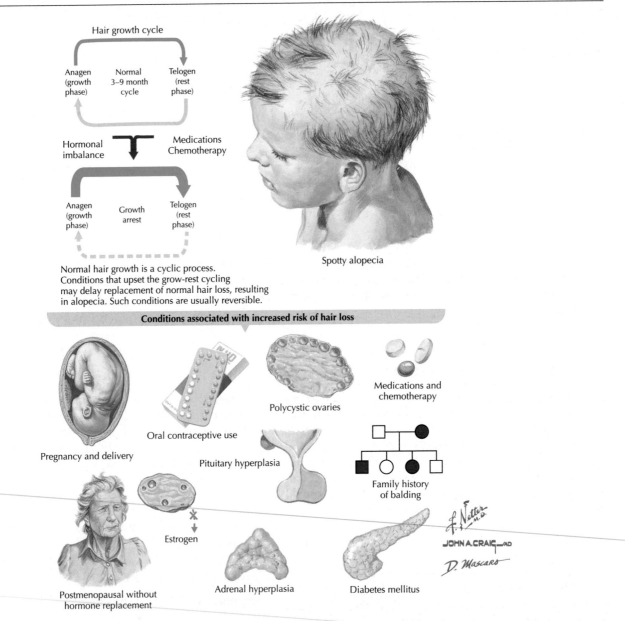

Hair growth cycle

Anagen (growth phase) — Normal 3–9 month cycle — Telogen (rest phase)

Hormonal imbalance | Medications Chemotherapy

Anagen (growth phase) — Growth arrest — Telogen (rest phase)

Normal hair growth is a cyclic process.
Conditions that upset the grow-rest cycling
may delay replacement of normal hair loss, resulting
in alopecia. Such conditions are usually reversible.

Spotty alopecia

Conditions associated with increased risk of hair loss

Pregnancy and delivery

Oral contraceptive use

Polycystic ovaries

Medications and chemotherapy

Pituitary hyperplasia

Family history of balding

Postmenopausal without hormone replacement

Estrogen

Adrenal hyperplasia

Diabetes mellitus

alternative, particularly in widespread disease and in children. Other treatment options include tacrolimus ointment, squaric acid, and topical minoxidil.

ANDROGENETIC ALOPECIA

Etiology and Pathogenesis

Androgenetic alopecia predisposes affected individuals to lose hair from androgen-sensitive follicles on the scalp. Proposed mechanisms include autosomal dominance with incomplete penetrance and polygenic inheritance.

Clinical Presentation

Affecting men and women equally, hair loss begins in the 20s and is fully expressed by middle age. Men have frontal recession, proceeding to loss of hair in the crown and sometimes to total hair loss in the central scalp. The terminal scalp hairs become vellus hairs. In advanced cases, the scalp is shiny and smooth. Women have miniaturized hairs, increased space between individual hairs, and preservation of the frontal hairline.

Differential Diagnosis

Alopecia areata and telogen effluvium are the two other conditions to consider.

Diagnostic Approach

A thorough history and examination are usually adequate. A careful medication history will exclude drug-induced alopecia. Medications associated with hair loss include

Box 176-1 Evaluation of the Patient with Hair Loss

History

- Determine whether the hair loss is abnormal. Hair counts distinguish pathologic from physiologic hair loss. Have patients collect shed hairs for 7 days for the evaluation. Loss of more than 50 to 100 hairs per day indicates pathologic processes.
- Determine the timing of hair loss. Is it acute or gradual? Has it been present since birth?
- Identify associated symptoms such as pain, tenderness, and pruritus.
- Determine whether there are other skin complaints.
- Elicit a history of recent illness, stress, or medication use.
- Identify associated medical problems.
- Identify affected family members.

Clinical Examination

- Determine whether the hair loss is scarring or nonscarring. Scarring alopecia is characterized by the permanent loss of hair follicles within the foci of alopecia.
- Determine whether the process is inflammatory or noninflammatory. Inflammatory processes present with erythema, pruritus, or pain.
- Assess the presence or absence of scale, pustules, and adenopathy.
- Determine the pattern of hair loss. Is it restricted to focal areas of the scalp, or does it involve other hair-bearing regions?

Laboratory Examination

- The hair-pull test identifies pathologic hair loss. About 50 hairs are gently pulled from the base of the hairs. Release of two or more hairs is abnormal.
- Examine the bulbs of the released hairs microscopically to determine the phase of the hair cycle. Telogen hairs have rounded, nonpigmented bulbs. Anagen hairs have a cylindrical or tapered pigmented bulb (see Fig. 176-2).
- Hair shaft examination identifies traumatic or genetic causes for hair loss.
- Punch biopsy aids in identifying underlying pathology, particularly in cases of scarring or permanent hair loss.
- Potassium hydroxide preparation and fungal cultures are performed for suspected cases of tinea capitis.

Figure 176-2 Telogen and Anagen Hair Bulbs.

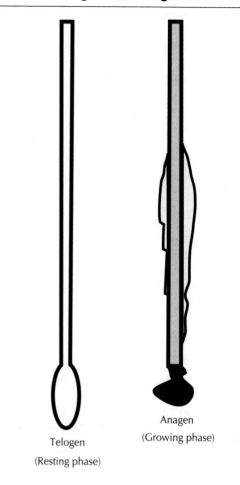

Telogen
(Resting phase)

Anagen
(Growing phase)

Figure 176-3 Alopecia Areata.
Short exclamation point hairs are visible within the patches of nonscarring hair loss.

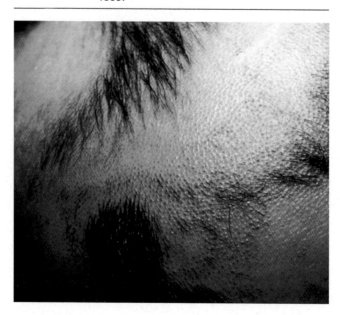

anticoagulants, angiotensin-converting enzyme inhibitors, β-blockers, lithium, oral contraceptives, retinoids, valproic acid, and vitamin A excess. In women, menstrual irregularity, hirsutism, severe acne, or infertility should prompt endocrinologic evaluation for a hyperandrogenetic state.

Management and Therapy

Optimum Treatment

Minoxidil, applied twice a day to a dry scalp, is the mainstay of therapy. It prevents further hair loss and provides moderate regrowth at the vertex of the scalp in 30% of patients. Results take at least 3 months to become evident. It must be used continually to preserve the beneficial effect. In men, finasteride (1 mg/day) used continuously to preserve regrowth is effective for hair loss at the crown. Decreased libido and erectile dysfunction occur in less than 2% of men. Finasteride is contraindicated in women. Minoxidil and finasteride may be used in combination. Advanced hair loss requires surgical intervention (hair transplantation or scalp reduction).

TELOGEN EFFLUVIUM

Etiology and Pathogenesis

A traumatic event (Box 176-2) can induce a large number of anagen (growing) hairs to prematurely enter catagen, then telogen (resting). Telogen hairs are shed 2 to 3 months after the event, with 50% of the hair affected.

Clinical Presentation

Telogen effluvium occurs in both sexes and all age groups with an abrupt onset of diffuse shedding. A precipitating event 3 months before the onset of the hair loss usually can be identified. Physical examination may appear unremarkable.

Differential Diagnosis

The differential diagnosis includes androgenetic alopecia, diffuse alopecia areata, and anagen effluvium. Anagen effluvium begins within 2 to 4 weeks after chemotherapy, produces much more marked hair loss, and is characterized by the presence of anagen hairs on the hair-pull test.

Diagnostic Approach

The characteristic history in a patient with a normal scalp is usually adequate. The hair-pull test is positive, revealing nondystrophic club telogen hairs. Biopsy is not indicated.

Management and Therapy

This condition spontaneously resolves in 6 to 12 months.

TINEA CAPITIS

Etiology and Pathogenesis

Tinea capitis is a contagious infection of the scalp and hair caused by superficial fungi (*Trichophyton tonsurans, Micros-*

Box 176-2 Causes of Telogen Effluvium

- Psychological stress
- Physical stress: systemic illness, surgery
- Anemia
- Endocrine: postpartum, perimenopausal or postmenopausal states, hypothyroidism or hyperthyroidism, oral contraceptives
- Nutritional: protein-calorie deprivation, essential fatty acid deficiency, zinc deficiency, biotin deficiency, iron deficiency, vitamin A excess
- Medications

---

porum canis). It is common in children and in patients chronically using topical corticosteroids in the scalp. Replication of fungi within and around the hair shaft leads to breakage as it exits the hair follicle, resulting in nonscarring hair loss. A vigorous inflammatory reaction called a *kerion* may develop. Chronic inflammation from the kerion or from secondary bacterial infection can lead to scalp fibrosis and permanent hair loss.

Clinical Presentation

Tinea capitis presents as single or multiple dry scaling patches, with numerous hairs broken off as they exit the follicle (black dot ringworm), with or without an inflammatory border. Kerion is characterized by boggy indurated plaques with pustules often associated with preauricular, postauricular, and cervical adenopathy.

Differential Diagnosis

Seborrheic dermatitis may also have this presentation.

Diagnostic Approach

Potassium hydroxide (KOH) preparation of plucked hairs and skin scrapings from the border of the lesion identifies spores within (endothrix) or outside (ectothrix) the hair shaft and hyphal elements. Fungal cultures are helpful in identifying suspicious KOH-negative cases. A punch biopsy with periodic acid–Schiff stain can demonstrate fungi.

Management and Therapy

Optimum Treatment

Griseofulvin, itraconazole, or terbinafine with adjunctive daily use of ketoconazole shampoo decreases the risk for infecting contacts. Concomitant use of systemic corticosteroids may reduce the inflammation and risk for fibrosis associated with kerion.

SCARRING (CICATRICIAL) ALOPECIA

Processes that lead to scarring alopecia result in irreversible hair loss. The hallmarks of scarring alopecia are visible loss of follicular ostia on clinical examination and destruction of the hair follicle on histopathology. The various conditions that lead to end-stage scarring alopecia can be distinguished by scalp biopsy. Two scalp biopsies for tranverse and vertical sectioning are recommended.

DISCOID LUPUS ERYTHEMATOSUS

Etiology and Pathogenesis

Discoid lupus erythematosus (DLE) is an autoimmune disorder of unclear etiology. Ultraviolet light and trauma are possible contributing factors. Five to 10% of patients with DLE have signs and symptoms of systemic lupus.

Figure 176-4 Discoid Lupus Erythematosus.
Note areas of scar formation and
complete absence of hair follicles.

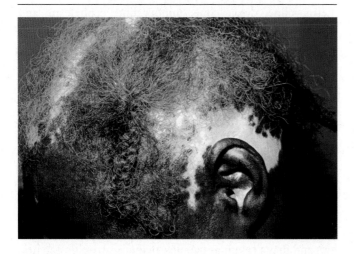

Clinical Presentation

Early lesions are erythematous to violaceous patches
and plaques with adherent scale and follicular plugging. A
hair-pull test may reveal anagen hairs. With progression,
patients develop mottled dyspigmentation, atrophy, telangiectasias, and fibrosis or scar (Fig. 176-4). Similar
appearing cutaneous lesions can be found in areas other
than the scalp. Often there are superficial ulcerations of
the palate as well as proximal nail-fold erythema and
telangiectasias.

Differential Diagnosis

Psoriasis, tinea capitis, and lichen planopilaris can be ruled
out by punch biopsy.

Diagnostic Approach

A punch biopsy specimen from the lesion border will demonstrate superficial and deep perivascular lymphocytic
infiltrate, interface dermatitis, follicular plugging, and
increased mucin deposition.

Management and Therapy

Optimum Treatment

Focal lesions can be treated with ultrapotent topical corticosteroids or intralesional triamcinolone acetonide to the
active inflammatory borders. Widespread disease often
requires the use of systemic agents (hydroxychloroquine,
quinacrine, chloroquine, or acitretin). End-stage fibrotic
lesions are not amenable to medical treatment. Cosmetics
may be useful in masking the atrophic hypopigmented
patches of end-stage lesions.

LICHEN PLANOPILARIS

Etiology and Pathogenesis

Lichen planopilaris is a progressive, scarring inflammatory
hair loss that may represent an autoimmune process. An
antigenic trigger may initiate the disease process.

Clinical Presentation

This condition typically affects middle-aged adults and is
more common in women. Patients present with focal
patches of hair loss with inflammatory violaceous to brown
keratotic papules at the lesion periphery. Tufts of three or
more hairs may remain within scarred foci. A hair-pull test
is positive for anagen hairs. Clinical lesions of lichen planus
may be seen at sites other than the scalp, including the
mucous membrane (lacy white reticulated Wickham's striae
of the oral cavity), skin (violaceous polygonal flat-topped
papules and plaques), and nail changes (pterygium).

Differential Diagnosis

DLE is the sole differential diagnosis.

Diagnostic Approach

Punch biopsy specimens reveal a lichenoid perifollicular
lymphocytic infiltrate. Giemsa stain demonstrates decreased
or absent perifollicular elastic fibers. Direct immunofluorescence studies show globular deposits of IgM and IgA at the
follicular basement membrane referred to as *cytoid bodies*.

Management and Therapy

Optimum Treatment

High-potency topical corticosteroids or intralesional triamcinolone acetonide can be used for local disease. Tapering courses of systemic corticosteroids over 3 months may
be effective in slowing or halting hair loss before use of
acitretin or hydroxychloroquine. Patients often experience
relapse after discontinuation of therapy.

ACNE KELOIDALIS

Etiology and Pathogenesis

Acne keloidalis is an inflammatory condition that may be
associated with the unique property of the pilosebaceous
unit, hair shaft, or scalp skin of African American people.
It may be precipitated by mechanical trauma, excoriation,
seborrhea, infection with *Demodex* or bacteria, and
autoimmunity.

Clinical Presentation

This condition occurs mostly in African American men
after adolescence. Patients present with firm, skin-colored

to erythematous follicular papules on the posterior neck and occipital scalp. These papules may coalesce to form keloidal nodules or plaques with associated hair loss. Symptoms include pruritus and burning.

Differential Diagnosis

Folliculitis is in the differential diagnosis.

Diagnostic Approach

The diagnosis is usually clinical. A punch biopsy shows perifollicular lymphocytes and plasma cells pronounced at the level of the sebaceous glands. Ongoing disease leads to complete follicular destruction.

Management and Therapy

Optimum Treatment

Mild disease can be controlled with high-potency topical steroids in combination with topical antibiotics. More severe disease is treated with monthly intralesional triamcinolone acetonide and oral antibiotics. Adjunctive use of antibacterial soaps is recommended.

DISSECTING CELLULITIS

Etiology and Pathogenesis

Dissecting cellulitis may represent an aberrant immune response to *Staphylococcus aureus* or *Propionibacterium acnes*; however, the etiology remains unknown.

Clinical Presentation

Active lesions present as a vigorous inflammatory reaction characterized by pustules, fluctuant abscesses, and sinus tracts. This painful, chronic, progressive, suppurative process commonly affects young African American men and eventually results in true scarring and permanent hair loss. When cultured, pustules are typically sterile or grow skin commensals.

Differential Diagnosis

Kerion and furunculosis are in the differential for the presentation of dissecting cellulitis.

Diagnostic Approach

Perform a culture to rule out fungal and bacterial pathogens. Punch biopsy specimens demonstrate follicular abscesses containing neutrophils. Lymphocytes, plasma cells, and foreign body giant cells may also be present. Late-stage lesions show destruction of follicles with true scarring. Special stains for microbial pathogens should be performed. Secondary bacterial infection is not uncommon.

Management and Therapy

Optimum Treatment

Tetracycline, doxycycline, minocycline, cephalexin, and isotretinoin are the mainstays of treatment. Tumor necrosis factor-α inhibitors such as etanercept and infliximab may be used for resistant disease.

SARCOID

Etiology and Pathogenesis

Granuloma formation may represent an immune response to a persistent antigen.

Clinical Presentation

This slowly progressive hair loss is more common in African American women. Sarcoid has variable morphologies and may present as papules, plaques, atrophic patches, or ulcerations with or without crust or scale, often in association with pulmonary sarcoid and other cutaneous sarcoidal lesions (erythema nodosum). Sarcoid causes true scarring (Fig. 176-5), although nonscarring sarcoidal alopecia has also been reported.

Differential Diagnosis

Discoid lupus erythematosus (DLE) can usually be ruled out by a punch biopsy.

Diagnostic Approach

A punch biopsy specimen reveals noncaseating granulomas and true scarring with decreased elastic fibers. Workup includes a full body examination for other cutaneous manifestations of sarcoid and chest radiographs to look for pulmonary disease.

Management and Therapy

Optimum Treatment

Ultrapotent topical corticosteroids, intralesional corticosteroids, systemic prednisone, hydroxychloroquine, and low-dose methotrexate are effective treatments.

PRIMARY OR METASTATIC NEOPLASMS

Etiology and Pathogenesis

Infiltrating tumor cells result in the destruction of normal skin architecture, including hair follicles.

Clinical Presentation

Examination reveals a firm nodule, plaque, or space-occupying mass that visibly replaces cutaneous appendageal structures.

Figure 176-5 Sarcoid.
No hair follicles are discernable in this plaque of alopecia.

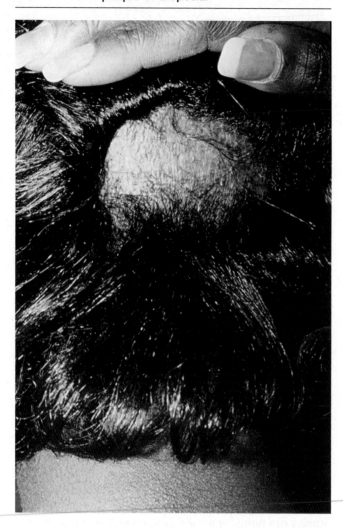

Differential Diagnosis

Common malignancies that infiltrate the scalp to cause hair loss include cutaneous T- or B-cell lymphomas and metastatic breast, lung, and prostate carcinoma.

Diagnostic Approach

Punch or incisional biopsy is essential to demonstrate the malignant histology.

Management and Therapy

Optimum Treatment

Treatment includes local excision and treatment of the underlying malignancy.

Avoiding Treatment Errors

For all types of alopecia, it is important to establish the correct diagnosis. If the etiology is unclear or the condition is not responding to treatment, a punch biopsy of the scalp may be indicated. Treatment with intralesional triamcinolone acetonide or ultrapotent topical corticosteroids on a long-term basis may cause atrophy of the skin.

Future Directions

Recent studies have shown that the nuclear receptor hairless (HR) controls the timing of Wnt signaling required for hair cycling. This observation raises the intriguing possibility that drugs could be designed to stimulate new hair growth by activation of this pathway. Such therapies would be useful in treating nonscarring hair loss, particularly androgenetic alopecia.

Additional Resources

American Academy of Dermatology. Available at: http://www.aad.org. Accessed December 9, 2006.
   This website provides accurate basic medical information about hair loss to patients.
National Alopecia Areata Foundation. Available at: http://www. alopeciaareata.com. Accessed December 9, 2006.
   This website is dedicated to alopecia areata and allows patients to form a support network.
Society for Investigative Dermatology. Available at: http://www.sidnet. org. Accessed December 9, 2006.
   This website is dedicated to basic science research of skin disease and provides links to various clinical resources for patients.

EVIDENCE

1. Chartier MB, Hoss DM, Grant-Kels JM: Approach to the adult female patient with diffuse nonscarring alopecia. J Am Acad Dermatol 47(6):809-818, 2002.
   This article provides an outline for diagnosing the primary causes of diffuse nonscarring hair loss in women.
2. Cotsarelis G: Epithelial stem cells: A folliculocentric view. J Invest Dermatol 126(7):1459-1468, 2006.
   The author explains the importance of bulge cells in the hair follicle as a potential target for developing future treatments for hair loss.
3. Olsen EA: Disorders of Hair Growth: Diagnosis and Treatment, 2nd ed. New York, McGraw-Hill, 2003.
   This book is written by one of the hair experts in dermatology and provides a comprehensive review of alopecia.
4. Ross EK, Tan E, Shapiro J: Update on primary cicatricial alopecias. J Am Acad Dermatol 53(1):1-37, 2005.
   This article reviews the etiology, diagnostic features, and therapeutic options for scarring hair loss.

177

Susan Riggs Runge • Craig Burkhart

Scabies and Pediculosis

SCABIES

Scabies is a contagious disease characterized by extreme pruritus. Severe outbreaks and complicated scabies are more common in institutions, such as nursing homes and hospitals, and among socially disadvantaged populations and immunocompromised hosts. Scabies occurs in all age groups, both sexes, all ethnic groups, and at all socioeconomic levels.

Etiology and Pathogenesis

Scabies results from the infestation of the skin with the mite *Sarcoptes scabiei* var. hominis. The mite completes its entire life cycle on human skin. The female mite burrows through the stratum corneum, laying three to four eggs a day for up to a month. The eggs hatch, and the larvae mature, perpetuating the cycle.

Although the predominant route of transmission is through close skin-to-skin contact, scabies can be transmitted indirectly through bedding and clothing. The likelihood of transmission of the infestation directly correlates with the number of mites harbored as in crusted scabies with hyperinfestation (see later).

Skin lesions result from a combination of infestation and a delayed hypersensitivity reaction to the mite, feces, and eggs in the skin. After initial infestation, there is usually a 3- to 6-week delay before the onset of pruritus and skin lesions. This delayed hypersensitivity reaction is the most likely reason that most patients continue to itch for 2 to 4 weeks after the mite is eradicated.

Clinical Presentation

Patients complain of pruritus that is usually worse at night. A history of pruritus in other members of the household is particularly suggestive.

Physical examination reveals inflammatory papules, which are often excoriated. There is a predilection for the finger webs, flexor aspects of the wrists, elbows, anterior axillary folds, buttocks, and genitalia (Fig. 177-1). The pathognomonic burrow is a 2- to 5-mm dirty white, slightly scaly, thread-like line found in the characteristic locations. Occasionally a black dot representing the mite is seen at the end of the burrow. Secondary impetiginization and eczematous change are common.

Scabies in infants and young children often presents as a widespread, pruritic eruption involving the face, scalp, palms, and soles. Elderly and immunosuppressed patients are less likely to develop a brisk inflammatory response and may present with pruritus and few skin lesions. Crusted (Norwegian) scabies is a hyperinfestation with thousands of mites that are present in exfoliating scales. This form of scabies is most often found in institutionalized elderly people or immunologically compromised hosts. Clinically, the skin lesions may resemble psoriasis, and pruritus is frequently absent.

Differential Diagnosis

In patients with few skin lesions, scabies can be misdiagnosed as a neurodermatosis with excoriations. Crusted scabies is easily confused with a papulosquamous disorder. Scabies can mimic many diseases, including atopic dermatitis, papular urticaria, pyoderma, insect bites, and dermatitis herpetiformis.

Diagnostic Approach

The clinical diagnosis of scabies in a patient with pruritus is based on finding the characteristic skin lesions in typical predilection sites or a history of exposure. A definitive diagnosis requires the identification of the mite, egg, or feces from a skin scraping (see Fig. 177-1). Because of the very low sensitivity of skin scrapings, the failure to find mites does not rule out scabies.

Management and Therapy

Scabies has traditionally been treated with topical scabicides (Fig. 177-2); however, oral therapy with ivermectin has evolved into a very useful alternative. Treatment of the index case as well as all household members and sexual contacts, even if asymptomatic, is the mainstay of therapy. The ease of transmission of crusted scabies necessitates the

Figure 177-1 Dermatoses Secondary to Ectoparasites.

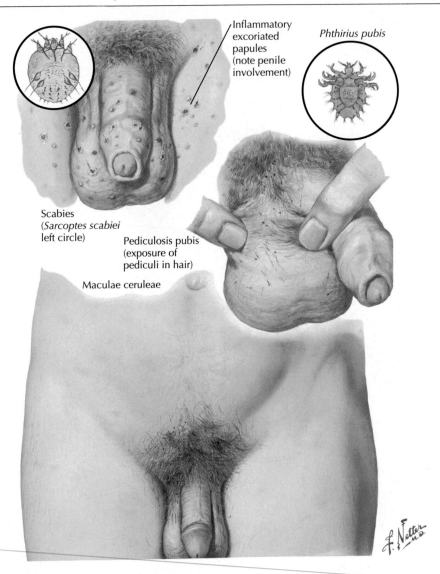

Inflammatory excoriated papules (note penile involvement)

Phthirius pubis

Scabies
(*Sarcoptes scabiei* left circle)

Pediculosis pubis (exposure of pediculi in hair)

Maculae ceruleae

treatment of all contacts, including patient care staff and support staff in institutional settings.

Scabicides should be applied in a thin layer from the head down to the soles of the feet, with special attention to the areas between the fingers and toes, under the nails, the umbilicus, genitalia, and between the buttocks. The medication should be washed off after 8 to 14 hours. After therapy, all linens, towels, bedclothes, and underwear should be washed in a washing machine with hot water (60° C). Children's plush toys, if not washable, should be put out of human contact for 72 hours, allowing the mite to die. For both oral and topical therapy, most experts advocate a second treatment 1 week to 14 days later.

Permethrin 5% cream is the first choice in topical scabicides because of its high efficacy and low potential for toxicity. Although not approved for infants younger than 2 months or pregnant or lactating women, 5% permethrin

is U.S. Food and Drug Administration pregnancy category B and safe for use on young children.

Lindane 1% cream has similar efficacy to permethrin but has much higher potential for central nervous system toxicity. Lindane should not be used in children younger than 3 years, in pregnant or lactating women, or in patients with underlying neurologic disorders. It should not be applied on broken skin or used in those with the potential for misuse of the medication.

Precipitated 6% sulfur in petrolatum is an alternative for infants younger than 2 months and in pregnant or lactating women. Crotamiton is also safe in children and infants but has questionable efficacy.

Ivermectin, an oral antiparasitic agent used extensively for several other parasitic infections, is safe and efficacious in the treatment of scabies in nonpregnant or lactating patients more than 15 kg in weight. Ivermectin is pre-

Figure 177-2 Sexually Transmitted Ectoparasites.

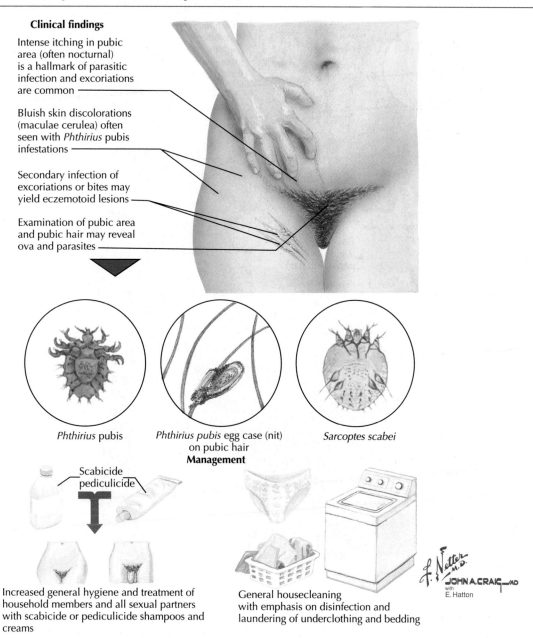

Clinical findings

Intense itching in pubic area (often nocturnal) is a hallmark of parasitic infection and excoriations are common

Bluish skin discolorations (maculae cerulea) often seen with *Phthirius* pubis infestations

Secondary infection of excoriations or bites may yield eczemotoid lesions

Examination of pubic area and pubic hair may reveal ova and parasites

Phthirius pubis

Phthirius pubis egg case (nit) on pubic hair

Sarcoptes scabei

Management

Scabicide pediculicide

Increased general hygiene and treatment of household members and all sexual partners with scabicide or pediculicide shampoos and creams

General housecleaning with emphasis on disinfection and laundering of underclothing and bedding

scribed at 200 μg/kg and repeated 7 to 14 days later. Patients who have no response to topical scabicides, who have generalized eczema, or who are unable to tolerate or comply with topical therapy are ideal candidates for ivermectin.

Oral antihistamines and medium-potency topical steroids provide symptomatic relief of the pruritus that often persists for up to 1 month after therapy.

Avoiding Treatment Errors

Treatment failure often results when other close contacts are not treated or when patients do not treat their entire skin surface. Even if asymptomatic, all household members and sexual contacts should be treated at the same time as the index case. As noted, patients should pay special attention to the areas between the fingers and toes, under the nails, the umbilicus, genitalia, and between the buttocks when applying topical scabicides.

PEDICULOSIS

Pediculosis is an infestation by *Pediculosis capitis* (head louse), *Pediculosis humanus* (body louse), or *Phthirius pubis* (pubic louse). Head lice are mainly found in children, and pubic lice in sexually active adults. Both head lice and pubic

lice are found in patients of all socioeconomic levels; in contrast, body lice are associated with poor hygiene, poverty, and overcrowding.

Head Lice

Head lice affect all levels of society and all races, with the exception of African Americans, in whom incidence is extremely low. The louse is transmitted by direct head-to-head contact or through shared towels or hair-grooming instruments. Head lice infestations are a common problem.

Clinical Presentation

The hallmark of head lice is intense scalp pruritus. Physical examination reveals nits and adult lice in the scalp hair. Nits are gray or brown oval egg capsules that adhere firmly to the hair shaft (see Fig. 177-2). Secondary changes resulting from immunologic response to lice saliva or excreta include scaling and erythema of the scalp with erythematous papules on the posterior neck and excoriations secondary to scratching. Intense scratching may lead to secondary infection of the scalp with associated honey-colored crusting over matted hair and lymphadenopathy.

Diagnosis

Active infestations are confirmed by observing live adult lice in the scalp or hair. Nits may be identified by their adherence to the hair shaft and microscopically by the presence of a breathing aperture at the superior aspect of the egg casing. The presence of nits alone does not confirm active infection. Because of their tight adherence to hair and resistance to degradation, hatched or nonviable nits may remain attached to hair for several weeks after resolution of an infestation.

Differential Diagnosis

Other causes of scalp pruritus, including tinea capitis and seborrheic dermatitis, should be considered, especially in children.

Management and Therapy

Permethrin cream rinse 1% and pyrethrin with piperonyl butoxide are available over the counter. Both are highly efficacious with a low toxicity profile. After treatment, nits can be removed with a fine-toothed comb. Despite instructions to the contrary on many package inserts, two applications 1 week apart are advised with all topical preparations. This approach ensures the killing of any surviving nits and decreases the risk for resistance.

Following therapy, all clothing, towels, bed linens, hair ribbons, and clothes should be machine washed and dried or dry-cleaned. Plush toys should be stored in plastic bags in a warm place for 2 weeks. Washing hair-grooming implements in hot, soapy water for 20 minutes is essential, and thorough vacuuming of floors and furniture is important to remove any shed hairs with viable eggs. Most practitioners recommend treating all family members with signs of active infection.

The increasing resistance to permethrin and pyrethrins with piperonyl butoxide has increased the need to use prescription products. Topical malathion applied overnight for 8 to 12 hours has not resulted in any reports of resistance in the United States. The use of topical lindane should be limited because of reports of central nervous system toxicity in patients who overused or misused the product. This drug is only recommended in patients who fail to respond to other approved lice therapies. One dose of oral ivermectin at 250 µg/kg with a repeat dose 7 to 10 days later has not been thoroughly studied in clinical trials, but appears very effective in resistant cases.

Treatment is successful when live lice can no longer be found within the scalp hair. Residual nits do not signify active infestation and should not be used to exclude a child from school.

Body Lice

Body lice are found where poor hygiene and crowded living conditions predominate. In the United States, body lice are usually seen in homeless people. The louse is spread through infested clothing and bedding.

Clinical Manifestations

The primary symptom is severe pruritus. These patients frequently have numerous linear excoriations over the trunk and neck due to intense scratching. Secondary bacterial superinfection is common. Close examination may reveal a few macules or papules at the sites where the louse has fed. Lice are rarely present on the patient, but both lice and nits are often found in the seams of clothing.

Diagnosis

The diagnosis should be suspected in indigent patients with severe pruritus and few primary skin lesions. Although the louse is rarely present on the infested individual, nits are present on the clothing, particularly the seams near the body folds. The identification of nits or live lice in clothing confirms the diagnosis.

Differential Diagnosis

Pediculosis corporis can easily be misdiagnosed as neurodermatitis unless the patient's clothing is examined.

Management and Therapy

The mainstay of therapy is deinfestation of clothing and bedding. The patient's clothing, towels, and bed linens should be laundered with hot, soapy water or dry-cleaned or boiled. One application of 5% permethrin cream is the usual therapy as described in the management of scabies.

Pubic (Crab) Lice

Pediculosis pubis is a sexually transmitted disease. Although it is found in all socioeconomic levels and ethnic groups, it is most common among homosexual men. The presence of pubic lice should elicit increased vigilance for other sexually transmitted diseases.

Clinical Manifestations

Pubic lice most commonly affect the pubis, but any hair, including the short hair in the inguinal area, perianal area, thighs, and trunk, may be affected. In children, the eyelashes and periphery of the scalp hair can be involved. Patients complain of pruritus in the affected area.

Patients most often present with pruritus of the pubic region. Close examination reveals lice and nits cemented to the pubic and perianal hair (see Fig 177-2). Excoriations, secondary bacterial infection, and lymphadenopathy may accompany the infestation.

Diagnosis

Diagnosis is confirmed by plucking an affected hair and examining it microscopically. The presence of nits suggests past or present infestation, whereas live lice confirm active infestation. It is important to examine all hair-bearing sites in infected patients because sites outside the pubic area are frequently involved.

Management and Therapy

Treatment consists of topical application of various preparations. The entire pubic area should be treated as well as the thighs, trunk, and axillary regions. The simultaneous treatment of sexual partners is essential. Unaffected household members do not require therapy. Following therapy, all underwear, clothing, linens, and towels that came into contact with the infested person should be washed in hot, soapy water.

As with head lice, therapy with all topical insecticides requires two applications, 1 week apart. The most commonly used agents are topical 1% permethrin, synergized pyrethrin shampoos, 5% permethrin cream, and 1% lindane shampoo. A fine-toothed comb may be used to remove residual nits and lice. When topical therapy is unsuccessful or undesirable, oral ivermectin is indicated at a dose of 250 µg/kg repeated in 7 days. Involvement of the eyelashes should be treated by oral ivermectin or by petrolatum applied twice daily for a week followed by removal of any remaining nits.

Avoiding Treatment Errors

Resistant cases of lice are most often due to improper application of pediculicides, reinfestation, or misdiagnosis. Pediculicides should be applied to dry hair or body surfaces and always reapplied after 7 to 10 days. Prevent reinfestation by treating all family members at the same time, washing bed sheets and clothing in hot water, and washing hair-grooming supplies in hot, soapy water for 20 minutes or storing them in plastic bags for 1 week. The presence of nits alone does not confirm active infestation, and one should search for live lice before diagnosing resistant lice.

Future Directions

Future management of pediculosis and scabies will likely involve changes in the diagnosis and management of these infestations. The detection of serum antibodies to scabies by enzyme-linked immunosorbent assay is available for domestic animals and will likely become commercially available to improve the detection of scabies infestation in humans. Treatment of pediculosis will continue to evolve to a more physician-managed disease as increasing resistance to over-the-counter medications leads more and more patients to seek prescription therapy.

Additional Resources

Meinking TL, Burkhart CN, Burkhart CG: Infestations. In Bolognia JL, Jorizzo JL, Rapini RP (eds): Dermatology. New York, Mosby, 2003.
   This text chapter provides a thorough review of common skin infestations.

EVIDENCE

1. Chosidow O: Clinical practices. Scabies. N Engl J Med 354(16):1718-1727, 2006.
   The author provides an extensive clinical review of the diagnosis and treatment of scabies.
2. Frankowski BL, Weiner LB; Committee on School Health, the Committee on Infectious Diseases, American Academy of Pediatrics: Head lice. Pediatrics 110(3):638-643, 2002.
   This is the consensus report of the American Academy of Pediatrics on diagnosis and management of lice infestations.
3. Heukelbach J, Feldmeier H: Scabies. Lancet 367(9525):1767-1774, 2006.
   The authors provide an excellent review of the etiology, pathology, and management of scabies.
4. Schachner LA: Treatment resistant head lice: alternative therapeutic approaches. Pediatr Dermatol 14(5):409-410, 1997.
   The author provides a review of the growing problem of resistant head lice.

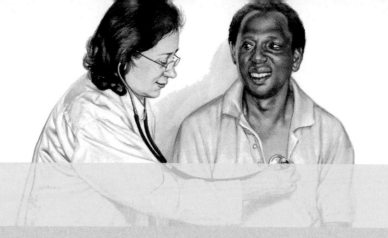
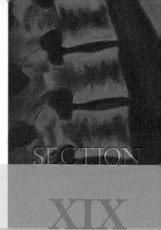

Geriatric Medicine

Drug Therapy in the Elderly: Appropriate Prescribing for the Older Patient

Introduction

With an increased concern for patient safety and error reduction has come the recognition that older patients are especially vulnerable to complications related to what is often inappropriate medication use. Surveys demonstrate that older patients use the most prescription medications; the older the person, the higher the number of medications. More than 90% of community-dwelling women take at least one medication, and more than 10% take more than 10 medications. Those who live in assisted living or skilled nursing facilities are more likely to take even more medications. As the population ages, this problem will become an even more significant public health issue. The challenge for the physician is to balance the need to treat elderly patients who may benefit from evidence-based drug regimens with the risks. Nearly one third of all elders have an adverse drug event necessitating medical intervention yearly—a risk directly related to the number of medications being taken.

Etiology and Pathogenesis

The etiology of polypharmacy and adverse drug events is complex. Even the definition is not clear—what entails *polypharmacy?* Is it simply the number of medications a patient is taking? How many is too many? With an aging society, chronic diseases such as diabetes, heart failure, and hypertension are increasingly common. There are evidence-based standards of care for each problem that often support the use of multiple medications. We now recognize that older patients who have a very high risk for a bad outcome with a certain diagnosis may actually gain the most from treatment. Moreover, we are less commonly using age alone as a reason not to treat a given condition. To complicate matters, patients today are more likely to receive their medications from multiple prescribers, multiple settings, and multiple pharmacies. Pharmaceutical companies now directly market to patients, including older

adults, as consumers. The use of herbal agents and over-the-counter medications has increased in elderly people. Nearly 25% of older patients in some surveys use an herbal medication, and more than half of those never report it to their primary physician.

The pathogenesis of adverse drug events in older patients is just as complex. Several major factors make older patients more susceptible to bad outcomes:

1. The pharmacokinetic changes of aging include the altered distribution, metabolism, and excretion of drugs. The volume of drug distribution in elderly people is altered by a decrease in lean body mass and an increase in body fat. Hepatic clearance is often decreased, and there is a well-documented decline in renal blood flow and glomerular filtration rate, increasing the half-life and decreasing the excretion of many drugs. Because of the decreased production of creatinine associated with

a decreased lean body mass in many older adults, a normal creatinine may actually represent a significant impairment in renal function.

2. Pharmacodynamic changes produce variances in the effect a given drug has on an individual. The fact that a therapeutic level of a certain drug may still have adverse effects mandates lower initial doses and careful titration of most drugs.

3. Drug-drug interactions are more common in older patients who take more medications.

4. Drug-disease interactions are also more common in older patients because of an increased prevalence of comorbidities. An older person with underlying cognitive impairment may become completely delirious after receiving a small dose of diphenhydramine, in contrast to a younger patient who merely becomes sedated for the night. A younger patient may become slightly hypotensive and lightheaded after receiving a tricyclic antidepressant, whereas an older person may have a syncopal episode and, because of underlying osteoporosis, sustain a hip fracture.

5. The use of multiple prescription drugs, polypharmacy, is more likely in older patients because of an increased prevalence of significant chronic diseases. The absolute risk for an adverse drug event is directly related to the number of drugs one takes—the higher the number of medications, the higher the risk. This is the major risk factor for having an adverse medication effect, even when controlling for other comorbidities and confounders.

6. Failure to recognize an adverse drug event is common in older patients. Side effects such as dizziness, confusion, and constipation are often attributed to other disease processes. When a symptom is not recognized as a side effect and then treated with an additional pharmacologic agent, the "prescribing cascade" may begin. There are many examples of the prescribing cascade—consider the older woman who is taking over-the-counter naproxen and has an elevation in her blood pressure for which she is prescribed hydrochlorothiazide. She perceives an increase in her urinary incontinence, sees her physician, and is then prescribed an agent such as oxybutynin. She later presents with constipation and is given polyethylene glycol. The story, of course, could continue.

Clinical Presentation

Unfortunately, the clinical presentation for inappropriate prescribing in the older adult is too often a significant adverse drug event that results in significant morbidity and mortality. Common adverse events include delirium, falls, fractures, orthostasis, constipation, and urinary retention. Care must be taken to identify such outcomes as possible adverse drug events and to target the underlying cause for

the problem in order to avoid falling into the prescribing cascade. Simply stated, it is always important to "first think drugs" in the case of elderly patients who present with new symptoms.

Management

Optimum Treatment

Optimum appropriate prescribing in older adults primarily requires awareness and vigilance in balancing adequate treatment and the potential for harm from the side effects of treatment. There are some basic strategies that are helpful:

1. Recognize and avoid potentially inappropriate medications (PIMs). A complete list of high-risk medications is included in the updated Beers criteria, a well-known document that addresses the issue of inappropriate medications in older patients. The Beers group reviewed medications that generally should be avoided or that should be avoided in certain medical conditions based on their level of risk for adverse outcomes, their lack of established effectiveness, and whether safer alternatives exist. Major offenders on the list include many muscle relaxants, tricyclic antidepressants, long-acting benzodiazepines, antispasmodic drugs such as dicyclomine and belladonna, anticholinergic agents such as diphenhydramine, narcotics such as meperidine and propoxyphene/acetaminophen, and many of the nonsteroidal anti-inflammatory agents.

   It is important to recognize that the PIM is not an absolute—there are often exceptions that need to be considered. For example, a severely anxious patient who is actively dying and requesting an anxiolytic may benefit from a low dose of a short-acting benzodiazepine. Making treatment plans based on the individual and recognizing the potential negative outcomes are the most important issues.

2. Recognize negative outcomes as possible adverse drug events and discontinue the drug instead of falling into the prescribing cascade.

3. Routinely ask about the use of over-the-counter medications, herbal agents, and vitamins and other supplements, and document their use.

4. Consider the use of databases that identify common drug-drug interactions.

5. Establish quality improvement–based protocols for monitoring levels, hepatic and renal function, anticoagulation effect, and so forth.

6. Record and report suspected adverse drug events.

7. Use generic drug names whenever possible. The use of both generic and trade names may result in confusion, even leading to patients' taking multiple agents that are similar or identical.

8. Educate patients regarding their medications, including the indications for each agent.

9. Have patients carry an updated medication list with them at all times. This is particularly helpful when patients are admitted and for medication "reconciliation" at the time of discharge.

10. Consider medication weaning as part of routine diagnostic decision making. This is especially important if goals of care have shifted to a more comfort-based approach or other changes have occurred such as weight loss, development of dementia, or a return from an admission to the hospital. Agents such as proton pump inhibitors may have been started in the hospital, and the patient may have no indication for their continued use. Steroids may be started for an acute problem and never weaned. Psychotropic medications may have unclear goals and effectiveness. The basic point: if an agent has not provided any significant benefit, consider discontinuation.

11. Have patients bring in pill bottles, not just a list, to the clinic for review. Errors can include pharmacy errors, patient-related errors, or prescribing errors that will otherwise not be identified.

12. Identify individual patient factors that may increase the risk for a negative outcome with prescription medications. These include literacy, visual loss, arthritis, and cognitive decline.

Avoiding Treatment Errors

The goal is to achieve an optimal balance between the indications for therapy and the potential negative side effects that come with the use of any medication. Older patients may have significant benefit from treatment of chronic disease states. It is especially important to avoid undertreatment based on age alone.

Future Directions

Prescribing medications for elderly patients is challenging and will become a problem faced by physicians in nearly every field as this segment of the population continues to grow. Clinical trials, which have traditionally excluded elderly people, need to continue to expand eligibility requirements and even specifically focus on this population. The balance between too much and too little in the older patient is something that will become increasingly challenging as the numbers of our elders, as well as our therapeutic options, continue to expand.

Additional Resource

Institute of Medicine. Available at: http://www.iom.edu.
   This is the home page for the Institute of Medicine, with links to programs aimed at reduction of medication errors and other quality improvement initiatives.

EVIDENCE

1. Fick DM, Cooper JW, Wade WE, et al: Updating the Beers criteria for potentially inappropriate medication use in older adults: Results of a U.S. consensus panel of experts. Arch Intern Med 163:2716-2724, 2003.
   This article expands on the work done in the original Beers review of inappropriate medications in older patients. The review looks at medications that should be limited or never used based on high rates of side effects, lack of utility, or better alternative medications.
2. Petrone K, Katz P: Approaches to appropriate drug prescribing for the older adult. Prim Care 32:755-775, 2005.
   This article provides a review for rational drug prescribing for older patients.

Nurum F. Erdem

Falls

Introduction

Falling is a common and serious problem in older people. A fall occurs when a person comes to rest inadvertently on the ground or a lower level. About 35% to 40% of community-dwelling adults older than 65 years and more than 50% of those in nursing homes and hospitals will fall each year. Falls are associated with considerable mortality, morbidity, and premature nursing home admission. Twenty-five percent of those who fall will die within 6 months, 60% have restricted mobility, and 25% remain functionally more dependent. Additionally, the fear of falling can result in decreased activity, isolation, and further decline. Medical costs of falling exceed $2 billion annually and account for 6% of all medical expenditures for persons age 65 years and older in the United States.

Etiology and Pathogenesis

The cause of falling is multifactorial and frequently preventable. There are intrinsic factors, such as medical conditions and normal age-related changes, and extrinsic factors, such as medications or environment. These factors may either predispose or precipitate a fall. Conditions such as arthritis; depressive symptoms; orthostasis; impaired cognition, vision, balance, gait, or muscle strength; and the use of four or more prescription medications have been shown to increase the risk for falling in two or more observational studies.

Several studies document strong correlations between exercise, strength and balance retraining, and decreased incidence of falls in the elderly. More specifically, hip abductor strength has been studied as a strong indicator of fall risk in the elderly population. Decreased hip abductor strength impairs protective extension and postural correction response time, which can increase fall risk.

Polypharmacy alone (taking four or more prescription medications) can predispose to falling. Medications commonly associated with falling in the elderly include sedative-hypnotics, especially long-acting benzodiazepines, and neuroleptic agents. Serotonin reuptake inhibitors and tricyclic antidepressants are also associated with an increase in falls. Cardiac medications such as digoxin, diuretics, and type 1A antiarrhythmics are weakly associated with falls.

Several studies suggest that the risk for falling increases dramatically as the number of risk factors increases. One study reported the percentage of community-dwelling older adults falling increased from 27% for those with no or one risk factor to 78% for those with four or more risk factors.

It is the combination of high degree of susceptibility to falls, because of multiple risk factors, and propensity to fall-related injury, caused by comorbidities such as osteoporosis and age-related changes, that makes falling a major problem in older adults.

Clinical Presentation

Falls in the community commonly present in association with accidents or environmental factors (37%). They can also result from weakness and balance or gait problems (12%). Drop attacks (11%), dizziness or vertigo (8%), and orthostatic hypotension (5%) also contribute to a significant proportion of falls. Eighteen percent of falls are caused by acute illness, confusion, drugs, or decreased vision, and many people fall for unknown reasons (8%).

In long-term care, the most common causes of falls are generalized weakness (31%) and environmental hazards (27%). Orthostatic hypotension causes about 16% of falls. Acute illness (5%), gait or balance disorders (4%), and drugs (5%) contribute to falls as well. In about 10%, the reason for falling in the nursing home is unknown.

Most falls result in some type of injury, usually soft tissue injury such as bruises or skin tears. About 10% to 15% result in fracture or other serious injury.

Figure 179-1 Clinical Approach to the Prevention of Falls.
From Tinetti M: Clinical Practice. Preventing falls in elderly persons. N Engl J Med 348(1):42-49, 2003.

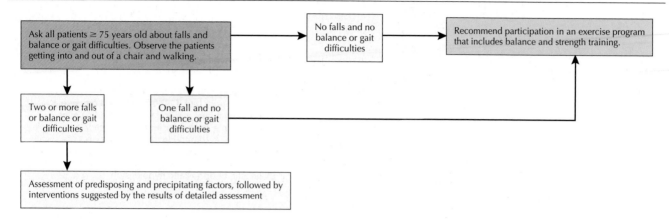

Of those who fall, only half are able to get up without help, thus experiencing the *found-down syndrome*, which is associated with decline in functional status and can complicate fall-related injuries.

Differential Diagnosis

Although falling is considered a common geriatric syndrome by itself, falls can also occur in association with other clinical diagnoses. Falls associated with loss of consciousness should lead to a workup for syncope (see Chapter 38). Falls can also occur in the setting of acute illness such as urinary tract infection or pneumonia. A diagnosis of Parkinson's disease can sometimes be made on the initial presentation to a physician after a fall. It is important to have a high index of clinical suspicion for these problems as well as other factors contributing to falls and fall risk.

Diagnostic Approach

The clinical approach to the prevention of falls is presented in Figure 179-1.

History

Although some patients present with fall as the chief complaint, many older adults may not give a history of falls unless inquiry is made. Therefore, eliciting a history of falls and balance or gait difficulties is an important component of the review of systems and should be performed at least once per year in all patients 75 years or older.

The previous history of falling should include the location and circumstances (including a witness account), associated symptoms, history of previous falls, risk factors for falls such as medications (prescription and over-the-counter), functional status, and injury (if presenting after fall).

The medication list should be reviewed for total number of drugs and specific high-risk medications. For those who are taking four or more medications, reduction of the total number should be strongly considered. The balance of risk and benefit for medications such as benzodiazepines, other sleep agents, neuroleptics, antidepressants, anticonvulsants, or class 1A antiarrhythmics should be considered, and appropriate tapering should be attempted.

Physical Examination

Especially in those patients who present with presyncope symptoms or syncope associated with fall, orthostatic blood pressure (Fig. 179-2) should be assessed along with targeted cardiovascular and neurologic examination. In addition to heart rate and rhythm, the cardiovascular exam should include carotid sinus massage with assessment of pulse. Many unexplained nonaccidental falls can be explained by carotid sinus hypersensitivity and potentially treated with pacemaker placement. The examiner should only perform carotid sinus massage in a controlled environment with access to cardiac monitoring and resuscitation equipment.

The ability for patients to maintain their center of mass within their base of support is crucial to preventing a fall. The three major receptive senses involved in balance are the visual, proprioceptive, and vestibular systems. The neurologic exam should focus on testing for impaired vision, sensation, vestibular dysfunction, and cognition. Visual acuity can be tested with a Snellen eye chart or grossly by asking the patient to read any available print in the examination room. In the older population, vibration sense is a more sensitive marker of neuropathy than impaired proprioception. Vibration can be tested using a low-pitched tuning fork of 128 Hz or 256 Hz and asking patients when they feel the vibration stop. Vestibular function can be evaluated by performing the Dix-Hallpike maneuver and assessing extraocular movements for

Figure 179-2 Orthostatic Hypotension.

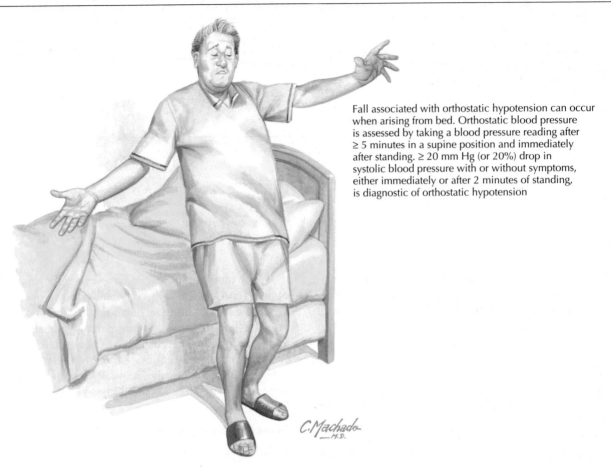

Fall associated with orthostatic hypotension can occur when arising from bed. Orthostatic blood pressure is assessed by taking a blood pressure reading after ≥ 5 minutes in a supine position and immediately after standing. ≥ 20 mm Hg (or 20%) drop in systolic blood pressure with or without symptoms, either immediately or after 2 minutes of standing, is diagnostic of orthostatic hypotension

nystagmus. The neurologic exam should also test cognition and look for changes associated with Parkinson's disease. Assessment for Parkinson's disease can be made by observing for festinating gait, tremor, muscle rigidity or cogwheeling, and bradykinesia (Fig. 179-3).

Musculoskeletal examination should focus on lower extremity joint abnormalities and dysfunction, such as limitation in range of motion as a result of arthritic change, and strength. With aging, skeletal muscles decrease in bulk, as evidenced by atrophy; however, muscle strength can be relatively well maintained.

If a fall is reported, further assessment of gait and balance should be performed. This can easily be done in the clinic by performing a "get up and go test." Patients are observed standing up from a chair without using their arms, walking 10 feet, turning, then walking back and sitting down in the chair. This should be accomplished in 10 to 20 seconds. Those patients who take longer than 20 seconds are at high risk for falling. The get up and go test can easily be used to screen for gait and balance problems even in the setting of a busy outpatient practice.

Balance can be assessed by having the patient hold a prolonged side-by-side stance, semi-tandem stance, and full tandem stance. The patient should be able to stand in all three positions for 10 seconds. The ability to withstand a nudge on the sternum without falling backward can also be used to assess balance. Because many people fall while reaching for objects on the floor, another clinical test of balance is observation as a patient tries to pick up an object from the floor such as a set of keys.

Laboratory Testing and Imaging

Although there is no standard laboratory testing for falls, complete blood count and basic chemistry can be helpful to rule out anemia, dehydration, and hyperglycemia as etiologies of falling. As well, vitamin B_{12} and thyroid function tests can be useful in ruling out reversible problems with gait and balance. More costly tests such as magnetic resonance imaging of the head, echocardiogram, or Holter monitoring should be reserved for patients in whom an abnormality is suggested based on findings obtained during the history or physical exam.

Home Hazard Assessment

Because environment is frequently a factor in falls that occur in the home, a home safety evaluation by a nurse,

Figure 179-3 Changes in Gait with Progression of Parkinson's Disease.

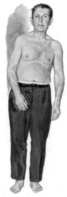
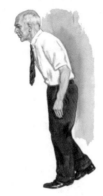
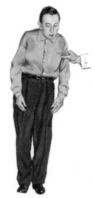

Stage 1: unilateral involvement; blank facies; affected arm in semiflexed position with tremor; patient leans to unaffected side

Stage 2: bilateral involvement with early postural changes; slow, shuffling gait with decreased excursion of legs

Stage 3: pronounced gait disturbances and moderate generalized disability; postural instability with tendency to fall

occupational therapist, or physical therapist is essential. Specifically assessing the environment for clutter, lighting, stairs, cords, or throw rugs is important. Other considerations include the placement of grab bars in the bathroom and shower. Shoes should be evaluated for appropriateness in the home and outside. Flat hard-sole shoes are considered the safest footwear. Footwear should also be evaluated for proper fit because poorly sized shoes may increase fall risk by providing poor support and increased risk for tripping.

Risk Factors for Injury

Assessment for risk factors for injury should include a bone density scan and considerations for anticoagulation.

Management and Therapy

Management is important not just for those who have recently fallen but also for those at high risk for falling because of the presence of a known risk factor for falling or a history of falls. Both single- and multifactorial-intervention strategies have been studied for the management of falls.

A systematic review of randomized trials of interventions designed to minimize the effect of, or exposure to, risk factors for falling in elderly people was conducted in association with the Cochrane Collaboration of systematic reviews. Main outcomes of interest were the number of fallers, or falls. Trials reporting only intermediate outcomes were excluded. Sixty-two trials involving 21,668 people were included. Single-intervention strategies that have been shown to be effective include a professionally supervised program of balance and gait training and muscle-strengthening; withdrawal of psychotropic medications (benzodiazepines, other sleep agents, neuroleptic agents, and antidepressants); Tai Chi group exercise intervention; home hazard assessment and modification that is professionally prescribed for older people with a history of falling; and cardiac pacing for fallers with cardioinhibitory carotid sinus hypersensitivity.

Multidisciplinary, multifactorial risk factor screening and intervention programs in the community for older people with and without a history of falling, or risk factors for falling, were shown to be beneficial. This was also true for those patients in residential care facilities. This finding was supported by another study performed with the Cochrane Collaboration of systematic reviews, which showed that the rate of injuries caused by falls decreased after population-based programs were introduced. This conclusion was qualified by the reviewers by stating that more studies of better quality are still needed to back up this conclusion.

Assistive devices such as canes and walkers seen in Figure 179-4 can help support weight and provide greater balance by increasing the patient's base of support. They must be prescribed and used correctly to achieve maximum safety. Physical therapists are helpful in instructing patients in the appropriate and safe use of such devices. Patients may benefit from learning about various types of assistive devices, such as three- and four-wheeled walkers, that can improve mobility safety without significantly limiting ambulation speed or outdoor mobility over varied terrain.

Fall management relies heavily on prevention of falls and the complications of falls. Evaluation and treatment of osteoporosis to prevent fracture in case of fall is an important consideration. Hip protectors are padded undergarments used to prevent hip fractures associated with fall. Although the data are controversial, earlier studies of hip protectors showed benefit in preventing hip fractures in

Figure 179-4 Canes, Crutches, and Walkers.

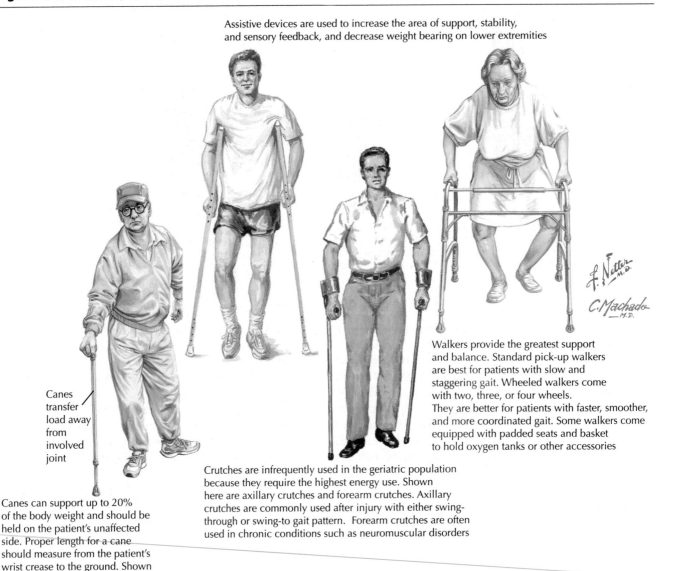

Assistive devices are used to increase the area of support, stability, and sensory feedback, and decrease weight bearing on lower extremities

Canes transfer load away from involved joint

Canes can support up to 20% of the body weight and should be held on the patient's unaffected side. Proper length for a cane should measure from the patient's wrist crease to the ground. Shown here is a standard cane. Canes come in a variety of handles and up to four tips (quad cane)

Crutches are infrequently used in the geriatric population because they require the highest energy use. Shown here are axillary crutches and forearm crutches. Axillary crutches are commonly used after injury with either swing-through or swing-to gait pattern. Forearm crutches are often used in chronic conditions such as neuromuscular disorders

Walkers provide the greatest support and balance. Standard pick-up walkers are best for patients with slow and staggering gait. Wheeled walkers come with two, three, or four wheels. They are better for patients with faster, smoother, and more coordinated gait. Some walkers come equipped with padded seats and basket to hold oxygen tanks or other accessories

those patients who wear them. This was not substantiated in later meta-analyses of randomized trials. Further, the lack of efficacy of hip protectors may be caused by low compliance and poor patient acceptance.

Anticoagulation in patients with atrial fibrillation is another important consideration in those patients who have a history of fall or are at high risk for falling. Although potential head trauma and subsequent subdural hematoma is an important complication of anticoagulation, recent studies have shown that the benefits of anticoagulation warrant the risks. Specifically, persons with an average risk for stroke from atrial fibrillation must fall about 300 times in 1 year for the risks of anticoagulation to outweigh its benefits.

Found-down syndrome can complicate injuries resulting from falls. Prevention of this includes placement of lifeline or accessible telephones in the home. Isolated elderly persons can benefit from friendly phone calls or visitors on a daily basis. In addition, teaching patients how to properly rise from the floor after a fall can be helpful in preventing found-down syndrome.

Optimum Treatment

Given that the etiology of falls is multifactorial and multifaceted, optimum treatment must be tailored to each individual. Even if a practitioner has experience in evaluating and treating falls, frequently referral to specialty services is necessary to optimize management. A geriatric medicine specialist may be necessary to assist with assessment of patients who have fallen or are at high risk for falls. Similarly, referral to physical therapy and occupational therapy is very important not only for assessment of the patient and home, but also in directing and implementing a treatment plan. These initial referrals are usually covered by Medicare; however, documentation of progress is necessary for ongoing coverage of therapy services.

Avoiding Treatment Errors

In managing a problem in which prevention and treatment are enmeshed, the key to avoiding treatment errors is in the clinical interview. Unless a patient presents with an injury related to a fall, many falls do not come to clinical attention because either the health care provider may not inquire or the patients do not report a fall. Patients may be reluctant to discuss a recent fall because of embarrassment, or the invalid assumption that falls are an inevitable part of aging. The American Geriatrics Society, the British Geriatrics Society, and the American Academy of Orthopaedic Surgeons, in a joint evidence-based guideline for prevention of falls, recommend that all elderly patients be asked about any falls that have occurred during the previous year and that they undergo a quick test of gait and balance. Additionally, the U.S. Preventive Services Task Force recommends that all persons 75 years or older, as well as those 70 to 74 years of age who have a known risk factor, be counseled about specific measures to prevent falls. It also recommends individualized multifactorial interventions for elderly persons at high risk for falling.

By identifying those patients at high risk and intervening appropriately, we can decrease the morbidity and mortality caused by falls, and subsequent complications.

Future Directions

There are several high priority issues identified for future research and analysis by the American Geriatrics Society Panel on Falls Prevention. Cost-effectiveness of recommended strategies and specific elements of successful strategies need to be evaluated to streamline management. For example, what are the effective elements of exercise programs (type, duration, intensity, and frequency), or can fall-prone individuals be risk-stratified in terms of who will benefit most from assessment and interventions? Because the etiology of falls is multifactorial and the elderly population is heterogeneous, these questions will prove challenging to answer.

Acknowledgment

Thank you to Jan Busby-Whitehead, MD, Anthony Caprio, MD, and Joshua Cohen, PT, MS for their assistance in reviewing this chapter.

Additional Resources

Leipzig RM, Cumming RG, Tinetti MD: Drugs and falls in older people: A systematic review and meta-analysis. II. Cardiac and analgesic drugs. J Am Geriatr Soc 47:40-50, 1999.

This meta-analysis critically evaluates the evidence regarding cardiac and analgesic drugs and the risk for falls in older people. Although the evidence to date is based solely on observational data, there is a weak association between the use of digoxin, type IA antiarrhythmic, and diuretic and falls in older adults. Also noted is that older adults taking more than three or four medications were at increased risk for recurrent falls.

Leipzig RM, Cumming RG, Tinetti ME: Drugs and falls in older people: A systematic review and meta-analysis. I. Psychotropic drugs. J Am Geriatr Soc 47:30-39, 1999.

This meta-analysis critically evaluated the evidence regarding psychotropic drugs and the risk for falls in older people. Although the evidence to date is based solely on observational data, there is a consistent association between the use of most classes of psychotropic drugs and falls.

Thapa PB, Gideon P, Cost TW, et al: Antidepressants and the risk of falls among nursing home residents. N Engl J Med 339:875-872, 1998.

This article reviews the risk for falls associated with selective serotonin reuptake inhibitor antidepressants versus tricyclic and other heterocyclic antidepressants. The authors find little difference in rates of falls between those treated with tricyclic antidepressants and those treated with selective serotonin reuptake inhibitors.

Tinetti ME, Speechley M, Ginter SF: Risk factors for falls among elderly persons living in the community. N Engl J Med 319:1701, 1988.

A one-year prospective investigation to study risk factors for falling in community dwelling persons 75 years of age or older noted that the risk for falling increased linearly with the number of risk factors. Falls among older persons in the community are common, and clinical assessment can identify the elderly persons at greatest risk.

Rubenstein LZ, Robbins AS, Josephson KR, et al: The value of assessing falls in an elderly population. Ann Intern Med 113(4):308-316, 1990.

A randomized controlled trial of elderly persons in long-term care assigned to either comprehensive postfall assessment or usual care found that through assessment, many remediable problems were detected that led to a statistically significant decrease in hospitalizations and reduction in hospital days.

EVIDENCE

1. Assessing Care of Vulnerable Elders (ACOVE) Physician Education Program for Falls and Mobility Disorders. Santa Monica, CA, RAND Corporation, 2004.

   This is a CD-ROM physician education program produced by Pfizer, the RAND Corporation, and the American Geriatrics Society to improve the quality care for older adults. It is an interactive program with printable forms and educational materials for the physician and patient.

2. Center for Disease Control and Prevention National Center for Injury Prevention and Control Web Site. Available at: http://www.cdc.gov/ncipc/pub-res/toolkit/toolkit.htm. Accessed October 14, 2006.

   This is a website from the Centers for Disease Control and Prevention and National Center for Injury Prevention and Control. The site has fact sheets for physicians as well as patient education materials. There are links to other fall-related websites.

3. Cummings RG, Thomas M, Szony G, et al: Home visits by an occupational therapist for assessment and modification of environmental hazards: A randomized trial of falls prevention. J Am Geriatr Soc 47(12):1397-1402, 1999.

   This randomized controlled trial was the first to show the effectiveness of a trained occupational therapist home visit to assess and modify the environment. There were limitations of this study because of potential confounding factors. The fact that falls away from home were also reduced in the treatment group suggested that the intervention influenced not only the environment but also the individual.

4. Gillespie LD, Gillespie WJ, Robertson MC, et al: Interventions for preventing falls in elderly people. Cochrane Database Syst Rev (4):CD000340, 2003.

   This is a comprehensive systematic review of randomized trials to assess the effects of interventions designed to minimize the effect of, or exposure to, risk factors for falling in elderly people. The review is extensive and serves as a good reference.

5. Guideline for the prevention of falls in older persons. American Geriatrics Society, British Geriatrics Society, and American Academy of Orthopaedic Surgeons Panel on Falls Prevention. J Am Geriatr Soc 49(5):664-672, 2001.

   The webpage from the American Geriatrics Society (http://www. americangeriatrics.org/news/media_adv_5.shtml.) also contains a link to the Falls Intervention Evidence Tables (PDF). The evidence tables are a comprehensive list of studies leading up to the 2001 meeting and commentary regarding the strength of the evidence. There is also a Consumer Pamphlet (PDF) for patients to review and list all of their medications to discuss with the physician at their next visit.

6. Man-Son-Hing M, Laupacis A: Anticoagulant-related bleeding in older persons with atrial fibrillation: Physicians' fears often unfounded. Arch Intern Med 14;163(13):1580-1586, 2003.

   This systematic review of the literature critically appraised whether the presence of clinical factors that increase the risk for bleeding affect the chance of anticoagulant-related hemorrhage. They found that many factors that are purported to be barriers in older patients, such as predisposition to falls and old age itself, should not influence the choice of stroke prophylaxis.

7. McClure R, Turner C, Peel N, et al: Population-based interventions for the prevention of fall-related injuries in older people. Cochrane Database Syst Rev (1):CD004441, 2005.

   This systematic review assesses the effectiveness of population-based interventions for reducing fall-related injuries among older people. The authors include studies that report changes in medically treated fall-related injuries among older people following the implementation of a controlled population-based intervention. In all of the five studies that met inclusion criteria, none of which were randomized controlled trials, they find significant decreases or downward trends in fall-related injuries with relative reduction of 6% to 33%. The conclusions are limited because of the quality of the studies reviewed.

8. Parker MJ, Gillespie WJ, Gillespie LD: Hip protectors for preventing hip fractures in the elderly. Cochrane Database Syst Rev (3):CD001266, 2005.

   This comprehensive systematic review of all randomized or quasi-randomized controlled trials compare the use of hip protectors with a control group to determine whether external hip protectors reduce the incidence of hip fractures in older people following a fall. The 15 trials include data from nursing homes and community-dwelling participants. Although earlier evidence shows that in institutions with high rates of hip fracture, the use of hip protectors may reduce the risk for a hip fracture, new evidence shows the effect may be less certain. There is no evidence of any benefit for older people living in the community. Long-term compliance overall is poor because of discomfort and practicality.

9. Tinetti M: Clinical practice: Preventing falls in elderly persons. N Engl J Med 2;348(1):42-49, 2003.

   This Clinical Practice review begins with a case vignette followed by evidence supporting various strategies for evaluation and management of falls in elderly persons. It is concise and well written, with an extensive list of references.

Hypertension in the Elderly

Introduction

As more of us are getting older and older, we are facing the risks associated with hypertension. By 2025, it is estimated that 20% of the U.S. population will be older than 65 years. The subgroup of people older than 80 years is one of the fastest growing segments of the population. It is now recognized that hypertension, especially isolated systolic hypertension, is indeed connected to age. Up to 50% of people ages 60 to 69 years have hypertension, but nearly 75% of those older than 70 years have some degree of hypertension. More startling is the finding that the risk for developing hypertension if one lives to the age of 85 years is 80% to 90%. In older patients, it is clear that the systolic blood pressure is a more important predictor of future cardiovascular events than the diastolic blood pressure. And the risk for developing hypertension and future cardiovascular disease is also increased in those with blood pressures in the range of 120 to 139 mm Hg, levels previously considered normal. Multiple trials have demonstrated a reduction in mortality, cardiovascular mortality, stroke, and congestive heart failure with treatment. Despite this, systolic hypertension in elderly people is often inadequately treated. There are multiple reasons for this: reaching goal blood pressure usually requires multiple medications; patients and physicians may have negative attitudes regarding treatment in this age group; and older patients may have more complications with orthostasis and other side effects.

Etiology and Pathogenesis

Most cases of combined systolic and diastolic hypertension occur by the age of 55 years. Systolic hypertension, defined as a systolic blood pressure of more than 140 mm Hg with a diastolic blood pressure of less than 90 mm Hg, is principally associated with aging. Other differences seen in elderly people include lower renin levels, higher sensitivity to sodium loads, and increased peripheral vascular resistance.

Clinical Presentation

Most patients do not have symptoms, which contributes to the lack of recognition of this problem and the associated public health epidemic. Patients may present with symptoms of cardiovascular disease, heart failure, stroke, or renal failure. The physical exam may reveal evidence of left ventricular hypertrophy, indicating an increased risk for cardiovascular disease (Fig. 180-1).

Differential Diagnosis

Pseudohypertension, falsely high sphygmomanometer readings secondary to decreased arterial wall compliance and increased vascular stiffness, should be considered in older persons with persistently elevated blood pressure measurements, no evidence of end-organ damage, near-syncopal symptoms with therapy, or a discrepancy in blood pressure readings between arms.

White-coat hypertension, with blood pressure readings taken during clinic visits that greatly exceed those taken at home or after the patient has had time to relax, is more commonly seen in older patients. The noncompliant vascular tree probably makes elders more susceptible to labile blood pressure swings. Ambulatory blood pressure monitoring can be helpful to identify this and is reimbursed by Medicare. In addition to identifying lower blood pressures that may correlate better with future cardiovascular events than clinic readings, the lack of a decrease in blood

Figure 180-1 Hypertension in the Elderly.

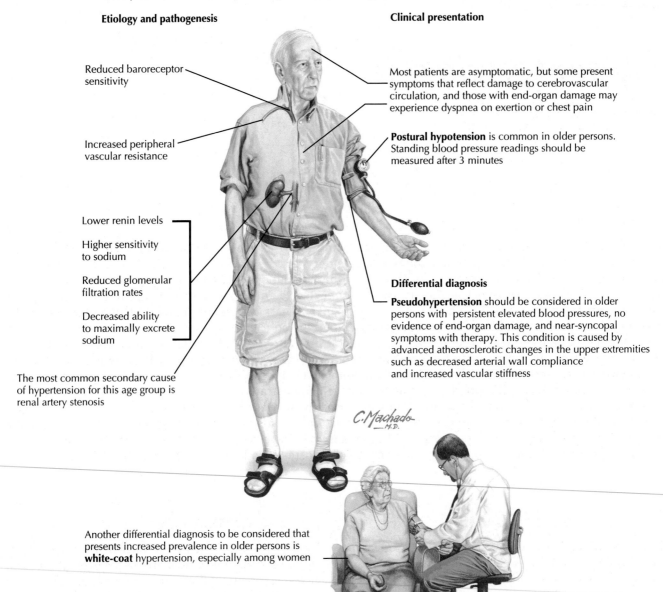

The diagnosis of hypertension for all adults is based on the finding of systolic blood pressure of more than 140 mm Hg with diastolic blood pressure of more than 90 mm Hg, after two or more readings. Each reading must be performed after the person has been sitting for 3 minutes. A single reading with systolic blood pressure of more than 210 mm Hg or diastolic blood pressure of more than 120 mm Hg is consistent with hypertension

Etiology and pathogenesis

Reduced baroreceptor sensitivity

Increased peripheral vascular resistance

Lower renin levels

Higher sensitivity to sodium

Reduced glomerular filtration rates

Decreased ability to maximally excrete sodium

The most common secondary cause of hypertension for this age group is renal artery stenosis

Clinical presentation

Most patients are asymptomatic, but some present symptoms that reflect damage to cerebrovascular circulation, and those with end-organ damage may experience dyspnea on exertion or chest pain

Postural hypotension is common in older persons. Standing blood pressure readings should be measured after 3 minutes

Differential diagnosis

Pseudohypertension should be considered in older persons with persistent elevated blood pressures, no evidence of end-organ damage, and near-syncopal symptoms with therapy. This condition is caused by advanced atherosclerotic changes in the upper extremities such as decreased arterial wall compliance and increased vascular stiffness

Another differential diagnosis to be considered that presents increased prevalence in older persons is **white-coat** hypertension, especially among women

C. Machado
—M.D.

pressure at night may identify patients who are particularly high risk for future cardiovascular events.

Secondary causes of hypertension are far less common in older patients, and further evaluation is indicated only with documented new onset and pronounced hypertension or new difficulty in controlling blood pressure. Renal artery stenosis is the most common secondary cause of elevated blood pressures in this age group (Fig. 180-2). The challenge is that many patients in this age group also have underlying diffuse small vessel disease because of atherosclerosis, and any correction of stenosis at the level

of the renal artery does not necessarily correct the underlying renovascular compromise.

Diagnostic Approach

The diagnosis of hypertension is based on the classification system used by the Joint National Committee on Prevention, Detection, Evaluation, and Treatment of High Blood Pressure for all adults (systolic blood pressure greater than 140 mm Hg or diastolic blood pressure greater than 90 mm Hg). Systolic hypertension, previously known as

Figure 180-2 Varieties of Renal Artery Disease that May Induce Hypertension.

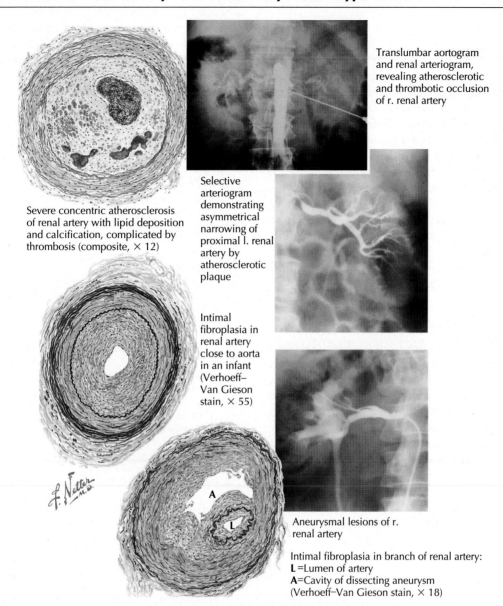

Severe concentric atherosclerosis of renal artery with lipid deposition and calcification, complicated by thrombosis (composite, × 12)

Translumbar aortogram and renal arteriogram, revealing atherosclerotic and thrombotic occlusion of r. renal artery

Selective arteriogram demonstrating asymmetrical narrowing of proximal l. renal artery by atherosclerotic plaque

Intimal fibroplasia in renal artery close to aorta in an infant (Verhoeff–Van Gieson stain, × 55)

Aneurysmal lesions of r. renal artery

Intimal fibroplasia in branch of renal artery:
L = Lumen of artery
A = Cavity of dissecting aneurysm
(Verhoeff–Van Gieson stain, × 18)

isolated systolic hypertension, is defined as a systolic blood pressure of more than 140 mm Hg with a diastolic blood pressure of less than 90 mm Hg. Hypertension is diagnosed based on two or more readings with an appropriately sized cuff, after the person has been sitting for 3 minutes. Because blood pressure variability is more common in elderly people, multiple readings are of great importance. Postural hypotension is common in elderly people; so, before initiating or altering treatment, blood pressure should be measured after the patient has been standing for 3 minutes.

Management and Therapy

Why Treat?

There is strong evidence that pharmacologic treatment of systolic hypertension in older patients reduces cardiovas-

cular events, including strokes and heart failure. Studies have consistently demonstrated a 35% reduction in stroke, 50% reduction in congestive heart failure, and 30% reduction in overall cardiovascular events in older patients who are treated. One meta-analysis examining the risks and benefits of treatment for isolated systolic hypertension in elderly people found that treatment decreased total mortality by 13%, cardiovascular mortality by 18%, all cardiovascular complications by 26%, and stroke by 30%. Greater benefits were seen in men, patients older than 70 years, and patients with prior cardiovascular complications. Notably, benefits are seen in the oldest patients, those older than 80 years, with 22% reductions in cardiovascular events and 39% reductions in heart failure. Whether treatment in very elderly patients improves mortality is less clear; however, there is significant benefit in improved quality of life and a reduction in stroke and heart failure in this age group.

Optimum Treatment

Treatment guidelines for older and younger patients are similar. Thiazide-type diuretics should be considered first line—these are the agents that were used in the major trials for the treatment of systolic hypertension in elderly patients. In addition, these agents are inexpensive, are usually well tolerated, and recently were demonstrated to be of equal or better effectiveness in reducing future cardiovascular events. Most older patients with systolic hypertension require more than one drug—many will need three medications to reach goal blood pressure. Other agents such as β-blockers, angiotensin-converting enzyme inhibitors, and calcium channel blockers are also effective and should be added depending on specific patient comorbidities like congestive heart failure.

Avoiding Treatment Errors

Older patients are much more likely to have orthostatic drops in blood pressure, labile blood pressures, and white-coat hypertension. Standing blood pressure readings should be checked in all older patients, and treatment should be based on these readings. Ambulatory blood pressure monitoring is often useful in patients who experience significant side effects and symptoms of orthostasis on therapy despite normal or even high blood pressure readings in clinic.

Age alone or fear of negative side effects should not lead to the avoidance of treatment. Good data document that older patients tolerate treatment with little or no impact on quality of life.

Future Directions

More focus is being directed toward decreasing the risk for dementia. Increasing evidence from multiple large trials of the treatment of systolic hypertension in elderly people documents the association of dementia with prior hypertension. The risk appears to include not only vascular dementia but also Alzheimer's-type dementia. Can we prevent or modify the development of dementia by more aggressively treating hypertension? Given the intricate ties among age, dementia, and hypertension, coupled with the aging of adults in the United States, this question is of great public health importance.

Knowledge about the treatment of hypertension in elderly people will grow as the prevalence of the disease within this age group is recognized and trials are designed specifically for these patients. In the past, there was a ten-

dency to undertreat older patients for fear of causing harm. Because older patients are at high risk for cardiovascular disease, any intervention that is of benefit actually stands to be of greater absolute benefit. Will we begin to recognize age as the new cardiovascular equivalent and aim to treat hypertension in older patients more aggressively?

Additional Resources

Seventh Report of the Joint National Committee on Prevention, Detection, Evaluation, and Treatment of High Blood Pressure (JNC 7). Available at: http://www.nhlbi.nih.gov/guidelines/hypertension/jnc7full.htm.

This report was sponsored by the National Heart, Lung, and Blood Institute and provides information for patients, public, and health professionals. A complete review of data and summary of recommendations are provided.

EVIDENCE

1. Forette F, Seux ML, Staessen JA, Thijs L: Prevention of dementia in randomized double-blind placebo-controlled Systolic in Europe (Syst-Eur) Trial. Lancet 352 1347-1351, 1998; and SHEP Cooperative Research Group: Prevention of stroke by antihypertensive drug treatment in older persons with isolated systolic hypertension. Final results of the Systolic Hypertension in the Elderly Program (SHEP). JAMA 265:3255-3264, 1991.

    The follow-up studies from the original work looking at treating systolic hypertension in the elderly demonstrates that older patients in the original treatment groups have a significant reduction in future risk for developing cognitive impairment when compared with those patients in the original placebo groups. One of the more interesting caveats to this is that all causes of dementia, vascular and Alzheimer's, were less in the original treatment groups.

2. Gueyffier F, Bulpitt C, Boissel JP, et al: Antihypertensive drugs in very old people: A subgroup meta-analysis of randomized controlled trials. INDANA Group. Lancet 353:793-796, 1999.

    This study addressed the issue of treating very elderly people, the fastest growing population in the United States, and found that even in this group, treatment of systolic hypertension appears to be of benefit in reducing heart failure and stroke. Although no clear mortality benefit is demonstrated, it is thought that the significant morbidity benefit of stroke reduction in very elderly people justifies therapy.

3. Hansson L, Lindholm LH, Ekbom T, et al: Randomised trial of old and new antihypertensive drugs in elderly patients: Cardiovascular mortality and morbidity. The Swedish Trial in Old Patients with Hypertension-2 Study. Lancet 354:1751-1756, 1999.

    This landmark study addresses the issue of which antihypertensive is best and found that the older agents such as thiazide diuretics are of equal, if not better, efficacy in preventing negative cardiovascular outcomes when compared with the newer agents often used and promoted today.

4. Straessen JA, Fagard R, Thijs L, et al: A randomised double-blind companison of placeso and active treatment for older patrents with isolated systolic hypetension. The Systolic Hypertension in Europe (Syst-Eur) Trial Investigators. Lancet 350:757-764, 1997.

    This and other large trials of this time period look at older patients with isolated systolic hypertension and clearly demonstrate that treatment of systolic hypertension leads to a decrease in cardiovascular events, strokes, and heart failure.

Delirium

Introduction

Delirium is a bilateral, physiologic disturbance of cortical function associated with disturbances of consciousness, attention, cognition, and perception that develops acutely or subacutely and characteristically fluctuates during the course of a day. Other terms for delirium include acute organic brain syndrome, metabolic or toxic encephalopathy, toxic brain syndrome, and acute confusional state. This potentially life-threatening condition often goes unrecognized or is misdiagnosed by health care professionals, making the recognition of the condition and the search for and mitigation of causative factors the central treatment goals.

Historically, a lack of clear criteria for defining delirium has confounded prevalence estimates, but it is a common condition, by any measure. Costs are estimated to be greater than $8 billion annually. Delirium is very common in hospitalized patients (10% to 30%), with the numbers being particularly notable in special populations, such as elderly patients (up to 50%), AIDS patients (30% to 40%), postsurgical patients (up to 50%), and burn unit patients. Prevalence rates in terminally ill patients can be as high as 80%. Additionally, 6% to 7% of nursing home patients, 5% to 10% of elderly emergency department admissions, and 1% to 2% of community populations suffer from delirium as well.

Risk factors include advanced age, cognitive impairment (especially dementia), preexisting brain injury, chronic medical illnesses, and drug intoxication. Dementia is a particularly important risk factor for delirium in hospitalized patients. Almost half of all dementia patients admitted to the hospital will have or will develop a delirium. Conversely, 25% to 80% of hospitalized patients with delirium will be found to have a preexisting dementia. Dementia is such a strong risk factor for delirium that all sudden mental status changes in a demented individual should be considered a delirium until proven otherwise. Other predictive risks for inpatients include use of physical restraints, malnutrition, more than three new medications, use of bladder catheter, hearing and vision impairment, high number of room changes, postoperative pain levels, use of meperidine, and any iatrogenic event.

Etiology and Pathogenesis

Potential causes of delirium can be predicted based on an understanding of the physical and metabolic needs of the brain to maintain optimal functioning. Essential factors include adequate oxygenation and nutrition, avoidance of toxins and infection, tight temperature regulation, and proper hydration. Thus, causes are varied and usually include combinations of factors that upset this delicate physiologic balance (Table 181-1). The exact pathogenesis remains unclear, but impairments in the reticular activating system and in cholinergic transmission may be present in most deliria. Ultimately, delirium can be seen as an early sign of impending brain failure, with those areas of the brain less immediately essential to life (i.e., the cortex) faltering while more essential regions (midbrain and brainstem) hang on. Seen from this perspective, the seriousness of this disorder can be better appreciated.

Using *Diagnostic and Statistical Manual of Mental Disorders*, 4th edition (*DSM-IV*) diagnostic criteria, causes can be grossly classified as attributed to a general medical condition, caused by substance abuse or withdrawal, because of multiple etiologies, or having an unspecified etiology.

International Statistical Classification of Diseases and Related Health Problems, 10th revision (ICD-10) choices include: delirium not induced by alcohol and other psychoactive substances; delirium not superimposed on Dementia,

Table 181-1 Potential Causes of Delirium

Potential Causes of Delirium	Examples (Partial List)
Drug induced	Neuroleptic malignant syndrome (NMS), anticholinergic toxicity, idiosyncratic neurotoxicity, allergic reactions, combination effects (e.g., narcotics plus antihistamines)
Metabolic abnormalities	Hypoxia, anemias, hypoglycemia, electrolyte imbalances, water imbalance (including dehydration), uremia, hepatic encephalopathy
Infectious processes	Intracranial (encephalopathy, meningitis) Systemic (pneumonia, sepsis, hepatitis, influenza)
Central nervous system disorders	Head trauma, space-occupying lesions, degenerative disorders, cerebrovascular disease, vasculitides
Acute vitamin deficiencies	Thiamine (Wernicke's encephalopathy), cyanocobalamin
Toxins	Organophosphates, CO, organic solvents, ethylene glycol, heavy metals
Intoxications	Stimulants, anticholinergics, hallucinogens, phencyclidine
Withdrawal states	Alcohol (delirium tremens), sedative-hypnotics, opiates
Miscellaneous	Seizures (partial-status, postictal delirium) Sensory deprivation Rapid-eye-movement sleep deprivation Temperature dysregulation (high fevers)

Box 181-1 Common Symptoms and Signs of Delirium

Common Symptoms of Delirium

Disorientation to time, place, and situation (and occasionally person)

Impaired recent memory, confused recall, visuospatial impairments

Perceptual disturbances (misinterpretations, illusions, hallucinations)

Disorganized thinking and speech, irrelevant conversation, delusions

Emotional lability, especially fearfulness (which can lead to aggression and escape behaviors)

Common Signs of Delirium

Psychomotor disturbances, including hyperactivity (often with psychosis), hypoactivity with somnolence, and mixed states

Electroencephalogram with generalized slowing (except sedative-hypnotic or ethanol withdrawal states)

Dysarthria, aphasia, dysgraphia, dysnomia

Specific physical examination findings: asterixis in hepatic encephalopathy and cranial nerve palsies in Wernicke's encephalopathy

Delirium, Superimposed on Dementia, and Other Delirium (including delirium of mixed origin, and subacute confusional states).

Clinical Presentation

The essential feature of delirium is a reduced level of consciousness with impaired ability to sustain, shift, or focus attention (Fig. 181-1). Because of this core deficit, a host of other signs and symptoms can be expected (Box 181-1). Typically, symptoms fluctuate over time and are often worse at night (*sundowning*). Onset may be acute or subacute, with prodromal symptoms of restlessness, anxiety, irritability, distractibility, or sleep disturbance progressing to delirium over 24 to 72 hours. Symptoms may last from less than 1 week to many months, with most resolving within 10 to 12 days; 15% last longer than 30 days, and symptoms often persist after discharge. A persistent cognitive deficit after maximal recovery is common in elderly patients and in patients with AIDS and may represent an unmasking of dementia. Delirium in the medically ill is associated with significant morbidity, including pneumonia, decubitus ulcers, longer hospital stays, and increased postoperative complications; 25% die within 6 months, and the mortality rate for hospitalized patients with delirium is 3 to 7 times higher than for patients without delirium (matched for age and illness severity). The general presentation can be hyperactive (most commonly recognized), hypoactive (frequently missed), and mixed states (most common). A quiet delirium may be more serious because of increased risk for dehydration, malnourishment, and misdiagnosis.

Differential Diagnosis

Delirium is most frequently confused with dementia, severe depression, or other functional psychotic disorders; however, it is critical not to let psychiatric symptoms lead to reduced medical surveillance. An evolving dementia may look like a delirium, especially in advanced cases in which reliable history is hard to obtain, but most acute mental status changes in dementia patients are caused by delirium (although not uncommonly, when the delirium resolves, the dementia will be seen to have progressed). In the case of mood disorders, cognitive impairment is usually a result of lack of effort rather than true deficits. Psychosis with severe cognitive disorganization can look like delirium with disorientation, memory impairments, and general confusion. However, a decrease in level of consciousness

Figure 181-1 Delirium.

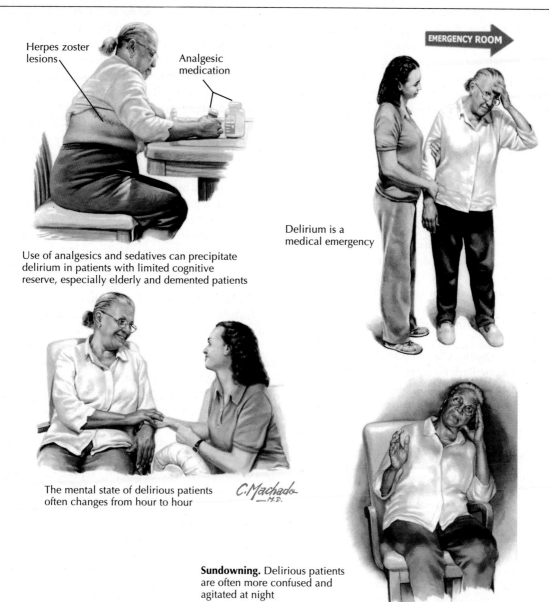

Herpes zoster lesions

Analgesic medication

EMERGENCY ROOM

Use of analgesics and sedatives can precipitate delirium in patients with limited cognitive reserve, especially elderly and demented patients

Delirium is a medical emergency

The mental state of delirious patients often changes from hour to hour

C. Machado —M.D.

Sundowning. Delirious patients are often more confused and agitated at night

is not seen with psychosis alone, and a normal electroencephalogram is most consistent with a nondelirious psychosis. *Although the symptoms of all these conditions can overlap at times, the fluctuating pattern of symptom expression in conjunction with reduced conscious awareness is unique to delirium.*

Diagnostic Approach

All patients with delirium of *uncertain etiology* require blood chemistries (electrolytes, glucose, calcium, albumin, blood urea nitrogen, aspartate transaminase, alanine transaminase, bilirubin, alkaline phosphatase, magnesium, PO_4), complete blood count with differential, electrocardiogram, chest x-ray, measurement of O_2 saturation or arterial blood gases, urinalysis with culture and sensitivity, and urine drug-toxicology screen.

When clinically indicated, consider specific blood tests: VDRL or fluorescent treponemal antibody, heavy metal screen, vitamin B_{12} and folate, antinuclear antibodies, urine porphyrins, blood ammonia, HIV, thyroid-stimulating hormone, blood cultures, medication blood levels (e.g., digoxin, lithium, phenobarbital, diphenylhydantoin [phenytoin], theophylline, tricyclics), lumbar puncture, and neuroimaging (computed tomography or magnetic resonance imaging). An electroencephalogram is probably more helpful in ruling out (when normal) than ruling in delirium.

A careful history can identify precipitating factors or predisposing conditions, whereas the physical exam can be useful in identifying contributing disorders. Most important, perhaps, is the need for a careful medication review, including all over-the-counter medications and nutraceuticals, concentrating in particular on anticholinergic agents and central nervous system depressants. For hospitalized patients, it is important to note that the cause of a delirium is frequently multifactorial, *so the search for a cause should not stop at the first identifiable factor.*

Management and Therapy

Optimum Treatment

Optimum treatment requires that a delirium be identified when present and that an aggressive search for *all* modifiable medical causes be undertaken. Early recognition of delirium may offer significant opportunities to prevent disability and irreversible deterioration. However, by one estimate, 32% to 67% of all deliria go undetected. While the search for causes is in progress, efforts to reduce patient distress and ensure safety should be initiated. Strategies for accomplishing both are listed in Box 181-2.

Medications can sometimes be useful to control symptoms or to increase patient comfort but should never detract from the main goal of identifying and mitigating causative factors. Antipsychotics and benzodiazepines have

been the mainstays of pharmacologic treatment, although other agents are sometimes useful for specific conditions.

Antipsychotics can be useful for the psychosis, agitation, and emotional lability seen with delirium. They have been shown to be superior to benzodiazepines in effectiveness, with fewer side effects in most studies except for sedative-hypnotic or ethanol withdrawal syndromes. High-potency agents are preferred because of minimal anticholinergic effects and sedation. Extrapyramidal side effects, although possible with these agents, are generally not a contraindication to short-term use in delirium. Anticholinergic antidotes should be avoided. Antipsychotics are absolutely contraindicated in neuroleptic malignant syndrome (NMS). If the QTc is greater than 450 msec, further assess cardiac status before beginning or continuing use of these agents.

Traditional choices include *haloperidol*, 1 to 2 mg every 4 hours orally, intramuscularly, or intravenously (0.25 to 0.50 mg for elderly patients), with titration to higher doses as indicated for continued agitation (intravenous dosing should be no more than 1 mg/min to reduce cardiac complications), and *droperidol* (more rapid onset of action, more sedating, similar dosing guidelines, but can prolong QTc).

There are few empirical data concerning the use of the newer atypical antipsychotic agents in delirium, and the better side-effect profile for long-term use of these agents in primary psychotic disorders may not be relevant for delirium. Nevertheless, newer agents such as *risperidone* (0.25 to 1 mg every 6 hours orally) and *olanzapine* (2.5 to 5 mg once or twice per day, orally or intramuscularly) have been effective in small open studies and case reports. *Quetiapine* may also be useful, especially in hyperactive delirium when sedation is needed (*25 to 50 mg PO two to three times per day*).

Benzodiazepines can be useful for agitation and fearfulness. Use as monotherapy for sedative-hypnotic or ethanol withdrawal delirium or adjunctively with antipsychotics if antipsychotics alone are not working for agitation. Lorazepam is the drug of choice because it is short acting and has no active metabolites. Avoid its use in patients with hepatic encephalopathy. Remember that benzodiazepines can promote amnesia and respiratory depression, which might worsen confusion.

Anticholinesterases (physostigmine, donepezil, rivastigmine) can be useful in anticholinergic delirium, and may work for other types of delirium as well, because brainstem cholinergic neurons support cortical activation, and many deliria may result from underactivity in this system (although, in alcohol withdrawal, the problem may be catecholaminergic overactivation). An example of dosing is as follows: physostigmine, 0.50 to 2 mg intravenously or intramuscularly or by continuous intravenous infusion at 3 mg/hour; donepezil: 5 to 10 mg once per day; or rivastigmine, 1.5 mg orally twice a day, maximum dosage 6 mg twice a day.

Additional treatment strategies include mitigating specific causes (such as *thiamine* for Wernicke's encepha-

---

Box 181-2 General Treatment Strategies

- Identify causative factors and mitigate if possible.
- Ensure safety and comfort of the patient and others.
- Avoid restraints if possible, but use if necessary for safety.
- Improve function and decrease symptoms (consider medications for severe symptoms).
- Reduce factors that may exacerbate delirium (such as anticholinergic medicines).
- Provide an optimal level of environmental stimulation: The room should be adequately lighted, including the use of night lights in the evening.
- Avoid overstimulation and understimulation. Keep exposure to chaotic environments to a minimum because many delirious patients are hyperresponsive to stimuli.
- Reduce sensory impairments (let patients use glasses and hearing aids if the clinical state allows).
- Provide environmental cues to facilitate orientation: The room should have a large, easily viewable calendar and clock.
- Staff and family should make the effort to remind the patient of the day, date, and situation frequently. Reminders of who people are may be necessary as well.
- If possible, familiar items from home should be brought into the room.
- Encourage frequent interactions with staff and family.
- Consider telling the patient that he (or she) is confused and disoriented.
- Eliminate nonessential medications and ensure adequate hydration and nutrition.

lopathy) or attenuating cortical dysfunction (such as *electroconvulsive therapy* for refractory NMS or prolonged delirium).

Avoiding Treatment Errors

The most common mistake in the treatment of delirium is the misidentification of the syndrome or failure to recognize it altogether. This prevents the appropriate mitigating interventions and can lead to the prescription of medications (such as anticholinergic antipsychotics or benzodiazepines) that can worsen the condition.

Future Directions

For delirium, the improvement in treatment will likely parallel advances in the recognition and management of the medical conditions that are etiologic. Concurrently, further work targeting the neurochemical disturbances in delirium will be needed to examine whether memory-enhancing agents that work through cholinergic mechanisms to reverse the symptoms of anticholinergic delirium or excitotoxic modulators such as memantine can be beneficial in other types of delirium as well. Along this same line of thought, research into efforts to prevent or reduce the likelihood of a delirium in high-risk situations, including the use of prophylactic anticholinesterases, is warranted.

Additional Resources

American Family Physician. Available at: http://www.aafp.org/afp/20030301/1027.html.
> *This website provides an overview of delirium and its treatment for family practitioners.*

American Geriatrics Society. Available at: http://www.americangeriatrics.org/.
> *Patient and family education materials on many geriatric conditions including delirium are available.*

American Psychiatric Association. Available at: http://www.psych.org/.
> *The latest delirium practice guidelines can be found here as well as patient and family guides to delirium.*

Sage Journals Online: Journal of Geriatric Psychiatry and Neurology. Available at: http://jgp.sagepub.com/cgi/content/abstract/19/2/83.
> *Note the 2006 article entitled "Delirium in Older Patients Admitted to General Internal Medicine."*

EVIDENCE

1. American Psychiatric Association: Practice guidelines for the treatment of patients with delirium. Am J Psychiatry 156:5(Suppl):1-20, 1999.
   > *These guidelines were last updated in August 2004 and provide the best review of the topic currently available.*
2. Boettger S, Breitbart W: Atypical antipsychotics in the management of delirium: A review of the empirical literature. Palliat Support Care 3(3):227-237, 2003.
   > *This article addresses use of new antipsychotic agents for treatment of agitation and psychosis in delirium.*
3. Coffey CE, Cummings JL (eds): Textbook of Geriatric Neuropsychiatry, 2nd ed. Arlington, VA, American Psychiatric Publishing, 2000.
   > *This is the most comprehensive and up-to-date, currently available textbook covering geriatric neuropsychiatric issues.*
4. Cole MG: Delirium in elderly patients. Am J Geriatr Psychiatry 12(1):7-21, 2004.
   > *This review focuses on systematic detection and preventive strategies for hospitalized patients.*
5. Dautzenberg PL, Mulder LJ, Olde Rikkert MG, et al: Delirium in elderly hospitalised patients: Protective effects of chronic rivastigmine usage. Int J Geriatr Psychiatry 19:641-644, 2004.
   > *This article addresses the issue of whether anticholinesterases might be useful in general delirium.*
6. Lipowski ZJ: Delirium in the elderly patient. N Engl J Med 325(9):578-582, 1989.
   > *This was the seminal article on delirium in this population.*
7. Wilber ST: Altered mental status in older emergency department patients. Emerg Med Clin North Am 24(2):299-316, 2006.
   > *Specific diagnoses are discussed, including delirium, stupor and coma, and dementia, along with an approach to all older patients that should result in increased clinician comfort with these patients.*

Dementia

Michael A. Hill

Introduction

Dementia is an acquired syndrome characterized by multiple cognitive deficits leading to reduced intellectual capacity and impairments in social or occupational functioning. Deficits always include short-term memory impairment and one or more of the following: impaired language skills (aphasia), motor planning difficulties (apraxia), sensory deficits (agnosia), and difficulties in judgment, planning, or abstract thinking (executive function).

The prevalence of dementia increases dramatically with age. Although exact numbers are not known, it is estimated that 4.5 million individuals in the United States suffer from Alzheimer's disease (AD) alone. Incidence and prevalence figures accelerate dramatically in people older than 85 years, with prevalence rates for AD approaching 50% in this population (Table 182-1). Besides AD, the most common dementias include vascular (VaD), Lewy-body (LBD), and alcohol-related dementias.

Dementias can be broadly classified as primary versus secondary, based on the pathophysiology leading to damaged brain tissue; cortical versus subcortical, depending on the location of the primary deficits; reversible versus irreversible, depending on optimal treatment expectations; and early versus late onset, depending on age of onset. Frontotemporal dementias, familial AD, and some VaDs are the most common early-onset dementias, whereas AD is the most common late-onset dementia. HIV is the most common cause of dementias beginning before age 55 years.

Most dementias have an insidious onset with progressive decline over many years. Some dementias have a more fulminate course (Creutzfeldt-Jacob disease [CJD]), and others may remit spontaneously or with treatment (vitamin B_{12} deficiency). Despite initial differences in presentation, late-stage dementias often look alike. Common causes of death in advanced dementia include aspiration pneumonia, sepsis from stasis ulcers, dehydration, and urinary tract infections.

Etiology and Pathogenesis

AD is the most common dementia and accounts for 50% to 75% of the total cases (with an even higher percentage of cases beginning after age 80 years). It has a predictable progression that can be reliably staged. Cognitive and social skills are often lost in the reverse order of development, and individuals may appear to function well on a superficial social level long after they have become incompetent to handle complex decision making such as financial planning. Alzheimer's patients typically live 8 to 10 years after diagnosis, and diagnosis often occurs 3 to 4 years after symptoms first appear.

Pathophysiology consists of higher than expected concentrations of neuritic (senile) plaques (abnormal insoluble amyloid protein fragments) and neurofibrillary tangles (disturbed tau-microtubule complexes), especially in hippocampal and posterior temporoparietal areas (Fig. 182-1). There is cholinergic system degeneration with decreased acetylcholine (ACh) levels and significant loss of neurons in areas such as the nucleus basalis of Meynert. Decreases in serotonin and norepinephrine and increases in glutamine activity have also been reported in AD.

Well-established risk factors include age, family history, Down syndrome, head trauma, female gender, and genetics. The apolipoprotein E-4 (APO E-4) allele on chromosome 19 has been associated with late-onset disease, and multiple autosomal dominant gene mutations on chromosomes 1, 14, and 21 have been associated with early-onset cases. Additional risk factors include ethnicity (African

Figure 182-1 Microscopic Pathology in Alzheimer's Disease.

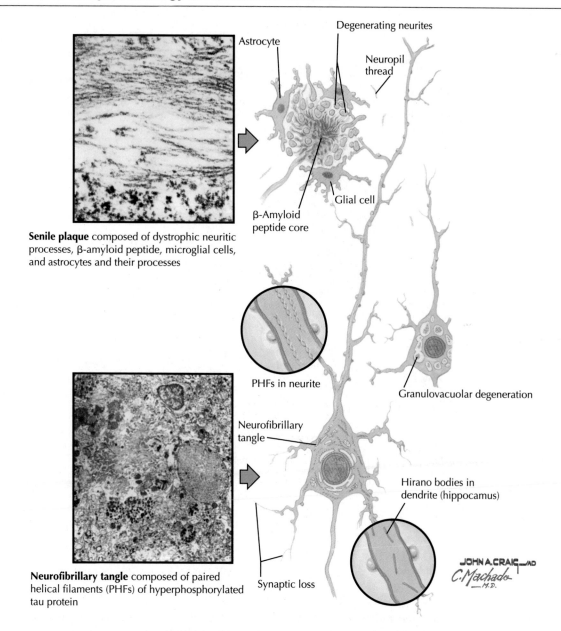

Senile plaque composed of dystrophic neuritic processes, β-amyloid peptide, microglial cells, and astrocytes and their processes

Astrocyte

Degenerating neurites

Neuropil thread

β-Amyloid peptide core

Glial cell

PHFs in neurite

Granulovacuolar degeneration

Neurofibrillary tangle

Hirano bodies in dendrite (hippocamus)

Neurofibrillary tangle composed of paired helical filaments (PHFs) of hyperphosphorylated tau protein

Synaptic loss

JOHN A. CRAIG—AD
C. Machado—M.D.

Age	Prevalence Estimates for Dementia*	Age (yr)	Incidence Estimates for Dementia
>65	5%-10%	65-74	0.5%-1%
>75	10%-20%	75-84	2%-4%
>85	25%-50%	85-95	6%-8%
>95	40%-70%	100+	May level off or decline after age 100 yr

Table 182-1 Prevalence Estimates for Dementia

* Lower numbers reflect prevalence of moderate to severe dementias.

Americans more than whites), late-onset depression, diabetes, and cerebrovascular disease. Possible protective factors include education, use of some anti-inflammatory agents, estrogen replacement, antioxidants, statins, and APO E-3 genotypes (Fig. 182-2).

VaD is the second most common dementia (15%-20%) and includes Binswanger's disease, multi-infarct dementia, anoxic damage, postcoronary artery bypass graft conditions, and inflammatory diseases. Age, hypertension, diabetes, and hyperlipidemia are the documented risk factors.

Figure 182-2 Risk Factors for Alzheimer's Disease.

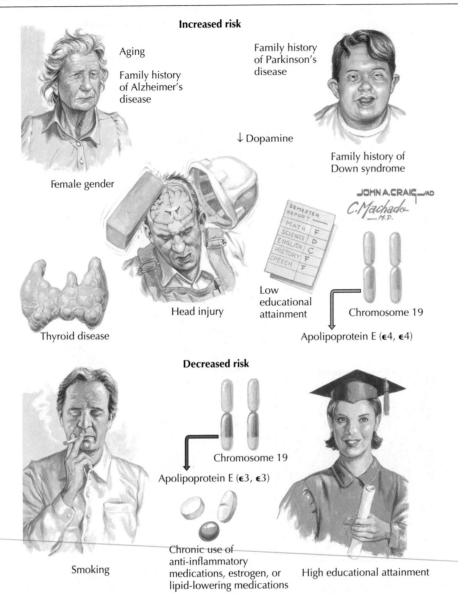

VaDs may show a stepwise progression and are frequently associated with focal neurologic findings. Cortical atrophy and periventricular white matter changes consistent with microvascular disease are the most common findings on head imaging. VaD typically has a shorter course and earlier onset than AD, but the two frequently coexist (mixed dementia). LBDs can have a presentation similar to AD, although subcortical symptoms, higher frequency of visual hallucinations, sensitivity to antipsychotic medications, and fluctuating symptoms can often distinguish the two clinically (Fig. 182-3). Alcohol-related dementias are also common (Box 182-1).

Clinical Presentation

Dementia is always associated with cognitive disturbances and functional impairments, whereas visuospatial deficits and behavioral disturbances are frequently seen as well. Initial presentations can vary depending on the type of dementia, stage of illness, willingness to seek help, and cultural tolerance for certain types of symptoms. Memory and language impairments include difficulty retaining new information (learning failure); information retrieval deficits (name or word-finding difficulties); personal episodic memory impairment (misplacing items); list generation deficits; and impairments in declarative memory (what) greater than procedural memory (how). Typically sentence structure becomes less complex, whereas auditory comprehension and social conversation are usually preserved. Visuospatial impairments can lead to not recognizing relatives, getting lost in familiar surroundings, and three-dimensional drawing deficits.

Behavioral symptoms are nearly universal and are often the main focus of families' concerns and complaints.

Figure 182-3 Vascular Dementia and Dementia with Lewy Bodies.

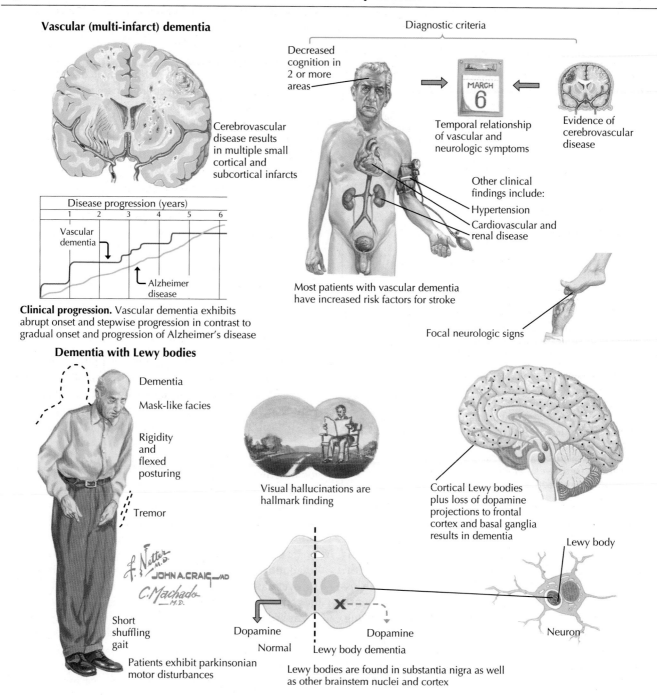

Vascular (multi-infarct) dementia

Cerebrovascular disease results in multiple small cortical and subcortical infarcts

Disease progression (years)

Vascular dementia

Alzheimer disease

Clinical progression. Vascular dementia exhibits abrupt onset and stepwise progression in contrast to gradual onset and progression of Alzheimer's disease

Diagnostic criteria

Decreased cognition in 2 or more areas

Temporal relationship of vascular and neurologic symptoms

Evidence of cerebrovascular disease

Other clinical findings include:

Hypertension

Cardiovascular and renal disease

Most patients with vascular dementia have increased risk factors for stroke

Focal neurologic signs

Dementia with Lewy bodies

Dementia

Mask-like facies

Rigidity and flexed posturing

Tremor

Short shuffling gait

Patients exhibit parkinsonian motor disturbances

Visual hallucinations are hallmark finding

Cortical Lewy bodies plus loss of dopamine projections to frontal cortex and basal ganglia results in dementia

Lewy body

Neuron

Dopamine

Normal

Dopamine

Lewy body dementia

Lewy bodies are found in substantia nigra as well as other brainstem nuclei and cortex

---

Inability to manage these types of symptoms is highly correlated with the need for institutional placement. Personality change occurs early and includes passivity (e.g., apathy, social withdrawal), disinhibition (e.g., inappropriate sexual behavior or language), and self-centered behaviors (e.g., childishness and loss of generosity). Agitation is very common and frequently worsens as the illness progresses. It includes verbal (25%) and physical (30%) aggression and nonaggressive behaviors such as wandering and pacing

(25% to 50%). Aggression strongly correlates with caregiver burnout, especially when wandering is also present.

Associated features of dementia include depression (often occurs early, common in AD and VaD); delusions (typically paranoia about theft, infidelity); hallucinations (often visual, particularly common in LBD); and sleep problems (insomnia, sleep-wake cycle disturbances).

Functional impairment and performance on cognitive testing may not correlate strongly early in the course of

---

Box 182-1 Less Common Dementias

Primary Degenerative Dementias

Frontotemporal dementias (Pick's disease) amyotrophic lateral sclerosis dementias, Huntington's disease

Neurologic Disorders Associated with Dementia

Progressive supranuclear palsy (profound apathy, downward eye gaze paralysis)

Dementia due to Parkinson's disease (20%-60% of patients)

Normal-pressure hydrocephalus (dementia, incontinence, ataxia)

Neoplasms (frontal and temporal tumors especially)

Head trauma (e.g., dementia pugilistica)

Subdural hematoma (chronic), central nervous system vasculitis, lupus

Demyelinating disorders

Infectious Causes of Dementia

Neurosyphilis, Lyme disease, HIV

Viral, parasitic, bacterial, and fungal meningitis or encephalitis

Postencephalitic dementia (especially following herpes encephalitis)

Opportunistic infections or brain abscess

Human prion disease (transmissible spongiform encephalopathies including Creutzfeldt-Jacob disease [CJD], variant CJD [mad cow disease] and kuru)

General Medical Causes of Dementia

Alcohol-related (Korsakoff's syndrome)

Thyroid and adrenal disease

Vitamin deficiency states (thiamine, niacin, or B_{12})

Metabolic derangements (dialysis dementia, hepatic encephalopathy, hypercalcemia, glucose dysregulation, electrolyte disturbances, posthypoxia)

Medications (sedatives, antihypertensives, cardiac medications, narcotics, anticholinergics)

Whipple's disease, sarcoidosis, Wilson's disease

Toxins (heavy metals, organic poisons)

---

dementia because an individual may function reasonably well in many areas despite deficits on testing early in the illness or vice versa. The rate and specific pattern of loss will vary by individual. Deficits appear first in instrumental activities of daily living such as managing finances, driving, using the telephone, taking medications, and keeping appointments. Eventually deficits appear in more basic skills such as feeding, grooming, dressing, eating, and toileting (activities of daily living).

Differential Diagnosis

Mild impairments in memory without clear-cut functional decline are referred to as *mild cognitive impairment* (MCI). With Mini Mental State Examination (MMSE) scores typically in the 24 to 30 range, many of these individuals are in the premorbid stage of a dementia, and about 15% per year progress to the full dementia syndrome. However, others remain stable or remit completely over time.

In a pure amnestic syndrome, short-term memory is impaired without significant impairments in other cognitive domains (e.g., alcohol amnestic syndrome), whereas the essential impairment in delirium is a reduced level of consciousness and attention along with rapidly fluctuating symptoms (although most of the symptoms of dementia are present as well).

Mental retardation is a developmental disorder associated with impaired intellectual capacities that may or may not affect memory. *Pseudodementia* refers to cognitive impairment in the context of another psychiatric disorder, such as depression, that is often attributed to decreased concentration or poor effort during testing. Finally, a receptive aphasia may be confused with dementia because of impaired cognitive testing secondary to comprehension failure.

Interestingly, many of these conditions have an association with dementia: For example, Down syndrome patients are at high risk for developing AD at a young age; pseudodementia and MCI often herald the onset of a true dementia; and delirium is an extremely common complication of dementia.

Diagnostic Approach

A careful history from the patient and a reliable informant are critical for early detection with chronology of symptoms and functional impairments of particular importance. A thorough physical examination with particular focus on the neurologic exam is an important part of the initial workup. Cognitive screening tools are helpful for documenting deficits and for monitoring progression. Examples include the MMSE, or the Six-Item Blessed Orientation-Memory-Concentration Test. The MMSE is widely available and easy to use and should be considered in all new patients older than 65 years. Scores less then 24/30 are considered worrisome for individuals with at least a 6th grade education. The Clock Drawing Test is another easy to administer screen for dementia, particularly AD. Neuropsychological assessment or referral to a specialist should be considered when cognitive testing and functional assessment are at odds, when there is a strong suspicion of early dementia in a high-IQ individual with a normal MMSE, for competency assessments in legal proceedings, or if mild impairment is seen with any of the following: low IQ or limited education, trouble with English, or minority racial or ethnic background.

The goal of the diagnostic workup is to rule out disorders besides dementia, to identify reversible (13%) dementias (such as NPH, B_{12} and folate deficiency, thyroid disease, psychiatric disorders), or to clarify the specific dementia syndrome (Table 182-2). Routine assessment includes complete blood count with differential, serum electrolytes, calcium, glucose, blood urea nitrogen, creatinine, liver function tests, thyroid function tests, B_{12} and folate, urinalysis, and syphilis serology. Consider sedimentation rate, HIV testing, chest x-ray, 24-hour urine for heavy metals, toxicology screen, neuroimaging, lumbar

Table 182-2 Dementia Types and Diagnosis

Dementia Type	Suggested by	Dementia Type	Suggested by
Alzheimer's disease	Insidious onset and progressive worsening Prominent memory retention deficits early in the course Onset after age 70 yr with no focal signs or gait disturbances Exclusion of reversible dementias List generation difficulties	Vascular dementia	Relatively abrupt onset and stepwise or fluctuating course History of stroke, hypertension, or diabetes Focal neurologic signs or symptoms Emotional lability, depression Somatic complaints with relative preservation of personality
Lewy body dementia	Executive function impairments greater than memory impairments early on Fluctuating deficits during the day Visual hallucinations Mild parkinsonism and sensitivity to antipsychotics	Dementia syndrome of depression (pseudodementia)	Memory, concentration impairments in the absence of apraxia, agnosia, and aphasia Apathy, low motivation, and other neurovegetative signs of depression Exaggerated complaints of memory impairment, poor effort in testing History of cognitive changes with depression
Frontotemporal dementia	Prominent early personality changes with apathy, disinhibition, and antisocial behavior Peculiar behavior and verbal stereotypes such as "let's go, let's go" Preserved visuospatial skills	HIV/AIDS dementia	Forgetfulness, psychomotor slowing, impaired problem solving, apathy Neurologic signs such as tremor, ataxia, hyperreflexia, frontal release signs Age <55 yr
Subcortical dementia	Psychomotor slowing, frontal systems dysfunction, short-term memory impairment Depression and apathy Neurologic findings such as parkinsonism, ataxia, and urinary incontinence Less pronounced language difficulties until late in course	Delirium (as opposed to dementia)	Acute or subacute onset Impaired consciousness and attention Fluctuating course Disorganized thinking Medical illness Mental status change in patient with preexisting dementia

puncture, electroencephalogram (EEG), functional imaging, Lyme titers, endocrine studies (other than thyroid), and rheumatologic studies when indicated. Neuroimaging should be considered in all new cases, although in individuals older than 80 years with no focal symptoms or signs, seizures, or gait disturbances, it can be considered optional. Magnetic resonance imaging (MRI) is preferred if the patient can tolerate it. A lumbar puncture is indicated for suspicion of metastatic cancer, central nervous system (CNS) infection, reactive serum syphilis serology, hydrocephalus, dementia before age 55 years, rapidly progressive dementias, immunosuppression, and suspicion of CNS vasculitis. EEG may be helpful in distinguishing delirium from dementia, diagnosing CJD, and identifying seizure disorders. If available, functional imaging (single-photon emission computed tomography, positron emission tomography [PET], magnetic resonance spectroscopy) may help clarify the type of dementia in diagnostically confusing cases. Staging identifies current care needs and predicts future requirements. Functional assessment scales such as the Functional Activities Questionnaire can be useful for clarifying impairments and tracking responses to interventions. Psychosocial assessment should address patient issues (such as safety and appropriateness of current living situation and presence of comorbid psychiatric conditions), caregiver issues (such as adequacy of support network, presence of depression, and need for financial planning), and environmental issues (such as home safety and driving concerns).

Management and Therapy

Optimum Treatment

Optimum treatment requires a systems approach that recognizes the needs of both the patient and the principal caregivers. The primary goal is to ensure the safety of patient and family, to improve the quality of life for the patient and caregivers, and ultimately to prevent caregiver burnout and forestall institutionalization. For the patient, attempts should be made to minimize cognitive symptoms, recognize and address behavioral and psychiatric comorbidities, and optimize functional adaptation. For caregivers, it is critical to recognize the need for emotional, physical, and financial support and to monitor carefully for

Figure 182-4 Pharmacologic Management Options in Alzheimer's Disease.

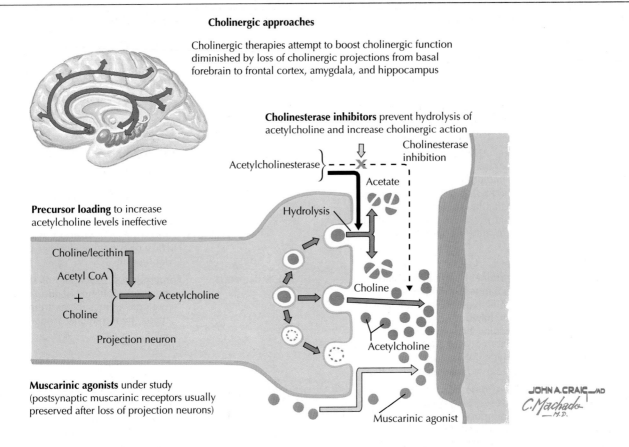

Cholinergic approaches

Cholinergic therapies attempt to boost cholinergic function diminished by loss of cholinergic projections from basal forebrain to frontal cortex, amygdala, and hippocampus

Cholinesterase inhibitors prevent hydrolysis of acetylcholine and increase cholinergic action

Acetylcholinesterase

Cholinesterase inhibition

Acetate

Hydrolysis

Precursor loading to increase acetylcholine levels ineffective

Choline/lecithin

Acetyl CoA

+

Choline

Acetylcholine

Choline

Projection neuron

Acetylcholine

Muscarinic agonists under study (postsynaptic muscarinic receptors usually preserved after loss of projection neurons)

Muscarinic agonist

JOHN A. CRAIG—MD
C. Machado—M.D.

Table 182-3	Cholinesterase Inhibitors		
Drug	**Starting Dose**	**Goal**	**Notes**
Tacrine	10 mg 4 times a day	120-160 mg/day	NOT FIRST LINE because of 4 times a day dosing and liver function test elevations
Donepezil	5 mg every day	10 mg every day	Maintain starting dose for 1-3 weeks to minimize side effects
Rivastigmine	1.5 mg twice a day	6-12 mg/day	Similar side effects to tacrine, donepezil, and galantamine: nausea, vomiting, bradycardia
Galantamine	4 mg twice a day	8-12 mg twice a day	Reversible anticholinesterase inhibitor plus modulation of receptors to increase acetylcholine release

the presence of clinical depression (which may occur in up to 50% of isolated caregivers). A referral to groups such as the Alzheimer's Association for support or to legal aid for competency questions can often be helpful.

Primary treatment strategies include efforts to mitigate or reverse cognitive symptoms, prevent progression of the illness, or optimize compensatory function. In some cases, specific therapies to reverse an underlying disease process (such as B₁₂ or thyroid replacement) may be all that is required. In most cases, however, the best practice is to try and mitigate the pathophysiologic dysfunction. In AD, (cholinergic dysfunction) excess glutaminergic activity, and the accumulation of abnormal amyloid protein have been the targets of medical intervention. Efforts to

increase cholinergic activity include precursor strategies (such as lecithin) to increase production of ACh, cholinergic agonists (not currently available) to mimic ACh, and cholinesterase inhibitors to prolong synaptic availability (Fig. 182-4). The latter has been most successful, and a number of anticholinesterases are available (Table 182-3). These agents may be useful in non-AD dementias as well. Currently evidence is strongest for VaDs and LBDs. Memantine, a weak antagonist of glutamate-gated NMDA receptor channels, has been shown to improve function in moderate to severe AD. By preventing overactivation during memory formation, it may also be useful in slowing progression of these disorders by preventing excitotoxic damage.

Figure 182-5 Amyloidogenesis in Alzheimer's Disease.

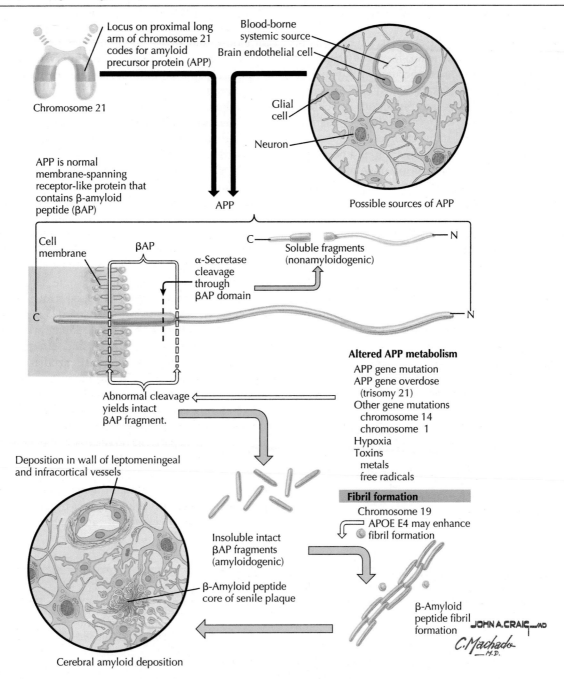

Locus on proximal long arm of chromosome 21 codes for amyloid precursor protein (APP)

Chromosome 21

Blood-borne systemic source
Brain endothelial cell
Glial cell
Neuron

APP is normal membrane-spanning receptor-like protein that contains β-amyloid peptide (βAP)

APP

Possible sources of APP

Cell membrane
βAP
α-Secretase cleavage through βAP domain

C
Soluble fragments (nonamyloidogenic)
N

C

N

Altered APP metabolism
APP gene mutation
APP gene overdose (trisomy 21)
Other gene mutations
chromosome 14
chromosome 1
Hypoxia
Toxins
metals
free radicals

Abnormal cleavage yields intact βAP fragment.

Deposition in wall of leptomeningeal and infracortical vessels

Fibril formation
Chromosome 19
APOE E4 may enhance fibril formation

Insoluble intact βAP fragments (amyloidogenic)

β-Amyloid peptide core of senile plaque

β-Amyloid peptide fibril formation

Cerebral amyloid deposition

JOHN A. CRAIG—AD
C. Machado —M.D.

Other promising therapies include gene replacement strategies, tissue transplantation, antiamyloid vaccines, and agents that interfere with abnormal amyloidogenesis (Fig. 182-5).

Strategies to prevent progression include controlling risk factors (hypertension and diabetes management, stroke prevention); treating underlying medical causes aggressively; and using cerebral shunts for normal-pressure hydrocephalus (which may also reverse symptoms). There is some limited evidence that antioxidants (vitamin E, gingko, selegiline), nonsteroidal anti-inflammatory agents, homocysteine reduction strategies, and other neuroprotective agents (acetyl carnitine) might be useful in progressive dementias. However, evidence is not strong enough to recommend any of these agents routinely, and the safety of even relatively nontoxic agents such as vitamin E has come into question.

Strategies to enhance CNS function (or to promote compensatory mechanisms) include estrogen replacement (which may be useful in delaying onset of AD in postmenopausal women), coping skills training (particularly for nonprogressive or slowly progressive dementias), and eliminating agents known to interfere with cognitive function such as anticholinergic agents and benzodiazepines (Box 182-2).

Treatment of the associated (secondary) symptoms of dementia often becomes the main focus of treatment because much of the morbidity associated with dementia (in both the patient and caregiver) is related to these symptoms, which include depression, agitation, psychosis, insomnia, and wandering. A careful medical evaluation, especially for sudden mental status changes, new-onset or worsening psychosis, or increased agitation, is a necessary first step. When satisfied that new or ongoing medical problems are being addressed appropriately, specific symptomatic interventions can be tried.

For psychosis, calm reassurance and distraction may be all that is required if there is little distress or danger. Although the atypical antipsychotics are quickly becoming the drugs of choice, haloperidol remains a good choice for the elderly patient owing to few side effects, proven efficacy, and low cost (Table 182-4). Orthostasis and anticholinergic effects are potential problems with both traditional neuroleptics and the new generation agents.

Maintain a low threshold for diagnosing depression because this condition is common and can make cognitive symptoms and overall functioning worse. Preservation of autonomy, supportive counseling, and encouragement of enjoyable activities can be useful interventions. Selective serotonin reuptake inhibitors are the first choice for medication treatment, but paroxetine should be avoided because of anticholinergic effects.

For agitation, responding in a direct and calm manner (rather than arguing), redirection, and determining what is upsetting the patient can be helpful. Medications, if needed, should target specific conditions first (e.g., antidepressants for agitation in the context of depression). Nonspecific antiagitation medications include antipsychotics, anticonvulsants, benzodiazepines, trazodone, and buspirone. Anticholinesterases may be effective for these and other secondary symptoms and should be considered if not already prescribed. Antipsychotics, although predictably effective, have come under some scrutiny recently because of the possibility of increased stroke risk in elderly dementia patients. Low-dose trazodone (25 mg every 6 hours as needed) or quetiapine (12.5 to 25 mg every 6 hours as needed) is often well tolerated and effective, although orthostasis can occur with both. Benzodiazepines should always be used cautiously in this population because of the potential for ataxia, worsened memory, and disinhibition.

Wandering can be minimized by secure, well-lit environments, dementia-proof locks, and environmental barriers such as grid patterns on the floor, and by determining whether the patient is anxious or restless. For insomnia, educate patients and caregivers about sleep hygiene measures and determine whether this symptom is a manifestation of another disorder such as depression. Avoid benzodiazepines because of ataxia and amnesia and

---

Box 182-2   Common Anticholinergic Agents

Antiparkinson drugs (benztropine, trihexyphenidyl)
Tricyclic antidepressants (especially amitriptyline and imipramine)
Traditional antipsychotics (especially low-potency drugs)
Atypical antipsychotics (especially clozapine and olanzapine)
Urinary agents for incontinence (tolterodine, oxybutynin)
Others (cimetidine, ranitidine, digoxin, furosemide, nifedipine, theophylline, paroxetine)
Sleep aids (diphenhydramine)

Table 182-4   Antipsychotics

Atypical Agent	Useful for	Pros	Cons*	Dose Range
Risperidone	Agitation, psychosis	Well studied, generally well tolerated	EPS common in elderly, prolactin elevations occur	0.25-2 mg twice a day
Olanzapine	Mania, psychosis, agitation	Weight gain can be a plus for some patients, dissolvable pill form available (Zydis)	Weight gain, hyperglycemia, anticholinergic effects	2.5-10 mg every day
Quetiapine	Psychosis, agitation, insomnia	Low doses useful for insomnia; not anticholinergic	Sedating, complicated dosing	12.5-200 mg twice a day
Ziprasidone	Psychosis, agitation	Low sedation and weight gain	Prolongs QTc interval	20-60 mg twice a day
Clozapine	Refractory psychosis (not for first line use)	Parkinson's disease patients may benefit	Sedation, bone marrow suppression, highly anticholinergic	12.5-300 mg every day
Haloperidol	Agitation, psychosis, mania	Best studied, well tolerated in elderly, few side effects, inexpensive, many dose forms	EPS (esp. akathisia); high TD risk with prolonged use	0.5-2 mg once or twice a day

* Potential orthostasis and high cost are problems with all these agents except haloperidol.
  EPS, extrapyramidal syndrome; TD, tardive dyskinesia.

diphenhydramine because of anticholinergic effects. Consider trazodone (25 to 100 mg) or quetiapine (25 to 50 mg) if medications are needed. Zolpidem (5 to 10 mg) or esopiclone (2 to 3 mg) may be useful for short periods.

Avoiding Treatment Errors

Ignoring the needs of the caregiver and not recognizing the presence of a delirium when mental status changes abruptly in a dementia patient are two common treatment errors. Additionally, failure to recognize treatable comorbidities such as depression and failure to minimize anticholinergic medications such as oxybutynin are also avoidable mistakes.

Future Directions

Research is progressing rapidly in the treatment of AD, the most common and fastest growing dementia. Antiamyloid vaccines, secretase inhibitors (plaque busters), anti-inflammatory strategies, and more specific memory enhancing agents are all being tested with encouraging early results. Gene manipulation and surgical implantation techniques are being investigated along with strategies that enhance the brain's ability to dispose of abnormal proteins. With justified excitement in the treatment realm, the need for accurate early detection strategies is of increasing importance, and the development of a safe, easy to use, and reliable screening test for Alzheimer's (and other degenerative dementias) will be a high priority. Currently, functional imaging, biologic markers, and genetic testing hold the most promise.

Additional Resources

Alzheimer's Association. Available at: http://www.alz.org/. Accessed November 17, 2006.

This website is a great resource for families and providers. The organization keeps abreast of current research, provides education for caregivers and patients, and provides links to support resources.

Alzheimer's Disease Education and Referral Center (ADEAR). Available at: http://www.nia.nih.gov/Alzheimers. Accessed November 17, 2006.

This site is an NIH resource for providers, patients, and families.

Alzheimer's Research Forum. Available at: http://www.alzforum.org/. Accessed November 17, 2006.

This site tracks the most current research and includes a section on new drug development.

American Association for Geriatric Psychiatry. Available at: http://www. aagpgpa.org/. Accessed November 17, 2006.

This website can be used to locate providers, track congressional action on geriatric topics, and obtain educational materials.

National Institute of Neurological Disorders and Stroke (NINDS). Available at: http://www.ninds.nih.gov/disorders/dementias/dementia. htm. Accessed November 17, 2006.

This NINDS dementia information page includes a listing of ongoing and recruiting studies.

EVIDENCE

1. American Psychiatric Association: Practice guidelines for the treatment of patients with Alzheimer's disease and other dementias of late life. Am J Psychiatry 154(5 Suppl):1-39, 1997.

   These summary recommendations for treating Alzheimer's disease patients describe evidence and rationales supporting best practice.

2. Blazer DG, Steffens DC, Busse EW (eds): Textbook of Geriatric Psychiatry, 3rd ed. Washington DC, American Psychiatric Press, 2004.

   This up-to-date review of geriatric psychiatry includes an overview of dementia diagnosis and treatment.

3. Feldman HH, Jacova C: Mild cognitive impairment. Am J Geriatr Psychiatry 13(8):645-655, 2005.

   The authors present an excellent review of this increasingly important topic.

4. Herrmann N, Mamdani M, Lanctot KL: Atypical antipsychotics and risk of cerebrovascular accidents. Am J Psychiatry 161(6):1113-1115, 2004.

   The authors provide an in-depth look at the data leading to the FDA's black-box warning about the use of these agents in AD.

5. Mayeux R, Sano M: Treatment of Alzheimer's disease. N Engl J Med 341(22):1670-1679, 1999.

   This is a good, concise review of the topic from a 1999 article, much of which is still relevant today.

6. Practice parameters for diagnosis and evaluation of dementia (summary statement). Report of the Quality Standards Subcommittee of the American Academy of Neurology. Neurology 44(11):2203-2206, 1994.

   This article provides the neurology perspective on diagnosis and treatment of dementia.

7. Rabins PV: Guideline watch: Practice guideline for the treatment of Alzheimer's disease and other dementias of late life. APA Practice Guidelines Update, 2006.

   This article updates the APA practice guidelines from 1997 (see reference 1).

8. Schulz R, Martire LM: Family caregiving of persons with dementia: Prevalence, health effects and support strategies. Am J Geriatr Psychiatry 12(3):240-249, 2004.

   The authors present a good overview of caregiver issues.

9. Small GW, Rabins PV, Barry PP, et al: Diagnosis and treatment of Alzheimer's disease and related disorders. Consensus statement of the American Association for Geriatric Psychiatry, the Alzheimer's Association, and the American Geriatrics Society. JAMA 278(16):1363-1371, 1997.

   This consensus statement on diagnosis and treatment predated the APA guidelines by 2 years and served as a model for the more recent guidelines.

Advance Directives

Introduction

Advance directives are documents that specify an individual's end-of-life care treatment preferences and designate surrogate decision makers if the person lacks decision-making capacity. The primary goal of advance directives, including living wills and health care proxy forms, is to promote respect for patients' treatment preferences when they cannot communicate. Despite a federal law enacted 15 years ago to increase the use of advance directives, low completion rates persist among adults—a fact of special note given prior studies that suggest that patients want physicians to discuss advance directives with them.

Background

The proliferation of life-saving treatments in the 1960s, such as cardiopulmonary resuscitation, mechanical ventilation, and hemodialysis, not only prolonged patients' lives but also prolonged the deaths of those left uncured. During the past three decades, the cases of three young women in persistent vegetative states—Karen Ann Quinlan in the 1970s, Nancy Cruzan in the 1980s, and Terri Schiavo in this decade—epitomize for many Americans the core problem with end-of-life care: dying patients who are unable to communicate their preferences are kept alive using medical technologies they may not want utilized at a time when they are powerless to determine their treatment. The legal conflicts involving these women have helped solidify dying patients' rights to determine their medical decisions, either themselves, through prior expression of their wishes, or through the voices of surrogate decision makers. The principle that respect for patient autonomy should be valued independent of patients' decision-making capacity is now well ingrained within the health care system.

Consensus that capable patients have the right to make their own medical decisions, even decisions that could hasten death, had been reached in the legal and medical communities before the Quinlan, Cruzan, and Schiavo cases. However, as with these women, most life-sustaining treatment withdrawal decisions affect patients who lack decision-making capacity and therefore cannot provide informed consent. Cognitive impairment from dementia, delirium, and serious illness prevents patients from understanding their condition, from weighing the risks and benefits of treatment decisions, and from expressing a treatment preference.

The decisions reached in these young women's cases established the ethical principles used to make medical decisions for incapacitated patients and provided the legal basis supporting the development of advance directives. In the Quinlan decision, a court supported her parents' request for decision-making authority based on the ethical principle of "substituted judgment," meaning that they could best represent the decisions that Ms. Quinlan would have made if conscious. This decision recognized that the use of a surrogate decision maker, usually a spouse or blood relative, could extend patients' decision-making autonomy to times when they are incapacitated. Physicians ask surrogate decision makers to consider any prior preferences expressed by the patient when making decisions, or to use judgment regarding the patient's best interests when specific instructions have not been given.

The Quinlan case demonstrated the need for incapacitated patients to have loved ones who could represent their treatment preferences. In response, patient advocates proposed advance directives as mechanisms for patients to specify treatment preferences and select preferred decision makers in advance of any condition associated with decision-making incapacity. A United States Supreme Court decision in the Cruzan case had the effect of promoting advance directive use by ruling that states could establish standards regarding the "clear and convincing"

evidence necessary to establish an incapacitated patient's treatment preferences. Based on this decision, all states have included advance directives as a mechanism to satisfy their evidentiary standards.

The nationally publicized Terri Schiavo case serves as the most recent reminder that advance directives can have an important role in end-of-life care decision making. Ms. Schiavo's protracted legal dispute would likely have been avoided if she had signed a living will or formally designated either her husband or one of her parents as her health care proxy.

Definitions and Legal Considerations

The two most commonly completed advance directives are *living wills* and *health care proxy* (or *health care power of attorney*) documents. Living wills can provide either general or specific information regarding patients' end-of-life care treatment preferences in the event of both decision-making incapacity and either a terminal illness or a persistent vegetative state. A living will may state that a person wishes to avoid receiving "extraordinary measures" without detailing the treatments considered by the patient as extraordinary. Other living wills provide a listing of treatment decisions ranging from mechanical ventilation to antibiotic use, and patients note whether or not they would be willing to receive each treatment.

Although living wills may provide information relevant to understanding patients' preferences regarding attempts at cardiopulmonary resuscitation, a separate Do Not Resuscitate order must be signed by a physician if patients wish to avoid cardiac resuscitative measures.

Health care proxy forms designate the individual who will serve as the surrogate decision maker in the event the patient becomes incapacitated. This form can also include the name of an alternate if the primary surrogate is unavailable. Physicians have an ethical and legal obligation to communicate with health care proxies to receive their consent for all medical decisions affecting patients. Although the scope of living wills is generally limited to end-of-life care decisions, the responsibility of health care proxies extends to all treatment considerations. The decision-making authority of health care proxies only pertains to medical decisions; other documents grant powers such as financial decision making when patients are incapacitated.

Patients may complete a living will, a health care proxy document, or both directives. Living wills and health care proxy documents become legally valid once signed in front of the required witnesses, which may include a notary public. A lawyer's assistance is not required to complete an advance directive. Advance directives do not expire unless specified by the patient and may be changed by a capable patient at any time. The laws governing advance directives vary from state to state, so it is important for patients to complete and sign directives that comply with their state's law. One state's advance directive may not be considered legally valid in other states. Some states honor directives from other states; others will honor out-of-state directives as long as they are in compliance with the state's own law; and some states do not provide clear guidance regarding the legal validity of out-of-state directives.

Although using a state-recognized form does have some advantages over use of other written documents or a physician's note that summarizes a discussion about a patient's stated treatment preferences, a written directive that does not satisfy all legal formalities can still help guide end-of-life care decision making. This document may represent the best evidence of a patient's wishes about life-sustaining treatment. In addition, oral statements previously made by the patient are also legally valid in some states.

A website sponsored by the National Hospice and Palliative Care Organization provides general information about advance directives and free access to the advance directive forms used in all 50 states and the District of Columbia along with completion instructions. A toll-free helpline is also available for patients with questions about advance directives (See Additional Resources). Figure 183-1 is the advance directive form used in North Carolina.

Clinical Implications

Multiple interventions have been implemented to increase advance directive completion rates, including the Patient Self-Determination Act. This Federal legislation enacted in 1991 requires all health care facilities receiving federal funding, including hospitals and nursing homes, to ask patients upon admission if they have an advance directive and to provide patients with help in completing a directive if requested. Unfortunately, this legislation and other efforts have not significantly affected completion rates—less than half of seriously ill patients have a signed directive. Also of note, prior research suggests that advance directives have had a limited impact on overall end-of-life care quality.

Studies have documented several factors that limit advance directive use and effect on end-of-life care decision making. There are significant differences in advance directive completion rates associated with race and ethnicity. Fewer African Americans and Latinos complete a living will or designate a proxy decision maker when compared with whites. Individuals from these minority groups are more likely to prefer continuation of life-sustaining treatments and perceive a living will, which is generally viewed as protecting patients against life prolongation, as antithetical to their interests. They also may be more accustomed to utilizing family consensus as the basis for their decisions and feel uncomfortable deciding on a single health care proxy, a legalistic standard that forces them to choose one decision maker among their loved ones.

Patients do not complete an advance directive for a variety of other reasons: they prefer to avoid contemplating

Figure 183-1 Example of a Living Will.
Note that this living will is the one used in North Carolina and that state laws vary.

North Carolina Statutory Form, N.C. Gen. Stat. § 90-321
Declaration of a Desire for a Natural Death (Living Will)

Declaration of a Desire for a Natural Death

STATE OF NORTH CAROLINA   COUNTY OF _____

I, _____, being of sound mind, desire that, as specified below, my life not be prolonged by extraordinary means or by artificial nutrition or hydration if my condition is determined to be terminal and incurable or if I am diagnosed as being in a persistent vegetative state. I am aware and understand that this writing authorizes a physician to withhold or discontinue extraordinary means or artificial nutrition or hydration, in accordance with my specifications set forth below:

(Initial any of the following, as desired):

_____ If my condition is determined to be terminal and incurable, I authorize the following:
     _____ My physician may withhold or discontinue extraordinary means only.
     _____ In addition to withholding or discontinuing extraordinary means if such means are necessary, my physician may withhold or discontinue either artificial nutrition or hydration, or both.
_____ If my physician determines that I am in a persistent vegetative state, I authorize the following:
     _____ My physician may withhold or discontinue extraordinary means only.
     _____ In addition to withholding or discontinuing extraordinary means if such means are necessary, my physician may withhold or discontinue either artificial nutrition or hydration, or both.

This the _____ day of _____, 20 _____

Signature _____, Declarant

I hereby state that the declarant, _____, being of sound mind signed the above declaration in my presence and that I am not related to the declarant by blood or marriage and that I do not know or have a reasonable expectation that I would be entitled to any portion of the estate of the declarant under any existing will or codicil of the declarant or as an heir under the Intestate Succession Act if the declarant died on this date without a will. I also state that I am not the declarant's attending physician or an employee of the declarant's attending physician, or an employee of a health facility in which the declarant is a patient or an employee of a nursing home or any group-care home where the declarant resides. I further state that I do not now have any claim against the declarant.

Witness _____

Witness _____

CERTIFICATE

STATE OF NORTH CAROLINA   COUNTY OF_____

I, _____, Notary Public for _____ County hereby certify that _____, the declarant, appeared before me and swore to me and to the witnesses in my presence that this instrument is his Declaration Of A Desire For A Natural Death, and that he had willingly and voluntarily made and executed it as his free act and deed for the purposes expressed in it.
I further certify that _____ and _____, witnesses, appeared before me and swore that they witnessed _____, declarant, sign the attached declaration, believing him to be of sound mind; and also swore that at the time they witnessed the declaration (i) they were not related within the third degree to the declarant or to the declarant's spouse, and (ii) they did not know or have a reasonable expectation that they would be entitled to any portion of the estate of the declarant upon the declarant's death under any will of the declarant or codicil thereto then existing or under the Intestate Succession Act as it provides at that time, and (iii) they were not a physician attending the declarant or an employee of an attending physician or an employee of a health facility in which the declarant was a patient or an employee of a nursing home or any group-care home in which the declarant resided, and (iv) they did not have a claim against the declarant. I further certify that I am satisfied as to the genuineness and due execution of the declaration.

This the _____ day of _____, 20 _____.

_____
Notary Public

(Notary Seal)

My Commission Expires: _____

their own mortality; they believe incorrectly that they must hire an attorney to complete a directive and cannot afford this cost; or they think that having a directive will limit their families' ability to make good decisions on their behalf. Patients may also have the misperception that advance directives are only for people who are very ill or very old.

Perhaps the most important factor limiting the use and impact of advance directives is the lack of physician participation when patients consider signing a directive or after they have completed a directive. Any advance directive is only as useful as the personal communication among patients, their physicians, and families that complements its completion. In one study, only 12% of patients with an advance directive had received input from their physicians in its development. Most physicians are unaware of whether their patients have signed a directive. If physicians do not communicate about a patient's motivations underlying the completion of a living will or the designation of a health care proxy, it is unlikely that the directive can constructively inform medical decisions.

There have been successful community-based programs to increase completion of advance directives. In La Crosse, Wisconsin, a relatively homogeneous community with a defined set of health care services, a community-based group developed the Respecting Choices initiative to promote completion of advance directives. Implementation of the Respecting Choices program was associated with almost complete consistency between patients' actual treatment decisions and their previously documented preferences and may have reduced hospital care at the end of life.

In the state of Oregon, public attention to advance directives was catalyzed by the debate around legalization of physician-assisted suicide. A group of health professionals and patient advocates designed a universal and portable set of end-of-life treatment orders that served as a binding directive regardless of the patient's health care setting. The Physician Orders for Life-Sustaining Treatment Program (POLST) is a physician's order regarding end-of-life treatment. It is available to patients in all settings but has primarily been used to increase documentation of nursing home residents' treatment preferences. Most Oregon nursing homes and hospices voluntarily participate in this program, with one study suggesting that no patients received unwanted intensive care, mechanical ventilation, or cardiopulmonary resuscitation. The successes of both the Respecting Choices and POLST programs have led other communities and states to implement these initiatives.

Physician Role

Patients value physician communication about advance directives (Box 183-1). Prior research demonstrates that patient-physician discussion about advance directives is

---

> **Box 183-1** Physician Communication Strategies Regarding Advance Directives
>
> 1. Ask whether the patient has completed an advance directive (living will and/or health care proxy).
> 2. If the patient has a directive, obtain a copy and confirm its legal validity according to state law. Also, ask about patient's motivations for completing a directive.
> 3. Ask whether the patient has any care preferences in the event of serious illness and inability to participate in the decision-making process.
> 4. Ask whether the patient has a preferred surrogate decision maker (or decision makers). Also, ask patients whether there are any individuals who they would prefer not participate in decision making.
> 5. Assess for any patient barriers to completing an advance directive.
> 6. Advise patients regarding the role and limitations of advance directives in end-of-life decision making, including that a separate document may need to be completed if a patient prefers to not have a cardiac resuscitation attempted.
> 7. Advise patients that an attorney's assistance is not required to complete an advance directive.
> 8. Assist patients by providing written information about advance directives, including access to websites with advance care planning resources, and by offering follow-up to answer questions that may arise after the visit.
> 9. Assure patients that advance directives may be changed at any time as long as they retain decision-making capacity.
> 10. Document the content of the communication in the patient's record.
> 11. Remind patients to discuss their preferences with their family members.

---

associated with increased patient satisfaction, decreased patient fear and anxiety about the end of life, and an increased patient belief that physicians understood their wishes. Patient-physician communication about end-of-life care also increases the likelihood that patients will sign advance directives. In one study, one-third of patients would discuss advance directives if physicians brought up the subject, suggesting that some patients will not complete a directive unless first asked by a physician.

Many opportunities exist for physicians to discuss advance directives with their patients, including routine office visits or when the patient experiences a change in health status such as an illness that requires a hospital admission. Although patients may fear that physicians who discuss advance directives in the hospital believe that they will die, office-based discussions can seem too theoretical to patients in the absence of a life-threatening illness.

Avoiding Errors

Perhaps the main error made by physicians regarding advance directives is to fail to ask patients whether they have a completed directive. Patients may sign a directive without ever informing their physicians, and they may not discuss their motivations for having a living will or health care proxy unless asked by physicians. These directives will certainly have no impact on decision making unless physicians know they exist, and will have greater influence if physicians use patients' completion of a directive as an opportunity to learn more about their end-of-life care goals and preferences.

Another error made by physicians and patients alike is to assume that living wills provide instructions regarding specific treatment preferences, including whether to attempt cardiopulmonary resuscitation. For patients who prefer to have a Do Not Resuscitate order, it may be necessary for their physicians to complete a separate document specifying the patients' preferences and capability to make the decision. Physicians should review their states' Do Not Resuscitate order policies. In addition, physicians should document the specific end-of-life care preferences expressed by patients, and patients should be encouraged to discuss these preferences with their families. When such family discussions do not occur, there is a high risk for misunderstanding and unwanted stress at the time that an advance directive is used.

Future Directions

Advance directives have an important yet limited role in end-of-life care decision making. Although interest in promoting advance directive completion has waned, efforts to improve physicians' end-of-life care communication skills are increasing given the evidence demonstrating the critical roles of physician-patient and physician-family communication in patients' end-of-life experiences. These programs include teaching physicians to communicate effectively about advance directives using culturally appropriate strategies but also provide broader education in areas such as eliciting care goals, fostering trust, and responding to patient and family emotions.

Additional Resources

Caring Connections. National Hospice and Palliative Care Organization (800-658-8898). Available at: http://www.caringinfo.org. Accessed February 2, 2007.

This website provides patients with a variety of free resources on end-of-life care topics, including advance care planning and access to state-specific advance directive documents and instructions.

End of Life/Palliative Education Resource Center (EPERC). Available at: http://www.eperc.mcw.edu . Accessed March 22, 2007.

This website provides health care professionals with peer-reviewed educational resources, including materials on communication and end-of-life decision making.

EVIDENCE

1. Kagawa-Singer M, Blackhall LJ: Negotiating cross-cultural issues at the end of life: "You got to go where he lives." JAMA 286:2993-3001, 2001.

   This article outlines some of the major issues in providing cross-cultural end of life care and recommends techniques for negotiating issues influenced by culture that are important in end-of-life care.

2. Kass-Bartelmes BL, Hughes R: Advance care planning: Preferences for care at the end of life. J Pain Palliat Care Pharmacother 18:87-109, 2004.

   This evidence-based review of research studies on advance care planning includes interventions to improve patient end-of-life decision making.

3. Meisel A, Snyder L, Quill T; American College of Physicians—American Society of Internal Medicine End-of-Life Care Consensus Panel: Seven legal barriers to end-of-life care: Myths, realities, and grains of truth. JAMA 284:2495-2501, 2000.

   The authors present legal myths about end-of-life care that can undermine good care and ethical medical practice as identified by a consensus panel of medical and bioethics experts. The panel concludes that physicians must know the law of the state in which they practice.

4. Teno JM, Gruneir A, Schwartz A, et al: Association between advance directives and quality of end-of-life care: A national study. J Am Geriatric Soc 55:189-194, 2007.

   This study completed a national survey of bereaved family members to examine the role of advance directives in end-of-life care and concludes that completion of an advance directive is associated with home deaths, hospice use, and fewer concerns with physician communication.

5. Teno J, Lynn J, Wenger N, et al: Advance directives for seriously ill hospitalized patients: Effectiveness with the patient self-determination act and the SUPPORT intervention. J Am Geriatr Soc 45:500-507, 1997.

   This article assesses the impact of advance directives on decision making about cardiac resuscitation in a clinical trial of seriously ill hospitalized patients that sought to improve end-of-life care decision making. The authors conclude that advance directives did not substantially enhance physician-patient communication or decision making about resuscitation despite their intervention and the implementation of the Patient Self-Determination Act.

6. Tulsky JA: Beyond advance directives: Importance of communication skills at the end of life. JAMA 294:359-365, 2005.

   This clinical review for practicing physicians addresses the challenge in creating and implementing advance directives and offers practical suggestions for improving end-of-life communication and decision making.

7. Winzelberg GS, Tulsky JA, Hanson LC: Beyond autonomy: Diversifying end-of-life decision-making approaches to better serve patients and families. J Am Geriatr Soc 53:1046-1050, 2005.

   This review offers end-of-life communication strategies to physicians when interacting with patients and family caregivers if advance directives have not been completed.

Index

Note: Page numbers followed by *f* and *t* indicate figures and tables, respectively. A *b* indicates boxed material.